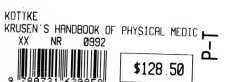

KRUSEN'S
H A N D B O O K   O F
PHYSICAL MEDICINE
and REHABILITATION

Fourth Edition

Frederic J. Kottke, M.D.

Professor Emeritus
Department of Physical Medicine and Rehabilitation
University of Minnesota Medical School
Minneapolis, Minnesota

Justus F. Lehmann, M.D.

Professor
Department of Rehabilitation Medicine
University of Washington School of Medicine
Seattle, Washington

1990

W.B. SAUNDERS
Harcourt Brace Jovanovich, Inc.

Philadelphia · London · Toronto · Montreal · Sydney · Tokyo

W. B. SAUNDERS COMPANY
Harcourt Brace Jovanovich, Inc.

The Curtis Center
Independence Square West
Philadelphia, PA 19106

Library of Congress Cataloging-in-Publication Data

Krusen's Handbook of physical medicine and rehabilitation.
—4th ed./[edited by] Frederic J. Kottke, Justus F. Lehmann.
p. cm.

Includes bibliographies and index.

ISBN 0–7216–2985–7

1. Medicine, Physical.   2. Physically handicapped—
   Rehabilitation.
   I. Krusen, Frank Hammond, 1898–1973. II. Kottke, Frederic
   J., 1917–   . III. Lehmann, Justus F. IV. Title. V. Title:
   Handbook of physical medicine and rehabilitation.
[DNLM: 1. Physical Medicine.   2. Rehabilitation.
WB 460 H233]

RM700.H36   1990   615.8—dc20

DNLM/DLC   89–10453

Editor: Edward H. Wickland, Jr.
Designer: Liz Schweber Doles
Production Manager: Peter Faber
Manuscript Editors: Carol DiBerardino and Janis Oppelt
Illustration Coordinator: Brett MacNaughton
Indexer: Mark Coyle
Cover Designer: Joanne Carroll

Krusen's Handbook of Physical Medicine and Rehabilitation   ISBN 0–7216–2985–7

Last digit is the print number: 9   8   7   6   5   4   3   2

Dedication

The title of the fourth edition of the Handbook continues to commemorate the name of Frank Hammond Krusen for his leadership in teaching, research and organizational activities during the development of physical medicine and rehabilitation as a medical specialty. He recognized that physical medicine and rehabilitation would become an integral part of medical practice only to the extent that the knowledge and skills of this specialty become incorporated in medical education. As a consequence, he devoted his time and energy mainly to research to increase knowledge of the specialty and to the education of physicians and others in the rehabilitation professions. In 1941, he authored *Physical Medicine* (Philadelphia, W. B. Saunders Co.) as the first general textbook on physical medicine in this country. Over the next six years he worked with John S. Coulter, Walter J. Zeiter, Kristian G. Hansson, Howard A. Rusk, and others to establish the American Board of Physical Medicine and Rehabilitation under the auspices of the American Board of Medical Specialties in 1947. These founders of the medical specialty emphasized that physical medicine and rehabilitation are essential components of comprehensive medicine and that handicapped patients have not had full treatment until they have been rehabilitated to their optimal level of performance.

Under Dr. Krusen's leadership in 1958 a number of academic physiatrists, many of whom had been students of his, began to meet periodically and formed a policy advisory group called the American Rehabilitation Foundation (ARF) Medical Committee. The Handbook first evolved in 1965 from the deliberations of this committee. The ARF Medical Committee has continued to meet each year to consider current issues related to educational needs in rehabilitation medicine.

Contributors

James C. Agre, M.D., Ph.D.
Assistant Professor, Department of Rehabilitation Medicine, University of Wisconsin, Madison, Wisconsin. Rehabilitation Medicine Service, University of Wisconsin Hospital and Clinics, Madison, Wisconsin.
Physiatry in Sports Medicine

Thomas P. Anderson, M.D.
Emeritus Professor, University of Minnesota Medical School, Minneapolis, Minnesota; Clinical Professor of Physical Medicine and Rehabilitation, Tufts University, Boston, Massachusetts. Senior Physiatrist, Spaulding Rehabilitation Hospital, Boston, Massachusetts.
Rehabilitation of Patients with Completed Stroke

Gary T. Athelstan, Ph.D.
Professor, Physical Medicine and Rehabilitation, and Psychology, University of Minnesota Medical School, Minneapolis, Minnesota. Counseling Psychologist, University of Minnesota Hospital, Minneapolis, Minnesota.
Vocational Assessment and Management

Essam A. Awad, M.D., Ph.D.
Professor and Clinical Chief, Department of Physical Medicine and Rehabilitation, University of Minnesota Medical School, Minneapolis, Minnesota. Clinical Chief, Department of Physical Medicine and Rehabilitation, University of Minnesota Hospital, Minneapolis, Minnesota. Attending Staff, United Hospitals, St. Paul, Minnesota.
Treatment of Spasticity by Neurolysis

Daniel T. Barry, M.D., Ph.D.
Assistant Professor, Department of Physical Medicine and Rehabilitation and the Bioengineering Program, University of Michigan. Attending Physician, Department of Physical Medicine and Rehabilitation, University of Michigan Medical Center, Ann Arbor, Michigan.
Measurement of Musculoskeletal Function

Jeffrey R. Basford, M.D., Ph.D.
Assistant Professor, Mayo Medical School, Rochester, Minnesota. Consultant, Department of Physical Medicine and Rehabilitation, Mayo Clinic and Mayo Foundation, Rochester, Minnesota.
Ultraviolet Therapy; Electrical Therapy

Kathleen R. Bell, M.D.
Clinical Instructor, University of Washington, Seattle, Washington. Providence Hospital Medical Center, Everett, Washington.
Rehabilitation's Relationship to Inactivity

Leonard F. Bender, M.D., M.S.
Professor and Chairman, Department of Physical Medicine and Rehabilitation, Wayne State University School of Medicine, Detroit, Michigan. President and Chief Executive Officer, Rehabilitation Institute, Detroit, Michigan. Chief of Service, Department of Physical Medicine and Rehabilitation, Detroit Receiving Hospital and University Health Center, Detroit, Michigan; Medical Staff, Harper-Grace Hospital, Detroit, Michigan; Consultant, Sinai Hospital and Children's Hospital of Detroit, and Veterans Administration Hospital, Ellen Park, Michigan.
Upper Extremity Orthotics; Upper Extremity Prosthetics

David R. Beukelman, Ph.D.
Barkley Professor, Special Education and Communication Disorders, University of Nebraska, Lincoln, Nebraska.
Speech and Language Disorders

Rita Bistevins, M.D., Ph.D., F.R.C.P.(C)
Clinical Assistant Professor, Department of Physical Medicine and Rehabilitation, University of Minnesota Medical School, Minneapolis, Minnesota. Clinical Physiatrist, University of Minnesota Hospital and Clinic; Attending Physiatrist, Minneapolis VA Medical Center.
Footwear and Footwear Modifications

Catherine W. Britell, M.D.
Assistant Professor, Department of Rehabilitation Medicine, University of Washington, Seattle, Washington. Assistant Chief, Spinal Cord Injury Service, VA Medical Center, Seattle, Washington.
Wheelchair Prescription

Jo Ann Brockway, Ph.D.
Assistant Professor, Department of Rehabilitation Medicine, University of Washington, Seattle, Washington. Adjunct Medical Staff, University of Washington Medical Center and Harborview Medical Center, Seattle, Washington.
Psychological Assessment and Management

Rene Cailliet, M.D.
Clinical Professor, Department of Rehabilitation Medicine, University of Southern California School of Medicine, Los Angeles, California. Director

of Rehabilitation, Santa Monica Hospital Medical Center, Santa Monica, California.
Spine: Disorders and Deformities

Diana D. Cardenas, M.D.

Associate Professor, Department of Rehabilitation Medicine, University of Washington, School of Medicine, Seattle, Washington. Director, Rehabilitation Medicine Clinic; Attending Physician, Multidisciplinary Pain Center, Rehabilitation Medicine Service, University of Washington Medical Center, Seattle, Washington.
Management of Chronic Pain

Sandra S. Cole, C.S.E., C.S.C.

Clinical Professor, Director of Sexuality Curriculum, University of Michigan Medical School, Ann Arbor, Michigan. Clinical Professor, Director, Sexuality Training Center; Director, Sexuality Evaluation Clinic, Department of Physical Medicine and Rehabilitation, University of Michigan Medical Center, Ann Arbor, Michigan.
Rehabilitation of Problems of Sexuality in Physical Disability

Theodore M. Cole, M.D.

Professor and Chairman, Department of Physical Medicine and Rehabilitation, University of Michigan Medical Center, Ann Arbor, Michigan. Chairman, Department of Physical Medicine and Rehabilitation, University of Michigan Hospitals, Ann Arbor, Michigan.
Measurement of Musculoskeletal Function; Rehabilitation of Problems of Sexuality in Physical Disability

D. Nathan Cope, M.D.

Vice President for Medical Affairs, NeuroCare, Inc., Concord, California.
The Rehabilitation of Traumatic Brain Injury

Darinka Dekanic, M.D., Ph.D.

Associate Research Professor and Chief, Laboratory for Human Metabolism, Institute for Medical Research, Zagreb, Croatia, Yugoslavia.
Osteoporosis

Barbara J. De Lateur, M.D.

Professor, Department of Rehabilitation Medicine, University of Washington School of Medicine, Seattle, Washington. Physiatrist-in-Chief, Harborview Medical Center, Seattle, Washington.
Gait Analysis: Diagnosis and Management; Diathermy and Superficial Heat, Laser, and Cold Therapy; Therapeutic Exercise to Develop Strength and Endurance; Lower Extremity Orthotics

Margaret M. Doucette, D.O.
Assistant Professor, Department of Physical Medicine and Rehabilitation, University of Minnesota Medical School, Minneapolis, Minnesota; Attending Physiatrist, University of Minnesota Hospital and Clinic.
Rehabilitation of the Patient with Heart Disease

Dennis D. Dykstra, M.D., Ph.D.
Assistant Professor, Department of Physical Medicine and Rehabilitation; Assistant Professor, Department of Urologic Surgery, University of Minnesota, Minneapolis, Minnesota.
Treatment of Spasticity by Neurolysis

Kelly J. Egan, Ph.D.
Assistant Professor, Department of Anesthesiology, University of Washington; University of Washington Medical Center, Seattle, Washington. Attending Psychologist, U.W. Multidisciplinary Pain Center, Seattle, Washington.
Management of Chronic Pain

Paul M. Ellwood, Jr., M.D.
Clinical Professor of Pediatrics, Neurology, and Physical Medicine and Rehabilitation, University of Minnesota Medical School, Minneapolis, Minnesota: President, Interstudy, Minneapolis, Minnesota.
Bed Positioning; Transfers—Method, Equipment, and Preparation

Gary Fell, M.D.
Second Assistant, University of Melbourne, Melbourne, Australia. Consultant Surgeon, Austin Hospital, Melbourne, Australia.
Management of Vascular Disease

Steven V. Fisher, M.D.
Assistant Professor, Department of Physical Medicine and Rehabilitation, University of Minnesota, Minneapolis, Minnesota. Medical Director, Upper Midwest Rehabilitation Institute, St. Paul, Minnesota; Burn Center Consultant and Staff Physician, Ramsey Medical Center, St. Paul, Minnesota.
Spinal Orthoses; Rehabilitation for Burn Patients

Wilbert E. Fordyce, Ph.D.
Professor Emeritus, Departments of Rehabilitation Medicine and Pain Service, University of Washington, Seattle, Washington.
Psychological Assessment and Management

Murray M. Freed, M.D.
Professor and Chairman, Department of Rehabilitation Medicine, Boston University School of Medicine, Boston, Massachusetts. Director of Rehabilitation Medicine; Director, New England Regional Spinal Cord Injury Center, The University Hospital, Boston, Massachusetts.
Traumatic and Congenital Lesions of the Spinal Cord

Lawrence W. Friedmann, M.D., F.A.C.A., F.I.C.A.
Professor of Rehabilitation Medicine, State University of New York at Stony Brook, East Meadow, New York. Chairman and Physiatrist-in-Chief, Department of Rehabilitation Medicine, Nassau County Medical Center, East Meadow, New York.
Rehabilitation of the Lower Extremity Amputee

Gail L. Gamble, M.D., FAAPMR
Assistant Professor, Physical Medicine and Rehabilitation, Mayo Medical School, Rochester, Minnesota. Consultant, Department of Physical Medicine and Rehabilitation, Mayo Clinic, Rochester, Minnesota.
Prescription Writing in Physical Medicine and Rehabilitation

Jerome W. Gersten, M.D.
Professor, Rehabilitation Medicine, University of Colorado School of Medicine, Denver, Colorado. Attending Physiatrist, University Hospital, University of Colorado Health Sciences Center; Attending Physiatrist; Rose Medical Center; Consulting Staff, Craig Hospital; Honorary Staff, Spalding Rehabilitation Hospital, Denver, Colorado.
Degenerative Diseases of the Central Nervous System

Carl V. Granger, M.D.
Professor of Rehabilitation Medicine, State University of New York at Buffalo, School of Medicine and Biomedical Sciences, Buffalo, New York. Head, Rehabilitation Medicine, The Buffalo General Hospital, Buffalo, New York.
Health Accounting—Functional Assessment of the Long-Term Patient

Eugen M. Halar, M.D.
Professor, Department of Rehabilitation Medicine, School of Medicine, University of Washington, Seattle, Washington. Chief of Rehabilitation Medicine, Veterans Administration Medical Center, Seattle, Washington.
Rehabilitation's Relationship to Inactivity

Daniel Halpern, M.D.
Clinical Professor, Department of Rehabilitation Medicine, Tufts-New England Medical Center. Consultant, Rehabilitation Medicine, Worcester City Hospital, Worcester, Massachusetts.
Rehabilitation of Children with Brain Damage

Therese J. Haney, B.S., O.T.
Clinical Faculty for Occupational Therapy School, University of Minnesota, Minneapolis, Minnesota. Clinician for Cardiac Rehabilitation, University of Minnesota Hospital and Clinic.
Rehabilitation of the Patient with Heart Disease

Ross M. Hays, M.D.
Assistant Professor, Rehabilitation Medicine and Pediatrics, University of Washington School of Medicine, Seattle, Washington. Associate Director, Department of Rehabilitation Medicine, Children's Hospital and Medical Center, Seattle, Washington.
Evaluation of the Patient

H. Frederic Helmholz, Jr., M.D.
Associate Professor Emeritus, Mayo Graduate School of Medicine, Rochester, Minnesota.
Rehabilitation of Respiratory Function

Chang-Zern Hong, M.D.
Assistant Professor, Department of Physical Medicine and Rehabilitation, University of California, Irvine, California. Clinical Director, Department of Physical Medicine and Rehabilitation, University of California Medical Center, Orange, California; Co-Director, Electrodiagnostic Section, Rehabilitation Medicine Service, VA Medical Center, Long Beach, California.
Measurement of Musculoskeletal Function; Physiatric Rehabilitation and Maintenance of the Geriatric Patient

David L. Hooks, Ph.D., CRC
Director of Vocational Services, Sacred Heart Medical Center, Spokane, Washington.
Prevocational Evaluation

Masayoshi Itoh, M.D., M.P.H.
Associate Professor of Clinical Rehabilitation Medicine; New York University Medical School, New York, New York. Associate Deputy Director, Department of Rehabilitation Medicine, Goldwater Memorial Hospital, New York University Medical Center, New York, New York.
The Epidemiology of Disability as Related to Rehabilitation Medicine

Rebecca D. Jackson, M.D.
Assistant Professor, Department of Medicine (Endocrinology) and Department of Physical Medicine, Ohio State University, Columbus, Ohio.
Osteoporosis

Ernest W. Johnson, M.D.
Professor, Department of Physical Medicine, The Ohio State University, Columbus, Ohio. Attending Staff, The Ohio State University Hospitals, Columbus, Ohio; Consulting Staff, The Children's Hospital, Columbus, Ohio.
Electrodiagnosis; Rehabilitation Management of Diseases of the Motor Unit

Miland E. Knapp, B.S., M.S., M.D.
Professor Emeritus, University of Minnesota Medical School, Minneapolis, Minnesota. Former Member of Staff, Metropolitan Medical Center and Hennepin County Medical Center, Minneapolis, Minnesota.
Massage; Aftercare of Fractures

Michael Kosiak, M.D.
Assistant Professor, Department of Physical Medicine and Rehabilitation, University of Minnesota, Minneapolis, Minnesota. Director, Department of Physical Medicine and Rehabilitation, St. Paul-Ramsey Hospital, St. Paul, Minnesota.
Prevention and Rehabilitation of Ischemic Ulcers

Frederic J. Kottke, M.D., Ph.D.
Professor Emeritus, Department of Physical Medicine and Rehabilitation, University of Minnesota Medical School, Minneapolis, Minnesota. Emeritus Member of Medical Staff, University of Minnesota Hospital and Clinics, Minneapolis, Minnesota.
The Neurophysiology of Motor Function; Therapeutic Exercise to Maintain Mobility; Therapeutic Exercise to Develop Neuromuscular Coordination; Prevention and Rehabilitation of Ischemic Ulcers

Myron M. LaBan, M.D., M.M.Sc.
Associate Clinical Professor, Physical Medicine and Rehabilitation, Wayne State University, Detroit, Michigan; Clinical Professor, Oakland University, Rochester, Michigan. Chairman, Department of Physical Medicine and Rehabilitation; Director, Residency Training, William Beaumont Hospital, Royal Oak, Michigan.
Rehabilitation of Patients with Cancer

Mathew H. M. Lee, M.D., M.P.H., F.A.C.P.
Professor of Clinical Rehabilitation Medicine, New York University School of Medicine, New York, New York; Clinical Professor of Oral and Maxillo-Facial Surgery, New York University College of Dentistry, New York, New York. Acting Chairman and Director, Rusk Institute of Rehabilitation Medicine, New York University Medical Center, New York, New York.
The Epidemiology of Disability as Related to Rehabilitation Medicine; Acupuncture in Physiatry

Justus F. Lehmann, M.D.
Professor, Department of Rehabilitation Medicine, University of Washington School of Medicine, Seattle, Washington. Co-Director, Brain Injury Clinic, University Hospital, Seattle, Washington.
Gait Analysis: Diagnosis and Management; Diathermy and Superficial Heat, Laser, and Cold Therapy; Therapeutic Exercise to Develop Strength and Endurance; Lower Extremity Orthotics

Loren R. Leslie, M.D.
Assistant Professor, University of Minnesota Medical School, Minneapolis, Minnesota. Chief, Rehabilitation Medicine Service, Minneapolis Veterans Administration Medical Center, Minneapolis, Minnesota.
Training for Functional Independence; Training in Homemaking Activities

Sung J. Liao, M.D., D.P.H.
Clinical Professor of Oral and Maxillo-Facial Surgery, New York University College of Dentistry, New York, New York; Former Chairman, Ad Hoc Committee on Acupuncture, Connecticut State Medical Society; Former Consultant, Rhode Island State Board of Acupuncture, Providence, Rhode Island. Attending Physiatrist, Waterbury Hospital, Waterbury Connecticut.
Acupuncture in Physiatry

Gordon M. Martin, M.D.
Emeritus Professor, Physical Medicine and Rehabilitation, Mayo Medical School, Rochester, Minnesota.
Prescription Writing in Physical Medicine and Rehabilitation

Velimir Matkovic, M.D., Ph.D.
Assistant Professor, Department of Physical Medicine and Department of Internal Medicine, Ohio State University, Columbus, Ohio.
Osteoporosis

Maurice H. Miller, Ph.D.
Professor of Audiology, New York University, New York, New York. Chief of Audiology, Center for Communication Disorders, Lenox Hill Hospital, New York, New York.
Diagnosis and Rehabilitation of Auditory Disorders

Walter J. Mysiw, M.D.
Assistant Professor, Department of Physical Medicine, Ohio State University, Columbus, Ohio.
Osteoporosis

Paul A. Nelson, M.D.
Resident Emeritus Staff, Cleveland Clinic Foundation, Cleveland, Ohio.
Rehabilitation of Patients with Lymphedema

Joachim L. Opitz, M.D.
Associate Professor of Physical Medicine and Rehabilitation, Mayo Medical School, Rochester, Minnesota. Consultant, Department of Physical Medicine

and Rehabilitation, Mayo Clinic and Mayo Foundation, Rochester, Minnesota.
Reconstructive Surgery of the Extremities

William S. Pease, M.D.
Assistant Professor, Department of Physical Medicine, The Ohio State University College of Medicine, Columbus, Ohio. Attending Staff, Ohio State University Hospitals, Columbus, Ohio.
Rehabilitation Management of Diseases of the Motor Unit

Inder Perkash, M.D., M.S., F.R.C.S.
Professor of Surgery and Paralyzed Veterans of America Professor of Spinal Cord Injuries, Stanford University Medical Center, Stanford, California. Chief, Spinal Cord Injury Center, Department of Veterans Affairs Medical Center, Palo Alto, California.
Management of Neurogenic Dysfunction of the Bladder and Bowel

Elizabeth A. Rivers, O.T.R., R.N.
Part-time Clinical Instructor, University of Minnesota and College of St. Catherine, St. Paul, Minnesota. Burn Rehabilitation Specialist, The Burn Center at St. Paul Ramsey Hospital, St. Paul, Minnesota.
Rehabilitation for Burn Patients

Mary D. Romano, M.S.W.
Adjunct Instructor, Virginia Commonwealth University, Richmond, Virginia. Director of Social Work, National Rehabilitation Hospital.
Psychosocial Diagnosis and Social Work Services

Jerome D. Schein, Ph.D.
Chair of Deafness Studies, University of Alberta, Edmonton, Alberta; Emeritus Professor of Sensory Rehabilitation, New York University, New York, New York.
Diagnosis and Rehabilitation of Auditory Disorders

Arthur A. Siebens, M.D.
Richard B. Darnell Professor of Rehabilitation Medicine and Surgery, The Johns Hopkins School of Medicine, Baltimore, Maryland; Director, Department of Rehabilitation Medicine, The Johns Hopkins Hospital, Baltimore, Maryland; Chief of Rehabilitation Medicine, The Good Samaritan Hospital, Baltimore, Maryland.
Rehabilitation for Swallowing Impairment

Walter C. Stolov, M.D.
Professor and Chairman, Department of Rehabilitation Medicine, University of Washington School of Medicine, Seattle, Washington. Attending Physi-

cian, Harborview Medical Center, University Hospital, and Veterans Administration Hospital, Seattle, Washington.
Evaluation of the Patient; Prevocational Evaluation

Henry H. Stonnington, M.B.B.S., M.S., F.R.C.P.
Professor, Department of Physical Medicine and Rehabilitation, Medical College of Virginia, Richmond, Virginia.
Rehabilitation for Respiratory Function

D. E. Strandness, Jr., M.D.
Professor, Department of Surgery, University of Washington, Seattle, Washington.
Management of Vascular Disease

Robert L. Swezey, M.D., F.A.C.P., F.A.C.R.
Clinical Professor of Medicine, UCLA, Los Angeles, California. Staff, St. John's Hospital, Santa Monica, California; Staff, Santa Monica Hospital, Santa Monica, California.
Rehabilitation in Arthritis and Allied Conditions

Jerome S. Tobis, M.D.
Professor Emeritus, Department of Physical Medicine and Rehabilitation, University of California, Irvine Medical Center, Irvine, California.
Measurement of Musculoskeletal Function; Physiatric Rehabilitation and Maintenance of the Geriatric Patient

Jay M. Uomoto, Ph.D.
Assistant Professor, Department of Rehabilitation Medicine, University of Washington School of Medicine, Seattle, Washington. Director, Brain Injury Clinic, University of Washington Medical Center, Seattle, Washington.
Neuropsychological Assessment and Training in Acute Brain Injury

Alan Howard Welner, M.D., M.P.H.
Researcher, Department of Environmental Science and Physiology, Harvard University School of Public Health, Boston, Massachusetts; Lecturer on Physical Medicine and Rehabilitation, University of Pennsylvania School of Medicine, Philadelphia, Pennsylvania.
Environmental Accessibility for Physically Disabled People

Robert Whitten, M.D.
Senior Resident, Department of Physical Medicine, Ohio State University, Columbus, Ohio. Attending Physician, Riverside Methodist Hospital, Columbus, Ohio.
Osteoporosis

David O. Wiechers, M.D.
Clinical Assistant Professor, Department of Physical Medicine and Rehabilitation, Ohio State University, Columbus, Ohio.
Electrodiagnosis

Kathryn M. Yorkston, Ph.D.
Professor, Department of Rehabilitation Medicine, University of Washington, Seattle, Washington.
Speech and Language Disorders

Preface to the Fourth Edition

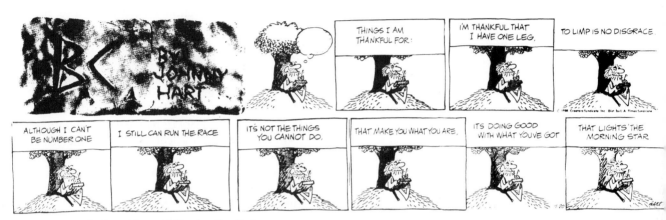

By permission of Johnny Hart and Creators Syndicate.

As the fourth edition of *Krusen's Handbook of Physical Medicine and Rehabilitation* goes to press, we find the medical specialty of physiatry is continuing to develop in line with the concepts of Frank H. Krusen, Howard A. Rusk, and the other founders of this specialty 50 years ago.[7, 8] In some respects, the advances have been most encouraging. In others, we continue to be faced with serious barriers and pitfalls. The most rapid growth of rehabilitation continues to be in the demand for services as the public recognizes the great benefits to be obtained. That demand still greatly exceeds both the supply of physiatrists and also the financial support available through health insurance and other health care financing to pay for rehabilitation. The availability of rehabilitation services has not been great enough to have an impact on the backlog of disabled persons currently being maintained in a state of dependency and needing treatment. The magnitude of the need for rehabilitation remains the same as it has been for at least the past 30 years.[2, 10] (See Figure 1 of the Preface to the Third Edition, which has been republished following this preface.) An estimated 2 to 3 per cent of the population, approximately five million persons, with chronic diseases and disabilities need physiatric services at this time. There is also an increasing demand for rehabilitation services for all kinds of medical problems proportional to the increasing awareness among the general public that restoration of a satisfactorily high quality of life of the physically impaired patient is dependent on timely provision of the appropriate rehabilitation services.

Medicine, as a whole, has been making highly significant progress in providing better health services. Acute medical and surgical services have successfully decreased mortality and extended life expectancy. As the success of acute surgical and medical care increases, the proportion of patients surviving with chronic diseases and disabilities that require more rehabilitation also increases. Therefore, the need for rehabilitation services to reduce the number of persons with dysmobility will continue into the next century. People are living longer. Life expectancy has increased, especially for older adults, and the cohort of survivors after 50 years of age has been increasing rapidly.[5] When rehabilitation restores functional capacity, those people remain significantly more independent until their near-terminal illnesses. If they receive that high quality health care for both their acute medical problems and also the necessary rehabilitation to maintain their functonal independence, their life curve of performance approaches the optimal as illustrated in Figure 5 of the Preface to the Third Edition.

The rate of growth of the concepts, knowledge, and application of rehabilitation also has been rapid. The concept of medical rehabilitation has continued to expand, and with it the concept of comprehensive medicine, as the potential for successful interventions has developed.[6] Rehabilitation is a complex process of the integrated application of many procedures to achieve the restoration of the individual to his or her optimal functional status at home and in the community that the appropriate utilization of all of that patient's residual assets allows. The fourth edition integrates these advances with the contents of the third edition in a focused form, which imparts the essential information, skills, techniques, and clinical application in an orderly manner to conserve the reader's time.

The first 12 chapters present the various components of evaluation of the patient for rehabilitation. Chapters 13 through 29 present the underlying knowledge and techniques of application of the methods used by physical medicine and rehabilitation. In the third section are 32 chapters dealing with the application of physical medicine and rehabilitation for specific kinds of disabilities that need therapy.

It is gratifying to know that physiatry has been recognized as a method that can restore the functional capacities of patients with disabilities or chronic diseases to become participants in their homes and communities, and that this recognition has had a highly significant influence, resulting in the broadening of the concept of comprehensive medical care. Comprehensive medical care today includes rehabilitation whenever necessary, to provide for the restoration of the patient with a disease or disability to return to his or her optimal functioning in his or her normal societal environment, with a *quality of life* as close to that of persons in normal society as is reasonably possible (see Chapter 12: Health Accounting—Functional Assessment of the Long-Term Patient). This expansion of the role of comprehensive medicine to maintain health at its highest level (see Fig. 4 in the Preface to the Third Edition), or when illness supervenes and to restore it as completely as possible (Fig. 5 in the Preface to the Third Edition) is of great benefit to all patients. Likewise, it benefits the economy of this country because it decreases the total costs of care and of dependency that result from disability and chronic disease (Figs. 2 and 3 in the Preface to the Third Edition), and it will increase productivity as more of these patients return to their communities and participate to increase the productivity of our economy.

As is indicated at the head of this Preface by Johnny Hart's cartoon, the wish of every patient is that his medical care will restore him to a quality of life that is highly satisfactory. We have now begun to recognize that comprehensive medicine, including rehabilitation whenever necessary, has the same goal of restoration of each patient to a high quality of life. The thinking of patients and doctors is on the same wavelength when they have the same goals. Quality of life for patients should be measured in the same way as the quality of life for others in the community.[6] For reasons that are now hard to understand, prior to the emergence of the concept that medical services should restore each patient to that quality of life that is optimal for him or her by utilizing all of the available assets that contribute to healthy functioning, it appears to have been generally held that medical services and the right to medical services stopped far short of that goal. Limited objectives such as relief of pain, restoration of the ability of the patient to survive outside of the hospital, the ability to live (exist) in a skilled nursing facility or extended care facility, or the ability to exist at home, dependent on members of the family for personal care and financial support, were considered points at which medical services might justifiably be stopped, regardless of the potential abilities of the patient to achieve a more independent role with a higher quality of life.

The various medical specialties always have had different goals for the services that they render, many of which leave the patient only partially restored. Certain medical interventions are provided with the objective to restore the patient only partially toward a full life, i.e., a high quality of life, whereas others are more comprehensive in design.[8] For example, the goals of certain types of interventions are focused on preventing potentially impending death by ensuring survival of an essential organ. Other interventions use procedures specifically for the relief of pain. If such limited interventions are not followed by other appropriate treatment, comprehensive medical care remains incomplete and a significant amount of a high quality of life remains unrestored. In the treatment of the chronic diseases and disabilities, this state of affairs, unfortunately, is still more frequent than not, as five million persons in immediate need of rehabilitation services today attest. Depending on the medical condition of the patient, the successful application of a medical intervention may do little to reestablish a high quality of life.[6] There are a number of factors that rank in both chronological and functional succession that determine the level of rehabilitation and the quality of life attained (Table 1).

The highest quality of life attainable for any normal person is the achievement of optimal function, resulting in using all of the assets that each person has. For the disabled patient, this means the rehabilitation to optimal functional performance. The restoration of hope and the will to aspire to try to achieve self-set goals is the highest level of quality of any life.[1, 3, 6] When the patient reaches this level of hope and expectation of achievement, life blooms to its greatest extent. A significant level of quality of life begins to develop as the result of comprehensive medical care only as the patient

TABLE 1. Component Factors
Contributing to Quality of Life*

Highest level of attainment

Aspiration for personal
   achievement and creativity
Vocational capability and performance
Social interaction
Communicative abilities
   Writing
   Reading
   Speaking
Activities of daily living
Mobility
   Ambulation and transfers
   Manipulative skills
   Posture
Sensory perception

Moderate level of attainment

   Hearing
   Vision
   Touch
   Spatial orientation
Enjoyment—satisfaction
Sense of self-worth
Comfort versus pain
Awareness—cognition
Survival of essential organs
Supportive environment
Food, shelter, clothing, personal safety

Lowest level of attainment

*The component factors underlying quality of
life are arrayed in this table, from the bottom
upward, in ascending order of attainment during
rehabilitation. Restoration to each level requires
the prior attainment of the functional capabilities of subordinate levels.

becomes reintegrated internally so that he or she is able to begin to carry
out meaningful activities. The person's quality of life expands further as he
or she reestablishes interaction with others and with his or her environment.
Hope, will, and aspiration to again attempt to achieve self-set goals are the
characteristics of achievement of the highest quality of life.

As the result of the maturation of the concept of comprehensive medical
care, it is now beginning to be recognized that the goal of medicine is to
restore the optimal quality of life that is possible by utilizing the residual
resources of the patient. Each medical intervention, therefore, should have
as its objective the improvement of the patient toward that goal. Outcome,
which is evaluated by change in function as the result of the medical
intervention, is the only true measure of the value of that medical care.[9] It
is pleasing that both the criteria for evaluation by outcome and the goal of
therapy to restore quality of life are the same today for comprehensive
medicine as they are for medical rehabilitation. This demonstrates that today
rehabilitation has become fully integrated into the best of medical practice,

just as physiatry has been advocating over the past 30 years. Evaluation of the benefits of medical care by outcome is in stark contrast to the currently used method of evaluation of medical acceptability by review of the kind, quality, and appropriateness of the professional services (PSRO) that the patient received, based on the prior establishment by decisions of a committee of the appropriate processes of evaluation and treatment for each diagnostic category or group. This emerging concept portends a change in the way in which medical services will be reevaluated: on the basis of outcome or change of functional status of the patient rather than being based on an evaluation of the quality and acceptability of the rendered services. Evaluation of health care by outcome will increase the demand for physiatry further as it becomes more apparent that health and optimal functioning are not restored to the greatest possible level without the appropriate rehabilitative services.

Successful rehabilitation to the level at which the individual can participate in society provides the basis for the restoration of hope and the aspiration for creativity, to try to achieve whatever self-determined goals that person has set for himself or herself. Whether a person is normal or handicapped, physiological survival of the individual is essential, of course, as the basis for establishing a functional life of quality, but physiological survival of the vegetative functions only, provides no quality of life. It is only after the person becomes integrated internally and with the world around him that the quality of life develops increasingly to provide the satisfactions that all of us desire. Some persons may protest that this ultimate goal of aspiration for creativity is far beyond the scope of medicine because complete satisfaction depends on financial and social factors that medical care can neither guarantee nor provide.[4] However, such an interpretation is a misunderstanding of the goal of rehabilitation, which is the restoration of the available assets of the impaired patient in order to optimize his or her capabilities to such a level that he or she develops the will to attempt to achieve rather than the guarantee that all aspects of success (personal, social, and environmental) will result from rehabilitation.

The health services necessary for the optimal functional rehabilitation of these disabling conditions just referred to above are not universally available through legislated medical programs or private medical insurance. In part, this situation is related to the persistence of an antiquated and retrogressive understanding of the role of medicine that in the past had focused almost exclusively on prevention of death from acute causes and on relief of pain. In the 19th century and the early decades of the 20th century, there were very few specific medical treatments that produced cures, and both surgery and anesthesia entailed high risks. At that time, the emphasis of the teaching in the medical schools was on the identification of pathology and the diagnosis of disease. The teaching of therapeutic management other than surgery was minimal because of this limited specific armamentarium. In the middle of this century through the explosion of medical information through research, the antibacterials, antibiotics, and many other specific treatments for diseases became available. At the same time, there was rapidly expanding knowledge in pathology and diagnosis. Teaching intensified, especially regarding those pathologic conditions that threaten immediate death, and the knowledge that had to be taught easily filled all of the teaching time available. Location and specification of the pathology has become the ultimate goal in the teaching of acute diseases. Even our standard classification of disease is by location and pathological cause, whereas no consideration is given in that classification to the disturbances of the functions of the body.

As a consequence, in the very limited time for teaching, inadequate consideration has been given to the components of comprehensive treatment for chronic diseases and multiple disabilities. In addition, there is a major difference between acute disease with an abrupt onset and most chronic diseases. In acute disease, there is usually only one pathology, and when that pathology is corrected, the patient is restored to health. Therefore, medical teaching has been conducted on the precept that the multiple symptoms in an acute disease should have a unitary cause. The use of multiple diagnoses to explain such an illness is discouraged because the approach may mask that identity of the unitary cause. On the other hand, in chronic diseases and disabilities there are usually multiple problems resulting from disturbances of multiple organ systems, each with an individual cause that must be identified and treated. This difference in the concept of acute and chronic disease makes it more difficult for individuals trained in the evaluation and treatment of acute unitary diseases to become interested in chronic disabilities of multiple organ systems, none of which carries the urgent threat of death and, also, none of which has such overall importance that appropriate treatment of that single problem will restore the patient to optimal function. For chronic disabilities, adequate management requires much time and attention to the many details of the management of many problems. This emphasis in teaching, skewed to focus on acute disease, has carried over into clinical practice, resulting too frequently in incomplete attention to patients with multiple problems, and, with it, incomplete restoration of such patients to their potential for a high quality of life. Patients with diseases and disabilities that severely impair the quality of life but that are not acutely lethal are not receiving the necessary medical care, even though the impaired quality of life may last for years or decades. This lack of provision of the needed health services for chronic nonlethal conditions relegates patients to a lifetime of greatly reduced quality, especially those geriatric patients with chronic impairments (Chapter 58), children with congenital disabilities (Chapter 39), and patients with arthritic conditions (Chapter 31) and a wide variety of post-traumatic and other prolonged neuromusculoskeletal conditions, which are discussed in Chapters 30 to 44.

There is, also, a negative side to this story of maturation of the concept of comprehensive medical care. This negative side relates to the efforts of the payers for health services to cut back the comprehensiveness of many health services as the costs of acute surgical, medical, and hospital care increase at the same time that more and more patients are requesting the exceptionally expensive services developed for medical intervention, such as organ transplants and prolonged intensive care. Similarly, as the knowledge of the benefits of comprehensive health care spread, more people who have chronic disabilities will seek those rehabilitative services that will restore them to the optimal level of functioning again. The consequence is that the cost of requested care exceeds the financial resources available, and the insurance providers and the government have cut back services to decrease costs to match the level of current resources. It makes no difference today whether health care is provided by governmental programs such as Medicare and Medicaid, private medical insurance, employment-linked group insurance, capitation health plans, or personal resources. With the rare exception of the extremely wealthy, none of these health-financing systems is funded adequately to be able to pay the cost of all the comprehensive medical services that could be provided. This situation, then, has led to demands to reduce health expenditures to the finances available by some form of rationing of health care. Triage results. Who shall be denied the medical services he or she seeks and why? Today, the urgency of the demand for provision of medical and surgical services for the acutely ill has prevailed, driving the decisions of providers to support the treatment of the potentially lethal acute conditions and defer or deny less urgent health care as elective. These decisions have placed the greatest restrictions on the development of adequate rehabilitation programs as the result of this severe underfunding, even though today patients with inadequately treated chronic diseases and disabilities constitute the majority of patients needing health services. Other health programs, for example, those in Canada and Oregon, have not made the same decisions. They have decided that those excessively expensive acute interventions cannot be supported regardless of the lethal risk to the individual. The decision has been made that the deprivation of needed medical care for so many other patients because of diversion of huge sums of money for the excesssively costly care to one individual cannot be justified. As long as urgency drives decision-making and diverts all available funds to excessively expensive care for a few, it jeopardizes the goal of restoring persons with chronic diseases and disabilities to the high quality of life available to them if each were rehabilitated to his or her optimal level of function. Only the wealthy few who have the financial resources to purchase the necessary rehabilitative services to restore each person to his or her optimal function can achieve the desired quality of life until a national attitude develops that supports the policy that a high quality of life should be the goal for all patients and should be obtained through the institution of adequate programs of comprehensive health care.

Hospitals and skilled nursing facilities recognize that they cannot provide high quality medical care to restore their patients to the optimal level of functioning of which each is capable unless each institution receives the necessary physiatric prescription and the direction of rehabilitative services. Yet each of the medical insurance programs severely restricts physiatric participation and continuing supervision. Rehabilitative services that will restore optimal function do not result from the general application of standard formulae but, rather, depend upon a precise evaluation of functional assets and impairments and precise prescriptions based on knowledge gained from physiatric training as presented in *Krusen's Handbook of Physical Medicine and Rehabilitation.* It is unfortunate for persons impaired by physical handicaps that, as more and more hospitals, skilled nursing facilities, and extended care facilities establish components of rehabilitation services, there are not enough qualified physiatrists available to provide the evaluations and supervision that result in the best outcomes.

Even more disturbing is the fact that the programs for financing medical care do not provide for the delivery of full physiatric supervision to the patient as needed. The greatest professional deficiency among all of the medical specialties today is this shortage of physiatrists, with the demand for physiatrists being at least 50 per cent higher than the total number in practice. Health insurance today is focused primarily, and in some cases solely, on those aspects of medical care that attempt to ensure survival, since without survival more advanced levels of human performance are not possible. However, survival alone provides only the biological basis for higher levels of performance while contributing little to the sense that there is any quality to that life (see Chapter 12). One of the results of federalization of health insurance was the expansion of the health services provided beyond emergency and acute care, to include the element of rehabilitation for certain kinds of diseases and disabilities but not for others. Primarily, the focus of health insurance has been on short-term in-hospital care, which represents by far the most expensive daily cost.

Insurance has always concentrated on dramatic medical interventions for urgent risk, which requires prompt diagnosis of the pathology followed by prompt short-term intervention. The extent of coverage of the costs usually has been proportional to the urgency of the intervention. Instead of comprehensive evaluation and treatment with restoration to optimal function as is needed for chronic conditions, provision under legislative programs as well as private insurance frequently has been made only for evaluation when the problems do not threaten immediate death. Evaluation without the necessary subsequent treatment is valueless for the patient. Those patients remain the same as they were before that evaluation. They have received a service that has had no impact on their quality of life, i.e., an activity that is really a nonservice to the individual. Only when we recognize, adopt, and institute management according to the concepts of comprehensive medical care will we begin to serve the totality of health needs of the types of prolonged conditions discussed in this text.

The editors wish to express their profound appreciation to each of the contributors of the chapters that make up *Krusen's Handbook of Physical Medicine and Rehabilitation.* These authors have become authorities on the material of the chapters on which they write. They know the literature, past and present, and from it select the most pertinent knowledge, applications, and techniques to aid the reader to carry out the most pertinent activities in the field of physical medicine and rehabilitation, using the methods which are of optimal benefit for the patients. For this diligent effort, the principal compensation that each of the chapter authors receives is the awareness that each has made a personal contribution to the education of young physicians and other professionals in rehabilitation by making the principles and application of rehabilitation more available in a form that is easy to study. The eventual beneficiaries are the handicapped patients who receive the most effective, improved, and extended rehabilitation services. The wide distribution and general use of *Krusen's Handbook of Physical Medicine and Rehabilitation* in its past editions indicates that the Expert Physiatric Committee of the American Rehabilitation Foundation, which, under the chairmanship of Dr. Frank H. Krusen 30 years ago initiated the planning, development, and publication of the First Edition, was successful in achieving the goal of writing a general textbook of physical medicine and rehabilitation directed toward the needs of the postgraduate resident, the young physiatrist beginning his practice, and the undergraduate medical student.

New knowledge in physiatry has required that the text be brought up to date every 6 to 8 years so that physiatric practitioners may keep abreast of advancing knowledge. The knowledge in physiatry, like that in other medical specialties, expands ever more rapidly. As a consequence, the chapters of the Fourth Edition are longer, and the list of carefully selected references at the end of each chapter also is longer. In a textbook that presents concepts, knowledge based on research and clinical experience, and techniques of application, if it is to meet the needs of its student readers, the content cannot be too condensed or it becomes too generalized to be applicable. On the other hand, for that reader who wishes to study a topic in great detail, this textbook may be used as a guide to the breadth of material that may be found in the biomedical literature. For that purpose, the references listed aid the reader to enter the biomedical literature in a meaningful way and follow the streams of development of ideas back to their sources. Such reading also stimulates new ideas and helps to induce transmutation of associations and concepts, leading to more profound understanding of the phenomena of physiatry.[6]

We wish to express our appreciation to Joan Odegard and Ruth Giaconi for their extensive assistance in preparation and correction of the manuscripts and galleys. Finally, we wish to thank Mr. Edward H. Wickland, Jr., Senior Medical Editor, and his staff and the W. B. Saunders Company for the willing collaboration and excellent support that we have received in the editing and publishing of this book.

FREDERIC J. KOTTKE
JUSTUS F. LEHMANN

References

1. Crewe, N. M.: Quality of life. The ultimate goal in rehabilitation. Minnesota Med., 63:586–589, 1980.
2. England, G. W., and Lofquist, L. L.: A survey of the physically handicapped in Minnesota. Minnesota Studies in Vocational Rehabilitation Bulletin 26, pp. 1–54, Industrial Relations Center, University of Minnesota, 1958.
3. Flanagan, J. C.: A research approach to improving our quality of life. Am. Psychol., 33:138–147, 1978.
4. Friedlieb, O. P.: Letter to editor. J.A.M.A., 242:1490, 1979.
5. Katz, S., Branch, L. G., Branson, M. H., Papsidero, J. A., Beck, J. C., and Greer, D. S.: Active life expectancy. N. Engl. J. Med., 309:1218–1224, 1983.
6. Kottke, F. J.: Philosophic considerations of quality of life for the disabled. Arch. Phys. Med. Rehabil., 63:60–62, 1982.
7. Krusen, F. H.: The expanding field of physical medicine. Arch. Phys. Med., 27:201, 1946.
8. Rusk, H. A.: Rehabilitation. J.A.M.A., 140:286–292, 1949.
9. Schoening, H. A., and Iversen, I. A.: Numerical scoring and self-care status: A study of the Kenny self-care evaluation. Arch. Phys. Med. Rehabil., 49:221–229, 1968.
10. White, K. L.: Life and death in medicine. Sci. Am., 229:23–33, 1973.

Preface to the Third Edition

When physical medicine and rehabilitation, or physiatry, was recognized formally as a medical specialty in 1947 by the establishment of the American Board of Physical Medicine and Rehabilitation, comprehensive rehabilitation was not being taught in our medical schools and was practiced in very few civilian centers in the United States. At that time, only four years had elapsed since Dr. Howard A. Rusk had conclusively demonstrated to the Army that rehabilitation rather than convalescence was essential to restore soldiers to fitness for return to duty. Only three years previously, because of a nationwide demonstration under the auspices of the American Medical Association of the benefits of early ambulation, doctors in civilian hospitals were just beginning to abandon the time-honored custom of keeping patients bedfast for two to three weeks after abdominal surgery. Although the benefits of early ambulation were striking and patients were beginning to be mobilized more rapidly, physicians were still focusing almost exclusively on identification and eradication of acute pathology, after which patients were allowed to convalesce for weeks or months, and all too frequently to stagnate for years. At that time Dr. Rusk began to refer to rehabilitation as "the third phase of medical care" to be instituted following the first phase, preventive medicine, and the second phase, curative medicine and surgery.[1] He emphasized that "in that period when the 'fever is down and the stitches are out,' in the period 'between the bed and the job,' " the patient should be engaged in an active rehabilitation program rather than in passive convalescence.[2] When rehabilitation was applied in this way it represented a great stride forward. However, only a small minority of chronically disabled patients received rehabilitation as a part of the plan of medical management. All too frequently patients experienced further deterioration rather than recovery of neuromusculoskeletal function during a stage of inactive convalescence. Many months and often years would go by with no evidence of improvement of function. In the mid-1950's the Office of Vocational Rehabilitation reported that the average interval from the onset of a stroke to the referral for rehabilitation services was still four years (compared to experience today that the average time for *completion* of the rehabilitation program after the onset of a stroke is approximately two months).

Much progress has been made because of the teaching and advocacy of Drs. Krusen and Rusk and their students. Rehabilitation medicine is recognized today as a necessary and integral part of the management of chronic diseases and disabilities.[3] Rehabilitation services are being paid for increasingly under the various insurance systems for financing health care. Hospitals, extended care facilities, and nursing homes are seeking rehabilitation services for the chronically ill and disabled. The demands for rehabilitation services are growing faster than professional personnel are being trained. As Dr. Rusk has said, "Rehabilitation of the chronically ill and the chronically disabled is not just a series of restorative techniques; it is a philosophy of medical responsibility. Failure to assume this responsibility means to guarantee the continued deterioration of many less-severely disabled persons until they, too, reach the severely disabled and totally dependent category." The neglect of disability in its early stages is far more costly than an early aggressive program of rehabilitation which will restore the individual "to optimal self-sufficiency and functional performance."[4] The American public—that is, the relatives and friends of the chronically ill and disabled—has accepted this philosophy and seeks its application as a part of standard medical care.

That demand for rehabilitation services as indicated by the shortage of rehabilitation personnel appears most promising until it is compared with the relative effort devoted to the teaching of rehabilitation by our medical schools at the present time. Although in numbers more persons need rehabilitation services for significant handicaps resulting from chronic diseases and disabilities than are being admitted to hospitals for treatment of acute diseases, chronic diseases receive only a tiny fraction of the emphasis placed on diagnosis, clinical pathology, and treatment of acute diseases by our medical schools (Fig. 1). Rehabilitation still has not achieved sufficient stature to become an essential part of the education of the medical student. It suffers from the "one-down" effect described by Forman and Hetznecker.[5]

The medical establishment thrives on short term care and dramatic cures. Sophisticated drug regimens and surgical interventions—the essentials of (acute) medical methodology—are of limited usefulness in the treatment of a handicap. At bottom, the handicapped patient is not particularly attractive in terms of the medical challenge and opportunities he presents. But not only is the handicapped patient "one-down"; so is his physician. . . . The status of the physician is determined, to a major extent, by the status of his patient, and this phenomenon may be described as the "status rub-off effect."

This "one-down" phenomenon pervades the policies of medical education also, so that rehabilitation of the handicapped, although a major problem of our society today, receives only minor attention in the medical curriculum. Only half of the medical schools in the United States have organized departments of physical medicine and rehabilitation. Even those departments are allowed very little time in the curriculum to teach concepts of rehabilitation medicine or procedures and skills. Only 0.5 per cent of medical graduates have been selecting physical medicine and rehabilitation as a specialty for practice. Currently there are only 2200 physiatrists in practice, although 5 to 10 per cent of the total population are estimated to be in need of physical medicine and rehabilitation services at this time. At least three times as many physiatrists would be needed to provide those services. Most other physicians have had little or no training to enable them to use physiatry knowledgeably. Therefore, while the need is great and still increasing, the rate of training of physiatrists and other physicians to practice rehabilitation medicine at present does not indicate that the supply of services will begin to approach the need for services within the next two decades unless a major increase in education in rehabilitation medicine can be achieved.

In the face of this changing pattern of need with the rapid ascendency of

Major Disease Categories
Ranked According to Limitation of Activity

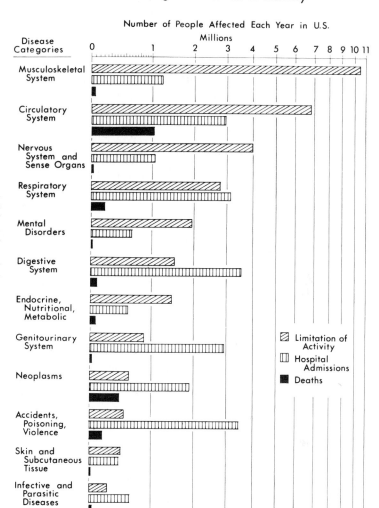

FIGURE 1. Two thirds of the persons with limitation of activity, which means significant impairment of self-care, ambulation, or ability to carry on the usual daily activities, have diseases of the musculoskeletal, circulatory, or nervous systems. The incidence of dependency-producing disabilities is not proportional either to annual mortality or to hospital usage by persons in each of the 12 major disease categories.

chronic diseases and disabilities as major problems, rehabilitation to restore the disabled to optimal levels of performance in society will test the efficiency of medical care in the foreseeable future. However, achievement of efficiency in medical care will require better organization of the resources for provision of health services so that those services are directed toward the return of individuals to the community at optimal functional levels, whether they are disabled by acute illness or by chronic dysfunction. Over the last 50 years medicine and surgery have prevented the deaths of countless persons who were critically ill. Many have been cured. However, there also have been a progressively increasing number left with chronic disabilities. A high proportion of these have not been restored to their optimal levels of functioning in relation to their remaining abilities; multiple sample surveys have estimated that between 5 and 10 per cent of the total population fall into this category of disability. These disabled persons have greatly increased costs for maintenance in addition to the costs of medical care required because of the continuing disability. The costs of dependency resulting from such disabilities have a negative effect on the economy, whether those costs are paid by private or by public funds. In either case dependency consumes resources without enhancing productivity or quality of life for the patient.

The development of rehabilitation as an integral part of comprehensive medical care and its application to restore persons with continuing impairments to the optimal level of performance in their homes and communities will increase the efficiency of our system of health care, as measured by cost-benefit analysis. Just as we do for other modern industries and services, we need to relate the costs involved to the product obtained from medical care. This product is the outcome of medical care as measured by the effect on the life of the patient. There is an economic efficiency to be considered and also a human efficiency.

$$\text{Economic Efficiency} = \frac{\text{Benefits Obtained}}{\text{Investment}}$$

$$= \frac{(P + C_{\overline{S}R} - C_{\overline{P}R})\,T - C_R}{C_R}$$

where P = vocational productivity
$C_{\overline{S}R}$ = cost of care and maintenance without rehabilitation
$C_{\overline{P}R}$ = cost of care and maintenance after rehabilitation
C_R = cost of rehabilitation
T = time of survival in years

$$\text{Human Efficiency} = \frac{\text{Actual Performance}}{\text{Optimal Performance}}$$

Too often when economic efficiency of rehabilitation is considered, only vocational productivity rather than savings in the cost of maintenance is taken into account. It is nearly impossible to obtain data regarding the full cost of the unrehabilitated handicapped because support must come from so many sources. However, the data that have become available demonstrate the high efficiency of rehabilitation as a newly emerging component of medical care.[6] The reduction of dependency through rehabilitation is cost effective.

The best measure of the value of medical services is the outcome, measured by the degree of improvement of function and the quality of life of the patient. Outcome should be measured by parameters of patient performance throughout the life span rather than by length of survival. Anderson et al.[7] have developed a general scale of functional outcome of rehabilitation modified from Williamson[8] to assess levels of performance across the entire range from normal to death, as shown in Table 1.

This scale focuses on the change of functioning performance of the patient as increasing illness or disability increases dependency until death super-

TABLE 1. Scale of Functional Outcome
of Rehabilitation

1. Normal or asymptomatic
2. Symptomatic
3. Partially independent (more than 50 per cent
   independent)
4. Partially dependent (more than 50 per cent
   dependent)
5. Totally dependent
6. Death

venes. Conversely, with rehabilitation the patient moves upward through stages of increasing independence to the optimal level of functional performance. Although the assumption often is true in acute episodic diseases that if patients survive they will return to normal activity, the 30 million persons in the United States with chronic disabilities that influence their life styles attest to the fact that commonly cited statistics on mortality and survival do not present an adequate evaluation of healthfulness or of the need for health services. The development of quantitative scales of functional outcome of medical care which define smaller changes in function would make it possible to provide more precise evaluation of patients throughout the entire range of performance. For all patients the assessment of changes in functional performance should be used to define the benefits of therapy. Programs for health services should be designed to restore patients to the optimal levels of function that they can achieve and sustain in relation to the intrinsic and extrinsic resources available to them.

What is the economic cost of dependency? Currently in the United States 10 million people receive disability payments for assistance in maintaining themselves.[9] This represents 7 per cent of the Gross National Product being devoted to disability payments made to approximately 5 per cent of the population. Among the working population, ages 20 to 65, the disability payments amount to $47.6 billion annually. In addition, medical program expenditures for this same group amount to $13 billion annually. Beyond that, the direct services provided to this group cost $2.4 billion annually. Therefore, the total federal disability-related expenditures for the adult working-age population were $63 billion in 1977 and have been increasing about 35 per cent per year—faster than the cost-of-living increases due to inflation. To understand the full cost of disability we must also add the increased costs of care and maintenance of handicapped children and of the disabled among the geriatric population. For disabled persons the costs of maintenance represent approximately 75 per cent of the direct cost of disability (disregarding loss of earned income).

Maintenance of the disabled has been recognized as a major part of the cost of disability for many years. In 1949, in Hennepin County, Minnesota, Stinson studied the distribution of payments by the county welfare program.[10] Forty-nine per cent of the costs were payments to nursing homes for maintenance of the disabled. Twenty-five per cent of the cost was for acute hospital care. Fifteen per cent of the cost was for physician services, and 10 per cent of the cost was for pharmaceutical and other supplies.

In 1980 the Minnesota Department of Public Welfare reported spending

$566 million for Medicaid. Fifty-three per cent of the expenditures went for nursing home care, 14 per cent for care in state hospitals, 14 per cent for acute hospital care, and 2 per cent for hospital outpatient services (Fig. 2). Sixty-seven per cent of these costs were spent on institutional maintenance services. If acute hospital care, physicians, dentists, and pharmacy costs are included as a therapeutic group, 28 per cent of the costs went for those therapeutic services. Usually when costs of illnesses are calculated, only the costs of therapeutic services are considered and the much higher costs of maintenance services are ignored because, in general, they are paid from other sources. This separation of costs has caused us to fail to recognize the magnitude of potential savings to be obtained through rehabilitation.

Who received these Medicaid services? (Fig. 3). Forty-six per cent of the dollars spent for Medicaid in Minnesota went to the geriatric population. Thirty-five per cent of Medicaid was paid out for services to the disabled and blind of the state. Fourteen per cent of Medicaid was spent for medical services to families with dependent children. In each of these groups there were many individuals who could be made independent or less dependent so that the costs of dependency would be reduced.

The major disease categories leading to dependency have not changed significantly over the last 20 years. Therefore, data from the National Center for Health Statistics in 1972 provide a reasonable representation of our status today. The top 12 major disease categories presented in Figure 1 are arranged in descending order by (1) prevalence of limitation of activity, and also

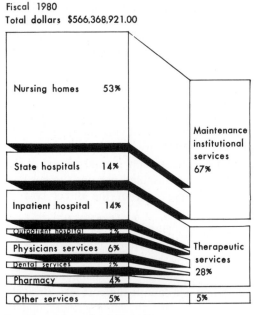

Minnesota medicaid expenditures

Fiscal 1980
Total dollars $566,368,921.00

Nursing homes 53%	
State hospitals 14%	Maintenance institutional services 67%
Inpatient hospital 14%	
Outpatient hospital 2%	
Physicians services 6%	Therapeutic services 28%
Dental services 2%	
Pharmacy 4%	
Other services 5%	5%

Data: Department of Public Welfare

FIGURE 2. Sixty-seven per cent of expenditures by the state of Minnesota through Medicaid in 1980 were for maintenance of the chronically ill and disabled in nursing homes or chronic care hospitals. (Republished with permission from the Star Tribune, Dec., 1981.)

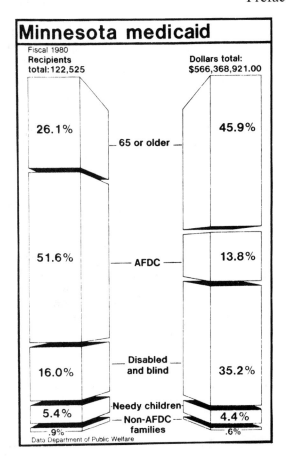

FIGURE 3. Seventy-one per cent of Medicaid expenditures by Minnesota in 1980 provided chronic care for geriatric patients or disabled younger persons. (Republished with permission from the Star Tribune, Dec., 1981.)

showing (2) hospital admissions annually and (3) deaths annually. Limitation of activity is defined as significant impairment of ability for self-care, ambulation, or ability to carry on the usual daily activities. Hospital admissions are an approximation of the relative costs of hospital care for these major disease categories. Limitation of activity shows no relationship either to deaths annually or to hospital costs. Note that one third of all disabilities are due to conditions of the musculoskeletal system, especially back problems and disabilities of the joints. Back injury is the most common disability in industry and also the most common of all disabilities in the United States. Limitation of activity due to heart disease, stroke, and peripheral vascular disease is considered under diseases of the circulatory system, which constitute about 21 per cent of all significant disabilities. Disabilities due to diseases of the nervous system and sense organs constitute 12 per cent of all limitation of activity. Disabilities in these three categories of diseases constitute two thirds of all of the disability as measured by limitation of activity in the United States. The physiatrist has been concentrating on and should continue to concentrate on this group of disabilities. However, since physiatrists constitute only 0.5 per cent of physicians in the United States, the impact of rehabilitation services on disabilities is far below the need for services.

Limitation of activity has a highly significant societal impact because it carries with it the major economic costs of dependency maintenance and loss of productivity. However, limitation of activity has not been a major focus of medical education which has concentrated its attention on the major causes of death, the pathologic aspects of disease, and the diagnostic processes by which pathology is identified. Neither has dependency resulting from disability been of major concern for acute medical care services nor for acute hospital care. These resources have been focused on the eradication of pathology that jeopardizes survival or limits the ability to live outside of the hospital, but they have not been committed to carrying the patient through to full restoration.

Why have we not used our health care resources for restoration of patients to optimal functional performance? The reasons are not obvious. In part, it may relate to the historical perspective that less than 100 years ago medical attention was directed almost entirely to survival or relief of pain. Not until about 60 years ago did we begin to develop specific cures for diseases. The development of antibiotics and physiological support systems over the past 40 years has increased the number of disabled persons who survive for many years. Health maintenance has changed from an abstraction to a process for application over the past 15 years. However, we are groping for parameters to measure the changes that can be achieved in the process of rehabilitating the patient to optimal performance (see Chap. 12). Until we can measure meaningful changes in performance and establish relationships between the health services provided and the improvement of performance achieved, we will not be able to establish systematic servicing programs. Until such time we will continue to have fractionated, disorganized, and unfocused health services.

Comprehensive rehabilitation needs to become outcome oriented, by developing means to measure outcome and then providing the guidance that is necessary so that the application of the entirety of medical services is oriented toward the optimal outcome for the individual. This goal should be optimal functional performance in the home and community throughout life. A simple illustrative diagram of human performance plotting the Scale of Functional Outcome of Rehabilitation against life span is shown in Figure 4. From birth there is a progressive increase of function through childhood up to a peak performance in early adulthood. If good health is maintained throughout life, function should persist near maximal until far into old age,

Human Performance as the Measure of Health Throughout Life

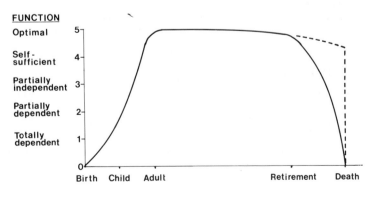

FIGURE 4. The functional performance of the normal, healthy person develops during childhood and is maintained through adult life.

and death would terminate that high level of function. We might liken that possibility to Oliver Wendell Holmes' "one-hoss shay," which fell apart "all at once and nothing first, just as a bubble when it bursts."

A functional life history when severe disability intervenes in adulthood is illustrated in Figure 5. Illness suddenly decreases functional capacity to total dependency. Medical care alone may ensure survival (curve A) but may leave patients totally or partially dependent throughout the remainder of their lives. Acute medical care plus limited rehabilitation may restore individuals to a higher level of function, but if the rehabilitation is not followed by an adequate maintenance program, there may be progressive loss of function to the level of dependency (curve B). The goal of every rehabilitation program should be to restore patients to a level of independent living so that at the end of the rehabilitation program they have adequate training and understanding to use available resources to maintain their functional levels throughout life. An optimal outcome of such a program is indicated by curve C.

One indication of the success that may be attained in the maintenance of function is indicated by the maintenance of mobility of a group of 80 stroke patients who underwent rehabilitation[11] (Fig. 6). An assessment of these patients at an average of 6 years (range 3 to 10 years) after rehabilitation showed that while 25 per cent of these patients had become nonambulatory or required supervision during walking, 75 per cent had maintained the functional ability that they had gained through rehabilitation. All of our services should be assessed by evaluation of outcome similar to this.

The potential functional outcome curves of children with developmental disabilities are illustrated in Figure 7. Children without rehabilitation remain very severely dependent, highly expensive invalids who survive for decades today in complete dependency. Inadequate or incomplete rehabilitation may raise the level of performance for a variable period of time but leave the individual with significant dependency needs. In many cases this is the best outcome that can be achieved today. A great deal of research is needed in rehabilitation of developmentally disabled children. Again, the goal for restoration and maintenance for these children should be self-sufficiency, independent living, education, and productivity throughout a normal life span.

Human Performance of Adult Disabled as the Measure of Rehabilitation

FIGURE 5. The functional performance of an adult who becomes disabled may remain at the level of dependency or be only partially restored without adequate rehabilitation followed by an appropriate program for maintenance.

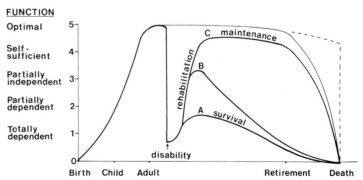

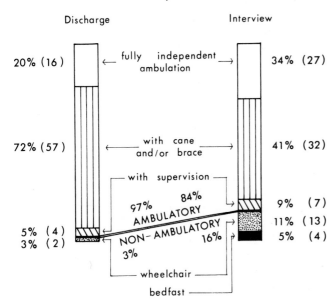

Mobility Level

FIGURE 6. Rehabilitation followed by appropriate maintenance can preserve a high level of function for years, as indicated by the maintenance of independent walking in patients for 3 to 10 years following a stroke. (From Anderson, E., Anderson, T. P., and Kottke, F. J.: Stroke rehabilitation: Maintenance of achieved gains. Arch. Phys. Med. Rehabil., 58:345–352, 1977.)

This third edition of *Krusen's Handbook* presents the concepts and practices of comprehensive rehabilitation and continuing maintenance of patients with disabilities, consistent with the needs described above. Since comprehensive rehabilitation has not been fully integrated into the medical curriculum, many medical students and practicing physicians lack knowledge of both principles and techniques of physical medicine and rehabilitation. Both aspects are presented here, so that *Krusen's Handbook* is a textbook for medical students, residents, and therapists as well as a ready reference for physicians in practice.

The book is organized into three general sections: evaluation, therapy, and rehabilitation of the major disabling conditions. The 12 chapters of the first section present the components of evaluation that provide the basis for comprehensive rehabilitation. Chapters 1 and 2 explain clinical evaluation of the patient for rehabilitation, and succeeding chapters discuss special techniques of performance evaluation, including electrodiagnosis and elec-

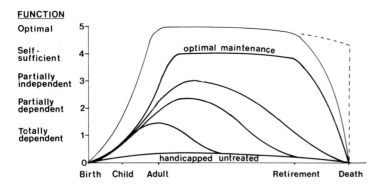

Human Performance of Developmentally Disabled as the Measure of Rehabilitation

FIGURE 7. Rehabilitation of disabled children is especially important, since without it they do not have an opportunity to develop and may remain severely dependent throughout a survival time of many decades.

tromyography, gait analysis, evaluation of speech and communication, psychological assessment and management, prevocational evaluation, epidemiology of disability, and reflex evaluation to assess neuromuscular function. Chapter 12 presents a system for health accounting in which systematic organization and recording of the ongoing rehabilitation process help to define the patient's status on admission and to evaluate the response to rehabilitation.

The second section, on therapeutics, consists of 17 chapters. Those dealing with standard aspects of therapy which have been of proven value for more than 50 years—thermotherapy, ultraviolet therapy, electrotherapy, massage, and exercise—have been updated to present recent innovations and newly developed techniques in addition to well-established principles and practices. Significant advances of the past decade in techniques of exercise for mobility, coordination, strength, and endurance are presented. A chapter has been devoted to the newly emerging application of functional electrical stimulation for patients with neuromuscular impairments. The following aspects of rehabilitation training have been updated: bed positioning, transfer training, wheelchair use, training for functional independence, and training for homemaking. Three chapters are devoted to the principles of design and application of orthotics for the upper extremities, the neck and trunk, and the lower extremities. One chapter considers specific aspects of the prescription of physical and occupational therapy by the physician.

The third section consists of 23 chapters dealing with the evaluation and rehabilitation management of disabling conditions that are encountered in physical medicine and rehabilitation. Arthritis and back disorders are most frequently encountered, with 5 per cent of the population significantly limited in daily self-care, ambulation, or vocational activity and many affected individuals homebound or sequestered in nursing homes. Therefore, knowledge of the rehabilitation management of arthritis and back disorders is important to all physicians in primary care as well as to physiatrists. Another large category of disability for which specific techniques of rehabilitation management are presented includes neurologic problems: stroke, closed head injuries, spinal cord injuries, cranial palsies, and traumatic and degenerative diseases of the nervous system. Rehabilitation management of cerebral palsy and other neurologic diseases of childhood involves consideration of the developmental aspects of childhood, both physical and psychosocial, as well as the specific aspects of therapy for motor and intellectual impairments. The techniques of rehabilitation of the cardiac patient either in the acute phase or in the convalescent phase of recovery are presented. Two chapters deal with the selection of prosthetics for upper extremity amputation and for lower extremity amputation and the fitting and training of the patient in their use. Chapters on specific organ sytstem management discusss neurogenic bowel and bladder, prevention of ischemic ulcers, care of the feet, problems of sexual function and disability, and deafness. Each is presented from the aspect of comprehensive rehabilitation. Finally, new chapters have been included in this third edition of *Krusen's Handbook* on rehabilitation of patients with cancer and on the response of the body to immobility.

The editors wish to express their deep appreciation to each of the authors who made a contribution to *Krusen's Handbook*. The major recompense that the authors receive is their awareness that they are making a significant contribution to the training of young physicians and others in the rehabilitation professions in the principles and application of physical medicine and rehabilitation. The eventual benefits are the improved and extended rehabilitation services that are made available to handicapped persons. However, in addition to that, the wide acceptance and use of this text in its first two editions indicate that many readers have appreciated the contributions of these authors. The contributing authors have been picked because they are authorities on their subjects, who not only select but also interpret and present from the literature the most pertinent information in a manner most meaningful to the reader. This careful preparation of each chapter with selected references provides the basis for entry into the biomedical literature by any reader who wishes to study a subject in greater depth.

We wish to thank Edna Maneval for her extensive editorial assistance, Jean Magney for her excellent illustrations, and, for secretarial help, especially Joan Odegard and Marion Hunter.

Grateful appreciation is expressed to the staff of the W. B. Saunders Company for their willing collaboration and excellent support in the editing and publishing of this book.

FREDERIC J. KOTTKE
JUSTUS F. LEHMANN
G. KEITH STILLWELL

References

1. Rusk, H. A.: Rehabilitation. JAMA, 140:286–292, 1949.
2. Rusk, H. A.: Advances in rehabilitation. Practitioner, 183:505–512, 1959.
3. Krusen, F. H.: Concepts in Rehabilitation of the Handicapped. Philadelphia, W. B. Saunders Company, 1964.
4. Rusk, H. A.: Preventive medicine, curative medicine–then rehabilitation. New Phys., 13:165–167, 1964.
5. Forman, M. A., and Hetznecker, W.: The physician and the handicapped child. JAMA, 247:3325–3326, 1982.
6. Kottke, F. J.: Historia, obscura hemiplegiae. Arch. Phys. Med. Rehabil., 55:4–13, 1974.
7. Anderson, T. P., McClure, W. J., Athelstan, G., Anderson, E., Crewe, N., Arndts, L., Ferguson, M. B., Baldridge, M., Gullickson, G., and Kottke, F. J.: Stroke rehabilitation: Evaluation of its quality by assessing patient outcomes. Arch. Phys. Med. Rehabil., 59:170–175, 1978.
8. Williamson, J. W.: Assessing and Improving Health Care Outcomes: The Health Accounting Approach to Quality Assurance. Cambridge, Ballinger, 1978.
9. Joe, T. C.: Professionalism: A new challenge for rehabilitation. Arch. Phys. Med. Rehabil., 62:245–250, 1981.
10. Stinson, M. B.: Medical care and rehabilitation for the aged. Geriatrics, 8:226–229, 1953.
11. Anderson, E., Anderson, T. P., and Kottke, F. J.: Stroke rehabilitation: Maintenance of achieved gains. Arch. Phys. Med. Rehabil. 58:345–352, 1977.

Contents

xxxix

1

Evaluation of the Patient

WALTER C. STOLOV   ROSS M. HAYS

Readers might ask why the need for a chapter on patient evaluation in a textbook on physical medicine and rehabilitation. They have, after all, learned and gained experience on how to elicit symptoms and signs from the history and physical examination of a patient. They already know how to use these data to establish a diagnosis of a patient's disease. Why not get on with the special therapeutics?

The reason is simple. *The symptoms and signs required for the diagnosis of disability are not synonymous with those required for the diagnosis of disease.*

Consider the following example:

A 22-year-old medical student in a skiing accident fractures his left humerus. As the history is being taken, he complains, "I can't raise my hand." "I can't straighten my fingers." "My grip is weak." Examination reveals paralysis of the wrist and finger extensors, and hypesthesia over the dorsum of the first digit.

The diagnosis of the *disease* is clear. The patient has, in addition to a fracture, a radial nerve palsy. The *disability,* however, is not clear and has not yet been diagnosed. One question must yet be asked: "With which hand do you usually write?" If the answer is "The left," one additional examination finding must be elicited. After the fracture is reduced and the arm placed in a cast, the patient's writing skill must be assessed. If the patient is unable to write, then at least part of the disability diagnosis (tnere may be other functions interrupted) includes the *inability to write.*

Neither the question, "With which hand do you usually write?" nor the examination of the patient's writing skill after casting was necessary to make the diagnosis of the disease, but both were necessary to diagnose the disability. The history and physical examination required for the two diagnoses were different.

Consider further the possibility that the patient may have answered, "I write with my right hand." The writing disability would therefore not be present, yet the disease would still be the same. This illustrates:

There is no one-to-one correlation between a disease and the spectrum of disability problems that may be associated with it. The disability is dependent on the patient's total requirements.

Consider further that our patient with the writing disability is advised that the radial nerve will not regrow successfully. As a result, the patient enters a deliberate systematic training program to develop writing ability with the normal right arm, and succeeds. The patient then has removed the disability, although the radial nerve palsy that caused it in the first place is still present. This illustrates:

There is no one-to-one relationship between a disease and the amount of residual disability. Disability problems can be removed even though the disease is unchanged.

This principle further points out a second important reason for a chapter on patient evaluation in a textbook on rehabilitation.

The ability of a patient and a physician to remove disability in the face of chronic disease is dependent on the residual capacity of the patient for physiological and psychological adaptation. The patient's residual strengths must be evaluated and built upon to "work around" impairment to remove disability.

Disability means lost function. Our initial example dealt with the loss of a physical function, writing. Other kinds of functional losses can occur:

A 55-year-old male outdoor construction worker complained of "shortness of breath" and "weakness." His-

WALTER C. STOLOV AND ROSS M. HAYS

tory and physical examination along with laboratory data confirmed the diagnosis of chronic obstructive pulmonary disease.

What, however, of the disability? Inquiry about employment revealed the patient was fired from a job because of a gradual reduction in work output. The patient confirmed that energy for the work was gone. The physician indicated that response to treatment of the lung disease would not be sufficient to allow for a return to outdoor construction work. The disability diagnosis will then include the problem of *unemployment.*

Were the same patient engaged in a white-collar job requiring minimal physical energy, unemployment would not be a problem. On the other hand, a white-collar worker with chronic obstructive pulmonary disease, although not disabled from work, may have the disability problem of loss of the major avocational pursuit (e.g., hunting) because of the disease.

The examples indicate the character of those diseases that produce disability. They are either diseases in which part or all of the pathological process is irreversible and hence are always present, i.e., chronic diseases, or they are diseases in which a significant period of time must elapse before the pathological process can be reversed. In either class, they may produce problems of dependency on others in activities of basic *physical function.* They may produce problems that relate to *social* functions in the home and with the family unit. They may produce problems in *vocational* functions and in the ability to engage in *avocational* pursuits. And finally, they may produce chronic emotional stresses that may lead to *psychological* problems requiring adjustments not only by the patient but by the family unit as well.

A host of conditions exist for which diagnosis of disease alone without including the diagnosis of disability will lead to insufficient treatment. The disabilities must first be identified. The spectrum of disability problems that occur depends upon the interaction of the patient with the environment. This interaction is shown schematically in Figure 1–1. It indicates that the total disability (i.e., the disability diagnosis—the total list of disability problems) derives from factors specific to the patient and specific to the environment.

Weed's problem-oriented approach[17] to the process of patient care is particularly suited to the evaluation of a patient with chronic illness and disability. The reader will profit by reviewing his monograph. He divides the patient treatment proc-

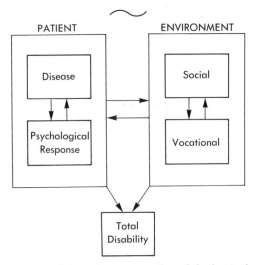

FIGURE 1–1. Schematic representation of the interaction of the patient with his environment. On the left, disease factors are reciprocally influenced by psychological factors. On the right, social factors are mutually influenced by vocational factors. The patient and his environment mutually influence each other. The Total Disability is fed by all areas.

ess into four phases. *Phase 1* includes the history, physical examination, and the initial laboratory studies as a data base. *Phase 2* identifies a specific problem list from the data base. *Phase 3* identifies a specific treatment plan for each of the problems. *Phase 4* describes the effectiveness of each of the plans and describes subsequent alterations in each, depending on the patient's progress.

The data base, therefore, goes beyond diagnosis determination. While a problem list will include known diagnoses, it will also include physiological syndromes, symptoms, signs, and laboratory abnormalities for which a disease diagnosis is as yet undetermined. The problem list also includes the specific impairments of function in the basic physical self-care skills, and those specific problems in social, vocational, and psychological function either secondary to or concurrent with the diseases. The individual identification of these functional problems leads to a plan for their solution, and hence for the removal of disability.

In this chapter are discussed specific methods of patient evaluation that will create the appropriate data base necessary to allow the physician to achieve a diagnosis of disability. History and physical examination data pertinent to an evaluation of lost function are described, and problem list formulation is introduced. A section on the disabled child is also included.

History

Historical data of prime importance in diagnosing disability are obtained from the *Chief Complaint, Present Illness,* and *Social and Vocational History* sections of the usual patient work-up. The nature of the *Chief Complaint* may provide a hint to the existence of disability. The *Present Illness* data can determine the extent of lost function in basic self-care activities. The *Social and Vocational History* evaluates the environment and provides insight into the psychological make-up of the patient. The *Review of Systems* and *Past Medical History* contribute to the assessment of residual capacity.

Chief Complaint

All chief complaints or main reasons a patient may seek the assistance of a physician derive from changes in health or in well-being. These changes create within the patient either (1) fear or anxiety, (2) discomfort, or (3) an inability to function. Chief complaints in which information on inability to function is included are the ones most apt to be associated with chronic illness and are those most likely to indicate that disability is present. The classes of diseases most likely to produce complaints of loss of function are those that involve the *musculoskeletal system*, the *neurological system,* or the *cardiovascular system*.[7]

The list of chief complaints and final discharge diagnoses presented in Table 1–1 was extracted from a series of charts.* In this list, the statements referring to function are in italics.

Although the majority of chief complaints related to loss of function are associated with chronic diseases of the musculoskeletal, neurological, or cardiovascular system, diseases in other systems also may yield statements related to loss of function (Table 1–2).

In these illustrations, the chronic diseases were in the pulmonary and gastrointestinal systems.

Complaints related to loss of function are presented also by patients with psychiatric disease and without organic pathological changes, as in the following examples extracted from charts of patients hospitalized on a psychiatric ward:

"Unable to *take care of myself*"
"Fear of going places"
"*Incapable of doing* job"
"Continuous ache in neck made worse by *movement and exercise*"
"I just can't *work, eat, or sleep*"
"I have had a *terrible family life*"

These examples illustrate that psychological responses to the stress of chronic disease may aggravate disability from organic pathological changes.

---

*The charts from which the statements have been abstracted are those of 50 patients consecutively discharged from a Veterans Administration hospital in 1967—10 each from a medical, surgical, neurological, psychiatric, and rehabilitation medicine service.

TABLE 1–1. Examples of Chief Complaints Associated with Diagnoses in Neurological, Musculoskeletal, and Cardiovascular System Diseases

CHIEF COMPLAINT	DISCHARGE DIAGNOSIS
"Pain in calves after *walking* several blocks"	Peripheral vascular disease
"Can't *control* right leg"	Stroke
"Right-sided *clumsiness,* trouble with *balance*"	Multiple sclerosis
"Inability to *use* legs well"	Multiple sclerosis
"Can't *walk* or *talk* well"	Parkinsonism
"Leg weakness, unable to *stand* alone"	Transverse myelitis
"Pain in back and left leg. The more I *do physically*, the more I hurt"	Herniated disc
"*Walking* and *bladder trouble*"	Parkinsonism
"Low back pain increased by *walking* and *sitting*"	Lumbar disc disease
"Difficulty *walking*"	Musculoskeletal trauma
"Unable to *stand* up"	Stroke
"Aching wrist aggravated by *activity*"	Degenerative joint disease
"Difficulty with *ambulation* control"	Brain trauma

TABLE 1–2. Examples of Chief Complaints Related to Diagnoses of Diseases in Other Systems

CHIEF COMPLAINT	DISCHARGE DIAGNOSIS
"Severe chest pain while *driving car*"	Chronic lung disease
"Pain after *eating*"	Peptic esophagitis
"Trouble *breathing* after *exercise*"	Obstructive pulmonary disease
"*Weakness*"	Carcinoma of the lung

When, therefore, chief complaints contain statements related to loss of function, the physician is alerted to pursue carefully a search for disability. The physician must search for the dependency of the patient on others to carry out basic self-care skills. The physician must search for problems in social functions in the home and family unit, problems of employment, and problems secondary to chronic psychological stress. The physician is further alerted to the need for careful study of the musculoskeletal, neurological, and cardiovascular systems.

Present Illness

One of the hallmarks of disability is a dependency on others for the performance of basic self-care activities, sometimes termed activities of daily living. Historical information about this dependency is best included under the category of *Present Illness*. Such data are really part of the symptom complex of the disease and are the essence of the disability the disease is producing. For example, it is not so much weakness that a patient is concerned about but the reduced ambulation that results. It is not the tremor that worries a patient, but the lost ability to hold a cup of coffee. Similarly, it is not so much the reduction in shoulder and elbow range or motion that a patient wishes to correct, but rather the lost ability to comb the hair or attend to his perineal hygiene after defecation.

The basic activities for which inquiry should be made as part of the *Present Illness* review can be divided into six categories: (1) ambulation, (2) transfer activities, (3) dressing activities, (4) eating skills, (5) personal hygiene, and (6) communication activities. The quantification of dependency in the performance of any of these activities of daily living is achieved by determining from the patient who in the family unit provides the assistance and the nature of the assistance provided. Assistance is in one of the following categories:

1. *Standby* assistance. As the activity is being performed by the patient, the individual may not always do it safely or correctly. The assistant then is "standing by" to guard against the occurrence of accidents and to ensure the correctness and completeness of performance by pointing out errors or omissions.

2. *Partial physical assistance*. As the activity is being performed, the patient is able to do a good part but not all of it alone. The assistant then provides partial physical assistance. For example, the assistant may buckle the patient's belt after the patient puts on pants or may hold the wheelchair stationary while the patient is transferring into bed.

3. *Total physical assistance*. For the activity to be accomplished, the assistant has to do all of it because the patient can contribute little or nothing toward its execution. The patient is, therefore, totally dependent.

Ambulation History. Ambulation may be defined in the broadest sense as *travel from one place to another over a finite distance*. Ambulation thus includes not only walking but also wheelchair travel and even crawling. To assess the extent of disability with regard to ambulation, the patient's capacity for ambulation in different environments must be obtained.

The environments of significance are the home, its immediate vicinity, and the community at large. A patient may, for example, be totally independent in walking within and around the house but not in the community. The environments found in theaters, restaurants, subways, or downtown stores may require that the patient have partial physical assistance in order to negotiate them safely. The disability diagnosis for such a patient will therefore include the problem of *decreased community ambulation*.

If a patient is not walking but uses a wheelchair, the extent of his independence in its use needs to be known. For example, the examiner should determine whether the patient is able to maneuver it independently within the home, whether he is also independent in its use outside his home, and if he can take it successfully into the community at large without assistance.

Sample questions in an exploration of ambulation skill are:

1. Can you walk without assistance?
2. Do you use equipment (canes, crutches, braces)?
3. Do you use a wheelchair?
4. Is there a limit to how far you can walk (or use your wheelchair) outside the home?
5. Can and do you go out visiting friends, or to restaurants, theaters, or stores?
6. Do you have falls?
7. Do you drive a car?
8. Can you climb stairs?

Transfer History. Transfers are movements that involve *changes of position in place.* They include such activities as going from a bed to a wheelchair or regular chair; going from a wheelchair to a toilet, bathtub, shower, or car; and going from a wheelchair, regular chair, or toilet seat to a standing position. These activities are more basic than ambulation. For example, while independent in walking, the patient may be physically dependent on others to get out of his chair into a standing posture. Independent ambulation therefore is not always available to the patient if the assistance for the transfer into the upright posture is not always present.

Sample questions to begin on assessment of disability in transfer abilities are:

1. Can you get in and out of bed unaided?
2. Can you get on and off a toilet unaided?
3. Can you get in and out of the tub unaided?

Dressing History. A disabled patient's ability to put on and take off clothes must be carefully assessed. If a patient is not independent in dressing, the person is less likely to leave the home and is less likely to receive guests other than the immediate family. Dressing dependency therefore greatly restricts the environments available to the patient.

In obtaining a history of performance in dressing skills, it is not sufficient merely to ask, "Do you dress yourself?" An untrained disabled patient may have for some time abandoned the use of those garments more difficult to put on. Typically abandoned are shoes, socks, pants, clothes with buttons, and close-fitting undergarments. A patient therefore may answer "Yes" to such a question without realizing how few clothes are still worn. A more complete probe is therefore necessary to gain insight into his performance.

Sample questions that may be asked to explore competence in dressing are:

1. Do you dress in street clothes daily?
2. Can you put on without assistance your shirt, pants, dress, undergarments, and so forth?
3. Do you need help with shoes and socks?

Eating History. The loss of independence in a patient's capacity for self-feeding can be most devastating to the self-image. Unlike the activities already discussed, it is the one activity that *must still go on even if total physical assistance is necessary.* A patient who is dependent on others for feeding is literally reduced to the level of an infant.

Eating skills include the use of a fork, spoon, and knife, and the handling of cups and glasses.

Sample questions in an exploration of this area include:

1. Can you feed yourself unassisted?
2. Can you cut meat?
3. Do you have trouble holding glasses and cups?

Personal Hygiene History. Personal hygiene activities include the spectrum of skills concerned with cleaning and grooming: toothbrushing, hair combing, shaving, the use of tub and shower, perineal care, and the successful handling of bowel and bladder elimination. Loss of independence in the performance of these skills is severely disabling to the patient. This is particularly so when the patient cannot handle bowel and bladder elimination in a socially acceptable manner. If a patient must be concerned with the possibility that the trousers or the bed or someone's car may be soiled with feces or urine, the emotional stresses placed on the patient and the family can be quite severe. The adult who requires that the spouse help clean up after defecation may soon be dealing with a strained marriage. Efforts at increasing social functioning and directed toward vocational rehabilitation will be unsuccessful until the patient can develop a system of elimination that is consistently successful.

Socially acceptable elimination does not necessarily require that the systems be physiologically normal. Patients with catheters can develop a successful system if they can handle the emptying of collecting bags and can satisfactorily hide the collecting system under trousers or skirts.

Sample questions to explore the personal hygiene area include:

1. Can you shave (use make-up) and comb your hair unaided?
2. Can you shower or bathe without assistance?

WALTER C. STOLOV AND ROSS M. HAYS

3. Can you use a toilet unaided?

4. Do you need help in cleaning up after a bowel movement?

5. Are bladder and bowel accidents a problem for you?

Communication History. Communication activities include the spectrum of skills associated with listening, speaking, reading, and writing. This area demonstrates the breadth and depth of language function. It is therefore, in part, dependent upon the patient's education and intellectual level. Further, listening and reading skills are also dependent upon the integrity of the auditory and visual organs, and speaking and writing skills are dependent upon the integrity of the motor functions associated with articulation and hand dexterity.

To achieve a historical understanding of these skills, the examiner may need to direct the inquiry to family members or others who have a recent and a long-standing relationship with the patient. For deficits that are not stable, the time course of deterioration should also be assessed.

Sample questions to explore the communication area include:

1. Do people have trouble understanding your speech?

2. Do you have trouble understanding what other people are saying?

3. Do you have difficulty reading newspapers or magazines?

4. Is writing difficult for you?

5. Do you have or use any special methods to improve your ability to communicate either in writing or speech?

General Principles in Determining Disability in Basic Functions. In exploring for disability in the five basic functions of ambulation, transfers, dressing, eating, and personal hygiene, several principles should be kept in mind:

1. When the patient reports the loss of independence, determine the type of assistance: standby, partial physical, or total physical.

2. Determine who is supplying the assistance.

3. Separately interview the people (usually family members) who are supplying the assistance. The assistant may indicate that the degree of assistance is actually greater than that reported by the patient. The two may not interpret in the same way what is actually occurring. A significant difference in the context of their remarks may indicate that neither is satisfied with what is going on.

4. When it is expected or anticipated that the patient may be dependent, questions of the "Can you . . ." or "Do you . . ." type should be rephrased to "Who helps you. . . ." Questions asked in this way may yield more information. Patients may wish initially to appear more independent than they actually are.

5. When the disability is of acute onset, the inquiry should also include the pre-morbid level of independence. This is particularly important in the older patient. Earlier disease or trauma may have left some residual dependency. Therapeutics brought to bear on the new problems are not likely to result in a degree of independence greater than pre-morbid levels.

6. If dependency is present and the disease is of a chronic progressive type, determine the time course of the loss of independence. Therapeutics are more likely to remove disability in more recently lost functions rather than in those lost many years previously.

7. For some patients, the answers to certain of the preceding sample questions may be obvious and hence need not be asked. It is best, however, to assume less and inquire more, thereby avoiding omissions of significant data.

When an inquiry into the basic self-care functions of ambulation, transfers, dressing, eating, and personal hygiene is complete, specific disability problems become identified. They need to be identified separately in the patient's list of problems even though they are secondary to a specific disease. Since the pathological condition may be irreversible in part or in whole, these functional problems will not be eliminated by reversal of the disease process and will have to be attacked individually. Before therapeutics can be applied, however, problems must be identified.

Review of Systems

As already indicated, the ability of a patient and the physician to remove disability is dependent on the patient's residual capacity. Often, specific exercise and training activities are required to remove disability and restore function. The status of four systems in particular must be evaluated to assess the patient's capacity for this training. The *Review of Systems* inquiry, therefore, requires careful study of the cardiovascular, respiratory, neurological, and musculoskeletal systems. The cardinal symptoms in each of these systems are

Cardiovascular. Dyspnea, orthopnea, chest pain, limb claudication, palpitation, and cough.

Respiratory. Cough, sputum, hemoptysis, chest pain, and dyspnea.

Neurological. Numbness, weakness, fainting or loss of consciousness, dizziness, pain, headache, and defective memory or thinking.

Musculoskeletal. Pain, deformity, weakness, limitation of movement, and stiffness.

Past Medical History

Like the *Review of Systems,* the *Past Medical History* provides information on the residual capacity of the patient. Concurrent disease or previous trauma and surgery may have produced residual impairments. Although these impairments no longer produce disability themselves, they may compound the disability of the present illness when added to the new impairments.

A few examples may help clarify this principle:

A patient suffered a severe left brachial plexus injury, which resulted in paralysis of the triceps and the muscles of the wrist and hand. The past medical history revealed an earlier right hip fracture. Although the hip fracture had healed well, residual hip abductor muscle weakness required the use of a cane in the left hand for safe ambulation. Prior to the brachial plexus injury, the patient had not been disabled, since ambulation needs could be handled with the cane.

The profound paralysis of the left arm, as a result of the brachial plexus injury, has now disabled the patient for ambulation.

Loss of ambulation is never a consequence of a brachial plexus injury alone. The past medical problem has compounded the disability.

A patient in an automobile accident suffered a complete paraplegia as a result of injury at the level of the tenth thoracic vertebra. The past medical history revealed a problem of recurrent shoulder dislocation, which was successfully repaired by surgery. The patient, after paraplegia occurred, began a heavy exercise program for the upper extremities in preparation for training in transfer activities. During a bout of exercise, shoulder dislocation occurred. After reduction, immobilization of the arm for six weeks was recommended.

The patient, therefore, became disabled for transfer activities not as a result of paraplegia but because of the compounding effect of his previously dormant past medical problem.

A careful *Past Medical History* review is therefore an essential component of the evaluation of a patient with disability. A simple recitation of past or concurrent disease or trauma may not be enough. The inquiry requires an understanding of residuals, however slight they may seem.

Social and Vocational History

The social and vocational history of the patient is the source for the necessary data about the environment with which the patient must interact. A careful review will identify environmental problems secondary to or concurrent with the disease. It also provides insight into the personality of the patient. Information on his ability to adjust to the stress of chronic disability can be obtained, and the psychological problems that may need to be dealt with can therefore be identified early.

It is convenient to divide the personal history data of the patient into three categories: *social, vocational,* and *psychological.*

Social History. When dependency on others for the performance of basic self-care skills occurs, or if a job is lost because of disease, the patient's family unit is compromised. The need to help the disabled person perform the activities of daily living and the loss of income may force some family members to alter their own plans greatly. A major disability of one member of a family unit will create problems of adjustment for all and even threaten the integrity of the unit. Superimposition of a major disability on a family unit already beset with social problems is particularly threatening. Identification of secondary and concurrent social issues as *patient problems* and inclusion of them in the patient's problem list allows the physician to begin to attack the environmental problems at the same time that the physician attacks problems directly related to organic pathological processes.

The assessment of social impairment is obtained from inquiries into the stability of the family unit, the history of the unit, the resources within the unit, the responsibilities of the patient within the unit, and the physical environment of the home and the community.

The physical environments are important because independence or dependence in the performance of an activity is directly related to where the activity is being carried out. The following examples illustrate the influence of physical environments on independence:

A patient who is independent in wheelchair travel may require physical assistance to transfer from toilet to wheelchair if the toilet seat is too low. Similarly, a patient may be dependent in bed

WALTER C. STOLOV AND ROSS M. HAYS

transfers if the bed is too high. On the other hand, a patient who is independent in wheelchair travel and in transfers, regardless of the toilet seat height, may still be dependent on others for bathroom activities if the door to the bathroom is too narrow to allow for entrance of the wheelchair.

A patient who lives in a large city may be totally confined to the home and be unable to go downtown or to a store because such a trip may require the use of the subway and hence the ability to negotiate three flights of stairs. If he is not independent in such stairclimbing skills, subway travel will be beyond reach and downtown inaccessible. On the other hand, a patient with identical skills who lives in a smaller city or in a suburban or rural community and who can perform automobile transfers and knows how to drive or has someone who can drive will have accessibility to downtown.

Sample questions to begin a search for problems in social functioning can include:

1. Where do you live? (Urban? Suburban? Rural?)

2. Do you rent or own your residence?

3. Are the bedroom, bathroom, kitchen on the same floor?

4. Are there entrance stairs or stairs within the home or apartment?

5. Who else is at home? (Wife, husband, children [ages], and friends?) Do any of them go to work or school? Are they in good health? Are the children having trouble in school?

6. Do your parents, brothers, and sisters live in the area? Do you maintain any contact with them?

7. Are you (how long have you been) married? Is this your first marriage?

8. What activities and functions did you do at home for the family that you no longer can do? (Examples are discipline of children, financial management, chores, sexual functions, avocational activities.) How are these functions now handled?

9. Where were you born?

10. Where else have you lived?

11. What did (or do) your father and siblings do for a living?

12. When did you leave your parents' home?

13. What was your family life as a child like?

The answers to these questions will provide information on the patient's social background and current resources, as well as suggest current or potential problems. "Abnormal" responses to these questions should be pursued. For example, if a patient has been married before, inquiry into

the number of previous marriages, their lengths, reasons for break-up, other children, and financial obligations will yield further insight.

Vocational History. A patient's disease may also produce the disability of unemployment. Whether there is or will be a problem in this area requires an understanding of the physical, intellectual, and interpersonal requirements of the patient's job.

Sample questions to determine if the disease and the lost function in the activities of daily living will be compatible with employment are:

1. When did you last work?

2. For whom did (do) you work?

3. How long did you (have you) work(ed) for them?

4. Describe what you did (do) on the job. Be specific. Start with what you do when you first arrive.

5. Was (is) your income sufficient to support your family or do you have other sources? Do you have debts?

If job instability is suspected—for example, if the last (current) job was held for less than two years, or if the last (current) job seems to be incompatible with the current illness even after rehabilitation treatment—then more information is needed:

1. Inquire about what kind of work is planned for the future.

2. Obtain chronological history of employment, job requirements, and reasons for change.

3. Inquire about special skills, licenses, union memberships, and ratings received.

4. Inquire about highest attained educational level, age at time schooling was completed, and level of school performance.

These additional facts will indicate whether there have been work adjustment problems. The strengths in the patient's vocational background on which one can build will also become clear. If the patient has not been working, inquire into the current sources of financial support and their sufficiency.

For the homemaker who is not employed outside the home, inquire:

1. When did you last do the cooking? Shopping? Light housekeeping? Heavy cleaning?

2. Who does these things now?

3. Is this arrangement satisfactory for you and your family?

Avocational activities are also an important aspect of a patient's function. Many patients derive more of their enjoyment of life from their avocational pursuits than from vocational activities. *To seek for problems in this area, the following sample questions are useful:*

1. What do you do with your leisure time after work and on weekends by yourself? With your family?

2. What organizations or religious groups are you active in?

3. When did you last participate in these activities?

Psychological History. Psychological function needs to be assessed in patients with a chronic illness or physical disability for several reasons: (1) Since the organic pathological changes may be incompletely reversible, the stress of the disease is always present. This stress may be of great magnitude. For example, a patient who loses a leg has to adjust not only to this loss but also perhaps to the secondary stress of loss of a job. The physical requirements of the job may be incompatible with activity limits of an artificial limb. (2) The patient and the family may have to relinquish established goals and old ways of doing things. The patient may have to learn new ways of self-maintenance that are not at all consistent with the patient's personality. These new modes of behavior are usually not the patient's preferred way of doing things, and often not society's preferred way. (3) The patient's psychological make-up needs to be understood, for if new learning is to be facilitated in treatment, an understanding of what is likely to motivate the patient and reinforce new learning is necessary. (4) For patients with brain damage from trauma or disease, an understanding of intellectual function will be required if they are to be trained successfully in the removal of disability in the basic functions.

Psychological problems should be included in the patient's problem list when the reaction to the stress of the disease is inappropriate or insufficient and when new learning is not occurring during treatment. While the *Mental Status* examination can assess current function, the social and vocational history data will yield a great deal of information about the patient's basic personality.

Interpretation of social and vocational data to yield psychological characteristics is a relatively simple matter when organized into four categories:

1. The patient's previous life style.

2. The patient's past history or response to ordinary life stresses.

3. The patient's current response to the stress of the disease.

4. The activities likely to motivate the patient to "train around" the disability.

Life Style. Characterization of a patient's life style is an attempt to identify a common thread in his social, vocational, and avocational activities. A *symbol-oriented* person is concerned predominantly with the world of ideas, abstract concepts, words, and numbers. A *motor-oriented* person is concerned with the world of objects or physical movement. An *interpersonally oriented* person's life is dominated by activities involving close personal contact with others.

For many people, their usual style is heavily invested in only one of these areas. If such a person suffers a loss of function that interferes with the ability to maintain a preferred mode of living, the psychological burden the disease produces will be great. For example, a professional athlete whose illness produces lower limb paralysis will have a greater psychological burden to adjust to than will a bookkeeper with the identical paralysis. If, however, the bookkeeper's major source of enjoyment of life was derived from hunting, fishing, and camping activities, the burden may be as great as the athlete's. Those whose life style is well balanced among these three areas will be more likely to adjust to disability that affects only one of the areas.

Knowledge of the patient's usual life style and the effect of his disease will yield insight into the psychological response and the problems the patient may have.

The following sample groupings of vocational and avocational data obtained from the history will assist in this determination:

SYMBOL-ORIENTED *concerned c̄ ideas, abstract concepts, words + #'s*

Vocations: Law, accounting, science, clerical fields.

Avocations: Reading, conversation, theater, museums.

MOTOR-ORIENTED *concerned c̄ objects or physical movement*

Vocations: Manual labor, tools, machinery, athletics.

Avocations: Active sports, hobby shop, hiking, camping.

INTERPERSONALLY ORIENTED *activities c̄ others*

Vocations: Sales, service, teaching.

Avocations: Church groups, clubs, meetings, parties.

WALTER C. STOLOV AND ROSS M. HAYS

Past Response to "Ordinary" Life Stresses. For some people, the simple business of living produces stresses that they are unable to handle successfully. For these people, it can be anticipated that the superimposition of the stress of disability may be overwhelming. Such patients may actually be more psychologically comfortable with the state of dependency the disability creates. To successfully remove the disability for such patients may be a difficult task.

The physician is alerted to this potential problem when the social and vocational data reveal such things as multiple marriages, multiple vocational and business failures, alcoholism, psychiatric hospitalization, police involvement, delinquent children, and excessive debts.

When, however, the history is devoid of such social and vocational events, the patient may be more likely to be successful in removing the disability and regaining independence.

Current Response to the Disease Stress. If a patient is being evaluated some time after the onset of the disability-producing disease, insight into the patient's ability to handle stress can be obtained from what has transpired. If the social history and present illness data reveal that the patient has been getting prescriptions filled, taking medicine, keeping appointments, altering habits, monitoring diet, and avoiding preventable secondary complications, then the patient is exhibiting a satisfactory adjustment. Such a patient is more likely to be able to remove disability and achieve independence.

Motivational Factors. The same social and vocational data that identify the patient's life style will also identify the type of activities that can be used as goals toward which the patient works as he strives to remove dependency during treatment. The likelihood of success in an activity consistent with the patient's pre-morbid life style will serve as a motivational factor, even if the work the patient must perform to achieve his goals includes activities that are in themselves alien to the patient's usual style.

For example, an interpersonally oriented individual may be motivated to perform certain heavy exercises important for health if, on achieving a required level of strength, increased visitation with others is permitted. Similarly, a symbol-oriented individual may be motivated to develop transfer skill independence (a motor-oriented task) if, on success, the opportunity to attend a play or concert is made available.

Thus, the social and vocational data provide information that will allow the physician to build on the patient's strengths as the physician attempts to assist the patient in the removal of disability.

Summary

When the classic approach to the history is elaborated in certain key areas, a patient's total disability can be properly diagnosed.

If the *Present Illness* is studied with regard to the patient's status in ambulation, transfers, eating, dressing, and personal hygiene, the spectrum of problems in self-care functions can be identified.

Study of the *Review of Systems* and the *Past Medical History* provides information on the residual capacity of the patient.

If the *Personal History* is elaborated to include careful study of the *Social and Vocational History,* then the problems within the environment can be identified. When such data are also scrutinized with regard to the psychology of the disabled patient, then problems of the patient's reaction to the stress of the incompletely reversible pathological condition can also be identified.

Not until these four classes of problems (*physical, social, vocational,* and *psychological*) are identified can the rehabilitation treatment process begin.

The Physical Examination

The information obtained from the physical examination of a patient whose history reveals the presence of disability serves three functions. First of all, the examination searches for the signs that signify deviations from normal structure and function. Correlation of these signs with the patient's history and laboratory data will yield the disease diagnoses. Second, in the examination of a disabled patient the physician searches for those signs that signify secondary problems that are not a necessary direct consequence of the disease. Such secondary problems may occur either as a result of treatment of the disease or as a result of lack of institution of appropriate preventive measures. Finally, the third main function of the physical examination is to assess the residual strengths in the systems or parts of systems unaffected by the disease. It is on these strengths that the patient and the physician build to remove the disability and reestablish the lost functional skills. These residual abilities are what the patient uses to "train around" the impairment induced by the chronic disease.

Some examples of secondary problems that occur as a result of treatment are as follows:

The arm of a patient with Colles' fracture of the wrist is placed in a cast. To prevent motion of the proximal fragment, the elbow is incorporated into the cast in a position of flexion. When the cast is finally removed, elbow flexion contracture is observed. Such a contracture is not a natural consequence of the wrist fracture but is secondary to correct treatment.

An elderly patient has a severely comminuted hip fracture for which operative reduction and internal immobilization are not feasible. A hip spica cast is applied. As a result of total bed immobilization, the secondary problems of generalized disuse weakness, urinary retention, and postural hypotension develop. These problems are natural direct consequences not of the fracture but of the appropriate treatment.

Examples of secondary problems that result from inappropriate preventive measures are:

A patient develops a partial radial nerve palsy secondary to trauma. The strength of the wrist dorsiflexors is insufficient to produce a full active range of wrist dorsiflexion. The patient is later found to have a wrist flexion contracture with shortening of wrist and finger flexor muscles. These contractures are not natural consequences of radial nerve palsy but are secondary to the omission of the preventive measure of regularly performed passive range of motion exercises of the wrist and fingers.

A patient suffers a fracture-dislocation of the seventh thoracic vertebra with resultant total paraplegia. During the patient's hospitalization, a decubitus ulcer develops over the sacrum. Such an ulcer is not a direct natural consequence of the paraplegia. Although the anesthesia over the sacrum is a direct consequence, the ulcer itself is secondary to omission of the preventive measure of periodic relief of pressure on the sacrum.

The major importance of secondary problems, whether treatment-induced or secondary to omission of preventive measures, is that they add to the patient's disability and they lengthen the treatment time necessary to remove the disabilities induced by the primary disease process. For example, the elbow flexion contracture will need to be treated before the patient can get full use of the healed fractured wrist and hand. Disuse weakness and postural hypotension will need to be treated before the patient with the healed hip fracture can achieve meaningful ambulation. The sacral ulcer has to heal before the paraplegic

patient can begin to learn dressing skills or begin to sit for long periods.

The particular areas of the physical examination that need close consideration in the search for secondary problems and for the evaluation of residual strengths are *skin, eyes, ears, mouth and throat, and genitalia and rectum; and cardiovascular, respiratory, neurological, musculoskeletal, functional neuromuscular,* and *mental status.*

What follows is not an exhaustive description of the examination of these areas. Pertinent highlights only are given.

Skin

Examine the skin over bony prominences in patients with anesthetic areas or those who have been on prolonged bed rest. Look for vasomotor changes in the skin of the hands and the feet in patients with arm and leg weakness, joint contractures, or pain.

Eyes

Carefully assess for near and far visual acuity, for visual field defects, diplopia, and adequacy of glasses. Since the patient may need to relearn new motor acts to eliminate disability in basic self-care skills or may require vocational alterations, visual skills may need to be maximized.

Ears

Assess hearing acuity. Impaired acuity will impair relearning.

Mouth and Throat

To ensure adequate nutrition, disabling factors that interfere with mastication and swallowing will need attention. Status of teeth, gums, and dentures should be made optimal.

Cardiovascular System

Retraining to restore basic self-care skills that are lost as a result of musculoskeletal and neurological disease usually requires specific therapeutic exercise regimens. An adequate cardiovascular reserve and optimized cardiovascular function are therefore essential.

Examination of the patient's blood pressure (in the supine, sitting, and standing positions), liver size, peripheral pulses, carotid pulses, venous return systems, peripheral skin temperature, peripheral skin hair, and peripheral edema should therefore be done. Cardiac size, cardiac rhythms, and cardiac sounds will need correct interpretations. All treatable abnormalities need to be identified.

Respiratory System

Much like the cardiovascular system, the respirtory reserve needs to be assessed in the evaluation of exercise tolerance.

Examination of the respiratory rate and rhythm, the chest shape, the fingers for clubbing, the facies for cyanosis, and the lungs for congestion and obstruction is essential. Pulmonary function laboratory tests may also be needed to supplement the physical examination of the respiratory system.

Genitalia and Rectum

Particularly critical for patients with diseases affecting functions of micturition and defecation are examinations for cystocele and rectocele, prostate size, sphincter tone, anal wink reflexes, perineal sensation, the presence of orchitis and epididymitis, and the presence of the bulbocavernosus reflex.

The bulbocavernosus reflex, if present, means that the sacral conus of the spinal cord at the level of S_2 to S_4 is intact. The afferent sensory stimulus is elicited by pressure on the clitoris or glans. For patients with catheters, a tug on the catheter will stimulate the afferent response. The efferent response is contraction of the external sphincter. A finger in the anus will detect this response.

Neurological Examination

This examination should be performed with the same care as is exercised by the neurologist searching for signs in a patient with a difficult diagnostic problem.[8] All 12 cranial nerves must be reviewed. Sensory examination should include superficial touch and pain, deep pain, position sense (large joints as well as small), vibration sense, stereog-

nosis, two-point discrimination, hot and cold perception, and the presence or absence of extinction to bilateral confrontation. Cerebellar and coordination functions need careful review, as do the deep tendon and pathological reflexes.

Communication skills are conveniently assessed during the neurological examination either as part of or following a broad assessment of the optic and auditory cranial nerves. All communication functions that were assessed during the interview need to be examined. Speech assessment includes evaluating articulation as well as the content of expression. The listening (i.e., receptive) skill can be assessed by presenting concrete instructions and abstract ideas of increasing complexity that require responses by the patient. Similar performance requirements will help assess reading and writing skills.

Musculoskeletal System

The functional unit of the musculoskeletal system is the joint and its associated structures: synovial membrane and the capsule, ligaments, and muscles that cross it. Examination of this complex anywhere in the body cannot be completed unless the underlying anatomy is known. A screening examination is useful in localizing abnormalities when the disability problems are minor.[13] For conditions that may result in major disability, individual joint examinations are necessary. Such examinations include *Inspection, Palpation, Passive Range of Motion, Stability, Active Range of Motion,* and *Muscle Strength.*

Inspection. The two sides of the body should be observed for symmetry in contour and size and differences measured. Atrophy, masses, swellings, and skin color changes must be noted.

Palpation. The origin of a pain symptom may be localized by palpation of the various anatomical structures about the joint. Palpation of the bones can determine their continuity in fracture assessment. Palpation of masses and swellings for consistency can allow the physician to distinguish between bone masses, edema, and joint effusions. To determine the presence of muscle spasm, muscle palpation when the patient is at rest can detect a sustained involuntary reflex contraction usually secondary to pain.

Passive Range of Motion. These tests are performed by the examiner while the patient is relaxed. When range of motion is limited, the examiner must determine if the limitation is due to joint surface incongruities; joint fluid excess or loose bodies; or capsule, ligament, or muscle contractures. Methods of measurement of passive range of motion and normal values for all of the various joints are described in the next chapter.

Stability. These tests assess whether a pathological condition of the bone, capsule, or ligament is causing abnormal movement (subluxations or dislocations). The joint should be moved under stress in the direction it is not supposed to move by virtue of its contour, ligaments and capsule, with the patient at rest. Tears in ligaments or laxity of the capsule will result in abnormal mobility. During movement, joint stability is also supported by active muscle contraction.

Active Range of Motion. These tests should be performed prior to strength tests in the event pain is a problem. Muscle tension and joint compressions induced by an active movement are less stressful than in a strength test. If pain is minimal in an active range of motion test, the examiner can more easily proceed with a strength test. When active range of motion is less than passive range of motion, the examiner must decide between true weakness, hysterical weakness, joint stability, pain, or malingering as possible causes.

Muscle Strength. Muscle strength can be tested if the prime action of a muscle is known. The body part can then be positioned to allow this prime action to occur. Grading systems are based on the ability of the muscle to move, against the force of gravity, the part to which it is attached.

GRADE 5. *Normal strength.* The muscle can move the joint it crosses through a full range of motion against gravity and against "full" resistance applied by the examiner.

GRADE 4. *Good strength.* The muscle can move the joint it crosses through a full range of motion against gravity with only "moderate" resistance applied by the examiner.

GRADE 3. *Fair strength.* The muscle can move the joint it crosses through a full range of motion against gravity only.

GRADE 2. *Poor strength.* The muscle can move the joint it crosses through a full range of motion only if the part is positioned so that the force of gravity is not acting to resist the motion.

GRADE 1. *Trace strength.* Muscle contraction can be seen or palpated but strength is insufficient to produce motion even with gravity eliminated.

GRADE 0. *Zero strength.* Complete paralysis. No visible or palpable contraction.

The key muscle grade with regard to disability assessment is grade 3. Since any activity a patient may perform is done in a gravity field, if at least grade 3 function is present, then the involved body part can be used. For grades less than 3, external support may be necessary to make the involved part useful to the patient. In addition, joints having muscles across them with less than grade 3 strength are prone to develop contractures.

Different examiners should agree on whether a muscle should be graded 0, 1, 2, or 3. For grades 4 and 5, there may be differences among examiners, depending on their expectations of different age groups and the amount of resistance they apply. As an examiner's experience increases, so will accuracy. For asymmetrical problems, grades 4 and 5 are useful even for inexperienced examiners as the two sides of the body are compared.

For conditions in which weakness is associated with spasticity, the grading system described is not as useful in predicting how much use the patient may get out of the muscle for the performance of his basic skill needs.

The next chapter discusses the major muscles in the body and describes how they are best tested, as well as their innervations.

Functional Neuromuscular Examination

The functional examination is the actual translation of the objective neurological and musculoskeletal examinations into performance. It defines at a given point in time the skill of the patient in the execution of the activities of daily living. It is the starting point from which improvement can occur through treatment even if the objective neurological and musculoskeletal signs may not be alterable owing to the nature of the disease.

The functional examination confirms the skill status reported by the patient in the history under *Present Illness* with regard to ambulation, transfers, eating, dressing, and personal hygiene. The functions to be tested are as follows:

Sitting Balance. This is a necessary prerequisite for most transfer skills. Test by placing the patient in the sitting posture, with feet on the floor, back unsupported, and hands in the lap. If the patient can hold this position, then nudge the person in various directions and observe the ability to recover.

Transfers. Abilities to be examined include turning from supine to prone and back, rising to a

WALTER C. STOLOV AND ROSS M. HAYS

sitting position, rising from sitting to standing, and moving from a bed or low examining table to a chair.

Standing Balance. This is a necessary prerequisite for safe ambulation. It should be assessed without support and, if balance is present, nudging from side to side should then be done to assess the patient's ability to recover.

Eating Skills. These can be assessed by demonstration of hand-to-mouth abilities utilizing various examining room objects or by means of actual observation at mealtime.

Dressing Skills. These skills are easily assessed in the examining room if the examiner is present at the time the patient removes the clothes prior to the examination and puts them on at the conclusion. If the examiner remains in the examining room while the patient undresses and does not leave before the patient dresses, much information on patient skill and patient family interaction can be gained.

Personal Hygiene Skills. The motions necessary for face, perineal, and back care can usually be mimicked in the examining room. Direct observation of the specific task when actually performed may be necessary if personal hygiene functions are significant disability problems.

Ambulation. Walking should be observed if the patient has standing balance. The patient should be essentially unclothed. Walking should be inspected with and without street shoes, and from the front and back as well as from the side. Abnormalities should be described in relation to the phase of the gait at which they occur. If pain is present, it, too, should be related to the phase of the gait.

Observation and description should be systematically performed and recorded:

Cadence: Symmetrical? Asymmetrical? Consistent?

Trunk: Fixed abnormal posture? Abnormal anterior, posterior, or lateral movements?

Arm Swing: Symmetrical?

Pelvis: Fixed abnormal posture? Abnormal pelvic tilt or drop?

Base: Narrow? Broad?

Stride Length: Short? Asymmetrical?

Heel Strike and Push Off: Present?

Swing Phase: Knee flexion? Circumduction?

Chapter 4 elaborates on gait evaluation, Chapter 28 describes lower extremity braces, and Chapter 49 describes prostheses for the lower extremity.

If the patient is unable to walk, *wheelchair ambulation* should be evaluated. The patient's ability to produce straight line travel and to negotiate turns should be observed.

Mental Status

The mental status examination, coupled with the psychological history, provides the data base for understanding the patient's basic personality structure and current emotional reactions to the disease and disability.

In addition, since removal of disability is a retraining and hence a relearning process for the patient, the mental status examination can be used to assess his learning potential. The examination becomes particularly pertinent in patients whose disease or trauma has produced brain damage.

Mental status examinations as they appear in psychiatric textbooks are oriented specifically toward the patient with psychiatric disease. When performed on the patient with physical disability, some of the areas investigated need to be elaborated upon.

For psychiatric patients, the outline described by Storrow[16] includes:
1. Appearance and general behavior
2. Intellectual functions
   a. Orientation
   b. Level of consciousness
   c. Memory
   d. General information
   e. Numerical ability
3. Perception
4. Speech and thinking
5. Affect
6. Insight
7. Judgment

The reader should consult Storrow's textbook[16] for the specific techniques he recommends to evaluate these areas.

For the disabled patient, additional evaluation beyond these usual techniques is necessary in the areas of *Recent Memory, Perception, Affect,* and *Judgment.*

Recent Memory. An understanding of recent memory function in a disabled patient is necessary because the patient's rehabilitation treatment will require learning new ways of performing those functions that were lost. The patient may, for example, need to learn a specific technique to execute a safe transfer or to coordinate crutch and leg movements for ambulation.

Teaching of these skills requires that the patient assimilate, retain, and reproduce new material not previously learned.

Recent memory functions with regard to language information may be assessed by asking the patient to remember, for example, an address that is given. Retention is then evaluated when the patient is asked to reproduce the address later and perhaps the next day. With regard to nonlanguage inputs, the patient can be taught a simple new motor task during the examination. Retention of this motor skill can then be assessed by later calling for its performance.

The emphasis should be on memory for totally new information. Asking the patient to recall what was eaten for breakfast; although in a sense a recent memory check, is not really new material for him.

When recent memory functions are decreased, the physician is alerted to the fact that much repetition should be used when the patient is in training to remove disability.

Perception. Perception includes the process by which the patient organizes sensory inputs into information about the environment. This term, as used in the context of the psychiatric interview, refers to statements by patients that represent either gross misinterpretations of observable stimuli or hallucinations. Disturbances of this nature are gross departures from reality and are easily detected. Interpretation of wallpaper designs as ants crawling on the wall, the hearing of voices in a quiet room, and the interpretation of radiator noises as special communication codes are examples of disturbed perception associated with psychiatric disease.

More subtle disturbances in perception are not associated with psychiatric disease, and these must be evaluated when retraining of motor skills is to be considered in a brain-damaged disabled patient. These disturbances deal with the interpretation of visual inputs of form, space, and distance. Such visual inputs require correct interpretation for the patient to be able to make a correct motor response based on them. For example, a patient in a wheelchair about to make a transfer onto a bed needs to interpret correctly first that both of the feet are on the floor, that the bed is close enough, and that nothing is in the way that will interfere with performance. Similarly, a patient about to put on a shirt needs first to interpret correctly the inside and outside parts of the shirt and that both sleeves are right side out.

Disturbances in perception of this type are more likely to occur in brain damage that affects the right cerebral hemisphere. They can be tested for by asking the patient to copy figures such as a square, a triangle, and a Maltese cross. The patient can also be asked to reproduce a clock face from memory. When disturbances in perception of form exist, these reproductions are distorted.[6] Asking a patient to put on a shirt that is presented rolled up with one sleeve inside out is also a useful test.

When perception disturbances exist, the examiner will recognize that the teaching of basic self-care skills by demonstration will not be as successful as verbal instruction.

Affect. A reactive depression is common following acute onset of a major disability in a previously normal patient, or following a relatively sudden additional functional loss in a patient with long-standing disease. It is a healthy response and indicates that the patient is at least able to recognize his losses. With such a recognition, he is more likely to be successful in removing disability.

A reactive depression requires remedial action if it is associated with disturbances of vegetative function or interferes with the patient's ability to respond to treatment. Judging whether such interference exists comes from observing patient participation during treatment rather than from what he says he is or will be doing.

The absence of a reactive depression may be a disturbing sign. If the patient is unable to face the loss, the ability to overcome the disability created by the loss may be reduced.

Mood swings are another feature of affect to consider. Rapid transitions from laughter to tears and back can represent the lability of an emotionally ill patient. Organic lability secondary to brain damage may show similar mood changes. Organic lability can, however, be more easily interrupted. Vigorously changing the subject matter of the conversation or sometimes a simple snapping of the fingers more easily curtails a flood of tears when such a lability is of organic origin. The presence of pseudobulbar neurological signs will also suggest that the lability of mood is of organic origin.

Judgment. Judgment factors in brain damage relate to difficulties that the patient may have in self-monitoring behavior. In manner of dress or activities of physical function, the patient may fail to detect errors and be unaware of mistakes. These problems need to be distinguished from simple apathy, carelessness, or sloppiness. If such behav-

WALTER C. STOLOV AND ROSS M. HAYS

ior is observed in the general assessment of the patient's appearance and the various activities performed during the course of the examination, judgment problems may exist. Insight into judgment can also be obtained during observation of the patient as the various tasks given are performed as part of the intellectual function inquiry. Family reports of exposure of genitals and other evidence of embarrassing behavior imply poor judgment. When such behavior represents changes in the patient's personality that are associated in time with the disease or the trauma, an organic origin is possible. When judgment problems are present, standby assistance may have to be provided for the patient as various basic functional activities are performed.

Summary

The physical examination of the disabled patient, as for any patient, is combined with the history and the laboratory data to achieve diagnosis of disease. In the disabled patient, it also reveals secondary physical problems that are not direct consequences of the disease and indicates the residual strengths on which the physician and patient must build to remove disability and reestablish function. It also verifies the functional self-care historical data discussed in the *Present Illness* part of the history. This section has emphasized the specific features to be considered when an examination is performed on a patient with disability.

The Problem List

The problem-oriented approach to medical management is a helpful technique in the management of patients with disability, as the following example illustrates.[15]

A 19-year-old woman fractured her cervical spine, which resulted in quadriplegia, in a small plane accident. Her male companion, with whom she had been living for the previous year and a half, was killed in the crash. Their relationship had been close and family oriented, since she served as "stepmother" for her companion's two small children from a prior marriage. Following the accident, responsibility for the children was legally assumed by their natural mother.

The patient was hospitalized for a short period on an acute neurosurgical service and then transferred to a comprehensive rehabilitation center for inpatient care. Her problem list following a complete comprehensive evaluation shortly after admission to the rehabilitation center included:

1. C_7 fracture dislocation
2. C_7 complete quadriplegia
3. Ambulation dependent
4. Transfer skills dependent
5. Eating, dressing, personal hygiene skills dependent
6. Neurogenic bowel dysfunction
7. Neurogenic bladder dysfunction
8. Decreased respiratory function
9. Potential for pressure sore
10. Potential for thrombophlebitis
11. Immature personality
12. Reactive depression
13. Home architecture incompatible with paralysis
14. Financially dependent
15. Estranged from parents
16. Unemployed, no prior work history
17. Homemaking skills deficient
18. Transportation dependent

Eighteen problems make for an impressive list, and one might argue that it need not be this long because nearly all are secondary to the first, C_7 *fracture dislocation,* and hence this one alone should be sufficient. Such an approach would be valid if there were a therapeutic technique that could reverse the spinal cord damage and restore full nervous system function. Unfortunately, such a technique does not exist. There does exist, however, a set of techniques for each of the 18 individual problems. These techniques can be used in minimizing the severity of the problems and in fully solving some of them—hence the importance of their identification.

Referring to the scheme in Figure 1–1 reveals problems 1, 2, 6, 7, 8, 9, and 10 to be of the character of "classic" medical problems. Problems 3, 4, 5, and 18, while also a direct result of the trauma, relate to the patient's physical disabilities. Problems 11 and 12 relate to the patient's psychological condition and problems 13, 14, 15, and 17 to the social sphere. Problem 16 succinctly identifies the vocational disability.

The problem-oriented approach to tracing the course of a problem includes:

1. The recording of subjective (S) data (patient symptoms and personal impressions).

2. The recording of objective (O) data (patient physical signs, laboratory and other test data, and quantified progress).

3. The assessment (A) of the problem (the interpretation of subjective and objective data into an impression of the status of the problem).

4. The plan (P) (the necessary additional consultations, diagnostics, therapeutics, or patient education required).

Thus the acronym SOAP serves as a means of organizing continuing management. The utilization of the problem-oriented approach to patients with significant disability by personnel in rehabilitation wards and centers has led to several suggested modifications and variations. The reader should consult other sources listed in the reference section for additional information.[1–3, 5, 10]

The Disabled Child

The infectious diseases that dominated the morbidity and mortality patterns of children in 1900 have now been decreased by 98 per cent.[4] Chronic illness is now the major threat to health for children. It has been estimated that 10 to 15 per cent of children in the United States have some form of chronic disease, and many of these have a disability severe enough to interfere with activities of daily living.[12] The majority of these children will live to adulthood because of innovations in both acute medical care and health care delivery. Therefore, all health care professionals must have some understanding of the evaluation and management of the child with chronic disease and disability.

There are many differences between the disabled child and the disabled adult with similar underlying diagnoses because children are undergoing rapid development. Proper evaluation of the patient must therefore take into account the appropriate developmental level of the child and the consequences the disability will have on the orderly acquisition of skills and experiences. The adult who acquires a disability suffers a loss of independence. The child who has or acquires a disability suffers a loss in *his potential* to obtain independence.

The goals to be achieved in the evaluation of the pediatric patient are (1) to accurately assess all aspects of the child's abilities and limitations within the context of normal growth and development; (2) to determine the potential for independent self-reliant behavior in the future; and (3) to ascertain family, educational, and community resources available to the child. This evaluation will produce treatment strategies that will be appropriate for the child's developmental and chronological age, that will minimize the tendency to create iatrogenic handicaps, and that will use medical intervention to improve function without sacrificing positive family relationships. The changing nature of the child requires continual reevaluation in order to modify treatment strategies as growth occurs.

History

The medical history for infants and young children will be provided by the responsible care providers, who are usually the parents. School-age children may be able to participate in the interview. Adolescents will not only be able to provide their own present medical history but will be able to describe their activities and limitations. The history for the handicapped child will incorporate the general pediatric history with special attention to the neuromuscular system. It will therefore include a medical diagnostic inquiry and a functional inventory to document current accomplishments and to elucidate all aspects of the child's disability.

A large number of disabling disorders in childhood are inherited. For this reason, it is useful to enlarge the interview to include a family history. The association of central nervous system injury with prenatal and perinatal complications necessitates a recounting of the mother's pregnancy and the child's perinatal and early history.

The review of systems may provide clues helpful for medical diagnosis and severity of disability. For example, oral-motor dysfunction is frequently reported as feeding difficulty. The nature of the feeding difficulty may indicate the type of neurological disorder. The pseudobulbar palsy in cerebral palsy often becomes manifest as difficulty in swallowing solids, whereas the more difficult task of swallowing liquids is associated with the true bulbar palsy of lower motor neuron disease. A report of recurrent fevers may be associated with urinary tract infections and a neurogenic bladder or, perhaps, impairment of respiratory function and respiratory tract infection. The child's nutritional status must also be reviewed, as children with disability may have difficulty acquiring adequate calories for normal growth. Visual and auditory function warrant careful attention in the history, for deficits in these areas have great impact on the potential for language and personal/social self-care development.

The core of the functional history in the disabled child is the assessment of development. The logical culmination of the developmental history is a survey of the child's current accomplishments. It is clear that the unique nature of the developing child is the major difference between assessment of the disabled child and the disabled adult. The six categories of ambulation, transfer activities, dressing activities, eating skills, personal hygiene activities, and communication are analogous to the gross motor, fine motor, adaptive skill, language,

WALTER C. STOLOV AND ROSS M. HAYS

and personal/social assessment areas of the developmental evaluation. The report of accomplishments in these areas must then be compared to the landmarks associated with acquisition of skills in normal children. An accurate understanding of the developmental sequence is necessary. With skillful evaluation in these defined areas, it is possible to distinguish between delayed development and the possibility of actual regression in pediatric handicapping disorders.

The corollary to the vocational evaluation in the adult is the educational inquiry in the child. With Public Law 94-142, the public education system is mandated to provide an appropriate educational experience for all children ages 3 to 21, regardless of disability. Frequently, objective evaluations that are helpful in the assessment of the disabled child can be provided through school records. A careful understanding of the child's past performance and the opportunities available in the school system will aid in the planning of an appropriate educational program. This is especially important in the child with an acquired central nervous system injury who, like the adult, has suffered loss of function and will require reintegration into an existing educational program.

A thorough assessment of behavior is necessary in view of the impact of behavior on the success of a rehabilitation program. Disabled children of normal or above average intelligence may exhibit abnormal behaviors associated with the adjustment to the disability. Children with impaired cognition may also have behavioral difficulties that require management in order to optimize their medical care.

The disabled child must be assessed in the context of the family setting. The family's ability to serve as an advocate for the child; their compliance with medical advice; their access to resources, both intellectual and financial; and their ability to mobilize community aid for the child must be carefully determined. The success of any pediatric rehabilitation program is only as good as the ability of the family to organize resources to meet the needs of the disabled child.

Physical Examination

The nature of the physical examination of the disabled child depends upon the age of the patient. In the infant and the very young child, observation may provide as much or more information than actual manipulation by the examiner. The skilled evaluator can interpret spontaneous activity in the infant and the young child and compare that with recognized patterns in normally developing children.

It is often impossible to perform an active range of motion evaluation on an infant or uncooperative young child. This information can be obtained more practically by a careful incorporation of postural changes to elicit primitive reflex patterns and thus evaluate the child's ability to move in comparison to the norm for that age.

Standard muscle grading must be adjusted for the size and age of the child. Frequently, children with muscular disorders will develop compensatory strategies for movement. The possibility of these compensatory strategies must be anticipated in the accurate assessment of muscle strength. Assessment of muscular strength is not usually accurate using standard evaluation techniques in the child under age five.[9] Quantitative testing is therefore recommended for children old enough to participate in standardized evaluations.

The correlates of central nervous system pathology are the same in children and adults. For example, ataxia on examination suggests cerebellar disease, dyskinetic movement is associated with basal ganglia involvement, and spastic incoordination accompanies cortical injury. It may require some experience to recognize the actual manifestation of these movement abnormalities in the very young child. The more traditional examination will be helpful in the school-age and adolescent child.

The musculoskeletal examination must be modified to account for the normal changes that occur in the developing child. Specific examples include the normal association of hip and elbow flexion contracture with intrauterine positioning. The 30-degree hip extension limitation and 25-degree elbow extension limitation found in normal newborn infants would be abnormal in the older child or adult. Similarly, a working knowledge of the development of gait and normal evolution of hip rotation is necessary to assess abnormalities in the gross motor examination of the developing toddler.[11] Musculoskeletal anatomical changes continue to occur into adolescence; therefore, all assessments of joint range movement limitations and gait must be weighed against norms for age.[14] Standardized developmental screening tools may be used as gross guides to obtain useful information in an efficient manner.[11]

Conclusion

It is essential for us to stress those parts of the classic history and physical examination on which special emphasis and elaboration are necessary when evaluating the disabled patient. Application of the techniques described will yield the diagnosis of disability.

Diagnosis of disease alone is insufficient for the planning of a comprehensive rehabilitation treatment program. The symptoms and signs required to diagnose disease are *not* synonymous with the symptoms and signs required to diagnose disability. To diagnose the disability—that is, the specific losses in physical, social, vocational, and psychological functions—requires investigations not ordinarily considered in the treatment of acute short-term disease.

The techniques described also identify those medical problems that are secondary but not natural consequences of a chronic impairment. To achieve a successful treatment program that removes disability, the physician must understand his patient's residual strengths. The methods to achieve this understanding have also been emphasized.

The adoption of systematic, problem-oriented record keeping is especially important for the care of physically disabled patients because almost always they have multiple problems that require continuing management. Following an appropriate evaluation, the physician is then able to list all of his patient's problems. Such a problem list will include disease diagnoses and secondary abnormalities. It must also include the specific losses in *physical* basic self-care functions, *social* functions, *vocational* functions, and *psychological* functions.

Once the problem list is established, the rehabilitation treatment process can begin. It begins with a specific plan for each of the problems on the list. It succeeds when each of the problems is solved to the highest degree obtainable by available therapeutic techniques.

Some of the other chapters in this book deal with further elaboration of methods of evaluation and the therapeutics that can be brought to bear on the solution of disability problems. The reader will find that the therapeutic techniques described fall within one of six general areas: (1) methods to prevent or correct secondary problems, (2) methods to enhance the capability of systems unaffected by the disease, (3) methods to enhance the functional capacity of affected systems, (4) methods to promote function through the use of adaptive equipment, (5) methods to modify the social and vocational environment, and (6) methods from psychological theory to enhance patient performance.

References

1. Abrams, K. S., Neville, R., and Becker, M. C.: Problem-oriented recording of psychosocial problems. Arch. Phys. Med. Rehabil., 54:316–319, 1973.
2. Dinsdale, S. M., Gent, M., Kline G., and Milner, R.: Problem-oriented medical records: Their impact on staff communication, attitudes and decision making. Arch. Phys. Med. Rehabil., 56:269–274, 1975.
3. Dinsdale, S. M., Mossman, P. L., Gullickson, G., Jr., and Anderson, T. P.: The problem-oriented medical record in rehabilitation. Arch. Phys. Med. Rehabil., 51:488–492, 1970.
4. Fries, J. F.: Aging, natural death and the compression of morbidity. N. Engl. J. Med., 303:130–135, 1980.
5. Grabois, M.: The problem-oriented medical record: Modification and simplification for rehabilitation medicine. South. Med. J., 70:1383–1385, 1977.
6. Heimburger, R. F., and Reitan, R. M.: Easily administered written test for lateralizing brain lesions. J. Neurosurg., 18:301–312, 1961.
7. Lehmann, J. F.: Patient care needs as a basis for development of objectives of physical medicine and rehabilitation teaching in undergraduate medical schools. J. Chronic Dis., 21:3–12, 1968.
8. Mayo Clinic: Clinical Examinations in Neurology, 4th Ed. Philadelphia, W. B. Saunders Company, 1976.
9. McDonald, C. M., Jaffe, K. M., and Shurtleff, D. B.: Assessment of muscle strength in children with myelomeningocele: Accuracy and stability of measurements over time. Arch. Phys. Med. Rehabil., 67:855–861, 1986.
10. Milhous, R. L.: The problem-oriented medical record in rehabilitation management and training. Arch. Phys. Med. Rehabil., 53:182–185, 1972.
11. Molnar, G. E., and Kellerman, W. C.: History and examination in pediatric rehabilitation. *In* Molnar, G. E. (Ed.): Pediatric Rehabilitation. Baltimore, Williams & Wilkins, 1985.
12. Perrin, J.: The Preface. *In* Hobbs, N., and Perrin, J. M. (Eds.): Issues in the Care of Children with Chronic Illness. San Francisco, Jossey-Bass Publishers, 1985.
13. Rosse, C., and Clawson, D. K.: The Musculoskeletal System in Health and Disease. New York, Harper and Row, 1980.
14. Staheli, L. T.: Medial, femoral torsion. Orthop. Clin. North Am., 11(1):39–50, 1980.
15. Stolov, W. C., and Clowers, M. R. (Eds.): Handbook of Severe Disability. Washington, D.C., U.S. Government Printing Office, 1981.
16. Storrow, J. A.: Outline of Clinical Psychiatry. New York, Appleton-Century-Crofts, 1969.
17. Weed, L. L.: Medical Records, Medical Education and Patient Care: The Problem-Oriented Record as a Basic Tool. Cleveland, Ohio, Case Western Reserve University Press, 1969.

2 Measurement of Musculoskeletal Function

THEODORE M. COLE   JEROME S. TOBIS

Goniometry

THEODORE M. COLE

Goniometry is the measurement of joint motion. It is an essential step in the evaluation of function in a patient with muscular, neurological, or skeletal disability. The diagnosis of the way in which a patient functions in daily life and how one moves about or manipulates the environment physically may depend heavily upon the degree to which the parts of his body can tolerate passive or active motion. The presence of voluntary muscular contraction, the application of a prosthetic or orthotic device, or the preservation of sensation in a part of the body may be of little value to the patient if the joints of that part are unable to be moved through all or part of their normal range of motion. In other cases—for example, when limitation of joint motion may still permit the patient to walk—endurance may be greatly hampered by the fatiguing effect of muscles exerting their forces at a biomechanical disadvantage.

In addition to helping the physician make a diagnosis of the patient's functional loss, the careful examination of joint motion can reveal the extension of a disease process or provide objective criteria for determining the effectiveness of a treatment program. Without such evaluation, not only is the patient's care impaired but legal determination of disability,[12] which in some cases depends upon joint motion, may be muddled and the extent of feasible rehabilitation misjudged.

An accurate medical record is not possible without accurate measurement. Should there be a change in the patient's therapist, should subsequent follow-up of a patient's disease be necessary, or should a dormant disease become reactivated, correct treatment depends upon accurate clinical measurement. If review of data from a patient's record should become necessary for purposes of research, the study will be meaningful only to the extent that procedures such as goniometry were performed and recorded correctly.

The reader setting out to learn the skillful employment of goniometry may have little interest in the accumulated years of controversy over tools and methods to measure the motion of joints. The reader will, however, be interested in readily acquiring the skill and applying it to patients so that they may benefit. One should also want to learn how to communicate findings accurately to colleagues and how to understand their records. To that end the physician should be acquainted with some of the more commonly used tools and techniques.

Tools and Instruments

Although many types of goniometers or arthrometers have been described,[11] the instrument most commonly used in the clinic is the universal goniometer, examples of which are shown in Figure 2–1. The two arms of the goniometer, with a pointer on one and a protractor scale on the other, are joined by a pivot, which provides enough friction so that the instrument remains stable when picked up and held for reading. Some goniometers are made with full-circle scales and others with

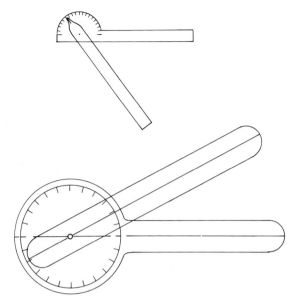

FIGURE 2–1. Two examples of universal goniometers commonly used by the clinician.

by Moore,[9, 10] who argues strongly that, whatever method is selected for use, it would be wise for everyone working in the same hospital, department, or clinic to utilize the same system of notation. The method put forth in this chapter is an adaptation of the system used by Knapp and West[6] and is based upon relating the range of motion of a joint to a full circle, or 360 degrees. Since the bones of the body may be considered as levers or systems of levers, they may be thought of as moving in a rotary fashion about an axis of rotation located in the center of their joints. When motion occurs about a joint, every point in the moving bone must describe an arc of a circle, the center of which lies on the axis of rotation.

It is important to correctly locate the axis of rotation of a joint to perform accurate goniometry. In almost all joints, the axis of a goniometer can be placed so as to coincide with the axis of rotation of the joint. The angle thus formed by the two arms of the goniometer corresponds to the angle formed by the two members of the joint.

The 0-degree position of a circle superimposed upon the joint has been arbitrarily assigned. With the patient in the anatomical position, 0 degrees is designated as the point directly over the patient's head, with 180 degrees toward the patient's feet. As shown in Figure 2–2, when the proximal member of a joint is moved from the anatomical position, the 0-degree position moves accordingly and will no longer lie over the patient's head. In the full-circle system, almost all joint motions can be considered as rotating away from or toward the overhead zero point in the frontal or the sagittal planes. Thus, in the sagittal plane, flexion is motion that rotates the distal member toward the 0-degree position on the circle and extension rotates it away from 0 degrees. Abduction is motion toward and adduction motion away from the 0-degree position in the frontal plane.

The horizontal or transverse plane applies to certain joints that rotate about the longitudinal axis of the body. Neck rotation is an example of such a configuration. The 0-degree position is designated on the superimposed circle as that point directly in front of the tip of the patient's nose.

Since the 0-degree position is defined in terms of one of the joint members, expressing the position of a joint in degrees signifies a definite relationship between the two members of the joint. Thus, when two arms of the goniometer are laid along the longitudinal axes of two joint members, and a measurement is made at the two extremes of motion, the examiner at once defines the limits

half-circle scales, but all should be clearly marked in degrees so that the scale may be easily read by the unaided eye at 18 in. The length of the arms of an easily portable goniometer is usually about 6 in. However, if more accurate measurements are required for joints of very large[1] or very small members, then longer or shorter arms may be preferred. The tool should also be lightweight, durable, and washable to ensure that it will be carried in the examiner's pocket or bag often enough to allow its frequent use.

Only rarely are other joint-measuring tools useful for the bedside examination. The exception to this generalization is the spine: meaningful measurements of joint motion in the spine are confounded by the multiplicity of participating joints, the paucity of reliable landmarks, and the bulk of soft tissue overlying the joints being measured. Spinal x-ray studies in extremes of motion offer more useful, readily available, and easily understood information. Bubble goniometers, plumb lines, electronic devices, and certain other tools are used only in special settings and will not be discussed here.[2, 3, 8]

Systems of Measurement

Many of the systems suggested for recording measurements of range of motion were reviewed

THEODORE M. COLE AND JEROME S. TOBIS

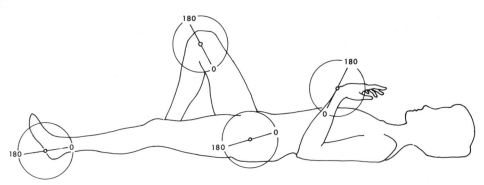

FIGURE 2–2. The full-circle or 360-degree system of goniometry applied to several joints of the body, illustrating the locations of the zero degree (0°) position.

of motion, the range of motion, and the many angles that may be formed at that joint.

Other systems of recording joint motion are based upon a different set of numerical figures attached to the zero points or starting points. Some argue for defining the anatomical position as 0 degrees and recording motion as deviation from 0 degrees. Others suggest modifications of this depending upon the joint and the motion being measured. Still other systems require the joining of positive and negative values to compute a range for the entire motion in question. Some workers argue for the use of small numbers, 180 degrees or less for a single motion, believing that smaller numbers can be more easily visualized.

When used consistently, the method of recording joint motion offered here has been found to be readily understood by therapists, nurses, and physicians. Examiners have been able to learn quickly where the zero or starting point is located. The notion that large numbers are difficult to visualize has not been borne out by examiners who use this method of recording in their daily work. Indeed, the 360-degree system was employed years ago by Knapp to facilitate quick learning by persons without medical or anatomical training.[7]

The 360-degree system has an added advantage. A flexion contracture, which produces an inability to move the part to its normal position of extension, or a recurvatum deformity, which is present when there is an excessive laxness of a joint permitting motion beyond normal extension, can be easily recorded. There is no need for awkward expressions. Further, there is no need to add or subtract numbers to arrive at the limits of motion.

Terminology

As in almost all other areas of medical communication, agreement on goniometric terminology has not been universal. The problem of communication is made worse by the insistence of some persons that the nomenclature should not include such terms as *dorsiflexion* or *radial deviation* but should utilize the "purer" terms of *flexion, extension, abduction, adduction,* and *medial* and *lateral rotation.* However, the choice of words should depend wholly upon whether or not they accurately communicate what the writer intends. The following glossary lists many of the terms commonly used in the language of goniometry.

Glossary of Goniometric Terms

Goniometer: an instrument for measuring angles.

Sagittal plane: the vertical, anteroposterior plane through the longitudinal axis of the trunk, dividing the body into right and left halves.

Frontal or *coronal plane:* any vertical plane at right angles to the sagittal plane, dividing the body into ventral and dorsal portions.

Horizontal or *transverse plane:* any plane through the body parallel with the horizon.

Flexion: bending of a joint so that the two adjacent segments approach each other and the joint angle is decreased.

Extension: straightening of the joint so that the two adjacent segments are moved apart and the joint angle is increased.

Rotation: turning or moving of a part around its axis.

Supination: rotating the forearm so that the palm is up (anterior in the anatomical position).

Pronation: rotating the forearm so that the palm of the hand is down (posterior in the anatomical position).

Deviation: moving away from a starting position; frequently to denote abduction or adduction relative to the midline, or rotation from a starting point.

Inversion: turning inward; turning the sole of the foot so it tends to face medially.

Eversion: turning outward; turning the sole of the foot so it tends to face laterally.

Abduction: motion at a joint so that a segment is moved laterally away from the midline.

Adduction: motion at a joint so that a segment is moved medially toward the midline.

Dorsiflexion: flexing or bending of the foot toward the leg so that the angle between the dorsum of the foot and leg is decreased.

Plantar flexion: flexing or bending the foot in the direction of the sole so that the angle between the dorsum of the foot and the leg is increased.

Opposition: moving the thumb away from the palm in a direction perpendicular to the plane of the hand.

Axis of rotation: a line at right angles to the plane in which adjacent limb segments move and about which all moving parts of the segments describe circular arcs.

Longitudinal axis: a line passing through a bone or segment, around which the parts are symmetrically arranged, and lying in both frontal and sagittal planes.

Accuracy

Accuracy is an objective of all measurement techniques. However, like other aspects of the clinical examination, accuracy is a relative term implying careful training and attention to technique, thereby keeping the variability of measurements to an acceptable minimum while making observations and compiling data that closely approximate the true state of affairs. The ultimate test of the data that are recorded is in their interpretation and utilization. Interpretation, in turn, depends upon the level of expectation of the interpreter, who must have a realistic understanding as to just how accurate the data really are. Unless goniometry is carried out by a highly trained examiner using specialized equipment in a time-consuming method, measurement of joint motion cannot be expected to yield figures closer to true value than 3 to 5 degrees.

Hellebrandt[4] found that the mean error for an average trained physical therapist was 4.75 degrees. For a thoroughly experienced physical therapist, it was 3.76 degrees. Since the average physician measures joint motion less frequently than the average physical therapist, a 5-degree error seems reasonable if the equipment is reliable and careful attention is given to technique.

In some cases, previous disease or surgical intervention alters the usual bone landmarks so as to render measurements less reliable. For example, the chronically dislocated hip makes the measurement of hip flexion-extension unreliable, as would the presence of an Austin-Moore prosthesis.

Conditions Affecting Measurement of Joint Motion

The examiner must indicate the conditions under which range of motion was measured. Was it done passively or actively; that is, did the patient move the part or did the examiner position the part? Was motion achieved with or without forcing the part through some portion of its total range? Did the patient experience pain during motion? Was motion opposed by voluntary or involuntary resistance? If resistance was detected, did it yield to sustained force exerted by the examiner or was the resistance unyielding? Was the patient able to cooperate with the examiner or was the examination carried out, for example, on a disoriented or confused patient who attempted to oppose the examiner? Was the patient under tension and anxious or was he relaxed? Was the examination encumbered by such things as a restrictive cast, a surgical wound, an appliance, or hypertrophied musculature? In addition to all these aspects, the patient's sex and age are known to influence the variability of normal joint motion.

Thus, many factors can influence the results of the examination, and since one or another of them may be present on one day and absent on the next, including such pertinent information is essential to an accurate interpretation of the data. Interpretation, of course, is the basis for decision-making.

General Principles in Measurement of Joint Motion

All motions that are commonly measured are carried out in one of three geometric planes (Table 2–1). In the sagittal plane, the following motions take place: flexion-extension and rotation at the shoulders, flexion-extension at the elbows, wrists, and fingers, and flexion-extension at the hips, knees, and ankles. Motions in the frontal or coronal plane are abduction and adduction at the shoulders and hips. Rotation of the hips and the cervical spine, which occurs in the horizontal plane of the body, radial and ulnar deviation at the fingers and wrists, and pronation-supination of the forearms are exceptions to the full-circle, 360-degree system.

Not all possible joint motions are measured in the usual clinical examination, because not all of the body's possible joint motions are important to the patient's pathological or functional diagnoses

THEODORE M. COLE AND JEROME S. TOBIS

TABLE 2–1. Joints and Motions That Can Be Measured According to Full-Circle or 360-Degree Goniometry and Exceptions to the System

JOINTS AND MOTIONS MEASURED ON A FULL CIRCLE (360 Degrees)		EXCEPTIONS TO THE FULL-CIRCLE SYSTEM
Sagittal Plane	**Frontal Plane**	
Shoulder: flexion-extension, rotation	Shoulder: abduction-adduction	
Elbow: flexion-extension		
Wrist: flexion-extension		Forearm: supination-pronation (abduction-adduction)
		Wrist: ulnar and radial deviation (abduction-adduction)
Finger: flexion-extension		
Hip: flexion-extension	Hip: abduction-adduction	Hip: rotation
Knee: flexion-extension		
Ankle: dorsiflexion-plantar flexion		Ankle: inversion-eversion

or to the treatment plan. Also, some joint motions can be only crudely measured, and efforts at accurate representation are not warranted. Instead, motions such as toe flexion-extension or back rotation are recorded descriptively in those cases in which their examination is germane to the patient's problem.

The examiner should become familiar with the normal ranges of motion for each joint. In many cases, the patient's unaffected, contralateral extremity can be measured to establish a normal value for that patient.

Technique of Joint Measurement

Joint—Shoulder

Motion
Flexion-extension (Fig. 2–3)

Plane of Motion
Sagittal

Positioning the Patient
The arm is at the patient's side.

How to Measure
The goniometer is centered on the shoulder just below the acromion. One arm of the goniometer is placed parallel to the midaxillary line of the

trunk; the other arm of the goniometer is placed parallel to the longitudinal axis of the humerus along the lateral side of the patient's arm. The patient's arm moves anteriorly in flexion or posteriorly in extension. Readings are taken at the completion of motion.

Normal Limits and Range of Motion
10 degrees—240 degrees

Motion
Abduction-adduction (Fig. 2–4)

Plane of Motion
Frontal

Positioning the Patient
The arm is at the patient's side with the palm toward the body. The arm is raised in the frontal

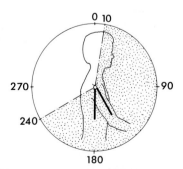

FIGURE 2–3. Shoulder: flexion-extension.

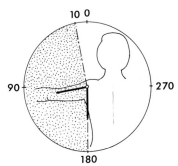

FIGURE 2–4. Shoulder: abduction-adduction.

plane to 90 degrees. As it continues upward, the arm is externally rotated so that the palm faces the midline at completion of movement. The greater tuberosity of the humerus is a limiting factor in abduction, and by rotating the arm it is partially removed from the line of action.

How to Measure
The goniometer is centered on the posterior aspect of the shoulder joint (on a level with a line projected posteriorly from below the acromion). One arm of the goniometer is aligned parallel to the midline of the body (vertebral column). The other arm of the goniometer is aligned with the longitudinal axis of the humerus, posteriorly, after the patient's arm is moved.

Normal Limits and Range of Motion
10 degrees—180 degrees

Motion
External and internal rotation (Fig. 2–5)

Plane of Motion
Sagittal

Positioning the Patient
The humerus is abducted to 90 degrees; the elbow is flexed to 90 degrees. The forearm is

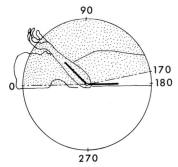

FIGURE 2–5. Shoulder: external and internal rotation.

positioned in pronation with the palm facing the feet.

How to Measure
The goniometer is centered on the elbow joint. One arm of the goniometer is held parallel to the midaxillary line of the thorax. The other arm of the goniometer is aligned with the longitudinal axis of the forearm. Measurements are made in extremes of external and internal rotation.

Normal Limits and Range of Motion
External rotation, 0 degrees
Internal rotation, 170 degrees

Joint—Elbow

Motion
Flexion-extension (Fig. 2–6)

Plane of Motion
Sagittal

Positioning the Patient
The arm is held at the side in the anatomical position. For the convenience of the sitting patient, the shoulder may be flexed.

How to Measure
The goniometer is centered over the elbow joint laterally. The forearm is maintained in supination. One arm of the goniometer is parallel to the longitudinal axis of the humerus, and the other arm is parallel to the longitudinal axis of the radius. Measurements are made in extremes of flexion and extension.

Normal Limits and Range of Motion
30 degrees—180 degrees

Joint—Radioulnar Joint

Motion
Pronation-supination (Figs. 2–7, 2–8)

Plane of Motion
This motion is an exception to the full-circle or 360-degree system of measurement. Motion takes place in the frontal plane.

Positioning the Patient
The humerus is adducted to the thorax and the elbow flexes to 90 degrees, with the radial aspect of the forearm directed toward the patient's head. This is the 0-degree position.

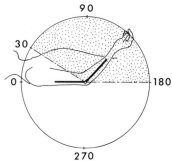

FIGURE 2–6. Elbow: flexion-extension.

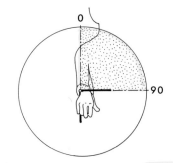

FIGURE 2–7. Radioulnar joint: pronation.

How to Measure

To measure pronation (see Fig. 2–7), the forearm is first fully pronated. The goniometer is held against the dorsal surface of the wrist and centered over the ulnar styloid; one arm of the goniometer is placed parallel to the longitudinal axis of the humerus. The other arm of the goniometer remains across the dorsum of the wrist.

To measure supination (see Fig. 2–8), the forearm is first fully supinated. The goniometer is held against the volar surface of the wrist and centered on the ulnar styloid. One arm of the goniometer remains across the volar surface of the wrist while the other is aligned with the longitudinal axis of the humerus.

Normal Limits and Range of Motion

The 0-degree reading is as described in *Positioning the Patient*. The normal limits of pronation and supination are 90 degrees in each direction, totaling 180 degrees of range.

Joint—Wrist

Motion
Flexion-extension (Fig. 2–9)

Plane of Motion
Sagittal

Positioning the Patient
The forearm and hand are held in pronation.

How to Measure
The goniometer is centered on the ulnar styloid; one arm of the goniometer is parallel with the longitudinal axis of the forearm along the ulnar border; the other arm is parallel with the longitudinal axis of the fifth metacarpal and is moved with

the fifth metacarpal to measure flexion or extension.

Normal Limits and Range of Motion
90 degrees—250 degrees

Motion
Radioulnar deviation (abduction-adduction) (Fig. 2–10)

Plane of Motion
This motion is an exception to the full-circle or 360-degree system of measurement. Motion takes place in the horizontal plane.

Positioning the Patient
With the elbow at 90 degrees of flexion-extension, the forearm is held in pronation and the wrist at 180 degrees of flexion-extension.

How to Measure
The goniometer is placed over the dorsum of the hand and centered over the proximal portion of the third metacarpal bone; one arm of the goniometer is placed along the midline of the forearm, the other is placed parallel to the longitudinal axis of the third metacarpal bone. Meas-

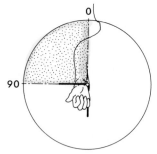

FIGURE 2–8. Radioulnar joint: supination.

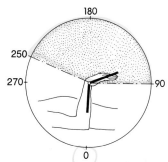

FIGURE 2–9. Wrist: flexion-extension.

urements are made when the hand completes maximum deviation to the radial (abduction) and ulnar (adduction) sides.

Normal Limits and Range of Motion
Since this motion is an exception to the full-circle or 360-degree system of measurement, the 0-degree position is as described in *Positioning of Patient* above. Normal motion is 20 degrees of radial deviation and 30 degrees of ulnar deviation, totaling 50 degrees.

Joint—Metacarpophalangeal Joints

Motion
Flexion-extension (including the thumb) (Fig. 2–11)

Plane of Motion
Sagittal

Positioning the Patient
The hand is held in any restful position, and the thumb and fingers are extended.

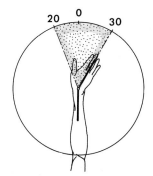

FIGURE 2–10. Wrist: radioulnar deviation.

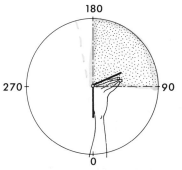

FIGURE 2–11. Metacarpophalangeal joint: flexion-extension.

How to Measure
The patient flexes each finger at the metacarpophalangeal joint. The goniometer is centered over the metacarpophalangeal joint being measured. One arm of the goniometer is placed on the dorsum of the hand and the other arm is placed on the dorsum and parallel to the longitudinal axis of the finger being measured. Measurements are made at maximum flexion and extension.

Normal Limits and Range of Motion
90 degrees—180 degrees

Joint—Interphalangeal Joints (Including Thumb)

Motion
Flexion-extension (Fig. 2–12)

Plane of Motion
Sagittal

Positioning the Patient
The hand is held in any restful position.

How to Measure
The goniometer is centered over the joint to be measured. One arm of the goniometer is placed

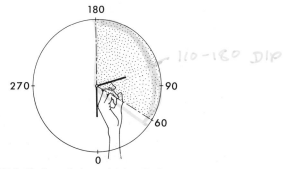

FIGURE 2–12. Interphalangeal joint: flexion-extension.

THEODORE M. COLE AND JEROME S. TOBIS

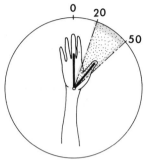

FIGURE 2–13. First metacarpophalangeal joint: abduction-adduction of the thumb.

on the dorsal surface of the proximal phalanx and the other arm is placed over the dorsal surface of the distal phalanx. Readings are taken at positions of maximum flexion and extension.

Normal Limits and Range of Motion
Proximal interphalangeal joints, 60 degrees—180 degrees

Distal interphalangeal joints, 110 degrees—180 degrees

Joint—First Metacarpophalangeal Joint

Motion
Abduction-adduction of the thumb (Fig. 2–13)

Plane of Motion
This joint is an exception to the full-circle or 360-degree system. Motion is in a plane parallel to the palm of the hand.

Positioning the Patient
The hand is in any restful position and the fingers are extended.

How to Measure
The goniometer is centered over the volar aspect of the first carpal-metacarpal joint. One arm of the goniometer is placed parallel to the longitudinal axis of the third metacarpal; the other arm is aligned with the longitudinal axis of the first metacarpal. Readings are made in maximum abduction and adduction of the thumb.

Normal Limits and Range of Motion
20 degrees—50 degrees

Motion
Opposition of the thumb (Fig. 2–14)

Plane of Motion
This motion is an exception to the full-circle or 360-degree system of measurement. The motion is made in a plane perpendicular to the plane of the palm.

Positioning the Patient
The hand is in any restful position with the fingers extended.

How to Measure
The goniometer is centered over the radial aspect of the first carpometacarpal joint. One arm of the goniometer is placed on the radial surface of the hand parallel to the longitudinal axis of the second metacarpal; the other arm is aligned parallel to the longitudinal axis of the first metacarpal. Measurements are made when the thumb is maximally approximated to and opposed from the palm.

Normal Limits and Range of Motion
0 degrees—35 degrees

Joint—Hip

Motion
Flexion-extension (Fig. 2–15)

Plane of Motion
Sagittal

Positioning the Patient
The patient may be supine, lying on the side, or standing.

How to Measure
Draw a line on the patient's skin from the anterosuperior iliac spine to the posterosuperior iliac spine. Drop a perpendicular from this line to a point on the skin overlying the anterosuperior

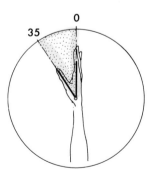

FIGURE 2–14. First metacarpophalangeal joint: opposition of the thumb.

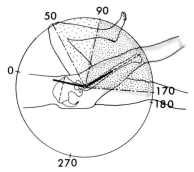

FIGURE 2–15. Hip: flexion-extension.

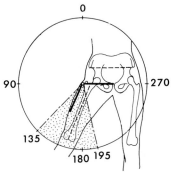

FIGURE 2–17. Hip: abduction-adduction (Method No. 2).

aspect of the greater trochanter. One arm of the goniometer is placed on this line with the center of the goniometer placed over the anterosuperior aspect of the greater trochanter. The other arm is placed parallel to the longitudinal axis of the femur on the lateral surface of the thigh. Caution must be taken to ensure that the marks drawn on the skin continue to overlie their bony landmarks as the hip is moved into positions of flexion and extension. If they do not, draw new ones.

Normal Limits and Range of Motion
With the knee extended, 90 degrees—170 degrees
With the knee flexed, 50 degrees—170 degrees

Motion
Abduction-adduction (Figs. 2–16, 2–17)

Plane of Motion
Frontal

Positioning the Patient
Patient supine or standing

How to Measure
Draw a line on the skin connecting the antero-superior iliac spines (see Fig. 2–16). Place one arm

of the goniometer on this line. Align the other arm so that it falls on a line parallel to and overlying the midline of the anterior thigh.

An alternate method (see Fig. 2–17) uses the same reference line between the anterosuperior iliac spines, but one arm of the goniometer is placed parallel to and below the reference line rather than on the line, and the goniometer is centered over the trochanter of the hip being measured. The other arm lies parallel to the long axis of the thigh.

Normal Limits and Range of Motion
135 degrees–195 degrees

Motion
External and internal rotation (Figs. 2–18, 2–19)

Plane of Motion
This joint is an exception to the full-circle or 360-degree system of measurement. Motion takes place on the horizontal or transverse plane and is measured as deviation in the direction of internal or external rotation from the neutral or anatomical position of the lower extremity.

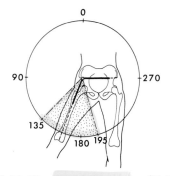

FIGURE 2–16. Hip: abduction-adduction (Method No. 1).

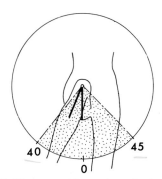

FIGURE 2–18. Hip: external-internal rotation in the hip (flexed position).

THEODORE M. COLE AND JEROME S. TOBIS

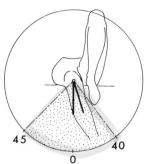

FIGURE 2–19. Hip: external-internal rotation in the hip (extended position).

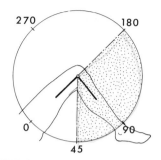

FIGURE 2–20. Knee: flexion-extension.

Positioning the Patient

The patient is supine. To measure motion in the hip-flexed position (see Fig. 2–18), the hip and knee are flexed to approximately 90 degrees each. To measure motion in the hip-extended position (see Fig. 2–19), the thigh is flat on the table but the lower leg hangs over the end and the knee is flexed to 90 degrees.

How to Measure

The goniometer is centered on the knee joint. Both arms of the goniometer are placed parallel to the longitudinal axis of the tibia on its anterior surface. One arm is moved to overlie the anterior surface of the tibia after it swings laterally or medially, whereas the other arm remains held in the position where the tibia had been prior to hip rotation.

Normal Limits and Range of Motion

External rotation (hip flexed, 40 degrees)
External rotation (hip extended, 45 degrees)
Internal rotation (hip flexed, 45 degrees)
Internal rotation (hip extended, 40 degrees)

Joint—Knee

Motion

Flexion-extension (Fig. 2–20)

Plane of Motion

Sagittal

Positioning the Patient

The patient may be supine or sitting on the edge of a chair or table.

How to Measure

The goniometer is centered over the knee joint laterally; one arm is parallel to the longitudinal

axis of the femur on the lateral surface of the thigh; the other arm is parallel to the longitudinal axis of the tibia on the lateral surface of the leg and pointing toward the ankle just anterior to the lateral malleolus.

Normal Limits and Range of Motion

45 degrees—180 degrees

Joint—Ankle

Motion

Dorsiflexion-plantar flexion (flexion-extension) (Fig. 2–21)

Plane of Motion

Sagittal

Positioning the Patient

The patient may be sitting or supine, but the knee should be flexed to permit maximum dorsiflexion of the ankle.

How to Measure

One arm of the goniometer is placed on a line parallel to the longitudinal axis of the fibula on the lateral aspect of the leg. The goniometer is cen-

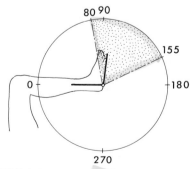

FIGURE 2–21. Ankle: dorsiflexion-plantar flexion.

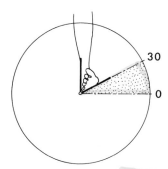

FIGURE 2–22. Ankle: inversion.

tered on the sole of the foot in line with the longitudinal axis of the fibula. The other arm of the goniometer is placed parallel to the longitudinal axis of the fifth metatarsal. Care should be taken to avoid forced dorsiflexion or plantar flexion of the forefoot.

Normal Limits and Range of Motion
80 degrees—155 degrees

Motion
Inversion-eversion (Figs. 2–22, 2–23)

Plane of Motion
This motion is an exception to the full-circle or 360-degree system of measurement. Movement takes place in the frontal plane.

Positioning the Patient
The patient may be sitting or supine. If patient is sitting, the knee should be flexed over the end of the table and the sole parallel to the floor. If patient is supine, the sole of the foot should be perpendicular to the longitudinal axis of the trunk (vertebral column).

How to Measure
The goniometer is set at 90 degrees. This position is considered 0 degrees. One arm is placed

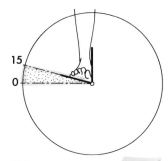

FIGURE 2–23. Ankle: eversion.

parallel to the longitudinal axis of the lower leg. The goniometer is held laterally to measure inversion (Fig. 2–22) and medially to measure eversion (Fig. 2–23). The other arm is held parallel to the plantar surface of the forefoot behind the head of the first metatarsal.

Normal Limits and Range of Motion
Movement is recorded as deviation from the 0-degree position at which the sole of the foot is either parallel to the floor or perpendicular to the longitudinal axis of the trunk, depending upon whether the patient is sitting or supine.
Inversion, 30 degrees (see Fig. 2–22)
Eversion, 15 degrees (see Fig. 2–23)

Joint—Cervical Spine

The clinical measurement of motion in the cervical spine is probably the least accurate of all common measurements of the joints of the body because of the paucity of available landmarks and the depth of the soft tissues overlying the bony segments. Kottke and Mundale[5] believe that measurement should be made by an x-ray study of the specific joints involved.[4] However, approximations of cervical flexion, extension, internal and external rotation, and right and left lateral bending can be made by using the universal goniometer. For more precise measurements, however, roentgenographic examination of the cervical spine will be necessary.

Motion
Flexion-extension (Figs. 2–24, 2–25)

Plane of Motion
Sagittal

Positioning the Patient
The patient should sit erect. (Measurements made in the supine position, with the weight of the head removed from its compressive position, show increased range of motion.) The head is vertical, the eyes are forward in a "natural" position, and the shoulder girdle is relaxed. The patient holds the end of a tongue depressor blade firmly between the molars on the same side that the examiner is standing.

How to Measure
The examiner opens the goniometer about 60 degrees and grasps that corner of the protractor that is at the furthermost end of the goniometer arm. In order to steady the goniometer, the examiner braces one forearm against the patient's

THEODORE M. COLE AND JEROME S. TOBIS

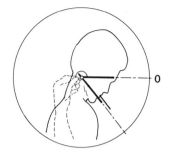

FIGURE 2–24. Cervical spine: flexion.

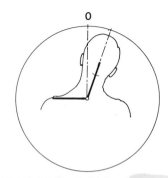

FIGURE 2–26. Cervical spine: lateral bending.

shoulder. The goniometer is centered over the angle of the jaw. The protractor arm should be parallel to the long axis of the protruding tongue depressor. The other arm is pointing in the direction of the motion to be measured. During flexion or extension, the pointer arm is adjusted to lie parallel to the new position of the tongue depressor.

Motion
Lateral bending (Fig. 2–26)

Plane of Motion
Frontal

Positioning the Patient
The position is the same as for neck flexion-extension except that a tongue depressor is not used.

How to Measure
The goniometer is centered at the spinous process of the seventh cervical vertebra; one arm of the goniometer is held in a position parallel with the floor; the other, or moving arm, is aligned with the external occipital protuberance. As the neck flexes from right to left, the movable arm records right and left lateral bending.

Motion
Rotation (Fig. 2–27)

Plane of Motion
This motion is an exception to the full-circle or 360-degree measurement. The motion takes place in the transverse or horizontal plane and is recorded as deviation from the zero position, which is achieved when the head is vertical with the eyes forward in a "natural" position. Rotation is recorded as deviation from zero to the right or left.

Positioning the Patient
The position is the same as for neck bending, above.

How to Measure
The examiner should stand on a low stool directly behind the patient. The goniometer is set at 90 degrees and is centered over the vertex of the head. One arm of the goniometer is held steady in a line with the acromion process on the side being tested. The other, or moving arm, is in line with the tip of the nose. The movable arm follows the tip of the nose as the head is rotated from side to side. Readings are taken at the points of maximum rotation.

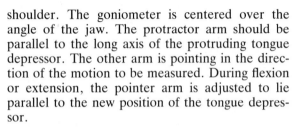

FIGURE 2–25. Cervical spine: extension.

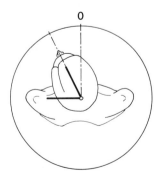

FIGURE 2–27. Cervical spine: rotation.

Muscle Testing

JEROME S. TOBIS
CHANG-ZERN HONG

Classification of Muscle Tests

Manual muscle testing provides very valuable information in clinical practice. However, it is usually not sufficient to describe muscle function in rehabilitation practice. The current concept of *muscle function,* which includes strength, endurance, and motor skills, should be applied to test the muscle.

Tests of Muscle Strength

MANUAL MUSCLE TEST

Grading System. Muscle strength can be graded using the scales shown in Table 2–2.[11] This is the most popularly used system. It is simple, fast, and convenient. However, it is nonlinear, somewhat subjective, and may produce variable results from one time to another, being influenced by motivation, fatigue, and pain. Muscle weakness of mild degree in a very muscular individual may not be detected on manual muscle testing if the examiner is weaker than the patient.

Based upon extensive experimental data, Beasley found the grading scales in a manual muscle test were inconsistent among different muscle groups when they were evaluated by a quantitative method[1-5] for lower motor neuron lesions. Figures 2–28 and 2–29 show the variability of the average percentage level of "fair" grade of a manual muscle test in different muscle groups from Beasley's studies. The muscle strength graded as "fair" varied from less than 2 to 42 per cent of average

normal force as measured with quantitative methods.

In the presence of an upper motor neuron lesion, the traditional manual muscle test has limited value. It may only give the examiner a gross estimate of the severity of the motor loss in a hemiplegic patient. Spasticity does not permit voluntary movements to be performed with ease and may mask the motor power that the patient possesses for a given movement. The recovery of strength after the occurrence of an upper motor neuron lesion usually follows certain patterns (especially in the case of a middle cerebral artery infarction). When the recovery of muscle strength occurs, it usually appears in the following sequence: (1) flaccid paralysis, (2) spastic paralysis, (3) synergic movement, (4) isolated movement of some muscle groups, and (5) complete control of each individual muscle group.

The description of muscle strength therefore cannot be based only on the manual muscle test but should also include the stage of recovery of the muscle group.

Measurement Using Instruments. Some devices are designed for a more objective measurement of muscle strength. Various types of dynamometers can be used to measure the muscle strength of certain muscle groups. The absolute strength can be read from the numerical value. Beasley[1-5] developed a quantitative muscle testing technique using instrumentation, including an electronic myodynagraph. Normal muscle contraction controlled by voluntary effort was recorded as a *tensive impulse curve* with a broad flat top throughout the trial period, which was usually timed by metronome at 5, 10, or 15 sec. Based on this curve, muscular strength can be measured as the maximum instantaneous tension attained in a trial, or the average tension for the whole trial. Resnick and co-workers demonstrated that quantitative evaluation by Beasley's method of ankle plantar flexor strength in patients with dermatomyositis provided a better criterion for the clinical status of the patient than any of the other laboratory tests studied.[13]

The Cybex dynamometer is an isokinetic exercise machine and can also be used to measure either isokinetic or isometric muscle strength (see Tables 2–5 and 2–6).

TABLE 2–2. Grading of Manual Muscle Test

GRADE	LOVETT METHOD (1916)
5/5	Normal (N)
4/5	Good (G)
3/5	Fair (F)
2/5	Poor (P)
1/5	Trace (T)
0/5	Zero (Z)

THEODORE M. COLE AND JEROME S. TOBIS

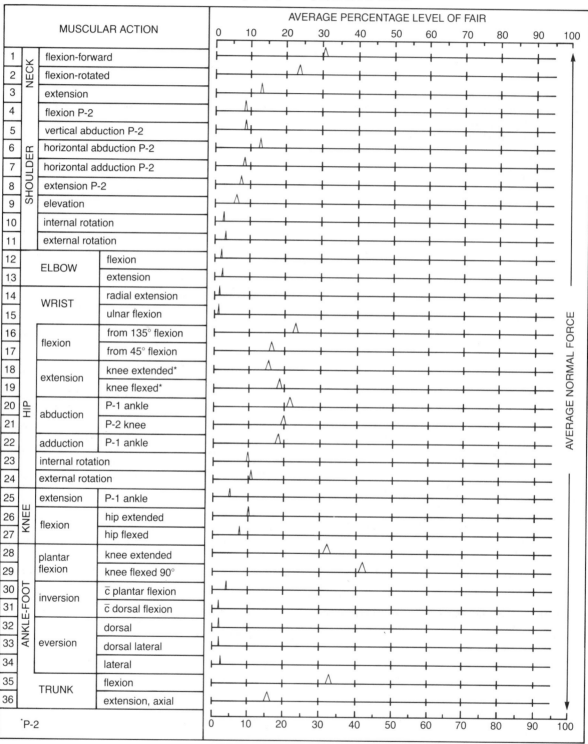

FIGURE 2–28. The percentage level of "fair" in various muscle groups. (Used by permission from Beasley, W. C.: Normal and fair muscle systems: quantitative standards for children 10 to 12 years of age: 36 muscular actions. An exhibit shown at the 39th Annual Scientific and Clinical Session, American Congress of Physical Medicine and Rehabilitation, Cleveland, 1961).

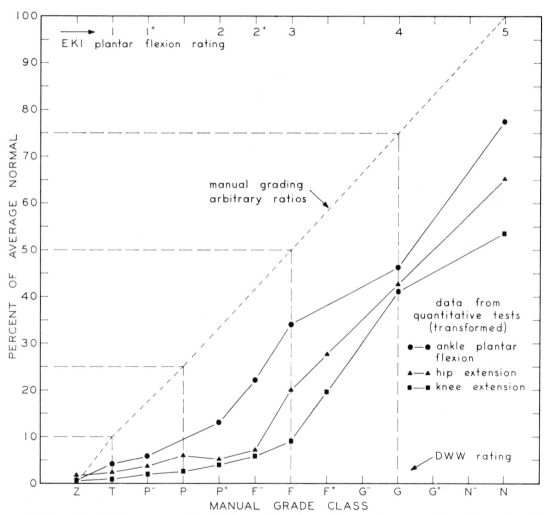

FIGURE 2–29. Relationship between manual grade classifications of muscular strength among patients after poliomyelitis and quantified ratings based upon measurements of muscular force on normal subjects and on the same patients. (Used by permission from Beasley, W. C.: Quantitative muscle testing: Principles and applications to research and clinical services. Arch. Phys. Med. Rehab., 42:398–425, 1961.)

THEODORE M. COLE AND JEROME S. TOBIS

Test of Muscle Endurance

Muscular endurance means the ability of muscular strength to persist. It is defined and measured as the repetition of submaximal contractions (dynamic endurance) or submaximal holding time (static endurance). Muscular endurance is essential for performing activities of daily living. Once one has the strength to perform a repetitive task, additional improvement in performance depends on muscular endurance.

Test of Muscle Skill

Muscle skills include many parameters, such as speed of muscle contraction, agility, coordination, and balance. The detailed evaluation of motor skills is described in several areas of this book.

Before obtaining a more detailed evaluation of motor skill, a routine neurological examination should be performed to evaluate the total clinical picture. For example, the presence of a sensory deficit will increase a motor disability. Hemianopsia may add to the difficulties of a hemiplegic patient in receiving adequate visual cues. The presence of spasticity or rigidity will impair motor skill. Thus, determination of the neurological deficits is important not only because of their diagnostic implications but in order to develop an effective program of management. In evaluating the patient's performance, one must test not only for range of motion and strength, but also the patient's capacity to perform various tasks must be determined. Such testing may consist of an inventory of the activities that are routinely performed in daily life. It may consist of evaluating the transfer activities from bed to wheelchair, or the ability to ambulate and take care of one's personal hygiene and dressing. In Table 12–1, a method is shown for recording such an inventory of motor skills.

Since so many of the patients who are treated by physiatric techniques suffer from locomotor disturbances, it is incumbent upon the examiner to study the patient's posture and gait (see Chapter 4).

Figure 2–30 provides a rapid means of analyzing the capacity of disabled patients to be responsible for their own housekeeping.

Test of Muscle Tone

Evaluation of muscle tone is important in rehabilitation medicine, since it may affect the other components of muscle function. Abnormal muscle tone can display either hypotonicity (as occurs in a lower motor neuron lesion or peripheral neuropathy) or hypertonicity. There are two main types of hypertonicity. *Rigidity* is hypertonicity from prolonged discharge of the alpha motor neurons. *Spasticity,* on the other hand, is hypertonicity from overdischarge of the gamma-1 motor neurons, which excite the annulospinal sensory endings on nuclear bag fibers of the muscle spindles and thereby makes the muscle spindle hypersensitive to sudden stretch. Table 2–3 shows the difference between rigidity and spasticity, both physiologically and clinically. However, it is not unusual to see both spasticity and rigidity at the same time in a patient with a head injury or other central nervous system lesions. In such a case, it is difficult to distinguish which type of hypertonicity is involved. Muscle tone can be tested manually by feeling the resistance, or by a myotonometer[9] or a tissue compliance meter.[7] Clinically, spasticity is assessed by resistance to movement as well as by the degree of hyperactivity of tendon reflexes. A reflexogram is the performance of electromyographic recording of muscle activity in response to a well-controlled tendon tap.

Manual muscle testing permits one to evaluate the strength of a movement. The strength of an individual muscle cannot be routinely isolated and tested unless it is solely responsible for moving the body part in the performance of a particular movement. For example, the gastrocnemius and soleus muscles are the plantar flexors of the ankle. Since the heads of the gastrocnemius attach to the condyles of the femur, it is possible to reduce the role of the muscle markedly by testing plantar flexion with the knee flexed. In this way, the strength of the soleus can be tested. However, the gastrocnemius still makes some contribution in this posture.

It is important that substitution be avoided in evaluating the strength of a muscle responsible for a movement. Thus, in the presence of a paretic muscle or group of muscles, a movement may be performed by a muscle that ordinarily does not serve in that role. For example, the hamstrings flex the knee. In full extension, as in standing with the foot fixed on the floor, the hamstrings may permit the knee to be fully extended even though the quadriceps—the prime extensor of the knee—is paralyzed.

Manual muscle testing is of value in the peripheral neuropathies and may be helpful in differentiating injury of the peripheral nerves from radicular damage. The peripheral and radicular innervations of skeletal muscles and their actions

Normal Daily Household Activities

Is patient able to meet the following activity requirements? (Write "N" if not necessary.)

Meal preparation, serving and clean-up _____

Work heights_____ Dominance_____

Marketing_____

Washing and hanging clothes_____

Ironing_____

Bedmaking_____

Light housekeeping (dusting, sweeping, etc.)_____

Heavy household activities (washing floors, windows, etc.)_____

Hobbies and special interests_____

Number of stairs_____ Family members_____

Child care: number of children_____ Ages_____

Will patient be alone for long periods of time?_____

Available help in family and outside_____

Limitations and contraindications for working _____

_____

Budget: Supported_____ Self-sustaining_____ Middle_____ High_____

Ambulation status:_____

Assistive devices:_____

_____

Comments:

FIGURE 2–30. Household activities information.

THEODORE M. COLE AND JEROME S. TOBIS

TABLE 2–3. Rigidity and Spasticity

	RIGIDITY	SPASTICITY
Physiology		
Overdischarge of motor neuron	Alpha motor neuron	Gamma motor neuron
Influence from higher center	Extrapyramidal	Pyramidal
Influence from peripheral afferents	Limited	Important
Temperature changes	Less sensitive	More sensitive
Sleep	Less changes	Released
Clinical Test		
Range of hypertonicity	Whole ROM*	Initial movement
	Lead pipe resistance	Clasp knife release
Deep tendon reflexes	Unchanged or decreased	Increased
Selective involvement	Diffuse	Antigravity muscles
Affected by postural change	Less	More
Treatment: drugs	Anticholinergic dopamine	Spasmolytic
Motor point block less effective (intramuscular neurolysis not practical neurolysis)		

*ROM = range of motion.

and tests are shown in Table 2–4 and Figures 2–31 to 2–58 and the following outline, which is from the Mayo Clinic's *Clinical Examinations in Neurology*.[12]

In the following descriptions of the tests, the name of each muscle is followed in parentheses by the peripheral nerve and spinal segmental supply. There is considerable variability in segmental supply, particularly to certain muscles, as given by different authorities. Furthermore, there is some anatomical variation both in the plexus and in the peripheral nerves. The segments listed cannot, therefore, be regarded as absolute. The principal and usual supply is underlined. Under "Action" are listed only the principal and important secondary or accessory functions—those particularly useful in testing and those that may cause confusion by substituting for the activity of other muscles. In the description of the test itself, the position and movement given first refer to the patient unless otherwise clearly stated. In some instances, the movement is adequately indicated by the action of the muscle and, hence, is omitted here. The term "resistance," unless otherwise specifically stated, refers to the pressure applied by the examiner, and this is in the direction opposite to that of the movement. For brevity and uniformity in description of the tests, the method of testing in which the patient initiates action against the resistance of the examiner is given except when the other method is distinctly more applicable. However, *this concession to uniformity and brevity of description is not meant to imply a preference for the method of testing in which the patient initiates action.* The location of the belly of the muscle and its tendon is often given to stress the importance of observation and palpation in identifying function of that particular muscle. As participating muscles, only those are listed that have a definite action in the movement being tested and that may substitute at least in part for the muscle being discussed.

Individual Manual Muscle Tests

Trapezius (Figs. 2–31 and 2–32). (Spinal accessory nerve)

ACTION
Elevation, retraction (adduction) and rotation (lateral angle upward) of scapula, providing fixation of scapula during many movements of arm.

TEST
Elevation (shrugging) of shoulder against resistance tests upper portion, which is readily visible.

Bracing shoulder (backward movement and adduction of scapula) tests chiefly middle portion.

Abduction of arm against resistance intensifies winging of scapula.

TABLE 2—4. Neurological Muscle Chart

FASCICUL.	TONE	SIZE	STRENGTH	R MUSCLES L		STRENGTH	SIZE	TONE	FASCICUL.
				Cranial Nerves					
				Temporal	Cr. V				
				Masseter	Cr. V				
				Pterygoid	Cr. V				
				Forehead	Cr. VII				
				Orbicularis oculi	Cr. VII				
				Mouth	Cr. VII				
				Platysma	Cr. VII				
				Soft palate	Cr. X				
				Pharynx	Cr. X				
				Sternomastoid	Cr. XI				
				Trapezius	Cr. XI				
				Tongue	Cr. XII				
				Cervical Nerves					
				Neck, flexor	C 1 to 6				
				Neck, extensor	C 1 to T 1				
				Diaphragm	C 3,4,5				
				Levator scapulae	C 3,4,5				
				Rhomboids	C 4,5				
				Serratus anterior	C 5,6,7				
				Supraspinatus	C 4,5,6				
				Infraspinatus	C 4,5,6				
				Pectoralis major (clavicle)	C 5,6,7				
				Pectoralis major (sternum)	C 6,7,8,T 1				
				Subscapularis	C 5,6,7				
				Latissimus dorsi	C 7,8				
				Teres major	C 5,6,7				
				Deltoid	C 5,6				
				Biceps, Brachialis	C 5,6				
				Radial Nerves					
				Triceps	C 6,7,8				
				Brachioradialis	C 5,6				
				Extensor carpi radialis longus	C 6,7,8				
				Extensor carpi radialis brevis	C 6,7,8				
				Supinator	C 5,6,7				
				Extensor digitorum	C 6,7,8				
				Extensor digiti quinti	C 7,8				

Table continued on following page

THEODORE M. COLE AND JEROME S. TOBIS

TABLE 2–4. Neurological Muscle Chart *(Continued)*

FASCICUL.	TONE	SIZE	STRENGTH	R MUSCLES L	STRENGTH	SIZE	TONE	FASCICUL.
				Extensor carpi ulnaris C 7,8				
				Abductor pollicis longus C 7,8				
				Extensor pollicis longus C 7,8				
				Extensor pollicis brevis C 7,8				
				Extensor indicis C 7,8				
				Median Nerve				
				Pronator teres C 6,7				
				Flexor carpi radialis C 6,7				
				Palmaris longus C 7,8, T1				
				Flexor digitorum sublimis C 7,8, T1				
				Flexor digitorum profundus I, II C 7,8, T1				
				Flexor pollicis longus C 7,8, T1				
				Pronator quadratus C 7,8, T1				
				Abductor pollicis brevis C 8, T1				
				Opponens pollicis C 8, T1				
				Flexor pollicis brevis (superficial) C 8, T1				
				Ulnar Nerve				
				Flexor carpi ulnaris C 7,8, T1				
				Flexor digitorum profundis IV, V C 7,8, T1				
				Hypothenar C 8, T1				
				Interossei C 8, T1				
				Flexor pollicis brevis (deep) C 8, T1				
				Adductor pollicis C 8, T1				
				Thoracic Nerves				
				Back				
				Abdomen (upper) T 6 to 9				
				Abdomen (lower) T 10 to L 1				
				Femoral Nerve				
				Iliopsoas L 1,2,3,4				
				Sartorius L 2,3,4				
				Quadriceps L 2,3,4				
				Pectineus L 2,3,4				

TABLE 2–4. Neurological Muscle Chart *(Continued)*

FASCICUL.	TONE	SIZE	STRENGTH	R MUSCLES L	STRENGTH	SIZE	TONE	FASCICUL.
				Obturator Nerve				
				Adductor longus L 2,3,4				
				Adductor brevis L 2,3,4				
				Adductor magnus L 2,3,4				
				Gracilis L 2,3,4				
				Obturator external L 2,3,4				
				Superior Gluteal Nerve				
				Gluteus medius L 4,5, S1				
				Gluteus minimus L 4,5, S1				
				Tensor fasciae latae L 4,5, S1				
				Inferior Gluteal Nerve				
				Gluteus maximus L 5, S1,2				
				Peroneal Nerve				
				Tibialis anterior L 4,5, S1				
				Extensor digitorum longus L 4,5, S1				
				Extensor hallucis longus L 4,5, S1				
				Peronei L 4,5, S1				
				Extensor digitorum brevis L 4,5, S1				
				Tibial Nerves				
				Gastrocnemius, Soleus L 5, S1,2				
				Tibialis posterior L 5, S1				
				Toes, flexors L 5, S1,2				
				Foot, intrinsic; medial L 5, S1				
				Foot, intrinsic, lateral L 5, S1,2				

THEODORE M. COLE AND JEROME S. TOBIS

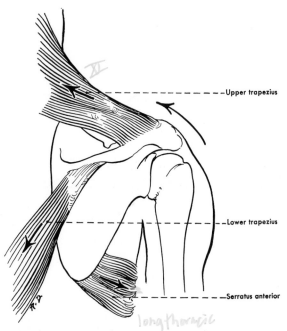

FIGURE 2–31. Upward rotators of the scapula. (Redrawn from Hollinshead, W. H., and Jenkins, D. B.: Functional Anatomy of the Limbs and Back, 5th Ed. Philadelphia, W. B. Saunders Company, 1981.)

Participating Muscles
Elevation—Levator scapulae (cervical nerves 3 and 4 and dorsal scapular nerves, C 3 4 5).
Retraction—Rhomboids.
Upward rotation—Serratus anterior.

In isolated trapezius palsy with the shoulder girdle at rest, the scapula is displaced downward and laterally and is rotated so that the superior angle is farther from the spine than the inferior angle. The lateral displacement is due in part to the unopposed action of the serratus anterior. The vertebral border, particularly at the inferior angle, is flared. These changes are accentuated when the arm is abducted from the side against resistance. On flexion (forward elevation) of the arm, however, the flaring of the inferior angle virtually disappears. These features are important in distinguishing trapezius palsy from serratus anterior palsy, which produces an equally characteristic winging of the scapula but in which movement of the arm in these two planes has the opposite effect. Atrophy of the trapezius is evident chiefly in the upper portion.

Rhomboids (Fig. 2–32). (Dorsal scapular nerve from anterior ramus, C 4 5)

ACTION
Retraction (adduction) of scapula and elevation of its vertebral border.

TEST
Hand on hip, arm held backward and medially. Examiner attempts to force elbow laterally and forward, observing and palpating muscle bellies medial to scapula.

Participating Muscles
Trapezius; levator scapulae—elevation of medial border of scapula.

Serratus Anterior (Fig. 2–31). (Long thoracic nerve from anterior rami, C 5 6 7)

ACTION
Protraction (lateral and forward movement) of scapula, keeping it closely applied to thorax.
Assistance in upward rotation of scapula.

TEST
Forward thrust of outstretched arm against wall or against resistance by examiner.

Isolated palsy results in comparatively little change in the appearance of the shoulder girdle at

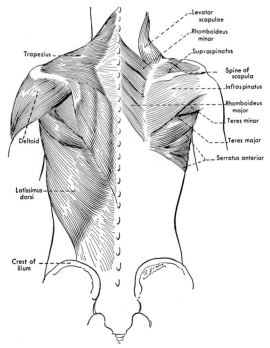

FIGURE 2–32. Musculature of the shoulder from behind. (From Hollinshead, W. H., and Jenkins, D. B.: Functional Anatomy of the Limbs and Back, 5th Ed. Philadelphia, W. B. Saunders Company, 1981.)

rest. There is, however, slight winging of the inferior angle of the scapula and slight shift medially toward the spine. When the outstretched arm is thrust forward, the entire scapula, particularly its inferior angle, shifts backward away from the thorax, producing the characteristic wing effect. Abduction of the arm laterally, however, produces comparatively little winging, demonstrating again an important difference in comparison with the manifestations of paralysis of the trapezius.

Supraspinatus (Fig. 2–33). (Suprascapular nerve from upper trunk of brachial plexus, C 4 5 6)

ACTION
Initiation of abduction of arm from side of body.

TEST
Above action against resistance.
Atrophy may be detected just above the spine of the scapula, but the trapezius overlies the supraspinatus, and atrophy of either muscle will produce a depression in this area. Scapular fixation is important in this test.

Participating Muscle
Deltoid.

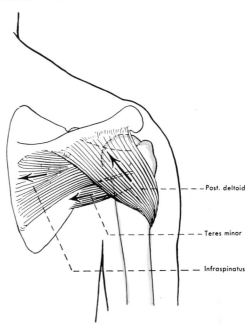

FIGURE 2–34. The chief external rotators of the humerus. (Redrawn from Hollinshead, W. H., and Jenkins, D. B.: Functional Anatomy of the Limbs and Back, 5th Ed. Philadelphia, W. B. Saunders Company, 1981.)

Infraspinatus (Fig. 2–34). (Suprascapular nerve from upper trunk of brachial plexus, C 4 5 6)

ACTION
Lateral (external) rotation of arm at shoulder.

TEST
Elbow at side and flexed 90 degrees. Patient resists examiner's attempt to push the hand medially toward the abdomen.
The muscle is palpable, and atrophy may be visible below the spine of the scapula.

Participating Muscles
Teres minor (axillary nerve); deltoid—posterior fibers.

Pectoralis Major (Fig. 2–35). Clavicular portion (lateral pectoral nerve from lateral cord of plexus, C 5 6 7)
Sternal portion (medial pectoral nerve from medial cord of plexus, lateral pectoral nerve C 6 7 8 T 1)

ACTION
Adduction and medial rotation of arm.
Clavicular portion—assistance in flexion of arm.

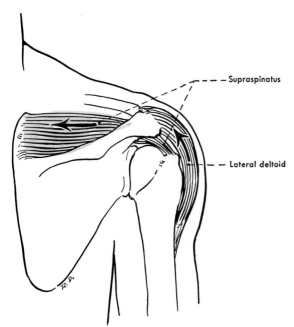

FIGURE 2–33. Abductors of the humerus. (From Hollinshead, W. H., and Jenkins, D. B.: Functional Anatomy of the Limbs and Back, 5th Ed. Philadelphia, W. B. Saunders Company, 1981.)

THEODORE M. COLE AND JEROME S. TOBIS

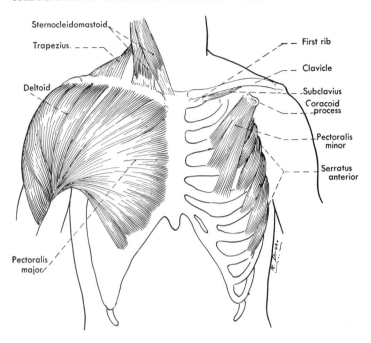

FIGURE 2–35. Muscles of the pectoral region. (Redrawn from Hollinshead, W. H., and Jenkins, D. B.: Functional Anatomy of the Limbs and Back, 5th Ed. Philadelphia, W. B. Saunders Company, 1981.)

TEST

Arm in front of body. Patient resists attempt by examiner to force it laterally.

The two portions of the muscle are visible and palpable.

Latissimus Dorsi (Fig. 2–36). (Thoracodorsal nerve from posterior cord of plexus, C 6 7 8)

ACTION

Adduction, extension, and medial rotation of arm.

TEST

Arm in abduction to horizontal position. Downward and backward movement against resistance applied under elbow.

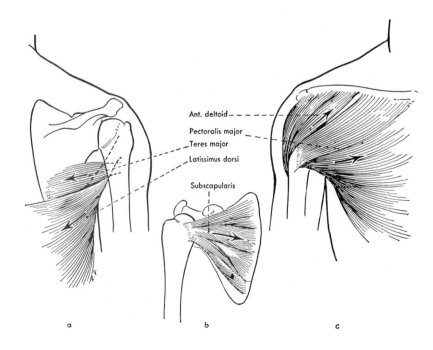

FIGURE 2–36. The chief internal rotators of the humerus. *a,* Posterior view. *b* and *c,* Anterior views. (From Hollinshead, W. H., and Jenkins, D. B.: Functional Anatomy of the Limbs and Back, 5th Ed. Philadelphia, W. B. Saunders Company, 1981.)

The muscle should be observed and palpated in and below the posterior axillary fold. When the patient coughs, a brisk contraction of the normal latissimus dorsi can be felt at the inferior angle of the scapula.

Teres Major (Fig. 2–36a). (Lower subscapular nerve from posterior cord plexus, C 5 6 7)

ACTION and TEST are the same as for latissimus dorsi. The muscle is visible and palpable at the lower lateral border of the scapula.

Deltoid (Figs. 2–35 and 2–36b). (Axillary nerve from posterior cord of plexus, C 5 6)

ACTION
Abduction of arm.
Flexion (forward movement) and medial rotation of arm—anterior fibers.
Extension (backward movement) and lateral rotation of arm—posterior fibers.

TEST
Arm in abduction almost to horizontal position. Patient resists effort of examiner to depress elbow.

Paralysis of the deltoid leads to conspicuous atrophy and serious disability, since the other muscles that participate in abduction of the arm (the supraspinatus, trapezius and serratus anterior—the last two by rotating the scapula) cannot compensate for lack of function of the deltoid.

Flexion and extension of the arm against resistance.

Participating Muscles
Abduction—given above.
Flexion—pectoralis major—clavicular portion; biceps.
Extension—latissimus dorsi; teres major.

Subscapularis (Fig. 2–36b). Upper and lower subscapular nerves from posterior cord of plexus, C 5 6 7)

ACTION
Medial (internal) rotation of arm at shoulder.

TEST
Elbow at side and flexed 90 degrees. Patient resists examiner's attempt to pull the hand laterally.

Since this muscle is not accessible to observation or palpation, it is necessary to gauge the activity

of other muscles that produce this movement. The pectoralis major is the most powerful medial rotator of the arm; hence, paralysis of the subscapularis alone results in relatively little weakness of this movement.

Participating Muscles
Pectoralis major; deltoid—anterior fibers; teres major; latissimus dorsi.

Biceps; Brachialis (Fig. 2–37). (Musculocutaneous nerve from lateral cord of plexus, C 5 6)

ACTION
Biceps—flexion and supination of forearm.
Assistance in flexion of arm at shoulder.
Brachialis—flexion of forearm at elbow.

TEST
Flexion of forearm against resistance. Forearm should be in supination to decrease participation of brachioradialis.

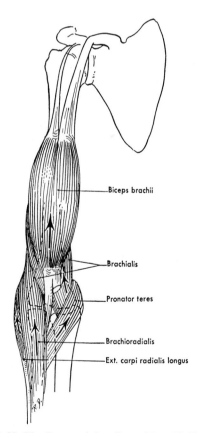

Biceps brachii

Brachialis

Pronator teres

Brachioradialis

Ext. carpi radialis longus

FIGURE 2–37. The flexors of the elbow. (From Hollinshead, W. H., and Jenkins, D. B.: Functional Anatomy of the Limbs and Back, 5th Ed. Philadelphia, W. B. Saunders Company, 1981.)

THEODORE M. COLE AND JEROME S. TOBIS

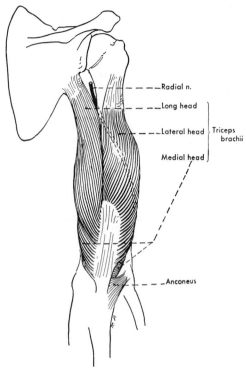

FIGURE 2–38. Muscles of the extensor (posterior) surface of the right arm. (From Hollinshead, W. H., and Jenkins, D. B.: Functional Anatomy of the Limbs and Back, 5th Ed. Philadelphia, W. B. Saunders Company, 1981.)

Triceps (Fig. 2–38). (Radial nerve, which is continuation of posterior cord of plexus, C 6 7 8)

ACTION
Extension of forearm at elbow.

TEST
Forearm in flexion to varying degree. Patient resists effort of examiner to flex forearm further. Slight weakness is more easily detected when starting with forearm almost completely flexed.

Brachioradialis (Fig. 2–39). (Radial nerve, C 5 6)

ACTION
Flexion of forearm at elbow.

TEST
Flexion of forearm against resistance with forearm midway between pronation and supination.

The belly of the muscle stands out prominently on the upper surface of the forearm, tending to bridge the angle between the forearm and arm.

Participating Muscles
Biceps; brachialis.

Supinator (Fig. 2–39). (Posterior interosseous nerve from radial nerve, C 5 6 7)

ACTION
Supination of forearm.

TEST
Forearm in full extension and supination. Patient attempts to maintain supination while examiner attempts to pronate the forearm and palpates biceps.

Resistance to pronation by the intact supinator can usually be felt before there is appreciable contraction of the biceps.

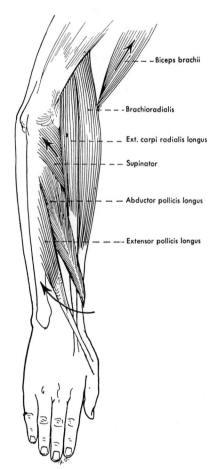

FIGURE 2–39. The chief supinators of the forearm. (From Hollinshead, W. H., and Jenkins, D. B.: Functional Anatomy of the Limbs and Back, 5th Ed. Philadelphia, W. B. Saunders Company, 1981.)

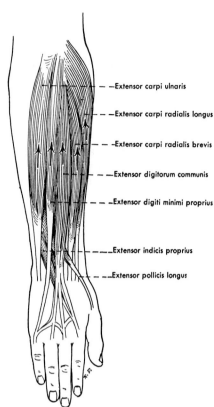

- —Extensor carpi ulnaris
- —Extensor carpi radialis longus
- -Extensor carpi radialis brevis
- —Extensor digitorum communis
- —Extensor digiti minimi proprius
- —Extensor indicis proprius
- —Extensor pollicis longus

FIGURE 2–40. The chief extensors of the wrist. (From Hollinshead, W. H., and Jenkins, D. B.: Functional Anatomy of the Limbs and Back, 5th Ed. Philadelphia, W. B. Saunders Company, 1981.)

Extensor Carpi Radialis Longus (Fig. 2–40). (Radial nerve, C 6 7 8)

ACTION
Extension (dorsiflexion) and radial abduction of hand at wrist.

TEST
Forearm in almost complete pronation. Dorsiflexion of wrist against resistance applied to dorsum of hand downward and toward ulnar side.

The tendon is palpable just above its insertion into the base of the second metacarpal bone. The fingers and thumb should be relaxed and somewhat flexed to minimize participation of the extensors of the digits.

Extensor Carpi Radialis Brevis (Fig. 2–40). (Posterior interosseous nerve from radial nerve, C 6 7 8)

Measurement of Musculoskeletal Function

ACTION
Extension (dorsiflexion) of hand at wrist.

TEST
Forearm in complete pronation. Dorsiflexion of wrist against resistance applied to dorsum of hand straight downward.

The tendon is palpable just proximal to the base of the third metacarpal bone. The fingers and thumb should be relaxed and somewhat flexed to minimize participation of the extensors of the digits.

Extensor Carpi Ulnaris (Fig. 2–40). (Posterior interosseous nerve from radial nerve, C 7 8)

ACTION
Extension (dorsiflexion) and ulnar deviation of hand at wrist.

TEST
The forearm is in pronation. Dorsiflexion and ulnar deviation of wrist against resistance applied to dorsum of hand downward and toward radial side.

The tendon is palpable just below or above the distal end of the ulna. The fingers should be relaxed and somewhat flexed to minimize participation of the extensors of the digits.

Extensor Digitorum (Fig. 2–40). (Posterior interosseous nerve from radial nerve, C 6 7 8)

ACTION
Extension of the fingers, principally at metacarpophalangeal joints. Assistance in extension (dorsiflexion) of wrist.

TEST
Forearm is in pronation. Wrist is stabilized in straight position. Extension of fingers at metacarpophalangeal joints against resistance applied to proximal phalanges.

The distal portions of the fingers may be somewhat relaxed and in slight flexion. The tendons are visible and palpable over the dorsum of the hand.

Extension at the interphalangeal joints is a function primarily of the interossei (ulnar nerve) and lumbricals (median and ulnar nerves).

The extensor digiti quinti and extensor indicis (posterior interosseous nerve, C 7 8), proper extensors of the little and index fingers, respectively, can be tested individually while the other fingers are in flexion to minimize the action of the common

THEODORE M. COLE AND JEROME S. TOBIS

extensor. In a thin person's hand, the tendons can usually be identified.

Abductor Pollicis Longus (Fig. 2–39). (Posterior interosseous nerve from radial nerve, C 7 8)

ACTION
Radial abduction of thumb (in same plane as that of palm, in contradistinction to palmar abduction, which is movement perpendicular to plane of palm).
Assistance in radial abduction and flexion of hand at wrist.

TEST
Hand on edge (forearm midway between pronation and supination).
Radial abduction of thumb against resistance applied to metacarpal.

The tendon is palpable just above its insertion into the base of the metacarpal bone and forms the anterior (volar) boundary of the "anatomical snuffbox."

Participating Muscle
Extensor pollicis brevis.

Extensor Pollicis Brevis. (Posterior interosseous nerve from radial nerve, C 7 8)

ACTION
Extension of proximal phalanx of thumb.
Assistance in radial abduction and extension of metacarpal of thumb.

TEST
Hand is on edge. Wrist and particularly metacarpal of thumb is stabilized by examiner. Extension of proximal phalanx against resistance applied to that phalanx while distal phalanx is in flexion to minimize action of extensor pollicis longus.

At the wrist, the tendon lies just posterior (dorsal) to the tendon of the abductor pollicis longus.

Participating Muscle
Extensor pollicis longus.

Extensor Pollicis Longus (Fig. 2–40). (Posterior interosseous nerve from radial nerve, C 7 8)

ACTION
Extension of all parts of thumb but specifically extension of distal phalanx.
Assistance in adduction of thumb.

TEST
Hand is on edge. Wrist, metacarpal, and proximal phalanx of thumb are stabilized by examiner

with thumb close to palm at its radial border. Extension of distal phalanx against resistance.

If the patient is permitted to flex the wrist or abduct the thumb away from the palm, some extension of the phalanges results simply from lengthening the path of the extensor tendon. At the wrist, the tendon forms the posterior (dorsal) boundary of the "anatomical snuffbox."

The characteristic result of radial nerve palsy is wristdrop. Extension of the fingers at the interphalangeal joints is still possible by virture of the action of the intertossei and lumbricals, but extension of the thumb is lost.

The next group of muscles examined is that supplied by the median nerve, which is formed by the union of its lateral root, from the lateral cord of the brachial plexus, and its medial root, from the medial cord of the plexus. Then the muscles supplied by the ulnar nerve (arising from the medial cord of the brachial plexus) are tested. However, for convenience in order of examination, some of the muscles in the ulnar group are tested with the median group.

Pronator Teres (Fig. 2–41). (Median C 6 7)

ACTION
Pronation of forearm.

TEST
Elbow at side of trunk, forearm in flexion to right angle, and arm in lateral rotation at shoulder to eliminate effect of gravity, which, in most positions, favors pronation. Pronation of forearm against resistance, starting from a position of moderate supination.

Participating Muscle
Pronator quadratus (anterior interosseous branch of median nerve C 7 8 T 1)

Flexor Carpi Radialis (Figs. 2–41 and 2–42). (Median nerve, C 6 7)

ACTION
Flexion (palmar flexion) of hand at wrist.
Assistance in radial abduction of hand.

TEST
Flexion of hand against resistance applied to palm. Fingers should be relaxed to minimize participation of their flexors.

The tendon is the more lateral (radial) one of the two conspicuous tendons on the volar aspect of the wrist.

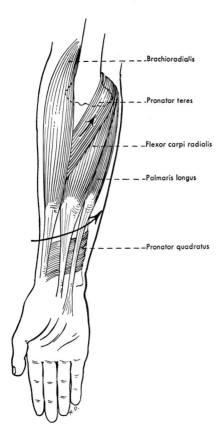

FIGURE 2–41. Pronators of the forearm. (From Hollinshead, W. H., and Jenkins, D. B.: Functional Anatomy of the Limbs and Back, 5th Ed. Philadelphia, W. B. Saunders Company, 1981.)

In complete median nerve palsy, flexion of the wrist is considerably weakened but can still be performed by the flexor carpi ulnaris (ulnar nerve) assisted to some extent by the abductor pollicis longus (radial nerve). In this event, ulnar deviation of the hand usually accompanies flexion.

Palmaris Longus (Figs. 2–41 and 2–42). (Median nerve, C 7 8 T 1)

ACTION
Flexion of hand at wrist

TEST
Same as for flexor carpi radialis.

The tendon is palpable at the ulnar side of the tendon of the flexor carpi radialis.

Flexor Carpi Ulnaris (Fig. 2–42). (Ulnar nerve, C 7 8 T 1)

Measurement of Musculoskeletal Function

ACTION
Flexion and ulnar deviation of hand at wrist. Fixation of pisiform bone during contraction of abductor digiti quinti.

TEST
Flexion and ulnar deviation of hand against resistance applied to ulnar side of palm in direction of extension and radial abduction. Fingers should be relaxed.

The tendon is palpable proximal to the pisiform bone.

Flexor Digitorum Sublimis (Fig. 2–42). (Median nerve, C 7 8 T 1)

ACTION
Flexion of middle phalanges of fingers, at first interphalangeal joints primarily; flexion of proximal phalanges at metacarpophalangeal joints secondarily.
Assistance in flexion of hand at wrist.

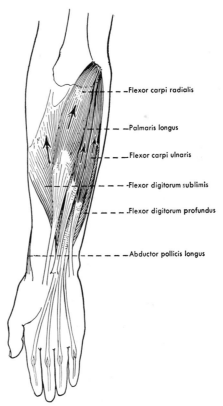

FIGURE 2–42. The chief flexors of the wrist. (From Hollinshead, W. H., and Jenkins, D. B.: Functional Anatomy of the Limbs and Back, 5th Ed. Philadelphia, W. B. Saunders Company, 1981.)

THEODORE M. COLE AND JEROME S. TOBIS

TEST

Wrist in neutral position, proximal phalanges are stabilized. Flexion of middle phalanx of each finger against resistance applied to that phalanx, with distal phalanx relaxed.

Flexor Digitorum Profundus (Fig. 2–42). Radial portion—usually to digits II and III (median nerve and its anterior interosseous branch, C 7 8 T 1)

Ulnar portion—usually to digits IV and V (ulnar nerve, C 7 8 T 1)

ACTION

Flexion of distal phalanges of fingers specifically; flexion of other phalanges secondarily.

Assistance in flexion of hand at wrist.

TEST

Flexion of distal phalanges against resistance with proximal and middle phalanges stabilized in extension.

With middle and distal phalanges folded over edge of examiner's hand, patient resists attempt by examiner to extend distal phalanges.

Flexor Pollicis Longus (Fig. 2–43). (Anterior interosseous branch of median nerve, C 7 8 T 1).

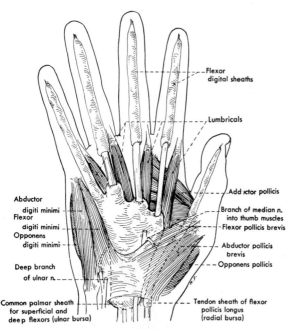

FIGURE 2–43. Short muscles of the thumb and little finger. (Redrawn from Hollinshead, W. H., and Jenkins, D. B.: Functional Anatomy of the Limbs and Back, 5th Ed. Philadelphia, W. B. Saunders Company, 1981.)

ACTION

Flexion of thumb, particularly distal phalanx.

Assistance in ulnar adduction of thumb.

TEST

Flexion of distal phalanx against resistance with thumb in position of palmar adduction and with stabilization of metacarpal and proximal phalanges.

Abductor Pollicis Brevis (Fig. 2–43). (Median nerve, C 8 T 1)

ACTION

Palmar abduction of thumb (perpendicular to plane of palm).

Assistance in opposition and in flexion of proximal phalanx of thumb.

TEST

Palmar abduction of thumb against resistance applied at metacarpophalangeal joint.

The muscle is readily visible and palpable in the thenar eminence.

Participating Muscle

Flexor pollicis brevis (superficial head).

Opponens Pollicis (Fig. 2–43). (Median nerve, C 8 T 1)

ACTION

Movement of first metacarpal across palm, rotating it into opposition.

TEST

Thumb in opposition. Examiner attempts to rotate and draw thumb back to its usual position.

Participating Muscles

Abductor pollicis brevis; flexor pollicis brevis.

Flexor Pollicis Brevis (Fig. 2–43). Superficial head (median nerve, C 8 T 1), deep head (ulnar nerve, C 8 T 1)

ACTION

Flexion of proximal phalanx of thumb.

Assistance in opposition, ulnar adduction (entire muscle), and palmar abduction (superficial head) of thumb.

TEST

Thumb in position of palmar adduction with stabilization of metacarpal. Flexion of proximal phalanx against resistance applied to that phalanx while distal phalanx is as relaxed as possible.

Participating Muscles

Flexor pollicis longus; abductor pollicis brevis; adductor pollicis.

Severe median nerve palsy produces the "simian" hand, wherein the thumb tends to lie in the same plane as the palm with the volar surface facing more anteriorly than normal. Atrophy of the muscles of the thenar eminence is usually conspicuous.

Three muscles supplied, at least in part, by the ulnar nerve have already been described: flexor carpi ulnaris, flexor digitorum profundus, and flexor pollicis brevis. The remaining muscles supplied by this nerve follow.

Hypothenar Muscles. (Ulnar nerve, C 8 T 1)

ACTION

Abductor digiti quinti

Flexor digiti quinti—abduction and flexion (proximal phalanx) of little finger.

Opponens digiti quinti—opposition of little finger toward thumb.

All three muscles—palmar elevation of head of fifth metacarpal, helping to cup palm.

TEST

Action usually tested is abduction of little finger (against resistance).

The abductor digiti quinti is readily observed and palpated at the ulnar border of the palm. Opposition of the thumb and little finger can be tested together by gauging the force required to separate the tips of the two digits when opposed, or by attempting to withdraw a piece of paper clasped between the tips of the digits.

Interossei (Figs. 2–44 and 2–45). (Ulnar nerve, C 8 T 1)

ACTION

Dorsal—abduction of index, middle, and ring fingers from middle line of middle finger (double action on middle finger—both radial and ulnar abduction, radial abduction of index finger, ulnar abduction of ring finger).

First dorsal—adduction (especially palmar adduction) of thumb.

Palmar—adduction of index, ring, and little fingers toward middle finger.

Both sets—flexion of metacarpophalangeal joints and simultaneous extension of interphalangeal joints.

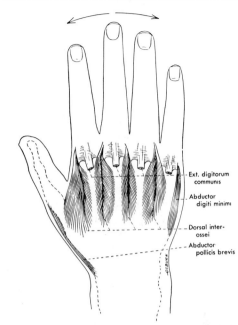

FIGURE 2–44. Dorsal view of the chief abductors of the digits. (Redrawn from Hollinshead, W. H., and Jenkins, D. B.: Functional Anatomy of the Limbs and Back, 5th Ed. Philadelphia, W. B. Saunders Company, 1981.)

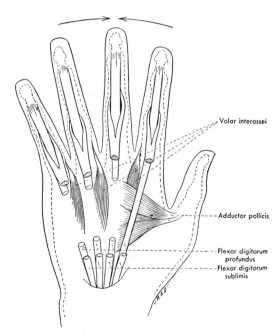

FIGURE 2–45. The chief adductors of the digits. (From Hollinshead, W. H., and Jenkins, D. B.: Functional Anatomy of the Limbs and Back, 5th Ed. Philadelphia, W. B. Saunders Company, 1981.)

THEODORE M. COLE AND JEROME S. TOBIS

Test

Abduction and adduction of individual fingers against resistance with fingers extended. Adduction can be tested by retention of a slip of paper between fingers, and between thumb and index finger, as examiner attempts to withdraw it.

Ability of patient to flex proximal phalanges and simultaneously extend distal phalanges.

Extension of middle phalanges of fingers against resistance while examiner stabilizes proximal phalanges in hyperextension.

The long extensors of the fingers (radial nerve) and the lumbrical muscles (median and ulnar nerves) assist in extension of the middle and distal phalanges. The first dorsal interosseous is readily observed and palpated in the space between the index finger and the thumb.

Adductor Pollicis. (Ulnar nerve, C 8 T 1)

Action

Adduction of thumb in both ulnar and palmar directions (in plane of palm and perpendicular to palm, respectively).

Assistance in flexion of proximal phalanx.

Test

Adduction in each plane against resistance.

Retention of slip of paper between thumb and radial border of hand and between thumb and palm, without flexion of distal phalanx.

It is often possible to palpate the edge of the adductor pollicis just volar to the proximal part of the first dorsal interosseous.

Participating Muscles

Ulnar adduction—first dorsal interosseous, flexor pollicis longus, extensor pollicis longus, flexor pollicis brevis.

Palmar adduction—first dorsal interosseous particularly; extensor pollicis longus.

In severe ulnar nerve palsy, atrophy is evident between the thumb and index finger, between the extensor tendons on the dorsum of the hand, and in the hypothenar eminence. The little finger is separated from the ring finger and cannot be brought into contact with it. The little and ring fingers especially are hyperextended at the metacarpophalangeal joints and flexed at the interphalangeal joints. The index and middle fingers are much less affected because of the intact lumbricals of these fingers (supplied by the median nerve). The true "clawhand" (*main en griffe*) is found only in combined median and ulnar nerve palsy. Attempt to adduct the thumb is usually accompanied by flexion of the distal phalanx, indicating activity of the flexor pollicis longus (median nerve) in an effort to compensate for paralysis of the adductor. Froment's sign of ulnar palsy is an application of this phenomenon (Fig. 2–46). The patient grasps a piece of cardboard firmly with the thumb and index finger of each hand and pulls vigorously. If flexion of the distal phalanx of the thumb occurs, the test is positive and indicative of ulnar palsy.

Localization of lesions of the brachial plexus (Fig. 2–47) is based on the pattern of muscular weakness (and the distribution of sensory impairment).

Damage to the most proximal elements of the plexus (anterior primary rami) is manifested by weakness or paralysis of one or more of the muscles deriving nerve supply from the rami, such as the rhomboids and the serratus anterior, as well as by segmental distribution of muscular weakness (and sensory deficit) in the more distal portions of the upper extremity. Injury to the anterior ramus T 1 produces Horner's syndrome.

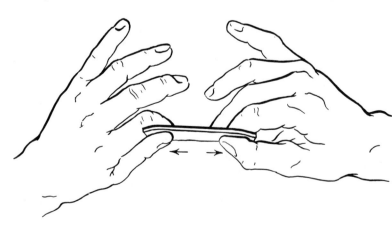

FIGURE 2–46. Froment's sign of ulnar palsy. Positive in the left hand, as indicated by flexion of the terminal phalanx of the thumb. (From Mayo Clinic: Clinical Examinations in Neurology.)

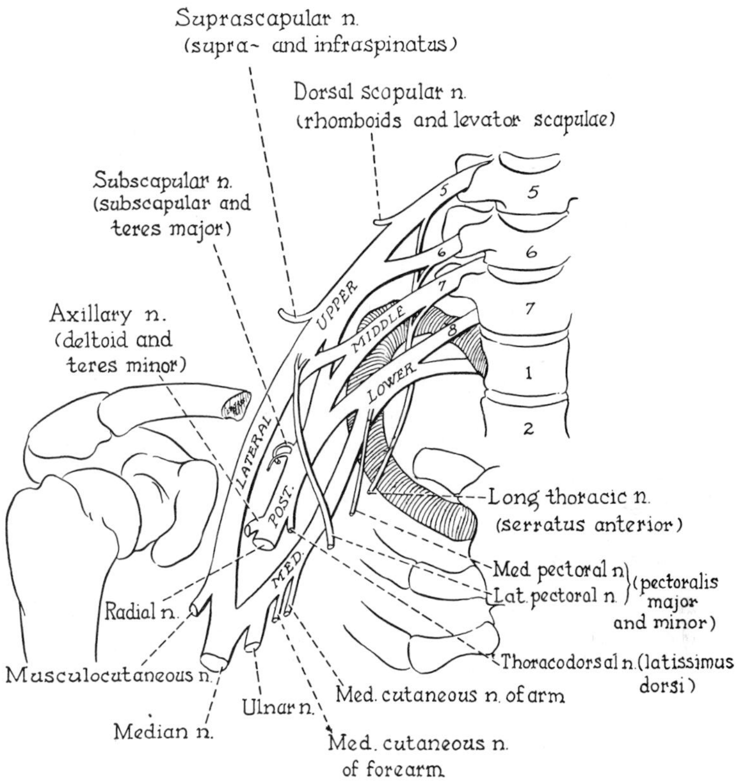

FIGURE 2–47. The brachial plexus. The muscles supplied by the various nerves are in parentheses. (From Mayo Clinic: Clinical Examinations in Neurology.)

Suprascapular n. (supra- and infraspinatus)

Dorsal scapular n. (rhomboids and levator scapulae)

Subscapular n. (subscapular and teres major)

Axillary n. (deltoid and teres minor)

Long thoracic n. (serratus anterior)

Med. pectoral n.
Lat. pectoral n. }(pectoralis major and minor)

Thoracodorsal n. (latissimus dorsi)

Radial n.

Musculocutaneous n.

Median n.

Ulnar n.

Med. cutaneous n. of arm

Med. cutaneous n. of forearm

Lesions involving the most distal parts of the plexus spare some of the muscles of the shoulder girdle, and the pattern of muscular weakness (and sensory impairment) is more like that due to peripheral nerve injuries.

Lesions affecting the upper portion of the plexus, such as the upper trunk, impair the function of muscles supplied by segments C 5 and C 6 (syndrome of Duchenne-Erb) such as the supraspinatus, infraspinatus, deltoid, biceps, brachialis, brachioradialis, and supinator. The arm tends to hang limply at the side, medially rotated and pronated.

Injuries of the lower elements of the plexus, such as the lower trunk, C 8 and T 1 (syndrome of Klumpke), produce disability chiefly of the intrinsic muscles of the hand and flexors of the digits.

These examples illustrate the general principles of localization of lesions on the basis of examination of muscular strength.

The muscles of the neck and trunk may be examined in groups in most instances.

Flexors of Neck. (Cervical nerves, C 1 to C 6)

TEST
Sitting or supine. Flexion of neck, with chin on chest, against resistance applied to forehead.

Extensors of Neck. (Cervical nerves, C1 to T 1)

TEST
Sitting or prone. Extension of neck against resistance applied to occiput.

Diaphragm. (Phrenic nerves, C 3 4 5)

ACTION
Abdominal respiration (inspiration), as distinguished from thoracic respiration (inspiration), which is produced principally by the intercostal muscles.

TEST
Observation of patient for protrusion of upper portion of abdomen during deep inspiration when thoracic cage is splinted.
Ability of patient to sniff.
Litten's sign—successive retraction of lower intercostal spaces during inspiration.
Fluoroscopic observation of diaphragmatic movements.

THEODORE M. COLE AND JEROME S. TOBIS

Weakness of the diaphragm should be suspected in diseases of the spinal cord, when the deltoid or biceps is paralyzed, for these muscles are supplied by neurons situated very near those innervating the diaphragm.

Intercostal Muscles. (Intercostal nerves, T 1 to T 11)

ACTION
Expansion of thorax anteroposteriorly and transversely, producing thoracic inspiration.

TEST
Observation and palpation of expansion of thoracic cage during deep inspiration while maintaining pressure against thorax.
Observation for asymmetry of movement of thorax, particularly during deep inspiration.

Other more general tests of function of the respiratory muscles are
Observation of patient for rapid shallow respiration, flaring of alae nasi, and use of accessory muscles of respiration.
Observation of ability of patient to repeat three or four numbers without pausing for breath.
Observation of ability of patient to hold his breath for 15 sec.

Anterior Abdominal Muscles. Upper (T 6 to T 9) Lower (T 10 to L 1)

TEST
Supine—flexion of neck against resistance applied to forehead by examiner.

Contraction of the abdominal muscles can be observed and palpated. Upward movement of the umbilicus is associated with weakness of the lower abdominal muscles (Beevor's sign).
Supine—hands on occiput. Flexion of trunk by anterior abdominal muscles followed by flexion of pelvis on thighs by hip flexors (chiefly iliopsoas) to reach sitting position. Examiner holds legs down.

Completion of this test excludes significant weakness of either the abdominal muscles or the flexors of the hips. Weak abdominal muscles, in the presence of strong hip flexors, result in hyperextension of the lumbar spine during attempts to elevate the legs or rise to a sitting position.

Extensors of Back

TEST
Prone with hands clasped over buttocks. The head and shoulders should be elevated away from the table while examiner holds legs down.

The gluteal and hamstring muscles fix the pelvis on the thigh.

The movements of the lower extremities are not as complex as those of the upper extremities; hence the examination is somewhat simpler. Since the muscles of the pelvic girdle and thigh do not lend themselves as well to a sequence of examination based on the anatomy of the lumbosacral plexus (Fig. 2–48) as do the muscles of the upper extremities, the order is determined largely by clinical convenience with some considerations given to segmental innervation.

Many of the muscles are so powerful that when little or no weakness is present they can be tested profitably by certain maneuvers performed by the

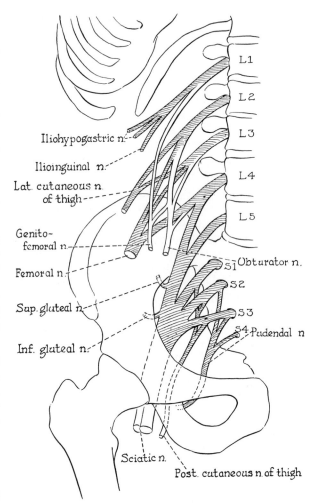

FIGURE 2–48. The lumbosacral plexus. (From Mayo Clinic: Clinical Examinations in Neurology.)

patient in a standing position. Observations of the patient's gait reveals weakness of certain muscles, and atrophy may be visible:

Iliopsoas—difficulty in bringing affected leg forward.

Abductors of thigh (chiefly gluteus medius and gluteus minimus)—sagging opposite side of pelvis and lateral displacement of pelvis to affected side when weight is on that leg.

Quadriceps—keeping knee locked when weight is placed on affected leg.

Tibialis anterior and extensors of toes—varying degrees of "steppage gait" and footdrop.

Gastrocnemius and soleus—limp produced by difficulty in raising heel from floor.

Certain maneuvers by the patient will make muscular weakness more apparent. The principal muscles involved are given:

Stepping up on a step

Raising leg up to step—Iliopsoas.
Raising body—gluteus maximus and quadriceps.
Squatting and rising—quadriceps particularly.
Walking on heels—tibialis anterior and extensors of toes.
Walking on toes—gastrocnemius and soleus.

When there is little or no weakness, it is feasible to conduct the more detailed examination of the muscles of the lower extremities with the patient in the sitting posture throughout. However, the action of certain muscles is somewhat different in the sitting posture as compared with the supine or prone position. In particular, some of the lateral rotators of the thigh function also as abductors. Furthermore, the sitting posture interferes seriously with observation and palpation of some muscles—particularly the gluteus maximus and to a lesser extent the hamstrings. The muscles mentioned are therefore more accurately tested in the prone position.

In some instances it is convenient and advantageous to test the corresponding muscles of the two sides simultaneously for comparison. Examples are the adductors and abductors of the thighs and the extensors (dorsiflexors) and flexors (plantar flexors) of the feet and toes.

Iliopsoas (Fig. 2–49). Psoas major (lumbar plexus [Fig. 2–45], L 1 2 3 4); iliacus (femoral nerve, L 2 3 4)

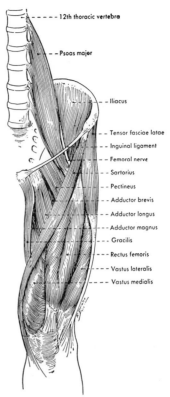

FIGURE 2–49. The more superficial muscles of the anterior aspect of the thigh. (From Hollinshead, W. H., and Jenkins, D. B.: Functional Anatomy of the Limbs and Back, 5th Ed. Philadelphia, W. B. Saunders Company, 1981.)

ACTION
Flexion of thigh at hip.

TEST
Sitting—flexion of thigh, raising knee against resistance by examiner.
Supine—raising extended leg off table and maintaining it against downward pressure applied by examiner just above knee.

Participating Muscles
Rectus femoris and sartorius (both—femoral nerve, L 2 3 4); tensor fasciae latae (superior gluteal nerve, L 4 5 S 1).

Adductor Magnus, Longus, Brevis (Fig. 2–49). (Obturator nerve, L 2 3 4. Part of adductor magnus is supplied by sciatic nerve, L 5, and functions with hamstrings.)

ACTION
Principally adduction of thigh.

THEODORE M. COLE AND JEROME S. TOBIS

TEST

Sitting or supine. Holding knees together while examiner attempts to separate them.

The two legs can also be tested separately and the muscles palpated.

Participating Muscles
Gluteus maximus; gracilis (obturator nerve, L 2 3 4).

Abductors of Thigh (Fig. 2–50). (Superior gluteal nerve, L 4 5 S 1)

Gluteus medius and gluteus minimus principally. Tensor fasciae latae is important only if hip is flexed.

ACTION

Abduction and medial rotation of thigh.
Tensor fasciae latae assists in flexion of the thigh at the hip.

TEST

Sitting—separation of knees against resistance by examiner.

In this position, the gluteus maximus and some of the other lateral rotators of the thigh function as abductors, hence diminishing the accuracy of the test.

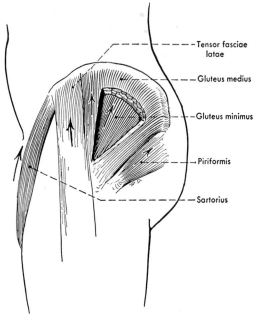

FIGURE 2–50. The abductors of the thigh. (From Hollinshead, W. H., and Jenkins, D. B.: Functional Anatomy of the Limbs and Back, 5th Ed. Philadelphia, W. B. Saunders Company, 1981.)

Supine—same test as above. More exact.
Lying on opposite side—abduction of hip (upward movement) while examiner presses downward on lower leg and stabilizes pelvis.
The tensor fasciae latae and to a lesser extent the gluteus medius can be palpated.

Medial Rotators of Thigh. Same as abductors.

TEST

Sitting or prone—knee flexed to 90 degrees. Medial rotation of thigh against resistance applied by examiner at knee and ankle in attempt to rotate thigh laterally.

Lateral Rotators of Thigh (Fig. 2–51). (L 4 5 S 1 2)

Gluteus maximus (inferior gluteal nerve, L 5 S 1 2) chiefly
Obturator internus and gemellus superior (nerve to obturator internus, L 5 S 1 2)
Quadratus femoris and gemellus inferior (nerve to quadratus femoris, L 4 5 S 1)

TEST

Sitting or prone—Knee flexed to 90 degrees. Lateral rotation of thigh against attempt by examiner to rotate thigh medially.

The gluteus maximus is the muscle principally tested and can be observed and palpated in the prone position.

Gluteus Maximus (Fig. 2–51). (Inferior gluteal nerve, L 5 S 1 2)

ACTION

Extension of thigh at hip.
Lateral rotation of thigh.
Assistance in adduction of thigh.

TEST

Sitting or supine—starting with thigh slightly raised, extension (downward movement) of thigh against resistance by examiner applied under distal part of thigh.

This is a rather crude test and the muscle cannot be observed or readily palpated.

Prone—knee well flexed to minimize participation of hamstrings. Extension of thigh, raising knee from table against downward pressure by examiner applied to distal part of thigh.

The muscle is accessible to observation and palpation in this position.

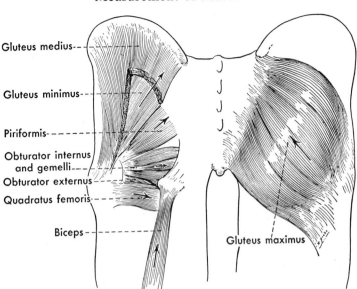

FIGURE 2–51. The posteriorly placed external rotators of the thigh. (From Hollinshead, W. H., and Jenkins, D. B.: Functional Anatomy of the Limbs and Back, 5th Ed. Philadelphia, W. B. Saunders Company, 1981.)

Labels on figure: Gluteus medius, Gluteus minimus, Piriformis, Obturator internus and gemelli, Obturator externus, Quadratus femoris, Biceps, Gluteus maximus

Quadriceps Femoris (Fig. 2–52). (Femoral nerve, L 2 $\underline{3}$ 4)

ACTION

Extension of leg at knee.
Rectus femoris assists in flexion of thigh at hip.

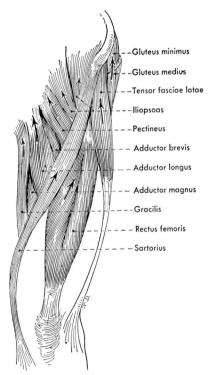

FIGURE 2–52. Flexors of the thigh. (From Hollinshead, W. H., and Jenkins, D. B.: Functional Anatomy of the Limbs and Back, 5th Ed. Philadelphia, W. B. Saunders Company, 1981.)

Labels on figure: Gluteus minimus, Gluteus medius, Tensor fasciae latae, Iliopsoas, Pectineus, Adductor brevis, Adductor longus, Adductor magnus, Gracilis, Rectus femoris, Sartorius

TEST

Sitting or supine—lower leg in moderate extension. Maintenance of extension against effort of examiner to flex leg at knee.
Atrophy is easily noted.

Hamstrings (Fig. 2–53). (Sciatic nerve, L 4 $\underline{5}$ S $\underline{1}$ 2)

Biceps femoris—external hamstring (L 5 S $\underline{1}$ 2)
Semitendinosus—internal hamstrings (L 4 $\underline{5}$ S $\underline{1}$ 2)
Semimembranosus (L 4 $\underline{5}$ S 1 2)

ACTION

Flexion of leg at knee.
All but short head of biceps femoris assist in extension of thigh at hip.

TEST

Sitting—flexion of lower leg against resistance.
Prone—knee partly flexed. Further flexion against resistance.
Observation and palpation of the muscles and tendons are important for proper interpretation.

Tibialis Anterior (Figs. 2–54, 2–55, and 2–56). (Deep peroneal nerve, L $\underline{4}$ 5 S 1)

ACTION

Dorsiflexion and inversion (particularly in dorsiflexed position) of foot.

TEST

Dorsiflexion of foot against resistance applied to dorsum of foot downward and toward eversion.

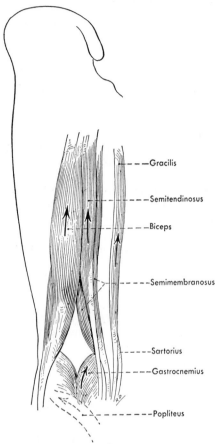

FIGURE 2–53. The flexors of the knee. (From Hollinshead, W. H., and Jenkins, D. B.: Functional Anatomy of the Limbs and Back, 5th Ed. Philadelphia, W. B. Saunders Company, 1981.)

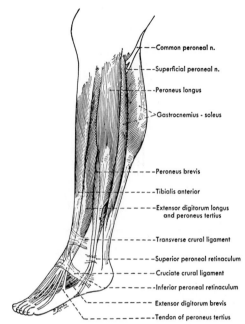

FIGURE 2–54. The lateral muscles of the leg. (From Hollinshead, W. H., and Jenkins, D. B.: Functional Anatomy of the Limbs and Back, 5th Ed. Philadelphia, W. B. Saunders Company, 1981.)

The belly of the muscle just lateral to the shin, and the tendon medially on the dorsal aspect of the ankle should be observed and palpated. Atrophy is conspicuous.

Participating Muscles
Dorsiflexion—extensor hallucis longus; extensor digitorum longus.
Inversion—tibialis posterior.

Extensor Hallucis Longus (Fig. 2–55). (Deep peroneal nerve, L 4 5 S 1)

ACTION
Extension of great toe and dorsiflexion of foot.

TEST
Extension of great toe against resistance while foot is stabilized in neutral position.

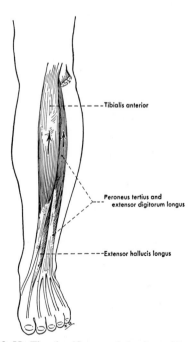

FIGURE 2–55. The dorsiflexors of the foot. (From Hollinshead, W. H., and Jenkins, D. B.: Functional Anatomy of the Limbs and Back, 5th Ed. Philadelphia, W. B. Saunders Company, 1981.)

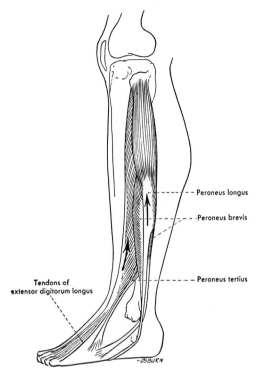

FIGURE 2–56. Evertors of the foot. (From Hollinshead, W. H., and Jenkins, D. B.: Functional Anatomy of the Limbs and Back, 5th Ed. Philadelphia, W. B. Saunders Company, 1981.)

The tendon is palpable between those of the tibialis anterior and the extensor digitorum longus.

Extensor Digitorum Longus (Figs. 2–54 and 2–55). (Deep peroneal nerve, L 4 5 S 1)

ACTION
Extension of lateral four toes and dorsiflexion of foot.

TEST
Similar to above.

The tendons are visible and palpable on the dorsal aspect of the ankle and foot lateral to that of the extensor hallucis longus.

Extensor Digitorum Brevis (Fig. 2–54). (Deep peroneal nerve, L 4 5 S 1)

ACTION
Assists in extension of all toes except little toe.

TEST
Observe and palpate belly of muscle on lateral aspect of dorsum of foot.

Peroneus Longus, Brevis (Fig. 2–56). (Superficial peroneal nerve, L 4 5 S 1)

ACTION
Eversion of foot.
Assistance in plantar flexion of foot.

TEST
Foot in plantar flexion. Eversion against resistance applied by examiner to lateral border of foot.

The tendons are palpable just above and behind the external malleolus. Atrophy may be visible over the anterolateral aspect of the lower leg.

Gastrocnemius; Soleus (Fig. 2–57). (Tibial nerve, L 5 S 1 2)

ACTION
Plantar flexion of foot.
The gastrocnemius also flexes the knee and cannot act effectively in plantar flexion of the foot when the knee is well flexed.

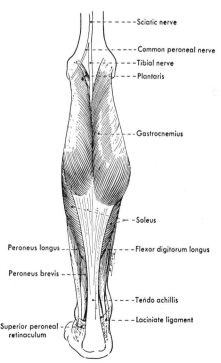

FIGURE 2–57. The musculature of the calf of the leg, first layer. (From Hollinshead, W. H., and Jenkins, D. B.: Functional Anatomy of the Limbs and Back, 5th Ed. Philadelphia, W. B. Saunders Company, 1981.)

THEODORE M. COLE AND JEROME S. TOBIS

TEST

Knee extended to test both muscles. Knee flexed to test principally the soleus. Plantar flexion of foot against resistance.

The muscles and tendon should be observed and palpated. Atrophy is readily visible. The gastrocnemius and soleus are very strong muscles, and leverage in testing favors the patient rather than the examiner. For this reason, slight weakness is difficult to detect by resisting flexion of the ankle or by pressing against the flexed foot in the direction of extension. Consequently, it is advisable to test the strength of these muscles against the weight of the patient's body. Have the patient stand on one foot and flex the foot so as to lift the body directly and fully upward. Sometimes it is necessary for the examiner to hold the patient steady as this test is performed.

Participating Muscles

Long flexors of toes; tibialis posterior and peroneus longus and brevis (particularly near extreme plantar flexion).

Tibialis Posterior (Fig. 2–58). (Posterior tibial nerve, L 5 S 1)

ACTION

Inversion of foot.
Assistance in plantar flexion of foot.

TEST

Foot in complete plantar flexion. Inversion against resistance applied to medial border of foot and directed toward eversion and slightly toward dorsiflexion.

This maneuver virtually eliminates participation of the tibialis anterior in inversion. The toes should be relaxed to prevent participation of the long flexors of the toes.

Long Flexors of Toes (Fig. 2–58). (Posterior tibial nerve, L 5 S 1 2)
Flexor digitorum longus
Flexor hallucis longus

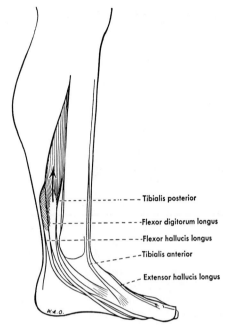

FIGURE 2–58. Invertors of the foot. (From Hollinshead, W. H., and Jenkins, D. B.: Functional Anatomy of the Limbs and Back, 5th Ed. Philadelphia, W. B. Saunders Company, 1981.)

ACTION

Plantar flexion of toes, especially at distal interphalangeal joints.
Assistance in plantar flexion and inversion of foot.

TEST

Foot stabilized in neutral position. Plantar flexion of toes against resistance applied particularly to distal phalanges.

Intrinsic Muscles of Foot. Virtually all except extensor digitorum brevis (Medial plantar nerve, L 5 S 1; lateral plantar nerve, S 1 S 2)

ACTION

Somewhat comparable to that of intrinsic muscles of the hand. Many people have very poor individual function of these muscles.

TEST

Cupping the sole of the foot is an adequate test for most clinical purposes.

Quantitative Assessment of Physical Performance

DANIEL T. BARRY

To provide a complete description of even a single individual's physical abilities, including functional abilities and task performance, is an immense project. The project can be made manageable by identifying specific questions to be answered by the evaluation. The specific questions usually relate to task performance, e.g., can an individual return to work full-time, or will an athlete be capable of a record performance? Task performance is difficult to measure directly, particularly when details of the task and the environment vary from day to day. The general assessment of physical performance therefore relies heavily on parameters that underlie the performance of each task.

Quantification of physical parameters, such as strength and sensation, is essential if accurate comparisons are to be made over time and among individuals. Accurate and concrete measures of progress rely on quantified measures, such as number of pounds lifted or number of repetitions completed. Using a standardized method of quantifying parameters permits different observers in different locations to compare data in a straightforward manner. In addition to improving reliability and reproducibility, quantification can produce a record that reflects the full sensitivity of a particular test. Furthermore, quantified parameters allow standards of performance to be established for a population of individuals. Comparisons among individuals permit the important parameters for a particular task to be identified. Eventually, minimal levels of achievement in certain parameters may be determined as necessary for successful performance of a particular task.

Routine evaluations usually do not require highly accurate measures of performance. There is no need for testing strength by a Cybex machine to determine if a healthy child can participate in standard sports. However, even routine tests can be made more accurate and reproducible by habitually using quantified measures of performance. There are general parameters, such as strength and sensation, that are important for almost all tasks.

For each parameter discussed below, there are techniques for quick, routine evaluation and the discovery of alternatives when detailed, accurate assessment is needed.

Range of Motion

Routine range of motion examination of the extremities results in angles that are accurate to about 5 degrees. The first part of Chapter 2 of this handbook describes methods and conventions of range of motion measurements in detail. Spinal range of motion measurements can be made more accurate by using spinal x-ray studies; this technique has been used to establish the proper cervical orthosis when a particular level of cervical spine immobilization is desired.[18] Tucci and co-workers[60] describe a simple modification of a gravity goniometer to allow reliable assessment of cervical range of motion.

Strength and Power

Strength may be quantified by the manual method according to the Medical Research Council scale,[9, 40] or by more precise quantitative methods. Table 2–5 shows normal values of isometric strength for adults employed in manual jobs.[6] These values were obtained using specific body postures and isometric conditions. Table 2–6 displays normal values for isometric lifting, pushing, and pulling—an attempt to address strength in functional activity. Figure 2–59 shows the positions used to obtain data in Table 2–6.

Accurate measurements of strength can be easily and reliably obtained if torque production is monitored from a motivated patient, who is in a comfortable position, with standardized joint angles and measured limb lengths. The answer to the question of whether to measure concentric, isometric, eccentric, isotonic, isokinetic, or some

THEODORE M. COLE AND JEROME S. TOBIS

TABLE 2–5. Static Muscle Strength Moment Data (Nm) for 25 Men and 22 Women Employed in Manual Jobs in Industry*

MUSCLE FUNCTION	JOINT ANGLES	MALE (PERCENTILE)			FEMALE (PERCENTILE)		
		5	50	95	5	50	95
Elbow flexion	90° Included to arm (arm at side)	42	77	111	16	41	55
Elbow extension	70° Included to arm (arm at side)	31	46	67	9	27	39
Medial humeral (shoulder) rotation	90° Vertical shoulder (abducted)	28	52	83	9	21	33
Lateral humeral (shoulder) rotation	5° Vertical shoulder (at side)	23	33	51	13	19	28
Shoulder horizontal flexion	90° Vertical shoulder (abducted)	44	92	119	12	40	60
Shoulder horizontal extension	90° Vertical shoulder (abducted)	43	67	103	19	33	57
Shoulder vertical adduction	90° Vertical shoulder (abducted)	35	67	115	13	30	54
Shoulder vertical abduction	90° Vertical shoulder (abducted)	43	71	101	15	37	57
Ankle extension (plantar flexion)	90° Included to shank	69	126	237	31	81	131
Knee extension	120° Included to thigh (seated)	84	168	318	52	106	219
Knee flexion	135° Included to thigh (seated)	58	100	157	22	62	104
Hip extension	100° Included to torso (seated)	94	190	419	38	97	180
Hip flexion	110° Included to torso (seated)	118	185	342	57	126	177
Torso extension	100° Included to thigh (seated)	164	234	503	71	184	348
Torso flexion	100° Included to thigh (seated)	89	143	216	49	75	161
Torso lateral flexion	Sitting erect	95	159	261	50	94	162

*Chaffin, D. B., and Andersson, G.: Occupational Biomechanics. New York, John Wiley and Sons, 1984, p. 100. Reprinted with permission, all rights reserved.

other contraction protocol is dependent on the outcome goals. For example, if the goal is to achieve improved performance in a sport requiring rapid contractions, then high-velocity isokinetic strength is a more important parameter than isometric strength. In this example, power, or the rate of work performance, is likely to be an important parameter. High maximum power implies an ability to generate bursts of energy.

Reduced motivation or reduction in voluntary control can make accurate assessment of muscle strength difficult. However, the maximal force that a nerve-muscle system can generate can be determined for some muscles by percutaneous nerve stimulation. This technique has been applied in the evaluation of fatigue (see Fig. 2–60 and later) and has the additional feature of providing a measurement that is independent of factors such as motor unit synchronization or learned increased activation. The technique must be used with care, since sudden, maximal contractions of some muscles, particularly the quadriceps, can cause tendon damage or even avulsion. In these cases submaximal stimulation can be used.[2]

Hand-held myometers provide quantitative measures of strength with good interrater and test-retest reliability, although the reliability is dependent on the particular muscle group tested.[32, 33] There are several commercially available, fixed-site devices that can accurately measure torque and power over a wide range of velocities and joint angles. The Cybex II dynamometer is described in Chapter 20 of this handbook. The devices of Kin-Com and Loredan systems are versatile in that they can be programmed to perform and monitor a wide variety of exercise protocols and range of motion measurements.

Quantitative monitoring of force production can also be accomplished with surface electromyography and/or acoustic myography under certain conditions. Both the integrated surface electromyographic (EMG) signal and the root-mean–

squared acoustic signal provide reasonably linear indications of force production from a muscle at moderate levels of contraction, provided that no fatigue occurs. The EMG signal does not decline in amplitude with the decline in force in fatigue, although there is a shift in peak frequency. The root-mean–squared value of the surface acoustic signal does decline linearly with fatigue[1] (Fig. 2–61).

Endurance and Fatigue

A good definition of fatigue is suggested by Bigland-Ritchie and Woods[4]—". . . any reduction in the force generating capacity of the total neuromuscular system regardless of the force required in any given situation . . ." as a result of prior metabolic activity. This definition implies that fatigue originates at more than one level of the neuromuscular system. "Central fatigue" is due to decreased excitation of motor neurons, whereas "peripheral fatigue" results from processes within motor units (motor neuron, synapse, and muscle fibers). Central fatigue can be distinguished from peripheral fatigue by applying maximal peripheral nerve stimulation while measuring force production. The difference between the voluntary force level and the force produced by the shock is a measure of the degree of central fatigue (Fig. 2–61).

The function of the neuromuscular junction in producing muscle fiber action potentials is readily assessed by measuring EMG signals while inducing fatigue. Several investigators[1, 4, 13, 41] have found that the surface EMG signal amplitude does not decline with the decay of force in fatigue from voluntary contractions. There are reports of EMG and force signals declining in parallel[58] so that, under some circumstances with high firing rates,

TABLE 2–6. Static Strengths Demonstrated by Workers when Lifting, Pushing, and Pulling with Both Hands on a Handle Placed at Different Locations Relative to the Midpoint Between the Ankles on Floor*

	HANDLE LOCATION (cm)†		MALE STRENGTHS (N)			FEMALE STRENGTHS (N)		
TEST DESCRIPTION	Vertical	Horizontal	Sample Size	Mean	Standard Deviation	Sample Size	Mean	Standard Deviation
Lift—leg partial squat‡	38	0	673	903	325	165	427	187
Lift—torso stooped over‡	38	38	1141	480	205	246	271	125
Lift—arms flexed‡	114	38	1276	383	125	234	214	93
Lift—shoulder high and arms out	152	51	309	227	71	35	129	36
Lift—shoulder high and arms flexed	152	38	119	529	222	20	240	84
Lift—shoulder high and arms close	152	25	309	538	156	35	285	102
Lift—floor level-close (squat)	15	25	309	890	245	35	547	182
Lift—floor level-out (stoop)	15	38	170	320	125	20	200	71
Pull down—waist level	118	38	309	432	93	35	325	71
Pull down—above shoulders	178	33	309	605	102	35	449	107
Pull in—shoulder level, arms out	157	33	309	311	80	35	244	53
Pull in—shoulder level, arms in	140	0	205	253	62	52	209	62
Push out—waist level, stand erect	101	35	54	311	195	27	226	76
Push-out—chest level, stand erect	124	25	309	303	76	35	214	49
Push-out—shoulder level, lean forward	140	64	205	418	178	52	276	120

*Chaffin, D. B., and Andersson, G.: Occupational Biomechanics. New York, John Wiley and Sons, 1984, p. 102. Reprinted with permission, all rights reserved.

†Handle locations are measured in midsagittal plane, vertical from floor and horizontal from the midpoint between the ankles.

‡See Figure 2–59 for illustrations of these positions.

THEODORE M. COLE AND JEROME S. TOBIS

MUSCLE STRENGTH EVALUATION

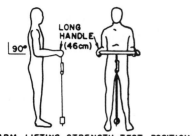

ARM LIFTING STRENGTH TEST POSITION

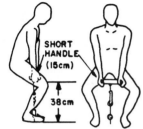

LEG LIFTING STRENGTH TEST POSITION

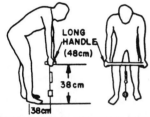

TORSO LIFTING STRENGTH TEST POSITION

FIGURE 2–59. The postures used to obtain static strength data presented in Table 2–7. (Chaffin, D. B. and Anderson G.: Occupational Biomechanics. John Wiley and Sons, New York, 1984, p. 105, reproduced with permission, all rights reserved.)

neuromuscular junction failure may occur and contribute to fatigue. The biochemical changes that occur in contracting muscle fibers may interfere with excitation-contraction coupling and produce fatigue. Nuclear magnetic resonance techniques demonstrate a drop in phosphocreatine levels that parallels the decline of force in a fatiguing muscle.[42] Adenosine triphosphate (ATP) remains constant until extreme fatigue occurs and then is only moderately reduced. Lactic acid, adenosine diphosphate (ADP), inorganic phosphate, and hydrogen ion concentrations all increase with fatigue; the difficulty is determining which parameters induce the reduction in force and which are just byproducts. The rate of resynthesis of phosphocreatine after a fatiguing contraction may be a useful way of measuring oxidative metabolism. Of course, the ultimate limitation of endurance is the supply of glucose and fatty acids that are normally stored as glycogen (in muscle and liver) and adipose tissue triglycerides, respectively.

As a clinical complaint, fatigue encompasses a broad range of symptoms, and the first step of evaluation is to determine what the patient means by the term "fatigue." Frequently, patients describe a sense of increased effort to accomplish daily tasks. Actual muscle weakness may not be a component of the complaint. Once the symptom is understood, one can assess the degree of central fatigue. One should keep in mind the possibilities of hormonal or cardiopulmonary pathology and central nervous system lesions in addition to pain, depression, decreased motivation, and neurasthenia as etiologies for central fatigue. If a standard physical examination does not determine whether the fatigue is central or peripheral, then specialized tests can be performed.

Examples of specialized tests include:

1. Applying maximal peripheral stimulation during voluntary contraction while measuring force output. As described above and in Figure 2–60, the difference between voluntary force and stimulated force is a measure of central fatigue.

2. Monitoring EMG and acoustic signals from a muscle as the patient voluntarily contracts the muscle.[1] The ratio of acoustic signal amplitude to EMG amplitude is a measure of peripheral fatigue (Fig. 2–61).

3. Monitoring the change in surface EMG signal frequency. The median frequency declines with fatigue.

4. Using bicycle ergometry to measure the rate of fatigue. Ergometry can be combined with oxygen uptake measurements to quantitate metabolic coefficients of energy production. The threshold for performance without fatigue can be determined and should be about 15 per cent of a maximal voluntary contraction.

5. Using nuclear magnetic resonance (NMR) measurements of metabolites to document the biochemical changes that accompany the fatigue symptoms.

Before initiating treatment of fatigue, one must remember that normal peripheral fatigue serves a protective function for muscles. Fatigue prevents the muscle from completely exhausting all metabolic reserves and limits the build-up of toxic metabolites. Bicycle ergometry is useful to quantify the actual amount of work performed in a training session and can be used to demonstrate improve-

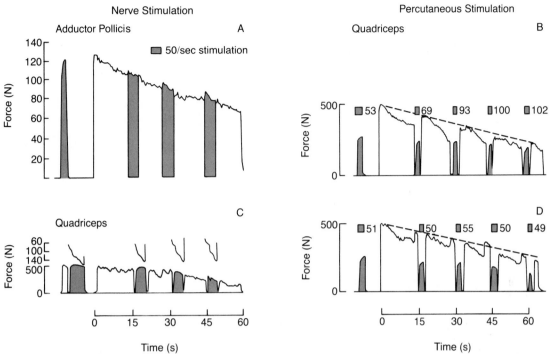

FIGURE 2–60. Sustained maximal voluntary contractions of adductor pollicis and quadriceps muscles interrupted periodically by maximal tetanic stimulation of the nerve *(A and B)*, or 53 per cent *(C)* and 51 per cent *(D)* of the total quadriceps muscles by percutaneous stimulation of intramuscular nerve endings. The contraction in *C* shows evidence of central fatigue. In *D*, the same subject was asked to make an "extra effort" just before each stimulation period. The ratio between stimulated and voluntary force then remained unchanged as force declined. The waveforms above the force in *B* and the boxes above the forces in *A, C*, and *D* indicate the stimulation rates used. The rates were slightly above the value needed for a fully fused tetanic contraction. (From Bigland-Ritchie, B.: EMG and fatigue of human voluntary and stimulated contractions. CIBA Found. Symp., 82:130–156, 1981. Copyrighted 1981. CIBA-Geigy Corp. Reproduced with permission from the CIBA collection of medical illustrations by Frank H. Netter, M.D. All rights reserved.)

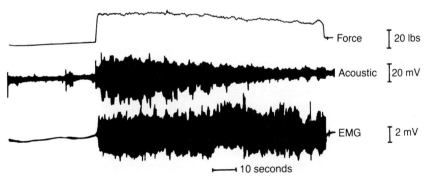

FIGURE 2–61. An example of simultaneous recording of acoustic myography, surface electromyography, and force with the high initial force (75 per cent of maximal voluntary contraction) held as long as possible. Statistical analysis of 14 experiments demonstrated a linear relationship of acoustic amplitude to force during fatigue. (From Barry D. T., et al.: Acoustic myography: A noninvasive monitor of motor unit fatigue. Muscle Nerve, 8(3):189–194, 1985. Reproduced with permission, all rights reserved.)

THEODORE M. COLE AND JEROME S. TOBIS

ments with time. Effectiveness of the exercise can be monitored by the Karvonen method of a target heart rate equal to the resting heart rate plus 60 to 90 per cent of the heart rate reserve (age-predicted maximum heart rate − resting heart rate = heart rate reserve). Of course, patients with cardiovascular or pulmonary disease will need modified criteria. Another measure of exercise is oxygen use; endurance training requires the achievement of approximately 60 to 80 per cent of VO_2 max.

Sensation

Quantification of the sensory examination is a straightforward approach to increasing the sensitivity and reproducibility of the general physical examination. Although the highest resolution measurements of sensation are obtained with fixed-location devices in specially constructed rooms and computerized protocols, bedside examination can be improved with some simple techniques:

1. Vibration testing is a sensitive test for large fiber neuropathies: count the number of seconds from the time the patient reports no sensation until the examiner can no longer hear the tuning fork. If the examiner has a hearing deficit, then the time can be counted until the examiner can no longer feel the vibration. However, this variation suffers from the problem that vibration sense declines more rapidly than the low frequency (128 Hz) hearing threshold as individuals age.[24] Another variation, useful in peripheral neuropathies, involves counting the seconds between absent sensation in the toes and absent sensation in the fingers of the patient. More accurate testing requires instruments that control for pressure, waveform, area, location, and method of stimulation. The Bio-Thesiometer (Bio-Medical Instruments, Co., Newbury, OH) meets some of these requirements but still has the inaccuracies inherent in a hand-operated device.

2. Tactile or touch sensation is traditionally quantified by testing the threshold to response of various thickness horsehairs (von Frey hairs). Again, the inaccuracies of a hand-held device without control of pressure are apparent. Sensitivity to various grades of sandpaper have also been used as a measure of tactile sensation.[12] Renfrew[49] describes a simple "depth-sense" esthesiometer that quantifies tactile sense by determining the threshold for detection of an edge. Renfrew also describes a simple, easy-to-use device to measure two-point discrimination sense, which is a quantitative measure of tactile resolution.

3. Temperature sensation can be quantified by using Minnesota thermal disks.[12] Disks of four different thermal conductivities (copper, stainless steel, glass, and polyvinyl chloride) are sequentially placed on the skin. The materials with higher thermal conductivity feel colder because they conduct more heat away from the skin when the disks are applied for a short time.

4. Pain sensation is routinely tested by the patient's response to a sharp pinprick. Hardy[29] describes a dolorimeter for quantifying the pinprick pain threshold. Painful responses to deep pressure over trigger points have been quantified by measuring the depth of skin dimpling that produces the pain, the pressure that produces pain,[17] or skin compliance.[16] Thermography may eventually become a quantified tool for evaluating local areas of pain that have altered blood flow.

Coordination

Good coordination requires complex interplay among many physiological systems. Reflexes, tone, proprioception, balance, and reaction time all play critical roles in performing coordinated movements.

Muscle tone can be quantified by measuring the elastic and viscous properties of muscle. Mechanical properties of muscle are revealed by torque-frequency relationships. A typical test monitors the force required to passively range the wrist sinusoidally at various frequencies.[23, 30, 32, 38, 61] At low frequencies elastic forces dominate, whereas at high frequencies forces due to mass and viscosity dominate. The phase relationships of position to force are distinct (0 degrees elastic, 90 degrees viscous, 180 degrees mass) and are used to separate the various force components. The viscous component of spasticity is reflected by the well-known phenomenon that the force required to range a spastic limb increases with the velocity of ranging. An adjunct to muscle tone testing is reflex quantification that can be accomplished with tendon-tapping with measured forces[21] or with H-reflex recovery curves.[59]

Ambulatory monitors of muscle activity can be used to document muscle activity for a continuous 24-hour period and then, in spastic patients, to quantitate the number and severity of spasms.[57] The extent of reflex overflow to adjacent muscles and lack of inhibition of muscle groups can be documented with electromyography. Control of individual motor units can be achieved with appropriate biofeedback.[52] Recovery stages have been quantified in some syndromes (e.g., Brunnstrom's stages).

Balance can be quantified at the bedside by simple methods, such as the time that balance can be maintained in various positions (e.g., with the patient standing on both feet, standing on one foot, standing on toes, sitting with hands in the lap). Dynamic balance is quantified by parameters, such as the number of tandem steps or the ability to recover from a measured perturbing push. Dependence on visual cues is important and forms the basis for the Romberg test. More sensitive testing is accomplished with tilt platforms combined with measurements of body sway.[46]

Reaction time is easily measured by measuring the distance a yardstick drops before the patient catches it between thumb and forefinger. Typical stimulus-response times are about 0.3 sec,[37] corresponding to about a 40-cm drop of the yardstick.

Generalized coordination activities are hard to quantify, but a few techniques can be employed. A joystick control can be used to follow a dot on a video screen while the computer calculates a cumulative error. Standardized objects (e.g., a baseball bat) can be balanced in the hand for measured lengths of time. Reaching motions can be analyzed to plot speed of movement and distance moved over time.[37] Uncoordinated activity yields erratic curves that can be quantified by the size of the error in a second-order fit of a least mean squared curve.

Gait Analysis

Gait analysis encompasses many levels of neuromuscular functioning. Strength and coordination are combined to produce a statically unstable, dynamically stable state. Quantification includes measurement of muscle activity from many muscles throughout the gait cycle; position of ankle, knee, and hip joints and center of gravity; foot placement; force transmission through the limbs and spine; and the energy required to ambulate under various conditions. More global assessments include mechanical energy measurements[47] and oxygen consumption measurements during gait. Recent quantitative analysis of power generation and absorption has demonstrated that "energy-return" prostheses are capable of reducing forces at the knee and hip that are normally encountered by prosthetic wearers.[7, 8]

Hand Function

Hand function is quantified by a series of timed tasks, such as buttoning, block placement, and lacing, combined with measurements, such as range of motion and grip strength.[34, 54] Normal values have been established, and progress is indicated by a reduction in time needed to perform the tasks. Of course, performance times improve as individuals simply gain practice with the test, so it is important to not test too frequently with the same tasks. The format of the test has been modified to allow testing and comparison of upper extremity prosthetic devices.[56]

Overall Measures of Performance

Functional Scales

Many functional assessment scales must be considered when attempting to quantitate performance. The key is to pick a scale that is sensitive to the patient's particular disabilities, that measures functions important to the patient, and that has been shown to be valid and reliable.[25, 36] In some cases, such as complete spinal cord injury, expected physical performance levels are well documented and are based on the level of the lesion.[20] In most cases, however, a general functional scale is needed. The Barthal index,[26, 39] the PULSES profile,[26, 43, 44] the functional independence measure, the ESCROW scale, the Tufts Assessment of Motor Performance,[22] and the Occupational Therapy Comprehensive Functional Assessment[55] are examples of functional scales—for details, refer to the chapter on *Functional Assessment*. These scales measure function, and as Moskowitz[43] points out, disability evaluation and functional assessment are not the same entity. The functional scales are designed to assess changes in patients with chronic disease, and they do not directly lead to an assignment of a disability level for medicolegal purposes.

Many scales have been developed for particular injuries or diseases. In particular, several scales for functional status following head injury have been developed. The Glasgow Coma Scale tracks emergence from coma, whereas the Glasgow Outcome scale,[35] the Extended Glasgow Outcome scale,[54] the Disability Rating Scale,[48] and the Levels of Cognitive Function Scale[28] rate levels of functional recovery later during the healing process.

Another approach to functional evaluation is to

THEODORE M. COLE AND JEROME S. TOBIS

assess the energy output that a patient can sustain for various lengths of time. Cardiac rehabilitation routinely uses metabolic power requirements (METS) to assess progress and provide guidance regarding safe activities (see the chapter "Common Cardiovascular Problems in Rehabilitation" in this handbook). The total energy required to perform a physical task can be divided by the length of time the task is performed to determine the continuous power needed while performing the task—the power can then be interpreted in MET levels.

Disability

Disability is not the same as physical impairment. Consider the following definitions from the American Medical Association's (AMA) Guides to Permanent Impairment:[27]

1. Disability is the limiting loss or absence of the capacity of an individual to meet personal, social, or occupational demands, or to meet statutory or regulatory requirements.

2. Impairment is the loss of, loss of use of, or derangement of any body part, system, or function.

These definitions imply that impairment is a medical condition that can be determined by a qualified physician, whereas disability is dependent on many circumstances beyond the altered health status. The existence of an impairment does not guarantee the existence of a disability.

Impairment ratings are expressed in terms of a percentage of total impairment. The guidelines used to determine impairment percentages can include the AMA's Guides to Permanent Impairment,[27] the VA Physician's Guide to Disability Evaluation Examination, or HEW's Disability Evaluation Under Social Security. The guidelines explicitly define percentages of impairment for various medical conditions. For example, the chapter on extremities, spine and pelvis in the AMA's Guides to Permanent Impairment[27] lists the percentage of impairment resulting from altered range of motion at any particular joint. Also, explicit tables are included for the cumulative effects of multiple separate impairments into one final "whole person" impairment rating. The objective is to have a system that results in consistent impairment rating to within 5 per cent.

Ergonomic centers, such as the one at the University of Michigan,[6, 45] are developing new, more objective techniques to measure work capacity. Monitoring forces exerted in repetitive tasks can potentially reveal reduced effort by analysis of the variation of effort from one repetition to the next. Maximal efforts produce only small variations. Workplace simulations and evaluations at the actual workplace increase the relevence of the data for a particular individual.

Summary

Quantitative assessments of range of motion, strength, endurance, sensation, coordination, task performance, and functional abilities provide increased reliability, reproducibility, and sensitivity in the assessment of physical performance. These measurements are essential to the scientific basis of rehabilitation medicine; quantified performance allows valid comparisons among various treatment protocols and the establishment of standards of performance. Many quantitative techniques can be employed as part of the routine physical examination, and specialized devices can be used when more accurate data are needed.

ACKNOWLEDGMENTS

This chapter is, in part, based on research supported by grant NS01017 from National Institute for Neurological and Communicable Diseases and Stroke (NINCDS) of the National Institutes of Health. Parts of the section on *Fatigue and Endurance* were previously published as a course handout at the American Academy of Physical Medicine and Rehabilitation (AAPMR) meetings in Orlando, FL, 1987.

References

Goniometry

1. Clayson, S. J., Mundale, M. O., and Kottke, F. J.: Goniometer adaptation for measuring hip extension. Arch. Phys. Med., 47:255, 1966.
2. Defibaugh, J. J.: Measurement of head motion, Part I: A review of methods of measuring joint motion. J. Am. Phys. Ther. Assoc., 44:157, 1964.
3. Defibaugh, J. J.: Measurement of head motion, Part II: An experimental study of head motion in adult males. J. Am. Phys. Ther. Assoc. 44:163, 1964.
4. Hellebrandt, F. A., Duvall, E. N., and Moore, M. L.: The measurement of joint motion, Part III: Reliability of goniometry. Phys. Ther. Rev., 29:302, 1949.
5. Kottke, F. J., and Mundale, M. O.: Range of mobility of the cervical spine. Arch. Phys. Med., 40:379, 1959.

6. Knapp, M. E.: Measurement of joint motion. Univ. Minn. Med. Bull., 15:405–412, 1944.

7. Knapp, M. E.: Measuring range of motion. Postgrad. Med., 42:123, 1967.

8. Leighton, J. R.: An instrument and technique for the measurement of range of joint motion. Arch. Phys. Med., 36:571, 1955.

9. Moore, M. L.: The measurement of joint motion, Part I: Introductory review of the literature. Phys. Ther. Rev., 29:195, 1949.

10. Moore, M. L.: The measurement of joint motion, Part II: The technic of goniometry. Phys. Ther. Rev., 29:256, 1949.

11. Moore, M. L.: Clinical assessment of joint motion. In Licht, S.: Therapeutic Exercise, 2nd Ed., Revised. New Haven, Elizabeth Licht, Publisher, 1965, p. 128.

12. The Committee on Rating of Medical and of Physical Impairment: A Guide to the Evaluation of Permanent Impairment of the Extremities and Back. J.A.M.A. (Special Edition), Feb. 15, 1958, pp. 1–112.

Muscle Testing

1. Beasley, W. C.: Influence of method on estimates of normal knee extension force among normal and postpolio children. Phys. Therapy Rev., 36(1):21–41, 1956.

2. Beasley, W. C.: Instrumentation and equipment for quantitative clinical muscle testing. Arch. Phys. Med. Rehabil., 37:604–621, 1956.

3. Beasley, W. C.: Quantitative clinical muscle testing—with emphasis upon estimating level of paresis relative to a standardized normal value. An exhibit shown at the 3rd International Congress of Physical Medicine, Washington, D.C., 1960.

4. Beasley, W. C.: Normal and fair muscle systems: quantitative standards for children 10 to 12 years of age: 36 muscular actions. An exhibit shown at the 39th Annual Scientific and Clinical Session, American Congress of Physical Medicine and Rehabilitation, Cleveland, 1961.

5. Beasley, W. C.: Quantitative muscle testing: Principles and applications to research and clinical services. Arch. Phys. Med. Rehabil., 42:398–425, 1961.

6. Chusid, J. G., and McDonald, J. J.: Correlative Neuroanatomy and Functional Neurology. Los Altos, CA, Lange Medical Publications, 1962.

7. Fisher, A. A.: Tissue compliance meter for objective and quantitative documentation of soft tissue consistency and pathology. Arch. Phys. Med. Rehabil., 68:122–125, 1987.

8. Glathe, J. P., and Achor, R. W. P.: Frequency of cardiac disease in patients with strokes. Proc. Mayo Clin., 33:417–422, 1958.

9. Gordon, A. H.: Method to measure muscle firmness or tone. Res. Q., 35:482–490, 1964.

10. Haymaker, W., and Woodhall, B.: Peripheral Nerve Injuries, 2nd Ed. Philadelphia, W. B. Saunders Company, 1953.

11. Lovett, R., and Martin, E. G.: Certain aspects of infantile paralysis: With a description of a method of muscle testing. J.A.M.A., 66(Mar):729–733, 1916.

12. Mayo Clinic: Clinical Examinations in Neurology, 4th Ed. Philadelphia, W. B. Saunders Company, 1976.

13. Resnick, J. S., Mammel, M., Mundale, M. O., and Kottke, F. J.: Muscular strength as an index of response to therapy in childhood dermatomyositis. Arch. Phys. Med. Rehabil., 62:12–19, 1981.

Quantitative Assessment

1. Barry, D. T., Geiringer, S. R., and Ball, R. D.: Acoustic myography: A noninvasive monitor of motor unit fatigue. Muscle Nerve, 8:189–194, 1985.

2. Bigland-Ritchie, B.: EMG and fatigue of human voluntary and stimulated contractions. CIBA Found. Symp., 82:130–156, 1981.

3. Bigland-Ritchie, B., Kukulka, C. G., and Hippold, O. C. J.: The absence of neuromuscular transmission failure in sustained maximal voluntary contractions. J. Physiol. 330:265–278, 1982.

4. Bigland-Ritchie, B., and Woods, J. J.: Changes in muscle contractile properties and neural control during human muscle fatigue. Muscle Nerve, 7:691–699, 1984.

5. Carroll, J. E., Hagberg, J. M., Brooke, M. H., and Shumate, J. B.: Bicycle ergometry and gas exchange measurements in neuromuscular diseases. Arch. Neurol. 36:457–461, 1979.

6. Chaffin, D. B., Andersson, G.: Occupational Biomechanics. New York, John Wiley and Sons, Inc., 1984.

7. Czerniecki, J. M., Gitter, A., and Munro, C. F.: Muscular power output characteristics of amputee running gait. Arch. Phys. Med. Rehabil., 68:636, 1987.

8. Czerniecki, J. M., Munro, C. F., Gitter, A.: A comparison of the power generation/absorption characteristics of prosthetic feet during running. Arch. Phys. Med. Rehabil., 68:636, 1987.

9. Daniels, L., and Worthingham, C.: Muscle testing techniques of manual examination, 5th Ed. Philadelphia, W. B. Saunders Company, 1986.

10. DeLateur, B. J., Lehmann, J. F., and Giaconi, R.: Mechanical work and fatigue: Their roles in the development of muscle work capacity. Arch. Phys. Med. Rehabil., 57:319–324, 1976.

11. DeLorme, T. L.: Restoration of muscle power by heavy resistance exercises. J. Bone Joint Surg., 27:645–667, 1945.

12. Dyck, P. J., Karnes, J., O'Brien, P. C., and Zimmerman, I. R.: Detection thresholds of cutaneous

sensation in humans. *In* Dyck, P. J., Thomas, P. K., Lambert, E. H., and Bunge, R. (Eds.): Peripheral Neuropathy, Vol. I, 2nd Ed. Philadelphia, W. B. Saunders Company, 1984, pp. 1103–1138.

13. Edwards, R. G., and Lippold, O. C. J.: The relation between force and integrated electrical activity in fatigued muscle. J. Physiol., 132:677–681, 1956.

14. Edwards, R. H. T., and McDonnell, M.: Hand-held dynamometer for evaluating voluntary muscle function. Lancet, 2:757–758, 1974.

15. Edwards, R. H. T., Wiles, C. M., and Mills, K. R.: Quantitation of muscle contraction and strength. *In* Dyck, P. J., Thomas, P. K., Lambert, E. H., Bunge, R. (Eds.): Peripheral Neuropathy, Vol. I, 2nd Ed. Philadelphia, W. B. Saunders Company, 1984, pp. 1093–1102.

16. Fischer, A.: Tissue compliance meter for objective, quantitative assessment of soft tissue consistency and pathology. Arch. Phys. Med. Rehabil., 68:122–125, 1987.

17. Fischer, A. A.: Pressure threshold meter: Its use for quantification of tender spots. Arch. Phys. Med. Rehabil., 67:836–838, 1986.

18. Fisher, S. V., Bowar, J. F., Awad, E. A., and Gullickson, G.: Cervical orthoses effect on cervical spine motion: Roentgenographic and goniometric method of study. Arch. Phys. Med. Rehabil., 58:109–115, 1977.

19. Fortinsky, R. H., Granger, C. V., and Seltzer, G. B.: Use of functional assessment in understanding home care needs. Med. Care, 19:489–497, 1981.

20. Freed, M. M.: Traumatic and congenital lesions of the spinal cord. *In* Kottke, F. J., Stillwell, G. K., and Lehmann, J. F. (Eds.): Krusen's Handbook of Physical Medicine and Rehabilitation, 3rd edition. Philadelphia, W. B. Saunders Company, 1982, pp. 643–673.

21. Frollo, I., Kneppo, P., Krizik, M., and Rosik, V.: Microprocessor-based instrument for Achilles tendon reflex measurements. Med. Biol. Eng. Comput., 19:695–700, 1981.

22. Gans, B. M., Haley, S. M., Inacio, C. A.: Concurrent validity of the Tufts Assessment of Motor Performance. Arch. Phys. Med. Rehabil., 68:638, 1987.

23. Gielen, C. C., and Houk, J. C.: Nonlinear viscosity of human wrist. J. Neurophys., 52:553–569, 1984.

24. Goldberg, J. M., and Lindblom, U.: Standardized method of determining vibratory perception thresholds for diagnosis and screening in neurological investigation. J. Neurol. Neurosurg. Psychiatry, 42:793–803, 1979.

25. Gouvier, W. M., Blanton, P. D., Laporte, K. K., and Nepomuceno, C.: Reliability and validity of the Disability Rating Scale and the Levels of Cognitive Functioning Scale in monitoring recovery from severe head injury. Arch. Phys. Med. Rehabil., 68:94–97, 1987.

26. Granger, C. V., Albrecht, G. L., and Hamilton, B. B.: Outcome of comprehensive medical rehabilitation: Measurement by PULSES profile and Barthal index. Arch. Phys. Med. Rehabil., 60:145–154, 1979.

27. Guides to the Evaluation of Permanent Impairment, 2nd Ed. Chicago, American Medical Association, 1984.

28. Hagan, C., Malkmus, D., and Durham, P. Levels of cognitive functions. *In* Professional Staff Association for Rancho Los Amigos Hospital, Inc.: Rehabilitation of the head injured adult: comprehensive physical management. Downey, CA, Professional Staff Association of Rancho Los Amigos Hospital, Inc., 1979.

29. Hardy, J. D., Wolff, H. G., and Goodell, H.: Pain sensations and reactions. Baltimore, Williams & Wilkins Co., 1952.

30. Hayes, K. C., Newell, E., Sinclair, P., and Ageranioti, S.: Quantitative characteristics of hypertonia in spastic hemiplegia. Arch. Phys. Med. Rehab., 68(9):644, 1987.

31. Hinderer, K. A., Dietz, J., Jaffee, K., and McMillan, J. A.: Reliability of the myometer in muscle testing children and young adults with myelodysplasia. Arch. Phys. Med. Rehabil., 68:665, 1987.

32. Hinderer, K. A., and Gutierrez, T.: Myometry measurements of children using isometric and eccentric methods of muscle testing. Arch. Phys. Med. Rehabil., 68:586, 1987.

33. Hinderer, S. R., Lehmann, J. F., de Lateur, B. J., White, O. R., and Deitz, J. L.: Spasticity in spinal cord injured persons; quantitative effects of Baclofen and placebo treatments. Arch. Phys. Med. Rehab. 68(9):654, 1987.

34. Jebsen, R. H., Taylor, N., Trieschmann, R. B., Trotter, M. J., and Howard, L. A.: Objective and standardized test of hand function. Arch. Phys. Med. Rehabil., 50:311–319, 1969.

35. Jennett, B., Snoek, J., Bond, M. R., and Brooks, N.: Disability after severe head injury: observations on use of the Glasgow Outcome Scale. J. Neurol. Neurosurg. Psychiatry, 44:285–293, 1981.

36. Kaufert, J. M.: Functional ability indices: Measurement problems in assessing their validity. Arch. Phys. Med. Rehabil., 64:260–267, 1983.

37. Kottke, F. J.: Therapeutic exercise to develop neuromuscular coordination. *In* Kottke, F. J., Stillwell, G. K., Lehmann, J. F. (Eds.): Krusen's Handbook of Physical Medicine and Rehabilitation, 3rd edition. Philadelphia, W. B. Saunders Company, 1982, pp. 403–426.

38. Lakie, M., Walsh, E. G., and Wright, G. W.: Resonance at the wrist demonstrated by the use of a torque motor: An instrumental analysis of muscle tone in man. J. Physiol. (Lond.), 353:265–285, 1984.

39. Mahoney, F. I., Barthal, D. W.: Functional evaluation: Barthal index. Md. Med. J., 14:61–65, 1965.

40. Medical Research Council: Aids to the Examination of the Peripheral Nervous System. Memorandum

No. 45. Her Majesty's Stationary Office, London, 1976.

41. Merton, P. A.: Voluntary strength and fatigue. J. Physiol., 123:553–564, 1954.

42. Miller, R. G., Milner-Brown, S., Layzer, R. B., Hooper, D., and Weiner, M.: A new method of studying human muscle fatigue: Correlation of force/EMG and nuclear magnetic resonance spectroscopy. Muscle Nerve, 8:623, 1985.

43. Moskowitz, E.: PULSES Profile in retrospect. Arch. Phys. Med. Rehabil., 66:647, 1985.

44. Moskowitz, E., and McCann, C. B.: Classification of disability in chronically ill and aging. J. Chronic Dis., 5:342–346, 1957.

45. National Institute for Occupational Safety and Health: A Work Practices Study Guide. Tech. Report 81-122. Cincinnati, OH, US Dept. Health and Human Services, 1981.

46. Newton, R. A., and Cromwell, S.: Testing standing balance in normal subjects. Arch. Phys. Med. Rehabil., 68:638, 1987.

47. Olney, S. J., Monga, T. N., and Costigan, P. A.: Mechanical energy of walking of stroke patients. Arch. Phys. Med. Rehabil., 67:92–98, 1986.

48. Rappaport, M., Hall, K., Hopkins, K., Belleza, T., Berrol, S., and Reynolds, G.: Evoked brain potentials and disability in brain-damaged patients. Arch. Phys. Med. Rehabil., 58:333–338, 1977.

49. Renfrew, S.: Fingertip sensation. A routine neurological test. Lancet, 1:396–397, 1969.

50. Resnick, J. S., Mammel, M., Mundale, M. O., Kottke, F. J.: Muscular strength as an index of response to therapy in childhood dermatomyositis. Arch. Phys. Med. Rehabil., 62:12, 1981.

51. Sekular, R., Nash, D., and Armstrong, R.: Sensitive objective procedure for evaluating response to light touch. Neurology, 23:1282–1291, 1973.

52. Simard, T. G., and Basmajian, J. V.: Methods in training conscious control of motor units. Arch. Phys. Med. Rehabil., 48:12–19, 1967.

53. Smith, H. B.: Smith hand function evaluation. J. Occup. Ther., 27:244–251, 1973.

54. Smith, R. M., Fields, F. R., et al.: Functional scale of recovery from severe head trauma. Clin. Neuropsychol., 1:48–50, 1979.

55. Smith, R. O.: The Occupational Therapy Comprehensive Functional Assessment: pilot test results and the implications for rehabilitation medicine. Arch. Phys. Med. Rehabil., 68:638, 1987.

56. Stein, R. B., Walley, M.: Functional comparison of upper extremity amputees using myoelectric and conventional prostheses. Arch. Phys. Med. Rehabil., 64:243–248, 1983.

57. Stenehjem, J., Grange, T., and Swenson, J. R.: Ambulatory monitoring of spasticity in SCI. Arch. Phys. Med. Rehabil., 68:604, 1987.

58. Stephens, J. A., and Taylor, A.: Fatigue of maintained voluntary muscle contraction in man. J. Physiol., 220:1–18, 1972.

59. Tardieu, C., Lacert, P., Lombard, M., Truscelli, D., and Tardieu, G.: H reflex and recovery cycle in spastic and normal children: Intra- and inter-individual and inter-group comparisons. Arch. Phys. Med. Rehabil., 58:561–567, 1977.

60. Tucci, S. M., Hicks, J. E., Gross, E. G., Campbell, W., and Danoff, J.: Cervical motion assessment: A new, simple, and accurate method. Arch. Phys. Med. Rehabil., 67:225–230, 1986.

61. Walsh, E. G.: A torque-induced motion analyzer. J. Physiol. (Lond.), 244:14P–15P, 1974.

62. Walton, J. A.: Clinical examination of the neuromuscular system. In Walton, J. A. (Ed.): Disorders of Voluntary Muscle, 4th edition. Edinburgh, Churchill Livingstone, 1981, pp. 448–480.

63. Wilkie, D. R.: Shortage of chemical fuel as a cause of fatigue: Studies by nuclear magnetic resonance and bicycle ergometry. In Porter, R., and Whelan, J., (Eds.): Human muscle fatigue: physiological mechanisms. CIBA Symp. 82. London, Pitman Medical Ltd., 1981, pp. 102–119.

3 Electrodiagnosis

DAVID O. WIECHERS
ERNEST W. JOHNSON

Electromyography and Nerve Stimulation Techniques

Neurophysiology

The motor unit is composed of a motor neuron located in the anterior horn of the spinal cord, its axon, and all the individual muscle fibers supplied by its terminal axon branches. All the muscle fibers of one motor unit are of the same histochemical fiber type. The number of muscle fibers belonging to one motor neuron varies directly with its size and inversely with its threshold of activation. Different muscles have different populations of motor units dependent on the muscle's functional characteristics.

Activation of the motor neuron results in a wave of depolarization traveling down the axon at a rate of 30 to 80 meters per second. Once the wave of depolarization has arrived in the many nerve terminals, a chemical mediator, acetylcholine, is released, which diffuses across the synaptic cleft in about 10 to 50 μsec. The acetylcholine is picked up by receptors on the postsynaptic end plate, usually located in the middle of the muscle fiber. If enough acetylcholine is picked up, the end plate is depolarized and a wave of depolarization is propagated down the muscle fiber in both directions at 1.5 to 6.5 m/sec[43] (Fig. 3–1). Recovery to the resting state proceeds immediately following the wave of excitation. The short delay immediately before this recovery is termed the refractory period. The first 0.2 msec of this delay is termed the absolute refractory period because no stimulus, no matter how intense, will excite the cell. A longer period following this is the relative refractory period, since a stronger stimulus than normal is necessary to cause excitation. It takes about 1 msec after electrical depolarization for the muscle fiber to physically contract. If a small recording electrode of about one half the muscle fiber's diameter (approximately 25 μ in diameter) is placed within 300 μ of an active muscle fiber, a biphasic wave with an initial positive deflection will be recorded.[43] This is a single-fiber recording. If a larger electrode, such as a concentric or monopolar, with a recording surface of 0.07 to 0.1 mm² is utilized to record the depolarization of a motor unit, a composite recording that is the

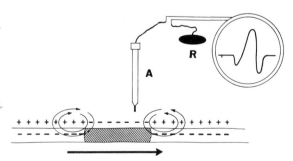

WAVE OF EXCITATION PASSING ALONG A MUSCLE FIBER

FIGURE 3–1. The wave of excitation passes along each muscle fiber. The monopolar electrode records the motor unit action potential, which is the algebraic summation of the depolarizations of each individual muscle fiber.

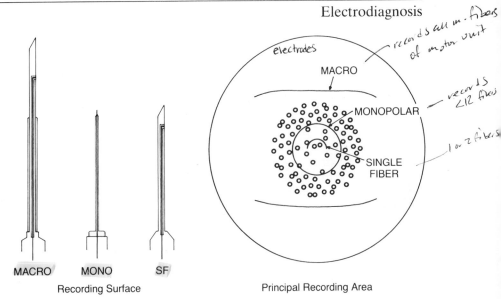

FIGURE 3–2. The macro electrode records from all the muscle fibers of the motor unit. The monopolar electrode records from less than 12, and the single-fiber (SF) electrode records from one or two muscle fibers belonging to the same motor unit.

algebraic summation of 2 to 12 biphasic single-fiber discharges will be recorded.[46] This recording is biphasic in shape if it is recorded near the end plate zone of the muscle, or it can be triphasic if it is recorded away from the end plate zone. This recording is referred to as the motor unit action potential (MUAP). If an even larger recording surface of 15 mm in length is placed in the area of the active motor unit, all the muscle fibers belonging to the motor unit will be recorded.[41] This is referred to as a "macro" motor unit potential (Fig. 3–2).

Electromyography is the study of the electrical recordings of a part of or of the whole motor unit. Motor nerve conduction studies are the studies of the speed of conduction along the axon of the motor unit.

Instrumentation

The voluntarily elicited electrical activity of the motor unit can be recorded by electrodes placed within or upon a muscle. This electrical activity can be amplified and converted from analogue to digital records for subsequent visual and audio display, electronic manipulation, or storage on paper, tape, or disk. The electrical activity of the muscle can also be elicited by nerve stimulation. Recordings are made with a differential amplifier

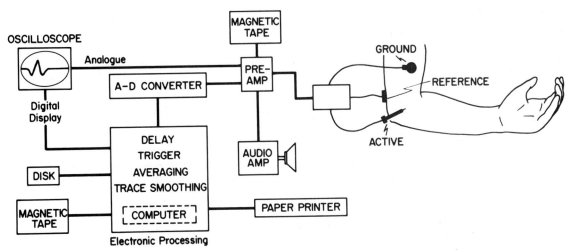

FIGURE 3–3. Diagrammatic representation of the modern electromyograph.

DAVID O. WIECHERS AND ERNEST W. JOHNSON

that records and intensifies the differences between two separate electrodes (Fig. 3–3).

ELECTRODES

Surface. The surface electrodes vary in size but for routine motor and sensory recordings with nerve stimulation are 0.5 cm to several centimeters in diameter. To record the compound muscle action potential with nerve stimulation, one of the active electrodes is placed over the motor point while a second, or reference electrode, is placed over the tendon. This same-sized electrode is frequently used as a reference for recording with intramuscular monopolar electrodes.

Monopolar. Monopolar electrodes are sharpened pieces of stainless steel wires coated with an insulating material, such as Teflon, excepting a small area of approximately 0.1 mm² at the tip. A surface electrode, or another subcutaneous monopolar electrode, is necessary for a reference. The slippery characteristics of the insulating material make repetitive insertions within the muscle almost painless. The insulating material does tend to peel with repetitive use and sterilization, and therefore the electrode is not permanent and should be visually and electrically checked periodically (Figs. 3–4 and 3–5).

Concentric. The concentric electrode is a hollow needle with a platinum wire inserted and insulated

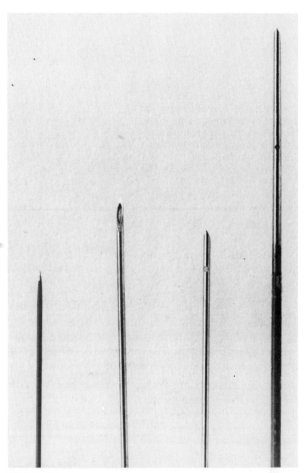

FIGURE 3–5. Photomicrograph of the recording surfaces of the monopolar, concentric, single fiber, and macro electrodes.

from the shaft. The platinum wire is cut on a 15-degree angle and has an exposure surface of 0.07 mm². The shaft of the needle is used as the reference electrode. The angle of the recording surface gives this electrode directional properties. Consequently, it records from fewer muscle fibers of a motor unit than does a monopolar electrode, and as a result, the recorded amplitudes are about 50 per cent less. The advantage of this electrode is that the recording surface remains stable over time (Figs. 3–4 and 3–5).

Single-Fiber. This concentric electrode is used to record depolarizations of individual muscle fibers and is therefore very selective. The inner platinum wire is 25 μ in diameter and is led off the cutting side of the hollow needle 4 mm from the tip (Fig. 3–6).

Macro. The macro electrode is actually two electrodes in one. A hollow needle is insulated

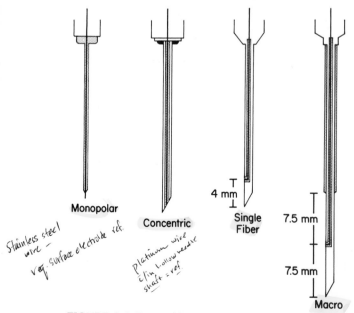

FIGURE 3–4. Types of intramuscular electrodes used in electromyography.

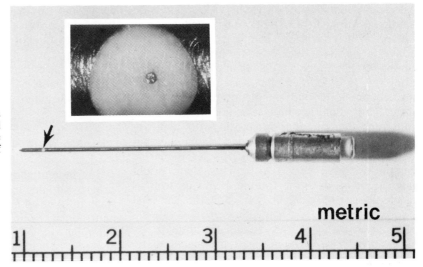

FIGURE 3–6. Photomicrograph of a single fiber electrode. Note the small 25-μ diameter lead-off surface of the single fiber electrode in the center of the insulation material.

with Teflon except for 15 mm at the tip. This large lead-off surface is referenced to a surface or a subcutaneous needle electrode to record the macro or whole motor unit potential. A 25-μ platinum wire is inserted within the hollow needle and is then led out a side port 7.5 mm from the tip. This single-fiber recording surface is referenced to the cannula and is used to activate an electronic trigger, which then records epochs of data from the large recording macro surface (Fig. 3–7).

PREAMPLIFIER

The amplifier should have a uniform response for frequencies from 2 to 10,000 Hz for routine recordings and as high as 20 to 32 KHz for special applications. The input impedance should be at least 50 megOhms or 10 times the impedance of the active electrode. The amplifier is a differential or push-pull type, amplifying the difference re-corded between two input signals. The ability of the amplifier to reject signals that are common to both inputs is referred to as the common mode rejection ratio and should be at least 100,000:1 for use in general hospital surroundings. Filters should be available to allow the removal of unwanted frequencies to improve recordings. Removing low frequencies of 500 Hz and lower removes un-wanted baseline fluctuations from distant muscle fibers when recording single-fiber discharges. Re-moving high frequencies above 8 KHz will some-times improve sensory recordings, since the sen-sory response does not normally have any component frequencies above 3 to 5 KHz.

A-D CONVERTERS AND SAMPLING RATE

Once the analogue signal is obtained, it can be displayed or digitized and then further electroni-

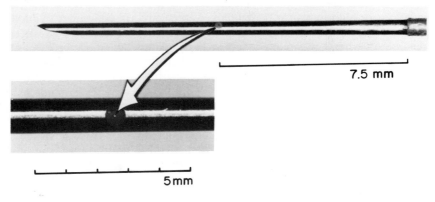

FIGURE 3–7. Photomicrograph of a macro electrode. The small 25-μ single-fiber surface is used as a trigger to record epochs of data from the large 15-mm macro re-cording surface.

DAVID O. WIECHERS AND ERNEST W. JOHNSON

cally manipulated prior to display. The conversion to digital format is usually accomplished by an 8-bit or 12-bit converter. The speed at which the converter works is referred to as the sampling rate or sampling frequency. For example, if the sampling rate is 10 K, then 10,000 samples per second are obtained, or one sample of data every 100 μsec. This would not be fast enough to give accurate reproduction of a waveform with high-frequency components as is recorded in some myopathies. If the sampling rate is 100 K, then one sample is taken every 1 μsec. This, then, would give accurate data for routine EMG as well as single-fiber EMG calculation. For the minimal accuracy of digital reproduction of an analogue signal, the sampling rate should be at least 2½ times the highest frequency of the signal to be analyzed. This is referred to as the Nyquest frequency. For routine EMG recordings, sampling frequencies of 25 K to 50 K are employed. The sampling rate in some instruments varies with the sweep speed and may limit the instrument's applications.

VISUAL DISPLAY

An oscilloscope provides a vector display of the analogue signal and is the best display for the study of spontaneous or insertional activity. The oscilloscope allows the best simultaneous visual to audio display and assures accurate reproduction. The signal, once digitized, can be displayed on a oscilloscope or on a raster display or TV monitor. With a raster display, the number of dots across the screen (pixels) should be such that the waveform can be accurately reproduced; 1000 pixels or greater assures good reproducibility. The speed of the A-D converter, however, is most critical, because if an insufficient number of data points are sampled, the display may plot three or four dots for each data point actually taken. This can result in a less than smooth waveform. Arithmetic calculations or algorithms can be employed to calculate the direction of data movement between two data points when not enough data have been taken by the A-D converter. These algorithms then fill in the dots between data points. This gives the incorrect impression that more genuine data have been sampled and fills in the visual display dots to make the waveforms smooth.

An oscilloscope can display an analogue signal of 6 to 8 mV while recording at 1 mV/cm. If this is attempted with a digitized signal, a waveform of only 3.5 to 4 mV is seen and a straight line extends across the top of the potential. This occurs when the A-D converter is saturated with data points. To display the entire digitized signal, the gain must be reduced to 2 mV or 5 mV/cm. This saturation of the A-D converter may necessitate using several different gains to obtain the total voltage as well as accurate take-off and returns to the baseline.

The Normal Electromyogram

The patient should be comfortable and the procedure should be thoroughly explained before starting. A brief history and a short but systematic neurological examination is absolutely necessary in planning the electromyogram. If the diagnostic question being asked of the electromyographer is complicated, a complete consultation may be necessary in order to perform an adequate examination. The electromyographical examination, after all, is simply an extension of the history and physical examination (Fig. 3–8).

There are five basic steps to the electromyographical examination. The needle electrode is inserted, and the patient is asked to contract the desired muscle to ensure that the electrode is in the correct muscle.

Muscle at Rest

Sweep speed is usually set at 10 msec/cm and the gain at 50 to 100 μV/cm. When normal muscle is at rest, there is electrical silence.

Insertional Activity

Sweep speed is usually 10 msec/cm and the gain 50 to 100 μV/cm. Movement of the needle electrode in muscle provokes electrical activity or insertional activity. Normally this electrical activity starts and stops abruptly with needle movement. The duration of this burst of activity, which usually has an initial positive deflection, is based primarily upon the distance and velocity of needle movement.[55, 60] In muscle in which there has been fibrosis and little or no functional muscle remains, the duration of insertional activity is reduced. In pathological states such as nerve injury or section, the duration of the insertional potentials does not actually increase, but abnormal potentials, such as positive sharp waves, follow so closely that it gives

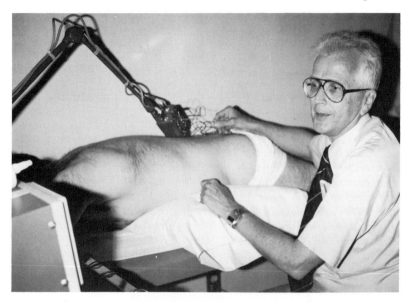

FIGURE 3–8. Electromyographic examination of the lumbosacral paraspinals.

the impression of increased insertional activity.[54] If the tip of the exploring electrode is near the motor end plate, two distinct types of electrical activity can be recorded, either together or individually (Fig. 3–9). Most prominent is a high-frequency monophasic potential of 10 to 30 μV in amplitude and 0.5 to 1 msec in duration. This has the characteristic sound of a seashell murmur and is called miniature end plate potentials (MEPPs). MEPPs are nonpropagated depolarizations of portions of the end plate and are the result of the release of acetylcholine quanta. Associated with MEPPs are sputtering diphasic spikes with an initial negative deflection. These spikes are 100 to 300 μV in amplitude, are 2 to 4 msec in duration, and fire with an irregular frequency of 5 to 50 Hz. The patient usually complains of pain as end plate potentials are elicited. These potentials are more likely to be encountered in the middle third of the muscle and particularly in the small muscles of the hands and feet. If the needle is advanced slightly farther, these single muscle fiber diphasic spikes

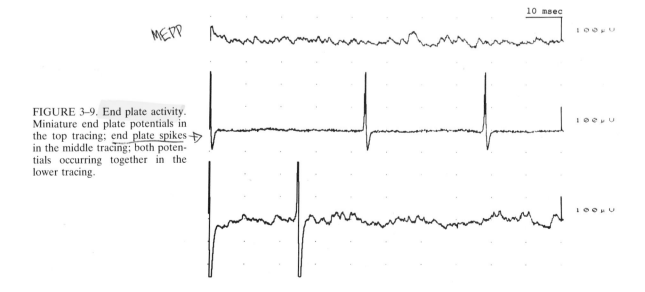

MEPP

10 msec

100 μV

100 μV

100 μV

FIGURE 3–9. End plate activity. Miniature end plate potentials in the top tracing; end plate spikes in the middle tracing; both potentials occurring together in the lower tracing.

DAVID O. WIECHERS AND ERNEST W. JOHNSON

may be recorded as positive-shaped potentials that may be confused with positive sharp waves seen in pathological conditions.

Minimal Muscle Contraction

Sweep speed is usually 2 msec/cm or 5 msec/cm and the gain 200 μV to 1 mV/cm. A single low threshold MUAP is elicited by asking the patient just to think of contracting the desired muscle and then carefully moving the needle electrode toward the firing unit. The sound becomes louder and the amplitude increases as the tip of the exploring electrode nears the electrical center of the motor unit, which usually extends 5 to 10 mm.[8] When the electrical center is found, the peak to peak amplitude of the potential is maximal and the rise time of the negatively directed spike less than 500 μsec. Only in this position can the size and shape of the MUAP be analyzed. The parameters of amplitude measured peak to peak, duration measured from the take-off to the return to the baseline, shape or phases expressed as the number of baseline crosses minus one, and stability or variability of the MUAP size and shape with repetitive discharge are measured for each unit[36, 56] (Fig. 3–10). The normal MUAP should be stable in size and shape with repetitive discharge. The parameters of amplitude, duration, and shape vary with the electrode and recording system, the muscle being studied, the strength of contraction, the intramuscular temperature, and the age of the patient.[7, 9] It is therefore imperative that normal values be established for each laboratory. At least 20 MUAPs are visually examined in an "impressionistic" inspection, or they can be quantified if there is a question about their normalcy.

The recruitment interval or the time between firings of the same potential at the point when the next higher threshold MUAP is recruited should be noted.[38] The steady recruitment of higher threshold MUAPs of increasing amplitude should be observed and related to strength of contraction.

Maximal Muscle Contraction

Sweep speed employed is 5 to 10 msec/cm and the gain 1 mV to 5 mV/cm. As the strength of contraction increases, additional MUAPs are recruited. After about four or five low-threshold MUAPs are systematically recruited, it becomes very difficult to isolate individual MUAPs and study their parameters. In normal and near-normal conditions, only the parameter of amplitude can be accurately studied with higher threshold potentials. The needle electrode is placed superficially to reduce discomfort, and the patient is asked to contract the muscle against maximal resistance by the examiner. The needle electrode is then reinserted into different positions of the muscle, and the maximum amplitude of different high-threshold MUAPs is determined.

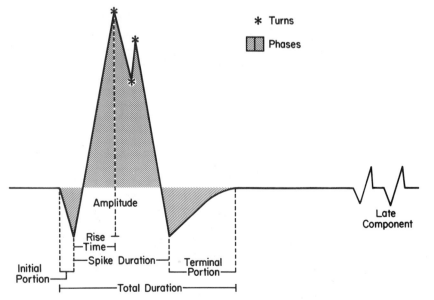

FIGURE 3–10. Motor unit action potential parameters.

An estimate of the number of MUAPs functioning can be determined as the patient increases the strength of contraction. With normal recruitment of higher threshold MUAPs, the display becomes increasingly full until the screen is blotted out. Sampling several areas of muscle can give an estimate as to whether a normal number of MUAPs are functioning or whether they are mildly, moderately, or markedly decreased in number per strength of contraction. Normal low-threshold motor units initiate contraction at 4 to 5 Hz and increase to 6 to 10 Hz before the next threshold MUAP is activated. High-threshold MUAPs fire at 30 to 50 Hz. The audio display is frequently more helpful than is the visual in estimating the number of MUAPs recruited per strength of contraction.

Distribution of Abnormalities

If abnormal potentials are recorded in a muscle, it is necessary to integrate this information with the history and physical to determine which muscle to next study to identify an anatomical distribution. Is it a branch of a nerve, a peripheral nerve, a portion of a plexus or a root or cord segment, or is it diffuse?

It is imperative that the electromyogram be performed by a physician for three reasons. First, a neurological history and examination are necessary to plan the electromyogram, and this plan must usually be modified as the electromyographic findings unfold. Second, the displayed electrical activity depends on each discrete action of the electromyographer as well as on the precise location of the electrode. Consequently, recording of an electromyogram for later interpretation by the physician is inappropriate. Third, the physician can and should interpret electromyographical findings immediately in conjunction with those of the history and neurological examination.

Children and Electromyograms

In most cases, testing can be more easily accomplished when children are separated from their parents. Explain the procedure to all above the age of four years. Often a few words, such as "You're going to see your muscles on television," will put the youngster at ease. Always refer to the electrode as a pin or mosquito bite and avoid showing the child the needle electrode if at all possible. Using the smallest possible diameter and length needle electrode, the pin should be inserted concomitantly with a slap or pinch on the thigh or arm, particularly if the room is semidarkened.

Careful physical examination and planning are necessary to ensure that the minimal number of muscles is examined to render an accurate diagnosis. Anesthesia is rarely necessary, but for children under the age of four years, chloral hydrate or assistance with restraining the child, or both, may be necessary.

Obtaining muscle relaxation is the difficult part of the examination, but it may be done by forcibly positioning the muscle at its shortest length. For example, to investigate the anterior tibial muscle in an uncooperative child, the foot should be dorsiflexed as much as possible.

Nerve Stimulation Techniques

Electrical Stimulation of Nerve

Peripheral nerves can be stimulated with surface electrodes usually 0.5 to 1.0 cm in diameter or with needle electrodes. The current flows from the anode (positive pole) to the cathode (negative pole). The negative charges accumulate beneath the cathode and are most effective in depolarizing the nerve. The stimulus is usually delivered as a square wave of 0.05 to 0.5 msec in duration and 0 to 300 V in amplitude. The surface-stimulating electrodes are usually mounted 2 to 3 cm apart. When stimulating with a needle as the cathode, the anode may be a second needle or a surface electrode. To ensure supramaximal stimulation of a nerve, the stimulus is increased by 25 to 30 per cent once the maximal response is obtained.

Normal Motor Nerve Stimulation

Electrical stimulation of a peripheral nerve containing motor axons results in a depolarization of its innervated muscles. With a supramaximal stimulation, all of the motor axons are depolarized and an "M"-shaped wave or compound muscle action potential is recorded with a surface-active electrode over the motor point and a reference electrode over the tendon of the muscle (Figs. 3–11 and 3–12). The recording electrodes are usually

DAVID O. WIECHERS AND ERNEST W. JOHNSON

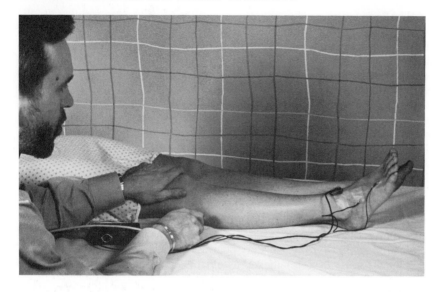

FIGURE 3–11. Peroneal motor nerve conduction study. The bipolar stimulating electrode is at the fibular head, the active electrode is over the motor point of the extensor digitorum brevis, and the reference electrode is on the tendon.

0.5 to 1 cm diameter silver disks. A ground electrode is placed between the stimulation site on the nerve and the recording site on the muscle. The time from stimulation, identified by the stimulation artifact, which triggers the sweep of the display to the onset of the "M" wave, is referred to as the latency. The conduction velocity in meters per second of the fastest conducting motor units supplying the muscle can then be calculated[23, 52] (Fig. 3–13). The distance between a proximal and distal site of stimulation measured on the skin divided by the difference of the latencies obtained from each stimulation site results in a conduction velocity. If a peripheral motor nerve is stimulated most distally at the site where it enters the muscle, there is a conduction delay of several milliseconds. This latency represents the delay at the neuromuscular junction (0.2 to 0.5 msec) and the prolonged conductivity along the terminal axon twigs, which are small in diameter and unmyelinated at their endings. This delay is referred to as the *terminal conduction delay*. The difference between this delay and the expected delay (i.e., calculated from the observed velocity along the more proximal nerve trunk) is referred to as *residual latency*.

There is faster (5 to 10 m/sec) conduction velocity in more proximal nerve segments. However, measurement errors are more likely in the proximal segments of the limbs. The error in measurement along the skin is such that the conduction

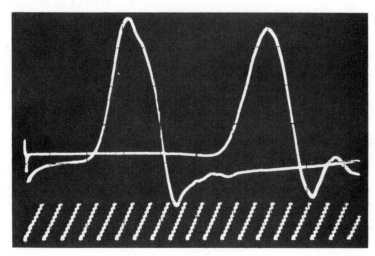

FIGURE 3–12. Recording of peroneal motor nerve conduction velocity (49 m/s). Calibration signal is 1 mV in amplitude; duration of one vertical line is 1 msec.

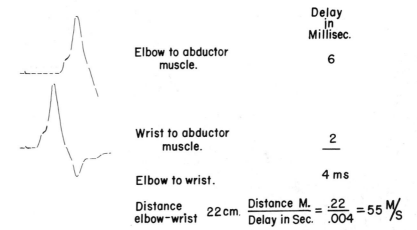

	Delay in Millisec.
Elbow to abductor muscle.	6
Wrist to abductor muscle.	2
Elbow to wrist.	4 ms

Distance elbow-wrist 22 cm. $\dfrac{\text{Distance M.}}{\text{Delay in Sec.}} = \dfrac{.22}{.004} = 55 \text{ M/S}$

FIGURE 3–13. Sample of calculation of the conduction velocity of the ulnar nerve.

velocity can be statistically significant only to the nearest meter per second. Recording the motor "M" response with surface electrodes allows calculations of its amplitude, duration, and area for comparison with proximal or distal sites of stimulation. Recording the motor response with a needle electrode within the muscle does not give a reflection of the total number of motor units or muscle fibers within the muscle as is seen with the surface-recorded "M" wave. It does, however, give the conduction velocity of the fastest conducting motor units whose muscle fibers are within the recording area of the recording needle electrode.

Normal Sensory Nerve Stimulation

Sensory conduction studies can be performed in a similar manner on almost any pure sensory peripheral nerve or on the sensory fibers of mixed nerves.[21, 52] Orthodromic techniques employ surface electrodes placed over the distal sensory branches of the nerve that are used for stimulation with recording electrodes placed proximally over the nerve trunk. Antidromic techniques can also be employed with stimulation over the proximal nerve trunk and recording over the sensory distal branches. The recording electrodes are placed approximately 4 cm apart. This 4 cm separation of recording electrodes ensures maximal amplitude of the nerve action potential (Fig. 3–14).

In most routine recordings, the negative spike of the evoked sensory response is approximately 5 to 60 μV in amplitude, and under 2 msec in duration, using either orthodromic or antidromic

techniques. By convention, latencies in sensory studies are measured to the peak of the negative spike (Fig. 3–15).

Conduction velocities may be determined by stimulating the nerve at two sites and dividing the distance between the sites by the difference in latencies. This value also can be determined by dividing the latency into the distance of a single stimulation. To be more accurate, especially for short distances, 0.1 msec should be subtracted before calculation to correct for latency of activation.

"F" Wave

Supramaximal stimulation of a motor nerve, preferably with the cathode proximal, will frequently result in a late response referred to as the "F" wave.[25, 52] This late response recorded from the muscle occurs after the "M" wave and is lower in amplitude. With successive supramaximal stimulation, the "F" wave latency and its size and shape change repetitively. The "F" wave is the result of antidromic conduction along the motor fiber that results in a backfiring or recurrent discharge of the motor neuron and then orthodromic conduction along the motor unit. Not every motor neuron is capable of recurrent activation.[51] The recorded "F" wave then represents the recurrent discharge of different groups of motor neurons with successvie supramaximal stimulation. Usually 20 to 100 supramaximal stimulations are recorded, and the shortest latency is reported as the "F" wave latency (Fig. 3–16).

DAVID O. WIECHERS AND ERNEST W. JOHNSON

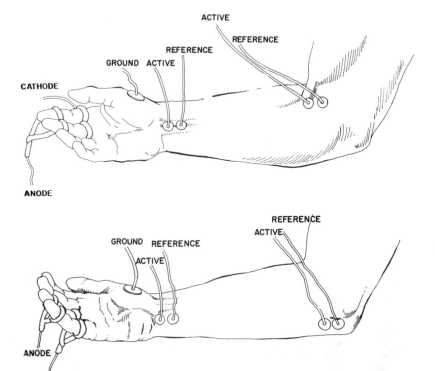

FIGURE 3–14. Placement of electrodes for sensory conduction studies of median nerve (upper) and ulnar nerve (lower). Antidromic technique is done by recording on the fingers and stimulating at the wrist.

"H" Reflexes

If the tibial nerve is stimulated with the cathode proximal in the popliteal space with low voltage and recording electrodes placed over the soleus, an initial "M" wave is recorded and then 20 to 35 msec later a second response or "H" reflex may be recorded.[3, 4] If the intensity of the stimulus is increased, the "M" wave will increase while the "H" reflex will decrease in amplitude. If the stimulus is increased further to supramaximal, the "H" reflex will disappear and the "F" wave will appear

(Fig. 3–17). The "H" reflex is the electrical recording of the muscle stretch reflex. Unlike the tendon tap stimulus-induced reflex, the muscle spindle is bypassed and the Ia afferent fibers are stimulated directly. The impulse travels into the cord through the Ia sensory fibers and to the anterior horn where it synapses with the motor neuron. Those motor neurons that are not in a state of depolarization as a result of contributing an "M" wave are available to be activated and produce an "H" reflex. The "H" reflex is facilitated by stimulation of low voltage and long du-

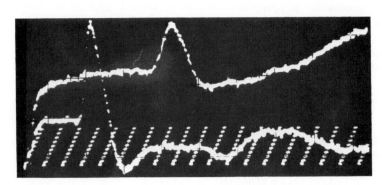

FIGURE 3–15. Normal median sensory conduction study (59 msec), antidromic. Latency is 3.4 msec. Calibration signal is 20 μV in amplitude; duration of one vertical line is 1 msec.

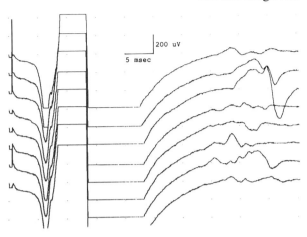

FIGURE 3–16. Normal "F" waves following the large "M" wave, which has saturated the A-D converter and is not fully displayed. Each of the eight "F" waves recorded is different in size, shape, and latency. The shortest latency is 32.5 msec.

ration (1.0 msec) (so as not to activate the motor axon directly and produce an "M" wave), and slow rates (one per 2 to 3 seconds).

The "H" reflex may also be normally demonstrated in the vastus medialis and the flexor carpi radialis of adults at rest and in any peripheral nerve of infants under one year of age. If found in relaxed muscles of adults by stimulation of the radial, ulnar, or peroneal nerves, the "H" reflex may indicate upper motor neuron disease due to injury below the mid-brain. However, it has been demonstrated in apparently normal adults by having the individual contract the muscle slightly, a maneuver that results in facilitation of the muscle stretch reflex.

Root Stimulation

Stimulation of the C8 spinal nerve can be performed with the antidromic technique by insertion of a stimulating electrode (cathode) one fingerbreadth lateral from the spinous process of the C7 vertebra, and in contact with the transverse process of C7.[34] The evoked response may be an "M" wave from a distal C8 innervated muscle or a nerve action potential recorded over a measured distance along a nerve trunk, e.g., ulnar nerve, or along the course of the peripheral nerve. Comparison from side to side in normals should reveal a latency difference of less than 1.0 msec. The latency is usually half of the "F" wave from the abductor digiti quinti. Other cervical, thoracic, and lumbar nerve roots can be stimulated with similar techniques.

Somatosensory Evoked Potentials

The electrical excitation of peripheral sensory nerves produces impulses that ascend posterior

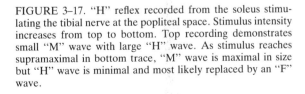

FIGURE 3–17. "H" reflex recorded from the soleus stimulating the tibial nerve at the popliteal space. Stimulus intensity increases from top to bottom. Top recording demonstrates small "M" wave with large "H" wave. As stimulus reaches supramaximal in bottom trace, "M" wave is maximal in size but "H" wave is minimal and most likely replaced by an "F" wave.

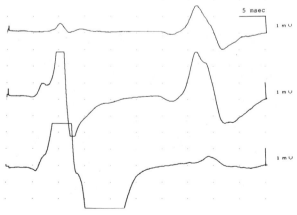

DAVID O. WIECHERS AND ERNEST W. JOHNSON

columns, medial lemniscus, and thalamocortical projections to the somatosensory cortex. These afferent volleys can also be recorded over the proximal nerve trunks, spinal cord, and scalp using various surface electrode placement locations referred to as montages.[12] The potentials recorded from the scalp and spinal cord are frequently less than 1 mV in amplitude and must be discerned from background EEG and myoelectrical activity and therefore require averaging 100 to 1000 stimulations to obtain an accurate result. The recording electrodes can be conventional EEG 0.5-cm surface or 1-cm stainless steel subdermal electrodes. The skin must be prepared with a pumice paste to minimize impedance when using surface electrodes. A frequency band width of 10 to 5000 Hz is adequate for most recordings. In the upper extremity, the median, ulnar, or radial nerve can be stimulated at the wrist with the cathode proximal at an intensity 1.5 times the motor threshold and a rate of 2 to 5 Hz. The potential is recorded from an active electrode near Erb's point, over the midpoint of the clavicle, over the spinous processes of C7 and C2, and over the contralateral cortex at C3' or C4' (international 10–20 system); each electrode is referenced to an electrode at F_z. Absolute latency measurements will vary with arm length, but this four-channel recording results in a negative wave at approximately 9 msec, 13 msec,

and 19 msec and a positive-directed wave at approximately 22 msec (Fig. 3–18).

Absolute latencies and amplitude as well as interpeak latencies of these major components are recorded. Comparison with studies obtained from stimulation of the opposite side may also be helpful. In a similar manner, the tibial, peroneal, saphenous, or sural nerves can be stimulated and recorded over the popliteal fossa, the spinous process of L 4, T 12, and the scalp at C z.[2] The popliteal electrode is placed over the nerve and its reference is placed over the medial joint line.

The L 4 and T 12 electrodes are referenced to electrodes over L 1 and T 10 respectively. The C z electrode is referenced to F pz. The potential recorded from the scalp is a wave with an initial positive deflection or P_1 followed by a negative deflection N_1 and then another positive or P_2 and negative N_2. The absolute values vary, but for tibial nerves the approximate values are P_1 38, N_1 48, P_2 60, N_2 80 msec (Fig. 3–19).

Factors Affecting Nerve Conduction Measurement

The effect of reduced temperature on slowing nerve conduction velocity is so significant in distal segments of peripheral nerve that either patients

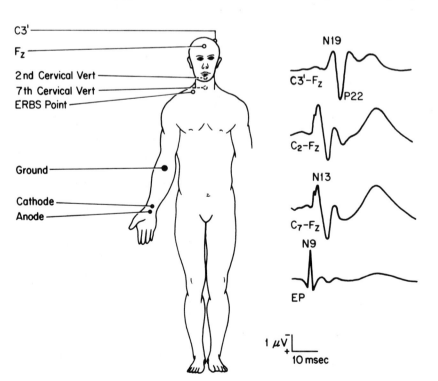

FIGURE 3–18. Somatosensory evoked potentials recorded with median nerve stimulation.

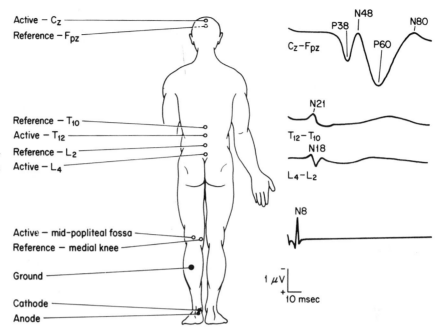

FIGURE 3–19. Somatosensory evoked potentials recorded with tibial nerve stimulation.

should be warmed to a constant temperature or temperature should be recorded and a correction calculated. The conduction velocity reduces almost linearly by approximately 5 per cent or 1.8 to 4 m/ sec per degree centrigrade.[19, 23]

At birth, the conduction velocity is almost half the adult values.[48] By age two to three years, it reaches low adult values, and by four or five years it averages adult values. In premature infants, the conduction correlates well with the degree of prematurity.[11] The conduction velocity reduces with age beginning after the fourth decade and falls approximately 10 m/sec by the age of 60 years.

The anomalous innervation of specific muscles that are used for recording nerve conduction studies, if not understood, can lead to confusion and erroneous conclusions. The most common of these is the Martin-Gruber anastomosis of median nerve fibers crossing over into the ulnar nerve in the forearm occurring in as many as 30 per cent of individuals[29, 61] (Fig. 3–20). This most commonly involves fibers supplying the ulnar intrinsic hand muscles that for some reason begin in the median nerve and then cross over in the forearm. When the median nerve is compromised at the wrist and then stimulated at the elbow, the median fibers that cross over to the ulnar nerve pass into the hand unimpeded. This results in a fictitiously fast calculated forearm conduction velocity. This can frequently be detected by observing an initial pos-

itive deflection of the "M" wave when stimulating at the elbow. Another anomalous connection frequently encountered is the accessory branch of the deep peroneal nerve.[30] This additional branch passes beneath the lateral malleolus in up to 20 per cent of individuals and innervates the extensor digitorum brevis.

Pathophysiology

Types of Nerve Injuries

For classification, three degrees of nerve injuries have been described: (1) focal conduction block, which can be transient (neurapraxia) or more persistent with demyelination or axonal constriction (axonostenosis); (2) axonotmesis; and (3) neurotmesis.[50] Since these conditions occur in individual axons, it is common to find in peripheral nerve injuries some fibers within the affected nerve demonstrating each different type. Neurapraxia is the temporary loss of excitability. It is a physiological block of conduction without anatomical abnormality. Conduction is blocked at the site of compromise, but stimulation distal to the compromise is normal. If not all the fibers in a nerve are affected or if there is localized demyelination, then temporary conduction across the lesion may be slowed and the size of the "M" wave reduced. Axonot-

DAVID O. WIECHERS AND ERNEST W. JOHNSON

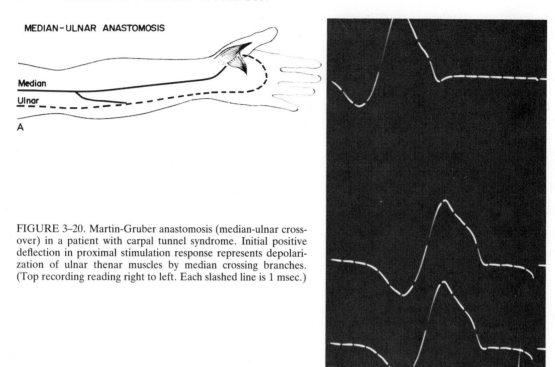

FIGURE 3–20. Martin-Gruber anastomosis (median-ulnar cross-over) in a patient with carpal tunnel syndrome. Initial positive deflection in proximal stimulation response represents depolarization of ulnar thenar muscles by median crossing branches. (Top recording reading right to left. Each slashed line is 1 msec.)

mesis occurs when there is a loss of continuity of the axon and subsequent wallerian degeneration. The distal segment of the nerve will retain its excitability for approximately 72 hours. Anatomically distal to the lesion there is a loss of the myelin sheath and then disintegration of the axis cylinder. Ordinarily, it takes 18 to 21 days before the once innervated muscle fibers become hyperexcitable enough to fibrillate. Regeneration of the nerve axon along its intact nerve sheath occurs at 1 to 3 mm per day or about 1 inch per month. Neurotmesis occurs when not only the axon is severed but also its supporting connective tissue. Wallerian degeneration occurs, but regeneration of the axon in the absence of its supportive structures, if it does occur, is very poor. These lesions require surgical correction and frequently grafting.

Reinnervation by Terminal Axon Sprouting

This process is also referred to as collateral reinnervation.[62] With motor neuron death, axonotmesis, or neurotmesis, the resulting denervated muscle fibers may become reinnervated by the surviving motor units. Terminal axon sprouts of the surviving motor unit will grow toward and connect with nearby denervated muscle fibers. It takes three to four weeks for this process to begin and make initial contact.[18] The site of nerve sprout contact with the denervated muscle fiber becomes the new motor end plate. The reinnervated muscle fiber will change histochemical fiber type to comply with the reinnervating motor unit. Transmission of the impulse from the surviving motor unit to the new muscle fiber may take 6 to 12 months to become normal, and in some instances may never normalize.[56]

Abnormal Potentials in Electromyography

Fibrillation Potentials

Recording with a monopolar electrode, the amplitude of fibrillation potentials is 50 to 300 mV, the duration 0.5 to 2 msec with a regular rhythm and a frequency of 2 to 10 per second (Fig. 3–21). They are usually diphasic or triphasic, with the initial phase positive. Their sound resembles that of eggs frying or cellophane paper being crumpled. This is the electrical activity associated with the spontaneous discharge of a single muscle fiber, the result of abnormal muscle membrane irritability produced in a variety of circumstances, such as denervation, inflammation, degeneration, electrolyte disturbances, trauma, and upper motor neuron disease. Single muscle fiber contractions are not visible grossly through intact skin or mucous membrane. Their appearance is enhanced by heat, cholinergic drugs, and mechanical stimulation.

Positive Sharp Waves

Positive sharp waves are potentials having a sharp positive deflection followed by a long-duration negative phase of lower amplitude. The amplitude and duration vary considerably, as does the frequency. These potentials may appear as trains of discharges at the rate of 50 to 100 per second. They occur spontaneously but are usually provoked by needle electrode insertion (Fig. 3–21). They are abnormal only if they persist after needle electrode movement stops, since the potentials provoked with electrode movement in muscle are also usually of an initial positive deflection. They occur when the needle electrode tip is in the injured or diseased area of the muscle fiber. The resultant provoked wave of depolarization moving away from the electrode tip produces the initial positive deflection. These potentials are seen prior

to the development of fibrillation potentials following nerve section.[54] Like fibrillation potentials, they imply that an abnormality of the muscle membrane's electrical stability has occurred.

Fasciculation Potentials

Fasciculation potentials are due to the spontaneous depolarization of a group of muscle fibers or a whole motor unit. They can frequently be observed through the skin as a twitching. They may be of any size or shape and usually occur singly, firing at rates slower than one per second. They may occasionally fire in groups or in a repetitive burst. Fasciculation potentials can originate from the motor neuron or anywhere along the axon, including a terminal branch[53] (Fig. 3–22).

They are seen in normal individuals and are enhanced by fatigue and stimulants such as caffeine. They occur in all types of disorders affecting the motor neuron and axon. They are so common in disorders affecting the motor neurons that one is reluctant to make that diagnosis in their absence.

Complex Repetitive Discharge

This group of potentials, usually polyphasic or complex in shape, with an amplitude of 0.1 to 1 mV, begins spontaneously or after needle movement. They fire repetitively at slow or fast rates

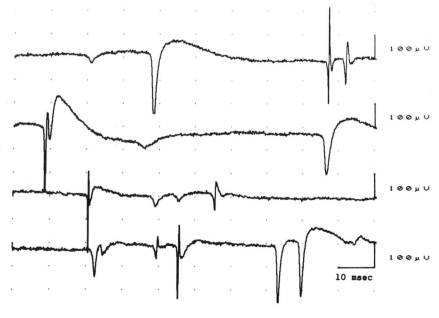

FIGURE 3–21. Positive sharp waves and fibrillation potentials.

DAVID O. WIECHERS AND ERNEST W. JOHNSON

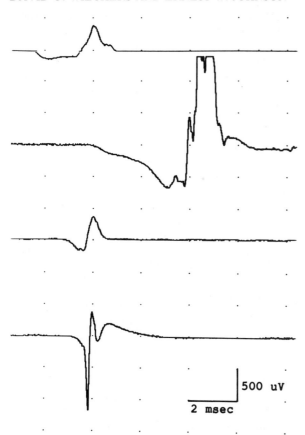

500 uV

2 msec

FIGURE 3–22. Fasciculation potentials of various sizes and shapes all recorded from the same area of the vastus lateralis muscle in a patient 32 years after polio.

FIGURE 3–23. Complex repetitive discharge recorded from a patient with Duchenne muscular dystrophy.

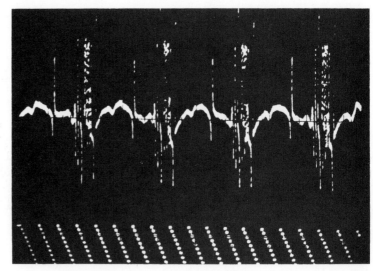

from 5 to 100 Hz with a uniform frequency. They are recorded in a localized area of a muscle and start and stop abruptly. They occur primarily in muscle where a loop of discharge has developed in a group of fibers when side by side muscle fibers activate each other ephaptically.[43] These potentials occur in myopathies and neuropathies and chronic radiculopathies (Fig. 3–23).

Myotonic Discharges

This repetitive discharge of 20 to 80 Hz is composed of biphasic (positive-negative) spikes of less than 5 msec in duration or positive waves that vary in both frequency and amplitude. They have been likened audibly, as they wax and wane in frequency and amplitude, to a diving airplane that pulls out only to dive again. They are not specific for myotonia dystrophica or myotonia congenita, but are recorded in other conditions such as myotubular myopathy, hyperkalemic periodic paralysis, and hyperthyroidism (Fig. 3–24).

Motor Units in Pathological Conditions

In disorders that affect the motor neuron or axon there is a loss of functioning motor units, and orphaned or denervated muscle fibers develop throughout areas of the muscle. Some and possibly all of the denervated muscle fibers will be reinnervated by either terminal axon sprouting or regrowth of the axon back to the muscle.[62] The result of reinnervation by sprouting from the terminal axon is that there will be more muscle fibers per motor unit. The resultant new composite MUAP will reflect an increased number of biphasic spikes generated by each additional muscle fiber. The MUAP will then be of increased amplitude and direction and have polyphasic shapes and possibly some late components. During the first 6 to 12 months of reinnervation there will be increased delays in transmission of the impulses to the reinnervated muscle fibers as the newly formed axon sprouts and end plates mature.[18] This maturation will result in instability or variability of the MUAP in size and shape with repetitive discharge (Fig. 3–25).

In disorders affecting the muscle directly, there can be an actual loss of muscle fibers per motor unit or problems with transmission down the muscle fiber's membrane. The loss of muscle fibers produces an MUAP that has fewer biphasic spikes to contribute to the composite MUAP and is lower in amplitude, shorter in duration, and polyphasic in shape. As many of these myopathic disorders progress there is a reinnervation of fragments or lost segments of muscle fibers. Many functioning muscle fibers split but maintain one motor end plate. Transmission down the compromised muscle membrane can also become very slow. The end result of these various restorative processes is a polyphasic MUAP of very long duration, usually with many late components[59] (Fig. 3–26).

In disorders affecting the neuromuscular junction, the delays and failure of impulse transmission to individual muscle fibers within a motor unit change its size and shape with repetitive discharge. If the disease process is severe, individual muscle fibers will not depolarize and the resultant MUAP will reflect a loss of muscle fibers and be of reduced amplitude and duration as seen in some myopathies.[40]

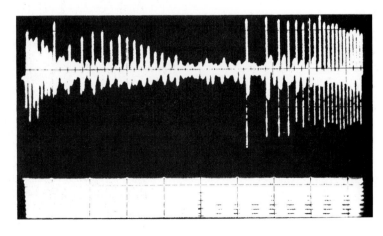

FIGURE 3–24. Myotonic discharge recorded from a patient with myotonia congenita, elicited by needle electrode movement. Calibration signal is 1 mV in amplitude; duration of the entire sweep is 2 sec.

DAVID O. WIECHERS AND ERNEST W. JOHNSON

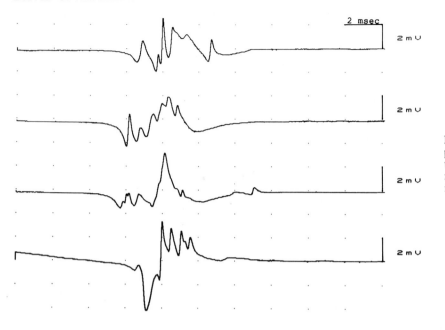

FIGURE 3–25. Motor unit action potential instability recorded from the extensor digitorum communis muscle following a severe radial nerve injury.

Single-Fiber Electromyography

Recording the Single-Fiber Discharge

Single-fiber EMG (SFEMG) is a technique to record from individual muscle fibers. The recording surface of the single-fiber EMG electrode is 25 μ in diameter and about ½ the diameter of a muscle fiber[15, 43] (Fig. 3–6). The electrode records from a hemispheric area within the muscle of about 300 to 350 μ in diameter. To avoid unwanted fluctuations in the baseline from discharging muscle fibers outside of the 300- to 350-μ range, the low-frequency filter is raised to 500 Hz. The electrode is inserted perpendicular to the muscle to be studied. The patient is asked to voluntarily contract the muscle, and the electrode is moved to an electrically active site. Recordings can be made with electrical stimulation of the nerve supplying the muscle or more directly by motor point stimulation with a monopolar electrode. With stimu-

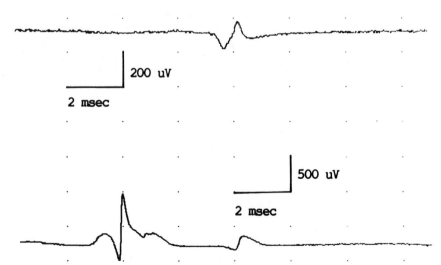

FIGURE 3–26. Two MUAPs recorded from the same area of muscle in a patient with limb-girdle muscular dystrophy demonstrating the great variability seen in size, shape, and duration.

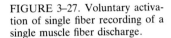

FIGURE 3–27. Voluntary activation of single fiber recording of a single muscle fiber discharge.

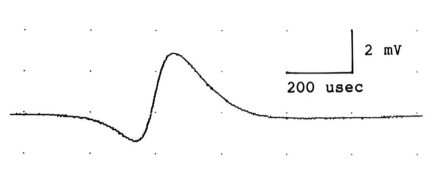

2 mV

200 usec

lation techniques, care must be taken to ensure that the stimulus is well above threshold to avoid introducing variabilities in depolarization. The single-fiber discharge is a biphasic spike (positive-negative) with a rise time of less than 300 μsec and a duration of less than 2 msec and a peak to peak amplitude of 200 μV to 7 mV (Fig. 3–27).

Fiber Density

With 70 per cent of insertions of the single-fiber electrode and moving toward a voluntarily activated motor unit, a single-fiber discharge is recorded. In about 25 per cent of recordings, two single-fiber discharges will be elicited, usually by less than a 2-msec interval. To be sure that both fibers belong to the same motor unit, the patient is asked to change the rate of activation or to even stop, ensuring that both potentials are linked together in time. With four or five separate skin insertions, 20 different recordings are made, and the number of single-fiber discharges that are greater than 200 μV with a rise time of less than 300 μsec is counted. The mean number of fibers for the 20 insertions is calculated and becomes the fiber density.[47] Normal fiber density is approximately 1.5 but varies from muscle to muscle and increases over the age of 60 years. Fiber density is then a very good indicator of the anatomical arrangement of muscle fibers within the motor unit. An increase in fiber density is many times the first indicator of reinnervation and can be seen as early as three to four weeks after nerve injury.[18]

Jitter

When holding the electrode perfectly still and watching the repetitive discharge of a recording from two single fibers that belong to the same motor unit, a variability in the time between the two potentials is seen. This variability in the time between the two single-fiber potentials or interpotential interval (IPI) with repetitive discharge is referred to as jitter (Fig. 3–28). The jitter is expressed statistically as the mean of the consecutive differences (MCD) of the IPIs for 50 to 200 consecutive discharges.[16] Normal jitter is 45 to 65 μsec but varies from muscle to muscle and increases over the age of 60 years.

Jitter represents the variability of transmission within an individual motor unit. There are three determinants of jitter: (1) transmission within the terminal axon; (2) transmission across the neuromuscular junction; and (3) transmission along the muscle fiber membrane to the recording electrode. Normal jitter is primarily a reflection of neuromuscular transmission. An abnormal increase in jitter can be the result of abnormalities at any of the three determinant sites (Fig. 3–29). For routine studies, 20 different recordings are made and an MCD for each is calculated.

Blocking

Transmission of the impulse within a motor unit may be very severely impeded, such that the impulse on occasion may fail to depolarize the muscle

DAVID O. WIECHERS AND ERNEST W. JOHNSON

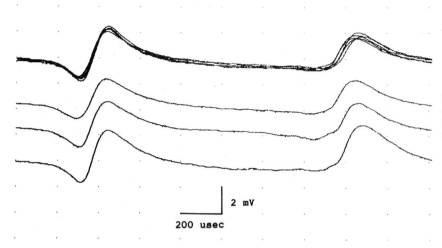

FIGURE 3–28. Normal jitter in a single fiber pair. Five superimposed discharges in the top recording.

2 mV

200 usec

1 mV

500 usec

FIGURE 3–29. Ten superimposed discharges of a single fiber pair demonstrating an increase in jitter.

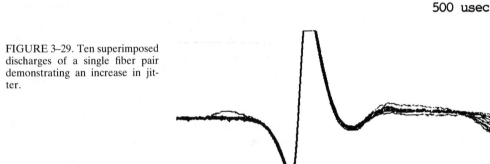

1 mV

500 usec

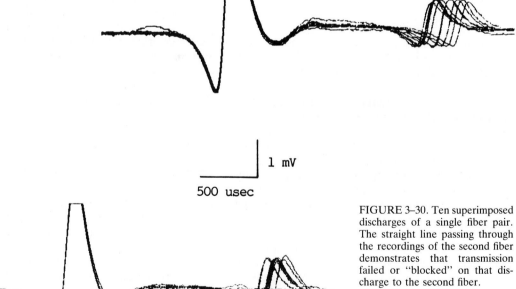

FIGURE 3–30. Ten superimposed discharges of a single fiber pair. The straight line passing through the recordings of the second fiber demonstrates that transmission failed or "blocked" on that discharge to the second fiber.

fiber. This failed transmission to a muscle fiber is referred to as blocking[42] (Fig. 3–30). Blocking does not normally occur unless the MCD is quite abnormal and usually above 80 μsec. Transmission can also break down at the site of branching of a terminal axon. This is encountered in reinnervated muscle in which there may be many muscle fibers established on one branch of an axon. With this failure of transmission, a group of muscle fibers blocks in an all or none fashion. This is referred to as *neurogenic blocking* to emphasize the location of the abnormality of transmission.

Reporting

Since the jitter represents the variability of transmission between two motor end plates, a completed study of 20 recordings has studied 40 motor end plates. After 20 different recordings are performed and the MCD has been calculated for each, the number of normal recordings is presented first. The number of recordings with mild abnormalities of transmission as identified by an increase in jitter is then reported. Finally, those recordings with severe abnormalities of transmission as demonstrated by blocking are reported. A mean for all the MCDs, or the mean jitter, is calculated. The fiber density value is presented separately from the jitter studies.

Macro Electromyography

Recording the Macro Potential

Macro EMG is a technique used to record the electrical activity of the entire motor unit.[41] The macro needle electrode has a large recording surface extending over 15 mm and should therefore record from all the muscle fibers within the motor unit (Fig. 3–2). The electrode is actually a modified single-fiber EMG electrode with the single-fiber recording surface placed 7.5 mm from the tip. The electrode shaft or cannula, which is the macro recording surface, is insulated with Teflon to within 15 mm of the tip (Fig. 3–7). One channel records the signal difference between the single-fiber EMG surface and the cannula. The second channel records the signal difference between the cannula and a small surface electrode or monopolar electrode inserted subcutaneously. The single-fiber EMG recording is used as a trigger to activate an averager that takes data of epochs from the macro recording surface. In this manner, action potentials of the asynchronously firing motor units are extracted. The resultant averaged potential is referred to as the macro motor unit action potential (macro MUAP) (Fig. 3–31).

The single-fiber EMG recording is displayed at 0.5 msec/cm (usually on a separate oscilloscope) and can also provide fiber density data. It is carefully monitored throughout the recording to be sure the electrode does not change position. The macro recording is delayed about 40 msec and the potentials during a total epoch of at least 80 msec are recorded, from which the middle 60 msec portion is used for analysis. The macro MUAP is usually displayed at 5 or 10 msec/cm at a gain of 50 to 200 μV/cm. Twenty different macro MUAPs are obtained from four or five different skin insertions at least 2 cm from the end plate zone.

Macro EMG in Normal Muscles

Macro MUAP shape varies from muscle to muscle. In biceps, the shape tends to be simple with single or double peaks. In tibialis anterior potentials, two or more peaks occur frequently. In vastus lateralis, complex potentials are common (Fig. 3–32). The normal distribution of values of amplitude and area is not always gaussian, and the median value is therefore reported. Individual normal values of upper and lower limits for amplitude are obtained after discarding the extreme values at each end. In this way the study is abnormal either if the median value is abnormal or if more than one macro amplitude or area is outside the minimum or maximum limits for the decade.

Clinical Application

Anterior Horn Cell Disease

Disorders that affect the motor neuron in the anterior horn of the spinal cord include poliomyelitis, amyotrophic lateral sclerosis or motor neuron disease, progressive spinomuscular atrophy, myelopathies (such as syringomyelia and radiation), and intermedullary spinal cord tumors. The electrical abnormalities in these disorders reflect the extent of involvement and the speed of progression of the disorder. There are no pathognomonic potentials characteristic of any of these

DAVID O. WIECHERS AND ERNEST W. JOHNSON

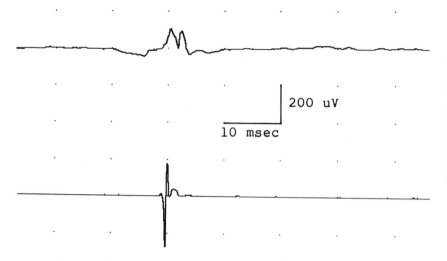

200 uV

10 msec

FIGURE 3–31. Top recording is of a macro motor unit action potential. This is the averaged recording from the 15-mm recording surface. Bottom recording is the single-fiber recording from the 25-μ record surface used to trigger the averager to take samples of data for the above macro recording.

disorders and electrically they are all essentially identical.

Fasciculation potentials of any size or shape are so very frequent in these disorders that it is difficult to make the diagnosis in their absence. With the death of the motor neuron, fibrillations and positive sharp waves appear within 18 to 21 days. The denervation of muscle fibers results in the process of reinnervation by sprouting of the terminal axons. During voluntary contraction, the affected muscles demonstrate a drop-out or loss of motor units per strength of contraction. The surviving MUAPs now reflect the process of reinnervation and are increased in amplitude (low threshold 6 to 10 mV and high threshold 15 to 30 mV) and duration (12 to 25 msec) as recorded with monopolar electrodes. The number of unstable poly-

phasic MUAPs is increased and late components are quite common. With time the MUAPs become less polyphasic and again more triphasic in shape, but they remain unstable (Fig. 3–33). As the disease progresses, more and more denervation occurs and the presence of positive sharp waves and fibrillation potentials becomes profound.

The motor nerve conduction velocity is normal or low-normal in anterior horn cell disorders and reflects the speed of conduction in the surviving motor units.[32] Temperature of the affected limb may be reduced, and the limb frequently has to be warmed to obtain accurate results.

Single-fiber EMG demonstrates an increase in fiber density and an increase in jitter with neurogenic blocking.[44] The more acute and rapidly progressive the disorder, the greater the abnormality

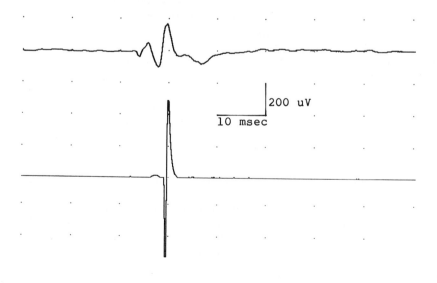

200 uV

10 msec

FIGURE 3–32. Top recording is a macro motor unit action potential recorded from the vastus lateralis. Bottom recording is the single-fiber recording used as the trigger.

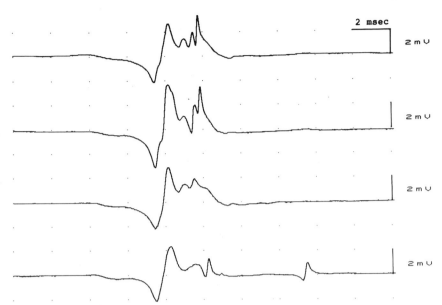

FIGURE 3–33. Low threshold MUAP of increased amplitude and duration recorded from a patient with a motor neuron disorder. Note instability of shape with repetitive discharge.

in jitter and the less abnormal the fiber density. The more slowly progressive or chronic and long-standing the reinnervation, the less abnormal the jitter and blocking and the higher the fiber density.[43]

Macro EMG demonstrates increased amplitude especially in slowly progressive forms in which amplitude can be increased 15 to 20 times normal. In rapidly progressive forms, macro MUAPs may be normal or slightly increased in amplitude. In end stage motor neuron disease, the MUAP tends to revert back toward more normal size.

Peripheral Nerve Disease

Disorders affecting primarily the axon of the motor unit include diabetic and alcoholic peripheral neuropathy, acute inflammatory demyelinating polyradiculoneuropathy (Guillain-Barré syndrome), hereditary motor and sensory neuropathy (Charcot-Marie-Tooth disease), and toxic neuropathies. Examples of focal axonal problems include carpal tunnel syndrome, cubital tunnel syndrome (tardy ulnar nerve palsy), peroneal nerve compromise at the fibular head (cross leg palsy), and radiculopathies. Nontraumatic disorders affecting the peripheral nerves have been classified into "axonal" if the primary process affects the axon directly or "demyelinating" if the primary process affects the Schwann cell.

In "axonal" conditions, the axon is lost and the muscle fibers become denervated. The process of reinnervation by sprouting of terminal axons follows. The resultant MUAPs are of increased amplitude, duration, and percentage of polyphasics. If the disease process is ongoing, then the MUAPs remain unstable as the process of reinnervation continues. Recruitment becomes abnormal and there is a loss of motor units per strength of contraction. The first recruited motor unit may be very large, reflecting either the results of reinnervation or the selective loss of motor units of lower threshold.

Axonal disease is differentiated from anterior horn cell disease by the reduced motor nerve conduction velocity. In a slowly progressive peripheral neuropathy it can be many months or years before the conduction velocity is slowed. In this instance, the electrodiagnostic abnormalities are then based on the finding of loss of motor units and reinnervation bilaterally only in distal muscles. In peripheral neuropathies, single-fiber EMG abnormalities of increased fiber density may be seen in some more proximal muscles that appear normal with routine studies.

In demyelinating conditions, the myelin sheath is affected, slowing conduction velocity over a localized segment of the nerve by usually greater than 40 per cent. Conduction can fail or be blocked at this demyelinated segment. This conduction block is noted on nerve conduction studies when

DAVID O. WIECHERS AND ERNEST W. JOHNSON

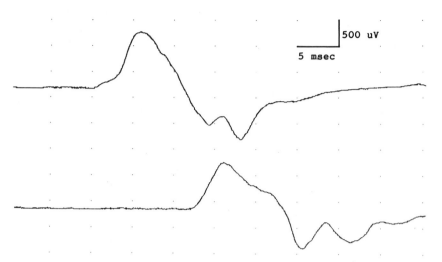

500 uV

5 msec

FIGURE 3–34. Median motor nerve conduction velocity across the forearm of 15 m/sec in a patient with Charcot-Marie-Tooth disease or HMSN type I.

the amplitude and/or area of the compound muscle action potential falls significantly with stimulation above and below the demyelinated segment. If the demyelination process is ongoing or severe, the axon itself may die and the process of reinnervation by terminal axon sprouting will proceed. As more axons are lost, it becomes difficult to determine whether the disease process is demyelinating or axonal or both (Fig. 3–34).

Localized traumatic areas of nerve compromise may be identified by stimulating proximal and distal to the site of compromise and noting a prolonged latency across the diseased segment. A reduced amplitude and/or area of the compound muscle action potential when stimulation is proximal to the compromise is usually also observed. Injury to a peripheral nerve and compression of a nerve root produce EMGs characterized by abnormal insertional activity, loss of motor units, and reinnervated MUAPs. The distribution of abnormalities permits the localization of the compromise. For example, fibrillation or fasciculation potentials or an increased proportion of polyphasic potentials of long duration in the anterior tibial, peroneal, and flexor digitorum longus muscles, as well as in the paraspinal muscle at the L 5 level, indicate a compromise at or proximal to the L 5 root level. The motor and sensory roots join and leave the spinal canal via the intervertebral foramen as a mixed nerve, then split into the posterior primary ramus that goes to the muscle and skin of the back and the anterior primary ramus. The anterior primary ramus is distributed through the plexus to the extremity. Thus an electromyograph-

ical abnormality in the muscles of the extremity, as well as in the paraspinal muscles at the appropriate level, indicates a compromise of the spinal nerve before it divides into the anterior and posterior primary rami.

Neuromuscular Junctional Disease

Myasthenia gravis is the most common disorder affecting neuromuscular transmission. Disorders that even mildly affect the transmission of the impulse across the neuromuscular junction result in an increase in jitter on single-fiber EMG.[43] As the jitter becomes increasingly abnormal, blocking begins to occur and the abnormality can be seen on routine EMG as a variation in size and shape of the MUAP with repetitive discharge. As the number of muscle fibers with severe abnormalities of transmission or blocking increases and approaches 10 per cent of a muscle, an abnormality of repetitive motor nerve stimulation may start to develop. Repetitive stimulation is performed by recording the amplitude and/or area of the compound muscle action potential with supramaximal stimulation at two to three per second. The test is considered positive if the area and/or amplitude between the first and fourth or fifth stimulation falls by at least 10 per cent. To make the test more sensitive, the neuromuscular junction can be sensitized with exercises or curare. Injection of Tensilon will tend to repair the defect in transmission.

Since myasthenia gravis is a postsynaptic disorder that results in a destruction of receptor proteins for acetylcholine on the postsynaptic membrane, the defect in transmission is accentuated by an increased rate of discharge.[40] Myasthenic syndrome is a condition in which a presynaptic abnormality develops that results in a reduced number of acetylcholine quanta released with each nerve impulse.[31] This condition is most frequently seen in association with small cell carcinoma of the lung.[14] Here the abnormality in transmission occurs most markedly with slow rates of discharge or stimulation and is improved at rapid firing rates.

Diseases of Muscle

Disorders that primarily affect the muscle include the muscular dystrophies, inflammatory myopathies, endocrine and metabolic myopathies, and congenital myopathies. In these conditions, some or all of the muscle fibers of a motor unit do not function properly and additional motor units are recruited to provide a specific strength of contraction. Nerve conduction velocities are normal, although the compound muscle action potential may be reduced in amplitude and area. The electrical abnormalities in these disorders vary greatly, not only between different diseases, but also with the course of the specific disorder.

In the inflammatory myopathies of dermatomyositis and polymyositis, there is segmental necrosis of the muscle cell. As a result of this process, a single muscle fiber can be divided into many individual segments, only one of which is innervated. The result is profuse positive sharp waves and fibrillation potentials.[13] This is followed by reinnervation of the individual segments. The MUAPs can then be of normal or low amplitude, of short or long duration, and polyphasic in shape. Macro MUAP amplitudes likewise initially may be low. In more chronic or long-standing cases, some macro MUAP amplitudes may be normal or slightly increased.

Early in the muscular dystrophies, positive sharp waves and fibrillation potentials may be common. The MUAPs initially are of low amplitude, of short duration, and polyphasic in shape. There is a marked increase in the number of low-threshold motor units recruited for contractions of mild strength. As the disease approaches end stage and much of the muscle becomes nonfunctional and electrically silent, there is a loss of motor units per strength of contraction, especially at maximal contraction. Positive sharp waves and fibrillation potentials are not usually found and the surviving motor units can become extremely long in duration (40 to 50 msec) with many late components.[58] The MUAP amplitude may remain reduced or approach normal values. As with most myopathies, the MUAPs in the muscular dystrophies are relatively stable. Single-fiber EMG demonstrates a mild increase in jitter with very little blocking. Fiber density is increased and reflects localized areas of reinnervation, fiber splitting, and muscle cell regeneration. Macro EMG amplitude may be normal or slightly reduced. Those with normal amplitude tend to demonstrate complex shapes and increased duration.

In the congenital myopathies, the EMG abnormalities may be minimal. Insertional abnormalities of positive sharp waves and fibrillation potentials may not be seen. The only abnormality may be a mild increase in polyphasic potentials seen only with quantitative motor unit analysis.

Upper Motor Neuronal Disorders

Electrodiagnostic tests can be helpful in the differential diagnosis of disorders of upper motor neurons. Delayed or absent evoked potentials, especially from stimulation of nerves of the lower extremity, are frequently seen in multiple sclerosis. The EMG in multiple sclerosis is normal with the exception of weak muscles that frequently demonstrate a decreased number of motor units recruited at maximal contraction. Eighteen to 21 days following a stroke, positive sharp waves and fibrillation potentials appear in the affected arm and leg. These abnormal potentials, however, start to resolve once spasticity or voluntary activity returns.[24] This finding in stroke patients implies that failure of excitation of the motor unit produces denervation-like hypersensitivity of the muscle fibers in the same way as actual denervation. It is the lack of frequent excitation of each muscle fiber that is responsible for the progressive decrease in the threshold of that muscle fiber until we begin to see "spontaneous" potentials, which we have called in the past denervation potentials.

Specific Applications

Carpal Tunnel Syndrome

This condition is the most common disorder studied in the clinical practice of EMG. The median nerve is located within the rigid tunnel at the

DAVID O. WIECHERS AND ERNEST W. JOHNSON

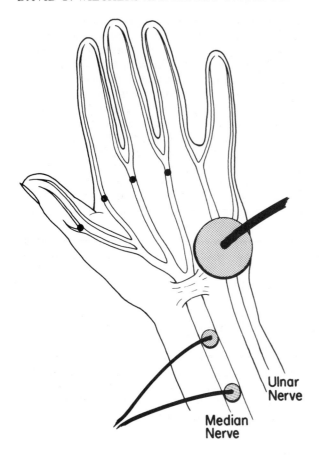

FIGURE 3–35. An 8-cm orthodromic recording of median nerve action potential from median sensory branches from thumb and first, second, and third common palmar branches.

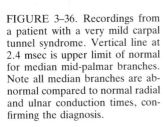

FIGURE 3–36. Recordings from a patient with a very mild carpal tunnel syndrome. Vertical line at 2.4 msec is upper limit of normal for median mid-palmar branches. Note all median branches are abnormal compared to normal radial and ulnar conduction times, confirming the diagnosis.

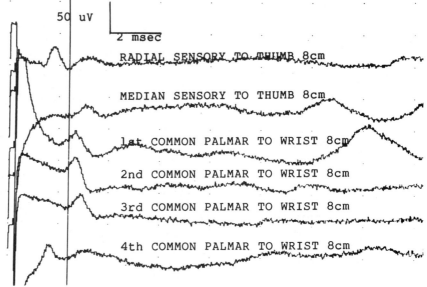

50 uV

2 msec

RADIAL SENSORY TO THUMB 8cm

MEDIAN SENSORY TO THUMB 8cm

1st COMMON PALMAR TO WRIST 8cm

2nd COMMON PALMAR TO WRIST 8cm

3rd COMMON PALMAR TO WRIST 8cm

4th COMMON PALMAR TO WRIST 8cm

wrist. Any disease or injury that increases the volume of the tunnel's contents or distorts its structure may thus compromise the median nerve. The electrodiagnosis is based on slowing of normal conduction across the tunnel.[27] Studies of nerve conduction in the hand are extremely sensitive to temperature; hands are routinely warmed to above 32° C as measured in the distal palm. The 8-cm distal median motor latency across the tunnel is normally less than 4.3 msec.[37] In mild carpal tunnel syndrome it is normal, and abnormalities are seen only in sensory conductions. An 8-cm orthodromic mixed sensory and motor conduction recording over the median nerve at the wrist with stimulation in the mid-palm of the first, second, or third common palmar branches is normally less than 2.4 msec[45, 57] (Fig. 3–35). Comparison of the median mid-palmar latencies can also be made to 8-cm orthodromic radial and ulnar (fourth common palmar) branches. Comparison of latencies of the median branch to the thumb with the radial branch to the thumb, and median midpalmar branch with the fourth common palmar branch should show discrepancies of less than 0.4 msec in normals (Fig. 3–36). In extremely mild cases of carpal tunnel syndrome, the only abnormality may be in an individual branch, and most commonly the third common palmar.[57] In other very mild cases, the latency values may all be normal and only the comparisons with the radial and ulnar values are found to be abnormal. Except in severe or long-standing cases, it is rare to see positive sharp waves and fibrillation potentials in the median intrinsic muscles of the hand. In long-standing cases of moderate severity, there may be a loss of high-threshold motor units with MUAPs demonstrating reinnervation.

Syndrome of Root Compression

Compromise of a lumbosacral nerve root is the second most common disorder in the clinical practice of EMG. The electrical abnormalities in cervical, thoracic, or lumbosacral radiculopathies are totally dependent on the severity of the compromise to the sensory and motor fibers that travel in the nerve root.[22] Most commonly, both sensory and motor fibers are affected. With a significant compromise of at least 50 per cent of the motor axons, a loss or drop-out of motor units can be seen immediately in the muscles supplied by the compressed root. If S 1 is the compromised root, then abnormalities in the "H" reflex can also be seen immediately.[39] If the sensory axons are sufficiently compromised, abnormalities of the somatosensory evoked potentials may be detected. After about 72 hours, the distal segments of the axons that are not neurapraxic will no longer conduct, and a fall in the amplitude and area of the compound muscle and/or sensory action potential can be recorded from an affected muscle or peripheral nerve. By 18 to 21 days, positive sharp waves and then fibrillation potentials will start to appear in the muscles supplied by the anterior primary ramus (limb, chest, or abdominal muscles) and usually earlier in the posterior primary ramus muscles (paraspinals). In many mild radiculopathies, the presence of insertion abnormalities in the muscles is the first reproducible indicator that confirms the radicular compromise. Within a month, the motor unit of those axons that survived and did not undergo wallerian degeneration will begin the process of reinnervation by sprouting terminal axons. Single-fiber EMG will demonstrate an increase in fiber density and increased jitter and blocking. MUAPs over the next several months will show the signs of reinnervation with unstable MUAPs of increased duration, amplitude, and percentage of polyphasics.[56]

Injury to Peripheral Nerves

As in root level injury of nerves following compromise, the distal segment of the injured axon, which will subsequently undergo wallerian degeneration, will conduct an impulse for about 72 hours. After this time the size of the "M" wave will be proportional to the number of surviving motor units. The time until onset of provokable positive sharp waves in those motor units undergoing degeneration is dependent on the length of the axon from the site of compromise. It takes approximately 18 to 21 days for abnormalities to develop in the hand when the C8 root is compromised in the cervical spine, but only five to seven days when the median nerve is cut at the wrist. Reinnervation will proceed by two methods. Sprouting terminal axons will be detectable first at three to four weeks by an increase in fiber density with single-fiber EMG. Surviving motor units will begin to take on more muscle fibers, and unstable MUAPs of increased duration and polyphasic shape will be seen. With time, if the compromise

DAVID O. WIECHERS AND ERNEST W. JOHNSON

has not been severe, the MUAPs will stabilize and the amplitude increase. The durations will usually remain prolonged but not as increased as seen early in reinnervation.

A second type of reinnervation or regrowth of the proximal axon to the denervated muscle will also occur. When the peripheral nerve has been completely severed high in the arm and the nerve has to be surgically repaired, the reinnervation process may take many months before functional activity is again seen in the hand. When the axon regrows to the denervated muscle, the initial MUAPs will be unstable, of low amplitude, and polyphasic in shape. The duration, amplitude, and degree of polyphasics will increase for a period of time as more and more muscle fibers are reinnervated by the single axon.

The size of the "M" wave in the recovered nerve reflects the number of muscle fibers reinnervated. The speed of conduction in the regrowing smaller diameter axon will initially be very slow and may be only 50 per cent of normal values. Whereas this may improve with time as more axons regrow, the speed of conduction rarely reaches preinjury rate.

After a prolonged period of denervation, muscle fibers may be replaced by fibrous tissue, a condition that reduces the number of fibrillation potentials as well as the amount of insertional activity.

Compromise of the Ulnar Nerve

In clinical practice, the ulnar nerve is frequently found to be compromised at the elbow. In this condition, stimulation of the ulnar nerve above the elbow will demonstrate a prolonged delay and a reduced amplitude of the "M" wave of the abductor digiti quinti and the sensory nerve action potential recorded from digit V. Stimulation below the site of compromise will typically show normal motor and sensory conduction velocity and a normal amplitude "M" wave and sensory nerve action potential. EMG in clinically significant cases will show varying degrees of positive sharp waves and fibrillation potentials with motor unit loss and reinnervation in ulnar intrinsic muscles.

Diabetic Peripheral Neuropathy

This is the most common peripheral neuropathy encountered in clinical practice. It most commonly presents as a distal symmetrical primarily sensory neuropathy, although it can present as a proximal asymmetrical painful motor neuropathy, an autonomic neuropathy, or a mononeuropathy.[1] The neuropathy can affect predominantly small fibers with axon loss or large fibers with demyelination and remyelination being more prominent than axonal loss.[49] Typically, the first conduction velocities to be altered are the "H" reflex, which contain the largest diameter Ia afferent fibers. The distal sensory sural conduction will first lose amplitude and then the velocity will become slow. Finally, many years after the onset of diabetes, the motor conduction velocity will start to demonstrate mild slowing, first in the peroneal, and then followed by the facial, ulnar, and median. With time, the conduction velocity continues to decrease to approximately 20 m/sec, at which time it becomes difficult to record a response from the distal muscle. Long before abnormalities of conduction velocity can be detected, mild abnormalities of MUAP indicative of reinnervation can be demonstrated in distal muscles of the foot and leg. Single-fiber EMG will demonstrate an increase in fiber density in the more proximal muscles, such as the anterior tibial, before routine EMG abnormalities can be detected.[5] Patients with diabetic peripheral neuropathy frequently have symmetrical involvement of the lumbosacral paraspinal muscles to a mild degree. Confirming electrically the diagnosis of a superimposed lumbosacral radiculopathy in a diabetic with peripheral neuropathy necessitates the study of most proximal muscles of the hip and leg innervated by L 5 and S 1.

Acute Inflammatory Demyelinating Polyradiculoneuropathy

This condition, frequently referred to as Guillain-Barré syndrome, is a demyelinating disorder that classically begins at the motor root, involving motor axons. Sensory axons and autonomic axons also can be affected. Not all nerves are affected equally. The sural nerve is commonly spared. Since, in many cases, the initial lesion is proximal at the radicular level, prolongation of the "H" reflex and "F" wave may be the first abnormality.[26] The distal latency becomes prolonged and there is usually temporal dispersion of the "M" wave when the nerve is stimulated proximally within the first two weeks. Reduction in nerve conduction velocity may appear as early as 10 to 14 days and may drop 75 to 80 per cent of normal.[10] Conduction block is

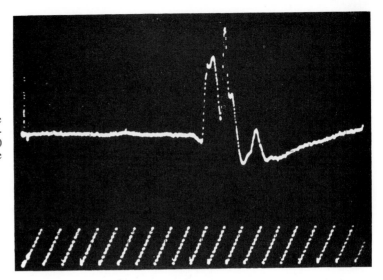

FIGURE 3–37. Motor unit recorded in the anterior tibialis two months after onset of Guillain-Barré syndrome. Calibration signal is 200 μV in amplitude; duration of one vertical line is 1 msec.

common when the stimulation crosses the demyelinated segments of the nerve. Positive sharp waves, fibrillation potentials, and fasciculation potentials are seen and MUAPs reflect the stage of reinnervation (Fig. 3–37). With recovery, the conduction velocity improves but lags behind the clinical improvement.

Facial Paralysis

The prognosis for outcome of paralysis of the seventh cranial nerve as first described by Sir William Bell, or "Bell's palsy," can be improved by electrodiagnostic testing. The facial nerve can be stimulated under the tip of the ear lobe and an "M" wave recorded from the frontalis, orbicularis oculi, nasalis, orbicularis oris, or other facial innervated muscles. This stimulation is below the site of the lesion so the response will remain normal in those axons about to undergo wallerian degeneration for about 72 hours after compromise. Following this time, the change in amplitude and area reflects the number of motor units that are not neurapraxic. If the latency is prolonged, the prognosis is less favorable. Needle studies will demonstrate positive sharp waves and fibrillation potentials as early as 10 to 12 days. The number and extent of innervated muscles by the facial nerve that maintain voluntary activity in the first 10 days of onset is probably of greatest prognostic significance.[17] The more individual muscles that maintain voluntary activity, the better the prognosis for complete functional recovery. The blink

reflex, or stimulating the fifth cranial nerve via the supraorbital nerve, will result in two responses recorded from the orbicularis oculi that can be helpful in following the course of paralysis[28] (Fig. 3–38). The first response, or R_1, is evoked only on the side of stimulation with a latency of less than 13 msec. The second response, or R_2, is variable

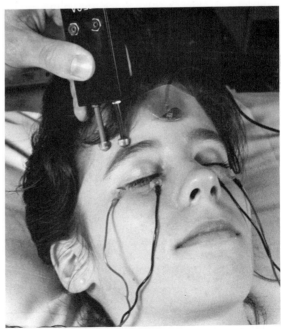

FIGURE 3–38. Blink reflex is elicited by stimulating the fifth cranial nerve in the supraorbital foramen and recording bilaterally from the orbicularis oculi.

DAVID O. WIECHERS AND ERNEST W. JOHNSON

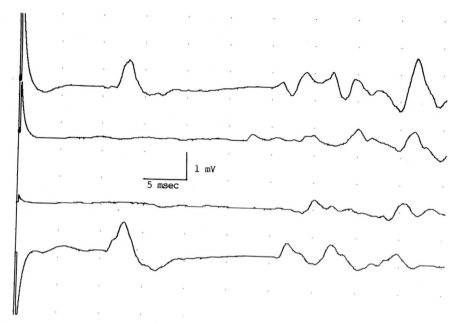

FIGURE 3–39. Normal blink reflex recordings. The top two recordings were produced by stimulating the right fifth cranial nerve, the lower two recordings by stimulating the left. The first recording is from the right orbicularis oculi. Latency to the first component, or R_1, is 11.5 msec. Latency to the second component, or R_2, is 29.9 msec. The second recording from the left orbicularis oculi has an R_2 at only 26.9 msec. The third recording from the right orbicularis oculi has an R_2 of 34.1 msec. The last recording from the left orbicularis oculi has an R_1 of 10.5 msec and an R_2 of 30.8 msec.

but less than 41 msec ipsilateral and 44 msec contralateral (Fig. 3–39). Since the blink reflex reflects conduction along the entire length of the facial nerve, it is affected in all but the very mildest forms of Bell's palsy. On the affected side, the R_1 is prolonged or absent in essentially all patients and the R_2 in most patients. On the nonaffected side the R_2 remains normal. The recovery of the blink reflex, usually the R_2 response, and then the R_1 is a good prognostic sign and generally occurs before the return of the direct facial nerve response.

Duchenne Muscular Dystrophy

The EMG recordings in this X-linked recessive disorder of little boys changes greatly over the course of the disease. At the time of the initial diagnosis, complex repetitive potentials are frequently recorded at rest. Positive sharp waves and fibrillation potentials are found with searching. Low-threshold MUAPs are of low amplitude, 50 to 200 μV, with high-threshold MUAPs 1000 to 2500 μV. The duration may be very short, 1 to 3 msec, and many if not most will be polyphasic in shape. Most prominent is the increased number of motor units recruited for just mild strengths of contraction. As the disease progresses, areas of the muscle become nonfunctional and electrically silent. MUAPs become very long in duration with late components making the overall duration 30 to 40 msec[58] (Fig. 3–40). The amplitude of the few remaining motor units may actually increase to normal values. Prominent at this state is the loss of high-threshold motor units. Jitter is increased in 20 to 40 per cent of recordings but blocking is uncommon, occurring in less than 10 per cent of recordings.

Facioscapulohumeral Muscular Dystrophy

This dystrophy affecting the muscles of the face, shoulder girdle, and ankle dorsiflexors is an autosomal dominant disorder that has marked variation in expression from generation to generation. The EMG abnormalities may be minimal and the weak muscles should be studied first. Positive sharp waves and fibrillation potentials may or may not be found. Early in the disease or at the time of diagnosis, MUAPs are of low amplitude, of short duration, and polyphasic in shape. Recruitment reveals an increased number per strength of contraction.

Limb-Girdle Muscular Dystrophy

This slowly progressive autosomal recessive disorder affecting the proximal muscles can have its onset in the second or third decade or later in life. Like facioscapulohumeral dystrophy, the abnormalities are variable and the weak muscles should be studied. Positive sharp waves and fibrillations are uncommon. Polyphasic MUAPs of low amplitude and short duration are most common (Fig. 3–26). As the disease progresses, the increased number of motor units recruited at a contraction of a given strength are smaller, low-threshold motor units. In end-stage disease at a similar strength of contraction high-threshold motor units may be entirely lacking.

Myotonic Muscular Dystrophy

Myotonia is the painless delay in muscle relaxation recorded electrically as the repetitive discharge of a single muscle fiber following activation (myotonic discharge). Myotonic discharges occur in a variety of disorders and in myotonic muscular dystrophy. This disease is an autosomal dominant multisystem disorder characterized by frontal balding, ptosis, and weakness of neck flexors and distal muscles. Myotonic discharges are most common in distal muscles. Abnormalities of MUAPs may be seen only in distal muscles and are of low amplitude, short duration, and increased polyphasia. The rapid recruitment of additional motor units may be difficult to evaluate in some muscles because of ongoing myotonic discharges.

Inflammatory Myopathies

These acquired myopathies include polymyositis and dermatomyositis. The EMG abnormalities change dramatically with the course of the disease.[6] Before treatment with steroids, positive sharp waves and fibrillation potentials are usually exuberant. As the various segments of the muscle fibers that have been denervated due to the underlying process of segmental muscle neurosis become reinnervated, the MUAPs progressively change. Initially, polyphasic shape and short duration potentials become normal and then long in duration as the reinnervation proceeds. The MUAPs remain of normal to low amplitude. Single-fiber EMG can follow the course of the disease by studying the process of reinnervation.[20] Initially there is a lot of blocking with increased jitter, and with time, if the disease process is slowing, the blocking stops and the jitter reverts toward normal.

Amyotrophic Lateral Sclerosis

The electrical abnormalities of this disorder, frequently referred to as ALS or motor neuron

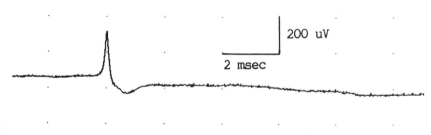

200 uV

2 msec

FIGURE 3–40. A low amplitude short duration MUAP and a long duration polyphasic MUAP recorded from a patient with Duchenne muscular dystrophy.

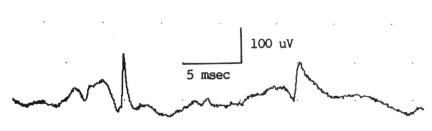

100 uV

5 msec

DAVID O. WIECHERS AND ERNEST W. JOHNSON

disease, vary greatly with the course of the disease. Very early in the disease there may be very few positive sharp waves and fibrillation potentials and few muscles with MUAPs of increased amplitude, duration, and percentage of polyphasics. As the disease progresses, the positive sharp waves and fibrillation potentials become profuse and involve almost all muscles whether clinically weak or not. Fasciculation potentials are prominent. Motor unit loss is progressive and the MUAPs remain unstable.[44] Nerve conduction velocity remains normal or low-normal, but with time, the "M" wave becomes reduced.[32] The amplitude of the MUAPs can become extremely large and 30 to 40 mV is not uncommon. The diagnosis is based on abnormal findings in multiple limbs and cranial innervated muscles, such as the tongue, digastric, and sternocleidomastoid.

Reporting the Electromyogram

Many different types of forms can be employed to report the findings of the electromyogram. They vary from a strictly narrative report to a chartlike form with areas in which to check abnormalities and conclusions. Most forms incorporate characteristics of both. The form we employ is presented

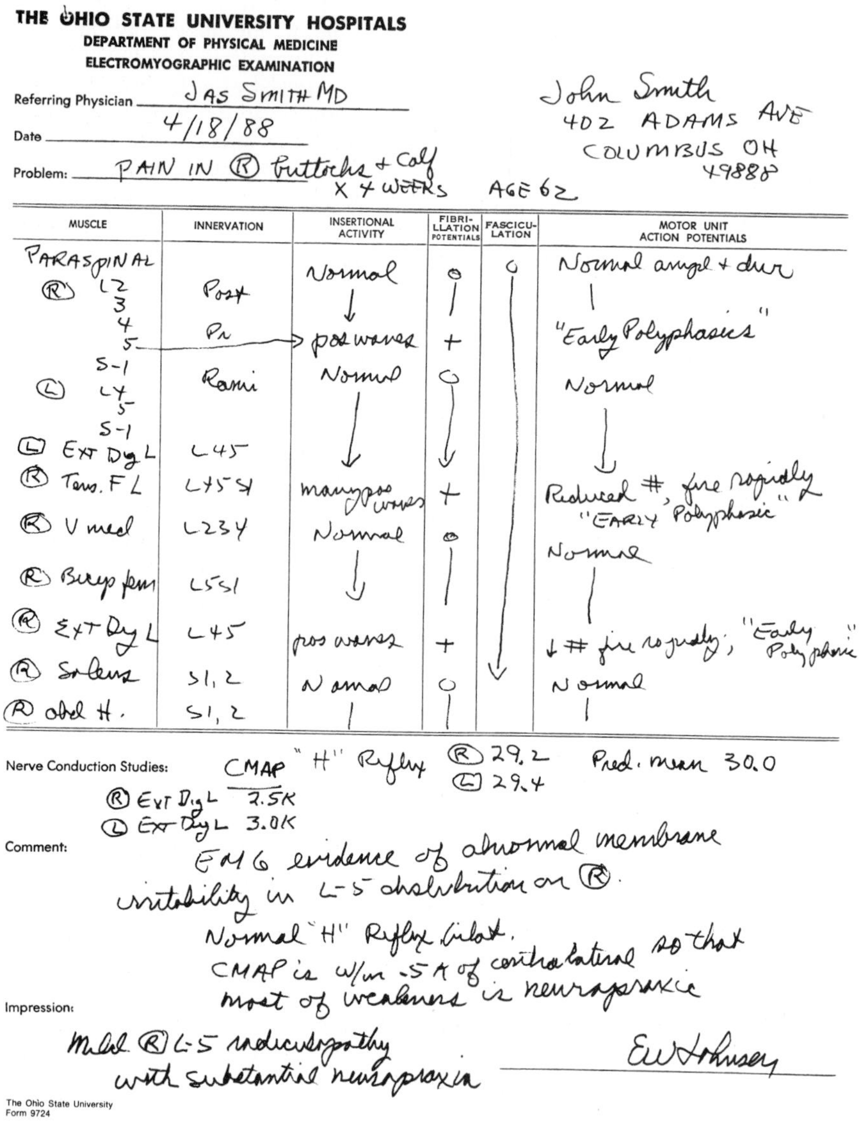

FIGURE 3–41. Sample EMG report.

in Figure 3–41. There are certain minimum requirements that should be a part of all reports, not only for the referring physician, but also for comparison with future electromyograms.

Muscles Examined

The specific muscles examined should be identified along with the innervating peripheral nerve and its cord levels. If the differential diagnosis involves a branch of a plexus or a very distal branch of a peripheral nerve, more specific identification of the nerve supply is indicated.

Insertional Activity

The report should include the presence or absence of positive sharp waves and whether these are found in localized pockets or diffusely throughout the entire muscle. Positive sharp waves and fibrillation potentials are graded according to the number present on a scale from 1 to 4. Grade 1 implies that they are difficult to find but definitely reproducible. Grade 4 indicates the display screen is filled horizontally with the potentials. Grades 2 and 3 represent the in-between stages of a few to a moderate amount. The presence of high- or low-frequency complex repetitive potentials and myotonic potentials and their frequency of appearance is noted. A reduced amount of provoked electrical activity or a mechanical resistance with needle electrode movement as is frequently seen in end stage myopathies and neuropathies with fibrosis is reported.

Spontaneous Activity

Fibrillation potentials are graded on a scale of 1 to 4 as discussed with positive sharp waves. It is also of importance to note whether they occur diffusely throughout the muscle or in localized areas. Fasciculation potentials may be reported on a scale of 1 to 4 also but frequently are reported as rare, occasional, few, or many. The configuration should be noted, whether simple or complex. The waveform should be followed over multiple discharges to note the stability of the complex. When there is clinical suspicion, quiet muscle should be observed for at least one minute before concluding no fasciculations are present.

Recruitment

The number of MUAPs recruited per strength of contraction is reported as increased, normal, or reduced. If the number of MUAPs recruited is increased or reduced, then it is further classified as mild, moderate, or marked.

Motor Unit Action Potentials

At least the parameters of amplitude, duration, shape, and stability should be reported for each muscle. If quantitative analysis is performed, then the mean of the amplitude and duration should be reported along with the percentage of polyphasic and unstable MUAPs. If the impressionistic or qualitative technique is employed, then a range of values for amplitude and duration and the approximate percentage of polyphasic and unstable motor units is reported. Both of these methods study primarily low-threshold motor units. Routinely, the only parameter of high-threshold motor units reported is amplitude.

Nerve Stimulation Studies

The distal latency and conduction velocity of stimulated motor and sensory nerves should be presented. The amplitude, duration, and area of the evoked response at each site of stimulation can be extremely important and can be reported in tabular form. If the temperature of the studied limb is not constantly maintained, then the temperature should be reported so that necessary corrections can be performed. This is most crucial for the study of distal sensory latencies.

Comment

Finally, the electromyographic findings should be summarized and then translated into a specific clinical diagnosis. Not uncommonly, the findings are compatible with several disorders. In this situation, the findings are interpreted as being most compatible with a specific diagnosis and a differential diagnosis is included. An electromyogram without a clinical impression is of little value to the practicing physician.

DAVID O. WIECHERS AND ERNEST W. JOHNSON

References

1. Asbury, A. K., and Johnson, P. C.: Pathology of Peripheral Nerve. Philadelphia, W. B. Saunders Company, 1978.
2. Baran, E.: Somatosensory Evoked Potentials from Lower Extremity Nerve Stimulation, Course Supplement Vol. 3. Meeting of the American Academy of Physical Medicine and Rehabilitation, 1987, p. 1161.
3. Braddom, R., and Johnson, E. W.: H reflex: Review and classification with suggested clinical uses. Arch. Phys. Med. Rehabil., 55:412, 1974.
4. Braddom, R., and Johnson, E. W.: Standardization of H reflex and diagnostic use in S_1 radiculopathy. Arch. Phys. Med. Rehabil., 55:161, 1974.
5. Bril, V., and Werb, M.: SFEMG in tibialis anterior muscles of patients with diabetic peripheral neuropathy. Muscle Nerve, 9:563, 1986.
6. Buchthal, F., and Pinelli, P.: Muscle action potentials in polymyositis. Neurology, 3:424, 1953.
7. Buchthal, F., Guld, C., and Rosenfalck, P.: Action potential parameters in normal human muscle and their dependence on physical variables. Acta Physiol. Scand., 32:200, 1954.
8. Buchthal, F., Guld, C., and Rosenfalck, P.: Multielectrode study of the territory of a motor unit. Acta Physiol. Scand., 39:83, 1957.
9. Buchthal, F., Pinelli, P., and Rosenfalck, P.: Action potential parameters in normal human muscle and their physiological determinants. Acta Physiol. Scand., 32:219, 1954.
10. Cerra, D., and Johnson, E. W.: Motor nerve conduction velocity in "idiopathic" polyneuritis. Arch. Phys. Med. Rehabil., 42:159, 1961.
11. Cerra, D., and Johnson, E. W.: Motor nerve conduction velocity in premature infants. Arch. Phys. Med. Rehabil., 43:160, 1962.
12. Chiappa, K. H.: Evoked Potentials in Clinical Medicine. New York, Raven Press, 1983.
13. Desmedt, J., and Borenstein, S.: Relationship of spontaneous fibrillation potentials to muscle fiber segmentation in human muscular dystrophy. Nature, 258:531, 1975.
14. Eaton, L., and Lambert, E.: Electromyography and electric stimulation of nerves in diseases of motor units. Observations on myasthenic syndrome associated with malignant tumors. J.A.M.A., 163:1117, 1957.
15. Ekstedt, J., and Stalberg, E.: How the size of the needle electrode lead-off surface influences the shape of the single muscle fiber action potential in electromyography. Comput. Programs Med., 3:204, 1973.
16. Ekstedt, J., Nilsson, G., and Stalberg, E.: Calculation of the electromyographic jitter. J. Neurol. Neurosurg. Psychiatry, 37:526, 1974.
17. Granger, C.: Prognosis in Bell's palsy. Arch. Phys. Med. Rehabil., 57:33, 1976.
18. Hakelius, I., and Stalberg, E.: Electromyographical studies of free autogenous muscle transplant in man. Scand. J. Plast. Reconstr. Surg., 8:211, 1974.
19. Hendriksen, J. D.: Conduction Velocity of Motor Nerves in Normal Subjects and Patients with Neuromuscular Disorders. Thesis, University of Minnesota, 1956.
20. Henriksson, K., and Stalberg, E.: The terminal innervation pattern in polymyositis: A histochemical and SFEMG study. Muscle Nerve, 1:3, 1978.
21. Johnson, E. W., and Melvin, J.: Sensory conduction studies of median and ulnar nerves. Arch. Phys. Med. Rehabil., 48:25, 1967.
22. Johnson, E. W., and Melvin, J. L.: Value of electromyography in lumbar radiculopathy. Arch. Phys. Med. Rehabil., 52:239, 1971.
23. Johnson, E. W., and Olsen, K. J.: Clinical value of motor nerve conduction velocity determination. J.A.M.A., 172:2030, 1960.
24. Johnson, E. W., Denny, S. T., and Kelly, J. P.: Sequence of electromyographic abnormalities in stroke syndrome. Arch. Phys. Med. Rehabil., 56:468, 1975.
25. Kimura, J.: F-wave velocity in the central segment of the median and ulnar nerves. A study in normal subjects and in patients with Charcot-Marie-Tooth disease. Neurology, 24:539, 1974.
26. Kimura, J.: Proximal versus distal slowing of motor nerve conduction velocity in the Guillain-Barré syndrome. Ann. Neurol., 3:344, 1978.
27. Kimura, J.: The carpal tunnel syndrome, localization of conduction abnormalities within the distal segment of the median nerve. Brain, 102:619, 1979.
28. Kimura, J., Giron, L., and Young, S.: Electrophysiological study of Bell palsy. Electrically elicited blink reflex in assessment of prognosis. Arch. Otolaryngol., 102:140, 1976.
29. Kimura, J., Murphy, M., and Varda, D.: Electrophyiological study of anomalous innervation of intrinsic hand muscles. Arch. Neurol., 33:842, 1976.
30. Lambert, E.: The accessory deep peroneal nerve. A common variation in innervation of extensor digitorum brevis. Neurology, 19:1169, 1969.
31. Lambert, E., and Elmquist, D.: Quantal components of end-plate potentials in myasthenic syndrome. Ann. N.Y. Acad. Sci., 183:183, 1971.
32. Lambert, E., and Mulder, D.: Electromyographic studies in amyotrophic lateral sclerosis. Proc. Staff Meet. Mayo Clin., 32:441, 1957.
33. Lindstrom, J., and Lambert, E.: Content of acetylcholine receptor and antibodies bound to receptor in myasthenia gravis, experimental autoimmune myasthenia gravis, and Eaton Lambert syndrome. Neurology (N.Y.), 28:130, 1978.
34. MacLean, I., and Taylor, R. S.: Nerve root stimulation to evaluate brachial plexus conduction. Abstracts of Communications of the Fifth International Congress of Electromyography, Rochester, Minnesota, 1975, p. 47.

35. Magladery, J., Ward, D., and McDougal, B. Jr.: Electrophysiologic studies of nerve and reflex activity in normal man. 1. Identification of certain reflexes in the EMG and conduction velocity of peripheral nerve fibers. Bull. Johns Hopkins Hosp., 86:265, 1950.

36. Melvin, J., and Wiechers, D.: Measurement of motor unit action potentials. Arch. Phys. Med. Rehabil., 57:325, 1976.

37. Melvin, J., Schuchmann, J., and Lanese, R.: Diagnostic specificity of motor and sensory nerve conduction variables in the carpal tunnel syndrome. Arch. Phys. Med. Rehabil., 54:69, 1973.

38. Petatan, J.: Clinical electromyographic studies of diseases of the motor unit. Electroenceph. Clin. Neurophysiol., 36:395, 1974.

39. Schuchmann, J. A.: Evaluation of the H-reflex latency in radiculopathy. Arch. Phys. Med. Rehabil., 58:560, 1976.

40. Stalberg, E.: Clinical electrophysiology in myasthenia gravis. J. Neurol. Neurosurg. Psychiatry, 43:522, 1980.

41. Stalberg, E.: Macro. EMG, a new recording technique. J. Neurol. Neurosurg. Psychiatry, 43:475, 1980.

42. Stalberg, E., and Thiele, B.: Transmission block in terminal nerve twigs: A single fiber electromyographic finding in man. J. Neurol. Neurosurg. Psychiatry, 35:52, 1972.

43. Stalberg, E., and Trontelj, J.: Single Fiber Electromyography. Woking, U.K., Mirvalle Press, 1979

44. Stalberg, E., Schwartz, M., and Trontelj, J.: Single fiber electromyography in various processes affecting the anterior horn cell. J. Neurol. Sci., 24:403, 1975.

45. Stevens, J. C.: The electrodiagnosis of carpal tunnel syndrome. Muscle Nerve, 2:99, 1987.

46. Thiele, B., and Boehl, A.: Anzhal der Spike-komponenten im motor-unit potential. EEG EMG, 9:125, 1978.

47. Thiele, B., and Stalberg, E.: Fiber density of the motor unit in the extensor digitorum communis muscles in man. J. Neurol. Neurosurg. Psychiatry, 37:874, 1975.

48. Thomas, J., and Lambert, E.: Ulner nerve conduction velocity and H-reflex in infants and children. J. Appl. Physiol., 15:1, 1960.

49. Thomas, P. K., and Eliasson, S. G.: Diabetic neuropathy. In Dyck, P. J., Thomas, P. K., Lambert, E. H., and Bunge, R. (Eds.): Peripheral Neuropathy, Vol. 2. Philadelphia, W. B. Saunders Company, 1984.

50. Thomas, P. K., and Holdorff, B.: Neuropathy due to physical agents. In Dyck, P., Thomas, P. K., Lambert, E., and Bunge, R. (Eds.): Peripheral Neuropathy, Vol. 2. Philadelphia, W. B. Saunders Company, 1984, p. 1479.

51. Trontelj, J.: A study of the F-response by single fiber EMG. In Desmedt, J. (Ed.): New Developments in Electromyography and Clinical Neurophysiology, Vol. 3. Basel, Kargen, 1973, p. 318.

52. Weber, R.: Motor and sensory conduction and entrapment syndromes. In Johnson, E. W. (Ed.): Practical Electromyography, 2nd Ed. Baltimore, Williams & Wilkins, 1988.

53. Wettstein, A.: The origin of fasciculations in motor neuron disease. Ann. Neurol., 5:295, 1979.

54. Wiechers, D.: Mechanically provoked insertional activity before and after nerve section in rats. Arch. Phys. Med. Rehabil., 58:402, 1977.

55. Wiechers, D.: Electromyographic insertional activity in normal limb muscles. Arch. Phys. Med. Rehabil., 60:359, 1979.

56. Wiechers, D.: Single fiber EMG with a standard monopolar electrode. Arch. Phys. Med. Rehabil., 66:47, 1985.

57. Wiechers, D.: A simple comprehensive electrodiagnostic study for the difficult carpal tunnel diagnosis. Muscle Nerve, 10:647, 1987.

58. Wiechers, D.: Motor unit potentials in disease. In Johnson, E. W. (Ed.): Practical Electromyography, 2nd Ed. Baltimore, Williams & Wilkins, 1988.

59. Wiechers, D.: Normal and abnormal motor unit potentials. In Johnson, E. W. (Ed.): Practical Electromyography, 2nd Ed. Baltimore, Williams & Wilkins, 1988.

60. Wiechers, D., Stow, R., and Johnson, E. W.: Electromyographic insertional activity mechanically provoked in biceps brachii. Arch. Phys. Med. Rehabil., 58:573, 1977.

61. Wilbourn, A., and Lambert, E.: The forearm median-to-ulnar nerve communication: Electrodiagnostic aspects. Neurology, 26:368, 1976.

62. Wohlfart, G.: Collateral regeneration from residual motor nerve fibers in amyotrophic lateral sclerosis. Neurology, 7:124, 1957.

4 Gait Analysis: Diagnosis and Management

JUSTUS F. LEHMANN
BARBARA J. DE LATEUR

Gait Pattern

In order to analyze a gait pattern, to diagnose pathological changes, and to understand therapeutic interventions such as braces and prostheses, it is essential to understand the biomechanics and physiology of normal gait.[12, 38, 39]

Points of the Gait Cycle

The cycle from heel strike on one leg to the next heel strike on the same leg equals 100 per cent of a total gait cycle. One can identify specific points in time during this gait cycle. At 0 per cent, the heel strikes at the beginning of the stance phase. At 15 per cent, the forefoot is also in contact with the floor; therefore, it is called "foot flat." At 30 per cent, the heel leaves the ground, called "heel off"; at 45 per cent, the knee and hip bend to accelerate the leg forward in anticipation of the swing phase, and this is called "knee bend." At 60 per cent, the toe leaves the ground, which also signals the end of the stance phase and the beginning of the swing phase. This is called "toe off."

At mid-swing, foot dorsiflexion provides toe clearance. No accurate percentile can be attributed to this event. At 100 per cent, heel strike again occurs with the same leg. Thus, by definition, the duration of the stance is 60 per cent of the total gait cycle and the swing phase is 40 per cent of the total.

Phases of the Gait Cycle

The terms for the phases from point to point of the gait cycle are as follows: The period from 0 to 15 per cent is called the *heel strike phase*; from 15 to 30 per cent, *mid-stance*; from 30 to 45 per cent, *push off*; from 45 to 60 per cent, *acceleration of the swing leg*. The swing phase is subdivided into the swing-through portion and deceleration of the swinging leg at the end of the period.

Near the end of the stance phase of one leg and at the beginning of the stance phase of the other, there is a time of double support of the body by both legs. This phase of double support extends over approximately 11 per cent of the gait cycle.

Energy is consumed in two ways. For example, when the leg is decelerated during the end of the swing phase, a swinging mass is decelerated and a forward movement is transmitted to the body so that it is actually accelerated. Energy is also consumed during the shock absorption of heel strike. The body's center of gravity tends to continue forward owing to inertia and downward owing to gravity. The restraint exerted by muscles is called *shock absorption*. Energy is also required for propulsion during push off when the center of gravity is actually propelled up and forward. The ratio of energy consumption of the two activities is 5:8 between propulsion on the one hand and shock absorption/deceleration on the other.[19] Thus, biologically, more energy is actually consumed in controlling forward movement than in moving forward.[23]

To further clarify terminology, Figure 4–1 shows stride length, defined as the length extending from heel strike to heel strike of the same foot; step length is from heel strike of one foot to heel strike of the other foot. Stride width is determined by the distance between the midline of one foot and the midline of the other foot. On the average, these values are approximately 156 cm for stride length and half that value for step length. Stride width is 8 cm ± 3.5, and the angle at which we normally toe out from the line of progression is about 6.7 to 6.8 degrees. The mean duration of the total gait cycle is slightly over one second (1.03 ± 0.10). Cadence, the number of steps per minute, is approximately 117, or not quite 60 strides per minute. However, for all these measures there is some variation.[22, 34-37]

The most important variable influencing energy consumption is the character of the movements of the center of gravity. The center of gravity moves up and down and right and left, and the amplitude of these excursions essentially determines the amount of energy consumption during walking activity. The center of gravity pathway requiring the least energy consumption would be a straight line parallel to the ground. Such a line is possible only with wheels, and our translatory motion during ambulation occurs as a result of angular changes at the two ends of stick levers. Since a straight line is not feasible, the next best trajectory would be a sinusoidal curve of the least possible amplitude.

Determinants of Gait

Translatory movement of the body, as in walking, is brought about by alternating angular changes at the upper and lower end of the stick levers that constitute the lower limbs.[42] If the leg consisted of a single lever with mobility only at

foot and hip, a "compass" gait would result. If the pivot point were the contact area with the ground, the arc described by the center of gravity would have a vertical excursion of approximately 3 inches. At the low end of the center of gravity curve, an abrupt change of direction as well as a deceleration and subsequent acceleration would occur, both energy-consuming processes. This center of gravity pathway curve is modified in reality by six determinants.[41]

The first modification of this inefficient compass gait is *pelvic rotation* of 4 degrees in either direction, a total of 8 degrees (Fig. 4–2). The rotation occurs maximally to one side at the phase of double support, that is, when both legs are on the ground and the center of gravity is at the low end of the pathway curve. Thus, the length of the supporting leg is effectively increased and the lowest point of the center of gravity pathway curve is elevated. As the other leg swings forward, the pelvis rotates 4 degrees in the opposite direction, with the same effect on the center of gravity pathway curve. This elevation of the low end of the center of gravity pathway curve reduces the total amplitude by 3/8 inch.

The second determinant is that of *pelvic tilt*. As one walks, the pelvis drops on the side of the swinging leg. This drop is controlled by the hip abductors (gluteus medius and minimus) of the stance leg. Since the center of gravity is midway between the hips, the pathway curve also drops. This reduces its greatest elevation from the floor during mid-stance. At about the same time, the swing leg must be foreshortened by hip and knee flexion and ankle dorsiflexion to provide toe clearance. This pelvic drop is about 5 degrees and saves 3/16 inch of vertical excursion at the top of the center of gravity pathway curve.

The third determinant is *knee flexion*, which occurs during the mid-stance. The knee is extended during heel strike, flexed to 15 degrees toward

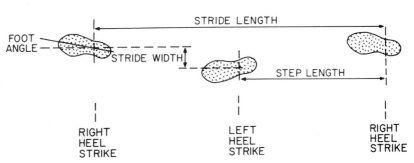

FIGURE 4–1. Schematic representation of stride dimensions: step and stride length, stride width, and foot angle. (Used with permission from Murray, M. P., et al.: Walking patterns of normal men. J. Bone Joint Surg., 46A:341, 1964.)

JUSTUS F. LEHMANN AND BARBARA J. DE LATEUR

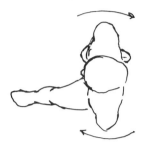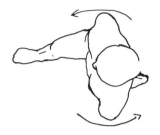

FIGURE 4–2. Pelvic rotation, 4 degrees in either direction.

mid-stance, and then extended toward push off. This effectively reduces leg length during mid-stance, when the center of gravity reaches its highest point. The reduction in leg length lowers the center of gravity at its highest point by 7/16 inch; thus, the sum of reductions in vertical excursion caused by the first, second, and third determinants is 1 inch, reducing total amplitude to less than 2 inches (1.7 inches), with considerable energy saving.

However, the abrupt change in direction and the deceleration and subsequent acceleration around the lower point of the center of gravity pathway have not yet been eliminated by these determinants. The fourth and fifth determinants are responsible for smoothing out this part of the curve. This is *knee and ankle motion*. The ankle motion (Fig. 4–3), in combination with the already described knee motion, produces a smooth sinusoidal pathway of the center of gravity. The ankle pivots on the posterior heel with a relatively short

radius of motion to the foot flat position. The ankle position then remains the same until the heel leaves the ground at the toe off position; during this phase, the ankle pivots over the ball of the foot with a much larger radius of the arc. The fourth and fifth determinants convert the vertical center of gravity pathway curve into a smooth sinusoidal curve of less than 2 inches amplitude.

The last determinant concerns the *motion of the center of gravity* in the horizontal plane. To be stable, the center of gravity must be brought over the supporting limb. A plumb line should fall over the supporting foot; thus, for one to stand on the left leg, one's center of gravity must shift toward the left side and then sway to the right side when one steps onto the right foot, a total excursion of 6 inches. This is an inefficient use of energy. The normal anatomical valgus at the knee brings the feet closer to the midline; therefore, less lateral sway is necessary. The excursion is again less than 2 inches, an average of about 1.7 inches for an adult. The center of gravity pathway describes a smooth sinusoidal pathway curve, not only up and down but also from side to side. Thus, the center of gravity is found in the midline and at its lowest point during the phase of double support. As weight is put on the right foot, it shifts to its highest and most lateral position toward the right during mid-stance. As the other heel strikes, the center of gravity is back at its lowest point in midline to move up and left laterally toward mid-stance on the left.

The limb also undergoes a considerable amount of rotation during the gait cycle; the pelvis rotates 8 degrees, the femur 8 degrees, and the tibia 9 degrees, a total of 25 degrees. Figure 4–4 shows the direction of rotation. From the beginning, at toe off, all the rotation moves in the direction of internal rotation until a peak is reached at mid-stance (15 to 20 per cent of the gait cycle). Then the rotation begins to reverse toward external rotation until push off. During push off, especially during the very last part of the stance, there is a

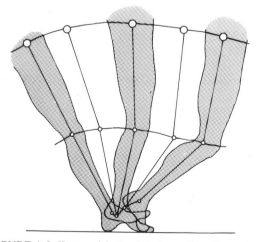

FIGURE 4–3. Knee and foot rotation smoothing the center of gravity pathway. (Redrawn from Saunders, J. B., Inman, V. T., and Eberhart, H. D.: The major determinants in normal and pathological gait. J. Bone Joint Surg., 35A:543, 1953.)

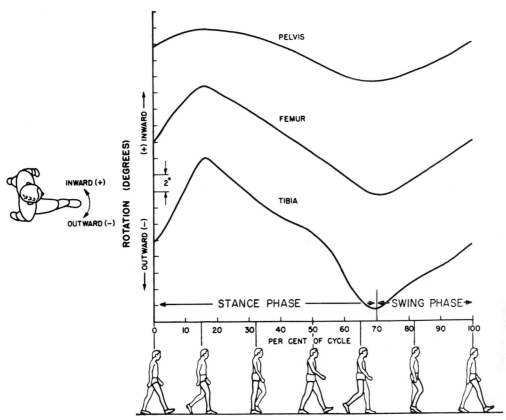

FIGURE 4–4. Relative rotations at knee and hip joints as viewed from above. Pin studies, average of 12 subjects. There is considerable variability in the stride length, step length, stride width, gait cycle duration, and cadence. (From Human Limbs and Their Substitutes by Klopsteg and Wilson. © 1954 by McGraw-Hill Book Company, Inc. Used with permission from the McGraw-Hill Book Co.)

more rapid change into external rotation, particularly of the tibia. If one walks on the wet sand at the beach, a cake of sand is thrown out at this point, indicating this rotation. This rotation is difficult to imitate in prosthetic replacement of the limb.

Muscle Activity in the Gait Cycle

If we examine the motor power that produces the motion of the limb segments in Figures 4–5 and 4–6, the pre-tibial group shown in the graph is most active during the heel strike phase, in which a lengthening contraction of the foot dorsiflexors lets the foot down from heel strike to the foot flat position slowly, in a controlled manner. The small activity during the rest of the stance phase is due to the fact that these same dorsiflexors are also invertors and evertors, a bridle to keep the foot stable in the mediolateral direction, together with the corresponding invertors and evertors in the calf. This is important for the stability of walking on rough ground or on a hillside.[30] The small activity during the swing phase results from picking up the toe for toe clearance.

The calf group, primarily the gastrocnemius and soleus, shows maximal peak activity during push off to propel the center of gravity up and forward. The quadriceps group is maximally active just after heel strike, acting as a shock absorber to control knee flexion to the allowed 15 degrees. It prevents the center of gravity from being driven down and forward by gravity and inertia. The rectus femoris again is active during the latter part of the stance phase when the hip is flexed and the leg is accelerated forward (to prevent excessive heel rise).

JUSTUS F. LEHMANN AND BARBARA J. DE LATEUR

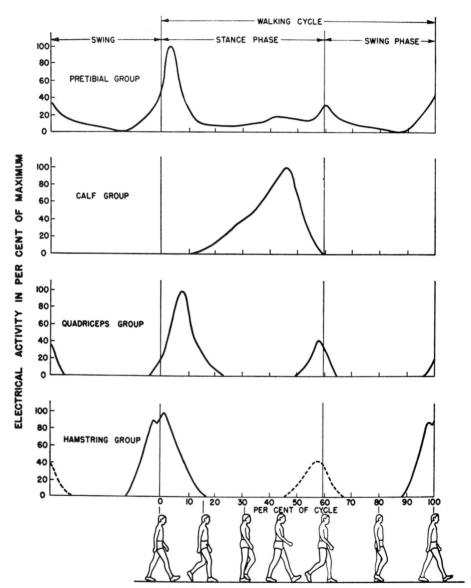

FIGURE 4–5. Phasic action of major muscle groups during level walking. Electromyograph studies, 10 adult males. (From Human Limbs and Their Substitutes by Klopsteg and Wilson. © 1954 by McGraw-Hill Book Company, Inc. Used with permission from the McGraw-Hill Book Co.)

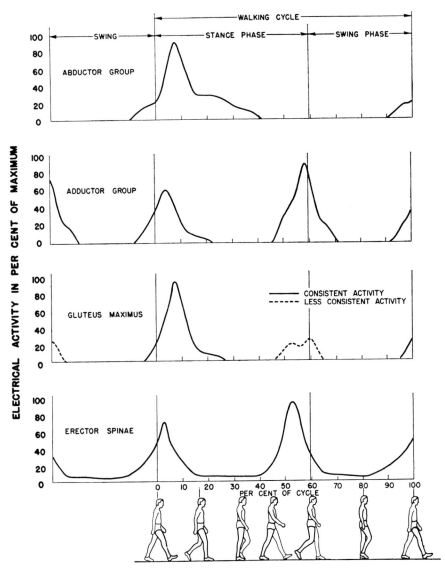

FIGURE 4–6. Phasic action of major muscle groups during level walking. Electromyograph studies, 10 adult males. (From Human Limbs and Their Substitutes by Klopsteg and Wilson. © 1954 by McGraw-Hill Book Company, Inc. Used with permission from the McGraw-Hill Book Co.)

The quadriceps is also active in producing adequate forward swing of the leg below the knee while the hip is flexed. This is an extension action to make the leg follow the thigh segment. The hamstrings have a double peak just before and after heel strike. The first peak occurs during the swing when there is an open kinetic chain—that is, when the foot is not firmly planted on the ground—and this peak decelerates the forward swing of the leg by its extension action across the hip and its flexion action across the knee. The moment the foot is planted firmly on the ground, the open kinetic chain is converted to a closed kinetic chain, and the hamstrings now keep the knee from buckling, that is, from going into further flexion. They act as shock absorbers and also keep the hip from buckling. With the quadriceps they act as knee extensors to limit knee flexion at 15 degrees. The hamstrings may show a second peak of activity at the termination of the stance phase, probably working toward hip and knee extension for push off.

JUSTUS F. LEHMANN AND BARBARA J. DE LATEUR

The abductor group, gluteus medius and minimus, is primarily active during heel strike and the early stance phase to stabilize the pelvis tilt to 5 degrees.

The adductor group's first peak of activity occurs right after heel strike. In part, this peak may be explained by the hamstring portion of the adductor magnus controlling hip flexion as do the other hamstrings. This is also the time when the femur moves toward internal rotation. The adductor group may assist in this motion. Whereas the adductors are external rotators when the limb is free (open kinetic chain), they allegedly reverse their function and act as internal rotators with the foot planted on the ground (closed kinetic chain).[4, 18] Klopsteg states that they "stabilize the pelvis."[23] The second peak occurs at the end of the stance phase. The explanation may be that they work together with other hip flexors to accelerate the limb forward in preparation for the swing. It is also noted that at this time the limb segments move toward maximal external rotation.

The gluteus maximus is most active during the heel strike phase when the maximus acts as a shock absorber. Its extension function across the hip and knee keeps both joints from buckling and keeps the person from folding down during heel strike. Again there is a peak of activity during the push off, when it works with the hamstrings and the adductor magnus portion of the hamstrings to extend hip and knee for propulsion of the center of gravity. Its function may also add to the external rotation of the limb segments.

The erector of the spine becomes active during heel strike of each leg. This activity is necessary to keep the trunk from folding forward from the forces of inertia and gravity at heel strike. It also stabilizes the trunk mediolaterally.

These functions taken together show that the muscles work during the gait cycle only for short and limited periods of time. For instance, the shock absorbers, like the quadriceps and the foot dorsiflexors, work early during the stance phase, and the plantar flexors, gastrocnemius, and soleus work during the push off phase. The muscles cannot sustain a strong contraction for long periods of time. There must be relaxation between contractions to allow the blood flow to restore itself fully for the resupply of oxygen and nutrients and the removal of waste and carbon dioxide. In an activity like walking, which we can maintain for long if not indefinite periods of time, it is essential that muscles work "on" and "off."

Force Transmission Through the Limb

Figure 4–7 shows the forces exerted against the ground. During heel strike the force vector slants down and forward. This vector is the sum of a vector shearing forward, parallel to the ground, and another perpendicular. During push off the resultant force is down and backward. It is the sum of a posterior shear vector and vertical force, shown in Figure 4–7. The horizontal, dotted line

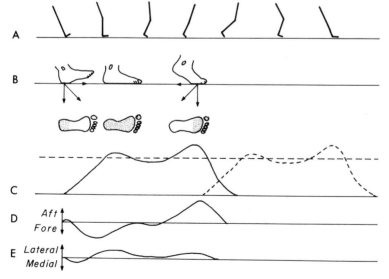

FIGURE 4–7. Forces during phases of the gait cycle. *A*, Points: heel strike, foot flat, heel off, toe off, knee bend, foot dorsiflexion, heel strike. *B*, Force vectors at heel strike and push off. *C*, Vertical ground reactive force. Horizontal dotted line indicates body weight; dotted curve indicates same phases on opposite leg. *D*, Fore and aft shear. *E*, Mediolateral shear. (Redrawn from Klopsteg, P. E., and Wilson, P. D. [Eds.]: Human Limbs and Their Substitutes. New York, McGraw-Hill Book Co., Inc., 1954.)

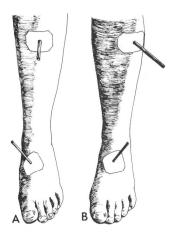

FIGURE 4–8. Pins fixed to the tibia and first metatarsal show the following: *A*, With foot planted on the ground, the tibial pin points straight ahead. *B*, When the tibia rotates externally, the foot is inverted, stiffening the arch. (Redrawn from Inman, V. T.: The Joints of the Ankle. Baltimore, Williams and Wilkins, 1976.)

indicates body weight (vertical force): it is exceeded during the shock absorption phase when the dynamic deceleration of the center of gravity produces a force against the ground. Then inertia carries the body forward; therefore, the force against the ground vertically is less than body weight. Finally, during push off, when we actually push against the ground to propel ourselves up and forward, the vertical loading on the ground may go up to 120 per cent of body weight as a result of acceleration (force = mass × acceleration). The ground reactive force declines, and the dotted line indicates when the other leg takes up the force during the phase of double support.

The fore and aft shear is shown in Figure 4–7. At heel strike there is a small kick backward as the curve indicates.[8, 9, 23] Then through the heel strike phase there is a primarily forward shear. If we step on a banana peel at that time, the leg slides out in front. Then, during push off, shear is reversed to the posterior direction; if we then step on the banana peel, the foot slips out from under us backward.

On heel strike, there is a short period of medial shear, followed by lateral shear throughout most of the stance. The lateral shear is produced by the action of gluteus medius and minimus, which act to stabilize the pelvis and limit pelvic tilt. Normative data of this type have been reviewed by Chao et al.[11] Ground reaction forces in running have been studied by Munro et al.[33]

Inman[20] found that the subtalar joint complex functions essentially as a mitered hinge to allow force transmission through the foot during push off. When the tibia rotates externally, the arch is increased and the foot is inverted, stiffening the foot for better force transmission (Fig. 4–8*A*,*B*). Push off occurs just when the maximal rate and degree of external rotation are reached in the tibia (see Fig. 4–4).

Energy Cost of Ambulation

Efficiency is best illustrated by the number of calories consumed to propel the body over a given distance (e.g., 1 meter), prorated per kilogram of body weight. This figure has been found by many authors to be very close to 0.8 calorie per meter per kilogram for normal ambulation at a comfortable speed[13] (Table 4–1). Whenever a pathological process disturbs normal ambulation, this figure is markedly elevated. In Figure 4–9, for normal per-

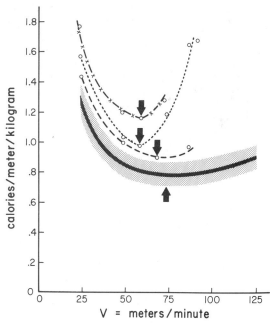

FIGURE 4–9. Energy expenditure in calories/meter/kilogram of normal subjects (heavy curve). Stippled area, one standard deviation. Broken line, amputee walking with suction-socket prosthesis. Dotted line, same, using pylon. **x-x-x**, same using forearm crutches. (Used with permission from Bard, G., and Ralston, H. J.: Measurement of energy expenditure during ambulation, with special reference to evaluation of assistive devices. Arch. Phys. Med. Rehabil., 40:417, 1959.)

JUSTUS F. LEHMANN AND BARBARA J. DE LATEUR

TABLE 4–1. Energy Requirements in Normal Ambulation*

RESEARCHER, DATE	N	TYPE OF DISABILITY	SPEED (Meters/Min)	ENERGY EXPENDITURE kcal/min/kg	ENERGY EXPENDITURE kcal × 10⁻³/m/kg
McDonald, 1961	583	Normals (F)	80	0.067[b]	0.83
		Normals (M)	80	0.061[b]	0.76
Ralston, 1958	19	Normals (M&F)	74[c]	0.058[b]	0.78
Corcoran, 1970	32	Normals (M&F)	83[c, d]	0.063[b]	0.76
Waters, 1976	25	Normals (M&F)	82[d]	0.063[b]	0.77
Ganguli, 1973	16	Normals (M)	50[e]	0.044	0.88[a]
Bobbert, 1960	2	Normals (M)	81[e]	0.063[f]	0.78[a]
Peizer, 1969	?	Normals (?)	80[g]	0.043[g]	0.54

*Modified from Fisher, S. V., and Gullickson, G.: Energy cost of ambulation in health and disability: A literature review. Arch. Phys. Med. Rehabil., 59:124–133, 1978. Used with permission.
[a]Calculated knowing kcal/min, m/min, and weight.
[b]Calculated knowing kcal/meter, m/min, and weight.
[c]Most efficient speed of ambulation.
[d]Speed chosen by the subjects.
[e]Speed chosen by researcher (the only speed or a representative speed).
[f]Calculation from author's equation and/or percentage figure.
[g]Approximated from a graph.

sons, energy consumption is minimal at a certain comfortable walking speed.[3] This speed is approximately 60 to 75 meters per minute; at slower speeds, relatively more energy is consumed for stabilization without increase in propulsion. As one walks faster than the comfortable walking speed, the curve of energy consumption increases at a more rapid rate. When the phase of double support is lost, walking turns to running. As Figure 4–9 shows, when a pathological alteration such as amputation produces a gait abnormality, there is an upward shift of the total curve; at any given speed, energy consumption will be greater. The comfortable walking speed—that speed at which the patient moves over a given distance with a minimal amount of energy consumption—will shift to slower walking speeds. The increase in oxygen consumption at speeds faster than comfortable speed occurs at a much more rapid rate; the curve rises more steeply. It also ends abruptly at higher speeds, representing the maximum speeds these people can walk safely. Maximal walking speed is reduced; in practical terms, patients with significant limps are usually unable to run.

The efficiency of the total gait mechanism can be measured by determining the ratio of metabolic expenditure in calories per minute over mechanical work, as shown in Table 4–2. This efficiency ratio, according to Ralston,[40] is between 0.21 and 0.24 at the speed of 73.2 meters per minute. Engineers tell us that this is approximately the maximum

efficiency that can be achieved by moving a stick-lever system through angular changes to produce the translatory motion of our anatomical system. Aura and Komi[2] estimated the mechanical efficiency of pure positive work of locomotion to be on the average 19.8 ± 1.2 per cent for female subjects and 17.4 ± 1.2 per cent for male subjects. The mechanical efficiency for pure negative work was 59.3 ± 14.4 per cent versus 75.6 ± 29.3 per cent for men and women respectively.

In designing devices such as orthoses and prostheses, it is important to realize that adding weight to the body increases metabolic demand, but the amount of increase depends on where the weight is added.[7] If we add a load equal to 17 per cent of body weight to the trunk, metabolic de-

TABLE 4–2. Metabolic Expenditure and External Positive Work: Gross Efficiency of Two Females and One Male Walking at 73.2 Meters/min*

SUBJECT	METABOLIC EXPENDITURE (cal/min)	POSITIVE WORK (cal/min)	RATIO
PK	3010	713	0.24
JR	3450	716	0.21
JC	3780	863	0.23

*From Ralston, H. J., Lukin, L.: Energy levels of human body segments during level walking. Ergonomics, 12:45, 1969. Used with permission.

mand increases only 3 per cent. If we add the same load to the foot, there is a 31 per cent increase in metabolic expenditure.[40] Thus, the weight of lower extremity orthoses can make a significant difference. However, one must keep in mind the influence of design of the orthosis or prosthesis on the center of gravity pathway. It has an even greater role in influencing energy expenditure, because anything that alters the center of gravity pathway means that the total body weight has to be lifted and lowered by that much, therefore changing metabolic demand.

Gait Analysis

In analyzing a patient with a limp, it is most important to do a thorough, step-by-step appraisal. First one should look at symmetry and smoothness of movement. Stride length and width of the gait base should be observed. One should observe separately and deliberately each component part of the body: head, shoulders, arms, pelvis, hip, knees, ankles, and feet. Shoulders should be observed for dipping, elevation, depression, protraction, retraction, and ease of rotation. Listing of the trunk, asymmetrical armswings, abnormal tilting, hiking, dropping, or fixedness should be noted. Circumducting the hip is another sign to watch. The stability of the knee and excessive inversion or eversion of the foot are only some of the other indicators of gait abnormality.

Pathological Gaits

There may be several general causes of pathological gait: *structural*, including abnormal bone length or shape; *pathological changes of joint and soft tissue*, such as contractures; and *neuromuscular disorders*, which include the involvement of the central and peripheral nervous system and the musculature itself.

If one limb is involved, the hallmark of abnormality of gait is its asymmetry between the affected and unaffected sides, which is true of limps produced by stroke[44] as well as of limps produced by prostheses.[15, 16]

Common Abnormalities

Inequality of leg length is a common structural abnormality. If the shortening is moderate, less than 1½ inches, there is an apparent elevation of the shoulder on the opposite swing side and dipping of the shoulder on the affected side. Compensation is sought by dropping the pelvis on the affected side. One observes exaggerated flexion at the hip, knee, and ankle during swing phase of the opposite limb. If, on the other hand, the differential is more than 1½ inches, the patient usually switches to a different mode of compensation—that is, walking on tiptoe on the short leg to lengthen the limb.

If there is an *ankylosis* or *limitation of the joint range*—of the hip, for example—compensatory motion is usually present in the lumbar spine. Since the pelvis and trunk are tilted as a rigid unit to substitute for motion at the hip, excessive motion will be seen in the lumbar spine and in the unaffected hip joint.

Arthritic conditions of the knee such as rheumatoid arthritis or osteoarthritis produce a reduction of walking velocity, reduced knee flexion and extension rates, and reduced range of knee motion.[10] Waters et al.[46] studied the energy cost of walking with arthritis and found that the mean rate of oxygen uptake did not exceed normal. However, the energy cost per meter walked was elevated. Khodadadeh[24, 25] studied the deviation of ground reaction forces in degenerative joint disease.

If the knee is limited by contracture, the limb is shortened and all the hallmarks of a short leg limp will be present. Usually the problem is apparent only at higher walking speeds if the contracture is less than 30 degrees. If it is greater, it will also be apparent at slower speeds. If the contracture is in extension, the limb becomes too long. Circumduction, hip hiking, or tiptoeing on the unaffected side becomes necessary to swing the leg through. During the stance phase, the pelvis and center of gravity rise too far because the 15 degrees of knee flexion cannot occur. Heel strike is jarring because shock absorption requires knee flexion.

Equinus deformity of the foot produces a steppage gait, that is, excessive flexion of hip and knee because the leg segment is too long for the swing phase. *Calcaneal* deformity prevents an effective push off, and its absence is visible.

Joint instability shows up in excessive range of motion, abnormal motion, inability to support body weight, and sudden buckling.

Painful or antalgic gait is characterized by avoidance of weight-bearing on the involved side, shortening of the stance, and an attempt to unload the limb as much as possible. If there is a midline lesion in the spinal column, the gait is slow and symmetrical; the jarring of active heel strike is avoided on both sides. Short steps are taken to limit the weight-bearing period. In lumbar lesions one can see rigid guarding of the back musculature. The lumbar lordosis is often decreased or abolished. Unilateral lesions (for example, the impingement of nerve roots by the disk in the intervertebral foramen) are often relieved by bending the trunk forward to the unaffected side to open the foramen. Muscle guarding, small steps, and avoidance of heel strike are observed. The patient with hip pain reduces mechanical stress on the hip joint by shifting the center of gravity over the affected hip joint. Therefore, during the stance one sees a dipped shoulder on the affected side, a relative elevation of the shoulder on the unaffected side, and a sliding of the trunk over the stance leg. In the swing phase, especially if there is an effusion present, the limb is carried in a slightly flexed, externally rotated position that relaxes the capsule and ligaments. Heel strike is avoided because of the jarring. A painful knee is usually carried in slight flexion, especially when effused, to relieve the tension. The patient in this situation may walk on his or her toes. At the least, heel strike is avoided.

Gaits from Neurological Deficits

Gaits resulting from neurological deficits in the central control mechanism may vary greatly depending on the type and localization of the lesion. Only a few common patterns can be mentioned.

One of the most common problems is encountered in patients whose strokes result in hemiplegia. Most patients with *extensor synergies* will ambulate. The extensor synergy includes extension and internal rotation at the hip, extension at the knee, plantar flexion of the foot and toes, and inversion of the foot. The patient is more likely to ambulate if this is not associated with severe sensory loss, especially of joint position sense; unilateral neglect; or equilibrium difficulties. Hemiparetic gait is characterized by slow speed and poorly coordinated movements.[29] Consistent with this finding, Mizrahi et al.[31, 32] felt that the best way to monitor improvement of gait was to check the improvement of walking speed. Because the values of gait parameters vary with changes in speed, the slow speed that is typical of hemiparetic gait necessitates applying controls for the influence of speed when comparing hemiparetic and able-bodied persons.[29] Hemiparetic persons ambulating had a shorter step length, longer duration of stance, and shorter duration of swing phase on the affected side than normal. They displayed a greater than normal flexion of the affected hip during midstance, which by putting the center of mass farther in front of the knee may explain the increased knee extension moment due to vertical force components. The increased flexion during mid-stance may be related to the difficulties the patient has advancing the center of gravity during the latter part of the stance because the foot remains in plantar flexion and the knee extended. In severe cases the patient appears to walk up to the affected foot but not through to the next step (step-to pattern). As a result of the straight knee, there may also be an excessive rise of the hip and center of gravity. Affected hip adduction during single support was less in hemiparetic persons than in able-bodied persons, indicating a decreased lateral shift to the paretic side. During the swing phase, the affected limbs of hemiparetic persons were in less knee flexion and less dorsiflexion at the ankle than normal, necessitating circumduction to achieve toe clearance. This also may lead to a shortened heel strike phase, and sometimes the forefoot may strike before the heel. In cases of more flaccid paralysis, especially in the presence of reduced sensory feedback, knee instability may be pronounced. As part of hemiparetic gait, the arm is held in adduction and internal rotation at the shoulder. The elbow, wrist, and fingers are flexed. In addition, Bohannon and Larkin[6] found that there is reduced weight-bearing on the paretic side compared with the intact extremity when bilateral standing is attempted.

Other lesions, such as those in cerebral palsy, may lead to adductor spasms with scissoring.

The *ataxic gait* that occurs in cerebellar lesions shows a typical dysmetria and incoordination. Staggering and lack of smooth motion are compensated for by a wide-based gait.

Lack of sensory feedback—for example, in posterior column disease (e.g., tabes dorsalis)—produces an uncontrolled motion. Commonly, innervation of the hamstrings and other muscles is not timed appropriately because of lack of sensory feedback. The knee is forcefully extended against the ligaments, which may ultimately be damaged, producing a Charcot joint with genu recurvatum and additional mediolateral instability. Jerky movements during the end of the swing phase and improper placement of the feet on the ground are observed. The gait abnormalities are increased if visual feedback is removed.

Basal ganglia disease such as Parkinson's disease produces a *festinating or propulsive gait*. Noticeable are the lack of armswing and the short quick steps with increasing speed, as if the patient were trying to race after his or her center of gravity. Ultimately the patient may fall. He or she cannot stop abruptly or change direction without danger of falling. Changes in ground reaction forces have been studied by Koozekanani et al.[26] Characteristically, the second vertical force peak was reduced.

Gaits from Lower Motor Neuron Lesions

The gaits produced by lower motor neuron lesions are characteristic in their effect on specific muscle groups. An understanding of these limps and compensatory mechanisms is essential for remediation.

If weakness is suspected in the accelerator group of muscles used in push off, the physician should direct the patient to walk up an incline; this activity will demonstrate a pronounced deficit in these accelerator muscles. The functioning of the shock absorbers that work during heel strike are more distinct when the patient walks down an incline. Almost all limps, with the exception of the gluteus medius limp, are more exaggerated on fast walking than on slow walking. The gluteus medius limp is obscured because inertia carries the body through, making the gluteus medius limp less visible.

Hip extensor gait, or weakness of the gluteus maximus, is striking because the trunk and pelvis are suddenly thrown backward after heel strike on the affected side, and the affected hip seems to protrude owing to the trunk motion. The knee is tightly extended in mid-stance, which slightly elevates the hip on that side. At heel strike the shock absorption function of the gluteus maximus is missing; hip flexion cannot be controlled unless the trunk is thrown farther back so that the center of gravity force line to the supporting foot falls well behind the hip joint. This action creates a rotatory moment rotating the hip in extension and locking it against tight extensor check ligaments, thus making it stable. The knee must be kept tightly extended because if the knee is flexed when the foot is on the ground, the hip is unavoidably flexed as well. This gait cannot be corrected by braces, and a pelvic band is awkward. The best intervention is probably two crutches or canes with a three-point gait if the lesion is unilateral; if the lesion is bilateral, using crutches with an alternating two-point or four-point gait is best.

The uncompensated gluteus medius limp occurs in moderate weakness of the gluteus medius when it can only partly control the pelvic drop on the opposite swing side. In this case one sees a greater dropping of the pelvis on the unaffected swing side and an apparent lateral protrusion of the stance hip; if necessary, the patient may use a steppage gait to clear the swing leg. The best remedy for this limp is a cane in the opposite hand. If the gluteus medius is still weaker or entirely absent, the patient uses another gait pattern, the *compensated gluteus medius limp*. To prevent the pelvis from dropping too far on the opposite swing leg, the patient shifts the trunk so that the center of gravity is balanced over the stance hip joint. This maneuver produces less drop of the pelvis on the affected side than does the uncompensated gluteus medius limp. There is a medial deviation (rather than a lateral protrusion) of the affected hip because of the shift of the trunk. There is lateral bending of the trunk and dipping of the shoulder toward the affected side. The steppage gait on the unaffected swing leg is usually absent or less pronounced, since the hip does not drop as much.

Hip flexor paralysis is demonstrated by a limp that starts at push off, lasts throughout the rest of stance, and continues during the swing phase. The limb is swung forward solely by the musculature of the opposite hip throwing the trunk backward. The affected hip on the swing side becomes tightly extended against the check ligaments. Trunk rotation is transmitted via the ligaments to the swing leg, accelerating the leg forward. When the trunk stops moving, the leg continues forward by inertia into hip flexion.

The *quadriceps gait* pattern appears most obvious during the heel strike phase, the shock absorption phase, but it also shows during the swing phase. The knee is forcibly thrown into extension at or preceding heel strike and is associated with a smooth lurch of the trunk forward immediately following the heel strike. This is done in order to manipulate the center of gravity force line to the ground in front of the tightly extended knee joint, safely maintained in extension against the posterior capsule and ligaments. During rapid walking, the quadriceps is needed to accelerate the lower limb forward, motion that does not occur in the absence

JUSTUS F. LEHMANN AND BARBARA J. DE LATEUR

of the quadriceps. The leg lags behind by inertia, and an excessive heel rise results.

Gastrocnemius-soleus dysfunction is frequently the result of cauda equina lesions, peripheral neuropathies, stroke, or brain injury.[28] As the center of pressure (that is, the location of the ground reaction force) moves forward of the ankle, a dorsiflexion moment is created that is normally stabilized by the contraction of gastrocnemius and soleus. This starts long before the heel comes off (Figs. 4–10 and 4–11). In cases of paralysis, the center of gravity of the body and therefore the location of the ground reaction force is held back in order to avoid an unstable collapse of the ankle into dorsiflexion. The forward movement does not occur until after the opposite heel strike. As a result, the ground reaction force line is found well behind the knee center, creating a posterior moment arm that in turn produces a major bending moment at the knee and knee instability. This bending moment has to be counteracted by vol-

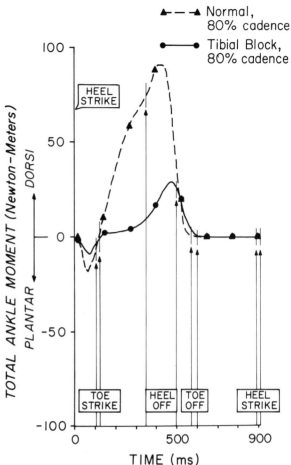

FIGURE 4–11. Total ankle moment versus time. Curves represent the mean of six trials of one subject. (From Lehmann, J. F., Condon, S. M., de Lateur, B. J., and Smith, J. C.: Gait abnormalities in tibial nerve paralysis: A biomechanical study. Arch. Phys. Med. Rehabil., 66:80–85, 1985.)

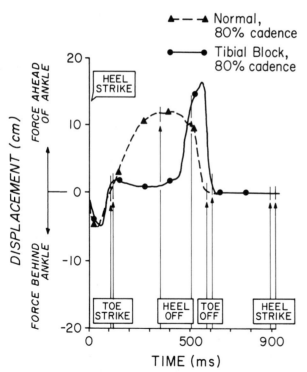

FIGURE 4–10. Vertical force moment arm with respect to the ankle versus time. Curves represent the mean of six trials of one subject. (From Lehmann, J. F., Condon, S. M., de Lateur, B. J., and Smith, J. C.: Gait abnormalities in tibial nerve paralysis: A biomechanical study. Arch. Phys. Med. Rehabil., 66:80–85, 1985.)

untary knee extensor effort (Fig. 4–12). In addition to the lack of forward movement of the center of gravity, the whole pelvis lags behind the normal position (Fig. 28–19), which leads to a short step on the opposite side and therefore a reduction in speed. Clinically, one observes the lack of forward movement of the pelvis during the push off phase and the late heel rise. The weakness of gastrocnemius and soleus is shown best when the patient walks up an incline.

In paralysis of the foot dorsiflexors due to peroneal palsy paralysis, the following abnormalities were observed to be significant.[27] The abnormalities involved both the stance and swing phases. There was a decrease in the duration of the heel

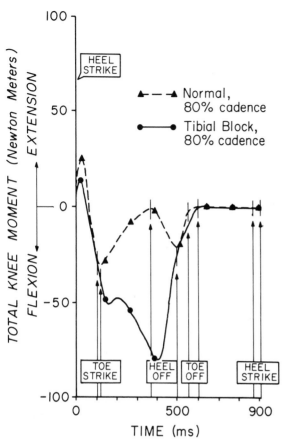

FIGURE 4–12. Total knee moment versus time. Curves represent the mean of six trials of one subject. (From Lehmann, J. F., Condon, S. M., de Lateur, B. J., and Smith, J. C.: Gait abnormalities in tibial nerve paralysis: A biomechanical study. Arch. Phys. Med. Rehabil., 66:80–85, 1985.)

and no slap will be heard after heel strike because the patient no longer strikes the ground with his or her heel. Rather, the patient lands on the ball of the foot. During the swing phase the toe hangs down, requiring a steppage gait for ground clearance.

Walking Aids

Stability when walking and standing depends on the location of the center of gravity. The center of gravity plumb line or force line to the ground must fall into the area of support to make the stance stable. The area of support can be increased if the

strike phase (Fig. 28–16) and a reduction in the peak plantar flexion moment. During mid-stance, there was an increase in the range of inversion-eversion, suggesting medial-lateral instability. The second vertical force peak and the aftershear force peak were reduced. These reductions are believed to be due to medial-lateral instability during push off. During the swing phase, a steppage gait was observed. In mild partial paralysis of the foot dorsiflexors, the lengthening contraction during the heel strike phase is inadequate (Fig. 4–13). The patient comes down to foot flat too fast, producing an audible slapping of the foot against the ground. During the swing phase, these muscles may be still strong enough to pick up the patient's foot for toe clearance. However, if the muscles are very weak or absent, there will be a "drop foot" during swing

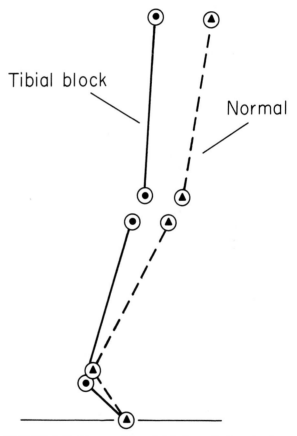

FIGURE 4–13. Mean position of right lower limb at the time of left heel strike. Stick figures represent the mean of six trials of one subject. Circles represent markers placed on the greater trochanter, lateral epicondyle, fibular head, lateral malleolus, and fifth metatarsal head. (From Lehmann, J. F., Condon, S. M., de Lateur, B. J., and Smith, J. C.: Gait abnormalities in tibial nerve paralysis: A biomechanical study. Arch. Phys. Med. Rehabil., 66:80–85, 1985.)

JUSTUS F. LEHMANN AND BARBARA J. DE LATEUR

patient has difficulties maintaining the center of gravity safely over the support area. The patient automatically assumes a wide-base gait if he or she cannot control the sway of the center of gravity.

The base of support can be increased by appliances such as a cane (Fig. 4–14) or crutches (Fig. 4–15). The triangular area between the crutches and the feet is the base of support that makes the patient stable. A four-legged cane increases the base of support beyond that of a simple cane. A walkerette not only maximally enlarges the area of support but also increases stability beyond that provided by crutches.

The cane is always used in the hand opposite to the leg with muscular weakness or pathological joint changes in order to provide a normal pathway for the center of gravity. If the cane is carried on the same side, it produces an unnecessary and exaggerated trunk sway. In bilateral disease, two canes may be used, usually with an alternating two-point gait. In an alternating two-point gait pattern, cane and opposite leg are advanced at the same time. The cane is commonly used in patients with lesions such as gluteus medius weakness or pathological joint changes at knee or ankle. The maximum weight that can be put on the cane is approximately 25 per cent of body weight.[45] Forearm crutches may be used in the same fashion as a cane. Maximal loading of the forearm crutches can be up to 45 per cent of body weight if a single forearm crutch is used.[45]

The following gait patterns are commonly in use: (1) A forearm crutch or a cane is used on the

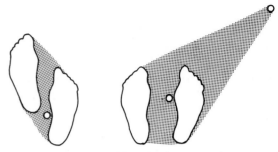

FIGURE 4–14. Foot position showing supporting area and location of center of gravity force line, and its enlargement with the use of a cane. (Redrawn from Williams, M., and Lissner, H. R.: Biomechanics of Human Motion. Philadelphia, W. B. Saunders Company, 1962.)

side opposite the affected limb, or an alternating two-point gait is used. These approaches only partially relieve weight-bearing of the legs. (2) A three-point gait can completely eliminate weight-bearing on one extremity. In this case, when the affected leg is on the ground, the patient puts all weight on the two forearm crutches. This gait pattern can be used in amputees. The intact limb is fully weighted without the support of the crutches. During the stance phase of this leg, the crutches are swung forward together with the affected limb. The energy cost of ambulation with crutches with a three-point gait is twice as great as normal,[13, 14] a finding confirmed by Hinton and Cullen.[17] (3) The other gait pattern used with forearm crutches is the four-point gait. In this case there are always three points of support, either

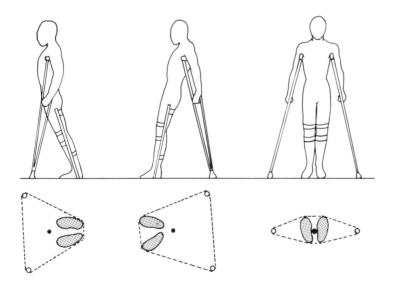

FIGURE 4–15. Different bases of support offering varying amounts of stability. (Redrawn from Williams, M., and Lissner, H. R.: Biomechanics of Human Motion. Philadelphia, W. B. Saunders Company, 1962.)

two crutches plus one leg or two legs plus one crutch; that is, the right crutch is moved while both legs and the left crutch are on the ground. Subsequently the left leg is moved forward while the two crutches and the right leg are on the ground. Then the left crutch moves while two legs and the right crutch are on the ground. Then the right leg moves while the two crutches and the left leg are on the ground, and so forth. First a crutch, then the opposite limb, is always moved. Although this gait pattern is slower than the other patterns described, it distributes weight over three points of support at all times, either through the upper extremities to the crutches and one leg or to two legs and one crutch and upper extremity. This pattern is commonly indicated to reduce weight-bearing by any one extremity to a minimum, for instance, in rheumatoid arthritis involving both upper and lower extremities.

Axillary crutches are used more commonly in such conditions as paraplegia. However, in some lower levels of the lesion, forearm crutches may be used. Axillary crutches can be used with an alternating two-point gait, or three-point or four-point gaits. In paraplegia, a swing-to or swing-through pattern may be used. The swing-to pattern reduces the triangle of support represented by the two crutches and the feet by lifting the body with the arms and sliding the feet forward closer to but never to the same level as the crutches, because anterior-posterior instability would result (Fig. 4–15). The crutches are then moved forward to enlarge the triangle of support and this maneuver is repeated. The patient must be braced at knee and ankle for either swing-to or swing-through patterns.

In the swing-through pattern, at the start the patient leans forward on the crutches and lifts and swings the legs through to a heel strike in front of the crutches. Since the ankle and knee are braced, arching the back makes this position stable. The hip is extended against ligaments that lock in extension because the center of gravity force line to the ground falls behind the hip joint, creating an extension moment. Subsequently the patient swings the crutches forward and again is stable because the center of gravity force line falls in the triangle of support. Gravity acting on the trunk will extend the hip. With this gait pattern the patient is stable twice: once with the crutches in front and once with the crutches behind. This is a mechanically effective gait pattern that produces a brisk speed of walking. Because the center of gravity pathway amplitude is large and not smooth,

this pattern is very energy-consuming. Depending on the level of the lesion, energy expenditure may be between three and four times as much as that in normal ambulation, and in higher lesion levels it may even exceed 10 times normal energy requirements.[13]

In the injured or diseased hip joint, a three-point gait pattern can be used with partial or complete weight-bearing relief. However, a special consideration should be given to the effectiveness of a single cane or crutch in the opposite hand, or an alternating two-point gait in the case of bilateral disease. The loading on the hip of a patient standing on both legs is 50 per cent of body weight on each side. As the patient walks or stands on one leg, pelvic drop is controlled by the force of the gluteus medius on the stance side (Fig. 4–16). This counteracts the gravitational force on the center of gravity. The fulcrum is the hip. The approximate length of the levers is 1 inch for gluteus medius force (F) and 3 inches for the gravitational force (W) on the center of gravity of the body. The rotatory moment created by the gravitational force is three times 165 inch-pounds if the body weight is 165 pounds. Thus it must be counterbalanced by the rotatory moment of the gluteus medius contraction (F). The moment arm is 1 inch; therefore, the gluteus medius force must be equal to 3×165 pounds or 495 inch-pounds. Therefore, the reactive force on the fulcrum of the hip (H) must be gluteus

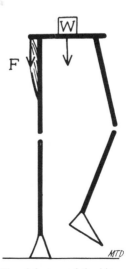

FIGURE 4–16. The abductors of the hip on one side balance the pelvis when the opposite leg is lifted. F is the force exerted by these muscles and operates at the hip in addition to W. (Used by permission from Harper & Row for Rosse, C., and Clawson, D. K.: Introduction to the Musculoskeletal System. New York, Harper & Row, 1970.)

JUSTUS F. LEHMANN AND BARBARA J. DE LATEUR

medius force (F) plus gravitation force (W), or four times body weight.

If a cane is used (Fig. 4–17), the force put on the cane (C) is multiplied by a moment arm of a total of 8 inches, creating an elevation of the pelvis on the swing side. In addition, the gluteus medius force (F) creates a rotatory moment in the same direction. Thus the sum of the counterclockwise rotatory moment is (F × 1 inch) + (C × 8 inches). The clockwise rotatory moment is created by the gravitational force acting on center of gravity (W) multiplied by 3 inches (W × 3). Clockwise and counterclockwise moments must therefore be in equilibrium:

$$W \times 3 = (F \times 1) + (C \times 8)$$
$$165 \times 3 = F + (60 \times 8)$$
$$F = 15 \text{ lb}$$

assuming 60 pounds force is put on the cane.

The force on the hip is therefore the sum of the vertical forces down (F + W) minus the vertical force up on the cane (H = W + F − C) or H = 165 + 15 − 60 = 120 pounds. Thus, because of its leverage, the cane eliminates necessary gluteus

medius force and reduces the compressional force on the hip. A more accurate and detailed account has been given by Blount.[5]

In summary, understanding normal and abnormal gait is an essential basis for corrective action.

ACKNOWLEDGMENT

This chapter is based in part on research supported by Research Grant #G00830076 from the National Institute of Disability and Rehabilitation Research, Department of Education, Washington, DC 20202.

References

1. Anderson, M. H., Bray, J. J., and Hennessy, C. A.: Prosthetic Principles—Above Knee Amputations. Springfield, Illinois, Charles C Thomas, Publisher, 1960.
2. Aura, O., and Komi, P. V.: The mechanical efficiency of locomotion in men and women with special emphasis on stretch-shortening cycle exercises. Eur. J. Appl. Physiol., 55:37–43, 1986.
3. Bard, G., and Ralston, H. J.: Measurement of energy expenditure during ambulation, with special reference to evaluation of assistive devices. Arch. Phys. Med. Rehabil., 40:415–418, 1958.
4. Basmajian, J. V.: Muscles Alive. Baltimore, Williams & Wilkins, 1962.
5. Blount, W. P.: Don't throw away the cane. J. Bone Joint Surg., 38A:695–708, 1956.
6. Bohannon, R. W., and Larkin, P. A.: Lower extremity weight bearing under various standing conditions in independently ambulatory patients with hemiparesis. Phys. Ther., 65:1323–1325, 1985.
7. Braune, W., and Fischer, O.: Über den Schwerpunkt des menschlichen Körpers unter Rucksicht auf die Ausrüstung des deutschen Infanteristen. Abhandl. König. Sachs. Ges. Wiss. (Leipzig), 15:559–672, 1889.
8. Bresler, B., and Berry, F. R.: Energy and power in the leg during normal level walking. University of California (Berkeley) Prosthetic Research Project Report, Series 11, Issue 15, May 1951.
9. Bresler, B., and Frankel, J. P.: The forces and moments in the leg during normal level walking. University of California (Berkeley) Prosthetic Research Project Report, Series 11, Issue 6, June 1948.
10. Brinkmann, J. R., and Perry, J.: Rate and range of knee motion during ambulation in healthy and arthritic subjects. Phys. Ther., 65:1055–1060, 1985.
11. Chao, E. Y., Laughman, R. K., Schneider, E., and Stauffer, R. N.: Normative data of knee joint motion and ground reaction forces in adult level walking. J. Biomech., 18:219–233, 1983.
12. Eberhart, H. D., Inman, V. T., and Bresler, B.: The principal element in human locomotion. In Klopsteg, P. E., and Wilson, P. D. (Eds.): Human

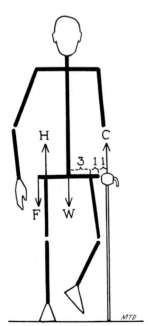

FIGURE 4–17. Schematic representation of forces acting on the hip with the use of a cane. F = gluteus medius force; C = force on cane; W = gravitational force acting on center of gravity; H = reactive force on hip fulcrum. (Used with permission from Harper & Row for Rosse, C., and Clawson, D. K.: Introduction to the Musculoskeletal System. New York, Harper & Row, 1970.)

Limbs and Their Substitutes. New York, McGraw-Hill Book Company, 1954.

13. Fisher, S. V., and Gullickson, G., Jr.: Energy cost of ambulation in health and disability: A literature review. Arch. Phys. Med. Rehabil., 59:124–133, 1978.

14. Fisher, S. V., and Patterson, R. P.: Energy cost of ambulation with crutches. Arch. Phys. Med. Rehabil., 62:250–256, 1981.

15. Hannah, R. E., Morrison, J. B., and Chapman, A. E.: Kinematic symmetry of the lower limbs. Arch. Phys. Med. Rehabil., 65:155–158, 1984.

16. Hannah, R. E., Morrison, J. B., and Chapman, A. E.: Prostheses alignment: Effect on gait of persons with below-knee amputations. Arch. Phys. Med. Rehabil., 65:159–162, 1984.

17. Hinton, C. A., and Cullen, K. E.: Energy expenditure during ambulation with ortho crutches and axillary crutches. Phys. Ther., 62:813–819, 1982.

18. Hollinshead, W. H., and Jenkins, D. B.: Functional Anatomy of the Limbs and Back, 5th Ed. Philadelphia, W. B. Saunders Company, 1981.

19. Inman, V. T.: Conservation of energy in ambulation. Arch. Phys. Med. Rehabil., 47:484–488, 1967.

20. Inman, V. T.: The Joints of the Ankle. Baltimore, Williams & Wilkins, 1976.

21. Inman, V. T., and Mann, R. A.: Biomechanics of foot and ankle. In Inman, V. T. (Ed.): DuVries Surgery of the Foot, 3rd Ed. St. Louis, C. V. Mosby Company, 1973.

22. Jansen, E. C., Vittas, D., Hellberg, S., and Hansen, J.: Normal gait of young and old men and women. Acta Orthop. Scand., 53:193–196, 1982.

23. Klopsteg, P. E., and Wilson, P. D. (Eds.): Human Limbs and Their Substitutes. New York, McGraw-Hill Book Company, 1954.

24. Khodadadeh, S.: Osteoarthritic gait dynamics from forceplate measurements. J. Biomed. Eng., 6:315–317, 1984.

25. Khodadadeh, S.: Legendre polynomial coefficients in the analysis of the force plate measurements from an osteoarthritic gait. J. Biomed. Eng., 7:318–320, 1985.

26. Koozekanani, S. H., Balmaseda, M. T. Jr., Fatehi, M. T., and Lowney, E. D.: Ground reaction forces during ambulation in parkinsonism: Pilot study. Arch. Phys. Med. Rehabil., 68:28–30, 1987.

27. Lehmann, J. F., Condon, S. M., de Lateur, B. J., and Price, R.: Gait abnormalities in peroneal nerve paralysis and their corrections by orthoses: A biomechanical study. Arch. Phys. Med. Rehabil., 67:380–386, 1986.

28. Lehmann, J. F., Condon, S. M., de Lateur, B. J., and Smith, J. C.: Gait abnormalities in tibial nerve paralysis: A biomechanical study. Arch. Phys. Med. Rehabil., 66:80–85, 1985.

29. Lehmann, J. F., Condon, S. M., Price, R., and de Lateur, B. J.: Gait abnormalities in hemiplegia: Their correction by ankle-foot orthoses. Arch. Phys. Med. Rehabil., 68:673–771, 1987.

30. Matsusaka, N.: Control of the medial-lateral balance in walking. Acta Orthop. Scand., 57:555–559, 1986.

31. Mizrahi, J., Susak, Z., Heller, L., and Najenson, T.: Objective expression of gait improvement of hemiplegics during rehabilitation by time-distance parameters of the stride. Med. Biol. Eng. Comput., 20:628–634, 1982.

32. Mizrahi, J., Susak, Z., Heller, L., and Najenson, T.: Variation of time-distance parameters of the stride as related to clinical gait improvements in hemiplegics. Scand. J. Rehabil. Med., 14:133–140, 1982.

33. Munro, C. F., Miller, D. I., and Fuglevand, A. J.: Ground reaction forces in running: A reexamination. J. Biomech., 20:147–155, 1987.

34. Murray, M. P., et al.: Walking patterns of normal men. J. Bone Joint Surg., 46A:341, 1964.

35. Murray, M. P., Kory, R. C., and Clarkson, B. H.: Walking patterns in healthy old men. J. Gerontol., 24:169–178, 1969.

36. Murray, M. P., Kory, R. C., Clarkson, B. H., and Sepic, S. B.: Comparisons of free and fast speed walking patterns of normal men. Am. J. Phys. Med., 45:8–24, 1966.

37. Murray, M. P., Kory, R. C., and Sepic, S. B.: Walking patterns of normal women. Arch. Phys. Med. Rehabil., 51:637–650, 1970.

38. Normal human locomotion. In Lower Limb Orthotics, 1974 Revision. New York University, Post Graduate Medical School, Prosthetics and Orthotics, pp. 19–52.

39. Perry, J.: The mechanics of walking. In Perry, J., and Hislop, H. (Eds.): Principles of Lower Extremity Bracing. New York, American Physical Therapy Association, 1967.

40. Ralston, H. J., and Lukin, L.: Energy levels of human body segments during level walking. Ergonomics, 12:45, 1969.

41. Saunders, J. B., Inman, V. T., and Eberhart, H. D.: The major determinants in normal and pathological gait. J. Bone Joint Surg., 35A:543, 1953.

42. Steindler, A.: Kinesiology of the Human Body. Springfield, Illinois, Charles C Thomas, Publisher, 1955.

43. Stolov, W. C.: The lower extremity. In Rosse, C., and Clawson, D. K. (Eds.): Introduction to the Musculoskeletal System. New York, Harper & Row, 1970.

44. Wall, J., and Turnbull, G. I.: Gait asymmetries in residual paraplegia. Arch. Phys. Med. Rehabil., 67:550–553, 1986.

45. Warren, C. G.: Personal communication, 1979.

46. Waters, R. L., Perry, J., Conaty, P., Lunsford, B., and O'Meara, P.: The energy cost of walking with arthritis of the hip and knee. Clin. Orthop., 214:278–284, 1987.

47. Williams, M., and Lissner, H. R.: Biomechanics of Human Motion. Philadelphia, W. B. Saunders Company, 1962.

5 Speech and Language Disorders

KATHRYN M. YORKSTON
DAVID R. BEUKELMAN

The primary goal of human communication is accurate and rapid transfer of information through the spoken, written, or gestural modes. The ability to do such things as share daily experiences, draw up legal agreements, and record history is dependent on an extensively developed communication system. Since most of us acquire our native verbal language with little voluntary effort, we are unaware of the complexities of acquisition until we attempt to learn a second language or to write clear, concise term papers, or until we experience a communication impairment.

Communication impairment may involve any aspect of the hearing, language, or speech processes. Discussion of all possible communication disorders in this chapter would lead to superficial descriptions of each. Therefore, only those speech and language disorders clearly having a physical basis are discussed. Because of the number of patients with neurogenic speech and language problems served by physical medicine and rehabilitation teams, additional emphasis is placed on these disorders. In preparation for the discussion of communication disorders, a brief review of normal language and speech processes is presented.

Normal Language and Speech Processes

Language

Verbal language is an arbitrary code that symbolically associates sound and meaning in patterns that are produced and understood by members of a linguistic community. The notion of a "code" implies that verbal language involves numerous symbols and rules that are unique to a specific language (e.g., English, Japanese, and Spanish). Although reading and writing heavily involve language processes, the written form of a language is usually derived from its spoken form. Verbal language may be divided into four subdivisions—phonology, semantics, syntax, and pragmatics.

Phonology is the area of linguistic study dealing with the relationships among sounds. Humans are able to produce many different sounds, but only a few of them are used as speech sounds. For example, the English language system makes use of only about 45 different sound elements (phonemes), which can be differentiated from each other because they change the meaning of a sound sequence. For example, the words *bat* and *cat* have different meanings in English. The *b* and *c* are distinct sound elements (phonemes) because they signal these differences in meaning.

Semantics is the study of linguistic units of meaning. As children, we learn that certain sound sequences consistently symbolize specific meanings. As children's language systems mature, the quantity and specificity of their vocabularies increase. For example, a child initially may label all animals *dogs*. However, in time, the label *dog* is attached to a specific animal and the words *cat, horse, cow, mouse,* and *elephant* are added to the vocabulary. As normal adults speak, appropriate words are selected and produced rapidly (approximately 160 to 180 words per minute).

Syntax refers to the rules used to establish structured word relationships in forming phrases and sentences. Such rules are complex and numerous. For example, a change in word order can result in a change in meaning ("The dog bit the boy" versus "The boy bit the dog"). Children learn to generate sentences using most syntactic rules accurately by the time they enter school. However, only during the school years do they learn the most complex rules of syntax and to verbalize the specific grammatical rules of our language. Eventually, errors of usage are eliminated as older children learn exceptions to grammatical rules. Language development has been studied extensively.[16, 38, 145] A detailed review is beyond the scope of this chapter. However, Cohen and Cross[33] have edited a resource book describing many aspects of child development, including language development.

Pragmatics refers to the rules regarding the function of language in social contexts. For example, language can be used for such functions as to demand, command, request, protest, threaten, impress, placate, or regulate. The rules of pragmatics also apply to dialogue strategies and to conversational interactions that occur in human communication. This relatively new field of study is receiving increased attention in both adult and child language research.[8, 38]

Speech

Speech is the motor activity by which the oral, laryngeal, and respiratory structures produce the sound patterns of a language. Speech production involves the dynamic interaction of various components of the speaking mechanism. Despite the complex interactions among the various components of the speech mechanism, each is discussed separately. Selected speech mechanism muscles and their motor innervations are listed in Table 5–1.

RESPIRATION

Respiration is the energy source for speech. The respiratory system is responsible for generating subglottal air pressure below the vocal folds. This pressure is maintained or varied depending on the loudness level the speaker wishes to achieve. Normal speech is produced during the exhalation phase of respiration. Speech loudness (intensity) in-

TABLE 5–1. Selected Muscles of Speech Mechanism with Motor Innervation*

MUSCLES	MOTOR INNERVATION
Respiration	
Diaphragm	Phrenic
Sternomastoid	Accessory (XI)
External intercostals	Intercostals T_2 through T_{12}
Internal intercostals	Intercostals T_2 through T_{12}
External and internal oblique	Intercostals T_6 through T_{12}
Transversus abdominis	Intercostals T_7 through T_{12}
Phonation	
Interarytenoid	Vagus (X), inferior
Lateral cricoarytenoid	Vagus (X), recurrent branch
Posterior cricoarytenoid	Vagus (X), recurrent branch
Thyroarytenoid	Vagus (X), recurrent branch
Cricothyroid	Vagus (X), recurrent branch
Articulation	
Tongue	
Superior longitudinal	Hypoglossal (XII)
Inferior longitudinal	Hypoglossal (XII)
Transversus	Hypoglossal (XII)
Styloglossus	Hypoglossal (XII)
Palatoglossus	Accessory (XI)
Hypoglossus	Hypoglossal (XII)
Genioglossus	Hypoglossal (XII)
Mandible	
Masseter	Trigeminal (V), anterior
Temporalis	Trunk of mandibular branch
Internal, external, and pterygoid	Trunk of mandibular branch
Velopharyngeal mechanism	
Levator palatini	Vagus (X)
Tensor palatini	Trigeminal (V)
Palatoglossus	Accessory (XI)
Pharyngeal constrictor	Vagus (X)

*After Zemlin, W.: Speech and Hearing Sciences: Anatomy and Physiology. 3rd ed., Englewood Cliffs, NJ, Prentice-Hall, 1968, pp. 403, 404, 405.

creases in proportion to the increase in subglottal air pressure. Since the average utterance varies minimally in loudness, the respiratory mechanism must ensure that a relatively constant level of subglottal air pressure is maintained throughout the utterance even though the lung volume level changes and the relative contributions of the elastic recoil forces of the structure of the lungs and thorax and the inspiratory and expiratory muscles change. This interaction between muscle activity and lung volume level during speech has been studied extensively[80] and is summarized as follows:

KATHRYN M. YORKSTON AND DAVID R. BEUKELMAN

The amount of muscular pressure required at a given instant during speech depends upon the alveolar pressure (subglottal air pressure) needed and the relaxation pressure available at the prevailing lung volume.[79]

During "high" lung volumes, the pressure bias of the muscles of the respiratory system is inspiratory in nature, thus checking the combined recoil forces of the lungs and thorax. During "low" lung volume levels, the combined recoil forces of the lungs and thorax are supplemented increasingly by the net expiratory muscular pressure. Recent research[81] suggests slightly different speech breathing behavior from a senescent client than from a young adult client. Specifically, when contrasting young adult speakers (approximately 25 years of age) with elderly speakers (approximately 75 years of age), older speakers might be expected to speak using (1) high lung volume and rib cage initiations, (2) larger lung volume and rib cage volume excursions, (3) fewer syllables per breath, and (4) greater average lung volume expended per syllable.

PHONATION

Phonation refers to laryngeal sound production in speech. Two types of phonation occur during speech, voicing and whispering. Generally, voiced phonation occurs during the normal production of all vowels and voiced consonant sounds. Voicing is achieved by adducting the vocal folds to constrict the glottis, thereby momentarily interrupting the flow of air from the trachea through the larynx. The build-up of subglottal air pressure below the adducted folds causes the folds to be "blown apart," and a puff of air escapes into the upper vocal tract. A combination of the elastic recoil and muscle force of the laryngeal structures and the Bernoulli effect draws the vocal folds once again into the adducted position. This pattern is repeated many times per second, with an average fundamental frequency of around 125 Hz for men and 200 Hz for women.

Fundamental frequency (pitch) and intensity (loudness) are two speech parameters controlled primarily by the interaction of the laryngeal and respiratory systems. Fundamental frequency is controlled by changes in vocal fold thickness, mass, length, and tension.[85, 86] Generally, an increasing fundamental frequency contour is associated with increase of (1) vocal fold length, and with it the longitudinal tension of the folds (stretching the folds), or (2) medial compression (adductory squeeze), or a decrease in vocal fold thickness and

mass. With other factors constant, an increase in subglottal air pressure results in an increase in fundamental frequency.

Intensity adjustments are controlled by subtle interactions between the respiratory and laryngeal systems. There appears to be a close relationship between subglottal air pressure and voice intensity. A doubling of subglottal air pressure is associated with a 9 to 12 decibel increase in voice intensity.[27] Usually, the pattern of vocal fold movement changes as intensity is increased. The duration of the closed phase (time that the vocal folds are approximated) is increased, and the duration of the open phase of each vibratory cycle of the folds is decreased. This change probably occurs because of an increase in medial compression of the folds associated with increases in intensity.

ARTICULATION

The vocal tract is a dynamic tubelike series of cavities beginning at the vocal folds and ending at the lips. The soft palate and pharynx, tongue, lips, cheeks, and mandible are the primary structures of articulation whose movements influence the shape and configuration of the vocal tract. Individual speech sounds are acoustic events that are made of a combination of acoustic vibration and silent intervals that occur when the air within the vocal tract is set into vibration, is impeded, or is modified in some other way (e.g., fricated between the teeth and tongue or lips). The major source of energy for speech sound production is the flow of air from the lungs. When specific speech sounds are produced in isolation, the speaker produces an ideal configuration of the vocal tract. During running speech in casual conversation, ideal targets are rarely met.

Speech sounds have been divided into two categories, vowels and consonants. Vowels include a family of sounds that are produced with a relatively open oral tract. The sound source is at the level of the larynx, and the distinct identity of each vowel depends on the shape and size of various cavities in the vocal tract. The critical factors in vowel production are the height of the dorsum of the tongue, the front-to-back position of the high point of the tongue in the oral cavity, and the degree of lip opening. The consonant category includes a group of sounds in which the vocal tract is completely or closely constricted during sound production. The sound source for these consonants may be a turbulent source in the oral cavity, e.g., /s/ and /f/, with no laryngeal sound source (voiceless consonants); a combination of a turbulent sound source in the oral cavity and a laryngeal sound source, e.g., /z/ and /v/ (voiced consonants); or sounds with only a laryngeal sound source, e.g., /l/.

The articulatory targets of most vowel and consonant sounds include a complete or nearly complete closure of the velopharyngeal port (the passage from the oral into the nasal cavity). The nasal consonants (/m/, /n/, and /ng/) are exceptions to this pattern, as these sounds involve the radiation of acoustic energy through the nasal cavity. The degree of velopharyngeal closure that a speaker achieves during the production of a vowel may vary to some extent depending on the adjacent sounds. If the adjacent sounds require complete velopharyngeal closure, the port will probably be closed during the production of the intervening vowel. If one or both of the adjacent sounds is a nasal consonant, the velopharyngeal port may not be completely closed during the production of the intervening vowel.

PROSODY

Prosody encompasses the rate, rhythm, loudness, and pitch contours that signal stress and therefore carry additional meaning beyond individual speech sounds, words, or sequences of words. It is an overall dimension of verbal communication that cannot be ascribed to any of the speech mechanism components described earlier. Overall prosodic patterns are produced by a complex interaction of all of the speech components. A normal speaker will produce the sentence "Show Sam some snow" differently depending on whether it is in response to the question "To whom should I show the snow?" or to "What should I show Sam?" Normal stressing patterns are achieved by subtle changes in fundamental frequency, loudness, and duration.[109]

Aphasia

Aphasia is defined as an impairment in the ability to interpret and formulate language symbols as a result of brain damage.[32, 43, 47, 101] Darley[40] describes aphasia as a disorder of the "central language process" that underlies the various language modalities, such as comprehension of verbal material, reading, speaking, and writing. The most common cause of aphasia (85 per cent) is left cerebral vascular accident.[87, 104] Although specific prevalence figures for aphasia are not available, it has been estimated that two million Americans are handicapped to some degree by stroke.[181] Other common causes of aphasia are arteriovenous malformation, tumor, and head injury.

Terminology

Aphasia is not restricted to one language process; rather, an aphasic individual has reduced ability in all language modalities, including speaking, auditory comprehension, reading, writing, and expression through pantomime. Patients exhibit a variety of different patterns of deficits. For example, some patients exhibit auditory comprehension problems that are disproportionately severe when compared with problems exhibited in naming or other verbal tasks. Other patients may have relatively severe word-finding problems yet perform fairly well on auditory comprehension tasks. These differences in patterns of deficits seen in behavioral examination form the basis for classifying aphasic patients.

One widely used descriptive system to classify aphasic speakers is based on the patients' verbal output.[58] The fluent aphasias are associated with lesions that are posterior to the rolandic fissure. These aphasias are characterized by effortless, well-articulated speech with normal speech rhythm and melody. Failure to use the correct word is common. Words devoid of content, nonspecific words, and circumlocutions frequently occur. The verbal output of a severely involved, fluent speaker may contain jargon or nonsense words as well as meaningful ones. Fluent aphasics often do not recognize their errors. The nonfluent aphasias, on the other hand, are associated with lesions anterior to the rolandic fissure. They are characterized by limited speech that is uttered slowly, with great effort, and may often be telegraphic in nature, containing only the information-bearing words and excluding the words necessary for complete grammatical structure, such as prepositions and conjunctions. Patients with nonfluent aphasia generally have less difficulty comprehending than formulating language, but they do have difficulty comprehending language that involves lengthy, syntactically complex sentences.

Within the broad fluent/nonfluent dichotomy, more specific subtypes of aphasia can be identified by including other language processes such as auditory comprehension, naming ability, and the ability to repeat (Fig. 5–1).

KATHRYN M. YORKSTON AND DAVID R. BEUKELMAN

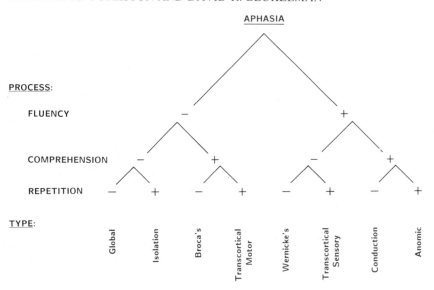

FIGURE 5–1. The pattern of deficits for varying types of aphasia. (For a description of terms, see Aphasia and Associated Disorders: Taxonomy, Localization, and Recovery. New York, Grune & Stratton, 1979.)

Global Aphasia: Severe deficits are found in all language processes, including speech production, auditory comprehension, reading, and writing.

Isolation Aphasia: All language processes are poor, except for the ability to repeat.

Broca's Aphasia: Speech is effortful and halting, with impaired articulation and reduced grammar. Comprehension is relatively good except for syntactically complex sentences, and reading is superior to writing.

Transcortical Motor Aphasia: Speech, in some ways, is similar to Broca's aphasia. However, the cardinal feature of this rare syndrome of aphasia is the preserved ability to repeat fluently to a degree that would not be expected from observing spontaneous speech.

Wernicke's Aphasia: Speech is fluent with paraphasic errors (sounds in words may be substituted for one another; order may be reversed). Auditory comprehension, reading, and writing are also impaired.

Transcortical Sensory Aphasia: This rare syndrome is similar to Wernicke's aphasia; however, the ability to repeat is remarkably preserved.

Conduction Aphasia: Spontaneous speech is relatively fluent with good comprehension, but there is selective loss of the ability to repeat.

Anomic Aphasia: Speech is well-articulated, grammatical, and fluent, but it is marked by severe word-finding difficulties and circumlocutionary attempts. Auditory comprehension is good, and reading and writing are variable.

With the availability of CT scan information regarding localization of lesion, a number of subcortical lesion sites with specific patterns of speech and language behavior are being identified.[14, 15, 76, 77, 154] For example, in thalamic aphasia,[14, 154] spontaneous speech is minimal. Verbal output is characterized by word-finding problems, perseveration, neologisms, and fading volume. Auditory comprehension and word repetition are intact. Three subcortical syndromes have been identified,[137] one with features resembling Broca's aphasia, one resembling Wernicke's aphasia, and one resembling global aphasia.

Neurological Correlates

For most people, the language centers are in the left cerebral hemisphere. The reported incidence of aphasia with right cerebral insult varied up to 10 per cent in right-handed individuals and from 10 to 20 per cent in left-handed individuals.[131] Within the left hemisphere, fluent aphasia is usually associated with damage in the posterior parietal and temporal lobes, and nonfluent aphasia is associated with more anterior lesions in the left hemisphere.

Studies of localization of language function have a long history. For 100 years, attempts have been made to specify areas of cortical function via autopsy findings of aphasic individuals who exhibited typical behavioral patterns.[172] This type of investigation has several obvious disadvantages, not the least of which is the fact that long periods of time often elapsed between onset of the disorder and the postmortem examination. Localization of language function in the left hemisphere has also been explored via cortical mapping of neurosurgical patients undergoing resection for medically intractable focal epilepsy.[148] During these experiments, weak electrical currents were applied to the cortex during a naming task. In a study of 11 patients, results indicated that the extent of the language cortex in an individual can be wider than that traditionally proposed. Only a narrow band of posterior inferior frontal lobe, immediately anterior to the motor strip, showed involvement in all patients. Within the larger language areas, language is discretely localized, with different sites variably committed to the naming function.

With the onset of a number of new brain-imaging techniques, our knowledge of the neurological correlates of aphasia has expanded rapidly. The following review is designed to provide a brief introduction to the topic with references provided for more in-depth investigation.

Naeser and his colleagues[139] reported that four kinds of *computed axial tomography* (CT) data are essential to predict severity of aphasia: the number of slices on which a lesion appears, the size of lesion on each slice, the average CT number of the lesion, and the neuroanatomical locus of the lesion. CT scans have provided an excellent technique for examination of the relationship between nature of lesions and type/severity of aphasia, and they have confirmed some traditional concepts. For example, Kertesz et al.,[105] in a blind research design, compared localization results obtained from CT scans with classifications derived from clinical testing. Results indicate that there are

. . . distinct areas of Broca's, conduction and Wernicke's aphasia along the parasylvian axis of the lateral templates. Lesion of global aphasics covered all of these areas, while transcorticals were outside of them. Lesion size and severity of aphasia showed significant correlations.

Other studies have necessitated the revision of traditional concepts regarding aphasia.[7] For example, Mohr et al.[133] used autopsy reports, arteriograms, and CT scans to compare anatomical and clinical findings of Broca's aphasia. They found that when damage was limited to Broca's area, the clinical symptoms were not those of Broca's aphasia but rather were characterized by mutism replaced by a rapidly improving dyspraxia and effortful articulation. Further, the speech disorder clinically labeled Broca's aphasia results from damage extending outside Broca's area. Studies of global aphasia have also been revealing, with various studies suggesting that it does not necessarily result from large lesions involving both Broca's and Wernicke's areas[123] and that lesions resulting in global aphasia may be large or small, anterior or posterior, single or multiple.[151] Data from CT scans have also led to a revision of the concept that aphasia is exclusively a cortical disorder.[39, 137] Because individuals with aphasia may "pass through" a number of differential types of aphasia as they improve, literature relating CT scan information to the evolution of aphasia is also available.[107, 138, 150, 194]

Positron emission tomography (PET) scans have been used to study local cerebral metabolic rates of glucose in various types of aphasia.[71, 72, 99, 125] Results of this work have suggested metabolic depression extending beyond the zone of infarction, implying that function in nonstructurally damaged tissue was not normal.[124, 126, 127]

Cerebral blood flow techniques in which radioisotopes are infused into the brain are also being used to study aphasia.[88] Although studies report different rCBF patterns for motor, sensory, and global aphasia, most do not find a close correspondence between rCBF patterns and classical localization models.[173] Several studies have found right hemisphere increase in lieu of increases in the damaged left hemisphere in aphasia patients.[128, 193]

Assessment

Extensive and systematic language assessment can serve a variety of purposes. One of the primary goals of assessment is to arrive at a differential diagnosis of the type of aphasia. In order to do this, systematic samples of a variety of language tasks, including speaking, listening, reading, and writing, must be obtained. This allows the clinician to identify the pattern of deficits in order to differentiate aphasia from other neurogenic communication disorders or to classify subtypes of aphasia.

A second major purpose for assessment of aphasia is to measure the severity of the disorder. The broad classification of aphasia is not sufficient to describe fully the language capabilities of an aphasic individual. Because a wide range of sever-

KATHRYN M. YORKSTON AND DAVID R. BEUKELMAN

ity levels are possible, some measure of the degree of processing deficits is also necessary. In the area of auditory comprehension, the most severe deficits may be characterized by an inability to understand any verbal message. With less severe deficits, the patient may be able to comprehend single words or single-stage directions and to respond to brief yes/no questions. In the mild range of impairment, an aphasic patient may be able to understand ordinary conversations with only occasional repetition. In the area of verbal output, a patient with severe deficits may not speak or may produce only jargon. With less severe deficits, the patient may produce automatic phrases or name simple objects and actions. In the mild range of impairment, the patient may convey information slowly with some word-finding, grammatical, or articulatory problems. Reading and writing disorders range in severity from an inability to read or write single words to slowness in handling adult-level material.

The third major function of assessment is to establish a prognosis for recovery of language skills. Both severity and type of aphasia have important prognostic implications. Kertesz et al.,[106] in a long-term follow-up study, found that global aphasic patients frequently exhibited good recovery. Severity of the overall impairment at one, three, and six months after onset can also be used to predict performance at points later in the recovery.[153] For those patients with severe language deficits, recovery is not expected to be as great as for those with moderate or mild deficits. For the severely aphasic patient, changes that occur in communication performance, as measured by standardized tests, may not be reflected in increasing ability to perform functionally in other communication situations. This point can be illustrated with the example of a severely aphasic speaker who may show improvement in test performance on easier tasks, such as matching identical objects or matching pictures of objects with actual objects, but whose functional communication ability remains severely impaired.

The fourth major function served by the assessment process is the identification of realistic treatment goals and appropriate treatment tasks. Selection of appropriate treatment tasks involves identification of tasks that have functional relevance and are at an appropriate level of difficulty. The difficulty level varies from patient to patient and is defined by that individual's unique skills and needs. Generally, a level is selected at which the patient is able to achieve a high success rate. With

a success rate of approximately 80 per cent, the patient does not experience excessive frustration, yet errors are frequent enough that the patient is continually forced to actively process the stimulus and monitor the response for possible errors. Because standardized aphasia tests typically sample many tasks, they allow the clinician to select tasks at the appropriate difficulty levels for each of the language areas. Routine administration of standardized tests allows the monitoring of performance. Decisions to continue or terminate treatment often are based on this information.

The standardized tests commonly used by speech/language pathologists to evaluate language disturbances in adult-injured individuals are listed with a brief description of each.

Minnesota Test for Differential Diagnosis of Aphasia:[167] This test includes 47 different subtests that focus on five disorder areas, including (1) auditory disturbances, (2) visual and reading disturbances, (3) speech and language disturbances, (4) visual, motor, and handwriting disturbances, and (5) disturbances of numerical relationships and arithmetic processes. The responses are scored as either correct or incorrect.

Boston Diagnostic Aphasia Examination:[63] This test evaluates auditory comprehension, oral expression, understanding of written language, and writing. Responses are scored either in a plus-minus fashion, on a rating scale, or with longhand notation, depending on the subtest. Test results are arranged on a profile of characteristics according to subtest scores. These profiles are particularly useful in classifying patients into the various subtypes of aphasia.

Porch Index of Communicative Ability:[152] This test contains 18 10-item subtests measuring communicative behavior in the gestural, verbal, and graphic output modalities. Responses are scored according to a 16-point multidimensional system based on accuracy, responsiveness, completeness, and promptness. Because of the multidimensional scoring and standardized administration techniques, special training is required in administering and interpreting this test. Results are reported in percentiles comparing the patient's performance with a large group of left hemisphere–damaged individuals. This test can be readministered on a monthly basis and can be used to establish a prognosis and to assess therapeutic progress.

Western Aphasia Battery:[103, 106, 170] This test is sensitive to fluency, information content, comprehension, repetition, and naming ability. Responses are scored on a 1- to 10- to 100-point scale depending on the subtest. Patterns of performance among the subtests categorize the patient according to the type of aphasia.

Token Test:[22, 51] This is not a comprehensive test but focuses on auditory comprehension skills. The test contains 20 unique tokens of various sizes, shapes, and colors. The patient is asked to follow 36 orally presented commands at various difficulty levels. This test is particularly sensitive to mild auditory comprehension deficits. Cutoff scores separate "normal" from "aphasic" performance. Scores can be adjusted for educational level.

The Functional Communication Profile:[163] This profile consists of 45 communication behaviors that are rated on a 9-point scale. Behaviors are divided into five major groups: movement (gesture), speaking, understanding, reading, and other (handling money, and so on). Data are collected in an interview format.

Communicative Abilities in Daily Living:[83] This test consists of 68 items incorporating everyday language activities presented in a natural style to approximate normal communication. Responses are scored on a 3-point scoring system—wrong, adequate, or correct. Results yield information about the functional communications skills of aphasic patients.

Boston Naming Test:[97] This test consists of 60 pictures, ordered from easiest to most difficult. If patients are unable to name the objects, they are first given "stimulus" cues (e.g., it's something to eat) and later given "phonemic" cues (e.g., the first sound of the word). Norms are available for children, normal adults, and adult aphasic patients.

Treatment Goals

The speech/language pathologist's major goal is to establish the most effective means of communication by which aphasic individuals can relate meaningfully to those around them. Treatment tasks and goals depend on the nature and severity of the language disorder and may vary from patient to patient.[121] For example, goals for a patient with aphasia characterized by severe comprehension deficits and speech consisting largely of jargon are quite different from goals for a patient with fair comprehension and limited but appropriate speech. The following treatment approaches reflect a variety of techniques utilized by speech/language pathologists in dealing with aphasic individuals at different severity levels.

For severely involved patients, direct speech treatment involving drill and repetitive practice has not met with success.[120, 166] Tasks easy enough to ensure some success may not be functionally relevant. For example, a person's ability to match identical objects does not translate into "real-life" communication skills. For this reason, tasks at the appropriate difficulty level for the severely aphasic patient are often not tolerated by the patient. With the exception of a small number of highly structured programs,[75, 76, 78] little direct treatment is employed. However, a good deal of time is devoted to managing the patient's communication environment by counseling the family and training family members in techniques to optimize communication potential. The direct treatment of the severely involved aphasic patient may be limited to construction of an individualized "communication book" that includes photographs of the patient's family along with those who are currently providing care for him or her. Photographs illustrating needs, activities, and locations may also be incorporated. Experience has shown that severely involved aphasic patients tend to respond better to photographs, which are more concrete than symbolic line drawings. The aphasic patient can point to the communication book to indicate specific needs or a general topic. If necessary, the communication partner can obtain more specific information by asking a series of questions. Often patients and their communication partners need training in order to use such a system.

With aphasic individuals in the moderately severe to mild range, more direct speech treatment can be carried out and a variety of approaches can be taken.[32] The stimulation approach[168] stresses the repetitive presentation of stimuli designed to increase the patient's ability to organize, store, and retrieve language patterns formerly used. The speech/language pathologist functions not as a teacher but as a stimulator. This approach is based on the notion that the aphasic patient has not lost words but has lost the ability to retrieve, select, and sequence them. Stimuli of sufficient intensity are used so that responses are elicited, not forced. For example, rather than using a difficult confrontation naming task ("Tell me the name of the object.") with a patient who is experiencing word-finding difficulties, a sentence completion task ("You drink coffee out of a _____.") may be more appropriate.

Another widely used approach to direct treatment of moderately aphasic individuals is the programmed approach.[82] This approach centers on the application of learning principles, particularly those of shaping and differential reinforcement, to prompt reacquisition of language behavior. This approach is based on principles of programmed learning in which stimuli are controlled; as the patient improves, tasks are gradually made more difficult.

Promoting Aphasic's Communicative Effectiveness[47, 48] or PACE therapy is an approach to treatment designed to mimic a number of aspects of real face-to-face communication in structured clinical interactions. PACE is based on the following principles: (1) the clinician and patient participate equally as senders and receivers of messages, (2) there is an exchange of new information between the clinician and the patient, (3) the patient has a free choice as to which communication channels he or she may use to convey new information, and (4) feedback is provided by the clinician, as a receiver, in response to the patient's success in conveying the message.

With mildly aphasic patients, the speech/language pathologist must consider a new set of treatment strategies. The context-centered approach,[185] although not restricted exclusively to mild aphasia, is particularly useful with this group of patients. This approach deemphasizes direct language treatment and moves away from the search for specific words into the realm of ideas and thoughts. This technique is often used with high-level aphasics, who are encouraged to embellish and enrich content and move from concrete to more abstract and complete communication.

With the mildly aphasic patient, emphasis is placed on identification and remediation of specific vocational problems that might arise as a result of the communication disorder. Mildly aphasic individuals often are taught compensatory strategies to handle difficult communication tasks. For example, a mildly aphasic patient may be taught to create a detailed outline of business correspondence before actually writing a letter. The outline may contain not only a series of points that the writer wishes to make but also a system for logically organizing and sequencing them. The mildly aphasic speaker is often taught to make his or her communication partners aware of potential communication breakdowns. Mild language deficits may not be readily apparent, yet may cause the speaker a good deal of frustration.

Efficacy of Treatment

With any ongoing treatment program, regardless of severity or type of aphasia, the speech/language pathologist must be able to document the effectiveness of therapeutic intervention. Progress can be measured by readministering standardized tests and comparing current results with those of earlier testing sessions. The Porch Index of Communicative Ability (PICA)[152] is particularly sensitive to small changes in performance. This test not only gives an overall indication of change but also allows the clinician to identify changes in specific language areas such as verbal output, auditory comprehension, and graphic skills. Another way of monitoring progress is by maintaining careful records of scores on treatment tasks. In this way, the speech/language pathologist can identify trends in performance and document changing skills. Regardless of how it is obtained, a measure of progress is needed to justify continued treatment.

Predicting the pattern of recovery for a patient with aphasia is a complex process. Davis[47] presents some of the factors that must be considered:

Etiology: A traumatic injury may result in greater and more rapid recovery than an ischemic cerebral vascular accident (CVA).

Site of Lesions: Damage to marginal areas produces more complete and more rapid rate of recovery than damage to primary language areas.

Type of Aphasia: Broca's and conduction aphasia demonstrate the largest amount of recovery. Anomic aphasia results in best outcome. Wernicke's aphasia has demonstrated a mixture of poor and good recovery that may occur at a slower rate. Global has a poor prognosis for improvement of verbal expression, but auditory comprehension does improve with treatment as late as 6 to 12 months after onset.

Initial Severity: There appears to be a nonlinear relationship to amount, with the most severe and mild forms resulting in less recovery than moderate aphasias. Severity of auditory comprehension deficit may be predictive of overall recovery.

Age at Onset: Although some studies indicate that it is not an important predictor, chronological age may still make a difference because of the medical, psychological, and social complications that can accompany aging.

Lateralization: There may be more rapid recovery in left-handed patients and patients with a tendency toward left-handedness.

Time Since Onset: A later observation after onset means that less recovery can be expected subsequently.

Treatment: It has a favorable impact on recovery no matter when it occurs after onset of aphasia.

In addition to documenting or predicting changes in individual aphasic patients as treatment progresses and as recovery occurs, the question of efficacy of treatment has also been studied by examining changes in groups of treated and untreated patients. In this way, the issue of the contribution of spontaneous recovery to changing performance can be addressed. Darley[42] discussed a variety of research design problems, including the need to match groups in terms of age, etiology, site of lesion, initial severity, and so on. Despite these methodological problems, the literature contains several examples of group design efficacy studies. Basso et al.[6] studied the influence of language rehabilitation on 281 aphasic patients (162 treated and 119 untreated). They wrote that "rehabilitation had a significant positive effect on improvement in all language skills." Hagen[68] studied a group of 20 men with aphasia and found that several parameters changed more in treated than in untreated groups, including functional reading comprehension, language formulation, speech production, spelling, and arithmetic abilities. Vignolo[180] found that consistent improvement was noted if treatment was started between two and six months after onset and lasted longer than six months. Shewan and Kertesz[171] found that treated patients made significantly more improvement than did patients who were unable or who refused to participate in treatment.

Results of a large, well-controlled study of treatment efficiency were reported by Wertz and his colleagues.[189] Subjects were males between the ages of 40 and 80 years with pre-morbid reading and writing skills. They were aphasic as a result of a first thromboembolic CVA with damage localized to the left hemisphere and had no coexisting major medical complications. Time after onset at entry into the project was over four weeks. Severity levels ranged from the 15th to 75th overall percentile of the PICA. Subjects were randomly assigned to either traditional, individual stimulus-response type treatment of specific language deficits or group therapy designed to improve communication through group interaction and discussion. Results indicated that both groups improved significantly. The authors state,

If the traditional belief is correct, that significant spontaneous recovery is complete by three to six months post-onset, significant improvement in both groups beyond 26 weeks post-onset indicates both individual and group treatment are efficacious methods for managing aphasic patients.

In the second phase of their treatment efficacy study, Wertz and his colleagues[192] found patients treated in the clinic did better than a group of patients whose treatment was deferred. Patients whose treatment was deferred for 12 weeks ultimately improved as much as the early treatment group.

Right Hemisphere Lesions

Recently speech/language pathologists have become increasingly interested in the role played by the right hemisphere in communication and communication disorders. However, the research results as yet provide incomplete information.[29, 59, 134–136, 182, 184] A review of literature[57, 129, 169] leads to the conclusion that the right hemisphere possesses a far greater capacity to comprehend than to produce speech and language. In addition, Levine and Mohr[115] concluded from a study of the language of individuals with bilateral cerebral infarctions that the right hemisphere may also have some role in normal articulation. Myers[136] argues that the most significant advances of research in right hemisphere communication disorders have been in the areas of describing and delineating the deficits themselves. Communication-related impairment associated with right hemisphere damage includes (1) lower-order perceptual problems, which include left-sided neglect and various visuospatial deficits; (2) problems with affect and prosody; (3) linguistic disorders; and (4) higher-order perceptual and cognitive deficits, including those impairments that result in general communicative inefficiency.[135]

Traumatic Brain Injury

Nature of the Problem

Although head injury is the major cause of death in persons under the age of 35 years,[96] an increasing number of patients are surviving with residual deficits that bring them to the attention of rehabilitation teams. A growing literature exists describing the cognitive and linguistic sequelae of traumatic brain injury in children* and adults.† A number of features distinguish head-injured patients from other patients with neurogenic com-

---

*See references 26, 28, 30, 31, 55, 60, and 161.
†See references 52, 66, 67, 111, 113, 116, 140, 160, 176, and 177.

munication disorders. First, the typical head-injured patient has an onset at a much younger age than does a post-stroke patient, thus necessitating long-term follow-up. Second, head injuries, especially closed head injuries, tend to produce diffuse rather than focal deficits, thus necessitating a multidisciplinary rehabilitation effort in order to address the complex cognitive, communicative, physical, social, and vocational problems faced by this population.

Communication Problems

A wide variety of communication problems may occur as the result of traumatic brain injury. Perhaps the most frequently occurring are language deficits called by various authors "subclinical aphasia,"[164, 165] "latent aphasia,"[22] "cognitive-language disorganization,"[69] and "confused language."[187] These deficits are different from aphasia[1, 84] in that language may be disrupted as part of a complex constellation of memory and cognitive deficits rather than as an isolated deficit as in aphasia. Characteristics of confused language[70] include reduced recognition of, understanding of, and responsiveness to the environment. Other sequelae of the disorder are disorientation to time and place, short-term memory loss, difficulty "tuning in" to novel tasks, impaired comprehension, rambling and incoherent speech, and inability to function on an abstract level. Traumatically brain-injured patients exhibit a unique pattern of language deficits as compared with aphasic individuals.[18, 66, 70] Other communication disorders experienced by traumatically brain-injured patients include classical aphasia,[165] dysarthria,[198] apraxia of speech, speechlessness resulting from persistent vegetative state,[92] and akinetic mutism.[114, 162]

Course of Recovery

Studies of the long-term outcome following traumatic brain injury are available[91, 94, 112, 175] and may be helpful in prognosis. The following levels of cognitive functioning were developed at Ranchos Los Amigos[69] as a behavioral rating scale to describe the progression of recovery of cognitive and communication function:

Level I: No response: Patient is completely unresponsive to any stimuli.

Level II: Generalized response: Patient reacts inconsistently and nonpurposefully to stimuli in a nonspecific manner. Responses may be physiological changes, gross body movements, and vocalization.

Level III: Localized response: Patient reacts specifically but inconsistently to stimuli presented, as in turning head toward a sound.

Level IV: Confused-agitated: Patient is in a heightened state of activity with severely decreased ability to process information. Behavior is frequently bizarre and out of proportion to stimuli.

Level V: Confused-inappropriate: Patient appears alert and is able to respond to simple commands fairly consistently. However, with increased complexity of commands, responses are nonpurposeful.

Level VI: Confused-appropriate: Patient shows goal-directed behavior, but is dependent on external input for directions. Responses may be incorrect owing to memory problems but are appropriate to the situation.

Level VII: Automatic-appropriate: Patient appears appropriate and oriented within hospital and home settings, goes through daily routine automatically but robot-like, with minimal to absent confusion, and has shallow recall of what he or she has been doing.

Level VIII: Purposeful-appropriate: Patient is alert and oriented, is able to recall and integrate past and recent events, and is aware of and responsive to his or her culture. The patient may continue to show decreases relative to pre-morbid ability in quality and rate of processing and abstract reasoning.

Treatment

Although the literature contains a growing number of descriptions of management programs,* well-controlled treatment efficacy studies are not yet available. The following are representative of the several approaches currently used with traumatically head-injured patients. *Cognitive process retraining* involves identifying cognitive components that are deficient, e.g., sequencing, memory, attention, and attempting to improve patient performance by drills. It is assumed that generalization to other tasks will follow. *Task-specific teaching* involves specifying behaviors that patients need to learn, systematically teaching that behavior, and monitoring changing performance. Examples of

---

*See references 2, 54, 93, 119, 132, 155, 194, and 196.

tasks might be teaching the patient to use a written sequence of grooming activities in the morning. *Environmental organization* involves imposing enough structure to enable the patient to function successfully. For example, an agitated patient might be put in an active environment as a spectator and successful performance defined as being nondisruptive. *Training self-coaching*[74, 196] involves teaching self-awareness and goal-setting. For example, video-recorded samples of the patient interactions may be reviewed as a means of identifying and reducing inappropriate behaviors.

Language Disorders Associated with Dementia

Dementia is a condition resulting in a chronic progressive deterioration of intellect, memory, and communication function resulting from organic brain disease.[3, 9–12, 35] The cardinal features of dementia are disorientation, impaired memory, defective calculation, and labile affect. Etiological factors may include Alzheimer's disease, multi-infarct dementia, Pick's disease, Parkinson's disease, Huntington's disease, and Korsakoff's disease. The language problems associated with dementia are beginning to receive considerable attention.[11, 13, 146, 147] The following description has been offered for the language disorders associated with generalized intellectual impairment:[41, 187]

Deterioration of performance on more difficult language tasks; reduced efficiency in all modes; greater impairment evident in language tasks requiring better retention, closer attention, and powers of abstraction and generalization; degree of language impairment roughly proportionate to deterioration of other mental functions.

The language disorders associated with dementia change as a function of the course of the disease. The following chronology of dementia is offered by Bayles:[10]

Early Stages: Language impairment is likely to go unnoticed in casual conversation. Although the content of conversation may be somewhat inappropriate because of word boundary erosion, the patient adheres to rules of syntax and phonology.

Middle Stages: The patient may be disoriented for time and place, but oriented for person. Language impairment is apparent, and conversation is vague, empty, and often irrelevant. Utterances are well formed in terms of phonological rule, but syntactic errors may be present.

Late Stages: The patient may be disoriented for time, place, and person, and may not recognize family members. Patients may be mute, be echolalic, or produce bizarre nonsensical utterances. Semantics, syntax, and phonology are all grossly disrupted.

The management of demented patients is a topic of some debate among speech/language pathologists. Golper and Rau[61] express a commonly held opinion when they write:

Nothing we have observed from working with patients who have generalized intellectual deficits, their families, or nursing staff personnel would cause us to feel that persons diagnosed as "demented" are particularly good candidates for learning adaptive or compensatory strategies to aid their communication.

Despite the fact that direct treatment focusing on reducing the impairment may not be appropriate, a number of indirect intervention approaches have been suggested,[23, 61, 141] including prosthetic aids, environmental adjustments and stimulation therapies, and spouse/family counseling.

Apraxia of Speech

Apraxia of speech is a sensorimotor disorder of articulation and prosody that frequently accompanies nonfluent aphasia and may also coexist with dysarthria.[187] Some writers disagree with the use of the term apraxia, feeling that the disorder is too closely associated with aphasia to be considered a separate entity.[122] However, because apraxia of speech includes some characteristics that distinguish it from other neurogenic language and speech disorders and because the treatment strategies typically employed are unique, apraxia of speech will be considered as a separate disorder. Apraxia of speech occurs in the absence of significant weakness or incoordination when performing reflexive or automatic movements.[49] It is characterized by impaired ability to program the positioning of the speech musculature and to sequence the movements for volitional production of speech. The physiological,[56, 89, 90, 178] acoustic,[179] and linguistic aspects of apraxia have also been investigated.[159]

Assessment

Because apraxia almost always appears concomitantly with aphasia, the speech/language pathologist will routinely administer standardized aphasia

KATHRYN M. YORKSTON AND DAVID R. BEUKELMAN

tests. With the apraxic speaker, these test results will usually indicate relatively intact auditory and reading comprehension skills. Writing skills are better than speaking skills. Tests specifically focusing on apraxia are also available.[36] The pattern of articulatory breakdown in apraxia is characteristic[95] in that articulatory errors include omissions, substitutions, distortions, additions, and repetition of speech sounds. Many of these errors appear to be off-target approximations made in an effortful manner. Apraxic speakers often appear to be groping for the proper articulatory position or sequence of positions. Errors are highly inconsistent, varying with the complexity of the sound patterns and length of the target words. There is a discrepancy between the accuracy of automatic-reactive speech and inaccuracy of volitional-purposeful speech. The speaker is often aware of errors but is usually unable to anticipate or correct them. If the patient attempts to monitor his or her speech, anticipation of errors often leads to a slowed rate and even stress and pacing.

Treatment

Treatment of apraxia of speech typically involves highly structured, controlled, and intensive practice of sound patterns and speech.[37, 156] Rosenbek and associates[158] suggest the use of an eight-step task continuum ranging from maximum cueing (simultaneous production with the clinician after having heard and seen the phrase being produced) to eliciting responses in a role-playing situation. Another approach often used with nonfluent aphasics who exhibit apraxia is Melodic Intonation Therapy.[174] This is a four-level program in which natural melody patterns are used to facilitate speech. Phrases are accompanied by exaggerated natural melody and rhythm patterns. As the patient progresses through the program, the melody and rhythm cues are gradually faded. Candidates for this treatment procedure have good auditory comprehension and good error recognition in the presence of severe articulatory deficits and poor ability to repeat.

Efficacy of speech treatment for apraxia has been documented for both single case and group studies.[50, 158, 186] Wertz[186] summarized the results of the Veterans' Administration Cooperative Study in which 19 subjects with apraxia of speech received treatment. The majority (74 per cent) improved. Results indicated that the type of treatment influenced whether improvement occurred, with four of five patients who did not improve receiving group treatment with no direct focus on motor speech practice.

Dysarthria

Differential Diagnosis

Dysarthria is a term that refers to a group of speech disorders resulting from a disturbance of motor control—weakness, slowness, or incoordination—of the speech mechanism due to damage to the central or peripheral nervous system.[46] Dysarthric speakers usually have normal auditory comprehension and can select words correctly and order them in grammatical strings without difficulty. However, they experience difficulty saying words and sounds precisely with appropriate stress, loudness, and pitch control.

The pattern of speech characteristics produced by a specific dysarthric individual depends on the site of neurological lesion and the severity of speech impairment.[46]

Flaccid Dysarthria: Damage to the nerves (or their nuclei) will result in speech characterized by breathy voice, hypernasality, imprecisely produced consonants, reduced speech loudness, and air escape through the nose (nasal emission). Flaccid dysarthria occurs in patients with a low brain stem stroke, polio, or myasthenia gravis.

Spastic Dysarthria: If the site of neurological lesion involves the upper motor neurons, a spastic condition may result in a speech pattern characterized by imprecise consonant production, monopitch, a strained-strangled voice quality, hypernasality, and occasional pitch breaks. Spastic dysarthric patterns are observed with spastic cerebral palsy and pseudobulbar palsy. Patients with amyotrophic lateral sclerosis will often exhibit a combination of flaccid and spastic dysarthria.

Ataxic Dysarthria: Patients with cerebellar disorders produce a characteristic speech pattern that includes irregular breakdowns and distortions of speech articulation. Prosodic patterns are unusual, in that some patients stress nearly all syllables equally, while others stress words and syllables inappropriately. These dysarthric speakers usually exhibit irregular, imprecise consonant production, distorted vowel production, excessive loudness variation, and occasional harsh voice. Ataxic dysarthria is found in patients with Friedreich's ataxia, some patients with multiple sclerosis, and some patients with severe head injury.

Hypokinetic Dysarthria: Patients with movement disorders also demonstrate unique dysarthric patterns. Parkinsonism is a neurological disorder of the basal ganglia, and the movements of these speakers are often reduced in rate. Hypokinetic dysarthric individuals usually speak with monopitch, reduced speech stress, short rushes of speech, inappropriate silences, and reduced speech loudness.

Hyperkinetic Dysarthria: Patients with movement disorders resulting in excessive motor activity, such as dystonia and chorea, exhibit hyperkinetic dysarthria. In dystonia, the dyskinesia is characterized by muscle contractions building slowly, distorting posture, and subsiding gradually. The dysarthric pattern includes imprecise consonant production, prolonged and distorted vowels, harsh voice, irregular articulation breakdowns, excessive loudness variations, and voice stoppages. Chorea, on the other hand, results in quick hyperkinesis with irregular, random, and unpatterned movements. Speech symptoms include imprecise speech articulation, speech sounds that are abnormally prolonged, variable speaking rate, and harsh voice.

Assessment

Assessment of dysarthric speech has taken a variety of forms, including overall assessment of the communication disability, and perceptual and component assessment of speech performance. Each of these approaches provides unique information. In *overall assessments* of the communication disability, the overall indicators of dysarthric speech performance are evaluated. The measurement of *speech intelligibility* provides an overall index of the speech disorder, which takes into account many different neuromuscular factors along with whatever compensatory strategies the dysarthric speaker may have adopted.[197, 199] Intelligibility measures are closely associated with other functional measures of communication such as the amount of information transferred.[19] Generally, intelligibility measures are a widely used index of speakers' disability level as they try to meet their communication needs of daily living. In addition to speech intelligibility, *speaking rate* is also an important overall measure. Taken together, speech intelligibility and speaking rate are used to provide an index of overall communication efficiency. In other words, a speaker who is 90 per cent intelligible who speaks at 70 words per minute is a less

efficient speaker than one with an intelligibility of 90 per cent who speaks at 140 words per minute. A third overall measure is *speech naturalness*. Speech is natural if it conforms to the listener's standards of rate, rhythm, intonation, and stress patterning, and if it conforms to the grammatical structure of the utterance being produced. It is considered unnatural or bizarre if it deviates from the expected or is unconventional.

The assessment of speech impairment is accomplished by both perceptual and physiological approaches. In perceptual assessment, Darley and co-workers[44, 45] rated dysarthric speech along 38 dimensions. Many of these perceptual dimensions were specific to one aspect of speech; for example, imprecise consonants, irregular articulatory breakdowns, and distorted vowels are all closely related to articulation. Other dimensions were more general—for example, intelligibility, bizarreness, and reduced stress. Results of this research revealed that clusters of deviant speech dimensions were associated with specific neurological disorders. This descriptive, perceptually based tool allows the speech/language pathologist to distinguish the various dysarthrias on the basis of a series of speech dimensions.

The physiological approach to assessing dysarthric speakers is described by Netsell[142–144] and Rosenbek and LaPointe.[157] The functional components of an individual's speech mechanism are systematically evaluated to determine the type and locus of breakdowns at points along the vocal tract where speech activities occur. For example, some speakers demonstrate their neuromotor deficits by failing to shorten the inhalation phase and lengthen the exhalation phase of respiration during speech. Others are unable to maintain relatively stable subglottal air pressure, and the loudness of their speech is abnormally variable or tends to decay toward the end of an utterance. Still others are unable to generate levels of subglottal air pressure (5 to 10 cm H_2O) needed to speak with appropriate loudness. Impairment of phonation may result in aphonia (absence of sound), dysphonia (distortions of sound quality), or disorders of pitch and loudness control. Neurogenic articulatory disorders may result in the inability to accurately achieve the movement patterns associated with target posture of various sounds. Imprecise sound production, substitution of one sound for another, or complete omission of sounds may result. If velopharyngeal mechanism control is deficient, hypernasality and nasal emission (air escape through the nose) will be present. Rosenbek and LaPointe[157] use the evaluation process to focus treatment. Abnormal function of speech mechanism components is identified so that treatment can be organized into a hierarchy based on the contribution of various symptoms to reduced intelligibility.

Treatment

The treatment hierarchy for dysarthric speakers who are recovering from a neurogenic impairment secondary to stroke, trauma, or surgery includes the following goals and procedures depending on severity level.[198] Initially, an early communication system is developed for the patient who is unable to speak functionally. Augmentative communication systems for these severely dysarthric individuals are discussed later in this chapter.

If a severely dysarthric speaker shows the potential for verbal communication, it is necessary to develop the motor skills involved in functional speech. This phase of treatment includes muscle strengthening and control exercises necessary for the production of single sounds. Next, the transition of speech mechanism movement from the target position for one sound to another sound is developed. All through this phase of the dysarthria treatment program, it is important that the speaker produce sounds that can be distinguished from one another by the listener. The next goal in treatment is to have the dysarthric speaker make the transition from producing single words and phrases in the treatment session to functional use of speech for communication for his or her daily needs. The authors commonly have their patients achieve this transition by teaching the dysarthric individuals to point to the first letter of each word on an alphabet board as they "speak." In this way, listeners are provided with additional information about the word that the dysarthric speaker is attempting to say. The use of this technique has allowed many dysarthric persons to begin to communicate verbally long before their speech intelligibility level without assistance would have permitted.

After the dysarthric person develops functional verbal communication supplemented by the alphabet board, the focus of treatment shifts to maximizing the intelligibility of speech. This involves training in specific skills or prosthetic management, or both. In an attempt to improve speech intelligibility, patients are taught to modify speaking rate, emphasize consonant sounds in important words, control the number of words per breath, and stress important words. Some patients need to be fitted with palatal lifts to reduce hypernasality and nasal emission.[62] The palatal lift consists of a dental retainer that is secured to the teeth (Fig. 5–2). A shelf attached to the retainer elevates the soft palate to the height necessary to reduce abnormal speech characteristics.

Once the recovering dysarthric speaker is intelligible, the last step in the treatment program is to increase the naturalness of speech. This is accomplished by teaching appropriate stress, loudness, and pitch patterns with consistently accurate articulation at a rate that allows intelligible speech.

The treatment hierarchy for dysarthria secondary to progressive diseases and conditions such as Parkinson's disease, multiple sclerosis, and amyotrophic lateral sclerosis is different from that for the recovering dysarthric individual. Initially, patients with progressive disorders are encouraged to maximize their level of functional communication by paying special attention to the clarity and precision of their speech. At some point, such patients will need to modify their speaking patterns by controlling rate, consonant emphasis, and number of words per breath. Some patients with progressive dysarthria make the adjustments in their speech pattern without specific treatment; others may need to practice these modifications with a speech/language pathologist or trained family member before the changes become habitual. In severe cases, communication augmentation systems may need to be considered. These systems are usually chosen or designed to accommodate most easily to the life styles of patients while serving their communicative needs over the longest period of time possible.

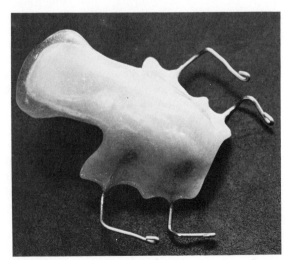

FIGURE 5–2. A palatal lift appliance for management of velopharyngeal dysfunction in dysarthria.

Reading Disorders in Neurologically Impaired Adults

The following discussion focuses on adult-onset, neurogenic reading deficits, which will be discussed in three broad categories. The first category includes reading disorders associated with aphasia. Since aphasia is defined as a language deficit that crosses all communication modalities, aphasic individuals will typically experience difficulty with oral and silent reading. These deficits are usually associated with left hemisphere lesions and are more prominent with posterior rather than anterior lesions. Severity can range from the inability to recognize simple words to mild reduction in the speech and efficiency with which adult-level material is read.

The second category includes reading disorders associated with perceptual problems. These reading deficits are typically associated with right hemisphere lesions and may be accompanied by left-sided neglect or visual field cuts. Individuals with perceptual problems will (1) experience difficulty scanning the line of print, (2) fail to return to the left margin of the page, and (3) skip lines of print. Reading rate is often significantly reduced, at times to the point where the individual is unable to understand the material. Difficulties are exaggerated by reducing the print size.

The third category includes reading disorders associated with confused language. Confused language has been characterized by Halpern and associates[70] as the reduced recognition and understanding of and responsiveness to the environment, faulty short-term memory, mistaken reasoning, and disorientation in the time and place. Reading deficits are often characterized by severely reduced comprehension in the face of relatively intact oral reading.

Assessment

When specific reading deficits are suspected, such as language-based (aphasias) or perceptually based problems, a variety of standardized and informal assessment techniques are available. Many standard aphasia test batteries sample reading performance with a variety of tasks that are graded in difficulty. For example, the Minnesota Test for Differential Diagnosis of Aphasia[167] contains a series of reading tasks ranging from matching shapes to the reading of paragraph length passages. LaPointe and Horner[108] have developed a reading battery entitled *Reading Comprehension Battery for Aphasia*, specifically designed to assess and monitor recovery of reading abilities in aphasic individuals. Perceptual deficits may be assessed using a series of written passages graded in perceptual difficulty. This series may range from large print and color-cued margins to standard newspaper print with multiple columns. Performance can be assessed by noting the number of tracking or scanning errors and reading rate as the patient reads the passage orally.

When the clinician is concerned with the extent to which reading deficits interfere with ordinary activities of living, a variety of functional tasks can be tested. A list of functional reading activities might include medicine bottle labels, bus and television schedules, and the like. These tasks are typically selected for patients on an individual basis depending on their communication needs. When considering the potential for return to educational or vocational settings, the reading performance of individuals with relatively mild reading deficits should be compared with that of the normal population. Standardized tests that have been normed on high-school and college students can be used for this purpose.

Treatment

With neurogenic reading disorders, treatment varies depending on the type of disorder. Reading deficits seen in aphasic patients are typically addressed as part of the normal course of treatment. Reading tasks can be ordered into a hierarchy of difficulty based on language-related variables including word frequency, grammatical complexity, and so on. As the patient improves, treatment progressively focuses on more difficult tasks.

Like the treatment of language-based reading deficits, the treatment of perceptually based deficits progresses through the hierarchy of tasks. Tasks can be ordered in terms of perceptual difficulty from easy tasks (large print, colored margins, markers to underscore lines of print) to more difficult tasks (small print, multiple columns, hyphenated words). The research of Weinberg and co-workers[183] indicated that this approach to remediating visual scanning difficulties is effective.

Reading treatment of severely confused patients is not typically undertaken for a variety of reasons. First, the combination of decreased error recognition and memory makes these patients poor treat-

KATHRYN M. YORKSTON AND DAVID R. BEUKELMAN

ment candidates. Second, traumatically caused confusion often clears during the initial phases of recovery. At the point in recovery when the confusion seems to have cleared, treatment of specific language or perceptually based reading deficits can be complete.

Voice Disorders

Phonation is a complex neuromotor activity; therefore, disorders of phonation may take several forms. Aphonia refers to an absence of phonation due to either hysterical problems or central or peripheral neurological problems interfering with the approximation of the vocal folds. Dysphonia refers to a number of phonatory disorders of sound quality that have a variety of causes. Vocal nodules are a callous formation at the anterior–middle third of the vocal folds. Laryngitis is an inflammation of the vocal folds, and vocal polyps are enlarged structures of a small blood vessel. Contact ulcers are an ulceration of the vocal folds on the free approximating margins of the vocal processes. Dysphonia may also result from forms of vocal fold paralysis or cancer of the larynx. In addition to dysfunction of the true vocal folds, adduction of the ventricular or false vocal folds during speech may occur as part of a disordered phonatory pattern. Spasmodic dysphonia refers to an intermittent strained, harsh voice with voice stoppage.

The primary objectives of the voice evaluation[4, 5, 24, 110] are (1) a detailed history of the phonatory problem, (2) a physical evaluation of the laryngeal structures by a laryngologist, (3) a description of current phonatory function, (4) the identification of use and abuse patterns that are contributing to the disorder, and (5) the determination of the patient's potential ability to modify phonatory patterns.

If the phonatory problem does not require medical treatment, a careful description of phonatory function includes an evaluation of pitch, quality, and loudness control. At times there is an interaction among these three parameters. For example, phonatory quality of some patients is dependent on the pitch range at which they are speaking. If the pitch is too low, the phonatory quality may be excessively harsh. The interaction between the phonatory and respiratory system is also important. Clavicular respiratory patterns are not conducive to clear, flexible, strong phonation; however, no particular pattern of breathing has been shown to be the best.

The speech treatment of noncancerous, nonparalytic voice problems usually involves several steps. First, an active program to minimize vocal abuse and at least temporarily decrease vocal use is initiated. Vocal abuse patterns of concern include such behaviors as smoking, excessive coughing and throat clearing, and talking or shouting over crowds or machine noise. Second, optimal pitch and loudness ranges for efficient phonatory production are selected. Third, the focus of sound resonance is shifted anteriorly from the pharyngeal to oral and nasal areas. Fourth, hard vocal fold approximations are replaced with easy, gentle approximations. Fifth, if present, abnormal respiratory patterns are modified.

Motor paralysis of the vocal folds can be unilateral or bilateral and may leave the folds in the adducted position or in several stages of abduction. A complete discussion of the causes of the various patterns of paralysis can be found in Hart[73] and Luchsinger and Arnold.[118] In case of complete abductor paralysis (folds in adducted position), the patient usually requires a tracheostomy initially to maintain a functional airway. Phonation may be achieved by plugging the tracheostomy tube with a finger and exhaling for speech. Eventually one of the folds may be surgically repositioned laterally in a somewhat abducted position, and thus establish an airway. However, this surgery results in phonatory quality that is breathy with reduced intensity. Recently, attempts to reinnervate the abductor muscle with a muscle pedicle transplant have shown some promise in restoring an airway and maintaining quality phonation in patients with abductor paralysis.[179] In the case of adductor paralysis (folds in abducted position), several surgical procedures may be employed, including surgically repositioning of a fold medially or implanting or injecting material into the fold to displace it toward the midline. Speech treatment for patients with motor paralysis of the vocal folds usually occurs in conjunction with the medical management program. The goal is to assist these patients to develop the most functional voice possible given the physical condition of the laryngeal mechanism.

Laryngeal cancer may initially be reflected in a phonatory disorder. The term "laryngectomy" refers to the partial or total removal of the larynx. An incomplete laryngectomy may or may not influence voice quality, depending on whether vocal fold tissue has been removed. The total laryngectomy results in complete loss of voice and most audible aspects of whisper. Depending on the type and extent of total laryngectomy surgery, three different speaking options may be available to the laryngectomee. First, a pseudoglottis or shunt constructed of human tissue or prosthetic material allows air to pass from the trachea into the esophagus, and sound is produced by vibrating esophageal tissue. Second, in laryngectomy patients without shunt, esophageal voice is produced by vibration of the upper narrow portion of the esophagus when air is injected into the esophagus and released. Third, a neck type or intraoral type of electrolarynx serves as a sound source and the laryngectomee "mouths" the messages. Nearly all laryngectomees can learn to use some form of electrolarynx. For detailed discussion of management of laryngeal cancer and related communication issues, the interested reader is referred to Diedrich and Youngstrom[53] and Keith and Darley.[98]

Cleft Palate

The congenital orofacial deformity of cleft palate with or without cleft lip occurs in approximately 1 of 600 to 900 caucasian births and 1 of 1500 to 2000 black births in the United States.[130] Cleft patterns for the individual children may involve the primary palate (lip and premaxillary or alveolar process anterior to the incisive foramen), the secondary palate, or both the primary and secondary palates.[17, 117] Clefts may be unilateral or bilateral as well as incomplete or complete.

Surgical repair for cleft lip and palate is usually staged as follows. Labial clefts are typically closed first, often within the first month of life. Primary surgical repair of the palate is completed later, with the timing dependent on the philosophy of the cleft palate management team. Prior to surgical repair of the palate, orthodontic appliances often are fitted to maintain or restore the contour of the maxillary arch and to occlude, at least partially, the cleft of the hard palate.

Some individuals with cleft palate remain velopharyngeally incompetent, unable to occlude the port between the oral and nasal cavity. Velopharyngeal incompetence following palatal surgery might be managed in one of several ways. An obturator may be fitted to occlude the velopharyngeal port. Secondary surgery might involve a "push-back" procedure with or without a pharyngeal flap attached to the soft palate. Detailed discussions of primary and secondary procedures

can be found in Cooper and co-workers[34] and Grabb and associates.[65]

Speech disorders may result from several factors related to orofacial deformity. Velopharyngeal incompetence results in the escape of air through the nasal cavity (nasal emission) during the production of sounds requiring the impounding of intraoral air pressure (s, p, b, f, v). Hypernasality during consonant sound production also results from velopharyngeal incompetency. Dental and occlusal abnormalities may hinder the development of normal articulation by the child with cleft palate. Children with cleft palate have demonstrated a greater than average occurrence of mild to moderate conductive hearing loss. This hearing impairment may contribute to delays in language and speech development in some children.

The communication management of the child with cleft palate focuses on the areas of hearing, language, and speech. Due to increased occurrence of hearing loss in cleft palate as compared with normal children, regular hearing assessments are scheduled. Depending on the outcome of the dental, orthodontic, and surgical management to achieve velopharyngeal competence and maxillary/mandibular arch alignment, the speech problems vary from child to child. Thorough speech evaluations are required to determine the error patterns and plan instruction programs appropriate to the individual. Because language development delays might occur in children with cleft palate, their language skills regularly should be assessed and additional instruction provided when delays are found.

Augmentative Communication

The term "augmentative communication" refers to any approach designed to support, enhance, or augment the communication of individuals who are not independent verbal communicators in all situations. As a result of cerebral palsy, brain trauma, cerebral circulation disorders, degenerative neurological diseases, severe hearing loss, or severe language or developmental disorders, some individuals are speechless, whereas others can be understood only by persons very familiar with them. In the past 15 years an increasing number of techniques for augmenting communication have been developed. Some of these approaches include electronic or mechanical devices; others, such as hand signing and gesturing, do not.

KATHRYN M. YORKSTON AND DAVID R. BEUKELMAN

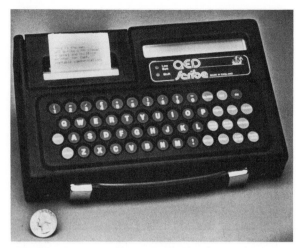

FIGURE 5–3. The Scribe Augmentative Communication device, available through Zygo Industries, Inc., Portland, OR 97207.

The augmentative communication process is usually divided into four basic components—message, symbols, transmission modes, and listener. As with speaking individuals, the messages of persons with severe communication disorders vary depending on the intent of the interaction. Some messages are designed to request wants and needs; others are intended to share information. Some messages are conveyed to establish social closeness; others conform to the requirements of social etiquette. The types of messages produced by individuals are dependent on their age, their cognitive and social capability, and their life style. All individuals, whether speaking or nonspeaking, select symbols to convey their messages. For the nonimpaired individual, messages are communicated through spoken words or on a letter-by-letter basis when these words are written. However, with the severely, communicatively impaired individual, literacy skills may be very limited. Therefore, messages must be symbolized using objects, photographs, or line drawings, depending on the capability of the individual. Other persons who are unable to speak have the literacy skills to engage in spontaneous writing using an augmentative communication technique.

The transmission component of the augmentative communication model refers to those techniques that are used by the individual to convey the message to a listener. These techniques can be as common as a picture board, as nonspeaking individuals point to a photograph or line drawing in a way that can be observed or recognized by their listeners. At other times, the transmission of the message is managed by a sophisticated electronic system that provides the nonspeaking person with a variety of control, system process, and

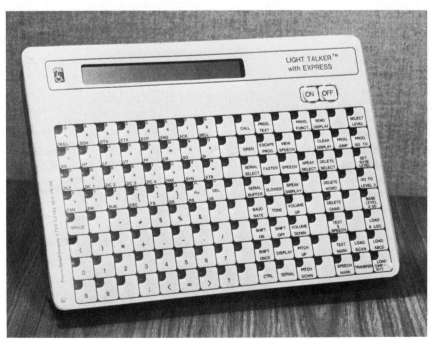

FIGURE 5–4. The Light Talker augmentative communication device, available through Prentke Romich Company, Wooster, OH 44691.

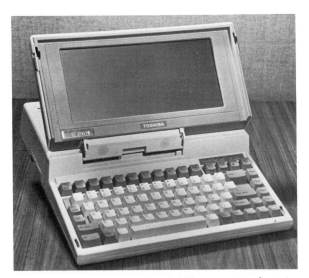

FIGURE 5–5. Photograph of the EZ Keys augmentative communication device, available through Adaptive Communication Systems, Inc., Coraopolis, PA 15108.

KATHRYN M. YORKSTON AND DAVID R. BEUKELMAN

ing, with consultation from medical, psychological, and seating experts. Of course, nonspeaking individuals and their family members are involved in the selection process. Symbol selection usually requires extensive information about the linguistic, motor control, cognitive, and visual abilities of the impaired individual, along with a detailed analysis of current and future communication needs. Extensive training is required to prepare individuals to use augmentative communication systems effectively. The augmentative communication field is changing rapidly; therefore, the following references are provided for interested readers.[20, 21, 64]

ACKNOWLEDGMENT

Preparation of this chapter was supported in part by Grant #G008200020 from the National Institute of Disability and Rehabilitation Research, Department of Education, Washington, DC 20202. We wish to acknowledge the assistance of Nickola Wolf Nelson in reviewing this manuscript.

References

1. Adamovich, B. B.: Language vs. cognition: The speech/language pathologist's role. *In* Brookshire, R. (Ed.): Clinical Aphasiology: Conference Proceedings. Minneapolis, BRK Publishers, 1981.
2. Adamovich, B. B., Henderson, J. A., and Auerback, S.: Cognitive Rehabilitation of Closed Head Injury Patients. San Diego, College-Hill Press, 1985.
3. Albert, M. L.: Changes in language with aging. Semin. Neurol., 1:43–46, 1981.
4. Andrews, M., and Summers, A.: Voice Therapy for Adolescents. San Diego, College-Hill Press, 1987.
5. Aronson, A. E.: Clinical Voice Disorders: An Interdisciplinary Approach. New York, Thieme-Stratton, 1980.
6. Basso, A., Capitani, E., and Vignolo, L. A.: Influence of rehabilitation on language skills in aphasic patients. Arch. Neurol., 36:190, 1979.
7. Basso, A., Roch Lecours, A., Moraschini, S., and Vanier, M.: Anatomoclinical correlations of the aphasia as defined through computerized tomography: Exceptions. Brain Lang., 26:201–229, 1985.
8. Bates, E.: Language and Context. New York, Academic Press, 1976.
9. Bayles, K. A.: Language function in senile dementia. Brain Lang., 16:265–280, 1982.
10. Bayles, K. A.: Language and dementia. *In* Holland, A. L. (Ed.): Language Disorders in Adults. San Diego, College-Hill Press, 1984.
11. Bayles, K. A., and Boone, D.: The potential of language tasks for identifying senile dementia. J. Speech Hear. Disord., 47:210, 1982.
12. Bayles, K. A., and Kaszniak, A. W.: Communication and Cognition in Normal Aging and Dementia. San Diego, College-Hill Press, 1987.
13. Bayles, K. A., and Tomoeda, C. K.: Confrontation naming impairment in dementia. Brain Lang., 19:98–114, 1983.
14. Bell, D. S.: Speech functions of the thalamus inferred from the effects of thalamotomy. Brain, 91:619–638, 1968.
15. Benson, D. F.: Aphasia, Alexia, and Agraphia. New York, Churchill Livingstone, 1979.
16. Berko Gleason, J.: The Development of Language. Columbus, OH, Charles E. Merrill Publishing Company, 1985.
17. Berlin, A.: Classification of Cleft Lip and Palate. Boston, Little, Brown & Company, 1971.
18. Bernstein-Ellis, E., Wertz, R. T., Dronkers, N. F., and Milton, S. B.: PICA performance by traumatically brain injured and left hemisphere CVA patients. *In* Brookshire, R. (Ed.): Clinical Aphasiology: Conference Proceedings. Minneapolis, BRK Publishers, 1985.
19. Beukelman, D. R., and Yorkston, K. M.: The relationship between information transfer and speech intelligibility of dysarthric speakers. J. Commun. Dis., 12:189–196, 1976.
20. Beukelman, D., Yorkston, K. M., and Dowden, P.: Communication Augmentation: A Casebook of Clinical Management. San Diego, College-Hill Press, 1985.
21. Blackstone, S. (Ed.): Augmentative Communication: An Introduction. Rockville, MD, American Speech-Language-Hearing Association, 1986.
22. Boller, F., and Vignolo, L. A.: Latent sensory aphasia in hemisphere-damaged patients: An experimental study with the Token Test. Brain, 89:815, 1966.
23. Bollinger, R. L., Waugh, P. F., and Zatz, A. F.: Communication Management of the Geriatric Patient. Danville, IL, The Interstate Printers and Publishers, Inc., 1977.
24. Boone, D.: The Voice and Voice Therapy. Englewood Cliffs, NJ, Prentice-Hall, 1977.
25. Brandenberg, S., and Vanderheiden, G.: Communication Aids: Resourcebook I. San Diego, College-Hill Press, 1987.
26. Brink, J. S., Imbus, C., and Woo-Sam, J.: Physical recovery after severe closed head trauma in children and adolescents. J. Pediatr., 97:721–727, 1980.
27. Broad, D. J.: Phonation. *In* Minifie, F. (Ed.): Aspects of Speech, Hearing and Language. Englewood Cliffs, NJ, Prentice-Hall, 1973, pp. 127–168.
28. Brown, G., Chadwick, O., Shaffer, D., Rutter, M., and Traub, M.: A prospective study of children with head injuries. 3. Psychiatric sequelae. Psychol. Med., 11:63–78, 1981.

29. Burns, M. S., Halper, A. S., and Mogil, S. I.: Clinical Management of Right Hemisphere Dysfunction. Rockville, MD, Aspen System Corp., 1985.

30. Chadwick, O., Rutter, M., Brown, G., Shaffer, D., and Traub, M.: A prospective study of children with head injuries. 2. Cognitive sequelae. Psychol. Med., 11:49–61, 1981.

31. Chadwick, O., Rutter, M., Shaffer, D., and Shrout, P. E.: A prospective study of children with head injuries. 4. Specific cognitive deficits. J. Clin. Neuropsychol., 3:101–120, 1981.

32. Chapey, R. (Ed.): Language Intervention Strategies in Adult Aphasia. Baltimore, Williams & Wilkins, 1981.

33. Cohen, M., and Cross, P.: The Development Resource: Behavioral Sequences for Assessment and Program Planning. New York, Grune & Stratton, 1979.

34. Cooper, H. K., Harding, R. L., Krogman, W. M., Mazaheri, M., Millard, R. T., and Spencer, S. M.: Cleft Palate and Cleft Lip: A Team Approach to Clinical Management and Rehabilitation of the Patient. Philadelphia, W. B. Saunders Company, 1979.

35. Cummings, J. L., and Benson, D. F.: Dementia: A Clinical Approach. Boston, Butterworth, 1983.

36. Dabul, B.: Apraxia Battery for Adults. Tigard, OR, C. C. Publications, 1979.

37. Dabul, B., and Bollier, B.: Therapeutic approaches to apraxia. J. Speech Hear. Disord., 41:268–276, 1976.

38. Dale, P. S.: Language Development Structure and Function, 2nd Ed. New York, Holt, Rinehart & Winston, 1976.

39. Damasio, A., Damasio, H., Rizzo, M., Varney, N., and Gersh, F.: Aphasia with nonhemorrhagic lesions in the basal ganglia and internal capsule. Arch. Neurol., 39:15–20, 1982.

40. Darley, F. L.: Diagnosis and Appraisal of Communication Disorders. Englewood Cliffs, NJ, Prentice-Hall, 1964.

41. Darley, F. L.: Aphasia: Input and output disturbances in speech and language processing. Presented in dual session on aphasia to the American Speech and Hearing Association, Chicago, IL, 1969.

42. Darley, F. L.: The efficiency of language rehabilitation in aphasia. J. Speech Hear. Disord., 37:3–21, 1972.

43. Darley, F. L.: Aphasia. Philadelphia, W. B. Saunders Company, 1983.

44. Darley, F. L., Aronson, A. E., and Brown, J. R.: Clusters of deviant speech dimensions in the dysarthrias. J. Speech Hear. Res., 12:462–496, 1969.

45. Darley, F. L., Aronson, A. E., and Brown, J. R.: Differential diagnostic patterns of dysarthria. J. Speech Hear. Res., 12:246–269, 1969.

46. Darley, F. L., Aronson, A. E., and Brown, J. R.: Motor Speech Disorders. Philadelphia, W. B. Saunders Company, 1975.

47. Davis, G. A.: A Survey of Adult Aphasia. Englewood Cliffs, NJ, Prentice-Hall, 1983.

48. Davis, G. A., and Wilcox, M. J.: Incorporating parameters of natural conversation in aphasia treatment. In Chapey, R. (Ed.): Language Intervention Strategies in Adult Aphasia. Baltimore, Williams & Wilkins, 1981.

49. Deal, J.: Consistency and adaptation in apraxia of speech. J. Commun. Dis., 7:135–140, 1974.

50. Deal, J. L., and Florance, C. L.: Modification of the eight-step continuum for treatment of apraxia of speech in adults. J. Speech Hear. Disord., 43:89–95, 1978.

51. DeRenzi, E., and Faglioni, P.: Normative data and screening power of a shortened version of the Token Test. Cortex, 14:41–49, 1978.

52. DeRuyter, F., and Lafontaine, L. M.: The non-speaking brain-injured: A clinical and demographic database report. Augment. Altern. Commun., 3:18–25, 1987.

53. Diedrich, W., and Youngstrom, K.: Alaryngeal Speech. Springfield, IL, Charles C Thomas, 1966.

54. Diller, L., and Gordon, W. D.: Interventions for cognitive deficits in brain injured adults. J. Consult. Clini. Psychol., 49:822–834, 1981.

55. Eiben, C. F., Anderson, T. P., Lockman, L., Mathews, D. J., Dryja, R., Martin, J., Burrill, C., Gottesman, N., O'Brian, P., and Witte, L.: Functional outcome of closed head injury in children and young adults. Arch. Phys. Med. Rehabil., 65:168–170, 1984.

56. Fromm, D., Abbs, J., McNeil, M., and Rosenbek, J.: Simultaneous perceptual-physiological method for studying apraxia of speech. In Brookshire, R. (Ed.): Clinical Aphasiology: Conference Proceedings. Minneapolis, BRK Publishers, 1982.

57. Gardner, H., Brownell, H., Wapner, W., and Michelow, D.: Missing the point: The role of the right hemisphere in the processing of complex linguistic material. In Perecman, E., (Ed.): Cognitive Processing in the Right Hemisphere. New York, Academic Press, 1983.

58. Geschwind, N.: Current concepts, aphasia. N. Engl. J. Med., 12:284, 1971.

59. Gianotti, G., Caltagirone, C., Miceli, G., and Masullo, C.: Selective semantic-lexical impairment of language comprehension in right-brain damaged patients. Brain Lang., 13:201–211, 1976.

60. Gilchrist, E., and Wilkinson, M.: Some factors determining prognosis in young people with severe head injuries. Arch. Neurol., 36:355–359, 1979.

61. Golper, L. C., and Rau, M.: Treatment of communication disorders associated with generalized intellectual deficits in adults. In Perkins, W. (Ed.): Language Handicaps in Adults. New York, Thieme-Stratton, 1983.

62. Gonzalez, J. B., and Aronson, A. E.: Palatal lift prosthesis for treatment of anatomic and neurologic

palatopharyngeal insufficiency. Cleft Palate J., 7:91–104, 1969.

63. Goodglass, H., and Kaplan, E.: The Assessment of Aphasia and Related Disorders, 2nd Ed. Philadelphia, Lea & Febiger, 1983.

64. Goosens, C., and Crain, S.: Augmentative Communication: Intervention Resource. Lake Zurich, IL, Don Johnston Developmental Equipment, 1987.

65. Grabb, W., Rosenstein, S. W., and Bzoch, K. R.: Cleft Lip and Palate. Boston, Little, Brown & Company, 1971.

66. Groher, M.: Language and memory disorders following closed head trauma. J. Speech Hear. Res., 20:212, 1977.

67. Groher, M.: Communication disorders. In Rosenthal, M., Griffith, E., Bond, M., Miller, J. D. (Eds.): Rehabilitation of the Head Injured Adult. Philadelphia, F. A. Davis, 1983.

68. Hagen, C.: Communication abilities in hemiplegia: The effect of speech therapy. Arch. Phys. Med. Rehabil., 35:377, 1970.

69. Hagen, C.: Language disorders in head trauma. In Holland, A. L. (Ed.): Language Disorders in Adults. San Diego, College-Hill Press, 1984.

70. Halpern, H., Darley, F. L., and Brown, J. R.: Differential language and neurologic characteristics in cerebral involvement. J. Speech Hear. Dis., 38:162–173, 1973.

71. Hanson, W. R., Metter, E. J., Riege, W. H., Kempler, D., Jackson, C. A., Mazziotta, J. C., and Phelps, M. E.: Comparison of regional cerebral metabolism (PET), structure (x-ray CT), and language in categories of chronic aphasia. In Brookshire, R. (Ed.): Clinical Aphasiology: Conference Proceedings. Minneapolis, BRK Publishers, 1986.

72. Hanson, W. R., Metter, E. J., Riege, W. H., Kuhl, D. E., and Phelps, M. E.: Positron emission tomography. In Brookshire, R. (Ed.): Clinical Aphasiology: Conference Proceedings. Minneapolis, BRK Publishers, 1984.

73. Hart, C. W.: Functional and neurological problems of the larynx. Otolaryngol. Clin. North Am., 3:609–623, 1970.

74. Helffenstein, D. A., and Wechsler, F. S.: The use of Interpersonal Process Recall (IPR) in the remediation of interpersonal and communication skill deficits in the newly brain-injured. Clin. Neuropsychol., 4:139, 1982.

75. Helm, N., and Barresi, B.: Voluntary control of involuntary utterances: A treatment approach for severe aphasia. In Brookshire, R. (Ed.): Clinical Aphasiology: Conference Proceedings. Minneapolis, BRK Publishers, 1980.

76. Helm-Estabrooks, N.: Treatment of subcortical aphasias. In Perkins, W. H. (Ed.): Language Handicaps in Adults. New York, Thieme-Stratton, 1983.

77. Helm-Estabrooks, N.: Severe aphasia. In Holland,

A. L. (Ed.): Language Disorders in Adults. San Diego, College-Hill Press, 1983.

78. Helm-Estabrooks, N., Fitzpatrick, P., and Barresi, B.: Visual action therapy for global aphasia. J. Speech Hear. Disord., 47:385–389, 1982.

79. Hixon, T.: Respiratory function in speech. In Minifie, F., Hixon, T., and Williams, F. (Eds.): Normal Aspects of Speech, Hearing, and Language. Englewood Cliffs, NJ, Prentice-Hall, 1973, pp. 73–122.

80. Hixon, T.: Respiratory Function in Speech and Song. San Diego, College-Hill Press, 1987.

81. Hoit, J., and Hixon, T.: Age and speech breathing. J. Speech Hear. Res., 30:351–366, 1987.

82. Holland, A. L.: Case studies in aphasia using programmed instruction. J. Speech Hear. Disord., 35:377–390, 1970.

83. Holland, A.: Communicative Abilities in Daily Living. Baltimore, University Park Press, 1980.

84. Holland, A. L.: When is aphasia aphasia? The problem of closed head injury. In Brookshire, R. (Ed.): Clinical Aphasiology: Conference Proceedings. Minneapolis, BRK Publishers, 1982.

85. Hollien, H.: Vocal pitch variation related to changes in vocal fold length. J. Speech Hear. Res., 3:150–156, 1960.

86. Hollien, H.: Vocal fold thickness and fundamental frequency of phonation. J. Speech Hear. Res., 5:237–243, 1962.

87. Hook, O.: Aphasia and related communication disorders after brain damage. Lecture presented at the Second Annual Conference: Head Trauma Rehabilitation Coma to Community. San Jose, California, 1979.

88. Horner, J., and Chacko, R.: Cerebral blood flow. In Brookshire, R. (Ed.): Clinical Aphasiology: Conference Proceedings. Minneapolis, BRK Publishers, 1984.

89. Itoh, M., Sasanuma, S., Tatsumi, I. F., Murakami, S., Fukasaki, Y., and Suzuki, T.: Voice onset time characteristics in apraxia of speech. Brain Lang., 17:193, 1982.

90. Itoh, M., Sasanuma, S., and Ushijima, T.: Velar movements during speech in a patient with apraxia of speech. Brain Lang., 7:227–239, 1979.

91. Jennett, B.: Prognosis after severe head injury. Clin. Neurosurg., 19:200–207, 1971.

92. Jennett, B., and Plum, F.: Persistent vegetative state after brain damage. Lancet, 1:734–737, 1982.

93. Jennett, B., and Teasdale, G.: Management of Head Injuries. Philadelphia, F. A. Davis, 1981.

94. Jennett, B., Teasdale, G., Braakman, R., Minderhoud, J., and Khill-Jones, R.: Predicting outcome in individual patients after severe head injury. Lancet, 1:1031–1034, 1976.

95. Johns, D., and Darley, F.: Phonemic variability in apraxia of speech. J. Speech Hear. Res., 13:556–583, 1970.

96. Kalsbeek, W. D., McLaurin, R. L., Harris, B. S., and Miller, J. D.: The national head and spinal

cord injury survey: Major findings. J. Neurosurg., 53:519–531, 1980.

97. Kaplan, E., Goodglass, H., and Weintraub, S.: Boston Naming Test. Philadelphia, Lea & Febiger, 1983.

98. Keith, R. L., and Darley, F. L.: Laryngectomee Rehabilitation. Houston, College-Hill Press, 1986.

99. Kempler, D., Metter, E. J., Jackson, C. A., Hanson, W. R., Phelps, M., and Mazziotta, J.: Conduction aphasia: Subgroups based on behavior, anatomy and physiology. *In* Brookshire, R. (Ed.): Clinical Aphasiology: Conference Proceedings. Minneapolis, BRK Publishers, 1986.

100. Kent, R. D., and Rosenbek, J. C.: Acoustic patterns of apraxia of speech. J. Speech Hear. Res., 26:231–249, 1983.

101. Kertesz, A.: Aphasia and Associated Disorders: Taxonomy, Localization, and Recovery. New York, Grune & Stratton, 1979.

102. Kertesz, A.: Western Aphasia Battery. New York, Grune & Stratton, 1982.

103. Kertesz, A., and Poole, E.: The aphasia quotient: The taxonomic approach to measurement of aphasia disability. Can. J. Neurol. Sci., 1:7–16, 1974.

104. Kertesz, A., and Sheppard, A.: The epidemiology of aphasic and cognitive impairment in stroke: Age, sex, aphasia type and laterality differences. Brain, 104:117–128, 1981.

105. Kertesz, A., Lesk, D., and McCabe, P.: Isotope localization of infarcts in aphasia. Arch. Neurol., 34:590–601, 1977.

106. Kertesz, A., Harlock, W., and Coates, R.: Computer tomographic localization, lesion size, and prognosis in aphasia and nonverbal impairment. Brain Lang., 8:34–50, 1979.

107. Knopman, D. S., Selnes, O. A., Niccum, N., Rubens, A., Yock, D., and Larson, D.: A longitudinal study of speech fluency in aphasia: CT correlates of recovery and persistent nonfluency. Neurology, 33:1170–1178, 1983.

108. LaPointe, L., and Horner, J.: Reading Comprehension Battery for Aphasia. Tigard, OR, C. C. Publications, 1979.

109. Lehiste, I.: Suprasegmentals. Cambridge, MIT Press, 1970.

110. Leith, W., and Johnston, R.: Handbook of Voice Therapy for School Clinicians. San Diego, College-Hill Press, 1986.

111. Levin, H., Benton, A., and Grossman, R.: Neurobehavioral Consequences of Closed Head Injury. New York, Oxford University Press, 1982.

112. Levin, H. S., Grossman, R. G., Rose, J. E., and Teasdale, J.: Long term neuropsychological outcome of closed head injury. J. Neurosurg., 50:412–422, 1979.

113. Levin, H. S., Grossman, R. G., Sarwar, M., and Meyers, C. A.: Linguistic recovery after closed head injury. Brain Lang., 12:360–374, 1981.

114. Levin, H. S., Madison, C. F., Bailey, C. B., Meyers, C. A., Eisenberg, H. M., and Guinto, F. C.: Mutism after closed head injury. Arch. Neurol., 40:601–606, 1983.

115. Levine, D. N., and Mohr, J. P.: Language after bilateral cerebral infarctions: Role of the minor hemisphere in speech. Neurology, 29:927–938, 1974.

116. Lezak, M. D.: Recovery of memory and learning functions following traumatic brain injury. Cortex, 15:63–72, 1979.

117. Logemann, J. (Ed.): Cleft Palate and Other Maxillofacial Disorders. San Diego, College-Hill Press, 1987.

118. Luchsinger, R., and Arnold, G.: Voice-Speech-Language. Belmont, CA, Wadsworth Publishing Company, 1965.

119. Malkmus, D., Booth, G., and Kodimer, C.: Rehabilitation of the Head Injured Adult: Comprehensive Cognitive Management. Downey, CA, Rancho Los Amigos Hospital, 1980.

120. Marks, M., Taylor, M., and Rusk, H.: Rehabilitation of the aphasic patient: A survey of three years experience in a rehabilitation setting. Neurology, 7:837–843, 1957.

121. Marshall, R. C.: Case Studies in Aphasia Rehabilitation. Austin, ProEd, 1986.

122. Martin, A. D.: Some objections to the term "apraxia of speech." J. Speech Hear. Dis., 39:53, 1974.

123. Mazzochi, R., and Vignolo, L. A.: Localization of lesions in aphasia. Clinical-CT scan correlations in stroke patients. Cortex, 15:627–654, 1979.

124. Metter, E. J., Hanson, W. R., Riege, W. H., Kuhl, D. E., and Phelps, M. E.: The use of (F18) fluorodeoxyglucose positron computed tomography in the study of aphasia: A review. *In* Brookshire, R. (Ed.): Clinical Aphasiology: Conference Proceedings. Minneapolis, BRK Publishers, 1983.

125. Metter, E. J., Riege, W. H., Hanson, W. R., Camras, L., Kuhl, D. E., and Phelps, M. E.: Correlations of cerebral glucose metabolism and structural damage to language function in aphasia. Brain Lang., 21:187–207, 1984.

126. Metter, E. J., Riege, W. H., Hanson, W. R., Kuhl, D. E., Phelps, M. E., Squire, L. R., Wasterlain, C. G., and Benson, D. F.: Comparison of metabolic rates, language, and memory in subcortical aphasias. Brain Lang., 19:33–47, 1983.

127. Metter, E. J., Wasterlain, C. G., Kuhl, D. E., Hanson, W. R., and Phelps, M. E.: FDG positron emission computed tomography in a study of aphasia. Ann. Neurol., 10:173–183, 1981.

128. Meyer, J. L., Sakai, F., Yamaguchi, R., Yamamoto, M., and Shaw, T.: Regional changes in cerebral blood flow during standard behavioral activation in patients with disorders of speech and mentation compared to normal volunteers. Brain Lang., 9:61–77, 1980.

129. Millar, J. M., and Whittaker, H. A.: The right hemisphere's contribution to language: A review

KATHRYN M. YORKSTON AND DAVID R. BEUKELMAN

of the evidence from brain-damaged subjects. *In* Segalowitz, S. (Ed.): Language Functions and Brain Organization. New York, Academic Press, 1983.

130. Millard, D. R.: Cleft Craft: The Evaluation of its Surgery #1. The Unilateral Deformity. Boston, Little, Brown & Company, 1976.

131. Milner, B., Branch, C., and Rasmussen, T.: Observation of cerebral dominance. *In* DeReuck, A., and O'Connor, M. (Eds.): Disorders of Language. London, Churchill Livingstone, 1964, pp. 200–222.

132. Milton, S., and Wertz, R. T.: Management of persisting communication deficits in patients with traumatic brain injury. *In* Uzzell, B., and Gross, Y. (Eds.): Clinical Neuropsychology of Intervention. Boston, Martinus Nijhuff, 1986.

133. Mohr, J. P., Pessin, M. S., Finkelstein, S., Funkenstein, H. H., Duncan, G. W., and Davis, K. R.: Broca aphasia: Pathologic and clinical. Neurology, 28:311–324, 1978.

134. Myers, P. S.: Profiles of communication deficits in patients with right cerebral hemisphere damage. *In* Brookshire, R. (Ed.): Clinical Aphasiology: Conference Proceedings. Minneapolis, BRK Publishers, 1979.

135. Myers, P. S.: Right hemisphere communication disorder. *In* Perkins, W. H. (Ed.): Current Therapy in Communication Disorders. New York, Thieme-Stratton, 1983.

136. Myers, P. S.: Right hemisphere impairment. *In* Holland, A. (Ed.): Language Disorders in Adults. San Diego, College-Hill Press, 1984.

137. Naeser, M. A., Alexander, M. P., Helm-Estabrooks, N., Levine, H., Laughlin, S., and Geschwind, N.: Aphasia with predominantly subcortical lesion sites: Description of three capsular/putaminal aphasia syndromes. Arch. Neurol., 39:2–14, 1982.

138. Naeser, M. A., Hayward, R. W., Laughlin, S. E., Becker, J. M. T., Jernigan, T. L., and Zataz, L. M.: Quantitative CT scan studies in aphasia. II. Comparison of the right and left hemispheres. Brain Lang., 12:165–189, 1981.

139. Naeser, M., Hayward, R., Laughlin, S., and Zatz, L.: Quantitative CT scan studies in aphasia. I. Infarct size and CT numbers. Brain Lang., 12:140–164, 1981.

140. Najenson, T., Saxbon, L., Fiselson, J., Becker, E., and Schechter, I.: Recovery of communicative functions after prolonged traumatic coma. Scand. J. Rehabil. Med., 10:15–21, 1978.

141. National Institute of Aging Task Force: Senility reconsidered: Treatment possibilities for mental impairment in the elderly. J.A.M.A., 244:259–263, 1980.

142. Netsell, R.: Speech physiology. *In* Minifie, F. D., Hixon, T. J., and Williams, F. (Eds.): Normal Aspects of Speech, Hearing and Language. Englewood Cliffs, NJ, Prentice-Hall, 1973.

143. Netsell, R.: Physiological studies of dysarthria and their relevance to treatment. Semin. Lang., 5:279–292, 1984.

144. Netsell, R.: A Neurobiological View of Speech Production and the Dysarthrias. San Diego, College-Hill Press, 1986.

145. Nippold, M. A.: The Normal Development of Language: Ages Nine Through Nineteen. San Diego, College-Hill Press, 1988.

146. Obler, L. K., and Albert, M. L.: Language in the elderly aphasic and the dementing patient. *In* Sarno, M. T. (Ed.): Acquired Aphasia. New York, Academic Press, 1977.

147. Obler, L. K., and Albert, M. L.: Language and aging: A neurobehavioral analysis. *In* Beasley, D. S., and Davis, G. A. (Eds.): Aging Communication Processes and Disorders. New York, Grune & Stratton, 1981.

148. Ojemann, G. A., and Whitaker, H. A.: Language localization and variability. Brain Lang., 6:239–260, 1978.

149. Owens, R.: Normal Language Development: An Introduction, 2nd Ed. Columbus, OH, Charles E. Merrill Publishing Company, 1988.

150. Pieniadz, J., Naeser, M., Koff, E., and Levine, H.: CT scan cerebral hemispheric asymmetry measurements in stroke cases with global aphasia: Atypical asymmetries associated with improved recovery. Cortex, 19:371–391, 1983.

151. Poech, K., DeBleser, R., and Graf von Keyserlingk, D.: Neurolinguistic status and localization of lesion in aphasic patients with exclusively consonant-vowel recurring utterances. Brain, 107:199–217, 1984.

152. Porch, B. E.: Porch Index of Communicative Abilities, 3rd Ed. Palo Alto, CA, Consulting Psychologists Press, 1981.

153. Porch, B., Collins, M., Wertz, R. T., and Frieden, T. P.: Statistical prediction of change in aphasia. J. Speech Hear. Res., 23:312–321, 1980.

154. Reynolds, A. F., Turner, P. T., Harris, A. B., Ojemann, G. A., and Davis, L. F.: Left thalamic hemorrhage with dysphonia: A report of five cases. Brain Lang., 7(1):62–73, 1979.

155. Rosen, C. D., and Gerring, J. P.: Head Trauma: Educational Reintegration. San Diego, College-Hill Press, 1986.

156. Rosenbek, J. C.: Treating apraxia of speech. *In* Johns, D. F. (Ed.): Clinical Management of Neurogenic Communication Disorders. Boston, Little, Brown & Company, 1985.

157. Rosenbek, J. C., and LaPointe, L. L.: The dysarthrias: Description, diagnosis, and treatment. *In* Johns, D. F. (Ed.): Clinical Management of Neurogenic Communication Disorders. Boston, Little, Brown & Company, 1985.

158. Rosenbek, J. C., Lemme, M. L., Ahern, M. B., Harris, E. H., and Wertz, R. T.: A treatment for apraxia of speech in adults. J. Speech Hear. Disord., 38:462–472, 1973.

159. Rosenbek, J. C., McNeil, M. R., and Aronson, A. E. (Eds.): Apraxia of Speech: Physiology, Acoustics, Linguistics, Management. San Diego, College-Hill Press, 1984.

160. Rusk, H., Block, J., and Lowmann, E.: Rehabilitation of the brain injured patient: A report of 157 cases with long term follow-up of 118. *In* Walker, E., Caveness, W., and Critchley, M. (Eds.): The Late Effects of Head Injury. Springfield, IL, Charles C Thomas, 1969.

161. Rutter, M.: Psychological sequelae of brain damage in children. Am. J. Psychiatry, 138:1533–1544, 1981.

162. Sapir, S., and Aronson, A. E.: Aphonia after closed head injury: Aetiology considerations. Br. J. Disord. Commun., 20:289–296, 1985.

163. Sarno, M. T.: The Functional Communication Profile Manual of Directions. Rehabilitation Monograph 42, New York Institute of Rehabilitation Medicine, New York University Center, 1969.

164. Sarno, M. T.: The nature of verbal impairment after closed head injury. J. Nerv. Ment. Dis., 168:685–692, 1980.

165. Sarno, M. T., Buonagura, A., and Levita, E.: Characteristics of verbal impairment in closed head injured patients. Arch. Phys. Med. Rehabil., 67:400–405, 1986.

166. Sarno, M. T., Silverman, M., and Sands, E.: Speech therapy and language recovery in severe aphasia. J. Speech Hear. Res., 13:607–623, 1970.

167. Schuell, H. M.: Minnesota Test for Differential Diagnosis of Aphasia. Minneapolis, University of Minnesota Press, 1955.

168. Schuell, H., Jenkins, J. J., and Jiménez-Pabón, E.: Aphasia in Adults. New York, Harper & Row, 1964.

169. Searleman, A.: A review of right hemisphere linguistic capabilities. Psychol. Bull., 84:503–528, 1977.

170. Shewan, C. M., and Kertesz, A.: Reliability and validity characteristics of the Western Aphasia Battery. J. Speech Hear. Disord., 45:300, 1980.

171. Shewan, C. M., and Kertesz, A.: Effects of speech and language treatment on recovery from aphasia. Brain Lang., 23:272–299, 1984.

172. Sies, L. F. (Ed.): Aphasia Theory and Therapy: Selected Lectures and Papers of Hidred Schuell. Baltimore, University Park Press, 1974.

173. Soh, K., Larsen, B., Skinhoj, E., and Lassen, N. A.: Regional cerebral blood flow in aphasia. Arch. Neurol., 35:625–632, 1978.

174. Sparks, R., and Holland, A.: Melodic intonation therapy for aphasia. J. Speech Hear. Disord., 41:287–297, 1976.

175. Teasdale, G., and Jennett, B.: Assessment and prognosis of coma after head injury. Acta Neurosurg., 34:45–55, 1976.

176. Thomsen, I. V.: The speech pathologist's approach to the patient with severe head injury. Folia Phoniatr. (Basel), 214:281–286, 1969.

177. Thomsen, I. V., and Skinhaj, E.: Regressive language in severe head injury. Acta Neurol. Scand., 54:219–226, 1976.

178. Tognola, G., and Vignolo, L.: Brain lesions associated with oral apraxia in stroke patients: A clinio-neuroradiological investigation with CT scan. Neuropsychologia, 18:257–272, 1980.

179. Tucker, H.: Human laryngeal reinnervation. Laryngoscope, 86:769–778, 1976.

180. Vignolo, L. A.: Evaluation of aphasia in language rehabilitation: A retrospective exploratory study. Cortex, 1:344, 1964.

181. The Vocational Rehabilitation Problems of the Patient with Aphasia. A workshop sponsored by Western Michigan University, U.S. Dept. of Health, Education and Welfare, Social and Rehabilitation Services Administration, Washington, DC, 1967.

182. Wapner, W., Hamby, S., and Gardner, H.: The role of the right hemisphere in the appreciation of complex linguistic material. Brain Lang., 14:15–33, 1981.

183. Weinberg, J., Diller, L., Gordon, W. A., Gerstman, L. J., Lieberman, A., Lakin, P., Hodges, G., and Ezrachi, O.: Visual scanning training effect on reading-related tasks in acquired right brain damage. Arch. Phys. Med. Rehabil., 58:479, 1977.

184. Weintraub, S., Mesulam, M., and Kramer, L.: Disturbances in prosody: A right-hemisphere contribution to language. Arch. Neurol., 38:742–744, 1981.

185. Wepman, J. M.: Aphasia therapy: A new look. J. Speech Hear. Disord., 37:203–214, 1972.

186. Wertz, R. T.: Response to treatment in patients with apraxia of speech. *In* Rosenbek, J. C., McNeil, M. R., and Aronson, A. E. (Eds.): Apraxia of Speech: Physiology, Acoustics, Linguistics, Management. San Diego, College-Hill Press, 1984.

187. Wertz, R. T.: Neuropathologies of speech and language: An introduction to patient management. *In* Johns, D. F. (Ed.): Clinical Management of Neurogenic Communication Disorders. Boston, Little, Brown & Company, 1985.

188. Wertz, R. T., Bronkers, N. F., and Deal, J. L.: Language and localization: A comparison of left, right, and bilaterally brain-damaged patients. *In* Brookshire, R. (Ed.): Clinical Aphasiology: Conference Proceedings. Minneapolis, BRK Publishers, 1985.

189. Wertz, R. T., Collins, M., Weiss, D., Kurtzke, J., Friden, T., Brookshire, R., Pierce, J., Holtzapple, P., Hubbard, D., Porch, B., West, J., Davis, L., Matovitch, V., Morley, G., and Resurreccion, E.: Veterans Administration cooperative study on aphasia: A comparison of individual and group treatment. J. Speech Hear. Res., 24:580, 1981.

190. Wertz, R. T., Deal, J. L., and Robinson, A. J.: Classifying the aphasias: A comparison of the Boston Diagnostic aphasia examination and the Western Aphasia Battery. *In* Brookshire, R. (Ed.):

Clinical Aphasiology: Conference Proceedings. Minneapolis, BRK Publishers, 1984.

191. Wertz, R. T., LaPointe, L. L., and Rosenbek, J. C.: Apraxia of Speech in Adults: The Disorder and Its Management. New York, Grune & Stratton, 1984.

192. Wertz, R. T., Weiss, D. G., Aten, J. L., Brookshire, R. H., Garcia-Bunuel, L., Holland, A. L., Kurtzke, J. F., LaPointe, L. L., Milianti, F. J., Brannegan, R., Greenbaum, H., Marshall, R. C., Vogel, D., Carter, J., Barnes, N. S., and Goodman, R.: Comparison of clinic, home and deferred language treatment for aphasia. Arch. Neurol., 43:653–658, 1986.

193. Yamaguchi, R., Meyer, A., Sakai, F., and Yamamoto, M.: Case reports of three dysphasic patients to illustrate rCBF responses during behavioral activation. Brain Lang., 9:145–148, 1980.

194. Yarnell, P., Monroe, M., and Sobel, L.: Aphasia outcome in stroke: A clinical and neuroradiological correlation. Stroke, 7:516–522, 1976.

195. Ylvisaker, M. (Ed.): Head Injury Rehabilitation: Children and Adolescents. San Diego, College-Hill Press, 1985.

196. Ylvisaker, M. S., and Holland, A. L.: Coaching, self-coaching, and rehabilitation of head injury. *In* Johns, D. F. (Ed.): Clinical Management of Neurogenic Communication Disorders. Boston, Little, Brown & Company, 1985.

197. Yorkston, K. M., and Beukelman, D. R.: Assessment of Intelligibility of Dysarthric Speech. Austin, ProEd, 1981.

198. Yorkston, K. M., Beukelman, D. R., and Bell, K. R.: Clinical Management of Dysarthria Speakers. San Diego, College-Hill Press, 1988.

199. Yorkston, K. M., Beukelman, D. R., and Traynor, C. D.: Computerized Assessment of Intelligibility of Dysarthric Speech. Austin, ProEd, 1984.

200. Zemlin, W.: Speech and Hearing Sciences: Anatomy and Physiology. Englewood Cliffs, NJ, Prentice-Hall, 1968.

6

Psychological Assessment and Management

JO ANN BROCKWAY
WILBERT E. FORDYCE

The purpose of this chapter is to analyze the medical rehabilitation process in cognitive/behavioral terms to provide a framework for conceptualizing the so-called psychological or motivational problems that medical staff observe in dealing with patients in the rehabilitation setting. The major objectives are to provide the physician and other health care professionals with an appreciation of (1) the nature of these patient management problems; (2) the methods of assessing the problems; and (3) the strategies for working with patients to increase the benefits they derive from medical rehabilitation.

The clientele of medical rehabilitation practitioners are primarily individuals who are at a functional disadvantage in our society, as a consequence of physical disability, in the performance of at least some of life's tasks. Depending upon the nature of the medical problem, medical rehabilitation is concerned with limiting, reducing, or eliminating the functional impairment or with slowing its progression. *Comprehensive* medical rehabilitation is also concerned with assisting the individual to increase functional performance in the face of impairment by reestablishing prior skills and by developing compensatory skills if needed, and with assisting the disabled individual to become re-engaged in the affairs of society and daily living at a level at which the patient can achieve a satisfactory quality of life. Comprehensive medical rehabilitation attempts to improve the patient's medical or physical status, whatever that status may be, and to increase the efficacy of the patient's performance. The former of those two areas of

concern focuses primarily on medical problems, in a broadly defined sense. The latter area involves problems of learning and behavior. This chapter is primarily concerned with the latter area and addresses this issue from a broadly based behavioral perspective.

Several characteristics of the behavioral approach[17] suggest that it is an appropriate perspective from which to view comprehensive medical rehabilitation. First, the behavioral approach is based on learning concepts; comprehensive medical rehabilitation is a learning process. At the onset of a physical disability, some immediate changes take place in the behavior potential or the response repertoire of the individual who has been disabled. For example, the patient who sustains an injury to the spinal cord undergoes significant change in a host of behaviors, e.g., the ability to relieve pressure on the skin and the ability to ambulate. The disability will change the patient's needs as well as how the patient can fulfill those needs. But the new behaviors will not occur until the patient has learned them. Effective learning consists of both acquiring the skill or ability to do something and using the skill when it is appropriate. Both skill acquisition and appropriate use of the skill are part of the learning process.

Second, the behavioral perspective views normal and abnormal behavior as quantitatively rather than qualitatively different, i.e., behaviors are not inherently "sick" or "healthy." Instead, types of behavior represent points on a continuum to which psychological principles apply at all points. This is a useful approach to take in viewing the "behav-

JO ANN BROCKWAY AND WILBERT E. FORDYCE

ioral" or "adjustment" problems that are seen in the medical rehabilitation setting. It may be best to view the clientele of medical rehabilitation as normal individuals who have undergone an abnormal event (i.e., the onset of a physical disability). If the patient's reactions to the onset of disability are viewed as being subject to the principles of psychology and are thus understood in the context in which they occur, these reactions may be seen by staff as more manageable and as less disruptive to the rehabilitation program.

Third, the behavioral approach focuses directly on maladaptive behavior. Behavior is viewed not as a sign of some underlying pathological condition, but as the focus of treatment in itself. Traditionally, problems of adjustment have been viewed from a medical or medically oriented conceptional model. That is, those behaviors in which the individual engages that cause others to identify him as either adjusted or not adjusted have been seen as under the control of intrapsychic factors within the individual. This approach has evolved from traditional medical concepts in which symptoms are identified as being under the control of underlying pathological conditions. The medical frame of reference (Fig. 6–1) has been applied by analogy to problems of adjustment. The behavioral perspective (Fig. 6–2) used here views those behaviors defined as indicative of adjustment or maladjustment as subject to the influence of learning processes. The behavioral perspective applies appropriate learning principles directly to the behavior to be changed rather than trying to change inferred underlying attitudes or feeling states so that a behavior change may occur. In essence, the major distinction between the medical model and the learning model, in the context of assimilation of disability, is that the approach of the medical

1. Observe "illness behavior" (symptom).
2. Identify "illness behavior"-consequence relationships.
3. Change behavior by rearranging behavior-consequence relationships.

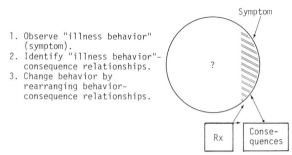

FIGURE 6–2. The learning model.

model emphasizes the change of underlying attitudes and feeling states so that new behaviors may occur. In contrast, the learning model aims at changing these behaviors directly. Treating behavior directly does not mean, in a broad-based learning view, that internal states are necessarily ignored or rejected. The cognitive behavioral approach focuses on beliefs and thought processes when these elements are seen as problems in and of themselves.

A fourth characteristic of the behavioral approach is the emphasis on the assessment of behavior and the evaluation of treatment. The problem is carefully defined so that the target behavior and the conditions under which it occurs can be specified. Such specificity facilitates evaluation of the effectiveness of the intervention. Such a focus is particularly appropriate for providing feedback to patients, families, and staff in the rehabilitation setting. One of the major differences between rehabilitation medicine and most other medical fields is that rehabilitation medicine focuses on medical problems of a chronic nature. Disability usually cannot be totally eliminated or resolved and residual impairments persist. In contrast to acute, time-limited medical problems, which ordinarily do not require the patient to make a lasting behavior change, chronic disease problems, as with physical disability, usually do require major and permanent behavior changes. In addition, many behavior changes that are required owing to the disability are low-frequency, low-strength, low-value behaviors, having minimal inherent attractiveness to the patient or to the family, thereby complicating the learning process. Finally, it is generally the case that the rate of progress in rehabilitation is relatively slow in comparison with the time frame of acute illness. As a consequence, the learning process may be further burdened by a dearth of the rewards for rapid progress, not only for the patient and the family but for the staff as well. By specifying and quantifying appropriate

1. Observe symptoms ("illness behavior").
2. Try to identify underlying pathology ("diagnosis").
3. Treat by attacking underlying pathology.

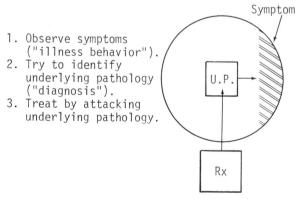

FIGURE 6–1. The disease-medical model.

target behaviors, progress in rehabilitation therapy activities can be documented and can become part of the client's and the family's reinforcement systems, as well as part of the staff's reinforcement system.

Although a behavioral perspective has much to offer as a viewpoint for patient behaviors of concern to medical rehabilitation staff, it is important to establish an appropriate perspective with regard to the use of behavioral methods. At one extreme, the more psychodynamic (e.g., Freudian) approaches to understanding human behavior have postulated the emergence of a basic personality or set of attitudes, i.e., a configuration of traits, that direct or guide behavior. The emphasis is on inferred inner or underlying psychological mechanisms. That view has tended to attach little importance either to discriminative stimuli or to contingent consequences in either the present or the future environment. At the other extreme, cumbersome doctrinaire behavioral approaches state that behavior is controlled strictly by discriminative stimuli or contingent consequences, thereby underemphasizing the contributions of the meaning of the stimuli to the individual, and of prior experience or learning. Both are oversimplifications. The position taken here is an "interactionist" one. Behavior is seen as a complex function of biological predisposition, meaning,* prior experience, and present stimuli. Previous learning has helped to determine which stimuli in the environment will be discriminated and responded to and which contingencies are likely to prevail as consequences of alternative behaviors. At the same time, the present environment will provide cues or indicators of probable consequences of alternative behaviors.

Learning Principles

The learning principles underlying the behavioral perspective are described briefly. It is not possible to develop mastery over their application by study of the summary statements and illustrations provided here. It should be possible, however, to develop an understanding of the principles involved and an appreciation of basic methods sufficient to participate with the behavioral psychologist in their application.

There are essentially two types of learning, clas-

---

*Meaning also implies anticipation of consequences and, as such, points to the role of both cognitive and behavioral factors.

sical and operant conditioning, which have been demonstrated in the laboratory.[17] Classical conditioning occurs when a previously neutral stimulus (the conditioned stimulus) is temporally paired with a stimulus (the unconditioned stimulus) known to automatically elicit a particular response (the unconditioned response). After a number of pairings, presentation of the conditioned stimulus alone will elicit a response (conditioned response) that is similar to the unconditioned response. The principles underlying operant conditioning are the principal focus of this chapter. Operant conditioning principles derive from the work of B. F. Skinner.[31, 32] Concise treatment of operant principles and illustrations of applications are found, for example, in Berni and Fordyce,[6] Marr and Means,[23] Ince,[16] Krasner and Ullmann,[18] Michael,[24] Patterson and Guillion,[26] and Reese.[28] The brief statement of the principles given here draws heavily on the work of Michael[24] and of Lindsley and Skinner.[22]

A distinction is drawn between respondent and operant behavior. Respondents are responses of the organism involving glandular, smooth muscle, or reflex phenomena. They are under the control of antecedent stimulation—that is to say, upon occurrence of an adequate stimulus, the respondent follows automatically. Operants are behaviors involving striated muscles or voluntary actions. Operants may be elicited by an antecedent stimulus. However, the strength of an operant response (i.e., the probability that it will occur in a given situation) is subject to influence by consequences. Manipulation of consequences is the critical operation in operant conditioning. When an operant is followed by a positive consequence (reinforcer), its frequency tends to increase. When an operant is followed by a negative or aversive reinforcer (punisher), its rate tends to decrease, although this effect is generally temporary. When positive reinforcers are withdrawn from an operant, its rate will diminish and ultimately disappear, a process termed extinction.

The effectiveness of a reinforcer on an operant is related to prior stimulus situations in which the operant has occurred contiguous to that reinforcer. A reinforcer will have more effect on an operant when it is delivered or withheld in the same stimulus setting as has occurred previously. The more the setting in which the stimulus has occurred has changed, the less is the effect of the reinforcer. As behavior occurs and is reinforced or punished in changing stimulus situations, the new stimuli will tend to act as reinforcers, i.e., they become conditioned reinforcers or conditioned punishers.

JO ANN BROCKWAY AND WILBERT E. FORDYCE

A given consequence can be identified as a reinforcer or punisher only by observation of its effects on the behavior it follows. One cannot assume that a given consequence is a positive reinforcer. One may accept the hypothesis and experiment with it. Having done so, if in fact the behavior the consequence follows increases in rate, it may be inferred that the consequence is a positive reinforcer for that person.

In order to be effective, reinforcers must be delivered as soon as possible following the behavior they are designed to influence. The longer the delay, the less effective the reinforcer will be. Schedules of reinforcement play an important role. When starting a new behavior or increasing the rate of occurrence of a behavior that previously rarely occurred, it is advantageous to reinforce as many occurrences of the behavior as possible (continuous reinforcement), i.e., one approaches a 1:1 response-reinforcement ratio. When a behavior becomes established, it will become more durable if the reinforcement schedule is reduced (intermittent reinforcement), i.e., a decreasing proportion of occurrences of the response receives reinforcement.

The most important principle to remember in regard to selection and programming of reinforcers is the Premack principle.[27] It states that ". . . high-frequency behavior can be used to strengthen low-frequency behavior . . ." That idea can be paraphrased as, "What a person does repeatedly can, when appropriately programmed, be a powerful means of increasing actions that the person usually does not do, i.e., the behavior that needs to be strengthened." One implication of this principle is that a potentially effective reinforcer will always be available in any situation; the person is sure to be doing something constantly, even if it is only insisting on remaining in bed instead of getting up for treatment.

New and complex responses are acquired by shaping. In shaping, successive approximations of the desired response are reinforced. Systematically varying the stimulus situations for an established response (stimulus fading) helps bring the response under control of increasingly complex or remote stimuli, thereby making it more durable. Certain rules should be kept in mind in applying these principles:

1. It is not effective simply to try to eliminate a behavior. An alternative response must be available; if one is not, the person should be helped to acquire an alternative.

2. It is easier to accelerate than to decelerate a response. This means that when trying to help a person eliminate or reduce some behavior, it is usually easier to focus on increasing a response incompatible with the one to be reduced rather than only trying to extinguish the undesired behavior.

3. Reinforcers or consequences naturally occurring in the treatment environment are usually more effective and easier to program than a consequence found outside that environment. Rest or time-out from arduous activity and praise, attention, or social reinforcement are the more common examples.

The sequence for initiating operant-based behavior change is as follows: (1) The behavior to be increased or decreased is pinpointed. (2) Measurable units of that behavior are defined, e.g., the beginning and the end of the cycle of movements constituting the behavior. A movement cycle may be said to have occurred when the organism is in a position to repeat the behavior. (3) The rate at which the behavior occurs is recorded. Rate is always defined as the number of movement cycles over a unit of time. (4) Reinforcers that are anticipated to be effective are identified. Reinforcers should not be used unless they can be made contingent upon the behavior to be influenced. If a reinforcer cannot be available to a patient, the process should not be used. (5) A schedule of reinforcement is specified. (6) The program is tried. If the rate of the behavior in question does not change following a reasonable number of trials, each of the preceding steps needs to be reexamined. As progress occurs, it is usually desirable to decrease the rate of reinforcement, i.e., to expect increasing amounts of performance for each unit of reinforcement. In later portions of this chapter, examples will be given of applications of these methods to specific problems in patient management.

The behavioral analysis and contingency management systems for modifying behavior described here represent a departure from more traditional approaches. Behavioral methods can be very effective in bringing about behavior change, but their use requires appropriate training and experience. Their use also raises a number of ethical questions that deserve at least brief consideration here. Further discussion of ethical issues can be found in Berni and Fordyce[6] and in Ulrich and co-workers.[35, 36]

Contingency management methods involve the manipulation of behavior-consequence relationships. When these manipulations are handled correctly, behavior change probably will ensue. The question rightfully should be raised as to whether one is arbitrarily manipulating a patient when these techniques are being applied. Concern about manipulation of patients should be directed toward any treatment approach that fails to specify methods and goals as well as to provide an opportunity for the patient to decide whether or not to participate.

There is every reason to explain to the patient in detail the design and objectives of a contingency management program. It is sometimes mistakenly inferred that telling the patient about a contingency management program will somehow compromise its effectiveness. Quite to the contrary, a well-planned program involves the patient to a much greater degree than frequently is true of more traditional approaches. Behaviors that are expected by the end of the program, i.e., the program's goals, should be specified. Those goals should be formulated with the patient. The patient should also participate, when possible, in the selection of reinforcers. The only exceptions to this procedure are those situations in which the patient is not able to participate because of youth (preschool age) or because of an intellectual impairment from a cortical deficit.

Adjustment to Disability

In a sense, the process of adjustment to disability begins at birth. This may be obvious in the context of the individual whose disability is congenital. It is less obvious in but equally true of the individual with a later onset of disability. An individual's adjustment to disability is a function of the behavioral repertoire acquired prior to the onset of the disability, the behavioral repertoire remaining to the patient after the onset of the disability, the meaning or value of the disability and losses to the patient, and the response of the environment to the patient with respect to the disability (Fig. 6–3).

The individual's behavioral repertoire before the onset of the disability is itself a complex function of biological predispositions, learning history, and environmental stimuli. As discussed in an earlier section, behavior is influenced by its consequences. An individual's behavioral repertoire is maintained by some kind of reinforcement. The onset of disability usually results in a decrease in or elimination of at least some of the individual's abilities and requires the acquisition of new behaviors that

are often undesired by the individual. These changes entail a modification of the pattern of the individual's behavior and the environmental consequences of such behavior.

The newly disabled individual, then, will likely experience a decrease in reinforcement because the patient can no longer engage in behaviors that were supported by the earlier types of reinforcement. After the onset of disability, the individual's opportunities for obtaining reinforcement may be significantly diminished. If the patient needs hospitalization for acute or rehabilitative care at a distance from the home community, the patient is separated from the family and the social support network. New limitations in physical activity may result in at least a temporary loss of reinforcement previously derived from vocational endeavors or from recreational activities. Similarly, the individual who derived reinforcement from what were felt to be attractive physical attributes may perceive a loss of reinforcement owing to undesired changes in the body that may accompany the onset of disability.

The acquired disability often not only results in a loss of reinforcement but also may result in the onset of aversive consequences. Pain, for example, may accompany the onset of the disability. The early lack of control over bodily functions, such as urination or defecation; the inability to perform seemingly simple, previously routine tasks such as eating or dressing; and the fatigue at the end of the day are other aversive consequences of physical disability.

Perhaps even more aversive and more problematic for many newly disabled individuals are their own negative emotional reactions to acquiring a disability, emotions that may be intensified by the patient's cognitive abilities. The individual's negative emotional reactions to the disability are related to the social and verbal history. The individual very likely has a pre-disability perception, perhaps in part incorrect, of what changes in life style the disability might entail. In addition, the patient has been exposed to and probably shares the widespread negative stereotype of the disabled and the negative attitude toward the abilities and worth of people with disabilities.[29, 30, 38] All of these elements can be experienced, not once, but repeatedly. As Michael[25] put it, the individual, ". . . because of his verbal skills, can react to the situation all at once, as soon as the verbal stimuli are appropriate. Furthermore, he/she can react to it again and again as he/she and others provide further stimuli, related to the irreversible change, and this reaction

JO ANN BROCKWAY AND WILBERT E. FORDYCE

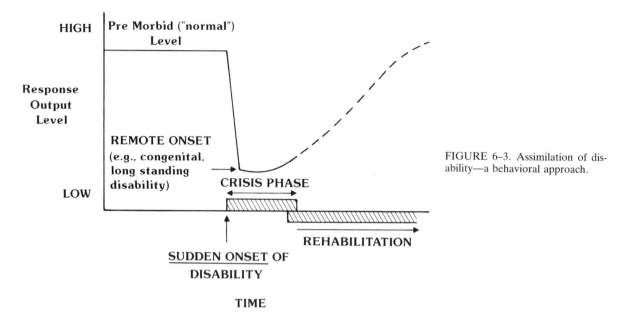

FIGURE 6–3. Assimilation of disability—a behavioral approach.

. . . consists of negative emotional conditions plus his operant repertoire of escape and avoidance behaviors."

The loss of reinforcement resulting from the limitations imposed by the new disability on a wide range of life's activities, the aversive sequelae of disability such as pain and fatigue, the individual's cognitions regarding the negative aspects of disability, and the negative attitudes of others toward the disabled can combine to result in emotional catastrophe.[25] The individual's reaction to such a catastrophe may include a variety of escape and avoidance behaviors, such as refusal to participate in therapy, lack of interaction with staff or other patients, and exhibition of verbally or physically aggressive behaviors. Such reactions from the newly disabled individual, although they are by no means universal, should not be surprising if one conceptualizes the newly acquired disability as punishment.

As noted previously, *punishment* refers to any stimulus change, when it is contingent on a behavior, that serves to decrease the strength or rate of occurrence of that behavior or strengthens behavior designed to avoid or escape the punishing stimulus.[7] Another way of stating the same idea is that punishment may be thought of as either the withdrawal of positive reinforcers or the application of aversive stimuli, both of which can occur as a result of the onset of physical disability. The concept of the onset of disability as punishment does not imply physical punishment or even the

activity of another person. Rather, the patient's loss of access to the positive reinforcers previously sustaining work and leisure activities, the onset of pain, physical distress, difficulty in accomplishing tasks, and negative cognitions may all be conceptualized as punishment.

The result of punishment is generally either a decrease in strength of the behavior it follows or an increase in behaviors designed to escape or avoid the punishment. Participation in rehabilitation activities, such as physical therapy or catheterizing, may lead to the onset of physical discomfort or negative cognitions or, expressed another way, to punishment. Thus, one should not be surprised if the individual who is newly disabled engages in withdrawal behavior at times that allows the avoidance of therapy activities that may be painful or frustrating or may engender negative cognitions. Similarly, the behavior of the individual who is at times verbally abusive to staff and thus temporarily interrupting (escaping) an aversive activity may be seen in a less adversarial light. Such behaviors may serve to decrease the punishing aspects of disability by providing time-out from having to actively engage in disability-related behavior, or by providing time-out from acknowledging the reality of the disability. Although such behaviors are frustrating for staff and maladaptive in terms of the patient's achieving optimal function, they may be understandable as psychologically lawful and predictable responses, given the conceptualization of the onset of disability as punishment. With this perspective in mind, the rehabilitation professional may be able to respond to such behaviors in a more productive manner.

The response of the social environment toward the patient is important in the individual's adjustment to disability. Within the acute care and rehabilitation period, the response of the immediate environment, i.e., family, friends, and rehabilitation team, may play a large part in the patient's progress toward rehabilitation goals. Most recently disabled patients have not yet learned ineffective behaviors related to their disabilities, and their families have not yet evolved a pattern of reinforcing such behaviors. If rehabilitation-appropriate behaviors are reinforced by the rehabilitation team, if rehabilitation-inappropriate behaviors are not reinforced, and if family members can be taught to do the same, good adjustment is facilitated.

A host of issues related to the response of the larger environment, i.e., the social, cultural and political environment, to individuals with disability has a bearing on the patient's long-term adjustment to disability. Although it is not the focus of this chapter to review these issues, the rehabilitation professional should be cognizant of them. The reader is referred to Vash for further reading.[37]

Evaluation

The objectives of psychological evaluation in rehabilitation are to predict what the patient is likely to do in rehabilitation and in relevant situations in the future and to identify stimulus situations and reinforcers likely to influence patient behavior. Fulfilling these objectives can provide a basis for planning rehabilitation.

It was noted in an earlier section that an individual's adjustment to disability is related to the following: the behavioral repertoire the patient had prior to onset of the disability, the behavioral repertoire remaining to the patient after the onset of the disability, the meaning or value of the disability and the ensuing life changes to the patient, and the environment's response to the disability. The greater the similarity between the patient's past behavior and the patient's capabilities after disability, the less likely it is that the ensuing behavior changes will be perceived by her as low frequency, low strength, and low value. In addition, the better the patient's coping skills are prior to the onset of the disability, the better equipped the patient will be to make the needed

changes in behavior. It is important, therefore, to identify what the patient has done in the past to assess whether special intervention will be needed to establish new behaviors.

Evaluation may include a combination of history-taking in the form of an interview with the patient and/or the family, psychometric testing, and obtaining current behavior samples from the patient in the form of direct observation. The interview may elicit information regarding the patient's understanding and expectations of the medical nature and functional outcome of the disability, the patient's goals for participation in the rehabilitation process, and the patient's cognitions regarding the disability. The best estimate of an individual's future behavior is derived from knowledge of the patient's past behavior. Information about the patient's vocation, recreation, and leisure-time pursuits should tell much about what is likely to be a reinforcing factor in the future. Information regarding coping skills, substance abuse, and risk-taking is useful in predicting future behavior. Nonetheless, there are many reasons why the patient's past behavior may not be an adequate prologue for future behavior. Youthfulness of the patient, a vague or incomplete picture of what the patient had done, or radical changes in what is possible for the patient in the future all make additional information essential.

An additional and frequently very rich source of information for providing estimates of future activities that are likely to be reinforcing is the group of activities in which the patient's early models—usually parents or older siblings—have engaged. Personality and modes of self-expression and coping are, in large measure, learned. They are learned by a combination of the influence of consequences of behaviors practiced in a particular environment and by modeling or learning by social imitation.[2-4] It frequently proves fruitful, therefore, to obtain a detailed picture of the leisure and vocational activities of those who have served as significant models for the patient.

The use of psychological testing in patient evaluation needs some consideration. Which tests are used and how frequently they are used varies markedly from psychologist to psychologist. That variability and the sometimes seemingly inexplicable relationship between the stimulus materials in a test and the inferential comments made about test responses make it difficult to maintain a clear perspective as to what psychological testing is all about. Psychological tests are one kind of behavior sample designed to provide a basis for predicting how the tested person will behave in nontest situations.

Sometimes psychological tests, like x-ray studies, are seen as revealing underlying characteristics that, when understood, permit rather precise predictions of future behaviors. That view, however, is of questionable validity. It implies that personality steers the individual into actions somewhat independently of the context in which the individual functions. It is more accurate to recognize that human behavior is governed by a combination of the repertoire of the individual and influences from the immediate environment. Psychological test responses are one kind of behavior. What the person will do in some other situation is another kind of behavior. The degree to which these two behaviors do correlate in fact cannot exceed the degree of comparability of test stimuli and future situations. As future situations depart more and more from stimuli surrounding the testing and the test itself, the predictive efficiency of the test data is correspondingly diminished.

The accuracy of predictions that a psychologist may make based on test data depends in part upon the extent to which the test has been standardized for comparable populations. This point is illustrated by the obvious fallacy of trying to predict subsequent academic performance of an English-speaking native of upper Sudan based on scores derived from intelligence tests standardized on middle-class American normative groups. Some tests have normative data based on reference populations about which much is known. When the rehabilitation clients being tested are from comparable reference populations, the normative data are directly relevant and few interpretative problems exist. When standardization is carried out on a different type of population or when very limited standardization is carried out, as frequently is the case in many psychological tests, reliance on the extrapolating acumen of the psychologist is increased.

Rehabilitation programs are confronted with many evaluation problems for which few, if any, standardization data are available. The compromise imposed by necessity is to ask the psychologist to make estimates or predictions according to the psychologist's best judgment and experience based on the test data accumulated. The psychologist must therefore have latitude in selecting the tests to be used so that, given the assessment question and the particular patient to be assessed, instruments can be used that are most appropriate psychometrically and with which the psychologist has had the most experience. Under these conditions, the utility of the psychological test report will be correspondingly greater as the psychologist becomes better acquainted with the stimulus situations in which the behavior the psychologist is trying to predict will occur. The psychologist's contribution will be enhanced if the specialist is well acquainted with the rehabilitation process, the specific style of the rehabilitation team, and the literature regarding the use of the test instruments in relevant populations. The rehabilitation physician can enhance the contribution of the psychologist by encouraging continuing functional exposure to the rehabilitation team and by providing feedback to the psychologist about the accuracy of the predictions.

The direct observation of behavior is a valuable method of assessing what are often called "behavioral" or "motivational" problems. If done appropriately, such observation can help define target behavior, determine the antecedent stimuli and consequences of the behavior at issue, and identify potential reinforcers for alternative behavior.

Unfortunately, at times the environment provides reinforcers that are contingent on rehabilitation-inappropriate behaviors, such as withdrawal or aggressiveness. For example, during the initial period after injury when the patient can do very little independently, the patient may receive considerable attention and sympathy from family, friends, and staff. Even after becoming more active and beginning to participate in rehabilitation activities, the patient may receive considerable attention for withdrawal or dependent behaviors. On some occasions, attention may be given by the staff contingent on inappropriate behavior. That is, the patient who engages in appropriate behaviors may receive little social attention. When the patient refuses to attend therapy or does not drink enough liquids, the staff may offer considerable attention by verbalizing the necessity of engaging in the desired behavior, by encouraging the patient to engage in the desired behavior, and perhaps even by pleading with or cajoling the patient. Likewise, the patient who is verbally or physically aggressive may receive considerable attention for this behavior.

In addition, the family, friends, and staff sometimes actively, although perhaps unwittingly, discourage rehabilitation-appropriate behavior. In an attempt to express love, concern, or support, the family may offer unneeded assistance or may interrupt the patient's attempts at some activity by doing it themselves. To save time, the staff may administer care in which the patient could participate but that would take more time with the patient's participation. Behavioral assessment can be of particular importance in evaluating such problem behaviors. Careful observation can shed light on the antecedent conditions preceding the problem behavior and the consequences of the behavior. The specification and subsequent understanding of these relationships leads to the development of the strategy for altering the consequences of the problem behavior and thus modifying the patient's response.

Management Issues

A number of general principles, if followed, will decrease the frequency of patient-management problems. The principles are rather simple and appear almost too obvious to mention. Perhaps for those reasons they are often forgotten. First, the rehabilitation professional should treat the patient with respect. This may mean respecting privacy by knocking on the door before entering and by discussing patient problems in an area where others cannot hear the discussion; it may mean listening to the patient's concerns. Second, the patient should be actively involved in the rehabilitation process. Providing the patient with a clear rationale for treatment, discussing treatment alternatives with the patient, and requesting patient input into the decision-making process are important. Too often the team expects the patient to be able to manage self-care and to direct an attendant after discharge but responds negatively to patient assertiveness and direction during the rehabilitation process.

Third, it is important for the team to specify expectations and treatment goals. The rehabilitation team's evaluation of the patient should lead to a specification of the skills required in the environment in which the client will be placed and an understanding of the behaviors likely to be reinforced or punished by that environment. The rehabilitation team sometimes conceptualizes its goals in broad generalities, e.g., helping the patient to gain greater independence and more mobility. Eventually, a concept like independence must be translated into terms that specify the operations or behaviors in which the patient, the rehabilitation team, and the family are to engage. Failure of the rehabilitation team to arrive at those specifications leads to two kinds of problems. One is that individual therapists may be unclear as to what it is they are to do. What they do may even come into conflict with other aspects of the program. Failure to specify the target behaviors of the program also makes it difficult to realistically identify the extent to which the program has succeeded or failed. The failure to specify goals in concrete operational terms risks fostering the continuation of procedures that are ineffectual or inefficient.

Fourth, family members, like everyone else, need positive reinforcement for their behavior. Often, it is not sufficient to provide them with relevant information. The social worker and others on the rehabilitation team can make important contributions to patient progress through systematic contact with family members. These contacts should be designed to help the family anticipate the reinforcers that will become available to the patient and to themselves as the rehabilitation program progresses. Once communication and working relationships are well established, the focus can shift more toward working out details of what the patient and family will be doing upon completion of the rehabilitation program.

The patient who has had the disability for a long time may come from an environment that evolved effective reinforcement patterns for ineffectual or disability-inappropriate behavior. If substantial ineffectual behavior has been exhibited, the behavior must have been receiving reinforcement. If such a patient were to leave the rehabilitation program precipitately, the patient would return to an environment that would sustain the existing behavioral repertoire. If the patient successfully completes the rehabilitation program, the patient may return to an environment that will fail to reinforce the new behaviors and may resume reinforcing the previously ineffectual behaviors reduced by rehabilitation. It should be evident that those planning rehabilitation programs for patients who have had their disabilities for long periods of time need to be particularly concerned with analyzing the home situation. If a program concerns itself only with the patient's behavioral repertoire and ignores that of the family, behavioral changes brought about in rehabilitation may not persist.

The tactical steps for helping family members to change their behavior are the same as those for helping the patient. Family members need aid to pinpoint their own and the patient's behavior, to be aware of the rate of these behaviors, and to establish patterns of desired behaviors through the use of contingent rewards.

JO ANN BROCKWAY AND WILBERT E. FORDYCE

Crisis Management

Most rehabilitation facilities admit patients a few weeks or even a few months following the onset of an illness or trauma. As a consequence, the process of assimilation of what has happened by the patient will have already begun, whether purposefully or simply in the natural course of events. Sometimes rehabilitation begins soon after onset. In such cases, crisis management issues are important in early work with the recently disabled patient.

The radical change in the physical state of the body that accompanies significant disability of sudden onset (e.g., spinal cord injury, stroke, amputation) inherently provides a situation analogous to the work of Hebb of many years ago. Hebb noted that subjecting a person to a radical alteration in sensory input nearly always leads to disorganized behavior.[15] A case in which the lower half of a person's body is suddenly deprived of sensation represents a prototype of Hebb's concept because that person's central nervous system suddenly receives a quite different configuration of kinesthetic, tactile, and proprioceptive inputs. In addition to the neurophysiological sensory changes occasioned by severe injury, the move to a hospital bed and the subsequent changes in mobility and environment provide sudden and dramatic alterations in sensory input.

For the first several days or weeks following the onset of a disability, confusion and disorganization are to be expected. Familiar faces may be unrecognized. Temper outbursts may occur with little or no provocation. Intellectual confusion and misunderstanding of even simple communications may occur. This in itself does not imply disintegration of coping mechanisms or personality functioning. For some people, the stress of assimilating the fact of serious injury is more than they can readily handle, and indeed they become disorganized. However, virtually everyone with serious disability initially will show periods of confusion that do not presage lingering disorganization.

The theory of crisis management can be divided into two parts. The first is the recognition that the patient's difficulty will tend to improve if those responsible for the patient's care use reasonable skill. Hanford has noted that people in a crisis situation tend to be suggestible.[13] Therefore, the first rule of thumb in crisis management is to establish and maintain a calm environment as much as possible. This does not mean that sensory deprivation should be increased by keeping the patient isolated. To do that would likely aggravate the problem. It means to ensure that those working with the patient go about their business in a calm, deliberate, and supportive way. Members of the immediate family should also be helped to recognize that if they remain calm the patient will benefit.

The second part of the theory of crisis management takes us back to one of the basic principles of behavioral management, namely, that if one wishes a person to reduce some behavior (in this case, crisis-related behaviors) it is important to ensure that alternative behaviors are available. One of the more helpful crisis management tactics is to identify a concrete "life-on-the-ward" issue of relevance to the patient and then to enhance the patient's skill in coping with the problem. For example, it might be noted that an individual who is newly disabled with quadriplegia is not effective in asking for help in ways that make it easier for the helper to give help. The patient's frequent disorganized requests to the nursing staff to provide a service, particularly immediately after the nurse has just fulfilled a previous request and left the patient's room, are not well designed to enhance nurse support. If, however, a person such as the ward psychologist began working with the patient on organizing requests and on improving social skills with respect to assertiveness (e.g., ways of asking for help), two goals might be reached. One is the improvement of the patient's skill at developing optimal working relationships specifically with the treatment staff and the more general ability to foster and maintain needed assistance. The other goal is building the patient's sense of mastery of an immediately relevant problem and helping the patient to develop behavior alternatives to ruminating or daydreaming, or random and scattered mentation. A similar approach is also useful in the management of family members in a crisis situation. Identifying a concrete relevant task in which the family member can be involved will provide a focus for the person's attention and energy, a sense of contribution, and a sense of accomplishment.

Denial

Often, the patient with a recent onset of disability verbalizes after admission to the rehabilitation unit the expectation that "everything will return to normal," a notion that may be contrary to the rehabilitation team's perception of the prognosis. Rehabilitation staff often label this type of thinking denial. Often, people around the patient reinforce this behavior by making unrealistic statements indicating that the disability is temporary. If the patient verbalizes these feelings and yet continues to participate fully in the rehabilitation program, no problem should evolve. The denial can, in fact, be an adaptive behavior if it serves as a reinforcer of rehabilitation-appropriate behavior by providing the patient with the goal of improved function toward which to work. However, if the patient refuses to participate in various activities that are of importance, the rehabilitation team should take action.

The optimal conditions for extinction of refusal behavior are as follows: response occurs, it is not reinforced, an alternative response is available, and the alternative is effectively reinforced. The rehabilitation team should seek to reduce the direct reinforcement of unrealistic fantasies. The rehabilitation team should also move as rapidly as possible to shape alternative, rehabilitation-appropriate behaviors under optimal conditions of reinforcement. At all costs, the team should avoid punishing withdrawal or denial of disability. Punishment of the patient makes it more likely that the punisher will become a conditioned aversive stimulus, and the caretaker will thereby lose effectiveness as a source of support and reinforcement. At the same time, the punishment of denial behaviors risks suppressing the behavior to be extinguished. That factor, in turn, will inhibit extinction.

The patient's family may also need help with problems relating to the extinction of rehabilitation-inappropriate behavior. One reason families engage in unrealistic denial and reassuring behavior with the patient is that they lack viable alternatives. Providing families with information about what the patient is going to be able to do at the end of the program and about the patient's progress helps to give them alternatives that can be communicated to the patient. The use of performance graphs at the patient's bedside is one illustration of how this goal may be accomplished.

Depression and Grieving

Symptoms of depression are commonly exhibited by patients in the rehabilitation process. Two general behavioral conceptualizations of depression are recognized. The reinforcement view postulates that depression is a result of the reduction in the rate of response-contingent positive re-

inforcement,[20, 21] a condition that occurs at the onset of disability. The intervention strategy is to help the patient gain access to an increased rate of response-contingent reinforcement.

The second category of behavioral conceptualization of depression is the cognitive view of depression.[5] This view posits that depression is the result of negative cognitions; depressed people have negative views of themselves, the world, and the future. Intervention strategies focus on changing negative cognitions. Both conceptualizations have something to offer to the rehabilitation professional in dealing with the depressed patient.

The evaluation process will have provided information regarding previously reinforcing activities. Efforts should be made to ensure that some of those activities are available in the rehabilitation setting. Efforts also should be made to immediately provide tasks related to treatment that elicit reinforceable responses from the patient. Tasks should be broken down into small, manageable, reinforceable steps. Reinforcement should be provided for the accomplishment of each step. This may be done by social reinforcement or by providing access to some desired activity. Visual feedback in the form of performance graphs may both provide positive reinforcement and attack negative cognitions regarding inability. The team should focus on what the patient can do, pointing out the patient's skills and assets, and providing information on what kinds of things people with similar disabilities do (e.g., skiing, basketball, jobs). Individual or group counseling that focuses on changing negative cognitions is appropriate.

Chemotherapeutic intervention with antidepressant medication is sometimes indicated. Some depressive patterns are so severe that they leave the patient virtually incapable of producing reinforceable responses. Psychiatric consultation is certainly indicated in this kind of situation. Chemotherapeutic intervention should not be seen as incompatible in any way with the behavioral approaches just described. On the contrary, when chemotherapy is used, it should be coupled with the graded introduction of treatment-related tasks and the application of the appropriate reinforcing contingencies.

Motivation

The occurrence of rehabilitation-inappropriate behavior and the lack of rehabilitation-appropriate behavior have often been conceptualized as result-

JO ANN BROCKWAY AND WILBERT E. FORDYCE

ing from some sort of deficit within the patient, e.g., a lack of motivation. Goldiamond, a psychologist who sustained a spinal cord injury, described the reactions of the rehabilitation staff to his fellow patients who showed minimal rehabilitation-appropriate behavior:

Such cases puzzled the hospital staff. After all, people should want to get better, should want to stay alive longer. The staff knew how to make them better; so the patients should *want* to cooperate. When they did not, the staff would give them pep talks or scare talks, warning of the dire consequences of degeneration, show them movies, reason with them, etc. None of these tactics helped. The staff ascribed the negative attitudes of such patients to hostility, depression, or some underlying psychodynamic problem. But none of these labels were relevant to the problem, namely, the absence of consequences important enough to sustain the difficult responses necessary for producing and maintaining them.[12]

There is little doubt that the most frequently mentioned psychological problem in the context of disability and rehabilitation concerns patient motivation. Fishman[8] states: "Empirical evidence substantiates the theoretical consideration that the single most important problem facing the rehabilitation worker concerns the ways and means of implementing marginal motivation."

The conceptualization of motivation implicit in Goldiamond's description is based on the learning model; the management techniques derived from that model are quite different from the more traditional view based on a medical model.[9–11, 34] In the medical model, motivation is not an attribute of behavior but an inference about an inner state of the organism derived from observations of behavior. Used in that way, the concept of motivation adds nothing to information about the patient or to the clarification of courses for remedial action. Statements about the patient's motivation, although used characteristically as if they described some inner state of the organism, are in fact based on a relationship between what the patient has done and what observers thought the patient should do. That is, a patient is held to be "motivated" if engaged in the behaviors of interest at a rate acceptable to the rehabilitation team. If those behaviors do not occur at an acceptable rate, the patient is considered to be "unmotivated" or to be "motivated" for some less desirable goal.

Approaching the concept of motivation from the point of view of the learning model leads to a different formulation. Behavior is sensitive to consequences. If a behavior is occurring at an inade-

quate rate (i.e., the patient is "unmotivated"), some adjustment is needed in the contingencies to that behavior. If a patient is doing too much of something that interferes with performance of rehabilitation-appropriate behavior at a desired rate (i.e., the patient is "unmotivated" or "motivated" for the wrong reasons), the reinforcers to those undesired behaviors need to be withdrawn. To quote Michael,

From a behavioral point of view, however . . . marginal motivation seems merely to be a case of insufficient or poorly arranged reinforcement. The basic question that should be asked is 'What does the patient get out of his activity?' The problem of motivation is a simple one. One must merely arrange the environment so that its desirable features are only available contingent upon participation and accomplishment in the rehabilitation training activity.[24]

There are several reasons why motivation problems are so prominent in rehabilitation. The earlier discussion of punishment has shown how the onset of disability and the entrance into rehabilitation may initially be aversive. It is not surprising, therefore, that many patients fail to produce rehabilitation-appropriate behaviors at the desired rate.

There is another reason for the prominence of motivational problems. Staats[33] points out, "Discussions with therapists in rehabilitation suggest that much of their work, especially with children, involves training new behaviors under circumstances in which the reinforcers are weak. For example, prior to developing skills to deal with a prosthesis, the child secures reinforcement more easily for various previously learned substitution movements. Thus, some way must be found at first to supply 'prosthetic response,' in a competitive sense, since these responses are not in themselves 'naturally' reinforcing."

The essential features in the psychological management of motivation problems in rehabilitation consist of establishing treatment relationships that enhance the reinforcing value of interactions with rehabilitation professionals, of enhancing the value of long-term reinforcers for disability-appropriate behavior, and of carrying out the behavioral analysis and contingency management steps that promote acquisition of the new behaviors provided by effective rehabilitation.

Maintenance of Patient Performance

It is important to distinguish between the ability to do something and the probability that it will be done. It is easy to lose sight of the fact that these concepts are not the same. The knowledge that the patient has the ability to do something by no means ensures that, in fact, it will be done. If the rehabilitation program has given the patient the ability to do something that is subsequently not done, the program cannot be considered a success. The objectives of a rehabilitation program should be that the target behaviors occur at an appropriate rate in the environment in which they are supposed to occur and not only in the rehabilitation center. Obviously a rehabilitation program is limited in the extent to which it can influence the environment outside the treatment area to increase the probability of adequate patient performance. Nonetheless, the program should be considered incomplete if it has failed to assess the influence of the target environment on the behaviors being developed within rehabilitation and if actions have not been taken to influence the environment toward the end of increasing patient performance.

As noted earlier and by Staats,[33] rehabilitation may require the patient to perform tasks that are not intrinsically reinforcing and that, in fact, initially may be noxious, cumbersome, or unrewarding. The environment outside the rehabilitation program may not reinforce many newly acquired disability-relevant behaviors (e.g., ambulating by wheelchair, drinking large amounts of fluids, wearing an upper extremity prosthesis) at the same rate that it did for previous, nondisability-related behaviors. That means that special efforts must be made to provide contingencies in the environment that will maintain disability-relevant behaviors. If that effort is not made and the natural environment fails to reinforce disability-relevant behaviors acceptably, those behaviors will fade or be carried out at a rate that is lower than desirable.

The maintenance of disability-relevant behaviors following departure from the formal rehabilitation program is essentially a problem of generalization. Generalization in this context refers to the extent to which behavior that occurs in rehabilitation will also occur in the natural environment.

Two major strategies should be considered in promoting generalization. One is to bring disability-relevant behaviors under the control of reinforcers naturally occurring in the target environment. The other is to make a special effort to reprogram the natural environment so that it will deliver appropriate reinforcement contingent upon performance of these behaviors.

The first of these strategies, that is, relating the disability behaviors to naturally occurring reinforcers, provides the major conceptual basis for the importance of social and vocational programs in physical or medical rehabilitation. When a patient is effectively employed, for example, the reinforcers available in the work situation are likely to maintain behaviors immediately elicited by the job and other work-related behaviors, such as effective self-care, mobility, and fluid intake. The reinforcers provided by work may be money, status and prestige, socialization, sense of accomplishment, or other factors. One or more of those reinforcers may effectively maintain work behavior. For some people, they will not maintain work behavior at an adequate rate. In either case, alternative reinforcers may be available in the home environment to maintain essential disability-related behaviors. Stimulating recreational and leisure-time activities, for example, may provide sufficient reinforcement to maintain both the behaviors immediately elicited by those kinds of activities and related self-care behaviors.

A rehabilitation program can also enhance generalization by providing for gradual and systematic rehearsal of disability-relevant behaviors in environments closely approximating the natural environments in which they are to be carried out following rehabilitation. When a patient is provided the opportunity to exercise his new disability-related skills outside the treatment setting, it is more likely that those behaviors will come under the influence of reinforcers available in the nontreatment environment.

Excellent discussions of the principles of generalization and some illustrative applications are found in an article by Baer, Wolf, and Risley.[1]

CASE EXAMPLES

The following case studies illustrate some of the management problems seen in rehabilitation, the assessment of such problems, and management strategies. The first two cases illustrate the behavioral management approach in general procedural terms; the second two cases illustrate specific contingency management methods.

Case A

Ms. J. was a 22-year-old woman who was severely disabled with multiple sclerosis. She was unable to speak owing to dysarthria and had very poor trunk control, balance, and motor coordination. She was able, however, to communicate with others, using hand signals for "yes" and "no" responses.

In the psychologist's initial evaluation, an attempt was

made to administer tests of cognitive abilities that required no speech and limited hand function, but Ms. J. refused to complete the testing. Thus, no estimate of intellectual ability was obtained. Among the initial goals of the rehabilitation program were the development of a more practical communication system, independent wheelchair ambulation, and increased independence in activities of daily living. Although Ms. J. was improving her function in all areas, her progress was somewhat less than expected. The therapists noticed that she frequently cried in the therapy situation. The primary nurse observed that Ms. J. seemed to enjoy visits from her family but would begin to cry when the family members began to get ready to leave. In addition, the primary nurse noted that Ms. J.'s mother and sister frequently did things for her that she was able to do for herself.

It was decided to evaluate the problem further. Each staff member who worked with the patient was assigned the task of recording the number of times per therapy session or nursing contact that she cried, the duration of each crying spell, what activity preceded the crying, and what the staff member and others did in response to her crying. The primary nurse had, in addition, the responsibility for recording the same observations for the patient's interactions with her family.

After a one-week evaluation period, the staff met to discuss their findings. They found that Ms. J. cried in therapy when asked to attempt an activity that was either new or difficult for her, or when the therapist was attending to another patient. If the former were the case, the therapist would frequently encourage Ms. J. and tell her how well she was doing; if the crying persisted, the therapy session might be terminated. If the latter were the case, the therapist spent a great deal of time with Ms. J., encouraging her to attempt the difficult activity, talking with her in an attempt to find out what the problem was, or telling her that she could do the activity herself and that it was important that she do so. The primary nurse noted that when Ms. J. asked her family to do something for her, they would most often do it and then no crying would occur. The nurse also noted that when family members said they were leaving, or prepared to leave by doing such things as putting on coats or picking up packages, Ms. J. would begin to cry, an action that would result in the family's delaying their departure.

It was decided to propose a behavior modification program to Ms. J. and her parents.* It was explained to

*Ms. J.'s parents were involved in the consent primarily for two reasons. First, Ms. J.'s capacity to give informed consent was in question. Second, the parents were heavily involved in her care; thus they were a large part of the system of reinforcing appropriate or inappropriate behavior.

Ms. J. and her parents that her crying interfered with her rehabilitation program. The observed relationship between antecedent conditions (such as Ms. J.'s attempting a difficult task, or her parents' preparations to leave her room), Ms. J.'s crying, and the consequences of her crying (e.g., avoidance of the difficult task, her parents' delaying their departure) was explained in layman's terms. The method by which the team proposed to rearrange the patient behavior-consequence contingencies in an attempt to decrease crying and to increase independence was explained. The following program was implemented with the consent of Ms. J. and her parents. When Ms. J. cried in the therapy session after being asked to do something, the therapist said, "I'd like to work with you, but we can't accomplish anything when you are crying. I'll check back with you in a few minutes. If you are calm then, we can continue." The therapist then walked a short distance away and became busy with some other task, then returned to re-attempt the previous activity. The therapist also attempted to break down each activity into small, manageable steps and delivered social reinforcement, such as praise or social interaction, for the accomplishment of each step. If Ms. J. cried while the therapist was interacting with another patient, the therapist would walk over to Ms. J. and tell her that he would not return until Ms. J. regained her composure.

The primary nurse applied similar techniques when Ms. J. requested that the nurse do something for her that she could have done herself. The nurse refused, but said that she would visit with her while Ms. J. did the activity herself. The nurse also made a point of stopping by Ms. J.'s room for five minutes every half hour when Ms. J. was not crying. If she did cry, the nurse would enter her room and tell her that she'd return when Ms. J. was calmer and able to communicate.

The most difficult part of the intervention was training the family to respond in a manner similar to that of the staff. The psychologist met with the family and explained the rationale for the approach and the specifics of the approach. The family had to learn to leave when they said they had to go instead of staying longer, even though the patient cried. The family also role-played with the psychologist in responding to the patient's request for aid by telling her to take care of the matter herself and indicating that they would stay and chat while she did it. The primary nurse instructed the family as to what the patient could do for herself, so that they would know when her requests were legitimate. The primary nurse also gave the family positive reinforcement when appropriate for their nonreinforcement of Ms. J.'s crying and for their reinforcement of her independence.

The therapists and the nurse kept records of the

frequency and duration of crying over a six-week period, including the baseline or evaluation period. They found that crying episodes decreased in frequency from an average of six times a day, with a mean duration of three minutes during the base line period, to an average of twice a week, with a mean duration of 30 seconds by the end of the third week of the intervention, and that they became less frequent thereafter.

Case B

Mr. C. was a 34-year-old married man with no children who became a C 7 to C 8 quadriplegic as a result of a motor vehicle accident. He was admitted to the rehabilitation medicine service approximately three weeks after the injury. He had graduated from high school and had attended one year of college in an art-related field. Prior to his injury, he worked at two construction jobs and was in the process of building a home.

During the initial evaluation, Mr. C. was given the Wechsler Adult Intelligence Scale (WAIS) and the Minnesota Multiphasic Personality Inventory (MMPI) and was interviewed by the psychologist. He indicated in the interview that he was a "gimp" (i.e., a cripple), useless, and a burden to his wife. He said that he would not be able to do any of the things that he enjoyed, such as drawing, playing guitar, building his home, or walking in the woods. He expressed a considerable amount of anger and self-deprecation. On the WAIS he obtained a verbal IQ score within the high average range of intellectual function, a score that indicated that he was a bright man with good intellectual skills. The performance subtests were not given at that time because of his limited hand function. The MMPI profile suggested that Mr. C. was an active and energetic man who minimized emotional or interpersonal conflicts and who was concerned about somatic problems. The profile also suggested that he was likely to be somewhat manipulative and angry and tended to blame others for his difficulties. These results were communicated to the team.

After about two months, the primary nurse noted that Mr. C. increasingly complained of nausea and illness that at times prevented him from attending therapies. The nurse further noted that he often became angry during his wife's visits, that he told her to "go find a whole man," and that he made other angry, self-deprecating remarks. It was decided in a team conference to assess the problems by observation and by requesting that the psychologist interview the patient. The nursing staff and therapists were to record each time Mr. C. complained of illness and/or said he could not go to therapy because of illness, as well as to record their own behavior in response to his complaints and his declining to participate in treatment. In addition, the nursing staff was to record the frequency of Mr. C.'s angry outbursts

at his wife, the context and frequency of his self-deprecating comments to her, and her response to both. The psychologist interviewed Mr. C. regarding what goals he had set for himself, what reinforcers he perceived as no longer available, what reinforcers were available, and his cognitions regarding his disability.

It was found that Mr. C. complained of feeling ill primarily in the evenings and immediately before a scheduled therapy session that was preceded by his being in bed. He rarely complained of discomfort once he was up and in the therapy session. The staff noted that they responded to his complaints and refusals to come to therapy by encouraging him to get up; he generally responded with an angry outburst, after which he was left alone. His primary nurse noted that when his wife came to visit in the evenings, he was often in bed; she would encourage him to get up, or talk with him about what he had done or she had done during the day. Mr. C. often responded with anger, stating that he was not interested in what she did and that he could do nothing. She would then tell him how much luckier he was than some of the other patients, at which point he would generally make comments such as "go away and leave me alone," or "go find someone else who's not a gimp." She would then, typically, reassure him that nothing in their relationship had changed.

Mr. C. indicated in his interview with the psychologist that he felt that he had no goals and that he did not think he could do anything worthwhile. The things he had liked about himself were no longer accessible to him, and there was nothing that he liked about himself now. For example, he had liked himself for his mechanical ability, which had enabled him to do many of his own car repairs; he was no longer physically able to repair his car.

The rehabilitation team felt that at least two significant problems were identifiable. One involved Mr. C.'s negative cognitions about himself as a disabled person. He saw himself as unable to do anything worthwhile. The second was an inability to perceive that he was making any gains. He was still unable to do an independent transfer; therefore, he had made no progress in transfers.

The team decided to make several changes in Mr. C.'s program. These changes were designed to provide increased feedback to him regarding progress and to focus on what he could do rather than what he could not do. Each staff member compiled a list of concrete activities that Mr. C. should be able to accomplish before he was discharged. Each activity was broken down into a sequence of individual steps so that progress could be seen as each step was accomplished. For example, the activity of dressing included putting on T-shirts, putting on short-sleeved shirts with buttons, putting on long-sleeved shirts with buttons, taking off long-sleeved shirts

JO ANN BROCKWAY AND WILBERT E. FORDYCE

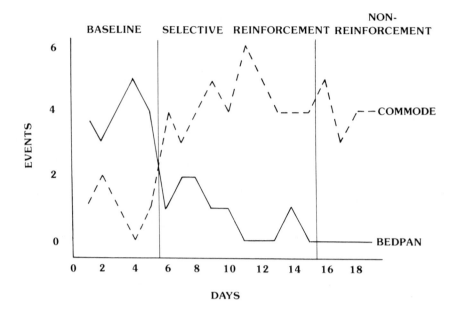

FIGURE 6–4. Improving self-care performance with social reinforcement.

with buttons, putting on pants, and so on. Each item was checked off as it was accomplished. Graphs were made of Mr. C.'s progressive resistance exercises, wheelchair ambulation distance and times, and other appropriate activities to show his progress visually. It was felt that feedback enabling Mr. C. to see his progress would be reinforcing in itself. Complaints of fatigue and illness were to be responded to in a neutral manner by staff; Mr. C. was simply told in a matter-of-fact way that he was expected in therapy.

In addition to the above, the psychologist worked individually with Mr. C. for several sessions, explored his cognitions regarding disability, and attempted to focus on what he *could* do rather than what he *could*

not do. For example, the psychologist pointed out that although Mr. C. might not be able to get under the hood of his car and work on the engine, he still had the intellectual skill to diagnose the car's problem and tell someone else what to do about it. The psychologist also worked with Mr. C.'s wife to help her learn to look at his records of progress and reinforce his specific accomplishments, to respond to his self-deprecating remarks in a neutral way, and to share with him her reactions to his behavior as well as her concerns about their future.

Mr. C. was encouraged to participate in the decision-making process in his rehabilitation program. As he began to be aware of his progress and to focus on his skills rather than his limitations, his complaints of nausea

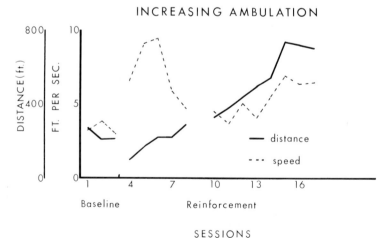

FIGURE 6–5. Increasing ambulation.

and illness decreased sharply. He became more active in his rehabilitation program and began to accept the process of devising better methods of doing things as a challenge. For example, he suggested a modification of a splint that resulted in increased hand function for himself.

Case C

The patient was a 62-year-old woman who had a resection of the left head and neck of the femur because of infection. Postoperatively, she had hyponatremia, a myocardial infarction, acute tubular necrosis, and anemia. Three weeks after the myocardial infarction, she began rehabilitation for ambulation. She was emaciated and weak and had a painful left hip. She rapidly learned transfers and gained strength. However, routinely she requested a bedpan rather than transferring to a commode. The target behavior was to increase use of the commode. The movement cycle was to transfer to the commode and to return to bed or to the wheelchair.

Reinforcers. It was observed that the patient engaged the staff in conversation at any opportunity and that she seemed to get a great deal of pleasure from these conversations. Therefore, chatting and interacting with the staff were chosen as the reinforcers.

Procedure. (1) Base line: Requests for bedpan or commode were honored without comment and the nursing staff continued to chat with the patient at those times. In general, the patient used the commode once daily and the bedpan the rest of the time. (2) Selective reinforcement: As before, the bedpan or commode was supplied upon request. The nurse would stay to chat only when the commode was used. The patient was not informed of this. Nonetheless, within three days use of the bedpan had fallen essentially to zero. On the 16th day, the selective reinforcement program was terminated in order to assess how well the new behavior was established. (3) Result: Use of the bedpan remained at zero. Behavioral data are found in Figure 6–4.

Case D

The patient was a 28-year-old male who had sustained an L 5–S 1 fracture-dislocation that resulted in incomplete paraplegia. Owing to the seriousness of the injury, many additional procedures were necessary, including diversionary colostomy, and multiple graft and skin flap rotations to repair massive soft tissue injury. Sequelae included multiple surgeries for recurrent renal stone formation associated with primary renal failure at the time of injury, immobilization, hypercalcemia, and recurrent urinary tract infections. In addition to these many setbacks, the patient had been under psychiatric care for four years prior to the injury and was described as having a schizoid personality. For the patient, the

result was apprehension, mistrust, and the conviction that his injury was a form of punishment.

The immediate treatment task considered here was to increase ambulation with a walker and with the use of short leg braces, the goal being independence in mobility. The target was ambulation, and the movement cycle was the number of laps walked, expressed in the number of feet traversed. In addition, the speed of walking was recorded.

After full discussions by the psychologist with the patient and in collaboration with the physical therapist, a contingency management plan was set up. The reinforcers were praise by the therapist, rest (two minutes following achievement of a quota), and a cup of ice chips, which the patient had been observed to enjoy. For three days, from twice daily sessions and two trials per session, baseline values were obtained without reinforcement. Thereafter, the contingency arrangements went into effect. One additional trial was added to each session. Thus, additional trials and additional distance constituted a fading of reinforcement, because attainment of the rewards of praise, rest, and ice chips required increasingly greater amounts of performance. Behavioral data are shown in Figure 6–5.

References

1. Baer, D., Wolf, M., and Risley, T.: Some current dimensions of applied behavior analysis. J. Appl. Behav. Anal., 1:91–97, 1968.
2. Bandura, A.: Psychotherapy Conceptualized as a Social-Learning Process. Unpublished manuscript, Stanford University, 1964.
3. Bandura, A.: Behavioral Modification through modeling procedures. In Krasner, L., and Ulllmann, L. (Eds.): Research in Behavior Modification. New York, Holt, Rinehart and Winston, 1966, pp. 310–340.
4. Bandura, A., and Walters, R.: Social Learning and Personality Development. New York, Holt, Rinehart and Winston, 1963.
5. Beck, A. T., Rush, A. J., Shaw, B. F., and Emery, G.: Cognitive Therapy of Depression. New York, Guilford Press, 1979.
6. Berni, R., and Fordyce, W.: Behavior Modification and the Nursing Process, 2nd Ed. St. Louis, C. V. Mosby Co., 1977.
7. Ferster, C.: Classification of behavioral pathology. In Krasner, L., and Ullmann, L. (Eds.): Research in Behavior Modification. New York, Holt, Rinehart and Winston, 1966, pp. 6–26.
8. Fishman, S.: Amputation. In Garrett, J., and Levine, E. (Eds.): Psychological Practices with the Physically Disabled. New York, Columbia University Press, 1962, pp. 1–50.

9. Fordyce, W. E.: Behavioral Methods in Rehabilitation. Washington, D.C., American Psychological Association, 1970.
10. Fordyce, W.: Research on influencing level of patient participation in the rehabilitation process. *In* Fuhrer, M. (Ed.): Selected Research Topics in Spinal Cord Injury Rehabilitation. Rehab. Serv. Admin. Washington, D.C., Department of Health, Education, and Welfare, 1975, pp. 55–69.
11. Fordyce, W.: Behavioral methods in the rehabilitation process. *In* Eisenberg, M., and Falconer, J. (Eds.): Treatment of the Spinal Cord Injured: An Interdisciplinary Perspective. Springfield, Ill., Charles C Thomas, Publisher, 1979, pp. 82–100.
12. Goldiamond, I.: A diary of self-modification. Psychology Today, 7(6):95–102, 1973.
13. Hanford, D.: Life crisis viewed as opportunity. The Bulletin, Division of Mental Health, State of Washington, 9(2):87, 1965.
14. Hathaway, S. R., and McKinley, J. C.: The Minnesota Multiphasic Personality Inventory Manual (Revised). New York, Psychological Corporation, 1967.
15. Hebb, D.: The Organization of Behavior. New York, John Wiley and Sons, 1949.
16. Ince, L.: Behavior Modification in Rehabilitation Medicine. Springfield, Ill., Charles C Thomas, Publisher, 1976.
17. Kazdin, A. E.: History of Behavior Modification. *In* Bellack, A. S., Hersen, M., and Kazdin, A. E. (Eds.): International Handbook of Behavioral Modification and Therapy. New York, Plenum Press, 1982.
18. Krasner, L., and Ullmann, L. (Eds.): Research in Behavior Modification. New York, Holt, Rinehart and Winston, 1966.
19. Krasner, L.: Applications of token economy in chronic populations. *In* Token Economies: Current Status—Future Directions. Symposium presented at the Meeting of the American Psychological Association, San Francisco, September, 1968.
20. Lewinsohn, P. M., and Amenson, C. S.: Some relations between pleasant and unpleasant mood-related events and depression. J. Abnorm. Psychol., 87:651–654, 1978.
21. Lewinsohn, P. M., and Graff, M.: Pleasant activities and depression. J. Consult. Clin. Psychol., 41:271–278, 1978.
22. Lindsley, O., and Skinner, B.: A method for the experimental analysis of the behavior of psychotic patients. Am. Psychol., 9:419–420, 1954.
23. Marr, J., and Means, B.: Behavior Management Manual: Procedures for Psychosocial Problems in Rehabilitation. Hot Springs, Ark., Arkansas Rehabilitation Research Training Center, 1981.
24. Michael, J.: Management of Behavioral Consequences in Education. Inglewood, CA, Southwest Regional Laboratory for Educational Research and Development, 1967.
25. Michael, J.: Rehabilitation. *In* Neuringer, D., and Michael, J. (Eds.): Behavior Modification in Clinical Psychology. New York, Appleton-Century-Crofts, 1970.
26. Patterson, G., and Guillion, M.: Living with Children. Champaign, Ill., Research Press, 1968.
27. Premack, D.: Toward empirical behavior laws: I. Positive reinforcement. Psychol. Rev., 66:219–233, 1959.
28. Reese, E.: The Analysis of Human Operant Behavior. Dubuque, Iowa, William C. Brown, 1966.
29. Siller, J., and Chipman, A.: Attitudes of the Nondisabled Toward the Physically Disabled. New York University School of Education, 1967.
30. Siller, J., Ferguson, L., Vann, D., and Holland, B.: Studies in reaction to disability. *In* Siller, J., Ferguson, L. T., Vann, D. H., Holland, B., Leff, W., and Bradley, P.: Structure of Attitudes Toward the Physically Disabled: Disability Factor Scales—Amputation, Blindness, Cosmetic Conditions. Vol. XII. New York, New York University School of Education, 1967.
31. Skinner, B.: The Technology of Teaching. New York, Appleton-Century-Crofts, 1968.
32. Skinner, B.: Verbal Behavior. New York, Appleton-Century-Crofts, 1957.
33. Staats, A.: A case in and a strategy for the extension of learning principles to problems of human behavior. *In* Krasner, L., and Ullmann, L. (Eds.): Research in Behavior Modification. New York, Holt, Rinehart and Winston, 1966, pp. 27–55.
34. Trieschmann, R.: The psychological, social, and vocational adjustment in spinal cord injury: A strategy for future research. Final Report, RSA, 13–P59011/9–01, April, 1978.
35. Ulrich, R., Stachnick, T., and Mabry, J.: Control of Human Behavior. Glenview, Ill., Scott, Foresman and Company, 1966.
36. Ulrich, R., Wolfe, M., and Dulaney, S.: Punishment of shock-induced aggression. J. Exp. Anal. Behav., 112:1009–1015, 1969.
37. Vash, C. L.: The Psychology of Disability. New York, Springer Publishing Company, 1981.
38. Wright, B.: Disabling Myths About Disability. Paper presented at the meeting of the National Society for Crippled Children and Adults, Denver, September, 1963.

7
Psychosocial Diagnosis and Social Work Services

MARY D. ROMANO

Rationale for Psychosocial Concerns in Rehabilitation

Rehabilitation as both a field and a process has long recognized the unity of body and mind. Inherent in the nature of the impairments treated by rehabilitation specialists are their profound effects upon multiple areas of function.[16] For example, a spinal cord–injured quadriplegic may lack more than volitional movement of and sensation in the extremities; bowel and bladder control and a host of other behaviors that had been acquired in early childhood and that, in our society, are deemed necessary to the socialization and civilizing process may be compromised. Thus, for consumers of rehabilitation services, organic impairment has an impact on social and emotional function, and we can no more separate an individual patient from familial, cultural, and social contexts than we can separate the body from the mind.

The nature of the rehabilitation process is one of learning rather than treating; that is, the rehabilitation specialist works with people, not on them. This learning model separates rehabilitation from many other medical specialties. Because, as of this writing, cure is not an option for most of the impairments seen in rehabilitation settings, the ultimate goals of rehabilitation involve teaching functionally impaired persons to live with and in spite of their impairments through remastering and maximization of functional performance and social and emotional abilities so that they can resume some degree of control over their bodies, minds, and environments.

Moreover, to a degree perhaps greater than in other medical specialties, the rehabilitation process is grounded in an interdisciplinary team approach. The many disciplines involved in the rehabilitation process share roles, although each may have designated primary responsibilities in the overall process. This inherent role diffusion, in contrast to role discretion, makes the rehabilitation setting a therapeutic milieu in which all disciplines have an opportunity for behavioral and attitudinal modeling.[25]

Rehabilitation takes place in a variety of settings, such as hospital-based or independent specialty programs; clinics and comprehensive outpatient rehabilitation facilities; some skilled nursing and other long-term care facilities; and schools and other community-based settings, including patients' homes. That these settings have longer lengths of stay and/or lengths of treatment than do acute general medical and surgical settings results in rehabilitation specialists knowing their consumers far better than do providers in short-term settings; duration of care alone allows a more intimate knowledge of the patient, the family, and friends and the duration as well as the nature of the process itself fosters a remarkable degree of involvement between the staff, the patient, and the family, resulting in rehabilitative care being more closely tied to the community than many other types of specialty-based care. Our holistic, community-oriented approach leads the rehabilitation specialist to view patients as "real" people, like us, rather than as passive recipients of ministrations; thus, the rehabilitation specialist expects patients to wear street clothes, not hospital gowns, and to be active participants in the rehabilitation process.[15, 27]

171

MARY D. ROMANO

As Trieschmann[27] suggests, the behavioral outcomes of rehabilitation are a function of personal and environmental variables in addition to organic ones. Inherent in the nature and duration of the rehabilitation process, in its settings, and in its goals is the opportunity to recognize and understand the interaction of the multiplicity of variables that influence rehabilitation outcome. This chapter will address psychosocial rehabilitation and the social worker's participation in that process.

What Is Psychosocial Rehabilitation?

Colloquially, psychosocial rehabilitation involves the patient's adaptation or adjustment to impairment. By definition, adaptation or adjustment assumes a process, the duration of which may vary greatly among individuals.[23, 27] The process itself implies an acknowledgment of an onerous reality, the reality of the impairment itself. Acknowledgment of this reality, however, does not suggest the abandonment of hope, nor should it suggest that its goal is ecstasy at being disabled. Although some persons who have lived with and in spite of disabling impairments for many years may report that the presence of the impairment has had beneficial effects on some aspects of their lives, most people would have preferred even more to gain those positive effects without the impairment. Rehabilitation specialists may practice for a lifetime without hearing a consumer tell them that a spinal cord injury was the best thing that ever happened or without a family telling them how wonderful it is that Aunt Millie had a stroke.

The reality is that most disabling impairments are uninvited and unwelcome events in people's lives. Onset is typically sudden and unanticipated, and initial outcome may be ambiguous. As much for the family and community as for the designated patient, disabling impairments affect what people do, how people live, and what people feel. These impairments confront people with their own mortality and with the potential ephemerality of function and behavior that may be taken for granted.

To the extent that onset of disability disrupts usual means of coping and previously held expectations about the way one's life will be, it may be defined as a major life crisis. Homeostasis is altered. Stress is experienced not only by the designated patient but by those in the usual environment, i.e., family, friends, and co-workers. This sudden and unwelcome disruption of homeostasis may result in overwhelming and aversive feelings, including but not limited to fear, anxiety, guilt, blame, and shame. It may also result in significant situational concerns, such as how money will be earned, how food will be obtained and prepared, how the children will be cared for.

As with other crises, the onset of impairment may be perceived as a threat, a loss, or a challenge. As with other crises, restoration of homeostasis occurs through the accomplishment of crisis- or impairment-specific tasks.[21] In rehabilitation, organic tasks may be related to stabilization and to functional performance, e.g., regaining bowel and bladder regulation and remastering daily living and mobility skills. The psychological tasks involved in restoring homeostasis may include minimizing learned helplessness, fostering an internal locus of control, remastering social skills, reframing dichotomous thinking of independence versus dependence into the more adaptive concept of interdependence, and integrating the impairment itself as just one aspect of a person's self-concept. Social tasks deal with resolving whatever situational problems affect or are affected by the impairment; preserving the integrity of the family unit; planning for continuing care needs; and understanding the impacts of one's cultural, ethnic, and spiritual belief systems on one's response to the impairment and its implications.

The crisis of the onset of disability does not have a limited time frame within which it is "normal" to have homeostasis restored. For some people the process may take six weeks, and for others it may take six years. The recognition of this point is important for two reasons, one having to do with professionals' expectations of outcome and the second relating to the psychosocial adaptation process itself.

What the rehabilitation team sees during initial acute rehabilitation is just a ripple in time in the course of a person's life.[9] Too often, however, rehabilitation specialists in acute settings generalize their observations of patient-family function and assume that the situation will remain the same in perpetuity. They assume that discharge from rehabilitation for an acute illness or trauma is the end of the process when, in reality, for many it is the beginning of life with and in spite of disability. Some patients and families who impress the team as doing well first acknowledge the onerous reality of disability only upon discharge when the security and predictability of institutional supports are no longer available. Other patients and families who appear chaotic or overly hopeful to the team pull together after discharge from the rehabilitation center. And still other patients and families move ahead in goal-directed ways, both during and after acute rehabilitation.

Contributing to the misapprehension that psychosocial rehabilitation should be completed by the time of discharge from acute rehabilitation is an often-held belief among rehabilitation specialists that persons with impairments and their families must pass through an orderly process of adjustment characterized by specific stages. Perhaps the most widely accepted example of these stage models is the one described by Kubler-Ross[17] in which the individual moves from denial to anger, followed by bargaining and then depression, and ultimately to acceptance. Bray[1] describes a somewhat analogous progression for families: fear, denial, bargaining, depression, mourning, and rapprochement. A third model, elucidated by Vash,[28] suggests three stages: recognition of detestable facts, acceptance of their inconvenience, and transcendence through embracing the experience of impairment as a growth opportunity.

Such models have benefits as well as burdens. One benefit is that they allow providers to create order out of what may be experienced as chaos; thus, they encourage staff to see angry and abusive patients as normal instead of mean and bad. Second, stage models provide staff with hope that things will improve, e.g., that an angry patient will not stay angry forever.

Among the burdens of stage models, however, is that their necessity for psychosocial adaptation has not been empirically proved. In establishing an orderly conceptual framework for staff, such models can lead staff to become rigid in their approach by forcing the patient/family into the model, by overdiagnosing psychopathology, and by undermining adaptive defenses and hope rather than supporting them.[7-8, 14] Particularly in the acute phases of rehabilitation, when patients may perceive their continued existence as dependent upon the goodwill of staff, the overreliance by staff on orderly stages of adjustment may force patients to hide their real feelings and to tell the staff what they want to hear. An example of this situation is the patient whom the staff expect to be depressed; if the patient says that he feels good, then the staff accuses him of denial. Similarly, denial and hope may be confused in minds of the staff. The patient who is actively participating in the rehabilitation program but who says, "I know someday I'm going to walk!" is not necessarily denying; instead, the patient is probably hoping for a better tomorrow,

yet staff will negatively label such a patient as a denier because the patient hopes that the disability is not irrevocable. Such rigidity of expectations by the staff can be destructive to the patient and the family and to the collaboration between the consumer and the team, which is seen as essential to the rehabilitation process. Whether it is based on the staff's projection of their own imagined feelings onto patients and families or the staff's need for order in caring for a patient with an overwhelming impairment, the replacement of valuable direct observation and honest exchange with the expectation of conceptual uniformity is dysfunctional to all participants and to the process itself.

Psychosocial Rehabilitation in Pediatric and Geriatric Populations

Although the foregoing material can be applied to all consumer populations, it should be recognized that potentially disabling impairments can occur at any point in the life cycle from birth to old age. Psychosocial rehabilitation in pediatric or geriatric populations, however, may present special issues not as commonly seen in young adult and mid-life groups, related, among other things, to human developmental issues of childhood and old age and to children's and older people's relationships to their families and the larger society.

I am the mother of this child. While it is she who must bear the trauma, the pain, and the limitations, it is I who suffers with her and sometimes, truthfully, because of her. . . . At first the attention a family gets in these circumstances is unbelievable. You're special, everyone wants to help, and there is a certain amount of glory or martyrdom involved . . . you do it because you have to. There is no one else to do it for you. . . . It's almost as if this child will be mine forever—in the sense that I will always be responsible for her. While this may sound selfish, I can't imagine any parent wanting to keep their children with them for the rest of their lives. . . . It was a long time before I could say that sometimes I hate her for all the problems she presents. A parent cannot easily voice this emotion regarding a child, especially a handicapped child. Karen's sisters could say "hate" much easier. . . . Sometimes I feel pity. . . . Often I feel compassion. . . . I always feel guilty. . . . What will Karen be when she grows up? My head knows that there's a place for her somewhere—my heart wonders if she'll find it.[20]

Parents, siblings, extended family, and disabled children themselves struggle with a multitude of psychosocial issues.[6, 10, 11, 18, 19, 29, 30] From birth through adolescence, children move through five of Erikson's[12] eight stages of man—trust versus mistrust, autonomy versus doubt, initiative versus guilt, industry versus inferiority, and identity versus role diffusion—in healthy ego development, achieving an approximation of the first words in each of these dyads. For the child with a disability, the potential difficulties in this developmental process are evident, as are the concerns of the child's family who are trying to balance normal developmental expectations against the nature of the impairment: to foster trust and autonomy in the presence of possibly painful and intrusive therapeutic procedures and in spite of possibly prolonged dependence; to reward initiative and industry regardless of parental guilt feelings, secondary overprotectiveness, and anxiety; and, at the same time, to maintain a family unit in which the disabled child is but one member, in which the parents avoid exhaustion, and in which the other children in the household can also flourish. This formidable agenda demands the sensitivity of rehabilitation specialists who can see beyond their focus on the disabled child as designated patient, who can minimize the burdens of care and treatment on family members, and who can value parents as experts on their child.

In geriatric psychosocial rehabilitation, the older person, balancing the acceptance of life as the person knows it against fears of dying, is confronted with the rehabilitative demand to change the ways things are done in the context of precipitating events that may have made fears of dying all too real. The presence of significant physical impairment can compound the gradual functional losses that often accompany the aging process (e.g., diminished vision, hearing, and smell) coupled with common social losses (e.g., retirement from job, geographical distance from children, death of friends). It can be difficult for the rehabilitation specialist to identify those rewards that will reinforce patient participation in the functional tasks of rehabilitation, not to mention its psychosocial tasks. Rehabilitative goals for geriatric patients may also be different from those of younger consumers. For example, return to work and independent living may not be realistic outcomes of the rehabilitation process. Rehabilitation specialists who define successful outcome in these terms may have trouble making empathic connections with geriatric patients, and some may even believe that geriatric rehabilitation is a wasted effort. Humanitarian philosophy suggests that one is never too old for dignity or for control over one's life; at the same time, limited rehabilitation and community resources and fiscal scarcity raise ethical questions about utilization of rehabilitation services that have yet to be widely considered but that may serve to exclude geriatric consumers from access to comprehensive rehabilitation services.

Psychosocial Assessment

Psychosocial assessment represents the first phase of psychosocial rehabilitation. It involves information-seeking, direct observation, and information-giving. It culminates in an integration of information and observation with theoretical knowledge of human personality development/deviation/behavior, sociology, economics, and anthropology: these are synthesized into a clinical impression and plan of care. Through the process of performing the psychosocial assessment, a therapeutic alliance is established between the staff member, the patient, and the family as they begin to recognize that the rehabilitation specialist is interested in learning about them as individuals and as a family unit: how they function, how they feel, what they believe and expect, what they understand about the nature of the impairment, what past significant experiences have influenced their current states of being, how they live, and their strengths as well as their perceived problems. Both through the questions asked in the psychosocial assessment and through information provided, the rehabilitation specialist initiates an educational process designed to facilitate the successful completion of the social and psychological tasks of crisis resolution.

Rarely in rehabilitation settings do we have the opportunity to know our patients prior to the onset of their impairments. In consequence, much of the information obtained in psychosocial assessment is retrospective in nature. Information obtained from the patient is validated, expanded, and balanced by information obtained from family and significant others as well as by direct observation of the patient, family, and significant others as they give information and of their interaction when they are seen together.

Within the psychosocial assessment, there are four major areas of inquiry:

1. Situational information: This includes factual data about the patient's living situation; source and amount of income, resources, expenses, and outstanding debts; type and extent of health insurance

coverage; level of education and type of employment; avocational interests and activities prior to the onset of the disability; and the family group, including persons residing with or available to the patient.

2. Cultural information: This includes data on ethnocultural and religious identity, both that with which the patient was raised and that to which he still subscribes. However emancipated from one's background one believes oneself to be, people maintain shadows of ethnocultural values and belief systems, which affect their response to crisis. Such values and beliefs may provide a source of support and comfort, and they may also provide dysfunctional expectations that can complicate the rehabilitation process.

3. Interactional information: This area includes anecdotal and observational data on the patient's interpersonal relationships and about significant others' knowledge and understanding of the impairment and its implications. Noted here would be current and past marital issues, parent-child relationships, nature and extent of friendships, repertoire of social skills, sexual functioning, experiences and abilities in negotiating with complex social systems, relationships with pets, and so forth. Wherever possible, it is helpful to obtain behavior-specific information, e.g., by asking how the patient's family handles decision-making, how they communicate, how they fight, how they resolve conflict, and who has what jobs within the family.

4. Personal information: Included here are multiple areas of inquiry, including but not limited to how the person has dealt with stress in the past, what the person's understanding is of the impairment and its implications, whether the person has an internal or external locus of control (that is, a belief that the person's actions can influence subsequent events as opposed to the belief that the person is a victim of circumstance or beneficiary of luck), what feelings the person is currently experiencing and what questions the person has that have gone unanswered. The aim here is to acquire information about the patient's personality style, self-image, rewards, habits, coping mechanisms, and emotional state. Again, behavioral specificity is key.

Throughout the process of gathering this information, it is imperative to identify strengths as well as problems, for it is the strengths in the situational, cultural, interactional, and personal areas that will provide the hooks on which the psychosocial rehabilitation process hangs and that

will enable the patient and family to resolve the crisis of onset of disability and learn to live with and in spite of the impairment.

Many disciplines within the rehabilitation team may contribute information to the psychosocial assessment. For example, the recreation therapist may provide data on avocational and leisure activities, and the chaplain may provide assessment of the patient's religious and spiritual beliefs. Through home evaluation, physical and occupational therapists may provide direct observation of the living situation. The neuropsychologist may provide information about cognitive functioning, and the clinical psychologist may contribute information about past and current personality style. From intensive direct observation, the rehabilitation nurse may provide information about the patient's social and interactional skills, family relationships, and current emotional state.

However, it is the rehabilitation social worker's responsibility to independently gather data from the patient, family, and friends; to integrate this information with that provided by the other disciplines and with that obtained through the social worker's direct observation of the patient, family, friends and rehabilitation team and to synthesize these data into an overall assessment and plan of care. Within the plan of care, the social worker involves the patient and family in identifying short-term and long-term goals, setting priorities for these goals, and agreeing to measures for their achievement. Goals and priorities are seen as dynamic, not static, and may change in response to concerns that arise during the course of rehabilitation, thus reflecting the vicissitudes of everyday life with or without an impairment.[9]

What Is a Rehabilitation Social Worker?

Usually, a rehabilitation social worker has completed a Master's degree in social work from a graduate professional program accredited by the Council on Social Work Education. Social work education is essentially generic in nature, with specialization occurring after receipt of the graduate degree. For rehabilitation social workers, health care is their area of specialty and rehabilitation a subspecialty. The Master's level credential in social work has provided its recipient with theoretical grounding in the social sciences (particularly psychology and sociology) and with supervised clinical training in individual, family, and group assessment and treatment. In most contemporary social work curricula, there is a recognition of and emphasis on social systems as the context within which people live and with which they must deal. This appreciation of systems is brought to bear by the social worker in rehabilitation settings on the internal treatment milieu and on the patient-family-community triad. The latter involves not only treatment but teaching patients and their families to negotiate with community and social agency systems. This knowledge of communities, their resources, and how to gain access to them and make them work is a significant component of the rehabilitation social worker's expertise.

Rehabilitation social workers, then, are facilitators, educators, and advocates.[24] In addition to psychosocial assessment, they provide individual, family, and group treatment to facilitate completion of specific tasks and resolution of problems. As educators, they participate in teaching patients and their families about the nature of the specific impairment and its implications; they may do this in formal teaching settings, but they also do it through conscious use of themselves as models reflecting adaptive attitudes and behaviors and engaging patients and families in moving beyond the acknowledgment of disability as a threat and a loss to reframing the experience as a challenge. In their role as advocates, rehabilitation social workers work with and on behalf of consumers to effect change through the development of needed resources, by making internal and external systems more responsive to consumer needs and demands, and by advocating broad social policy changes.

As collaborators, rehabilitation social workers also function as facilitators, educators, and advocates within the rehabilitation team. They use their knowledge of systems to foster interdisciplinary collaboration and to develop and maintain a therapeutic milieu. They educate other team members about psychosocial issues, both specific and general. They act as advocates for patients and families within the health care service delivery system, but they also act as advocates for the system with patients and families.

Rehabilitation social work is not limited to acute inpatient settings. Because the social worker deals with both internal and external systems, the specialist provides consultation and ongoing treatment, education, and advocacy services to patients, their families and friends, community agencies, and the general public. These services may be provided through the auspices of a formal outpatient rehabilitation program, as an extension of inpatient community reintegration program activities, or from community-based settings themselves. Community reintegration requires not only that the patient and family be trained to manage physical care but that they be prepared to assert themselves socially, vocationally, and recreationally; that they understand their rights and responsibilities; and that they be taught such practical things as how to hire, train, and manage personal care attendants.[31] Because communities may be unprepared to meet the needs of disabled citizens, rehabilitation social workers may participate in educational sessions for prospective employers, consult with schools about special needs, work with landlords and local housing authorities to create accessible housing, consult with city planners to assess and reduce architectural barriers, and provide public education about attitudinal barriers.

Social Work Treatment

As was previously noted, the rehabilitation social worker uses individual, family, and group modalities to effect change in patients and their significant others. The focus of these modes of treatment may be reactive or proactive. Treatment will be reactive in relation to solving problems or resolving concerns identified by patients and families; examples here might include dealing with financial worries, child care problems, or anxiety secondary to sudden physical dependence on others. Treatment is proactive when it prepares people for situations as yet unmet and when it educates people about potential behavioral options, about the nature of their impairments, and so forth; examples of this type of treatment might include social skills training, re-education and counseling regarding sexuality, or preparing children for the acceptance of parental disability.[23]

Regardless of the modality used, the social worker employs a range of counseling skills, consciously employed to meet the needs of a given patient or significant others. Among these skills are attending (that is, listening carefully and providing verbal and nonverbal indications of listening); feeding back the words used; information-seeking; information-giving; universalization; verbal direction, including behavioral assignments; limit-setting; interpretation; confrontation; and the planned use of silence. These therapeutic intervention skills can be used in behavior-oriented as well as psychodynamically based treatment.

Again, regardless of modality used, social work treatment is based as much as possible on face-to-face contacts with patients and families. It must, however, be recognized that direct interviews are not always possible, e.g., when a patient is being treated in Florida and the family lives in Alaska. Nonetheless, direct interaction is preferable because it permits the observation and transmission of nonverbal as well as verbal behavior between consumer and social worker. Because the therapeutic process is a learning process, it is important for patients and families to see that the social worker accepts the changed physical bodies of the patients and their feelings; this modeling of acceptance by the social worker (and other members of the team) is critical to patients' attempts to learn to accept their own changed bodies and their emotional responses.

In addition to individual and family treatment, the use of groups as the means and context of treatment has rapidly grown in recent years. Groups are more than economically efficient; they provide opportunities for consumers to directly experience that others like themselves are coping with similar issues and feelings, and through planned and guided group processes, groups enable people to consider a broader variety of behavioral options than they might on an individual basis. Typically, social worker–led groups in rehabilitation fall into several broad categories:

1. Education and discussion groups: Included here are groups that provide orientation to a rehabilitation facility or program, groups that provide didactic content about an aspect or issue related to a specific impairment followed by general discussion (e.g., behavioral management following brain injury for the families of brain-injured persons), and so forth.

2. Training groups: These deal with specific issues and the behavioral skills to handle them, e.g., social skills training groups and groups on how to hire, train, and manage a personal care attendant.

3. Supportive therapy groups: In these groups, people come together to share feelings, problems, and possible solutions, perhaps gaining insight into their attitudes and behaviors through the supportive group process. Often groups of this type are composed of persons with similar diagnoses or of their families.

A fourth and different type of group available to rehabilitation patients and their families in some settings is the self-help group. By definition, this type of group is led by consumers rather than by professionals. Alcoholics Anonymous, Al-Anon, and Narcotics Anonymous are examples of this type of group. Self-help groups may combine features of educational and support groups; usually, they are community-based, but as rehabilitation specialists have increasingly recognized the prevalence of chemical use and abuse problems among their consumers and as they have come to acknowledge that the stresses of living with and in spite of impairment can be ameliorated to some degree by ongoing support, some settings are now bringing self-help groups into the treatment setting itself. Where such groups remain as community-based institutions, rehabilitation social workers may refer patients and families to them as a supportive resource adjunctive to the formal rehabilitation process.

If staffing is adequate in the setting, social workers like to involve members of other disciplines in their group treatment activities as resource people or co-leaders, or both. This interdisciplinary involvement fosters team-building and also increases the probability of consistent communication between team members and patients and among family members. Especially with training groups, it facilitates *in vivo* as well as *in vitro* learning. Members of a social skills training group, for example, can discuss potentially problematic social situations and identify and rehearse behavioral options within the group; if the group is co-led by a recreation therapist, group members can then planfully practice the options they have discussed on community outings, with resulting continuity and feedback from the learning situation to the real one and back again.

Discharge Planning in Rehabilitation

As hospitals, insurance carriers, and government agencies have become increasingly preoccupied with financial accountability in the utilization of health care resources, and as professionals have become more aware of the ethical issues associated with allocation of scarce health care resources, rehabilitation settings have found themselves needing to justify the care they are providing to patients. One manifestation of this situation is the recognition that goal-oriented care with associated outcome measures is an essential component of rehabilitation service delivery.

Directly tied to this issue are the need for and documentation of timely discharge planning. Discharge planning is defined as any activity or set of activities that facilitates the transition of the patient from one environment to another.[26] The very goals of rehabilitation suggest that it has always been concerned with such transitions; in its learning model, functional and psychosocial therapies are geared toward teaching people to remaster skills that will enable them to live in the least restrictive environment possible, ideally through reintegration into their communities. Because consumers of rehabilitation services are generally learning to live with and in spite of a lifetime of impairment, they must consider an ongoing continuum of health-related needs. In consequence, in rehabilitation, discharge planning might better be called "continued care planning."

The patient, the family, and all the professionals on the team are involved in this continued care planning process, and in order for the process to be maximally effective, they must work in synchrony rather than in parallel. To facilitate this process, coordination of continued care planning is essential, and often the rehabilitation social worker has primary responsibility for this coordination.

Continued care planning is not a set of activities separate from other aspects of psychosocial rehabilitation. It is interwoven through the psychosocial rehabilitation process. Based on the psychosocial assessment of the social, psychological, environmental, and financial impacts of impairment on patients and families, it is an integral theme of individual, family, and group treatment; of their education and training processes; and of their referral for entitlement benefits and other external resources. It may address financial needs, needs for home care services, special transportation services, special schooling, day care, and respite care; it may involve assistance in obtaining durable medical equipment, home modifications, and ongoing medical care; in some instances, it may involve the decision to proceed by placing the patient in a long-term care facility or transitional living establishment and providing assistance in locating suitable facilities. The rehabilitation social worker's orientation toward recognizing patients as part of family and community systems, coupled with the knowledge of these systems and of community resources, puts the social worker in a pivotal position in relation to this overall planning process.

Continued care planning takes time, and even though the process begins with psychosocial assessment, patients and families may not be able to contemplate their future needs at the point when the staff has begun to think about such needs, especially in inpatient rehabilitation settings for acute illness or trauma. Particularly for patients and families who are experiential as opposed to cognitive learners, full recognition of ongoing needs may not occur until after rehabilitation discharge. Thus, the rehabilitation social worker remains a consultant and a resource to patients and families, providing consultation, counseling, information and access to referral services, and interdisciplinary and interagency collaboration in order to effect environmental transitions with a minimal amount of disruption.

Social Work Research

Rarely in rehabilitation settings is social work research conducted in the absence of other disciplines. Instead, it is a component of interdisciplinary research. Social workers may participate in the development of research proposals and protocols, in the identification of suitable research participants, in the acquisition of informed consents, in the actual collection of data, and in the preparation and presentation of research findings.

Social Work Outcome Measures

Measurement of social work outcomes has unfortunately received little attention in social work education and in clinical practice, and in consequence, social work outcome measures have tended toward fuzzy subjectivity, except in those areas relating to situational problems where quantification is possible, e.g., numbers of patients discharged to their homes or to alternate care facilities, numbers of referrals for Social Security benefits, and numbers of special school placements. Social workers generally can readily report the volume of their clinical and nonclinical activities, but these volume figures are not themselves outcome related. To some degree, social workers can identify consumer satisfaction with their services by the presence or absence of verbal and written complaints and by responses to follow-up satisfaction instruments; consumer satisfaction, however, may not correlate to outcome itself.

None of these measures correlate with the critical, longitudinal issues of psychosocial rehabilitation. How, in fact, does one measure psychosocial adaptation to disability? It would seem that such measures could be based in self-observation and report by patients and their families: of their specific activities and of the frequency of their occurrence, of new ways of functioning in family and social interaction, of resolutions to situational problems, and of subjective satisfaction with their lives.[2-5, 13] Indeed, such measurement instruments exist, but their implementation by rehabilitation social workers in determining successful psychosocial rehabilitation remains an area for further work.

Summary

Psychosocial rehabilitation is integral to the comprehensive rehabilitation process, regardless of the setting in which rehabilitation takes place. It requires an understanding and appreciation of the interaction among personal, environmental, and organic variables that are highly individualized, and it is based in a framework that recognizes that people must function within systems.

The rehabilitation social worker shares significant roles in the psychosocial rehabilitation process with other disciplines but has primary responsibility for synthesizing the psychosocial assessment, for coordinating continued care planning, and for linking community resources with patients and families who need them. As a facilitator, educator, and advocate, the rehabilitation social worker uses individual, family, and group treatment modalities to help patients and families learn to deal with situational, cultural, interactional, and personal issues that affect or are affected by disability. In the broadest sense, the goal of the rehabilitation social worker is to enable people to regain control over their own lives so that they can truly own what they do and how they live in ways that are meaningful and satisfying to them.

References

1. Bray, G. P.: Family adaptation to chronic illness. *In* Caplan, B. (Ed.): Rehabilitation Psychology Desk Reference. Rockville, Aspen Publishers, 1987, pp. 171–183.
2. Brown, M., Gordon, W. A., and Ragnarsson, K.: Unhandicapping the disabled: What is possible? Arch. Phys. Med. Rehabil., 68:206–209, 1987.
3. Buck, F. M., and Hohmann, G. W.: Personality, behavior, values and family relations of children of fathers with spinal cord injury. Arch. Phys. Med. Rehabil., 62:432–438, 1981.
4. Buck, F. M., and Hohmann, G. W.: Child adjustment as related to severity of paternal disability. Arch. Phys. Med. Rehabil., 63:249–253, 1982.
5. Buck, F. M., and Hohmann, G. W.: Child adjustment as related to financial security and employment status of fathers with spinal cord injuries. Arch. Phys. Med. Rehabil., 65:327–333, 1984.
6. Capell, J. T., and Bensman, A.: Behavioral adaptations that may be problems in the management of children with handicaps. *In* Bishop, D. S. (Ed.): Behavioral Problems and the Disabled: Assessment and Management. Baltimore, Williams & Wilkins, 1980, pp. 434–453.
7. Caplan, B.: Staff and patient perception of patient mood. Rehabil. Psychol., 28:68–77, 1983.
8. Caplan, B., and Shechter, J.: Denial and depression in disabling illness. *In* Caplan, B. (Ed.): Rehabilitation Psychology Desk Reference. Rockville, Aspen Publishers, 1987, pp. 133–170.
9. Collins, L. B.: The role of the clinical social worker on the rehabilitation team. *In* Krueger, D. W. (Ed.): Rehabilitation Psychology. Rockville, Aspen Publishers, 1984, pp. 183–192.
10. Drotar, D., Baskiewicz, A., Irvin, N., Kennell, J., and Klaus, M.: The adaptation of parents to the birth of an infant with a congenital malformation: A hypothetical model. *In* Power, P. W., and Dell Orto, A. E. (Eds.): Role of the Family in the Rehabilitation of the Physically Disabled. Baltimore, University Park Press, 1980, pp. 195–207.
11. Enright, M. M.: Chronically ill child and the family. *In* Browne, J. A., Kirlin, B. A., and Watt, S. (Eds.): Rehabilitation Services and the Social Work Role: Challenge for Change. Baltimore, Williams & Wilkins, 1981, pp. 167–172.
12. Erikson, E. H.: Childhood and Society. New York, W. W. Norton and Company, 1950.
13. Evans, R. L., Bishop, D. S., Matlock, A. L., Stranahan, S., Halar, E. M., and Noonan, W. C.: Prestroke family interaction as a predictor of stroke outcome. Arch. Phys. Med. Rehabil., 68:508–512, 1987.
14. Gans, J. S.: Depression diagnosis in a rehabilitation hospital. Arch. Phys. Med. Rehabil., 62:386–389, 1981.
15. Goffman, E.: Asylums. Garden City, Doubleday & Co., 1961.
16. Goffman, E.: Stigma: Notes on the Management of Spoiled Identity. Englewood Cliffs, Prentice-Hall, Inc., 1963.
17. Kubler-Ross, E.: On Death and Dying. New York, Macmillan Publishing Co., 1969.
18. Mattsson, A.: Long-term physical illness in childhood: A challenge to psychosocial adaptation. *In* Power, P. W., and Dell Orto, A. E. (Eds.): Role of the Family in the Rehabilitation of the Physically Disabled. Baltimore, University Park Press, 1980, pp. 180–194.
19. Obetz, S. W.: The child with severe illness. *In* Krueger, D. W. (Ed.): Rehabilitation Psychology. Rockville, Aspen Publishers, 1984, pp. 345–354.

20. Personal Statement: Karen. *In* Power, P. W., and Dell Orto, A. E. (Eds.): Role of the Family in the Rehabilitation of the Physically Disabled. Baltimore, University Park Press, 1980, pp. 220–223.

21. Rapoport, L.: Crisis intervention as a mode of brief treatment. *In* Roberts, R. W., and Nee, R. H. (Eds.): Theories of Social Casework. Chicago, University of Chicago Press, 1970.

22. Romano, M. D.: Family response to traumatic head injury. Scand. J. Rehabil. Med., 6:1–4, 1974.

23. Romano, M. D.: Preparing children for parental disability. Soc. Work Health Care, 1:309–315, 1976.

24. Romano, M. D.: Social worker's role in rehabilitation: A review of the literature. *In* Browne, J. A., Kirlin, B. A., and Watt, S. (Eds.): Rehabilitation Services and the Social Work Role: Challenge for Change. Baltimore, Williams & Wilkins, 1981, pp. 13–21.

25. Romano, M. D.: The therapeutic milieu in the rehabilitation process. *In* Krueger, D. W. (Ed.): Rehabilitation Psychology. Rockville, Aspen Publishers, 1984, pp. 43–49.

26. Society for Hospital Social Work Directors of the American Hospital Association: The Role of the Social Worker in Discharge Planning. Chicago, American Hospital Association, 1985.

27. Trieschmann, R. B.: Spinal Cord Injury: Psychological, Social and Vocational Adjustment. New York, Pergamon Press, 1980.

28. Vash, C. L.: The Psychology of Disability. New York, Springer Publishing Company, 1981.

29. Voysey, M.: Impression management by parents with disabled children. *In* Power, P. W., and Dell Orto, A. E. (Eds.): Role of the Family in the Rehabilitation of the Physically Disabled. Baltimore, University Park Press, 1980, pp. 380–393.

30. Ziebell, B.: As Normal As Possible. Tucson, The Arthritis Foundation—Southern Arizona Chapter, 1976.

31. Zola, I. K.: Social and cultural disincentives to independent living. Arch. Phys. Med. Rehabil., 63:394–397, 1982.

8 Vocational Assessment and Management

GARY T. ATHELSTAN

Definition and Scope of Vocational Rehabilitation

Since rehabilitation services were first established in America by an Act of Congress in 1920, employment has been their primary goal. The Act defined rehabilitation as "the rendering of a person disabled fit to engage in a remunerative occupation."[1] Consequently, governmental support for rehabilitation services has been justified by a financial equation: rehabilitation saves more than it costs, since service recipients become taxpayers instead of tax consumers.

The vocational emphasis of rehabilitation programs was reaffirmed when the medical rehabilitation research and training centers were established in 1961 and placed under the direction of the Office of Vocational Rehabilitation.

Over the years, both the definition of disability and the goals of rehabilitation have broadened. The original act was concerned with disability "by reason of a physical defect or infirmity." Now disabilities due to mental illness, mental retardation, and certain social disadvantages are included. In the 1960s, the goals of rehabilitation were expanded to encompass "(restoration of) . . . the handicapped individual to the fullest physical, mental, social, vocational and economic usefulness of which he is capable."[2] Even within that broadened framework, however, the disabled person was required to show potential for work in order to be eligible for services.

The Comprehensive Rehabilitation Services Act of 1978 added independent living as a goal. Employment continued to be the desired outcome of rehabilitation services but did not need to be an immediate objective. Thus, persons who appeared initially to be too severely disabled to work were nevertheless eligible for government-supported rehabilitation services to help them live and function independently in their family or community. The growing concern with the quality of life of disabled persons[3] may further reduce the emphasis on the "vocational feasibility test" as a criterion of eligibility for services.

The Importance of Work

The importance of work is stressed in the economic goals of the state-federal vocational rehabilitation system. It is also reflected in the value our society attaches to productivity and the negative social and psychological consequences that unemployment has for the individual. Thus the welfare of the patient dictates that the physician consider employment as a possible goal of rehabilitation. Sir Ludwig Guttman, a British pioneer in the rehabilitation of patients after spinal cord injury, wrote:

> The most gratifying result of the return of a paraplegic to useful life, apart from the beneficial effect upon both physical condition and mental outlook, is the realization that employment is essential to human happiness. In this connection it may be noted that many paraplegics with military or industrial pensions, to whom employment may not be essential from a financial point of view, recognize that it is essential for their well being.[4]

Much has been said in the years since that statement about the declining importance of work

181

in our modern "leisure society." Nevertheless, in our society a person's identity, social status, and feelings of self-worth are still often based upon occupation. Prolonged unemployment can be psychologically and socially devastating, even when disability provides a socially acceptable excuse. For these reasons, the physician must always ask at the outset, "What is the effect of disability on this person's ability to work, and how can that effect be ameliorated?"

The Structure of Vocational Rehabilitation Services

State vocational rehabilitation agencies, variously called departments, divisions, or bureaus of vocational rehabilitation, are the primary sources of vocational services for handicapped people. Governed by federal legislation and state administrative plans, and funded mainly by federal money, the agencies in every state conduct rather similar programs of services under the direction of the Office of Special Education and Rehabilitative Services.

The principal service provider in the state agency is the vocational rehabilitation counselor, who usually has a master's degree or some graduate level training in that specialty. The counselor's functions include vocational evaluation, counseling, coordination of restorative and training services, and job placement. In many agencies, these functions may be divided among a number of specialists.

When a disabled person is referred to the state agency for services, the counselor must make a series of judgments about whether the disability constitutes a vocational handicap, the likelihood of benefit from services, and what can be done to help the individual achieve independent living or employment. These judgments require medical information, and the formulation of a vocational plan may depend upon medical consultation and further restorative or medical rehabilitation services.

To prevent delay in obtaining consultations and services, many hospitals and medical rehabilitation centers maintain an office for the state agency counselor. This can expedite referrals and permit early initiation of vocational planning. Medical and vocational rehabilitation services can also be closely coordinated. To further facilitate continuity of services, some treatment centers employ their own rehabilitation counselors.

Although the state-federal program is the main element in the rehabilitation system, there are also numerous voluntary agencies. The private sector has grown rapidly in recent years, as the carriers of worker's compensation and disability insurance have sought to reduce their costs by employing their own rehabilitation personnel or by contracting directly for services from private providers. Also, a number of large, self-insured business and manufacturing firms have developed their own in-house rehabilitation programs.

Most private rehabilitation agencies provide specialized vocationally oriented services, such as work evaluation, work adjustment training, long-term sheltered employment, and job placement. Many are subsidized by the state agencies and provide most of their services under contract to state agency counselors and insurance companies.

Vocational Assessment

Rehabilitation goals must be as specific as possible. If the patient is of working age, the goals should usually include employment. Consequently, accurate assessment of vocational capabilities and potential will frequently be an essential component of the medical rehabilitation process.

As soon as possible after the onset of disability, judgments must be made about whether the patient will be able to work and, if so, at what kind of job. Such judgments have implications for compensatory training, use of adaptive equipment, surgery, and other treatment procedures. Planning for employment will also influence the expectations of both the patient and the rehabilitation team. Patients who assume that they will work after completing rehabilitation and are reinforced in that assumption have the best prospects for success.

For the disabled worker who had been employed previously, it may be of critical importance to give the employer an early estimate of vocational potential. Such information can facilitate a return to the previous job or to a different job with the same employer.

The primary responsibility for determination of vocational disability and assessment of vocational potential belongs to a specialist such as the vocational rehabilitation counselor or counseling psychologist. However, it is clear that the physician and every other member of the rehabilitation team contribute to an accurate assessment. Moreover, the physician often plays a central role in deciding when a vocational expert is needed and how that person should be involved in the rehabilitation process.

Assessing the Whole Person

In general, the best predictor of future behavior is past behavior. Thus, vocational potential can be estimated best on the basis of past vocational achievement. However, a disability may impose so many limitations on the individual as to prevent or greatly change the application of skills and abilities that were previously vocationally useful. Moreover, the young rehabilitation patient may have very little history that relates to vocational questions.

For these reasons, assessment must include a thorough review of the patient's past nonvocational performance—in school, hobbies, sports, social groups, or any other activities involving behaviors that may relate to employment. Assessment must also include analysis of the person's abilities, skills, interests, and social and physical environment, and of the disability and the limitations it imposes. Attention must be given to the ways in which the limitations of a disability interact with all of the other characteristics of the individual and the environment.

In this connection, the physician must keep in mind the distinctions among impairment, disability, and handicap. An impairment is a residual limitation resulting from a congenital defect, a disease, or an injury. Evaluation of an impairment is primarily the function of the physician.

A disability exists when an impairment causes an inability to perform some major life function, such as self-care, mobility, communication, or employment. The judgment as to whether an impairment constitutes a disability is not exclusively a medical one, since that judgment requires consideration of the whole person, including such factors as abilities, skills, and the possibilities of adaptation. Unfortunately, the distinction between impairment and disability is not always recognized, and the existence of an impairment is sometimes taken as *prima facie* evidence of disability. This confusion leads to problems in the medicolegal system in connection with disability determination and compensation proceedings, and in the self-definitions of people with impairments who may be motivated to be considered disabled.

A handicap results when a disability interacts with the environment to impede the individual's functioning in some area of life, such as work, travel, or fulfilling family or other social roles. The importance of the environment in defining a handicap can be illustrated by considering the paraplegic who needs to use a wheelchair. Such a person has a disability but would not be handicapped at all with regard to mobility in an architecturally accessible environment.

Information Needed for Assessment

As indicated previously, an adequate vocational assessment requires information about all aspects of the individual and the immediate circumstances. However, some personal characteristics, such as abilities, skills, interests, and physical capacities, have special vocational relevance. In the sections that follow, these factors and the principal means of measuring them will be more fully discussed.

Abilities

Abilities are the presumably innate capacities for performance that relate to proficiency in a wide range of activities. They should be distinguished from skills, which are the demonstrated proficiencies in performance resulting from training or practice. Abilities represent a potential for performance in the future and may set limits on ultimate achievement in an activity; however, they relate mainly to the speed of acquisition of a new skill. Thus, the person with high ability in a particular area will generally learn a new skill more quickly than the person with low ability, as well as possibly attain a higher level of proficiency.

Abilities are measured to make predictions about the likelihood of success in training or in a job that requires the development of new skills. The relationship of ability to success in school or work is not a simple one in which more ability ensures more success; rather, it appears that most complex activities have an ability threshold. Success may demand that a person possess the relevant abilities beyond a certain minimum level, but once the minimum is surpassed, other factors, such as motivation, perseverance, or personality, are more important.

Two kinds of ability are considered to have vocational relevance. One is general ability, often referred to as general intelligence; the other is special ability, which is synonymous with aptitude. In common usage, the terms ability, aptitude, and skill are often used interchangeably to denote any indication of proficiency in an activity. However, the correct definitions are different and it is both meaningful and important in rehabilitation practice to maintain a clear distinction between skill on the one hand and ability or aptitude on the other.

Research on the structure of ability has not produced a consensus on the number and composition of different aptitudes. Vocational counselors are concerned mainly with those that have been demonstrated by empirical research to be relevant to job performance. Only about a dozen aptitudes meet this criterion.

One of the most widely accepted systems for classifying and measuring abilities has been developed by the United States Department of Labor. The Department's studies have found nine basic aptitudes to be important in training and job performance. These are measured by the General Aptitude Test Battery (GATB) in a testing program carried out by the Employment Service.

The Department of Labor has also analyzed a very large number of jobs with regard to their ability requirements. Continuing studies produce regularly updated information about the ability characteristics of workers in relation to their performance on the job. Thus, norms are available that enable the vocational counselor to evaluate a person's abilities in relation to a wide variety of different jobs.

The aptitudes measured by the GATB comprise the principal components of ability considered important in work.

Intelligence, or general learning ability, is the ability to "catch on" or understand instructions and underlying principles. It includes the ability to reason, to solve problems, and to make judgments, and is closely related to doing well in school.

Verbal aptitude is the ability to understand the meaning of words and to use them effectively. It includes the ability to comprehend language, to understand relationships between words, and to understand the meanings of whole sentences and paragraphs. Verbal aptitude is generally the most conspicuous or easily recognized ability and is frequently the basis for casual judgments about intelligence. However, its significance as a predictor of success is largely limited to performance in school and in highly verbal occupations.

Numerical aptitude is the ability to perform arithmetic operations quickly and accurately. Numerical and verbal aptitude together are the primary components of general intelligence as measured by the GATB.

Spatial aptitude is the ability to think visually of geometric forms and to comprehend the two-dimensional representation of three-dimensional objects. It includes the ability to recognize the relationships resulting from the movement of objects in space. Spatial aptitude is an important component of mechanical ability, which is not in itself considered a basic aptitude but has elements of several different basic abilities.

Form perception is the ability to perceive pertinent detail in objects or in pictorial or graphic material. It includes the ability to make visual comparisons and discriminations and to see slight differences in shapes and shadings of figures and widths and lengths of lines. Together with spatial aptitude, form perception is important in the skilled trades and many other occupations involving fabrication or assembly. This aptitude is probably also a component of mechanical ability.

Clerical perception is the ability to perceive pertinent detail in verbal or tabular material. It includes the ability to observe differences in copy, to proofread words and numbers, and to avoid perceptual errors in arithmetic computation.

Motor coordination is the ability to coordinate eyes and hands or fingers rapidly and accurately in making precise movements. It is also the capacity to make a movement response accurately and swiftly.

Finger dexterity is the ability to move the fingers and manipulate small objects rapidly and accurately.

Manual dexterity is the ability to move the hands easily and skillfully. It includes the ability to work with the hands in placing and turning motions that also involve the wrist.

There are other dimensions of ability, such as artistic, mechanical, and musical aptitude, which the counselor might assess for specific purposes. Many cognitive abilities, such as judgment, abstract reasoning, and several kinds of memory, may be important in job performance, but occupational norms have not been developed for them. Extensive research shows that the nine GATB aptitudes account for much of the variance in abilities for which vocational relevance has been established.

Whenever there are questions about a patient's capacity for vocational planning, the assessment of abilities must be thorough. Considerable variation is common in brain-damaged persons, and even the normal individual may possess widely varying levels of different abilities. Therefore, it is not safe to assume that either a very high or a very low level of functioning in one area, such as verbal ability, will be accompanied by similar levels in other areas.

Brain injury producing severe impairment of some aspect of ability that is critical in vocational functioning or in everyday life, but that leaves verbal ability intact, is especially frequent. Such cases are often difficult for the physician to detect, because the patient may communicate well and appear normal in a brief encounter but have memory, judgment, or other cognitive deficits that rule out competitive employment.

Skills

Skills are the learned proficiencies that comprise the major part of every person's repertoire of vocational behaviors. Abilities underlie and influence the development of skills, but skills represent an achieved level of performance.

The skills a person possesses at the time of assessment are among the most important factors in determining immediate employment prospects. However, disability often impairs skills or prevents the application of those that are still intact. For example, an auto mechanic who has become paraplegic may possess highly developed manual and mechanical problem-solving skills but be unable to employ them in his usual occupation because of the climbing, reaching, kneeling, and other gross bodily movements the work involves. In such cases, identification of transferable skills becomes crucial in vocational rehabilitation.

Whenever a disability requires a change of occupation or limits an initial occupational choice, retraining or special training is often considered. However, vocational assessment should focus first on skills that can be transferred from a prior job to a new one. After all, the goal of vocational rehabilitation is to return the person to productive activity as soon as possible. Even when retraining is feasible, the expense in time and money may not be justifiable if the patient already has skills that can be applied in a new combination or under different environmental circumstances in a new occupation.

Every job involves some skills that potentially can be transferred, even if they are as basic as the capacity to understand and follow instructions. With higher level intellectual skills, such as reading, writing, and oral communication, it is usually possible for a person with almost any physical disability to engage in some kind of remunerative employment.

Skills are assessed mainly by the history of an individual's accomplishments in school, in the labor market, and in other areas of life. Information about skills is thus usually obtained by interview or through review of written records. If useful information cannot be obtained by interview or from records, job tryouts in work evaluation may be necessary to accurately assess skills.

Most persons possess a wide variety of skills that they have acquired throughout life, not only in work, but in school, avocational activities, and everyday living. This fact has gained wide recognition in recent years as large numbers of homemakers have sought to re-enter the labor market after many years of not being employed outside the home. Such persons were long believed to be handicapped by lack of vocational qualifications, but economic necessity and improved vocational assessment have led to a greater appreciation of the value of the organizational and managerial skills acquired in homemaking. Equally sensitive assessment is needed with disabled persons.

Interests

Interests should be given as much attention as other factors in vocational assessment, but many rehabilitation professionals appear implicitly to discount interests when a person's options are restricted by disability. Limited alternatives do, indeed, reduce one's chances of obtaining satisfying employment. However, such assumptions should not limit the planning process. Disabled people should have just as much opportunity as the able-bodied to seek realization of their interests. Rehabilitation professionals should provide whatever resources will help make that possible.

The vocational significance of interests appears to reside primarily in their relationship to occupational choice and tenure. People tend to move toward and to stay longest in occupations that are consistent with their vocational interests.[5] They tend to move out of occupations that do not fit their interests, presumably because of the part that satisfaction plays in long-term vocational behaviors. Consequently, vocational planning that is guided by accurate assessment of interests can help the disabled make choices that will contribute to both occupational stability and self-fulfillment.

Interests must be measured in the same careful, professional manner as any of the other vocation-

GARY T. ATHELSTAN

ally relevant qualities of the individual. Most people are able to describe their interests specifically, and it is common practice to take such self-descriptions at face value. However, there is good evidence that stated interests are strongly influenced by limited or inaccurate information and by social and occupational stereotypes. As such, they are not necessarily accurate predictors of occupational satisfaction nor a valid basis for career choice. The vocational counselor tends to place more weight upon standardized measures of interests that correct for such influences and have had their validity established by empirical research.

Physical Capacities

Physical capacities should be assessed in functional terms rather than in medical or diagnostic terms. This serves several purposes. First, a functional analysis provides the kind of information the vocational counselor needs to determine whether the patient can meet the physical demands of particular jobs. For example, some counselors have a general idea of what a person with complete C 6 to C 7 quadriplegia can and cannot do, but it is necessary to know the extent of the person's independence in transfers and wheelchair use, sitting tolerance, nature and strength of grip, and other such details of physical functioning.[6]

Second, the lack of functional precision in even those diagnoses that have an air of exactness argues for a functional approach. A vocational counselor may be very familiar with C 6 to C 7 spinal cord injuries but still needs to know precisely where the patient falls in the widely varying distributions of specific physical capacities possessed by such quadriplegics.

Finally, a functionally oriented evaluation of the patient is likely to be less negative or restrictive in its implications than any other approach. A thorough functional assessment will indicate what the patient *can* do, as well as what limitations are present. Specification of remaining abilities is not merely an affirmation of a positive rehabilitation philosophy; it is absolutely essential to the provision of adequate vocational rehabilitation services.

Several systems have been devised to facilitate the physician's evaluation of physical capacities, but most yield information that is of limited value in vocational planning. Therefore, it is probably most helpful if the physician remembers to be thorough and to describe capacities and limitations in everyday language as they relate to common physical activities.

The physical functions that are important in many jobs include mobility, ambulation, upper extremity and hand function, coordination, motor speed, strength and endurance, and the ability to bend, lift, reach, handle, and feel. In quantifying these capacities, vocational relevance is more important than precision or the type of measure used. Thus, for example, it is more helpful for the vocational counselor to know how many yards or blocks the person can walk or propel a wheelchair without resting, and how long that takes, than to know walking speed in meters per minute. Strength might best be expressed as the ability to repetitively lift weights of 5, 25, or 50 lb, endurance as the ability to be up and active in a job for two hours, a half day, or a full day, and so on. Similarly, it is less useful for the counselor to learn the degrees of limitation of motion in a person's knee joint than to know that the particular limitation makes it impossible for the person to kneel or climb a ladder. The experienced counselor will often put questions to the physician in exactly these terms, but it is helpful for the physician to be oriented to these aspects of physical function at the time of evaluation.

Other Factors Affecting Vocational Potential

MOTIVATION FOR WORK

The patient's interest in employment is probably the most important single determinant of a return to work. In this connection, rehabilitation professionals often place great importance on the concept of "motivation." Patients are usually categorized as either "motivated" or "unmotivated," and the "unmotivated" patient may be subject to urgent exhortations aimed at increasing motivation. In fact, no patient is ever devoid of motivation. The problem arises when the patient's motivation is different from what the rehabilitation professionals believe it should be.

Most rehabilitation patients are motivated primarily to regain whatever physical function they have lost because of their disability. Patients may be concerned about the impact of disability on their earning capacity, social relationships, and many other areas of their life. However, usually their first wish is simply to recover. This is especially true during the early stages of rehabilitation, while the patient is still in the hospital and focusing all attention on medical treatment. In fact, at this stage of rehabilitation, the patient may not have grasped yet the permanence of the disability and its implications for psychosocial and vocational functioning. Although this can be a critical time for vocational intervention, the vocational counselor is often at a serious disadvantage in attempting to initiate vocational rehabilitation procedures.

Some patients remain uninterested in employment throughout the rehabilitation process. Indeed, it is not unusual to find that the person disabled by a work-related injury was in vocational trouble before the onset of disability. In such cases, it may appear that the disability provided a socially acceptable escape from an intolerable work situation, and it is possible that psychological factors contributed to the onset of the disability. This is sometimes especially evident in instances where unusual accident proneness appeared in the work setting or where psychological components are obvious in "functional overlay," which influences the type and extent of the disability.

Finally, despite the importance of employment to the identity and morale of most people, it is clear that many people simply do not enjoy working much. For some people, work is a major source of satisfaction; for others, it is a necessary unpleasantness. In general, people will work if they have to; but, in the absence of financial necessity, some people would prefer not to. In this connection, Social Security Disability Income, Worker's Compensation payment, and other sources of compensation or support for disabled persons often act as disincentives for employment.

FINANCIAL AND PSYCHOLOGICAL DISINCENTIVES

Much attention has been given in recent years to the various financial disincentives that work against effective rehabilitation. One of the major problems is that most of the compensation or support systems work with rigid definitions and criteria and according to inflexible rules. For example, until recently, a person had to be judged "totally and permanently disabled" for any remunerative employment in order to be eligible for Social Security payments. The concepts of permanence and totality seem unreasonable when both individual potential and the environmental circumstances that create a vocational handicap may change. Moreover, the psychological impact on the disabled individual of being labeled "totally and

permanently disabled" may contribute to a self-fulfilling prophecy.

Most of the services or financial benefits for disabled people place the burden of proof for eligibility on the applicant. Thus the individual is required to "prove" not only the existence of a disability but the extent of its limiting effects in order to obtain assistance. In behavioral terms, this creates a contingency in which a certain degree of helplessness is the most likely route to reward. Ongoing litigation concerning a personal injury or other cause of disability creates a similar contingency. The anticipated or real size of the settlement of the lawsuit may be directly related to the degree of disability demonstrated.

Another major problem with the sources of financial support for handicapped persons is that they are very difficult to use flexibly in conjunction with a positive program aimed at helping the individual get back to work. For example, benefits may be terminated very soon after return to work, thus creating a major financial risk if the job does not last. Also, financial support may be provided on an all-or-nothing basis that prevents its use to supplement a person's income or to help meet some of the expenses that may be part of the cost of employment for a severely disabled person. Recent federal legislation has only partially alleviated this problem in connection with the way that Social Security Disability payments are provided, but financial disincentives are still too frequently a barrier to vocational rehabilitation.

Age and prior work experience are factors influencing future vocational prospects. Up to a point, increasing age is an advantage, since the older person is considered more mature and, therefore, a better employment risk. However, both the very young and the older disabled person are likely to encounter employer prejudice despite the existence of laws forbidding age discrimination in employment.

Both the quantity and quality of prior work experience affect job prospects. The person who has a "spotty" job history, including frequent job changes and significant gaps between jobs, may be correctly regarded as a poor risk by the potential employer. Similarly, the person who has very little or no prior work experience and is further disadvantaged by a disability will have a much harder time finding an accepting employer than will the person with an ample work history.

Family attitudes and beliefs are important. For example, family members may profess to support rehabilitation goals but place subtle obstacles in the way of a return to work if their own needs are better met by having the disabled person remain at home. It is not unusual for family members to believe that the disabled person is too fragile or too disabled to work, or that working entails unreasonable risks to health. Such fears can sabotage the most carefully crafted vocational rehabilitation plan. On the other hand, if the family is psychologically supportive of employment and willing to contribute the time and assistance that may be necessary to facilitate work, most of the tasks of vocational rehabilitation will be much simpler.

The environment of the neighborhood and community must be considered in its relationship to vocational rehabilitation. Very few communities permit easy access by people in wheelchairs or with other mobility impairments. Problems in transportation discourage the kind of mobility needed in many jobs. If the home is not architecturally accessible, it may be easier to stay in it than to leave for work and return each day. In this connection, it may be necessary to evaluate the suitability of the home for home employment.

Small towns and rural areas lack the vocational rehabilitation facilities and services that can be of help to the disabled. They also are less likely to have a range of jobs in different settings, involving a variety of tasks, that might be suitable for handicapped workers.

Of perhaps even greater importance is the lack of social amenities in small towns. Very few offer much opportunity for contact with other handicapped people; social support systems, such as clubs or organizations for the handicapped, are rare. Because of the limited resources for disabled persons in rural areas, relocation may be necessary to permit realization of the individual's full potential.

Timing of vocational rehabilitation intervention is important in several respects. It can be difficult to engage the patient in effective vocational planning or other constructive steps toward re-employment when the patient's energies are focused on medical treatment. Furthermore, the patient must have achieved a reasonably accurate understanding of the nature of the disability and the limitations it imposes in order to formulate a sensible plan. It is unusual for such an understanding to be reached while the patient is still in the hospital. Some people, especially those with severe disabilities, require months of living at home, "getting used to being disabled," before they are ready to undertake vocational rehabilitation.

Because unemployment itself can constitute a

vocational handicap, the need to await patient readiness for vocational rehabilitation must always be balanced against the advantage of an early return to work. Conventional wisdom among vocational counselors maintains that prospects for re-employment diminish steadily over time, to a virtual zero point after five years. However, research on people with spinal cord injuries[7] has not supported this opinion, suggesting, in fact, that employment may never be a completely dead issue. Some persons studied re-entered the labor market after absences as long as 15 to 25 years. Nevertheless, it is clear that considerations of both employer acceptance and patient readiness dictate that re-employment be effected as soon as possible after the onset of disability.

Assessment Techniques

The Interview

A correct diagnosis and complete medical evaluation of any disabling condition require an understanding of its effects on every aspect of the patient's life. Therefore, vocational assessment begins during the first meeting between the physician and a new patient. The routine history and physical examination should give attention to the patient's educational and vocational background, socioeconomic status, life style, and leisure time activities. The individual's behavior in these areas may be related to the onset or to the nature of the medical problem and will certainly have implications for treatment. Moreover, the patient's vocational functioning can be indirectly affected by the impact of disability on other aspects of the patient's life.

Research shows that a work history obtained by interview cannot always be assumed to be accurate.[8] People tend to upgrade their job title, level of responsibility, and income when reporting work history data. In addition, patients tend to tell professionals what they believe professionals want to hear.

Information is more likely to be accurate and significant if it is obtained by narration and asking the patient to "tell your story." If answers to specific questions are needed, they can always be obtained by following up later, after the patient has made a narrative response to an open-ended question.

The physician should also recognize that work history information will not be very useful unless it includes some behavioral detail, not just a job title. Job titles are unreliable indicators of work activities, since the duties associated with a given job title may vary from one setting to another. For example, the physician might assume that a paraplegic could return to work as a shipping clerk unless it was known that the particular job included lifting and transporting large boxes of merchandise, climbing ladders while stocking and retrieving inventory, and loading and unloading trucks. After learning a patient's job title, the physician should always ask, "Just what do you do in that job? What is your work area like? How does your work come to you?" and other such questions.

Psychological Tests

The vocational rehabilitation counselor or counseling psychologist uses many different tests to evaluate patients' vocationally relevant characteristics as an adjunct to other assessment procedures. Psychological tests provide a basis for making inferences about patients' attributes or predictions about their future behaviors. Although tests measure directly only the behavior involved in taking the test, they substitute for more direct measures of the behavior in which the counselor is interested. At times, heavy reliance upon test data may be necessary because of the limited availability of direct information or because of significant change in the patient's attributes due to disability.

The range of tests used includes measures of abilities, skills, interests, and emotional state or personality.

The physician is unlikely to become involved directly in the choice of particular tests or in decisions concerning the timing of testing. However, it is important for the physician to know the purposes, values, and limitations of tests in order to help create appropriate patient expectations and to encourage cooperation with testing. The physician should also be familiar with the kind of information produced by tests and with the ways in which tests are related to the real world.

A psychological test can be defined as a sample of behavior obtained under standardized conditions, in which the individual's responses to standardized stimuli are recorded for subsequent evaluation. A person's performance is usually quantified in a numerical score, and the significance of an individual's score is determined by comparing it to the scores of other, similar people. This is known as the "normative" approach to evaluation of test performance, and it requires careful adherence to standardized procedures.

One of the best methods of normatively evaluating a test score is to determine its percentile rank in relation to a specific norm group. If a test measures an ability that is significantly related to performance in a training program or an occupation, the percentile rank immediately clarifies the meaning of a score. For example, a clerical aptitude score that stands at the 85th percentile in comparison to employed clerical workers has implications for success in clerical work that are very different from a score at the 10th percentile. A score at the 10th percentile does not necessarily predict failure in clerical work but would certainly place a person at a competitive disadvantage, since that score is surpassed by 90 per cent of clerical workers. Such a score would suggest careful examination of the specific tasks involved in any clerical job under consideration, followed by selective placement or possibly by special training in clerical skills.

Another advantage of the percentile rank is its uniform interpretation. A given percentile always denotes the same relative standing in a group, regardless of the attribute or the test used to assess it. This is not true of other measures of test performance, such as the IQ, in which interpretation may vary depending on the test and sometimes on the age of the individual tested. For these reasons test reports should usually include the percentile rank of any scores and specify the norms used.

The importance of using norms that are both specific and appropriate can be illustrated by referring to mechanical reasoning ability, for which some occupations are highly selective. For example, a mechanical reasoning score at the 50th percentile against general population norms (i.e., an "average" score) would fall below the 10th percentile on norms for mechanical engineers. Moreover, the difference would not result from the higher educational level or general intelligence of engineers in relation to the general population. In comparison to trade school students in auto mechanics or tool and die making, the percentile rank of such a score would be even lower.

Exactly appropriate norms are not always available, so it is sometimes necessary to approximate from the most relevant ones. For example, a patient's performance may be compared to the norms for students in an architectural drafting training program when norms for employed draftspersons cannot be obtained. However, it is important to remember that the levels of different norm groups may vary greatly, possibly making such substitutions misleading.

In addition to the available norms, the most important qualities of a psychological test are its reliability and validity. Reliability is the ability of a test to measure a patient's attributes consistently. Most psychological tests show some variation in their measure of a supposedly stable trait from one testing to another. However, if the psychologist is careful to adhere to standard conditions of administration, the extent of variability or unreliability in a test's scores can be rather precisely estimated. It is inappropriate to discuss test scores in terms that imply greater precision than they possess. For example, it is technically incorrect to describe an IQ of 113 as higher than one of 110, since both scores are in the "high average range." On the other hand, it is not reasonable to discount differences that are significant or to disregard test scores because of their modest reliability.

The validity of a psychological test is determined by the extent to which it measures what it is supposed to measure. Validity is usually expressed in terms of a coefficient of correlation between a test score and some external criterion, such as performance in school or on the job. The most important kind of validity for tests used in rehabilitation is predictive validity.

The validity of most psychological tests is even more modest than their reliability. However, limited validity should not cause test results to be ignored. Test results should not be used to prescribe what a patient *should* do, but they can help suggest alternatives and assist the patient in making decisions about the future.

Most vocational tests are designed for administration to groups in educational settings and personnel selection programs. Consequently, administration procedures make little provision for individual attention nor for adaptation to the limitations or special requirements of the disabled person. In addition, many vocational tests are timed, so that speed of performance may significantly influence a person's score. Both of these common characteristics of vocational tests limit their use in rehabilitation, especially in the medical setting.

The counselor can sometimes deal with these limitations of vocational tests by finding alternative measures. For example, it may be possible to substitute an untimed test for one with time limits. However, such options are generally limited, because the purposes of vocational testing usually require very specific norms that are seldom available for more than one test. As a rule, a test that lacks relevant norms is not very useful in vocational counseling, even if it accurately measures the attribute of interest to the counselor.

As alternatives, the counselor may delay testing until the patient's condition permits standardized administration, use a test with somewhat inappropriate norms, or rely on other assessment methods. Occasionally, testing may have to be foregone altogether. This need not block rehabilitation progress, but it can result in delays by forcing the patient to directly explore avenues that could be more quickly evaluated by tests.

Standardization of testing procedures is important because of the effect that conditions of administration can have on performance. If a test is administered under widely varying environmental conditions or with different time limits or instructions, the performance of individuals will obviously vary. The problem arises in attempting to determine how much of the variation is due to conditions of administration and how much to real differences among the people tested. Also, predictions based on test performance may be invalidated by failure to adhere to standard procedures. This is a frequent problem in rehabilitation, because a patient's physical, sensory, or intellectual limitations may interfere with standardized administration. For example, a test that is ordinarily self-administered may produce different results when the items must be read aloud by the examiner and the responses marked for the patient. Also, the patient's performance may vary from day to day owing to the effects of stress, pain, drugs, and other temporary factors.

These problems do not mean that valid vocational testing is impossible in a medical rehabilitation setting. However, they do impose some constraints on the choice of tests and on the timing of assessment. In addition, the psychologist is sometimes required to exercise special ingenuity to identify and assess the impact of factors that can cause inaccuracy in test results.

Tests Frequently Used in Vocational Assessment

The psychological test library in a comprehensive medical rehabilitation center may contain up to 80 different tests. In practice, however, the counselor will make frequent use of only a few. Many of the tests used in vocational assessment are designed as omnibus instruments that measure a number of traits simultaneously. For example, the GATB covers nine aptitudes; the Strong-Campbell Interest Inventory measures 23 "basic" interest dimensions and has scales for 207 different occupations; the Minnesota Multiphasic Personality Inventory evaluates 10 major traits and has over 500 special scales for specific aspects of personality or behavior.

Because the patients in a comprehensive medical rehabilitation center usually present a limited range of vocational assessment questions, perhaps 90 per cent of vocational testing makes use of 15 or so different tests, comprising six distinct types: (1) general ability or intelligence; (2) special ability or aptitude; (3) achievement or skill; (4) interests; (5) values or attitudes; and (6) personality. Brief descriptions of each type and examples of some specific tests follow.

GENERAL ABILITY OR INTELLIGENCE TESTS

The Wechsler Adult Intelligence Scale (WAIS) is the most widely used individually administered test of intelligence. It is designed for use throughout the adult age range above 16 years and is available in a similar version for children, the Wechsler Intelligence Scale for Children (WISC). Administration resembles a structured interview in which the subject answers questions, solves problems, and is given tasks to perform. The test must be given by a trained examiner and takes about one and one-half hours to complete, making it expensive to use. However, careful observation of the patient during this test may permit valuable inferences to be drawn about behavior and personality.

The WAIS consists of 11 scales or subtests containing different kinds of tasks. Six of the subtests yield a verbal IQ based on such tasks as information, comprehension, and vocabulary, whereas the remaining five, including block design, picture arrangement, and object assembly, produce a performance IQ. Overall ability is represented by the Full Scale IQ. Since educational deprivation, brain damage, or other impairments may affect verbal and performance abilities differently, it is often useful in rehabilitation to be able to evaluate them separately.

Scores can also be obtained on several basic factors that underlie intelligence, such as verbal comprehension, memory, freedom from distractibility, and perceptual organization. Variations among these factors and among the subtest scores are sometimes taken as diagnostic clues to central nervous system problems.

The unit of measurement for the WAIS is the IQ, which, on this test, is statistically designed to have a mean of 100 and a standard deviation of 15. Thus, IQ scores are easily translated into percentile ranks; an IQ of 115 stands near the 85th percentile; 130, at about the 98th; and an IQ of 85 ranks near the 15th percentile.

Because of frequent misunderstanding of the IQ among the general public, it is usually best to describe WAIS performance in terms of percentiles or broad zones, such as "average," "below average," or "above average." It is also desirable to avoid terms that have a value connotation, such as "subnormal," "borderline retarded," "superior," and "genius." The percentile rank is the clearest and most neutral indicator of performance on any ability test, and it should usually be used when discussing performance with a patient or family member.

Since there are no occupational norms for the WAIS, its application in vocational assessment is rather limited. However, WAIS scores are highly related to school performance and to speed of learning in the clinical setting. The test can also contribute to an understanding of the patient's personality, problem-solving style, and specific intellectual strengths and weaknesses. These uses of the test often outweigh its limitations for specific vocational purposes.

Several tests of intelligence have been designed for people with specific limitations, such as the Hayes adaptation of the Stanford-Binet test for the blind, the Revised Beta Examination for people with hearing impairment or non-native language background, and the Peabody Picture Vocabulary Test for aphasic and deaf people. A number of nonverbal and other special tests of intelligence also are available. Most of these instruments are rarely used in general rehabilitation practice, but the physician who expects frequent contact with patients having such problems should become familiar with the special tests.

SPECIAL ABILITY OR APTITUDE TESTS

Aptitudes may be tested either by selected single-aptitude tests or by a multi-aptitude test *battery*. The abilities that can be measured range from such complex ones, including computer programming, musical aptitude, and sales aptitude, to the more "basic," such as clerical, arithmetic, and spatial aptitude. Single-aptitude tests are used to answer specific questions concerning a person's chances of success in a particular occupation or training program. General occupational exploration has been completed and counseling is focusing on just one or two options. This allows the counselor to select a single-aptitude test having specific norms and validity that relate directly to the question at hand. Some aptitude tests, devised by large companies to help select workers for particular jobs, may be used before initiating job placement effort.

The principal application of the multi-aptitude test battery is in comprehensive vocational evaluation or initial vocational exploration, when information is needed about the range of the patient's alternatives. A major advantage of the multi-aptitude battery is the opportunity it affords of making intra-individual comparisons. Because all of the tests in a battery have been standardized with the same basic norm group, scores on the different aptitudes can be used to identify a patient's particular strengths and weaknesses.

The General Aptitude Test Battery (GATB) is not only the most widely used multi-aptitude battery; it is one of the most frequently used vocational tests of any kind. It measures intelligence; verbal, numerical, and spatial ability; form and clerical perception; motor coordination; and finger and manual dexterity, the nine basic aptitudes that were described earlier. The GATB has norms for people employed in more than 400 different specific occupations. The GATB tests are all timed, an important disadvantage in rehabilitation use, since patients are often slowed by pain, medications, or inactivity. However, careful attention to the patient's condition, with some flexibility in the scheduling of testing, can usually eliminate any problems with slowness. If a better measure of "power" is needed, a substitute can generally be found, usually in a single-aptitude test.

GATB scores can be evaluated in two different ways. First, the scores on each of the nine aptitudes can be examined and compared. The scores are standardized on the general working population, with a mean of 100 and a standard deviation of 20. Inspection of the "aptitude profile" or list of scores quickly reveals the individual's strongest and weakest abilities and the individual's standing on each ability in relation to the general population. A second means of evaluating an individual's scores is to compare them to the Occupational Aptitude Patterns (OAPs). OAPs are clusters of aptitudes that correlate with performance in occupations that have similar ability requirements. There are at present 66 different OAPs encompassing approximately 11,000 occupations to which GATB scores have been related. Each OAP has cutting scores for its aptitudes representing the minimum level of ability that is believed to be necessary for success in the occupations within that OAP group. The individual's aptitude profile can be compared with preferred OAP cutting scores, thus determining the families of jobs for which the person qualifies. Since the cutting scores for occupations within an OAP usually vary slightly, the suitability of a particular job can be checked by consulting the Specific Aptitude Test Battery (SATB) for that occupation.

The GATB does not assess factors other than ability, such as interests or skills, which may be important to success in an occupation. However, it can be very helpful in opening up possibilities not previously considered.

The Differential Aptitude Test (DAT) is another widely used multi-aptitude test. It has measures of verbal, abstract, and mechanical reasoning, numerical ability, clerical speed and accuracy, spatial relations, and language usage. However, the DAT is designed primarily for educational evaluation and planning in high schools. It emphasizes abilities that are important mainly in academic activities, and it has few norms for adults or for occupational groups. The principal applications of the DAT in rehabilitation would be in educational planning with high school–age patients or in evaluating adults who are considering trade school.

There are other multi-aptitude batteries, such as the Flanagan Aptitude Classification Test and the SRA Primary Mental Abilities, which are sometimes used in vocationally oriented agencies. Also, some agencies and individual vocational counselors have "favorite" tests that they use extensively because of the advantages of familiarity with one test, or because of the needs or characteristics of a particular clientele. However, none of the other tests approaches the GATB in its extensive norms and validation research or in its wide applicability.

ACHIEVEMENT OR SKILL TESTS

Large numbers of achievement tests have been developed, mainly for use in schools. Because their different purposes and specific applications are so numerous, no attempt will be made here to describe particular examples. Rather, this section will present the characteristics and uses of achievement tests in general.

Most achievement tests measure academic skills, such as reading comprehension, vocabulary, and arithmetic, or knowledge of specific content areas, such as science, history, and social studies. Some achievement tests have been designed to measure specific vocational skills, but in recent years such tests have been largely supplanted in rehabilitation by work samples or job tryouts in work evaluation.

The most frequent use of achievement tests in rehabilitation is to determine a patient's readiness for vocational training or further general education. Vocational training, even in semiskilled occupations, usually requires the ability to read at a 10th or 11th grade level. Mastery of 8th grade mathematics is also generally necessary. Training in a skilled trade is likely to demand high school graduate–level achievement in both of these areas.

Even if further training or education is not part of the rehabilitation plan, it may be important to assess a patient's academic skills, since many jobs require 8th to 10th grade literacy. Some jobs with no literacy requirements have application blanks that demand 12th grade reading ability. Surprisingly large numbers of rehabilitation patients do not possess educational skills at this level.

Academic or educational achievement tests are generally designed to measure skills at specific levels, for example, mathematical achievement among students in grades seven through nine. Because the normal range of achievement varies considerably in different grades, it is important to select the appropriate instrument for the specific testing purpose at hand. This is especially true when the patient is an adult, because adult achievement levels often do not correspond very closely to years of education completed.

Achievement test scores are usually reported in grade level equivalents. For example, a reading comprehension score of 11.2 denotes comprehension at a level that is average for students two months into the 11th grade in school. Sometimes a percentile rank within a specified grade level is given.

The physician should always ask for thorough interpretation of achievement test data, because the implications may not be obvious, even when the specific meaning is clear. For example, the practical importance of reading skill level is clarified by the fact that most newspapers, including the employment advertisements, are written at about an 11th grade level of difficulty.

VOCATIONAL INTEREST TESTS

Interest tests can contribute greatly to the quality of rehabilitation outcomes by objectively evaluating a patient's likes and dislikes. The information produced by tests can be helpful in exploring avocational possibilities, as well as in selecting an occupational goal.

Among the best known interest tests are the Strong-Campbell Interest Inventory (SCII), the Career Assessment Inventory (CAI), and the Kuder Occupational Interest Survey. Each of these tests has occupational scales, which compare the individual's likes and dislikes with those of people in selected occupations. The SCII and CAI also have basic interest scales, which measure an individual's *likes* in such general areas as science, nature, art, and athletics.

The Strong-Campbell Interest Inventory is the most extensively used and thoroughly researched of all interest tests. Description of this instrument will illustrate some of the principal features and uses of interest tests. The SCII has 325 items dealing with such things as occupations, school subjects, activities, amusements, and types of people. The individual responds "like," "indifferent," or "dislike" to each of the items, and the responses are scored on both occupational and basic interest scales. Only one form of the test is available for both sexes, but the norms for men and women differ. The 207 occupations represented on the SCII are strongly skewed in a professional direction, with many requiring college preparation. The instrument has been criticized for this limitation, but a recent revision has improved it. The Career Assessment Inventory, which is newer, uses the same measurement approach to provide better coverage of occupations with lower educational requirements.

The occupational scales of the SCII empirically score an individual's responses compared with the responses of various occupational groups. The more similar the individual's likes and dislikes are to those of people in an occupation, the higher will be the score on the scale for that occupation. The average score of an occupational group on its own scale is 50; the average score on that scale of people not in the occupation is about 25.

The SCII does not directly measure interest in an occupation. However, the relationship of interests measured in this way to long-term vocational behavior has been amply demonstrated by research. People tend to enter occupations for which they have high scores (45 and above), and to avoid fields in which they score low (25 or below). People who stay in an occupation that does not fit their interests tend to be engaged in atypical activities. For example, the physician with a low score on the physician's scale will probably be working as a medical administrator, researcher, or medical writer, or engaged in other nonmedical activities.

The SCII also measures a person's interests within broad categories or types, called occupational interest themes. Examples are the artistic, social, and enterprising themes, represented by such occupations as photographer, social worker, and life insurance agent, respectively. A person's occupational theme scores and basic interests provide a basis for extrapolating the test results to occupations that are not represented on the SCII profile. Thus, the SCII and similar instruments can be used very flexibly by the counselor to suggest directions for both vocational and leisure time planning.

VALUE OR ATTITUDE TESTS

Most tests of values or attitudes are used by counselors to provide a focus for discussion of personal matters and to assist their clients in gaining better self-understanding. These uses can enhance communication in counseling and facilitate progress in vocational planning. However, the vocational relevance of such tests is generally quite limited. The information they yield relates more to personality and life style than to vocational choice or to questions of vocational success. However, since values and attitudes may influence decisions and behaviors, they can have an indirect effect on the results of rehabilitation.

The Study of Values, developed by Allport, Vernon, and Lindzey and often referred to as the AVL, is one of the oldest and most widely used instruments in this category. It measures the relative strength in the individual of six basic motives or evaluative attitudes: *theoretical*, characterized by interest in discovery of truth and by an empirical, critical, rational, "intellectual" approach; *economic*, emphasizing useful and practical values typical of the businessman; *aesthetic, social, political*, and *religious*. The norms for this instrument are somewhat limited, but include high school and college students and several occupational groups. The value profiles of various samples show differences in the expected directions. For example, medical students score highest on the theoretical scale, and theology students in the religious area. Studies also show some relationship between value profiles and academic achievement in areas that correspond to the high value scores and between values and vocational interests.

The Internal-External Locus of Control (I-E

scale) by Rotter is not clearly a value or attitude scale. However, it measures some aspects of an individual's beliefs that are relevant to rehabilitation. The concept of a locus of control reflects the perceptions that people have of the relationship between their behavior and subsequent reinforcers. At one end of the continuum are people who believe that chance, luck, or fate is more important than their own behavior in determining what happens to them. At the other end of the continuum are those who perceive reinforcers as contingent mainly on their own behavior or personal characteristics. They believe in internal control.

The scale consists of a series of paired statements dealing with beliefs about the locus of control. For example: (a) In the long run, people get the respect they deserve in this world; (b) Unfortunately, an individual's worth often passes unrecognized no matter how hard he tries. The individual selects the one statement from each pair that more closely corresponds to the individual's own view. The inventory contains 29 similar items, and the score it yields will place the individual somewhere on the continuum of beliefs. Internal scorers are usually described as more active, independent, effective, and achieving than external scorers. Research on this inventory in rehabilitation settings suggests that internal scorers take more personal responsibility for their treatment and are likely to achieve better outcomes.

The Minnesota Importance Questionnaire (MIQ) is one of a small number of devices designed to measure values specifically related to work. It has 21 scales that measure such vocational needs as achievement, independence, recognition, security, and variety. The MIQ presents a series of statements describing what a person's "ideal job" would be like. The individual ranks the statements within each group to indicate which aspects of a job are most important. Examples of the statements are, "On my ideal job . . . the job could give me a feeling of accomplishment" (achievement), ". . . I could work alone on the job" (independence), ". . . I could do things for other people" (social service).

Scores on the MIQ indicate the relative strengths of the different values within the individual. Also, an individual's entire "need profile" can be compared to the profiles of various occupational groups. Similarity between an individual's profile and that of a particular occupational group is believed to predict "probable satisfaction" in that occupation. Extensive occupational norms are available for the MIQ, as well as norms for different groups of students and vocational rehabilitation clients.

PERSONALITY TESTS

The role of personality measures in vocational assessment is similar to that of most value and attitude measures. There are no vocational norms for personality tests, and the importance of personality in rehabilitation has more to do with overall personal effectiveness, coping skills, and behavior patterns than with questions of vocational choice or specific vocational performance. However, evaluation of coping skills and behaviors is frequently helpful in rehabilitation, and understanding a patient's personality can often facilitate progress in treatment.

There are two schools of thought in psychology concerning personality assessment. One view, held by those with a psychoanalytic or similar "psychodynamic" orientation, advocates the use of projective tests, such as the Rorschach test. The other view, sometimes characterized as "empirical," favors objective tests, such as the Minnesota Multiphasic Personality Inventory. The two approaches to assessment are quite different and reflect different concepts of the origins and structure of personality. The language employed by practitioners of these approaches to describe personality also differs. However, research shows that the inferences and predictions of behavior based on the different approaches are of similar accuracy and practical utility.

Because of their lower cost, objective tests are much more widely used in rehabilitation practice, although this varies in different regions of the United States. Most projective tests are individually administered, scored, and evaluated by a licensed psychologist, requiring several hours of professional time. Objective tests, on the other hand, may be administered to groups and can be given by a psychometrician or specially trained clerk. Scoring is entirely a clerical process and is often done by computer. Only evaluation requires the expertise of the psychologist.

Regardless of approach, there is an important caution to observe concerning the use of personality tests in rehabilitation. Most tests have been designed for use in psychiatric settings to facilitate diagnosis or evaluation of abnormal behaviors. The resulting emphasis on pathology in personality testing is due to habit rather than necessity. With a focus on assets, tests can help to identify the patient's strengths of personality as well as possible problems.

Patients in rehabilitation often experience emotional difficulties because of the stress of disability. However, their rate of mental illness and truly pathological behavior is the same as that of the normal population; they do not need the stigma of a personality description in psychiatric terms added to the burden of disability.

Because of this traditional bias in personality testing, a special effort may be required to balance its potentially negative effects. Therefore, when personality assessment is to be done by a consultant unfamiliar with rehabilitation, the physician should make a point of requesting an evaluation in nonpathological language that includes attention to assets as well as to problems.

The Minnesota Multiphasic Personality Inventory (MMPI) is not only the most widely used objective test of personality; it is the most frequently used and extensively researched psychological test of any kind. Originally designed as an aid to psychiatric diagnosis, it has nine basic scales that measure such psychiatrically defined traits as hypochondriasis, depression, hysteria, psychopathic deviation, and paranoia. The standard personality profile of the MMPI also includes the trait of introversion-extroversion. Many hundreds of special scales have been developed to assess various aspects of normal, as well as abnormal, behavior. For example, a scale for intellectual efficiency has been devised as a personality-based measure of intelligence.

The MMPI has 550 affirmative statements about one's physical and mental health, attitudes, behaviors, interests, beliefs, self-concept, and relationships with other people. The person responds "true" or "false" to each item to indicate whether it is usually or mostly true or false as applied to the person being tested. Examples of some items are, "I do not tire quickly," "I liked school," "I am happy most of the time," "I believe I am being plotted against," and "My sex life is satisfactory."

Items are grouped into scales on the basis of their ability to distinguish between a "criterion group" having certain defined characteristics or displaying certain distinctive behaviors and the general population. Thus, the hypochondriasis scale includes items to which hypochondriacs respond in a certain way more often than do normals. The original diagnostic or clinical scales, as they are called, were all based on the responses of patients with established psychiatric diagnoses.

Scores on the scales of the MMPI are determined by totaling the number of items to which the individual responds in the same way as people in a selected criterion group. Scores are standardized on the general population, yielding a mean of 50 and a standard deviation of 10. A standard score of 70, at the 98th percentile on general population norms, is usually the level where scores are considered significant in identifying a characteristic of personality, or "abnormal" in psychiatric evaluation.

Although some of the items have frankly abnormal or socially undesirable content and rather obvious intent, MMPI results are not easily distorted. The inventory includes several "validity" scales that measure openness, honesty, and other aspects of test-taking attitude. These scales are quite effective in identifying deliberate attempts at faking and they even provide a sensitive indicator of unconscious or other subtle distortions of responses. As a result, the MMPI can be successfully used in a wide variety of settings and circumstances, even when examinees have little motivation to provide accurate self-reports.

In the years since its original publication, the MMPI has been extensively used in schools, in health care and social service agencies, and in personnel selection efforts. Whenever people are being evaluated or selected for some purpose in which personality is relevant, the MMPI has been widely applied. At present, its use in assessment of normal personality characteristics is probably more frequent than its psychiatric or mental health applications.

Many of the special scales of the MMPI have been developed for use in some aspect of medical care: tendencies toward alcoholism or allergies, headache proneness, the "ulcer personality," and rehabilitation motivation. The ready availability of normative data and the established techniques of scale construction make it easy to create new scales for specific applications. In addition, there are extensive MMPI data on specific disability groups, such as patients with spinal cord injury and multiple sclerosis. These data indicate some of the personality characteristics associated with severe physical disability and have contributed greatly to an understanding of psychological reactions to disability.

The California Psychological Inventory (CPI) was derived from the MMPI. Many of the 480 items on the CPI came directly from the MMPI and are still used in their original form, calling for a "true" or "false" response. However, the CPI was designed from the outset to evaluate the normal personality. This is accomplished through the use of 15 scales measuring such traits as dominance, sociability, self-acceptance, and responsibility.

The scales of the CPI were empirically validated; the criterion groups were selected on the basis of displaying certain normal personality traits to an outstanding degree. Thus, the scale for sociability is composed of items that distinguish between students rated "most sociable" and students who lack that trait as rated by the students' peers and teachers. The basic validation of most of the scales proceeded in this fashion, contrasting the responses of people identified on the basis of conspicuous presence or absence of the traits evaluated.

In comparison with the MMPI, the CPI has the advantages of language and topics that are less "sensitive" to most people, and a focus on assessing the normal personality. It also has norms for people as young as 13, whereas the MMPI is of marginal suitability below age 18. The CPI has less research behind it and less information on its use in rehabilitation. However, it is potentially at least as flexible as the MMPI and it deserves to be included in any rehabilitation center's test library.

Referring the Patient for Testing

In preparing the patient for testing, the physician should keep in mind both the strengths and the limitations of tests. Too often, referrals for counseling are made with a statement like, "I am going to send you to the vocational counselor to take some tests and see what you can do." This places an inappropriate emphasis on one procedure when, in fact, tests are usually a small part of the assessment and counseling process. It also tends to subtly reinforce the expectation of many patients that the "magic" of tests will provide all the answers. This can lead to disillusionment with the entire counseling process when hard and fast answers are not forthcoming. Finally, submitting passively to testing and awaiting its "verdict" can diminish the patient's active involvement in other aspects of assessment and planning and contribute to a reduced sense of responsibility for both the process and outcome of rehabilitation counseling.

In keeping with the traditional rehabilitation emphasis on strengths rather than weaknesses, tests should be used in a positive vein, to expand possibilities rather than limit them. However, by specifying a deficit that may virtually rule out certain plans, tests can sometimes prevent frustration and loss of valuable time. For example, I was once asked to evaluate a 40-year-old physician with left-sided hemiplegia due to a stroke. Evaluation at another center had seemed to confirm the suitability of his plan to leave his previous practice, which he was physically unable to continue, and enter therapeutic radiology. His memory, verbal ability, and other obvious intellectual capacities appeared intact. However, testing revealed impairment of his mathematical ability, to the extent that he was completely unable to perform the operations involved in calculating radiation dosages. This proved to be irremediable. Unfortunately, he did not fully appreciate the significance of his deficit but was able to conceal it well enough to gain admittance to a residency program. His problem was discovered in time to avert disaster for his patients, but not soon enough to avoid a great deal of anguish for him and others concerned.

When test scores are evaluated by an experienced psychologist or vocational counselor and considered along with information from other sources, they can be highly accurate and meaningful. Their contribution to the planning process can be crucial.

Work Evaluation and Other Observational Techniques

Observation of the patient during participation in a rehabilitation treatment program will yield information regarding qualities such as cooperativeness, the ability to follow instructions, reliability in following schedules or keeping appointments, and ability to get along with others. Qualitative assessments of behavior as related to judgment, memory, impulsivity, and other possible problems can be made. Research on spinal cord–injured patients, for example, has shown that measures of independence, mobility, and diversity of behavior in the hospital are related to community involvement after discharge and to the incidence of medical complications requiring rehospitalization.[9]

Work evaluation is the main observational approach to assessment of rehabilitation patients. It usually consists of a series of situational tests designed to evaluate behaviors of the individual that are not measured effectively by psychological tests or casual observation. The principal uses of work evaluation are to assess work habits, readiness for employment, and tolerance for work. Occasionally, work evaluation is used to determine a patient's interests or skills in certain tasks when psychometrics are not satisfactory.

As indicated earlier, work evaluation is usually carried out in sheltered workshops or other specially designed facilities that can accommodate simulated work settings with a variety of business and manufacturing equipment. However, large, comprehensive medical rehabilitation centers often have work evaluation facilities, sometimes called prevocational evaluation units.

The work samples or tasks used in work evaluation are available in systems or "packages" that can be purchased commercially, such as the TOWER (Testing, Orientation and Work Evaluation in Rehabilitation) and the JEVS (Philadelphia Jewish Employment and Vocational Service Work Sample Battery). Such systems are usually "standardized," which means that there is a prescribed method of administration and "scoring," just as with traditional psychological tests. Also, there are usually norms that permit comparison of the patient's speed and quality of output with those of competitively employed workers, sheltered workers, and hospitalized patients.

The norms provided with commercial work evaluation systems are usually national or otherwise broadly based. However, most work evaluators eventually develop their own norms, which can be related to the standards of local industries that hire handicapped workers.

Work evaluation is often necessary as a supplement to, or substitute for, traditional psychological testing, especially when the patient's motor, intellectual, or behavioral limitations prevent adherence to standardized conditions. Since work evaluation requires individualized observation, it is usually possible to be flexible in changing time limits, physical arrangements, or other conditions of administration.

Work evaluation is not solely an assessment technique. It can also serve as a valuable tool in the management of the vocational rehabilitation process.

Management: The Process of Vocational Rehabilitation

If vocational assessment has been thorough and accurate, most patients will have a vocational objective before discharge from the inpatient rehabilitation service. Ideally, the objective should be clear enough and identified early enough to permit some progress toward it while the patient is still in the hospital. Vocational planning seems most likely to succeed if it starts early and sustains some momentum throughout the rehabilitation process. Such movement is facilitated if the initial steps are taken while the entire rehabilitation team is working with the patient.

Developing a Vocational Plan

The vocational plans made early in rehabilitation need not be firm. Indeed, many factors may preclude definite plans, such as an uncertain medical prognosis or the possibility of major change in financial status, family arrangements, or other aspects of the patient's life. Also, some patients resist planning as a way of denying the reality of their disability. However, plans are needed to guide the treatment program and to establish some landmarks for measuring progress aside from physical restoration.

One way to deal with an uncertain future or a patient's reluctance to plan is to sketch several "what if———?" scenarios with the patient. These can provide the frameworks for a series of alternative plans, with the choice of plan depending upon how the contingencies unfold. For example, a paraplegic with an incomplete spinal cord injury may wish to wait for maximum return of function before making plans to change occupation, even when it is clear that the greatest possible degree of recovery will still necessitate change. Refusing to plan allows the patient to maintain hope of recovery. The physician could confront such a patient with questions like, "What if you will need a wheelchair to get around after you leave the hospital? What will you do then about your job?" This approach can sometimes ease the implicit threat involved in planning and secure the patient's cooperation "just in case" plans for change are needed.

It is vital to success that the rehabilitation plan be the patient's rather than the treatment team's. Inevitably, there are differences, especially early in rehabilitation when the patient may be unwilling to work toward anything less than full recovery. However, these differences must and usually can be resolved through a combination of education, counseling, and negotiation.

Success in carrying out a rehabilitation plan is most likely if both the patient and family understand, accept, and actively support the plan. Serious problems can arise when the rehabilitation professionals have imposed their own judgments, values, and beliefs too strongly in planning. This is easy to do despite the best of intentions, since the balance of power and authority is so heavily on the side of the professionals. The danger is that the patient and family may accept the professionals' goals too readily because of unrecognized feelings of intimidation. When this happens, the plan that is launched with ease and enthusiasm by the treatment team may become a nightmare for everyone as it gradually breaks down without meeting anyone's expectations.

Identifying a suitable vocational goal and developing a plan to achieve it may be difficult and time consuming, but it usually requires the direct involvement of only the counselor and the patient. However, implementing the plan may involve the active participation of several members of the treatment team.

Implementing the Vocational Plan

A rehabilitation goal for the patient identifies the steps to be taken to reach the goal. The relationships among assessment, goal-setting, and progress in treatment are often complementary in that goals are identified and refined through a series of successive approximations as limitations become clear and as the patient's hopes and expectations evolve.

The key to successful implementation of a plan is to break it down into small steps, each of which can be easily achieved. This allows the patient to experience frequent success, thus helping to sustain momentum, and it simplifies the measurement of progress as successive steps are accomplished. This approach is especially important if the ultimate goal is unlikely to be reached within a few months of discharge from the inpatient rehabilitation program. Employment, in particular, is likely to be a long-term goal, often taking several years for severely disabled patients to achieve.

PSYCHOLOGICAL AND SOCIAL ADJUSTMENT

Delays in vocational rehabilitation result from the time needed for physical restoration and also from the slowness of psychological and social adaptation and relearning. In a study of paraplegics, Cogswell[10] found that their behavior during the first few months after discharge from initial hospitalization was characterized by a marked reduction in social contacts, in the frequency of entering community settings, and in the number of roles played.

may not be realistic owing to limitations of available resources in the labor market or in the patient's potential for work. The selection of a realistic goal must be based on a thorough assessment of all these factors. Suggesting specific outcomes for counseling narrows its focus unreasonably. Counseling could lead to other, even better, outcomes, but the patient with specific expectations may be unwilling to consider them. Inaccurate expectations for counseling create a likelihood of disappointment and failure. The physician can avoid such problems by simply encouraging participation in counseling. The patient's questions about possible outcomes should be referred to the counselor.

Unless good communication is established, working with a vocational counselor is often a frustrating experience for the physician because of the differing perspectives of the two professionals. The physician usually expects the counselor to secure employment for the disabled patient. The physician and counselor agree that this expectation is reasonable only for certain patients, but they often disagree on which ones. The patient who responds well to medical treatment is not necessarily a good candidate for employment. The hemiplegic, for example, may be a model patient for the physician but a source of exasperation for the counselor. Even when the patient has good potential for employment, the physician may be unaware of the obstacles that have to be overcome and of the time that takes before the patient can work. The physician may also think of employment as part of treatment, through which many of the patient's problems will be resolved.

Another source of difficulty is the tendency of physicians to measure employment in all-or-nothing terms; anything less than complete success is viewed as failure. On the other hand, the counselor may regard some degree of productive activity to be a highly successful outcome for certain patients and for others an intermediate step on the way to eventual full employment. Problems that stem from differences in the perspectives of the counselor and physician may be avoided if the counselor specifies an expected outcome of vocational rehabilitation and the steps and timetable needed to achieve that outcome. This defines vocational reality for the physician. The importance of effective communication to the smooth functioning of the treatment team makes it worth considerable effort.

The Counselor's Role

In general, the vocational counselor is responsible for initiating and directing the evaluation, planning, and treatment procedures that relate to the patient's vocational functioning. The details of what the counselor does may vary somewhat, depending upon the training of the individual. The vocational rehabilitation counselor is usually trained as a specialist whose expertise is in assessment of disability, vocational evaluation and planning, and coordination of rehabilitation services.

The counselor with a degree in psychology, although possessing some specialized training in rehabilitation, is primarily a psychologist. The practice of the counseling psychologist encompasses normal human development, including education, growth of the self, psychological adjustment, and career development. The psychologist may be expected to emphasize psychological assessment and the use of counseling or other psychological techniques to facilitate behavior change in patients. The psychologist will also generally be more interested in the patient's total psychological adjustment rather than with the more narrow concerns of vocational adjustment. When a psychological obstacle to rehabilitation arises, the rehabilitation counselor is likely to refer the patient, whereas the counseling psychologist is more likely to assume direct responsibility for working with the problem.

It is common practice to refer to the person who is filling the vocational rehabilitation role as the "vocational counselor," or simply the "counselor," regardless of the individual's academic background. Although some counseling psychologists, especially those with doctoral degrees may prefer to be identified as psychologists, the term *counselor* is practical and has been used throughout this chapter to denote both professionals. Outside the medical setting, the vocational rehabilitation counselor is usually considered "captain of the rehabilitation team." This is not merely an affirmation of the vocational emphasis of rehabilitation programs; it accurately reflects the central role played by the counselor in planning, directing, and coordinating all of the services included in vocational rehabilitation.

The counselor's interest in medical rehabilitation is usually limited to obtaining accurate medical information and ensuring that the patient will achieve maximum medical benefit before the vocational program is concluded. In addition, the counselor needs a medical evaluation to establish a patient's eligibility for services and to precisely determine physical capacities and limitations.

The counselor treats the patient's disability as only one of the several variables among the skills, abilities, and interests that need to be considered in vocational planning. The counselor's job is simplified if the patient's medical condition is as stable as any of these other variables. If the patient's physical functioning can be stabilized or improved by medical treatment, the counselor may contract with a physician for "physical restoration," which is the general term used by the vocational agencies to denote any medical rehabilitation treatment. Physical restoration may be just one of several specialized services that the counselor will seek from independent professionals, community agencies, and other "service vendors" to help achieve a vocational plan.

Because of the leading role played by counselors in vocational agencies, the counselor who takes a job in a medical rehabilitation setting may have difficulty adjusting to the change in emphasis. Being displaced by a new "captain" of the rehabilitation team and finding that vocational considerations are secondary in the hospital can be distressing to the counselor.

The responsibilities of the vocational counselor often overlap with those of other rehabilitation professionals. In particular, the social worker will share some of the counselor's interest in the patient's family relationships and functioning in the community. Similarly, the clinical psychologist may share the counselor's concern for the patient's psychological adjustment and an interest in the use of counseling and other psychological techniques to induce behavior change. When these other specialists are part of the treatment team, as they often are in a medical rehabilitation setting, frequent communication and careful coordination are needed to ensure that the overlap of professional domains is a source of strength, rather than a hindrance, to the rehabilitation plan.

The counselor is responsible for knowing what vocational services are available in the community, for referring patients to appropriate vocational agencies after discharge from the hospital, and for maintaining liaison with these agencies. The counselor is also usually the only member of the rehabilitation team who has any responsibility for job placement. Since placement involves securing employment that the patient can perform satisfactorily, it entails more than simply "finding a job" for the patient. Placement requires that the counselor know both the jobs and the patients well enough to make good matches between them. A placement must last long enough to give the patient a firm foothold in the labor market. The counselor must also maintain good working relationships with employers who can provide a range of jobs in different settings, suitable for people with a variety of abilities and limitations.

Placement often requires "selling" to the employer the handicapped applicant who is unable to make a convincing presentation of his or her qualifications for work. Few counselors have much taste or ability for sales work. Consequently, in the community vocational rehabilitation agencies, placement is usually handled by a specialist who works directly with employers. Only the largest medical rehabilitation centers can justify having their own placement specialist. However, it is reasonable to expect that the staff counselor will maintain effective liaison with placement services and handle the referral of patients who are ready for placement.

Including a vocational counselor on the inpatient medical rehabilitation team requires attention to effective communication for both the counselor and other team members. Nevertheless, significant benefits can result from early and continuous attention to vocational concerns throughout rehabilitation, and from having the counselor's advice and consultation readily available when treatment decisions are made that relate to a patient's prospects for employment. These benefits are worth the extra efforts required in communication and coordination among the professionals involved.

The Work Evaluator's Role

The work evaluator or prevocational therapist is another important figure in the vocational rehabilitation of some patients. In consultation with the counselor and the physician, the work evaluator takes direct responsibility for carrying out most work evaluation and work adjustment training. The work evaluator can be expected to contribute significant information not only about the patient's work habits, skills, and readiness for employment but also about the possibilities of modifying job duties or a job site to adapt to a patient's limitations. The work evaluator also shares with the counselor responsibility for having current knowledge of job opportunities and job performance standards in both competitive and sheltered employment that may be available to patients.

Work evaluators are trained in job analysis, human engineering, and performance analysis techniques. Their expertise includes observation, time sampling and other assessment techniques, and measurement and norming procedures. They must also have knowledge of the worker trait requirements of many different jobs. Traditionally, the background of the work evaluator has been in occupational therapy or industrial arts education. In recent years, however, many people have received special training in this field, and it is now possible to earn a graduate degree in work evaluation.

One of the special techniques the work evaluator may use to enhance readiness for employment is to arrange for trial work periods. Sometimes these involve tryouts in simulated jobs in the work evaluation unit, but work evaluators may also set up work stations in various departments of the hospital or institution where they work. Setting up such work stations may be difficult because of work rules, insurance complications, and the uncertain supply of patients capable of filling a job opening reserved for this purpose. This is especially true when work stations are established outside of the hospital. Nevertheless, such work stations can be of great value by providing a realistic setting and conditions to help bridge the gap between intensive rehabilitation care and actual employment.

Special Problems in Vocational Rehabilitation

The Progressive or Unstable Disability

Several problems arise in working with people whose disabiities fluctuate or tend to worsen. One of the most important is the difficulty of predicting functional limitations. Vocational plans that are predicated on specific functional capacities may be upset when those capacities diminish. Training to develop vocational skills may be entirely negated if any of the critical underlying abilities change. For example, a journeyman bricklayer was forced to change occupations after becoming paraplegic due to a spinal cord tumor. Because he had the interest and ability, he took training in architectural drafting. However, he had worked in his new job less than a year when progression of the tumor impaired the use of his hands and prevented him from continuing as a draftsman. A progressive disability of this sort may force several major, successive changes in a person's life.

The psychological impact of an unstable disability is another source of difficulty. For example, it is common for the patient with a condition such as

multiple sclerosis to insist that planning of any kind is futile, because "I don't know what I will be like tomorrow." Such patients often demonstrate an interplay between their psychological defense mechanisms and the nature of their disability, which is very resistant to intervention. On the one hand, their avoidance of planning makes it easier for them to deny the reality or seriousness of their condition. On the other hand, the very uncertainty of the disease provides a "reason" or socially acceptable excuse for not planning that psychologically legitimizes their strategy for coping with it.

Dealing with both the practical and the psychological implications of an unstable disability often requires highly skilled counseling. The denial and avoidance behavior that many patients exhibit is usually based on anxiety about the future, and the patient may need considerable assistance to cope with this anxiety.

Usually, direct confrontation of the possibilities is the most effective way of inducing constructive participation in planning. The patient must be informed, fully and clearly but in a supportive manner, how the condition may progress and what limitations will result. The patient can then be encouraged to work with the counselor on a series of alternative plans, each of which would seek, despite increasing limitations, to preserve something of importance to the patient. At one end of the continuum of disability, the plans may specify alternative job possibilities; at the other, counseling may focus on how to maintain satisfying social and family relationships. In between, options for various avocational activities may be considered.

From a practical viewpoint, it makes sense to take a somewhat conservative approach to planning so that the patient does not make too large an investment in alternatives that may later be impossible. Regardless of its focus, the very process of detailed planning can do much to promote a sense of mastery in the patient over the patient's destiny. In addition, making the possibilities known and helping the patient to understand how they may be dealt with can contribute greatly to alleviating anxiety about the future.

Vocational Planning for Young People

Vocational rehabilitation of the developmentally disabled or children with severe disabilities of early onset presents some special challenges. The main problem is that the need for special vocational plans may have implications for much of the child's educational program. Valuable time can be saved and consistent educational and vocational progress may be facilitated by making the right decisions about a child's education, sometimes as early as age 10 or 12. For example, if a child has the intellectual potential for a professional level career, many vocational possibilities are open that would be unavailable to the child with lesser ability. However, the need to gain access to such opportunities may dictate the choice of a college preparatory program in high school. In some instances, a college education may be possible, but only if certain deficits in educational skills can be corrected. Then, decisions about remedial education may have to be made early as part of a long-range educational-vocational plan.

Children who do not have the potential for primarily intellectual work may benefit from special attention to their social skills and general work-related skills. This can sometimes be facilitated through enrollment in a work-study program or a vocationally oriented high school curriculum.

The difficulty in making long-range plans for young people stems from the frequent unreliability of early judgments about potential. In the first place, tests of intelligence and special aptitudes are usually less reliable for children than for adults. The greater the distance in time spanned by a prediction based on test results, the less accurate the prediction is likely to be. Repeated measures of multiple predictors may be needed to compensate for the unreliability of tests in long-range predictions.

The unreliability of tests and other measures over time is sometimes compounded by the difficulty of accurate assessment on a single occasion. Because of the skewed social experience of many handicapped children, it is notoriously easy to either over- or underestimate their ability. Habitual avoidance of competitive or stressful situations, or a history of being catered to by overly solicitous parents, may prevent a child from making an optimum effort in testing. On the other hand, social and verbal skills may be overdeveloped in relation to other skills in children who have had extensive experience interacting with rehabilitation professionals. Moreover, sensory, perceptual, and motor impairments as well as widely varying rates of development of different abilities may also interfere with accurate assessment.

The resources available for dealing with the vocational needs of handicapped children are rather limited. For example, persons under age 16 are usually not eligible for services from the state vocational rehabilitation agency. Moreover, even when a vocational counselor is available, the counselor has usually had little experience with children. On the other hand, a child psychologist may be able to handle the assessment needed but know little about how to use the results for vocational purposes. Nevertheless, the comprehensive rehabilitation program does afford some possibilities. Frequently, the state agency counselor will provide consultation, even when the child cannot be accepted for direct services. Special education consultants and teachers can also be of help, as can the educational or child psychologist. Many large medical centers either employ such specialists or have reasonable access to them.

A team composed of the vocational counselor, the child psychologist, the teacher, the school counselor, and the physician is needed to develop a suitable long-range educational-vocational plan.

Alternatives to Employment

Some disabled people need an extended period of recuperation or adjustment following onset of a disability before they are ready to attempt work. For others, employment may never be feasible.

Some of the nonworking disabled welcome an opportunity to spend more time with their family. They are sometimes able, in new roles and relationships, to contribute significantly to the well-being of family members. However, others have difficulty adopting new roles or changing their relationships because of rigid views about the definition of roles. Also, value conflicts may arise from a sense of guilt over not working. All such people can benefit from rehabilitation services to increase their independence, improve their psychological and social adjustment, and help them constructively occupy their time. The physician should be alert to the need for such services and aware of what can be done to help achieve such goals.

If a disability not only prevents employment but also interferes with the pursuit of previous interests, counseling or occupational therapy may help the individual develop new avocations. In some cases, avocational rehabilitation may involve major changes in life style. For example, a person may be forced by disability to give up former avocations of a largely solitary nature and to depend more on interaction with others for recreation. Occasionally, substitute activities can be found that entail fewer physical demands but are psychologically similar to previous avocations or offer similar satisfactions. For example, the former recreational athlete may be restricted to sedentary activities but may learn to enjoy the contest of scrabble, chess, cards, or other intellectually competitive games. Accomplishing such changes, however, may require extensive assistance in the form of counseling, training, or guided recreation.

Alternative approaches to increasing constructive use of time among the nonworking disabled include participation in organized programs of day activities, work activities, independent living programs, or sheltered employment. Most metropolitan areas, and many smaller communities as well, offer some opportunities of this kind. The programs are usually operated by private rehabilitation agencies, such as the Easter Seal Society, Jewish Vocational Service, or United Cerebral Palsy, with subsidies from the state vocational rehabilitation agency. The activities programs usually have primarily social and recreational purposes, but they are often intended also to improve a person's ultimate prospects for employment through teaching of skills for social interaction and independent living. Sheltered workshops usually have a more explicit vocational orientation in that their services are intended to lead to competitive employment for those who have the potential, or to provide long-term sheltered work for those who do not.

Whether a disabled person has immediate prospects for employment or no apparent prospects at all, the physician must recognize the importance of constructive activity. Unemployment and inactivity inevitably carry some stigma for the individual, even if there is ostensibly a socially acceptable reason for it, such as severe disability. Also, the person who has activities and interests to fill time and provide a stimulating environment is likely to maintain better mental and physical health, not be a burden to others, and enjoy a better quality of life.

References

1. United States Statutes at Large, Vol. 41, Sixty-sixth Congress, 1920, p. 735.
2. McGowan, J. F., and Porter, T. L.: An Introduction to the Vocational Rehabilitation Process. Washington, D.C., United States Department of Health, Education and Welfare (Rehabilitation Services Administration), 1967, p. 4.
3. Crewe, N. M.: Quality of life: The ultimate goal in rehabilitation. Minnesota Med., 63:586–589, 1980.
4. Guttman, L.: Our paralyzed fellowmen at work. Rehabilitation, 43:9–17, 1962.
5. Strong, E. K., Jr.: Vocational Interests 18 Years After College. Minneapolis, University of Minnesota Press, 1955.
6. Crewe, N. M., and Athelstan, G. T.: Functional assessment in vocational rehabilitation: A systematic approach to diagnosis and goal setting. Arch. Phys. Med. Rehabil., 62:299–305, 1981.
7. Crewe, N. M., and Athelstan, G. T.: Employment after spinal cord injury: A handbook for counselors. Minneapolis, University of Minnesota Medical Rehabilitation Research and Training Center No. 2, 1978.
8. Keating, E., Paterson, D. G., and Stone, C. H.: Validity of work histories obtained by interview. J. Applied Psychol., 34:6–11, 1950.
9. Norris-Baker, C., et al.: Patient behavior as a predictor of outcomes in spinal cord injury. Arch. Phys. Med. Rehabil., 62:602–608, 1981.
10. Cogswell, B. E.: Rehabilitation of the paraplegic: Processes of socialization. Sociol. Inquiry, 37:11–26, 1967.
11. Dunn, M. E.: Social discomfort in the patient with spinal cord injury. Arch. Phys. Med. Rehabil., 58:257–260, 1977.
12. Mishel, M. H.: Assertion training with handicapped persons. J. Counseling Psychol., 25:238–241, 1978.

9 Prevocational Evaluation

WALTER C. STOLOV   DAVID L. HOOKS

A physician's commitment to comprehensive rehabilitation includes a determination to develop the maximum vocational potential of every patient. This commitment carries with it specific responsibilities. It is not sufficient for the physician simply to say, "I have diagnosed and provided the best of medical treatment, I have assisted my patient in achieving maximum ambulatory and self-care skills, and I have assisted the patient and the patient's family in developing a safe and satisfactory social interaction and psychological adjustment. I have therefore already maximized vocational potential, and all the patient need now do is look for a job as might any able-bodied person." Successful employment does not naturally follow the maximum achievement of physical, social, and psychological function. Specific therapeutic processes must be put into play to achieve the vocational goal.

A physician, and in particular a specialist in physical medicine and rehabilitation, has the obligation to include in the patient problem list the problem of *unemployment* when the patient is over 18 years of age (perhaps even as young as 16) and is unemployed, is not in school or in a training program, and has no direction toward achieving an employment goal. There exists a host of various professionals skilled specifically in vocational rehabilitation to whom the physician should refer, or better yet with whom the physician should become involved, to develop the therapeutic processes necessary to achieve the goal. For the patient who indicates a desire to move into employment, the initial steps may be easy ones. For the patient who makes no such request, the process is a little more difficult. The physician's obligation includes the initiation of a dialogue with the patient to raise the patient's level of awareness of the possibility

of employment. Such an educational function by the physician is as important as standard educational efforts in good health habits and in preventive medicine techniques.

Age Relationships

Patients who come under medical rehabilitation care with an unemployment problem and who are in the traditional vocational age range of 18 to 65 years usually fall into one of five categories:

1. There are those *disabled from birth*, or essentially within the first five to ten years of life, who by virtue of their disability did not receive the breadth of experiences that normal growth produces and who therefore come to adulthood ill-equipped to move smoothly into the labor market.

2. There are those who are *disabled in their teens*, at a most critical stage in their development, who not only also reach adulthood ill-equipped because of an impoverishment of experiences but are somewhat further handicapped by a keener awareness of their deficiencies when comparing themselves with their able-bodied friends.

3. There are those *disabled as young adults* who have yet a different set of problems with regard to vocational matters. Maturation for entry into the vocational world usually has already been achieved. They may already have been on a training path or perhaps in the work force. They usually, however, have not yet achieved an enduring, successful vocational history. They have accumulated some knowledge about the world of work, which may keenly point out to them the difficulties presented by their disability. When disability develops in the young adult, from a single traumatic insult, the burden of the shock of acute

onset is tempered by the relatively reduced stress of a stable disability not likely to further progress. A heavier burden of stress is borne by the young adult who acquires a chronic disease process, which by its nature has a progressive component. Whether such progression is continuous or is unpredictably intermittent, there is the stress of uncertainty. The set of vocational problems acquired by the latter subgroup within the young adult population is greater generally than of those with the acute stable lesion.

4. There are those *disabled as mature adults*, perhaps within the working age of 35 to 55 years, who have a vocational history that, perhaps more than anything else, describes them. They have a much greater sophistication and understanding of what the world of work is about and, if they have been successful, are perhaps in a better position than the young adult. They carry, however, by virtue of a more advanced age, the added burdens of greater financial responsibility and less adaptability.

5. Finally, there are those *disabled in late life* in the age range between 55 and 65 years who may well have the severest burden in readapting to the world of work, particularly if they had not been, during most of their prior life, in self-employed or professional fields.

All of these categories of patients present the same "unemployment" problem. These simple descriptions suggest that the therapeutic techniques and solutions are likely to be different for each group.[1] For each, nevertheless, the ultimate goal is the achievement of a stable, enduring vocational placement consistent with maximum potential and with opportunities for maximum growth.

The Process

Physicians in the past and unfortunately still in the present have treated the employment problem rather naively. The physician who tells a patient to "Get a different job" or "Learn a new skill" or "Get lighter work" simply is insufficiently sophisticated about the world of work. This type of "advice" has often been directed at the vocational rehabilitation counselor under relatively similar headings, namely, "Get my patient a different job" or "Teach him a new skill" or "Get my patient lighter work." All too often the physician wonders after a week or ten days have elapsed why the rehabilitation counselor has not yet been successful. Another concern is the advice of "You need

retraining." Retraining may not be realistic or may actually be constrained under law, as may occur in the case of Workman's Compensation or other legally involved situations. Primarily focused on acute medical care, the physician often finds it difficult to appreciate that some therapeutics take a little more time.

The vocational rehabilitation process can be divided into four stages:

1. The initial evaluation phase.
2. The prevocational (i.e., pre-employment) exploration.
3. The job-seeking and placement period.
4. The follow-up after placement.

Before discussing the prevocational component, it is useful to indicate the required information that the vocational professional needs from a patient's physician in order to establish an effective plan with the client, the physician's patient.

Medical Information

Simply passing on to the vocational counselor or prevocational professional a copy of the history and physical and the diagnostic impressions, or even, if the patient has recently been hospitalized, a discharge summary, does not provide the information essential for proper planning.

The Disease. The name of the disease is helpful for coding, categorizing, or classifying, but it does not tell the counselor very much. The physician must also include the *location of the pathology* and the systems involved. The physician must make clear the *necessary medications* and *health measures* the patient should be taking to sustain maximal function. The vocational professional must know from the physician whether the injury or the disease produces disability that is *stable* or has a *progressive component* and, if so, what additional systems may become involved. The physician must also communicate *complications* likely to develop if preventive health measures are not undertaken. This permits the counselor to plan in a way that will not contribute to the development of such complications. The physician must communicate to the counselor the patient's need for *continuing medical attention* to maintain health. Such information enlists the aid of the vocational professional in health maintenance. And finally, with regard to the disease, if impending death is a factor to be considered, the counselor should be permitted the physician's best guess (not some number derived from an average of such patients) whether the client being referred will survive two years, five years, or ten or more years. The counselor's approach may appropriately be different for the two-, five-, and ten-year categories.

The Function. The knowledgeable physician also transmits to the experienced counselor specific information on the breadth of *ambulatory skills*. Such data include needs for canes, crutches, braces, and wheelchairs, and whether ambulation skills include the community at large or are restricted. The physician communicates *stair-climbing abilities, transportation possibilities* within the community (be it public or automobile), special needs the patient may have with regard to *bowel and bladder function*, and the extent of independence in *transfer skills* and *activities of daily living*. All are useful to the counselor in understanding what it takes for the client to get up in the morning and prepare to go to employment and what needs the person may have during the working day.

Special Problems. Knowledgeable physicians communicate to the experienced counselor information that they have with regard to the strength and weaknesses of the patient in the areas of basic *intellect, personality, vision, hearing acuity*, written and oral *communication ability*, sense of *smell*, *memory* function, *learning skills*, and overall *cardiac* and *respiratory* function.

The physician must also be aware of significant differences in vocational counselor expertise. For some problems, referral to specialized centers is needed. This is especially true in dealing with complex problems found in some disability entities such as spinal cord injury and head injury. Traumatic brain injury with its myriad complexities can easily lead to errors in counselor judgment. Reduced attention can be attributed to "poor compliance and laziness." Memory deficits can be interpreted as "denial and lack of cooperation." Clear and explicit descriptions of expected client behavior will increase the probability of vocational success.

The Environment. The counselor must know and physicians must communicate their best guesses with regard to whether the patient can sustain *outdoor* as well as *indoor* employment, *temperature* and *humidity* extremes, *mobility* on rough terrain, and variations in *air quality*. Further, requirements with regard to *bathroom accessibility, quality of illumination* in a work environment, and *noise level* limitations, if any, must also be made known.

Environmental adaptation may also need to be supplemented by a *designated attendant* in the work place to assist if emergencies occur. This is necessary for something as mundane as transfers, as unpleasant as bowel and bladder problems, and as emergent and critical as dysreflexia.

Physical Work Categories. Finally, physician communications to the vocational professional must include an assessment of the physical capacity of the patient. These should be expressed in terms most often used by the vocational community in categorizing the physical demands of an employment activity. The category indicated may well be only the physician's best guess and might well be modified up or down as the prevocational process evolves. Nevertheless, the guidance is still helpful as a starting point. These categories include the following.[2]

SEDENTARY WORK. In this activity, the lifting requirements are of a magnitude of 10 pounds (4.5 kg) maximum and usually involve small objects. The work is usually done sitting, although some walking or standing may be required.

LIGHT WORK. This activity implies a lifting capacity of up to 20 pounds (9.0 kg), with significant walking or standing requirements. A heavy requirement for pushing, pulling, or leg control is also consistent with most sitting work in this category.

MEDIUM WORK. At this level, a lifting maximum of 50 pounds (22.7 kg) with a usual lifting requirement of about 25 pounds (11.4 kg) exists. This type of work and the two types that follow usually require walking and standing capacities.

HEAVY WORK. At this level, a lifting maximum of up to 100 pounds (45.5 kg) exists, with the usual requirement at the 50 pound (22.7 kg) level.

VERY HEAVY WORK. At this highest level of physical exertion, a lifting maximum of greater than 100 pounds (45.5 kg) exists, with a usual carrying capacity of 50 pounds (22.7 kg).

In addition to these categories, additional comments are useful that discuss any potential interferences in lower extremity functions such as *climbing, balancing, stooping,* and *kneeling*, and in upper extremity functions such as *reaching, handling, grasping,* and *feeling*.

Initial Evaluation

Successful employment, both for placement and for maintenance, requires the job candidate or employee to have proficiency in four primary skill sets: (1) interpersonal relationships, (2) work performance, (3) intellectual function, and (4) work behaviors. These four sets are not mutually exclusive, but for ease and clarity of analysis they are considered individually.

Interpersonal Skills

The ability to "get along with" others and good skills in interpersonal communication are often considered to be elements of personality. Concepts such as attitude, friendliness, cooperation, determination, and awareness are components of this set. These are the standards against which employees are measured when their interaction with the public, peers, and supervisors is assessed and evaluated. An employee must have mastery of these concepts simply to maintain the *status quo* and to avoid negative relationships. To advance and be considered for jobs of increasing responsibility, an employee must have a high level of competence in interpersonal skills. At an initial interview for employment, these skills have, with the exception of physical appearance, the highest initial impact on a prospective employer.

Performance Skills

These skills are those that affect the work product. They are measured by quantity and quality. Quantity is simply the total output of a worker (e.g., units). Quality is a measure of the acceptability of the units and is often expressed as a ratio of acceptable units completed to the total number of units attempted. This measurement system, although being "production line" oriented, can be generalized to human services and other work settings as well. There is always a balance between quantity and quality. Rarely are the two expected to be equal (e.g., the perfect worker). The employer sets the balance that is minimally acceptable.

An employee's physical capabilities impinge heavily in the area of work performance. Clearly, the ability to stoop, bend, stand, lift, or push, for example, may well affect performance. Depending on the product, interpersonal skills, intellectual skills, and work behaviors can affect performance. The ultimate measure in work evaluation still remains, "How much and how fast?"

Intellectual Function

These skills include, for example, problem-solving, innovation, and rate of knowledge communi-

cation. The degree of intellectual skills required varies greatly from job to job. While an employer seldom looks for people who function at low levels, the ability of a person to persevere at routine and repetitive tasks is generally inversely related to intelligence. Some employers are likely to screen out highly educated, highly intelligent candidates for repetitive tasks, especially if the job is to be permanent or long term.

Work Behaviors

This fourth category includes a large number of activities that also must be acceptable. Even those with superior interpersonal, performance, and intellectual skills will find little success in their vocational pursuits within our modern society if their work behaviors are not sufficiently acceptable. These are activities common to any job. The following lists examples of work behaviors critical to job success.

1. One's personal hygiene, grooming, and dressing habits must be appropriate to the work setting. Thus, whereas body odor is not a negative factor for a professional football player during competition, it is indeed a significant factor in a crowded office or where public interaction is required.

2. Personal habits must not be offensive to others. Although also highly variable to the setting, such things as nose-picking, groin-scratching, lack of handkerchief use, spitting on the floor, and constant humming or whistling are obvious examples of potential deterrents to successful employment. Even these, however, may be acceptable in some settings.

3. Punctuality and attendance records are obvious in their influence in determining work acceptability.

4. Communication skills directly related to work needs must also meet certain minimums. They are equal to performance skills in order of importance. Employees who cannot effectively communicate with their supervisors or co-workers with regard to their work needs or the work needs of others cannot succeed. Communication skills are an entity different from interpersonal skills (e.g., "He is really a very nice guy and tells great stories, but for the life of me, I can't understand his reports.") Most work-related communication is either written or oral. At least one must be mastered and the two should not conflict.

5. Coping ability refers to how well, when

WALTER C. STOLOV AND DAVID L. HOOKS

faced with a problem, the employee handles it until it is solved. "Frustration tolerance" is another way of indicating this work behavior. If frustration reaches a level that causes work performance to deteriorate, employability diminishes. Clearly, coping skills rank high in importance.

6. Endurance and vitality, although in a sense performance measures, refer to the ability to perform continually with expected quantity and quality, hour in and hour out, day in and day out, and week in and week out. Particularly for the disabled, the ability to sustain a four- or eight-hour day, day in and day out, is an important behavior to assess. Vitality is a measure that refers to whether performance levels sustain or deteriorate over time. Vitality deterioration usually occurs before the endurance level—the point at which the work quality becomes unacceptable—is reached and the worker must actually stop the activity.

7. Production consistency, although in part related to vitality and endurance, differs in that one must assess, even before the vitality and endurance end points are reached, whether the worker's output is predictable or varies from unit to unit; even in the early part of the day when endurance and vitality are not factors.

8. Distractibility, although in part related to consistency, differs in that one may have great vitality and consistency of output but be relatively less productive should neighboring extraneous factors not related to one's work, such as background noise, conversation, and visitors, cause relaxation of concentration and a decline in production.

9. Conformity to safety rules and practices is increasingly important. The high costs incurred by employers for injured workers and the high standards imposed by regulatory agencies may cause the unsafe and careless worker to lose a job in spite of high performance skills.

10. Adverse reactions to changes in work assignments or to the occasional or frequent monotonous task can also defeat successful employment. The worker who reacts with anger, hostility, or frustration to a less pleasant job assignment is not likely to endear himself or herself to a supervisor or to co-workers.

11. Work methods refer to how well one organizes tools and materials. This behavior may relate to personal habits and may, if deficient, affect quantity of output.

12. Supervision requirements, which in part relate to performance and intellectual skills, specifically measure how closely and how often a supervisor must monitor an employee after what may

be deemed a sufficient initial period of instruction. Related behaviors in connection with supervision include one's ability to accept the authority of the supervisor, to avoid becoming tense when close supervision is deemed necessary, and to be able to respond favorably to constructive criticism.

Initial Evaluation Phase

The client and counselor have as their ultimate goal a successful and enduring vocational placement with sufficient underpinnings for equally successful future advancement. The Dictionary of Occupational Titles lists 40,000 specific job titles.[2] Obviously, much work is necessary to reduce these options to an appropriate and manageable number and to maximize the four sets of skills previously described.

Armed, it is hoped, with appropriate medical information equally well understood by client and counselor, the two "go to work." This initial phase is an intense intellectual and personal exercise often stressful to both. Its function is to narrow down and select from the world of work those areas or directions in which it may appear that the client may have his or her best success. This exercise must be pursued with great skill. One must not be too broad and end with too many options that would take too long to pursue successfully. At the same time, one must not be too narrow and hence run the risk of no success. The assessment draws upon all that precedes. Included is prior education and training and prior employment work history (unsuccessful as well as successful). Previous work history provides one of the best predictors of vocational success. Verbalized personal preferences, clear understanding of physical limits, clear understanding of physical strengths, and an assessment of the four sets of skills required for successful employment are also necessary. Standard psychometric testing is often administered to supplement this assessment. The counselor has available, in addition, specific tests to evaluate, for example, eye-hand coordination, manual dexterity, spatial perceptual function, fine and gross motor skills, and reaction time.

Development of areas within the world of work that initially look promising for the client are further tempered with what may be available in the job market within the available geographical area. The geographical area open to the client is governed not only by the client's physical skill, but by social requirements and life style as well as the logistic constraints of housing and transportation. In certain situations, there may be legal constraints that preclude an optimal plan and require major compromises on the part of the client and the counselor.

Prevocational Exploration

The client and counselor are, after the initial evaluation phase, now ready to test out the initial assessment of potentially suitable work. In this prevocational exploration, the client is directly engaged in the performance of job units. Having the client engage in actual work samples or in a work performance setting allows an assessment of the best of alternative directions and also provides answers to questions not obtained by the initial phase. Depending on the work setting selected, prevocational exploration can also be therapeutic, in that solutions of work behavior problems that may have been present in the past can be found.

The amount and extent of the prevocational period is highly correlated with the client categories defined on page 209. Thus, what might be necessary for the client who is disabled from birth and has carried a disability throughout the formative years is entirely different from what might be required by the 55-year-old who has developed leukemia or perhaps lost a limb through peripheral vascular disease. Prevocational evaluation can be diagnostic as well as therapeutic. Some of the goals that can be achieved include the following.

1. Interests can be developed, particularly when no useful interests were generated by the initial vocational phase. Interest development may also be required even if interests do exist, for one may not be able to build upon them by virtue of the physical disability present. This is a critical process. The client is often required to make a major change in interests. There is often, as well, a grieving of loss, in terms of both function and limited choices. The counselor needs to be acutely aware of this grieving process and not simply provide a list of alternative vocational tasks.

2. Skill exploration is another goal of a prevocational program. Psychometric testing and even some of the more specific manual skill instruments may not be sufficient to assess if a client has potential skill in an area. Vocational samples can help assess whether there is inherent skill with certain tools, for example, sufficient to meet employment standards or to warrant specific training.

3. Confidence building is obtainable through a prevocational "on the job" performance without the consequences of failure. Within the protected confines of a prevocational sample, confidence can be created without much stress.

4. For the physically disabled who have achieved maximum levels of independence through rehabilitation in self-care and ambulation skills, the prevocational setting allows the generalization of achieved skills into the work setting.

5. Endurance is another important factor to be assessed, particularly for the physically disabled. It may not be possible to predict whether the patient can maintain a daily work schedule of four or six or eight hours without a prevocational evaluation that approaches the same levels of stress and duration. Caution must be used in evaluating endurance of clients with progressive diseases such as multiple sclerosis. What holds true for today may rapidly not be accurate in a few months or a year from now.

6. Growth in output, sometimes referred to as "work hardening," is another therapeutic goal achievable through prevocational activities. This is particularly useful for the younger age group who have not had much prior work experience. Prevocational activities can simply, through repetition and daily attention to work, increase work productivity.

7. A prevocational work period may be part of skill exploration in that it may help solidify a preliminary decision that specific training, be it at a school or through an apprenticeship, is a worthwhile possibility.

Prevocational explorations occur in quite variable settings. The mode selected is determined by the questions being asked or the goals that must be achieved. They extend from execution of standardized work samples performed in an artificial environment to placements in actual work settings alongside the able-bodied.

Work Samples

Various approaches to work sampling are used by work evaluators and counselors in rehabilitation facilities. The samples are often described as being standardized but may not always be statistically sound. Of the many work samples available, approximately 10 to 12 are consistently used. The most well known include the Philadelphia Jewish

Employment and Vocational Service Work Sample System (JEVS), the Singer Vocational Evaluation System (Singer), the Testing, Orientation and Work Evaluation in Rehabilitation System (TOWER), and the Valpar Component Work Sample Series (Valpar). A brief description of these work sample systems will indicate the differences in their approaches.

In using standardized work samples, it is important to remember the concept of standardization. The samples are based on norms, and the norms used must be considered carefully. Performance scores of severely disabled clients must *not* be compared with able-bodied workers. The key is to evaluate the client's work behaviors and focus on the behavioral correlates, not on a set of test scores.

The JEVS system, developed under sponsorship of the U.S. Department of Labor, was designed around various work traits that collectively constitute performance skills. There are 26 work samples that are formally administered to a client, and the work traits sampled include such characteristics as handling, sorting, manipulating, inspecting, and drafting. The system uses a realistic work atmosphere and requires six to seven days to complete. The JEVS is highly standardized. Essential to its use is a high level of accuracy of the observations made and the data collected. It is comprehensive and thorough in assessing client potential.

The Singer system, developed by the Singer Educational Division, Rochester, New York, utilizes over 20 different work samples drawn from the skilled trades and assesses potential for specific jobs. The client performs work typical of the job as opposed to the more abstract samples used in the JEVS. Each sample has its own work station, as opposed to some of the other systems in which the tasks are brought to a central work station. The Singer has a strong emphasis on career exploration from an information point of view but is weak in determining client potential.

The TOWER was developed by the Institute for the Crippled and Disabled, New York, and is one of the oldest systems. It consists of 93 work samples that are combined to assess 14 job-training areas such as clerical, drafting, jewelry making, mail clerk, sewing machine operator, and assembly. The TOWER is a complete work evaluation system and provides a realistic setting in which to evaluate and analyze job potential. Although comprehensive, it is somewhat narrow in focus and does not generalize well to other job areas. Both the dependence on written instructions and the relative complexity of the tasks may eliminate its use by the comparatively illiterate, mentally retarded, and severely disabled. The TOWER has been the "work horse" of work evaluators but has been for the most part replaced by newer systems that have better predictive value. The Valpar is representative of these new evaluation models. The norming groups have been expanded both in size and in the nature of the population sampled. Components still are often found in occupational therapy settings. Depending on the number of tests used, the TOWER can require up to three weeks to complete. Seldom are all tasks given.

The Valpar was developed by the Valpar Corporation in Phoenix and is one of the newer samples available. It was developed to assess performance of industrially injured workers. The Valpar is a trait and factor system and is based on task analysis. As each sample is self-contained, an evaluator might use any one or more of the 12 samples, such as small tools, problem-solving, and soldering, to assess a client. This ease of use also contributes to its major criticism, namely, that it lacks a unified analysis and reporting system. The behavioral observations are somewhat subjective, and therefore inter-rater reliability is low. On the positive side, it is rapidly administered (1 hour per sample) and appeals to clients. A recent concern is the misuse of Valpar components as a "work-hardening" tool. The test is given over and over ostensibly to increase endurance. This is an inappropriate use of any standard tool or measure.

The choice of the work sample evaluation system to be used is based on the patient's medical picture, the job market, and the objectives to be achieved. For further information on work evaluation systems, the comprehensive summaries prepared by the Stout Vocational Rehabilitation Institute at the University of Wisconsin should be consulted.[3]

Most work samples do not evaluate interpersonal skills or many of the varied work behaviors adequately, but they are useful for specific performance evaluation and also provide some measure of intellectual skills. Evaluation and assessment of interpersonal skills and work behaviors require other techniques, such as sheltered workshops and job stations.

Sheltered Workshops

Workshop settings are geared for "long-term" prevocational evaluations. They are "sheltered" by appropriate certification by the Federal or State

Departments of Labor to be outside general employment rules such as minimum wage regulations. They are further viewed as sheltered in that the quantity of acceptable units of production by its workers is generally below that considered minimum for industrially competitive employment. They are not, however, to be viewed as places for recreation or play. Sheltered workshops typically have specific contracts to produce specific outputs by a specific time for a specific customer. In many instances, the actual work one sees performed in a sheltered workshop is quite similar to what one might see in an ordinary industrially competitive setting. Many industries do not "tool up" for all their production needs and subcontract some of their work. Sheltered workshops often compete with traditional industrial companies for the same subcontract.

For certain clients, sheltered workshops end up as the final placement. For others, they serve as a transitional place of employment prior to entrance into the regular job market. For many, workshops are used for prevocational evaluation toward the goals enumerated earlier.

Job Stations

Perhaps more advanced than the sheltered workshop is the job station in an industrial setting. In this example, a vocational rehabilitation service program develops relationships with specific public or private industrial settings that permit clients to be placed for short periods in work positions alongside the able-bodied. Any one such individual placement is likely to be about one month in duration, although, depending on the setting and the disability, it may be longer. Appropriate relationships must first be established, both for the protection of the client and for the protection of the company that allows such placements to occur. Essential is the need for the supervisor at the job station to interact with the vocational counselor or work evaluator so that they, as well as the client, get the necessary feedback from the supervisors. This feedback helps to identify problems that the client and counselor must solve together. Direct behavioral observation by the counselor of the client is often utilized in the setting for detection of strengths on which to build or weaknesses in need of solution.

Whereas job stations of this type are obviously longer than job samples, they may not be as suitable as sheltered workshops when the prevo-

cational phase needs to extend into two, three, or four months or more. In the latter instance, the sheltered workshop may well be the more suitable placement. Volunteer work in public or private industrial settings, when well-evaluated, is akin to the formal job station. In addition, current federal legislation allows industrially competitive settings to engage in *job tryout*. The employer is able to apply for a special fund and to utilize these funds to pay salaries for a person to participate in a trial work period. If the worker proves to be successful, the trial period may lead to regular employment. If the trial period proves unsuccessful, the client and counselor have gained important information, and, at the same time, the employer has not sustained a financial loss.

Finally, one additional form of prevocational "job station" evaluation needs to be mentioned, although actually there is nothing prevocational about it. The client is simply returned to his or her previous employment. This method is suitable for people who were employed at the onset of illness or time of injury and for whom there is a probability of returning to their job following rehabilitation. Assuming that the client has achieved, in the past, a record of reliability and good performance, the employer is often willing to give it a try. In such a situation, the first few weeks or month in a job becomes the prevocational phase, when the person is actually already employed. Care must be used in this approach, because a poor performance may tarnish an otherwise good record. It should be used, perhaps, only when there is at least a 75 per cent probability of success.

Relationship of Prevocation Phase to Disability Onset

The discussion now allows some general statements with regard to what a prevocational exploration must accomplish for each of the categories enumerated on page 206.

Clearly, for those disabled from birth or in the first five to ten years of life, the prevocational phase may well be as much as 6 to 18 months long. Much must be accomplished. Such clients reach working age with very little in the way of experiences that normal growth produces to prepare them for the labor market. All aspects—performance skills, intellectual skills, interpersonal skills, and work behaviors—must be developed.

Clients with severe cognitive deficits from brain damage fall into similar categories. The length of the evaluation period is complicated by the length and unpredictability of the client's recovery curve. Many vocational rehabilitation systems are not well equipped to handle this category of client. They are not "compliant" and do not fit any current model of evaluation. They typically do not get served, and the physician should be aware of the need to refer and re-refer the client for services.

The same applies, but less so, to those disabled in the teens. Whereas maturation is only in part slowed, endurance testing, confidence building, and training might be the more important issues. The prevocational phase for this group is likely to be less than three months.

For those disabled in the young adult years, prevocational exploration needs are further reduced. Interest generation might be important, depending on the degree of disability, and a certain measure of endurance training and assessment may be necessary.

For those in the age range of 35 to 55 years, the prevocational phase, assuming a good prior work record, has perhaps as its main function the assessment of performance skills. This again does not require much time in a prevocational setting.

Finally, the adult in a late stage of vocational life, 55 to 65 years, either moves directly into a job tryout setting or more likely back to a prior job setting, if indeed possibilities for employment exist. If neither of these can be achieved, the likelihood of a return to employment is quite low.

References

1. Stolov, W. C., and Clowers, M. R. (Eds.): Handbook of Severe Disability. Rehabilitation Services Administration. Washington, DC, U.S. Government Printing Office, 1981.
2. Dictionary of Occupational Titles, Vol. 2, 3rd Ed. Washington, DC, U.S. Government Printing Office, 1965.
3. A Comparison of Vocational Evaluation Systems. Materials Development Center, Stout Vocational Rehabilitation Institute, Menomonie, WI, 1981.

10

The Epidemiology of Disability as Related to Rehabilitation Medicine

MASAYOSHI ITOH   MATHEW H. M. LEE

The word epidemiology is derived from the Greek *epidēmios*, meaning "among the people." Thus, it is no coincidence that in the early 20th century, C. O. Stallybrass defined epidemiology as "the science which considers infectious diseases—their course, propagation, and prevention."[89] This rather narrow and restricted definition, although obsolete, has a historic value, since it characterized epidemiology as a science.

Hippocrates stressed meteorological variations and seasonal characteristics as the fundamental elements that determine cyclic variations in epidemic diseases.[82] Until the 17th century this theory was widely accepted as the dominant concept for explaining the causes of transmissible disease. Few supported Fracastoro[28] in the 16th century when he theorized that infection was a cause and epidemics were a consequence. He further recognized three modes of contagion: (1) by direct contact from person to person; (2) by an intermediate agent; and (3) through the air. Sydenham in the 17th century suggested that there were intercurrent diseases that were dependent on the susceptibility of the human body.[82]

Beginning with ancient civilizations, the practitioners of medicine, the church, and governments struggled against epidemics by using theory, superstition, authority, and religion to compensate for lack of scientific knowledge. Throughout the medieval period, it was generally assumed that sorrow and suffering create a particularly favorable environment for the rise and spread of disease. The panic that erupted during epidemics was re-garded as furthering the spread of the disease. Thus, municipal authorities in many European cities felt it advisable to forbid tolling the customary death knell, as it would be ringing continuously night and day. Since epidemics were attributed to the sins of the people, elders of the church went from house to house hounding those suspected of religious irregularities and immoral conduct. Numerous men and women were expelled from the community in disgrace for minor offenses, since it was believed that eradication of sin and the sinful would halt an epidemic.[33]

As outrageous and primitive as it may sound, these and similar preventive measures were guided by contemporary medical beliefs and prevailed until the 20th century. Yet, we are not too far away from the day when tuberculosis and epilepsy were considered shameful afflictions. Even today, many still view venereal diseases as a sign of immorality; and superstition and fear doom patients with leprosy to life as social outcasts in many communities of the world. Because of such stigmatization, early discovery in these diseases remains extremely difficult. This is not meant to belittle or negate the tremendous amount of epidemiological knowledge that has been accumulated in this century. It does, however, suggest that in centuries to come, our present-day knowledge of causation and prevention of diseases and morbid conditions may be considered as primitive as the witch hunt or voodoo rite.

W. H. Welch defined epidemiology as a study of the natural history of disease.[104] Lilienfeld described it as the study of the distribution of a disease or condition in a population, and of the factors that influence this distribution.[59] In these definitions, epidemiology is not restricted solely to the study of transmissible diseases but can embrace all types of diseases as well as disabilities, whether physical or mental.

This chapter on epidemiology discusses conceptual aspects, the classic theory of the natural history of disease, and practical application of an epidemiological approach to the daily practice of rehabilitation medicine in the office, hospital, extended care facility, or home.

Spectrum of Health

The noted English biographer Izaak Walton stated in his famed *Compleat Angler*,

Look to your health; and if you have it, praise God, and value it next to a good conscience; for health is the second blessing that we mortals are capable of; a blessing that money cannot buy.

Benjamin Disraeli, the great English statesman, said in 1877,

The health of people is really the foundation upon which all their happiness and all their powers as a state depend.

Health is an essential preliminary to the best success in the best work, and to the highest attainment in the widest usefulness. Without it there is sadness at the hearthstone, silence and sorrow, instead of cheerful words and happy heart.[27]

Whether considered as personal treasure or national strength, health has long been regarded as the prime factor of human welfare. Therefore, prior to a discussion of disease and disabilities, some thought should be given to the concept of health.

One of the most frequently quoted and dynamic definitions of health was issued by the World Health Organization: "a state of complete physical, mental and social well-being and not merely the absence of disease or infirmity."[106] This rather simply phrased definition contains two distinct thoughts. The words "complete physical, mental and social well-being" imply an infinite number of variables relative to the present and to the ever-changing future. Rogers, in his Health Status Scale,[81] terms this state "Optimum Health" and notes that it is seldom maintained for a prolonged period. The second important aspect of the W.H.O. definition is the phrase "absence of dis-

ease or infirmity." This recognizes the existence of a state of health that is neither Optimum Health nor actual illness and that may be called Suboptimum Health. Suboptimum Health can best be illustrated by the patient undergoing the incubation period of bacterial or viral disease or the person with latent diabetes mellitus.

Usually it is not too difficult to recognize the state of Overt Illness or Disability. However, in those diseases with insidious onset, such as multiple sclerosis or arteriosclerosis, it is often difficult to detect this state. When the process of disease threatens life, the individual reaches the state of Approaching Death. Today, however, this state does not necessarily mean that a person is going to die. A cardiac pacemaker, organ transplantation, or exchange transfusion may bring a person back to Suboptimum Health.

In spite of advancements in scientific knowledge and technology, the individual reaches a state of Death, which is absolute and irreversible, when all vital organs cease to function. The fundamental goal of medical science is not to produce an immortal person but to maintain people in Optimum Health as long as possible, ideally until death.

The most important aspect of Rogers' Health Status Scale (Fig. 10–1) is that no person can stay in one particular spot on this scale for an indefinite period. If we assume that the sum of the word "health" is constant as is the word "weather," then ill health is discord, whereas health is concord. Thus, as a person's health status declines, a portion of health decreases and that of ill health increases. Like a train on a funicular railway, a person's health status constantly goes up and down from the peak of health to the edge of the valley of death.

This concept of health can be easily applied to the diseases or conditions that are observed in a rehabilitation service. Let us take as an example the case of a 60-year-old female who fell and sustained a subcapital fracture of the femur. Prior to the accident, this woman most likely had postmenopausal osteoporosis and possibly impairment of reflexes, of body balance, and of musculoskeletal coordination. Although the patient might have thought she was in perfect health, the presence of these conditions indicates that her health status classification at the time of the fall was, at best, Suboptimum.

Now she is obviously in a state of Overt Disability. If this case is mismanaged, i.e., with prolonged bed rest subsequent to traction, then hypostatic pneumonia and possibly decubiti may

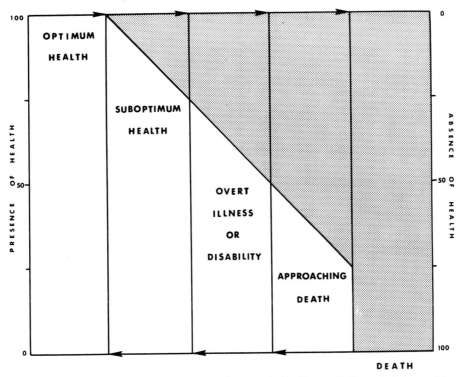

FIGURE 10–1. Health Status Scale. Arrows on the top and bottom of this diagram indicate declining and improving health, respectively. (Modified from Rogers, E. S.: Human Ecology and Health. New York, The Macmillan Company, 1960.)

develop. Thus, this woman's health enters the Approaching Death stage and may decline until it reaches Death. Not too long ago, this was the most commonly expected course after this type of accident.

The prognosis for subcapital fracture is poor if the fracture is treated with the Smith-Peterson nail, because the head of the femur will inevitably develop aseptic necrosis within a few months. In order to avoid this disaster and to bring the patient back to Suboptimum Health as rapidly as possible, replacement of the femoral head is the logical treatment.

Such surgical treatment, with proper restorative care, will return the patient to her normal state, Suboptimum Health, in a period of a few weeks. This model of the health status scale is applicable to every disabling condition, including loss of limbs or body organs.[43]

In the case just discussed, even the loss of the femoral head can be analyzed by the use of the health status scale. The femoral head initially was in Suboptimum Health. Trauma from the fall resulted in Approaching Death of the femoral head. Its removal by surgery, since it could no longer function, is tantamount to Death of the femoral head. Insertion of the prosthesis, although it does not restore any portion of health to the femoral head, does restore a portion of health to the patient. In fact, it restores the patient to the level of health she enjoyed prior to the accident. Thus, Death of the femoral head prevented the patient from sliding to a lower level on the Health Status Scale.

Natural History of Disease

In this concept of health, it is obvious that there is a specific mechanism by which health changes from one direction to the other. The history of medicine clearly indicates that our predecessors made a great effort to identify the causation of illness. In early times, strange reasons were advanced as the causes of disease. Virtually anything that was beyond human control was, at one time or another, considered the cause of some disease or affliction. Astrology and religions held that evil spirits and sins were responsible for the rise and fall of plagues. Evil spirits rising with the stench

MASAYOSHI ITOH AND MATHEW H. M. LEE

from sewage or stagnant water were thought to be the cause of epidemics. The initial use of smelling salts by European ladies may well have been an early but vague recognition of environment as a causative factor of disease.

It was not until the 17th century that the idea of human susceptibility emerged. During the onslaught of epidemics in the medieval period, the "sinful" people who fell victim to epidemics were obviously highly susceptible to the disease. Those who survived were naturally less susceptible but not necessarily any less sinful.

As early as the mid-17th century, existence of the microorganism as a causative agent of illness was suspected. It was not until the 19th century, however, that this obscure theory was proved. Identification and isolation of a specific microorganism as a responsible agent of a particular disease enforced the concept of a single cause of disease, and less attention was focused on causes related to the host and environment.[53]

In the early 20th century, various epidemiological investigations on outbreaks of transmissible diseases were conducted. These studies revealed that mere exposure of the human host to a specific agent did not inevitably produce the state of Overt Illness. Thus, the modern epidemiological concept that illness is caused by simultaneous interaction of host, agent, and environment was established.

In order to comprehend this triad theory, which is highly relevant to later discussions in this chapter, it is essential to analyze each causative factor. The host, being human, has various characteristics: age, sex, race, chromosomal variety, body constitution, immunity, marital status, education, occupation, habit and custom, psychological state, and so forth. Although certain behavioral patterns of a host have been categorized as part of the host characteristics, sexual orientation *per se* has not been so recognized. However, cumulative epidemiological data strongly indicate that male homosexual activity, particularly anal intercourse, places a person at high risk for transmission of human immunodeficiency virus (HIV), the causative organism of acquired immune deficiency syndrome (AIDS). The sharing of a needle or syringe among intravenous drug users, a known method of transmitting hepatitis B, has also been identified as high-risk behavior for the transmission of HIV. The significance of host characteristics may be illustrated by the fact that certain diseases or conditions are more prevalent in persons with similar characteristics than in others lacking those characteristics.

Biological, chemical, mechanical, genetic, nutrient, and physical elements are often cited as qualitative agent factors that may vary in their virulence. It is also important to note the value of the quantitative aspect of agent factors. Quantity may be understood in two categories: *dosage* and *frequency*. Frequent exposure to a low dosage of the agent could develop either of two opposing results: increased resistance or a cumulative effect.

Increased resistance is exemplified by tuberculosis in the New World. White settlers had been exposed to *M. tuberculosis* for centuries in Europe and thus had developed resistance. Despite many hardships in America, there was no marked increase of tuberculosis among the white settlers. At the same time, Native Americans and the imported black slaves in Argentina suffered greatly and some tribes and groups were virtually wiped out. Similarly, some childhood diseases may afflict adults who have had little exposure to them and thus offer low resistance.

The cumulative effect of frequent and/or prolonged exposure to a low dosage of agents is often associated with environmental pollution. "Black lung," which is produced only after years of silica dust inhalation, is commonly found among mining workers.[67] However, one visit to a coal mine cannot result in pulmonary silicosis. Similarly, inhalation of asbestos dust seems to be responsible for a high incidence of lung cancer among asbestos workers and ship pipefitters.[5, 36] Byssinosis results from chronic inhalation of fibers in a cotton mill.[6a]

The ill effects of pollutant agents are not limited to occupational exposure to toxic substances. A classic example is the tragic Minamata disease, which was caused by frequent consumption of fish contaminated by mercury compound.[29] While the ecological effect of DDT, fictionalized in *Silent Spring*,[16] is now a historical reality, contamination of drinking water with polychlorinated biphenyls (PCB) and other industrial chemical substances is a major problem today. Soil pollution, which necessitated evacuation of residents in the Love Canal section of Niagara County, New York, was traced back to industrial waste used for sanitary landfill in the area.[9]

It is important to differentiate between the epidemiological concept of environment as the third causative factor of a disease and environmental pollution in epidemiology. The environment is the vessel in which pollutant agents are contained.

Environment may be viewed in terms of physical, biological, socioeconomic, political, and other aspects. Physical environment may refer to the physical characteristics of the immediate sur-roundings or to atmospheric conditions such as climate, atmospheric pressure, gaseous composi-tion, and quality of air. Such characteristics of socioeconomical environment as education, cus-toms, and nutritional habits may greatly influence host susceptibility.

Paul[73] recognized two types of epidemiological climate: micro-climate, described as the social cli-mate and representing intimate living conditions within the home or place of work; and macro-climate, which represents climate in the ordinary meteorological sense of temperature, humidity, and rainfall. The concept of micro-climate is more individualized in its interpretation of environment and includes some host characteristics that are related to socioeconomical conditions. For exam-ple, certain political climates could make one group of hosts more or less deprived in a socio-economical sense.

When a disease or condition is analyzed, the factors of host, agent, and environment must be carefully considered. An acceptable and perhaps innocent clinical statement such as "Fracture of the neck of femur is commonly seen in elderly people, mostly women"[42] is far short of satisfactory in an epidemiological sense. Mere age and sex cannot accurately represent the host characteris-tics. Such characteristics in an aging female may involve body constitution—for example, post-menopausal osteoporosis, diminished vision, and a propensity for falling—in other words, an impaired sense of body balance. This could be caused by cerebral arteriosclerosis or by medications being administered for hypertension. But this is still a limited analysis. Custom and habit can also con-tribute to this injury and disability. Many women at home customarily wear house slippers, which cause a shuffling gait and make the wearer more susceptible to falling accidents. Some investiga-tors[7, 101] claim hip fracture is common among whites but another[80] disputes this by citing a large number of cases among blacks. Thus, even the racial factor must be considered when discussing the prevalence of this condition.

Since most hip fractures occur inside the home, the peculiarities of the environment must be stud-ied. Highly waxed or wet floors, slippery throw rugs, or a dangling telephone cord may become menacing obstacles. Cluttered floors, poor lighting, sagging floors or steps, defective handrails on stair-cases, or crowded housing indicating a hazardous physical environment may be host characteristics related to the socioeconomical and education fac-tors.

The agent in the accident discussed as an ex-ample is mechanical force, which exerted extreme stress to body structure.[18] Unsuccessful attempts to regain body balance resulted in the fall, and stress produced the fracture. However, one can easily ascertain that various host characteristics and environmental factors had existed for some time prior to this accident. Most likely, there had been episodes of loss of balance or near-accidents before this incident. The fact that injury did occur at this particular time indicates that the three causative factors—host, agent, and environment—sufficiently and simultaneously interacted and re-sulted in fracture.

The period when these three causative factors exist independently and have not completed inter-action is called the Prepathogenesis Period (Fig. 10–2). Upon completion of simultaneous interac-tion, a disease stimulus is produced. At this stage, Early Pathogenesis, a person's health status changes from Optimum to Suboptimum Health. However, until the disease process reaches above the Clinical Horizon, the presence of illness is not recognizable. Once reaching the state of Overt Illness, the individual may recover to Suboptimum and, hopefully, Optimum Health, at which time he or she returns to the Prepathogenesis Period and commences another cycle for other disease. This model of the natural history of disease is applicable to virtually all diseases and conditions and is the basis for the epidemiology of disability. A survey done by the Environmental Protection Agency after the Love Canal disaster found 32,254 sites in this country that may cause health hazards, and many may already be affecting the health of people in those areas.[4] The residents in these sites could be considered to be in their period of Pre-pathogenesis.

Levels of Prevention

Health care includes preventive and clinical medicine. Any health care that attempts to halt a person's slide down the slope of the health status scale is termed preventive and any attempt to push it up toward the peak, Optimum Health, is called therapeutic. This definition is essential to concep-tualization of the Levels of Prevention. Although activities in preventive medicine have no direct therapeutic value, every measure administered in therapeutic or clinical medicine has its preventive aspects. Vaccination or fluoridation of drinking water protects populations from disease but does

MASAYOSHI ITOH AND MATHEW H. M. LEE

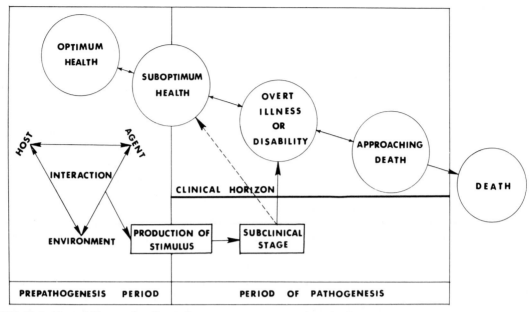

FIGURE 10–2. Natural history of a disease in a person as constructed on the Rogers' Health Status Scale shown in Figure 10–1. Not every disease appears above the clinical horizon. The individual may recover from the subclinical stages directly to Suboptimum Health.

not cure any disease. On the other hand, antibiotics are therapeutic agents that can also prevent septicemia and death. Similarly, internal fixation of hip fracture is a therapeutic surgical treatment but also prevents pulmonary and peripheral vascular complications.

Within this frame of reference, the total spectrum of health care is classified into three levels of prevention: Primary, Secondary, and Tertiary. Primary prevention is applicable during the Prepathogenesis or Optimum Health periods. The other two levels cover the period of pathogenesis or, let us say, all gradations of the health scale from Suboptimum Health to Approaching Death.

Each level of prevention consists of various representative activities. Table 10–1 shows a comparison of the activities at each level, as interpreted

by the authors of this chapter and by others. All the listed authors agree wholly on activities basic to Primary prevention and agree in part with our interpretation of Secondary prevention. Our interpretation of rehabilitation and limitation of disability activities differs from that of the other authors, and they also differ from each other in interpretation of these measures.

Rehabilitation is defined as "the ultimate restoration of a disabled person to his maximum capacity—physical, emotional, and vocational."[84] It is widely believed that rehabilitation must be started at the earliest possible time in order to ensure the best results. Thus, the diagnosis must be established in the earliest possible phase of disease, and all necessary treatment, including rehabilitation, must be initiated at that time. The belief that

TABLE 10–1. Levels of Prevention

AUTHORS	PRIMARY	SECONDARY	TERTIARY
Leavell and Clark[18]	Health promotion	Early diagnosis	Rehabilitation
	Specific protection	Proper treatment	
		Disability limitation	
Columbia University[24]	Health promotion	Early diagnosis	Disability limitation
	Specific protection	Proper treatment	Rehabilitation
Itoh and Lee[43]	Health promotion	Early diagnosis	Disability limitation
	Specific protection	Proper treatment	Custodial care
		Rehabilitation	

rehabilitation should commence after termination of specific treatment of a disease or condition that results in disability is the basis for classifying rehabilitation at the Tertiary prevention level. The writers admit that this idea is regrettably widespread, and such procedure is common practice. But this is obviously a misconception. Inasmuch as rehabilitation should be administered in conjunction with specific medical or surgical treatment of diseases or conditions that can result in disablement, rehabilitation should be considered an integral part of Secondary prevention.

Disability limitation (Table 10–1) refers to preventing an increase in the intensity or scope of an existing disability. This measure, therefore, becomes necessary after termination of active medical or surgical treatment and rehabilitation. Disability limitation is generally known as maintenan' treatment. It is particularly indispensable for those who are chronically ill or disabled and absolutely mandatory for geriatric patients. Another example of disability limitation is recreation therapy. Eventually, lack of stimuli, regimented daily life, and hopelessness can mold the population of a chronic disease institution into a depressed, docile, apathetic mass. Recreation therapy, through programs designed to stimulate both groups and individuals, can prevent this kind of psychological crippling.

One of the most important aspects of disability prevention is pain control. Regardless of its origin, intractable pain is an extremely debilitating symptom, emotionally as well as physically. Although the tolerance to pain may vary from one individual to another, no person is immune to pain. Often patients with chronic pain may state that they "have gotten used to pain" or "have learned to live with it." Such statements should not be taken literally as a sign of increased pain tolerance but should be considered a possible sign of resignation, which in itself can be destructive. Whereas there is no ideal analgesic, the discovery of enkephalins and endorphins[90, 91] may revolutionize the concept of and approach to pain management. Relationships between these opiate-like peptides and some old and new pain control techniques such as acupuncture, transcutaneous nerve stimulation, and behavior modification are currently under investigation.[14]

We have included custodial care in our table of health care. The purpose of custodial care is to make people as comfortable as possible for the last few years or days of their lives. When custodial care is indicated, there is usually no hope for reversal or cure. This does not mean that disability limitation is not indicated. It is warranted because it prolongs activity and comfort and it should be listed as an independent entity in tertiary prevention.

Management of the terminal cancer patient has always been a problem for health care systems and an agonizing experience for patients and their families. Recently, great attention has been focused on pain control and tertiary care for terminal cancer patients. This management of pain is not limited to somatic pain but encompasses social, emotional, and spiritual pain. Following the pioneer work by Saunders at St. Christopher's Hospice in London, the importance and need for hospice type care has been recognized and is gaining worldwide acceptance.[40, 58, 62, 75, 98] The basic concept of hospice care is to alleviate all kinds of pain for patients and their families so that they are able to maintain rewarding relationships and live as fully as possible during the final stages of the patient's illness.

The model of Levels of Prevention that is described here can be applied to each individual disease or condition. Thus, in reality, a person may be subjected to various levels of prevention simultaneously. For example, a 65-year-old man has had a cerebrovascular accident secondary to arteriosclerotic heart disease. He complains of fatigue and shortness of breath after exercise and experiences pitting edema. He was recently discharged to his home from a rehabilitation service and is able to ambulate with a short leg brace but his upper extremity is spastic and nonfunctional. The time is late November and the city health department predicts influenza epidemics during the coming winter.

The cardiac condition receives priority attention; early diagnosis and prompt treatment for cardiac decompensation are in order. This is secondary prevention. The patient is advised to wear the short leg brace daily and is given a static splint for his upper extremity. Further, ambulation commensurate with his tolerance is encouraged, and a visiting physical therapist gives passive exercise to his upper extremity to prevent contracture of fingers. These are disability limitation measures. The attending physician would probably give influenza vaccine to prevent any danger to the patient from the threatening epidemic. This is primary prevention.

Another example is cardiac surveillance of elderly disabled who are undergoing a rehabilitation program. Solomon and associates[94] found that over

25 per cent of geriatric lower extremity amputees who had no previous history of ischemic heart disease showed changes indicative of myocardial ischemia on telemetric dynamic electrocardiograms taken during ambulation exercise. This finding provides information necessary for regulating the patients' physical activity within the limits of cardiac tolerance so that ischemic heart disease might be prevented. Whereas these patients are obviously receiving rehabilitation, the Secondary preventive care, the surveillance program promotes the "specific protection" of Primary prevention.

The purpose of this epidemiological approach to patient care is to provide the tools that seek and analyze all factors contributing to disease and disability. It demonstrates a rational and individualized approach that assures that no factor is overlooked and no question remains unanswered.

Functional Diagnosis

Prevention consists of two interrelated processes: the anticipation of future events and the action to thwart occurrence. Anticipation is possible only if there is some recall from past experience. When experience is documented in detail and carefully analyzed, prognostication can be reasonable and accurate. Epidemiology systematically studies the process of a disease or condition and demonstrates a chain of events that is known as the natural history. Once the natural history of a disease is established, the weakest link in the chain of events is the point where the attack to prevent the disease should start.

In the early part of this century, epidemics of an unknown malady became prevalent in the southern part of the United States. An epidemiological investigation was launched and certain characteristics regarding the prevalence of the disease were uncovered. Thus, the disease caused by a deficiency of niacin and now known as pellagra was identified.[30][34] The methods used to discover the identity of pellagra were identical to the approach that previously had been applied only to transmissible diseases. The most important aspect of the pellagra investigation is that the whole epidemiological study was based solely upon accurate clinical documentation of the condition of each patient so afflicted.

Rehabilitation, one of the secondary levels of prevention, focuses its attention on disability. Other specialties in therapeutic medicine require early and precise diagnosis in order to institute the most effective treatment. The same logic applies to rehabilitation, and the disabled should be given early evaluation and intensive treatment to prevent permanent disability.[51] Dynamic rehabilitation care can be administered only when an explicit early diagnosis of the disability has been established.[95] The longer explicit diagnosis is delayed, the less effective the consequent restorative care becomes.

For example, right hemiplegia due to cerebral artery thrombosis is not sufficiently accurate as a diagnosis to be utilized in making an effective rehabilitation care plan. Because the ultimate goal of rehabilitation is total restoration, the total person, physically, emotionally, vocationally, and socially, must be considered in the diagnosis. Most medical records and case histories do not indicate the physical, mental, or socioeconomical ability of a person.[97] There are no two identical hemiplegics. The aforementioned diagnosis, although medicolegally acceptable, does not indicate the extent of brain damage or note cultural background, which will directly influence the patient's ability to comprehend, retain instruction, or respond to the rehabilitation process. Thus, the conventional non-illuminating diagnostic nomenclature for statistical purposes[107] is insufficient for dynamic rehabilitation care.

Diagnosis of disability may be expressed either in terms of the amount of disability or in terms of the amount of remaining function. The former category is commonly called the disability evaluation or rating. In the latter category, functional diagnosis is the preferred terminology. Regardless of choice, the sum of the results from either system remains constant. It is universally agreed that disability evaluation is, in reality, a quantitative diagnosis as contrasted with the more familiar qualitative diagnosis.[25, 49, 50, 108] Evaluation of disability has long been important in the legal field.[1, 49, 64, 102] Since no single standard wholly fulfills the specific needs of all programs concerned with disability,[77] various rating systems according to diagnostic groups have been reported.[2, 35, 74, 108] One of the most widely used is the cardiac classification ratings of the American Heart Association. A variety of disability scales to evaluate the injured in liability or workmen's compensation cases were developed in the first half of this century.[13, 15, 31, 66, 111]

Countless methods to assess the extent of disability pursuant to a treatment plan and to evaluate the progress of a patient in a rehabilitation program are in the literature. Some are more ingenious or sophisticated than others. Moskowitz and McCann[68] developed a physical profile called

PULSES that utilizes a set of ordinal scales. PULSES expresses general physical condition, the function of upper and lower extremities, sensory status, continency, and emotional status by six representative digits. The Sokolow method[93] rates physical, social, emotional, and vocational capacity, but a national field trial[92] revealed that this method contributes little of significant value to vocational counseling. For the past two decades, numerous Activities of Daily Living (ADL) scales have been reported.* Although ADL scales are mainly in the domain of the occupational therapist, Pool and Brown[76] selected certain activities that a physical therapist could evaluate.

A large volume of data must be collected in order to produce one comprehensive functional diagnosis. The accumulation of voluminous information inadvertently necessitates involvement with the problem of effective format and storage that will permit easy retrieval of all the data. In this regard, electronic data processing techniques have been found to be most advantageous.[93, 95]

The expression of disability evaluation or functional diagnosis varies according to the method. The most common method is a numerical presentation in either percentage or digit based on a specific scale. The other common method is a graphic presentation. Unlike Lawton's method[52] for ADL, Huddleston and colleagues[39] produced a graph called the Patient Profile Chart on which the value of muscle power and comparative functional capacities were arranged. In reviewing all these methods, there are more numerical presentations than descriptive ones. This tendency is perhaps due to the fact that the use of digits gives simplicity and provides mathematical advantages such as weighting.

The ordinal scale is becoming more popular than the nominal scale. However, one must recognize that a well-conceived nominal scale is superior to a haphazard ordinal scale despite the use of digits. One pitfall in the nominal scale is that innovators sometimes become trapped in their own jargon. There is a need to eliminate or replace vague stereotyped expression with more realistic and accurate terminology.[10] A good example of this type of ambiguous phraseology is "partial independent" or "minimum assistance." Ideally, a classification scheme should meet the following three criteria: (1) its classes must be mutually exclusive; (2) it should be exhaustive; and (3) there should

*See references 8, 11, 15, 21, 32, 37, 38, 48, 52, 60, 63, 86, and 109.

be a reasonable number of classes as well as a reasonable frequency of cases in each class.[39a] The ideal functional diagnosis should be

1. Simple enough so that rapid evaluation is possible.

2. Reproducible so that constancy may be maintained.

3. Objective and using measurable factors so that the results are statistically more reliable.

4. Descriptive so that the actual situation is accurately reflected.

5. Comprehensive so that the diagnosis is completely and specifically utilizable in the direct care of patients and is practicable for epidemiological investigation.

To date there is no single standard that measures disability with precision, nor is there any set of precise biological units, free of subjective influences, that uniformly conveys universally acceptable measuring criteria.[49]

In relation to functional diagnosis, Wylie and White[110] stated:

In each field of knowledge, such as medicine or public health, a new measuring instrument commonly results in new studies and observation: from these we evolve new hypotheses, and further instruments are invented to test these ideas. . . . When the field of knowledge is still in a rudimentary stage, often a scarcity of measuring instruments delays this cycle.

Thus, the use of epidemiology in rehabilitation can aid in defining the natural history of physical disabilities in mankind and it is well recognized that there is a gap in our knowledge of human incapacitation. Better "instrument" or better functional diagnosis means that new studies, new observation, and new hypotheses will emerge.

Secondary Disability

In the daily practice of rehabilitation medicine in a hospital-based service or private office, there is a tendency to view disability in a simplistic or superficial way. Excluding iatrogenic disability and physical disability due to psychiatric illness,[56] two types of disabilities exist. Disabilities that are direct consequences of a disease or condition are called primary disability. Paraplegia, quadriplegia following spinal cord injury, hemiplegia, hemianopia, aphasia due to cerebral vascular accident, or traumatic fracture are examples of primary disability. On the other hand, disabilities that did not exist at the onset of the primary disability but subsequently developed are called secondary disabilities.[85] The secondary disability is indirectly related to the disease or condition that is responsible for the primary disability. Examples are joint contracture, subluxation of shoulder joint in hemiplegia, disuse muscle atrophy, and decubiti.

The epidemiology of primary disability, a subject outside the province of conventional rehabilitation medicine, is discussed later in this chapter under *Preventive Rehabilitation*. Since the secondary disability develops while the patient is under the physiatrist's care, it is important to discuss it in depth. However, literature related to the epidemiology of secondary disability is minimal. Abramson and colleagues[1] claimed that among injured workers there is a correlation between the degree of disability, the circumstances of injury, and the sex, age, employment status, economical status, and place of residence of the injured. This finding should not be interpreted as proof of the existence of malingering among workers covered by workmen's compensation but rather as proof that many complex factors are responsible for disablement. The group of secondary disabilities commonly found in cases of Hansen's disease has received intensive epidemiological study,[70, 96] perhaps because the nature of the illness requires that a large number of epidemiologists be engaged in control of the disease.

An epidemiological analysis of secondary disability reveals certain characteristics in the causative factors. Elderly people and those who have had a primary disability for an extended period are more susceptible to a secondary disability. Further, when the disease or condition causing the primary disability is accompanied by pain or spasticity, the prevalence of secondary disability increases. The frequency of flexion contracture in the hip joint of above-knee amputees or the multiple contractures in rheumatoid arthritis or multiple sclerosis are examples of these. On the other hand, if the original disease diminishes skin sensation, particularly pain or temperature, the patient is also predisposed to the secondary disability. Decubiti in paraplegics, plantar ulcers in patients with diabetes, and plantar ulcers and absorption of fingers in patients with Hansen's disease are representative. When nutrition is poor, certain disabilities such as decubiti are more easily developed. Socioeconomical and vocational factors may have indirect relationship to the causation of secondary disability. The level of intelligence, often related to cultural and educational background, and individual motivation are other indirect causative factors.

The environmental factor involved in the development of secondary disability is simply the position of the body itself. The idea of considering body position as an environmental factor may be unorthodox. However, positioning of either hemiplegic extremities or the stump after an amputation is external to the host and thus constitutes a contrived manmade environment. Negligence or ignorance on the part of paramedical personnel or family members results in placing the disabled in positions that foster secondary disability. Certain body positions that involve maintaining a particular position for a prolonged period may well prevent one disability but inadvertently cause another. Placing elderly patients with above-knee amputations or fractured hips on wheelchairs during the day is an effective measure to prevent pneumonia but tends to result in flexion contracture of the hip joint.

Another important factor affecting the "environmental body" is the condition of the objects with which it has direct contact. Materials that are rough surfaced, rigid, and minimally ventilated also predispose the host to secondary disability.

The most intriguing part in epidemiological observation of secondary disability is identification of the agent. The agent is sometimes mechanical force, which may be either excessive or totally absent. Excessive and concentrated force to the skin area may result in decubitus, and the absence of force may cause demineralization of bone or disuse atrophy of muscle. At times this force may simply be the natural presence of gravity. Equinus deformity in flaccid footdrop and subluxation of the shoulder joint in hemiplegics are some examples of secondary disability related to gravity. The concept of the natural history of secondary disability specifies that the three causative factors (agent, host, and environment) must interact frequently or for a prolonged period. The time element is perhaps the key to the occurrence of disability stimuli.

The characteristics of secondary disability in the period of pathogenesis are always insidious and the symptoms are nonspecific, regardless of the primary disability and its causative disease or condition. The process is always progressive and if not checked can at some point become irreversible. The secondary disability is usually painless but may sometimes be fatal if allowed to develop to the ultimate. The most usual result is a severe curtailment of function. There seems to be little seasonal variation and there is no known immunity to this condition.

Immobilization

One universally recognized condition that severely damages the disabled is immobilization. According to the United States Public Health Service, disability due to immobilization was one of 10 leading preventable health problems in 1960. Merely by utilization of present knowledge, such disability in the United States could be reduced by 50 to 75 per cent.[78] Correlation between the amount of damage from immobilization and the duration of the immobilization is a controversial subject.[72, 88] In general, the greater the size of the body segment and the longer the period of immobilization, the greater the intensity of the pathological condition and the number of organ systems that become involved.

The discussion of the agent factor provides the basis for understanding the mechanism of immobilization as one of the causes of secondary disability. Undoubtedly, immobilization is associated with the absence of mechanical force, the one stimulus so essential to maintenance of proper body function. Osteoporosis, the loss of bone density, is the most commonly known pathological change due to immobilization. This change is often detected in patients after a long-term plaster cast immobilization and is also found in the lower extremities of paraplegics. If the absence of force as a stimulus is the agent factor for osteoporosis, then it should be possible to produce this pathological condition in normal individuals in a simulated environment. This hypothesis was proved correct by the distinct decrease in bone density and increase in calcium excretion in the astronauts during the 14-day Gemini VII voyage.[61, 105]

Many experimental immobilizations have revealed similar results. Mechanical stress, such as is produced by weight-bearing and muscle tension, is necessary for maintenance of the normal skeletal mass. During prolonged bed rest or extended conditions of zero gravity, the static stress distribution and its metabolic requirements are altered. The absence of normal mechanical stress on the skeletal system removes some of the stimuli necessary to bone formation.[47] Moreover, previously discussed causative factors of secondary disablement are also applicable to immobilization. The deleterious effect of immobilization cannot be considered a primary disability.

Every pathophysiological change starts its development at the onset of immobilization, just as the aging processes begin at birth. It is interesting to review the literature that seeks to establish the exact point wherein these changes become recognizable. The cardiac rate at rest increases approximately 0.5 beat per minute per each day of immobilization, and the loss of muscle tone resulting from complete disuse is estimated to be 10 to 15 per cent of strength per week.[99] After a few days of immobilization, an increase in bone blood flow was detected by means of radioactive strontium uptake and it was suggested that this may favor bone atrophy.[87] Similarly, within six to ten days following immobilization, the nitrogen balance of healthy male subjects reverses to a negative balance.[20] Significantly, the tendon capillary bed decreases after a six-week period of immobilization, but nothing of significance was observed in the muscle capillary bed. Because of this finding it is advisable to mobilize the recently repaired or reconstructed tendon as soon as possible, consistent with the limits of healing tensile strength.[83]

Events resulting in immobilization may be classified in various ways. Inadvertent and therapeutic immobilizations[44] are probably the most inclusive classifications. Bed rest and confinement to chair or wheelchair belong to the former category. Posttraumatic or postsurgical states, acute infection or inflammation, and the convalescent period from nonsurgical ailments, for example, constitute the latter category. In either group, immobilization is artificially forced upon the patients. On the other hand, there may also occur unavoidable immobilization, such as is caused by severe pain, neuromuscular impairment, or psychiatric illness. Irrespective of the reason, the pathophysiological changes and clinical symptoms of immobilization are nonspecific.

These changes and symptoms continue progressively throughout the immobilization, and reversal is not always spontaneous upon termination of the restriction. Even if the changes are reversible, the period of recovery from these effects is much longer than the period of immobilization. An experiment determined that young healthy men confined in bed for three weeks need five weeks after resumption of normal activity to regain normal cardiovascular response to the upright position.[99] It is conceivable that those who have deteriorated physically, particularly the elderly, need a longer recovery period. Besides the time element, the cost in manpower and money required for restoration is enormous. Pathological changes of immobilization superimposed upon the primary disability often create totally dependent persons out of patients who initially would have been self-sufficient. This can be devastating to the families

MASAYOSHI ITOH AND MATHEW H. M. LEE

and the socioeconomical well-being of a community. Since total immunization against the ill effects of immobilization has not been developed, simulation of mechanical stimuli to the human body during immobilization is the most effective preventive measure.

Primary Disability—Past, Present, and Future

Incidence and type of primary disabilities are often a reflection of contemporary technology and the political and social cultures of the society in which the population at risk resides.

For thousands of years the simple societies of our ancestors presented few risks to life and limb. In one century we have enriched our lives through technology and we have also increased our risks a thousand-fold. The endless drive for more speed, more products, and more power has created more comfort, more leisure, and more problems.

In a primitive society, a person depends solely on his or her two legs for locomotion. Thus, paraplegia due to locomotive activity in such a society is most likely caused either by a falling object or by the person's falling. Since the development of the wheel, there has been continuous evolution in locomotive devices for comfort, convenience, and efficiency. Thus, invention of the internal combustion engine produced the automobile. As the automobile became larger, heavier, and faster, a vast network of highway systems became a part of American life. The net result was drastic increases in highway accidents, which often resulted in fatalities or left the survivors with severe disabilities. We cannot go back in time and abolish the wheel, because the quadriplegic who was a victim of wheels and technology regains his mobility by using a motorized wheelchair, which is also a product of wheels and technology.

Major political decisions are seldom made on the basis of humanity or health. However, the Federal Government reduced the speed limit on highways to 55 miles per hour to decrease fuel consumption. Inadvertently, this economical decision dramatically decreased the incidence of highway accidents. In addition, future automobiles are expected to be equipped with less powerful engines, again a measure to save fuel. Since these engines will be unable to attain high speeds, we can hope for further reduction in the number of serious accidents. In 1986, again for political reasons, the U.S. Congress raised the speed limit on rural sections of highway to 65 miles per hour, the final decision resting with each state. An increase in highway mortality and morbidity can be expected.

Almost daily a new machine replaces some type of skilled or unskilled labor. The skilled and educated are usually able to adapt to other occupations. The unskilled and undereducated add to the ever-increasing group of chronically unemployed. Many others learn to live by their wits, sometimes within the law and sometimes not.

An observation at a municipal hospital in New York City shows that two decades ago the major causes of traumatic paraplegia and quadriplegia were automobiles, falling, and industrial and swimming accidents. The current most common cause is the gunshot wound.[55] The circumstances that lead to this injury are often obscured, but they are usually related to some kind of illegal activity, particularly drugs.

However, the drug problem is not confined to the impoverished ghetto. Middle and upper income communities complain of drugs in their schools. Colleges report greater usage on their campuses, and physicians acknowledge an increase in rhinoplasty due to a growing number of wealthy cocaine addicts. Cerebral anoxia due to overdose is commonly seen in hospital emergency rooms everywhere in this country.

Mental health has long been involved in treatment of addiction, and rehabilitation medicine has treated the victims of drug-related accidents and violence. However, if the prevalence of drug addiction persists, we can expect myriad physical disabilities in these addicts if they live to reach middle age.

Technology and culture are constantly changing for better or for worse. These changes directly or indirectly influence morbidity. Whereas some disabilities that were prevalent in the past become nonexistent, disabilities due to new causes emerge. Examples of the former are disabilities caused by infections such as poliomyelitis or gonorrhea. Some examples of the latter have already been discussed. Trauma to upper and lower extremities due to skateboarding and severe injuries due to snowmobile accidents are new types of injury.

A spinal cord injury at the level of C2, C3 has been considered a fatal injury. However, improvement of emergency medical services and new medical and surgical techniques[3, 12] are now able to save these patients and keep them alive with the aid of a respirator. If this trend continues, an increase in the number of high quadriplegics must be expected.

The cumulative effects of low dosage but frequent and/or prolonged exposure to an agent are insidious. Noise notch, a hearing deficit at a specific frequency of sound, has been known as an occupational disability. Thus, noise control in work environments and mandatory use of earmuffs and plugs in certain occupations are a part of occupational safety measures. Ultraloud music in the discotheque and blasting hard rock music on radios and record players are part of today's youth culture. It is reasonable to assume that this will create noise notch in many of these young people.

Jogging has become very popular among all age groups in the United States in the past few years. This activity may be of benefit to cardiopulmonary function,[100] but a sedentary middle-age person may injure various organ systems[22, 65] by daily jogging on paved streets or by starting this sport without sufficient preparation. Disorders of the nipples of the breasts due to jogging have already been reported.[57, 69]

High-heel shoes are known to cause various foot disorders in women. Recent fashion promotes high-heel shoes and cowboy boots for men. The high-heel shoe simply adds one or more inches to the regular broad heel of a man's shoe. The cowboy boot, however, has a slanted narrow high heel and sharply pointed toe. Originally custom-made and fitted to the wearer by a skilled boot-maker, it was designed to hook into the stirrups of a saddle and to maintain a foothold on unpaved ground. Today, thousands of young men wear a mass-produced variety on city sidewalks instead of regular shoes. It is hard to believe that men are immune to foot disorders, and we can expect to see men with the same foot problems that have heretofore been confined to women.

Contraceptive devices and pills are effective tools for population control programs that are fundamentally socioeconomical and ecological measures. Today their widespread use in industrialized countries has created the potential for an increase in disability among young women. It is well known that intrauterine devices can penetrate the uterine wall and cause catastrophic infections, whereas the pill appears relatively harmless. But now when a young woman is brought into an emergency room with symptoms of cerebral vascular accident, we suspect rupture of congenital aneurysm, embolism due to rheumatic heart disease, or prolonged intake of contraceptive pills.[19, 45]

Some say the use or misuse of population control tools and the moral implications are not within the province of medicine. Wherever the life and health of the population is involved, all the questions that arise should be our concern. We know that the health and survival of the individual are related to the total population that this earth can support. Medicine concerned with the future health and survival of the people cannot ignore any phase of any effort to preserve earth so that it can continue to nurture the human race.

We must be concerned with earth and its population, with rehabilitation of that which has been destroyed or contaminated, and with prevention of future destruction and contamination that maims people and deforms infants, whether by nuclear war or other means. We must contribute our expertise to every dialogue and every plan to preserve the health of people and earth for future generations. We cannot limit ourselves to rehabilitation of the victims of manmade disabilities and disasters. We must also use our expertise to prevent their occurrence.

A history is taken from the patient in order to make a diagnosis and prognosis. Our future patients are living their history today. If we are alert to what is happening in their and our world, we can often predict future outcomes. We need to anticipate and be prepared to cope with the disabilities of the future and prevent those that can be prevented. It is reasonable to assume that new causes of disability that cannot be imagined today will be identified in the decades to come, and we must develop our science to meet that challenge.

Preventive Rehabilitation

All clinical specialties focus their interest and effort toward restoration of health from the state of Overt Illness to Optimum Health. In this sense, if the definition of rehabilitation is accepted, all clinicians practice "the act of rehabilitation."[43] Care provided through rehabilitation medicine consists of restoration of function and prevention of disability. Diverse therapeutic exercises are instrumental in anatomical and physiological restoration of function. Although this type of physical rehabilitation is ideal, the outcome depends heavily on natural recovery from the lesion responsible for the disability, and this goal is not always attainable. When anatomical and physiological restoration has failed, a compensatory body mechanism or an orthotic or prosthetic device substitutes for the lost function. Although the goals of nursing and physical and occupational therapy are primarily directed toward complete restoration or func-

MASAYOSHI ITOH AND MATHEW H. M. LEE

tional substitution, in actuality this may mean that they predominantly engage in prevention of secondary disability. As the greater portion of the time and energy of rehabilitation professionals is devoted, intentionally or unintentionally, to prevention of secondary disability, rehabilitation medicine should certainly become more emphatically involved in the epidemiological approach and its application to preventive measures.

The term "Preventive Rehabilitation" has been introduced in response to this need.[41, 43, 46] Until the mid-20th century, the stigmatizing deformities commonly seen in patients with Hansen's disease were believed to be primary disabilities. Careful and painstaking clinical investigation and epidemiological analysis revealed the natural history of these disabilities: they are secondary disabilities caused by trauma and infection. They result from the neglect and ignorance of both patients and medical professionals. Modifications in activities of daily living, simple self-administered daily exercise, early case finding, and regular, adequate specific chemotherapy can prevent these disabilities. Heretofore, the only alternative was reconstruction by skilled plastic surgery after these disabilities had become irreversible. "Preventive Rehabilitation" became a component of conventional rehabilitation in leprosy-control programs.[71]

In recent years epidemiologists have become progressively involved in the clinical epidemiology of diseases that result in physical disabilities, and clinicians have become increasingly aware of the epidemiological approach to clinical problems. Feinstein[26] characterized clinical epidemiology as being not restricted by type of disease, age, locale, or any particular form of data collection. Clinical epidemiology may be viewed as ecological medicine, social medicine, or community medicine. The concept of health and the model for the natural history of disease were derived from experience in transmissible disease, and they are essential to any analysis of noninfectious diseases or conditions such as disability. The fundamental purpose of epidemiology is the prevention and eradication of diseases and conditions through a better understanding of causation. If complete prevention or total eradication is not possible, containment is the second choice.

In pursuit of the philosophy of Preventive Rehabilitation, medical and paramedical specialists in rehabilitation must develop keen sensitivity to the relationship between social, economical, cultural, and political environment and disability. Recreational use of motorcycles and mopeds is increasing, and unchecked operation of these vehicles may cause primary disability not only to the drivers but also to pedestrians.[6] Motorcycles are becoming a popular mode of transportation among the young population. In many states, drivers are obliged to wear a crash helmet to prevent fatal head injury in an accident. The helmet may decrease fatality but does not necessarily prevent spinal cord injury.

In December 1984, a malfunction in a Union Carbide Corporation pesticide plant in Bhopal, India, accidentally released methyl isocyanate (MIC) gas over an area of 40 square kilometers. The Bhopal Working Group of the American Public Health Association[6b] stated, "The well publicized number of 2500 deaths is conceded by many to be grossly underestimated. Although the real number may never be known, most observers place it between 6000 to 20,000 dead and at least 15,000 injured. An estimated 100,000 to 200,000 people were exposed to a toxic plume of MIC." Many survivors have permanent disabilities, such as respiratory dysfunction and blindness.

In April 1986, an explosion at the Chernobyl nuclear power plant in the U.S.S.R. resulted in 31 deaths and necessitated the semipermanent evacuation of over 135,000 residents from the surrounding communities.[105a] Although the official casualty figures are relatively small, radioactive fallout was observed throughout the entire northern hemisphere. The effects of this increase in atmospheric radioactivity on human health are not immediately measurable, requiring observation for decades to come.

Many industrial accidents that have injured workers in plants have occurred in the past, but extraordinary environmental contamination events such as these, involving a large number of the general population in the surrounding communities, or on a global scale, have never been experienced. Although the great number of deaths caused by these accidents is lamentable, the greater number of those injured and becoming disabled is the lasting catastrophe. In a highly technological and industrialized society, one can speculate that disasters of greater magnitude involving toxic substances will occur. It is now almost certain that these accidents were caused by human error. In order to prevent primary disabilities such as these, the intensification of training of industrial workers and the development of technology that precludes human error are essential.

Various investigators have estimated the cost of care for decubitus ulcers. Calculation of the cost differs from one study to another, and the more recent the study, the higher the cost because the inflationary factor is taken into consideration. Weinstein[103] estimated that a minimum cost for prevention and treatment of the ulcer in the United States was 357 million dollars as of 1970 to 1973. Lee,[54] on the other hand, calculated the total cost of treatment of decubitus ulcers in the United States at a minimum of 883 million dollars in 1977.

Public education is often offered as a method of preventing disability. Instituting educational programs does not necessarily mean that the intended goal is achieved. For example, high-school driver education has not decreased the incidence of fatal automobile accidents.[79] What are needed now are aggressive public relations programs rather than educational programs.

The pioneers of rehabilitation utilized the public relations technique, presenting successfully rehabilitated cases and the economical value of rehabilitation programs in order to justify expenditures for this new specialty. Whereas this campaign was obviously effective, the public began to place too much trust in the capability of the rehabilitation program. People are often careless and take unnecessary risks believing that surgery and rehabilitation can correct any injury or disability. There is a tendency to believe that rehabilitation can work miracles. Glorification of rehabilitation medicine is no longer necessary. Rather, the public must be informed of the not-so-glamorous parts of rehabilitation—the high cost, the plight of the disabled, and the grim statistics of unsuccessful cases. The emphasis of the new public relations campaign must be placed on prevention of primary disability. In doing so, we must learn to reach business, government, economists, legislators, bureaucrats, and the general public.

In this new concept of Preventive Rehabilitation, the scope of expertise and the role of the physiatrist must be enlarged. Prevention of disability does not start at birth or after a primary disability occurs. Disability due to genetic defects or genetic incompatibility can be prevented by means of genetic counseling. The prevention of diseases caused by genetic abnormalities will soon become reality through gene line therapy.[4a] However, the ethical implications of gene therapy must be thoroughly explored prior to the use of such genetic engineering techniques in humans. During the early gestation period, expectant mothers must be protected from rubella and from certain pharmaceutical products. Amniotic fluid analysis may provide vital information pertinent to the discovery of potentially disabling diseases in the newborn. These are measures to prevent primary disability. However, artificial termination of pregnancy to eliminate the fetus with suspected deformities should not be considered as prevention of primary disability. The justification for advocating artificial abortion in these cases is preponderantly psychosocial and economical, not medical. Cerebral palsy due to intracranial damage in a high forceps delivery should concern the physiatrist as much as it involves the obstetrician. Although modern health care provides many deterrents to primary disability (Fig. 10–3), prevention has mainly involved public health specialists and allied health professionals but not the physiatrist.

Current population growth, particularly a rapid increase of the aged, predicts a sharp rise in our disabled population in the near future. It is well documented that there is a great shortage of medical and paramedical professionals to care for the disabled, and we cannot even meet present demands.

In recent years, specialists in neurology, orthopedic surgery, and pediatrics are increasingly involved and have a vital role in the field of rehabilitation medicine. This phenomenon should not be interpreted as an invasion of the field by other specialists, but rather it signifies recognition of the importance of rehabilitation medicine. The additional expertise of specialists in public health and preventive medicine is also a welcome contribution to the further enrichment of rehabilitation medicine.

Unless more effective methods of specific prevention are developed to protect the population from primary disability in the future, the newly disabled will face a critical situation. The cumulative shortage of health manpower will cause them to be without benefit of rehabilitation services, and superimposed secondary disabilities will render them totally dependent. This will result not only in insurmountable personal tragedy, but will create infinite economical problems for families, communities, and nations.

Exploration into the epidemiology of disability, the causative factors, the natural history of secondary disability, the epidemiology of immobilization, and the importance of functional diagnosis exposes the urgency for a reassessment of rehabilitation medicine. Our professionals, medical and paramedical, have played rather passive roles in clinical medicine and comprehensive health care.*

---

*Comprehensive health care is defined as care that is provided to patients according to their needs in appropriate, continuous, and dynamic patterns.[23]

MASAYOSHI ITOH AND MATHEW H. M. LEE

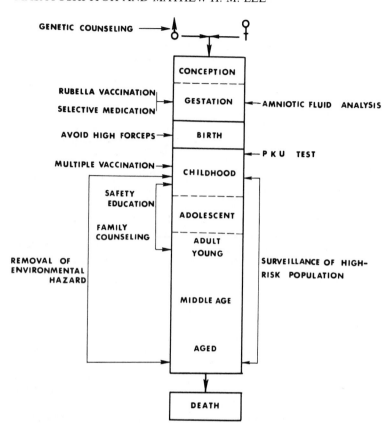

FIGURE 10–3. Prevention of primary disability in the life of a person. Items on the left side of the column indicate specific protection against primary disability. Measures on the right side are for early detection and probable prevention of potential primary disability.

Although rehabilitation medicine has pioneered in vocational and legislative areas and contributed immeasurably to the welfare of the handicapped, it has not played the same spectacular role in the delivery of health care. Further, we need to focus our attention on research, health planning, and health education. Laymen, through the efforts of rehabilitation medicine, are now sensitive to and aware of the social and vocational needs of the disabled, and many laymen are now capable of furthering the principles that we initiated. It is now time for the science-oriented medical rehabilitation community to develop and promote its more scientific aspects, to explore every phase of disability and disability prevention, and to contribute epidemiological investigation that will make it possible for those engaged in rehabilitation to prevent epidemics of disability in much the same manner that we are now able to prevent communicable disease.

References

1. Abramson, J. H., Mann, K. J., Nizan, A., and Goldberg, R.: Epidemiology of disability after work injuries. Arch. Environ. Health, 9:572–580, 1964.
2. Alba, A., Trainor, F. S., Ritter, W., and Dacso, M. M.: A clinical disability rating for Parkinson patients. J. Chron. Dis., 21:507–522, 1968.
3. Albin, M. S.: Resuscitation of spinal cord. Crit. Care Med., 6:270–276, 1978.
4. American Public Health Association: Report after Love Canal—Thousand areas are potential hazard. Nation's Health, 8:1–6, 1978.
4a. Anderson, W. F.: Human gene therapy: Scientific and ethical considerations. Recomb. DNA Tech. Bull., 8:55–62, 1985.
5. Askergreen, A., and Szamosi, A.: Relation between radiological pleuropulmonary changes, clinical history and weight index of construction workers. Scand. J. Work Environ. Health, 4:179–183, 1978.
6. Balcerak, J. C., Pancione, K. L., and States, J. D.: Moped, minibike and motorcycle accidents. Associated injury problems. N.Y. State J. Med., 78:628–633, 1978.
6a. Banhuys, A., Schoenberg, J. B., Beck, G. J., and Schilling, R. S. F.: Epidemiology of chronic lung disease in a cotton mill community. Lung, 154:167–186, 1977.
6b. Bhopal Working Group: The public health implications of the Bhopal Disaster. Report to the

Program Development Board, American Public Health Association. Am. J. Public Health, 77:230–236, 1987.

7. Boyd, H. B., and George, I. L.: Fracture of the hip. Result following treatment. J.A.M.A., 137:1196–1199, 1948.

8. Brown, M. E.: Daily activity inventory and progress record for those with atypical movement. I. Am. J. Occup. Ther., 4:195–204, 1950.

9. Brown, M. H.: Love Canal, U.S.A. New York Times Magazine, pp. 23, 38, 41–44, 21 Jan., 1979.

10. Bruett, T. L., and Overs, R. P.: A critical review of 12 ADL scales. Phys. Ther., 49:857–862, 1969.

11. Buchwald, E.: Physical Rehabilitation for Daily Living. New York, McGraw-Hill Book Company, 1952.

12. Burke, D. C.: Early management of spinal cord injury. Med. J. Aust., 1:145–148, 1978.

13. Burns, R. M.: Rating of industrial disabilities. Lancet, 58:17–20, 1939.

14. Carbone, A.: Agonist-antagonist theory: New pain killer. Hosp. Formulary, 13:877–881, 1978.

15. Carroll, D.: The disability in hemiplegia caused by cerebrovascular disease. J. Chron. Dis., 15:179–188, 1962.

16. Carson, R.: Silent Spring. Boston, Houghton Mifflin Company, 1962.

17. Carter, R. M.: Estimation of disability. Industr. Med., 8:52–54, 1939.

18. Clark, E. G.: The epidemiological approach and contribution to preventive medicine. In Leavell, H. R., and Clark, E. G. (Eds.): Preventive Medicine for the Doctor in His Community. New York, McGraw-Hill Book Company, 1965.

19. Collaborative Group for Study of Stroke in Young Women: Oral contraception and increased risk of cerebral ischemia or thrombosis. N. Engl. J. Med., 288:871–878, 1973.

20. Deitrick, J. E., Whedon, G. D., and Shorr, E.: Effects of immobilization upon various metabolic and physiologic functions of normal men. Am. J. Med., 4:3–32, 1948.

21. Dennerstein, A. S., Lowenthal, M., and Dexter, M.: Evaluation of a rating scale of ability in activities of daily living. Arch. Phys. Med., 46:579–584, 1965.

22. Deutsch, M. E.: More on jogger's ailment. N. Engl. J. Med., 298:405, 1978.

23. Division of Chronic Disease, Public Health Service: The concept of comprehensive care. In Lilienfeld, A. M., and Gifford, A. J. (Eds.): Chronic Disease and Public Health. Baltimore, Johns Hopkins Press, 1966.

24. Division of Epidemiology, Columbia University, School of Public Health and Administrative Medicine: Principles, Methods and Uses of Epidemiology. New York, 1965.

25. Dristine, M. J.: Disability evaluation. Principles of quantitative diagnosis. Northwest Med., 61:1041–1042, 1962.

26. Feinstein, A. R.: Clinical epidemiology. I. The populational experiments of nature and of man in human illness. Ann. Intern. Med., 69:807–820, 1968.

27. Fowler, C. H., and DePuy, W. H.: Home and Health and Home Economics. New York, Phillips and Hunt, 1880.

28. Fracastoro, G.: De contagione et contagiosis morbis et eorum cruratine, Libri III. Translated and notes by Wilmer Cave Wright. New York, G. P. Putnam's Sons, 1930.

29. Fukuji, M.: Studies of the causative agent of Minamata disease, especially on the accumulation of the mercury compound in the fish and shellfish of Minamata Bay. J. Kumamoto Med. Soc., 37:494–521, 1963.

30. Goldberger, J., Wheeler, G. A., and Sydenstricker, W.: A study of the relation of diet to pellagra incidence in seven textile-mill communities of South Carolina in 1916. Public Health Rep., 35:648–713, 1920.

31. Goodwin, W. M.: Meaning of functional disabilities. Int. J. Surg., 37:540–548, 1924.

32. Gorden, E. E., and Kohn, K. H.: Evaluation of rehabilitation methods in the hemiplegic patient. J. Chron. Dis., 19:3–16, 1966.

33. Gordon, B. L.: Medieval and Renaissance Medicine. Chapter XXII. New York, Philosophical Library, Inc., 1959.

34. Gordon, J. E., and LeRiche, H.: The epidemiologic method applied to nutrition. Am. J. Med. Sci., 219:312–345, 1950.

35. Greenseid, D. Z., and McCormack, R. M.: Functional hand testing. A profile evaluation. Plast. Reconstr. Surg., 42:567–571, 1968.

36. Hammond, E. C., Selikoff, I. J., and Churg, J.: Neoplasia among insulation workers in USA with special reference to intra-abdominal neoplasia. Ann. N.Y. Acad. Sci., 132:519–525, 1965.

37. Hoberman, M., Cicenia, E. F., and Stephenson, G. R.: Daily activity testing in physical therapy and rehabilitation. Arch. Phys. Med., 33:99–108, 1952.

38. Hoff, W. I., and Mead, S.: Evaluation of rehabilitation outcome. An objective assessment of the physically disabled. Am. J. Phys. Med., 44:113–121, 1965.

39. Huddleston, O. L., Moore, R. W., Rubin, D., Humphrey, T. L., Campbell, J. W., and Balanchetter, R.: Evaluation of physical disabilities by means of patient profile chart. Arch. Phys. Med., 42:250–257, 1961.

39a. Ibrahim, M. A.: Epidemiology and Health Policy. Rockville, MD, Aspen Systems Corp., 1985, p. 15.

40. Ingles, T.: St. Christopher's Hospice. Nursing Outlook, 22:759–763, 1974.

41. Itoh, M.: Preventive rehabilitation for leprosy—A new approach to an old problem. Rehab. Rev., 19:13–14, 1968.

42. Itoh, M., and Dacso, M. M.: Rehabilitation of

MASAYOSHI ITOH AND MATHEW H. M. LEE

patients with hip fracture. A clinical study of 126 cases. Postgrad. Med., 28:134–139, 1960.

43. Itoh, M., and Lee, M. H.: The future role of rehabilitation medicine in community health. Med. Clin. North Am., 53:719–733, 1969.

44. Jebsen, R. H.: Therapeutic exercise in motion problems. I. Northwest Med., 65:742–747, 1966.

45. Jick, H., Porter, J., and Rothman, J.: Oral contraceptives and non-fatal stroke in healthy young women. Ann. Intern. Med., 89:58–60, 1978.

46. Karat, S.: Preventive rehabilitation in leprosy. Leprosy Rev., 39:39–44, 1968.

47. Kazasian, L. E., and Von Gierker, H. E.: Bone loss as a result of immobilization and chelation. Preliminary results in *Macaca mulatta*. Clin. Orthop., 65:67–75, 1969.

48. Kelman, H. R., and Muller, J. N.: Rehabilitation of nursing home residents. Geriatrics, 17:402–411, 1962.

49. Knapp, M. E.: Disability evaluation. I. Postgrad. Med., 46:184–186, 1969.

50. Knapp, M. E.: Disability evaluation. 2. Postgrad. Med., 46:201–203, 1969.

51. Krusen, E. M.: Rehabilitation of the elderly. South. Med. J., 51:225–228, 1958.

52. Lawton, E. B.: Activities of daily living: Testing, training and equipment. New York, Institute of Physical Medicine and Rehabilitation. New York University Bellevue Medical Center, Monograph No. 10, 1956.

53. Leavell, H. R., and Clark, E. G.: Levels of application of preventive medicine. *In* Leavell, H. R., and Clark, E. G. (Eds.): Preventive Medicine for the Doctor in His Community. New York, McGraw-Hill Book Company, 1965.

54. Lee, M.: The decubitus ulcer patient—Statement of the problem. Presented at the Conference on Current Trends in the Care and Treatment of Decubitus Ulcer. Goldwater Memorial Hospital, New York, Oct. 4, 1977.

55. Lee, M. H., Novey, J., and Rusk, H. A.: An experiment in the care and rehabilitation of severely disabled young adults in a long term hospital. Paper presented at Amer. Cong. Rehab. Med., Nov., 1978. Also appeared in RT-1 Report 1978, New York Univ. Med. Center.

56. Lerner, J.: Disability evaluation in psychiatric illness and the concept of hysteria. Can. Psychiatr. Assoc. J., 11:350–355, 1966.

57. Levit, F.: Jogger's nipples. N. Engl. J. Med., 297:1127, 1977.

58. Liegner, L. M.: St. Christopher's Hospice, 1974. Care of dying patient. J.A.M.A., 234:1047–1048, 1975.

59. Lilienfeld, B. E.: Epidemiologic methods and inferences. *In* Hilleboe, H. E., and Larimore, G. W. (Eds.): Preventive Medicine. Philadelphia, W. B. Saunders Company, 1965.

60. Linn, M. W.: A rapid disability rating scale. J. Am. Geriatr. Soc., 15:211–214, 1967.

61. Lutwak, L.: Chemical analysis of diet. Urine, feces and sweat parameters relating to the calcium and nitrogen balance studies during Gemini VII flight (Exp. M7). NASA Contractor Report, NAS 9–5375, 1966.

62. Lysman, A. G.: Drug therapy in terminally ill patients. Am. J. Hosp. Pharm., 32:270–276, 1975.

63. Mahoney, F. I., Wood, O. H., and Barthel, D. W.: Rehabilitation of chronically ill patients. Influence of complication of chronically ill patients. South. Med. J., 51:605–609, 1958.

64. Mann, K. J., Abramson, J. H., Nizan, A., and Goldberg, R.: Epidemiology of disabling work injuries in Israel. Arch. Environ. Health (Chicago), 9:505–513, 1964.

65. Massey, E. W., and Pleet, A. B.: Neuropathy in joggers. Am. J. Sports Med., 6:209–211, 1978.

66. McBride, E. D.: Disability evaluation—Principles of treatment of compensable injuries, 4th Ed. Philadelphia, J. B. Lippincott Company, 1942.

67. Milby, T. H.: Pneumoconioses. *In* Occupational Diseases, A Guide to Their Recognition. Washington, DC, U.S. Dept. of Health, Education and Welfare, Public Health Service. Public Health Service Publication No. 1097, 1964, Section V.

68. Moskowitz, E., and McCann, C. B.: Classification of disability in chronically ill and aging. J. Chron. Dis., 5:342–346, 1957.

69. Nequin, N. D.: More on jogger's ailment. N. Engl. J. Med., 298:405–406, 1978.

70. Noordeen, S. K., and Srinivasan, H.: Epidemiology of disability in leprosy. I. A general study of disability among male patients above fifteen years of age. Int. J. Leprosy, 34:159–169, 1966.

71. Pan American Health Organization: Consolidated Report on Item III, Determination of Objectives and Preparation of Timetables, 1968.

72. Patel, A. N.: Disuse atrophy of human skeletal muscles. Arch. Neurol., 20:413–421, 1969.

73. Paul, J. R.: Clinical Epidemiology. Chicago, The University of Chicago Press, 1966.

74. Pederson, E.: A rating system for neurological impairment in multiple sclerosis. Acta Neurol. Scand., 41[Suppl. 13]:557–558, 1965.

75. Plant, J.: Finding a home for hospice care in the United States. Hospitals, 51:53, 55, 57–58, 1977.

76. Pool, D. A., and Brown, R. A.: A functional rating scale for research in physical therapy. Texas Rep. Biol. Med., 26:133–136, 1968.

77. Price, L.: Medical disability standards. J. Occup. Med., 8:542–547, 1966.

78. Public Health Service: Public Health Service Hearing before the House Subcommittee on Appropriations, Eighty-sixth Congress, Second Session, 1960, pp. 1205–1212.

79. Robertson, L. S., and Zador, P. L.: Driver education and fatal crash involvement of teenaged drivers. Am. J. Public Health, 68:959–965, 1978.

80. Robey, L. R.: Intertrochanteric and subtrochan-

teric fracture of the femur in the Negro. J. Bone Joint Surg., 38A:1301–1312, 1956.

81. Rogers, E. S.: Human Ecology and Health. Introduction for Administrators. New York, Macmillan Company, 1960.

82. Rosen, G.: A History of Public Health. New York, MD Publications, 1958.

83. Rothman, R. H., and Slogoff, S.: The effect of immobilization on the vascular bed of tendon. Surg. Gynecol. Obstet., 124:1064–1066, 1967.

84. Rusk, H. A., and Hilleboe, H. E.: Rehabilitation. In Hilleboe, H. E., and Larimore, G. W. (Eds.): Preventive Medicine. Philadelphia, W. B. Saunders Company, 1965.

85. Ryder, C. F., and Daitz, B.: Prevention of disability. In Selle, W. A. (Ed.): Restorative Medicine in Geriatrics. Springfield, Illinois, Charles C Thomas, Publisher, 1963.

86. Schoening, H. A., and Iverson, I. A.: The Kenny Selfcare Evaluation: A Numerical Measure of Independence in Activity of Daily Living. Minneapolis, Kenny Rehabilitation Institute, 1965.

87. Semb, H.: Effect of immobilization on bone blood flow estimated by initial uptake of radioactive strontium. Surg. Gynecol. Obstet., 127:275–281, 1968.

88. Sevitt, S., and Gallagher, N.: Venous thrombosis and pulmonary embolism. Br. J. Surg., 48:475–489, 1961.

89. Smillie, W. G.: Preventive Medicine and Public Health. Chapter 18. New York, Macmillan Company, 1952.

90. Snyder, H.: Opiate receptors and internal opiates. Sci. Am., 236:43–56, 1977.

91. Snyder, H.: The opiate receptor and morphine-like peptides in the brain. Am. J. Psychiatry, 135:645–652, 1978.

92. Sokolow, J., and Taylor, E. J.: Report of a national field trial of a method for functional disability evaluation. J. Chron. Dis., 20:896–909, 1967.

93. Sokolow, J., Silson, J., Taylor, E. J., Anderson, E. T., and Rusk, H. A.: A method for the functional evaluation of disability. Arch. Phys. Med. Rehabil., 40:421–428, 1959.

94. Solomon, M., Itoh, M., Clarke, C. P., and Goldstein, J. M.: Telemetric electrocardiogram as a tool for dynamic cardiac evaluation in physical therapy. Arch. Phys. Med. Rehabil., 15:730, 1970.

95. Spencer, W. A., and Vallbona, C.: A preliminary report on the use of electronic data processing technics in the description and evaluation of disability. Arch. Phys. Med., 43:22–35, 1962.

96. Srinivasan, H., and Noordeen, S. K.: Epidemiology of disability in leprosy. Int. J. Leprosy, 34:170–174, 1966.

97. Stinson, M.: Medical care and rehabilitation of the aged. Geriatrics, 8:266–299, 1953.

98. Stoddard, S.: The Hospice Movement. A Better Way of Caring for the Dying. New York, Random House, 1978.

99. Taylor, H. L., Henschel, A., Brozek, J., and Key, A.: Effects of bedrest on cardiovascular function and work performance. J. Appl. Physiol., 2:223–239, 1949.

100. Vaisrub, S.: Joyful jogging (editorial). J.A.M.A., 240:1385, 1978.

101. Van Demark, E. G., and Van Demark, R. E.: Hip nailing in patients of eighty years or older. Am. J. Surg., 85:664–668, 1953.

102. Vorwald, A. J., Robin, E. D., Gordon, B. L., Moteley, L., and Noonan, T. B.: Evaluation of disability. Arch. Environ. Health, 8:889–897, 1964.

103. Weinstein, B.: The cost of decubitus ulcer. A statistical approximation (mimeographed report). Personal communication. Rehab. Unit, University of Rochester, New York.

104. Welch, W. H.: Institute of hygiene. In Rockefeller Foundation Annual Report. New York, 1916, pp. 415–427.

105. Whedon, C. D., Lutwak, L., and Neuman, W.: Calcium and Nitrogen Balance. In a review of medical results of Gemini VII and related flights. J. F. Kennedy Space Center, Florida, NASA SP–121, 1967.

105a. Wilson, R.: A visit to Chernobyl. Science, 239:1636–1640, 1987.

106. World Health Organization: Constitution of the World Health Organization. Geneva, World Health Organization, 1964.

107. World Health Organization: Manual of the International Statistical Classification of Diseases, Injuries and Causes of Death. 1965 Revision, Vol. 1. Geneva, World Health Organization, 1967.

108. World Health Organization: Classification of disabilities resulting from leprosy, for use in control program. Bull. W.H.O., 40:609–612, 1969.

109. Wylie, C. M.: Administrative research in the rehabilitation of stroke patient. Rehab. Lit., 25:2–7, 1964.

110. Wylie, C. M., and White, B. K.: A measure of disability. Arch. Environ. Health, 8:834–839, 1964.

111. Yamshon, L. T.: Industrial injury. Practical need for evaluation of capacity. J.A.M.A., 165:934–938, 1957.

11

The Neurophysiology of Motor Function

FREDERIC J. KOTTKE

There is a lack of agreement regarding the neurophysiological mechanisms resulting in the organization of motor function in humans.* The differences in interpretation of existing scientific data are profound. For this reason, at the outset it is worth emphasizing that essentially the same data are interpreted quite differently by different authorities depending on each individual's concept of the organization of the nervous system. An overly simplistic summary of the conventional presentation is that voluntary muscular coordination is initiated in the motor cortex and transmitted over uninterrupted axons that cross through the medullary pyramids to synapse on motor neurons in the contralateral anterior horn of the spinal cord and provide a direct connection for control of each of the muscles in the coordination pattern. Most textbooks of physiology imply, even if they do not directly state, that movements originate in a limited region of the cortex or arise there in response to stimuli from other regions of the brain, and that each movement is encoded in the cortex as a pattern of nerve impulses transmitted over the corticospinal tract to the appropriate motor neurons to produce the desired motor pattern.[67] It was even suggested very early that each neuron of the premotor cortex contains a pattern of coordination and that this area of the cortex serves as a keyboard from which appropriate combinations of activities are selected by some unidentified area of the brain to produce the desired coordination[18] (Fig. 11–1).

Another hypothesis is that subcortical structures in the basal ganglia, thalamus, and brain stem ganglia act as the organizers or integrators to combine into coordinated patterns the sensorimotor relationships stored in the cortex.[60] Still others hypothesize that the pyramidal system and the

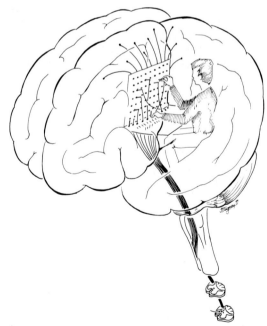

FIGURE 11–1. Coordination is far more complex than selecting and exciting neurons in the motor cortex that have genetically encoded patterns of motor activity. (From Kottke, F. J., Halpern, D., Easton, J. K. M., Ozel, A. T., and Burrill, C. A.: Training of coordination. Arch. Phys. Med. Rehabil., 59:567–572, 1978.)

---

*See references 3, 9, 16, 21, 26, 37, 39, 42, 60, 66, and 67.

extrapyramidal system monitor motor activities in different segments of the extremities, or that the pyramidal tract is responsible for fast actions and the extrapyramidal tract for initiating slow or postural responses.

Likewise there are markedly different concepts regarding the involvement of the reflexes in normal coordination. One concept is that reflexes are residuals of an ancient nervous system and are redundant because of the more direct pathways that have developed from the brain. Another hypothesis is that the reflexes exist in a parallel relationship to motor coordination so that initiation of reflexes can facilitate and amplify the magnitude of the voluntary response.[21, 39] Still another hypothesis, which is the thesis of this chapter, is

that the reflexes form the basic organized pathways in the spinal cord, and regulation from higher centers is accomplished by excitation and inhibition imposed on these reflex pathways[42] (Fig. 11–2). To prevent undesired activity, the higher centers must maintain an inhibitory control over the spinal reflexes. To produce motor activity, the higher centers must release the inhibition or stimulate excitation. Without the millions of sensory impulses entering the central nervous system each instant, the level of irritability of the internuncial neurons and anterior horn cells will not be high enough to allow any excitation from supraspinal motor centers. Over 100 years ago, Hughlings Jackson hypothesized this concept as the application of the theory of evolution to the nervous system.[37] A

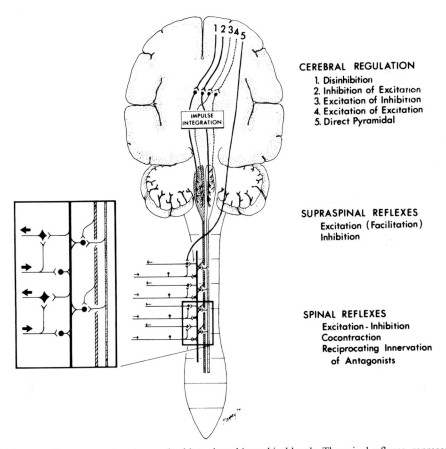

CEREBRAL REGULATION
1. Disinhibition
2. Inhibition of Excitation
3. Excitation of Inhibition
4. Excitation of Excitation
5. Direct Pyramidal

SUPRASPINAL REFLEXES
Excitation (Facilitation)
Inhibition

SPINAL REFLEXES
Excitation - Inhibition
Cocontraction
Reciprocating Innervation
of Antagonists

FIGURE 11–2. The central nervous system is organized into three hierarchical levels. The spinal reflexes, representing the lowest level, have stereotyped pathways in which only the degree of spread of activity varies according to the intensity of excitation and inhibition. The supraspinal reflexes and the reticular facilitatory and inhibitory centers at the middle level act by modifying the spinal reflexes. Cerebral regulation at the highest level also acts through modification of the activities of the lower levels. Cerebral coordination is achieved by activating engrams of facilitation and inhibition transmitted in the extrapyramidal system through the middle and lowest levels. Direct corticospinal control makes variation of the activity of one prime mover at a time possible by localized excitation directly on the lowest level. (Modified from Kottke, F. J.: From reflex to skill: The training of coordination. Arch. Phys. Med. Rehabil., 61:551–561, 1980.)

FREDERIC J. KOTTKE

scientific basis for this hypothesis was laid with the fundamental studies of the spinal and supraspinal reflexes by Sherrington.[64] Subsequent research has added further details. Today this hypothesis appears to provide the best fit for the data developed from the research of many investigators.

Organization of the Spinal Cord

The spinal reflexes are the basic units in the organization of the nervous system. These reflex pathways are activated and maintained by external stimuli, which initiate millions of sensory impulses each instant. There is a continual interaction between the sensory inflow, internuncial excitation through spinal and supraspinal pathways, and motor outflow (Fig. 11–3). These basic sensorimotor

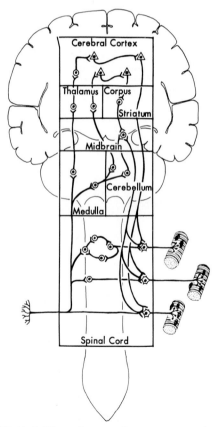

FIGURE 11–3. The entire central nervous system is a sensorimotor system at all levels with all activity driven by sensory excitation. In these schematic diagrams, internuncial neurons of the spinal cord and brain are represented by circles; major cells of the cortices of the cerebrum and cerebellum are represented by pyramids; and anterior horn cells are represented as stellate.

units continue throughout life as the units of neurological function. The effect of the activities of the higher centers is to modify and regulate the activities of the spinal reflexes but not to displace them.

The typical spinal reflex arc consists of a sensory neuron, one or more internuncial neurons, and the motor neuron with an axon and branches to the muscle fibers of the motor unit. The reflex pathway can become increasingly more complex at spinal and supraspinal levels to produce complex rather than simple responses. The greater the number of internuncial neurons in the pathway, the slower will be the spread of excitation through that pathway and the more complex the pathway may become. Since internuncial neurons have many dendritic synapses for excitation and many axonal branches for transmission, recirculation of impulses through an internuncial pool occurs and provides a mechanism for prolonged reexcitation as well as for maintenance of a *high level of activity at all times* in the central nervous system[47] (Fig. 11–4).

This high level of activity is important because each neuron reaches its excitatory threshold only when it is stimulated by a large number of excitatory stimuli. Each neuron has many dendritic synapses, some of which transmit excitatory impulses and others of which transmit inhibitory impulses. The sum of the excitatory impulses must exceed the number of inhibitory impulses sufficiently so that the threshold of excitability of that neuron is exceeded in order for it to discharge an impulse over its axon. When motor neurons are investigated eletrophysiologically, it is found that the intraneuronal potential at rest is approximately 70 mV of negative potential in relation to the extracellular fluid. Each excitatory impulse decreases this negative potential, whereas each inhibitory impulse increases the negative potential (Fig. 11–5). In nature there is a continual flow both of excitatory impulses and of inhibitory impulses to each neuron. When the excitatory impulses exceed the arriving inhibitory impulses so that the intraneuronal negative potential is reduced to the excitatory threshold, which is at about −50 mV, the neuron discharges an impulse. When the threshold is exceeded, there is an abrupt rise of positive charges within the neuron, caused by inflow of sodium ions through the cell membrane. The neuron becomes positively charged to approximately +30 mV, and an impulse is generated that is transmitted over the axon and all of its branches to excite the axonal synaptic endings. Electro-

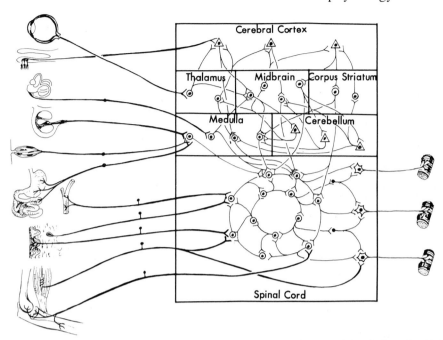

FIGURE 11–4. The many excitatory and inhibitory synapses of neurons create an internuncial pool through which nerve impulses may recirculate repeatedly. Sensory impulses from all types of receptors contribute to the high level of activity of the internuncial pool in proportion to the intensity of excitation. Sensory input is essential to maintain internuncial activity at a continually high level. The primary inhibitory center in the brain stem modulates the activity of internuncial neurons and decreases the excitability of motor neurons in the anterior horn below the discharge threshold so that a few more impulses of reflex or volitional origin are sufficient to excite a motor response.

FIGURE 11–5. A neuron at rest has an intracellular potential of −70 mV in relation to that of the extracellular fluid. Excitatory stimuli reduce this potential; when it falls below the threshold, there is reversal of the intraneuronal potential, and an axonal impulse is generated.

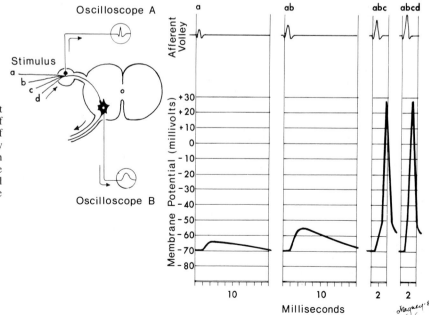

FREDERIC J. KOTTKE

physiologically, therefore, the level of activity of each neuron in the neuron pool can be described in terms of positive and negative charges associated with excitation, quiescence, or inhibition of that neuron.

There are three aspects of neuron inhibition that influence spinal reflexes. Postsynaptic inhibition occurs when an axonal ending makes an inhibitory synapse with the cell membrane of another neuron. Transmission of an impulse across this inhibitory synapse increases the intracellular or postsynaptic negative potential and decreases the excitability of that neuron (Fig. 11–6). Presynaptic inhibition, which occurs in reciprocal excitation-inhibition of spinal reflexes, apparently acts proximal to the synaptic junction on the presynaptic axon terminal, preventing it from discharging to excite the dendritic receptor.[26] This blocking action isolates the neuron from excitation without depression of excitability. Instead, the temporary isolation of the neuron from excitation because of presynaptic inhibition results in increasing membrane instability. Therefore, postsynaptic inhibition decreases the excitability of a neuron, whereas presynaptic inhibition increases the subsequent excitability of that neuron. Recurrent inhibition occurs when an impulse transmitted over an axon spreads through a collateral branch and back through a Renshaw cell to inhibit the excited motor neuron and adjacent motor neurons. Recurrent inhibition is a physiological mechanism that produces self-monitoring inhibition of motor neurons and by doing so limits the maximal rate of discharge. In the same way there can be recurrent inhibition of inhibition to antagonists so that excitation of an impulse in an agonist motor neuron spreads through the recurrent collaterals to block inhibitor impulses to the antagonist.

The net result of the continuous sensory inflow into the central nervous system is the establishment of a very high level of continual activity in the internuncial pool. All excitation of the central nervous system is derived from these external sensory stimuli. No cells have been identified in the central nervous system that can spontaneously generate impulses. Fundamentally, therefore, the entire nervous system is built on and dependent on reflex activity. The background of activity of the internuncial pool, derived from sensory stimuli, raises the level of excitability of the motor neurons, and in the normal central nervous system a mechanism is present through which inhibition is adequate to suppress the level of excitability of each motor neuron below its threshold until that activity

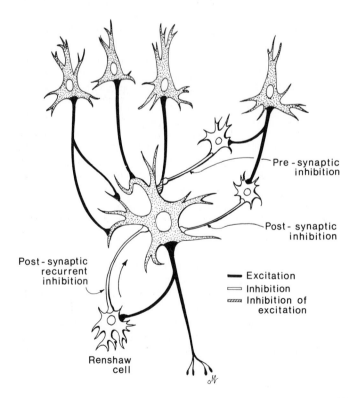

Pre-synaptic inhibition

Post-synaptic inhibition

Post-synaptic recurrent inhibition

━━ Excitation
═══ Inhibition
▨▨▨ Inhibition of excitation

Renshaw cell

FIGURE 11–6. Inhibition is a positive neurophysiological phenomenon. Presynaptic inhibition prevents excitatory impulses from reaching the neuron but does not decrease neuronal excitability. Postsynaptic inhibition increases the internal negative potential of the neuron and decreases neuronal excitability. Recurrent inhibition results after excitation of a motor neuron as impulses are conducted through axon collaterals to the Renshaw cell, which imposes postsynaptic inhibition on the excited motor neuron.

is required. Therefore, although a person may remain motionless, the activity of the nervous system is continually at an extremely high level and needs very little change in excitation in order to generate muscular activity. In conditions such as spinal shock in which the flow of impulses to the internuncial pool is suddenly reduced, excitability of motor neurons soon falls far below the threshold level and the person becomes flaccid and areflexic.

Internuncial circuits are organized unilaterally. They probably are organized in even more restricted arrangements than that, but these have not been successfully identified (Fig. 11–7). As a result of the unilateral organization, however, patients may show unilateral hypotonia or hypertonia. When the activity of the internuncial pool is reduced, a diffuse increase of sensory input is effective to increase the level of excitability.[9] Conversely, if there is excessive stimulation, e.g., nociceptive stimulation from skin irritation such as ulcers, tight shoes, rubbing braces, bladder infections, fractures, or sprains, there is an increase of uncontrolled reflex activity.

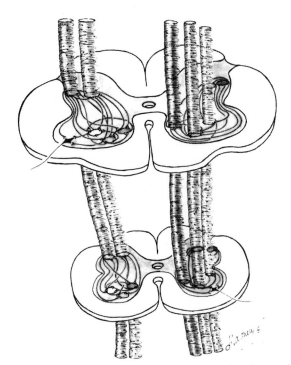

FIGURE 11–7. Internuncial pools in the dorsal and ventral horns of the spinal cord provide preferential reverberating connections between neurons at segmental and intersegmental levels.

The Muscle Spindle

The muscle spindle is an elaborate and complex sensory mechanism[2, 52] (Fig. 11–8). It is composed of two specialized types of muscle fibers enclosed in a fibrous capsule, innervated by two types of sensory fibers and two types of gamma motor neurons. Muscle spindles are usually located at or near the ends of fascicles in the muscle, attaching to tendon, aponeurosis, or perimysium at one end and running parallel to the extrafusal muscle fibers to attach to the connective tissue surrounding those muscle fibers at the other end. The nuclear bag intrafusal muscle fibers have all of their nuclei collected at the equatorial region of the fiber, and although this concentration of nuclei results in little or no enlargement of the muscle fiber, it still has been labeled a nuclear bag. Myofibrils run through the two polar ends but not through the nuclear bag. Consequently, the nuclear bag is more distensible than the rest of the fiber and is stretched when the myofibrils of that cell contract. Approximately the central one sixth of the nuclear bag fiber is surrounded by the connective tissue capsule of the spindle, which is filled with a lymphlike fluid. There may be from one to six nuclear bag fibers in a muscle spindle.

The nuclear chain muscle fibers are much smaller than the nuclear bag fibers, are contained entirely within the spindle capsule, and are attached to the spindle capsule at either end of the muscle fiber. The number of nuclear chain muscle fibers is more variable than is the number of nuclear bag fibers per spindle. From none to ten nuclear chain fibers may be found in a muscle spindle. The row of nuclei scattered along the central portion of the fiber gives the nuclear chain fiber its name. There are myofibrils concentrated in the polar regions of the nuclear chain fiber but also running through the central portion where the nuclei are located. The arrangement of myofibrils in the nuclear chain muscle fibers has not been demonstrated, but it appears that contraction of the nuclear chain fiber stretches and discharges the sensory endings surrounding it.[2]

The muscle spindle is innervated by two types of sensory fibers. The group I afferent or Ia fiber is a large myelinated fiber conducting impulses at 70 to 100 m/sec. It has large annulospiral endings around the bag portion of nuclear bag muscle fibers and partially if not completely encircling endings around the central portion of nuclear chain muscle fibers in an arrangement that responds to disten-

FREDERIC J. KOTTKE

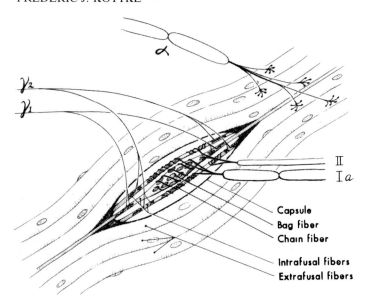

FIGURE 11–8. Schematic representation of the components of a typical muscle spindle. Group Ia sensory fibers have stretch sensitive endings on both the nuclear bag and the nuclear chain muscle fibers. Group II sensory fibers have stretch sensitive endings on the nuclear chain muscle fibers and a flower spray ending of unknown function on the region adjacent to the nuclear bag of the nuclear bag muscle fibers. Gamma-1 axons innervate nuclear bag fibers; gamma-2 axons innervate nuclear chain muscle fibers. The motor end plates of the alpha motor neurons, which innervate the extrafusal muscle fibers, are located at the midregion of those fibers rather than close to the muscle spindle, as the illustration suggests.

tion by generation of a sensory impulse. It appears that the tension necessary to discharge the annulospiral endings on a nuclear bag is only about 40 per cent of that necessary to discharge the endings on nuclear chain fibers. There is only one Ia sensory fiber per muscle spindle. This fiber branches so that there may be sensory endings on multiple nuclear bag and nuclear chain muscle fibers within that spindle, but all are branches from the same Ia sensory neuron. Each muscle spindle, therefore, initiates impulses in only one Ia sensory neuron. There is no evidence that Ia sensory neurons have endings on more than one muscle spindle.[52]

The other type of sensory fiber on muscle spindles is the group II or secondary sensory fiber. Two types of endings have been described for this fiber also. The more complex ending is a partially circumferential, stretch-sensitive ending on the nuclear chain muscle fibers. There is another plaque-like or flower-spray ending on the nuclear bag fiber adjacent to the region of the bag but overlying myofibrils; it is not clear what function is played by this flower-spray ending. The group II afferent fibers are smaller and less myelinated than the Ia fibers and conduct impulses at 40 to 70 m/sec. Their endings are less sensitive to stretch but appear to produce a more prolonged discharge when they are excited.

Each type of intrafusal muscle fiber appears to have innervation from a specialized gamma motor neuron.[2] Gamma-1 axons innervate the nuclear bag muscle fibers. The axons to the nuclear chain

muscle fibers, labeled gamma-2 axons, appear to be slightly smaller and conduct more slowly than the gamma-1 axons to the nuclear bag fibers. On these intrafusal muscle fibers it has been reported that there are some well-developed, large, space-occupying motor end plates similar to those found on extrafusal muscle fibers, which would appear to cause spreading excitation and contraction of the entire intrafusal muscle fiber. There are also small multiple endings in a line or trail, similar to endings of autonomic nerve fibers on smooth muscle, which may be small enough to cause only localized rather than spreading excitation. The possibility that trail-ending excitation might cause localized and sustained partial contraction such as occurs in smooth muscle fibers adds a further dimension of flexibility to the potential responses of the muscle spindle.

The two types of intrafusal muscle fibers, each with two types of motor innervation and two types of sensory innervation, provide the muscle spindle with the possibility for multiple complex responses in the excitation of reflex activity of the muscle.

The Spinal Reflexes

The Primary Stretch Reflex

The muscle spindle stretch reflexes can be divided into the primary sensory fiber stretch reflex, the secondary sensory fiber stretch reflex, and the fusimotor reflexes. The primary stretch reflex, the

Ia sensory fiber reflex, can be subdivided again into the dynamic response, also called the phasic or clonic stretch reflex response, which appears to arise from stretch of the highly sensitive annulospiral endings on the nuclear bag, as opposed to the static, tonic, or tetanic reflex response arising from stretching the endings of the Ia sensory fiber located on the nuclear chain muscle fibers. Both of these endings will be stretched if the entire muscle is stretched. If the nuclear bag fibers are stimulated to contract by the gamma-1 motor neurons, the sensitivity of the endings on the nuclear bags will be enhanced. On the other hand, if the nuclear chain muscle fibers are contracted in response to stimuli from the gamma-2 motor neurons, discharge from the static endings will be increased.[4] In order for the muscle spindle to be effective to facilitate the contraction of a muscle, it is necessary that the intrafusal muscle fibers contract as much as or to a greater extent than the contraction of the extrafusal motor units. This generally occurs in muscular contractions from resting fiber length down to about 70 per cent of resting length. As muscles shorten to less than 70 per cent of their resting length, it is observed that strength falls off rapidly, owing, in part, to loss of facilitation from the muscle spindles[52] (Fig. 11–9).

The pathway in the central nervous system for the primary stretch reflex (the Ia sensory neuron reflex) will be the same whether impulses arise from sensory endings of that neuron on the nuclear bag or on the nuclear chain fibers (Fig. 11–10). If the stimulus is minimal, only the monosynaptic pathways will be excited. Whether an alpha motor neuron with a monosynaptic pathway from a Ia spindle sensory fiber reaches the threshold of excitation depends on the number of excitatory synaptic terminals converging on the motor neuron from that sensory neuron.[14, 31, 32, 56] When a stronger stimulus results in a greater discharge of impulses, multisynaptic pathways will also be excited. The extent of spread of the muscular response will depend on the intensity of excitation and relates to the number of synaptic resistances that must be overcome. There are monosynaptic or short multisynaptic connections to other motor units in the muscle stretched, to a few motor units in synergists of the muscle stretched, and a few even to the antagonists. The longer multisynaptic connections are to other motor units in the synergists and antagonists and to motor neurons on the opposite side of the cord, where there is a reversal of pattern so that the homologous muscle is inhibited and its antagonist is facilitated. In every neuron, the excitatory threshold must be exceeded before an impulse is discharged over the axon. However, a lesser number of stimuli that do not reach the threshold level still increase the excitability of that neuron, or facilitate it, so that fewer excitatory stimuli from other sources become adequate to achieve threshold excitation. Conversely, inhibitory stimuli decrease neuronal excitability and increase the number of excitatory stimuli necessary to exceed the threshold level. The summation at any instant of excitatory stimuli from all sources minus the inhibitory stimuli that reduce excitability

FIGURE 11–9. The major function of gamma motor neurons is to excite contraction of the intrafusal muscle fibers to maintain or increase tension on the stretch-sensitive endings of the muscle spindle so that spindle activity continues to facilitate the strength of contraction as the muscle shortens.

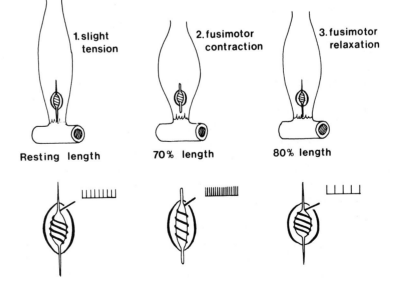

FREDERIC J. KOTTKE

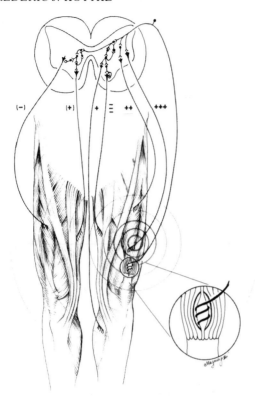

FIGURE 11–10. Representation of the field of distribution of the primary sensory stretch reflex, Ia. It is monosynaptic and strongest to motor units lying close to the muscle spindle in the muscle. It has more synapses in the pathways and, therefore, is less excitable to more distant motor units or to synergists. The intensity of inhibition of antagonists also depends on the number of synapses in the pathway. The pathway crosses to the opposite side to produce a reversal of the pattern. The intensity of excitation decreases from maximal muscle response $+++$ to minimal facilitation of neuron excitability $(+)$. The intensity of inhibition decreases from complete blocking of muscular excitation $\equiv$ to decreasing the threshold of excitation of the motor neuron $(-)$.

determines whether the threshold of excitation will be exceeded and an impulse generated over the axon. This reflex is centripetal in that the greatest effect is centered close to the excited muscle spindle and the intensity of response diminishes progressively with the distance from the point of excitation. Stretching of the nuclear bag ending produces a burst of impulses that accommodates rapidly. On the other hand, the Ia endings on the nuclear chain muscle fibers have a higher threshold so that they do not begin to discharge until a certain degree of stretch has been exceeded, and then they continue to discharge for the duration of the stretch at a rate that increases slowly with any

further increase in stretch. It is evident, therefore, that because of the functional organization of the spindle, the primary sensory fiber may generate either dynamic (clonic) or static (tetanic) discharges. A change of the response can be produced by varying the rate of discharge of the gamma-1 motor neurons or of the gamma-2 motor neurons. Often it is possible during the examination of a patient to vary spasticity from clonus to rigidity or the reverse merely by manipulation of an extremity, which changes the relative excitability of the gamma motor neurons and therefore the relative amount of contraction of the nuclear bag fibers compared with the nuclear chain fibers.[4, 11, 52]

Secondary Sensory Neuron Reflex

The reflexes initiated from the muscle spindle over the secondary sensory neuron (secondary spindle reflexes) are not nearly as well understood as the primary sensory reflexes. It has proved to be much more difficult to isolate and study them. As a result there is disagreement and confusion surrounding this topic. On the basis of his research, Hunt[35] postulated that the secondary spindle reflexes caused contraction only in the flexor muscles regardless of whether that spindle was located in a flexor or an extensor. On other less direct bases, it has been hypothesized that the broadly responsive multiextremity postural reflexes described by Sherrington,[64] Marie and Foix,[51] and others are initiated by stimulation of the sensory endings of the secondary sensory fibers in muscle spindles.[41]

The effective stimulus for initiation of the secondary spindle reflexes is the stretch of the secondary sensory nerve endings on the nuclear chain intrafusal fibers by stretch of the whole muscle, by stretch of the nuclear chain fibers when contraction of the extrafusal muscle fibers compresses the spindle capsule (Fig. 11–11), and by contraction of nuclear chain myofibrils in response to gamma-2 motor neuron stimulation. The pathway of this reflex is multisynaptic, slowing recruiting, and long-persisting, and spreads broadly to cause patterns of flexion synergies or patterns of extension synergies. Stimulation of secondary sensory endings in flexors initiates flexion synergies. Stimulation of secondary sensory endings in extensors causes extensor synergies. The reflex spreads by multisynaptic segmental pathways to alpha and gamma motor neurons and also has a pathway up

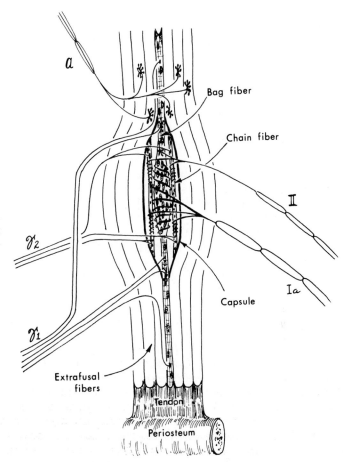

FIGURE 11–11. Compression of the spindle capsule as a muscle contracts may stretch the sensory ending on nuclear chain fibers of the muscle spindle and increase their rate of discharge.

the spinal cord to the reticular formation of the brain stem, which results in marked augmentation due to the excitation returning through the reticulospinal pathway. This recurrent reticulospinal excitation enters the internuncial pool of the spinal cord to cause alpha and gamma motor neuron activation of the stretched muscle and its synergists and overflow of impulses to cause some co-contraction of antagonists. This strong contraction of synergists with weaker co-contraction of antagonists is typical of supraspinal facilitation.[19]

The patterns produced by the secondary spindle reflexes were described during early studies of the spinal reflexes, although at that time they were not specifically identified as originating from muscle spindles. Unfortunately, because the original investigators in describing these responses used terminology relating to the position of the joints, these reflexes often are considered to originate from the joints rather than from the muscles.[64] As a consequence, the semantics of the statement that

"extension of a joint causes a flexion reflex" becomes confusing in its implications, whereas the explanation that *stretch of the secondary sensory endings of muscle spindles in flexors initiates a flexor synergy and stretch of secondary endings in spindles of extensors produces an extensor synergy* identifies the separateness of these flexor and extensor multimuscular, multiextremity reflexes. The reflexes that make up these synergies are the contractions of the synergic muscles of the local extremity (the extremity in which the stimulus is initiated), the long spinal reflex, the crossed extension-flexion reflex, and the extensor thrust reflex, all described by Sherrington[64] and the flexion reflex of Marie and Foix.[51] These reflexes might also be identified as the proximal muscle synergies and the distal muscle synergies in the terminology used by Brunnstrom[5] and other therapists. The long spinal reflex and the crossed extension-flexion reflex together with the contraction of synergists in the stimulated extremity are all parts of the same

FREDERIC J. KOTTKE

proximal muscle synergy, whereas the extensor thrust reflex represents a distal muscle extensor synergy, and the Marie-Foix reflex represents a distal muscle flexor synergy. When the secondary sensory endings of muscle spindles in flexors are stretched, the spread of excitation is to flexor muscles in the synergic distribution. When the secondary sensory endings of muscle spindles in extensor muscles are stretched, there is spread of excitation to the extensor muscles in the synergic distribution.

The proximal muscle flexor synergy is excited when secondary muscle spindle endings are stretched in flexor muscles of the hip or knee and result in reflex activation of the flexors of that extremity, the flexors of the hip and knee of the opposite extremity, and the flexors of the shoulder and elbow of the same side (Fig. 11–12). The same response occurs if there is stretch of the secondary sensory endings of the proximal flexor muscles (shoulder and elbow) of the upper extremity—excitation of flexion in that extremity, in the opposite extremity, and in the ipsilateral lower extremity. Stretch of the secondary sensory endings in any of the extensor muscles of the proximal joints of the upper or lower extremity causes reflex excitation of extensors of that extremity, of the extensor muscles of the contralateral extremity,

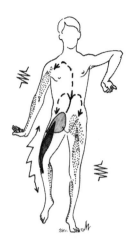

■ Extensor muscle spindles stretched
▒ Extensor reflex contraction

FIGURE 11–13. Stretch of the secondary sensory endings in any of the extensor muscles of proximal joints produces reflex contraction of extensor muscles (1) of the same extremity, local synergies; (2) of the ipsilateral extremity, long spinal component; and (3) of the opposite extremity, crossed extension component.

and of the extensors of the ipsilateral extremity (Fig. 11–13).

The long spinal reflex refers to the response of the secondary spindle reflex in muscles of the ipsilateral extremity, whereas the crossed extension-flexion reflex refers to the response seen in the contralateral extremity. The long spinal reflex is a part of the unilateral component of the secondary spindle stretch reflex, in that stretch of proximal extensor muscles in the upper extremity generates impulses that cause contraction of the ipsilateral extensor muscles in the lower extremity and vice versa. The same rule applies to the stretching of flexor muscles of the proximal joints in one extremity to cause reflex flexion in the other extremity on the same side. This long spinal reflex component of the secondary spindle reflex augments interaction between the two extremities on the same side and is seen with increasing clarity as a person progresses from a slow walk to a fast walk, to running, to hurdling (Fig. 11–14).

The other component of the secondary sensory fiber reflex synergy of the muscle spindles of the proximal muscles was called the crossed extension-flexion reflex by Sherrington. When an extensor muscle of a proximal joint is stretched, there is reflex contraction of the extensors in the same extremity and simultaneously reflex contraction of extensors in the contralateral extremity. The same

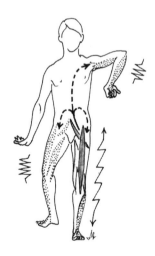

□ Flexor muscle spindles stretched
▒ Flexor reflex contraction

FIGURE 11–12. When any of the flexor muscles of the proximal joints are stretched, impulses from the secondary sensory endings produce reflex contractions of the flexor muscles (1) of the same extremity, local reflex components; (2) of the ipsilateral extremity, long spinal component; and (3) of the opposite extremity, crossed flexion component.

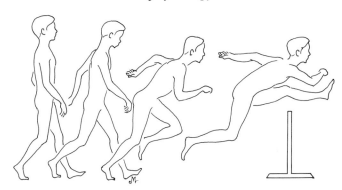

FIGURE 11–14. The secondary sensory spindle reflex posture becomes more evident both in its long spinal and in its crossed extension-flexion components as intensity of effort increases from slow walking to running to hurdling.

rule applies to flexor muscles: stretch of secondary endings of muscle spindles of flexors causes the contraction of flexor muscles in the extremity stretched and in the contralateral extremity. This applies both to the upper and to the lower extremities. When the flexor synergy is inadequately inhibited, stretch of the hip flexors or knee flexors not only increases contraction in the flexors on the same side of the body but also increases contraction of the flexors of the hip and knee on the opposite side of the body, which interferes with full extension of both hips and both knees during standing. In the absence of inhibition, this reflex synergy interferes with normal relaxed standing with minimal effort because it causes partial flexion of the hips and of the knees bilaterally, and continual muscular contraction is necessary to counteract the force of gravity. This reflex produces flexion of the hips and of the knees to an angle of approximately 135 degrees, which is the angle at which joint flexors and joint extensors receive equal reflex excitation.[28] This reflex interferes seriously with prolonged standing and walking in patients with loss of secondary spindle reflex inhibition (Fig. 11–15). Any assumption that extension of the hips to the normal maximal angle of 170 degrees[58] and extension of the knees to 180 degrees is the physiologically neutral and quiescent position not requiring constant inhibition of the secondary spindle proximal reflexes is not correct. Since this synergy also spreads to the contralateral extremity, flexion of one hip or knee will decrease the flexor tone and increase the extensor tone in the muscles of the opposite extremity. This fact has been applied practically for thousands of years by societies all over the world in using a variety of stances in which the hip and knee on one side are flexed to facilitate full extension for easy standing on the opposite extremity (Fig. 11–16).

The major difference between the distal synergic reflexes arising from the secondary sensory endings

of muscle spindles and the proximal synergies is that the distal synergic responses appear to be limited to the extremity to which the stimulus is applied. Secondary spindle reflexes arising from extensor (elongator or plantar-extensor) muscles of the toes or ankle produce reflex contraction of the toe plantar flexors, ankle plantar flexors, knee and hip extensors, adductors, and internal rotators of that extremity in the patient with a transected spinal cord (Fig. 11–17). If the gamma loop to the reticular formation is intact, the reflex pattern, called the positive supporting reaction, occurs in which there is weak co-contraction of the flexor antagonists together with the strong contraction of the extensors, changing the lower extremity into a solid pillar of support. The distal flexor synergy has been called the Marie-Foix reflex[51] (Fig. 11–18). It is initiated by stretching the muscle spindles in the dorsiflexor muscles of the toes and results

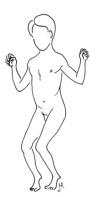

FIGURE 11–15. The activation of hip and knee flexors vs. extensors resulting from the secondary spindle reflexes of the muscles of the proximal joints is equivalent at an angle of 135° at the hip and at the knee. This prevents the person with uninhibited secondary spindle reflexes of the lower extremities from standing with full hip extension and full knee extension. Therefore, considerable muscular effort must be exerted to support the weight of the body against the force of gravity whenever the person attempts to stand.

FREDERIC J. KOTTKE

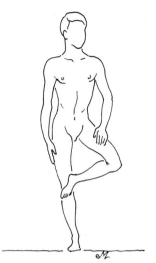

FIGURE 11–16. Nomadic plainsmen have developed the habit of standing on one leg with the opposite foot on the knee. The stretch of proximal extensors in the flexed extremity facilitates extension of the supporting extremity through the secondary spindle reflex.

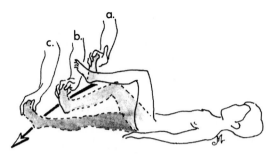

FIGURE 11–17. The extensor thrust reflex is produced by stretch of the plantar extensor muscles of the toes and ankle. This is the distal synergic reflex from the secondary sensory endings of muscle spindles in those muscles, causing toe and ankle plantar extension, knee extension, and hip extension, adduction, and internal rotation.

in synergic contraction of the dorsiflexors of the toes, dorsiflexors of the ankle, flexors of the knee, and flexors, abductors, and external rotators of the hip. Marie and Foix also reported that pressure on the ball of the foot facilitates this reflex. Pressure on the ball of the foot initiates the cutaneous-gamma reflex to cause intrafusal fiber contraction in the muscle spindles of the dorsiflexors of the toe which increases the discharge of impulses over the secondary sensory fibers from those muscle

spindles. Bechterew also described a component of this reflex synergy: stretch of the dorsiflexors of the ankle facilitates the flexor synergy at the hip and knee.

The extensor thrust and Marie-Foix reflexes operate in the upper extremities also. Stretch of secondary sensory endings of muscle spindles of the flexors of the fingers and of the wrist (which phylogenetically are elongators of the upper extremity) produces reflex contraction of the muscles of the distal extensor synergy, the extensors of the elbow, and the protractors of the shoulder (Fig. 11–19). The Marie-Foix maneuver of the upper extremity is produced by stretching the finger and wrist dorsiflexors (which are phylogenetic shorteners or flexors) resulting in co-contraction of those muscles, the flexors of the elbow, and the flexors

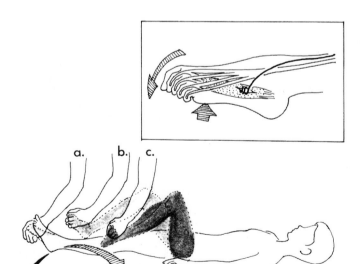

FIGURE 11–18. The Marie-Foix flexion reflex is produced by stretch of the toe dorsiflexors and initiates a flexor response of the ankle, knee, and hip.

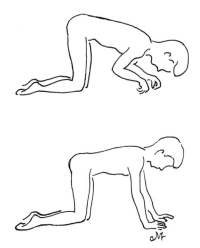

FIGURE 11–19. In the upper extremities, the extensor thrust reflex is initiated by stretching secondary spindle endings in the flexors of the wrist and fingers (phylogenetically volar extensors) and causes contraction of the protractors of the shoulder, extensors of the elbow, and volar flexors of the wrist and fingers.

rule exists that excitation of secondary sensory endings in muscle spindles of flexors (shorteners) spreads to flexors, and excitation of secondary spindle reflexes in extensors (elongators) spreads to extensors.

The neural pathway postulated for the secondary sensory fiber reflex from the muscle spindles appears to have a spinal intersegmental component and also a supraspinal component through the reticular formation of the brain stem (Fig. 11–21). The spinal intersegmental pathway is multisynaptic, long, and slow. Stretch of flexors radiates reflex activity to flexors in the synergic distribution. Stretch of extensors radiates reflex activity to extensors in the synergic distribution. The spinal intersegmental pathway appears to extend to both alpha and gamma motor neurons in that synergic pattern. Impulses that travel upward to synapse in the reticular formation result in a much stronger outflow to the internuncial pool of the spinal cord, producing a slower but much more prolonged and powerful reflex response with much stronger activation of agonists in the pattern and also some overflow of excitation to antagonists. If this postulated pathway from the secondary endings of muscle spindles back to gamma motor neurons is correct, it represents a positive feedback mechanism that should progressively and increasingly reexcite itself unless there is continuous inhibition

and retractors of the shoulder (Fig. 11–20). Terminology and adapted anatomy for prehension make these muscle synergies confusing if one forgets that the relationships developed phylogenetically when the extremities were used for support, at which time the muscles of the wrist and hand that we now call flexors were elongators of the extremity and the muscles that we now call extensors were used to shorten or withdraw the extremity. If that relationship is kept in mind, then the

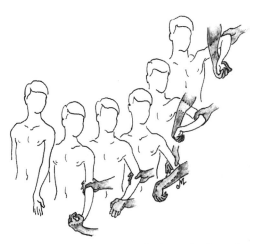

FIGURE 11–20. The Marie-Foix flexion reflex is produced in the upper extremity by flexing the fingers and wrist and causes flexion of the elbow, pronation of the forearm, and flexion, abduction, and internal rotation of the shoulder.

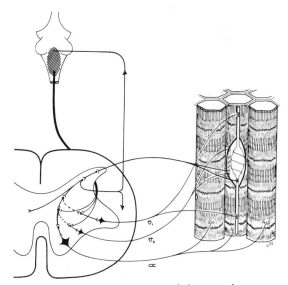

FIGURE 11–21. The components of the secondary sensory fiber reflex from the muscle spindle appear to be a spinal intersegmental multisynaptic pathway to alpha and gamma motor neurons and a stronger but slower supraspinal pathway through the reticular formation.

FREDERIC J. KOTTKE

to control and regulate the system. It is of interest that athetoid patients who show inability to inhibit these reflex patterns also frequently show a progression from areflexia or hyporeflexia to normal reflexia, to hyperreflexia, and finally to a dystonia in this posture as inhibition becomes progressively less adequate.

The feedback of excitation to intrafusal muscle fibers through gamma motor neurons causes activation of the primary sensory neurons of the muscle spindle as well as the secondary sensory neurons, and consequently the Ia stretch reflex will be superimposed on the pattern of the group II spindle reflex.

The reflexes from the secondary sensory neurons of muscle spindles become very complex in their patterns of response because of the regional spread of excitation to the many muscles of the synergic distribution rather than being concentrically specific to one or very few muscles. Whereas the primary stretch reflex has its major impact on motor units of the muscle that is stretched (Fig. 11–10), the response to stimulation of the secondary spindle reflex is a generalized diffuse regional response. Moreover, the spindles of all muscles have secondary sensory endings that discharge impulses when stretched to produce these diffuse synergic reflex responses. Contraction of a flexor muscle results in stretch of the extensor antagonists with stimulation of the secondary spindle endings in those extensors, which initiates competing extensor reflexes. As a consequence, a large number of augmenting or competing reflexes are set up in the muscles of each joint as they deviate from the physiologically neutral position, with the result that a pure flexor or pure extensor reflex pattern rarely occurs throughout the whole extremity. Rather, the posture assumed is the summation of multiple flexor and extensor synergies. In any pathological state in which normal inhibition is diminished, the result of these competing reflexes will be an agonist-antagonist hypertonia with shifting dominance depending on the relative amounts of stimulation summated from the multiple sensory endings. When inhibition is lacking, these competing secondary spindle flexion and extension synergies result in prolonged dystonic postures.

Each secondary sensory spindle reflex, when maximally stimulated and not opposed, produces a target posture of the body because it activates multiple muscles across multiple joints. For the secondary spindle reflex, in contradistinction to the primary spindle reflex, it is not sufficient to think merely of contraction of the stretched muscle, but rather one must consider the posture produced by contraction of all muscles in that flexion synergy or extension synergy. If there is maximally effective stimulation of a proximal flexion synergy without competing or interfering extensor reflex contractions, what will be the posture produced by that reflex, i.e., the "target posture" of that reflex synergy? Such a maximal "target posture" does not occur as a persisting attitude because the position imposed by the target posture stretches the antagonist muscles, causing strong stimulation of the secondary spindle endings of those muscles, which initiates competing or interfering muscular contractions. On occasion one may see the maximal target posture for a fleeting period before it is modified by the opposing reflexes that are initiated. As the reflex response diminishes in intensity or is opposed by other reflexes, one or more of the muscles will be insufficiently excited to produce a maximal response and therefore the posture will show a progressive deviation from the target position as the intensity of the reflex diminishes. It is necessary to know the target posture produced by maximal effective stimulation of a reflex in order to recognize the various components of that reflex. In a number of joints we are dealing not only with flexion and extension but also with abduction, adduction, internal rotation, and external rotation. We need to know how these other motions also are involved in the reflex patterns. Kabat[38] pointed out in 1952, as have others, that many joint motions involve rotation and abduction or adduction as well as flexion and extension, producing what he called diagonal patterns. However, previous investigators have not defined the maximal reflex posture or "target posture" produced by each of the secondary spindle reflex synergies when acting in isolation.

In the secondary spindle reflex flexion synergy of the upper extremity, flexion of the shoulder is associated with abduction and internal rotation so that the maximal target posture is flexion, abduction, and internal rotation of the shoulder. Flexion of the elbow is associated with pronation of the forearm. The reflex is completed by flexion of the wrist and flexion of the fingers, producing a posture similar to that which results if one attempts to tuck the fist into the axilla (Fig. 11–22). Logic suggests that the posture of the "extension" reflex synergy should be essentially opposite the flexion posture, and investigation demonstrates that to be the case. In the extension synergy of the upper extremity

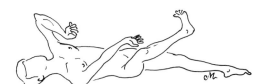

FIGURE 11–22. The target postures produced when the responses of the extremities to the secondary spindle flexor or extensor reflexes of the muscles of the proximal joints are unopposed. In this figure, the flexed extremities show the unopposed flexion synergic posture and the extended extremities show the unopposed extension synergy. (From Kottke, F. J.: Neurophysiologic therapy for stroke. *In* Licht, S. [Ed.]: Stroke and Its Rehabilitation. Baltimore, E. Licht, Publisher, 1975.)

the shoulder is extended, adducted, and externally rotated. If extension occurs before adduction the arm will be behind the plane of the torso, but if the adduction component is initiated before the extension component the torso will block and maintain the adducted, extended, and externally rotated arm crossing diagonally in front of the body. The elbow is extended with the forearm in supination. The wrist and fingers are extended. Components of these reflex synergies can be seen in any part of the range from full extension to full flexion. In athetoid and dystonic patients, there is simultaneous activation of components of both extensor synergies and flexor synergies, since activation of one will stretch and excite muscle spindles in the antagonists, and the resulting posture will shift along the range depending on the relative excitation of the opposing antagonists. Therefore, it is only rarely and fleetingly that the maximal target posture of either synergy will be seen. Kabat[39] and Brunnstrom[5] have advocated the use of these synergies in retraining of upper extremity function. When a synergy is in its maximal target posture, the muscle spindles of the muscles of that synergy will be at minimal length with minimal stimulation to maintain that position. As the extremity deviates from the target posture, the spindle endings will be stretched progressively, augmenting the discharge of impulses to increase the strength of the reflex contraction to return the extremity to the target posture. The position assumed, therefore, will be at the point of balance between the forces produced by reflex activation of the synergy in one direction and the opposing forces produced by gravity, opposing reflexes, or other muscular contractions tending to move the extremity away from the target posture. Similarly, the abductor, adductor, and rotator muscles also contain spindles that contribute to the reflex syn-

ergies just as the spindles of the extensors and flexors do. Consequently, stretching an adductor or an external rotator of the shoulder will facilitate extension of the shoulder and elbow. Conversely, stretching an abductor or internal rotator will facilitate the flexion synergy in the upper extremity. This reflex excitation will also be exerted in the lower extremity as the long spinal reflex and in the contralateral extremity as the crossed extension-flexion reflex. Because of the multiple muscles from which muscle spindles initiate these synergies and the multiple muscles that respond to each secondary spindle discharge from any muscle, a reflex contraction in a given muscle may be maintained strongly in spite of any procedures performed to block the pathways from the spindles of that muscle. General rather than local inhibition of secondary spindle reflexes is necessary because of the multiextremity pattern of responses, both for flexor synergies and for extensor synergies. Within an extremity it may be observed that full flexion of one joint will cause stretch of spindles in the extensor muscles to produce reflex extension at the next joint, and that extension in turn stretches flexor spindles, which then produce flexion in the joint beyond. For that reason in athetoid and dystonic patients in whom the secondary sensory reflex synergies frequently are evident, it is not unusual to see alternating flexion and extension in successive joints in an extremity.

There are similar target postures in the lower extremity resulting from the secondary spindle reflexes. The maximal target posture of the flexion synergy consists of flexion, abduction, external rotation of the hip, flexion of the knee, dorsiflexion and eversion of the ankle, and dorsiflexion of the toes. The extension synergy consists of extension, adduction, internal rotation of the hip, extension of the knee, plantar flexion and inversion of the ankle, and plantar flexion of the toes. The toe dorsiflexors are part of the flexion synergy, and the toe plantar flexors are part of the extension synergy. Gellhorn observed that the same synergic combinations of muscular responses were elicited by electrical stimulation of the premotor cortex as were elicited by excitation of a reflex from its sensory receptor, i.e., cortical stimulation excited the existing spinal reflex patterns.[20] The total reflex pattern in the maximal target position in humans resulting from the secondary sensory fiber reflex of the proximal muscle spindles is illustrated both for flexor synergies and for extensor synergies in Figure 11–22. Since these extreme postures of the extremities initiate counterreflexes by stretch of the muscle spindles of antagonist muscles, we rarely and only fleetingly see a near-maximal response; however, components of these responses occur regularly in normal individual activities and become more evident in persons who have impairment of inhibition.

Fusimotor Reflexes

The fusimotor reflexes cause contraction of the intrafusal muscle fibers. These reflexes are mediated through the gamma motor neurons, which apparently can activate the nuclear bag fibers or the nuclear chain fibers separately and, by doing so, selectively increase the response of the sensory endings on the respective fibers.[2] When the gamma-1 neurons discharge, causing contraction of nuclear bag fibers, there is an increase in the dynamic response of the primary spindle reflex and little if any change of response of the secondary spindle reflex. On the other hand, when the gamma-2 motor neurons excite contraction of the nuclear chain muscle fibers, there is a prolonged static response of the primary stretch reflex and excitation of the secondary spindle reflex synergy. Since the muscle spindle reflexes are the major facilitators of voluntary muscular contractions, the major fusimotor function is to cause co-contraction of intrafusal muscle fibers equal to or exceeding the contraction of extrafusal motor units so that reflex facilitation from the muscle spindle is maintained throughout the period of voluntary contractions of muscles.[26] Intrafusal muscle fiber contraction can maintain stretch on the sensory endings, causing reflex facilitation of motor units, until shortening of the muscle reaches approximately 70 per cent of its resting length. When a muscle contracts to less than 70 per cent of its resting length, the muscle spindle discharge falls off rapidly. When a muscle shortens maximally to 60 per cent of resting length, the sensory endings of the spindle are scarcely stimulated and reflex facilitation from the muscle spindles essentially ceases.

Although in some cases reflexes are defined by the sites or types of the sensory receptors, in the case of the fusimotor reflexes we are classifying reflex activity of a specific group of motor neurons, the gamma motor neurons, to cause contraction of intrafusal muscle fibers. All of the teleceptors—the retina, olfactory organ, taste endings, organ of Corti, labyrinths—supply sensory input to activate the fusimotor reflexes. Much of this activity is through multisynaptic pathways into the excitatory center of the reticular formation of the brain stem and is referred to generally as reticular excitation because of the difficulty in isolating specific pathways from the multiple sensory endings through the reticular formation to the gamma motor neurons (Fig. 11–23). Supraspinal excitation into the reticular formation is mingled with cutaneous and proprioceptive spinal excitation. However, excitation of gamma motor neurons occurs from the excitatory center of the reticular formation and persists even after all of the dorsal roots of the spinal cord of the cat are cut, demonstrating the great influence of the supraspinal input to raise the level of excitation of the internuncial pool of the spinal cord through which impulses flow to the alpha motor neurons. In addition to the diffuse reticular excitation, specific reflex stimulation of fusimotor activity can also be demonstrated. The static labyrinthine reflex has been demonstrated to activate gamma motor neurons of the antigravity flexor muscles of the upper extremities and the extensor muscles of the lower extremities and back when the head is upright or supine.[24]

The cutaneous fusimotor reflex demonstrated first on human patients by Kenny[40] and verified by Hagbarth[27] in the animal laboratory is initiated by stimulating the skin overlying the belly of the muscle and the tendon of insertion (Fig. 11–24).

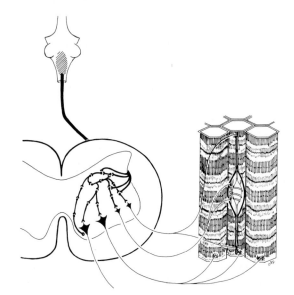

FIGURE 11–23. Reticulospinal excitation from the primary excitatory center in the brain stem causes strong facilitation of fusimotor reflexes.

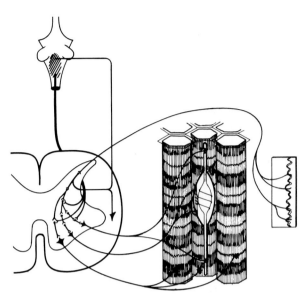

FIGURE 11–24. The cutaneous fusimotor reflex is initiated by stimulation of the skin overlying the belly of the muscle and the tendon of insertion and results in localized facilitation.

37° C until the cold blocks axonal transmission at about 2° to 4° C. Therefore, moderate cooling increases reflex activity, whereas intense cooling inhibits it. Ice packs, immersion in ice water, and ice massage all have been used to block pain and relax muscle spasm after injury. The reported results have been variable, from excellent to ineffective and even to increasing the strength of maximal voluntary muscular contraction after ice massage.[54, 61] Fusimotor activity is initiated also by the tonic neck reflexes. Finally, it appears that fusimotor activity is increased by stimulation of the secondary sensory fiber endings on the nuclear chain muscle fibers of the muscle spindle.

Tendon Organ of Golgi Reflex

Golgi described specialized sensory endings at the musculotendinous junction that enfold a number of collagen bundles in such a way that tension in the muscle causes stretch of these endings. Stretching of the Golgi tendon organ causes inhibition of the alpha and gamma motor neurons to the muscle stretched and release from inhibition of the antagonist[25] (Fig. 11–25). The response of these tendon organ endings is reported to be about 1/10 to 1/30 as sensitive to stretch as are the sensory endings in muscle spindles. Inhibition induced by stretching has been used by many therapists for treatment of hypertonia and represents the initiation of this tendon organ inhibitory reflex to decrease undesired muscular contraction.[1] Tendon organ endings are sensitive enough that they are activated by normal muscular contractions that are of greater than moderate intensity, but require a tension of longer duration than the sensory endings on the muscle spindles do. Moreover, a very prolonged stretch provides inhibition for a much longer time than does a stretch of relatively short duration. It is probable that they provide a reflex mechanism to protect the body from mechanical disruption by preventing excessively strong muscular contractions.

Irritation of the skin by stroking, touching, pulling hairs, pricking, slapping, or icing results in a cutaneous-gamma activity proportional to the intensity of the stimulation.[10, 15, 27, 62, 63] This reflex is localized, producing alpha motor neuron and fusimotor activity and reflex activation of the muscle underlying the stimulated skin. The cutaneous-gamma motor neuron reflex appears to have a weak, multisynaptic spinal segmental pathway and a much slower but stronger supraspinal pathway. This reflex may be confused with or obscured by the nociceptive flexion reflex. In the spinal or decerebrate cat or in normal humans, both gamma and alpha motor neurons are activated by cutaneous stimulation, but the fusimotor activity has a lower threshold than does the pathway directly to the alpha motor neuron.[15] When there is loss of supraspinal inhibition, the nociceptive flexion reflex becomes more sensitive with prolonged and dominant muscular contractions that may also extend to the opposite side of the body.[10] When there is loss of supraspinal excitation of the muscle spindles, such as after cord transection, the cutaneous-gamma superficial abdominal reflexes are lost. This shows that cutaneous-gamma reflexes alone in the absence of supraspinal facilitation are inadequate to activate the muscle spindles sufficiently to cause reflex contraction. The sensory endings initiating the cutaneous-gamma reflex are stimulated progressively as temperature falls below

Nociceptive Flexion Reflex

The nociceptive flexion reflex was described by Sherrington.[64] In response to a noxious stimulus of the distal part of the extremity there is contraction of flexor muscles and inhibition of extensors proportional to the intensity of the stimulus. If the

FREDERIC J. KOTTKE

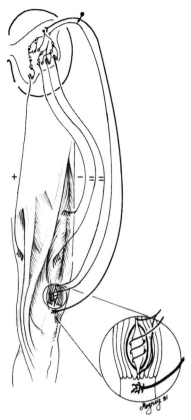

FIGURE 11–25. The inhibitory tendon organ reflex of Golgi produces inhibition of alpha and gamma motor neurons to the stretched muscle and facilitation of the antagonist. It also facilitates reversal of the pattern on the opposite side of the body.

stimulus is slight, the response is localized. As the stimulus becomes stronger, the response spreads progressively to the muscles of the more proximal joints, and the speed of flexion withdrawal increases. The reflex pathway extends to alpha motor neurons as well as to gamma motor neurons, although the reflex time is longer than that of the monosynaptic stretch reflex. Megirian restudied the reflex response to a noxious stimulus from multiple skin sites.[55] He found that when the stimulus was applied to the skin of the proximal part of the extremity rather than the distal, the contraction occurred in the muscles underlying the area of stimulated skin and served to move the part away from the source of the stimulus (Fig. 11–26). If the stimulus was on an extensor surface, the underlying extensor muscles contracted, arching the body away. If the stimulus was on a flexor surface, the flexor muscles contracted. This again appears to be the mixing of the more sensitive

cutaneous-gamma reflex with the less sensitive nociceptive flexion reflex.[10] As the noxious stimulus becomes strong, the nociceptive flexion reflex becomes predominant and the cutaneous-fusimotor reflex is no longer seen. The Babinski reflex represents the release of the nociceptive flexion reflex from inhibition when there has been damage to the inhibitory center or pathways. When there is severe loss of inhibition and of extensor facilitation from the supraspinal centers, nociceptive stimulation may cause the mass flexion reflex of Riddoch with simultaneous flexion bilaterally of extremities, neck, and trunk, spreading to autonomic discharge with evacuation of bowel and bladder, flushing of the skin, sweating, and piloerection (Fig. 11–27).

Motor activity begins first in the fetus at 7.5 weeks after conception as contralateral contraction of cervical flexors in response to exteroceptive stimulation of the nose-mouth area.[33] This relatively distant reflex is probably the earliest nociceptive reflex. Very rapidly, reflex activity spreads both rostrally and caudally from the muscles in-

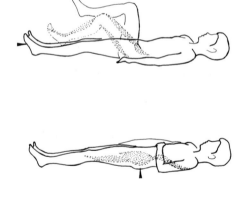

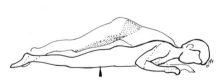

FIGURE 11–26. The nociceptive flexion reflex or withdrawal reflex shows a flexor response proportional to the intensity of the stimulus when the extremity is stimulated distally. When the skin of a proximal part of an extremity is stimulated using a weak or mild stimulus, the reflex contraction occurs in the muscles underlying the area of stimulation, the cutaneous-fusimotor reflex. As the stimulus is increased to become strong, the nociceptive flexion reflex becomes predominant, obscuring any cutaneous-fusimotor response.

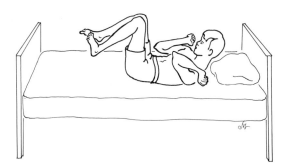

FIGURE 11-27. The mass flexion reflex of Riddoch.

nervated by the upper cervical segments. At 8.5 weeks of menstrual age, the human fetus responds with cervical flexion, brachial extension, and forward rotation of the rump[34] (beginning of Moro reflex?).

It appears that this list of reflexes is relatively limited until one considers all of the possible combinations of responses that may be accomplished by manipulation of portions or all of these reflexes. It then becomes apparent that any muscular function may be activated by one or more of these reflexes. As will be discussed in detail later, it appears that activities of the higher centers of the nervous system are superimposed on the existing spinal reflexes so that supraspinal motor responses are achieved by the changes that are induced through the spinal reflexes. The one exception to this is the pyramidal pathway from Brodmann's area 4 gamma in the precentral cortex with each axon extending down through the spinal cord to the region of the motor neurons of prime movers, which allows excitation of individual or very small groups of motor neurons under direct, conscious supervision.

The Supraspinal Reflexes

The supraspinal reflexes consist of the tonic neck reflexes, both symmetrical and asymmetrical, and the static and kinetic labyrinthine reflexes. The positive supporting reaction and negative supporting reaction, which are frequently listed as supraspinal reflexes, are merely reticular facilitation of the extensor thrust and Marie-Foix spinal reflexes. The righting reflexes[48] are not separate reflexes, but rather combinations of the previously listed reflexes that assist the patient to assume and maintain the upright position.

Tonic Neck Reflexes

The tonic neck reflexes originate from sensory endings located beneath the ligaments around the joints between the occiput, the atlas, and the axis.[48] The sensory fibers enter the central nervous system through the first, second, and third posterior cervical roots of the spinal cord to centers in the upper two cervical segments and the lower medullary reticulum. The reflex activity appears to be initiated through the gamma neurons to increase spindle activity in the muscles stimulated.

The asymmetrical tonic neck reflex is initiated when the head is rotated or tilted to one side.[30] The side toward which the head is rotated or tilted is referred to as the chin side, and the opposite is called the skull side. On rotation of the head, the chin shoulder is abducted and the elbow extended; the chin lower extremity also is extended (Fig. 11-28). The skull shoulder is abducted and the elbow flexed. The skull lower extremity also flexes. The tonic neck reflexes are not affected directly by gravity. However, when the head is erect so that the labyrinthine reflexes are active, the latter may oppose and therefore diminish or mask the tonic neck reflex response. Although some of the literature reports that the tonic neck reflexes are aberrant in cerebral palsied children, Hellebrandt[29] found that the responses were consistent during strong effort. The aberrations that have been reported apparently have been due to confusion of the effects of the tonic neck reflexes with effects produced by other reflexes. The tonic neck reflexes

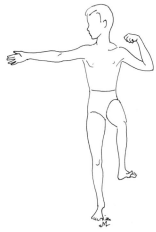

FIGURE 11-28. The asymmetrical tonic neck reflex, caused by turning or tilting the head to one side, produces extension in the chin extremities and flexion in the skull extremities.

FREDERIC J. KOTTKE

were considered to be abnormal and found only in decerebrate animals[48] or brain-damaged humans[49, 68] until the 1940s, when Wells,[69] Ikai,[36] and Hellebrandt and co-workers[30] demonstrated the appearance of these reflexes in normal humans proportional to the intensity of effort. These reflex patterns clearly are used to facilitate the stronger muscular contractions.

The symmetrical tonic neck flexion reflex is produced by flexing the neck forward in the sagittal plane. This reflex is unaffected by gravity, but the static labyrinthine reflex (see below) may interfere with its response when the head is oriented in a position that stimulates the latter. Neck flexion increases flexor tone and grasp and decreases extensor tone in the upper extremities[48] (Fig. 11–29). It also decreases the activity of the erector spinae muscles. Neck flexion increases the extensor muscle activity and decreases flexor activity in the lower extremities. Conversely, neck extension increases the activity of the extensor muscles in the upper extremities and trunk and decreases flexor tone and grasp in the upper extremities, whereas it increases flexor tone and decreases extensor tone in the lower extremities (Fig. 11–30).

When the patient is in the quadruped position, there is usually a mixed response with reflex activ-

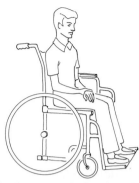

FIGURE 11–30. The symmetrical tonic neck extension reflex increases the tone of the extensor muscles of the upper extremities and back and of the flexor muscles of the hips, knees, and ankles.

ity from the tonic neck reflexes competing with static labyrinthine reflexes. In the quadruped position, neck flexion causes the arms to be brought to the sides with flexion of the elbows, wrists, and fingers (Fig. 11–31). In the lower extremities, extensor tone is increased. The erector spinae relax and the back flexes. When the neck is extended, this produces extension of the shoulder to 90 degrees, with protraction of the scapulae, extension of the elbows, and increased extensor tone in the wrists and fingers. There is increased erector spinae contraction with increasing lordosis. The hips, knees, and ankles are flexed. When the

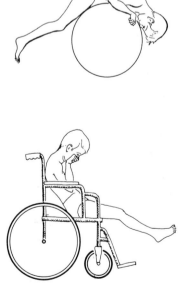

FIGURE 11–29. The symmetrical tonic neck flexion reflex produces flexion in the upper extremities with the fists under the chin, flexion of the back, and extension of the lower extremities without relationship to the orientation of the head to gravity.

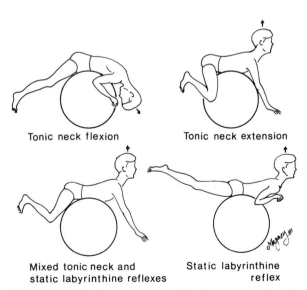

Tonic neck flexion

Tonic neck extension

Mixed tonic neck and static labyrinthine reflexes

Static labyrinthine reflex

FIGURE 11–31. Postures produced by the unopposed tonic neck flexion, tonic neck extension, and static labyrinthine reflexes compared with the posture resulting from the competing tonic neck extension and static labyrinthine reflexes.

patient is on hands and knees with neck extended, the symmetrical neck extension reflex plus the extensor thrust reflex from stretch of the finger flexors produces a stronger extensor response in the upper extremities than the flexor response produced by the static labyrinthine reflex. In the lower extremities, the competing reflexes produce incomplete flexion of the hips and knees.

The tonic neck reflexes extend to the jaw and face in responses that are less well recognized. Extension of the neck causes opening of the lower jaw, whereas flexion of the neck is associated with clenching of the jaw. The asymmetrical tonic neck reflexes appear to cause asymmetrical changes in facial muscle responses that have not been precisely defined.

The tonic neck reflexes can act only on a background of spinal reflex activity. Unless the central nervous system excitation is great enough to approach the threshold for motor response, the tonic neck reflexes will not be manifest. During the practice of relaxation training or during sleep, the general level of excitation in the central nervous system will be reduced enough so that the tonic neck reflexes may not be evident. However, as soon as the patient assumes antigravity activity or other activity that increases excitation in the internuncial pool, the tonic neck reflexes will reappear. Prolonged relaxation training does not develop the capacity for inhibition of the tonic neck reflexes during activity, i.e., generalized relaxation and specific inhibition of undesired reflex activity during voluntary muscular contraction are not the same phenomena.

Static Labyrinthine Reflexes

The labyrinthine reflexes or vestibular reflexes (the terms will be used as synonyms in this chapter) may be divided into the static labyrinthine reflexes and the kinetic labyrinthine reflexes. The static labyrinthine reflexes are produced by the force of gravity acting on the receptors in the utricle of the inner ear.[46] The maximal effect occurs when the head is tilted back in the supine, semireclining position at an angle of 60 degrees to the horizontal (Fig. 11–32). Minimal stimulation occurs when the head is in the diametrically opposite position, prone with the head down 60 degrees below the horizontal. Stimulation of the static labyrinthine reflex produces increased flexor tone in the upper extremities with the shoulders abducted to 90 degrees and externally rotated, the elbows flexed, and the fingers flexed so that the hands are up beside the head. The back is extended. The lower extremities are extended in competition with the crossed extension-flexion component of the secondary spindle reflex. As a consequence of these competitive reflexes, if the person is suspended in

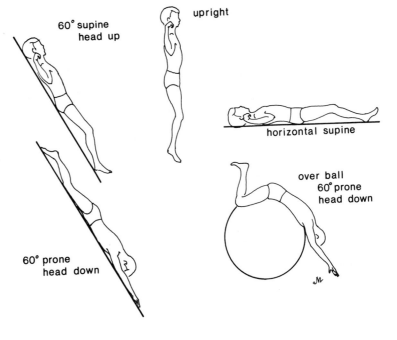

FIGURE 11–32. The static labyrinthine reflex is maximal in the upright 60-degree semireclining position and diminishes to minimal effect when the head is prone and down 60 degrees.

60° supine head up

upright

horizontal supine

over ball 60° prone head down

60° prone head down

FREDERIC J. KOTTKE

the upright position there is incomplete extension of hip and knee. If the feet are in firm contact with the floor, the static vestibular reflex plus the extensor thrust reflex results in full extension of hip and knee. The static vestibular reflex, therefore, assists the upright standing position by facilitating lower extremity extension, back extension, and neck extension. When extensor contraction is weak, maintaining the head in the upright position rather than allowing the patient to look at the feet increases extension in the lower extremities. Conversely, if there is inadequate inhibitory control, the overactive static labyrinthine reflex causes bilateral extension of the lower extremities and interferes with the walking pattern. Since adduction and internal rotation are components of the extensor synergy of the hip, an inadequately inhibited static labyrinthine reflex will activate extension, adduction, and internal rotation at the hip, producing the scissoring pattern during standing and walking.

When the patient is upright, the static labyrinthine reflex facilitates abduction, flexion, and external rotation of the arm, bringing the hand up beside the head and out of the line of sight. This interferes seriously with hand activity, since the patient cannot bring the hands down in front into the line of vision nor to the midline for hand-to-hand activities. It appears that the static labyrinthine reflex is the major reflex interfering with bringing the hand to the midline or across the midline. The static labyrinthine reflex also interferes with moving the hand down to the side so that the patient may push down on the arm of a chair or push down on the handle of a crutch or cane for support (Fig. 11–33). The static labyrinthine reflex is responsible for the floating hand that is held out to the side in midair rather than relaxing onto a supporting surface or hanging at the side.

The so-called aversive reaction is a manifestation of an inadequately inhibited static labyrinthine reflex. Reflexes are dynamic and exert their effect in proportion to the distance that the extremity is from the target position. Consequently, the farther toward the midline or the farther toward the floor the patient attempts to reach, the stronger will be the dynamic effect of the labyrinthine reflex. As a person reaches toward an object, the initial ballistic motion is strong and fast, exceeding the strength of the static labyrinthine reflex. The final approach, however, is under direct volitional control and is relatively weak as well as precise. At the transition between the forceful ballistic engram and the less

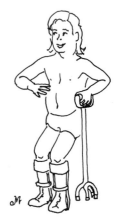

FIGURE 11–33. The effect of the static labyrinthine reflex to flex and abduct the upper extremities makes it difficult for the patient to push down on the handle of a crutch or cane for support.

forceful final directed approach, the static labyrinthine reflex becomes stronger than the volitional effort, and the patient's hand is withdrawn reflexly (Fig. 11–34). The farther the hand is moved from the target position of the labyrinthine reflex, the stronger the aversive response becomes. The response occurs repeatedly without any apparent compensatory learning because the person does not perceive any sensory change prior to the reflex withdrawal. Training a patient with an aversive reaction due to the static labyrinthine reflex to perform the appropriate precise motion to make the correct contact with a target object is difficult.

During sitting, the increased extensor tone at the hips and knees due to the static labyrinthine reflex causes the patient to slide forward in the wheelchair or to stand on the foot plates of the chair. If the patient is startled, which overloads the capacity to inhibit the static labyrinthine reflex response, the sudden extension of the lower extremities and back may cause "vaulting" backward over the back of the chair (Fig. 11–35).

When the patient is lying in the supine position, there is strong stimulation of the static labyrinthine reflex, approximately 50 per cent as strong as when the head is upright. When the patient lies prone, the labyrinthine reflexes are markedly diminished in proportion to the vector force of the size of the angle of deviation of the orientation of the head from the 60-degree semireclining supine position (Fig. 11–32). The strength of the reflex response diminishes progressively to a minimum when the patient is prone and head-down at an angle of 60

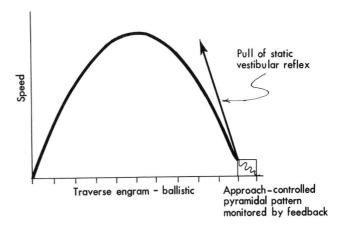

FIGURE 11–34. The aversive reaction causing withdrawal of the reaching hand occurs at the point where the pull of the static vestibular reflex becomes stronger than the precisely directed but relatively weak volitional approach to the target.

degrees. There is a misconception expressed in some of the literature that there is a prone labyrinthine reflex. That is incorrect. There is merely absence of the static labyrinthine reflex, which is stimulated when the head is in the upright position. If the patient is prone with the neck extended so that the head is upright, then the static labyrinthine reflex will again appear in proportion to the approach of the head to the orientation for maximal stimulation. When the patient lies on the side, the labyrinthine reflex appears to be as much reduced as when the patient lies prone. It is of interest to speculate whether people normally sleep on one side or turn on the side or face down as they fall asleep to diminish the stimulation of the static labyrinthine reflex on the excitatory center in the reticular formation.

When a patient is on hands and knees with the head up, or over a beach ball with the head up, the net result of competition for dominance by the tonic neck extension reflex and the static labyrinthine reflex is to cause extension and protraction of the upper extremities supporting the quadruped position, strong extension of the back, flexion of the hips to approximately 110 degrees (which is inadequate for stable support), strong flexion of the knees to less than 90 degrees, and sharp dorsiflexion of the ankles (Fig. 11–31). This posture is multiply unstable in that the knees are in contact with the floor caudad to the hips and the lower extremities force the torso forward so that the patient tends to pitch forward on his or her face. In addition, the strongly flexed knees hold the legs and feet in midair so that they cannot provide lateral stability to the position of the hips. If the vestibular reflex is inadequately inhibited, the legs tend to suddenly extend out behind the

patient in a "vestibular shoot" as the head comes up (Fig. 11–36).

The equilibrium reaction or response to slow tilt is a mixture of the static labyrinthine reflex effected through the gamma system on muscle spindle sensitivity and a proprioceptive response to stretch. As a person tilts in one direction, the static labyrinthine receptors on the "down side" increase their discharge to antigravity muscle spindles on that side with an increased antigravity response in the extremities of extension and adduction. On the "up side" the diminished labyrinthine activation of the muscle extensor spindles results in flexion and abduction (Fig. 11–37). When the sitting person

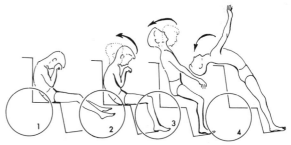

FIGURE 11–35. Inadequate inhibition of the static labyrinthine reflex, which originates from the utricle, interferes with normal sitting. Patients learn to keep the neck flexed (1) to reduce neck, back, and lower extremity extension caused by static labyrinthine stimulation. When the head is lifted in response to a command (2) or to look at an object of interest, the back and lower extremities extend reflexly and the patient stands on the foot plates, rising out of the seat of the wheelchair (3). If a patient is startled (4), the sudden overloading of the inhibitory mechanism by the sharply increased sensory input allows the static labyrinthine reflex to escape this inadequate inhibition, resulting in extension of neck, back, and lower extremities that is vigorous enough to cause "vaulting" backward over the back of the chair.

FREDERIC J. KOTTKE

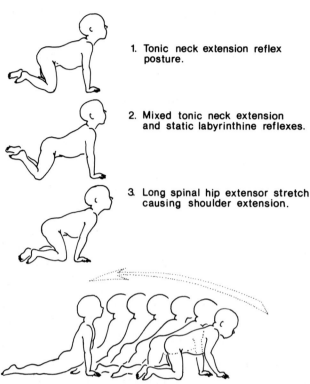

1. Tonic neck extension reflex posture.

2. Mixed tonic neck extension and static labyrinthine reflexes.

3. Long spinal hip extensor stretch causing shoulder extension.

FIGURE 11–36. Variations of kneeling posture influenced by reflexes. (1) The tonic neck extension reflex causes flexion of the knees to an angle less than 90 degrees, lifting the feet and legs off the floor and reducing lateral stability of the hip. (2) The mixed tonic neck extension and static vestibular posture result in hip extension beyond 90 degrees so that the patient is likely to go into a vestibular shoot (4). (3) The long spinal reflex interferes with flexion of the shoulder when the hip extensors are stretched.

4. Vestibular shoot from hand-knee posture due to inadequately inhibited static vestibular reflex as head is raised to erect position.

tilts forward, the back and neck extend and the arms and legs are retracted toward the body, which maintains the center of gravity over the center of the base of support (Fig. 11–38). When a sitting person tilts backward, the opposite reaction occurs with flexion of the neck and back and extension forward of the extremities, which again maintains the center of gravity over the center of the base of support.

When a person on hands and knees is tilted forward, the neck and back extend, the upper extremities extend, and the lower extremities flex, pushing the person backward toward the center of the base of support (Fig. 11–39). When the person tilts backward, the neck, back, and upper extrem-

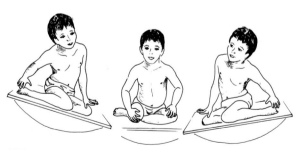

FIGURE 11–37. The reaction to slow tilt is a mixture of static labyrinthine and proprioceptive stretch reflexes. Slow tilt sideward causes extension and adduction of the arm and leg on the downtilting side and flexion and abduction of the uptilting side with rotation of the head and trunk toward the uptilting side.

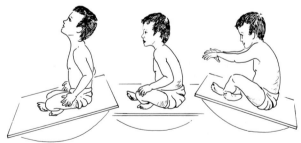

FIGURE 11–38. Forward tilt in the sitting position causes extension of the trunk and neck, with retraction of the upper and lower extremities. Backward tilt causes flexion of the neck and trunk and forward thrusting of the upper and lower extremities. (From Kottke, F. J.: Neurophysiologic therapy for stroke. *In* Licht, S. [Ed.]: Stroke and Its Rehabilitation. Baltimore, E. Licht, Publisher, 1975.)

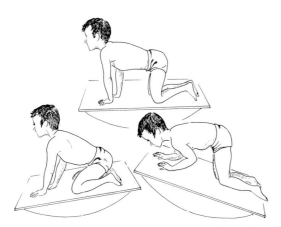

FIGURE 11–39. When the patient is on hands and knees, forward tilt causes extension of neck, back, and upper extremities and flexion of the lower extremities in the tonic neck extension reflex posture. Backward tilt causes flexion of the neck, back, and upper extremities and extension of the lower extremities, the tonic neck flexion reflex posture. (From Kottke, F. J.: Neurophysiologic therapy for stroke. *In* Licht, S. [Ed.]: Stroke and Its Rehabilitation. Baltimore, E. Licht, Publisher, 1975.)

ities flex and the hips and knees extend, moving the center of gravity toward the center of the base of support. These are typical symmetrical tonic neck reflexes.

When there is damage to one labyrinth, there is decreased antigravity tone in the upper and lower extremity on the side of damage, and even tilting of the head toward that side is not performed to the extent that bilaterally equal antigravity tone is restored. The equilibrium reactions are seen only when the shift in position is slow, since if the shift occurs rapidly enough to stimulate the kinetic labyrinthine reflexes, then movements of protective extension become predominant.

Kinetic Labyrinthine Reflexes

The kinetic labyrinthine reflexes are initiated by angular acceleration of the head, stimulating the acceleration-sensitive mechanism of the semicircular canals. These kinetic labyrinthine reflexes produce upper and lower extremity responses, which are referred to clinically as protective extension. The three pairs of semicircular canals initiate reflex responses in the muscles of the extremities and trunk of the same side of the body in response to rotation occurring in the plane of each canal. The horizontal semicircular canals are oriented in the head in such a position that they are horizontal

when the normal line of sight is directed 30 degrees below the horizontal plane. Rotation of the head around a vertical axis causes maximal stimulation of the horizontal semicircular canals, with flexion of the arm, trunk, and leg on the side toward which the head is rotating, i.e., the axial side, and extension of the arm, trunk, and leg on the side away from which the head is rotating, i.e., the peripheral side (Fig. 11–40). The strong reflex response occurs rapidly and reverses as soon as the head ceases turning. The stimulus is produced by the inertia of the fluid in the semicircular canals distorting the neural cristae in the direction opposite to the rotation of the head. When the head stops after rotation, inertia causes the fluid in the semicircular canals to continue rotation in the same direction, which distorts the cristae in the opposite direction and produces a reversal of the pattern. Therefore, it is important to recognize whether any description of the effect of stimulation of a canal is a response occurring during angular acceleration or the response after angular acceleration has ceased because opposite responses will be described in the two cases. Unfortunately, these opposing descriptions have occurred many times in the clinical literature without identifying whether the observation was made during rotation or after cessation of rotation. Temple Fay[17] recognized that flexion of the arm and leg was facilitated on the side toward which the head was turning and that extension was facilitated on the

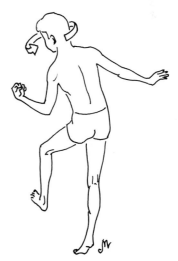

FIGURE 11–40. Rotation of the head around the axis through the vertex stimulates the horizontal semicircular canals, causing flexion of the arm, trunk, and leg on the axial side and extension on the peripheral side.

opposite side and referred to this as the salamander crawling pattern or the homologous crawling pattern. It should be noted that the rapid reflex response from the horizontal semicircular canal when the head is turned is just the reverse of the slower response initiated by the asymmetrical tonic neck reflex. Consequently, when the head is rotated on the neck, during rotation the kinetic labyrinthine reflex from the horizontal semicircular canals will cause flexion on the axial side and extension on the peripheral side, but several seconds after rotation has stopped, the slowly recruiting asymmetrical tonic neck reflex will produce the opposite posture of extension of the chin arm and leg (which was the axial side) and flexion of the skull arm and leg (which was the peripheral side).

The plane of each anterior or superior semicircular canal is oriented vertically and directed forward and outward at an angle of 45 degrees to the sagittal plane. Any vector motion in the forward direction rotating around a transverse axis will stimulate the cristae of these canals bilaterally. Maximal stimulation occurs when rotation is in the plane of the canal and diminishes as the rotation deviates from that plane. However, falling directly forward stimulates the cristae of both of the superior canals, causing reflex elevation of the arms above the head, with extension of the elbows, extension of the neck and back, and flexion of the lower extremities in the typical "belly flop" dive (Fig. 11–41). The plane of the posterior semicircular canals is oriented vertically, projecting backward and outward 45 degrees from the sagittal plane. Motion of the head rotating backward around a transverse axis stimulates the cristae of these canals. When a person falls backward, the kinetic reflex of the posterior semicircular canals

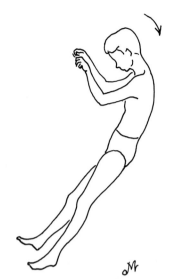

FIGURE 11–42. Falling backward stimulates the posterior semicircular canals, causing flexion of the upper extremities, neck, and trunk and extension of the lower extremities.

causes flexion of the upper extremities, flexion of the neck and back, and extension of the lower extremities (Fig. 11–42).

When a person falls sideward, there is excitation of the superior and posterior semicircular canals on the side toward which the person is falling and diminution of stimulation on the opposite side. The stimulation of the superior semicircular canal causes reflex extension of the arm, whereas stimulation of the posterior semicircular canal causes reflex extension of the leg on the side toward which the person is falling, with flexion of the arm and leg occurring on the side away from which the person is falling (Fig. 11–43).

All of the postures just described can be recognized as the protective extension responses of the extremities to rapid motion of the head. The effect of these responses is to broaden the base of support and protect against a fall. It is not known why protective extension, based on these reflexes, increases with practice.

Positive and Negative Supporting Reactions

The positive supporting reaction is provided by reticular facilitation of the spinal extensor thrust reflex. Although this has been described as a brain stem reflex, it appears that facilitation, resulting in a stronger response of the extensor thrust reflex

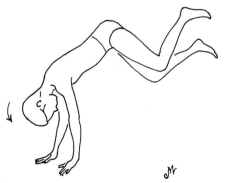

FIGURE 11–41. Forward falling stimulates the superior semicircular canals, causing extension of the upper extremities, neck, and back and flexion of the lower extremities.

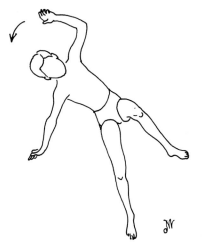

FIGURE 11–43. Falling sideways stimulates both the superior and posterior semicircular canals on the side toward which one falls, producing extension of the arm and leg on that side and flexion of the arm and leg on the opposite side.

plus some supraspinal overflow causing co-contraction of the flexors of the hips and knees to convert the lower extremity into a rigid pillar of support, is the only change that occurs (see Fig. 11–17). This reflex has also been called the magnetic reaction, since pressure properly applied to the ball of the foot initiates the positive supporting reaction and then slow withdrawal of the hand allows the reflex extension in the lower extremity to keep up with the stimulating hand as though drawn by a magnet. The negative supporting reaction represents facilitation from the reticular formation of the brain stem of the Marie-Foix flexion reflex (see Fig. 11–18). The stretch of the toe dorsiflexors is more effective to produce dorsiflexion of the toes and ankles, flexion of the knees, and flexion, abduction, and external rotation of the hip when there is also strong excitation from the reticular formation to the gamma motor neurons to increase the sensitivity of the secondary sensory endings of the muscle spindles. The negative supporting reaction, therefore, often appears considerably stronger than the Marie-Foix spinal flexion reflex.

Righting Reflexes

The righting reflexes were studied and described by Magnus in 1924.[48] He was looking for those reflexes or combinations of reflexes that assist an animal to assume and maintain the upright position. He described these responses as reflexes prior to the time that some of the other reflexes had been fully defined. It will be seen as these reflexes are reviewed that most of them are combinations of the reflexes that have just been discussed.

The optical righting reaction is not a reflex but rather a conscious learned reaction of orienting the head upright in response to visual recognition of the surrounding environment (Fig. 11–44). It is necessary that the pathway to the visual cortex be intact and that the animal be conscious and able to recognize objects in the environment for this reaction to occur. In the environment there are numerous cues signifying vertical and horizontal orientation. Through experience the normal individual learns to recognize from these cues whether or not the head is in the vertical position and observes the relationships that are seen in this position. The person learns through proprioceptive and other perception that it is easier and less fatiguing to maintain the head in the upright position than to maintain it in any position that deviates from upright. From this, the person learns to use the visual righting reaction. On the other hand, an environment that does not provide vertical and horizontal cues makes this optical righting reaction useless. A person in complete darkness, in a dense fog, or in any other situation in which orienting cues are absent cannot use the optical righting reaction. The learned response to visual cues is used in the amusement park funhouse where a room is built so that the apparently vertical and horizontal cues do not coincide with the pull of gravity. In that case, the optical righting reaction

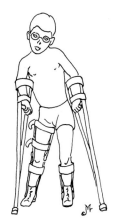

FIGURE 11–44. The optical-righting reaction requires conscious recognition of cues in the environment by which to orient the head in the upright position. When visual perception is distorted, causing the head to be tilted, the entire balance is disturbed.

FREDERIC J. KOTTKE

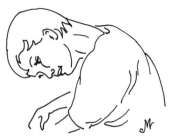

FIGURE 11–45. The labyrinthine righting reflex allows the head to be held upright automatically. When this reflex pathway is damaged, patients can maintain the head erect only by conscious effort and then cannot attend to other activities simultaneously.

and the labyrinthine righting reflex provide contradictory information, in which case the observer becomes confused and loses balance. In the same way, when there is damage to the visual system so that perception of the upright position is distorted, the patient tries to correct for this by tilting the head, which in turn competes with the responses of the labyrinthine reflexes.

The labyrinthine righting reflex is produced by the stimulation of the force of gravity on the receptor endings in the utricle. This reflex requires an intact pathway through centers in the mid-brain. In response to stimulation, the head is oriented upright in space regardless of the orientation of the body (Fig. 11–45). If there is damage to the labyrinth on one side, there is less stimulation from that side and the head tilts toward that side, apparently to balance the input from the two sets of receptor organs. Damage to the labyrinthine

righting reflex diminishes the sense of verticality and makes it difficult for the patient to maintain the head easily oriented in the upright position. Patients lacking the labyrinthine righting reflex have to concentrate on holding the head upright. When they pay attention to another complex task they are unable to simultaneously hold the head erect and carry out the complex activity. A partially damaged labyrinthine righting reflex appears to be trainable to increase its responsivity. On the other hand, it may be that the training results in improved proprioception rather than a change in the response of the labyrinthine righting reflex.

The body-righting reflex acting on the body can occur when there is a pathway only as high as the medulla. The effective stimulus is pressure on the underside of the body as it lies on one side. The response is a cutaneous fusimotor reflex with extension of the arm and leg on the side of pressure and flexion of the trunk, arm, and leg on the upper or unstimulated side (Fig. 11–46). This results in overbalancing the body forward so that the patient rolls face down. Stimulation of the skin over the thighs and lower abdomen causes flexion of the hips and knees so that the body is raised rear end first. In this case the lack of facilitation from the mid-brain prevents effective use of the tonic neck reflexes to raise the shoulders. Consequently the individual rises to the hand-knee position by flexing hips and knees to shift the weight of the torso backward below the knees and then balancing on the knees and legs while extending the hips enough to lift the trunk and shoulders to a horizontal crawling position.

Stimulus - unilateral pressure of body lying on one side.
Center - medulla.

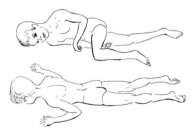

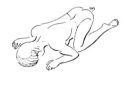

FIGURE 11–46. Body-righting reflex acting on the body. (From Kottke, F. J.: Neurophysiologic therapy for stroke. *In* Licht, S. [Ed.]: Stroke and Its Rehabilitation. Baltimore, E. Licht, Publisher, 1975.)

Normal response - uppermost leg and arm flexed; lowermost leg and arm extended.
Rotation of uppermost side of pelvis forward toward prone position.
Successive rotation of pelvis, lumbar trunk, thoracic trunk and fore-quarters to prone position.

In the absence of ability to extend the neck, patient pulls knees under hips and gets up rear end first.

Stimulus - unilateral pressure of body lying
on one side.
Center - midbrain.

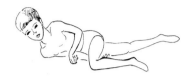

Response - head lifted and rotated to upright
position.

FIGURE 11–47. Body-righting reflex acting on the head. (From Kottke, F. J.: Neurophysiologic therapy for stroke. *In* Licht, S. [Ed.]: Stroke and Its Rehabilitation. Baltimore, E. Licht, Publisher, 1975.)

The body-righting reflex acting on the head arises from stimulation of cutaneous receptors and requires a pathway to a center in the mid-brain. When the body is lying on one side so that there is stimulation from pressure only on one side of the body, the response is the lifting of the head away from the side of pressure and rotating it toward the upright position (Fig. 11–47).

The neck-righting reflex acting on the body requires an intact pathway as high as the mid-brain. When the body is recumbent, because of the labyrinthine reflex the head is raised erect so that there is rotation or tilting of the neck, and a sequence of responses occurs that appear to be typical tonic neck reflex responses (Fig. 11–48). The chin shoulder retracts and extends. The skull shoulder protracts and flexes, which rotates the shoulders into the neutral position in relation to the head. The rotation of the shoulders produces stretch reflex responses in the muscles of the thorax so that the thorax rotates to a balanced position under the shoulders. The lumbar muscles rotate to a balanced position under the thorax. The pelvis rotates to a balanced position below the lumbar spine. The chin leg is extended and the skull leg is flexed as a result of the asymmetrical tonic neck reflex, which assists to orient the pelvis and the lower extremities in a prone and straight position in relation to the head. Then as the labyrinthine righting reflex orients the head in an upright position, which extends the neck, the tonic neck extension reflex causes extension of the upper extremities, extension of the trunk, and flexion of the lower extremities, bringing the patient to the squatting position. All of these responses are consistent with a progressive display of the asymmetrical tonic neck reflex, the muscle spindle stretch reflexes, and the tonic neck extension reflex under the persistently upright head.

Reflexes to the Muscles of the Face and Tongue

There are a number of reflexes affecting the face that are seen particularly in the young infant or in the brain-damaged patient. Generally these are cutaneous reflexes and probably exert their function by cutaneous fusimotor facilitation. The rooting reflex is initiated by touching the skin around

FIGURE 11–48. Neck-righting reflex acting on the body. (From Kottke, F. J.: Neurophysiologic therapy for stroke. *In* Licht, S. [Ed.]: Stroke and Its Rehabilitation. Baltimore, E. Licht, Publisher, 1975.)

Stimulus - neck rotated or bent (with head in normal position).
Center - midbrain

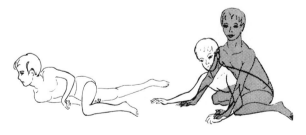

Normal response -
Chin shoulder retracted and extended; skull shoulder protracted and flexed.

Rotates thorax into neutral position vs. head with neck straight.
Contraction of lumbar muscles to rotate lumbar spine and pelvis to neutral vs. thorax. Chin leg extended and skull leg flexed to orient lower extremities to neutral vs. thorax and head.

FREDERIC J. KOTTKE

the mouth of the infant, causing the infant to turn toward the side of stimulation. In this case we see activation of neck muscles for head-turning as well as activation of muscles of the face. The snout reflex is another cutaneous, probably fusimotor, reflex arising from stimulation of the skin of the lips that causes contraction of the orbicularis oris and protrusion of the lips. Pressure on the gums or on the teeth causes the response of closing the jaw and tongue retraction, which produces sucking. Whether this is a superficial fusimotor reflex or a stretch reflex of the muscles of mastication has not been fully investigated. Touching the tip of the tongue produces the spitting reflex with tongue protrusion. When this reflex is uninhibited, the tongue is protruded when it is touched and consequently feeding is impaired.

The jaw responses to neck or head motions may interfere with feeding or speaking functions. When the neck is extended, the jaw opens. When the neck is flexed, the jaw is closed and the teeth are gritted together while the lips are compressed in a grinning grimace. Jaw motion and facial motion also occur when the head is turned. It has not been identified whether these responses are secondary to motion in the neck or to stimulation of the semicircular canals. However, in patients with athetosis, motion of the head and neck is associated with involuntary motion of the muscles of the face.

The onset of reflexes in the muscles of the neck, face, and tongue begins at 7.5 weeks of fetal age in the human with contralateral neck flexion in response to cutaneous stimulation around the nose and mouth.[33] At 9.5 weeks, the first local response to perioral cutaneous stimulation is active mouth opening.[34] The deglutition reflex becomes functional at 10.5 weeks, lip closure at 12.5 weeks, and tongue movements not until 14 weeks. The early development and activation of facial cutaneous reflexes allows more than 20 weeks of reflex activities of these muscles of the anterior neck and face before birth. This prolonged intrauterine exercise prepares these muscles for the essential activity of nursing and swallowing well before the normal 40-week gestation ends. It also indicates why a very premature delivery leaves that child ill-prepared for nursing.

Cerebral Coordination of Motor Function

The organization of the forebrain for coordination of neuromuscular function is not understood, and every concept that has been proposed is open to challenge. The tremendous complexity of the system, which has a capacity exceeding by a number of magnitudes that of even the largest computer, has made all hypotheses of consciousness, thought-processing, motor-planning, and motor execution impossible to verify up to the present time. Recent research in neurophysiology seems increasingly to support the hypothesis of Jackson[37] that higher centers produce motor action by modifying the lower centers to increase or decrease performance. According to this schema in which the higher centers can function only by modification of the lower centers, the basic spinal reflexes provide the foundation for all motor function. Sensorimotor interaction occurs continually at the lowest level of function in the nervous system. Spinal reflexes are maintained at a level of activity just below threshold by supraspinal inhibition in order that excitatory impulses from supraspinal centers can act on them to produce movement.[45, 50] Cerebral regulation is accomplished by modifying the supraspinal or spinal activity. Even the pyramidal tract running directly from the motor cortex to the region of the anterior horn cells is not truly independently active but rather facilitates a highly localized response only because the anterior horn cells have been aroused to the subthreshold level of function by reflex activation. It appears, therefore, that the basis for all motion is modification of the basic reflex patterns.

The cerebrum regulates the lower centers through any combination of mechanisms, which can be placed in five categories: (1) disinhibition, or inhibition of supraspinal inhibition, releases spinal reflex activity so that motion occurs; (2) inhibition of supraspinal excitation decreases spinal reflex activity and decreases the motor response; (3) excitation of supraspinal inhibition decreases reflex activity and decreases motor response; (4) excitation of supraspinal excitation increases spinal reflex activity and increases the motor response. These four mechanisms all are integrated through the basal ganglia of the cerebrum and the brain stem nuclei through the extrapyramidal system. It is through this mechanism for integration of components of excitation and inhibition that engrams of activity can be formed, developed, and by repetition made automatic so they do not require constant conscious monitoring. The highest level of motor coordination—if by highest we mean the most complex, quickest, most specific, and strongest responses developed as patterns of multimuscular activity—is, therefore, extrapyramidal. Normal coordination appears to be extrapyramidal automatic activity. Patterns of neuromuscular activity are programmed in the extrapyramidal system by repetition millions of times in the course of development.[7] Development of these programs of activity requires that a fifth pathway be used, (5) the corticospinal pyramidal pathway running from Brodmann's area 4 gamma motor cortex to the immediate region of the motor neurons in the anterior horn of the spinal cord. This direct corticospinal tract is used to excite the desired activity repeatedly, which programs extrapyramidal pathways until those patterns become automatic engrams. In normal infants this programming begins in utero, for the face and neck perhaps as early as the fifth fetal week after fertilization,[33] and engrams develop only as the result of repeated practice of the correct pattern. At first only simple patterns can be performed and those with frequent errors. As they are perfected by repetition into engram units, those units can be combined or chained and then the more complex patterns can be practiced. Although in many ways this need to practice patterns of activity has been noted in our society, the concept of maturation of genetic potential with age[6, 23] has caused many investigators to ignore the importance of this practice as "only play." Moreover, the tacit acceptance by investigators that cognitive recognition of an activity was the major component of motor learning and that the remaining factor in the development of automatic motor engrams was maturation has caused them to overlook the fact that hundreds of thousands or millions of repetitions are necessary to develop each automatic motor engram.[7, 43] Improvement of skills is usually tested after 10 to 100 repetitions, rarely after many hundreds, and practically never after thousands. Yet that is only the beginning of the formation of an engram.[42] This beginning of training might be thought of as the facilitation and modification of a specific reflex activity by the corticospinal pyramidal tract until the extrapyramidal engram begins to develop.

In addition, the pyramidal tract can impose single pathway modification on established extrapyramidal engrams as they are being carried out but only at a maximal rate of shift of attention of two to three per second.[44, 65] However, the ability to impose pyramidal influence on extrapyramidal engrams results in an ability to produce a whole spectrum of performances of a trained coordinated activity.

Consciousness, initiation of neuromuscular function, and coordination of neuromuscular function all arise from subcortical regions in the forebrain rather than being initiated in some area of the cortex. Penfield[60] and others demonstrated that any portion of the cerebral cortex can be extirpated without abolition of the functions listed above. The cortical switchboard, hypothesized by Ferrier[18] to contain patterns of activity localized in the neurons of the precentral cortex, with each neuron or neuron group producing a coordinated pattern of performance when it was excited, has never been demonstrated to exist even after nearly a century of exquisitely precise investigation by numerous neurophysiologists. There is no center in the premotor cortex that when stimulated will produce a highly coordinated performance of a neuromuscular pattern. Rather, what emerges is the elicitation of relatively primitive excitation of spinal and supraspinal reflexes. Although the patterns emerging appear to have a somewhat purposeful appearance, there is never the highly precise and coordinated multimuscular pattern and sequence that any normal person can very easily produce.[60] These data collectively provide the basis for the concept that coordination is not a function localized in the neurons of the cerebral cortex.

Consciousness was localized by Penfield in a subcortical area that he called the centrencephalic center but did not otherwise define anatomically.[60] It probably includes the forebrain structures of the thalamus, basal ganglia, and possibly hypothalamus. From that center emanate impulses that activate the sensorimotor associations stored in the neurons of the motor and premotor cortices to produce activity coordinated through the integrating function of the cerebral basal ganglia and the brain stem ganglia. Just how this integration of coordination occurs still must be defined. Nevertheless, the observation in athetoid cerebral palsy that damage to the cerebral basal ganglia results in inability to develop engrams of motor coordination supports the hypothesis that the integrative action occurs at that level.[8, 59] The studies of Magoun,[50] Moruzzi,[57] and others demonstrated that the primary inhibitory center is located in the brain stem reticular formation and the paleocerebellum intermingled with the cells of the primary excitatory or arousal center. Impulses integrated through the basal ganglia apparently act selectively on this excitatory-inhibitory system to evoke the patterns of coordination that are produced.

In the discussions of neuromuscular function, the terms *control* and *coordination* are used with different meanings by different authors and often without meaningful distinction. Since physiologi-

FREDERIC J. KOTTKE

cally there are two distinct mechanisms of neuromuscular excitation, these terms will be applied specifically to differentiate these mechanisms. Control refers to the excitation of the corticospinal pathway from the 4 gamma motor cortex under direct attention and volition to activate a few motor units of a single muscle in the anterior horn of the spinal cord to produce an isolated contraction of that selected muscle. Since this is a purely excitatory pathway, there is no inhibition of other neurons, and the conscious activity can occur in isolation only if the person is otherwise relaxed and adequately supported and the excitation is maintained at a noneffortful level by carrying out the activity slowly and against minimal resistance. A person cannot monitor a control activity to cause isolated contraction of a prime mover and maintain relaxation of all other muscles unless the activity is slow. If the activity is rapid or against increased resistance, the increased effort causes irradiation of impulses transcerebrally and through internuncial synapses to produce co-contraction of other muscles. Control, therefore, is the activation imposed on one muscle voluntarily through the corticospinal pyramidal pathway.

Coordination refers to a more complex neuromuscular activity in which some muscles are excited and others are inhibited in patterns and sequences to produce the functional motions of the body. Volition is required to excite, maintain, and discontinue the coordinated activity, but the individual elements of that activity are not consciously monitored. Coordination requires the integrating activity of the basal cerebral ganglia and the brain stem ganglia acting on the excitatory and inhibitory centers to produce these patterns. Coordination develops only as the result of prolonged precise practice of the elementary units of each pattern of activity. The neuromuscular phenomenon involved in the development of each pattern is called an engram. Simple engrams, as they are developed by practice, can be combined by further practice to produce larger and more complex engrams. When an engram has been developed, it can be executed faster than the person can perceive all of the activity that is occurring. It has been reported that the muscular activities in an engram can be performed three to ten times as fast as they can be directed by pyramidal control.[13] One essential component of coordination is the capacity to inhibit those muscles that should not be activated at the same time that the desired muscles are contracting. With continued correct practice, the capacity for inhibition increases and then the effort to produce a faster, stronger, more complex engram can be increased without irradiation of excitation to muscles that should not be active. Normal activity is mainly coordination on which control of one prime mover at a time can be imposed by directed attention to provide almost infinite variations of performance.

Both the learning of control and the learning of coordination require sensory feedback. It appears that the major pathway for sensory feedback is through the spinocerebellar system. The most important proprioceptive and stereognostic feedback arise from sensory endings around the joints. Small motions or change in tension on joints produces spinocerebellar-cerebral feedback, which produces awareness of the relationship between activation of the corticospinal pathway and the response obtained. In the same way, as patterns of activity evolve, the spinocerebellar feedback reports how accurately the pattern is performed. Modifications of excitation make corrections for errors that have occurred. In addition there is interaction between the cerebellum and the basal ganglia to automatically adjust for errors of performance without that correction coming to consciousness.

The conscious control of motor activity is limited. We can consciously attend to only one activity, one position, one movement, or one muscle at a time and shift our attention only two to three times per second. Stimulus-response time to a naive performance is about 300 msec when a person is rested and slows to about 500 msec per stimulus-response as the activity is prolonged.[31]

The fastest stimulus-response time to patterns of activity integrated into engrams is only about 100 to 150 msec. However, the greater value of the extrapyramidal engram mechanism is that multiple channels can be utilized simultaneously so that complex performances of trained engrams may be carried out. Conscious monitoring of engrams consists of retrospective recognition that an error has occurred. Engrams are preprogrammed in a feed-forward pattern. Automatic sensorimotor integration provides for automatic maintenance of patterns. When the performer wishes to consciously monitor the components of an activity, that activity must be slowed down to allow the attention to be shifted from one component to another at a rate no faster than three times per second. In normal skilled performers we always see this slowing in the performance when there is conscious checking of the components of the performance.

The cerebral cortex, instead of being the central ganglion for the initiation of all of the patterns of activity that occur in coordinated functions, is, rather, an association storage site for sensory and sensorimotor relationships that can be called upon by the center for initiation of activity and the center for integration of performance. The integrative center for neuromuscular performance may be likened to a computer. The mechanism for integration is complex but need not be massive in size. On the other hand, the size of a computer must enlarge as the number of "bytes" of information stored there is increased. The great expansion of the cerebral cortex in the human relates to the capacity to store and recall the billions of sensorimotor associations that can be used in integrated performance. If we compare humans to other animals, we find that it is not the speed of performance that is increased in people; there are many animals that can run faster or carry out muscular activity with greater speed or skill. However, people are unique in the vast variety of performances that they can consistently execute in a coordinated manner, especially the performance required for speech and for manual manipulation. The variability of the repertory of humans is vastly superior to that of other animals, and the capacity for expanding that repertory by training is likewise very great due to the capacity for storage of sensorimotor relationships in the cerebral cortex.

References

1. Bobath, K., and Bobath, D.: Spastic paralysis: Treatment by use of reflex inhibition. Br. J. Phys. Med., 13:121–127, 1950.
2. Boyd, I. A.: Nuclear-bag fibre and nuclear-chain fibre systems in muscle spindles of cat. *In* Barker, D. (Ed.): Symposium on Muscle Receptors: Proceedings of a Meeting Held in September 1961 as Part of the Golden Jubilee Congress of the University of Hong Kong. Hong Kong, Hong Kong University Press, 1962, pp. 185–188.
3. Brooks, V. B., and Stoney, S. D.: Motor mechanisms: The role of the pyramidal system in motor control. Annu. Rev. Physiol., 33:337, 1971.
4. Brown, M. C., and Matthews, P. B. C.: On the subdivision of the efferent fibres to muscle spindles into static and dynamic fusimotor fibers. *In* Andrew, B. L. (Ed.): Control and Innervation of Skeletal Muscle. Dundee, Thomson, 1966.
5. Brunnstrom, S.: Movement Therapy in Hemiplegia. A Neurophysiological Approach. New York, Harper & Row, 1970.
6. Coghill, G. E.: Anatomy and the Problem of Behavior. Cambridge, Cambridge University Press, 1929.
7. Crossman, E. R. F. W.: A theory of acquisition of speed-skill. Ergonomics, 2:153–166, 1959.
8. Denny-Brown, D.: Diseases of the Basal Ganglia and Subthalamic Nuclei. Oxford, Oxford University Press, 1946.
9. Denny-Brown, D.: The Cerebral Control of Movement. Liverpool, Liverpool University Press, 1966.
10. Dimitrijevic, M. R., and Nathan, P. W.: Studies of spasticity in man. 3. Analysis of reflex activity evoked by noxious cutaneous stimulation. Brain, 91:349–368, 1968.
11. Eccles, J. C.: Central connections of muscle afferent fibers. *In* Barker, D. (Ed.): Symposium on Muscle Receptors. Hong Kong, Hong Kong University Press, 1962.
12. Eccles, J. C.: Presynaptic inhibition in the spinal cord. Prog. Brain Res., 12:65–91, 1964.
13. Eccles, J. C.: The dynamic loop hypothesis of movement control. *In* Leibovic, K. N. (Ed.): Information Processing in the Nervous System. New York, Springer, 1969, pp. 245–269.
14. Eccles, J. C., Eccles, R. M., and Lundberg, A.: The convergence of monosynaptic excitatory afferents onto many different species of alpha motor neurones. J. Physiol., 137:22–50, 1957.
15. Eldred, E., and Hagbarth, K. E.: Facilitation and inhibition of gamma efferents by stimulation of certain skin areas. J. Neurophysiol., 17:59–65, 1954.
16. Evarts, E. V.: Representation of movements and muscles by pyramidal tract neurons of the precentral motor cortex. *In* Yahr, M. D., and Purpura, D. (Eds.): Neurophysiologic Basis of Normal and Abnormal Motor Activities. Hewlett, NY, Raven Press, 1967, pp. 215–251.
17. Fay, T.: The neurophysical aspects of therapy in cerebral palsy. Arch. Phys. Med. Rehabil., 29:327–334, 1948.
18. Ferrier, D.: The Functions of the Brain. New York, G. P. Putnam's Sons, 1876.
19. Fulton, J. F.: Physiology of the Nervous System, 3rd Ed. New York, Oxford University Press, 1949, p. 179.
20. Gellhorn, E.: The validity of the concept of multiplicity of representation in the motor cortex under conditions of threshold stimulation. Brain, 73:267–274, 1950.
21. Gellhorn, E.: Physiological Foundations of Neurology and Psychiatry. Minneapolis, University of Minnesota Press, 1953.
22. Gellhorn, E., Riggle, C. M., and Ballin, H. M.: Summation, inhibition and proprioceptive reinforcement under conditions of stimulation of the motor cortex and their influence on activities of single motor units. J. Cell Comp. Physiol., 43:405–414, 1954.

FREDERIC J. KOTTKE

23. Gesell, A.: The Embryology of Behavior. New York, Harper & Brothers, Publishers, 1945.

24. Gilman, S., and Van Der Meulen, J. P.: Muscle spindle activity in dystonic and spastic monkeys. Arch. Neurol., 14:553–563, 1966.

25. Granit, R.: Receptors and Sensory Perception. New Haven, Yale University Press, 1955.

26. Granit, R.: The Purposive Brain. Cambridge, MA, MIT Press, 1977.

27. Hagbarth, K. E.: Excitatory and inhibitory skin areas for flexor and extensor motoneurones. Acta Physiol. Scand., 26[Suppl. 94]:1–58, 1952.

28. Halpern, D.: Unpublished data.

29. Hellebrandt, F. A., and Waterland, J. C.: Expansion of motor patterning under exercise stress. Am. J. Phys. Med., 41:56–66, 1962.

30. Hellebrandt, F. A., Houtz, S. J., Partridge, M. J., and Walters, C. E.: Tonic neck reflexes in exercises of stress in man. Am. J. Phys. Med., 35:144–159, 1956.

31. Henneman, E., Somgen, G., and Carpenter, D. O.: Excitability and inhibitability of motoneurons of different sizes. J. Neurophysiol., 28:599–620, 1965.

32. Henneman, E., Somgen, G., and Carpenter, D. O.: Functional significance of cell size in spinal motoneurons. J. Neurophysiol., 28:560–580, 1965.

33. Hooker, D.: Early human fetal behavior with a preliminary note on double simultaneous fetal stimulation. Res. Publ. Assoc. Nerv. Ment. Dis., 33:98–113, 1954.

34. Humphrey, T.: The trigeminal nerve in relation to early fetal activity. Proc. Assoc. Res. Nerv. Ment. Dis., 33:127–154, 1954.

35. Hunt, C. C., and Perl, E. R.: Spinal reflex mechanisms concerned with skeletal muscle. Physiol. Rev., 40:538–579, 1960.

36. Ikai, M.: Tonic neck reflex in normal persons. Jpn. J. Physiol., 1:118–124, 1950.

37. Jackson, J. H.: On some implications of dissolution of nervous system. Med. Press Circular (London), 2:411, 433, 1882.

38. Kabat, H.: Studies on neuromuscular dysfunction. XV. The role of central facilitation in restoration of motor function in paralysis. Arch. Phys. Med. Rehabil., 33:521–533, 1952.

39. Kabat, H.: Proprioceptive facilitation in therapeutic exercise. In Licht, S. (Ed.): Therapeutic Exercise, 2nd Ed. New Haven, E. Licht, Publisher, 1961.

40. Knapp, M. E.: Exercises for poliomyelitis. In Licht, S.: Therapeutic Exercise, 2nd Ed. New Haven, E. Licht, Publisher, 1965.

41. Kottke, F. J.: Reflex patterns initiated by secondary sensory fiber endings of muscle spindles: Proposal. Arch. Phys. Med. Rehabil., 56:1–7, 1975.

42. Kottke, F. J.: From reflex to skill: The training of coordination. Arch. Phys. Med. Rehabil., 61:551–561, 1980.

43. Kottke, F. J., Halpern, D., Easton, J. K. M., Ozel, A. T., and Burrill, C. A.: Training of coordination. Arch. Phys. Med. Rehabil., 59:567–572, 1978.

44. Lancing, R. W., Schwartz, E., and Lindsley, D. B.: Reaction time and EEG activation under alerted and nonalerted conditions. J. Exp. Psychol., 58:1–7, 1959.

45. Llinos, R., and Terzuolo, C. A.: Mechanism of supraspinal actions upon spinal cord activities. Reticular inhibition mechanism on alpha extensor motoneurons. J. Neurophysiol., 27:579–591, 1964.

46. Lorente de No, R.: Ausgewahlte Kapitel aus der vergluchenden Physiologie des Labyrinthes. Die Augenmuskelnreflexe beim Kaninchen und ihre Grundlagen. Ergeb. Physiol., 32:75–237, 1931.

47. Lorente de No, R.: A Study of Nerve Physiology. Parts I and II. Studies from the Rockefeller Institute for Medical Research, Monograph 131, 1947; Monograph 132, 1947.

48. Magnus, R.: Cameron prize lectures on some results of studies in physiology of posture. Lancet, 2:531–536, 1926.

49. Magnus, R., and de Kleign, A.: Weitere Beobachturgen uber Hals und Labyrinthreflexes auf die Gliedermuskeln des Menschen. Arch. Physiol., 160:429, 1915.

50. Magoun, H. W., and Rhines, R.: Spasticity. The Stretch Reflex and Extrapyramidal Systems. Springfield, Illinois, Charles C Thomas, Publishers, 1947.

51. Marie, P., and Foix, C.: Reflexes d'automatisme medullaire et reflexes dits de defense. Le phenomene des raccourcisseurs. La Semaine Medicale, 33:505–508, 1913.

52. Matthews, P. B. C.: Mammalian Muscle Receptors and Their Central Actions. Baltimore, Williams & Wilkins, 1972.

53. McCouch, G. P., Deering, I. D., and Ling, T. H.: Location of receptors for tonic neck reflexes. J. Neurophysiol., 14:191–195, 1951.

54. McGown, H. L.: Effects of cold application on maximal isometric contraction. J. Am. Phys. Ther. Assoc., 47:185–192, 1967.

55. Megirian, D.: Bilateral facilitatory and inhibitory skin areas of spinal motoneurons of cat. J. Neurophysiol., 25:127–137, 1962.

56. Mendell, L. M., and Henneman, E.: Terminals of single Ia fibers: Location, density and distribution within a pool of 300 homonymous motoneurons. J. Neurophysiol., 34:171–187, 1971.

57. Moruzzi, G.: Problems in Cerebellar Physiology. Springfield, Illinois, Charles C Thomas, Publisher, 1950.

58. Mundale, M. O., Hislop, H. J., Rabideau, R. J., and Kottke, F. J.: Evaluation of extension of the hip. Arch. Phys. Med. Rehabil., 37:75–80, 1956.

59. Oppenheim, H., and Vogt, C.: Nature et localization de la paralysie pseudobulbaire congenetale et infantile. Psychol. Neurol., 18:293–300, 1911.

60. Penfield, W.: Mechanisms of voluntary movement. Brain, 77:1–17, 1954.
61. Petajon, J. H., and Watts, N.: Effects of cooling on triceps surae reflex. Am. J. Phys. Med., 41:240–251, 1962.
62. Rood, M. S.: Neurophysiological reactions as a basis for physical therapy. Phys. Ther. Rev., 34:444–449, 1954.
63. Rood, M. S.: Neurophysiological mechanisms utilized in the treatment of neuromuscular dysfunction. Am. J. Occup. Ther., 10:220–225, 1956.
64. Sherrington, C. S.: The Integrative Action of the Nervous System. New York, Charles Scribner's Sons, 1906; 2nd Ed., New Haven, Yale University Press, 1947.
65. Stark, L.: Neurological Control Systems—Studies in Bioengineering. New York, Plenum, 1968.
66. Teyler, T. J., Roemer, R. A., Wheeler, W., Metzler, J., and Thompson, R. F.: The pyramidal motor system: A site of sensori-motor integration. *In* Buerger, A. A., and Tobis, J. S. (Eds.): Neurophysiological Aspects of Rehabilitation Medicine. Springfield, Illinois, Charles C Thomas, Publisher, 1976, pp. 105–148.
67. Towe, A. L.: Motor cortex and the pyramidal system. *In* Moser, J. D. (Ed.): Efferent Organization and Integration of Behavior. New York, Academic Press, 1973, pp. 67–97.
68. Walshe, F. M. R.: The decerebrate rigidity of Sherrington in man. Arch. Neurol. Psychiatry, 10:1–23, 1923.
69. Wells, H. S.: Demonstration of tonic neck and labyrinthine reflexes and positive heliotropic responses in normal human subjects. Science, 99:36–37, 1944.

12
Health Accounting—Functional Assessment of the Long-Term Patient

CARL V. GRANGER

Definition of Functional Assessment

Functional assessment is a method for describing abilities and limitations to measure an individual's use of the variety of skills included in performing tasks necessary to daily living, leisure activities, vocational pursuits, social interactions, and other required behaviors. For a comprehensive functional assessment, selected diagnostic descriptors, performance (skill/task) descriptors, and social role descriptors are used to assemble the information desired. The technique includes coding the component skills and tasks according to categories of activities required in daily living. The data are used to help formulate judgments as to how well these essential skills are used and to gauge the degree to which tasks are accomplished and social role expectations are being met. A clinician who is proficient in using functional assessment can obtain a performance-oriented data base that can be analyzed with diagnostic descriptions of pathological conditions and impairment states. This integration of medical status, status in performance of tasks and fulfillment of social roles, together with knowledge of the individual's level of social supports, allows for the construction of a set of data that profiles the whole person. Given this profile derived from analysis of data about function, problems and areas of need can be identified more accurately and interventions and long-range coordination strategies (e.g., case management) can be developed that maximize personal independence and well-being. This type of data base provides a framework for an orderly review of needs at the physical, individual, and societal level, which is important for development of skills, accomplishment of tasks, and fulfillment of social roles and for a satisfactory quality of life.

It is possible to compare changes in status over periods of time by assessing function at appropriate intervals to determine whether social roles have been influenced by the professional interventions of health care, rehabilitation, education, or psychological and social counseling. The measures can describe changes both for individuals and for groups of individuals.

Utilizing the example of the problem-oriented medical record described by Weed,[1, 2] functional assessment represents the extension of the defined data base beyond the traditional components of the history, the physical examination, and the laboratory data. Functional assessment provides a framework for an orderly review of those biological and psychological, as well as physical and social, environmental systems, that are important to the fulfillment of social roles and for a satisfactory quality of life. Conceptual underpinnings for functional assessment are provided through the "disability models" proposed by Nagi[3, 4] and Wood.[5, 6] Nagi proposes that the process is outlined by the following pattern: PATHOLOGY → IMPAIRMENT → FUNCTIONAL LIMITATIONS → DISABILITY. Pathology is the interruption of normal processes and the simultaneous efforts of the organism to restore a normal state. Impairment is the anatomical, physiological, mental, or psychological loss or abnormality. Functional limitations reflect reductions in functioning of the whole person to account for ways in which impairment contributes to disability. Disability is used to mean inability or limitation in performing activities related to social roles, such as in work, family, or independent living.

Wood proposes that the process is shown in the following pattern: IMPAIRMENT → DISABILITY → HANDICAP. Wood and Nagi agree on the use of the term impairment. Wood considers disability to be the representation of reductions in composite activities and behaviors that are generally considered to be essential components of everyday life. Wood thus considers functional limitations to be manifestations of impairment. Handicap is used to represent the values attached to an individual's situation when it departs from the social norm. Social norms are defined in the World Health Organization (WHO) document[7] within six key roles or dimensions of experiences in which competence is expected of the individual for survival: orientation, physical independence, mobility, occupation, social integration, and economic self-sufficiency. To satisfy these social roles, the individual employs a variety of functional skills that result in complex behaviors and performances of tasks.

Certain fundamental accomplishments or behaviors related to the existence and survival of people as social beings are expected of the individual in virtually every culture:

1. The individual is expected to receive signals from surroundings (such as seeing, listening, smelling, or touching), to assimilate these signals, and to express a response to what is assimilated.

2. The individual is expected to maintain a customarily effective independent existence in regard to the more immediate physical needs of the body, including feeding, personal hygiene, and various other activities of daily living.

3. The individual is expected to move around effectively in the environment.

4. The individual is expected to occupy the time in a fashion appropriate to his or her sex, age, and culture, including following an occupation, such as tilling the soil, laboring for others, running a household, bringing up children, and carrying out activities such as play or recreation.

5. The individual is expected to participate in and maintain social relationships with others.

6. The individual is expected to sustain socioeconomic activity and independence by virtue of labor or exploitation of material possessions, such as natural resources, livestock, or crops. This economic self-sufficiency customarily includes obligations to sustain others, such as members of the family.

Chronic diseases have increased in prevalence as prime public health problems. Estimation of health status relies on symptoms, signs, and other indicators more directly related to those biological responses that are associated with morbidity or proneness to morbid conditions. Measurement of health and well-being of a population must include mental health, social health, and functional limitations as related to disability.[8-10] Until 1984, measures used by the National Center for Health Statistics (NCHS) to account for disability were life years, institutional days, activity limitation days, presence of acute or chronic illnesses, bed disability days, and days lost from work due to illness.[11] Yet these measures rely upon symptoms and rates of utilization of health and medical services by the population and are, therefore, still measuring health status or morbidity rather than disability. Measures of disability for a population are difficult to construct, since they require descriptions of task performances and behaviors in the context of "normally" expected social roles, which themselves are difficult to define precisely. However, in 1987, NCHS reported the results of household interviews covering 10 tasks about mobility, endurance, lifting or carrying, upper and lower body strength, reaching, and grasping. Subjects were asked of their ability to perform, or else the degree of difficulty, or their inability to accomplish the tasks.[11] Questions about actual task performance explain disability more accurately than questions about symptoms or utilization of health or medical services.

Stewart and co-workers[8, 9] studied functional limitations in a household sample using domains of mobility or traveling, physical activity including working and bending, and social activity including work, play, self-care, and leisure time activities. They found strong associations between all three scales; in particular, social dysfunction nearly always occurred along with mobility limitations, whereas the opposite was not true. A major weakness of population studies was noted in this study in that 90 per cent or more of individuals did not have functional limitations on most of the items and scales. Thus, it would require very large samples to detect any differences in health according to functional limitation assessments. The authors also noted in their study that considerable overlap was present in the measures that they used.

Desirable Features of a Functional Assessment Instrument

A functional assessment instrument should meet certain objectives, such as those summarized by

Donaldson and co-workers:[12] (1) objective description of functional status at a given point in time, (2) serial repetition allowing detection of changed functional status, (3) data collected through observation relevant to and useful in monitoring the treatment program, (4) enhancement of communication among treatment team members and between referral agencies, and (5) comparable clinical observations compatible with research questions. Other researchers (1) emphasize using a classification that is "composed of a set of descriptive terms that are patient-oriented, multidimensional in content, objectively stated, precisely defined, and relative to the goals of long-term care"[13]; (2) stress compacting a wide range of data "that is unobtrusive to the service provider, is adaptable to the particular clinical setting, that reinforces the goals of the service program by identifying problems and needs and by aiding comprehensive planning, and that utilizes standard expressions"[14]; and (3) advocate methods for quality assurance by using the data to perform program evaluation, program audit, and analyses of outcomes and benefits as well as cost-effectiveness.[15, 16]

Development of Functional Assessment Instruments

Deaver and Brown[17] summarize the basic goals of medical rehabilitation as (1) maximum use of the hands, (2) ambulation, (3) independence in self-care, (4) communication, and (5) the appearance of being normal. Lists of tasks have been compiled by many rehabilitation workers and are called the activities of daily living (ADL). They are usually used for teaching patients how to take care of themselves.[18] Over the past 35 years many different scales have emerged to tabulate those activities performed independently versus those performed through assistance of another person or with a mechanical aid. These are used as measures of functional independence. Donaldson and co-workers[12] performed a survey of the English language literature from 1950 to 1970 and determined that 25 scales met two of three criteria: (1) they had a mechanism for scoring, (2) they had been used in a survey or other type of research, and (3) they were applicable to a general rehabilitation population. These researchers devised and tested a new, expanded instrument that permitted concurrent scoring of the Katz, Barthel, and Kenny scales.[19–21] Their conclusions were that (1) the new

scale was more useful than prior scales because of clear criteria for mutually exclusive categories, and (2) 92 of 100 pairs of pre-test and post-test scores showed comparability of Kenny, Barthel, and Katz scores, with the Kenny being the most sensitive to change and the Katz the least sensitive.

The Functional Life Scale (FLS), developed by Sarno and colleagues,[22] recognizes that knowing the actual performance of skills is a better measure of degree of disability than knowing the elements that constitute performance. For example, a scale should indicate the adequacy of locomotion rather than whether range of motion and muscle power of the legs are normal or not. The FLS as reported in 1973 is composed of 44 items designed for application outside of the hospital setting based upon an interview technique. Normal behavior is used as the standard for comparison. Items assessed were judged for self-initiation, frequency, speed, and overall efficiency and were numerically rated along a continuum from 0 to 4, yielding a series of subscores. Test-retest reliability, inter-rater reliability, internal consistency, and validity testing were generally satisfactory and in some cases yielded high correlation values.

The Long-Range Evaluation System (LRES) developed by Granger and others[14] has some features in common with other ADL scales. In the first place, it incorporates the scoring methodology of the Barthel index and the PULSES profile,[23] and as such, the domain of personal care depends heavily upon independent functioning in self-care, mobility and bladder and bowel sphincter control. Abilities in active use of the limbs; in communication and vision; the need for physician or nursing services, or both; and the level of social supports are described through the ESCROW profile.[24] The three scales together form the backbone of the LRES.

Other functional assessment scales have been developed.[25–27] A summary of functional assessment scales and bibliography up to 1979 appeared in *Functional Limitations: A State of the Art Review*.[28]

In 1983, the American Academy of Physical Medicine and Rehabilitation and the American Congress of Rehabilitation Medicine jointly sponsored an effort to meet the long-standing need to document the severity of patient disability and the outcomes of medical rehabilitation. The result is the Uniform Data System for Medical Rehabilitation (UDSMR),[29–31] which incorporates a minimum data set for uniformly describing and communicating information about disability. The UDSMR is endorsed or participated in by 11 other national rehabilitation professional organizations. Developmental work was supported in part through a grant from the U.S. Department of Education, National Institute of Handicapped Research (now National Institute for Disability and Rehabilitation Research).

Included in the UDSMR is the Functional Independence Measure (FIM) (Fig. 12–1), which is a discipline-free, easily administered, valid, and reliable measure to be used for periodic assessment of changes in patient performance over time and

outcomes of rehabilitation. The data set, including the FIM, is a tool to facilitate treatment management and monitoring, quality assurance, program evaluation, determination of cost-effectiveness of processes and resources used, and care policy decision-making. The Data Management Service (DMS) provides a subscription service for medical rehabilitation facilities to enter their data into the system and receive feedback reports. A *Guide for Use of the Uniform Data Set for Medical Rehabilitation* is available from The Buffalo General Hospital/State University of New York at Buffalo.[32]

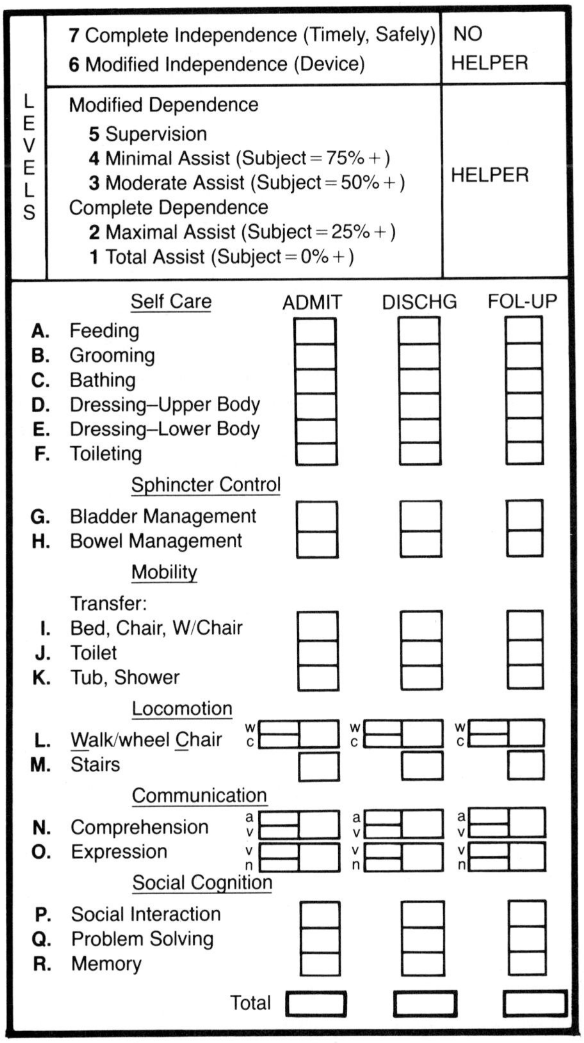

Uniform Data System for Medical Rehabilitation (UDSMR)

In clinical medicine we have the thermometer to measure body temperature, which we know indicates degrees of heat. Because we lacked the equivalent of the clinical thermometer or a uniformly applied measure of function to indicate levels of dependency in clinical rehabilitation, the FIM was developed.

The FIM is the component of the UDSMR that measures the functional level of a patient. The conceptual basis of the FIM is that the degree of disability is an indicator of the "burden of care." Thus, the burden that disability represents is the substituted time and energy that must be brought to serve the needs of the dependent individual in order that a certain quality of life is achieved or maintained. Since dependency can be related to social and economic consequences, the FIM is a way to represent the "cost" of an individual's disability. Use of a validated dependency measurement instrument for estimating degree of disability and outcome of medical rehabilitation is expected to improve the effectiveness and efficiency of services rendered to people with disabilities.

The FIM is constructed with seven levels of function, two in which no human helper is required, and five in which progressive degrees of help are required. Eighteen items are defined within six areas of functioning: self-care, sphincter control, mobility, locomotion, communication, and social cognition. All basic life activities are not measured, only the more critical ones. The FIM measures levels of disability regardless of the nature or extent of the underlying pathology or impairment. The FIM is not designed for use with individuals with mental impairment alone, although it does report on certain important cogni-

FIGURE 12–1. Functional independence measure (FIM). (Copyright 1987, Research Foundation—State University of New York.)

tive and behavioral activities. The FIM can be used in multiple settings, including a hospital, a clinic, a nursing home, or an individual's private home.

Purposes and Uses of Functional Assessment

Functional assessment is primarily a method for integrating data on diagnostic descriptions of pathological conditions and impairment states with data related to limitations or residual abilities in the performance of social roles. By constructing a set of data that profiles the whole person, it becomes possible to understand better how a person with a disability functions. Given this understanding, problems and areas of need can be identified more accurately and interventions can be developed that are more appropriate for enhancing personal independence and autonomy in fulfilling social roles.

In particular, functional assessment and analysis are useful in the following ways:

1. Systematically developing a patient problem list that includes limitations in functioning.

2. Determining clinical care changes in patients or clients by comparing measures of function before and after treatment interventions.

3. Relating needs of a defined population through assessment and analysis of function measured from samples of individuals representative of that population.

4. Determining the benefits of clinical care in analyzing cost-benefits and cost-effectiveness.

5. Providing manpower studies that can relate needs for various numbers and kinds of health care personnel to levels of severity of disability in the patients being served.

6. Providing utilization review for necessity of given levels of care and alternative levels of care and to justify costs.

7. Setting priorities of needs should it become necessary to ration scarce resources.

8. Providing program evaluation, quality assurance, and medical care audit studies in order to detect deficiencies in care and then to improve care.

9. Tracking patients through a system of care in order to determine the strengths and weaknesses of the system.

10. Establishing comparability of groups of patients for research studies and for policy planning.

11. Facilitating case management in order to assure that a program of care is addressing issues that are most likely to increase the quality of life for the disabled person.

Kottke[33] presents a spectrum of the stages of recovery (Figs. 12–2 and 12–3) based on a scheme of growth and development. This scheme can guide the responses of the rehabilitation team professionals toward helping the patient achieve and maintain an optimal quality of life. The survival of organs is the first concern of acute medical care. The hazard is that, in preserving an organ, the physician may lose sight of the whole patient and thus unwittingly continue to reinforce the patient's passive ("sick") role in the recovery process. The activities of the rehabilitation professionals are

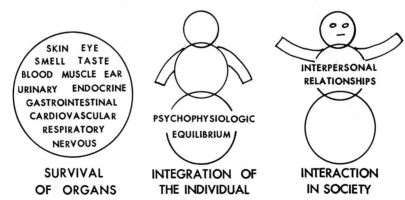

FIGURE 12–2. The stages of recovery based on a scheme of growth and development. The survival of organs is the first concern of acute medical care. The activities of the rehabilitation professionals are most intense during establishment of psychophysiological equilibrium and reintegration. They continue support through interpersonal relationships in order to enhance interactions with society. (From Kottke, F. J.: Philosophical Considerations of Quality of Life for the Disabled. Presented at the 56th Annual Session of the American Congress of Rehabilitation Medicine, November 11, 1979, Honolulu, Hawaii.)

FIGURE 12–3. Further stages of recovery. The patient moves away from overdependence upon professional help and organizes his or her life toward productive and constructive efforts. Finally, the patient participates in creative performances, being less dependent upon routine endeavors. (From Kottke, F. J.: Philosophical Considerations of Quality of Life for the Disabled. Presented at the 56th Annual Session of the American Congress of Rehabilitation Medicine, November 11, 1979, Honolulu, Hawaii.)

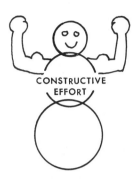

CONSTRUCTIVE EFFORT

PRODUCTIVE CAREER

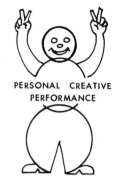

PERSONAL CREATIVE PERFORMANCE

PARTICIPATION

most intense during the establishment of psychophysiological equilibrium and reintegration. Their strategy includes reintegrating the patient as a total being. The rehabilitation professionals continue to support and encourage the patient through the next stage. At the same time, the personality of the patient takes on a more important role if the patient is to be more effective in interpersonal relationships and interactions with society. The following stage (Fig. 12–3) requires that the patient "dare to succeed," meaning that the patient moves away from comfortable supports and overdependence on professional help. By now the patient should have learned how to utilize most self-help resources and begun to organize life toward productive and constructive efforts. The final growth stage is represented by less dependence on routine productive endeavors and more participation in creative performances. In actuality the final stage is also the first stage because all along the way, medical and rehabilitation professionals should be encouraging the patient to assume personal responsibility for activities and to move forward constructively toward personal goals. Application of functional assessment through the stages of recovery can document the recognized accomplishments of the rehabilitation process. Through feedback to the patient, motivation and personal progress can be enhanced.

The uses of functional assessment are applicable to medical rehabilitation inpatient and outpatient programs, nursing home care, and other long-term care facilities, day hospital and day care programs, vocational rehabilitation programs, home care programs, and other service programs for people with disabilities. In addition, functional assessment is the means for estimating levels of disability within a community population for purposes of epidemiological studies related to judging needs and for allocation of manpower and other resources.

In hospital rehabilitation programs, the majority of patients are discharged to home settings in the community, whereas the minority are discharged to long-term nursing home care facilities. One of the major aims of hospital rehabilitation programs[34] is to increase the percentage of patients discharged home. A number of studies have assessed the usefulness of functional assessment and other patient data for predicting the course of rehabilitation treatment. High assessment scores in physical functioning at discharge for populations with multiple diagnoses and with stroke were found to be important correlates[14, 35–37] with the private home for discharge placement and continued living site. Such areas as self-care, mobility, and sphincter control were components of the overall functional assessments. Age appeared as a predictor of placement in several studies, younger patients tending to be sent home rather than to institutions,[14, 35, 37–39] with the qualification that family support may be an intervening variable.[37, 38] Other predictors of home rather than institutional placement for stroke patients were absence of associated heart, pulmonary, and vascular disease; absence of intellectual, emotional, and perceptual deficits; presence of spouse or other family member; and competent family support and involvement.[35, 37, 38] Functional status as measured by admission and discharge scores on functional assessment instruments (Barthel index and PULSES profile), together with hospital length of stay for stroke patients, predicted whether patients returned home or were placed in long-term care facilities.[40]

Application of the Uniform Data System for Medical Rehabilitation (UDSMR)

The Uniform Data System for Medical Rehabilitation (UDSMR), with the component Functional

CARL V. GRANGER

Independence Measure (FIM), has been developed with the following issues foremost in consideration: comprehensiveness, effectiveness, efficiency, comparability, and predictability. Comprehensiveness reveals whether those aspects of disability that represent "burden of care" are covered according to the major functional and behavioral activities accounted for in the FIM. Effectiveness demonstrates, through changes in the FIM, that a person's recovery from disability follows the direction sought by the program. Efficiency is an analysis of whether the intensity (cost and duration) of a program is appropriate to the person's levels of function both before and after the onset of disability. Comparability is facilitated by the use of the UDSMR because outcomes of programs are described in a uniform manner. Since the same functional elements are in the FIM as are in the Barthel index, both FIM and Barthel scores can be derived from a single assessment.

Use of the UDSMR will allow facility administrators and clinicians to compile a data base to predict which persons are served best by the program, the kinds and amounts of services needed, and the likelihood of obtaining the desired results. These attributes make the UDSMR suitable for program evaluation and quality assurance and make it likely that the UDSMR or some component of the evaluation will be a potent determinant of how a prospective payment system for medical rehabilitation will be shaped.

Rationale for Quality Assurance and Program Evaluation

Codman[41] first described auditing to improve quality of medical care in what he described as "end result analysis." Donabedian[42-44] expressed the differences between measures of quality of medical care based upon judging (1) input or structural characteristics, (2) process characteristics, and (3) outcome characteristics or results. For example, input characteristics include certification of professional health care providers, and process characteristics include adherence to accredited treatment procedures. It has been assumed that the quality of treatment results could be approximated by assuring conformity to standards according to input or process features, or both. With rising costs of medical care and other human service programs, it has become necessary to measure, or at least estimate, efficacy, effectiveness, and efficiency. Of course, none of these factors are measurable without agreement on the benefits of care that has been rendered. Determination of outcomes is not only more difficult than documenting input or process characteristics but is essential to do in order to measure benefits.

In the report of a study by the Institute of Medicine, in reference to long-term care it is stated that "methods for assessing the quality of care should include all sources of care and should consider the impact of care on the patient's expected and actual ability to function in daily life." It also stated that "an assessment of quality based on diagnostic-specific criteria is often inappropriate, and functional status is a more relevant measure."[45]

Two volumes are recommended to the reader on this topic—*Assessing and Improving Health Care Outcomes* by J. W. Williamson and *Health Program Evaluation* by S. M. Shortell and W. C. Richardson. Williamson[15] suggests the following operational definitions:

1. Efficacy: the extent to which health care intervention can be shown to be beneficial under optimal conditions of care.

2. Effectiveness: the extent to which benefits achievable under optimal conditions of care are actually achieved in clinical practice. (Lack of effectiveness would be identified when achievable benefits were not obtained.)

3. Efficiency: the proportion of total cost (e.g., money, scarce resources, and time) that can be related to actual benefits achieved.

He further suggests prerequisites for measuring outcomes:

1. Outcomes should be defined clearly and objectively, including the process used and the time duration of the process. (Broadly speaking, outcomes are not solely confined to patient function or health status but can encompass any aspect of the patient and the patient's health problems or of providers and their interactions. Choosing the most relevant outcome for measurement is a basic requirement.

2. A causal relationship between outcome and process should be made explicit and be analyzed for validity. (Reasonable attribution of outcome to the care provided should be noted, even though in most situations medical care is based upon implicit assumptions of causality. The validity of these

assumptions must be supported by reasonable evidence, including consideration of the several factors involved, such as compliance of the patient.)

3. The value of the outcome should be analyzed for helpful and harmful effects—for the individual and for the social group—within a given time and under given circumstances. (Since life is a continuum and its several phases are subject to intrinsic influences as well as any medical care interventions, the number of different outcomes is almost infinite. Therefore, the time range over which change is expected to occur must be specified.)

Williamson summarizes by stating "the first can be established by consensual definition; the second requires valid scientific evidence; and the third requires value clarification."

Shortell and Richardson[16] state that:

. . . attempting to evaluate a social program is at best risky and at worst treacherous. In few other activities are the ambivalent tendencies of society so clearly revealed. On the one hand is society's desire to learn more so that the quality of life may be improved, while on the other hand is the ubiquitous fear of what might be found.

They identify the following deficits that characterized early efforts to evaluate the process of service delivery:

1. Neglect of outcome measures of program effectiveness.

2. Use of objectives based on untested, unstated, and frequently erroneous assumptions.

3. Reliance on biased data and samples of unknown representation.

4. Failure to follow principles of sound experimental design.

5. Inadequate attention given to the accuracy, reliability, and validity of measurement.

6. Inability to draw causal inferences regarding program effects.

They summarize that:

. . . program evaluation helps to answer basic questions concerning whether the program is any good; helps to ensure accountability to oneself, one's staff and one's clients; helps to keep the emphasis on end-results; contributes to the development of analytical processes; promotes the training of staff, and fosters the development of professional attitudes and behavior.

The medical rehabilitation facility or any facility providing long-term care for the patient or client that uses a reliable and valid functional assessment method has a tool that will greatly assist in accomplishing quality assurance and program evaluation.

Techniques for Functional Assessment and Program Evaluation

The functional assessment must cull out appropriate descriptors (often by proxy) that address relevancies within the concepts of pathology, impairment, functional limitations, disability, and handicap as defined by Nagi[3, 4] and Wood.[5-7] Diagnosis of pathology is usually considered to be the linchpin of medical characterization and classification; however, it may not necessarily be the most important variable to describe various states of disability. As noted by Sherwood and co-workers,[46] diagnostic classification for those with chronic illness is not simple. Diagnostic data come from several sources—the physician, a hospital record, and the patient. The physician-specialist may emphasize certain terms and omit others more distant to the sphere of interest of that physician. Hospital data may be distorted by the need to satisfy third-party requirements for reimbursement. The patient may not be fully informed of important diagnoses, may have been supplied with euphemistic terms, or may have suppressed discomforting information. Diagnoses tend to wax and wane in importance with the passage of time; a stroke that occurred 20 years ago has different implications than one that occurred one month previously. As one condition appears, others may become less important or may be resolved. Diagnostic designations, therefore, often are not permanent, nor does the same diagnosis necessarily have the same implication in different circumstances. Identical diagnoses may have variable impacts on the patient; in the absence of assessment of functional status, that impact cannot be quantified. A diagnosis of rheumatoid arthritis may reflect mild stiffness in a few joints or total incapacitation, requiring a bed-to-chair existence. With regard to diagnostic terminology, one must realize the following points:

1. Diagnosis may be serving a labeling function rather than transmitting real information.

2. Severity and prognosis cannot be presumed from most diagnoses alone but may require accurate descriptions of functional status.

3. Psychosocial implications and needs consequent to diagnostic conditions may be entirely missed without supplying specific supplemental information.

4. Diagnostic terminology may not be relevant

TABLE 12–1. Uniform Data System Impairment-Group Codes

STROKE

01.	Unspecified
01.1	Left body involvement
01.2	Right body involvement
01.3	Bilateral involvement
01.4	Without paresis

BRAIN DYSFUNCTION

02.	Unspecified
02.1	Nontraumatic, unspecified
02.11	Toxins: Anoxic brain damage
02.12	Infections: Encephalitis
02.13	Tumors: Malignant or benign neoplasm of brain, cranial nerves, cerebral meninges
02.14	Other
02.2	Traumatic (open or closed not specified)
02.21	Traumatic, open injury
02.22	Traumatic, closed injury

NEUROLOGICAL CONDITIONS

03.	Unspecified
03.1	Infections; Guillain-Barré syndrome, acute neuropathy, poliomyelitis
03.2	Demyelinating: Multiple sclerosis
03.3	Neurological: Parkinson's disease, peripheral neuropathy
03.4	Degenerative: ALS, Friedreich's ataxia, muscular dystrophy
03.5	Other

SPINAL CORD DYSFUNCTION

04.	Unspecified
04.1	Nontraumatic (paraplegia or quadriplegia, complete or incomplete not specified)
04.11	Nontraumatic paraplegia (complete or incomplete not specified)
04.111	Nontraumatic paraplegia, incomplete
04.112	Nontraumatic paraplegia, complete
04.12	Nontraumatic quadriplegia (complete or incomplete not specified)
04.121	Nontraumatic quadriplegia, incomplete
04.122	Nontraumatic quadriplegia, complete
04.2	Traumatic (paraplegia or quadriplegia complete or incomplete not specified—due to fracture, surgical, gunshot)
04.21	Traumatic paraplegia (complete or incomplete not specified)
04.211	Traumatic paraplegia, incomplete
04.212	Traumatic paraplegia, complete
04.22	Traumatic quadriplegia (complete or incomplete not specified)
04.221	Traumatic quadriplegia, incomplete
04.222	Traumatic quadriplegia, complete

AMPUTATION OF LIMB

05.	Unspecified
05.1	Single upper AE*
05.2	Single upper BE*
05.3	Single lower AK*
05.4	Single lower BK*
05.5	Double AK/AK
05.6	Double AK/BK
05.7	Double BK/BK
05.8	Other combinations

ARTHRITIS

06.	Unspecified
06.1	Rheumatoid
06.2	Osteoarthritis
06.3	Other

PAIN SYNDROMES

07.	Unspecified
07.1	Neck pain
07.2	Back pain
07.3	Extremity pain
07.4	Abdominal pain
07.5	Pelvic pain
07.6	Facial pain
07.7	Headache
07.8	Other pain

ORTHOPEDIC CONDITIONS

08.	Unspecified (fractures, bone or joint replacements)

CARDIAC CONDITIONS

09.	Unspecified (hypertension, CHF,* arrhythmia, congenital)

PULMONARY CONDITIONS

10.	Unspecified (bronchitis, emphysema, asthma, COPD*)

BURNS

11.	Unspecified

CONGENITAL DEFORMITIES

12.	Unspecified (CP,* spina bifida)
13.	Unspecified

*AE = above the elbow, BE = below the elbow, AK = above the knee, and BK = below the knee, CHF = congestive heart failure, COPD = chronic obstructive pulmonary disease, and CP = cerebral palsy.

to the cluster of problems to be resolved from the perspective of functions of daily living.

The standard International Classification of Diseases, 9th Revision—Clinical Modification (ICD9–CM)[47] coding is widely used by hospital medical record departments to describe the pathology and etiologies of various conditions and is sometimes useful to identify impairments. Wood[7] has proposed an exhaustive classification scheme that details each of the three concepts of impairment, disability, and handicap that he has outlined. These proposals to supplement the International Classification of Diseases are intended as a way to code data to reduce the amount of detail of a case into a standardized numerical form. This would facilitate retrieval of records and analysis of statistical data. The UDSMR uses a coding system for major impairments to identify types of organic deficits that are mainly responsible for the patient's need for rehabilitation or long-term care. A version of the classification system for coding the impairment groups is shown in Table 12–1.

Aggregated data representing all patients served by a rehabilitation facility may be displayed in many different ways. Such a display should be useful for understanding the performance of a rehabilitation program and would be doubly useful if it also met the requirements for program evaluation. The key elements of program evaluation are a written statement of purpose for the facility and knowledge of the program's specific goals and objectives. The objectives must be measurable and must be related to intake, process, and results. The Commission on Accreditation of Rehabilitation Facilities (CARF) requires that accredited facilities have an ongoing system of program evaluation.[48]

Program evaluation measures the results achieved by patients after they have received the services of the rehabilitation program. By a process of consensus among members of the facility staff, measurable objectives must be determined and a standard value set for each objective. The next step is to assign a weight value to each objective, apportioned in such a way that the sum of the weight values equals 100. It is important to realize that the assignment of standard values to the objective and the weighted scores is arbitrary and is not arrived at scientifically (at least not in this stage of development). Nevertheless, an illustration of the methodology is presented to reflect results at discharge; a more advanced modification will incorporate follow-up data to reflect results some time after receipt of services (Tables 12–2 and 12–3).

For the program evaluation model, four measurable objectives have been designated: (1) returning a high percentage of patients back to the community, (2) significantly improving the functional independence of patients, (3) successfully serving severely disabled patients, and (4) accomplishing program goals in the shortest time possible. The first objective rewards returning a high percentage of patients back to the community. The second objective rewards significantly improving the functional independence of patients. The third objective rewards successfully serving the severely disabled. The objective is attained, for example, if one half of the patients admitted have FIM scores <71 and one half of those with the lower FIM scores on admission are discharged with FIM scores >70. The fourth objective rewards accomplishing the goals in the shortest length of stay.

The data in the model are simulated. "HOSPX" not only may be compared with a standard index but also compared with a simultaneous sample of "ALL" hospitals. EXPECTANCIES are the values that are arbitrarily set to meet program objectives. ACTUAL means the actual values for the

TABLE 12–2. Measurable Objectives for Program Evaluation for the Uniform Data System for Medical Rehabilitation

---

1. Maximize number of discharges to the community.

2. Maximize ratio of effectiveness of rehabilitation of each patient.

3. Maximize rehabilitation of severely disabled patients by evaluating the change of the FIM scores of the program:

ADD
Per cent admission FIM scores < 71
and
Per cent discharge FIM scores > 70

SUBTRACT
Per cent admission FIM scores > 70
and
Per cent discharge FIM scores < 71

and MULTIPLY by TWO (2)

As a formula, it appears as:
(per cent adm FIM < 71 + per cent dis FIM > 70)

− (per cent adm FIM > 70 + per cent dis FIM < 71) × 2

= Functional improvement index for the severely disabled.

4. Minimize length of stay

FIM = Functional Independence Measurement

CARL V. GRANGER

TABLE 12–3. Values Used in the Program Evaluation Model for the Uniform Data System
for Medical Rehabilitation*

PROGRAM OBJECTIVES	EXPECTANCIES†	ACTUAL‡		PER CENT OF EXPECTANCIES§		WEIGHT‖	PERFORMANCE INDEX¶	
		HOSPX	All	HOSPX	All		HOSPX	All
1. Patients discharged to the community	80	85	76	1.06	.95	40	42.4	38
2. Effectiveness	.2	.14	.22	.70	1.10	20	14	22
3. Severely disabled	100	40	125	.40	1.25	20	8	25
4. Length of stay	32	36	28	.89	1.14	20	17.8	22.8
TOTALS						100	82.2	107.8

*Values in this table are simulated.
†EXPECTANCIES are the values that are arbitrarily set to meet program objectives.
‡ACTUAL means the actual values for the objectives.
§PER CENT OF EXPECTANCIES is the ACTUAL value divided by the EXPECTANCY, except for the fourth objective (length of stay), which is EXPECTANCY divided by ACTUAL.
‖WEIGHTs are arbitrarily assigned according to priorities of the objectives.
¶PERFORMANCE INDEX is the PER CENT OF EXPECTANCY multiplied by the WEIGHT.

objectives. PER CENT OF EXPECTANCIES is the ACTUAL value divided by the EXPECTANCY, except for the fourth objective (length of stay), which is EXPECTANCY divided by ACTUAL. WEIGHTs are arbitrarily assigned according to priorities of the objectives. The PERFORMANCE INDEX is the PER CENT OF EXPECTANCY multiplied by the WEIGHT.

For the first objective, the performance index exceeded the standard weight for HOSPX but did not meet it for ALL. For the second to the fourth objectives, the performance indexes did not meet the standard weights for HOSPX but exceeded them for ALL. The cumulative performance index did not meet the standard of 100 for HOSPX (82.2) but exceeded it for ALL (107.8). The program evaluation model provides a succinct display of the performance of HOSPX in comparison with ALL hospitals, using a few basic objectives. The format is easy to read, and the analysis can be repeated for comparison over time.

When an evaluation system of a program is first begun, initial results may be disappointing. However, with continued use and increased staff experience, the facility should soon approach maximum results. A program that is both effective and efficient in achieving its goals is beneficial to the patients served by that rehabilitation facility. The patients achieve significant improvements following discharge. Also, with program evaluation it is possible to have a meaningful presentation of a report that reflects the total program effort. The

report measures actual results against expected objectives. In this way, it becomes an invaluable tool for the manager of the facility. The person making the decisions needs information, and this method provides the raw material for decisions and actions. The manager will know whether or not a program is achieving its objectives, and any possible problem areas are highlighted. The facility that can show better information on results achieved can successfully compete for the limited monies that are available to conduct rehabilitation service programs. That facility is in a better position to justify, maintain, or expand funding and to gain community support.

This type of evaluation method is based upon outcomes of care and provides a measure of benefits derived from medical rehabilitation. Given data of this type about a facility, the managers and staff of a facility have the means to objectively study effectiveness and efficiency, monitor quality of care in an ongoing and complete fashion, and obtain objective data to support decisions for improving care or for containing costs.

References

1. Weed, L.: Medical Records, Medical Education and Patient Care. Cleveland, Case Western Reserve University, 1970.
2. Weed, L.: Medical records that guide and teach. N. Engl. J. Med., 278:593–600, 652–657, 1968.
3. Nagi, S. Z.: Disability concepts and prevalence.

Mershon Center, Ohio State University. Presented at the First Mary Switzer Memorial Seminar, Cleveland, Ohio, May, 1975.

4. Nagi, S. Z.: An epidemiology of disability among adults in the United States. Milbank Q., 54(4):439–467, 1976.

5. Wood, P. H. N., and Badley, E. M.: An epidemiological appraisal of disablement. *In* Bennett, A. E. (Ed.): Recent Advances in Community Medicine. Edinburgh, Churchill Livingstone, 1978.

6. Wood, P. H. N., and Badley, E. M.: Setting disablement in perspective. Int. Rehabil. Med., 1:32–37, 1978.

7. World Health Organization (WHO): International Classification of Impairments, Disabilities, and Handicaps. Geneva, World Health Organization, 1980, p. 184.

8. Stewart, A., Ware, J. E., and Brook, R. H.: The meaning of health: Understanding functional limitations. Medical Care, 15:939–952, 1977.

9. Stewart, A., Ware, J. E., and Brook, R. H.: The meaning of health: Understanding functional limitations. Unpublished manuscript.

10. Ware, J. E.: Health status scales for evaluation of medical outcomes. Health Serv. Res., 11:396–415, 1976.

11. Kovar, M. G., and LaCroix, A. Z.: Aging in the eighties, ability to perform work-related activities. Data from the Supplement on Aging to the National Health Interview Survey, United States, 1984. Advance Data From Vital and Health Statistics. No. 136. DHHS Pub. No. (PHS) 87–1250. Public Health Service. Hyattsville, MD., National Center for Health Statistics, May 8, 1987.

12. Donaldson, S. W., Wagner, C. C., and Gresham, G. E.: Unified ADL evaluation form. Arch. Phys. Med. Rehabil., 54:175–179, 185, 1973.

13. Jones, E. W.: Patient Classification for Long-term Care: User's Manual. DHEW Publication No. HRA 74–3107, Washington, D.C., U.S. Government Printing Office, 1973.

14. Granger, C. V., and Greer, D. S.: Functional status measurement and medical rehabilitation outcomes. Arch. Phys. Med. Rehabil., 57:103–109, 1976.

15. Williamson, J. W.: Assessing and Improving Health Care Outcomes: The Health Accounting Approach to Quality Assurance. Cambridge, Mass., Ballinger Publishing Company, 1978.

16. Shortell, S. M., and Richardson, W. C.: Health Program Evaluation. St. Louis, C. V. Mosby Company, 1978.

17. Deaver, G. G., and Brown, M. E.: Physical Demands of Daily Life. New York, Institute for the Crippled and Disabled, 1945.

18. Lawton, E. B.: Activities of Daily Living for Physical Rehabilitation. New York, McGraw-Hill Book Company, 1963.

19. Katz, S., Downs, T. D., Cash, H. R., et al.: Progress in development of index of ADL. Gerontologist, 10:20–30, 1970.

20. Mahoney, F. I., and Barthel, D. W.: Functional evaluation: Barthel index. Md. State Med. J., 14:61–65, 1965.

21. Schoening, H. A., and Iversen, I. A.: Numerical scoring of self-care status: A study of Kenny self-care evaluation. Arch. Phys. Med. Rehabil., 49:221–229, 1968.

22. Sarno, J. E., Sarno, M. T., and Levitz, E.: The functional life scale. Arch. Phys. Med. Rehabil., 54:214–220, 1973.

23. Moskowitz, E., and McCann, C. B.: Classification of disability in the chronically ill and aging. J. Chronic Dis., 5:324–346, 1957.

24. Fortinsky, R. H., Granger, C. V., and Seltzer, G. B.: The use of functional assessment in understanding home care needs. Medical Care, 19:489–497, 1981.

25. Breckenridge, K.: Medical rehabilitation program evaluation. Arch. Phys. Med. Rehabil., 59:419–423, 1978.

26. Grauer, H., and Birnbom, F.: A geriatric functional rating scale to determine the need for institutional care. J. Am. Geriatrics Soc., 23:472–476, 1975.

27. Duke University Center for the Study of Aging and Human Development: Multidimensional functional assessment. The OARS methodology, 2nd Ed. Durham, N. C., Duke University, 1978.

28. Muzzio, T. C., and Burris, C. T.: Functional Limitations: A State of the Art Review. 1979 Indices Inc., 5827 Columbia Pike, Falls Church, VA 22041.

29. Granger, C. V., Hamilton, B. B., Keith, R. A., Zielezny, M., and Sherwin, F. S.: Advances in functional assessment for medical rehabilitation. Top. Geriatr. Rehabil., 1(3):59–74, 1986.

30. Keith, R. A., Granger, C. V., Hamilton, B. B., and Sherwin, F. S.: The functional independence measure: a new tool for rehabilitation. *In* Eisenberg, M. G., and Grzesiak, R. C. (Eds): Advances in Clinical Rehabilitation. New York, Springer-Verlag, 1987, p. 6–18.

31. Hamilton, B. B., Granger, C. V., Sherwin, F. S., Zielezny, M., and Tashman, J. S.: A uniform national data system for medical rehabilitation. *In* Fuhrer, M. J. (Ed): Rehabilitation Outcomes: Analysis and Measurement. Baltimore, Brookes, 1987, p. 137–147.

32. Data Management Service: Guide for the use of the Uniform Data Set for Medical Rehabilitation. The Buffalo General Hospital/State University of New York at Buffalo, September 1, 1987.

33. Kottke, F. J.: Philosophical Considerations of Quality of Life for the Disabled. Arch. Phys. Med. Rehabil., 63:60–62, 1982.

34. Granger, C. V., Kaplan, M., Barrett, J., and Lunger, D.: Trends in outcome analysis: A program evaluation model. *In* Proceedings of the Seminar on

Medical Rehabilitation Model Delivery Systems. February 23–24, 1978, Association of Rehabilitation Facilities, 5530 Wisconsin Ave., Suite 955, Wash., D.C. 20015.

35. Granger, C. V., Greer, D. S., Liset, E., Coulombe, J., and O'Brien, E.: Measurement of outcomes of care for stroke patients. Stroke, 6:34–41, 1975.

36. Scranton, J. A., Fogel, M. L., and Erdman, W. J., II: Evaluation of functional levels of patients during and following rehabilitation. Arch. Phys. Med. Rehabil., 51:1–21, 1970.

37. Eggert, G. M., Granger, C. V., Morris, R., and Pendleton, S. F.: Caring for the patient with long-term disability. Geriatrics, 32:102–114, 1977.

38. Lehmann, J. F., Delateur, B. J., Fowler, R. S., et al.: Stroke rehabilitation: Outcome and prediction. Arch. Phys. Med. Rehabil., 56:383–389, 1975.

39. Kerstein, M. D., Zimmer, H., Dugdale, F. E., and Lerner, E.: What influence does age have on rehabilitation of amputees? Geriatrics, 30:67–71, 1975.

40. Granger, C. V., Sherwood, C. C., and Greer, D. S.: Functional status measures in a comprehensive stroke care program. Arch. Phys. Med. Rehabil., 58:555–561, 1977.

41. Codman, E. A.: A Study in Hospital Efficiency: As Demonstrated by the Case Report of the First Five Years of a Private Hospital. Boston, Thomas Todd Company, 1916. (This work was reproduced in 1972 by University Microfilms, Ann Arbor, MI.) See also Christoffel, J. D.: Medical care evaluation: An old new idea. Hosp. Med. Staff, 5(10):11–16, 1976.

42. Donabedian, A.: A Guide to Medical Administration, Volume II: Medical Care Appraisal—Quality and Utilization. New York (now Washington): American Public Health Association, 1969. (176 pages plus Annotated Selected Bibliography by A. J. Anderson.)

43. Donabedian, A.: Needed Research in the Assessment and Monitoring of Quality of Medical Care. DHEW publication No. (PHS) 78–3219. Research Report Series, 1978.

44. Donabedian, A.: Evaluating the quality of medical care. Milbank Memorial Fund Quarterly, 44(Suppl.):166–206, 1966.

45. Institute of Medicine: Assessing Quality in Health Care: An Evaluation. National Academy of Science, Washington, D.C., 1976.

46. Sherwood, S., Greer, D. S., Morris, J. N., Mor, V., et al.: An Alternative to Institutionalization: The Highland Heights Experiment. Cambridge, MA, Ballinger Publishing Company, 1981, p. 86.

47. International Classification of Diseases, 9th Edition—Clinical Modification (ICD9–CM). Commission on Professional and Hospital Activities, Ann Arbor, MI, 48105, July, 1978.

48. Commission on Accreditation of Rehabilitation Facilities: Program Evaluation in Inpatient Medical Rehabilitation Facilities. Tucson, Arizona, 1979.

13

Diathermy and Superficial Heat, Laser, and Cold Therapy

JUSTUS F. LEHMANN
BARBARA J. DE LATEUR

Therapeutic Heat

The following discussion is limited to local applications of heat. The various types of heating modalities used in therapy can be subdivided into those that heat the superficial tissues and those that heat the deeper structures (Table 13–1). They can also be subdivided according to the primary modes of heat transfer into the tissues, which are conduction, convection, and the conversion of other forms of energy into heat by absorption. Heat therapy by conversion of other forms of energy includes radiant heat and the three deep-heating modalities: short waves, microwaves, and ultrasound. Not every modality that heats by conversion is a deep-heating modality. It should be noted that radiant heat is a superficial heating agent in spite of the fact that it heats by converting photons into heat by absorption. However, the photons penetrate only into the more superficial layers of the tissues. Although all heating modalities produce the desirable therapeutic responses primarily by temperature elevation, the rationale for their use is derived from the fact that they selectively heat different areas in the body, with the peak temperatures in different locations. Therapeutic heat application is not a cure for any one of the indications for which it is used but is, rather, a valuable adjunct to other therapies if properly used with adequate equipment

TABLE 13–1. Therapeutic Heating Modalities*

PRIMARY MODE OF HEAT TRANSFER	MODALITY	DEPTH
Conduction	Hot packs Paraffin bath	Superficial Heat
Convection	Fluidotherapy Hydrotherapy Moist air	Superficial Heat
Conversion	Radiant heat Laser	Superficial Heat
	Microwaves Short waves Ultrasound	Deep heat

*From Lehmann, J. F., and de Lateur, B. J.: Therapeutic heat. *In* Lehmann, J. F. (Ed.): Therapeutic Heat and Cold, 3rd Ed. Baltimore, Williams & Wilkins, 1982.

Factors Determining the Extent of Biological Reactions

The temperature of the tissues is a most important factor in the physiological response to heat. Figure 13–1 shows the percentage of hyperemia plotted against the tissue temperature measured in a series of 560 experimental animals.[184] The duration of the tissue temperature elevation was kept constant. Below a certain temperature threshold, no reactions were observed. The curve of reactions is S-shaped, with the most rapid increase in reactions in the mid-range. In the upper portion of the curve, destructive changes are inevitably associated

JUSTUS F. LEHMANN AND BARBARA J. DE LATEUR

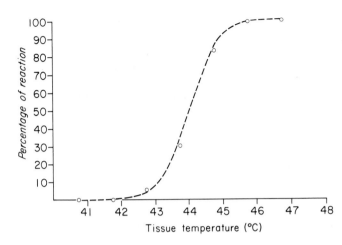

FIGURE 13–1. Dependence of hyperemia on tissue temperature. (From Lehmann, J. F.: The biophysical basis of biologic ultrasonic reactions with special reference to ultrasonic therapy. Arch. Phys. Med. Rehabil., 34:139–152, 1953.)

with the therapeutically desirable hyperemia. Thus, the therapeutic temperature range is a rather narrow one and extends in this particular reaction from approximately 43° C (109.4° F) to 45° C (113° F). It is apparent that, within the therapeutic range, a minor change in tissue temperature produces a major change in the degree of the physiological response and that the margin of effectiveness and safety is narrow. In order to produce a limited response, it is necessary to obtain tissue temperatures in the lower portion of the curve; if vigorous effects are desired, the temperatures have to be within the upper half of the effective range. Thus, the control of the technique of application and the use of available dosimetry are essential for success in the therapeutic situation.

In a similar type of experiment, it was found that the duration of the tissue temperature elevation was important in determining the extent of the biological reaction (Fig. 13–2).[184] For this reaction, a minimal effective duration of exposure was five minutes, whereas maximal reactions were obtained after exposure of approximately 30 minutes. The tissue temperature was kept constant throughout the experiment.

The rate of temperature increase also played a role in determining the extent of biological responses. Depending on the rate of increase, effective temperature levels will be reached sooner or later. Thus, a modality that rapidly raises the temperature to biologically effective levels will produce a more pronounced effect than a modality that raises the tissue temperature more slowly, provided that both modalities are applied over the same period of time.

In addition, it has been noted that some responses of temperature receptors seem to be more pronounced when the rate of the tissue tempera-

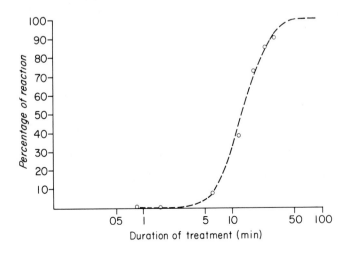

FIGURE 13–2. Dependence of hyperemia on duration of treatment. (From Lehmann, J. F.: The biophysical basis of biologic ultrasonic reactions with special reference to ultrasonic therapy. Arch. Phys. Med. Rehabil., 34:139–152, 1953.)

ture change is rapid.[67, 68, 134, 135, 191] The extent of reflex phenomena may also depend on the size of the area treated.[96]

In summary, the major factors determining the number and intensity of the physiological reactions to heat are

1. The level of tissue temperature. The approximate therapeutic range extends from 40 to 45.5° C (104 to 113.9° F).

2. The duration of the tissue temperature elevation. The approximate therapeutic range is 3 to 30 minutes.

3. The rate of temperature rise in the tissues.

4. The size of the area treated.

Physiological Effects of Therapeutic Significance

General Indications and Contraindications

In general, the physiological responses that are accepted as a basis for the most common therapeutic application of heat are as follows:

1. Heat increases the extensibility of collagen tissue.

2. Heat decreases joint stiffness.

3. Heat produces pain relief.

4. Heat relieves muscle spasm.

5. Heat increases blood flow.

6. Heat assists in the resolution of inflammatory infiltrates, edema, and exudates.

7. Heat has been used as part of cancer therapy.

Special safeguards must be observed when heat is applied. Heat application is either contraindicated or should be used with special precautions over anesthetized areas or in an obtunded patient. For most heat therapy, the sensation of pain is a warning signal that safe limits have been exceeded. In the absence of pain sensation, dosimetry is not accurate enough in most of the modalities to reliably avoid excessive temperatures. Heating of tissues with inadequate vascular supply is contraindicated, since the elevation of the temperature increases metabolic demand without adequate vascular response. The result may be an ischemic necrosis. Any bleeding tendency is markedly increased by heating because of the increase of blood flow and vascularity. If one suspects the presence of malignancy in the area to be heated, one generally should not apply heat, since temperatures below those therapeutic for cancer may accelerate

tumor growth[130] or increase the likelihood of formation of metastases resulting from the increase of blood flow and vascularity. At temperatures of 44 to 45° C, Child and co-workers[47] did not find an increase in the formation of metastases; these temperatures were produced by ultrasound application for 5 to 10 minutes. Also, heating of the gonads or the developing fetus should be avoided.*

Local Effects

Local effects are produced partly through a direct effect of the elevated temperature on the tissues. These physiological responses may occur to varying degrees, depending on the conditions of heating. In part, they are produced by direct action of the temperature elevation on tissue and cellular function, by the production and accumulation of metabolites and carbon dioxide, by the reduction of oxygen tension, and by the production of histamine-like substances and bradykinin. Temperature receptors may play an important role.[96]

With heat, there is a marked alteration of the physical properties of fibrous tissues as found in tendons, joint capsules, and scars;[103] these tissues yield much more readily to stretch when heated.[214] This effect is illustrated in Figure 13–3. In this experiment, the tendon was loaded with 73 gm in a 25° C (77° F) bath. The length of the tendon was maintained, and the tension decreased slightly. When the temperature of the bath changed from 25° C to 45° C (113° F), the tension deteriorated rapidly. Figure 13–4 shows the residual increase in length when various loads were applied at 45° C. It shows clearly that at 45° C a marked increase in length could be obtained, which increased in proportion to the load. Heat alone, without stretch, did not produce any length increase. In contrast to this, the controls at 25° C did not show such an elongation. It can be concluded, therefore, that heating produces a greater extensibility of fibrous collagen tissues. The optimal condition for obtaining this effect is the combination of heat and stretch application. Prolonged, steady stretch is more effective than intermittent or short-term stretch. This is of great significance in the management of joint contractures, as they occur as a result of tightness of the joint capsule and ligaments or fibrosis of muscle and scarring.

---

*See references 64, 65, 82–84, 105, 129, 243, 250, 256, 310.

JUSTUS F. LEHMANN AND BARBARA J. DE LATEUR

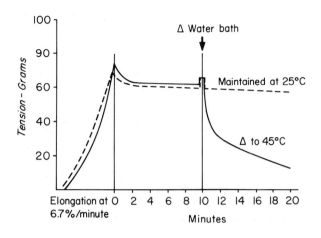

FIGURE 13–3. The effect of temperature elevation on tendon extensibility. (From Lehmann, J. F., Masock, A. J., Warren, C. G., and Koblanski, J. N.: Effect of therapeutic temperatures on tendon extensibility. Arch. Phys. Med. Rehabil., 51:481–487, 1970.)

Investigations by Bäcklund and Tiselius[13] and by Wright and Johns[157, 358, 359] have shown that the subjective complaints of stiffness on the part of the patient with rheumatoid arthritis coincide with changes in the measurements of the viscoelastic properties of joints.[13] The joint stiffness, assessed both subjectively and by objective measurement, could be influenced by treatment with drugs such as cortisone and by physical therapy such as the application of heat and cold. Heat application markedly decreases stiffness and the patient's dis-

comfort. Cold application increases stiffness and the patient's complaints.

Use of heat to relieve pain in a large variety of musculoskeletal conditions is widespread and empirically based.[2, 66, 126] In some cases, pain may be relieved by reducing the secondary muscle spasms. In tension syndromes, pain allegedly is related to ischemia, which, in turn, can be improved by the hyperemia that heat application produces. Heat has also been applied as a "counterirritant," that is, the thermal stimulus may affect pain sensation

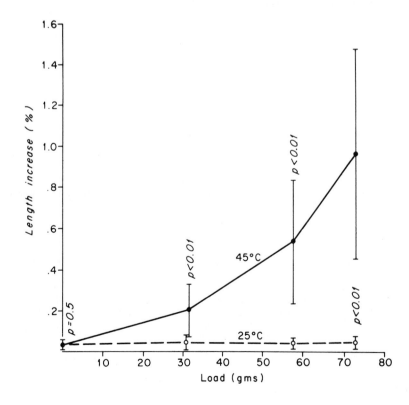

FIGURE 13–4. Residual tendon length as measured after loading at the indicated levels of 45° C and 25° C baths. (From Lehmann, J. F., Masock, A. J., Warren, C. G., and Koblanski, J. N.: Effect of therapeutic temperatures on tendon extensibility. Arch. Phys. Med. Rehabil., 51:481–487, 1970.)

as explained by the gate theory of Melzack and Wall.[241] Perhaps it could also be explained through the action of endorphins. Gammon and Starr[100] furnished limited support for the use of heat as a counterirritant. Heat ranked third in providing relief, as compared with other counterirritants. Application of heat to a peripheral nerve causes an increase in the pain threshold in the area supplied by the nerve without affecting the motor function. Also, one may elevate the pain threshold, as measured by the Hardy-Wolff-Goodell method,[125] by heating other tissues such as skin.[191]

Heating of tissues has been shown to affect the gamma fiber activity in muscle.[96] The resulting decrease in the sensitivity of the muscle spindle to stretch, as well as reflexes triggered through temperature receptors, may be the physiological basis for the clinically observed relaxation of muscle spasm following the use of heat. Mense[242] found that, in a prestretched muscle, warming increased the firing rate of the group 1A afferents. He distinguished between two types of secondary afferents; those with a high background discharge responded as the 1A afferents, whereas those with a low initial discharge rate showed a depression or cessation of firing by warming. The majority of the secondary endings showed the latter behavior when heated. Also, the Golgi tendon organs increased their firing rate when the temperature was increased. Therefore, one may speculate that if the secondary muscle spasm is a tonic phenomenon to a degree, the selective cessation of the firing from the secondary endings may reduce muscle tone, an effect that would be augmented by the greater inhibitory impulses from the Golgi tendon organs. Petajan and Eagan[271] showed that when heat was applied by external means with a resultant rise in muscle temperature, the relaxation time of the ankle jerk was decreased and little change in the rise time was noted. These observations extended only to temperatures below 40° C (104° F). Black and co-workers[29] found that ultrasound had no effect on ankle dorsiflexion isokinetic contractions at dynamometer velocities of 60 degrees per sec and 180 degrees per sec.

The blood flow is increased owing to arteriolar and capillary dilatation. These physiological changes are produced by a direct effect of the temperature elevation and by reflex mechanisms.[1, 2, 58, 120, 152, 274, 300] The reflex mechanisms range from simple axon reflexes to complex phenomena occurring as part of the core temperature control. The rate of filtration and of diffusion across biological membranes is increased. Thus, there may be a greater capillary membrane permeability with a resulting escape of plasma proteins. Vigorous heating may result in cellular responses associated with an inflammatory reaction, ranging from mild to severe.[184, 185] As a result of the temperature elevation, tissue metabolism is initially increased. However, if temperatures are elevated extensively for a prolonged period of time, tissue metabolism may be decreased.[209, 268, 361] Associated with the changes in metabolic rate are changes in enzyme reactions.[96] These may be speeded up by moderate tissue temperature elevation and gradually may be abolished at higher temperatures. This may be explained by the fact that the rate of chemical reaction is increased by temperature elevation, whereas the protein component of the enzyme system is destroyed at higher temperatures. Proteins may be denatured, and the resulting products, such as polypeptides and histamine-like substances, may in turn become biologically active.

A detailed review of hyperthermia as part of cancer therapy is presented elsewhere.[261] In malignancies, hyperthermia is primarily used in combination with other forms of therapy, for instance, where it increases the effectiveness of ionizing radiation or reduces the radiation dose required to obtain the same results. Figure 13–5 may serve as an example of this.

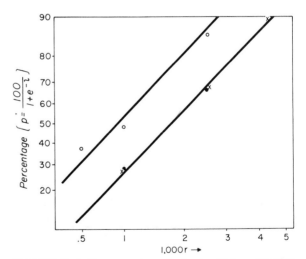

FIGURE 13–5. The percentage of mice in which a regression of tumor growth occurred is plotted against the dose of x-rays (scale according to Berkson[16]). Each point represents the percentage in 30 to 50 animals. Key: x's, treated with x-rays only; circles, treated with ultrasonic energy at 30° C and x-rays; and dots, treated with ultrasonic energy at 5 to 10° C and x-rays. (From Lehmann, J. F., and Krusen, F. H.: Biophysical effects of ultrasonic energy on carcinoma and their possible significance. Arch. Phys. Med. Rehabil., 36:452–459, 1955.)

JUSTUS F. LEHMANN AND BARBARA J. DE LATEUR

This brief review of the most significant local reactions to heat application indicates not only that a large number of physiological responses can be elicited but also that many of them can be produced to any desired degree, that is, vigorous responses can be readily produced.

Reactions Occurring Distant from the Site of Tissue Temperature Elevation

Reactions distant from the site of tissue temperature elevation are usually produced by elevating the surface temperature of the body.

If the skin of one part of the body (e.g., over one extremity) is heated, a consensual response in terms of blood flow increase is observed in other parts of the body (e.g., the opposite extremity). The consensual reaction is always less pronounced than the local response to heat application, and its intensity is dependent on the size of the area treated,[96] that is, on the extent of neural input.

If the skin is heated without heating the muscle, the vessels of the musculature beneath show no increase in diameter or may even show vasoconstriction,[96] which is consistent with the body temperature regulatory mechanism that diverts the flow to the skin for heat exchange and reduces flow to inactive organs.

If the skin of the abdominal wall is heated, it has been observed that a blanching of the gastric mucosa occurs and gastric acidity is reduced.

Relaxation of the smooth musculature of the gastrointestinal tract during the application of superficial heat has also been observed. This is evidenced by a decrease in peristalsis,[28, 96] which is the basis for relief of gastrointestinal cramps. Also, smooth musculature of the uterus relaxes, which in turn reduces menstrual cramps.

Heating of the superficial tissues produces marked relaxation of the skeletal muscles, and even protective muscle spasms may be resolved. The reaction may be reflex in nature and triggered by the effect on the temperature receptors in the skin. In addition, it has been shown[96] that stimulation of the skin in the neck region decreases gamma fiber activity, resulting in a decreased spindle excitability. This could explain why superficial heating agents decrease muscle spasm. Heating of the skin may have a psychological component as well.[96]

Some reactions may be produced by an elevation of the core temperature of the body, which in turn produces all those reactions commonly found as part of the mechanism regulating body temperature. Heat also has been applied as a counterirritant stimulus to the skin to provide pain relief. Again, the explanation for the pain relief may be based on the gate theory of Melzack and Wall[241] or on the action of endorphins.[100]

In summary, thermal reactions occurring distant from the site of temperature elevation are limited in number, site, and extent. They are always less pronounced than the corresponding reactions occurring locally at the site of temperature elevation.

Vigorous Versus Mild Heating

If vigorous heating effects are therapeutically desirable, the highest temperature must be produced at the site of the pathological lesion. Thus, vigorous local responses can be utilized. The tissue temperature is elevated close to tolerance level; the effective elevation of the tissue temperature is maintained for a relatively long period of time, and the rate of rise of the tissue temperature is rapid.

With mild heating, a relatively small temperature elevation is obtained in the tissues at the site of the pathological lesion, or the highest temperature is produced in a tissue that is superficial to, and therefore distant from, the site of the lesion. Effective local tissue temperature is usually maintained for a relatively short period of time, and the rate of increase of temperature in the tissues is often slow.

Vigorous heating is appropriately used for chronic disease processes. Mild heating may be used in subacute disease processes. The following examples may illustrate the use of vigorous heating versus mild heating. Vigorous heating is used for treatment of joint contractures when scarring and tightening of the joint capsule and the periarticular structures have occurred. It will increase the temperature in the scar tissues to a level at which they become more extensible and thus more amenable to therapy designed to increase the range of motion. However, with an acute synovial inflammatory response, such as occurs in rheumatoid arthritis, vigorous and selective heating of the area can aggravate the condition. Chronic pelvic inflammatory disease represents another indication for vigorous heating.[173, 174, 280] A marked increase in vascularity is produced that may assist in the resolution of the pathological process or may render antibiotic therapy more effective. On the other hand, vigorous heating is contraindicated in an acute inflammatory process, since it will superimpose another inflammatory reaction that ultimately may lead to undesirable effects, such as tissue necrosis or perforation of an abscess into the abdominal cavity.[302]

An example of a mechanical problem is an acutely protruded intervertebral disk impinging upon a nerve root in the intervertebral foramen. This condition represents a contraindication to vigorous heating, since any marked temperature elevation at the site of the encroachment will produce an increase in vascularity and edema, which are space-occupying processes and may aggravate the symptoms. On the other hand, superficial heating with resulting relief of secondary muscle spasm may subjectively benefit the patient without changing the pathological condition at the level of the nerve root.

Selection of Modality

In order to produce vigorous heating, the tissue temperature must be elevated close to tolerance levels at the site of the pathological lesion. This means that one must select the modality that will produce the highest temperature at the site of the lesion without exceeding tolerance levels in either the overlying or the underlying tissues. In order to select the proper modality for this purpose, it is important to know the temperature distribution produced by the available heating devices. In order to use the proper techniques of application with the selected modality, the factors that may modify this tissue temperature distribution and the actual temperature levels obtained must be understood.

If mild heating is desired in the depth of the tissues, there is a choice among superficial heating agents, such as infrared radiation, hot packs, paraffin baths, and others that produce only mild reflex responses in the deeper tissues, and a deep-heating modality that is applied in such a way as to limit the rise of the tissue temperature to moderate levels at the site of the lesion. However, if small parts of the body such as the fingers are treated, even a superficial heating agent may produce a marked elevation of the temperatures in the deeper tissues, resulting in vigorous heating effects that may or may not be desirable, depending upon whether the lesion is chronic or acute.

Deep-Heating or Diathermy Modalities

For therapeutic purposes, diathermy is defined as deep heating.

Factors Determining Temperature Distribution

The relative amount of energy converted into heat at any given point throughout the tissues is important and is called the pattern of "relative heating." The amount of energy converted into heat at the level of the interface between the subcutaneous fat and the musculature or at the interface between the musculature and the bone is customarily set as one. The pattern of relative heating depends on factors that will be discussed for the individual diathermy modalities, since these factors vary from one deep-heating agent to another.

The tissue temperature distribution depends not only upon the pattern of "relative heating" but upon such tissue properties as specific heat as well. The temperature distribution is also modified by the thermal conductivity of the tissues if heating extends over a period of time long enough to allow for heat exchange to occur.

A temperature distribution thus produced in tissues of a live organism will finally be modified by physiological factors such as pre-existing temperature distribution and blood flow changes. Usually, the skin surface is relatively cool and the core temperature relatively high. Any temperature elevation produced by diathermy application is superimposed upon this pre-existing physiological temperature distribution. As diathermy is applied, an increase in the blood flow may occur locally as a result of the tissue temperature elevation; since the blood temperature is usually cooler than that of the heated tissue, the inflowing blood may act as a cooling agent. A modification of the temperature distribution can be produced in this fashion.

Short Wave Diathermy

EQUIPMENT

Short wave diathermy is the therapeutic application of high-frequency currents. In spite of many variations, short wave diathermy machines have three basic components of the circuitry that are

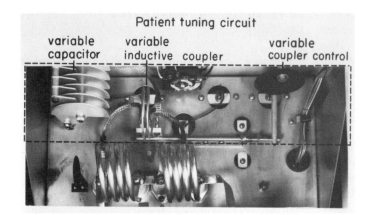

FIGURE 13–6. Patient tuning circuit of a typical short wave diathermy machine. (Courtesy of the Birtcher Corporation.)

common to all: power supply, oscillating circuit, and the patient's circuit. The frequency of the oscillating circuit, and thus that of the patient's circuit, is rigorously controlled to comply with the tolerance specified by the Federal Communications Commission (FCC). The frequencies that are allowed for short wave diathermy operations are 13.66, 27.33, and 40.98 MHz.[91] Wavelength is determined by the formula

$$\lambda = V/N$$

where λ is the wavelength, N is the frequency of oscillation, and V is the velocity of light. The wavelengths corresponding to the allowed frequencies are 22, 11, and 7.5 meters, respectively. Most of the commercially available diathermy machines operate at a frequency of 27.33 MHz and hence at a wavelength of 11 meters.

It is worth noting that in all machines, regardless of the technique of application, the patient's electrical impedance becomes part of the impedance of the patient's circuit. It is necessary for any given therapeutic application to retune the patient's circuit to resonance after the patient has been inserted into the circuit. Thus the frequency of the patient's circuit is made equal to the frequency of the oscillating circuit of the machine. Tuning is often accomplished by adjusting a variable capacitor (Figs. 13–6 and 13–7). The power meter on the panel of the machine will indicate maximal flow of current when the resonance frequency is obtained in the patient's circuit. The need for tuning has been eliminated in some machines by using an automatic device or by designing the machine so that the patient's electrical impedance has a negligible effect on the overall impedance of the patient's circuit. After the machine has been

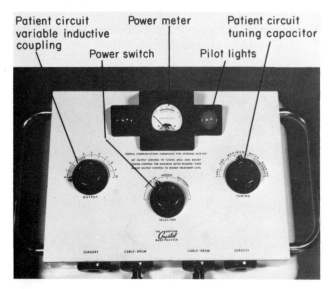

FIGURE 13–7. Typical control panel of a short wave diathermy machine. (Courtesy of the Birtcher Corporation.)

tuned, the current flow through the patient's circuit can be regulated. One way of doing this is to change the inductive coupling of the patient's and the high-frequency oscillating circuits.

The effectiveness of the equipment for deep-heating purposes largely depends on the quality of the mode of application, that is, application with induction coil or application with the condenser technique; the quality of the design of the applicator; and the various clinical modifications of the application. Lehmann and colleagues[215, 216] showed that the capability of the various induction coil applicators varies widely. The value of the deep-heating capability is best expressed by the ratio of the specific absorption rate (SAR) in muscle to SAR in fat. A larger ratio indicates better deep heating (Table 13–2). Electrostatic shielding of the applicator seems to produce better deep heating.

DOSIMETRY

At present, it is not possible to measure the high-frequency current flow through the body of the patient. The meter on the panel does not give this information. The dosimetry still depends largely on biological factors—the therapist is guided by the feeling of warmth on the part of the patient. When the dose applied is high, the patient's feeling of warmth goes up to tolerance; when the dose is medium, the patient feels comfortably warm; and when it is minimal, the patient just barely feels warmth. Although these are guidelines, it is obvious that they are unreliable for accurate dosimetry and depend on intact sensation and alertness on the part of the patient. However,

in the application of pelvic diathermy with an internal electrode, it is possible to obtain measurements of the biologically effective dose. Since the electrode is placed in the area of highest temperature elevation in the body, it rapidly assumes the tissue temperature owing to the high conductivity of the metal. Therefore, if a thermometer is inserted into the electrode, a reading of the tissue temperature elevation can be obtained. The duration of the tissue temperature elevation can be readily controlled by a timing device.

TECHNIQUES OF APPLICATION[298]

Condenser Technique

The affected part of the patient to be treated is placed between two capacitor plates. Four modifications of this technique are used: (1) Space plates are capacitor plates enclosed in rigid plastic material. A plastic ring surrounding the condenser plate is adjustable and provides proper spacing between body surface and condenser plates. (2) The capacitor plates are covered by a glass envelope. In order to avoid sweat accumulation and selective heating of the area, the glass cover should not be in direct contact with the skin. The position of the condenser plate within the glass envelope, and thus the distance between the body surface and the condenser plates, is adjustable. (3) The capacitor plates are flexible and are enclosed in rubber or plastic materials called condenser pads. Proper spacing between the skin and the electrode is provided by a 1- to 2-inch layer of terry cloth between the skin and the pads (Fig. 13–8). (4) Internal metal electrodes (Fig. 13–9) are inserted into the vagina or rectum after applying a water-soluble lubricant. The vaginal electrode is inserted so that the concave part comes to rest under the cervix and in the upper portion of the posterior fornix of the vagina. The rectal electrode is inserted to fit the slightly concave part over the prostate. A large belt-like electrode is applied over the abdomen, thus producing a high current density around the internal electrode. The largest internal electrodes that fit should be used so that complete contact is provided with the surrounding tissues. If the contact is partial, current concentrations may occur and lead to burns.

Techniques of Application to Specific Parts of the Body

—To the shoulder: Condenser plates may be used (Fig. 13–10).

—To the hip: The usual method is application with pads.

TABLE 13–2. Relative Heating Characteristics of Several Diathermy Applicators at 27.12 MHz*

| APPLICATOR | SAR MUSCLE/SAR FAT | |
	Peak Value	Average Value
Siemens Monode†	1.47	1.23
IME‡ round	1.83	1.75
IME pancake	2.15	2.29
IME square	2.27	2.67
IME Magnatherm 1000 head	1.41	1.48
Enraf Circuplode	1.48	1.58
ElMed Magnode*	0.39	0.39

*From Lehmann, J. F., McDougall, J. A., Guy, A. W., Warren, C. G., and Esselman, P. C.: Heating patterns produced by shortwave diathermy applicators in tissue substitute models. Arch. Phys. Med. Rehabil., 64:575–577, 1983.
†Applicator is not electrostatically shielded.
‡IME: International Medical Electronics.

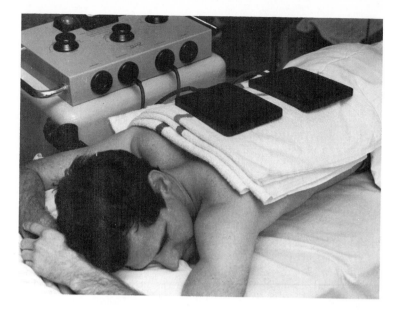

FIGURE 13–8. Short wave diathermy application with condenser pads to back, with spacing between skin and electrodes provided by layers of terry cloth.

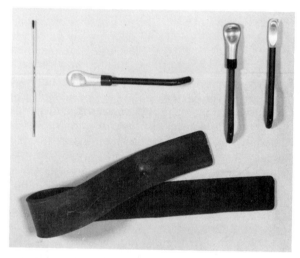

FIGURE 13–9. Internal vaginal and rectal electrodes with external belt and alcoholic thermometer. (Courtesy of the Burdick Corporation.)

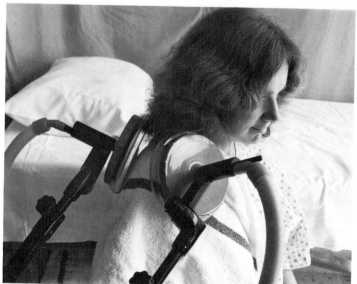

FIGURE 13–10. Condenser plates applied to the shoulder.

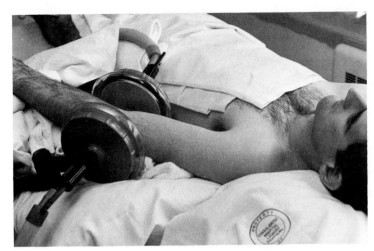

FIGURE 13–11. Condenser plates applied to the elbow.

—To the elbows, knees, ankles, arms, feet, and hands: Condenser plates and pads are commonly used (Figs. 13–11 and 13–12).

—To the hands: The method of choice is usually the application of condenser plates in the form of pads or space plates.

—To the back: Condenser plates or pads are used (see Fig. 13–8).

—To the neck: Condenser plates or pads are used.

—To the pelvic organs: The method of choice is application with internal electrodes.

The temperature elevation is measured with a thermometer inside the electrodes. Temperatures up to 45° C (113° F) have been recommended, and duration of application varies from 5 to 30 minutes. Often, it is advisable to start with a lower temperature and shorter duration and observe the tolerance of the patient. It is most important to realize that the more acute the process to be treated, the less the tissue temperature elevation should be and the shorter the duration of the treatment.

Induction Coil Application

Another mode of application is with the induction coil. The induction coil may be applied with the so-called "drum" (Fig. 13–13). The coil is enclosed in a plastic container that is flexible at the hinges and can be molded to fit the body. This plastic housing provides proper spacing between the skin and loops of the cable. Another applicator of this type is the "monode," which operates on the same basic principle but is not flexible (Fig. 13–14). Precautions should be taken to avoid direct contact between the plastic housing and the skin, since it interferes with the heat exchange. The result of direct contact application in human volunteers is shown in Figure 13–15, where the deepheating agent is converted into an agent that pro-

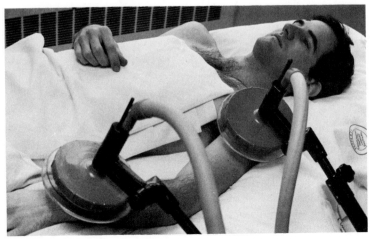

FIGURE 13–12. Short wave diathermy application to the arm with condenser plates. Spacing is provided by space plates.

JUSTUS F. LEHMANN AND BARBARA J. DE LATEUR

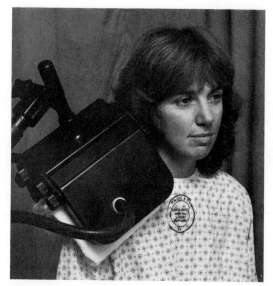

FIGURE 13–13. Short wave diathermy application with induction coil (drum applicator).

duces the highest temperature on the skin, whereas the same applicator with the appropriate air space of 2 cm between skin and plastic housing produces the highest temperatures in the superficial musculature (Fig. 13–16). A heavily insulated cable can be shaped to any desired form of applicator, such as the "pancake" coil (Fig. 13–17), or it may be wrapped around a joint (Fig. 13–18). Spacers are used to keep the loops apart. Special precautions must be taken to ensure that the cable turns do not cross each other; if this is inevitable, a special

separator must be inserted between the turns of the cable. In all these cases of cable application, the proper spacing between the skin and the loops of the cable is provided by an insertion of an approximately 2-inch thickness of terry cloth between the skin and the cable.

Techniques of Application to Specific Parts of the Body

—To the shoulder: The drum or monode may be used (see Fig. 13–13).

—To the elbows and knees: Wrap-around coils or the monode is used (see Fig. 13–18).

—To the hands and feet: The method of choice is usually the application of the monode or drum.

—To the back: The pancake coil or the drum is used (see Figs. 13–17 and 13–19).

—To the neck: The drum or monode (Fig. 13–20).

—To the hip: The drum or pancake coil.

—To the knees and ankles: Wrap-around coil.

TEMPERATURE DISTRIBUTION AS MODIFIED BY TECHNIQUE OF APPLICATION

For both the condenser type and induction coil applications, the specific absorption rate (H) is proportional to the square of the induced electrical current (I) and inversely proportional to the electrical conductivity of the tissues (G).[293]

$$H = I^2/G$$

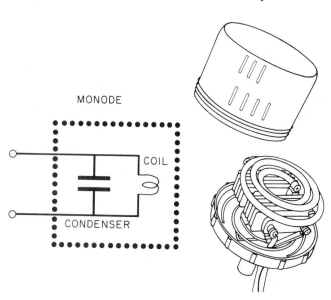

FIGURE 13–14. Monode applicator with wiring diagram. (Courtesy of Siemens-Reiniger Werke Ag.)

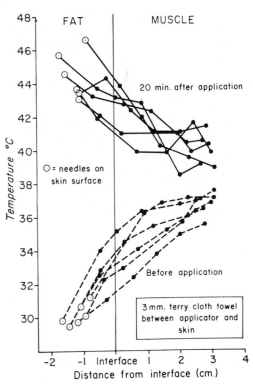

FIGURE 13–15. Temperature distribution in the human thigh at the completion of 20 minutes of exposure to short wave (27.12 MHz) applied with the monode with 3 mm of terry cloth inserted between applicator and skin. (From Lehmann, J. F., de Lateur, B. J., and Stonebridge, J. B.: Selective heating by short wave diathermy with a helical coil. Arch. Phys. Med. Rehabil., 50:117–123, 1969.)

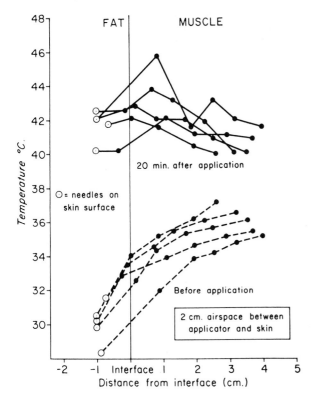

FIGURE 13–16. Temperature distribution in the human thigh at the completion of 20 minutes of exposure to short wave (27.12 MHz) applied with the monode with 2 cm of air space between applicator and skin. (From Lehmann, J. F., de Lateur, B. J., and Stonebridge, J. B.: Selective heating by short wave diathermy with a helical coil. Arch. Phys. Med. Rehabil., 50:117–123, 1969.)

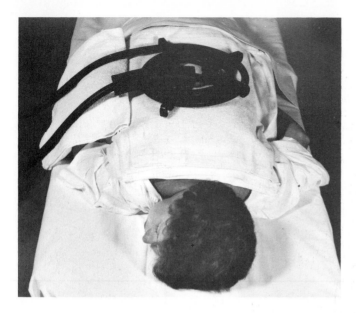

FIGURE 13–17. Short wave diathermy application to back with induction coil (pancake coil). Spacing between coil and skin is provided by layers of terry cloth. (Courtesy of the Burdick Corporation.)

FIGURE 13–18. Induction coil application to knee, with spacing provided by layers of terry cloth. (Courtesy of the Burdick Corporation.)

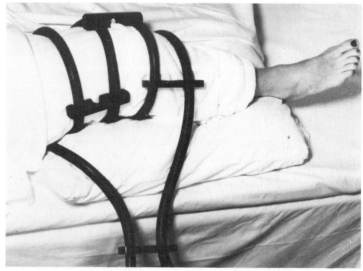
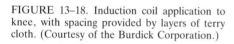

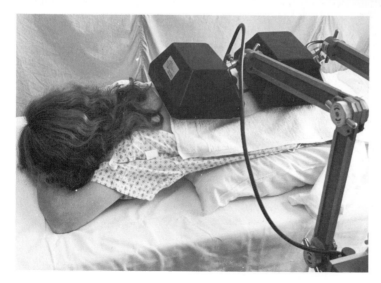

FIGURE 13–19. Induction coil applicators (IME) applied to the back.

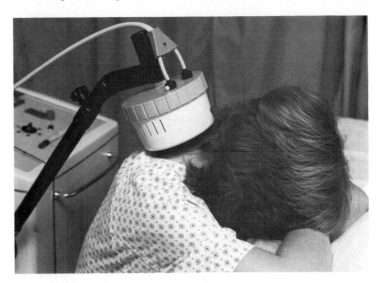

FIGURE 13–20. Monode applied to the neck.

The current distribution in a given part of the anatomy will depend on the mode of application and on the properties of the tissues, such as geometry (anatomy) and conductivity (reciprocal of resistance). Tissues can be considered to be in series or in parallel as they are traversed by the high-frequency current. If they are in parallel, it can be assumed that the greatest current flow occurs in the tissue with the greatest conductivity, that is, the tissues with the least resistance, and therefore this tissue is heated most, since heating occurs with the square of the current. If the tissues are in series, the tissue with the greatest resistance is heated most, since the current through all of them is the same and especially since the ratio of capacitance to resistance in each of the tissue layers is essentially constant. In this case, the heat is in direct proportion to the resistance. The conductivity of the tissues is closely related to the water content.

Capacitive Coupling

The higher the water content, the better the conductivity.[297] Guy and co-workers[120] reviewed the characteristics of short wave diathermy applicators. Capacitor (condenser) applicators have the fundamental characteristic of inducing greater power absorption in subcutaneous fat than in deep muscle tissue, except in situations in which capacitive fields need only pass through thin layers of fat. In some situations, however, capacitive electrodes can be effective in heating deeper tissues, that is, pelvic diathermy with internal electrodes. Figure 13–21 shows schematically the current density in the tissues as the capacitor plates are applied over the skin of the back. The greatest current density is found in the subcutaneous fat under the electrodes and in the superficial musculature between the electrodes. In the first location, the tissues are in series. In the second, they are resistors in parallel. Therefore, under the electrodes the subcutaneous fat is heated most, and between the electrodes the superficial musculature is heated most. Another example of how fields in the subcutaneous fat can be made significantly smaller in amplitude than in the deeper tissues to be treated is the use of capacitive applicators for heating the pelvic organs, using an internal electrode of small diameter and an external electrode of large surface area over the abdomen (Fig. 13–22). The resulting temperatures in the pelvic organs can be readily controlled and brought into the therapeutic range, whereas this is not possible when using microwave or ultrasound applicators (Fig. 13–23). Internal fields, which are much greater than those in the subcutaneous fat, can be produced because of the concentration of fields at the small electrode. Also, when small cylindrical, spherical, or ellipsoidal tissue shapes with thin fat layers, such as hands, wrists, ankles, and feet, are treated, relatively uniform heating due to the induced internal fields can be expected. It is a prerequisite that the parts of the body be small as compared with the wavelength. Finally, in areas where the subcutaneous fat thickness is minimal, a condenser applicator may be used for heating the deeper structures.

Inductive Coupling

Inductive coil applicators have been shown both theoretically and experimentally to produce higher

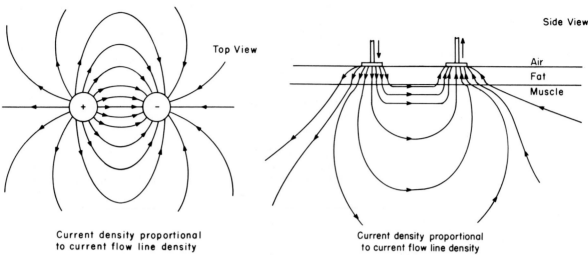

Top View

Side View

Air
Fat
Muscle

Current density proportional
to current flow line density

Current density proportional
to current flow line density

FIGURE 13–21. *A*, Schematic drawing of current flow lines in uniform tissues when short waves are applied with condenser plates (current density proportional to the current flow line density), top view. *B*, Schematic drawing of current flow lines in tissue layers when short waves are applied with condenser plates in one plane to fat-muscle-tissue layers, side view.

power absorption in the deeper high-water-content tissues than in the subcutaneous fat.[120] Circular electrical fields or eddy currents are induced in the tissues by the applied magnetic fields. If the magnetic field is directed normally (perpendicular) to the tissue interfaces, the electrical field is tangential to tissue interfaces and not as much modified by tissue boundaries as in the case of capacitive electrode applicators. Since the electrical conductivity of muscle is an order of magnitude greater than that of fat, the power absorption density will be an order of magnitude greater than in the fat.[295, 296] Thus, inductive applicators are preferred over condenser applicators if muscle heating is desired. Schematically, the anticipated current distribution in the tissues is shown in Figure 13–24, when the "pancake" coil is applied to the back. Pluses and minuses indicate the direction of current flow. Their density indicates the relative amount of

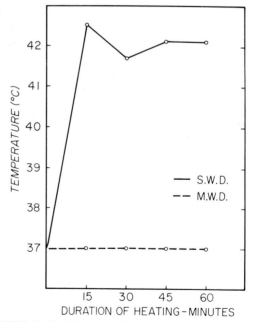

FIGURE 13–22. Field pattern that might be expected with the use of an internal electrode. (From Lehmann, J. F., and de Lateur, B. J.: Therapeutic heat. *In* Lehmann, J. F. [Ed.]: Therapeutic Heat and Cold, 3rd Ed. Baltimore, Williams and Wilkins, 1982.)

FIGURE 13–23. Mean rectal temperature during intrapelvic heating with short wave diathermy or low abdominal heating with microwave diathermy. (From Kottke, F. J.: Heat in pelvic diseases. *In* Licht, S. [Ed.]: Therapeutic Heat and Cold, 2nd Ed. Baltimore, Waverly Press, 1965, pp. 474–490.)

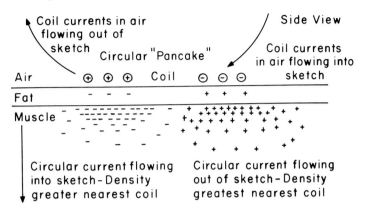

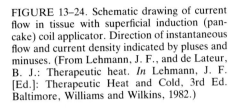

FIGURE 13–24. Schematic drawing of current flow in tissue with superficial induction (pancake) coil applicator. Direction of instantaneous flow and current density indicated by pluses and minuses. (From Lehmann, J. F., and de Lateur, B. J.: Therapeutic heat. *In* Lehmann, J. F. [Ed.]: Therapeutic Heat and Cold, 3rd Ed. Baltimore, Williams and Wilkins, 1982.)

current in a given area. Figure 13–25 shows the relative current distribution in the tissue layers when a wrap-around coil is used in the area of the thigh. The temperature distribution produced by the monode is shown in Figure 13–16.[196] Hollander and Horvath[145] observed temperature increases up to 38° C (101° F) when the knee joint was heated with a wrap-around coil. On the other hand, joints with a considerable amount of soft tissue cover, such as the hip joint, cannot be heated effectively by short wave diathermy application using the induction coil, even when the output of the equipment produces a first-degree burn and discomfort in the superficial tissue (see Fig. 13–47).[217]

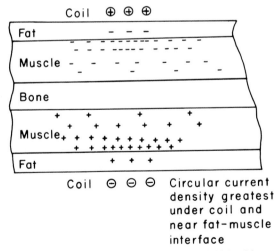

FIGURE 13–25. Longitudinal cross section of thigh with wrap-around coil showing current flow at coil and near fat-muscle interface. Direction of instantaneous flow and current density indicated by pluses and minuses. (From Lehmann, J. F., and de Lateur, B. J.: Therapeutic heat. *In* Lehmann, J. F. [Ed.]: Therapeutic Heat and Cold, 3rd Ed. Baltimore, Williams and Wilkins, 1982.)

NONTHERMAL EFFECTS

The potential use of pulsed short wave diathermy has been extensively reviewed.[206] Initially, pulsed short wave diathermy was used to minimize the heating effect, which is in proportion to the average output, in the hope that the peak intensities during the pulses may produce therapeutic nonthermal effects. Later, some other investigators* tried to show the existence of nonthermal effects to document their presence as potentially hazardous side effects of short wave diathermy application. The significance of the findings resulting from this type of investigative approach can be summarized as follows: although the existence of nonthermal effects can be documented, none of them has been proved to be clearly of therapeutic advantage over continuous wave application and none of them has been shown to produce any significant side effects during therapeutic application. The hope of distinguishing between thermal and nonthermal effects by comparing the responses obtained from pulsed wave application with those from continuous wave application has not been completely realized because, as in the pearl-chain formation of particles, many of the nonthermal effects respond to the average of the pulsed output, as do the heating effects, and not to the peak values during the pulses. Thus, at present, there is no specific therapeutic indication for the use of pulsed output.†

STANDARDS FOR EQUIPMENT

Standards need to be developed to assure effectiveness and safety of short wave diathermy equip-

*See references 11, 12, 133, 138, 139, 293, 318, and 322.
†See references 38, 53, 89, 92, 106, 132, 160, 193, 206, 225, 247, 254, 257, 284, 305, 306, 319, 320, 325, 348–350, 355.

JUSTUS F. LEHMANN AND BARBARA J. DE LATEUR

ment. The standard should, first, assure the user that the equipment is powerful enough to produce vigorous heating effects; second, that the user has adequate information as to where the highest temperature is produced in the tissues when the various available applicators are used; and third, that the equipment has been built to assure safety both to the patient treated and to the personnel administering the treatment.

Tissue substitute substances with electrical properties equal to those found in humans have been developed by Guy and associates[116, 120] and can be modeled to conform to comparable anatomical structures. The tissue substitute models allow identification of the location of the peak tissue temperature with different applicators without great difficulty. In pre-split models, the two halves can be readily separated for thermographic screening after short exposure. From the linear portion of the initial temperature rise in any part of the model, the specific absorption rate can be calculated and, on this basis, temperature distribution can be predicted in human application. Research is being developed to overcome the electromagnetic discontinuity at the site of the split of the model. On this basis, it has been predicted that in order to achieve a temperature increase adequate to produce vigorous therapeutic responses, an approximate absorbed power of the order of 170 watts per kg is required. Since at this point an increase in blood flow with resulting cooling is triggered, an additional absorbed power of more than 100 watts per kg is necessary to overcome the cooling effect of the blood flow. Therefore, the equipment should be powerful enough under those circumstances to produce, probably, an absorbed power in the tissues of more than 200 watts per kg. Much of the available equipment does not fulfill these requirements. Safety features of the equipment should include an adequate timer. Concern has also been voiced about stray radiation to which the therapist and parts of the patient's body that are not being treated are exposed.[193, 247]

PRECAUTIONS

Special precautions must be taken with all techniques of application. All metallic objects, such as watches or jewelry, should be removed. The patient should be positioned on a wooden plinth or chair. These precautions are necessary, since selective heating of metal parts could occur because of current concentration. For the same reason, the accumulation of sweat beads should be prevented by using terry cloth. Tuning of the patient circuit should always be done at the low output level to prevent excessive heating from an uncontrolled surge of current through the patient. The tuning of the patient circuit should be optimal. Then the output of the machine should be adjusted to the desired level. If this procedure is not followed, small movements of the patient may change the impedance of the circuit in such a fashion that resonance occurs and the current flow may be greatly increased without the therapist's being aware of it. An increase in dose, and possibly burns, may result.

Metallic implants, including surgical implants, cardiac pacemakers, and electrophysiological braces, should not be exposed to short wave diathermy because the implant may be destroyed, made to malfunction, or become selectively heated, resulting in a burn to the patient. Surgical implants, however, represent a contraindication only if it is anticipated that any significant current would reach the site of implant. Intrauterine devices (IUDs) containing copper or other metals should represent a contraindication to the use of short wave diathermy until proved otherwise.[289] Finally, contact lenses should be removed, since they may cause hot spots.

It should be noted that short wave diathermy applied to the lower back has been observed to increase menstrual flow, and patients should be advised of that possibility or therapy should be discontinued during the menstrual period. Pregnant women should not be treated with pelvic diathermy using internal electrodes because of possible damage to the fetus.[310] There is also some controversy about treatment of children around the bone growth zones and of the possibility of other side effects, which are summarized by Michaelson[247] and Lehmann.[193] By and large, for the short-term exposure as in therapy, the main concern should be to avoid temperatures that produce burns. The existence of stray radiation as an occupational hazard to the therapist is also controversial. Based on microwave studies, it has been suggested that in the absence of more accurate measures, intensity of long-term exposure should be held below 5 to 10 mW per cm^2.[193, 206]

Microwaves

Microwaves are a form of electromagnetic radiation,[97] with frequencies of 2456 and 915 MHz approved for medical use. As with other electro-magnetic waves, microwaves travel at the speed of light and can be propagated through a vacuum. They can be reflected, scattered, refracted, or absorbed. The medical use of microwaves is primarily based on the fact that they are selectively absorbed in tissues with high water content and thus allow selective heating of certain tissues such as the musculature.

EQUIPMENT

Therapeutic equipment ideally should be able to heat musculature selectively and evenly. The equipment should be able to raise the tissue temperature to tolerance levels and potentially to overcome the cooling resulting from increased blood flow. The equipment should be capable of demonstrating a vigorous physiological response with a minimum of stray radiation affecting sensitive organs of the patient and of the therapist. The meter should show, quantitatively, the flow of power into the tissues; that is, it should measure the total forward output minus reflected power. An accurate timer should be available. It has been shown that the use of the lower frequency of 915 MHz would be advantageous over 2456 MHz.[117, 119, 207] Direct-contact applicators provide better coupling and less stray radiation than the standard noncontact applicators. Such direct-contact applicators also can be equipped with air cooling with the air blown through a porous dielectric with which the cavity is loaded. A thin plastic radome with the proper distribution of air channels ensures even cooling of the skin and eliminates selective heating of the surface and of the applicator edges. Applicators may have a fixed direction of the E field vector; that is, they are linearly polarized (Fig. 13–26). Others are circularly polarized with the rotating E field vector (Fig. 13–27).

The noncontact applicators operating at 2456 MHz that are still in clinical use include the A, B, C, and E directors. The A director consists of an antenna with a hemispherical reflector (diameter 9.3 cm). The B director consists of an antenna rod with a hemispherical reflector with a diameter of 15.3 cm. Both produce a beam having a cross section pattern with the highest intensity in the shape of a ring, with the intensity in the center being approximately half of the value of the intensity in the ring. The size of the total therapeutic field is approximately equal to the diameter of the reflector. The C and E directors have an antenna rod with a corner reflector. The dipole antenna of

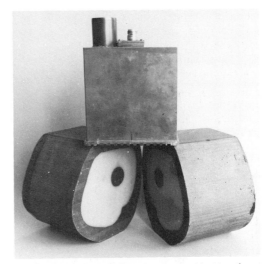

FIGURE 13–26. Phantom thigh model with 13-cm² contact microwave applicator with radome operating at 915 MHz. (From Lehmann, J. F., Guy, A. W., Stonebridge, J. B., and de Lateur, B. J.: Evaluation of a therapeutic direct-contact 915-MHz microwave applicator for effective deep-tissue heating in humans. IEEE Trans. Microwave Theory & Tech. MTT, 26:556–563, 1978.)

the C director has a length of half the wavelength. The E director has a full-wave, 12.2-cm dipole antenna. Both produce an oval high-intensity zone in the center of the cross section of the beam with a useful therapeutic field of a size approximately similar to that of the opening of the corner reflector. All of these applicators have poor beaming properties because the wavelength is comparable to the antenna size. Therefore, they should be applied at a distance of approximately 1 to 2 inches from the skin.

To assess the therapeutic effectiveness of the equipment, tissue substitute models, as described under *Short Wave Diathermy*[87] (Figs. 13–28 to 13–29), can be used to measure the linear transient of the temperature rise with short exposure from which absorbed power can be calculated at any given point in the model. Similar temperature measurements have been made in the human volunteer with temperature probes in place. Good agreement has been found between values of the specific absorption rate obtained in the model and those in the human volunteer (Fig. 13–30). In the human volunteer, also, the physiological responses in terms of blood flow can be estimated so that certain levels of specific absorption rates can be related to effectiveness, that is, to production of vigorous responses in terms of human blood flow

JUSTUS F. LEHMANN AND BARBARA J. DE LATEUR

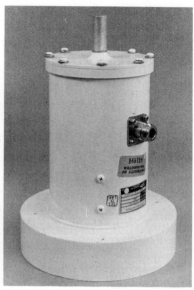
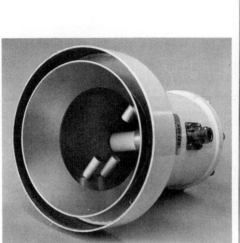

FIGURE 13–27. 2450 MHz Transco circularly polarized direct contact applicator with circular quarter wavelength choke around applicator edge. (From Lehmann, J. F., and de Lateur, B. J.: Therapeutic heat. *In* Lehmann, J. F. [Ed.]: Therapeutic Heat and Cold, 3rd Ed. Baltimore, Williams and Wilkins, 1982.)

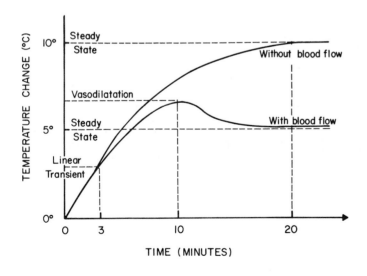

FIGURE 13–28. Schematic representation of linear transient and steady-state temperatures for a typical tissue under diathermy exposure. (From Lehmann, J. F., Guy, A. W., Stonebridge, J. B., and de Lateur, B. J.: Evaluation of a therapeutic direct-contact 915-MHz microwave applicator for effective deep-tissue heating in humans. IEEE Trans. Microwave Theory & Tech. MTT, 26:556–563, 1978.)

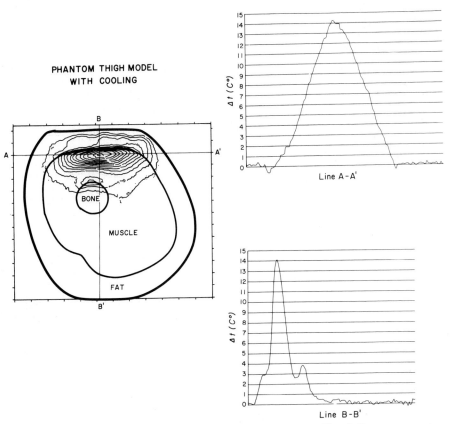

FIGURE 13–29. Isotherms produced in phantom thigh model after exposure to a 13-cm² direct-contact microwave applicator operating at 915 MHz with radome and cooling. (From Lehmann, J. F., Guy, A. W., Stonebridge, J. B., and de Lateur, B. J.: Evaluation of a therapeutic direct-contact 915-MHz microwave applicator for effective deep-tissue heating in humans. IEEE Trans. Microwave Theory & Tech. MTT, 26:556–563, 1978.)

JUSTUS F. LEHMANN AND BARBARA J. DE LATEUR

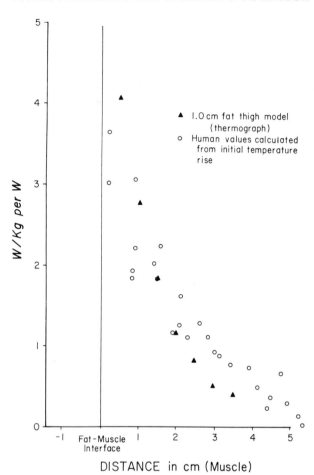

▲ 1.0 cm fat thigh model (thermograph)
○ Human values calculated from initial temperature rise

FIGURE 13–30. Comparison of the calculates of the SAR in thighs of human beings and models. (From Lehmann, J. F., Guy, A. W., Stonebridge, J. B., and de Lateur, B. J.: Evaluation of a therapeutic direct-contact 915-MHz microwave applicator for effective deep-tissue heating in humans. IEEE Trans. Microwave Theory & Tech. MTT, 26:556–563, 1978.)

change.[301] The values of specific absorption rates in the human thigh are shown and compared with the calculated change in blood flow rate they produce in Table 13–3. From these measurements it can be concluded that, at a specific absorption rate of up to 170 watts per kg, blood flow increases of up to 30 ml per 100 g tissue per minute were obtained. This increase in blood flow represents a vigorous physiological response, since blood flow increases under extensive exercise conditions are of the order of 30 to 35 ml per 100 g tissue per minute. With this information, tissue substitute models can be used for the quick determination of the maximum specific absorption rate in the muscle, and one can predict whether the absorption rate is adequate to produce a vigorous physiological response. It has been shown that direct-contact applicators can produce these vigorous responses with relatively little stray radiation (Fig. 13–31). Stray radiation was tested both in the model and in the human shoulder. It was found that stray radiation was considerably less with the direct-contact applicators.[222, 223] In addition, stray radiation was greatest in the area where the contact could not be maintained. If a linearly polarized applicator was used, the stray radiation was greatest in the direction of the E vector. That implies that one should avoid having the E field vector pointing at the sensitive organ and one should avoid losing contact in the direction of the sensitive organ.

PROPAGATION AND ABSORPTION OF MICROWAVES IN TISSUES

As with other modalities, most therapeutic effects of microwaves are due to heating; however, the temperature distribution in the tissues treated is specific for this modality and is influenced by the frequency used. It is on this basis that this modality is selected. The temperature distribution, in turn, depends on the propagation and absorp-

TABLE 13–3. Heat Therapy to Human Muscle

CALCULATED VALUES OF ABSORBED POWER IN HUMAN MUSCLE		CALCULATED VALUES FOR BLOOD FLOW IN HUMAN MUSCLE†	
Run	SAR*	Run	ml/100 g/min
1	121.60	1	28.90
2	78.17	2	28.91
3	118.70	3	25.00
4	75.27	4	23.64
5	167.93	5	29.69

*Specific Absorption Rate (SAR) in watts per kg in musculature (1–2 cm)—at 555.55 milliwatts per cm^2 maximum power density of incident radiation. (From Lehmann, J. F., Guy, A. W., Stonebridge, J. B., and de Lateur, B. J.: Evaluation of a therapeutic direct-contact 915 MHz microwave applicator for effective deep-tissue heating in humans. IEEE Trans. Microwave Theory & Tech. MTT, 26:556–563, 1978.)

†Calculated Blood-Flow Rate in Muscle. (From Lehmann, J. F., Guy, A. W., Stonebridge, J. B., and de Lateur, B. J.: Evaluation of a therapeutic direct-contact 915 MHz microwave applicator for effective deep-tissue heating in humans. IEEE Trans. Microwave Theory & Tech. MTT, 26:556–563, 1978.)

tion characteristics of the tissues traversed by the beam.[116–118, 144] Several workers have studied the absorption of microwave energy in biological media.[51, 54, 294, 296] It is apparent that the dielectric properties of the medium and the specific resistance or conductivity are responsible for the energy absorption. Tissues with high water content, such as musculature, and fluid media, such as found in the eye or in sweat beads, are likely to absorb more microwave energy than bone.

The reflection of microwaves at the body surface and at the tissue interfaces can be calculated if the dielectric properties and the conductivities of the tissues are known. Schwan[293] has pointed out that a large and variable amount of energy may be reflected at the skin surface under therapeutic conditions. It is possible to have variable losses of more than 50 per cent of the energy irradiated from the director, and thus it is difficult to reproduce the biological effects in a reliable fashion.

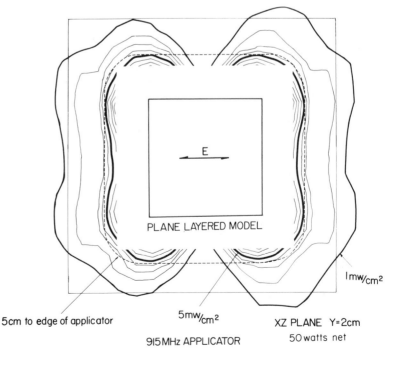

FIGURE 13–31. Stray radiation pattern for the XZ plane, with a 915-MHz direct-contact applicator on the plane-layered model. Graduated in 1 mW/cm^2 increments at 50 watts net input power. (From Lehmann, J. F., Stonebridge, J. B., and Guy, A. W.: A comparison of patterns of stray radiation from therapeutic microwave applicators measured near tissue-substitute models and human subjects. Radio Science, 14:271–283, 1979.)

This reflection is minimized by using the lower available frequency of 915 MHz and by using a direct-contact applicator, filling the cavity of the applicator with substances of matched dielectric properties.

Schwan[293] calculated a pattern of relative heating for homogeneous tissues with plane and parallel interfaces. Lehmann and associates[204] obtained the pattern of relative heating by actual measurements of the distribution throughout a specimen consisting of skin, subcutaneous fat, and musculature with typical anatomical and biological interfaces. They confirmed Schwan's calculations that an appreciable reflection of microwave energy occurred at the interface between subcutaneous fat and musculature, with the result that a large amount of energy was converted into heat in the subcutaneous tissues (Fig. 13–32A). Also, in agreement with Schwan, they found that the depth of penetration was poor in muscle tissues if the frequency of 2450 MHz was used. The intensity available at the surface of the muscle dropped to a 50 per cent level at a depth of approximately 1 cm. By contrast, the amount of energy converted into heat in the subcutaneous tissues was much less and the depth of penetration (approximately 3 cm) in the musculature was much better if microwave frequency of 900 MHz was used (Fig. 13–32B). The resulting temperature distribution in the live human was modified not only by such constants as specific heat, specific weight, and thermal conductivity but also by physiological responses such as change in the blood flow, as illustrated in Figure 13–33.[190] After a peak temperature is reached, blood flow cooling reduces tissue temperature in spite of continuous microwave application. As shown in Figure 13–33, the new experimental 915-MHz direct-contact applicator provides simultaneous cooling of the surface temperatures.[191] Even heating of the muscle can be obtained from the most superficial musculature to a depth of approximately 4 cm, that is, to the tissues adjacent to the bone (Fig. 13–34). Whereas the temperature distribution of microwaves operating at a frequency of 2456 MHz in most instances can be duplicated by short wave application, the 915 MHz direct-contact applicator is a unique tool for selective heating of the musculature.[207]

The conclusion for therapy is that the application of microwaves at the commercially available frequency of 2456 MHz would result in a relatively high, if not the highest, temperature in the subcutaneous tissues unless application is made to an area where skin and subcutaneous fat are of minimal thickness, as was demonstrated by Rae and co-workers[278] with dogs. Also, Hollander and Horvath[145] were able to elevate the joint temperature above the skin temperature in elbows and knees, both joints having a minimal soft-tissue cover. Their temperature differential was less pronounced in patients with rheumatoid arthritis. The application of microwaves around or below the frequency of 900 MHz to a person with a moderate amount of subcutaneous fat would result in a temperature distribution in which the highest temperature would occur in the muscle; also, the muscle could be evenly heated down to the bone.

Lehmann and associates[218] later studied a pattern of relative heating and the actual temperature distribution produced in specimens with more complex geometry, similar to that encountered in the treatment of joints, for the frequencies of 2456 and 900 MHz (Fig. 13–35). It was found that, during exposure to a frequency of 2456 MHz, a heating pattern indicative of energy reflection and production of a pattern of standing waves at the muscle-bone interface was observed. The development of undesirable "hot spots" can be the result. This possibility seems to be less around or below frequencies of 900 MHz. The difference between the frequencies with regard to the development of hot spots in front of the bone may be explained by the fact that the bone represents a reflecting obstacle for wave propagation at the higher frequency, since its diameter is relatively large as compared with the wavelength in muscle tissue. Thus, in Figure 13–35, the relation between bone diameter and wavelength is reversed at the low frequency, and the waves of high frequency are reflected to a greater extent than those of the low frequency. Consistent with these conclusions, Worden and co-workers[357] observed burns over the femurs of dogs (Fig. 13–36), which appeared to be the result of energy reflected at the bone surface. Engel and associates[88] reported that horse flesh was heated to a higher degree if bone was present under the flesh at a depth of 1 cm. Most recently, Addington and others[4] found that the hollow viscera heat differentially and that the stomach and liver may be considered hot spots. Selective burns in these areas were observed in dogs. Also, the tissues overlying the thoracic cage were selectively burned[148] and the anterior cardiac surface was selectively heated.[228, 237] Selective absorption can also occur if metallic implants are present in tissues that can be reached by an appreciable amount of microwave

Text continued on page 311

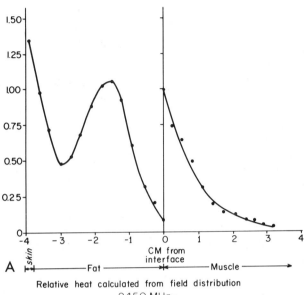

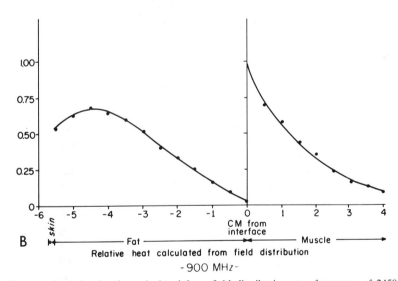

FIGURE 13–32. *A*, Pattern of relative heating calculated from field distribution at a frequency of 2450 MHz. *B*, Pattern of relative heating calculated from field distribution at a frequency of 900 MHz. (From Lehmann, J. F., Guy, A. W., Johnston, V. C., Brunner, G. D., and Bell, J. W.: Comparison of relative heating patterns produced in tissues by exposure to microwave energy at frequencies of 2,450 and 900 megacycles. Arch. Phys. Med. Rehabil., 43:69–76, 1962.)

JUSTUS F. LEHMANN AND BARBARA J. DE LATEUR

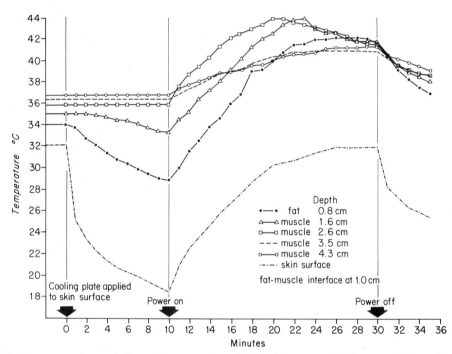

FIGURE 13–33. Temperature in a typical experiment at various depths of tissue resulting from application of microwave with a 915-MHz contact applicator. (From de Lateur, B. J., Lehmann, J. F., Stonebridge, J. B., Warren, C. G., and Guy, A. W.: Muscle heating in human subjects with 915 MHz microwave contact applicator. Arch. Phys. Med. Rehabil., 51:147–151, 1970.)

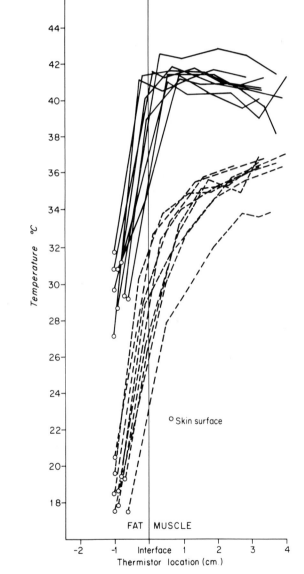

FIGURE 13–34. Temperature distribution in all volunteers with less than or equal to 1 cm of subcutaneous fat before (- - - -) and 20 minutes after (- - - -) microwave application. (From de Lateur, B. J., Lehmann, J. F., Stonebridge, J. B., Warren, C. G., and Guy, A. W.: Muscle heating in human subjects with 915 MHz microwave contact applicator. Arch. Phys. Med. Rehabil., 51:147–151, 1970.)

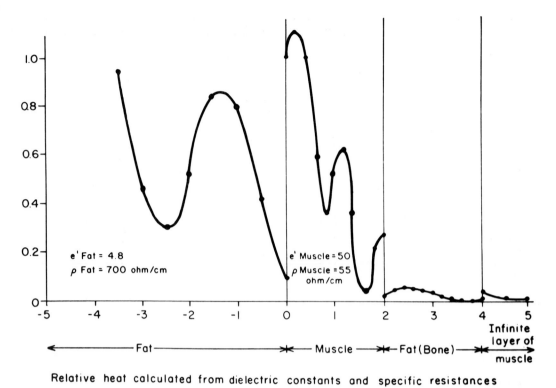

Relative heat calculated from dielectric constants and specific resistances
— 2 4 5 6 MC —

A

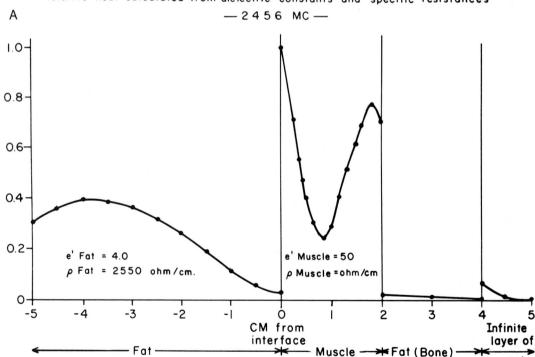

Relative heat calculated from dielectric constants and specific resistances
— 900 MC —

B

FIGURE 13–35. *A*, Pattern of relative heating calculated from dielectric constants and specific resistances in a complex specimen at a frequency of 2456 MHz. *B*, Pattern of relative heating calculated from dielectric constants and specific resistances in a complex specimen at a frequency of 900 MHz. (From Lehmann, J. F., McMillan, J. A., Brunner, G. D., and Guy, A. W.: A comparative evaluation of temperature distributions produced by microwaves at 2,456 and 900 megacycles in geometrically complex specimens. Arch. Phys. Med. Rehabil., 43:502–507, 1962.)

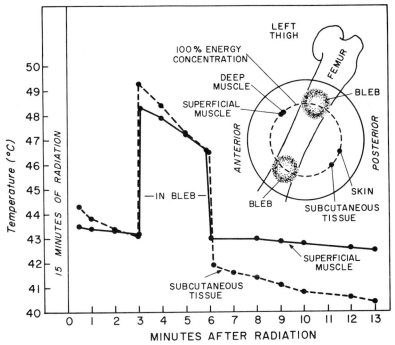

FIGURE 13–36. Development of burns from reflection, where high-intensity field crosses bone, and temperature measurement across the bleb. (From Worden, R. E., Herrick, J. F., Wakim, K. G., and Krusen, F. H.: The heating effects of microwaves with and without ischemia. Arch. Phys. Med., 29:751–758, 1948.)

energy.[93] A dramatic illustration of this can be given by igniting steel wool in the microwave field in air.

This review of the investigations using different frequencies strongly suggests that the microwave machines used at present do not operate at the most effective frequency. They were introduced into therapy because generators operating at these frequencies were available for medical application after World War II and not because 2456 MHz was considered to be the best frequency for medical use. The data now suggest that the optimal frequency would be at about 900 MHz or below, minimizing the heating effect in the subcutaneous tissues and heating the underlying tissues more adequately. The development of hot spots as a result of reflection from bone is prevented to a large degree. These frequencies also have a better depth of penetration. FCC regulations have allocated the frequency of 915 MHz for medical purposes.

These investigations also suggest that, because of the large amount of reflection at the bone surface, very little energy reaches the area beyond the bone at either frequency, 2456 or 900 MHz. This is indicated by the difference in temperature between the areas in front of and behind the bone when exposed to microwaves (Table 13–4). Though this difference is less when a frequency of 900 MHz is used, it is still too great to allow full therapeutic exposure of a joint through bone. If the purpose is to heat the entire joint, the joint should be exposed from all aspects, as is the case in ultrasonic therapy.[190, 282]

TABLE 13–4. Temperature Differences in Tissue Following Exposure to Microwaves*

2456 MHz	900 MHz
6.4° C	5.1° C
4.6° C	1.7° C
9.2° C	3.6° C
6.0° C	2.4° C

Difference in temperatures indicated by measurements in front of and behind bone after exposure to microwaves at frequencies of 2456 and 900 MHz.

*From Lehmann, J. F., McMillan, J. A., Brunner, G. D., and Guy, A. W.: A comparative evaluation of temperature distributions produced by microwaves at 2,456 and 900 megacycles in geometrically complex specimens. Arch. Phys. Med. Rehabil., 43:502–507, 1962.

JUSTUS F. LEHMANN AND BARBARA J. DE LATEUR

PHYSIOLOGICAL RESPONSES

Since microwave diathermy was introduced into physical medicine,[175, 279] extensive studies have been conducted on the physiological effects produced by this new type of radiation. A large number of physiological, pathological, and biochemical reactions were studied. In some instances the mechanisms by which they were produced were also investigated. A recent complete review of the literature has been done by Michaelson.[247] The result of these studies indicated that the microwave heating effects were responsible for the vast majority of the reactions of potential therapeutic significance. However, nonthermal reactions could also be demonstrated.

HEATING EFFECTS

Therapeutic Effects

Since microwave energy is absorbed in the body and is effective in elevating the tissue temperature, it is obvious that all reactions that can be produced by temperature elevation in the tissues can be observed after exposure to microwave energy of adequate power levels. From a therapeutic point of view, it is important to recognize that microwaves may selectively (see Fig. 13–34) and evenly heat the musculature. Microwaves also can selectively heat joints covered with little soft tissue.

Side Effects

The side effects of heating are also important, since they can create hazards if the temperature is raised selectively in sensitive organs. The effects of microwaves on the eye, among other organs, have been studied extensively.* It has been found that it may be possible to heat selectively the fluid media of the eye, including the lens. It is most likely that lenticular cataracts are produced by the heating effect of microwaves. Below a power density of 0.112 watt per cm^2, opacities have not been observed even after prolonged exposure.[40, 121] Other heat-sensitive organs include the testicles,[86, 110, 153, 247] which are easily exposed to stray radiation during therapeutic application. In contrast to the testicles, the ovaries are covered with such a thick layer of soft tissue that it is difficult to expose them to any significant amount of radiation.[168, 329] Other investigations have included the study of the effects of microwaves on bone growth. Wise and coworkers[351] found, after the application of high doses of microwaves, a decrease in bone growth,

---

*See references 39, 41, 59, 60, 244, 283, 346, and 362.

probably related to the heating effect. On the other hand, a lower dosage of short wave diathermy applied by Doyle and Smart[70] produced a stimulation of bone growth. Granberry and colleagues,[111] however, found no effect on bone growth without an associated sensation of pain. Finally, it has been established that temperature increases above 38.9° C (102° F)[129, 310] in the pregnant uterus may produce congenital anomalies in the fetus. Specifically, Rubin and Erdman[287] reported on four women treated with microwave diathermy for pelvic inflammatory diseases. These women were or became pregnant during the course of therapy. They were treated with frequencies around 2450 MHz and 100 W total output, using a nondirect-contact applicator. Three women delivered normal infants, and one aborted on day 67 but delivered a normal baby following a subsequent pregnancy, even though she again received microwave therapy. In these cases, however, it is doubtful that there was a significant temperature rise in the uterus. Microwaves were also used to ease parturition without injury to the newborns, who were followed for one year after delivery. As discussed also, reflection over bone may enhance energy levels to the point that burns occur, a point that should be considered in therapeutic application. Finally, selective heating of sweat beads may produce superficial skin burns, a problem totally avoided by air-cooled direct-current applicators.

Nonthermal Effects

Most of the biological reactions of therapeutic significance are due to the heating effect resulting from microwave absorption in the tissues. There are, however, some effects that are nonthermal in nature. The significance of these effects for therapeutic purposes is still inadequately understood. These effects have been reviewed by Michaelson[247] and Lehmann.[193] It is not known how many of these effects would actually occur in the live organism under therapeutic conditions. Therefore, for therapeutic purposes, this discussion is limited to the heating effect of microwave energy. However, it is possible that in the future some specific reactions that are nonthermal in nature and that may add to the specificity of the therapeutic results may be unveiled.

DOSIMETRY

The dose can be defined as the product of applied energy times duration of action. As in other types of diathermy, the actual tissue temperature is more important than the applied energy for determining the biological results, since most of the reactions to microwaves are thermal in nature. Even though we have information on the relative distribution of temperature in the organism exposed to microwaves, we do not at present have a way to assess the absolute level of the temperatures obtained in the tissue. However, major improvements in new equipment are possible. With direct contact applicators, the proposed federal Food and Drug Administration (FDA) standard for this equipment requires a meter indicating the forward power to the patient; that is, the total output minus the reflected power. From a previous study it can be anticipated that vigorous effects can be produced with forward power on the order of 50 watts,[212] with an average intensity of 500 mW/cm[2]. The air-cooled applicators are preferable because they avoid undesirable temperature increases in the skin and subcutaneous fat. However, to safeguard against exceeding tolerance levels, pain should still be used as a warning signal and vigorous exposure avoided in the absence of such a pain sensation.

Ultrasound

EQUIPMENT

The therapeutic ultrasound machine consists of a generator that produces a high-frequency alternating current of about 0.8 to 1 MHz. The high-frequency electric current is then converted by a transducer into mechanical, i.e., acoustic, vibra-

tions. The transducer consists basically of a crystal inserted between two electrodes. The conversion of the high-frequency alternating voltage into mechanical vibrations is accomplished by reversal of the piezoelectric effect, which is shown in Figure 13–37.[23] If an alternating electrical charge is applied to the surfaces of the crystal, the crystal will be deformed, depending on the sign of the charges. The three basic components of the electrical generator usually found in the therapeutic machines are the power supply, the oscillating circuit (radio frequency generator) producing the high-frequency current, and the transducer circuit. The power supply of therapeutically acceptable machines has full-wave rectification and filtering to provide for a steady output not appeciably (within 1 per cent) modified by the 60 Hz alternating line current. Federal standard proposes that variations exceeding ±20 per cent for all emanations greater than 10 per cent of the maximum emission are not acceptable. The capacitance and inductance of the oscillating circuit are selected to produce an alternating current of the same frequency as the mechanical resonance frequency of the quartz crystal in the transducer. Adjustment of the frequency is made possible by tuning, usually by adjusting a variable capacitor. Some manufacturers have eliminated the need for tuning by controlling the oscillating frequency.

The sound beams produced by therapeutic applicators are almost cylindrical in shape. The beaming properties of any sound applicator depend on its diameter and wavelength. The sine of the angle of divergence, γ, is in proportion to the ratio of the wavelength to the diameter of the applicator.

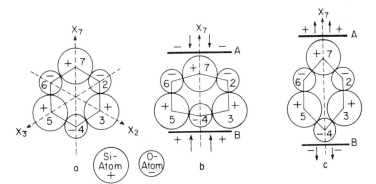

FIGURE 13–37. Quartz crystal lattice demonstrating the piezoelectric effect. *a*, Natural state of the crystal with electrical neutrality of the surfaces. *b*, Compressed crystal with greater proximity of the two negative charges to surface A and the two positive charges to surface B, producing corresponding changes of the surface charges. *c*, With crystal extended, proximity of the positive charge to the surface producing a positive charge at A and closer proximity of the negative charge producing negative surface charge at B. (From Bergmann, L.: Der Ultraschall und seine Anwendung in Wissenschaft und Technik. Stuttgart, S. Hirzel, Verlag, 1949.)

JUSTUS F. LEHMANN AND BARBARA J. DE LATEUR

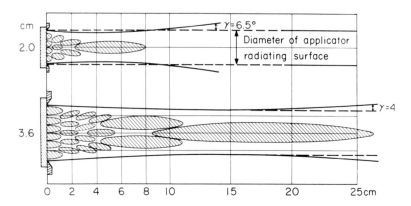

FIGURE 13–38. Schematic representation of ultrasound beam; γ is the angle of divergence of the beam; shaded areas are zones of high ultrasound intensity. (From Pohlman, R.: Die Ultraschalltherapie. Stuttgart, Georg Thieme Verlag, 1951.)

Thus, a transducer operating at therapeutic frequencies will produce a beam with a greater angle of divergence if the diameter of the transducer is small than if it is large (Fig. 13–38).[276]

The sound intensity across the beam produced by a therapeutic transducer is not uniform. If measurements are made of the sound intensity along the central axis of the beam produced by a therapeutic applicator, the intensity distribution shows maxima and minima near the applicator and then a gradual decline beyond the last maximum of intensity (Figs. 13–39 and 13–40).[210] The "interference" or "near field" is the area in the ultrasound beam extending from the applicator surface to the location of the most distant intensity maximum. In this area, maxima and minima of intensity are located close to each other. Beyond this point, the beam has a more uniform intensity, and this area is called the "far" or "distant field."[276] Figure 13–41 shows the distance between transducer surface and the last maximum intensity, dependent on the diameter of the radiating surface of the applicator.

The sound applicators produce an ultrasonic field in the vicinity of the applicator that shows a characteristic interference pattern. In the far field, the intensity distribution across the beam shows a bell-shaped distribution curve (Fig. 13–42).[210] The intensity of the sound field drops gradually to zero at the edge of the distribution. Therefore, a procedure has been developed to determine accurately the radiating surface of an applicator for comparison purposes. First, the total output of the applicator is determined, then baffles of decreasing diameter are used in front of the applicator that cut out the edge of the ultrasonic beam. The size of the opening of the baffle that cuts out 10 per cent of the total output of the applicator is equal to the radiating surface of the applicator. An arbitrary reduction of the total output to 10 per cent is commonly used to determine the radiating surface of the applicator for comparison purposes. A preferable applicator for therapeutic purposes should have a radiating surface area that is only slightly smaller than the total applicator surface. This minimizes the problem of maintaining full contact between the skin and the applicator surface, at the same time utilizing the total surface of the applicator for therapeutic irradiation. The ultrasonic intensity is expressed in watts per cm²,

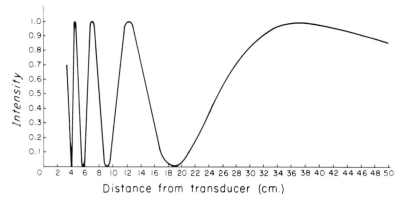

FIGURE 13–39. Calculated location of the maximum and minimum of intensity along the axis of the sound beam produced by a transducer with a diameter of 8 cm operating at a frequency of 0.35 MHz in water. (From Born, H.: Zur Frage der Absorptionsmessungen im Ultraschallgebiet. Zeitschrift Phys., 120: 383–396, 1943.)

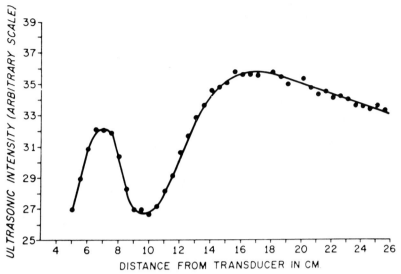

FIGURE 13–40. Measured intensity distribution along the central axis of the ultrasonic beam. (From Lehmann, J. F., and Johnson, E. W.: Some factors influencing the temperature distribution in thighs exposed to ultrasound. Arch. Phys. Med. Rehabil., 39:347–356, 1958.)

referring to the average intensity of the field. This average intensity is obtained by measuring the total output of the applicator (watts) and then dividing it by the size of the radiating surface of the applicator (cm²). In order to be able to produce

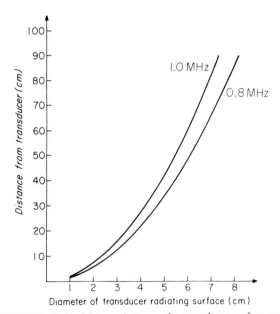

FIGURE 13–41. Distance between the transducer surface and the last interference maximum dependent on the diameter of the radiating surface of the applicator for the therapeutic frequencies of 0.8 and 1 MHz. (From Pohlman, R.: Die Ultraschalltherapie. Stuttgart, Georg Thieme Verlag, 1951.)

vigorous therapeutic effects in the depth of the tissues, the therapeutic applicator should be able to produce average ultrasonic intensities of 3 to 4 watts per cm². For an applicator with a radiating surface area of 10 cm², the maximal total output would be between 30 and 40 watts. The peak intensity, in the bell-shaped distribution curve, should be not more than approximately four times the average intensity. The peak intensity in the far field over average intensity is also a reasonable measure of the uniformity of the beam. This means that a therapeutically acceptable transducer has a broad-based, bell-shaped intensity distribution curve in contrast with an undesirable applicator, which produces a pencil-shaped type of beam with either one or several high-intensity peaks in the field distribution. Multiple high peaks with a non-uniform distribution are commonly encountered in so-called mosaic crystals. Therefore a single quartz or synthetic crystal is to be preferred. Machines with a nonuniform beam may be dangerous because undesirable side effects may be produced by the high intensities in the peaks of the distribution curve.

The losses in the therapeutic applicator should be kept to a minimum to avoid excessive heating during application, which may modify those therapeutic results dependent on temperature. Since the total output of an applicator is a product of average intensity (watts per cm²) and the total radiating surface area (cm²), it is desirable to have

JUSTUS F. LEHMANN AND BARBARA J. DE LATEUR

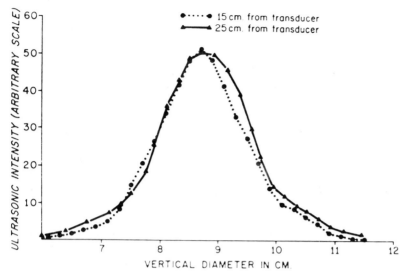

FIGURE 13–42. Intensity distribution in the vertical cross section of the ultrasonic far field. (From Lehmann, J. F., and Johnson, E. W.: Some factors influencing the temperature distribution in thighs exposed to ultrasound. Arch. Phys. Med. Rehabil., 39:347–356, 1958.)

larger applicators. The angle of divergence of the beam is less if an applicator with a large diameter is used. It is for this reason that applicators smaller than 5 cm^2 are not acceptable for therapeutic purposes. It is also difficult to treat the deep tissues in an area of limited size with a beam of small diameter. On the other hand, if the radiating surface of the applicator is too large, it may be difficult to maintain contact with the surface of the body at all times. Therefore, an applicator with a radiating surface of 7 to 13 cm^2 is most convenient and effective for therapeutic application. If the equipment produces pulsed output, the shape of the pulses should preferably be rectangular, with an accurate statement as to intensity during the

pulses, the rate of the pulses, and the duration of the pulses—that is, the duty cycle. The shape of the pulses should be known to avoid excessive temporal intensity peaks that may produce undesirable side effects.

MEASUREMENT OF ULTRASOUND[99]

If ultrasound is incident on a totally reflecting surface, pressure is exerted on the surface.[276] Figure 13–43 shows a schematic arrangement of the so-called sound-pressure balance. The balance is usually calibrated in watts. Similarly, if a floating reflector with its stem immersed in a heavier fluid such as carbon tetrachloride could be used, the

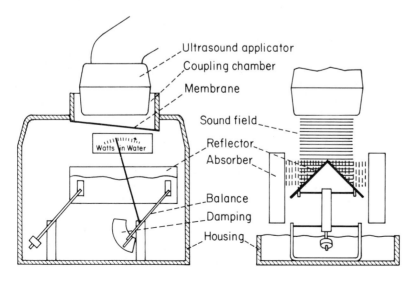

FIGURE 13–43. Schematic arrangement of a so-called sound-pressure balance. (From Pohlman, R.: Die Ultraschalltherapie. Stuttgart, Georg Thieme Verlag, 1951.)

stem would be calibrated, and as a result of the sound, pressure would be driven deeper into the heavy fluid. Also, small probes have been developed to determine sound intensities in small areas of the field.[23, 184, 276]

PHYSICS[23, 73, 99, 186, 193]

Ultrasound is defined as a form of acoustic vibration occurring at frequencies too high to be perceived by the human ear. Thus, frequencies under 17,000 Hz are usually called *sound*, whereas those above this level are designated *ultrasound*. With the exception of the differences in frequencies, the physics of ultrasound is in no way different from that of audible sound. Sound and ultrasound are propagated in the form of longitudinal compression waves. The movement of the particles in the medium occurs parallel to the direction of the wave propagation. In the case of a cylindrical ultrasound beam, the propagation also occurs parallel to the axis of the beam. Hence, the propagation of sound depends on the presence of a medium capable of being compressed. It follows that sound cannot be transmitted through a vacuum.

Ultrasonic frequencies used for therapeutic purposes range between 0.8 and 1 MHz. The sound velocity in water and in tissues is approximately 1.5×10^5 cm per sec. The wavelength is approximately 0.15 cm. Thus, many tissue structures are large as compared with the wavelength, although they are small as compared with the wavelength of audible sound. The result is that biological interfaces and structures that are transparent to audible sound waves may reflect or scatter ultrasound.

The primary reactions occurring within an ultrasonic beam at therapeutic intensities on the order of 1 to 4 watts per cm^2 are directly related to particle movement as a result of the wave propagation. It is possible to assess quantitatively the amplitude of the displacement of the particles in the medium as rarefaction and compression occur alternately. The amplitude of displacement is on the order of 1×10^{-6} to 6×10^{-6} cm. The maximum velocity of the particles is approximately 10 to 26 cm per sec. The accelerations to which the particles are subjected are about 5×10^7 to 16×10^7 cm per sec^2. This represents an acceleration that is approximately 100,000 times that of gravity. The pressure amplitude in the waves is approximately 1 to 4 atmospheres. It should be noted that the area of maximal pressure in the medium is separated by just one-half wavelength from the area of maximal rarefaction. Thus, a great difference in pressure occurs over a relatively short distance.

These powerful mechanical forces can create secondary reactions in the tissues. Since dissolved gases are always present in biological media, the phenomenon called gaseous cavitation may occur. Gas-filled cavities may be produced in the fluid medium during the phase of rarefaction in the sound waves. During the following phase of compression, these cavities may collapse, creating a high-energy concentration in the form of shock waves, or the gas bubbles may become larger. The growth of the bubbles can be explained by the following mechanism: During the phase of compression when the surface of the gas bubble is relatively small, the gas moves out of the bubble into the surrounding fluid. During the following phase of rarefaction when the bubble is expanded and its surface is relatively large, the gas moves out of the fluid into the cavity. The amount of gas passing into or out of the bubble is in proportion to the bubble surface; thus, there is a net gain of gas moving into the bubbles. Electrical and chemical phenomena have been described as results of cavitation. Mechanical destruction also may be produced when the cavities collapse or when gas bubbles grow large enough to vibrate in resonance with the sound waves.[182, 338, 343] The occurrence of gaseous cavitation can be prevented by application of external pressure of sufficient magnitude.

As sound is propagated through the tissues, it is gradually absorbed and converted into heat. The surface intensity is attenuated exponentially. The depth of penetration is commonly defined as that depth of the tissues at which the intensity drops to one half of its value at the surface.

The absorption of ultrasound in uniform tissues has been investigated by Hüter,[149, 150] Dussick and co-workers,[74] and Lehmann and Johnson.[210] Tissue with a very high coefficient of absorption will also show selective rise of temperature in its more superficial portion. Bone may serve as an example.

Carstensen and co-workers,[42] Piersol and colleagues,[275] and Smith[309] have demonstrated that ultrasonic absorption occurs primarily in the tissue proteins, although such structural elements as cellular membranes are responsible for a minor degree of absorption. Hüter[149, 150] has shown that attenuation of ultrasound in muscle tissue depends on whether or not the ultrasonic beam is parallel to myofascial interfaces, thus demonstrating a selective absorption at interfaces that can be explained on the basis of scattering, which, in turn,

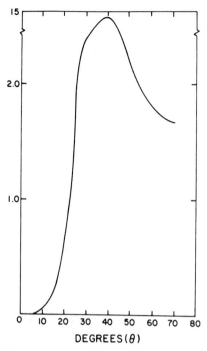

FIGURE 13–44. Ratio of heating due to shear wave to heating due to longitudinal wave. (From Chan, A. K., Sigelmann, R. A., and Guy, A. W.: Calculations of therapeutic heat generated by ultrasound in fat-muscle-bone layers. IEEE Trans. Biomed. Eng. BME, 21:280–284, 1973.)

results in an increased absorption at irregular surfaces. It is also possible that the longitudinal ultrasound waves may be converted into transverse, that is, shear waves, which are quickly attenuated. Chan and co-workers[43, 44] showed that the portion of ultrasonic heating resulting from shear waves is significant and depends on the angle of incidence (Fig. 13–44). In addition, as a result of absorbing ultrasound, a special gradient of acoustic energy is created, producing streaming in a viscous medium.

BIOPHYSICS[73, 247]

The propagation of ultrasonic energy in tissues depends mainly on two factors: absorption char-

acteristics of the biological media (Table 13–5) and reflection of ultrasonic energy at tissue interfaces (Table 13–6). Whole bone absorbs approximately 10 times more energy than skeletal muscle.

Reflection can occur at interfaces between tissues of different acoustic impedance. The impedance was measured and reflection at tissue interfaces determined by Lehmann and Johnson.[210] The results shown in Table 13–6 indicate that very little reflection occurs between soft tissues, but a great deal occurs at the surface of the bone, where up to 30 per cent of energy may be reflected. Surgical metallic implants constitute artificial interfaces. Acoustic impedance of stainless steel, vitallium, and titanium was found to be greatly different from that of bone or soft tissues. Thus, it could be anticipated that the major problem encountered with surgical metallic implants in the ultrasonic field might be that of reflection leading to an intense increase in ultrasonic energy due to the production of a pattern of standing waves and focusing.

THERAPEUTIC TEMPERATURE DISTRIBUTION

Once the absorption coefficient of the tissues and reflection at tissue interfaces are known, it is possible to calculate the so-called pattern of relative heating. This was done for therapeutic ultrasonic frequencies by Schwan[293] and Chan[43] (Fig. 13–45). The data indicate that relatively little energy is converted into heat in the subcutaneous fat and not much more energy is converted into heat in the musculature. The depth of penetration of the ultrasonic energy in the musculature is therefore very satisfactory. One half of the intensity at the muscle surface is still available at a depth of approximately 3 cm. Most of the energy is converted into heat at the bone interface.

The temperature distribution produced by ultrasound is unique among deep-heating modalities. Ultrasound causes comparatively little temperature elevation in the superficial tissues and has a greater

TABLE 13–5. Ultrasonic Attenuation in Pig Tissues*

TISSUE	NUMBER OF SAMPLES	ATTENUATION IN db/cm	STANDARD DEVIATION
Whole bone	13	8.4	± 1.2
Skeletal muscle	30	0.8	± 0.1
Subcutaneous fat	28	1.8	± 0.1

*From Lehmann, J. F., and Johnson, E. W.: Some factors influencing the temperature distribution in thighs exposed to ultrasound. Arch. Phys. Med. Rehabil., 39:347–356, 1958.

TABLE 13–6. Experimental and Calculated Reflection of
Ultrasonic Energy at Tissue Interfaces*

INTERFACE	OBSERVED REFLECTION (% OF INCIDENT ENERGY)	CALCULATED REFLECTION (% OF INCIDENT ENERGY)
Water-fat (pig)	0	0.2
Water-muscle (pig)	0	0.3
Fat-muscle (pig)	—	1.1
Water-bone (pig)	30	30
Muscle-bone (pig)	—	26.8

*From Lehmann, J. F., and Johnson, E. W.: Some factors influencing the temperature distribution in thighs exposed to ultrasound. Arch. Phys. Med. Rehabil., 39:347–356, 1958.

depth of penetration in the musculature and other soft tissues than do short wave and microwave diathermies. Ultrasound selectively heats interfaces between tissues of different acoustic impedance because of reflection, formation of shear waves, and the high selective absorption in the superficial layers of tissue with high coefficient of absorption. Thus, biophysical research suggests that ultrasound is the most effective deep-heating agent. The temperature in joints covered by heavy masses of soft tissues can be raised to therapeutic and even tolerance levels without any deleterious effects elsewhere in the tissues.[217] It was found by comparison that neither short wave nor microwave diathermy produced any therapeutic rise of temperature in the hip joint, even though a first-degree burn was obtained in the superficial tissues with either modality (Figs. 13–46 and 13–47). The high degree of reflection of ultrasound on the surface of the bone, as well as the high coefficient of absorption in bone tissue, eliminates the possibility of heating the distant side of the bone or joint.[217] A practical conclusion evolving from this research is that when treating an entire joint, one should utilize a multiple field technique, exposing all joint surfaces directly to the ultrasonic beam if the joint is to be heated uniformly throughout.

Experiments in pigs have shown that the structures of the knee joint can be selectively heated. As shown in Figure 13–48, the temperature was measured in the capsular tissues and bone just above the knee joint and at the level of the joint space through the capsular tissues and meniscus. The resulting temperature distributions are shown in Figure 13–49.[198]

It is characteristic of ultrasound that a selective increase in temperature may occur at the interface between tissues of different acoustic impedance. Such a selective temperature increase occurs in the human being as shown in Figure 13–50.[194] In ad-

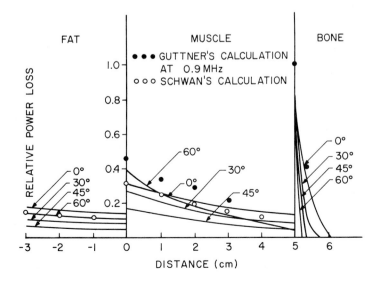

FIGURE 13–45. Relative heating pattern in a three-layered system (fat-muscle-bone). Frequency: 1 MHz. Schwan's and Guttner's calculated values are superimposed, but these values are renormalized. (From Chan, A. K., Sigelmann, R. A., and Guy, A. W.: Calculations of therapeutic heat generated by ultrasound in fat-muscle-bone layers. IEEE Trans. Biomed. Eng. BME, 21:280–284, 1973.)

JUSTUS F. LEHMANN AND BARBARA J. DE LATEUR

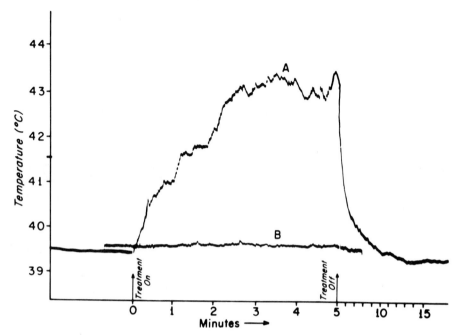

FIGURE 13–46. Change in temperature inside hip joint during exposure to *(A)* ultrasound and *(B)* microwave. (From Lehmann, J. F., McMillan, J. A., Brunner, G. D., and Blumberg, J. B.: Comparative study of the efficiency of short wave, microwave and ultrasonic diathermy in heating the hip joint. Arch. Phys. Med. Rehabil., 40:510–512. 1959.)

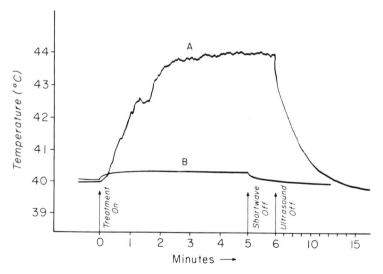

FIGURE 13–47. Change in temperature inside hip joint during exposure to *(A)* ultrasound and *(B)* short wave. (From Lehmann, J. F., McMillan, J. A., Brunner, G. D., and Blumberg, J. B.: Comparative study of the efficiency of short wave, microwave and ultrasonic diathermy in heating the hip joint. Arch. Phys. Med. Rehabil., 40:510–512, 1959.)

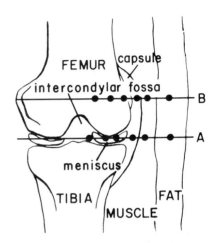

FIGURE 13–48. Needle location in the knee joint *(A)* and 2 cm proximal *(B)*. (From Lehmann, J. F., de Lateur, B. J., Warren, C. G., and Stonebridge, J. B.: Heating of joint structures by ultrasound. Arch. Phys. Med. Rehabil., 49:28–30, 1968.)

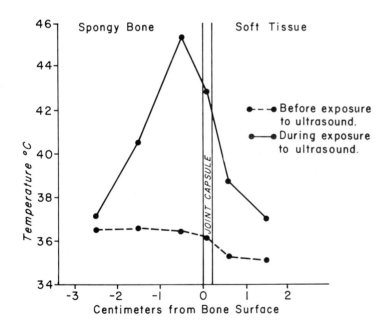

FIGURE 13–49. Temperature distribution 2 cm proximal to the joint space. (From Lehmann, J. F., de Lateur, B. J., Warren, C. G., and Stonebridge, J. B.: Heating of joint structures by ultrasound. Arch. Phys. Med. Rehabil., 49:28–30, 1968.)

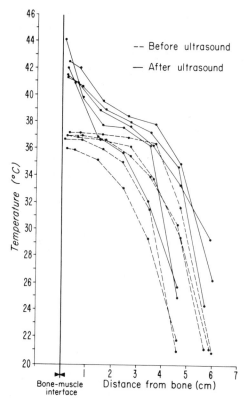

FIGURE 13–50. Comparison of temperature distribution in five human thighs before and after exposure to ultrasound, using a mineral oil coupling medium at 18° C. (From Lehmann, J. F., de Lateur, B. J., and Silverman, D. R.: Selective heating effects of ultrasound in human beings. Arch. Phys. Med. Rehabil., 47:331–339, 1966.)

If the therapeutic objective is to heat the capsular synovial tissues of the joint, the technique of application should be modified so as to minimize the difference between the peak temperature in the superficial bone and the temperature in the adjacent soft tissue structures.[197] This is illustrated in Figure 13–53, where the temperature was measured in front of the bone when the first pain was perceived. It should be noted that in individuals with less than 8 cm of soft tissue cover over the bone, higher temperatures were obtained at lower wattage. Also, at higher wattage the temperature in front of the bone, at pain, was markedly higher in the individual with a thick absorbing tissue cover over the bone than in the thin individual. This discrepancy was explained on the basis that if higher wattage was used in the thin individual the temperature of the superficial bone rose very rapidly and selectively, and thus insufficient time was available for thermal conduction to take place.

dition, it has been documented that the temperature distribution in the human largely depends on the type and temperature of the coupling medium used.[194] For instance, if water, which has a high thermal conductivity and high heat-carrying capacity, is used as a coupling medium, an adequate selective temperature increase in front of the bone still can be obtained at a temperature of 24° C (75° F) (Fig. 13–51). This is not so with the use of mineral oil (Fig. 13–52). Also, for practical purposes, the temperature of the applicator itself should be kept low. These studies, both in animals and in humans, indicate clearly that it is possible to selectively heat joint structures, such as capsules, synovia, and others, with ultrasound. However, it must also be recognized that the temperature obtained in the superficial bone will be slightly higher than that in the capsular tissues in front of the bone.[198]

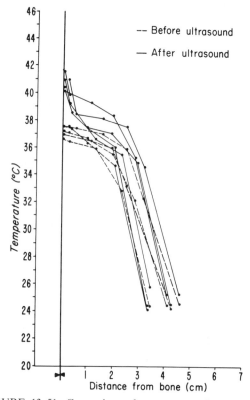

FIGURE 13–51. Comparison of temperature distribution in five human thighs before and after exposure to ultrasound, using degassed water coupling medium at 24° C. (From Lehmann, J. F., de Lateur, B. J., and Silverman, D. R.: Selective heating effects of ultrasound in human beings. Arch. Phys. Med. Rehabil., 47:331–339, 1966.)

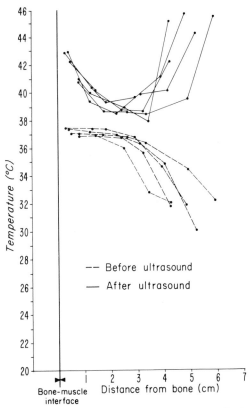

FIGURE 13–52. Comparison of temperature distribution in human thighs before and after exposure to ultrasound, using a mineral oil coupling medium at 24° C. (From Lehmann, J. F., de Lateur, B. J., and Silverman, D. R.: Selective heating effects of ultrasound in human beings. Arch. Phys. Med. Rehabil., 47:331–339, 1966.)

This would minimize the temperature difference between superficial bone and the site of measurement. Pain occurred earlier in these cases, whereas in the slim individual who received lower dosage the treatment was tolerated longer without pain; therefore, heat conduction from the superficial bone into the soft tissues in front of the bone substantially elevated the tissue temperature in front of the bone at the site of measurement. Similarly, at high wattages, temperature rose rapidly to the pain threshold in the superficial bone in the thin individual, and it took a longer period of time in the more obese individual.

The therapeutic application of these findings is that one should treat over a longer period of time, at least over 5 to 10 minutes per field, to obtain optimal heating of joint tissues located right in front of the bone.

There is also evidence that other biological interfaces are selectively heated by ultrasound.[137, 147, 219, 265, 285] Pätzold and Born[265] demonstrated that myofascial interfaces, as they occur in the musculature, are selectively heated. Rosenberger[285] found a selective rise of temperature in the sciatic nerve of experimental animals (Fig. 13–54). Herrick[137] and associates were able to destroy experimentally the sciatic nerve in dogs without affecting the histologic structure of surrounding musculature or the tissues.

On the other hand, ultrasound can be utilized safely in the presence of surgical metallic implants. Marked reflection occurs, resulting in the devel-

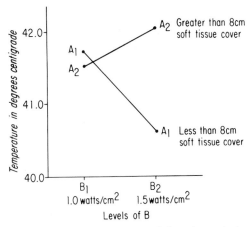

FIGURE 13–53. Temperature recorded at the periosteum of the femur at the moment of pain. (From Lehmann, J. F., de Lateur, B. J., Stonebridge, J. B., and Warren, C. G.: Therapeutic temperature distribution produced by ultrasound as modified by dosage and volume of tissue exposed. Arch. Phys. Med. Rehabil., 48:662–666, 1967.)

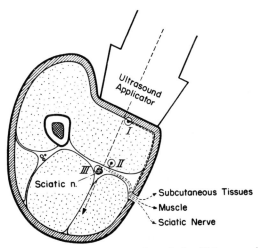

FIGURE 13–54. A cross section through the thigh exposed to ultrasound with thermocouples in I, subcutaneous tissues; II, muscle tissue; III, sciatic nerve. (From Rosenberger, H.: Über den Wirkungmechanismus der Ultraschallbehandlung, insbesondere bei Ischias und Neuralgien. Chirurg., 21:404–406, 1950.)

JUSTUS F. LEHMANN AND BARBARA J. DE LATEUR

opment of patterns of standing waves. Focal concentrations of energy may occur in the vicinity of the implant. This causes a large increase in ultrasonic intensity close to the metal (Table 13–7). Lehmann and colleagues[189] studied the distribution of temperature throughout specimens with metal implants and found that, when exposed to ultrasound, no selective rise of temperature occurred in these areas (Fig. 13–55). Often the temperature in the specimen close to metal was lower than the temperature measured in the same place without metal present. This was explained by the fact that the metal implants have a very high thermal conductivity. Thus, the heat energy is removed from the areas of increased intensity more rapidly than it is absorbed. The experimental findings obtained in specimens were later confirmed in live pigs.[188] Temperatures in the focal areas and in the standing waves close to the implants were within the therapeutic range and could be well controlled (Fig. 13–56). In another series, identical implants were inserted bilaterally into live pigs. One side served as a control and the other was exposed to ultrasound. After the pigs were killed, histological examinations showed no evidence of any retardation of the healing process or callus formation or any other untoward effects on the side treated with ultrasound. In conclusion, ultrasonic energy seems to be the only type of diathermy that can be used with metallic implants in the treatment field, a finding consistent with previous observations by Gersten.[102]

TABLE 13–7. Change of Ultrasonic Intensity Resulting from the Presence of Metallic Implants*

TYPE OF METAL IMPLANT	MODE OF APPLICATION OF ULTRASOUND AND LOCATION OF PROBE	FACTOR BY WHICH ULTRASONIC INTENSITY IS CHANGED (MEAN VALUE)	STANDARD DEVIATION OF THE MEAN
Stainless steel disk	Probe in front of disk, ultrasound beam incident at angle of 90°	1.9	± 0.06
Stainless steel disk	Probe behind disk, ultrasound beam incident at angle of 90°	0.03	± 0.22
Vitallium hip cup (diameter 5 cm)	Ultrasound beam incident perpendicularly at opening of cup, probe in focal area	6.2	± 0.10
Vitallium hip cup (diameter 5 cm)	Ultrasound beam incident at convex side of cup, measurements within cup	0.086	± 0.007
Vitallium hip cup (diameter 5 cm)	Ultrasound beam incident at side of cup, measurements within cup	0.1	± 0.00
Vitallium hip cup (diameter 3.1 cm)	Ultrasound beam incident perpendicularly at opening of cup, probe in focal area	6.4	± 0.06
Smith-Petersen nail	Ultrasound beam incident between two flanges of the nail, probe in focal area	2.7	± 0.07
Smith-Petersen nail	One flange pointing toward ultrasound applicator, probe in focal area	2.7	± 0.001
Küntscher nail	Ultrasound beam incident at groove of nail, probe in focal area	3.7	± 0.18

*From Lehmann, J. F., Lane, C. E., Bell, J. W., and Brunner, G. D.: Influence of surgical metal implants on distribution of the intensity in the ultrasonic field. Arch. Phys. Med. Rehabil., 39:756–760, 1958.

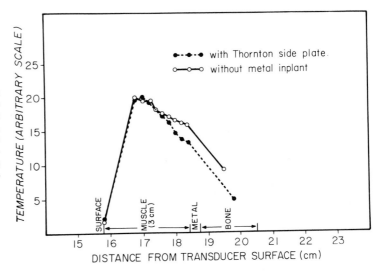

FIGURE 13–55. Temperature distribution in a specimen consisting of muscle and bones, with and without a Thornton side plate inserted in front of the bones. (From Lehmann, J. F., Brunner, G. D., and McMillan, J. A.: The influence of surgical implants on the temperature distribution in thigh specimens exposed to ultrasound. Arch. Phys. Med. Rehabil., 39:692–695, 1958.)

TECHNIQUE OF APPLICATION

Before ultrasound can be applied, the machine must be tuned and the output must be set. Proper coupling between the applicator and the skin surface must be provided. Coupling media that produce adequate transmission are shown in Figure 13–57.[335] Balmaseda and co-workers[14] studied the attenuation of ultrasound as a function of distance in various coupling media. They found that the commercially available gels had less attenuation and offered a better impedance match than other coupling media that have been used. However, it is important to realize that the effect of attenuation by absorption as studied in thick layers is minimized in the actual application of coupling media,

in which the coupling medium represents only a very thin film between applicator and skin. It is important, however, that the coupling media do not contain any gas bubbles that would significantly reflect and scatter ultrasound, with a resulting drop in transmission (Fig. 13–58). Also, gas bubbles may stick to the skin and produce a significant loss in transmission, according to Pätzold and associates.[266] These bubbles could be removed by using a wetting agent, such as a detergent, prior to treatment; the wetting agent must be carefully rinsed off to prevent skin irritation. The skin irritation is likely due to the fact that with ultrasound some of these agents may penetrate the skin.

Two types of application have been developed.

FIGURE 13–56. Change in temperature between flanges of stainless steel Smith-Petersen nail during exposure of a live pig to ultrasound. (From Lehmann, J. F., Brunner, G. D., Martinis, A. J., and McMillan, J. A.: Ultrasonic effects as demonstrated in live pigs with surgical metallic implants. Arch. Phys. Med. Rehabil., 40:483–488, 1959.)

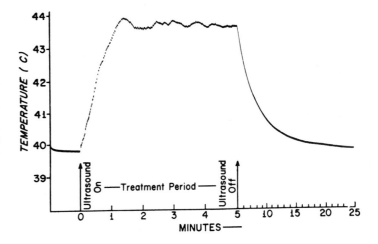

JUSTUS F. LEHMANN AND BARBARA J. DE LATEUR

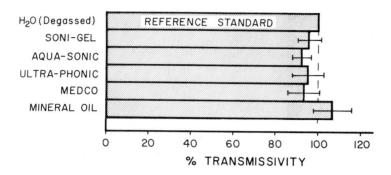

FIGURE 13–57. Per cent transmissivities of several coupling agents using ultrasound generator without transducer voltage control circuit. (From Warren, C. G., Koblanski, J. N., and Sigelmann, R. A.: Ultrasound coupling media: their relative transmissivity. Arch. Phys. Med. Rehabil., 57:218–222, 1976.)

The sound head may be held stationary, or it may be moved slowly in a back-and-forth stroking motion. The stationary technique is rarely used because it produces a rapid rise of temperature in a very small area, which is rather difficult to control. Hot spots are produced in the interference field and in the far field where the highest intensity is found in the center of the beam. These hot spots are likely to heat small areas excessively while the rest of the tissues are not heated adequately for therapeutic purposes.

The stroking technique is most commonly employed. Strokes are comparatively short, on the order of one inch in length, and each stroke partially overlaps the area of another, with the applicator gradually moving in a direction perpendicular to the strokes. Circular strokes may be used, but they are somewhat more difficult to control. The temperature increase produced by this technique is rather smooth with little ripples and can be well controlled, as seen in Figures 13–47 and 13–56. The temperatures obtained in the tissues depend on the total output of the applicator, the time of application, and the size of the field treated. For most therapeutic applicators, it is necessary to treat a field of approximately 3 to 4 sq in. If vigorous results are to be obtained, it is necessary to produce temperatures that are just below the maximally tolerated level. In order to find this level, it is advisable to continue until pain

is felt briefly by the patient and then either to reduce the output of the applicator slightly or to increase the field size, that is, the volume of tissue treated, maintaining the same output. With this procedure, one uses the warning signal of pain to test tolerance limits. However, the patient should be instructed to indicate pain immediately so that damage is avoided. Mild to moderate effects can be obtained by lowering the ultrasonic output substantially below the pain threshold.

The temperature distribution in the tissues is also modified by the temperature of the coupling medium or the temperature of the surface of the metal applicator.[194] The cooler the temperature of the coupling medium or the applicator, the greater the heat loss at the skin and the deeper the peak temperatures found in the tissues. These investigations suggest that if ultrasound is prescribed for deep-heating purposes, it is important to state the temperature of the coupling medium if water is used. Also, it is important to use an applicator with minimal electrical and mechanical losses that maintains a fairly constant temperature during treatment.[221] If the applicator warms up noticeably after one field is treated, it should be quickly placed in tap water to cool it before the next field is treated.

When a major joint covered with a large amount of soft tissue is treated with ultrasound, it has been shown in animal experimentation that the most

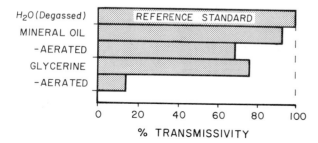

FIGURE 13–58. Per cent transmissivities for several common coupling media in aerated and nonaerated forms using ultrasound generator without voltage control circuit. (From Warren, C. G., Koblanski, J. N., and Sigelmann, R. A.: Ultrasound coupling media: their relative transmissivity. Arch. Phys. Med. Rehabil., 57:218–222, 1976.)

superficial bone is heated most.[194] In human volunteers, it was found that the temperature reached in the tissue in front of the bone—for example, joint structure—depended not only on the thickness of the soft tissue and the intensity of ultrasound but also on the interaction between these two factors. Thus, if the intensity is too high in a thin individual, tolerance levels in the superficial bone are exceeded before conduction of heat to the tissues in front of the bone can occur. The experimental evidence indicates that 5 to 10 minutes of ultrasound application per field is necessary to produce adequate heating of the joint structures in front of the bone.[197]

Joints such as the shoulder or the hip are typically treated with three fields of application: an anterior, a lateral, and a posterior field, since effective treatment through the interposed bone is not possible. In the case of the hip joint, special care should be taken to locate the lateral field of application so that one avoids aiming the sound beam at the greater trochanter.[217] It is also essential that any exercise or stretching procedure immediately follow the ultrasound treatment or be applied simultaneously with ultrasound; e.g., the anterior aspect of the hip joint could be treated with ultrasound and stretched in the Thomas position. A special technique has been developed so that one part of the shoulder joint is treated and subsequently stretched.[240] After this, another field is exposed and again the treated structures are stretched immediately, until the entire shoulder joint has been treated and stretched.

To avoid the occurrence of gaseous cavitation and its destructive effects,[193] the stroking technique can be used with intensities of up to 4 watts per cm² and a total output of 40 watts at a frequency of 1 MHz. Under those circumstances, cavitation is inhibited by the high viscosity of tissue fluids, such as blood serum, and the high volume concentration of cells in blood and tissues. However, cavitation can occur much more readily in the fluid media of the eye, the amniotic fluid, and the synovial fluid in joint effusions. Therefore, the eye, the pregnant uterus, and joints with effusions should not be treated with therapeutic intensities and frequencies.[185] For the stationary technique, the cavitation threshold is approximately between 1 and 2 watts per cm². These intensities applied in this fashion also produce burns. Because of the threshold for cavitation, ultrasonic equipment should not produce high temporal or spatial peak intensities that may exceed cavitation thresholds.

PULSED APPLICATION

The pulsing frequencies in most applications of pulsed ultrasound are so high that the temperature rise will be equal to that produced by continuous-wave application of the same average output. Therefore, all thermal reactions can be equally and less expensively produced by continuous-wave application. Also, the occurrence of many nonthermal reactions such as streaming are equal to the average output just as the thermal reactions are. There is no evidence that nonthermal reactions selectively produced by the high intensity during the pulses have any therapeutic significance.[193]

Equipment is also available that combines an electrical stimulator with an ultrasound generator. There is no evidence that this equipment has a greater therapeutic effect than when the two modalities are contained in separate pieces of equipment.

DOSIMETRY

The factors that determine the biological response to ultrasound are mainly the temperature obtained in the tissues and the duration of the temperature elevation. It would be ideal if it were possible to measure and control these factors accurately, permitting a quantitative control of the biological response. However, only the ultrasonic energy entering the tissues and the duration of the treatment can be measured, and thus the resulting tissue effect can only be estimated, provided that information is available on the temperature distribution in the organism as well as on how it can be modified by the technique of application. For therapeutic purposes, it is necessary to determine the total ultrasonic output (watts) and the average intensity (watts per cm²). Therapeutic machines can be tuned adequately in water and then applied to the patient without retuning. The output of the machine can be preset in a water bath utilizing a meter on the front panel of the machine that indicates total output (watts) and average intensity (watts per cm²). Some machines do not require tuning. The output can be preset by pressing a contact button, activating a simulated load. The output indicated on the meter will be transmitted to the tissues, provided that reflection at the skin surface is prevented by proper use of a coupling medium.

Some machines are equipped with a protective system. The moment that contact with the body is partially lost and the load of the applicator is therefore changed, a feedback to a control system reduces the output. This is indicated by the meter on the panel and a buzzing device. Its disadvantage is that no ultrasonic energy is applied to the body when poor coupling is inevitable because of uneven body surfaces where full contact cannot be maintained. Intensities found useful in therapy range from 0.5 to 4 watts per cm^2, usually applied with a moving applicator. If the applicator is kept stationary, intensities less than 1 watt per cm^2 are tolerated. The increase in temperature of the tissues is determined by the technique of application. The duration of the treatment is usually 5 to 10 minutes per field. Applications usually are repeated on a daily basis. Sometimes treatment is given twice a day or three times a week.

In order to obtain vigorous results in deep-heated structures such as the hip joint, intensities of up to 4 watts per cm^2 with a total output of 40 watts may be needed. For mild heating, intensities of 2 watts per cm^2 with a total output of 10 to 20 watts may be used. For applicators with smaller radiating surface area, allowances will have to be made. For very mild treatment or very superficial structures, average outputs of 0.1 to 1 watt per cm^2 are used, with a total output of 1 to 10 watts. Adjustment has to be made from these suggested outputs for more superficially located structures. The output should be reduced. It should be emphasized that the maximally tolerated output, which can be assessed by a brief occurrence of pain, can be used as a guide, especially for vigorous heating.

PHYSIOLOGICAL EFFECTS OF ULTRASOUND[193]

A large number of biological and therapeutic responses have been investigated.[186] In this chapter, the results of an extensive research effort in this area are summarized briefly. Reactions due to heating of the tissues and nonthermal reactions are discussed.

Reactions Due to Heating

Since physiologically effective temperature elevations can be produced in the tissues, it is logical to assume that all those reactions that are known to occur as a result of temperature elevation in the tissues will also be produced by ultrasound. Three groups of researchers[3, 25, 267] found that the peripheral arterial blood flow is increased as a result of ultrasound application. The tissue metabolism can be changed, according to Lehmann and co-workers[209] and Pauly and Hug.[268] Experimental evidence has been furnished that these reactions are quantitatively due to the heating effect of ultrasonic energy.[184, 185] It has been observed that reactions such as hyperemia and inflammatory responses characterized by an increase in vascularity, edema, and tissue necrosis all can be quantitatively explained on the basis of the heating effect of ultrasonic energy. It was also found experimentally that a marked increase in permeability of biological membranes and a change of membrane potentials can be produced and is, to a large degree, the result of the temperature elevation in the tissues during exposure to ultrasound.[184, 185, 187] However, part of the effect is also due to nonthermal mechanisms. The effects of ultrasonic energy on nerve tissues have been studied extensively, and most of them have been found to be due entirely to the heating effect.[151, 177, 182, 232] Recently, Kramer[169] found that ultrasound application increased nerve conduction velocities.

It is of interest for therapeutic purposes to note that conduction velocity in peripheral nerves can be altered and temporary blocks can be produced. Different types of fibers show differences in sensitivity to ultrasound; the smallest, C fibers, are the most sensitive. An increase or decrease of spinal reflexes can also be produced, depending on the dosage used.[6, 100, 303] Some of these effects on spinal cord function are nonthermal in nature.[103, 193] The pain threshold can be elevated by application of ultrasonic energy to the peripheral nerve or to the area of the free nerve endings.[191] "Muscle spasm" as found in poliomyelitis can be relieved by ultrasonic application.[98, 313] An increase in vascularity and skin temperature can be produced by ultrasonic radiation applied to the sympathetic nerves.[292, 316] Careful investigations of the action of ultrasonic energy on bone showed that if therapeutic dosage is applied, no detrimental effects are observed in either growing or adult bone.[15, 155] The use of ultrasound in the acceleration of fracture healing has been controversial.[9] In animal experiments, Corradi and Cozzolino[55, 56] found that healing of experimental fractures in rabbits was accelerated on the treated side compared with that of the untreated side. Intensities of 1.5 watts per cm^2 were applied daily for five minutes over a period of 15 days. Maintz,[233] on the other hand, found no improvement of callus formation as a result of ultrasound treatment. Hippe and Uhlmann[143] clinically described 181 cases of delayed fracture healing that they treated with 15 watts and intensities of 1.5 watts per cm² for five minutes every second to every third day, and observed improvement. On the other hand, whereas improved healing of fractures may be explained by a moderate increase in temperature, pathological fractures may be due to excessive heating. The length of time of application may also have an influence. In addition, Cochran and co-workers[50] showed experimental evidence that the application of ultrasound can produce a piezoelectric effect in bone that, in turn, may produce osteogenesis and an increased rate of fracture healing, which is especially useful in delayed union. Excessive dosage led to pathological fractures.[8]

Nonthermal Reactions

A review of the biological reactions indicates that most of these reactions clearly are due to the temperature elevation resulting from exposure to ultrasound.[332] In some instances, however, the entire reaction could not be explained on the basis of the heating effects of ultrasonic energy. The reaction was due in part to nonthermal effects. In only a few instances have nonthermal effects been studied in detail. It has been found that the permeability of biological membranes is altered not only by the heating effect of ultrasonic energy but also by nonthermal effects occurring during exposure to ultrasound that speed up the rate of diffusion of ions across the membrane.[226] Lehmann[184, 185] and Lehmann and Biegler[187] showed that this nonthermal reaction can be explained on the basis of streaming of fluids in the ultrasonic field and the resultant stirring effect; that is, an increase in the gradient of concentration of ions across the biolog-ical membrane that accelerates the rate of diffusion. Quantitatively, the thermal effect was definitely the dominant one. The stirring effect could also be demonstrated in living cells. Membrane potentials were similarly affected by the mechanical effect of ultrasonic energy. These experimental findings may be the basis for the type of clinical application of ultrasound called phonophoresis (see *The Clinical Use of Heat and Cold in Various Conditions*). Gersten[101, 103, 104] pointed out that neither the effect on tendon extensibility produced by ultrasound nor the effects on musculature or on the spinal cord could be explained entirely on the basis of thermal reactions alone.

Numerous reactions to gaseous cavitation are known; most of them, however, occur in the test tube only.[183] Typically destructive reactions such as hemolysis occur only if there is a low concentration of cells and the viscosity of the medium is low as compared with therapeutic conditions.[184, 185] Cavitation also was studied in the live organism.[208] The histological appearance of the cavitation reaction was characteristic: the destruction of cells was spotty and led to petechial hemorrhages. The appearance of the hemorrhages could be explained by the spotty occurrence of gas bubbles in the tissues (Fig. 13–59). Intensity thresholds of 1 to 2 watts per cm² were required to produce these lesions. The reactions could be prevented by the application of external pressure, proving that they were due to cavitation. It was noted that under conditions similar to those in therapy (i.e., at intensities of 1 watt per cm² or below applied with the stationary technique), the destructive effects

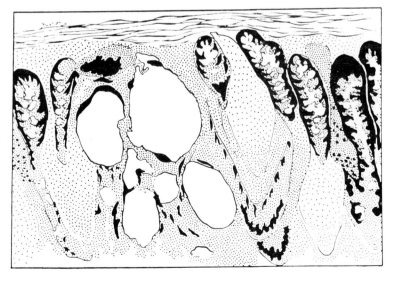

FIGURE 13–59. Destruction of mucous membrane in the intestine, with hemorrhage and formation of gas bubbles. (From Lehmann, J. F., and Herrick, J. F.: Biologic reactions to cavitation, a consideration for ultrasonic therapy. Arch. Phys. Med. Rehabil., 34:86–98, 1953.)

of cavitation did not occur. It was observed that when the stroking technique commonly used in therapy was simulated, intensities of up to 4 watts per cm^2 were tolerated without the appearance of destructive effects of cavitation. It also could be demonstrated that the danger of producing cavitation under therapeutic conditions is increased if unsuitable equipment is used. Animals were irradiated with the stationary applicator with an ultrasonic intensity of 1.5 watts per cm^2 and a total output of the applicator of 15 watts. The machine had a power supply with full-wave rectification. In one series of irradiations, filters were used to produce a steady ultrasonic output; in another series, the filters were removed, producing a greatly modulated ultrasonic output. In the animals treated with the steady output, a few reactions to cavitation were observed, whereas when ultrasound was applied with the same machine with the same average output but with the filtering removed, cavitation effects were observed in 55 per cent of the animals. These experiments demonstrate that peak ultrasonic intensities resulting from the lack of filtering of the rectified line voltage may be potentially dangerous.

Dyson and colleagues[75, 81] showed that if ultrasound was applied with the stationary technique, blood cell aggregates formed in the vessels in the wave nodes that occurred when a pattern of standing waves was set up; this led to a temporary stasis of blood flow. However, this effect could be avoided when the stroking technique was used.

Zarod and Williams,[363] Chater and Williams,[45] and Williams and co-workers[337, 340–342, 344, 345] observed *in vitro* platelet aggregation and an increase in the recalcification time of platelet-rich plasma; *in vivo* Zarod and co-workers found platelet aggregation following ultrasound exposure. The authors felt that hydrodynamic shear stresses, which can be produced by ultrasound, could be responsible. However, there is no evidence that the same phenomena occur under therapeutic conditions *in vivo*. These phenomena are less likely to be observed when the ultrasound is applied by the stroking technique. The mechanism is not clearly understood but is likely related to the occurrence of cavitation.

Dyson and associates[77] found clear evidence that varicose ulcers treated with ultrasound healed faster than those treated with mock insonation (Fig. 13–60). An ultrasonic frequency of 3 MHz with an average intensity of 1 watt per cm^2 and a duty cycle of 20 per cent was used. The mechanism

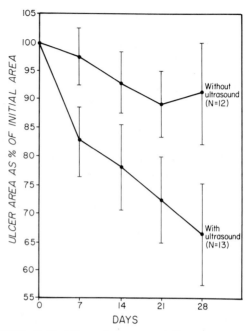

FIGURE 13–60. Effect of treatment with ultrasound on varicose ulcer area. (From Dyson, M., Franks, C., and Suckling, J.: Stimulation of healing of varicose ulcers by ultrasound. Ultrasonics, 14:232–236, 1976.)

by which ultrasound stimulates healing is uncertain. According to Dyson, the mechanism may be thermal or nonthermal. According to Dyson and Pond,[76, 78, 79] the therapeutic effect may be related to the stimulation of tissue regeneration and accelerated collagen deposition and also to remodeling of the scar collagen.

A large number of other effects have been investigated and are reviewed elsewhere.[73, 193] In most of the cases, the exact mechanism is unknown, and the conditions under which these physiological or destructive effects are observed are significantly different from those of therapeutic application.

In conclusion, this brief review of the physiological reactions to ultrasound indicates that those reactions of potential therapeutic significance are due primarily to the temperature elevation resulting from absorption of ultrasonic energy. In addition, a few nonthermal effects have been demonstrated, such as the acceleration of diffusion processes across biological membranes, which may be therapeutically useful. These effects are also dependent on temperature and occur at a faster rate if they are associated with temperature elevation. Fortunately, the destructive effects due to cavitation have not been observed under therapeutic conditions if the proper equipment is used and a therapeutic dosage is applied with the proper technique. A more detailed investigation of the nonthermal effects would be most desirable, since they could potentially lead to new specific indications for ultrasonic therapy. Investigation has also shown that there are marked differences between thermal reactions produced by ultrasound and those produced by other heating modalities. These discrepancies have been attributed mainly to the differences in temperature distribution produced by ultrasound and other heating modalities. Therefore, it is important to obtain information on those reactions that ultimately produce the temperature distribution characteristic of ultrasound application.

CONTRAINDICATIONS TO ULTRASOUND THERAPY

Ultrasound is a very powerful and effective heating agent. Therefore, it must be applied with the proper precautions, in the proper dosage, and with the correct technique. There are, however, only a very few specific contraindications.

Ultrasound should not be applied to the eye in therapeutic dosage range, since cavitation will most likely occur in the fluid media and may lead to irreversible damage.

The pregnant uterus should not be treated because of the possibility of cavitation in the amniotic fluid that may occur at therapeutic intensities and because of the danger of producing malformation of the fetus as a result of thermal damage.[73, 129, 310] Usually, this is not a problem, since the uterus is not reached by any appreciable amount of energy in any of the common therapeutic applications. Because of the good beaming properties of ultrasound applicators, it is also easy to avoid aiming the beam at the uterus.

Special precautions in adjusting the dosage should be taken when the area of the spinal cord is treated after laminectomy. After the covering tissues have been removed, it is likely that higher energy levels may be obtained in the spinal cord.[74] Again, because of the good beaming properties of most applicators, the facet joints, for instance, could be treated without exposing the spinal cord.

Ultrasound should be applied with caution over anesthetic areas. Since dosimetry is better developed in ultrasound than in short wave or microwave diathermy, it is possible to use ultrasound in such cases if special precautions are taken to ensure that the dose is below the damaging level.

Recent investigations determined that methyl methacrylate and high density polyethylene, materials commonly used in total joint replacements, absorb significantly more ultrasound than soft tissue. In addition, the absorption in methyl methacrylate depends largely on the conditions of mixing of the plastic and the ultimate air bubble content.[223] Whether or not this selective absorption by these materials would lead to overheating or even melting of the plastics has at the present time not been determined. Therefore, at present, materials of this type in the sound field should be considered a contraindication to therapy.

The heart should not be directly exposed to ultrasound because Mortimer[255] showed it would change the heart's action potential and contractile properties. Other investigators have shown changes in conduction properties. In addition, Williams[339, 341, 344] showed, in animal experiments, that hemolysis, probably through development of gas bubbles, may occur in the heart as a result of the turbulence of blood flow in that area.

Ultrasound should not be applied to areas where a malignant tumor could be reached by an unknown quantity of ultrasonic energy, since Hayashi[130] has shown that tumor growth may be accelerated both by such ultrasound and by short wave exposure. The increase or retardation of growth or the destruction of tumors by this type of heat therapy, according to Hayashi, depends on the dosage. Thus, if the dose is uncontrolled, hyperthermia may not necessarily have a beneficial effect.

Sound should not be applied over areas of vascular insufficiency because the blood supply would be unable to follow the increase in metabolic demand and necrosis might result. During the International Congress in Erlangen in 1949,[146, 281] it was agreed that ultrasonic energy could not be used for treatment of tumors, since a regression of growth could be obtained in a few cases only and the well-established x-ray therapy produced results far superior to those obtained with ultrasonic energy. In some cases, exposure to ultrasonic energy caused even more rapid growth, and such exposure was, therefore, considered to be potentially dangerous.[146, 273] Finally, all general contraindications to heat therapy should be observed carefully.

Superficial Heating Agents

The hallmark of all these modalities is that they produce temperature distributions, with the high-

JUSTUS F. LEHMANN AND BARBARA J. DE LATEUR

est temperature usually at the surface of the body. Consequently, these superficial heating agents may produce mild or vigorous therapeutic responses if the pathology is located in the most superficial tissues. The extent of the reaction will depend on the temperature at the site. For any pathology located deep in the tissue, these modalities can produce only a mild or moderate response. In the superficial tissue, they may produce physiological changes either by local changes of the tissue or cellular function or by triggering reflex mechanisms. Virtually all responses deep in the organism are produced indirectly through reflexes. The mode of heat transfer of these modalities, however, varies. They may heat by conversion, conduction, or convection.

Superficial Heat by Conversion: Radiant Heat

Mode of Heat Transfer. For heating purposes, the portion of the visible light from yellow to red and the near and far infrared are used. The portion of the visible light used for radiant heating purposes extends over the wavelength from 5500 to 7000 Å units and for the infrared, from 7000 to 120,000 Å. The infrared is subdivided into the near infrared, with wavelengths from 7000 to 14,000 Å, and the far infrared, with wavelengths from 14,000 to 120,000 Å.

The energy content of the photon is expressed by the formula

$$E = hF$$

where h represents Planck's constant and F is the frequency of radiation. Basically, the higher the energy content of the photon, the shorter the photon wavelength and, in turn, the greater the depth of penetration in the tissues.[195] However, practically, these differences have no significant influence on the temperature distribution. Once the photons have penetrated into the tissues, they are absorbed and converted into heat. However, all of them penetrate only into the most superficial tissues.

Technique of Application. One of the advantages of these modalities is that the heat can be applied without touching the body and the skin stays dry. Heat lamps are used for application. Heating elements are made out of carbon-metal alloys or special quartz tubes. Also, simple light bulbs with either carbon or tungsten filaments are used, such as a 250-watt Mazda lamp. A number of light bulbs are also used in the heat cradle. The quality of a single lamp should be judged primarily by how large the skin area is that is evenly heated. This, in turn, largely depends on the quality of the design of heating element and reflector. A simple test allows a check of the evenness of the heating effect. Carbon-blackened paraffin is poured into a pan and allowed to solidify. Once the lamp is turned on, the area where the paraffin begins to melt evenly is an indication of the area with similar intensity of the incident light (Fig. 13–61). The capability of such lamps to produce a vigorous effect over the area heated will depend on the total light output which, in turn, is most readily assessed by the electrical wattage rating of the heating elements. Finally, the quality of the stand, its versatility with regard to adjustment, and its stability are all features to be considered.

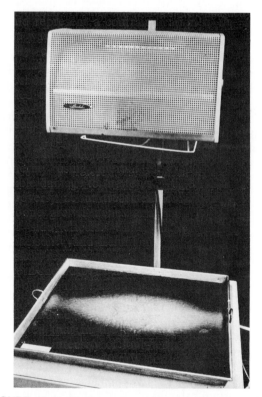

FIGURE 13–61. Heating pattern of lamp as demonstrated by melting of blackened paraffin. (From Lehmann, J. F., and de Lateur, B. J.: Therapeutic Heat. *In* Lehmann, J. F., [Ed.]: Therapeutic Heat and Cold, 3rd Ed. Baltimore, Williams and Wilkins, 1982.)

The large high-output commercial lamps usually produce more infrared than do light bulbs. As mentioned earlier, the differences in depth of penetration of various types of lamps with the difference in output in the visible light and the infrared spectrum is of no significance with regard to the temperature distributions they produce. Figure 13–62 shows clearly that the temperature distributions in the human are identical with three different lamps.

The advantage of the 250-watt bulb with a built-in reflector is that it is inexpensive, can be clamped onto chairs or other furniture, and can be used as a home heating device. However, its limitations are due to the fact that it heats only a very small area evenly and that it has a limited total wattage. The commercial lamps have a higher wattage on the order of 500 watts and heat a larger area evenly. Also, their stand is much more versatile. This is important, since it is preferred that the light be incident perpendicular to the skin. For heating a larger part of the body, the preferred apparatus is the heat cradle, which contains numerous light bulbs with either tungsten or carbon filaments, a switch to dial the number of bulbs to be lit, and a reflector. When two cradles are used, the trunk, arms, and legs can be covered. A blanket usually covers the cradle to retain the heat.

Dosimetry. Heat lamps may have switches to change the wattage output and thus the heat output. The light intensity can also be varied by varying the distance from the lamp to the skin. The lamps with reflectors produce a divergent beam. Increasing the distance reduces the light intensity to which the skin is exposed. Guidance is given by the subjective feeling of warmth. This physiological guide is adequate, since the skin, with its temperature receptors, is the area of highest temperature elevation. In the heat cradle, the number of bulbs lit may alter the heating effect. If two heat cradles are used, it should be remembered that under normal circumstances, the amount of heat the human body can transfer to the outside is 0.01 watt per cm^2 body surface. This may be raised about 10-fold under favorable circumstances, including evaporative cooling by sweating. The amount of radiant heat absorbed without causing a core temperature increase is possible only to the degree that the body, in turn, can lose the heat absorbed. This limit is reached if the heat input exceeds a value between 100 and 1000 watts. A normal heat cradle with an output of 300 watts is, therefore, not likely to raise body temperature. A double heat cradle, however, may do so. Studies by Evans and Mendelssohn[90] have shown that heat cradles and lamps do not reach maximum power output for one hour. The patient under the cradle, for instance, will receive three times as much radiation after one hour as at the beginning of the treatment. This is due to secondary radiation from bulb, envelope, and reflector.

Temperature Distribution. Temperature distribution is mentioned and is shown in Figure 13–62. The highest temperature values are found at the skin surface, with a rapid drop and no significant temperature elevation in the musculature.

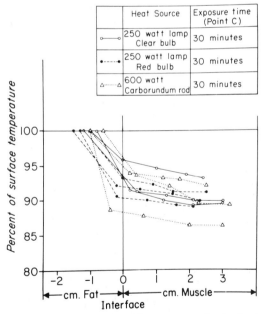

	Heat Source	Exposure time (Point C)
o——o	250 watt lamp Clear bulb	30 minutes
•----•	250 watt lamp Red bulb	30 minutes
△----△	600 watt Carborundum rod	30 minutes

FIGURE 13–62. Comparison of temperature distribution in the human thigh during exposure to infrared radiation in nine individuals using three modalities. (From Lehmann, J. F., Silverman, D. R., Baum, B. A., Kirk, N. L., and Johnston, V. C.: Temperature distributions in the human thigh, produced by infrared, hot pack and microwave applications. Arch. Phys. Med. Rehabil., 47:291–299, 1966.)

Superficial Heating by Conduction

Hydrocollator and Related Packs

Mode of Heat Transfer. The main mode of heat transfer is by conduction. Some additional heat transfer by infrared radiation and convection may occur. The amount of heat (H) that flows through the body by conduction is directly proportional to the time of flow (t), the area through which it flows (A), the temperature gradient (ΔT), and the thermal conductivity (k). It is inversely proportional to the thickness of the layer ΔL.

$$H = k \, At \, (\Delta T/\Delta L)$$

The practical application of this formula is that, in order to reduce the heat flow from the pack to the skin, the heat transfer can be slowed by inserting material with poor thermal conductivity, such as terry cloth toweling, between the pack and the skin. Slowdown of the heat flow, in turn, could be markedly reduced if the patient were lying on the pack and the water were coming out of the pack and thoroughly wetting the toweling, increasing the thermal conductivity. Even without the water seeping through the toweling, the thickness of the toweling would be compacted, reducing its insulating value.

Technique of Application. The most common commercially available packs are the Hydrocollator packs, which contain silicate gel in a cotton bag. They are heated in a thermostatically controlled water bath, where the gel absorbs and holds a large amount of water with its high heat content. The temperature of the pack when applied is about 71 to 79° C (160 to 175° F). Application is done drip-dry over layers of terry cloth for 20 to 30 minutes.

Dosimetry. Dosimetry with the pack at a constant temperature is done primarily by varying the thickness of the terry cloth, which, in turn, slows down the heat transfer. Temperatures produced by the pack are as shown in Figure 13–63. The highest temperatures were found in the skin of the human volunteer, with a rapid drop of the temperature to the subcutaneous fat. Deeper tissues such as musculature are not heated significantly.[193, 220] Repeated packing does not alter the temperature distribution significantly, since first the skin blood flow increase is triggered, which not only reduces the temperature in the skin but also creates an additional barrier for heat transfer into the deeper tissues.[220]

Hot Water Bottle

Frequently, a rubber hot water bottle can be used in the same fashion as the Hydrocollator pack. This heat application is preferred for home use. However, it must be realized that in this case the heat transfer into the tissues also depends on the temperature of the water in the bottle, which is not necessarily thermostatically controlled, as in

the Hydrocollator pack. For hospital use, hot packs of this type contain a thermostatically controlled fluid that is pumped through the pad to ensure the avoidance of burns. In this case, again the transfer is somewhat different, since the pack temperature remains constant in contrast to both the Hydrocollator pack and the hot water bottle.

Kenny Packs[98]

The Kenny pack was originally developed primarily for patients with polio to relieve muscle soreness and spasms. The pack consists of a woolen cloth that is steamed and then the surplus water content removed by spinning. The relatively dry pack is then applied quickly to the skin, usually at a temperature of 60° C (140° F). Since it contains little water and therefore has a low heat-carrying capacity, the temperature drops rapidly to 37.8° C (100° F) within 5 minutes. Thus this is a very short-term but vigorous heating application, producing a marked reflex response.

Electric Heating Pads

The electric heating pad can be used dry as a Hydrocollator pack. It may also be used, if properly insulated by plastic, over a moist cloth. The heat transfer is significantly greater to the skin using the moist pack application. The heat output of the electric heating pad can be adjusted by increasing or decreasing its wattage. The electric heating pad has one marked danger: the heat output steadily increases over a long period of time until finally equilibrium is reached. This is especially dangerous if the patient lies on the pad or falls asleep with the pad. The heat itself may be analgesic enough that severe burns may be produced.

Chemical Packs

Chemical packs currently available are in a flexible container in which, by moving the container, a compartment is broken. This allows the ingredients to come together and produce an elevation of temperature by an exothermic chemical reaction. All these packs are poorly controlled as to the temperature produced. The ingredients are irritating or harmful when the outer pack breaks and its content comes in contact with the skin. Therefore, this type of application is least desirable.

The Paraffin Bath

Technique of Application and Mode of Heat Transfer. For therapeutic purposes, paraffin wax with a melting point of approximately 51.7 to 54.5° C (125 to 130° F)[173, 314] is used. The thermostatically controlled container maintains the wax at its melting temperature. For safety reasons, a thermometer should be used to check the temperature.

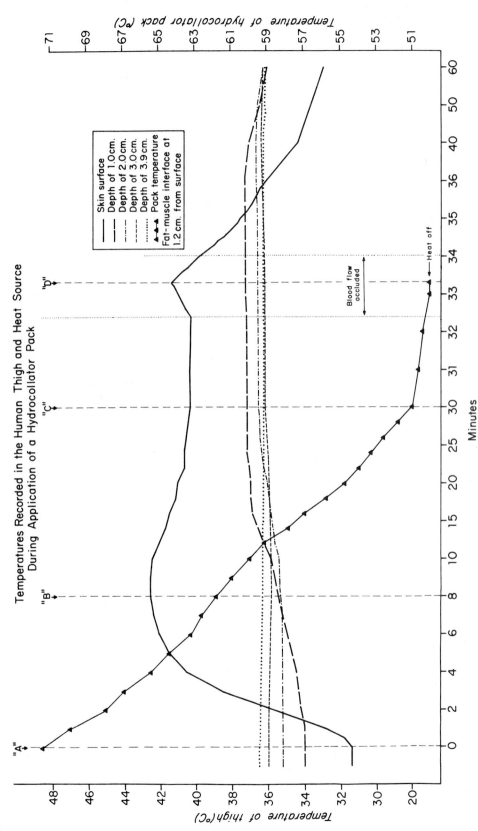

Temperatures Recorded in the Human Thigh and Heat Source During Application of a Hydrocollator Pack

FIGURE 13–63. Temperatures recorded in the human thigh during application of Hydrocollator hot packs. *A*, Temperature distribution before heat is applied. *B*, Peak temperature at skin surface. *C*, Temperature equilibrium approached throughout specimen. *D*, Blood flow obstructed by tourniquet just before heat is discontinued. (From Lehmann, J. F., Silverman, D. R., Baum, B. A., Kirk, N. L., and Johnston, V. C.: Temperature distributions in the human thigh produced by infrared, hot pack and microwave applications. Arch. Phys. Med. Rehabil., 47:291–299, 1966.)

JUSTUS F. LEHMANN AND BARBARA J. DE LATEUR

Another indication of the correct temperature is when melted and solid paraffin are found together in the container. Paraffin wax is most commonly used for application to hands, arms, and feet. The wax is applied by two methods. If the dip method is used, the patient inserts a hand, for instance, into the liquid paraffin, withdraws it when a thin layer of adherent solid paraffin is formed, and repeats the dipping until a thick glove of paraffin envelops the hand. The hand is then covered with terry cloth for another 10 to 20 minutes to retain the heat. Finally the glove of paraffin is peeled off. This produces a relatively mild heating effect, since the paraffin has a relatively low specific heat. Vigorous heating can be obtained by the immersion method where, for instance, the hand is immersed in the paraffin for a period of up to 20 to 30 minutes. The glove of solid paraffin forms around the immersed hand and, because of the low thermal conductivity of this layer of paraffin, the heat conduction into the hand is markedly slowed. Without this glove, the temperature of the liquid paraffin would be too hot to be tolerated over this period of time. This technique produces vigorous effects. It also produces a significant rise of temperature in the small joints, since the layer of soft tissue cover is thin. Thus this method also can be considered a vigorous method of heating these joints. The mode of heat transfer with either method of application is primarily through conduction.

Superficial Heating by Convection

Hydrotherapy

Mode of Heat Transfer. The mode of heat transfer is primarily through convection, since in most forms of hydrotherapy application the water is moved, achieving agitation, so that after the layer of water in contact with the skin has cooled off it is removed and replaced by another layer of higher temperature. Water has a high specific heat and, therefore, great heat-carrying capacity.

Technique of Application. For total immersion, hydrotherapy is usually done in a whirlpool bath. The water is usually agitated. The Hubbard tank, with its special configuration, allows exercising of arms and legs, with the buoyancy of the water eliminating the effects of gravity. The agitators, in turn, allow cleansing of wounds such as decubiti. However, the entire equipment has to be sterilized after such a procedure. This includes the agitator, which may be difficult to sterilize.[193] Special wading tanks and therapeutic pools are available in which ambulation is possible with the elimination of the force of gravity.

Temperature Distribution. The temperature distribution produces the highest temperature at the skin, with a rapid drop-off unless the core temperature is elevated and an artificial fever produced.

Dosimetry. With total body immersion, most of the temperature regulatory mechanisms of the body are disabled. An exchange from the skin to the surrounding environment by infrared radiation and sweating and convective cooling can occur only around the part that is not immersed. Panting, unlike its action in the dog, is not very effective in humans. In contrast to normal circumstances, the skin vasodilatation response to heating does not serve to transfer heat from the core to the outside, but rather picks up more heat from the surrounding water bath. Therefore, it is advisable under these circumstances to monitor the oral temperature. Such monitoring should occur with total body immersion at water temperatures above 37.8° C (100° F). Usually water temperatures above 40.6° C (105° F) are not used. For partial immersion, for instance, of a limb, temperatures up to 46.1° C (115° F) are applied.

Moist Air Cabinet

The moist air cabinet may apply heat to a part or to the entire body using water vapor–saturated air that is thermostatically controlled and blown over the patient. The recommended temperatures are the same as for Hubbard tank therapy. The possibilities of raising body core temperature also exist in this application.

Contrast Bath

A contrast bath produces hyperemia by alternating submersion in hot water and in cold water. The hot water is kept at a temperature between 40.6 and 43.3° C (105 and 110° F) and the cold water is between 15 and 20° C (59 and 68° F). This method has been used to treat rheumatoid arthritis of the fingers, feet, and ankles,[238, 277, 356] resulting in subjective relief of pain and stiffness. Hyperemia may be produced by submersing the affected part in hot water for 10 minutes, then in cold water for 1 minute, followed by cycles of 4 minutes in hot water and 1 minute in cold water, until a total of 30 minutes has elapsed.

Fluidotherapy

Mode of Heat Transfer and Technique of Application. The heat transfer occurs by convection. Thermostatically controlled hot air is blown through a pad of finely divided solids, e.g., glass beads.[34, 193] This produces a dry, warm semifluid mixture into which the hand, the foot, or part of the extremity can be immersed. The sterilization of the particles can be obtained by an auxiliary 300-watt heater that is used in addition to the 200-watt heater in the air line. In this type of application, the skin stays dry; heat exchange through sweating can occur.

Temperature Distribution. It must be assumed that the highest temperatures are found in the most superficial tissues, as in any type of convective heat therapy applied to part of the body.[35] Borrell, when he applied fluidotherapy at 47.8° C (118° F), observed temperature increases of 9° C (16.2° F) in the capsules of the small joints of the hands and feet. He compared these temperature increases with those obtained by mild application of heat with a dip method of paraffin wax and with the water bath treatment at 39° C (102° F). With these two methods, he found smaller temperature increases in the joints. However, the conclusion that therefore fluidotherapy is a more effective heating agent does not seem to be warranted by the experimentation, since the application of heat at higher water bath temperatures or with the immersion paraffin technique is also likely to produce higher temperatures in the joint. It is more likely that the joint temperatures will depend in this case not so much on the modality as on the temperature at which the modality is applied.

Laser Therapy

Definition and Biophysics

Lasers are light and, as such, have some characteristics in common with diffuse light. In contrast with the latter, however, a laser is a columnated beam of photons of the same frequency, with the wavelength in phase. In order to describe a laser, one must measure the wavelength in nanometers; the total pulse duration, repetition rate, and total exposure time; the energy and power intensity in joules per square centimeter; and the irradiance in watts per square centimeter. It is also important to know the beam divergence and the mode content, i.e., whether single or multiple. The mode describes the intensity along a cross section of the beam and may be a gaussian profile, with the maximum intensity in the center of the beam and cylindrically symmetrical. It is caused by the boundary conditions the laser cavity imposes on the electrical field of light. Photons of the same wavelength, whether in diffuse light or in laser, have basically the same interaction with tissue. As in diffuse light, a laser that produces photons of red or infrared heats the tissues, and photons of ultraviolet light in a laser produce photochemical reactions. As in diffuse light, the absorption and reflection characteristics of the tissues varies with the wavelength of the photon. A major difference from diffuse light is that, with lasers, it is possible to produce very high power intensities and irradiance in the laser beam. Nonthermal reactions may be produced even in the red and infrared spectrum. Phenomena that may be produced include pressure and elastic recoil; second harmonic generation; stimulated Raman and Brillouin scattering; inverse Bremstrahlung, in which "loosely bound electrons are accelerated by the strong electrical field associated with the laser pulse."[108] In this phenomenon, collisions with neighboring atoms and molecules can result in local thermal effects.[109] Other phenomena include free radical formation and double photon absorption that can produce a transitory excitation state and even cell death. The Raman and Brillouin effect is only of importance in diagnostic spectroscopy. The biological effects of the other phenomena have not clearly been demonstrated to be therapeutic.

Many forms of laser are available, and those that are frequently used in medicine include the following:
1. Helium-neon (HeNe) (632.3 nm)
2. Ruby (694.3 nm)
3. Argon (476.5–514.5 nm)
4. Krypton ion (476.1–647 nm)
5. Neodymium (Nd) (near infrared, 1060 nm)
6. Neodymium and yttrium-aluminum-garnet (Nd; YAG) (1060 nm)
7. Carbon dioxide (CO_2) (10,600 nm, infrared)

8. Helium cadmium (325–441.6 nm)
9. Nitrogen (337 nm)
10. Dye (tunable wavelength)

Lasers emit photons that can produce photo-thermal or photochemical reactions, as is the case with conventional (diffuse) light. Lasers differ from diffuse light in terms of their monochromaticity, coherence, and high intensity. In turn, the intensity of the biological reaction depends upon the absorption, reflection, and transmission of the wavelength; the power density; the time of exposure; and the blood flow.

Clinical Applications

Surgical applications of lasers are developing rapidly.* Lasers can be used to cut or to coagulate. As a knife, they can be used with great precision to extirpate even a few cells, as from the vocal cords. They can be directed through fiberoptic scopes and used, for example, to stop gastrointestinal bleeding. They can pass through the clear medium of the eye and be focused at a small treatment site. The application of lasers to hemangioma has led to the striking regression of such lesions, as it has with veruca, extensive basal cell carcinomas, infected breast tumors, and other tumors that are particularly difficult to manage and that have been resistant to other forms of treatment.[10] Not only can lasers be used for coagulation, they can also be used for recanalization of blood vessels.[48] In operations in which a large amount of blood loss would ordinarily be anticipated, use of lasers results in a striking reduction of blood loss.[161] Such precision and minimization of blood loss are also important in neurosurgery.[136] Jako[154] has summarized the advantages of laser surgery. Thus, the surgical applications are many and varied and often demonstrably effective.

The effectiveness of lasers in physical medicine or general nonsurgical applications has been less well documented. Attempts have been made to show benefits in wound healing, various arthritides, myofascial pain syndromes, and nerve conduction velocity. Reports are often anecdotal or, where controlled studies have been done, frequently fail to show benefit.

---

*See references 7, 10, 57, 94, 263, 286, 288, and 312.

Wound Healing

Basford and coworkers[17] conducted a randomized, blind, controlled study of the relative effects of ultraviolet light (cold quartz; two minimal erythemal doses [MED] twice daily, six days per week), low-energy laser (HeNe; 632.8 nm), and occlusion in the healing of wounds in six male pigs. Wounds were made with a router assembly and placed in an area next to the spine after povidone-iodine skin scrub. Wound separation was about 4 cm. The healing of all wounds, including that of controls, showed a similar trend; only wounds treated with occlusion healed significantly faster than those of controls.

Kahn[159] observed two patients in whom evidently improved wound healing made surgery unnecessary.

Mester and co-workers[246] studied complement activity, immunoglobulin levels, and circulating autoantibodies in the course of treatment of 20 patients with leg ulcers. They stated that a normalization of the humoral immune response was observed in patients with healing ulcers, whereas none was observed in patients in whom healing was stagnated.

Mester[245] also examined the tensile strength of healing wounds. Although the laser-treated wounds showed "significantly greater" tensile strength on the 8th day, they showed less strength than the controls by the 12th day. No statistical analysis was described.

Lane and Wynne[179–181] studied the course of incisions made by the krypton-fluoride excimer in guinea pig skin (as opposed to studying effects of laser application on pre-existing wounds). In these studies, which were essentially surgical, they demonstrated that tissue could be excised in a controllable fashion, following which there was good wound healing.

When Haina and co-workers[123] applied the HeNe laser to guinea pig wounds, they found 25 per cent more granulation tissue than in the controls. In contrast, Krikorian and co-workers[172] found no observable differences in the healing of laser-treated and untreated bruises in rats.

Anti-Inflammatory Action

Marhoffer and colleagues[236] studied the effect of HeNe low-power laser irradiation on three experimental models of inflammation. In a controlled study, they compared the effect of laser and diffuse red light of comparable wavelength. They concluded that, although there was a suggested change as compared with the control group in some cases, red light and laser were comparable in their effect.

The Arthritides

Goldman and co-workers[107] treated 30 patients with rheumatoid arthritis with a neodymium laser that operated at a wavelength of 1,060 nm with an output of 15 J per cm^2, a pulse duration of 30 nsec, and one pulse every five minutes. Patients were seen 13 times. Control evaluations were done during sessions 1 and 2; sessions 2 through 11 included the use of the laser. The duration of the laser exposure was not stated. Follow-up evaluations (sessions 12 and 13) were at one month and three months after the final laser treatment. One hand was treated at the proximal interphalangeal joint and the metacarpophalangeal joints, whereas the other hand received a sham exposure. They found that 21 patients noted improvement in both groups of joints in both hands. The hand that underwent laser treatment had a greater improvement in erythema and pain.

Laboratory data included the measurement of the titer of the rheumatoid factor antinuclear antibody or polyethylene glycol precipitates. Most of the results showed no differences. There was only a statistically significant difference between the first and the second platelet aggregation measurements.

In this group of patients, the first measurement was taken at the intake evaluation; the second was taken 10 weeks after laser treatment was initiated; and the third was taken three months after the last laser treatment. No controls were used.

In the physical examination, a lateral pinch was compared in the treated and the untreated hands. No difference was found in the lateral pinch or in range of flexion of the joints. Over time, a difference was found in both treated and untreated hands with regard to grasp strength. The increase was greater on the treated side. The only side effects noted were stinging during laser treatment; two patients noted erythema and hyperpigmentation at the laser impact site.

Discussed as possible mechanisms of the laser action were the heating effect, the laser shock wave, immunosuppression and immunostimulation, and stimulation of wound healing. The distal

effects beyond the treated area included pain relief. The condition of treatment did not make it likely that temperature elevation played a major role, but the authors concluded that the exact role of the laser irradiation upon the rheumatoid arthritis and its mechanism of action remains to be elucidated. This conclusion is important in light of the fact that there were no changes over time in both hands and that the only difference between the two hands was in grasp strength.

Osteoarthritis

Basford and co-workers[18] carried out a randomized controlled and double-blind study of the effects of low-energy (0.9 milliwat), continuous-wave HeNe laser treatment of osteoarthritis of the thumb. Eighty-one subjects (47 treated and 34 controls) completed the study and underwent nine treatment sessions (15-second laser or sham irradiation, three times a week for three weeks). The group that underwent laser treatment noted a slight but significant decrease in tenderness; however, the objective measures of pinch, grip, range of motion, activity level, and medication use showed no significant difference between the two groups. The authors concluded this treatment was safe but ineffective for osteoarthritis of the thumb.

Myofascial Pain Syndromes and Nerve Conduction Effects

Greathouse and co-workers[112] applied an infrared laser to the superficial radial nerve in humans. Twenty healthy adults were divided into three groups: group one contained five control subjects; group two contained 10 experimental subjects who received infrared laser irradiation for 20 sec to each of five 1 cm^2 segments of skin overlying the superficial radial nerve; and group three contained five experimental subjects who received the laser for 120 sec to each of the five 1 cm^2 segments. They found no elevation of subcutaneous temperature and no difference between treatment or control groups in distal sensory latency or amplitude of the evoked sensory response.

Snyder-Mackler and Bork[311] studied, in a randomized, double-blind study, the effect of the HeNe laser on latency of peripheral sensory nerves. They found a statistically significant increase in latency corresponding to a decrease in sensory nerve conduction velocity. The room temperature was maintained at 23° C (73.4° F). However, tissue temperatures were not taken, and there was a decrease in nerve conduction velocity in the placebo controls as well as in the treated areas.

Walker[333] used a low-power 1 mw HeNe laser over various nerves, such as the radial, the median, and the saphenous nerves, in the treatment of pain syndromes and studied the response to pain. Pain relief occurred only when the appropriate corresponding nerve site was treated. When patients with trigeminal neuralgia, postherpetic neuralgia, sciatica, and osteoarthritis were treated, 19 of 26 had relief of pain without medication, whereas those who received sham stimulation reported no analgesia. Nerve conduction and action potentials were not assessed, but those who experienced relief showed an increase in 24-hour urinary excretion of 5-hydroxyindoleacetic acid. Lasers have been used as a form of acupuncture, both in Europe and in the United States. Kleinkort and Foley[164] give a survey of such usage and describe three cases of patients with chronic pain who responded dramatically to laser application.

Walker and colleagues[334] also used the HeNe laser (1 mw, 20 Hz) to treat trigeminal neuralgia. The sites of application were the area of the skin overlying peripheral nerves and the skin overlying the painful facial areas. Control subjects received placebo treatment by an apparatus that looked identical to the laser but emitted no irradiation. The experimental group contained 18 patients, and the control group contained 17 patients. Assignment to the experimental group or control group was on a random basis. Assessment of pain was done subjectively on a scale from 0 to 100. The results suggested improvement with laser therapy.

In summary, the use of lasers in physical medicine and in rehabilitation and physical therapy has been advocated, but more controlled studies will be necessary to assess the efficacy of this new modality, and further studies are required to understand the mechanism of the interaction with biological tissues under therapeutic conditions.

Therapeutic Cold

Physiologic and Therapeutic Effects, Including Clinical Studies

The following does not deal with total body hypothermia; only local cold application for therapeutic purposes is discussed. This type of cold application is also frequently called cryotherapy. The rationale for the use of cryotherapy is primarily based on physiological changes that have been documented and supported by a few clinical studies. The details of these studies are reviewed elsewhere.[192]

The physiological and therapeutic effects in conjunction with some clinical studies form the rationale for the use of cold in (1) muscle spasm and spasticity, (2) mechanical trauma, (3) burns, (4) pain relief, and (5) arthritides.

The Use of Cold in Muscle Spasm, Spasticity, and Muscle Re-education

Physiologically, muscle tone and spasticity and muscle spasm seem to be reduced by an effect on the muscle spindle itself, provided that the muscle temperature is lowered.[85, 229, 248, 262]

These physiological observations are consistent with a documented reduction of spasticity and muscle clonus in patients (Fig. 13–64).[163, 270, 272]

Knutsson[166] found that not only was the clonus abolished but that the strength of the protagonist, freed from the influence of the hyperreflexic antagonist, was enhanced by more than 50 per cent in 11 of 29 cases. It is important to note that Miglietta[249] documented that the clonus disappeared only if the muscle temperature was lowered. Miglietta, as well as Hartviksen,[128] also demonstrated that the effect on the muscle temperature as well as on the spasticity lasted for a long period of time. The reason is that the insulating fat layer with the vasoconstriction slowed down the rewarming of the muscle from the outside, and, because of the vasoconstriction, the rewarming from the inside was also delayed. This is in contrast to the quick reversal of the temperature elevation with heating, in which increased blood flow rapidly

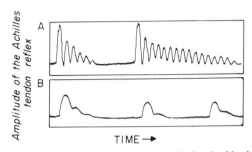

FIGURE 13–64. Effect of cooling on amplitude of ankle clonus recorded by photomotograph, *(A)* before and *(B)* after 20 minutes of cold application with water at 13° C in a spinal-cord-injured patient. (From Petajan, R. H., and Watts, N.: Effect of cooling on the triceps surae reflex. Am. J. Phys. Med., 41:240–251, 1962.)

cools the muscle. Thus the effect of the reduction on the muscle spasticity can be used for therapeutic purposes for range-of-motion exercises and for skill training, such as ambulation without interference of the spasticity. Temperatures that reduce spasticity do not affect sensory feedback to such a degree[192] that they would grossly interfere with skill training. In addition, cooling may affect the gamma fibers; the nerve conduction through the peripheral nerve, both sensory and motor; and the transmission of the nerve impulses through the myoneural junction. However, the sensitivity of these structures to the lower temperature is significantly less than that of the spindles; therefore, it is questionable how much the effect on these structures and their function contributes to the relief of spasticity.

Muscle spasms secondary to an underlying joint, skeletal lesion, or nerve root irritation are relieved by the same mechanism.

Knutsson and Mattsson[167] observed that, in some patients, an immediate temporary increase in the reflex muscle tone occurred after cold application. The Hoffman (H) response seemed to be enhanced in some cases. All the patients, however, showed ultimately a decline of the reflex muscle tone and tendon jerk. They attributed this effect to the influence of cold on the muscle and the peripheral nerve. They concluded that the initial increase in tone and H response may be produced by an increased excitability of the alpha motor neuron through stimulation of the exteroceptors of the skin. Hartviksen[128] also found in all his patients a decline in foot clonus which lasted for 1 to 1½ hours. However, he also observed, immediately after the ice pack application, a temporary increase in spasticity for about 15 to 30 seconds. Hartviksen

felt that spasticity disappeared while intramuscular temperature was still normal. However, the long-term effect was attributed by him to the lower intramuscular temperature, likely through an effect on the spindles.

Miglietta[249] found a decrease in clonus. However, he observed that the clonus was unchanged in the majority of cases (80 per cent) for the first 10 minutes of exposure to cold. It was evident that clonus started to decrease only after the intramuscular temperature started to drop. He concluded that the change in clonus was produced by a direct effect of cold on the spindle excitability. Trnavsky's[324] findings were consistent with the observation of Miglietta. It should be noted that the decreased muscle tone after cold application occurred only when the local muscle temperature was reduced. It should also be noted that Knutsson and Mattsson and Hartviksen spot-measured the temperature only at one place in the musculature and had no data available as to whether, at the time of earliest decreased reflex activity, another part of the muscle was already cooled. Knutsson and Mattsson found an increased H response during the first minutes of cold application, which is indicative of the facilitation of the alpha motor neuron discharge. Urbscheit and Bishop[327] also found an increase in the H response without significant change in the Achilles tendon reflex. Lightfoot and co-workers[227] found no significant change in the H/M (direct muscle response) ratio. They concluded that, in addition to an effect on the spindle, other factors were involved in reducing the reflex muscle tone, including slowing of contraction in muscle or motor nerve fiber and prolongation of twitch contraction and half-relaxation time.

Bell and Lehmann[21] measured skin and muscle temperature during cold application. The location of the temperature probe in the muscle was determined by soft tissue x-ray study. They found an average decrease in skin temperature of 18.4° C (65.2° F) and in muscle temperature of 12.1° C (53.6° F). Before, during, and after cold application, they examined the H response by a series of recruitment curves and related the maximal H response to the M response with supramaximal stimulation. They found that, in all 16 cases, the amplitude of the maximal M response decreased significantly in response to cooling. These changes in the recording of the compound action potentials should be considered when cooling experiments result in alterations in H or EMG response to tendon tap, since the changes in recording may affect all three potentials—the H wave, the M wave, and the tendon tap electromyogram (EMG). When using the M wave as a covariant in this analysis, no significant changes were noted in the H reflex amplitude. However, the tendon tap amplitude decreased significantly. Thus these findings do not support the claims that simple cooling facilitates the alpha motor neuron discharge measured by the H reflex. However, rubbing the skin over the muscle with ice may stimulate the mechanoreceptors. Hagbarth[122] has clearly shown that this may lead to facilitation of muscle tone. However, the study of Bell and Lehmann[21] confirms that tendon tap reflex is decreased by muscle cooling.

In the clinical use of ice application, one may conclude that cooling should be applied in such a way that the muscle temperature is lowered, spasticity is relieved, and muscle tone decreased. There is a consensus of all authors that, under those circumstances, reflex activity is diminished and the therapeutic effect on spasticity is achieved and maintained for an adequate period of time. In addition, the finding that stimulation of the exteroceptors of the skin may temporarily increase tone of the muscle may be the basis for ice massage as a technique for re-education of muscle function. The physiological effectiveness of this procedure is still open to question, and whether the mechanism of action is cooling or the stimulation of exteroceptors other than cold receptors is not known.

Use of Cold in Mechanical Trauma

Cold applied in acute but not severe trauma such as sprains produces desirable effects by vasoconstriction, which, in turn, reduces swelling and bleeding. Pain may be reduced directly through an effect on the sensory endings and pain fibers or by relieving muscle spasm. Indirectly, it may be reduced by prevention of swelling and bleeding. Pain also may be reduced indirectly by relieving muscle spasm. The vasoconstriction is produced reflexly via the sympathetic fibers and also by direct effect on the blood vessels by lowering the temperature.[270] Only Matsen[239] and Marek[234] found, contrary to the above, that in experimental fractures swelling was increased by cold application. However, Matsen's measured differences in swelling were not statistically significant. Schmidt's work[291] supported the traditional view; he reduced edema by application of ice and gel packs.

The physiological effect of cold application on mechanical trauma has been confirmed in a clinical study by Basur and co-workers,[19] who treated ankle sprains. Both in the control group and in the patients treated with ice compression, bandages were used. Exact outcome measures were not used. Nilsson[259] concluded on the basis of clinical trials of different treatment methods in acute ankle sprains that treatment should be conservative, using local cooling, anti-inflammatory medication, and elastic wrapping, regardless of severity of the injury. Stoller and co-workers[315] noted that the 14 per cent increase in laxity of the knee ligaments after exercise, which lasted on an average for 52.4 minutes, was reduced after ice application to the knee. However, the authors also observed that heat application in the form of ultrasound had the same effect. The clinical implications need further investigation. Hecht and associates[131] found that cold application decreases the swelling after total knee arthroplasty and partially alleviates the discomfort after exercise. In more serious injuries, Moore and Cardea[253] found a reduction of compartment pressures in the anterior, lateral, and posterior compartments of the leg. However, this study was not well controlled, since the treated group received not only ice application but also an intermittent compression program. Schaubel[290] found in postsurgical cases a reduction of swelling as indicated by the reduction of the need for cast splitting and also by reduction of pain as indicated by lesser usage of narcotics and sedatives as the occasion arises (prn).

Use of Cold in Burns

Zitowitz and Hardy[364] in animal experiments and Shulman[304] in patients with burns showed that immediate ice application reduced the effect of the burns only if required therapy was applied shortly after the thermal trauma. If it was applied later, it retarded healing or aggravated the tissue damage. Blomgren and associates[30] showed in animal experiments that cooling in water at 8° C (14.4° F) for 30 minutes after a burn reduced edema significantly, but not the ultimate necrosis. In a later study,[31] the authors found that there is a threshold temperature above which the skin is irreversibly injured, irrespective of the later cooling of the burn.

Use of Cold as an Analgesic

Cryotherapy not only relieves pain indirectly by reducing painful spasms, spasticity, or swelling from trauma or inflammatory reaction but can also be used as a counterirritant to relieve pain.[262] The experimental findings in which cold application to any part of the body increased the pain threshold when stimulating the tooth pulp can be explained either on the basis of the gate theory of Melzack and Wall[241] or by the production of endorphins (Fig. 13–65). In a recent experimental paper, Bini and co-workers[27] also concluded that activity in a low-threshold mechanoreceptor and cold sensitive units suppresses pain in the segmental levels.

Use of Cold in Arthritis

The benefit from cold application to a joint with inflammatory reaction or to the inflamed bursa is due in part to the vasoconstriction with reduction of edema. Pain is indirectly relieved in this way and also by direct effect on the nerve fibers. The application of ice to joints has been popularized by findings of Harris and McCroskery.[127] They showed that destructive enzyme activity such as that of collagenase was significantly lowered at 30 to 35° C (86 to 95° F), yet Wright and Johns[358, 359] and Bäcklund and Tiselius[13] clearly demonstrated by objective measurement that joint stiffness in patients with rheumatoid arthritis was increased by cold application and decreased by heat application. The subjective complaints of joint stiffness correlated highly with the objective measurements. Experimental studies in arthritis as performed by Schmidt and co-workers[291] showed variable results of application of heat and cold, depending on the experimental methodology used and especially depending on the mode of producing the joint inflammatory reaction. Clinical studies in humans unfortunately are all poorly controlled, with questionable outcome measurements. However, there seems to be a consensus that if painful joints are

cooled enough, pain will be reduced because the pain threshold is elevated.[264] Kirk and Kersley[163] found that when heat and cold were compared in a small number of patients with rheumatoid arthritis, both modalities alleviated pain and stiffness.

Similarly, Landon[178] found in 117 patients with low back pain an improvement with the use of both modalities. However, as measured by the length of hospital stay, patients with acute pain stayed for a shorter period in the hospital when treated with heat as compared with cold, whereas in the chronic pain patients the hospital stay was shorter when they were treated with cold. No differences between the hospital stay in patients treated with heat or cold were observed if the researcher did not differentiate between acute and chronic cases.

Techniques of Cold Application

The most commonly used technique of application is by melting ice together with water. The temperature of this mix is 0° C (32° F). The part may be treated by immersion in this ice water, or compresses may be used as applied to other parts of the body that cannot be easily submersed. Also, terry cloth, dipped in water with ice shavings then rung out and applied rapidly, is used for cooling larger portions of the body. Finally, ice massage, moving a block of ice over the surface to be cooled, has been used. The result of any one of these applications is a rapid drop in skin temperature and a much slower reduction of muscle temperature. The slowness of the drop of the muscle temperature depends largely on the thickness of fat. From the experiments shown in Figures 13–66 to 13–69, it becomes apparent that if the muscle is to be cooled—to reduce spasticity, for instance—it will take at least 10 minutes to begin to cool the muscle in a thin individual and probably half an hour to do the same in a more obese person. Clinically, one can best judge whether a desirable effect is obtained by checking, for instance, in case of spastic calf muscles, the ankle jerk. The therapeutic effect is achieved when the clonus or the tendon jerk is abolished. In other joints of the body, the decreased resistance to rapid motion will indicate that relief of spasticity is obtained. Short cooling with such a technique as ice massage affects only the skin and is frequently used for muscle reeducation, as described earlier. In this case, facil-

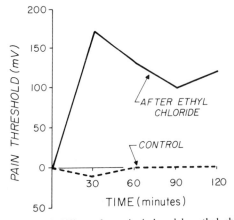

FIGURE 13–65. Effect of a pain induced by ethyl chloride spray on the pain threshold of normal human subjects. (From Parsons, C. M., and Goetzl, F. R.: Effect of induced pain on pain threshold. Proc. Soc. Exp. Biol. Med., 60:327–329, 1945.)

JUSTUS F. LEHMANN AND BARBARA J. DE LATEUR

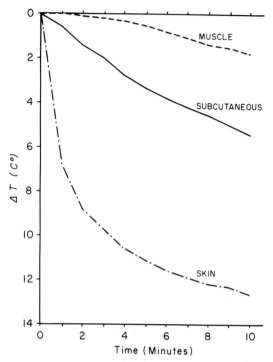

FIGURE 13–66. Change of skin, subcutaneous, and muscle temperatures during topical (thigh) ice application in a person with less than 1 cm of subcutaneous fat. (From Lehmann, J. F., and de Lateur, B. J.: Therapeutic heat. *In* Lehmann, J. F. [Ed.]: Therapeutic Heat and Cold, 3rd Ed. Baltimore, Williams and Wilkins, 1982.)

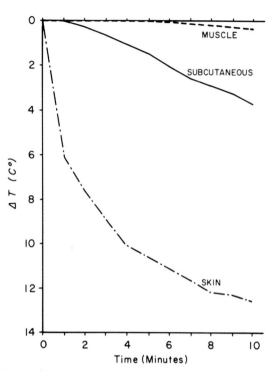

FIGURE 13–68. Change of skin, subcutaneous, and muscle temperatures during topical (thigh) ice application in a person with greater than 2 cm of subcutaneous fat. (From Lehmann, J. F., and de Lateur, B. J.: Therapeutic heat. *In* Lehmann, J. F. [Ed.]: Therapeutic Heat and Cold, 3rd Ed. Baltimore, Williams and Wilkins, 1982.)

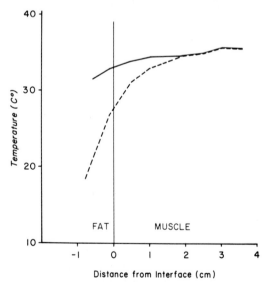

FIGURE 13–67. Temperature distribution before (solid line) and after (dashed line) topical (thigh) application for 10 minutes in a person with less than 1 cm of subcutaneous fat. (From Lehmann, J. F., and de Lateur, B. J.: Therapeutic heat. *In* Lehmann, J. F. [Ed.]: Therapeutic Heat and Cold, 3rd Ed. Baltimore, Williams and Wilkins, 1982.)

itation of the alpha motor neuron occurs only when the skin is cooled without significantly cooling the musculature.

Once the muscle is cooled enough to relieve spasticity, this effect usually lasts long enough to be of therapeutic value. When cooling is applied in trauma, it should be applied early before substantial swelling and hemorrhage have developed. This can be done with simultaneous compression of the injured part. This type of cooling is usually extended for four to six hours by renewing ice packing or adding ice to the water bath. Once swelling and bleeding are prevented and are not likely to recur, further cooling serves no purpose.

Lundgren and associates[231] have shown that cooling over an excessive period of time may retard healing. They showed that the retardation of wound healing seems to be secondary to the vasoconstriction. Sympathectomy in experimental animals prevented this retardation of wound healing.

Drez and co-workers[71] reported four cases in which ice application around the knee resulted in peroneal nerve damage with footdrop. In the case

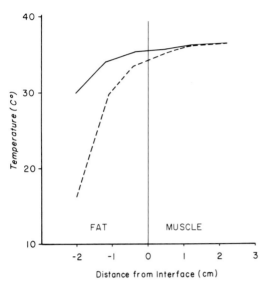

FIGURE 13–69. Temperature distribution before (solid line) and after (dashed line) topical (thigh) ice application for 10 minutes in a person with greater than 2 cm of subcutaneous fat. (From Lehmann, J. F. and de Lateur, B. J.: Therapeutic heat. *In* Lehmann, J. F. [Ed.]: Therapeutic Heat and Cold, 3rd Ed. Baltimore, Williams and Wilkins, 1982.)

of a two-hour application, EMG changes persisted over a period longer than 19 minutes. Collins and associates[52] described one case of peroneal nerve damage when the patient fell asleep during the application of ice around the knee. In all these cases, the ice application was not controlled, and the authors concluded that special precautions should be taken to prevent nerve damage, limiting ice application to 20 minutes and avoiding compression of the peroneal nerve. Also, gel packs, which produce temperatures below freezing, should not be used. Collins and associates considered a direct injury to the nodal membrane and neural edema, ischemia, suspension of axoplasmic transport, or a combination of these factors as possible mechanisms for this injury.[260]

The application of an evaporative cooling spray is done by spraying the skin with ethyl chloride from a distance of 1 m with a stroking motion.[26] Chlorofluoromethanes have been used[321] to replace the more flammable ethyl chloride. This type of cooling produces pain relief as a counterirritant via the mechanism described above.

Newer modalities of cold application use chemicals in an envelope that can be broken within the package to react with another agent to produce an endothermal reaction. These packs are not as effective and not as safe as the conventional meth-

ods of cooling, since the temperature they develop is poorly controlled, and if the outer envelope is broken the chemicals that come in contact with the skin may be irritating.

Refrigeration units used as cold applicators must be very well thermostatically controlled to prevent frostbite.[353, 354]

Comparison of Therapeutic Effects of Heat and Cold[192]

From the review of the literature on effects of heat and cold it becomes apparent that, in many cases, similar effects are obtained between the two ends of the temperature spectrum. In other cases, cold produces the opposite effect of that of heat application. There are a number of reactions in which heat and cold produce similar effects. Muscle spasm secondary to underlying joint or skeletal pathology can be effectively reduced by either modality. In this case, it is often necessary to break the vicious circle continuing the painful muscle spasm. In upper motor neuron lesions with spasticity, cold is very effective in reducing the spasticity, an effect that lasts long enough to be of therapeutic value. Although heat may also reduce spasticity, this effect is of very short duration, since the muscle tone is rapidly restored by the fact that the blood flow to the musculature is increased, cooling the heated tissue.

Pain may be reduced by both modalities if it is secondary to muscle spasms. The pain threshold also seems to be elevated by the direct effect of both heat and cold on the free nerve endings and of the pain-killing fibers.

Other reactions show a different behavior when the tissues are exposed to heat or cold. The blood flow is increased with heat application and decreased after cold application. Therefore, the tendency to bleed is increased with heat application and decreased with cold application. Edema resulting from trauma is increased with heat application, and most literature references claim it is decreased in its development by cold application. Swelling associated with inflammatory reactions shows the same behavior. Burns are aggravated by heat application, but the tissue damage is reduced with cold application immediately following the thermal trauma. Joint stiffness, as objectively measured, is decreased with heat application and increased with cold application.

JUSTUS F. LEHMANN AND BARBARA J. DE LATEUR

The Clinical Use of Heat and Cold in Various Conditions

In the following section, examples of some of the uses of heat and cold therapy in common clinical conditions are discussed. It should be remembered that therapeutic heat and cold are not curative in these disease entities but are a valuable adjunct when properly used in conjunction with other treatments. The other treatment procedures may include not only other physical therapy such as immobilization, stretch, and exercises but also medications and surgical procedures.

It is essential for successful therapeutic application of these modalities that the correct diagnosis be made first. The local condition to be treated is assessed and a judgment is made as to whether or not it is treatable with heat or cold. The localization of the pathological process is clearly identified, and, correspondingly, the modality is selected. It is essential that there is clear understanding of what physiological effect can be achieved, and finally it is equally important that the application be done with appropriate techniques.

The Treatment of Muscle Spasms and/or Muscle Pain

Skeletal Muscle[242]

Skeletal muscle spasms, often associated with a significant amount of pain, are frequently observed secondary to other pathological conditions. Muscle spasm and guarding may occur as a result of intervertebral disk protrusion, with or without nerve root irritation. In this type of condition, relaxation of the painful muscle spasm can be achieved by the use of various heating modalities. Specifically, short wave diathermy can be applied either with induction coil applicators or with condenser pads. Treatment should occur on a once- or twice-daily basis for 20 to 30 minutes. The advantage of short wave diathermy is that it is capable of heating the musculature itself as well as skin and subcutaneous tissues, and thus this application may have an effect directly on the spindle mechanism in addition to a muscle relaxation triggered reflexly through excitation of exteroceptors of the skin. For a more limited area of muscle spasm, specially designed induction coils like the International Medical Electronics (IME) applicator, the monode, and the microwave applicators can be used.

The relaxation of such muscle spasm can also be achieved by superficial heating agents including hot packs, such as Hydrocollator packs, or radiant heat application with the heat lamp or the heat cradle. Applications should be for a period of 20 to 30 minutes. With these modalities, muscle relaxation is achieved primarily through reflexes by heating the skin. Muscle spasm can also be relieved by cold application in the form of ice packs or ice massage. The objective is to cool the musculature and decrease the muscle spasm by reducing the spindle sensitivity. That implies that ice application probably should be continued for more than 10 minutes. The clinical study of Landon[178] on 117 patients with low back pain showed that heat and cold application were equally effective. However, there seemed to be a difference in the final result when these methods were used in either acute or chronic conditions. In the acute conditions, heat application reduced the hospital stay as compared with ice application. In chronic conditions, ice was more effective in reducing the hospital stay than was heat application. It should be noted that neither in the application of short waves or in superficial heating agents is the underlying pathologic condition, such as disk protrusion, affected at all. The treatment is symptomatic in that it reduces the painful muscle spasm. In contrast to the use of superficial heat, one should not use brief superficial ice application without cooling the muscle, since this may lead to facilitation of the alpha motor neuron discharges.[328] Secondary muscle spasm due to an underlying joint disease can be treated in the same fashion as described above.

In the acute or subacute phases of joint diseases such as rheumatoid arthritis, if heat is applied, the intent is not to heat the joint but to relieve the secondary symptoms. Therefore, in joints covered with relatively little soft tissue, such as the knee, ankle, small joints of hands and feet, and the elbow, short wave or microwave diathermy applications are frequently undesirable. Vigorous ultrasound treatment is contraindicated in such joints.

In myofibrositis or so-called trigger points, local application of both heat and cold can be used. Cold is frequently applied with an evaporative cooling spray.[32, 95, 170, 171, 307, 308, 323] Superficial heating modalities are often used in conjunction with friction massage. Ultrasound may be used in low doses such as 0.5 to 1.0 watts per cm^2, with a total output up to 5 to 10 watts. In contrast with these observations, Klemp and co-workers[165] found that the ^{133}Xe washout in the myofibrositic muscle was significantly reduced by ultrasound treatment, suggesting a decrease of blood flow.

In tension states with electromyographically documented increase of muscle activity, the discomfort and pain can be relieved by heat application either by short wave diathermy or by superficial heat application followed by radiant heat or hot packs. In these cases, the heat application should be followed with deep sedative massage. This treatment is also used in conjunction with biofeedback to relieve muscle tension.

The muscle soreness often called "spasm" in poliomyelitis responds very well to Kenny hot packs. Repeated packing of this type not only reduces the pain and soreness but also may eliminate to a large degree any need for analgesic drugs.

In all these cases in which heat or cold may be applied, it is likely that these applications produce pain relief not only by reducing the muscle tension but also through direct effect on the nerve fibers that transmit pain and on free nerve endings in the tissues.[69] There also is good evidence that these modalities may represent a counterirritant and would reduce pain as explained on the basis of the gate theory.[241, 264]

Smooth Muscle

Exaggerated peristalsis leads to cramping of the smooth musculature of the gastrointestinal tract and the onset of pain. These painful cramps are frequently observed in gastrointestinal upsets. The discomfort and the peristalsis can be reduced by superficial heat application in the form of hot packs or a hot water bottle to the abdominal wall. Also, an electric heating pad can be used with proper precautions. This leads to a measurable reduction of the peristalsis.[28, 96, 252] The reduction of the cramps is associated with reduction of blood flow to the mucous membranes of the gastrointestinal tract and reduction of hydrochloric acid secretion in the stomach. The mechanism is the result of reflex responses triggered by the heat receptors of the skin. Cold application to the abdominal wall does just the opposite of the heat application and aggravates the patient's condition.

Similarly, menstrual cramps respond well to superficial heat application.

Contractures

In the treatment of contractures in general, it is essential to selectively heat the fibrous tissues that limit motion. It is vital that the temperatures be brought close to tolerance levels. It is also important for a successful outcome that mobilization of the joint or other structures be done by stretch or range of motion exercise immediately after or, if possible, during heat application.

Fibrous Muscular Contractures

In fibrous contracture of the musculature it is desirable to heat the musculature evenly throughout and to elevate the temperature to tolerance levels while stretching the muscles.[62] The ideal heating modalities for this purpose are microwaves applied with direct contact applicators, preferably operating at a frequency of 915 MHz for 30 minutes. This modality is most effective if a diffuse fibrosis of the muscle is present. If the skin can be cooled at the same time, subcutaneous fat heating is essentially prevented. The temperature distribution that is achieved is shown in Figure 13–34. Skin cooling becomes even more important if the subcutaneous fat layer is greater than 1 cm. There is some limited evidence that this type of therapy is effective (Fig. 13–70). If microwaves are not available for this purpose, the best alternative is to use short wave induction coil applicators. However, uniform muscle heating cannot be achieved in this fashion; only the more superficial musculature will be heated selectively. If, for instance, due to electrical burns, a fibrous strand within the musculature produces the contracture, ultrasound would be the better heating modality, since it selectively heats such tissues. Application for at least 10 minutes per field would be necessary, best combined with simultaneous static stretching.

Joint Contractures

The treatment of joint contractures—whether the result of shortening of the capsular or periarticular tissues or of thickening and scarring of the synovium by a rheumatic process, the result of limitation of the joint range due to ligamentous and capsular tightness associated with degenerative joint disease, or the result of trauma or prolonged immobilization of the joint—is always the same. However, it is important to perform a careful clinical evaluation of the patient to rule out any persisting acute or subacute process or, in degenerative joint disease of the hip, for instance, a limitation of the range of motion resulting from bone spurs. In any one of these cases, the treatment involves selective heating of the contracted tissues, capsules, ligaments, and scarred synovium, raising the temperatures to maximally tolerated levels in conjunction with the use of either simultaneous or immediately applied stretch, range-of-motion exercises, or other joint mobilization tech-

JUSTUS F. LEHMANN AND BARBARA J. DE LATEUR

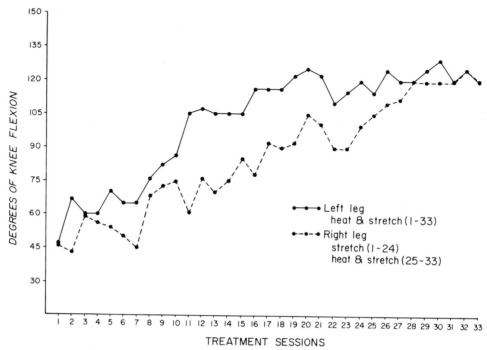

FIGURE 13–70. The degrees of knee flexion due to residual elongation of the right and left rectus femoris muscles before each treatment session. (From de Lateur, B. J., Stonebridge, J. B., and Lehmann, J. F.: Fibrous muscular contractures: treatment with a new direct contact microwave applicator operating at 915 MHz. Arch. Phys. Med. Rehabil., 59:488–490, 1978.)

niques. This type of approach would aggravate any persistent inflammatory reaction and would be totally ineffective in the presence of bone spurs limiting the motion.

In all joints covered with a significant amount of soft tissue, the modality of choice is ultrasound, usually applied with a multiple field technique at a relatively high dosage using stroking technique. Ultrasound can also be used for small joints, such as the interphalangeal joints of the fingers, toes, and the metacarpophalangeal or metatarsophalangeal joints. However, these joints also can be effectively heated by application of short wave, microwave, or paraffin wax using the immersion method. In larger joints with little soft tissue cover such as the elbow or the knee, the alternative to heating with ultrasound would be using induction coil applicators, including wrap-around coils for short wave diathermy, as a second choice.

A controlled clinical study of periarthritis of the shoulder[201] has shown that ultrasound is more effective than microwaves in gaining range of motion, since microwaves alleviate only the secondary muscle spasms (Table 13–8). Similarly, in a controlled clinical study it was shown that in patients with hip fractures treated with insertion of Rich-ard's screws, the gain in range of motion with ultrasound was greater than with infrared application, and the ambulatory potential of the patients improved (Table 13–9). Other studies had similar results. Hintzelmann[141, 142] found (Fig. 13–71) that in chronic ankylosing spondylitis ultrasound treatment to the costovertebral joints combined with deep breathing exercises increased chest expansion and vital capacity. No control subjects were presented in this study. Pain relief was an associated benefit. There is no reason why this type of treat-

TABLE 13–8. Gain in Range of Motion After Ultrasonic and Microwave Treatment*

	TREATMENT	
GAIN	Ultrasound	Microwaves
Forward flexion	27.4° ± 2.3°†	16.1° ± 1.5°
Abduction	32.6° ± 2.5°	21.2° ± 2.1°
Rotation	45.4° ± 2.8°	17.3° ± 4.0°

*From Lehmann, J. F., Erickson, D. J., Martin, G. M., and Krusen, F. H.: Comparison of ultrasonic and microwave diathermy in the physical treatment of periarthritis of the shoulder. Arch. Phys. Med. Rehabil., 35:627–634, 1954.

†Standard error of the mean.

Diathermy and Superficial Heat, Laser, and Cold Therapy

TABLE 13–9. Comparison of Amount of Change in Range of Motion After One Week of Treatment

	ULTRASOUND			INFRARED				
	N	Mean	S.D.	N	Mean	S.D.	t	p
Hip								
Flexion	15	21.67	9.7	15	5.40	11.4	4.057	0.01
Extension	15	10.40	8.2	15	−3.20‡	7.7	4.503	0.01
Abduction	15	6.33	7.4	15	−1.67‡	5.6	3.225	0.01
Adduction	15	9.67	6.6	15	−1.20‡	6.0	4.567	0.01
External Rotation	14	12.86	7.9	15	0.20	7.9	4.178	0.01
Internal Rotation	14	10.93	7.6	15	−1.60‡	8.8	3.965	0.01
Knee								
Flexion	15	18.33	14.9	15	10.33	13.3	1.498	0.20
Extension	15	3.60	3.9	15	−3.47‡	4.8	4.259	0.01

*From Lehmann, J. F., Fordyce, W. E., Rathbun, L. A., Larson, R. E., and Wood, D. H.: Clinical evaluation of a new approach in the treatment of contracture associated with hip fracture after internal fixation. Arch. Phys. Med. Rehabil., 42:95–100, 1961.

†Ultrasound and infrared groups compared using independent samples method.

‡When the mean is expressed as a negative value, range of motion has been lost during treatment.

ment could not be repeated frequently. Other clinical studies are reviewed elsewhere.[193]

Skin

In scleroderma, contractures may primarily be produced by the tightness of the skin rather than by the periarticular structures. The contracture most frequently involves the hands early in its development, limiting the range of motion at interphalangeal and metacarpophalangeal joints. Also, ischemic necrosis of the fingertips is observed. Ultrasound[326] has been used for this condition in conjunction with stretch and range-of-motion exercises. Also, temporary healing of the sores of the fingertips has been observed. However, since there were no controls and since the ultimate course of the disease was not changed, this is a condition in which ultrasound is of suggested value only. An alternative to the treatment of this condition is the use of the paraffin bath with either the dip or immersion method. Also, treatment with short wave diathermy and microwave could be tried.

Joint contractures as a result of superficial scars, for instance, due to electrical burns,[26] are usually

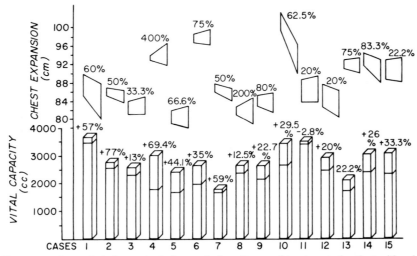

FIGURE 13–71. Chest expansion and vital capacity before and after ultrasound treatment of patient with ankylosing spondylitis. (From Hintzelmann, U.: Ultraschalltherapie rheumatischer Erkrankungen. Dtsch. Med. Wochenschr., 72:350–353, 1947; 74:869, 1949.)

treated with ultrasound in conjunction with exercise and stretching techniques.

Dupuytren's Disease

Dupuytren's disease is a contracture of the palmar fascia of unknown, probably in part genetic, origin. The nonsurgical treatment of the fibrous contracture of the palmar fascia is mostly done with ultrasound (Fig. 13–72).

Peyronie's Disease

Peyronie's disease is a condition associated with sclerosing lesions in the tunics of the corpora cavernosa of the penis, the septum, and Buck's fascia. Induration interferes with complete erection and often produces a lateral curvature of the penis. Patients complain of pain and interference with intercourse. The condition is self-limited, with resolution in approximately four years.[347] It is also associated with Dupuytren's contractures in 10 per cent of the cases. The condition has been treated with ultrasound at an intensity of approximately 1.5 watts per cm^2 with stroking technique over a period of five minutes. Several authors[72, 140, 158, 226, 299] suggest that daily treatments may reduce the time to resolution. Subjectively, patients noted better filling during erection and more satisfactory intercourse, with relief of erectile pain. No control studies are available, however.

Joint Stiffness and Pain

Joint Stiffness in Collagen Diseases

Stiffness and discomfort, especially in the morning, are common bothersome symptoms of patients with rheumatoid arthritis and other collagen diseases. Wright and Johns[157, 358, 359] and Bäcklund and Tiselius[13] were able to produce an objective measurement of joint stiffness and found a high correlation between measured stiffness and complaints on the part of the patient. They also found that heat as well as corticosteroids measurably reduced the joint stiffness. Cold application aggravated it. Heat was applied with superficial heating modalities. Clinically, both radiant heat and a hot tub bath are commonly used for this purpose. Modalities that selectively heat joints are usually not used in this condition, since it is frequently associated with activity of the rheumatoid process in the joint. For small joints in the hands and feet, a whirlpool bath or the mild heat application with the dip method of paraffin application is used. The use of immersion of small joints, i.e., hands and feet, in a water bath may be useful, but temperatures should not exceed 40.6° C (105° F) to produce a mild effect. If total immersion in a Hubbard tank or in a tub is used, it is equally important to limit the temperature to less than 38.9° C (102° F) and ensure avoidance of artificial fever by taking oral temperatures. Immersion of the limbs in the water eliminates most of the forces of gravity by buoyancy, and therefore range of motion exercises can be performed simultaneously with less pain and greater ease. Finally, for relief of stiffness in hands and feet the contrast bath is used. The measured benefit of this application is a very marked increase in blood flow to the part.[238]

If superficial heat application is used in the form of radiant heat, the heat lamp is used but can

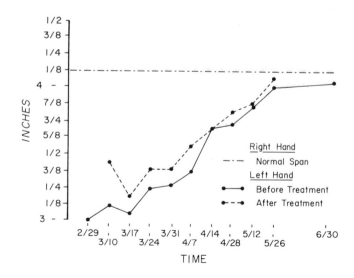

FIGURE 13–72. Influence of ultrasound on scar of left hand indicating span before and directly after each treatment. (From Bierman, W.: Ultrasound in the treatment of scars. Arch. Phys. Med. Rehabil., 35:209, 1954.)

cover only a limited number of joints. In more generalized stiffness, the heat cradle or double baker is recommended.

In spite of the fact that Johns and Wright[157] and Bäcklund and Tiselius[13] showed that joint stiffness is measurably increased by cold application, ice application to joints to relieve stiffness has been advocated. The suggestion to use ice has been based both on the fact that it numbs pain and on the findings of Harris and McCroskery[127] that the activity of destructive enzymes such as collagenase is reduced. Controlled clinical studies of enzyme activity or joint stiffness are not available, not even of medication schedules, which makes questionable any conclusion on therapeutic effectiveness in a disease such as rheumatoid arthritis.[269]

Reflex Sympathetic Dystrophy, Including Shoulder-Hand Syndrome and Sudeck's Atrophy

In the shoulder-hand syndrome, pain and joint stiffness can be treated in the same fashion as joint contractures in other conditions.[26, 179, 258, 331, 352] However, this type of therapy, which includes the selective heating of periarticular structures in combination with stretch and exercise to increase range of motion, has to be appropriately integrated with other therapeutic regimens. If sympathetic (that is, stellate) ganglion blocks are used, it is essential that the physical therapy with heat, stretch, and mobilization exercise follow the block immediately. Woeber[352] has also advocated treatment of the sympathetic outflow with ultrasound. Woeber claimed that ultrasound exposure of the sympathetics gave results similar to those obtained by stellate ganglion block. However, the study was not controlled. It is also important that this type of therapy be given in conjunction with therapeutic measures to reduce swelling; this would include elevation of the limb for postural drainage, manual or mechanical massage, and elastic wrapping, especially of fingers, from distal to proximal, and active exercise of the wrapped hand above the level of the heart.

Epicondylitis, Bursitis, and Tenosynovitis

In acute calcific bursitis, such as is commonly found in the subdeltoid or subacromial bursa, acute pain is present due to swelling pressure within the content of the bursa and an inflammatory reaction. Selective heating of the bursa is, therefore, contraindicated. Ice application may greatly alleviate

the acute pain, especially if used in conjunction with removal of the bursal content and injection of hydrocortisone preparations combined with a local anesthetic. Since this condition occurs frequently in combination with calcific tendinitis of the supraspinatus or biceps tendons and also is associated with tight capsules that limit the range of motion of the shoulder joint, treatment in the chronic stage is with ultrasound in conjunction with the corresponding stretch and range-of-motion exercises. There is no evidence, however, that large calcium deposits in the bursa, which may mechanically interfere with motion by impinging upon the greater tuberosity of the humerus or coracoacromial ligament, are more readily resolved with ultrasound treatment. As a matter of fact, it has been demonstrated that spontaneous resolution of the calcium deposit occurs as frequently with as without ultrasound.[5, 20, 360] In the rare instance of calcium deposits large enough to mechanically interfere with motion, surgical removal may be the only effective therapy.

As in the subacromial or subdeltoid bursa, closed sacs lined with cellular membranes resembling synovium are found in other locations to facilitate motion of tendons and muscles over bone prominences. Local pain and nonspecific inflammation are found as a result of friction or repeated trauma. Common sites of this type of bursitis include, in addition to the subdeltoid bursa, the olecranon, the trochanteric, the anserine, and several bursae in the patellar area. Treatment is as described under subdeltoid bursa. However, in these locales ice may be used. Often, injection of local anesthetics in combination with hydrocortisone preparations and with superficial heating and immobilization are preferred. Important elements of therapy are rest and the removal of the irritating factors. In all bursitis, the local therapy is used combined with systemic application of anti-inflammatory agents, such as nonsteroidal anti-inflammatory agents.[330]

In lateral epicondylitis, or tennis elbow, there is an inflammatory reaction in the area of the common origin of the extensor tendon upon the lateral epicondyle of the humerus. In the acute stage, treatment should be primarily that of rest and splinting combined with ice application.[251] If pain persists, superficial heat application may be useful. Mild short wave diathermy administration could also be used. This treatment is often combined with the injection of hydrocortisone preparations and of a local anesthetic. Ultrasound selectively raises the temperature of the common tendon of origin and the extensor aponeurosis. However, ultrasound is contraindicated in the acute stage but may be helpful in the presence of prolonged pain, especially when the patient is unable or unwilling to follow the prescribed regimen of immobilization. If in such cases ultrasound is used in the chronic stage, it should be given in a low dosage, approximately 0.5 watts per cm².

Tenosynovitis is treated in a similar fashion if it occurs as an overuse injury.[330]

The transmission of drugs through the skin using ultrasound, called phonophoresis, has been used for a number of indications. Griffin and co-workers[113] recommended treatment of common musculoskeletal diseases, such as degenerative joint disease, bursitis or capsulitis of the shoulder, epicondylitis, rheumatoid arthritis, and ankle strains, with hydrocortisone driven through the skin into the tissues. This therapy requires washing and rinsing of the skin and application of the ointment, which is used as a coupling medium for ultrasound; alternatively, submersion of the part in water can be used (water heated to 34.4° C [94° F]). In animal experiments, Griffin suggested that the active drug would penetrate through the skin into the tissues with this type of treatment regimen.[114, 115] However, the limitations of this therapy are that the dosimetry, as well as the control as to where the active drug will be deposited, cannot be controlled as effectively as using an injection of the active ingredient into the area to be treated.

Trauma

Surgical Trauma and Fractures

In major trauma such as in surgical procedures leading to subsequent casting Schaubel[290] found that cold application materially reduced the necessity for recasting due to swelling. He treated 207 patients with cooling and compared the results obtained in 312 patients without ice application. With ice application, the necessity for splitting the cast was reduced from 42.3 per cent to 5.3 per cent. Unfortunately, because of the nonuniformity of the surgical procedures and the presenting trauma, further clinical studies are needed to confirm the results. The procedures included knee surgery, surgery of the foot and the hip, repair of fractures, tendon repair, bone grafts, osteotomy, fusions, and others. Schaubel also found that the requirement for narcotics to produce pain relief was markedly decreased when ice was applied. In fractures of the distal tibia and fibula, Moore and Cardea[253] found measured increases in the anterior, lateral, superficial posterior, and deep posterior compartments. Five patients were treated conventionally and five patients were treated with the application of a water-cooled jacket that also produced intermittent compression. These authors observed a rapid return of the compartment pressures to normal as compared with the conventional treatment (Figs. 13–73 and 13–74). Only one contradictory study is available, which is by Matsen and associates.[239] They found that local cooling in femoral fractures of rabbits increased edema. However, the differences of the results were not statistically significant.

Minor Trauma

Minor trauma such as sprains has also been treated with cold application to produce vasoconstriction with reduction of swelling and bleeding. Basur and co-workers[19] treated 60 patients with ankle sprains without evidence of bone trauma. Two groups were compared. One group of patients was treated with compression bandages only. The

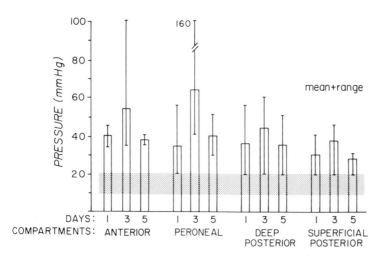

FIGURE 13–73. Compartment pressure changes in mm Hg (plotted as mean and range) after distal tibial fracture in 10 patients treated conventionally. Horizontal axis represents days after fracture. Shaded area represents range of normal values obtained from uninjured legs. (From Moore, C. D., and Cardea, J. A.: Vascular changes in leg trauma. South. Med. J., 70:1285–1286, 1977.)

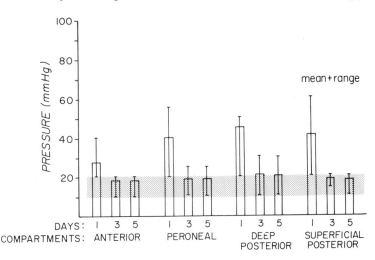

FIGURE 13–74. Compartment pressure changes in mm Hg (plotted as range and mean) during prototype boot application in five patients. Horizontal axis represents days after fracture. Shaded area represents range of normal values obtained from uninjured legs. (From Moore, C. D., and Cardea, J. A.: Vascular changes in leg trauma. South. Med. J., 70:1285–1286, 1977.)

other received additional ice therapy. The researchers found that recovery of function occurred earlier in the group treated with cold (Fig. 13–75). Hecht and co-workers[131] observed that swelling and discomfort were alleviated with ice application after total knee arthroplasty. Ice packs are used as the method of application.

Marek and associates[234, 235] treated post-traumatic edema with mild cooling, and Jezdinský[156] observed no inhibitory effect on the development of edema. In fact, he found a tendency toward an increase in edema after cold application. However, the standard procedure for such minor injuries usually combines cold application, compression, elevation, and immobilization. It must be remembered, however, that this application of ice should be extended only over a period long enough to prevent the swelling and the bleeding. Usually this can be accomplished with repeated ice packing for several hours, whereas prolonged ice application over more than one day may retard healing.[330]

During the subsequent phase of resolution, heat has been used more often. Basagoitia and co-workers[16] showed that inflammatory edema, as encountered after surgery, was better resolved with a combination of heat and cold application rather than by heat alone or by application of pressure. Pasila and colleagues suggested that diathermy application may reduce the swelling after the acute phase following ankle and foot sprains, whereas

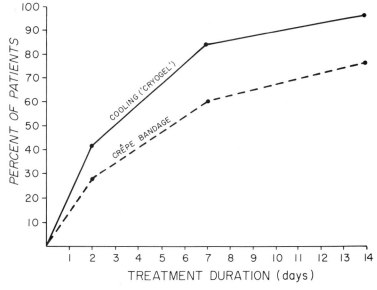

FIGURE 13–75. Percentage recovery at various stages of treatment with cooling and compression. (From Basur, R. L., Shepherd, E., and Mouzas, G. L.: A cooling method in the treatment of ankle sprains. Practitioner, 216:708–711, 1976.)

Stillwell[314] suggested that noninflammatory edema is aggravated by the use of either local or remote heating. Marek and co-workers[234, 235] studied the effect of various types of heat application on traumatic edema produced in the rat's hind paws by a quantified mechanical insult. They found that the edema was temporarily reduced as compared with the controls. However, after 24 hours, no significant difference was found in the edema, irrespective of treatment. On the other hand, these authors found no improvement of the edema when treated with radiant heat. In fact, a tendency toward increasing the edema was found. Hansen and colleagues[124] studied the ^{133}Xe clearance and found that, whereas massage temporarily increased the rate of clearance, short wave diathermy and ultrasound application did not produce significant changes. Injection of ^{133}Xe and subsequent clearance do not resemble the resolution of edema or clinical hematoma or that of any other clinical condition. Also, since no temperature measurements were made during short wave and ultrasound application, it is questionable as to whether the temperature changes were adequate to produce an increase of blood flow and, subsequently, an increase in the clearance. On the other hand, Brown[36] advocated heat for the treatment of subacute and chronic stages of trauma in which the resolution of hemorrhage and swelling is desired. Lehmann and associates[200] simulated intramuscular bleeding by injecting red blood cells labeled with radioisotope Cr[51] into the biceps femoris muscle of a pig. The site was treated with microwave diathermy and showed a more rapid resolution of the hematoma than the control side. The difference was statistically significant.

Thermal Trauma

Shulman[304] confirmed the results of animal experimentation by Zitowitz and Hardy[364] that, in superficial burns, ice pack application relieved pain and reduced the extent of redness and blistering if ice application occurred early after the thermal injury. These authors recommended that cooling be continued for several hours, and packs were reapplied if pain recurred after discontinuation of cold application. Shulman's findings were confirmed by Demling and co-workers.[63] In addition, Demling pointed out that timing of the ice application after thermal injury is critical. In his experiments, he found that cold treatment beginning two minutes after the burn did not decrease edema formation and did impair resorption.

Inflammation Associated With Infections

Furuncles and Other Skin Infections

The time-honored way to treat superficial skin infections, such as isolated folliculitis, furuncles, carbuncles, and paronychia, is with hot soaks or hot pack application with the intent to increase hyperemia and speed up abscess formation ("pointing"), pus evacuation, and healing. Obviously this method of treatment, although commonly used, is just an adjunct to other therapy.

Chronic Pelvic Inflammatory Disease

In chronic pelvic inflammatory disease, the pelvic diathermy applied with vaginal or rectal electrodes is capable of selectively heating this area, with full control of the temperature in the tissue surrounding the internal electrode. Treatment of this type increases blood flow and vascularity and thus assists the resolution of the process. Prior to the availability of antibiotics, Krusen and co-workers[173, 174, 280] found that in 86.5 per cent of a series of 37 patients with chronic pelvic inflammatory disease, the cultures became negative and remained so. An additional benefit may be derived from the therapy in that the poor vascularity in the inflamed tissues may prevent adequate antibiotic levels from reaching this area, a situation that potentially could be improved by the increase in vascularity and blood flow. In the acute stage of the disease, vigorous therapy with internal electrodes is contraindicated. Abscess formation and perforation of the tubal abscess, for instance, could be precipitated. Therefore, only chronic pelvic inflammatory disease should be treated, and it is imperative to start with short exposure at relatively low temperatures. The temperature and time of exposure may then be increased gradually as tolerated.

Vascular Disease

Peripheral Arterial Insufficiency

Peripheral arterial insufficiency is often caused by arteriosclerosis and is commonly found in the lower extremities. Heat application above the level of the lesion has resulted in increased blood flow below the level of the lesion. However, the measurements used to document the increase in flow may have been responsive primarily to changes in blood flow in the skin. There is no documentation that blood flow in the muscle is also increased.[2] Erdman[89] used short wave diathermy to the pelvic area to achieve an increase in vascularity in the lower extremity in normal subjects. Significantly increasing the temperature in the deep tissues below the level of the lesion is contraindicated. The increase in metabolic demand without the ability to increase the blood flow to fulfill this demand may lead to tissue necrosis.

Peripheral Venous Insufficiency and Varicose Ulcers

Dyson and co-workers[77, 80] showed in a controlled study that ultrasound improves the rate of healing of varicose ulcers (see Fig. 13–60). Dyson used an ultrasonic frequency of 3 MHz with average intensities of 1 watt per cm[2]. Some of the applications were pulsed, with a 20 per cent duty cycle. The duration of the pulses was 2 msec. The treatment was applied primarily to the edge of the healing ulcer with a commercial gel coupling medium. Treatments were repeated three times a week for a minimum of four weeks.

Pressure Sores

Decubiti resulting from vascular occlusion due to pressure in patients with loss of sensation or obtunded consciousness have been conventionally treated in the Hubbard tank. This therapy is especially helpful, since cleansing of the undermined edges can be readily obtained by the use of agitators. Water additives such as detergents and antibacterial agents, e.g., povidone-iodine (Betadine), have been advocated. It is most important to recognize that this treatment can be considered only as an adjunct to the relief of pressure and surgical debridement and repair through plastic surgery.

Ultrasound has also been tried as described in varicose ulcer therapy; however, no clinical study is available demonstrating any evidence that the therapy is of value in this case.

Thrombophlebitis

In superficial thrombophlebitis one adjunct to therapy may be the application of hot packs, hot moist packs, or both, or the heat cradle with resulting relief of inflammation and discomfort.

Raynaud's Disease

In Raynaud's disease, the digital arteries respond excessively to vasospastic stimuli, producing the characteristic bilateral symmetrical pallor and cyanosis of the skin of the digits followed by redness. The attack is precipitated usually by cold and relieved by warmth. Abnormalities of the sympathetic nervous system seem to play a role.

A number of authors[37, 317, 352] have advocated ultrasound application locally and to the sympathetics in an attempt to reduce the manifestations of the disease. Their empirical clinical findings seem to confirm this. However, more controlled clinical investigations are necessary. The treatment for Raynaud's phenomenon was similar.

Pain Syndromes

In the preceding discussion, it has been shown that heat or cold application may relieve pain in many conditions, either by a direct influence on pain fibers or free nerve endings or secondarily by relieving the painful conditions, such as inflammation, muscle spasm, and others. Ultrasound has been used specifically with two painful conditions: the painful amputation neuroma and postherpetic pain. In both cases, it has been documented that the peripheral nerve embedded in myofascial interfaces is selectively heated, and thus pain sensation could be altered.

Specifically in amputation neuromas, it is most important first to assess whether the pain actually originates in the amputation neuroma and to ensure that one is not dealing with a painful phantom limb resulting from other causes. If it is a local amputation neuroma that is irritated because of scarring, treatment should be with ultrasound applied over a very small field with relatively high intensities, with the intent to decrease the nerve function. Although there is no clear statistical evidence that this treatment is effective, clinical observations suggest its usefulness, and in the absence of any side effects it may be tried before surgical revision is considered.

The treatment of postherpetic pain is based on the same assumption and, since this is a condition difficult to deal with, a trial is worthwhile even though it is based purely on a clinical, empirical basis. In this case, the involved peripheral nerve should be treated.

Miscellaneous

There are a number of conditions in which ultrasound has been of suggested value empirically, and in the absence of side effects ultrasound could be given a trial.

In plantar warts,[46, 162] a relatively high dose of ultrasound is applied to the limited area of the wart on a daily basis. Since the plantar warts represent a difficult problem and ultrasound has no significant side effects in this application, a trial with this therapy may be worthwhile. Unlike ionizing radiation, this type of radiation can be repeated, and, unlike surgery, it does not produce scars.

Superficial radiant heat is also sometimes used as part of good nursing care, especially in paralyzed individuals, to dry out superficial lesions that occur with moisture accumulation in the perineal area. In this case it is most important that the heat application be very mild to prevent superficial burns.

In summary, although the various modes of heat and cold application can be used in many conditions, they are considered only an adjunct to proper therapy, but an adjunct that can significantly improve the therapeutic results and accelerate restoration to normal.

ACKNOWLEDGMENT

This chapter is based in part on research supported by Research Grant #G00830076 from the National Institute on Disability and Rehabilitation Research, Department of Education, Washington, D.C. 20202.

References

1. Abramson, D. I.: Physiologic basis for the use of physical agents in peripheral vascular disorders. Arch. Phys. Med. Rehabil., 46:216–244, 1965.
2. Abramson, D. I., Bell, Y., Tuck, S., Jr., Mitchell, R., and Chandrasekharappa, G.: Changes in blood flow, oxygen uptake and tissue temperatures produced by therapeutic physical agents: III. Effect of indirect or reflex vasodilatation. Am. J. Phys. Med., 40:5–13, 1961.
3. Abramson, D. I., Burnett, C., Bell, Y., Tuck, S., Jr., Rejal, H., and Fleischer, C. J.: Changes in blood flow, oxygen uptake and tissue temperatures produced by therapeutic physical agents: I. Effect of ultrasound. Am. J. Phys. Med., 39:51–62, 1960.
4. Addington, C. H., Osborn, C., Swartz, G., Fischer, F. P., Neubauer, R. A., and Sarkees, Y. T.: Biological effects of microwave energy at 200 mc. Biological Effects of Microwave Radiation. Proc. 4th Ann. Tri-Service Conf. on the Biological Effects of Microwave Radiation. New York, Plenum Press, 1961, vol. 1, pp. 177–186.
5. Aldes, J. H., and Klaras, T.: Use of ultrasonic radiation in the treatment of subdeltoid bursitis with and without calcareous deposits. West. J. Surg., 62:369–376, 1954.
6. Anderson, T. P., Wakim, K. G., Herrick, J. F., Bennett, W. A., and Krusen, F. H.: An experimental study of the effects of ultrasonic energy on the lower part of the spinal cord and peripheral nerves. Arch. Phys. Med. Rehabil., 32:71–83, 1951.
7. Apfelberg, D. B., Maser, M. R., Lash, H., and Rivers, J.: The argon laser for cutaneous lesions. J.A.M.A., 245:2073–2075, 1981.
8. Ardan, N. I., Janes, J. M., and Herrick, J. F.: Changes in bone after exposure to ultrasonic energy. Minn. Med., 37:415–420, 1954.
9. Ardan, N. I., Janes, J. M., and Herrick, J. F.: Ultrasonic energy and surgically produced defects in bone. J. Bone Joint Surg., 39A:394–402, 1957.
10. Aronoff, B. L.: The state of the art in general surgery and surgical oncology. Lasers Surg. Med., 6:376–382, 1986.
11. Bach, S. A.: Biological sensitivity to radiofrequency and microwave energy. Fed. Proc., 24(Suppl. 14):S-22-S-26, 1965.
12. Bach, S. A., Luzzio, A. J., and Brownell, A. S.: Effects of radio-frequency energy on human gamma globulin. Proc. 4th Ann. Tri-Service Conf. on the Biological Effects of Microwave Radiation, 1:117–133, 1960.
13. Bäcklund, L., and Tiselius, P.: Objective measurement of joint stiffness in rheumatoid arthritis. Acta Rheum. Scand., 13:275–288, 1967.
14. Balmaseda, M. T., Fatehi, M. T., Koozekanani, S. H., and Lee, A. L.: Ultrasound therapy: A comparative study of different coupling media. Arch. Phys. Med. Rehabil., 67:147–150, 1986.
15. Barth, G., and Bülow, H. A.: Frage der Ultraschallschädigung jugendlicher Knochen. Strahlentherapie, 79:271–280, 1949.
16. Basagoitia, F., Bolanos, O. R., Morse, D. R., and Furst, M. L.: The effect of hot and cold external application on experimentally induced inflammatory edema in guinea pigs: A pilot study. Ann. Dent., 44:16–20, 26, 1985.
17. Basford, J. R., Hallman, H. O., Sheffield, C. G., and Mackey, G. L.: Comparison of cold-quartz ultraviolet, low-energy laser, and occlusion in wound healing in a swine model. Arch. Phys. Med. Rehabil., 67:151–154, 1986.
18. Basford, J. R., Sheffield, C. G., Mair, S. D., and Ilstrup, D. M.: Low-energy helium neon laser treatment of thumb osteoarthritis. Arch. Phys. Med. Rehabil., 68:794–797, 1987.
19. Basur, R. L., Shephard, E., and Mouzas, G. L.: A cooling method in the treatment of ankle sprains. Practitioner, 216:708–711, 1976.
20. Bearzy, H. J.: Clinical applications of ultrasonic energy in treatment of acute and chronic subacromial bursitis. Arch. Phys. Med. Rehabil., 34:228–235, 1953.
21. Bell, K. R., and Lehmann, J. F.: Effects of cooling on H- and T-reflexes in normal subjects. Arch. Phys. Med. Rehabil., 68:490–493, 1987.

22. Bengston, R., and Warfield, C. A.: Physical therapy for pain relief. Hosp. Pract., (August):84E-84O, 1984.

23. Bergmann, L.: Der Ultraschall und seine Anwendung in Wissenschaft und Technik. Stuttgart, S. Hirzel Verlag, 1949.

24. Berkson, J.: A statistically precise and relatively simple method of estimating the bio-assay with quantal response, based on the logistic function. J. Am. Stat. Assoc., 48:565, 1953.

25. Bickford, R. H., and Duff, R. S.: Influences of ultrasonic radiation of temperature and blood flow in the human skeletal muscle. Circ. Res., 1:534–538, 1953.

26. Bierman, W.: Ultrasound in the treatment of scars. Arch. Phys. Med. Rehabil., 35:209–213, 1954.

27. Bini, G., Cruccu, G., Hagbarth, K.-E., Schady, W., and Torebjork, E.: Analgesic effect of vibration and cooling on pain induced by intraneural electrical stimulation. Pain, 18:239–248, 1984.

28. Bisgard, J. D., and Nye, D.: The influence of hot and cold application upon gastric and intestinal motor activity. Surg. Gynecol. Obstet., 71:172–180, 1940.

29. Black, K. D., Halverson, J. L., Majerus, K. A., and Soderberg, G. L.: Alterations in ankle dorsiflexion torque as a result of continuous ultrasound to the anterior tibial compartment. Phys. Ther., 64:910–913, 1984.

30. Blomgren, I., Bagge, U., and Johansson, B. R.: Effects of cooling after scald injury to a dorsal skin fold of mouse. Scand. J. Plast. Reconstr. Surg., 19:1–9, 1985.

31. Blomgren, I., Eriksson, E., and Bagge, U.: The effect of different cooling temperatures and immersion fluids on post-burn oedema and survival of the partially scalded hairy mouse ear. Burns, 11:161–165, 1985.

32. Bonica, J. J.: Management of myofascial pain syndromes in general practice. J.A.M.A., 164:732–738, 1957.

33. Born, H.: Zur Frage der Absorptionsmessungen im Ultraschallgebiet. Zeitschrift Phys., 120:383–396, 1943.

34. Borrell, R. M., Henley, E. J., Ho, P., and Hubbell, M. K.: Fluidotherapy: evaluation of a new heat modality. Arch. Phys. Med. Rehabil., 58:69–71, 1977.

35. Borrell, R. M., Parker, R., Henley, E. J., Masley, D., and Repinecz, M.: Comparison of in vivo temperatures produced by hydrotherapy, paraffin wax treatment, and Fluidotherapy. Phys. Ther., 60:1273–1976, 1980.

36. Brown, A. M.: Physical medicine in athletic rehabilitation. Md. Med. J., 19:61–64, 1970.

37. Buchtala, V.: The present state of ultrasonic therapy. Br. J. Phys. Med., 15:3–6, 18, 1952.

38. Cameron, B. M.: Experimental acceleration of wound healing. Am. J. Orthod., 3:336–343, 1961.

39. Carpenter, R. L.: Experimental radiation cataracts induced by microwave radiation. Proc. 2nd Tri-Serv. Conf. Biologic Effects Microwave Energy. Rome Air Dev. Center, Air Res. and Dev. Command, Rome, N.Y., ASTIA Doc. AD-131–477, July, 1958, p. 146.

40. Carpenter, R. L., Biddle, D. K., and van Ummerson, C. A.: Annual report of work in progress at Tufts University. January, 1958.

41. Carpenter, R. L., Biddle, D. K., and van Ummerson, C. A.: Progress report. Investigator's Conf. Biol. Effects of Electronic Radiating Equipment. Rome Air Dev. Center, Air Res. and Dev. Command, Rome, N.Y., ASTIA Doc. AD-214693, January, 1959, p. 12.

42. Carstensen, E. L., Li, K., and Schwan, H. P.: Determination of the acoustic properties of blood and its components. J. Acoust. Soc. Am., 25:286–289, 1953.

43. Chan, A. K., Sigelmann, R. A., and Guy, A. W.: Calculations of therapeutic heat generated by ultrasound in fat-muscle-bone layers. IEEE Trans. Biomed. Eng. BME, 21:280–284, 1973.

44. Chan, A. K., Sigelmann, R. A., Guy, A. W., and Lehmann, J. F.: Calculation by the method of finite differences of the temperature distribution in layered tissues. IEEE Trans. Biomed. Eng. BME, 20:86–90, 1973.

45. Chater, B. V., and Williams, A. R.: Platelet aggregation induced in vitro by therapeutic ultrasound. Thromb. Haemost., 38:640–651, 1977.

46. Cherup, N., and Bender, L. F.: Treatment of plantar warts with ultrasound. Arch. Phys. Med. Rehabil., 43:371, 1962.

47. Child, S. Z., Vives, B., Fridd, C. W., Hare, J. D., Linke, C. A., Davis, H. T., and Carstensen, E. L.: Ultrasonic treatment of tumors—II. Moderate hyperthermia. Ultrasound Med. Biol., 6:341–344, 1980.

48. Choy, D. S. J.: Laser revascularization, 1985: State of the art. Lasers Surg. Med., 6:408–411, 1986.

49. Clendenin, M. A., and Szumski, A. J.: Influence of cutaneous ice application on single motor units in humans. Phys. Ther., 57:166–175, 1971.

50. Cochran, G. V. B., Johnson, M. W., Kadaba, M. P., Vosburgh, F., Ferguson-Pell, M. W., and Palmieri, V. R.: Piezoelectric internal fixation devices: A new approach to electrical augmentation of osteogenesis. J. Orth. Res., 3:508–513, 1985.

51. Cole, K. S., and Cole, R. H.: Dispersion and absorption in dielectrics. I. Alternating current characteristics. J. Chem. Phys., 9:341, 1941.

52. Collins, K., Storey, M., and Peterson, K.: Peroneal nerve palsy after cryotherapy. Phys. Sports Med., 14:105–108, 1986.

53. Constable, J. D., Scapicchio, A. P., and Opitz, B.: Studies of the effects of diapulse treatment of various aspects of wound healing in experimental animals. J. Surg. Res., 11:254–257, 1971.

54. Cook, H. F.: A comparison of the dielectric behavior of pure water and human blood at microwave frequencies. Br. J. Appl. Phys., 3:249, 1952.

55. Corradi, C., and Cozzolino, A.: Azione degli ultrasuoni sulla evoluzione delle fratture sperimentali dei conigli. Minerva Ortop., 3:44–45, 1952.

56. Corradi, C., Cozzolino, A.: Gli ultrasuoni (U.S.) e l'evoluzione del callo osseo nei focolai di frattura. Arch. Ortop., 66:77–98, 1953.

57. Council on Scientific Affairs, Panel on Lasers in Medicine and Surgery, American Medical Association: Lasers in medicine and surgery. J.A.M.A., 256:900–907, 1986.

58. Crockford, G. W., and Hellon, R. F.: Vascular responses of human skin to infrared radiation. J. Physiol., 149:424–432, 1959.

59. Daily, L., Jr., Wakim, K. G., Herrick, J. F., and Parkhill, E. M.: The effects of microwave diathermy on the eye. Am. J. Physiol., 155:432, 1948.

60. Daily, L., Jr., Wakim, K. G., Herrick, J. F., Parkhill, E. M., and Benedict, W. L.: The effects of microwave diathermy on the eye of the rabbit. Am. J. Ophthalmol., 35:1001–1017, 1952.

61. de Lateur, B. J., Lehmann, J. F., Stonebridge, J. B., Warren, C. G., and Guy, A. W.: Muscle heating in human subjects with 915 MHz microwave contact applicator. Arch. Phys. Med. Rehabil., 51:147–151, 1970.

62. de Lateur, B. J., Stonebridge, J. B., and Lehmann, J. F.: Fibrous muscular contractures: treatment with a new direct contact microwave applicator operating at 915 MHz. Arch. Phys. Med. Rehabil., 59:488–490, 1978.

63. Demling, R. H., Mazess, R. B., and Wolberg, W.: The effect of immediate and delayed cold immersion on burn edema formation and resorption. J. Trauma, 17:56–60, 1979.

64. Dietzel, F., and Kern, W.: Kann hohes mütterliches Fieber beim Kind auslösen. Originalmitteilungen ist ausschliesslich der Verfasser verantwortlich. Naturwissenschaften, 2:24–26, 1971.

65. Dietzel, F., and Kern, W.: Kann hohes mütterliches Fieber Missbildungen beim Kind auslösen? Geburtshilfe Frauenheilkd., 31:1074–1079, 1971.

66. Dodi, G., Bogoni, F., Infantino, A., Pianon, P., Mortellaro, L. M., Lise, M.: Hot or cold in anal pain? A study of the changes in internal anal sphincter pressure profiles. Dis. Colon Rectum, 29:248–251, 1986.

67. Dodt, E., and Zotterman, Y.: Mode of action of warm receptors. Acta Physiol. Scand., 26:345–357, 1952.

68. Dodt, E., and Zotterman, Y.: The discharge of specific cold fibres at high temperatures (the paradoxical cold). Acta Physiol. Scand., 26:358–365, 1952.

69. Douglas, W. W., and Malcolm, J. L.: The effect of localized cooling on conduction in cat nerves. J. Physiol., 130:53–71, 1955.

70. Doyle, J. R., and Smart, B. W.: Stimulation of bone growth by shortwave diathermy. J. Bone Joint Surg., 45-A:15–24, 1963.

71. Drez, D., Faust, D. C., and Evans, J. P.: Cryotherapy and nerve palsy. Am. J. Sports Med., 9:256–257, 1981.

72. Dugois, P.: The action of ultrasonics in Peyronie's disease, accelerated by alpha-chymotrypsin. Lyon Med., 93:238, 1961.

73. Dunn, F., and Frizzell, L. A.: Bioeffects of ultrasound. In Lehmann, J. F. (Ed.): Therapeutic Heat and Cold, 4th Ed. Baltimore, Williams & Wilkins, 1989.

74. Dussick, C. T., Fritch, D. J., Kyraizidan, M., and Sear, R. S.: Measurement of articular tissues with ultrasound. Am. J. Phys. Med., 37:160–165, 1958.

75. Dyson, M.: Alterations in fibroblast activity in response to ultrasound. Presented 9/11/81 at "An International Symposium on Therapeutic Ultrasound," Winnipeg, Manitoba, Canada.

76. Dyson, M.: The effect of ultrasound on the rate of wound healing and the quality of scar tissue. Presented 9/11/81 at "An International Symposium on Therapeutic Ultrasound," Winnipeg, Manitoba, Canada.

77. Dyson, M., Franks, C., and Suckling, J.: Stimulation of healing of varicose ulcers by ultrasound. Ultrasonics, 14:232–236, 1976.

78. Dyson, M., and Pond, J. B.: The effect of pulsed ultrasound on tissue regeneration. Physiotherapy, 56:136–142, 1970.

79. Dyson, M., Pond, J. B., Joseph, J., and Warwick, R.: The stimulation of tissue regeneration by means of ultrasound. Clin. Sci., 35:273–285, 1968.

80. Dyson, M., and Suckling, J.: Stimulation of tissue repair by ultrasound: a survey of the mechanisms involved. Physiotherapy, 64:105–108, 1978.

81. Dyson, M., Woodward, B., and Pond, J. B.: Flow of red blood cells stopped by ultrasound. Nature, 232:572–573, 1971.

82. Edwards, M. J.: Congenital defects in guinea pigs. Arch. Pathol., 84:42–48, 1967.

83. Edwards, M. J.: Influenza, hyperthermia, and congenital malformation. Lancet, 1:320–321, 1972.

84. Edwards, M. J., Mulley, R., Ring, S., and Wanner, R. A.: Mitotic cell death and delay of mitotic activity in guinea-pig embryos following brief maternal hyperthermia. J. Embryol. Exp. Morphol., 32:593–602, 1974.

85. Eldred, E., Lindsley, D. E., and Buchwald, J. S.: The effect of cooling on mammalian muscle spindles. Exp. Neurol., 2:144–157, 1960.

86. Ely, T. S., Goldman, D., Hearon, J. Z., Williams, R. B., and Carpenter, H. M.: Heating Characteristics of Laboratory Animals Exposed to Ten Centimeter Microwaves. Bethesda, Md., U.S. Nav. Med. Res. Inst.(Res. Rep. Proj. NM 001–050. 13.02), IEEE Trans. Biomed. Eng., 11:123–137, 1964.

87. Emery, A. F., Stonebridge, J. B., Sekins, K. M., and Lehmann, J. F.: Experimental and numerical studies of the elevated temperatures induced in a human leg by microwave diathermy with surface cooling. Radio Science, 14(6S):297–314, 1979.

88. Engel, J. P., Herrick, J. F., Wakim, K. G., Grindlay, J. H., and Krusen, F. H.: The effect of microwaves on bone and bone marrow on adjacent tissues. Arch. Phys. Med. Rehabil., 31:453–461, 1950.

89. Erdman, W. J., II: Peripheral blood flow measurements during application of pulsed high-frequency currents. Am. J. Orthod., 2:196–197, 1960.

90. Evans, D. S., and Mendelssohn, K.: The physical basis of radiant heat therapy. Proc. R. Soc. Med., 38:578–586, 1945.

91. Federal Communications Commission: Rules and Regulations, vol. 2, subpart A, section 18.13, 1964.

92. Fenn, J. E.: Effect of pulsed electromagnetic energy (Diapulse) on experimental hematomas. Can. Med. Assoc. J., 100:251–254, 1969.

93. Feucht, B. L., Richardson, A. W., and Hines, H. M.: Effect of implanted metal on tissue hyperthermia produced by microwaves. Arch. Phys. Med. Rehabil., 30:164–169, 1949.

94. Finley, J. L., Barsky, S. H., Greer, D. E., Kamat, B. R., Noe, J. M., and Rosen, S.: Healing of portwine stains after argon laser therapy. Arch. Dermatol., 117:486–489, 1981.

95. Fischer, A. A.: Diagnosis and management of chronic pain in physical medicine and rehabilitation. In Ruskin, A. P. (Ed): Current Therapy in Physiatry. Philadelphia, W. B. Saunders, 1984.

96. Fischer, E., and Solomon, S.: Physiological responses to heat and cold. In Licht, S. (Ed.): Therapeutic Heat and Cold, 2nd Ed. Baltimore, Waverly Press, 1965.

97. Food and Drug Administration, US DHEW: Performance standard for microwave diathermy products. Fed. Reg., 40:23877–23878, 1975.

98. Fountain, F. P., Gersten, J. W., and Sengir, O.: Decrease in muscle spasm produced by ultrasound, hot packs, and infrared radiation. Arch. Phys. Med. Rehabil., 41:293–298, 1960.

99. Frizzell, L. A., and Dunn, F.: Biophysics of ultrasound. In Lehmann, J. F. (Ed.): Therapeutic Heat and Cold, 4th Ed. Baltimore, Williams & Wilkins, 1989.

100. Gammon, G. D., and Starr, I.: Studies on the relief of pain by counterirritation. J. Clin. Invest., 20:13–20, 1941.

101. Gersten, J. W.: Changes in spinal cord thresholds following the application of ultrasound. Paper given at Fourth Annual Conference, Amer. Inst. Ultrasonics in Med., Detroit, 1955.

102. Gersten, J. W.: Effect of metallic objects on temperature rises produced in tissues by ultrasound. Am. J. Phys. Med., 37:75–82, 1958.

103. Gersten, J. W.: Effect of ultrasound on tendon extensibility. Am. J. Phys. Med., 34:362–369, 1955.

104. Gersten, J. W.: Ultrasonics and muscle disease. Am. J. Phys. Med., 33:68–74, 1954.

105. Ghietti, A.: Embriopatia da onde corte. Minerva Nipiologica, 5:7–12, 1955.

106. Ginsberg, A. J.: Pulsed shortwave in the treatment of bursitis with calcification. Int. Record Med., 174:71–75, 1961.

107. Goldman, J. A., Chiapella, J., Casey, H., Bass, N., Graham, J., McClatchey, W., Dronavalli, R. V., Brown, R., Bennett, W. J., Miller, S. B., Wilson, C. H., Pearson, B., Haun, C., Persinski, L., Huey, H., and Muckerheide, M.: Laser therapy for rheumatoid arthritis. Lasers Surg. Med., 1:93–101, 1980.

108. Goldman, L.: Basic reactions in tissue. In Goldman, L. (Ed): The Biomedical Laser: Technology and Clinical Applications. New York, Springer-Verlag, 1981.

109. Goldman, L., and Rockwell, R. J.: Lasers in Medicine. New York, Gordon and Breach, 1971, p. 207.

110. Gorodetskaya, S. F.: The effect of centimeter radiowaves on mouse fertility. Fiziol. Zh., 9:394–395, 1963.

111. Granberry, W. M., and Janes, J. M.: The lack of effect of microwave diathermy on rate of growth of bone of the growing dog. J. Bone Joint Surg., 45A:4:773–777, 1963.

112. Greathouse, D. G., Currier, D. P., and Gilmore, R. L.: Effects of clinical infrared laser on superficial radial nerve conduction. Phys. Ther., 65:1184–1187, 1985.

113. Griffin, J. E., Echternach, J. L., Price, R. E., and Touchstone, J. C.: Patients treated with ultrasonic driven hydrocortisone and with ultrasound alone. Phys. Ther. 47:594–601, 1967.

114. Griffin, J. E., and Touchstone, J. C.: Ultrasonic movement of cortisol into pig tissues. I. Movement into skeletal muscle. Am. J. Phys. Med., 42:77–85, 1963.

115. Griffin, J. E., Touchstone, J. C., and Liu, A. C.-Y.: Ultrasonic movement of cortisol into pig tissues. II. Movement into paravertebral nerve. Am. J. Phys. Med., 44:20–25, 1965.

116. Guy, A. W.: Analyses of electromagnetic fields induced in biological tissues by thermographic studies on equivalent phantom models. IEEE MTT, 19:205–214, 1971.

117. Guy, A. W.: Electromagnetic fields and relative heating patterns due to a rectangular aperture source in direct contact with bilayered biological tissue. IEEE MTT, 19:214–223, 1971.

118. Guy, A. W., and Lehmann, J. F.: Comparative evaluation of electromagnetic diathermy modalities in 433 MHz to 2450 MHz. 21st ACEMB—Shamrock Hilton Hotel, Houston, Texas, Nov. 18–21, 1968.

119. Guy, A. W., and Lehmann, J. F.: On the determination of an optimum microwave diathermy frequency for a direct contact applicator. IEEE BME, 13:76–87, 1966.
120. Guy, A. W., Lehmann, J. F., and Stonebridge, J. B.: Therapeutic applications of electromagnetic power. Proc. IEEE, 62:55–75, 1974.
121. Guy, A. W., Lin, J. C., Kramar, P. O., and Emery, A. F.: Effect of 2450-MHz radiation on the rabbit eye. IEEE Trans. Microwave Theory Tech. MTT, 23:492–498, 1975.
122. Hagbarth, K.-E.: Excitatory and inhibitory skin areas for flexor and extensor motoneurones. Acta Physiol. Scand., 26(Suppl 94):1–58, 1952.
123. Haina, D., Brunner, R., Landthaler, M., Braun-Falco, O., and Waidelich, W.: Animal experiments on light-induced wound-healing. Laser Basic Biomed. Res., 4:22-1,–22-3, 1977.
124. Hansen, T. I., and Kristensen, J. H.: Effect of massage, shortwave diathermy and ultrasound upon ^{133}Xe disappearance rate from muscle and subcutaneous tissue in the human calf. Scand. J. Rehab. Med., 5:179–182, 1973.
125. Hardy, J. D., Wolff, H. G., and Goodell, H.: Studies on pain. A new method for measuring pain threshold: observations on spatial summation of pain. J. Clin. Invest., 19:649–657, 1940.
126. Hargreaves, A. S., and Wardle, J. J. M.: The use of physiotherapy in the treatment of temporomandibular disorders. Br. Dent. J., 155:121–124, 1983.
127. Harris, E., Jr., and McCroskery, P. A.: The influence of temperature and fibril stability on degradation of cartilage collagen by rheumatoid synovial collagenase. N. Engl. J. Med., 290:1–6, 1974.
128. Hartviksen, K.: Ice therapy in spasticity. Acta Neurol. Scand., 38(Suppl. 3):79–84, 1962.
129. Harvey, M. A. S., McRorie, M. M., and Smith, D. W.: Suggested limits of exposure in the hot tub and sauna for the pregnant woman. J. Can. Med. Assoc., 125:50–53, 1981.
130. Hayashi, S.: Der Einfluss der Ultraschallwellen und Ultrakurzwellen auf den maligen Tumor. J. Med. Sci. Biophysics Japan, 6:138, 1940.
131. Hecht, P. J., Bachmann, S., Booth, R. E., Jr., and Rothman, R. H.: Effects of thermal therapy on rehabilitation after total knee arthroplasty. A prospective randomized study. Clin. Orthop., (178):198–201, 1983.
132. Hedenius, P., Odeblad, E., and Wahlstroem, L.: Some preliminary investigations on the therapeutic effect of pulsed shortwaves in intermittent claudication. Curr. Ther. Res., 8:317–321, 1966.
133. Heller, J. H.: Reticuloendothelial Structure and Function. New York, The Roland Press Co., 1960, Chap. 12.
134. Hensel, H.: Temperaturempfindung und intracutane Wärmebewegung. Pflügers Arch., 252:165–215, 1950.
135. Hensel, H., and Zotterman, Y.: Quantitative Be-
ziehungen zwischen der Entladung einzelner Kaltefasern und der Temperatur. Acta Physiol. Scand., 23:291–319, 1951.
136. Heppner, F.: Neurosurgery: The state of the art. Lasers Surg. Med., 6:415–422, 1986.
137. Herrick, J. F.: Temperatures produced in tissues by ultrasound: experimental study using various technics. J. Acoust. Soc. Am., 25:12–16, 1953.
138. Herrick, J. F., Jelatis, D. G., and Lee, G. M.: Dielectric properties of tissues important in microwave diathermy. Fed. Proc., 9:60, 1950.
139. Herrick, J. F., and Krusen, F. H.: Certain physiologic and pathologic effects of microwaves. Elec. Eng., 72:239–244, 1953.
140. Heslop, R. W., Oakland, D. J., and Maddox, B. T.: Ultrasonic therapy in Peyronie's disease. Br. J. Urol., 39:415–419, 1967.
141. Hintzelmann, U.: Ultraschalltherapie rheumatischer Erkrankungen. Dtsch. Med. Wochenschr., 72:350–353, 1947.
142. Hintzelmann, U.: Ultraschalltherapie rheumatischer Erkrankungen. Dtsch. Med. Wochenschr., 74:869–870, 1949.
143. Hippe, H., and Uhlmann, J.: Die Anwendung des Ultraschalls bei schlecht heilenden Fracturen. Zentralblatt Chirurg., 28:1105–1110, 1959.
144. Ho, H. S., Guy, A. W., Sigelmann, R. A., and Lehmann, J. F.: Microwave heating of simulated human limbs by aperture sources. IEEE MTT, 19:224–231, 1971.
145. Hollander, J. L., and Horvath, S. M.: The influence of physical therapy procedures on the intra-articular temperature of normal and arthritic subjects. Am. J. Med. Sci., 218:543–548, 1949.
146. Horatz, K.: Erfahrungen bei der Tumorbeschallung. Ultraschall Med., 1:149–154, 1949.
147. Horvath, J.: Experimentelle Untersuchungen über die Verteilung der Ultraschallenergie im mensch lichen Gewebe. Ärztliche Forsch., 1:357–364, 1947.
148. Howland, J. W., Thomson, R. A. E., and Michaelson, S. M.: Biomedical aspects of microwave irradiation of mammals. Biological Effects of Microwave Radiation. Proc. 4th Ann. Tri-Service Conf. on the Biological Effects of Microwave Radiation, 1:261–285, 1961.
149. Hüter, T.: Messung der Ultraschallabsorption in tierischen Geweben und ihre Abhängigkeit von der Frequenz. Naturwissenschaften, 35:285, 1948.
150. Hüter, T., and Bolt, F. H.: An ultrasonic method for outlining the cerebral ventricles. J. Acoust. Soc. Am., 23:160–167, 1951.
151. Hüter, T., Dyer, J., Ludwig, G. D., and Kyrazia, D.: Thresholds of damage in nervous tissues. MIT Q. Prog. Rep., October, 1950.
152. Imig, C. J., Randall, B. F., and Hines, H. M.: Effect of ultrasonic energy on blood flow. Am. J. Phys. Med., 53:100–102, 1954.
153. Imig, C. J., Thomson, J. D., and Hines, H. M.:

Testicular degeneration as a result of microwave irradiation. Proc. Soc. Exp. Biol., 69:382–386, 1948.

154. Jako, G. J.: State of the art of otolaryngology. Lasers Surg. Med., 6:389, 1986.

155. Janes, J. M., Herrick, J. F., Kelly, P. J., and Peterson, L. F. A.: Long-term effect of ultrasonic energy on femora of the dog. Proc. Staff Meet. Mayo Clin., 35:663–671, 1960.

156. Jezdinský, J., Marek, J., and Ochonský, P.: Effects of local cold and heat therapy on traumatic oedema of the rat hind paw. I. Effects of cooling on the course of traumatic oedema. Acta Univ. Palacki. Olomuc. Fac. Med., 66:185–201, 1973.

157. Johns, R. J., and Wright, V.: Relative importance of various tissues in joint stiffness. J. Appl. Physiol., 17:824–828, 1962.

158. Kaczynski, A., Litwak, A., and Mika, T.: Remarques sur l'action de Pultrason et de la microonde dans le traitement de l'induration plastique du penis. Urol. Int., 20:236–245, 1965.

159. Kahn, J.: Case reports: Open wound management with the HeNe (6328 AU) cold laser. J. Orthop. Sports Phys. Ther., 6:203–204, 1984.

160. Kaplan, E. G., and Weinstock, R. E.: Clinical evaluation of Diapulse as adjunctive therapy following foot surgery. J. Am. Pod. Assoc., 58:218–221, 1968.

161. Kaplan, I.: The CO_2 laser in plastic surgery. Lasers Surg. Med., 6:385–386, 1986.

162. Kent, H.: Plantar wart treatment with ultrasound. Arch. Phys. Med. Rehabil., 40:15–18, 1959.

163. Kirk, J. A., and Kersley, G. D.: Heat and cold in the physical treatment of rheumatoid arthritis of the knee. Ann. Phys. Med., 9:270–274, 1968.

164. Kleinkort, J. A., and Foley, R. A.: Laser acupuncture: Its use in physical therapy. Am. J. Acupunct., 12:51–56, 1984.

165. Klemp, P., Staberg, B., Korsgård, J., Nielsen, H. V., and Crone, P.: Reduced blood flow in fibromyotic muscles during ultrasound therapy. Scand. J. Rehabil. Med., 15:21–23, 1982.

166. Knutsson, E.: Topical cryotherapy in spasticity. Scand. J. Rehabil. Med., 2:159–163, 1970.

167. Knutsson, E., and Mattsson, E.: Effects of local cooling on monosynaptic reflexes in man. Scand. J. Rehabil. Med., 1:126–132, 1969.

168. Kottke, F. J.: Heat in pelvic diseases. In Licht, S. (Ed.): Therapeutic Heat and Cold, 2nd Ed. Baltimore, Waverly Press, 1965, pp. 474–490.

169. Kramer, J. F.: Effect of therapeutic ultrasound intensity on subcutaneous tissue temperature and ulnar nerve conduction velocity. Am. J. Phys. Med., 64:1–9, 1985.

170. Kraus, H.: Clinical Treatment of Back and Neck Pain. New York, McGraw-Hill, 1970.

171. Kraus, H.: Treatment of myofascial pain. In Ruskin, A. P. (Ed.): Current Therapy in Physiatry. Philadelphia, W. B. Saunders, 1984.

172. Krikorian, D. J., Hartshorne, M. F., Stratton, S. A., and Nemmers, T. M.: Use of He-Ne laser for treatment of soft tissue trauma: Evaluation by gallium-67 citrate scanning. J. Orthop. Sports Phys. Ther., 8:93–96, 1986.

173. Krusen, F. H.: Physical Medicine. Philadelphia, W. B. Saunders Company, 1942.

174. Krusen, F. H., and Elkins, E. C.: Investigations in fever therapy. Arch. Phys. Ther., 20:77–84, 1939.

175. Krusen, F. H., Herrick, J. F., Leden, U., and Wakim, G.: Microkymatotherapy: preliminary report of experimental studies of the heating effect of microwaves ("radar") in living tissues. Proc. Staff Meet. Mayo Clin., 22:209–224, 1947.

176. Kubler, E.: Der Einfluss des Ultraschalls auf das Sudeck'sche Syndrome. Strahlentherapie, 87:575–584, 1952.

177. Lambert, E. H., Treanor, W. J., Herrick, J. F., and Krusen, F. H.: Comparative study of the effects of heat and ultrasound on nerve conduction. Fed. Proc., 10:78, 1951.

178. Landon, B. R.: Heat or cold for the relief of low back pain? Phys. Ther., 47:1126–1128, 1967.

179. Lane, R. J., Linsker, R., Wynne, J. J., Torres, A., and Geronemus, R. G.: Ultraviolet-laser ablation of skin. Arch. Dermatol., 121:609–617, 1985.

180. Lane, R. J., Wynne, J. J.: Medical applications of excimer lasers. Lasers Applications, 3 (November): 59–62, 1984.

181. Lane, R. J., Wynne, J. J., and Geronemus, R. G.: Ultraviolet laser ablation of skin: Healing studies and a thermal model. Lasers Surg. Med., 6:504–513, 1987.

182. Lehmann, J. F.: Beitrag zur Ultraschallhämolyse. Strahlentherapie, 70:533–542, 1950.

183. Lehmann, J. F.: Die Therapie mit Ultraschall und ihre Grundlagen. In Ergebnisse physikalischdiatetischen Therapie. Dresden, Verlag Steinkopff, 1951.

184. Lehmann, J. F.: The biophysical basis of biologic ultrasonic reactions with special reference to ultrasonic therapy. Arch. Phys. Med. Rehabil., 34:139–152, 1953.

185. Lehmann, J. F.: The biophysical mode of action of biologic and therapeutic ultrasonic reactions. J. Acoust. Soc. Am., 25:17–25, 1953.

186. Lehmann, J. F.: Ultrasound therapy. In Licht, S. (Ed.): Therapeutic Heat and Cold, 2nd Ed. Baltimore, Waverly Press, 1965, pp. 321–386.

187. Lehmann, J. F., and Biegler, R.: Changes of potentials and temperature gradients in membranes caused by ultrasound. Arch. Phys. Med. Rehabil., 35:287–295, 1954.

188. Lehmann, J. F., Brunner, G. D., Martinis, A. J., and McMillan, J. A.: Ultrasonic effects as demonstrated in live pigs with surgical metallic implants. Arch. Phys. Med. Rehabil., 40:483–488, 1959.

189. Lehmann, J. F., Brunner, G. D., and McMillan, J. A.: The influence of surgical implants on the temperature distribution in thigh specimens exposed to ultrasound. Arch. Phys. Med. Rehabil., 39:692–695, 1958.

190. Lehmann, J. F., Brunner, G. D., McMillan, J. A., Silverman, D. R., and Johnson, V. C.: Modification of heating patterns produced by microwaves at the frequencies of 2456 and 900 mc by physiologic factors in the human. Arch. Phys. Med. Rehabil., 45:555–563, 1964.

191. Lehmann, J. F., Brunner, G. D., and Stow, R. W.: Pain threshold measurements after therapeutic application of ultrasound, microwaves, and infrared. Arch. Phys. Med. Rehabil., 39:560–565, 1958.

192. Lehmann, J. F., and de Lateur, B. J.: Cryotherapy. In Lehmann, J. F. (Ed.): Therapeutic Heat and Cold, 4th Ed. Baltimore, Williams & Wilkins, 1989.

193. Lehmann, J. F., and de Lateur, B. J.: Therapeutic heat. In Lehmann, J. F. (Ed.): Therapeutic Heat and Cold, 4th Ed. Baltimore, Williams & Wilkins, 1989.

194. Lehmann, J. F., de Lateur, B. J., and Silverman, D. R.: Selective heating effects of ultrasound in human beings. Arch. Phys. Med. Rehabil., 47:331–339, 1966.

195. Lehmann, J. F., de Lateur, B. J., and Stonebridge, J. B.: Heating patterns produced in humans by 433.92 MHz round field applicator and 915 MHz contact applicator. Arch. Phys. Med. Rehabil., 56:442–448, 1975.

196. Lehmann, J. F., de Lateur, B. J., and Stonebridge, J. B.: Selective heating by shortwave diathermy with a helical coil. Arch. Phys. Med. Rehabil., 50:117–123, 1969.

197. Lehmann, J. F., de Lateur, B. J., Stonebridge, J. B., and Warren, C. G.: Therapeutic temperature distribution produced by ultrasound as modified by dosage and volume of tissue exposed. Arch. Phys. Med. Rehabil., 48:662–666, 1967.

198. Lehmann, J. F., de Lateur, B. J., Warren, C. G., and Stonebridge, J. B.: Heating of joint structures by ultrasound. Arch. Phys. Med. Rehabil., 49:28–30, 1968.

199. Lehmann, J. F., de Lateur, B. J., Warren, C. G., and Stonebridge, J. B.: Heating produced by ultrasound in bone and soft tissue. Arch. Phys. Med. Rehabil., 48:397–401, 1967.

200. Lehmann, J. F., Dundore, D. E., Esselman, P. C., Nelp, W. B.: Microwave diathermy: Effects on experimental muscle hematoma resolution. Arch. Phys. Med. Rehabil., 64:127–129, 1983.

201. Lehmann, J. F., Erickson, D. J., Martin, G. M., and Krusen, F. H.: Comparison of ultrasonic and microwave diathermy in the physical treatment of periarthritis of the shoulder. Arch. Phys. Med. Rehabil., 35:627–634, 1954.

202. Lehmann, J. F., Fordyce, W. E., Rathbun, L. A., Larson, R. E., and Wood, D. H.: Clinical evaluation of a new approach in the treatment of contracture associated with hip fracture after internal fixation. Arch. Phys. Med. Rehabil., 42:95–100, 1961.

203. Lehmann, J. F., Guy, A. W., de Lateur, B. J., Stonebridge, J. B., and Warren, C. G.: Heating patterns produced by shortwave diathermy using helical induction coil applicators. Arch. Phys. Med. Rehabil., 49:193–198, 1968.

204. Lehmann, J. F., Guy, A. W., Johnston, V. C., Brunner, G. D., and Bell, J. W.: Comparison of relative heating patterns produced in tissues by exposure to microwave energy at frequencies of 2,450 and 900 megacycles. Arch. Phys. Med. Rehabil., 43:69–76, 1962.

205. Lehmann, J. F., Guy, A. W., Stonebridge, J. B., and de Lateur, B. J.: Evaluation of a therapeutic direct-contact 915-MHz microwave applicator for effective deep-tissue heating in humans. IEEE Trans. Microwave Theory Tech. MTT, 26:556–563, 1978.

206. Lehmann, J. F., Guy, A. W., Stonebridge, J. B., and Warren, C. G.: Review of evidence for indications, techniques of application, contraindications, hazards, and clinical effectiveness of shortwave diathermy. Report No. FDA/HFK-75–1, to Office of DHEW/Public Health Service, Food and Drug Administration, 1/1/74 to 12/31/74, Contract Number FDA 74–32.

207. Lehmann, J. F., Guy, A. W., Warren, C. G., de Lateur, B. J., and Stonebridge, J. B.: Evaluation of microwave contact applicator. Arch. Phys. Med. Rehabil., 51:143–147, 1970.

208. Lehmann, J. F., and Herrick, J. F.: Biologic reactions to cavitation, a consideration for ultrasonic therapy. Arch. Phys. Med. Rehabil., 34:86–98, 1953.

209. Lehmann, J., and Hohlfeld, R.: Der Gewebestoffwechsel nach Ultraschall und Wärmeeinwirkung. Strahlentherapie, 87:544–549, 1952.

210. Lehmann, J. F., and Johnson, E. W.: Some factors influencing the temperature distribution in thighs exposed to ultrasound. Arch. Phys. Med. Rehabil., 39:347–356, 1958.

211. Lehmann, J. F., Johnston, V. C., McMillan, J. A., Silverman, D. R., Brunner, G. D., and Rathbun, L. A.: Comparison of deep heating by microwaves at frequencies 2456 and 900 megacycles. Arch. Phys. Med. Rehabil., 46:307–314, 1965.

212. Lehmann, J. F., and Krusen, F. H.: Biophysical effects of ultrasonic energy on carcinoma and their possible significance. 36:452–459, 1955.

213. Lehmann, J. F., Lane, C. E., Bell, J. W., and Brunner, G. D.: Influence of surgical metal implants on the distribution of the intensity in the ultrasonic field. Arch. Phys. Med. Rehabil., 39:756–760, 1958.

214. Lehmann, J. F., Masock, A. J., Warren, C. G.,

and Koblanski, J. N.: Effect of therapeutic temperatures on tendon extensibility. Arch. Phys. Med. Rehabil., 51:481–487, 1970.

215. Lehmann, J. F., McDougall, J. A., Guy, A. W., Chou, C. -K., Esselman, P. C., and Warren, C. G.: Electrical discontinuity of tissue substitute models at 27.12 MHz. Bioelectromagnetics, 4:257–265, 1983.

216. Lehmann, J. F., McDougall, J. A., Guy, A. W., Warren, C. G., Esselman, P. C.: Heating patterns produced by shortwave diathermy applicators in tissue substitute models. Arch. Phys. Med. Rehabil., 64:575–577, 1983.

217. Lehmann, J. F., McMillan, J. A., Brunner, G. D., and Blumberg, J. B.: Comparative study of the efficiency of shortwave, microwave and ultrasonic diathermy in heating the hip joint. Arch. Phys. Med. Rehabil., 40:510–512, 1959.

218. Lehmann, J. F., McMillan, J. A., Brunner, G. D., and Guy, A. W.: A comparative evaluation of temperature distributions produced by microwaves at 2,456 and 900 megacycles in geometrically complex specimens. Arch. Phys. Med. Rehabil., 43:502–507, 1962.

219. Lehmann, J. F., and Nitsch, W.: Über die Frequenzabhängigkeit biologischer Ultraschallreaktionen mit besonderer Berücksichtigung der spezifischen Temperaturverteilung im Organismus. Strahlentherapie, 85:606–614, 1951.

220. Lehmann, J. F., Silverman, D. R., Baum, B. A., Kirk, N. L., and Johnston, V. C.: Temperature distributions in the human thigh, produced by infrared, hot pack and microwave applications. Arch. Phys. Med. Rehabil., 47:291–299, 1966.

221. Lehmann, J. F., Stonebridge, J. B., de Lateur, B. J., Warren, C. G., and Halar, E.: Temperatures in human thighs after hot pack treatment followed by ultrasound. Arch. Phys. Med. Rehabil., 59:472–476, 1978.

222. Lehmann, J. F., Stonebridge, J. B., and Guy, A. W.: A comparison of patterns of stray radiation from therapeutic microwave applicators measured near tissue-substitute models and human subjects. Radio Science, 14:271–283, 1979.

223. Lehmann, J. F., Stonebridge, J. B., Wallace, J. E., Warren, C. G., and Guy, A. W.: Microwave therapy: stray radiation, safety and effectiveness. Arch. Phys. Med. Rehabil., 60:578–584, 1979.

224. Lehmann, J. F., Warren, C. G., Wallace, J. E., and Chan, A.: Ultrasound: Considerations for use in the presence of prosthetic joints. Arch. Phys. Med. Rehabil., 61:502, 1980.

225. Levy, H.: Pulsed shortwaves in sinus and allied conditions in childhood. West. J. Med., 2:246–250, 1961.

226. Liakhovitskii, N. S.: Experience in the use of ultrasonics in the therapy of plastic induration of the penis. Urology, 25:61, 1960.

227. Lightfoot, E., Verrier, M., and Ashby, P.: Neurophysiological effects of prolonged cooling of the calf in patients with complete spinal transection. Phys. Ther., 55:251–258, 1975.

228. Linke, C. A., Lounsberry, W., and Goldschmidt, V.: Effects of microwaves on normal tissues. J. Urol., 88:303–311, 1962.

229. Lippold, O. C. J., Nicholls, J. G., and Redfearn, J. W. T.: A study of the afferent discharge produced by cooling a mammalian muscle spindle. J. Physiol., 153:218–231, 1960.

230. Lota, M. J., and Darling, R. C.: Change in permeability of the red blood cell membrane in a homogeneous ultrasonic field. Arch. Phys. Med. Rehabil., 36:282–287, 1955.

231. Lundgren, C., Muren, A., and Zederfeldt, B.: Effect of cold vasoconstriction on wound healing in the rabbit. Acta Chir. Scand., 118:1–4, 1959.

232. Madsen, P. W., and Gersten, J. W.: The effect of ultrasound on conduction velocity of peripheral nerve. Arch. Phys. Med. Rehabil., 42:645–649, 1961.

233. Maintz, G.: Tierexperimentelle Untersuchungen über die Wirkung der Ultraschallwellen auf die Knochenregeneration. Strahlentherapie, 82:631–638, 1950.

234. Marek, J., Jezdinský, J., and Ochonský, P.: Effects of local cold and heat therapy on traumatic oedema of the rat hind paw. III. Effects of various kinds of compresses on the course of traumatic oedema. Acta Univ. Palacki. Olomuc. Fac., 66:203–228, 1973.

235. Marek, J., Jezdinský, J., and Ochonský, P.: Effects of local cold and heat therapy on traumatic oedema of the rat hind paw. III. The effect of heat radiation on the course of traumatic oedema. Acta Univ. Palacki. Olomuc. Fac. Med., 70:149–161, 1974.

236. Marhoffer, W., Marhoffer, E., Rusch, D., and Schmidt, K. L.: Untersuchungen zur Wirkung einer Soft-Laser-Bestrahlung (HeNe-Laser) auf experimentelle Entzündungen. Z. Phys. Med. Baln. Med. Klim., 16:389–393, 1987.

237. Marks, J., Carter, E. T., Scarpelli, D. G., and Eisen, J.: Microwave radiation to the anterior mediastinum of the dog (II). Ohio Med. J. 57:1132–1135, 1961.

238. Martin, G. M., Roth, G. M., Elkins, E. C., and Krusen, F. H.: Cutaneous temperature of the extremities of normal subjects and of patients with rheumatoid arthritis. Arch. Phys. Med., 27:665–682, 1946.

239. Matsen, F. A., III, Questad, K., and Matsen, A. L.: The effect of local cooling on post fracture swelling. Clin. Orthop., (109):201–206, 1975.

240. McGee, M., and Freshman, S.: Ultrasound and stretch: a decreased range of motion. A slide-tape presentation. Health Sciences Learning Resources Center, University of Washington, 1978.

241. Melzack, R., and Wall, P. D.: Pain mechanisms: a new theory. Science, 150:971–979, 1965.

242. Mense, S.: Effects of temperature on the discharges of muscle spindles and tendon organs. Pflügers Arch., 374:159–166, 1978.

243. Menser, M.: Does hyperthermia affect the human fetus? Med. J. Australia, 2:550, 1978.

244. Merola, L. O., and Kinoshita, J. H.: Changes in the ascorbic acid content in lenses of rabbit eyes exposed to microwave radiation. Proc. 4th Ann. Tri-Service Conf. on the Biological Effects of Microwave Radiation, 1:285–291, 1961.

245. Mester, E., Mester, A., and Toth, J.: Biostimulative effect of laser beams. In Atsumi, K. (Ed.): New Frontiers in Laser Medicine and Surgery. Amsterdam: Excerpta Medica, 1983.

246. Mester, E., Nagylucskay, S., Döklen, A., Tisza, S.: Laser stimulation of wound healing. II. Immunological tests. Acta Chirurg. Acad. Scient. Hungar., 17:49–55, 1976.

247. Michaelson, S. M.: Bioeffects of high frequency currents and electromagnetic radiation. In Lehmann, J. F. (Ed.): Therapeutic Heat and Cold, 4th Ed. Baltimore, Williams & Wilkins, 1989.

248. Michalski, W. J., and Seguin, J. J.: The effect of muscle cooling and stretch on muscle spindle secondary endings in the cat. J. Physiol., 253:341–356, 1975.

249. Miglietta, O.: Action of cold on spasticity. Am. J. Phys. Med., 52:198–205, 1973.

250. Moayer, M.: Die morphologischen Veränderungen der Plazenta unter dem Einfluss der Kurzwellendurchflutung. Tierexperimentelle Untersuchungen. Strahlentherapie, 142:609–614, 1971.

251. Modugno, P.: Sull'impiego della crioterapia locale nel trattamento dell'epicondilite omerale. Minerva Med., 74:703–706, 1983.

252. Molander, C. O.: Physiologic basis of heat. Arch. Phys. Ther., 22:335–340, 1941.

253. Moore, C. D., and Cardea, J. A.: Vascular changes in leg trauma. South Med. J., 70:1285–1286, 1977.

254. Morrissey, L. J.: Effect of pulsed short-wave diathermy upon volume blood flow through the calf of the leg: plethysmographic studies. J. Am. Phys. Ther. Assoc., 46:946–952, 1966.

255. Mortimer, A. J., Roy, O. Z., Taichman, G. C., Keon, W. J., and Trollope, B. J.: The effects of ultrasound on the mechanical properties of rat cardiac muscle. Ultrasonics, 16:179–182, 1978.

256. Mussa, B.: Embriopatie da cause fisiche. Minerva Nipiologica, 5:69–72, 1955.

257. Nadasdi, M.: Inhibition of experimental arthritis by athermic pulsing shortwave in rats. Am. J. Orthop., 2:105–107, 1960.

258. Newman, M. K., Kill, M., and Frampton, G.: Effects of ultrasound alone and combined with hydrocortisone injections by needle or hypospray. Am. J. Phys. Med., 37:206, 1958.

259. Nilsson, S.: Sprains of the lateral ankle ligaments. J. Oslo City Hosp., 33:13–36, 1983.

260. Nukada, H., Pollock, M., and Allpress, S.: Experimental cold injury to peripheral nerve. Brain, 104:779–811, 1981.

261. Oleson, J. R., and Gerner, E. W.: Hyperthermia in the treatment of malignancies. In Lehmann, J. F. (Ed.): Therapeutic Heat and Cold, 4th Ed. Baltimore, Williams & Wilkins, 1989.

262. Ottoson, D.: The effects of temperature on the isolated muscle spindle. J. Physiol., 180:636–648, 1965.

263. Parrish, J. A., Anderson, R. R., Harrist, T., Paul, B., and Murphy, G. F.: Selective thermal effects with pulsed irradiation from lasers: From organ to organelle. J. Invest. Dermatol., 80:75s–80s, 1983.

264. Parsons, C. M., and Goetzl, F. R.: Effect of induced pain on pain threshold. Proc. Soc. Exp. Biol. Med., 60:327–329, 1945.

264a. Pasila, M., Visuri, T., and Sundholm, A.: Pulsating shortwave diathermy: Value in treatment of recent ankle and foot sprains. Arch. Phys. Med. Rehabil., 59:383–386, 1978.

265. Pätzold, J., and Born, H.: Behandlung biologischer Gewebe mit gebundeltem Ultraschall. Strahlentherapie, 76:486–492, 1947.

266. Pätzold, J., Guttner, W., and Bastir, R.: Beitrag zum Dosisproblem in der Ultraschalltherapie. Strahlentherapie, 86:298–305, 1954.

267. Paul, W. D., and Imig, C. J.: Temperature and blood flow studies after ultrasonic irradiation. Am. J. Phys. Med., 34:370–375, 1955.

268. Pauly, H., and Hug, O.: Untersuchungen über den Einfluss von Ultraschallwellen und von Wärme auf den Stoffwechsel überlebender Gewebe. Strahlentherapie, 95:116–130, 1954.

269. Pegg, S. M. H., Littler, T. R., and Littler, E. N.: A trial of ice therapy and exercise in chronic arthritis. Physiotherapy, 55:51–56, 1969.

270. Perkins, J. F., Li, M.-C., Hoffman, F., et al.: Sudden vasoconstriction in denervated or sympathectomized paws exposed to cold. Am. J. Physiol., 155:165–178, 1948.

271. Petajan, J. H., Eagan, C. J.: Effect of temperature, exercise and physical fitness on the triceps surae reflex. J. Appl. Physiol., 25:16–20, 1968.

272. Petajan, R. H., and Watts, N.: Effect of cooling on the triceps surae reflex. Am. J. Phys. Med., 41:240–251, 1962.

273. Pezold, F. A.: Zur Frage des Ultraschallschadens. Ultraschall Med., 4:1–28, 1952.

274. Pickering, G. W.: The vasomotor regulation of heat loss from the human skin in relation to external temperature. Heart, 16:115–135, 1932.

275. Piersol, G. M., Schwan, H. P., Pennell, R. B., and Carstensen, E. L.: Mechanism of absorption of ultrasonic energy in blood. Arch. Phys. Med., 33:327–332, 1952.

276. Pohlman, R.: Die Ultraschalltherapie. Stuttgart, Georg Thieme Verlag, 1951.

277. Polley, H. F.: Physical treatment of arthritis. In Krusen, F. H. (Ed.): Physical Medicine and Re-

habilitation for the Clinician. Philadelphia, W. B. Saunders Company, 1951.

278. Rae, J. W., Jr., Herrick, J. F., Wakim, K. G., and Krusen, F. H.: A comparative study of the temperatures produced by microwave and short-wave diathermy. Arch. Phys. Med., 30:199–211, 1949.

279. Rae, J. W., Martin, G. M., Treaner, W. J., and Krusen, F. H.: Clinical experience with microwave diathermy. Proc. Staff Meet. Mayo Clin., 24:441, 1950.

280. Randall, L. M., and Krusen, F. H.: A consideration of the Elliott treatment of pelvic inflammatory disease of women. Arch. Phys. Ther., 18:283–287, 1937.

281. Rech, W., and Matthes, K.: Bericht über die medizinische Ultraschall-Arbeitstagung in Erlangen. Ultraschall Med., 1:366–368, 1949.

282. Reinike, A., and Alm, H.: Untersuchungen über die Tiefenwirkung der Mikrowellenbestrahlung im Bereich der Nasennebenhöhlen und des Ohres. Z. Laryn. Rhinol. Otol., 35:556–566, 1956.

283. Richardson, A. W., Duane, T. D., and Hines, H. M.: Experimental lenticular opacities produced by microwave irradiation. Arch. Phys. Med., 29:765–769, 1948.

284. Romero-Sierra, C., and Tanner, J. A.: Biological effects of nonionizing radiation: an outline of fundamental laws. Ann. N.Y. Acad. Sci., 238:263–272, 1974.

285. Rosenberger, H.: Über den Wirkungsmechanismus der Ultraschallbehandlung, insbesondere bei Ischias und Neuralgien. Chirurg, 21:404–406, 1950.

286. Rounds, D. E.: Laser applications in medicine. In Regan J. D., and Parrish, J. A. (Eds.): The Science of Photomedicine. New York, Plenum Press, 1982, pp. 533–543.

287. Rubin, A., and Erdman, W. J.: Microwave exposure of the human female pelvis during early pregnancy and prior to conception. Am. J. Phys. Med., 38:219–220, 1959.

288. Salmon, P. R.: The use of lasers in current surgical practice—an introduction. World J. Surg., 7:679–680, 1983.

289. Sandler, B.: Heat and the I.U.C.D. Br. Med. J., 25:458, 1973.

290. Schaubel, H. J.: The local use of ice after orthopedic procedures. Am. J. Surg., 72:711–714, 1946.

291. Schmidt, K. L., Ott, V. R., Rocher, G., et al.: Heat, cold and inflammation. Rheumatology, 38:391–404, 1979.

292. Schroeder, K. P.: Effect of ultrasound on the lumbar sympathetic nerves. Arch. Phys. Med. Rehabil., 43:182–185, 1962.

293. Schwan, H. P.: Biophysics of diathermy. In Licht, S. (Ed.): Therapeutic Heat and Cold, 2nd Ed. Baltimore, Waverly Press, 1965, pp. 63–125.

294. Schwan, H. P., and Li, K.: Hazards due to total body irradiation by radar. Proc. I. R. E., 44:1572, 1956.

295. Schwan, H. P., and Piersol, G. M.: The absorption of electromagnetic energy in body tissues. Part 1, Biophysical aspects. Am. J. Phys. Med., 33:371–404, 1954.

296. Schwan, H. P., and Piersol, G. M.: The absorption of electromagnetic energy in body tissues. Part 2, Physiological and clinical aspects. Am. J. Phys. Med., 34:425–448, 1955.

297. Scott, B. O.: Heating of fatty tissues in a shortwave field. Ann. Phys. Med., 2:48–52, 1952.

298. Scott, B. O.: Shortwave diathermy. In Licht, S. (Ed.): Therapeutic Heat and Cold, 2nd Ed. Baltimore, Waverly Press, 1965, pp. 279–309.

299. Scott, W. W., and Scardino, P. L.: A new concept in the treatment of Peyronie's disease. South. Med. J., 41:173–177, 1948.

300. Sekins, K. M., de Lateur, B. J., Dundore, D., Emery, A. F., Esselman, P., Lehmann, J. F., and Nelp, W. B.: Local muscle blood flow and temperature responses to 915 MHz diathermy as simultaneously measured and numerically predicted. Arch. Phys. Med. Rehabil., 65:1–7, 1982.

301. Sekins, K. M., Dundore, D., Emery, A. F., Lehmann, J. F., McGrath, P. W., and Nelp, W. B.: Muscle blood flow changes in response to 915 MHz diathermy with surface cooling as measured by Xe^{133} clearance. Arch. Phys. Med. Rehabil., 61:105–113, 1980.

302. Selke, O. O.: Complications of heat therapy. Am. J. Orth., 4:168–169, 1962.

303. Shealy, C. N., and Henneman, E.: Reversible effects of ultrasound on spinal reflexes. Arch. Neurol., 6:374–386, 1962.

304. Shulman, A. G.: Ice water as primary treatment of burns. J.A.M.A., 173:1916–1919, 1960.

305. Silverman, D. R.: A comparison of the continuous and pulsed shortwave diathermy resistance to bacterial infection of mice. Arch. Phys. Med. Rehabil., 45:491–499, 1964.

306. Silverman, D. R., and Pendleton, L.: A comparison on the effects of continuous and pulsed shortwave diathermy on peripheral circulation. Arch. Phys. Med. Rehabil., 49:429–436, 1968.

307. Simons, D. G.: Muscle pain syndromes—part I. Am. J. Phys. Med., 54:289–311, 1975.

308. Simons, D. G.: Muscle pain syndromes—part II. Am. J. Phys. Med., 55:15–42, 1976.

309. Smith, A., and Schwan, H. P.: Ultrasonic absorption and velocity of sound of cell nuclei. National Biophysics Conf., Columbus, 1957, Abstract, p. 66.

310. Smith, D. W., Clarren, S. K., and Harvey, M. A. S.: Hyperthermia as a possible teratogenic agent. J. Pediatr., 92:878–883, 1978.

311. Snyder-Mackler, L., and Bork, C. E.: Effect of helium-neon laser irradiation on peripheral sensory nerve latency. Phys. Ther., 68:223–225, 1988.

312. Solomon, H., and Goldman, L., Henderson, B., Richfield, D., Franzen, M.: Histopathology of the laser treatment of port-wine lesions. J. Invest. Dermatol., 50:141–146, 1968.

313. Stillwell, D. M., and Gersten, J. W.: Effect of ultrasound on spasticity. Am. Inst. Ultrasonics in Med. Proc. 4th Ann. Conf. on Ultrasonic Therapy, 124–131, 1955.

314. Stillwell, G. K.: General principles of thermotherapy. In Licht, S. (Ed.): Therapeutic Heat and Cold, 2nd Ed. Baltimore, Waverly Press, 1965, pp. 232–239.

315. Stoller, D. W., Markolf, K. L., Zager, S. A., and Shoemaker, S. C.: The effects of exercise, ice, ultrasonography on torsional laxity of the knee. Clin. Orthop., (174):172–180, 1983.

316. Stuhlfauth, K.: Neural effects of ultrasonic waves. Br. J. Phys. Med., 15:10–14, 1952.

317. Sulzberger, M. B., Wolf, J., Witten, V. H., and Kopf, A. W.: Dermatology, Diagnosis and Treatment. Chicago, Year Book Publishers, 1961.

318. Takashima, S.: Studies on the effect of radiofrequency waves on biological macromolecules. IEEE Trans. Biomed. Eng. BME, 13:28–31, 1966.

319. Taylor, K. J. W.: Ultrasonic damage to spinal cord and the synergistic effect of hypoxia. J. Pathol., 102:41–47, 1970.

320. Taylor, R. G.: The effect of diapulse (pulsed high frequency energy) on wound healing in humans. Cited by Lehmann, J. F., Guy, A. W., Stonebridge, J. B., and Warren, C. G.: Review of evidence for indications, techniques of application, contraindications, hazards, and clinical effectiveness of shortwave diathermy. Report No. FDA/HFK-75-1, to the Office of DHEW/Public Health Service, Food and Drug Administration, 1/1/74 to 12/31/74, Contract Number FDA 74–32.

321. Tennenbaum, J. I., and Lowney, E.: Localized heat and cold urticaria. J. Allergy Clin. Immunol., 51:57–59, 1973.

322. Texeira-Pinto, A. A., Nejelski, L. L., Cutler, J. L., and Heller, J. H.: The behavior of unicellular organisms in an electromagnetic field. Exp. Cell Res., 20:548–564, 1960.

323. Travell, J., and Rinzler, S. H.: Pain syndromes of the chest muscles: Resemblance to effort angina and myocardial infarction, and relief by local block. Can. Med. Assoc. J., 59:333–338, 1948.

324. Trnavsky, G.: Die Beeinflussung des Hoffmann-Reflexes durch Kryolangzeittherapie. Wien. Med. Wochenschr. 11:287–289, 1983.

325. Trojel, H., and Lebech, P. E.: Intermitterende kortbolge (Diapulse) i behandlingen af inflammatoriske underlivslidelser. Nordisk Med., 81:307–310, 1969.

326. Uchman, L. S.: Role of ultrasound in scleroderma. A preliminary report of two cases. Am. J. Phys. Med., 35:118, 1956.

327. Urbscheit, N., and Bishop, B.: Effects of cooling on the ankle jerk and H-response. Phys. Ther. 50:1041–1049, 1970.

328. Urbscheit, N., and Bishop, B.: Effects of cooling on the ankle jerk and H-response in hemiplegic patients. Phys. Ther., 51:983–988, 1971.

329. VanDemark, W. R., and Free, J. R.: Temperature effects. In Johnson, A. D., et al. (Eds.): The Testis, Vol. III. New York, Academic Press, Inc., 1973, pp. 233–312.

330. Vinger, P. F., and Hoerner, E. F. (Eds.): Sports Injuries, The Unthwarted Epidemic. Littleton, Mass., John Wright·PSG·Inc., 1982.

331. Wachsmuth, W.: Ultraschall bei Sudeckscher Krankheit. Ultraschall Med., Zurich, 1949.

332. Wakim, K. G.: Special review: ultrasonic energy as applied to medicine. Am. J. Phys. Med., 32:32–46, 1953.

333. Walker, J.: Relief from chronic pain by lower power laser irradiation. Neurosci. Lett., 43:339–344, 1983.

334. Walker, J. B., Akhanjee, L. K., Cooney, M. M., Goldstein, J., Tamayoshi, S., Segal-Gidan, F.: Laser therapy for pain of trigeminal neuralgia. Clin. J. Pain., 3:183–187, 1988.

335. Warren, C. G., Koblanski, J. N., and Sigelmann, R. A.: Ultrasound coupling media: their relative transmissivity. Arch. Phys. Med. Rehabil., 57:218–222, 1976.

336. Whyte, H. M., and Reader, S. P.: Effectiveness of different forms of heating. Ann. Rheum. Dis., 10:449–452, 1951.

337. Williams, A. R.: Intravascular mural thrombi produced by acoustic microstreaming. Ultrasound Med. Biol., 3:191–203, 1977.

338. Williams, A. R.: Release of serotonin from human platelets by acoustic microstreaming. J. Acoust. Soc. Am., 56:1640–1643, 1974.

339. Williams, A. R.: The effects of therapeutic ultrasound on platelets and the blood coagulation system. Presented 9/11/81 at "An International Symposium on Therapeutic Ultrasound." Winnipeg, Manitoba, Canada.

340. Williams, A. R., Chater, B. V., Allen, K. A., and Sanderson, J. H.: The use of β-thromboglobulin to detect platelet damage by therapeutic ultrasound in vivo. J. Clin. Ultrasound, 9:145–151, 1981.

341. Williams, A. R., Chater, B. V., Allen, K. A., Sherwood, M. R., and Sanderson, J. H.: Release of beta-thromboglobulin from human platelets by therapeutic intensities of ultrasound. Br. J. Haematol., 40:133–142, 1978.

342. Williams, A. R., Hughes, D. E., and Nyborg, W. L.: Hemolysis near a transversely oscillating wire. Science, 169:871–873, 1970.

343. Williams, A. R., and Miller, D. L.: Photometric detection of ATP release from human erythrocytes exposed to ultrasonically activated gas-filled pores. Ultrasound Med. Biol., 6:251–256, 1980.

344. Williams, A. R., O'Brien, W. D., and Coller, B.

S.: Exposure to ultrasound decreases the recalcification time of platelet rich plasma. Ultrasound Med. Biol., 2:113–118, 1976.

345. Williams, A. R., Sykes, S. M., and O'Brien, W. D., Jr.: Ultrasonic exposure modifies platelet morphology and function *in vitro*. Ultrasound Med. Biol., 2:311–317, 1976.

346. Williams, D. B., Monahan, J. P., Nicholson, W. J., and Aldrich, J. J.: Biologic effects of microwave radiation. USAF School of Aviation Medicine Report No. 55–94, Washington, 1955.

347. Williams, J. L., and Thomas, G. G.: The natural history of Peyronie's disease. J. Urol., 103:75–76, 1970.

348. Wilson, D. H.: Treatment of soft-tissue injuries by pulsed electrical energy. Br. Med. J., 2:269–270, 1972.

349. Wilson, D. H.: Comparison of shortwave diathermy and pulsed electromagnetic energy in treatment of soft tissue injuries. Physiotherapy, 60:309–310, 1974.

350. Wilson, D. H., Jagadeesh, P., Newman, P. P., and Harriman, D. G. F.: The effects of pulsed electromagnetic energy on peripheral nerve regeneration. Ann. N.Y. Acad. Sci., 238:575–585, 1974.

351. Wise, C. S., Castleman, B., and Watkins, A. L.: Effect of diathermy (shortwave and microwave) on bone growth on the albino rat. J. Bone Joint Surg., 31A:487–500, 1949.

352. Woeber, K.: Biological basis and application of ultrasound in medicine. Ultrasonics Biol. Med., 1:9, 1956.

353. Wolf, S. L., and Basmajian, J. V.: A rapid cooling device for controlled cutaneous stimulation. Phys. Ther., 53:25–27, 1973.

354. Wolf, S. L., and Basmajian, J. V.: Intramuscular temperature changes deep to localized cutaneous cold stimulation. Phys. Ther., 53:1284–1288, 1973.

355. Wong, C., and Ehrlich, H. P.: A preliminary report on pulsed high frequency energy (diapulse therapy) in wound healing. Cited by Lehmann, J. F., Fordyce, W. E., Rathbun, L. A., Larson, R. E., and Wood, D. H.: Clinical evaluation of a new approach in the treatment of contracture associated with hip fracture after interal fixation. Arch. Phys. Med. Rehabil., 42:95, 1961.

356. Woodmansey, A., Collins, D. H., and Ernst, M. M.: Vascular reactions to the contrast bath in health and in rheumatoid arthritis. Lancet, 2:1350–1353, 1938.

357. Worden, R. E., Herrick, J. F., Wakim, K. G., and Krusen, F. H.: The heating effects of microwaves with and without ischemia. Arch. Phys. Med., 29:751–758, 1948.

358. Wright, V., and Johns, R. J.: Physical factors concerned with the stiffness of normal and diseased joints. Bull. Johns Hopkins Hosp., 106:215–231, 1960.

359. Wright, V., and Johns, R. J.: Quantitative and qualitative analysis of joint stiffness in normal subjects and in patients with connective tissue diseases. Ann. Rheum. Dis., 20:36–46, 1961.

360. Wulff, D.: Behandlungsergebnisse mit Ultraschall. Ultraschall Med., 7:111, 1954.

361. Zankel, H. T.: Effect of ultrasound on leg blood flow. Scientific Proc. Seventh Ann. Conf. Am. Inst. Ultrasonics in Med., August 25, 1962, pp. 7–17.

362. Zaret, M. M., and Eisenbud, M.: Preliminary results of studies of the lenticular effects of microwaves among exposed personnel. Biological Effects of Microwave Radiation. Proc. 4th Ann. Tri-Service Conf. on the Biological Effects of Microwave Radiation, 1:293–308, 1961.

363. Zarod, A. P., and Williams, A. R.: Platelet aggregation *in vivo* by therapeutic ultrasound. Lancet, 1:1266, 1977.

364. Zitowitz, I., and Hardy, J. D.: Influence of cold exposure on thermal burns in the rat. J. Appl. Physiol., 12:147–154, 1958.

14

Ultraviolet Therapy

JEFFREY R. BASFORD

Most of the electromagnetic agents used in physical medicine rely for their effects on tissue heating. Ultraviolet (UV) light, on the other hand, owns its place in medicine because it produces direct photochemical reactions when it interacts with the body. Other agents such as low-energy lasers,[2] magnetic fields, and even monochromatic light may also have significant direct, nonthermal effects on the body. A number of these are being studied for a variety of analgesic and wound-healing indications. However, because their mechanisms of action are unknown, and their usefulness is unclear, they will not be pursued here.

Historical Background

Light, in the form of sunlight, has been used to treat arthritis, edema, jaundice, skin disorders, obesity, and even paralysis since at least the times of classical Greece and Rome.[7] Since infrared radiation makes up about 40 per cent of the energy in sunlight,[16] many of the therapies gained their effectiveness from heating rather than specific photochemical reactions. Nevertheless, some of the applications, such as the treatment of skin disease, may have had efficacy because of the presence of UV in the spectrum of sunlight.

Enthusiasm in Europe for light therapy declined following the classical period. However, by the end of the 18th century, the benefits of clean air and sunlight (frequently not distinguished) on indolent ulcers, tuberculosis, rickets, edema, and depression were again emphasized—with visits to the country recommended to those who could afford them.[7]

By the end of the 19th century, two important aspects of light were recognized: (1) sunlight was bactericidal and (2) the UV spectrum accounted for this property. In addition, and perhaps just as important, lamps that could provide intense and reliable sources of UV became available. Excesses undoubtedly occurred, but therapeutic alternatives to light therapy often did not exist; over the years, treatments for psoriasis, rickets, tuberculosis, and hyperbilirubinemia were developed.[7] Some of these, such as UV-based treatments of psoriasis, continue in use.

Background

Although the earth moves through a miasma of photons and subatomic particles, its major source of energy is the sun. In fact, an insolation of about 1350 W/m^2 of electromagnetic radiation is incident on the upper atmosphere. Much of this energy is scattered and attenuated as it passes through the atmosphere. Nevertheless, a large fraction, including about 30 W/m^2 of UV, reaches the earth at sea level.[8, 16]

About half the radiation incident on the atmosphere is in the visible range (0.40 to 0.80 μm), about 40 per cent is in the infrared, and about 8 per cent is UV.[16] The visible spectrum is central to our existence, and from this perspective conventional terminology makes sense: the infrared spectrum (0.8 μm to 15 μm) is "below" red and the ultraviolet spectrum (0.20 to 0.40 μm) is "above" violet (Table 14–1).

As a rule, infrared photons (energies of 0.8 to 1.6 eV [electron volts]) are not energetic enough

TABLE 14—1. Electromagnetic Spectrum

REGION	REPRESENTATIVE WAVELENGTHS	REPRESENTATIVE FREQUENCIES	ENERGY/PHOTON* (eV)
AM radio	300 m	1×10^6	4×10^{-9}
Short wave diathermy	11 m	27.33×10^6	1×10^{-7}
Therapeutic microwave	33 cm	915×10^6	3.8×10^{-6}
Infrared	0.8–15 μm	3.8–0.2×10^{14}	1.6–0.08
Visible			
Red	0.8 μm	3.8×10^{14}	1.6
Violet	0.4 μm	7.5×10^{14}	3.1
UV-A	0.32–0.40 μm	9.4–7.5×10^{14}	3.9–3.1
UV-B	0.29–0.32 μm	10.3–9.4×10^{14}	4.3–3.9
UV-C	0.20–0.29 μm	15.0–10.3×10^{14}	6.2–4.3

*Energy (joules) photon = hv = (6.63×10^{-34}) (frequency in hertz), where h is Planck's constant $(6.63 \times 10^{-34}$ joules sec) and v is frequency in H_2.

Energy (eV)/photon = hv = (4.14×10^{-15}) (frequency in hertz).

to alter the energy levels of atomic electrons. These photons produce only an increase in the random movement of the atoms and molecules of a material (i.e., heat). In distinction to the infrared situation, the energies of photons from the UV sources used in therapy (roughly 3 to 6 eV) are comparable to those separating atomic electronic energy levels. Thus, these photons can cause electronic transitions and produce excited or disassociated atoms capable of chemical reactions. This ability provides the rationale of UV therapy as well as the unwanted correlates of erythema, DNA damage, and skin cancer.

The biological effects of UV are wavelength-dependent (Table 14–2). As these variations are important, we will review the relative importance of the different UV spectra.

UV-A

UV-A (wavelength 0.32 to 0.40 μm, photon energy 3.1 to 3.9 eV) (Table 14–2) occupies the lowest energy portion of the UV spectrum and is important because of its ability to produce tanning with a minimum of skin erythema. It can, in fact, produce two types of tanning: immediate (Meirkowsky) and delayed. The first of these, immediate tanning, occurs in many but not all individuals, appears within an hour of exposure, and fades within a few days. This tan is probably due to the oxidation of melanin and is not due to a change in the number of melanocytes. The second of these tans, delayed tanning, occurs two to three days after exposure and will persist for two weeks. This latter tan is associated with a change in the distri-

TABLE 14—2. Effects of UV-A, UV-B, and UV-C

	UV-A 0.32–0.48 μm	UV-B 0.29–0.32 μm	UV-C 0.20–0.29 μm
Erythema			
Onset	Rapid	Delayed (1–2 hours)	Delayed (3–4 hours)
Dose	30 J/cm^2	30 mJ/cm^2	9 mJ/cm^2 (0.254 μm)
Peak	0–6 hours	18 hours	12–21 hours
Onset of pigmentation	Immediate (Meirkowsky) and delayed 18–24 hours	Delayed 48–72 hours	Minimal pigmentation
Oxygen dependency	O_2-dependent	O_2-independent	
Dose	Suberythemic	Erythemic	
Stratum corneum	± Increase in thickness following exposure	Thickens following exposure	
Melanin location	Basal cell layer	Entire epidermis	
Melanocyte number	Probably unchanged	Increased	

JEFFREY R. BASFORD

bution of melanin and increases in the number and size of melanocytes.[5, 11] UV-A is used commercially for tanning and medically for psoriasis (i.e., PUVA, psoralen–UV-A) treatment.

UV-B

UV-B (wavelength 0.29 to 0.32 μm, photon energy 3.9 to 4.3 eV) (Table 14–2) is on an "equal dose" basis 200 to 2000 times more likely to cause skin erythema and burning than is UV-A. This eliminates its usefulness for tanning. UV-B, however, is the UV adjunct to the Goeckerman treatment of psoriasis and has been reported to be effective in treating uremic pruritus.[1, 5]

UV-C

UV-C (wavelength 0.20 to 0.29 μm, photon energy 4.3 to 6.2 eV) occupies the most energetic part of the therapeutic UV spectrum. Although it is strongly scattered as it passes through the atmosphere and is absent at sea level, it is important because it is bactericidal. UV-C sources have been used for sterilization as well as to treat mycosis fungoides and decubitus ulcers.

Dose Response

The dose of ultraviolet that will produce, within a few hours, a minimal erythema in "Caucasian" skin is termed the minimal erythema dose (MED). This dose is established by exposing a subject's skin to increasing amounts of UV until a minimal erythema is noted to begin several hours after exposure. Variations in technique exist, but a common approach is to place a template with a number of holes over the volar forearm. The UV source is maintained at a fixed distance from the template, and exposures of various duration are made at the different openings. The lowest dose that produces minimal erythema four to eight hours later is the MED. It is important to note that the MED is an empirical value that has been determined with a *particular* source at a *fixed* distance from the skin of a *specific* individual. Most UV sources age, and the MED should be determined on a routine basis two or three times a year: an aged or abused lamp may emit heat and visible light but minimal UV.

Ultraviolet treatments are often prescribed in

TABLE 14–3. Adverse Effects of Ultraviolet Radiation

ADVERSE EFFECTS	PRECIPITATING FACTORS/ EXAMPLES
Sunburn	Sunlight, industrial or medical exposure to UV sources (particularly UV-B)
Light-induced/ aggravated	Polymorphous light reaction, solar urticaria, porphyria, melasma, freckles, systemic lupus erythematosus, sarcoid
Phototoxicity	Tetracycline, tricyclic antidepressants, phenothiazines, sulfonamides, psoralen, green soap, tar, some cosmetics and dyes
Photoallergy	Delayed onset following multiple exposures, rashes may occur distant from exposed area
Skin aging	"Farmer's neck"
Skin cancer	Basal cell carcinoma, squamous cell carcinoma, malignant melanoma

terms of a multiple of MEDs. As treatments continue, and as the patient's sensitivity decreases, it is usually possible to increase the number of MEDs in a session. As a rule of thumb, one MED, by definition, produces a first-degree (minimal) erythema. A second-degree erythema is produced by about 2.5 MEDs and has a latency of four to six hours. This erythema may be painful, and although it will subside in two to four days, it is followed by desquamation. A third-degree erythema is produced by about 5 MEDs and has latency as brief as two hours. This dose is associated with edema and marked desquamation, and treatment at this intensity must obviously be restricted to limited areas. Fourth-degree erythema is produced by about 10 MEDs and is characterized by blistering.

Precautions

The eyes of both the patient and the therapist must be shielded to prevent conjunctivitis, keratotic changes of the cornea, or even possibly lens damage. Shielding can be accomplished with protective goggles of ordinary glass or, in the case of the patient, cotton or gauze soaked in water and placed over the eyes.

If there is a significant difference in the distance between the UV source and the various parts of the body, excessive irradiation of the closer parts may occur. In general, it is good practice to drape

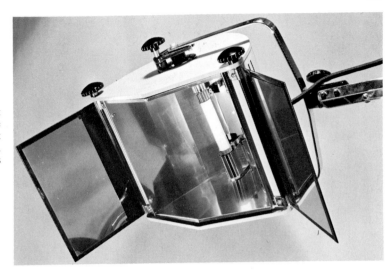

FIGURE 14–1. A "hot quartz" ultraviolet lamp, showing the burner and reflector. The wings of the reflector may be folded to limit the area of exposure. Radiation, however, may still escape, and the eyes should always be protected when using these lamps.

parts of the body not being treated. In addition, areas of atrophic skin, such as scars, and some skin grafts, are easily burned. These areas should be screened with wet towels or dressings.

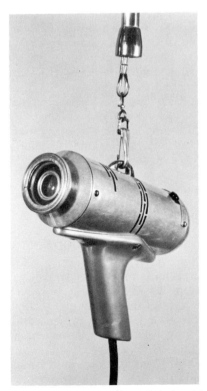

FIGURE 14–2. A "hot quartz" air-cooled ultraviolet source that may be used with orificial applicators or for small areas.

Erythema

The primary phenomenon in the production of erythema is believed to be absorption of UV photons by proteins in the prickle cell layer of the skin. Since this reaction, which denatures protein, is not affected by temperature, the threshold time of exposure is not temperature-dependent. Following irradiation, damaged cells release vasodilators, at a rate that *is* sensitive to temperature. The latent period for this release may be several hours, and the chemical mediators of the erythema from UV-A, UV-B, and UV-C exposure may not be the same.[12, 15] Combination of the erythema action spectrum and the solar spectrum suggests that the peak wavelength for erythema from sunlight is in the UV-B spectrum at 0.306 μm. However, because of the relatively large amount of UV-A in sunlight, about 15 per cent of solar erythemogenesis is due to UV-A.[12]

Adverse Effects

In the phototoxic situation (Table 14–3), UV radiation may be absorbed by a sensitizing chemical or compound and can then lead to oxidative reactions and cellular damage. Phototoxic reactions resemble sunburn and are localized to the area exposed to UV. Theoretically, anyone can suffer from them.

Photoallergy is relatively rare. It is mediated by immunological processes and may extend beyond the treated area. There is an incubation period

JEFFREY R. BASFORD

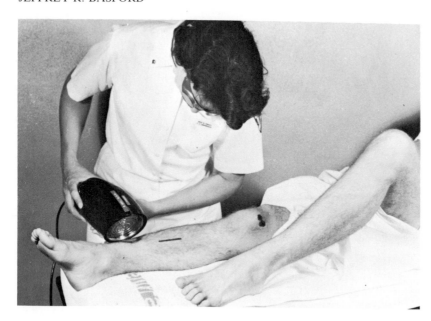

FIGURE 14–3. A "cold quartz" ultraviolet source being used in treatment of a chronic ulcer. (Courtesy of Dr. F. J. Kottke.)

following exposure to a chemical, and repeated exposures to the radiation are required.[3, 4]

UV is well established in the causation of basal cell carcinoma, squamous cell carcinoma, and malignant melanoma. This is mainly an effect of UV-B radiation and may be enhanced by phototoxic substances.[13]

Sources of Ultraviolet Irradiation

Therapeutic Devices

"Hot Quartz" Lamps. Hot quartz lamps (Figs. 14–1 and 14–2) operate with relatively high pressures of mercury and produce spectra with emission lines at 0.265, 0.297, 0.302, 0.313, and 0.366 μm, as well as some energy on each side of the 0.255 μm line. The MED of these lamps when in good condition may be about 15 seconds at a distance of 75 cm. Smaller lamps of this type may be cooled by a water jacket or an air blower (Kromayer type) and can be used close to the body without producing thermal burns (Fig. 14–2). These lamps can be adapted for orificial application, and in this situation their MEDs may be on the order of five seconds at a distance of 3 cm.

"Cold Quartz" Lamps. Cold quartz (germicidal) lamps (Fig. 14–3) have a relatively low mercury pressure and operate at temperatures of about 60° C. Almost all the transmitted ultraviolet from these lamps is at 0.254 μm.

"Sun Lamps." "Sun lamps" contain a tungsten filament to vaporize mercury so that an arc can be established. The envelope is a glass that will transmit ultraviolet radiation, and MEDs are usually measured in terms of minutes.

"Black-Light" Lamps. A glass filter may be used to prevent the emission of visible light from a UV source. This modification allows observation of UV-induced fluorescence and is useful in the diagnosis of a number of skin and eye conditions. Filters used have included black phosphate glass and Wood's nickel oxide glass.

Techniques of Application

The operator's manual for specific UV source should be reviewed before use. In general:

1. The eyes of the patient and therapist should be shielded with goggles or wet gauze from direct as well as scattered (from the patient, walls, and so on) radiation.

2. The MED of the source must be known. If it is not known, it should be determined.

3. Timing devices must be accurate and capable of measuring time in increments appropriate for

TABLE 14—4. Contraindications and Relative
Contraindications of UV Therapy

Albinism	Herpes simplex eruptions
Atrophic skin and scars	Skin carcinoma
Use of photosensitizing drugs and chemicals (see Table 14–3)	Sarcoid
	Systemic lupus erythematosus
Photosensitivity history	Xeroderma pigmentosum

the source (e.g., a second hand on a watch may be used if the MED is measured in seconds).

4. The distance from the source to the patient must be measured, not estimated.

5. Patient draping must be essentially identical from treatment to treatment. Scars and atrophic skin must be shielded. It is customary, although perhaps not essential, to drape the genital area.

6. Contraindications such as those in Table 14–4 must be kept in mind.

Indications for Ultraviolet Therapy

Table 14–5 shows that most of the diseases treated with UV fall within the domain of dermatology.[10] In the past, however, the physiatrist used UV to treat acne vulgaris and decubitus ulcers. Whereas cold quartz UV treatments of decubitus ulcers are still done at times, doubt exists about the effectiveness of either UV-A or UV-B on acne.[9]

Two MEDs of cold quartz ultraviolet will effectively kill motile bacteria.[6] (Although the bacteria in spore form are resistant to ultraviolet, they become susceptible when they become motile.) Since the bacteria in a wound are superficial, daily ultraviolet radiation is effective as a bactericidal agent for treatment of decubitus ulcers and superficial wounds. It should be noted that irradiation

TABLE 14—5. Therapeutic Uses of UV

DISEASE/CONDITION	POSSIBLE MECHANISMS
Psoriasis Mycosis fungoides	Phototoxicity
Hyperbilirubinemia Uremic pruritus Rickets	Photochemical effect
Vitiligo	Induced tanning
Soft tissue ulcers	Bactericidal

of up to 5 MEDs daily by a grid source, or an orificial applicator (for fistulas or undermined ulcers), does not destroy tissue. Irradiation at more than 5 MEDs, however, will delay epithelial formation, and irradiation at more than 10 MEDs may destroy viable tissue. UV produces vasodilation in intact epithelium at the margins of a wound; no vasodilation, however, has been observed in granulation tissue.[14]

References

1. Anderson, T. F., Waldinger, T. P., and Voorhees, J. J.: UV-B phototherapy. Arch. Dermatol., 120:1502–1507, 1984.

2. Basford, J. R.: Low energy laser treatment of pain and wounds: Hype, hope, or hokum? Mayo Clin. Proc., 61:671–675, 1986.

3. Emmett, E. A.: Drug photoallergy. Int. J. Dermatol., 17:370–379, 1978.

4. Epstein, J. H.: Photoallergy. Aust. J. Dermatol., 18:51–56, 1977.

5. Fitzpatrick, T. B.: Ultraviolet-induced pigmentary changes: Benefits and hazards. Curr. Probl. Dermatol., 15:25–38, 1986.

6. Koller, L. R.: Ultraviolet Radiation. New York, John Wiley & Sons, 1952.

7. Licht, S.: History of ultraviolet therapy. In Licht, S. (Ed.): Electricity and Ultraviolet Radiation. Baltimore, Waverly Press, 1967, pp. 31–53.

8. Nader, J. S.: Pilot study of ultraviolet radiation in Los Angeles. In Urbach, F. (Ed.): The Biologic Effects of Ultraviolet Radiation (With Emphasis on the Skin). London, Pergamon Press, 1969.

9. Mills, O. H., and Klikman, A. M.: Ultraviolet phototherapy and photochemotherapy of acne vulgaris. Arch. Dermatol., 114:221–223, 1978.

10. Parrish, J. A.: Phototherapy and photochemotherapy of skin diseases. J. Invest. Dermatol., 77:167–171, 1981.

11. Parrish, J. A., Anderson, R. R., Urbach, F., and Pitts, D.: Uses of UV-A involving exposure of humans. In Parrish, J. A., Anderson, R. R., Urbach, F., and Pitts, D.: UV-A Biological Effects of Ultraviolet Radiation with Emphasis on Human Responses to Longwave Ultraviolet. New York, Plenum Press, 1978.

12. Parrish, J. A., Anderson, R. R., Urbach, F., and Pitts, D.: Immediate and short-term biologic effects of ultraviolet radiation on normal skin. In Parrish, J. A., Anderson, R. R., Urbach, F., and Pitts, D.: UV-A: Biological Effects of Ultraviolet Radiation with Emphasis on Human Responses to Longwave Ultraviolet. New York, Plenum Press, 1978.

13. Parrish, J. A., Anderson, R. R., Urbach, F., and Pitts, D.: Skin aging and carcinogenesis due to ultraviolet radiation. In Parrish, J. A., Anderson,

JEFFREY R. BASFORD

R. R., Urbach, F., and Pitts, D.: UV-A Biological Effects of Ultraviolet Radiation with Emphasis on Human Responses to Longwave Ultraviolet. New York, Plenum Press, 1978.

14. Parrish, J. A., Anderson, R. R., Urbach, F., and Pitts, D.: Effects of ultraviolet radiation on microorganisms and animal cells. *In* Parrish, J. A., Anderson, R. R., Urbach, F., and Pitts, D.: UV-A: Biological Effects of Ultraviolet Radiation with Emphasis on Human Responses to Longwave Ultraviolet. New York, Plenum Press, 1978.

15. Warin, A. P.: The ultraviolet erythemas in man. Br. J. Dermatol., 98:473–477, 1978.

16. Weast, R. C.: CRC Handbook of Chemistry and Physics. Boca Raton, CRC Press, 1985.

15 Electrical Therapy

JEFFREY R. BASFORD

Electricity has a long history in medicine. Pliny, Aristotle, and Plutarch all knew that electric eels, rays, and catfish could produce numbness.[78] Unfortunately, knowledge increased slowly, and little of practical use was learned until after the Middle Ages. However, the rationalism of the Enlightenment in the 18th century brought an accelerated understanding; electrical generators and storage devices in the form of the rotary static generators and Leyden jars were in use by the mid-1700s. The battery soon followed and was developed by about 1800.[50] The theoretical understanding of electricity also grew: Ohm's law was discovered in 1827, and by the late 1860s Maxwell had developed his electromagnetic equations.

Medical exploration of electricity did not enjoy similar respect or success. Most of the early treatments, such as electrical "air baths," spark treatments, and localized as well as generalized "galvanism," were empirically developed and did not develop a scientific basis for their purported effects.[50] These faded from use. A few of the more restricted electrical therapies, such as cardioversion and electrocautery, have been refined and are still in use.

Modern electrical therapy developed from this past. As such, its growth has been hindered by disrepute as well as by ignorance about the interaction of electricity and the body. However, by early in this century, improving understanding and technological capabilities permitted the development of useful devices. This chapter considers only electrical therapies that utilize the direct effects of electrical stimulation on tissue. Other approaches, such as short wave diathermy, which converts electromagnetic energy to heat, are discussed elsewhere.

"Direct" electrical agents all apply some form of electricity to the body and are in many ways similar. Nevertheless, the clinical applications, such as analgesia, strengthening, wound healing, functional electrical stimulation, and iontophoresis, appear quite different. Whereas these distinctions are followed in this chapter, it should be remembered that once differing waveforms, frequencies, intensities, and techniques are taken into account, the treatments and equipment are often remarkably alike.

Analgesia

Transcutaneous electrical nerve stimulation produces analgesia in a wide range of medical conditions (Tables 15–1 and 15–2). Thus, whereas the term "transcutaneous electrical nerve stimulation" is not obviously restricted to analgesia alone, the analgesic effects are well known and the acronym TENS is now almost synonymous with electrical analgesia.

Despite widespread clinical use, TENS analgesia remains controversial. In particular, the mechanism of action is controversial, stimulating parameters are subjective, electrode placement is empirical, and its effectiveness is a subject of contention. Regardless of these uncertainties, the use of TENS is widespread (Tables 15–1 and 15–2); it is necessary to understand the more important theoretical bases and empirical findings on which this treatment is based.

Mechanism of Action

No single, widely accepted theory explains TENS analgesia. There are, however, a number

JEFFREY R. BASFORD

TABLE 15–1. TENS Analgesia—Surgery and Trauma

INDICATION*	NUMBER OF SUBJECTS	EXPERIMENTAL DESIGN	SUMMARY OF RESULTS
General Surgery			
Abdominal surgery (4, 30, 133)	40, 50, 12	Randomized	77% good or excellent results in TENS group; 50–67% reduction in medication usage in TENS group
Abdominal and thoracic surgery (64, 132)	213, 75	Randomized	TENS groups had less pain, improved pulmonary function, less ileus, and shorter ICU stays
Mixed surgery and trauma (120)	20	Uncontrolled	80% relieved of protracted ileus within 24 hours
Orthopedic Surgery			
Total hip replacement (124)	40	Randomized	Reduced medication use in TENS groups
Hand surgery (20)	44	Double-blind Controlled	23% reduction in anesthesia requirements in TENS group
Knee surgery (60)	34	Consecutive patients, no controls	Increased range of motion and reduced use of narcotics
Low back surgery (137)	52	Consecutive Randomized	TENS groups reduced narcotic consumption 57%
Podiatric surgery (5)	125	Controlled	TENS groups required fewer narcotics; 74% with TENS noted excellent pain relief compared with 17% of controls
Obstetrics			
Labor and delivery (10, 129, 145)	147, 67, 35	Variable	78–88% reported some relief, best relief in first stage; 70% required pudendal or epidural blocks
Postcesarean pain (142)	9	Controlled	50–60% reduction of pain with TENS; deep pain, such as uterine contractions, was not affected

*References are listed in parentheses.

of neurophysiological phenomena and theories that are important to its understanding. One of these, the gate theory, was developed by Melzack and Wall[105] and published in 1965. In it, the authors postulated that (1) cells within the substantia gelatinosa are stimulated by both small-diameter nociceptive and large-diameter sensory neurons and (2) these cells serve as gates by inhibiting the relaying of nociceptive information to the brain if nonpainful sensory stimuli are also present. Since TENS easily produces nonpainful sensory input, it became widely accepted following some successful trials.

The gate theory provides a rationale for electrical analgesia. Unfortunately, the theory does not explain a number of phenomena such as analgesia produced at unstimulated sites, delayed onset of analgesia, and analgesia continuing following cessation of stimulation. Alternative theories and modifications of the gate hypothesis have been proposed. One widely discussed alternative is that at least some forms of stimulation may produce

TABLE 15–2. TENS Analgesia—Miscellaneous Indicators

INDICATION*	NUMBER OF SUBJECTS	EXPERIMENTAL DESIGN	SUMMARY OF RESULTS
Acute rib fractures (141)	24	Randomized	Statistically significant increases in PaO_2 and peak expiratory flow rates in the TENS group
Brachial plexus avulsion (118)	58	Uncontrolled	60% with dramatic responses
Chronic interstitial cystitis (42)	23	Uncontrolled	78% good to excellent reduction of pain; 35% had urinary frequency return to normal
Rheumatoid arthritis (99)	20	Blinded	90% of patients doubled lifting endurance while using 70 Hz TENS
Burns (80)	24	Double-blind	TENS and morphine equally effective for analgesia during enzymatic burn debridement
Hemophiliac joint pain (131)	36	Controlled	71% of TENS patients *versus* 25% of controls reported at least 50% pain relief
Osteoarthritis (knee) (93)	30	Randomized Double-blind	TENS appeared more effective than paracetamol, but results were obscured by placebo effects
Angina (100)	10, 13, 21	Variable Multiple studies	Increased work capacity; decreased ST depression
Phantom limb pain (25)	3	Case reports	Contralateral electrode placement; all 3 patients felt TENS to be beneficial
Acute minor trauma (115)	100	Double-blind Controlled	TENS equivalent to acetomorphine-codeine
Dysmenorrhea (96)	21	Controlled	66% received some benefit from TENS, but majority felt Naprosyn to be equally or more effective
Spinal cord injury pain syndrome (35)	31	Uncontrolled	35% of treatments successful
Headache (musculoskeletal) (43)	60	Uncontrolled	70% of subjects received 60% reduction in headache severity and frequency

*References are listed in parentheses.

generalized, rather than just local and segmental, analgesic effects.

The discovery of CNS endorphins gives some support to this alternative. Nevertheless, controversy continues over whether TENS precipitates endorphin or other neurotransmitter release,[2, 6, 101] whether subjects with and without pain differ in response to stimulation,[63] and, if transmitters are released, what the most effective stimulation parameters are. Experimental findings are mixed. Many[2, 6, 63, 139, 140] but not all[1, 45, 58, 113, 153] studies find (1) evidence for CNS endorphin concentrations to

be elevated following stimulation and (2) the possibility that this release is more strongly associated with low-frequency–high-intensity stimulation (e.g., less than 10 Hz) than with the higher-frequency–lower-intensity (60 to 100 Hz) stimulation often used in clinical practice.

Pain threshold and pain tolerance studies could help clarify TENS theory and practice. Many studies have been done. Unfortunately, the results often disagree and the effects of differing noxious stimuli, such as ischemia and cold, are difficult to isolate. Some studies, for example, find that pain thresholds (the levels at which a painful stimulus is *perceived*) are either not altered by high-frequency (also known as "conventional") TENS[9, 13] or are increased by it.[130] Low-frequency TENS may also raise pain thresholds.[9] The relative effects high- and low-frequency TENS have on pain tolerance (the ability to *tolerate* a painful stimulus)[9, 13, 130] are not well understood, and it may be that the intensity of stimulation is important.

Other aspects of TENS are also controversial. In particular, reported benefits and effects are often poorly confirmed. For example, whereas one group reported that TENS produces vasodilation in subjects with chronic skin ulcers, Raynaud's phenomenon, and diabetic neuropathy,[70–74] other investigators find both similar and opposite effects in normal subjects.[26, 89, 152] The effects of stimulation location, intensity, and frequency as well as subject expectations and general health are potentially important and remain unclear.

Equipment

TENS units are routinely small, usually less than the size of a package of cigarettes, and are often programmable. Electronically, they are relatively simple devices and consist of a power source (usually a rechargeable battery), one or more signal generators, and a set of electrodes. Outputs vary depending on the unit and the choices of the therapist and patient. Typically, output currents are less than 100 mA, pulse rates are between 0.5 and 200 Hz, and pulse widths are from 10 to several hundred microseconds.

Pulse and wave train shape vary widely. Although monophasic pulses may be used, there is concern that since they transmit a net charge, they may produce irritation by altering skin pH[18, 112] or promoting iontophoresis. Experimental findings are mixed,[21, 56] and the FDA recommends limiting the charge delivered in a single phase of a TENS signal to 25 microcoulombs.[7] In practice, a variety of symmetrical, asymmetrical, monophasic, and biphasic outputs are available.

All TENS units allow adjustment of the stimulating intensity. Less expensive units may have fixed frequencies and waveforms, but most devices permit some variation of these parameters. Other options that may be present, absent, fixed, or modifiable include wave train "ramping" (i.e., allowing a train of pulses to gradually increase or decrease in amplitude) as well as alterations in pulse durations, interpulse separations, and frequency spectra.

Carbon-impregnated electrodes are sufficient for short-term use. These electrodes, however, must be taped to the body and require a conducting gel or moistened gauze to maintain good electrical contact. For longer-term use, more expensive self-adhesive electrodes are often used. Skin sensitivities to these materials vary, and it is not unusual that electrode types or placements may have to be altered because of limited skin tolerance.

Technique

Electrode placement and stimulation parameter choice remain more art than science. Electrodes are often placed over the painful area being treated. However, placement in paravertebral locations as well as over nerves proximal, distal, and even contralateral to a site of pain may be used. TENS is at times also used as a form of "electroacupuncture" either at traditional acupuncture points or at sites of high skin conductivity that have been isolated with a probe.[127] Other approaches, such as auricular therapy, in which TENS stimulation is applied to points on the auricle of the ear that are felt somatotopically related to the area of concern, are also possible.[114]

The success or failure of TENS cannot be established in a single therapy session. Even when a trial appears successful, a few therapy sessions and, ideally, an overnight trial or two are needed to establish the most effective stimulation parameters and eliminate some placebo effects. Nevertheless, TENS is frequently prescribed with little evaluation or patient instruction. When this is done, an unsuccessful trial is not necessarily a failure of TENS; it may be due to incorrect electrode placement or limited parameter adjustment. Thus, when TENS is reported as ineffective, it is necessary to ask in *detail* how the unit was used.

TENS units are expensive (often $500 or more), and once a patient feels that TENS is successful, the issue of cost must be faced. Fortunately, there are a number of ways to help control expenses. One of these is to survey the local vendors and use those that allow a free trial of a few days to a week for evaluation. Another is to prescribe a month's rental with the option to apply the rental fee to the purchase price if longer-term use seems necessary. A third way to make TENS use more cost-effective is to ask a patient who feels that TENS has been, or has become, ineffective how the unit was used. Often alternative parameters and placements need to be evaluated.

Stimulation parameters optimal for all patients do not exist. In practice, there is a division between high-frequency (~60 to 100 Hz) and low-frequency (~0.5 to 10 Hz) TENS. The high-frequency option is often termed "hi" or "conventional" TENS. The low-frequency approach is often simply called "lo" TENS. High-frequency treatments are routinely done at intensities ranging from the barely perceptible to two or three times the sensory threshold. Low-frequency treatments usually involve stronger intensities on the order of three to five times the sensory threshold. In distinction to high-frequency TENS (which can be tolerated for many hours), low-frequency stimulation is less comfortable and treatments usually last only 20 to 30 minutes. (Heuristically, stimulation frequency and intensity have a roughly inverse relationship; thus, high-frequency TENS implies a relatively low stimulation intensity, and low-frequency TENS implies a larger intensity stimulation.)

Although many therapists and physicians feel that certain stimuli are more effective than others, it is difficult to predict patient response, and parameter choice remains subjective. Thus, although specific choices may be made for specific situations, many routinely evaluate high-frequency TENS first and then proceed to the less comfortable low-frequency options if the first approach is not successful.

Indications

TENS is appropriate treatment for acute and chronic pain that cannot be treated less expensively, more safely, or more effectively by other means. Reported success rates (Tables 15–1 and 15–2) vary from placebo levels (~30 per cent) to as high as 80 to 95 per cent. It is, unfortunately, difficult to reconcile these variations because studies are seldom directly comparable and differences in outcomes may result from differences in (1) stimulating parameters, (2) electrode placement, (3) type of pain, (4) duration of pain, (5) concurrent medication, (6) previous treatment, (7) choice of controls, (8) patient expectations, and (9) length of follow-up.

Iontophoresis

Iontophoresis involves the introduction of electrically charged molecules or atoms (ions) into tissue using an electrical field. Since electrical field strength is determined by the voltage change per unit distance, the forces exerted on ions in a specific situation are proportional to the voltage applied. Current flow, on the other hand, is a measure of the movement of electrical charge. As such, it and the duration of treatment serve as a measure of the amount of material transferred.

Whether iontophoresis can deliver therapeutic concentrations of a medication at sites in or below the skin is controversial and must be dealt with on a drug-by-drug basis. In particular, parameters such as drug polarity and electrophoretic mobility must be known.

These measurements have been made for many substances at concentrations and pH levels appropriate for treatment. In some cases the situation seems quite clear; the HCl salts of local anesthetics (e.g., lidocaine) and epinephrine are known to have conductivities higher than that of a 5.0 mM NaCl solution.[47] In other cases the situation is less clear: several water-soluble corticosteroids (methylprednisolone sodium succinate [Solu-Medrol], hydrocortisone sodium succinate [Solu-Cortef], and hydrocortisone phosphate) have been reported as relatively highly conductive by one group,[47] whereas another group,[27] which also examined methylprednisolone sodium succinate and hydrocortisone sodium succinate, did not find significant electrophoretic mobility in a group of six corticosteroids. Other medications have been examined and a number of antiviral (e.g., vidarabine monophosphate) and chemotherapeutic drugs (e.g., methotrexate, cyclophosphamide) are highly conductive.[47]

Other restrictions on the applicability of a substance for iontophoresis exist. Among these are that the drug (and its vehicle, if any) must be nontoxic, soluble, and able to pass through the epidermis.

The clinical applications of iontophoresis are currently limited and are restricted to a number of "niches." There are several reasons for this, two of which are paramount. The first is that penetration beyond the skin surface is variable and drug-specific. The second is that even if a substance passes through the epidermis, local blood flow may rapidly remove it from the area to be treated and distribute it throughout the body—a situation more easily and cheaply produced by a pill or injection.

Technique

At its simplest, iontophoretic equipment consists of a direct current source and a pair of electrodes

JEFFREY R. BASFORD

covered with gauze pads moistened with a dilute (usually about 1 per cent) solution of the desired medication. In theory, a battery, a few wires, and pads should be all that is needed. In practice, a variety of refinements are available to improve efficiency, comfort, and safety: current limitation, power supply isolation, ammeters, and timers.

Sudden changes in current intensity can be uncomfortable. Iontophoretic units therefore either permit gradual changes in current flow manually or do this automatically. In addition, unidirectional current flow over prolonged periods can cause skin irritation due to effects such as pH changes; some units may take this into account and permit polarity reversal.

Current intensities and electrode areas depend on the treatment as well as patient tolerance. In general, however, currents can usually be estimated by multiplying the area of the active electrode (i.e., the phoresing electrode) by 0.1 to 0.5 mA/cm^2. The area of the inactive "dispersive" electrode, if larger than that of the active electrode, is immaterial, but is usually as large as convenient to minimize current intensity.

The polarity of a medication, and hence the choice of whether the positive or negative pole will be the active electrode, can be established from the chemical formula, the literature, the manufacturer's instructions, or a trial. Positive ions (such as many metals) are delivered by a positive electrode, and negative ions are delivered by a negative electrode. In particular, epinephrine, histamine, lidocaine, cocaine, dibucaine, prednisolone sodium phosphate, cisplatin, vincristine, and hyaluronidase are positively charged, and penicillin, acyclovir, indomethacin, insulin, and sulfonamide are negatively charged.[59, 68, 79, 88, 98, 125]

Complications and Contraindications

The goal of iontophoresis is the safe delivery of a therapeutic concentration of a drug to a limited area with minimal exposure of the rest of the body to the substance. If this goal is met, complications should be limited to the local toxicity of the drug, local hypersensitivity, and pain if the current intensity is too high. Unusual problems occasionally are reported. Iontophoresis over superficial nerves may produce prolonged blocks, and vertigo, nausea, and even facial palsy may occur following tympanic membrane iontophoresis with anesthetics.[15]

Indications

Multiple cutaneous, musculoskeletal, and neurological conditions have been treated with iontophoresis. Whereas laboratory and *in vitro* studies are often quantitative and well controlled, clinical studies are frequently inconclusive and subjective. With the exception of hyperhidrosis and diagnosis of cystic fibrosis, most procedures are controversial and have limited evaluation.

IDIOPATHIC HYPERHIDROSIS

Idiopathic hyperhidrosis is marked by palmar, plantar, or axillary sweating severe enough to be embarrassing as well as to damage clothing, irritate skin, and interfere with occupational activities. Treatment with concentrated antiperspirants such as aluminum chloride hexahydrate (Drysol) is effective in many cases. Tanning agents such as glutaraldehyde, tannic acid, and formaldehyde are also used, although they can stain and produce hypersensitivity.[54, 150] Iontophoresis provides an alternative to these approaches.

Iontophoretic treatment is the easiest for the hands and feet, for which success rates of 80 to 90 per cent are reported.[3] In these cases the patient either puts both hands or feet in a single container containing both a cathode and an anode, or places each extremity in a separate container, one of which contains a cathode and the other of which contains an anode.[32] Anticholinergic substances can be used, but tap water alone is effective.[3, 150] Since water produces neither sensitization nor systemic effects, it is often preferred. Treatment schedules may involve one or two treatments a day for a few weeks or until the hidrosis is reduced to an acceptable level. Subsequently, a less frequent maintenance schedule may be needed. Currents vary with the approach, but routinely range between 10 and 30 mA.

Axillary hyperhidrosis is more difficult to treat owing to body geometry. Nevertheless, electrodes covered with moist gauze pads can be placed in the axilla and treatment performed in a manner similar to that discussed for hands and feet.

The mechanism of action of iontophoresis in hyperhidrosis is not clear. It is reported that treatment produces no observable microscopic changes.[54] However, one theory that iontophoretic currents block sweat ducts is partially supported by the observations that (1) iontophoretic currents preferentially pass through the sweat ducts and (2) removal of the stratum corneum will reverse the effects of treatment.[54, 150]

TOOTH HYPERSENSITIVITY

Tooth hypersensitivity is a widespread problem that may be treated with iontophoresis. Treatments are usually done with sodium fluoride, and although some studies find iontophoresis effective in reducing hypersensitivity in about 75 to 80 per cent of cases,[97] others find topical application just as effective.[23] It is interesting that a proposed mechanism is again blockage of channels, this time dentinal tubules within the teeth.[97]

ANALGESIA

Iontophoretic analgesia has gained limited acceptance. It is reported, however, that lidocaine iontophoresis eliminates the pain of venipuncture and myringotomies.[8, 119] Iontophoretic vinca alkaloid treatments can also produce localized analgesia. Success rates of about 90 per cent in a variety of neuralgias including postherpetic neuralgia and trigeminal pain were reported by one group,[33] although benefits in patients with chronic postherpetic pain were limited in another study.[88]

ARTHRITIS

Corticosteroid and anesthetic iontophoresis is an intriguing alternative to intra-articular and soft tissue injections for musculoskeletal pain. Unfortunately, it is not established whether these agents are delivered to deep tissues. Some investigators report that corticosteroids such as triamcinolone-acetonide (Kenacort-A), prednisolone sodium tetrahydrophthalate, hydrocortisone sodium succinate (Solu-Cortef), dexamethasone sodium phosphate (Solu-Decadron), and methylprednisolone sodium succinate (Solu-Medrol) do not pass the skin during iontophoresis.[27] Others report that corticosteroid concentrations are not elevated in knee joint fluid following iontophoresis.[52] The issue is further confused by the findings of increased serum concentrations following iontophoresis by one group[68] and the report by another group that whereas no penetration of corticosteroids through the skin was detected, 56 per cent of the patients in a clinical trial reported remission of pain and reduced inflammation following iontophoresis.[27] These investigators suggested that the effects were due to the flow of electrical charge and not from the medications used.

CUTANEOUS DISEASE

Skin disease treatment often requires systemic or topical medication for prolonged periods. The allure of the rapid delivery of medication in high concentration to a limited area by iontophoresis is understandable. Antibiotics, in particular, have been studied. Investigations include the introduction of antibiotics into the eye (gentamicin, penicillin, and some sulfa-based drugs), ear cartilage and burns (gentamicin and penicillin), and middle ear (cefoxitin).[57, 62, 86, 119] Therapeutic concentrations are reported, but these approaches have gained limited clinical use.

MISCELLANEOUS

Other applications include iontophoretic delivery of pilocarpine for diagnosis of cystic fibrosis, chemotherapy for squamous cell and basal cell carcinoma,[98] silver ions for superficial and deep infection,[41, 135] mucolytic agents and antibiotics for otitis media,[119] insulin in diabetes mellitus,[79] salicylates and indomethacin for analgesia,[48, 125] iodine for tendon adhesions and scar reduction,[87, 146] acetic acid to aid resorption of calcium deposits,[75] zinc for ischemic ulcer treatment,[31] and vidarabine as well as idoxuridine for herpes simplex infections and aphthous ulcers.[46, 91] Corticosteroid iontophoresis has been recommended for Peyronie's disease[77] and facial pain.[76]

These applications are presented as an indication of potential uses of iontophoresis. In most cases, clinical use would require further evaluation.

Wound Healing

Low-intensity direct current (LIDC) was used to treat pressure sores and indolent ulcers in the 1960s and 1970s. Promising results were reported,[49, 151] but controlled evaluation was limited and electrical stimulation did not gain wide acceptance.

Interest in electrically stimulated wound healing is again increasing. Laboratory studies, for example, find many plant, animal, and human cell functions—such as orientation, collagen production, and protein synthesis—sensitive to physiologically tolerable electric fields.[17, 28, 128] In the clinical area, electrical stimulation is used as a treatment of nonunited fractures.[22, 102]

Electrically stimulated soft tissue wound healing is not as advanced as is the case for bone healing. However, some work is available. Uncontrolled experiments with milliampere currents find improved healing of indolent ulcers in nursing home patients following a program of low-intensity stimulation.[14] Other clinical studies, using a variety of waveforms and intensities, are under way that will provide additional information in the future.

Muscle Stimulation

Although there may be some exceptions, during normal volitional muscular activity, fatigue-resistant slow twitch (type I) fibers are recruited initially. As the level of exertion increases, stronger and more quickly exhausted fast twitch (types IIa and IIb) fibers are activated. During strenuous and prolonged activities, both fiber types fire at moderate rates; at maximal effort, all units fire at high frequencies.[37]

Muscles contracting as a result of electrical stimulation do not follow this pattern. In fact, muscle fibers that contract may be merely those (or those with the most sensitive motor neurons) near an electrode. The significance of this difference in contraction sequence is unknown but may be important in fine motor control and muscular endurance.

Four muscle conditions are frequently treated with electrical stimulation: normal muscle, immobilized and injured muscle, denervated muscle, and muscle affected by upper motor neuron injury. It is possible to make general statements about each of these situations.

Normal Muscle

Most electrical stimulation studies of normal muscle involve "normal, healthy" students and athletes. Training is often performed isometrically, and evaluation is usually done under isometric or isokinetic conditions. Less is known about strengthening under different conditions, and little is known about the middle-aged and elderly.

With these caveats in mind, it appears that in healthy, active men and women, (1) electrical stimulation does not strengthen muscles more rapidly than do traditional approaches, and (2) the combination of electrical stimulation and volitional contraction produces neither a stronger contraction nor a more rapid strength gain than does volitional contraction alone. These conclusions appear valid for both low-frequency (e.g., 25 Hz) and high-frequency (2500 Hz) stimulation programs.*

---

*See references 34, 40, 84, 85, 104, 106, 134, 138, and 144.

Immobilized and Injured Muscle

Electrical stimulation maintains isometric strength and, perhaps, myofibrillar ATPase during immobilization. However, bulk, speed, and glycogen stores are not protected.[29, 107, 143] Once immobilization is discontinued, the disparities between stimulated and nonstimulated muscle lessen, and by 8 to 12 weeks following immobilization, little difference can be found between stimulated and nonstimulated muscles.[107]

Sports clinics often use electrical stimulation to hasten recovery following musculoskeletal injury. A common example is an injury of the leg involving the quadriceps femoris muscle or the knee joint, in which recovery is typically slowed by pain, swelling, splinting, and limited range of motion—problems many therapists find lessened when electrical stimulation supplants or supplements volitional movement in the initial stages of postinjury training.

Denervated Muscle

Although electrical stimulation of denervated muscle has been in clinical use for more than 80 years, and studied for more than 140 years,[36, 95] its effects remain controversial. Much of the confusion may result from differing strengths, frequencies, and techniques of stimulation used in studies; strong, frequent stimulation with rest periods and resistance to muscle contraction may be the most effective.[83, 149] In particular, a number of small animal studies find that although stimulation retards muscle atrophy following denervation,[82, 83, 149] it may not promote reinnervation and may actually hinder terminal sprouting of motor axons.[24] Studies in humans, perhaps owing to small numbers and limited tolerance of high-intensity stimulation, are more mixed. Some studies find that stimulation retards atrophy following both neuronal injury from trauma and poliomyelitis.[66, 95, 116, 117] However, findings of improvement, much less accelerated recovery, are not universal,[19] and even investigators who find that stimulation has beneficial effects may feel that the primary benefit of stimulation may be in facilitating re-education of the impaired muscle.[36, 116] Even if atrophy retardation and strengthening effects are granted, it is possible that stimulation, particularly in the presence of sensory deficits, can result in overuse and damage of weakened muscles. Bell's palsy is a good example of the current situation: electrical stimulation is often prescribed, despite misgivings that it may not be effective.[108]

Upper Motor Neuron Injury

Electrical stimulation for muscle strengthening, cardiac conditioning, and possibly increasing bone mass is prescribed for general conditioning prior to beginning a program of functional electrical stimulation (FES) in patients with spinal cord injury. Effects can be graphic. In quadriplegics, for example, electrical stimulation programs increase strength, can increase resting blood pressure, and can lessen exercise-induced blood pressure elevation.[123]

Functional Electrical Stimulation (FES)

Functional electrical stimulation (FES) is the production of functional movement by electrical stimulation of muscles and nerves. Obvious benefits are the capabilities that injured people can gain with stimulation. Less obvious benefits may include reduction of spasticity and perhaps improved muscular control for a period following stimulation.[55, 148]

Liberson and colleagues[94] described in 1960 a peroneal nerve stimulator that was used to counteract hemiplegic footdrop. This marked the beginning of today's FES. Over the years, approaches have been refined, applications have been broadened, and technology has been improved. Nevertheless, the concept remains the same: using electrical stimulation to permit activities that would otherwise be impossible.

Most functional activities require an interplay of agonist, antagonist, and stabilizing muscles. Therefore, it is not surprising that whereas laboratory prototypes provide tantalizing looks at the potentials of FES, devices rugged and reliable enough to be clinically useful remain limited. A textbook cannot cover this area effectively, and an interested reader is directed to review articles[122, 148] that may, themselves, become rapidly dated.

Equipment

FES devices can be viewed as containing a power supply, a signal generator, a control circuit, a modulating circuit, an output circuit, and electrodes. The separate components are discussed in general terms.

Power Supply. Power supplies must be small, light, and reliable and should be able to power an FES device throughout at least a day of use. Rechargeable batteries are the *"de facto"* supplies. For single-channel devices, they suffice; for large multichannel systems, their endurance may be limiting.

Signal Generator. There is no ideal waveform, since stimulation parameters are a compromise between comfort, energy consumption, muscle fatigue, and the quality of the stimulated movement. Frequencies between 20 and 80 Hz and pulse widths from 0.05 to 1.0 msec are typically used for skeletal muscles.[148]

Control Circuit. The control circuit ultimately controls the form of the output of an FES system. Both "closed" and "open" circuits are used. "Closed" circuits use feedback (such as from switches, goniometers, pressure transducers, and EMG) to control the signal modulator. "Open" circuits, on the other hand, do not use feedback and merely deliver predetermined sequences of commands to the modulator.

Modulator Circuit. The modulator uses information from the input circuit to produce a wave train of a specific duration, amplitude, and shape. As would be expected, in a simple on-off feedback situation (e.g., a switch), the modulator is limited to producing a wave train of a specific duration with perhaps some signal ramping to improve comfort and function (Fig. 15–1). In proportional control devices, more complex engineering is needed to permit gradual changes in strength and speed.

Output Circuit. Both current-limited ("constant current") and voltage-limited ("constant voltage") output circuits are used. Each has advantages. Current limitation, as implied by the term, allows only a limited current to flow. This produces well-controlled stimulation but does not compensate for a situation such as a partially dislodged electrode, in which a current, while fixed at a nominally comfortable level, flows through a reduced area and produces a painful current intensity. Voltage limitation, on the other hand, limits the maximum stimulating voltage. This approach avoids the potential of painfully high current intensities, but stimulation effectiveness may be more variable than is the case for current-limited devices.[148]

Electrodes. Electrodes are usually placed at specific muscle motor points or over nerves (Figs. 15–2 to 15–8) and may be superficial, percutaneous, or implanted (Fig. 15–9). Each has advantages and disadvantages. Superficial electrodes (e.g., carbon-impregnated, metal, self-adhesive) are easily at-

Text continued on page 391

JEFFREY R. BASFORD

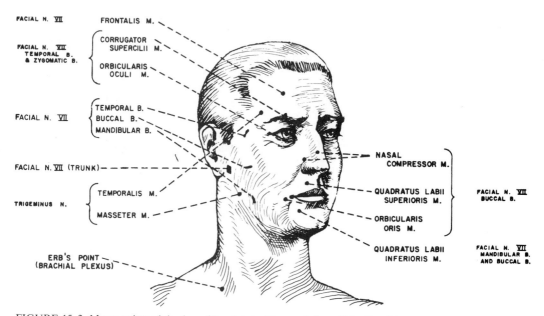

FIGURE 15–1. Amplitude modulation of a wave train produces smoother muscle contractions.

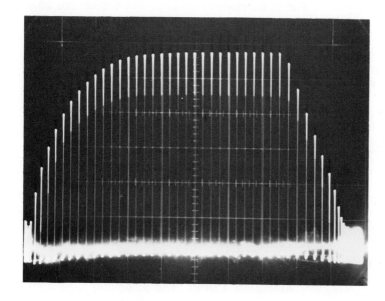

FIGURE 15–2. Motor points of the face. (Reprinted with permission of The Burdick Corporation, Milton, WI.)

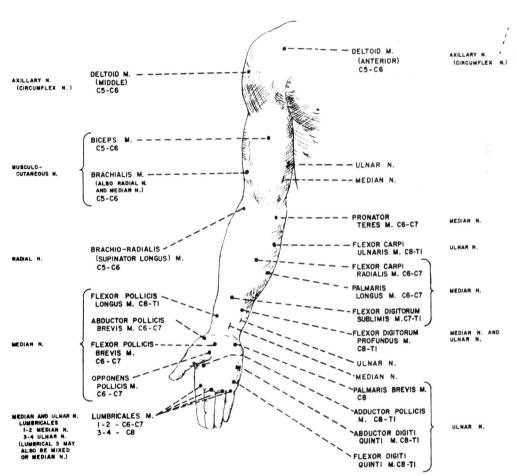

FIGURE 15–3. Motor points of the anterior upper extremity. (Reprinted with permission of The Burdick Corporation, Milton, WI.)

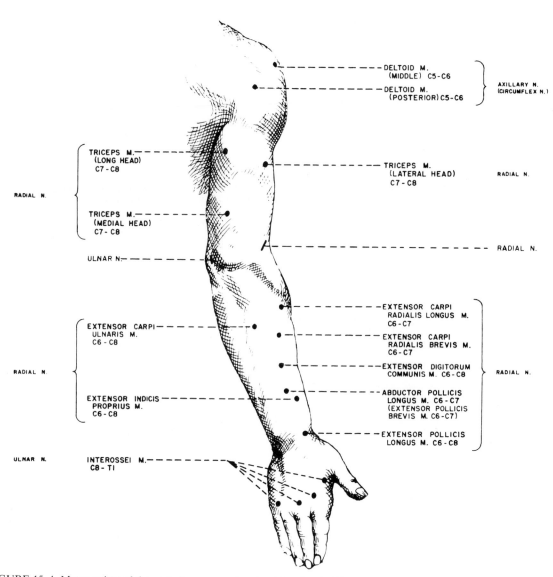

FIGURE 15–4. Motor points of the posterior upper extremity. (Reprinted with permission of The Burdick Corporation, Milton, WI.)

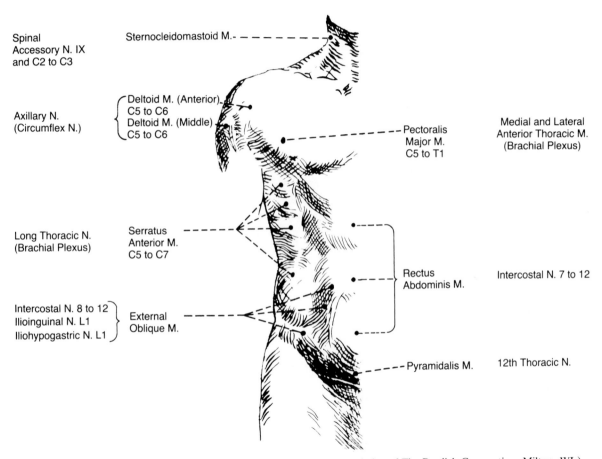

Spinal
Accessory N. IX
and C2 to C3

Sternocleidomastoid M.

Axillary N.
(Circumflex N.)

Deltoid M. (Anterior)
C5 to C6
Deltoid M. (Middle)
C5 to C6

Pectoralis
Major M.
C5 to T1

Medial and Lateral
Anterior Thoracic M.
(Brachial Plexus)

Long Thoracic N.
(Brachial Plexus)

Serratus
Anterior M.
C5 to C7

Rectus
Abdominis M.

Intercostal N. 7 to 12

Intercostal N. 8 to 12
Ilioinguinal N. L1
Iliohypogastric N. L1

External
Oblique M.

Pyramidalis M.

12th Thoracic N.

FIGURE 15–5. Motor points of the anterior trunk. (Reprinted with permission of The Burdick Corporation, Milton, WI.)

JEFFREY R. BASFORD

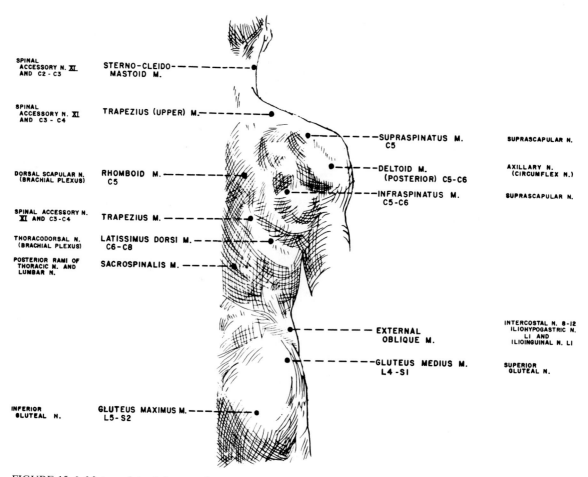

FIGURE 15–6. Motor points of the posterior trunk. (Reprinted with permission of The Burdick Corporation, Milton, WI.)

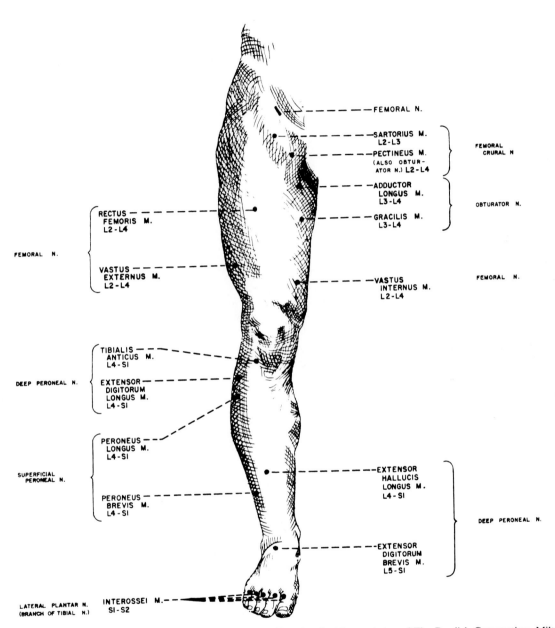

FIGURE 15–7. Motor points of the anterior lower extremity. (Reprinted with permission of The Burdick Corporation, Milton, WI.)

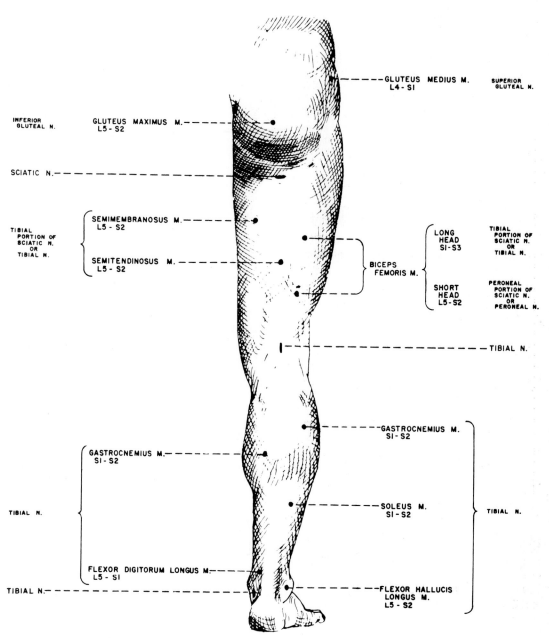

FIGURE 15–8. Motor points of the posterior lower extremity. (Reprinted with permission of The Burdick Corporation, Milton, WI.)

tached and adjusted. However, they may shift, may produce skin irritation, require high stimulation intensities, and are unsightly. Percutaneous electrodes permit more precise localization but penetrate the skin and require skilled insertion. As many as a third may fail within four months.[103] Implanted electrodes are located subcutaneously and are powered by signals transmitted through the skin. These electrodes are complex and require surgical placement. Although they have been used for peroneal nerve stimulation,[148] they are not in general use for FES.

Limitations

A major limitation of FES is that whereas it may be effective, the improvement over more traditional treatment may not be sufficient to warrant its use. Peroneal nerve stimulators demonstrate this well: gait is often improved with stimulation, but the improvement over an ankle-foot orthosis may not justify the increased cost and complexity.

FES use is also limited by patient capabilities and clinician skills. For example, the patient must desire to use FES, must understand how to use FES, and must be able to maintain and adjust the device. Similarly, the physician and therapist must understand the theory of FES and must have experience working with it.

There are also physiological restrictions on FES. Lower motor neuron disease is generally not treated with FES, and myopathic disease is usually a contraindication. Progressive diseases, such as multiple sclerosis, are relative contraindications depending on the rate of progression. Other physiological impediments include obesity (reducing motor point accessibility), joint contracture and instability, and uncontrollable spasticity. Disuse atrophy and osteoporosis must be taken into account, and strengthening programs are often needed before FES programs are begun.

Indications

Although a multitude of conditions should be appropriate for FES, two, hemiplegia and spinal cord injury, have received the most emphasis. These two uses, as well as a few of the less common, will be briefly outlined.

HEMIPLEGIA

Hemiplegia from these causes was one of the first areas of modern FES. In particular, peroneal nerve FES is well studied and provides an orthotic that reduces footdrop and improves the gait in 25 to 30 per cent of appropriate hemiplegic patients.[55] These orthotics, although refined over the years, routinely use a heel switch arrangement that was outlined[94] in 1960 (Figs. 15–9 to 15–11). FES of more proximal leg muscles in hemiplegia has had little development.

FES in the hemiplegic upper extremity is more complex and less studied than it is for the leg. In particular, the goal of an effective grasp remains elusive, even though FES of the finger and wrist extensors (Figs. 15–12 and 15–13) can complement residual finger flexor capabilities. FES, at times in association with neuromuscular blocks, may be used to facilitate neuromuscular re-education[81, 126] during therapy sessions and in home training programs.

SPINAL CORD INJURY

Although paraplegics and quadriplegics can ambulate with FES under controlled conditions, electrically stimulated walking (with or without braces) remains a laboratory exercise. Nevertheless, the technology that has developed has supported the development of more prosaic but possibly more immediately usable capabilities. Among these are unassisted standing and arising from a chair.[65, 67] Leg-propelled wheelchairs and tricycles,[51, 122] which may be useful for conditioning as well as, perhaps, transportation, have also been developed.

Spinal injury is likely to be accompanied by limitations of sensation and muscular control that are severe and bilateral. Thus, for these individuals to perform a function such as walking, it may be necessary to reproduce the entire function rather than improving only a portion of it, such as footdrop. Furthermore, sensory and motor deficits may make a spinal cord–injured person walking with FES incapable of either correcting balance after a stumble or of breaking a fall, once one has begun.

Severe deconditioning and atrophy is present in anyone with a long-term spinal cord injury. As a result, it is usually necessary to begin an electrical stimulation program to increase cardiovascular endurance, muscle strength, and bone density before attempting an FES program.[121, 123]

CEREBRAL PALSY

FES has been used to improve the gait of children with monoplegia, diplegia, bilateral hemiplegia, or quadriplegia as a result of cerebral palsy

Text continued on page 396

JEFFREY R. BASFORD

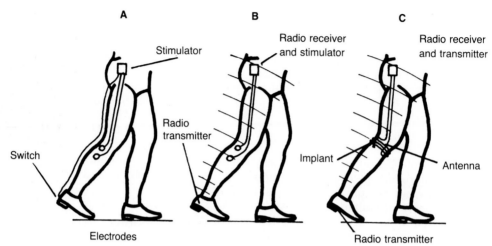

FIGURE 15–9. Various techniques for stimulation. *A*, Stimulation controlled by a switch in the heel of the shoe with wire connections to stimulator at hip and to surface electrodes. *B*, A radio link from a switch in the insole to stimulator with wire connections to surface electrodes. *C*, A radio link from a switch in the insole to implanted receiver, stimulator, and electrodes.

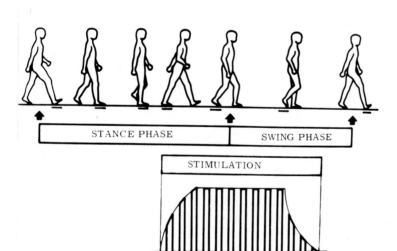

FIGURE 15–10. In this sequence, the peroneal nerve is stimulated by the closing of a switch as the ipsilateral heel breaks contact with the floor.

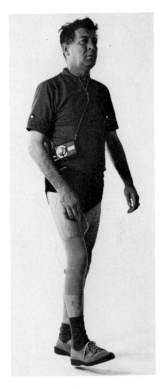

FIGURE 15–11. Gait of a patient with right hemiplegia, using FES to assist dorsiflexion. (From Vodovnik, L., Gračanin, F., and Strojnik, P.: Functional electrical stimulation for control of locomotor systems. CRC Crit. Rev. Bioeng., 6:63–131, 1981.)

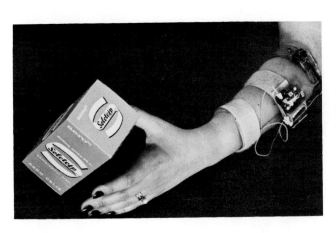

FIGURE 15–12. Stimulation of the finger and wrist extensors in a patient who has preserved ability for grasp enables her to use the hand for ADLs. The bracelet containing the control switch is seen near the elbow. The stimulator, batteries, and electrodes are attached to the arm by a Velcro tape.

JEFFREY R. BASFORD

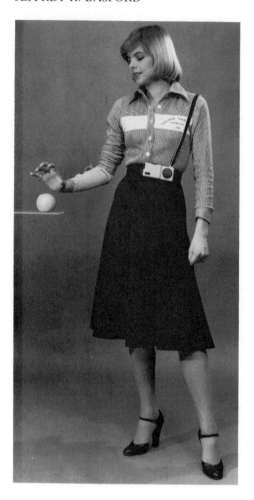

FIGURE 15–13. A system designed for the stimulation of finger and wrist extensors. Continuous control of the stimulus intensity is maintained through a slide potentiometer that is controlled by shoulder movements of the unaffected side. (From Vodovnik, L., Gračanin, F., and Strojnik, P.: Functional electrical stimulation for control of locomotor systems. CRC Crit. Rev. Bioeng. 6:63–131, 1981.)

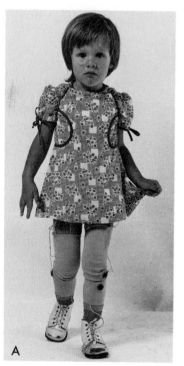
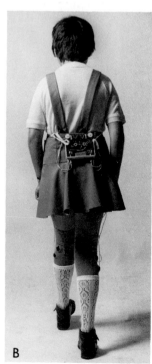

FIGURE 15–14. Two children with cerebral palsy using bilateral FES of the peroneal nerves. In both cases, successful prevention of equinus position of the foot and reduction of internal rotation and adduction at the hip were achieved. (From Vodovnik, L., Gračanin, F., and Strojnik, P.: Functional electrical stimulation for control of locomotor systems. CRC Crit. Rev. Bioeng., 6:63–131, 1981.)

TABLE 15–3. Electrical Stimulation—Miscellaneous Applications

INDICATION*	NUMBER OF SUBJECTS AND DESIGN	STIMULATION TECHNIQUE	SUMMARY OF RESULTS
Chronic constipation (136)	300 Uncontrolled	Over abdomen 200–300 msec, 1 Hz, 25 mA	85% with positive or excellent results
Urinary incontinence Frequency/urge (109, 110)	12, 22 Uncontrolled	Perianal: 0.5 msec, 20–100 Hz, 10–100 V Penile: 0.5 msec, 10–20 Hz, 5–50 V	45–75% showed post-stimulation improvement clinically
Stress, urgency (39)	46 Uncontrolled	Intravaginal stimulation 1–5 msec, 10–30 mA, 20–50 Hz	Average 25% increase in urethral pressure profile
Neurogenic bladder Incontinence (53)	11 Uncontrolled	Anal electrode 1 msec, 20 Hz, 10–15 mA	82% with lessening of incontinence following stimulation
Urinary retention (69)	11 Uncontrolled	Direct stimulation of bladder	Success difficult to evaluate; 63% failed or were removed by 3 years
Spastic and autonomic bladders (111)	11 Uncontrolled	Direct spinal cord stimulation 100–300 μsec, 15–40 Hz	Success difficult to evaluate; 73% with a "positive" therapeutic result
Shoulder subluxation in hemiplegia (12)	63 Controlled	Tetanizing stimulation 12–25 Hz, 6–7 hours/day	Subluxation reduced by 42% in the stimulated group at 6 weeks; no change in control group
Idiopathic scoliosis (16, 61)	236 (surface) 169 (implanted) Uncontrolled	Superficial electrodes (425 μsec, 50 Hz) Implanted electrodes (220 μsec, 33 Hz)	Effectiveness of electrical stimulation remains controversial, although some feel 70% of patients maintain improved curvature with treatment
Multiple sclerosis (44)	49 Uncontrolled	50 Hz, 0.25 msec	Decrease in symptoms and slight decrease in urinary frequency reported
Spasticity in spinal cord injury (11, 90, 92)	6, 27 Uncontrolled	Variable stimulation parameters	Variable results; duration of benefit may persist hours after stimulation
Hemifacial spasm (154)	21 Uncontrolled	1 Hz, 1 msec, 10–20 V above twitch threshold	In conjunction with muscle relaxants and minor tranquilizers, 81% found treatment effective
Tinnitus (38, 147)	50 Controlled	Multiple stimulation frequencies 0.5–2 Hz, 30 μA Auricular stimulation	Mixed results with 28–90% of subjects reporting improvement

*References are listed in parentheses.

JEFFREY R. BASFORD

(Fig. 15–14). Differences in pacing parameters exist between these children and adults, and flexion synergies complicate stimulation requirements.[55, 148]

Other Applications of Electrical Stimulation

Electrical stimulation has been used with variable success for a vast number of visceral and somatic applications. A number of these, such as bladder, cerebellar, scoliosis, and spinal cord stimulators, are summarized in Table 15–3.

References

1. Abram, S. E., Reynolds, A. C., and Cusick, J. F.: Failure of naloxone to reverse analgesia from transcutaneous electrical stimulation in patients with chronic pain. Anesth. Analg., 60:81–84, 1981.
2. Adams, J. E.: Naloxone reversal of analgesia produced by brain stimulation in the human. Pain, 2:161–166, 1976.
3. Akins, D. L., Meisenheimer, J. L., and Dobson, R. L.: Efficacy of the Drionic unit in the treatment of hyperhidrosis. J. Am. Acad. Dermatol., 16:828–832, 1987.
4. Ali, J., Yaffe, C. S., and Serratte, C.: The effect of transcutaneous electric nerve stimulation on postoperative pain and pulmonary function. Surgery, 89:507–512, 1981.
5. Alm, W. A., Gold, M. L., and Weil, L. S.: Evaluation of transcutaneous electrical nerve stimulation (TENS) in podiatric surgery. J. Am. Podiatry Assoc., 69:537–542, 1979.
6. Almay, B. G. L., Johansson, F., von Knorring, L., Sakurada, T., and Terenius, L.: Long-term high frequency transcutaneous electrical nerve stimulation (hi-TNS) in chronic pain. Clinical response and effects on CSF-endorphins, monoamine metabolites, substance P–like immunoreactivity (SPLI) and pain measures. J. Psychosom. Res., 29:247–257, 1985.
7. Alon, G., and De Domenico, G.: Therapeutic currents. In High Voltage Stimulation: An Integrated Approach to Clinical Electrotherapy. Chattanooga, Chattanooga Corp., 1987, pp. 31–56.
8. Arvidsson, S. B., Ekroth, R. H., Hansby, A. M. C., Lindholm, A. H., and William-Olsson, G.: Painless venipuncture. A clinical trial of iontophoresis of lidocaine for venipuncture in blood donors. Acta Anaesthesiol. Scand., 28:209–210, 1984.
9. Ashton, H., Ebenezer, I., Golding, J. F., and Thompson, J. W.: Effects of acupuncture and transcutaneous electrical nerve stimulation on cold-induced pain in normal subjects. J. Psychosom. Res., 28:301–308, 1984.
10. Augustinsson, L. E., Bohlin, P., Bundsen, P., Carlsson, C. A., Forssman, L., Sjoberg, P., and Tyreman, N. O.: Pain relief during delivery by transcutaneous electrical nerve stimulation. Pain, 4:59–65, 1977.
11. Bajd, T., Eng, D., Gregoric, M., Vodovnik, L., and Benko, H.: Electrical stimulation in treating spasticity resulting from spinal cord injury. Arch. Phys. Med. Rehabil., 66:515–517, 1985.
12. Baker, L. L., and Parker, K.: Neuromuscular electrical stimulation of the muscles surrounding the shoulder. Phys. Ther., 66:1930–1937, 1986.
13. Barr, J. O., Nielsen, D. H., and Soderberg, G. L.: Transcutaneous electrical nerve stimulation characteristics for altering pain perception. Phys. Ther., 66:1515–1521, 1986.
14. Barron, J. J., Jacobson, W. E., and Tidd, G.: Treatment of decubitus ulcers—a new approach. Minn. Med., 68:103–106, 1985.
15. Beauchamp, M. L., and Kemink, J. L.: Facial paralysis complicating iontophoresis of the tympanic membrane: A case report. Am. J. Otol., 4:93–94, 1982.
16. Benson, D. R.: Idiopathic scoliosis: The last ten years and state of the art. Orthopedics, 10:1691–1698, 1987.
17. Black, J.: Electrical stimulation of hard and soft tissues in animal models. Clin. Plast. Surg., 12:243–256, 1985.
18. Bolton, L., Foleno, T., Means, B., and Petrucelli, S.: Direct current bactericidal effect on intact skin. Antimicrob. Agents Chemother., 18:137–141, 1980.
19. Boonstra, A. M., van Weerden, T. W., Eisma, W. H., Pahlplatz, V. B. M., and Oosterhuis, H. J. G. H.: The effect of low-frequency electrical stimulation on denervation atrophy in man. Scand. J. Rehabil. Med., 19:127–134, 1987.
20. Bourke, D. L., Smith, B. A., Erickson, J., Gwartz, B., and Lessard, L.: TENS reduces halothane requirements during hand surgery. Anesthesiology, 61:769–772, 1984.
21. Bowman, B. R., and Baker, L. L.: Effects of waveform parameters on comfort during transcutaneous neuromuscular electrical stimulation. Ann. Biomed. Eng., 13:59–74, 1985.
22. Brighton, C. T.: Treatment of nonunion of the tibia with constant direct current (1980 Fitts Lecture, AAST). J. Trauma, 21:189–195, 1981.
23. Brough, K. M., Anderson, D. M., Love, J., and Overman, P. R.: The effectiveness of iontophoresis in reducing dentin hypersensitivity. J. Am. Dent. Assoc., 111:761–765, 1985.
24. Brown, M. C., and Holland, R. L.: A central role for denervated tissues in causing nerve sprouting. Nature, 282:724–726, 1979.

25. Carabelli, R. A., and Kellerman, W. C.: Phantom limb pain: Relief by application of TENS to contralateral extremity. Arch. Phys. Med. Rehabil., 66:466–467, 1985.

26. Casale, R., Gibellini, R., Bozzi, M., and Bonelli, S.: Changes in sympathetic activity during high frequency TENS. Acupunct. Electrother. Res., 10:169–175, 1985.

27. Chantraine, A., Ludy, J. P., Berger, D.: Is cortisone iontophoresis possible? Arch. Phys. Med. Rehabil., 67:38–40, 1986.

28. Cheng, N., Van Hoof, H., Bockx, E., Hoogmartens, M. J., Mulier, J. C., DeDijcker, F. J., Sansen, W. M., and DeLoecker, D.: The effects of electric currents on ATP generation, protein synthesis and membrane transport in rat skin. Clin. Orthop., 171:264–271, 1982.

29. Cole, B. G., and Gardiner, P. F.: Does electrical stimulation of denervated muscle, continued after reinnervation, influence recovery of contractile function? Exp. Neurol., 85:52–62, 1985.

30. Cooperman, A. M., Hall, B., Mikalacki, K., Hardy, R., and Sadar, E.: Use of transcutaneous electrical stimulation in the control of post-operative pain. Results of a prospective, randomized, controlled study. Am. J. Surg., 133:185–187, 1977.

31. Cornwall, M. W.: Zinc iontophoresis to treat ischemic skin ulcers. Phys. Ther., 61:359–360, 1981.

32. Craig, D. L., and Collie, J. W.: An iontophoresis unit for the treatment of hyperhidrosis. Australas. Phys. Eng. Sci. Med., 6:125–127, 1983.

33. Csillik, B., Knyihár-Csillik, E., and Szücs, A.: Treatment of chronic pain syndromes with iontophoresis of vinca alkaloids to the skin of patients. Neurosci. Lett., 31:87–90, 1982.

34. Currier, D. P., and Mann, R.: Muscular strength development by electrical stimulation in healthy individuals. Phys. Ther., 63:915–921, 1983.

35. Davis, R., and Lentini, R.: Transcutaneous nerve stimulation for treatment of pain in patients with spinal cord injury. Surg. Neurol., 4:100–101, 1975.

36. Doupe, J., Barnes, R., and Kerr, A. S.: Studies in denervation. H. The effect of electrical stimulation on the circulation and recovery of denervated muscle. J. Neurol. Psychiatry, 6:136–140, 1943.

37. Edström, L., and Grimby, L.: Effect of exercise on the motor unit. Muscle Nerve, 9:104–126, 1986.

38. Engelberg, M., and Bauer, W.: Transcutaneous electrical stimulation for tinnitus. Laryngoscope, 95:1167–1173, 1985.

39. Erlandson, B. J., Fall, M., and Sundin, T.: Intravaginal electrical stimulation, Part III, IVS: Clinical experiments on urethral closure. Nephrology [Suppl.] 44:31–39, 1977.

40. Fahey, T. D., Harvey, M., Schroeder, R. V., and Ferguson, F.: Influence of sex differences and knee joint position on electrical stimulation–modulated strength increases. Med. Sci. Sports Exerc., 17:144–147, 1985.

41. Falcone, A. E., and Spadaro, J. A.: Inhibitory effects of electrically activated silver material on cutaneous wound bacteria. Plast. Reconstr. Surg., 77:455–459, 1986.

42. Fall, M.: Conservative management of chronic interstitial cystitis: Transcutaneous electrical nerve stimulation and transurethral resection. J. Urol., 133:774–778, 1985.

43. Farina, S., Granella, F., Malferrari, G., and Manzoni, C.: Headache and cervical spine disorders: Classification and treatment with transcutaneous electrical nerve stimulation. Headache, 6:431–433, 1986.

44. Fredriksen, T. A., Bergmann, S., Hesselberg, J. P., Stolt-Nielsen, A., Ringkjoh, R., and Sjaastad, O.: Electrical stimulation in multiple sclerosis. Comparison of transcutaneous electrical stimulation and epidural spinal cord stimulation. Appl. Neurophysiol., 49:4–24, 1986.

45. Freeman, T. B., Campbell, J. N., and Long, D. M.: Naloxone does not affect pain relief induced by electrical stimulation in man. Pain, 17:189–195, 1983.

46. Gangarosa, L. P. Sr., Hill, J. M., Thompson, B. L., Leggett, C., and Rissing, J. P.: Iontophoresis of vidarabine monophosphate for herpes orolabialis. J. Infect. Dis., 154:930–934, 1986.

47. Gangarosa, L. P., Park, N. H., Fong, B. C., Scott, D. F., and Hill, J. M.: Conductivity of drugs used for iontophoresis. J. Pharm. Sci., 67:1439–1443, 1978.

48. Garzione, J. E.: Salicylate iontophoresis as an alternative treatment for persistent thigh pain following hip surgery. Phys. Ther., 58:570–571, 1978.

49. Gault, W. R., and Gatens, P. F. Jr.: Use of low intensity direct current in management of ischemic skin ulcers. Phys. Ther., 56:265–268, 1976.

50. Geddes, L. A.: A short history of the electrical stimulation of excitable tissue including electrotherapeutic applications. Physiologist, 27[Suppl.]:515–547, 1984.

51. Glaser, R. M., Gruner, J. A., Feinberg, S. D., and Collins, S. R.: Locomotion via paralyzed leg muscles: Feasibility study for a leg-propelled vehicle. J. Rehabil. Res. Dev., 38:87–92, 1983.

52. Gobelet, C., Follonier, A., Meyland, F., and Maeder, E.: Iontophorèse aux corticöides. Cinésiologie, 21:279–284, 1982.

53. Godec, C., and Cass, A.: Electrical stimulation for voiding dysfunction after spinal cord injury. J. Urol., 121:73–75, 1979.

54. Gordon, B. I., and Maibach, H. I.: Eccrine anhidrosis due to glutaraldehyde, formaldehyde, and iontophoresis. J. Invest. Dermatol., 53:436–439, 1969.

55. Gračanin, F.: Functional electrical stimulation. In Kottke, F. J., Stillwell, G. K., and Lehmann, J. F. (Eds.): Krusen's Handbook of Physical Medi-

cine and Rehabilitation, 3rd Ed. Philadelphia, W. B. Saunders Company, 1982, pp. 372–385.

56. Gračanin, F., and Trnkoczy, A.: Optimal stimulus parameters for minimum pain in the chronic stimulation of innervated muscle. Arch. Phys. Med. Rehabil., 56:243–249, 1975.

57. Greminger, R. F., Elliott, R. A., and Rapperport, A.: Antibiotic iontophoresis for the management of burned ear chondritis. Plast. Reconstr. Surg., 66:356–360, 1980.

58. Hansson, P., Ekblom, A., Thomsson, M., and Fjellner, B.: Influence of naloxone on relief of acute oro-facial pain by transcutaneous electrical nerve stimulation (TENS) or vibration. Pain, 24:323–329, 1986.

59. Harris, R.: Iontophoresis. In Licht, S. (Ed.): Therapeutic Electricity and Ultraviolet Radiation, 2nd Ed. New Haven, CT, Elizabeth Licht, Publisher, 1967, pp. 156–178.

60. Harvie, K. W.: A major advance in the control of postoperative knee pain. Orthopedics, 2:26–27, 1979.

61. Herbert, M. A., and Bobechko, W. P.: Paraspinal muscle stimulation for the treatment of idiopathic scoliosis in children. Orthopedics, 10:1125–1132, 1987.

62. Hughes, L., and Maurice, D. M.: A fresh look at iontophoresis. Arch. Ophthalmol., 102:1825–1829, 1984.

63. Hughes, G. S. Jr., Lichstein, P. R., Whitlock, D., and Harker, C.: Response of plasma beta-endorphins to transcutaneous electrical nerve stimulation in healthy subjects. Phys. Ther., 64:1062–1066, 1984.

64. Hymes, A. C., Yonehiro, E. G., Raab, D. E., Nelson, G. K., and Printy, A. L.: Electrical surface stimulation for treatment and prevention of ileus and atelectasis. Surg. Forum, 25:222–224, 1974.

65. Isakov, E., Mizrahi, J., and Najenson, T.: Biomechanical and physiological evaluation of FES-activated paraplegic patients. J. Rehabil. Res. Dev., 23:9–19, 1986.

66. Jackson, S.: The role of galvanism in the treatment of denervated voluntary muscle in man. Brain, 68:300–330, 1945.

67. Jaeger, R. J.: Design and simulation of closed-loop electrical stimulation orthoses for restoration of quiet standing in paraplegia. J. Biomech., 19:825–835, 1986.

68. James, M. P., Graham, R. M., and English, J.: Percutaneous iontophoresis of prednisolone—a pharmacokinetic study. Clin. Exp. Dermatol., 11:54–61, 1986.

69. Jonas, U., and Hohenfellner, R.: Late results of bladder stimulation in 11 patients: Followup to 4 years. J. Urol., 120:565–568, 1978.

70. Kaada, B.: Vasodilation induced by transcutaneous nerve stimulation in peripheral ischemia (Raynaud's phenomenon and diabetic polyneuropathy). Eur. Heart J., 3:303–314, 1982.

71. Kaada, B.: Promoted healing of chronic ulceration by transcutaneous nerve stimulation (TNS). Vasa, 12:262–269, 1983.

72. Kaada, B., and Eielsen, O.: In search of mediators of skin vasodilation induced by transcutaneous nerve stimulation: I. Failure to block the response by antagonists of endogenous vasodilators. Gen. Pharmacol., 14:623–633, 1983.

73. Kaada, B., and Eielsen, O.: In search of mediators of skin vasodilation induced by transcutaneous nerve stimulation: II. Serotonin implicated. Gen. Pharmacol., 14:635–641, 1983.

74. Kaada, B., and Helle, K. B.: In search of mediators of skin vasodilation induced by transcutaneous nerve stimulation: IV. In vitro bioassay of the vasoinhibitory activity of sera from patients suffering from peripheral ischemia. Gen. Pharmacol., 15:115–122, 1984.

75. Kahn, J.: Acetic acid iontophoresis for calcium deposits. Phys. Ther., 57:658–659, 1977.

76. Kahn, J.: Iontophoresis and ultrasound for postsurgical temporomandibular trismus and paresthesia. Phys. Ther., 60:307–308, 1980.

77. Kahn, J.: Use of iontophoresis in Peyronie's disease: A case report. Phys. Ther., 62:995–996, 1982.

78. Kane, K., and Taub, A.: A history of local electrical analgesia. Pain, 1:125–128, 1975.

79. Kari, B.: Control of blood glucose levels in Alloxan-diabetic rabbits by iontophoresis of insulin. Diabetes, 35:217–221, 1986.

80. Kimball, K. L., Drews, J. E., Walker, S., and Dimick, A. R.: Use of TENS for pain reduction in burn patients receiving travase. J. Burn Care Rehabil., 8:28–31, 1987.

81. Kiwerski, J.: New possibilities of improving the function of the hand of patients with spastic hemiplegia. Int. J. Rehab. Res., 7:293–298, 1984.

82. Kosman, A. J., Osborne, S. L., and Ivy, A. C.: The effect of electrical stimulation upon the course of atrophy and recovery of the gastrocnemius of the rat. Am. J. Phys., 145:447–451, 1946.

83. Kosman, A. J., Osborne, S. L., and Ivy, A. C.: The influence of duration and frequency of treatment in electrical stimulation of paralyzed muscle. Arch. Phys. Med., 28:12–17, 1947.

84. Kramer, J. F.: Effect of electrical stimulation current frequencies on isometric knee extension torque. Phys. Ther., 67:31–38, 1987.

85. Kramer, J., Lindsay, D., Magee, D., Mendryk, S., and Wall, T.: Comparison of voluntary and electrical stimulation contraction torques. J. Orth. Sports Phys. Ther., 5:324–331, 1984.

86. LaForest, N. T., and Cofrancesco, C.: Antibiotic iontophoresis in the treatment of ear chondritis. Phys. Ther., 58:32–34, 1978.

87. Langley, P. L.: Iontophoresis to aid in releasing

tendon adhesions. Suggestions from the field. Phys. Ther., 64:1395, 1984.

88. Layman, P. R., Argyras, E., and Glynn, C. J.: Iontophoresis of vincristine versus saline in postherpetic neuralgia. A controlled trial. Pain, 25:165–170, 1986.

89. Leandri, M., Brunetti, O., and Parodi, C. I.: Telethermographic findings after transcutaneous electrical nerve stimulation. Phys. Ther., 66:210–213, 1986.

90. Lee, W. J., McGovern, J. P., and Duvall, E. N.: Continuous tetanizing (low voltage) currents for relief of spasm: A clinical study of twenty-seven spinal cord injury patients. Arch. Phys. Med. Rehabil., 31:766–771, 1950.

91. Lekas, M. D.: Iontophoresis treatment. Otolaryngol. Head Neck Surg., 87:292–298, 1979.

92. Levine, M. G., Knott, M., and Kabat, H.: Relaxation of spasticity by electrical stimulation of antagonist muscles. Arch. Phys. Med. Rehabil., 33:668–673, 1952.

93. Lewis, D., Lewis, B., and Sturrock, R. D.: Transcutaneous electrical nerve stimulation in osteoarthrosis: A therapeutic alternative? Ann. Rheum. Dis., 43:47–49, 1984.

94. Liberson, W. T., Holmquest, H. J., Scot, D., and Dow, M.: Functional electrotherapy: Stimulation of the peroneal nerve synchronized with the swing phase of the gait of hemiplegic patients. Arch. Phys. Med. Rehabil., 42:101–105, 1961.

95. Liu, C. T., and Lewey, F. H.: The effect of surging currents of low frequency in man on atrophy of denervated muscles. J. Nerv. Ment. Dis., 105:571–581, 1947.

96. Lundeberg, T., Bondesson, L., and Lundstrom, V.: Relief of primary dysmenorrhea by transcutaneous electrical stimulation. Acta Obstet. Gynecol. Scand., 64:491–497, 1985.

97. Lutins, N. D., Greco, G. W., and McFall, W. T. Jr.: Effectiveness of sodium fluoride on tooth hypersensitivity with and without iontophoresis. J. Periodontol., 55:285–288, 1984.

98. Luxenberg, M. N., and Guthrie, T. H. Jr.: Chemotherapy of eyelid and periorbital tumors. Trans. Am. Ophthalmol. Soc., 83:162–180, 1985.

99. Mannheimer, C., and Carlsson, C.: The analgesic effect of transcutaneous electrical nerve stimulation (TNS) in patients with rheumatoid arthritis. A comparative study of different pulse patterns. Pain, 6:329–334, 1979.

100. Mannheimer, C., Carlsson, C., Vedin, A., and Wilhelmsson, C.: Transcutaneous electrical nerve stimulation (TENS) in angina pectoris. Pain, 26:291–300, 1986.

101. Mao, W., Ghia, J. N., Scott, D. S., Duncan, G. H., and Gregg, J. M.: High versus low intensity acupuncture analgesia for treatment of chronic pain: Effects on platelet serotonin. Pain, 8:331–342, 1980.

102. Marcer, M., Musatti, G., and Bassett, C. A. L.: Results of pulsed electromagnetic fields (PEMFs) in ununited fractures after external skeletal fixation. Clin. Orthop., 190:260–265, 1984.

103. Marsolais, E. B., and Kobetic, R.: Implantation techniques and experience with percutaneous intramuscular electrodes in the lower extremities. J. Rehabil. Res. Dev., 23:1–8, 1986.

104. Massey, B. H., Nelson, R. C., Sharkey, B. C., and Comden, T.: Effects of high frequency electrical stimulation on the size and strength of skeletal muscle. Sports Med. Phys. Fit., 5:136–144, 1965.

105. Melzack, R., and Wall, P. D.: Pain mechanisms: A new theory. Science, 150:971–979, 1965.

106. Mohr, T., Carlson, B., Sulentic, C., and Landry, R.: Comparison of isometric exercise and high volt galvanic stimulation on quadriceps femoris muscle strength. Phys. Ther., 65:606–612, 1985.

107. Morrissey, M. C., Brewster, C. E., Shields, C. L. Jr., and Brown, M.: The effects of electrical stimulation on the quadriceps during postoperative knee immobilization. Am. J. Sports Med., 13:40–45, 1985.

108. Mosforth, J., and Taverner, D.: Physiotherapy for Bell's palsy. Br. Med. J., 2:675–677, 1958.

109. Nakamura, M., and Sakurai, T.: Bladder inhibition by penile electrical stimulation. J. Urol., 56:413–415, 1984.

110. Nakamura, M., Sakurai, T., Tsujimoto, Y., and Tada, Y.: Bladder inhibition by electrical stimulation of the perianal skin. Urol. Int., 41:62–63, 1986.

111. Nashold, B. S. Jr., Grimes, J., Friedman, H., Semans, J., and Avery, R.: Operative stimulation of the neurogenic bladder. Neurosurgery, 1:218–220, 1977.

112. Newton, R. A., and Karselis, T. C.: Skin pH following high voltage pulsed galvanic stimulation. Phys. Ther., 63:1593–1596, 1983.

113. O'Brien, W. J., Rutan, F. M., Sanborn, C., and Omer, G. E.: Effect of transcutaneous electrical nerve stimulation on human blood beta-endorphin levels. Phys. Ther., 64:1367–1374, 1984.

114. Oleson, T. D., and Kroening, R. J.: A comparison of Chinese and Nogier auricular acupuncture points. Am. J. Acupunct., 11:205–223, 1983.

115. Ordog, G. J.: Transcutaneous electrical nerve stimulation versus oral analgesic: A randomized double-blind controlled study in acute traumatic pain. Am. J. Emerg. Med., 5:6–10, 1987.

116. Osborne, S. L.: The retardation of atrophy in man by electrical stimulation of muscles. Arch. Phys. Med., 32:523–528, 1951.

117. Osborne, S. L., Kosman, A. J., Bouman, H. D., McElvenny, R. T., and Ivy, A. C.: Anterior poliomyelitis; early and late electrical stimulation of the muscles. Surg. Gynaecol. Obstet., 88:243–253, 1949.

118. Parry, C. B. W.: Pain in avulsion of the brachial plexus. Neurosurgery, 15:960–965, 1984.

119. Passali, D., Bellussi, L., and Masieri, S.: Transtympanic iontophoresis: Personal experience. Laryngoscope, 94:802–806, 1984.

120. Perdikis, P.: Transcutaneous nerve stimulation in the treatment of protracted ileus. S. Afr. J. Surg., 15:81–86, 1977.

121. Petrofsky, J. S., and Phillips, C. A.: The use of functional electrical stimulation for rehabilitation of spinal cord injured patients. CNS Trauma, 1:57–74, 1984.

122. Petrofsky, J. S., and Phillips, C. A.: Closed-loop control of movement of skeletal muscle. CRC Crit. Rev. Biomed. Eng., 13:35–96, 1985.

123. Phillips, C. A., Petrofsky, J. S., Hendershot, D. M., and Stafford, D.: Functional electrical exercise. A comprehensive approach for physical conditioning of the spinal cord injured patient. Orthopedics, 7:1112–1123, 1984.

124. Pike, P. M. H.: Transcutaneous electrical stimulation. Its use in the management of postoperative pain. Anesthesia, 33:165–171, 1978.

125. Pratzel, H., Dittrich, P., and Kukovetz, W.: Spontaneous and forced cutaneous absorption of indomethacin in pigs and humans. J. Rheumatol., 13:1122–1125, 1986.

126. Rebersek, I. S., and Vodovnik, L.: Proportionally controlled functional electrical stimulation of hand. Arch. Phys. Med. Rehabil., 54:378–382, 1973.

127. Riley, L. H. Jr., and Richter, C. P.: Uses of the electrical skin resistance method in the study of patients with neck and upper extremity pain. Johns Hopkins Med. J., 137:69–74, 1975.

128. Robinson, K. R.: The responses of cells to electrical fields: A review. J. Cell Biol., 101:2023–2027, 1985.

129. Robson, J. E.: Forum, Transcutaneous nerve stimulation for pain relief in labour. Anesthesia, 34:357–360, 1979.

130. Roche, P. A., Gijsbers, K., Belch, J. J., and Forbes, C. D.: Modification of induced ischaemic pain by transcutaneous electrical nerve stimulation. Pain, 20:45–52, 1984.

131. Roche, P. A., Gijsbers, K., Belch, J. J. F., and Forbes, C. D.: Modification of haemophiliac haemorrhage pain by transcutaneous electrical nerve stimulation. Pain, 21:43–48, 1985.

132. Rooney, S. M., Jain, S., McCormack, P., Bains, M. S., Martini, N., and Goldiner, P. L.: A comparison of pulmonary function tests for postthoracotomy pain using cryoanalgesia and transcutaneous nerve stimulation. Ann. Thorac. Surg., 41:204–207, 1986.

133. Rosenberg, M., Curtis, L., and Bourke, D. L.: Transcutaneous electrical nerve stimulation for the relief of postoperative pain. Pain, 5:129–133, 1978.

134. St. Pierre, D., Taylor, A. W., Lavoie, M., Sellers, W., and Kotts, Y. M.: Effects of 2500 Hz sinusoidal current on fibre area and strength of the quadriceps femoris. J. Sports Med. Phys. Fit., 26:60–66, 1986.

135. Satyanand, E. I., Saxena, A. K., and Agarwal, A.: Silver iontophoresis in chronic osteomyelitis. J. Indian Med. Assoc., 84:134–136, 1986.

136. Scholz, H., and Schmidt, L.: Treatment of chronic constipation: Electrotherapy and diet. Br. J. Phys. Med., 15:254–256, 1952.

137. Schuster, G. K., and Infante, M. C.: Pain relief after low back surgery: The efficacy of transcutaneous electrical nerve stimulation. Pain, 8:299–302, 1980.

138. Selkowitz, D. M.: Improvement in isometric strength of the quadriceps femoris muscle after training with electrical stimulation. Phys. Ther., 65:186–196, 1985.

139. Sjölund, B. H., and Eriksson, M. B. E.: The influence of naloxone on analgesia produced by peripheral conditioning stimulation. Brain Res., 173:295–301, 1979.

140. Sjölund, B. H., Terenius, L., and Eriksson, M. B. E.: Increased cerebrospinal fluid levels of endorphins after electro-acupuncture. Acta Physiol. Scand., 10:382–384, 1977.

141. Sloan, J. P., Muwanga, C. L., Waters, E. A., Dove, A. F., and Dave, S. H.: Multiple rib fractures: Transcutaneous nerve stimulation versus conventional analgesia. J. Trauma, 26:1120–1122, 1986.

142. Smith, C. M., Guralnick, M. S., Gelfand, M. M., and Jeans, M. E.: The effects of transcutaneous electrical nerve stimulation of post-cesarean pain. Pain, 27:181–193, 1986.

143. Stanish, W. D., Valiant, G. A., Bonen, A., and Belcastro, A. N.: The effects of immobilization and of electrical stimulation on muscle glycogen and myofibrillar ATPase. Can. J. Appl. Sport Sci., 7:267–271, 1982.

144. Stefanovska, A., and Vodovnik, L.: Change in muscle force following electrical stimulation. Dependence on stimulation waveform and frequency. Scand. J. Rehabil. Med., 17:141–146, 1985.

145. Stewart, P.: Transcutaneous nerve stimulation as a method of analgesia in labour. Anesthesia, 34:361–364, 1979.

146. Tannebaum, M.: Iodine iontophoresis in reducing scar tissue. Phys. Ther., 60:792, 1980.

147. Vernon, J. A., and Fenwick, J. A.: Attempts to suppress tinnitus with transcutaneous electrical stimulation. Otolaryngol. Head Neck Surg., 93:385–389, 1985.

148. Vodovnik, L., Bajd, T., Kralj, A., Gračanin, F., and Strojnik, P.: Functional electrical stimulation for control of locomotor systems. CRC Crit. Rev. Bioeng., 6:63–131, 1981.

149. Wehrmacher, W. H., Thomson, J. D., and Hines, H. M.: Effects of electrical stimulation of dener-

vated skeletal muscle. Arch. Phys. Med., 26:261–266, 1945.

150. White, J. W. Jr.: Treatment of primary hyperhidrosis. Mayo Clin. Proc., 61:951–956, 1986.

151. Wolcott, L. E., Wheeler, P. C., Hardwicke, H. M., and Rowley, B. A.: Accelerated healing of skin ulcers by electrotherapy: Preliminary clinical results. South. Med. J., 62:795–801, 1969.

152. Wong, R. A., and Jette, D. U.: Changes in sympathetic tone associated with different forms of transcutaneous electrical nerve stimulation in healthy subjects. Phys. Ther., 64:478–482, 1984.

153. Woolf, C. J., Mitchell, D., Myers, R. A., and Barrett, G. D.: Failure of naloxone to reverse peripheral transcutaneous electro-analgesia in patients suffering from acute trauma. S. Afr. Med. J., 53:179–180, 1978.

154. Yamamoto, E., and Nishimura, H.: Treatment of hemifacial spasm with transcutaneous electrical stimulation. Laryngoscope, 97:458–460, 1987.

16 Acupuncture in Physiatry

MATHEW H. M. LEE   SUNG J. LIAO

In the past decade the concept of acupuncture has burst upon the Western mind as a potential therapeutic tool for the treatment of chronic pain. This development has brought with it the suggestion that there might be other dimensions to health care than had been visualized previously here in the Western world. Vaguely unsettling to our accustomed ways of thinking, this idea is both exciting and challenging.

As so often happens in history, political developments and the opening of new channels of communication between cultures result in serendipitous rewards that are totally unexpected. The recent rapprochement of the People's Republic of China and the United States is a prime example of this kind of interrelatedness between international politics and cultural interchange. Because of this development, Western medicine began to examine seriously the potentials of acupuncture as a mode of therapy while a small but advanced segment of Chinese medicine had already taken steps to explore acupuncture in the context of modern scientific methods.

A chapter on acupuncture as it relates particularly to the practicing physiatrist may be controversial, but there is persuasive evidence that it should be seriously considered among the therapeutic armamentarium of physiatry.

For the purpose of reviewing acupuncture for fellow physiatrists, we shall attempt to concentrate on its modern scientific bases and briefly discuss its clinical applications. To provide some background, we offer a short discourse on its history and its traditional pathophysiological or physiologic-alchemic theorems. Although acupuncture has been used for a vast variety of conditions, for the purpose of this book, we will confine our discussion to the clinical application of acupuncture to the *chronic painful conditions* commonly seen in physiatric practice. As is the case with many other physical modalities, there is a dearth of strict, statistically designed double-blind studies of the clinical efficacy of acupuncture in humans. In order to provide a better understanding of the similarities between Western and Eastern cultures, we have also listed some comparable Western medical events contemporaneous to those in the field of acupuncture whenever possible. In sharing our experience with the readers, we hope to stimulate them to apply this alternative healing art to complement and supplement other physiatric modalities.

Historical Development

The word "acupuncture," from two Latin words, *acus* (needle) and *punctura* (puncture), was probably coined by Jesuit missionaries in the 17th century who were impressed by its effectiveness. Acupuncture originated in China in prehistoric times and is as indigenous and unique as the Chinese language. Sharp flakes of flint stones were probably inserted for healing purposes originally, but as technology advanced, bamboo splinters, bronze, iron from the bit of a horse's bridle, gold, silver, and now stainless steel have been used to make the needles. The stone used for acupuncture was referred to in *San Hai Jing (Classic of Mountains and Seas)*, which dates from the fifth century B.C. Silk scrolls and wooden strips used for recording medical texts, including acupuncture, were found in the tomb of a marquise and that of her son (burial date, 168 B.C.) at Mawangdui in Hunan Province. Gold acupuncture needles were found in the tomb of a prince (burial date, 113 B.C.) near

Beijing. The entire body of medical knowledge was probably crystallized in the compilation of the first book, *Su Wen (Book of Common Questions,* dating back to the second century B.C.), and the second book, *Ling Shu (Book of Acupuncture,* dating back to the first century B.C.), of *Huang Di Nei Jing (Yellow Emperor's Classic of Internal Medicine).* According to the chapter "Unusual Modalities" in the *Book of Common Questions,* and the chapter "Jade Plates" in the *Book of Acupuncture,* stone needles were originally used for treating abscesses. The chapter "Nine Needles and Twelve Origins" in the *Book of Acupuncture* states that fine needles rather than stone needles were used to animate the meridians and to harmonize blood and *qi* for muscular or soft tissue conditions. (*Qi* may be roughly conceived as the vital forces that appear in a variety of forms, depending on the conditions involved, and that must be normalized to restore the healthy state.) Bas-relief stone carvings of a legendary physician practicing acupuncture existed in the first century A.D.

In the latter part of the 17th century, physicians of the Dutch East India Company, such as Jacob de Bondt, Andreas Cleyer, and Willem ten Rhijne, were most likely the first Europeans to write about acupuncture (including illustrations of points and meridians) after observing it in the Dutch Indies and Japan (possibly not having journeyed to China proper). Soulie de Morand reintroduced traditional Chinese acupuncture to France during the 1930s[28] and then to the rest of Europe.

It was known in this country as early as 1825 when Bache[1] published his own case reports and translated de Morand's case report from French to English.[117] By the 1860s its use had declined, for the most part because of infections due to unsterile techniques.[79] Osler (1849–1919), one of the greats of modern medicine, indicated its effectiveness in the treatment of lumbago, suggesting the use of sterilized "ordinary bonnet-needles" in his textbook[124] from its first edition (1892) through its 14th edition (1944). Osler was taught the use of acupuncture by Ringer (1835–1910) of Ringer's solution fame.[26] Subsequently, acupuncture was practically forgotten by the American medical profession until 1971, when acupuncture analgesia was demonstrated to two eminent American physician-educators by the Chinese[29] and James Reston reported on the relief acupuncture afforded him from post-appendectomy complications he suffered while in China.[142] In the spring and, again, in the summer of 1972, the first recent tutorials were organized by us in the field of acupuncture for physicians and dentists in this country.

Electroacupuncture

With the advent of Volta's pile in 1799, the stimulation of muscles with electricity became possible. In 1816, Berlioz, father of the famous composer Louis Hector Berlioz, recorded the use of electrified acupuncture for the treatment of pain. Sarlandiere coined the word "electropuncture," following the techniques of Japanese acupuncture, for treatment of rheumatism and pain, publishing a book on the subject in 1825. In 1834 da Camin used Leyden jars for electropuncture. Duchenne (1806–1875), the father of neurology, started to experiment with electroacupuncture in 1833 and eventually developed the electrical stimulation technique using skin electrodes (without piercing the skin),[105] which essentially formed the basic concept of modern electrotherapy as well as the currently popular transcutaneous electrical nerve stimulation technique. The cervical vertebrae of a patient were allegedly fractured when Duchenne used electroacupuncture for therapy.[105] The use of large needles, which caused pain, and the inability to fine-tune the current with the crude electrical instruments available at that time were the most likely contributing factors to the relative unpopularity of electroacupuncture or electropuncture at that time. In addition, with the controversial nature of acupuncture in Europe then, electroacupuncture was almost forgotten. Electroacupuncture was "rediscovered" by the Chinese in the 1950s.[24]

Auricular Acupuncture

In the traditional Chinese literature, scattered statements about the importance of the ear relative to health and disease can be found as early as the *Yellow Emperor's Classic of Internal Medicine.* However, no specific acupoints were indicated on the auricles, nor did any meridians specifically traverse them. Around 1956, reports appeared both in China and in France that the diagnosis and treatment of illnesses could be attained through needling or stimulating specific points on the auricles. The Chinese claimed that in 1956, patients with painful throats were successfully treated with auricular acupuncture in a rural health station. According to Lu and Needham,[106] around 1950 a

MATHEW H. M. LEE AND SUNG J. LIAO

rural healer in southeastern France cured sciatica by cauterizing the auricles. In 1956–1957, Nogier, also of France, first reported his techniques of auricular acupuncture, later refining them in 1972.[123]

Acupressure

In the early seventh century, China began to establish a medical education system. The Imperial Medical College, the hierarchy of the system, was organized in A.D. 624 with Departments of Medicine (i.e., Herbal Medicine), Acupuncture, Massage, and so on. The Massage Department had a larger teaching staff than the Acupuncture Department. Massage was applied to acupoints as one of many massage techniques rather than being singled out as something special, as acupressure and reflexology have been recently in this country. Incidentally, even to this day, the specialty of massage in traditional Chinese medicine also includes manipulation, termed "push-pull." At one time, massage was almost exclusively performed by the blind in China, since nudity, in the presence of a stranger, was considered indecent. In Japan, such massage techniques are termed *shiatsu*, literally translated as finger pressure.

Traditional Physiologico-Alchemic Theorems

Essentially philosophical in nature, the traditional pathophysiological or, rather, physiologico-alchemic theorems regarded the human body (the microcosm) as a miniature model of the universe (the macrocosm) with the laws that governed the former following those of the latter. Many ancient cultures held fairly similar views, although none elaborated on them as thoroughly as the ancient Chinese did more than two and one half millennia ago.[91] By that time, China already had an abundance of divergent philosophies.[41] Books written then are still quite comprehensible to this very day without having to resort to something like the Rosetta stone. Their recording of the acupuncture system was so methodical that it has been used as the foundation for practice throughout the millennia.

The Taoist religious philosophy, which included the concepts of eternal life, prevention of illness, and promotion of health based on the concept of continual harmonic balance of opposites in nature and in the human body, dominated the field of medicine in the ancient times. A master of Taoism was awarded the title of *Zhen Ren* (the "True Man," or an "Immortal"). Some of them became recluses or hermits so that they could concentrate on their practice of Tao without the disturbances of their worldly environs. They attempted to achieve immortality and eternity by practicing breathing exercises *(Qi Gong)*, sunbathing (heliotherapy), gymnastic exercises, sexual techniques, and dietary management. Incidentally, the Chinese therapeutic exercises that were publicized by the Jesuit missionary to China, Father J. M. Amiot (*Mémoires Concernant l'Histoire, les Sciences et les Arts des Chinois*, Paris, 1779, Vol. IV), apparently inspired Per Henrik Ling (1776–1839) of Sweden to introduce "movement and cure" and, thus, to lay the foundation of modern physical therapy.[121] Since they were also technocrats and physiological alchemists, they tended to adapt natural events to traditional acupuncture with Taoism's interpretations, sometimes compounding medicine with its mystique. They embraced the philosophy of the *Yin-Yang Jia* (the Naturalist School) as the basic principle of the practice of medicine. In nature, as there are moon and sun, night and day, darkness and brightness, grand void and supreme infinity, female and male, negative and positive, reaction and action, and so on, so there are *yin* and *yang*. These two opposite forces have always coexisted simultaneously in the universe, as well as in our bodies in various proportions, operating harmoniously. The basic premise is that an equilibrium exists between these two opposing forces *(yin* and *yang)* in the body. From endocrinological studies, we know that there are small amounts of female sex hormones in the male, and male hormones in the female, gynecomastia in a male patient with cirrhosis of the liver being an appropriate example. Our autonomic nervous system consists of two opposing parts: the sympathetic and the parasympathetic. It was stated in the *Yellow Emperor's Classic of Internal Medicine* that there exist 360 acupuncture points (acupoints) corresponding with the 360 days in a year (according to the Chinese lunar calendar); however, an actual count reveals only 295 acupoints. Apparently, the Chinese discovered acupuncture points first, and then later hypothesized the meridian system, which evolved out of the typical Chinese disposition to organize these acupuncture points into a comprehensible system. The points were organized, essentially according to their assumed clinical function, into 12 main meridians (or channels) to coincide with the ancient Chinese system of 12 time intervals in the day. An analogous method for the classification of Nature might be found, albeit on a grand scale, in the Linnaean botanical and zoological systems that appeared more than 700 years later. As a matter of fact, in veterinary acupuncture there are acupoints but no meridians.[93, 94, 102]

Over the years, acupuncture has been developed into an intricate and complex holistic system of *yin* and *yang*, circulation of *qi* and *blood*, interaction of the *five elements*, circadian rhythm, and so on. In addition to the maintenance of an equilibrium between the two opposing forces *(yin* and *yang)* in the body, there is free and incessant circulation of *qi* along the meridians in the outer layers of the body and blood in its inner parts. Sickness results from a disturbance of the balance between *yin* and *yang*. This emphasis on the necessity of a balance between two opposing forces *(yin* and *yang)* in our body in order to maintain good health has a modern equivalent in Cannon's (1871–1945) concept of equilibrium of the internal environment, homeostasis.[11, 12] Stagnation of *qi* or blood along the meridians also may cause illness. Thus, acupuncture would be used to bring *yin* and *yang* into balance or to release the stagnation of *qi* or blood. The concept of circulation of *qi* and blood was first recorded in the book *Guanzi*, dating from the latter part of the fourth century B.C. Whereas the importance of circadian rhythm was recognized as early as A.D. 124, the concept did not evolve into mathematical formulae to determine appropriate acupuncture points for treating certain conditions until 1418.

In a similar way, Hippocrates (c. 460–400 B.C.) and the Hippocratic school of ancient Greece taught that the humors—blood (air), black bile (earth), yellow bile (fire), and phlegm (water)—composed the essence of medicine. The Chinese counterparts of the same period in history can be found in the five elements (water, fire, wood, metal, and earth) of traditional Chinese acupuncture. The concept of the "five elements" first appeared in the chapter "Hung Fan" (the "Grand Norm") of the *Book of History* (dated to the fourth to third century B.C.). Zou Yan (c. 305–240 B.C.), a major exponent of the *yin-yang* school of philosophy, innovated the concept of the interaction of the five "elements," according to Sima Qian's (c. 145–86 B.C.) *Shi Ji* (or Historical Records). During the fourth and third centuries B.C., there was already extensive commercial traffic along the Silk Road between China and India, Persia, Arabia,

and Asia Minor. It is quite conceivable that at that time there were cultural exchanges among Chinese, Ayurvedic, Arabic, and Grecian medicine to account for their certain similarities. Incidentally, the original Chinese term for five "elements" is five *xing*, which means activity, function, power, to walk, or to act. It is dynamic and cannot really be represented by a static word, "element." Those who would like to explore this fascinating matter further may refer to Fung[41] and Huard and Wong.[58] Environmental elements, such as humidity and dryness, coldness and heat, were regarded as contributory, if not causative, determinants of an ailment. Biological factors such as age and sex were further taken into consideration in the diagnosis and treatment with acupuncture.

Although such concepts were regarded as quite scientific for their day 2500 years ago, in today's research, thus far, there has been no reproducible scientific evidence to confirm the actual anatomical existence of acupoints or meridians. Just as we do not practice medicine today as Hippocrates did, there seems to be no need to adhere to such antiquated concepts in this high-technology era.

We hasten to point out that the connotations of anatomical and physiological terminology used in traditional Chinese acupuncture are vastly different from those in current use in Western medicine. For example, "lung" in acupuncture relates to skin diseases; "kidney" is concerned with the genital system; "spleen" regulates digestive functions. Basically, since acupuncture is problem-oriented and *quasi* organ-oriented, some of the meridians originated from a viscus and were named after it (e.g., the Shaoyin Heart Meridian of the Hand); some terminated in a viscus (e.g., the Taiyang Small Intestine Meridian of the Hand); while others passed through a viscus (e.g., the Shaoyang Kidney Meridian of the Foot). The ancient Chinese even invented some nonexistent organs, such as Sanjiao (Triple Warmer), to complete their schematics. They divided the viscera into two broad categories: *Zang*, the parenchymatous ones; and *Fu*, the hollow ones. There were six parenchymatous organs: heart, liver, spleen, lung, kidney, and heart-envelope (or pericardium). There were six hollow organs: gallbladder, stomach, small intestine, large intestine, urinary bladder, and Sanjiao.[99] In addition, there is extensive overlapping of symptoms as represented by the meridian system. The meanings of many of the terms are not always clear-cut and, sometimes, are even confusing. For those who would like to pursue the fine points a bit more, please refer to Liao[87] and Lu and Needham.[106]

Coincidental with the intrusion of acupuncture into American medicine, interest in the scientific investigation of pain has been rekindled, which, in turn, has helped to advance the understanding of acupuncture.

Biological Equivalents of Acupoints and Meridians

Acupoints relevant to a particular condition are generally tender to palpation. It has been found that about 80 per cent of all acupoints coincide with *trigger points*.[88] Melzack, Stillwell, and Fox[115] also demonstrated "a remarkably high degree (71 per cent) of correspondence" between trigger points and acupuncture points. They commented, "this close correlation suggests that trigger points and acupuncture points for pain, though discovered independently and labelled differently, represent the same phenomenon and can be explained in terms of the underlying neural mechanism."

Many acupoints coincide with the motor points of skeletal muscles,[91] e.g., Hegu point* (Large Intestine 4 [LI 4]) with the motor point of the first dorsal interosseous muscle of the hand; Jianjing point (Gall Bladder 21 [GB 21]) with that of the upper trapezius muscle; and Zusanli point (Stomach 36 [ST 36]) with that of the tibialis anticus muscle. Only the smallest amount of electricity is required to evoke contractions of a muscle when applied to its acupuncture point. Acupoints do possess certain biological characteristics, such as having high electrical conductivity and emitting spontaneous electrical discharges.[87]

In addition to the Hegu, Jianjing, and Zusanli points, the following points might also be chosen:

JIACHE (ST 6):
masseter muscle

TIANZHONG (SI 11):
infraspinatus muscle

LIANGMEN (ST 21):
rectus abdominis muscle

XIAOLUO (T 12):
triceps muscle

---

*In order to conform to the current trend, the official Chinese Romanized spelling system, Hanyu Pinyin, is used for all the Chinese words in this presentation. The alphanumeric notations of the acupoints are appended for easy identification.

XIMEN (P 4):
flexor digitorum superficialis muscle

XUEHAI (SP 10):
vastus medialis muscle

JIMEN (SP 11):
sartorius muscle

These offer a wide distribution of such acupoints on the head, trunk, and limbs.

The skin around an acupoint may be erythematous after insertion of an acupuncture needle. This is probably a part of the triple response (i.e., the red reaction, the spreading flush or flare, and local edema or wheal) of the skin to local stimulation, although local edema or wheal is very rarely seen. This is probably attributable to the H-substance of Lewis[83] liberated by the injured cells of the epidermis between the horny layer and the papilla of the skin or of the deeper tissues. Due to hyperalgesia in cutaneous injury, as suggested by Hardy and colleagues,[53] the skin becomes erythematous in addition to painful. Thus, Lewis suggested the term "erythralgia."[83] H-substance or some histamine-like compound is said to be responsible for causing both pain and vasodilation.[143]

It is essential to obtain a *de qi* response, or needling sensation, while the needle is manipulated in order to attain a satisfactory therapeutic result. These sensations can be demonstrable only if the needle is inserted in the proper acupoint at an appropriate depth. The *de qi* responses are described as soreness, numbness, warmth, heaviness, and a distended feeling. Wang and associates[165] found that group II afferent fibers conveyed a numb feeling, group III fibers a heavy and distended feeling, and group IV fibers a sore feeling. We may find an analogy of the *de qi* response in Sherrington's designation of pain as nociceptive in the sense that it is a protective response to intensified or noxious stimuli.[144]

Patients with chronic pain tend to have lower temperature gradients in the affected areas than in the corresponding normal parts of the body when examined by thermography. The application of acupuncture at points distant from the affected areas not only reduces pain, but also increases temperature.[100] Clark[25] reported a hyperthermic effect of met-enkephalin in cats. Bloom and co-workers[5] found that beta-endorphins produce hypothermia and gamma-endorphins hyperthermia in rats. Lee and Ernst[77] attributed the change of temperature and reduction of pain to an involvement of the autonomic nervous system.

While we are discussing referred pain, it seems

appropriate to summarize briefly the segmental nature of the sensory dermatomes. Five major experimental methods have been employed for its determination: (1) Sherrington's remaining sensibility method, (2) Head's clinical observation of herpes eruptions and referred pain in visceral diseases, (3) Foerster's vasodilation method, (4) Lewis's injection of irritants, and (5) Keegan and Garrett's clinical observation of herniation of intervertebral nucleus pulposus.

Using the remaining sensibility technique in monkeys, Sherrington demonstrated experimentally extensive overlapping of the sensory innervation by the posterior spinal nerve roots, although in a segmental fashion.[156]

Head, Sherrington's contemporary, drew his conclusions from extensive and astute studies of the distribution of herpes zoster lesions and the cutaneous hyperesthesia of visceral diseases. He found rather little overlapping of the segmental nature of skin lesions and sensibility.[54–56]

Foerster[39] stimulated the distal part of a divided posterior spinal nerve root of his patients with the faradic current and observed the resultant vasodilation. He found the areas of vasodilation having little overlapping, similar to Head's zones. However, when he traced the areas of cutaneous sensory changes with his "constructive" technique, he found their distributions having extensive overlapping similar to Sherrington's dermatomes. He speculated that two separate sets of nerve fibers were involved: the very fine myelinated fibers for the vasodilation, and the thick myelinated fibers for the sensory changes.

Kellgren[69, 70] injected 6 per cent hypertonic saline into interspinous ligaments, causing irritation of the posterior spinal nerve root. He observed pain in a well-defined segmental pattern with overlapping. Lewis and Kellgren[83, 84] demonstrated in decapitated cats "no specific form of pain, referred or otherwise" and that "pain of visceral or somatic origin cannot be distinguished as such." They concluded, "deep somatic and certain visceral structures are supplied by a common set of afferent nerves (including pain nerves)." In decapitated cats, stimulation of a viscus, mesentery or bowel itself, caused a rise of blood pressure. This seems to represent additional evidence of an involvement of the autonomic nervous system.

Feinstein and associates' methodical experiment[37] demonstrated that the *deep somatic pain* from segmental injection of paravertebral muscles of humans with 6 per cent hypertonic saline was referred regionally to several dermatomes with extensive overlapping. This referred pain could not be inhibited by sympathetic ganglion block or by peripheral nerve plexus block. They also observed muscle spasm in the areas of referred pain. Contrary to the previously reported hyperesthesia as in Sherrington's monkeys, in Head's zones, and by Lewis's irritant, they observed hypalgesia in the areas of referred pain. This is quite analogous to acupuncture analgesia. They emphasized the concomitant autonomic reactions, including pallor, sweating (often generalized), bradycardia, fall in blood pressure, subjective "faintness," nausea but no vomiting, and rarely syncope. They ascribed their results to a central spinal integrative mechanism.

Keegan and Garrett[68] observed pain and weakness of the limbs in patients who had herniation of the intervertebral nuclei pulposus compressing a single spinal nerve too and who were relieved by surgical decompression, as well as the effects of procaine injection of single nerves in medical students. They demonstrated continuous nonoverlapping bands from the spine into the limbs.

Most of the reports mentioned in the preceding section not only mapped out the segmental sensory distribution, overlapping or otherwise, but, just as important, also commented on the evoked autonomic reactions. A better understanding of the involvement of the autonomic nervous system may indeed help us to explain the discrepancies of the results obtained by the different methods as well as to increase our knowledge of the mechanisms of acupuncture.

Head reported that a diseased organ that might produce a dull aching sensation locally would provoke a sharp or stabbing pain with marked localized tenderness at a distant part of the body.[54–56] He suggested a central inhibitory interaction between pain and other forms of sensation. It should be noted here that visceral pain is a deep sensation, may or may not be referred, and usually is not well localized. Angina-like pain is reproducible by injection of hypertonic saline into the first thoracic interspinous ligament.[83] This is an exception rather than the rule. It is well recognized but not well emphasized that pain of the deep somatic tissues, either pathologically evoked or experimentally induced, tends to be referred to more than one single dermatome or to contiguous parts of several dermatomes with wide individual differences.[143] It is fairly commonly accompanied by reflex sympathetic dysfunctions, such as cold perspiration, lightheadedness from bradycardia or hypotension, nausea, sustained and diffuse but spontaneous muscle contractions (variously described as muscle rigidity or muscle spasm), and less commonly vomiting. Although such referred pain is often designated as aberrant or nonclassical because it does not follow the conventional dermatome supplied by the particular superficial nerve of the involved segment, it does, in fact, spread in consistent patterns to the deeper tissues, the myotomes and sclerotomes, which are innervated from the same segmental level of the spinal cord. Since it is not explicable by the classical concepts of the decerebrated reflex physiology of Sherrington's tradition, clinicians tend to reject the patient's complaints of such symptoms as psychogenic or embellishment for secondary gains. Such a designation is unwarranted.

There is a divergence of the cutaneous sensory nerve distribution and the nerve supply of the underlying deeper tissues.[59] For example, the C 4 spinal nerve supplies the skin of the infraclavicular region and the top of the shoulder. For treating hiccups, the Jianjing point (GB 21) on top of the shoulder is sometimes used. In addition, one suspects that the autonomic nervous distribution may be much different from the sensory and motor distributions in the same area. The *de qi* response provoked from needling the acupoints in the shoulder may be experienced not only locally but also as far away as in the dorsum of the hand, although this relates to the sclerotome distribution of nerves rather than the dermatome distribution.[59] It is altogether plausible that the autonomic nervous system is implicated in the meridian system of acupuncture and that the stimuli of acupuncture share the same pathways as those of referred pain but in the opposite direction. The challenge of integrating these observations with recent discoveries in neuroanatomy and neuropharmacology of pain and acupuncture mechanisms awaits further investigation.

Acupuncture Analgesia

Neural Mechanisms

The analgesic or hypalgesic effects of acupuncture were not explained scientifically until the 1970s. In 1973 it was reported that local infiltration with procaine at acupoints impeded the analgesic effects of acupuncture, whereas subcutaneous infiltration of a local anesthetic at the same sites did not.[21, 127, 145] This implicated the sensory receptors at the acupoint and their group II and group III small myelinated muscle afferent fibers of the peripheral nerve in the transmission of the impulses as generated by needling.

Electrical stimulation at the Futu point of the Neck (Large Intestine 18 [LI 18], located at the midpoint along the posterior border of the sternocleidomastoid muscle) can induce sufficient analgesia for thyroidectomy in humans.[4] The Futu point of the Neck is supplied by the cervical cutaneous nerve, which receives fibers from the C 3 spinal nerve root. The capsule of the thyroid gland is also innervated by the C 3 spinal segment. By recording electrical discharges of the brain with microelectrodes, it was demonstrated that the impulses from noxious stimuli to the tail of a rabbit could be blocked by acupuncture at its hind leg but not at its front leg.[14] The hind leg of a rabbit shares with its tail the nerve supplies from the same spinal segments, whereas the front leg does not. From the observations of these experiments, it seems that the analgesic effects of acupuncture are transmitted segmentally. In addition, it was demonstrated that analgesic effects have not only a segmental but also a bilateral distribution.[21, 22]

In hemiplegic patients, needling at the Hegu point (LI 4) or Zusanli point (ST 36) of the affected limbs did not induce analgesia; however, a similar maneuver on the normal limbs did.[127] In paraplegic patients, acupuncture at the Hegu point (LI 4) of the hand generated analgesia, whereas needling at the Zusanli point (ST 36) of the leg did not.[127] Spinal anesthesia eliminated *de qi* responses (the needling sensations) and the evoked myoelectrical potentials at acupuncture points.[127] These observations suggested that the integrity of the central nervous system is mandatory for the achievement of acupuncture analgesia.

In 1975, Chiang and associates[22] reported that the acupuncture stimuli were transmitted cephalad along the extralemniscal system (the spinoreticular, spinomesocephalic, and paleospinothalamic tracts) in the ventral two thirds of the lateral funiculus of the spinal cord, projecting to the reticular formation, central gray matter, and medial thalamic nuclei. Wall and Drubner[164] found that group I afferent activities were transmitted in the dorsal and ventral spinocerebellar tracts, but groups II and III afferent activities were mainly transmitted in the spinoreticular tracts. Chang[14] found that electroacupuncture at a certain acupoint, squeezing the Achilles tendon, or weak electrical stimulation of a sensory nerve could inhibit the pain responses of the neurons in the nucleus parafascicularis and nucleus centralis lateralis of the thalamus. He suggested that the thalamus exerted an integrative influence on acupuncture analgesia. Destruction of the caudate nucleus seemed to reduce pain suppression by acupuncture, even though it is not located along any known pathway of pain sensation.[145]

In 1974, Melzack and Melinkoff[114] raised the pain threshold of cats by electrically stimulating the mid-brain reticular formation. The analgesic effect of their procedure developed gradually over a period of five minutes. They speculated that the analgesic effect evoked by needling distant acupoints in humans, for example, needling the Lieque point (Lung 7, at the radial styloid) to relieve pain of the cervical region, might very well be mediated through the widely projecting, pain-inhibitory reticular formation. In Bowsher's 1976 review,[8] he noted that the reticular formation neurons failed to respond to peripheral stimulation at a frequency higher than 3 Hz and that gigantocellular reticular formation could be activated only by peripheral A delta stimulation. He suggested an analogy between these factors involving the reticular formation and those required to induce adequate analgesia by electroacupuncture.

The evoked potentials of an animal's sensory cortex, produced by electrical stimulation of its cervical cutaneous nerve, could be blocked by acupuncture at the Hegu point (LI 4) and Neiguan point (Pericardium 6 [P 6], located over the median nerve about 4 cm proximal to the volar carpal crease). Similar cortical evoked sensory potentials generated by stimulating tooth pulp could also be suppressed by acupuncture at the Hegu point (LI 4).[127] In 1974, Liao conducted an experiment on a rhesus monkey in which measured amounts of electrical current were applied to its forearm while the cortical evoked potentials were recorded with computer-averaged transients. Then, while this stimulation on the forearm continued, electroacupuncture was applied at the Quchi point (Large Intestine 11) on the lateral aspect of the elbow and the Shaohai point (Heart 3) on the medial aspect of the elbow on the same limb. The previously visible cortical evoked potentials were completely eliminated.[96]

Induction Time

To achieve sufficient acupuncture analgesia in humans, an induction time of 15 to 30 minutes is required.[127] Pomeranz and associates, in 1976[135] and 1977,[136] took 20 to 40 minutes to induce

acupuncture analgesia in anesthetized and alert animals. In their experiments, the induced analgesia lasted for one hour after acupuncture was terminated and then gradually subsided. It was also demonstrated in 1973 that it took two to five minutes for electroacupuncture to reach its maximal inhibitory effect on the firing of the cells in the nucleus centralis lateralis of the thalamus.[146] From our personal clinical experience, five minutes were sufficient for tooth extraction, while 20 to 30 minutes were needed for a tonsillectomy. The stimulation should be continued throughout the entire surgical procedure. In 1972, a 21-year-old male who was undergoing a tonsillectomy with acupuncture experienced the analgesic effect for at least 24 hours after surgery. During surgery, the patient's gag reflex and touch sensation persisted without any diminution.[101] These observations are entirely consistent with the fact that acupuncture generates only analgesia or hypalgesia rather than anesthesia.[98]

In 1974, Vierck and associates[163] investigated the analgesic effects of electroacupuncture on monkeys and found the need for an induction time to generate analgesia. The effect of their procedure lasted up to 70 hours with peaks of pain attenuation, interspersed with almost normal pain threshold. They also noted the importance of the precise localization of the acupoints.

Naloxone and Other Opioid Blocking Agents

The transmissibility of the analgesic effect of acupuncture in rabbits was demonstrated in 1973[130] with the use of a cross-circulation technique. Acupuncture, which was applied to the donor animal only, raised the pain threshold not only in the donor animal but in the recipient as well. Peng and associates[129] speculated that the endorphins obtained from one animal under acupuncture analgesia could produce analgesic effects in a second animal when administered through blood transfusion and circulation. In 1974, another group[141] reported the transmission of the analgesic effect of acupuncture by transfusion of the cerebrospinal fluid taken from the cerebral ventricles of animals treated by acupuncture and administered to animals not receiving acupuncture. They further demonstrated that reserpine, which acted as an antagonist to morphine by eliminating catecholamines (such as dopamine, norepinephrine, and 5-hydroxytryptamine), enhanced the analgesic effect of acu-

MATHEW H. M. LEE AND SUNG J. LIAO

puncture. However, the side effects of reserpine on the animals in their experiment were not described in the report. They also found that atropine, by blocking the muscarinic effect of acetylcholine in the brain, markedly weakened the analgesic effect of acupuncture but did not affect that of morphine at all. Their results seemed to support the concept that one of the non-opiate monoaminergenic systems is evoked by acupuncture.

In 1977, Mayer, Price, and Rafii[112] demonstrated analgesia against acute tooth pain in human volunteers by inserting and twirling an acupuncture needle at the Hegu point (LI 4). Intravenous naloxone partially abolished the analgesic effect of acupuncture in their volunteers, whereas intravenous saline did not. They were probably the first to implicate endogenous opioids as a pharmacological foundation of acupuncture.

In 1976, Pomeranz and Chiu,[135] using electroacupuncture in alert mice, found that naloxone completely blocked the analgesic effect of acupuncture whereas saline did not, and that sham acupuncture did not generate analgesia.

In 1977, Pomeranz, Cheng, and Law[136] demonstrated the dependency of acupuncture analgesia on the presence of the pituitary, which stores a large amount of endorphins. In 1979, Cheng, Pomeranz, and Yu[18] found that dexamethasone partially reduced, and 2 per cent saline treatment abolished, electroacupuncture analgesia. Tang and co-workers,[153, 154] using a radioreceptor assay, found that dexamethasone reduced the amount of endorphin in the pituitary and a bilateral adrenalectomy enhanced acupuncture analgesia and increased the amount of endorphin in the pituitary. It seemed that during electroacupuncture, endorphin was released by the pituitary, which somehow found its way into the blood, effecting an analgesia reversible by naloxone.[18, 129, 153, 168]

In 1979, Cheng and co-workers[17] found that the antagonism of naloxone to acupuncture analgesia was dose-related, i.e., increasing doses increased its antagonistic effect to acupuncture. Recording the electrical discharges of the layer-5 cells in the cat's spinal cord demonstrated that the analgesic effect of electroacupuncture was blocked by naloxone.

Non-Opioid Systems

In 1977, McLennan and associates[113] reported that acupuncture analgesia could be reversed by bicuculline, strychnine, or other monoamine inhibitors and that interference with the tryptaminergic mechanism or destruction of the dorsal raphe nuclei prevented the development of acupuncture analgesia. They concluded that acupuncture analgesia probably depends on the postsynaptic inhibition of the afferent nociceptive impulses. These results suggest that a non-opiate (or tryptamine-related) system is responsible for acupuncture analgesia in addition to the opioid system.

Five-hydroxytryptamine (5-HT) is also implicated in acupuncture analgesia. Electrolytic lesions of the raphe magnus nucleus reduced the effectiveness of electroacupuncture. Chemical lesions with 5,6-dihydroxytryptamine leading to degeneration of the descending 5-HT fibers also interfered with acupuncture analgesia. This inhibition lasted about three days and was possibly overcome by some other mechanism. Destruction of the ascending 5-HT fibers also seemed to interfere with acupuncture analgesia. Reduction of the 5-HT content in the brain, or blockade of its receptors, tended to decrease the effectiveness of acupuncture in pain reduction. Inhibition of its degradation enhanced the analgesia. This enhancement could not be abolished by naloxone and was probably due to an increase in cerebral catecholamines. Such an increase of its cerebral content was induced by electroacupuncture together with the production of analgesia in certain rats.[48] The general implication here is that both the descending and ascending 5-HT pathways are eminently involved in acupuncture analgesia.

Release of serotonin centrally, in addition to that of enkephalin and endorphins, was noted by Li, Tang, and Han with electroacupuncture in rats.[86] It appears that there is a correlation between the opioid system and the 5-hydroxytryptamine system in acupuncture analgesia. Both endorphins and 5-HT were increased during electroacupuncture. When one of them was reduced by their respective antagonists or blockers, the other was increased.[48]

Lee and associates,[36] using the technique of electrical stimulation of the pulp of a tooth to generate pain, demonstrated a significant and long-lasting decrease of pain sensitivity at the levels of both detection (Fig. 16–1) and discomfort (Fig. 16–2) by acupuncture. This decrease was not affected by intramuscular injection of 1.2 mg naloxone. They suggested that their observation invoked a non-opioid system.

Ehrenpreis[32, 33] demonstrated a potentiation of acupuncture analgesia by inhibiting endorphin deg-

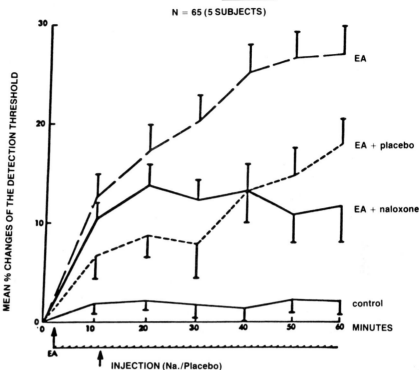

MEAN % CHANGES ± SE OF <u>DETECTION</u> THRESHOLD:

N = 65 (5 SUBJECTS)

FIGURE 16–1. Change of detection threshold for pain caused by electrical stimulation of pulp of tooth without and during electroacupuncture for 60 minutes recorded as mean percentage change from reference value ± standard error of the mean in 5 subjects. Experiments: EA = 22; EA + naloxone = 14; EA + placebo = 11; control = 11.

radation with D-phenylalanine or D-leucine. D-Phenylalanine and other met-enkephalin breakdown inhibitors could increase the efficacy of acupuncture in the treatment of patients with frozen shoulder or facial, neck, low back, and knee pain. The effectiveness of acupuncture analgesia in tooth extraction was also increased when applied in conjunction with D-phenylalanine. Similar potentiation of acupuncture analgesia could also be achieved in animals by bacitracin, another enkephalin degradation blocker. The bacitracin effect was reversible by naloxone.[163]

In 1982, Jenkins[62] studied 106 patients and found that the level of L-tryptophan (a precursor of serotonin) exerted a direct influence on serotonin's ability to transmit pain information to the neuroreceptor. Patients with low tryptophan levels would not respond to acupuncture or to other morphine analgesics. If given L-tryptophan, these patients would then respond to acupuncture satisfactorily.

The norepinephrine level in the rat brain was decreased by electroacupuncture.[122] The ascending norepinephrine pathway may exert a modulatory effect on acupuncture analgesia via the forebrain structures such as the habenula, periaqueductal gray, or nucleus accombens. The descending bulbospinal norepinephrine pathway may govern acupuncture effects at the spinal cord level.[48] Norepinephrine acts synergistically with serotonin in acupuncture analgesia.

Acetylcholine was found to have a facilitatory effect centrally in mediating acupuncture analgesia.[49, 139] The effect of atropine on acupuncture analgesia implied an involvement of the parasympathetic nervous system.[141]

Chu and associates[23] demonstrated in the thalamus and the cerebral cortex of mice an increase in glutamine and glutamate levels and a decrease of gamma-aminobutyric acid (GABA) content, together with an increase of gamma-aminobutyric acid transaminase activity when electroacupuncture achieved an analgesic effect. These changes were statistically significant. Glutamic acid enhanced neurotransmission, whereas GABA suppressed it. Their activities required the participation of Ca^{++} ions. GABA also was found to inhibit nociceptive neurons in the trigeminal nucleus of cats.[48]

In electroacupuncture analgesia, there was a decrease of Ca^{++} ions and an increase in Mg^{++} ions in the brain of mice. Intraventricular injection

MATHEW H. M. LEE AND SUNG J. LIAO

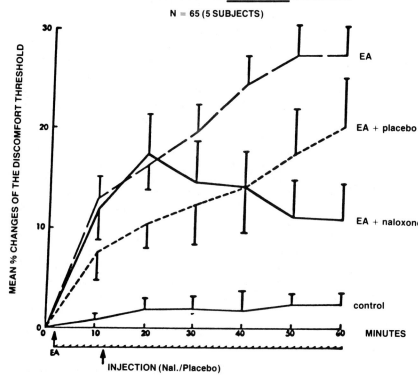

FIGURE 16–2. Change of discomfort threshold for pain caused by electrical stimulation of tooth pulp without and during electroacupuncture for 60 minutes in 5 subjects. Experiments: EA = 22; EA + naloxone = 14; EA + placebo = 11; control = 11.

of morphine caused similar changes. Ca^{++} ions exerted a suppressive effect like naloxone on morphine and on acupuncture analgesia.[48]

Autonomic Nervous System

Lee and associates[34–36, 77, 78] demonstrated a relationship between acupuncture and the autonomic nervous system by using thermography. Acupuncture was given at the Hegu point (LI 4) of one hand. There was an increase of the skin temperature not only in the treated hand but in the untreated one as well. They also found that manual acupuncture or electroacupuncture at either the Hegu point (LI 4) on the hand or Zusanli on the leg (ST 36) induced a nonsegmental long-lasting warming (sympatholytic) effect with a craniocaudal gradient in distribution (Fig. 16–3). This nonsegmental analgesia by electroacupuncture may be mediated through the reticular formation,[114] the activation of diffuse noxious inhibitory controls on the convergent cells of the dorsal horn of the spinal cord,[75] or some other yet-to-be-identified mechanism. Chiang and associates[21, 22] found diffuse an-

algesia of the body when acupuncture was applied to the acupoints on the arm. Lynn and Perl[107] also failed to produce localized analgesia. The effectiveness of acupuncture, as assessed by means of thermography, seemed to have a close correlation between its analgesic effect and an increase of temperature, especially of the areas of chronic pain, with a decreasing temperature gradient centrifugally.[100] Such findings were indicative of a possible activation of a central sympathetic inhibitory mechanism. These observations are compatible with the traditional acupuncture concept of using acupoints on the side opposite the painful site or those on the lower limbs to treat head or neck pain.

Experimental Design

In acupuncture research, the major difficulty of pain assessment in human subjects lies in the inconsistencies of the method. First, the commonly used instrumentation to measure pain leaves much to be desired. Second, few reports indicate the level of discomfort that the experimental subject

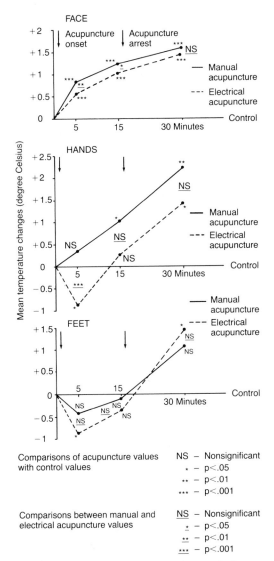

Comparisons of acupuncture values
with control values

NS	–	Nonsignificant
*	–	p<.05
**	–	p<.01
***	–	p<.001

Comparisons between manual and
electrical acupuncture values

NS	–	Nonsignificant
*	–	p<.05
**	–	p<.01
***	–	p<.001

FIGURE 16–3. Mean skin temperature changes during manual and electrical acupuncture of the Hegu hand point with the control values as reference (N = 19).

has reported as pain. Lee and associates[31] designed a precisely fitted electrode for stimulation of the pulp of the tooth that is molded to be fixed on an individual tooth to maintain a constant geometric relationship between the nerve of the pulp and the stimulating cathode (Figs. 16–4 and 16–5). The tooth pulp nerve is purely sensory and lends itself to such exacting studies. It is accurate, reliable, and comfortable for the subject and permits repeated measurements of pain at the same locus of the tooth during prolonged sessions and at intervals of months without any change of the baseline condition. Electroacupuncture was applied at the

Hegu point (LI 4) using constant-current stimulation to ensure consistency of the electrical current intensity. This nonsegmental analgesia by electroacupuncture may be mediated through the reticular formation,[114] the activation of the diffuse noxious inhibitory controls on the convergent cells in the dorsal horn of the spinal cord,[75] or some other yet-to-be-determined mechanism. Lee and Ernst[78] emphasized the need to determine the effect of acupuncture on the pain detection threshold and the pain discomfort threshold. They demonstrated the absence of a differential analgesic effect on low and high sensory levels of pain. A small dose (0.8 mg) of naloxone intramuscularly partially blocked the analgesic effect of acupuncture at both threshold levels whereas isotonic saline did not. This is not surprising, since the opioid-antagonist effect of naloxone is dose-related. It did implicate an endogenous opioid system in the delivery of acupuncture analgesia. However, it did not rule out the possible involvement of an additional endogenous non-opioid mechanism.

Hypnotizability

In 1976, 235 consecutive patients with various conditions of chronic pain were examined for their hypnotizability using Spiegel's eye roll test.[151] There was no statistically significant correlation between the patients' hypnotizability and the results of their acupuncture treatment.[103] In 1977, the analyses were repeated in one group of 200 patients with chronic head pain and another group

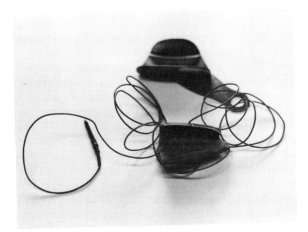

FIGURE 16–4. Silicone rubber mold for precise fit on an individual tooth showing electrode and Teflon-insulated connecting wire.

MATHEW H. M. LEE AND SUNG J. LIAO

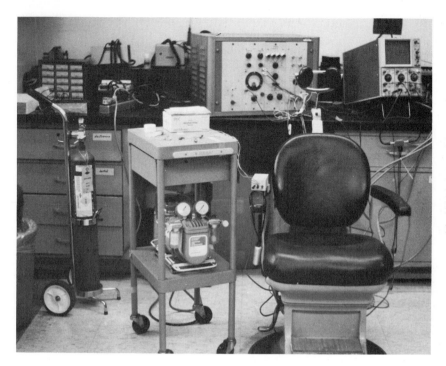

FIGURE 16–5. Experimental setting for study of acupuncture analgesia during stimulation of pulp of a tooth. The subject signals perception of the stimulus by pressing a button on either side that lights the experimenter's panel.

of 220 patients with chronic low back pain, and again, no statistically significant correlation was found between the patients' hypnotizability (as determined by Spiegel's eye roll test) and their response to acupuncture in the alleviation of these two types of syndromes of chronic pain.[45, 95] Among the three groups of patients, there seemed to exist a tendency for the patients who had a higher score on the eye roll test to be less responsive to acupuncture than those who had a lower eye roll score. In 1987, Peng and associates,[128] reporting on their double-blind evaluation of acupuncture results and hypnotic profile according to Spiegel's eye roll test, also failed to demonstrate a positive correlation between the two. It is interesting to note that the extent to which hypnosis produces total or partial anesthesia can be predetermined at the will of the hypnotist, whereas acupuncture can only alleviate the pain sensation while sparing the gag reflex, touch, and all the other cutaneous sensations. In addition, the resulting analgesia cannot be predetermined and varies tremendously among individuals, independent of age, sex, and the duration of the illness. Under hypnotic anesthesia the patient is in a trance and separated from reality, whereas with acupuncture analgesia the patient is fully awake and completely in touch with the real world. Furthermore, successful hypnotic anesthesia depends very much on prolonged and repeated contacts between the hypnotist and the patient in order to establish their relationship, whereas acupuncture analgesia does not demand any previous contact at all between the practitioner and the patient. In 1977, Mayer and associates[112] found that hypnosis in human subjects raised the pain threshold to a higher level than acupuncture did, that hypnotic anesthesia could not be reduced by naloxone while acupuncture analgesia could be, and that hypnotic anesthesia could be terminated immediately by a hypnotist while acupuncture analgesia would persist for a prolonged period of time after the removal of the needles. Goldstein and Hilgard[44] also reported the failure of naloxone to modify hypnotic analgesia. From these observations, acupuncture definitely cannot be considered a form of hypnosis.

Transcutaneous Electrical Nerve Stimulation (TENS)

The term "transcutaneous electrical nerve stimulation" first appeared around 1977 concomitant with the availability of commercial units used for the alleviation of pain. Basically, it is similar to the electrotherapy commonly used in physiatric practice. When it was initially introduced, a large chart explaining its use was sent to physicians showing lines drawn on the human figure that more or less traced the acupuncture meridians. The recommended loci for the placement of electrodes, as shown on the chart, also resembled traditional acupoints. The frequency of the electrical impulses is usually high, around 80 Hz or more. Since it is known that TENS does not really stimulate large nerves, but rather the endings of nerve fibers, the use of the term "transcutaneous electrical stimulation" or TES should really be substituted. It was reported that naloxone did not abolish high-frequency TENS–induced analgesia. Ernst and associates (Ernst and Lee; personal communication) demonstrated no significant alteration of skin temperature with TENS compared with sham TENS when using 80 Hz TENS units. Kaada[67] used low-frequency electrical stimulation at 2 Hz and produced a widespread and prolonged vasodilation that was not altered by naloxone, but was attenuated by a central serotonin blocker (cyproheptadine). However, electroacupuncture at low frequencies (such as 2 to 4 Hz) invokes the endogenous opioid system, whereas at high frequencies (as much as 200 Hz) the non-opioid–system, serotoninergic mechanisms are invoked.[16] A possible explanation is that TENS excites the sensory receptors in the skin and its effect is most likely transmitted via different afferent fibers to the spinal cord, depending on the intensity of the electrical stimulation. When the stimulus intensity is low, its effect is probably transmitted by the large myelinated A beta fibers, and when it is high, probably by the small myelinated A delta fibers or the smallest unmyelinated C fibers. Acupuncture activates the sensory receptors in the muscle, and its impulses are carried by the small myelinated groups II and III fibers to the spinal cord. Such a difference seems to indicate an evocation of different neuronal pathways in the alleviation of pain by these two different techniques.

Summation of Acupuncture Mechanisms

Watkins and Mayer[167] have proposed the possible existence of six different endogenous analgesic systems: neural opiate, hormonal opiate, neural non-opiate, hormonal non-opiate, unknown opiate, and unknown non-opiate. They believe that the mechanism of acupuncture analgesia is just on the hormonal opiate system.

We have constructed a table based on the essence of available information about the neuropharmacological mechanism of acupuncture analgesia (Table 16–1; see also Fig. 16–6).

In general, segmental application of acupuncture tends to have the strongest analgesic effect because the spinal cord is the final station at which all the neuropharmacological actions originating from all the levels of the central nervous system take place.

Acupuncture with low-frequency–high-intensity electrical stimulation tends to

1. Involve the endorphinergic mechanism.
2. Generate a slow-onset analgesia.
3. Have long-lasting results.
4. Have a cumulative effect.
5. Require usually only small doses of naloxone to inhibit its analgesic effect.

Acupuncture with high-frequency–low-intensity electrical stimulation tends to

1. Involve non-opioid monoaminergic systems.
2. Generate a rapid-onset analgesia.
3. Have short-lasting results.
4. Have no cumulative effect.
5. Require unusually large doses of naloxone to inhibit its analgesic effect.

Inhibition of degradation of met-enkephalin by D-phenylalanine or D-leucine may enhance the analgesic effect of acupuncture. Acupuncture could not generate analgesia in animals with genetically defective opiate receptors or endorphin deficiency.[126]

Acupoints are quite specific physiologically in the sense that de qi responses can be evoked only at the specified loci and are required to induce adequate analgesia. Acupuncture tends to produce diffuse, rather than strictly localized, analgesia. Such a lack of target specificity is basically compatible with the extensive involvement of the neuropharmacological systems, particularly at the hypothalamus-pituitary level. This aspect of the role of the autonomic nervous system awaits further investigation. The implication of the pathways of referred pain is still totally unknown relative to the effect of acupuncture. Nonetheless, acupuncture is probably the most thoroughly researched physical modality to date, particularly with regard to its neuropharmacology, although further extensive investigation is needed.

TABLE 16—1. Neuropharmacological Mechanism of Acupuncture Analgesia

Acupuncture → SKIN sensory receptors →
- A beta fibers large myelinated
- A delta fibers small myelinated

TENS ⟶

MUSCLE sensory receptors →

Acupuncture→
- C fibers smallest unmyelinated
- group II fibers small unmyelinated →numb feeling
- group III fibers small myelinated →heavy feeling
- group IV fibers smallest unmyelinated →sore feeling

→ dorsal root ganglion → SPINAL CORD

1. DORSAL HORN interneurons → a. presynaptic inhibition → ventrolateral lateral funiculus neurons

   b. postsynaptic inhibition

   (enkephalinergic, dynorphinergic, cholecystokinin-like)→inhibits pain sensation

2. along ventrolateral funiculus→reticular formation→raphe magnus nucleus in MEDULLA OBLONGATA (tryptaminergic)→ dorsolateral funiculus→dorsal horn interneurons→inhibiting pain sensation

3. along ventrolateral funiculus→periaqueductal gray in MESENCEPHALON (enkephalinergic)→neurons of dorsolateral funiculus (serotoninergic and norepinephrinergic)→dorsal horn interneurons in spinal cord→inhibits pain sensation

4. along ventrolateral funiculus→ventroventricular ARCUATE NUCLEUS (endorphinergic)→raphe nucleus→dorsolateral funiculus→dorsal horn interneurons in spinal cord→inhibiting pain sensation

5. along ventrolateral funiculus→reticular formation→ HYPOTHALAMUS→PITUITARY →release of lipoprotein→ACTH and beta-endorphin→cerebrospinal fluid and venous system→inhibiting pain sensation

416

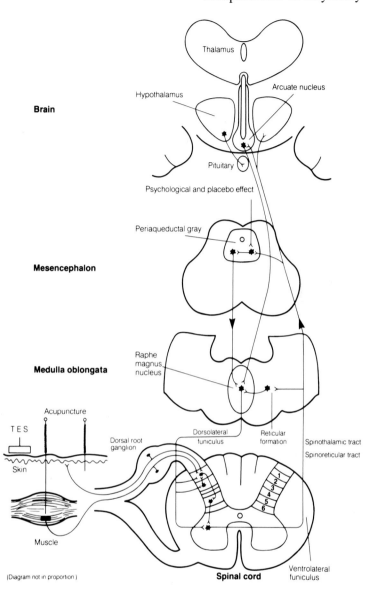

FIGURE 16–6. Diagram of the neuroanatomy of the essence of the available information about the neuropharmacological mechanism of acupuncture analgesia.

Clinical Applications

Like any other practice in the medical domain, acupuncture was originally developed empirically through astute bedside observation, and the continuation of its acceptance depends on its clinical effectiveness. Statistically designed investigations in recent years do, indeed, confirm its therapeutic efficacy in certain illnesses. One must also realize the difficulty in designing the research protocol for a blind study because of the very characteristics of this procedure.

Chronic Pain Unit—Rehabilitation Medicine Department, Goldwater Memorial Hospital

Projects involving the measurement of dental pain and dental acupuncture analgesia are being carried out at the Chronic Pain Unit of the Department of Rehabilitation Medicine at Goldwater Memorial Hospital. Over 200 dental procedures, including cavity preparation, deep gingival curet-

MATHEW H. M. LEE AND SUNG J. LIAO

tage, and extractions, have been performed with 80 per cent success in achieving clinically satisfactory analgesia. The management of pain due to other types of orofacial problems has proved promising as well (Table 16–2).

Since it has been shown that acupuncture produces an initial vasoconstriction followed by a marked vasodilation of the blood vessels, thermographic studies of conditions associated with chronic pain are also being performed to determine changes of thermographic pattern following acupuncture. Preliminary studies suggest that thermography offers a simple, objective, noninvasive technique to assess chronic pain qualitatively and to measure the effect of acupuncture on its alleviation.[76]

Acupuncture and Trigger Point Injection

In 1947, Travell and associates[155] demonstrated that injections of procaine or of physiologic saline,

TABLE 16–2. Milestones: Chronic Pain Unit of the Rehabilitation Medicine Department at Goldwater Memorial Hospital (established 1978)

Dental extraction of third molar	Dental acupuncture analgesia, 1973
Cumulative report 20 dental cases	Lee, M. H. M., Teng, P., Zaretsky, H. H., and Rubin, M.: Acupuncture anesthesia in dentistry. NY State Dent. J., 39:299–301, 1973
Development of precision tooth pulp stimulation technique	With Rockefeller University Dr. Barry Dworkin (31)
Tooth pulp stimulation Test for pain threshold and maximum tolerance	(36)
Naloxone challenge	Ernst, M., and Lee, M. H. M.: Influence of naloxone on electro-acupuncture analgesia using an experimental dental pain test. Review of possible mechanisms of action. Acupunct. Electrother. Res. Int. J., 12:5–22, 1987
Cerebral evoked potential Laser stimulation and treatment	With Dr. Ami Carmon, Technion-Israel Institute of Technology, Dept. of Bioengineering; Abstract presented at 2nd International Symposium on Pain, Montreal, 1978
Thermography	Sympatholytic effect (77) Cephalad-Caudal (34)

or "dry needling," were all effective for the alleviation of pain at trigger areas. Travell and Simons[156] report that "precise dry needling of trigger points without injecting any solution, approaches, but does not equal, the therapeutic effectiveness of injecting procaine into the trigger points." In Denmark in 1980, Frost and associates[40] reported their double-blind studies of mepivacaine injection *versus* saline injection for myofascial pain. They demonstrated that a physiological saline injection was statistically more effective than a mepivacaine injection and attributed the effectiveness to an irritation from the needling, concluding: "There is much to suggest that injection therapy of myofascial pain is one form of acupuncture."

Acupuncture and Arthritides

In the fall of 1973, the National Institute of Arthritis, Metabolism and Digestive Diseases, in cooperation with the Arthritis Foundation, sponsored a workshop on the "Use of Acupuncture in the Rheumatic Diseases." No substantial agreement or conclusion was reached, as reported by Plotz and colleagues.[133] This is not surprising, since at that time few physicians in this country had extensive experience in acupuncture. Shen and associates reported on a fairly comprehensive double-blind investigation including patients' subjective responses, functional levels, erythrocyte sedimentation rate, rheumatoid factor, x-ray examination of the joints, and psychological evaluation of the patients' susceptibility to suggestion of the effect of acupuncture on rheumatoid arthritis;[147] not surprisingly, their results were not remarkable. In general, it has been found that pain from osteoarthritis or degenerative arthritis responds much better than that due to rheumatoid arthritis. In early cases of degenerative arthritis of the hip, acupuncture also improves the range of motion of the affected joint by releasing the associated periarticular muscle spasm.[98] Gaw and associates[42] performed a double-blind investigation of acupuncture for relief of pain due to osteoarthritis of the finger, hip, knee, or cervical, lumbar, or thoracic spine, using loci adjacent to rather than at the classical acupoints for the control group, and found that significant pain reduction was achieved in both groups of patients. Thus, the question was raised whether the adjacent loci also are as capable of blockade of pain as are classical acupoints and whether the various affected parts of the body would respond uniformly to acupuncture, as a result of lack of target specificity that has been noted elsewhere in this chapter.

A significant decrease in circulating immune complexes (measured by platelet aggregation) after laser acupuncture has been found in the hands in rheumatoid arthritis. However, no other significant differences have been found in the titer of the rheumatoid factor, antinuclear antibody, polyethylene glycol precipitates, or Westergren erythrocyte sedimentation rate; the patients had some subjective improvement in activity and hand function.[43]

Man and associates[109, 110] treated a group of patients with rheumatoid arthritis of the knees, giving intra-articular steroids to one knee and electroacupuncture or placebo acupuncture to the other. The average duration of pain reduction was 4 to 12 weeks with electroacupuncture, 2 to 6 weeks with intra-articular steroids, and less than 10 hours with placebo acupuncture. The patients reported a 90 per cent moderate decrease of pain with acupuncture, 80 per cent with steroid injections, and 10 per cent with placebo. Range of motion of the knees was increased by 30 per cent with acupuncture and by 20 per cent with steroid injections, and no change was observed with placebo.

Guillemin[46] noted that acupuncture caused the pituitary to release beta-lipoprotein, the precursor of ACTH and beta-endorphin. Cheng and associates[17] reported that electroacupuncture elevated blood cortisol levels in naive horses, whereas sham treatment had no such effect. Using animal models, Sin[148] found that electroacupuncture suppressed exudate reaction, inhibited the early phase of increased vascular permeability, and impaired the leukocyte adherence to vascular endothelial cells just as well as oral nonsteroidal anti-inflammatory drugs (indomethacin, piroxicam, or aspirin). These studies suggest that the effectiveness of acupuncture in the treatment of arthritides may be through the anti-inflammatory effects of the released ACTH and cortisol. Lee and Yang[79] reviewed the available literature and recommended the consideration of acupuncture as an alternative treatment for arthritis because of its pain-alleviating and inflammation-suppressing effects.

Acupuncture for Painful Conditions

ACUPUNCTURE FOR CRANIAL PAIN

Hansen and Hansen[50] found that acupuncture was "significantly more pain relieving than placebo acupuncture" for chronic tension headache. Dowson and associates[30] used "mock transcutaneous electrical nerve stimulation" as a placebo to assess the efficacy of acupuncture in the relief of headache in 39 patients. They found that "at most, acupuncture appears to be approximately 20 per cent more effective than a placebo in alleviating headache but no statistically significant difference between these two treatments could be demonstrated." Over a two-year period, 217 patients with cranial pain were treated.[95] Forty-one per cent of the entire group experienced complete subsidence of pain and were able to completely abstain from all medication for at least three months without relapse.

ACUPUNCTURE FOR FACIAL PAIN

Facial pain due to trigeminal neuralgia is often unmanageable and very disabling. Bossy[7] tried to correlate the relationship of the spinal nucleus of the trigeminal nerve and the acupuncture points for treating trigeminal neuralgia. When conventional medical management fails to alleviate it, acupuncture may offer a 50 per cent chance.[98] The major difficulty in managing such patients is their very low tolerance of emotional and environmental stress.

Biedermann and associates[4] reported a case in which acupuncture treatment relieved facial pain in the temporomandibular region during the unmedicated stage but failed to relieve the pain after administration of a tricyclic antidepressant (doxepin). The question remains as to which of the mechanisms for relief of pain by acupuncture was blocked by this medication.

Facial pain due to temporomandibular joint dysfunction or arthritis is another quite disabling condition. Raustia[137] states that "acupuncture seems to be useful as a complementary treatment especially in cases of disorders of the temporomandibular joint with evidence of psychophysiological or neuromuscular disturbances but not so clearly where marked occlusal disturbances or joint damage are involved."

It is our general impression that the therapeutic effects of the common nonsteroid anti-inflammatory drugs are usually enhanced by acupuncture. This is indeed a very interesting field for further research.

At the recent NIH Consensus Development Meeting in 1986, acupuncture was recommended

MATHEW H. M. LEE AND SUNG J. LIAO

as an additional efficacious modality for the treatment of pain.*

ACUPUNCTURE FOR CERVICAL PAIN

Peng and associates[128] reported on a double-blind study of the long-term therapeutic effects of electroacupuncture for chronic neck and shoulder pain. Twenty-four of 37 patients (64.9 per cent) had significant long-term improvement. They attributed the effects of electroacupuncture to an increase in regional microcirculation, similar to a peripheral sympathetic nerve block. Petrie and Hazleman[131] compared "sham transcutaneous nerve stimulation" with acupuncture for the relief of neck pain. They used points GB 20 and GB 21 bilaterally and GV 14 on the midline. This raised the question as to whether the acupuncture treatments as given were really appropriate if only a few fixed acupoints were utilized without any regard to the individual status of each patient. To the patients, transcutaneous nerve stimulation, sham or real, is quite obviously different from acupuncture, thus nullifying the purpose of a blind design. In addition, the pharmacological effects of these two modalities are very different (Ernst and Lee: unpublished data). In a study of 195 cases of cervical spondylosis treated with acupuncture, 46 per cent experienced marked improvement after an average of five treatments.[92]

ACUPUNCTURE FOR EPICONDYLITIS

Brattberg[10] reported acupuncture to be an excellent alternative to steroid injections for epicondylitis, demonstrating statistically significantly better results with acupuncture than with steroid injections. Historically, Renton, in 1830, was probably the first to report treating pain of the extensor forearm with needling.[140] In a study of 156 patients with epicondylitis, approximately 85 per cent experienced satisfactory alleviation of their elbow pain after an average of five to six sessions of treatment by acupuncture.[98]

ACUPUNCTURE FOR LOW BACK PAIN SYNDROME

Of 220 patients with a chief complaint of the syndrome of low back pain due to various causes, after acupuncture 59 per cent had a reduction of pain to a barely perceptible or zero level lasting

---

*National Institutes of Health Consensus Development Conference: Integrated Approach to the Management of Pain. Washington, DC, May 19–21, 1986.

from a minimum of three months to no recurrence at all. Of the entire patient population, 20 per cent had undergone prior surgical procedures, such as laminectomy, diskectomy, and the like, but the intractable pain remained. As a subgroup, the level of improvement of the group who had prior surgery was less satisfactory at a statistically significant incidence than that of patients who had not undergone surgery.

PAINFUL CONDITIONS OF THE FOOT

Painful forefoot was first described in 1876 by Morton—thus, Morton's neuroma, Morton's neuralgia, or Morton's metatarsalgia.[119] He attributed its cause to a neuroma of the third digital nerve of the foot, formed by an anastomosis of a medial branch of the lateral plantar nerve and a lateral branch of the medial plantar nerve between the third and fourth metatarsal heads. It should not be confused with painful foot due to Morton's toe, a short and hypermobile first metatarsal, usually with hypertrophy of the cortex of the second metatarsal and callus formation underneath the second metatarsal head, described in 1928 by D. J. Morton.[118] Of 20 cases of Morton's neuroma, 17 had complete relief of pain for at least one year after acupuncture, and four of six cases of Morton's toe had similar relief.[98]

MISCELLANEOUS PAINFUL CONDITIONS

Many other conditions, such as postherpetic neuralgia, pain from cancer,[72] phantom limb pain, shoulder pain, and dysmenorrhea,[57] have been treated with acupuncture with variable results. Consideration of the use of D-phenylalanine, L-tryptophan, and so on for the enhancement of acupuncture has been proposed.

Clinical Principles, Significant Observations, and Techniques of Acupuncture Therapy for Pain

It is mandatory that each pain patient be medically assessed before acupuncture therapy is instituted. Caution should be observed in treating cardiac patients, hemophiliacs, epileptics, pregnant individuals, and those with infectious diseases.

It has been observed that the clinical effect of acupuncture is cumulative. Quite commonly, pain is gradually reduced during the course of acupuncture treatment and is, finally, completely eliminated. Only in less than 5 per cent of patients did one session of acupuncture treatment completely abolish pain.[98]

The New York Society of Acupuncture for Physicians and Dentists advocates a course of six treatments (given twice per week or once weekly) in order to determine its efficaciousness. Periodic boosters may be necessary to sustain a continued positive response.

A certain percentage of patients whose pain was not immediately affected by a short-term course (such as one to five sessions) of acupuncture became aware of its complete disappearance several days to four or five weeks after cessation of treatment and experienced no recurrence. This "delayed response" phenomenon has been observed frequently and was confirmed in personal communications with colleagues in China, although it has not yet been reported in published form.

Response to therapy should be recorded by both the patient and the physician. The reduction of medication and overall improvement in activities of daily living remain the principal yardsticks for measuring a positive response.

Most acupuncture needles are made of stainless steel. Popular sizes vary from 10 to 13 mils (thousandths of an inch) in diameter and 1 to 3 inches in length. For needle sterilization, autoclaving is recommended, and needles should be discarded after use in patients with a history of hepatitis, AIDS, or AIDS-related complex. Individual, sterilized, disposable needles are now available.

It is essential to evoke the *de qi* response at the acupoint after inserting the needle, since it is an indication that the proper acupoint is ascertained and the therapy should be effective. This can easily be done by gently twirling the needle. The needles should remain *in situ* for 15 to 20 minutes.

Before inserting a needle anywhere, you must know anatomy and be able to visualize the structures you are penetrating. Occasionally, muscle spasm might prevent a needle from being removed, and if so, massaging the surrounding area gently will relax the muscles, expediting its removal.

Often, a patient may feel drowsy, groggy, or even sleepy soon after acupuncture treatment, which is most likely a side effect of the endorphins produced. Much less frequently, a patient may feel "high" or "full of energy." Three patients independently reported that they giggled intermittently for several hours after each acupuncture treatment. Patients with these three types of reaction invariably tend to attain satisfactory alleviation of pain. Their psychological relationship in the personality inventory awaits investigation.[98]

Eight acupoints, probably the most commonly used for painful conditions, are illustrated (Figs. 16–7 to 16–15). Each acupoint is listed in Table 16–3 with its anatomical location, blood and nerve supply, and indications as determined empirically.

Statistical Design of Clinical Investigation

Several studies have reported the ineffectiveness of acupuncture. Because of the very nature of the procedure, it is difficult indeed to design a statistically competent double-blind cross-over experiment. For example, it is often observed that the insertion of a needle at an acupoint, whether superficially or deeply, may have the same therapeutic effect. Therefore, a "sham" acupoint may not really be sham. There are two volumes of "Extra-Meridian Odd Points"[51, 52] listing 1595 acupoints in addition to the 360 classical points. Recently, one of us (S. J. L.), in collaboration with Dr. Nguyen Van Nghi of Marseilles, translated 281 "odd" and "new" acupoints from Chinese into French.[157–162] Thus, it is quite possible that some

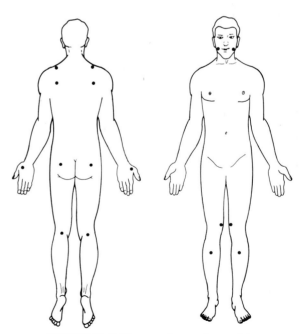

FIGURE 16–7. Diagram of general acupoints.

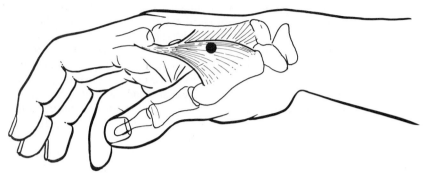

FIGURE 16–8. Hegu, LI 4.

of the so-called sham acupoints may have real therapeutic effect, whereas some supposedly effective acupoints may not be the appropriate ones for a particular patient. Taping a needle onto the skin, or utilizing sham or real TENS (or TES) as a placebo, nullifies the purpose of a blind design. The placebo effect of the attitude of the investigator in implicitly influencing the outcome of a human experiment cannot be dismissed lightly and is rarely, if ever, expressed in scientific reports. Lee and associates[80] demonstrated clearly that there was no statistically significant difference between the effectiveness of a lactose placebo and aspirin in the alleviation of experimentally induced tooth pulp pain. They attributed this to the suggestive power of the ritual of drug administration. They further emphasized the importance of psychological factors such as expectation in the perception and interpretation of noxious stimuli. In 1955, Betterman and Grossman,[3] while studying salicylamide for its analgesic and antirheumatic effects, also found that the double-blind technique

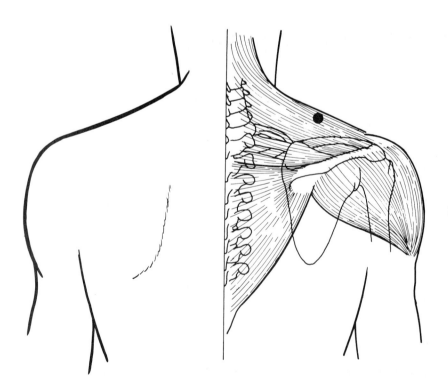

FIGURE 16–9. Jianjing, GB 21.

needle is introduced into areas such as the upper trapezius muscle or supraspinatus muscle is a significant concern. Similarly, Reinstein and associates reported a case of pneumothorax as a complication of needle electromyography.[138] However, with awareness and appropriate care, such incidents are rare among medical practitioners.

Hematoma formation can easily be induced by any needling procedure, especially in patients who are on anticoagulants, and acupuncture is no exception. Smith and co-workers[150] reported a case of deep hemorrhage resulting in anterior compartment syndrome after acupuncture treatment. Thus, such patients should be handled with appropriate caution if treated by acupuncture.

Cases of otitis externa[64] and of perichondritis or chondritis of the pinna were reported[27, 166] as a result of auricular acupuncture that entailed the insertion of a small metal studlike needle into the pinna. These reports did not state whether the acupuncture practitioners involved were nonphysicians or physicians. Also, a case of subacute

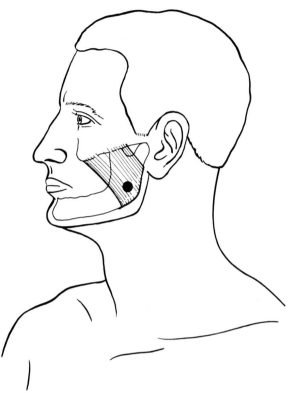

FIGURE 16–10. Jiache, ST 6.

was not a valid method for distinguishing the effectiveness of analgesic agents, although blind controls are widely considered an integral part of statistical design in medical research.

Precautions

Because the American public is so fearful of "needles," vasovagal episodes are not uncommon and can, occasionally, be quite severe. If one suspects a patient to be susceptible to such an episode, as a preventive measure it is well advised to have the patient in a recumbent position during acupuncture treatment. Of course, such incidents are not confined to acupuncture treatment alone, since they may occur under any circumstances in which a needle is inserted into a susceptible person.[76]

One case of pneumothorax and one case of hemothorax, complicated by pneumonia and wound infection following acupuncture performed by a nonphysician, have been reported.[13] The possibility of such complications occurring when a

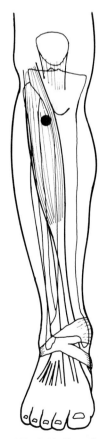

FIGURE 16–11. Zusanli, ST 36.

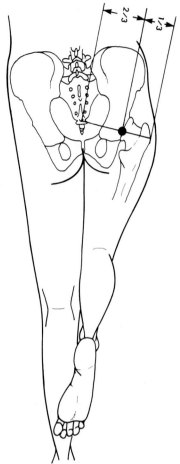

FIGURE 16–12. Huantiao, GB 30.

There was sufficient evidence to suggest that contaminated needles were repeatedly used from one patient to the next, and to indicate that the practitioner did not seem to understand or to observe the absolute necessity of sterile technique in the administration of therapy. There was also a distinct possibility that being a nonphysician, he might not have recognized the illness, since the epidemic appeared to have been started by treating an acute hepatitis patient who had obvious jaundice. The next 10 patients developed clinical hepatitis with jaundice. The Kent-Brondum epidemic was not an isolated episode. In 1977, a similar incident was reported by Boxall,[9] and in 1986, Stryker and associates[152] reported six patients with hepatitis who had been treated with needles insufficiently sterilized by using benzalkonium chloride solution. No known serological investigation for hepatitis infection was conducted in these two incidents.

bacterial endocarditis, or possible septicemia, was reported following acupuncture with a small metal stud inserted into the pinna of a patient's ear.[19, 20, 81] Staphylococcal septicemia was reported by Izatt and Fairman.[61]

Kent, Brondum, and associates[71] reported on their careful detective work concerning one of the largest, if not the largest, outbreaks of a hepatatis B epidemic stemming from a single nonphysician acupuncturist's office among patients treated between January 1 and November 30, 1984. It was probably the first time an epidemic of hepatitis was so definitively diagnosed, relying not only on clinical investigation, but on serological studies of the patient population as well. Thirty-five cases of hepatitis B out of 316 patients tested, an infection rate of 111 per thousand, were determined by detecting the presence of HBsAg or anti-HBc IgM in the patients' sera. In a general population, the positive rate is usually one to five per thousand.

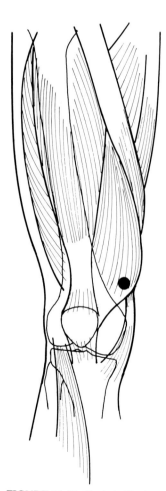

FIGURE 16–13. Xuehai, SP 10.

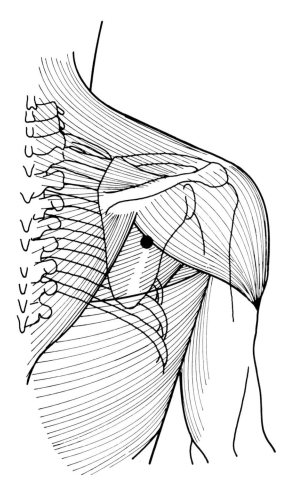

FIGURE 16–14. Tianzhong, SI 11.

allergic dermatitis from wearing costume earrings with stainless steel posts. Acupuncture needles are usually made of stainless steel in which nickel is an important ingredient, as it is in white gold. The first patient was treated with several yellow gold needles that were especially made for her; laser acupuncture was substituted in the subsequent two. Fisher[38] reported a similar case of allergic dermatitis from acupuncture needles and quoted two other cases. It is beneficial to question patients about such allergies during the routine history-taking.

Traditional Japanese acupuncture may entail "burying" thin gold needles in the soft tissue as a

Among the patients in the Kent-Brondum epidemic, three individuals were avowed homosexuals, yet no serological investigation of the HIV viral infection was conducted on the blood samples (Brondum: personal communication). The transmission of AIDS and other infectious diseases is an ever-present risk when contaminated needles are used. It is, therefore, prudent for the practitioner to take strict precautionary measures and exercise due judgment in the management of acute hepatitis patients or posthepatitis patients with painful conditions.[76] If patients are suspected of having hepatitis or AIDS, disposable needles should be utilized. For all other patients, needles must be sterilized using standard sterilization procedures.

During 15 years of clinical experience, only three patients have been encountered who are allergic to nickel.[98] All were females who had experienced

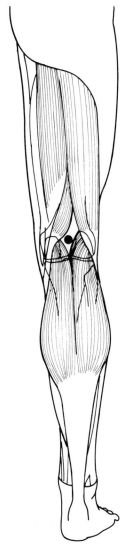

FIGURE 16–15. Weizhong, UB 40.

MATHEW H. M. LEE AND SUNG J. LIAO

TABLE 16–3. Acupoints

Acupoint	Hegu, LI 4 (Fig. 16–8)
Surface anatomy	At the prominence of the contracted first dorsal interosseous muscle, near the radial aspect of the second metacarpus
Nerve supply	Sensory: the superficial ramus of the radial nerve (C 6)
	Motor: the proper palmar digital ramus of the median nerve (C 7, 8, T 1) and the dorsal interosseous ramus of the ulnar nerve (C 8, T 1)
Blood supply	Dorsales pollicis artery of the radial artery
Physiatric indications	Headache, toothache, analgesia for head and neck surgery, analgesia for dental extraction and surgery, abdominal pain, facial palsy
Acupoint	Jianjing, GB 21 (Fig. 16–9)
Surface anatomy	In the upper trapezius muscle, midway between the C 7, T 1 interspinous space and the acromion
Nerve supply	Sensory: the lateral ramus of the supraclavicular nerve (C 4, 5, 6)
	Motor: accessory nerve (XI)
Blood supply	Suprascapular artery
Physiatric indications	Pain of neck, shoulder, upper back
Acupoint	Jiache, ST 6 (Fig. 16–10)
Surface anatomy	At the prominence of the contracted masseter muscle, about one fingerbreadth anterior and superior to the angle of the jaw
Nerve supply	Sensory: the third division (mandibular) of the trigeminal nerve (V)
	Motor: the cervicofacial ramus of the facial nerve (VII)
Blood supply	External maxillary artery of the facial artery
Physiatric indications	Trigeminal neuralgia, temporomandibular joint syndrome, toothache, facial palsy
Acupoint	Zusanli, ST 36 (Fig. 16–11)
Surface anatomy	In the tibialis anticus muscle. Place your thumb, pointing laterally and horizontally, just distal to the tibial tubercle with the interphalangeal joint on the tibial crest—the acupoint will be found where the tip of your thumb is.
Nerve supply	Sensory: the lateral sural cutaneous nerve (S 1, 2) and the cutaneous ramus of the saphenous nerve (L 3, 4)
	Motor: the deep peroneal nerve (L 4, 5, S 1)
Blood supply	Anterior tibial artery
Physiatric indications	Gastric pain, headache, pain of the knee joint and leg, hemiplegia
Acupoint	Huantiao, GB 30 (Fig. 16–12)
Surface anatomy	With the patient in the lateral recumbent position and hip semiflexed, this acupoint is located at the junction of the lateral and the middle thirds of a line drawn from the greater trochanter to the sacral hiatus
Nerve supply	Sensory: the inferior gluteal cutaneous nerve (S 1, 2)
	Motor: the sciatic nerve (L 4, 5, S 1, 2, 3) and the inferior gluteal nerve (L 5, S 1, 2)
Blood supply	Inferior gluteal artery
Physiatric indications	Pain of the lower back and hip region, pain and weakness of the lower limb, hemiplegia
Acupoint	Xuehai, SP 10 (Fig. 16–13)
Surface anatomy	At the prominence of the vastus medialis muscle. To locate the point, cup your right-hand palm on patient's left knee—the point is located where the tip of your semi-abducted thumb is. Use your left hand to locate this acupoint on the patient's right thigh.
Nerve supply	Sensory: the anterior femoral cutaneous nerve (L 3)
	Motor: the femoral nerve (L 2, 3, 4)
Blood supply	Femoral artery
Physiatric indications	Pain of the medial aspect of the thigh, dysmenorrhea
Acupoint	Tianzhong, SI 11 (Fig. 16–14)
Surface anatomy	In the infraspinatus muscle, at the junction of the superior and the middle thirds of the perpendicular line drawn from the inferior border of the scapular spine to the inferior angle of the scapula
Nerve supply	Sensory: the cutaneous ramus of the fourth intercostal nerve (D 4)
	Motor: the suprascapular nerve (C 5, 6)
Blood supply	Circumflex scapular branch of the subscapular artery
Physiatric indications	Pain of the scapular region, pain of the posterolateral aspects of the arm and elbow
Acupoint	Weizhong, UB 40 (Fig. 16–15)
Surface anatomy	At the midpoint of the transverse crease of the popliteal fossa, between the tendons of the semimembranosus and the biceps femoris muscles
Nerve supply	Sensory: the posterior femoral cutaneous nerve (S 2)
Blood supply	Popliteal artery
Physiatric indications	Low back pain, sciatic neuralgia, abdominal pain, hemiplegia

treatment for chronic painful conditions. These needles may migrate into the spinal canal, causing serious injuries to the spinal cord or spinal nerves.[60] The "buried needle" technique is peculiar to the Japanese practice of acupuncture.

Pregnancy is not an absolute contraindication; however, certain acupuncture points should be avoided, i.e., the Hegu point (LI 4), which tends to cause dilation of the cervix and initiate contraction of the uterus.[76]

Patients with pacemakers should not be treated with electroacupuncture, particularly in the upper half of the body, owing to the possibility of electrical interference.[76]

Legal Aspects of Acupuncture Practice

There is no uniform national legislation concerning the practice of acupuncture. Each state has its own set of rules and regulations governing acupuncture practice by physicians and nonphysicians. For example, in New York State, acupuncture is considered an experimental procedure; physicians must have 300 hours of didactic and clinical training in the field of acupuncture and must also practice under an approved research protocol. Physicians should check with the State Education Department or Division of Professional Licensing in their particular state for certification requirements.

In Rhode Island, in addition, there are certain educational requirements. A nonphysician practitioner must pass a bilingual written examination and an oral clinical examination in order to be licensed to practice acupuncture independently.

In Connecticut, the State Department of Health Services interprets the practice of acupuncture as the practice of medicine; thus, nonphysicians cannot legally practice acupuncture unless under a physician's personal and immediate supervision.

Physiatrists who wish to practice acupuncture should check with their state licensing authorities regarding its legality.

Summary

Although many Chinese publications have been reviewed, they have not been included in the references because of language and library accessibility, in addition to the fact that many were not germane to the subject of chronic pain.

Basic research in acupuncture for control of pain is discussed, and attempts are made to reconcile the clinical observations of acupuncture with neurophysiological observations.

The authors have presented their varied clinical applications of acupuncture for the treatment of chronic painful conditions commonly seen in a physiatric practice.

As we search for alternative therapies for management of chronic pain, acupuncture presents a fascinating challenge. We are confident that science will provide a logical explanation for many of our currently empirical findings.

Should this chapter help stimulate fellow physiatrists to evaluate the use of acupuncture in their own clinical practices and to share their experiences, then it will have provided an invaluable service.

References

1. Bache, F.: Cases illustrative of the remedial effects of acupuncture. North Am. Med. Surg. J., 1:311, 1825.
2. Best, C. H., and Taylor, N. B.: Physiologic Basis of Medical Practice, 2nd Ed. Baltimore, Williams & Wilkins, 1939.
3. Betterman, R. C., and Grossman, A. J.: Effectiveness of salicylamide as an analgesic and antirheumatic agent. Evaluation of the double-blind technique for studying analgesic drugs. J.A.M.A., 159:1619–1622, 1955.
4. Biedermann, H. J., Lapeer, G. L., Mauri, M., and McGhi, A.: Acupuncture and myofascial pain: Treatment failure after administration of tricyclic antidepressant. Med. Hypotheses, 19:397–402, 1986.
5. Bloom, F., Segal, D., Ling, N., et al.: Endorphins: Profound behavioral effects in rats suggest new etiological factors in mental illness. Science, 194:630–632, 1976.
6. Bossult, D. F., Leshin, L. B., and Stomberg, M. W.: Plasma cortisol and beta-endorphin in horses subjected to electroacupuncture for cutaneous analgesia. Peptides, 4:501–507, 1983.
7. Bossy, J.: Implication of the spinal nucleus of the trigeminal nerve in acupuncture. Acupunct. Electrother. Res. Int. J., 11:177–190, 1986.
8. Bowsher, D.: Role of the reticular formation in responses to noxious stimulation. Pain, 2:361–378, 1976.
9. Boxall, E. H.: Acupuncture hepatitis in West Midlands, 1977. J. Med. Virol., 2:377–379, 1978.
10. Brattberg, G.: Acupuncture therapy for tennis elbow. Pain, 16:285–288, 1983.
11. Cannon, W. B.: Bodily Changes in Pain, Hunger,

Fear and Rage, 2nd Ed. New York, D. Appleton & Company, 1929.

12. Cannon, W. B.: The Wisdom of the Body. New York, W. W. Norton & Company, 1939.

13. Carron, H., Epstein, B. S., and Grand, B.: Complications of acupuncture. J.A.M.A., 228:1552–1554, 1974.

14. Chang, H. T.: Integrative action of thalamus in the process of acupuncture for analgesia. Sci. Sin., 16:25–60, 1973.

15. Chang, S. H., and Dickenson, A.: Pain, enkephalin and acupuncture. Nature, 283:243–244, 1980.

16. Cheng, R., and Pomeranz, B.: Electroacupuncture analgesia could be mediated by at least two pain-relieving mechanisms; endorphin and non-endorphin systems. Life Sci., 25:1957–1962, 1979.

17. Cheng, R., McKibbin, L., Roy, B., et al.: Electroacupuncture elevates blood cortisol levels in naive horses, sham treatment has no effect. Int. J. Neurosci., 10:95–97, 1980.

18. Cheng, R., Pomeranz, B., and Yu, G.: Dexamethasone partially reduces and 2% saline treatment abolishes electroacupuncture analgesia: These findings implicate pituitary endorphins. Life Sci., 24:1481–1486, 1979.

19. Cheng, T. O.: Acupuncture needles as a cause of bacterial endocarditis. Br. Med. J., 287:689, 1983.

20. Cheng, T. O.: Letter to the editor. Int. J. Cardiol., 8:97, 1985.

21. Chiang, C. Y., Chiang, C. T., Chu, H. C., et al.: Peripheral afferent pathway for acupuncture analgesia. Sci. Sin., 16:210–217, 1973.

22. Chiang, C. Y., Liu, J. Y., Chu, T. H., et al.: Studies of spinal ascending pathways for effect of acupuncture analgesia in rabbits. Sci. Sin., 18:651–658, 1975.

23. Chu, C. C., Zong, Y. Y., Gong, M. E., Hong, Y. B., and Chen, J.: Effect of electro-acupuncture analgesia on free amino acid content in the brain of the mice. Kexue Tongbao, 24:45–46, 1979.

24. Chu, L. Y.: Electroacupuncture. Xian, Shenxi People's Publishers, 1957.

25. Clark, W. G.: Emetic and hyperthermic effects of centrally injected methionine-enkephalin in cats. Proc. Soc. Exp. Biol. Med., 154:540–542, 1977.

26. Cushing, H.: The Life of Sir William Osler. London, Oxford University Press, 1940.

27. Davis, O., and Powell, W.: Auricular perichondritis secondary to acupuncture. Arch. Otolaryngol., 111:770–771, 1985.

28. de Morant, G. S., and Ferreyrolles, P.: L'acupuncture en Chine et la reflexotherapie moderne. Homeopathie Francaise, Juin 1929.

29. Dimond, E. G.: Acupuncture anesthesia. Western medicine and Chinese traditional medicine. J.A.M.A., 218:1558–1563, 1971.

30. Dowson, D. I., Lewith, G. T., and Machin, D.: The effects of acupuncture versus placebo in the treatment of headache. Pain, 21:35–42, 1985.

31. Dworkin, B. R., Lee, M. H. M., Zaretsky, H. H., et al.: Instrumentation and techniques: A precision tooth-pulp stimulation technique for the assessment of pain threshold. Behav. Res. Methods Instrumentation, 9:463–465, 1977.

32. Ehrenpreis, S.: Potentiation of acupuncture analgesia by inhibition of endorphin degradation. Acupunct. Electrother. Res., 8:319, 1983.

33. Ehrenpreis, S.: Analgesic properties of enkephalinase inhibitors: Animal and human studies. Prog. Clin. Biol. Res., 192:363–370, 1985.

34. Ernst, M., and Lee, M. H. M.: Sympathetic vasomotor changes induced by manual and electrical acupuncture of the Hoku point visualized by thermography. Pain, 21:25–33, 1985.

35. Ernst, M., and Lee, M. H. M.: Sympathetic effects of manual and electrical acupuncture of the Tsusanli knee point: Compared with the Hoku hand point sympathetic effects. Exp. Neurol., 94:1–10, 1986.

36. Ernst, M., Lee, M. H. M., Dworkin, B., and Zaretsky, H. H.: Pain perception decrement produced through repeated stimulation. Pain, 26:221–231, 1986.

37. Feinstein, B., Langton, J. N., Jameson, R. M., and Schiller, F.: Experiments on pain referred from deep somatic tissues. J. Bone Jt. Surg., 36A:981–1007, 1954.

38. Fisher, A. A.: Allergic dermatitis from acupuncture needles. Cutis, 38:226, 1986.

39. Foerster, O.: The dermatomes in man. Brain, 56:1–39, 1933.

40. Frost, F. A., Jessen, B., and Siggaard-Andersen, J.: A control, double-blind comparison of mepivacaine injection versus saline injection for myofascial pain. Lancet, 1:499–501, 1980.

41. Fung, Y. L.: A Short History of Chinese Philosophy. New York, The Free Press, 1948.

42. Gaw, A. C., Chang, L. W., and Shaw, L. C.: Efficacy of acupuncture on osteoarthritic pain. A controlled double-blind study. N. Engl. J. Med., 293:375–378, 1975.

43. Goldman, J. A., Chiapella, J., Casey, H., et al.: Laser therapy of rheumatoid arthritis. Lasers Surg. Med., 1:93–101, 1980.

44. Goldstein, A., and Hilgard, E. R.: Failure of the opiate antagonist naloxone to modify hypnotic analgesia. Proc. Natl. Acad. Sci., 72:2041–2043, 1975.

45. Greenfield, M. E.: Acupuncture as a rehabilitation modality in chronic low back pain syndrome. Thesis for Master of Public Health Degree, Yale University Department of Epidemiology and Public Health, New Haven, Connecticut, 1977.

46. Guillemin, R.: Beta-lipoprotein and endorphins: Implications of current knowledge. Hosp. Pract., 13:53–60, 1978.

47. Hadden, W. A., and Swanson, A. J.: Spinal infection caused by acupuncture mimicking a prolapsed intervertebral disc. A case report. J. Bone Jt. Surg., 64:624–626, 1982.

48. Han, J. S., and Terenius, L.: Neurochemical basis

of acupuncture analgesia. Ann. Rev. Pharmacol. Toxicol., 22:193–220, 1982.

49. Han, J. S., Ren, M. F., Tang, J., et al.: The role of central catecholamines in acupuncture analgesia. Chin. Med. J., 92:793–800, 1979.

50. Hansen, P. E., and Hansen, J. H.: Acupuncture treatment of chronic tension headache—a controlled cross-over trial. Cephalalgia, 5:137–142, 1985.

51. Hao, J. K.: Zhen Jiu Jingwai Jixue Tupu (An Atlas of Extra-Meridian Odd Points of Acupuncture and Moxibustion). Xian, Shenxi People's Publishers, 1963.

52. Hao, J. K.: Zhen Jiu Jingwai Jixue Tupu Xuji (An Addendum to the Atlas of Extra-Meridian Odd Points of Acupuncture and Moxibustion). Xian, Shenxi People's Publishers, 1974.

53. Hardy, J. D., Wolff, H. G., and Goodell, H.: Experimental evidence on the nature of cutaneous hyperalgesia. J. Clin. Invest., 29:115–140, 1950.

54. Head, H.: On the disturbances of sensation with especial reference to the pain of visceral disease. Brain, 16:1–133, 1893.

55. Head, H.: On the disturbances of sensation with especial reference to the pain of visceral disease. Part II. Head and neck. Brain, 17:339–480, 1894.

56. Head, H.: On the disturbances of sensation with especial reference to the pain of visceral disease. Part III. Pain in diseases of heart and lungs. Brain, 19:153–276, 1896.

57. Helms, J. M.: Acupuncture for the management of primary dysmenorrhea. Obstet. Gynecol., 69:51–56, 1987.

58. Huard, P., and Wong, M.: Chinese Medicine. London, World University Library, 1968.

59. Inman, V. T., and Saunders, J. B. de C. M.: Referred pain from skeletal structures. J. Nerv. Ment. Dis., 99:660–667, 1944.

60. Isu, T., Iwasaki, Y., Sasaki, H., and Abe, H.: Spinal cord and root injuries due to glass fragments and acupuncture needles. Surg. Neurol., 23:255–260, 1985.

61. Izatt, E., and Fairman, M.: Staphylococcal septicemia with disseminated intravascular coagulation associated with acupuncture. Postgrad. Med., 53:285–286, 1977.

62. Jenkins, C.: On L-tryptophan. Acupunct. News, 10:3, 1982.

63. Johnson, E. W., and Parker, W. D.: Electromyography examination. In Johnson, E. W. (Ed.): Practical Electromyography. Baltimore, Williams & Wilkins, 1980.

64. Jones, H. S.: Case records. Auricular complications of acupuncture. J. Laryngol. Otol., 99:1143–1145, 1985.

65. Junnila, S. Y. T.: Acupuncture superior to Piroxicam in the treatment of osteoarthritis. Am. J. Acupunct., 10:341–346, 1982.

66. Kaada, B.: Mechanism of vasodilatation evoked by transcutaneous nerve stimulation (TNS). Acupunct. Electrother. Res. Int. J., 10:217–219, 1985.

67. Kaada, B., Jorum, E., and Sagvolden, T.: Analgesia induced by trigeminal nerve stimulation (electroacupuncture) abolished by nuclei raphe lesions in rats. Acupunct. Electrother. Res. Int. J., 4:221–234, 1979.

68. Keegan, J. J., and Garrett, F. D.: The segmental distribution of cutaneous nerves in the limbs in man. Anat. Rec., 102:409–437, 1948.

69. Kellgren, J. H.: On the distribution of pain arising from deep somatic structures with charts of segmental pain areas. Clin. Sci., 4:35–46, 1939.

70. Kellgren, J. H.: Deep pain sensibility. Lancet, 1:943–949, 1949.

71. Kent, G. P., Brondum, J., Keenlyside, R. A., LaFazia, L. M., and Scott, H. D.: A large outbreak of acupuncture-associated hepatitis B. Am. J. Epidemiol., 127:591–598, 1988.

72. Kerr, F. W. L.: Acupuncture and pain. The Pain Book. Englewood Cliffs, Prentice-Hall, 1981, pp. 155–171.

73. Kerr, F. W. L., Wilson, P. R., and Nijensohn, D.: Acupuncture reduces the trigeminal evoked response in decerebrated cats. Exp. Neurol., 61:84–95, 1978.

74. LeBars, D., Besson, J. M., et al.: Diffuse noxious inhibitory control (DNIC). II. Lack of effect on non-convergent neurones, supraspinal involvement and theoretical implications. Pain, 6:305–327, 1979.

75. LeBars, D., Dickenson, A. H., and Besson, J. M.: Diffuse noxious inhibitory controls (DNIC). I. Effects on dorsal horn convergent neurons in the rat. Pain, 6:283–304, 1979.

76. Lee, M. H. M.: Acupuncture for pain control. In Mark, L. C. (Ed.): Pain Control. Practical Aspects of Pain Care. New York, Masson Publishing, 1981, pp. 83–88.

77. Lee, M. H. M., and Ernst, M.: The sympatholytic effect of acupuncture as evidenced by thermography. A preliminary report. Orthop. Rev., 12:67–72, 1983.

78. Lee, M. H. M., and Ernst, M.: Clinical and research observations on acupuncture analgesia and thermography. Presented at Duesseldorfer Akupunktur Symposium, July 31, 1987.

79. Lee, M. H. M., and Yang, W. G. F.: The possible usefulness of acupuncture in rheumatic disease. Clin. Rheumatol., 3:237–247, 1985.

80. Lee, M. H. M., Zarestky, H. H., Ernst, M., Dworkin, B., and Jones, R.: The analgesia effects of aspirin and placebo on experimentally induced tooth pulp pain. J. Med., 16:417–428, 1985.

81. Lee, R. J. E., and McIlwain, J. C.: Subacute bacterial endocarditis following ear acupuncture. Int. J. Cardiol., 7:62–63, 1985.

82. Lee, S. C., Yin, S. J., Lee, M. L., and Tsai, W. J.: Effects of acupuncture on serum cortisol level and dopamine beta-hydroxylase activities in normal Chinese. Am. J. Chin. Med., 10:62–69, 1982.

83. Lewis, T.: Pain. New York, Macmillan, 1942.

84. Lewis, T., and Kellgren, J. H.: Observations related to referred pain, visceromotor reflexes and other associated phenomena. Clin. Sci., 4:47–71, 1939.

85. Li, F. P., and Shiang, E. L.: Acupuncture and possible hepatitis B infection (letter). J.A.M.A., 243:1423, 1980.

86. Li, S. J., Tang, J., and Han, J. S.: The implication of central serotonin in electroacupuncture tolerance in rat. Sci. Sin., 25:620–629, 1982.

87. Liao, S. J.: Acupuncture—an appraisal. Conn. Med., 37:506–510, 1973.

88. Liao, S. J.: Acupuncture points and trigger points. Am. Congress Rehab. Med., Eastern Section Annual Meeting, Washington, DC, March 1973.

89. Liao, S. J.: Der Gebrauch von Akupunktur bei chronischen Kreuzschmerzen. Akupunktur Theorie und Praxis 1:31–33, 1973.

90. Liao, S. J.: L'acupuncture dans la lombalgie persistante post-operatoire. Les Mensuel du Medecin Acupuncteur, No. 7, Janvier 1974, pp. 22–25.

91. Liao, S. J.: Acupuncture points: Coincidence with motor points of skeletal muscles (abstract). Arch. Phys. Med. Rehabil., 56:550, 1975.

92. Liao, S. J.: Acupuncture in cervical spondylosis. Acupunct. Electrother. Res. Int. J., 1:226, 1975.

93. Liao, S. J.: Acupuncture veterinaire. Les Mensuel du Medecin Acupuncteur, No. 31, Mai 1976, pp. 35–40.

94. Liao, S. J.: Acupuncture veterinaire. Les Mensuel du Medecin Acupuncteur, No. 32, Juin 1976, pp. 71–78.

95. Liao, S. J.: Use of acupuncture for relief of head pain. Presentation at Am. Dental Assn. 118th Annual Session, Miami Beach, FL, October 10, 1977.

96. Liao, S. J.: Recent advances in the understanding of acupuncture. Yale J. Biol. Med., 51:55–65, 1978.

97. Liao, S. J.: Questions and Answers about Acupuncture. Middlebury, CT, Research Institute of Acupuncture and Chinese Medicine, 1980.

98. Liao, S. J.: Unpublished data.

99. Liao, S. J. (English Editor): Hunan College of Traditional Chinese Medicine (the Compiler-Translator): Chinese-English Terminology of Traditional Chinese Medicine. Changsha, Hunan, Hunan Science & Technology Press, 1983.

100. Liao, S. J., and Liao, M. K.: Acupuncture and tele-electronic infra-red thermography. Acupunct. Electrother. Res. Int. J., 10:41–66, 1985.

101. Liao, S. J., and Merriman, H.: Unpublished case report, 1972.

102. Liao, S. J., and Van Nghi, N.: Les Mensuel du Medecin Acupuncteur, No. 34, Septembre 1976, pp. 151–157.

103. Liao, S. J., and Wen, K. K.: Patients' hypnotizability and their response to acupuncture treatments for pain-relief. A preliminary statistical study. Am. J. Acupunct., 4:263–268, 1976.

104. Liao, Y. Y., Seto, K., Saito, H., et al.: Effect of acupuncture on adrenocortical hormone production: Variation in the ability for adrenocortical hormone production in relation to the duration of acupuncture stimulation. Am. J. Chin. Med., 7:362–371, 1979.

105. Licht, S.: History of electrodiagnosis. In Licht, S. (Ed.): Electrodiagnosis and Electromyography, 3rd Ed. New Haven, CT, Elizabeth Licht, Publisher, 1971, pp. 6–7.

106. Lu, G. D., and Needham, J.: Celestial Lancets. A History and Rationale of Acupuncture and Moxa. Cambridge, Cambridge University Press, 1980.

107. Lynn, B., and Perl, E. R.: Failure of acupuncture to produce localized analgesia. Pain, 3:339–351, 1977.

108. Malizia, F., Paolucci, D., et al.: Electroacupuncture and peripheral beta-endorphin and ACTH levels. Lancet 2:535–536, 1979.

109. Man, S. C.: Preliminary clinical study of acupuncture in rheumatoid arthritis with painful knees (abstract). Arthritis Rheum., 16:558–559, 1973.

110. Man, S. C., and Baragar, F. D.: Preliminary study of acupuncture in rheumatoid arthritis. J. Rheumatol., 1:126–129, 1974.

111. Masala, A., Satta, G., Alagna, S., et al.: Suppression of electroacupuncture (EA)–induced beta-endorphin and ACTH release by hydrocortisone in man. Absence of effects on EA-induced anaesthesia. Acta Endocrinol. (Copenh.) 103:469–472, 1983.

112. Mayer, D. J., Price, D. D., and Rafii, A.: Antagonism of acupuncture hypalgesia in man by the narcotic antagonist naloxone. Brain Res., 121:368–372, 1977.

113. McLennan, H., Gilfillan, K., and Heap, Y.: Some pharmacological observations on the analgesia induced by acupuncture in rabbits. Pain, 3:229–238, 1977.

114. Melzack, R., and Melinkoff, R. F.: Analgesia produced by brain stimulation: Evidence of a prolonged onset period. Exp. Neurol., 43:369–374, 1974.

115. Melzack, R., Stillwell, D. M., and Fox, E. J.: Trigger points and acupuncture points for pain correlation and implications. Pain, 3:3–23, 1977.

116. Moore, M. E., and Berk, S. N.: Acupuncture on chronic shoulder pain. An experimental study with attention to the role of placebo and hypnotic susceptibility. Ann. Intern. Med., 84:381–384, 1976.

117. Morand, S.: Memoir on Acupuncturation, Embracing a Series of Cases Drawn up under the Inspection of M. Julius Cloquet. Translated from the French, by Franklin Bache. Philadelphia, Robert Desilver, 1825.

118. Morton, D. J.: Hypermobility of first metatarsal segment. J. Bone Jt. Surg., 10:187–196, 1928.

119. Morton, T. G.: Peculiar and painful affection of

fourth metatarso-phalangeal articulation. Am. J. Med. Sci., 71:37–45, 1876.

120. Nappi, G., Faccinetti, F., et al.: Different releasing effects of traditional manual acupuncture and electroacupuncture on propiocortin-related peptides. Acupunct. Electrother. Res. Int. J., 7:93–103, 1982.

121. Needham, J.: Science and Civilisation in China, Vol. 2. History of Scientific Thought. Cambridge, Cambridge University Press, 1956.

122. Ng, L. K. Y., Thoa, N. B., Dothitt, T. C., Albert, C. A., and Viktora, J.: Decrease in brain neurotransmitters and elevation of footshock-induced pain threshold following repeated electro-stimulation of putative acupuncture loci in rats. Am. J. Chin. Med., 2:236–237, 1974.

123. Nogier, P. F. M.: Treatise of Auriculotherapy. Paris, Maisonneuve, 1972.

124. Osler, W.: The Principles and Practice of Medicine. Edinburgh, Y. J. Pentland, 1892.

125. Peake, J. B., Roth, J. L., and Schuchmann, G. F.: Pneumothorax: Complication of nerve conduction studies using needle stimulation. Arch. Phys. Med. Rehabil., 63:187–188, 1982.

126. Peets, J., and Pomeranz, B.: CXBX mice deficient in opiate receptors show poor electroacupuncture analgesia. Nature, 273:675–676, 1978.

127. Peking Acupuncture Anesthesia Coordinating Group: Preliminary study on the mechanism of acupuncture anesthesia. Sci. Sin., 16:447–456, 1973.

128. Peng, A. T. C., Behar, S., and Yue, S. J.: Long term therapeutic effects of electroacupuncture for chronic neck and shoulder pain—a double blind study. Acupunct. Electrother. Res. Int. J., 12:37–44, 1987.

129. Peng, L. H. C., Yuang, M. M. P., Loh, S. H., et al.: Endorphin release. A possible mechanism of acupuncture analgesia. Comp. Med. East West, 6:57–60, 1978.

130. People's Republic of China: Acupuncture Anesthesia. Color movies, 1973.

131. Petrie, J. P., and Hazleman, B. L.: A controlled study of acupuncture in neck pain. Br. J. Rheumatol., 25:271–275, 1986.

132. Pierik, M. G.: Fatal staphylococcal septicemia following acupuncture. Report of two cases—Occurrence of staphylococcal septicemia following acupuncture emphasizes need for thorough medical evaluation before such procedures. RI Med. J., 65:251–253, 1982.

133. Plotz, G. M., Plotz, P. H., and Lamont-Havers, R. W.: Workshop on the use of acupuncture in the rheumatic diseases: Summary of proceedings. Arthritis Rheum., 17:939–942, 1974.

134. Pomeranz, B.: Scientific basis of acupuncture. In Stux, G., and Pomeranz, B.: Acupuncture. Textbook and Atlas. Berlin, Springer-Verlag, 1987, pp. 1–34.

135. Pomeranz, B., and Chiu, D.: Naloxone blockade of acupuncture analgesia. Endorphin implicated. Life Sci., 79:1757–1762, 1976.

136. Pomeranz, B., Cheng, R., and Law, P.: Acupuncture reduces electrophysiological and behavioral responses to noxious stimuli. Pituitary is implicated. Exp. Neurol., 54:172–178, 1977.

137. Raustia, A. M.: Diagnosis and treatment of temporomandibular joint dysfunction. Proc. Finn. Dent. Soc., 82[Suppl. X]:1–41, 1986.

138. Reinstein, L., Twardzik, F. G., and Mech, K. F.: Pneumothorax: A complication of needle electromyography of the supraspinatus muscle. Arch. Phys. Med. Rehabil., 68:561–562, 1987.

139. Ren, M. F., Tu, Z. P., and Han, J. S.: The effect of hemicholin, choline, eserin, and atropine on acupuncture analgesia in rat. In Advances in Acupuncture and Acupuncture Anesthesia. Beijing, People's Publishing House, 1980, pp. 439–440.

140. Renton, J.: Observations on acupuncturation. Edinb. Med. J., 34:100, 1830.

141. Research Group of Acupuncture Anesthesia, Peking Medical College, Peking: The role of some neurotransmitters of brain in finger-acupuncture analgesia. Sci. Sin., 17:112–113, 1974.

142. Reston, J.: Now about my operation in Peking. The New York Times, July 26, 1971.

143. Rosenthal, S. R., and Sonnenschein, R. R.: Histamine as a possible chemical mediator for cutaneous pain. Am. J. Physiol., 155:186–190, 1948.

144. Ruch, T. C., and Fulton, J. F.: Medical Physiology and Biophysics, Chapters 13, 14, and 15. Philadelphia, W. B. Saunders Company, 1960.

145. Section on Acupuncture Analgesia of the Second Laboratory of Shanghai Institute of Physiology: Knowing the mechanism of acupuncture anesthesia in practice. Kexue Tongbao (Scientia), 23:342–347, 1976.

146. Shanghai Institute of Physiology: Electric response to noxious stimulation and its inhibition in nucleus centralis lateralis of thalamus in rabbits. Chin. Med. J., 131:135, 1973.

147. Shen, A. C., Whitehouse, M. J., Powers, T. R., et al.: A pilot study of the effects of acupuncture in rheumatoid arthritis. Arthritis Rheum., 16:569–570, 1973.

148. Sin, Y. M.: Acupuncture and inflammation. Int. J. Chin. Med., 1:15–20, 1984.

149. Sjolund, B., and Eriksson, M.: Electroacupuncture and endogenous morphine. Lancet, 2:1085, 1976.

150. Smith, D. L., Walczyk, M. H., and Campbell, S.: Acupuncture-needle-induced compartment syndrome. West. J. Med., 144:478–479, 1986.

151. Spiegel, H.: Hypnosis: An adjunct to psychotherapy. In Freedman, A. M., Kaplan, H. I., and Sadock, B. J. (Eds.): Comprehensive Textbook of Psychiatry, 2nd Ed. Baltimore, Williams & Wilkins, 1975.

152. Stryker, W. S., Gunn, R. A., and Francis, D. P.: Outbreak of hepatitis B associated with acupuncture. J. Fam. Pract., 22:155–158, 1986.

153. Tang, J., and Han, J. S.: Changes in the morphine-like activity in the rat brain and pituitary gland during electroacupuncture analgesia. J. Beijing Med. Coll., 3:150–152, 1978.

154. Tang, J., Wang, Y., Yang, X. D., and Han, J. S.: The pituitary opioids in electroacupuncture analgesia in the rat. J. Beijing Med. Coll., 13:202–204, 1981.

155. Travell, J.: Office Hours: Day and Night. The Autobiography of Janet Travell, M.D. New York, The World Publishing Company, 1968, pp. 257–260.

156. Travell, J. G., and Simons, D. G.: Myofascial Pain and Dysfunction. The Trigger Point Manual. Baltimore, Williams & Wilkins, 1983, pp. 20 and 76.

157. Van Nghi, N., and Liao, S. J.: Etude des points d'acupuncture. A. Les points curieux. Les Mensuel du Medecin Acupuncteur, No. 1, Mai 1973, pp. 35–38.

158. Van Nghi, N., and Liao, S. J.: Etude des points d'acupuncture. A. Les points curieux. Les Mensuel du Medecin Acupuncteur, No. 2, Juin 1973, pp. 32–38.

159. Van Nghi, N., and Liao, S. J.: Etude des points d'acupuncture. A. Les points curieux. Les Mensuel du Medecin Acupuncteur, No. 3, Juillet 1973, pp. 31–36.

160. Van Nghi, N., and Liao, S. J.: Etude des points d'acupuncture. A. Les points curieux. Les Mensuel du Medecin Acupuncteur, No. 4, Septembre 1973, pp. 31–37.

161. Van Nghi, N., and Liao, S. J.: Etude des d'acupuncture. B. Les points couveaux. Les Mensuel du Medecin Acupuncteur, No. 5, Octobre 1973, pp. 31–35.

162. Van Nghi, N., and Liao, S. J.: Etude des d'acupuncture. B. Les points couveaux. Les Mensuel du Medecin Acupuncteur, No. 6, Novembre 1973, pp. 31–36.

163. Vierck, C. J. Jr., Lineberry, C. G., Lee, P. K., et al.: Prolonged hypalgesia following "acupuncture" in monkeys. Life Sci., 15:1277–1289, 1974.

164. Wall, P. D., and Drubner, R.: Somatosensory pathways. Ann. Rev. Physiol., 34:315–336, 1972.

165. Wang, K. M., Yao, S. M., Xian, Y. L., and Hou, Z. L.: A study on the receptive field of acupoints and the relationship between characteristics of needling sensation and groups of afferent fibers. Sci. Sin., 28:963–971, 1985.

166. Warwick-Brown, N. P., and Richards, A. E. S.: Perichondritis of the ear following acupuncture. J. Laryngol. Otol., 100:1177–1179, 1986.

167. Watkins, L. R., and Mayer, D. J.: Organization of endogenous opiate and non-opiate pain control systems. Science, 216:1185–1192, 1982.

168. Yi, C. C., Yu, Y. G., Ji, X. Q., and Zou, K.: Preliminary studies on the discharge of endorphin from pituitary after electro-acupuncture. Nat. Med. J. China, 7:397–398, 1978.

169. Zhou, K., Yi, Q. C., Wu, S. X., Lu, Y. X., Wang, F. S., Yu, Y. G., Ji, X. Q., Zhang, Z. X., and Zao, D. D.: Enkephalin involvement in acupuncture analgesia. Sci. Sin., 23:1197–1207, 1980.

17

Massage

MILAND E. KNAPP

Definition. *Massage* is a term used to signify a group of systematic and scientific manipulations of body tissues that are best performed with the hands "for the purpose of affecting the nervous and muscular system and the general circulation."

History

Massage is probably the oldest of all remedies, since it is instinctive not only in humans but in the lower animals as well. The oldest written record of massage was made 3000 years ago by the Chinese. The ancient Hindus, Persians, and Egyptians used manipulation in some form and some of the movements of massage for rheumatic ailments. The Greeks recognized gymnastics as an institution that was an auxiliary to the development of the people, both socially and politically. Hippocrates wrote important papers on massage, for instance, about the use of friction after sprains and dislocations and about kneading in case of constipation. About two centuries ago, the Chinese books on massage were translated into French, which accounts for the French terminology so common in massage texts. At the beginning of the 19th century, Peter Henry Ling, a fencing master of Stockholm, Sweden, introduced a system of movement that he had not originated but had systematized. It consists of, first, massage (manipulation of the soft tissues) and, second, medical gymnastics (exercise of the joints). During the last century, Lucas-Championnière championed treatment of fractures by mobilization, including massage and exercise. During the years 1917 to 1940, James B. Mennell of England systematized massage movements and applied them to the treatment of a great many conditions.

Physiological Effects of Massage

Unfortunately, most of the teaching of massage in the past had been done by lay persons who did not understand physiology in the modern sense; therefore, many statements made in massage texts are obviously untrue insofar as physiological effects of massage are concerned. The effects may be classified as reflex and mechanical.

Reflex Effects. Reflex effects are produced in the skin by stimulation of the peripheral receptors, which then transmit impulses through the spinal cord to the brain and produce sensations of pleasure or relaxation. Peripherally, these impulses cause relaxation of muscles and dilatation or constriction of arterioles. Sedation is one of the very important physiological effects of massage. It is obtained when the massage is given in a monotonously repetitive manner, without sharp variations in pressure or irritating changes in the method of application. These pleasant effects result in relaxation of muscle as well as reduction of mental tension.

Mechanical Effects. The mechanical effects consist of (1) measures that assist return flow circulation of blood and lymph because the massage is given with the greatest force in the centripetal direction and (2) measures that produce intramuscular motion. They may be effective in stretching adhesions between muscle fibers and mobilizing accumulations of fluid.

Massage does *not* develop muscle strength and

should *not* be used as a substitute for active exercise.

Technique

Proficiency in the performance of massage movements is not easily acquired. It requires long and diligent practice. Massage is an art rather than a science. One individual may learn to administer acceptable massage quickly and after only a minimum of practice, whereas another may never give acceptable massage even after many months of assiduous effort. Natural ability is an important factor. However, as with other arts, improvement will be gained by practice.

I am not in favor of trying to teach the patient or the family to give massage at home except under unusual circumstances, because this kind of training is usually inadequate and the resulting treatment may produce harmful effects as easily as it may produce helpful results.

Description of technique is difficult, but certain principles may be stated:

1. The patient must be relaxed and comfortable. Clothing should not be tight, especially proximal to the area to be treated. Clothing should be removed from the area to be treated, but, to avoid embarrassment and needless cooling, the patient should not be uncovered unnecessarily.

2. The therapist should also be relaxed and comfortable and should stand in a position so that the entire stroke can be performed without change of stance or undue movement.

3. Skill is required rather than strength. Pain and apprehension must not be produced if deep effects are desired. A relaxed muscle has the physical properties of a liquid enclosed in a membrane, and pressure exerted on any portion of it will be transmitted equally in all directions. Pressure is thus transmitted to the deeper muscles. On the other hand, a tense, contracted muscle has the properties of a solid and does not transmit the force evenly.

4. A lubricating oil, powder, or cream facilitates good technique. Heavy mineral oil is suitable.

Stroking (*Effleurage*). Stroking massage is performed by running the hand lightly over the surface of the skin. The force of the stroke starts distally and progresses proximally to assist return flow circulation. The hands may be lifted off the part at the end of the stroke and returned to the point of beginning if the motion is rhythmic and the contact and release are performed gently, without abruptness. It is probably better, however, to return to the point of beginning with the hands in contact with the skin but producing little or no actual pressure.

Stroking may be superficial or deep. In superficial stroking, the direction of the force is not important, since the pressure is so light that mechanical effects are not produced. In deep stroking, the direction of force is important because the usual major objective is to assist return flow circulation. Therefore, the force of the stroke definitely should be centripetal.

Compression (*Pétrissage*). Compression includes kneading, squeezing, and friction. Kneading may be described as a motion in which the soft tissues are picked up between the fingers and manipulated in an alternating fashion so that there is motion within the muscle itself. It does not proceed in any particular direction but is used to mobilize the tissue fluids and create intramuscular motion to stretch adhesions. Squeezing is performed with larger portions of the muscle, squeezing the part either between the two hands or between the hand and a solid object such as the table or bone. Friction is a circular motion performed by placing a small part of the hand on the area. This portion of the hand is usually the thumb, the heel of the hand, or the fingertips. The movement is in circular loops and is done fairly rapidly with increasing pressure.

Percussion (*Tapôtement*). Percussive movements are alternating movements performed to produce stimulation. Hacking is usually done with the outer border of the hand or the relaxed fingers, bouncing the hands alternately off the part to be treated. It may also be used in a kind of whipping motion using the fingers as the flexible portion of the whip. Clapping is done with the palms of the hand in a similar manner. If the hands are cupped, the deeper sound produced may be of some psychological benefit. Beating is performed by a similar technique with the fist clenched. The therapist produces vibration by placing the fingertips in contact with the skin and shaking the entire arm. This transmits a trembling movement to the patient. The therapeutic value of this type of movement is questionable, although it is pleasant when performed expertly.

The movements of massage are not done in sequence but are intermingled, using varying techniques for different purposes. The compression techniques are used to mobilize tissue deposits and to stretch adhesions. They may be followed by stroking massage to remove the deposits or edema fluid. Friction is used to treat very limited areas, particularly nodules such as fibrositic nodules, and this again is followed by stroking massage. The percussive movements are ordinarily used at the end of the treatment. It is my opinion that they are used primarily for their psychological effects rather than for any real physical benefit.

Numerous mechanical devices have been invented and manufactured for the application of massage movements. Rollers of various types operated manually or by electric motors have been used to simulate kneading and stroking types of massage. Perhaps the most common machines are those that produce vibration. They are attached to the hand or incorporated in pads of various kinds and on tables. Although they may produce pleasurable effects, it is generally conceded that they are not therapeutically effective.

Indications

Massage is useful in any condition in which relief of pain, reduction of swelling, or mobilization of contracted tissues is desired. Probably its greatest single indication is to overcome the swelling and induration that frequently follow trauma (see Chapter 33). Fractures, dislocations, joint injuries, sprains, strains, bruises, and tendon and nerve injuries may be benefited by massage at certain stages of recovery. Arthritis, periarthritis, bursitis, neuritis, fibrositis, low back pain, and paralytic conditions, such as hemiplegia, paraplegia, quadriplegia, cerebral palsy, and multiple sclerosis, may present problems that can be relieved by massage.

Psychoneurotic patients and occasionally even patients with psychoses may be helped by massage. However, such treatment should be prescribed only after careful consideration of its psychological effects, because harmful psychological trends may be intensified by physical treatment.

Abdominal massage has been advocated and described in the past but is not used to any great extent at the present time. It is also ineffective for weight reduction.

Massage is not a substitute for exercise. It does not increase muscle strength. Strength develops in muscles contracting actively, preferably against resistance.

A masseur once told me he was giving an alcoholic patient massage equivalent to a three-mile hike. Perhaps he was, but the hike was being performed by the masseur, on his hands. The patient was getting rest in bed.

Contraindications

The greatest contraindications to massage are infections, because of the likelihood of spreading the infection through the tissues and breaking down barriers to its spread; malignancies, because tumor tissues similarly may be spread beyond confined limits and promote metastases or extension of the malignancy; and skin diseases (which might be communicated to the masseur), when irritation is contraindicated or when lesions might be spread by contact. Massage should be given with caution in debilitated individuals and in areas where the skin has been damaged by burns or where it is thin for other reasons. In thrombophlebitis, massage may be dangerous, because thrombi may be broken into emboli.

References

1. Krusen, F. H.: Physical Medicine. Philadelphia, W. B. Saunders Co., 1941.
2. Mennell, J. B.: Physical Treatment by Movement, Manipulation and Massage, 4th Ed. Philadelphia, The Blakiston Co., 1940.
3. Tidy, N. M.: Massage and Remedial Exercises in Medical and Surgical Conditions, 3rd Ed. Baltimore, William Wood and Co., 1937.
4. Wood, E. C., and Becker, P. D.: Beard's Massage, 3rd Ed. Philadelphia, W. B. Saunders Company, 1981.

18

Therapeutic Exercise to Maintain Mobility

FREDERIC J. KOTTKE

Therapeutic exercise may be defined as the prescription of bodily movement to correct an impairment, improve musculoskeletal function, or maintain a state of well-being. Therapeutic exercise may vary from highly selected activities, restricted to specific muscles or parts of the body, to general and vigorous activities, used to restore a convalescing patient to the peak of physical condition. The prescription for therapeutic exercise varies with the purpose for which it is used. This, in turn, is directly dependent upon the condition of the patient. An adequate medical evaluation is essential before therapeutic exercise is prescribed. Therapeutic exercise prescribed without competent medical evaluation and supervision may not only be inadequate but actually detrimental to the patient.

Knowledge of the biophysical and physiological aspects of kinesiology and the basic principles of therapeutic exercise is needed by the physician who plans to prescribe and supervise a program of therapeutic exercise for a patient. Therapeutic exercises have local and general effects on the physiology of the body. These responses occur in the muscular, skeletal, nervous, circulatory, and endocrine systems in particular. Metabolism may be altered significantly. The prescription of an exercise to produce a desired response is just as specific as and often more involved than the prescription of a pharmaceutical compound. An adequate program of therapeutic exercise requires that the prescription be modified as the condition of the patient changes.

This chapter contains the principles of therapeutic exercise to maintain mobility and information concerning the general types of exercises used in medical practice. Because the exercise program for each patient is developed according to the patient's needs on the basis of the medical evaluation of the disability, no attempt is made here to provide a "cookbook" of exercises, since for any part of the body, exercises may be designed in a number of ways depending upon the desired goal and the equipment at hand.

Exercises to Increase or Maintain Mobility of Joints and Soft Tissues

Physiology of Fibrous Connective Tissue

There is a continual turnover of the components of connective tissue caused by breakdown and replacement and by reorganization of the attachments of the various components. The connective tissue of the body provides the connection between all cells and around and between all organs under the epidermis. The fibers are made up of reticulin and collagen, which do not appear to be essentially different in their ultramicroscopic structure; elastic fibers, which differ from collagen in their physical and chemical characteristics as well as their metabolic response; and fibrin, which is a temporary connective tissue element that is extremely important in the process of repair. In addition, there is the amorphous ground substance, which is structureless but which plays an important role in binding the structural elements together. It appears that the attachments between fibers produced by

436

the ground substance can shift as the result of prolonged tension or can develop as the result of prolonged contact.

Although metabolic studies have not clearly defined the rate at which collagen is removed, altered, or replaced under ordinary circumstances, considerable information is available regarding the rapid response of fibrous connective tissue in areas where trauma has occurred. Newly formed collagen fibrils are abundant around proliferating fibroblasts within five days.[3, 6, 25] Recent studies indicate that in normal connective tissue, a small percentage of collagen is turned over rapidly, whereas the remainder of the collagen fibers show a very slow rate of metabolic change.[17]

The collagen fibril is an aggregation of tropocollagen rods in staggered array, forming the characteristic 640 A bands. The most soluble collagen is that most recently formed. Chemical bonding between parallel tropocollagen molecules leads to increasing insolubility and increased tensile strength. However, the process may be reversible, and soluble collagen may result from the breakdown of insoluble collagen as well as from the synthesis of collagen.[13]

Connective tissue is usually described in relation to the arrangement of the fibrous elements.

Organized Connective Tissue. Tendons and ligaments are made up of organized connective tissue composed of dense bundles of coarse collagen between which columns of fibrocytes are interspersed (Fig. 18–1). The collagen bundles are arranged linearly in the long axis of the tendon or ligament and present a uniform appearance. Within these heavy bundles, parallel collagen fibers run through the entire length of the bundle without interruption from the musculotendinous junction to the bone attachment. It is this uninterrupted continuity of collagen fibers throughout their length that gives tendons and ligaments their great strength (Fig. 18–2). Collagen fibers are extracellular and nonliving. However, they are totally dependent on the enzymes produced by the metabolism of adjacent fibrocytes for maintenance and repair of disruptions caused by normal activity. Anything that reduces fibrocyte metabolism, such as impairment of circulation, decreases the capacity for repair and allows the progression of deterioration. With loss of local circulation, death of fibrocytes occurs followed by progressive destruction of collagen bundles without repair. This leads to a local infarct of the tendon and the accumulation of calcium in the debris, resulting in a typical calcified tendinitis. More fibrocytes are present in columnar arrangement in tendons than in ligaments. These fibrocytes are stellate with processes extending between the bundles of collagen fibers. It appears that this organization is a response to the tension produced by muscular contraction.[3, 6]

TENDON HEALING. Buck[3] sectioned the Achilles tendon of the rat and allowed it to retract without suturing (Fig. 18–3). A fibrin coagulum was laid down randomly in the defect between the cut ends of the tendon, becoming oriented longitudinally with the tendon by the slight tension placed on the coagulum by the repeated contractions of the muscle. Fibroblasts began to grow into the coagulum from the periphery within three days, and reticulin fibers and collagen fibers were laid down within four days. The collagen fibers were oriented parallel to the fibrin threads in the long axis of the tendon. Within two weeks, the entire length of the

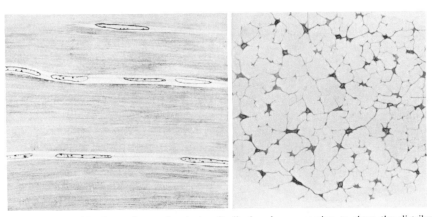

FIGURE 18–1. Drawing of the histology of a tendon in longitudinal and cross section to show the distribution of fibrocytes between the bundles of collagen fibers. (From Maximow, A. A., and Bloom, W.: A Textbook of Histology, 7th Ed. Philadelphia, W. B. Saunders Co., 1957.)

FREDERIC J. KOTTKE

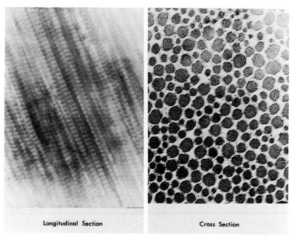

Longitudinal Section   Cross Section

FIGURE 18–2. Electron micrograph of longitudinal and transverse sections of a tendon showing bundles of coarse collagen fibers of various diameters running through the length of the tendon from muscle to bone without interruption, which gives the great tensile strength to tendon. Electron micrograph × 75,000. (Courtesy of William D. Paul.)

tendon up to the muscular insertion was invaded by fibroblasts. The reaction as indicated by proliferation of collagen and the persistence of fibroblasts throughout the length of the tendon lasted for four months. The healing reaction resulted in restoration of continuous linear collagen fibers from one end of the tendon to the other, except for minor irregularities of whorls of collagen along the line of the incision. It appears from this and other studies that a tendon 2 to 3 mm in diameter would redevelop near-normal strength in four to six months. In a tendon as large as the Achilles tendon in humans, reconstitution to near-normal strength requires 24 months if the circulation is normal.

When the muscle was denervated at the time the tendon was cut, the fibrin did not organize in a uniform longitudinal pattern and the collagen fibers, likewise, developed in a random orientation rather than in parallel bundles.

It appears that the regular pattern of fibers produced in the healing tendon is due to the exertion of tension on the fibrin coagulum to produce a linear pattern and that collagen is organized on this matrix.[1, 6]

ADHESION FORMATION. The increasing strength of new connective tissue is correlated with the formation and maturation of collagen fibers.[28] After injury, collagen fibrils can be detected by using the electron microscope as early as the second day, by biochemical means on the third day, and by use of the light microscope only a day or two later, when molecular accretion has occurred. Within four to five days, collagenous adhesions begin to form between a sutured tendon and the surrounding structures. Watson-Jones[30] observed collagen fibers at fracture sites within five days. Gentle passive motion of the sutured tendon begun

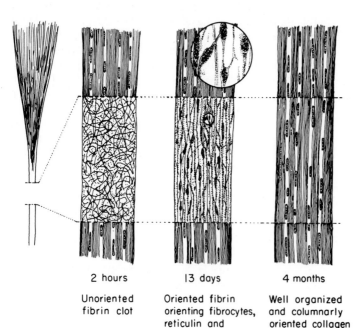

2 hours   13 days   4 months

Unoriented   Oriented fibrin   Well organized
fibrin clot   orienting fibrocytes,   and columnarly
                   reticulin and   oriented collagen
                   collagen   and fibrocytes

FIGURE 18–3. Diagram of healing of Achilles tendon of rat when cut and not sutured. (From data of Buck, R. C.: Regeneration of tendon. J. Pathol. Bacteriol., 66:1–18, 1953.)

the day after surgery will prevent adhesions to surrounding structures without producing significant tension on the suture. Gentle passive motion may be established in this manner in spite of the inflammation, which greatly reduces the tensile strength of the collagen bundles and the holding strength of any suture. The loss in tissue strength due to inflammation is greatest at two to three days. Tensile strength gradually increases so that, at 14 days, the tensile strength has recovered to become greater than that at the time that the sutures were first placed. This gentle passive motion prevents the formation of collagen fibers that extend from the inflamed tendon to the surrounding tissues and that immobilize the tendon in a dense scar, but since the invading fibrocytes produce new collagen, tensile strength begins to increase. This inflammatory reaction lasts for at least four months. Early gentle motion preserves the gliding motion of the tendon without force and shortens the functional recovery time, i.e., the time required for the tendon to be healed and to become free to move.[2]

Loose Connective Tissue. Loose or areolar connective tissue forms between organs and other structures, such as joint capsules, fascia, intermuscular layers, and subcutaneous tissue, where movement occurs repeatedly. It will allow movement through limited distances, adapt by shortening and fixation if there is no motion, or elongate slowly under prolonged or repeated tension.

Histologically, meshworks of collagen and reticular fibers run in all directions without a regular pattern, although there appears to be an increase in the number of fibers in the direction of repeated and strongest tension. These fibers form a loose mesh that can be distorted easily to allow flexibility for movement. When these fibers are laid down or replaced, their length and mobility between attachments depend upon the motion of the part during the period of formation. The recognition that it is a normal reaction of connective tissue to be laid down and to shrink in any immobilized area is the basis for the use of therapy to maintain mobility. Frequent daily exercises through the functional range of motion are necessary to maintain mobility. In the presence of inflammation, fibrosis occurs more rapidly. Each affected part needs to be moved through the range to be maintained at intervals shorter than the time required to lay down collagen.[23]

Thousands of reticular fibers, which appear to be single strands of collagen fibers, are attached over the entire external surface of the sarcolemma of each muscle fiber so that resistance to motion is provided not only through the heavy fibrous attachments at the ends of each muscle fiber but also through the reticular fibers to the surrounding connective tissue. The proportionate force of the muscular contraction transmitted through these reticular fibers is not known, but in conditions of intramuscular fibrosis it is increased significantly.

When a part is immobilized, the collagenous and reticular networks become contracted and the distance between attachments in the network is shortened so that the tissue becomes dense and hard and loses the suppleness of normal areolar tissue.

Dense Connective Tissue. In areas where motion does not occur, such as in fascial planes and the capsules of muscles or organs, collagen is laid down as dense meshworks, sheets, or bands. This type of connective tissue is also laid down in scars. If motion is maintained during healing of a wound, connective tissue of the areolar type develops. If the wound is immobilized, a dense contracted scar forms. In areas immobilized by edema, dense connective tissue will also develop. These densely packed collagen bundles not only restrict motion but also compress and cut off the capillary circulation so that the scar becomes ischemic and the capacity for remobilization is reduced. It is imperative if motion is to be maintained in a part that the motion be initiated early and carried on during the period of healing so that areolar rather than dense collagen networks form. Except in the case of necessary immobilization of a fracture or of an open draining wound, gentle passive or active assistive motion under proper supervision should be begun immediately after surgery or trauma to ensure that supple areolar connective tissue rather than dense scar develops in sites in which motion should occur.

Histological evidence of fibrosis may occur in as short a time period as four days.[3, 13] Gross evidence of restriction of motion begins to occur in approximately four days and develops progressively from that time. Immobilization of a normal joint for four weeks results in diminution or loss of motion because of formation of dense connective tissue. Immobilization of an injured joint for two weeks results in connective fiber fusion and loss of motion at that joint.

The following indicates the effect of limitation of motion on the development of restrictive connective tissue after injury to the shoulder.[23] If the shoulder is not immobilized, recovery occurs in 18 days. If the shoulder is immobilized for seven days, recovery occurs in 52 days. If the shoulder is

FREDERIC J. KOTTKE

immobilized for 14 days, recovery occurs in 121 days. If the shoulder is immobilized for 21 days, recovery occurs in 300 days.

Factors promoting the formation of dense fibrosis are immobilization, edema, trauma, and impaired circulation. *Immobilization* allows deposition of collagen and reticulin as a dense network instead of a loose areolar network. *Edema* increases the tendency toward fibrosis. Whether this is due to increased tissue fluid protein, impaired metabolism, increased metabolites, or other causes is not known. Probably all of these factors are important in the formation of both the edema and the fibrosis. *Trauma* causes capillary damage and increases the loss of protein into the tissue. Fibrinogen precipitates as a fibrin meshwork in the tissue spaces, forming a matrix on which collagen fibers are laid down. *Impaired circulation* appears to augment the rate of development of fibrosis. Coinciding with this phenomenon, the progressive decrease of circulation through the musculoskeletal system with age is associated with an increased rate of fibrosis, since restriction of motion develops rapidly as persons get older.

The Normal Maintenance of Mobility

Motion in joints and soft tissues is maintained by the normal movement of the parts of the body, including joint capsules, muscles, subcutaneous tissues, and ligaments, through full range of motion many times each day. In the course of the day, these movements traverse the full range of motion. If for any reason the range of daily motion is restricted, tightness develops and restricts the arc of motion.

It is easier to prevent tightness by frequently repeated activity than to correct it after it has developed.

Limitation of the range of motion is of the greatest importance when it interferes with habitual postures or activities. (For the normal range of motion of various joints see Chapter 2.)

Tightness that prevents normal standing without muscular support is disabling. In the normal relaxed standing posture, extension of the back, the hip, and the knee is maintained by positioning the center of gravity of the body above these joints so that the weight of the body holds the joints extended against restricting ligaments and the extensor muscles are relaxed.[14, 15, 24] Muscular activity is used for balance or motion rather than to support

the weight of the body. Electromyographic studies of patients during normal quiet standing reveal no continuously active contraction of the muscles in the back, the extensors of the hip, or the extensors of the knee.[14, 24] Maintenance of balance is provided mainly by activity of the soleus muscles and intermittent counterbalancing activity of the anterior tibial muscles. During relaxed standing, the center of gravity of the head, arms, and trunk falls slightly posterior (0.5 to 1.0 cm) to the center of motion of the acetabulum, far anterior (3 to 5 cm) to the center of motion of the knee, and through the center of the tarsal arch approximately midway between the points of contact of the heel and heads of the metatarsals[14] (Fig. 18–4).

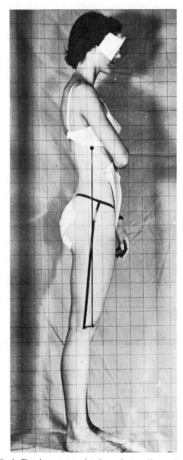

FIGURE 18–4. During normal relaxed standing, the hip is fully extended. The center of gravity falls just posterior to the center of the acetabulum, well in front of the knee and through the tarsal arch. The longitudinal and transverse axes of the pelvis and the longitudinal axis of the femur are marked. The subject is standing behind a two-inch grid. (From Kottke, F. J., and Kubicek, W. G.: Relationship of the tilt of the pelvis to stable posture. Arch. Phys. Med., 37:81–90, 1956.)

During relaxed standing, the hip and the knee are fully extended against restricting connective tissues. There is no free extension of the hip or knee beyond this standing position. Further extension is possible only to the extent that connective tissues can be stretched.[22]

Methods purporting to measure hyperextension of the hip beyond the standing position are erroneous because of inaccurate evaluation of the orientation of the innominate bone.

If tightness prevents complete extension of these weight-bearing joints, relaxed standing cannot occur. When the joints are not fully extended, muscles must support a part of the weight of the body during quiet standing. Therefore, the patient fatigues more rapidly and has less endurance for standing or ambulatory activity than does a person with normal mobility. In addition, the contraction of muscles to hold the body erect places more compressive stress on the joint surfaces, resulting in more rapid wear and more likelihood of joint pain.

Mechanics of Ambulation

HIP. During relaxed standing, the hip is fully extended, forming an angle of 160 to 175 degrees between the long axis of the pelvis and the femur[22] (Fig. 18–5). Maximal forced extension may add approximately 5 degrees to this angle. Therefore, it should be remembered that no free range of extension of the hip can occur beyond the position assumed during normal standing. The hyperextension that appears to occur is due to forward rotation of the pelvis with simultaneous extension of the lumbar spine and flexion of the opposite hip. If during this "hyperextension" the lumbar spine can extend in lordosis sufficiently so that the line of the center of gravity of head, arms, and trunk falls behind the center of the acetabulum, the patient can continue to stand relaxed without the need for muscular contraction to support any of the weight of the body except at the ankles (see Fig. 18–8).

The act of walking exerts repeated stretching on the ligaments, fascia, muscles, and connective tissue across the flexor aspect of the hip. Unless a person is standing and walking frequently each day, the normal reaction of fibrous connective tissue to shorten and fuse together results in a progressive limitation of extension. As extension of the hip becomes more limited, the extension of the lumbar trunk usually increases in a compensatory manner. Because of this compensatory ex-

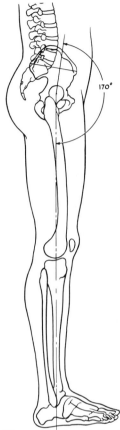

FIGURE 18–5. Diagram of the relationships of the lumbar spine, pelvis, and lower extremity in normal relaxed stance. The transverse axis of the pelvis is defined by a line drawn between the anterior and the posterior superior iliac spines. The longitudinal axis of the pelvis is perpendicular to this line dropped through the center of the acetabulum. The longitudinal axis of the femur is defined by a line from the center of the head of the femur to the center of weight-bearing at the knee. The pelvifemoral angle is formed by the longitudinal axes of the pelvis and the femur. (From Kottke, F. J., and Kubicek, W. G.: Relationship of the tilt of the pelvis to stable posture. Arch. Phys. Med., 37:81–90, 1956.)

tension in the trunk, the limitation of motion of the hip may develop insidiously until suddenly the patient is observed to stand and walk with an excessive lumbar lordosis or the patient loses the ability to stand (Fig. 18–6). Compensatory lordosis does not exceed the range of normal extension of the lumbar spine (Fig. 18–7). In children, who normally have lumbar extension of 80 to 90 degrees, compensatory lordosis may be that great. The range of lumbar extension is decreased in adulthood, and adults who develop flexion contractures of the hips do not develop as marked compensatory lumbar lordosis as is seen in children.[4]

FREDERIC J. KOTTKE

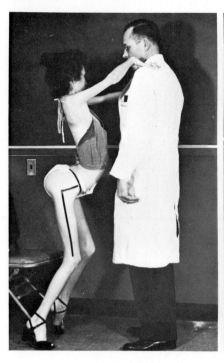 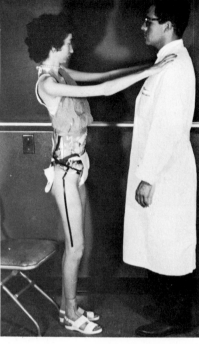

FIGURE 18–6. A patient with severe contractures of the hip flexors secondary to muscular dystrophy. Pelvifemoral angles have been marked as defined in Figure 18–5. Lumbar extension partially compensates for fixed hip flexion. Release of the contracted connective tissues and prolonged stretching increased the extension of the hips from 95 degrees to 150 degrees and made it possible for the patient to balance on her lower extremities again.

Habitual sitting makes flexion contractures of the hips likely unless they are prevented by appropriate stretching exercises. The difficulty in visualizing the change in position of the short innominate bone buried beneath thick soft tissues makes it possible for contractures of the flexors of the hips to develop to a severe degree before they are recognized.

During walking, in addition to full extension of the ipsilateral hip, the pelvis is tilted anteriorly and the lumbar spine is extended in order to bring the leg into the trailing position (Fig. 18–8). If the lumbar spine cannot extend enough to compensate for the anterior tilting of the pelvis, the center of gravity of the torso is shifted farther forward with the tilt of the pelvis and greater muscular work is required to support the weight of the body. The farther the center of gravity of the head, arms, and trunk is ahead of the acetabulum, the greater the muscular work required to support the torso.

Since the center of gravity falls ahead of the acetabulum during walking, weight can be borne on the trailing leg only if the extensor muscles of the hip are contracted. If the hip extensors are weak, the trailing leg may not be able to support the weight of the body. The amount of muscular strength needed to support the body on the trailing leg may be lessened by several compensatory mechanisms. The stride may be shortened. The lumbar spine may be extended farther to keep the center of gravity over the acetabulum. The knee may be flexed to allow the foot to trail farther behind the pelvis at the expense of a stronger contraction of the quadriceps femoris.

When a flexion contracture of the hip is present, one or more of the compensatory mechanisms must be utilized to allow stable walking. If lumbar extension is limited and the quadriceps femoris or hip extensors or both are weak, the hip becomes unstable in the trailing position. As the weight of the body moves ahead of the acetabulum, the knee flexes and collapses because the femur cannot extend further at the hip. Patients with a flexion contracture of the hip often can stand successfully when the leg on the side of the contracture is forward or in a mid-position but are unable to keep the knee extended when the leg is trailing during walking (Fig. 18–9). Consequently, the attention is directed toward the knee, and the conclusion may be drawn that the major problem is weakness of the quadriceps femoris or an abnormality of the knee when, in fact, the primary problem is the flexion contracture of the hip.

When a flexion contracture develops at the hip, the iliotibial band becomes progressively tighter, producing a flexion, abduction, external rotation deformity (Fig. 18–10). This progressive contracture may produce a pelvic obliquity and a secondary scoliosis.

When a patient lies on a flat, hard surface,

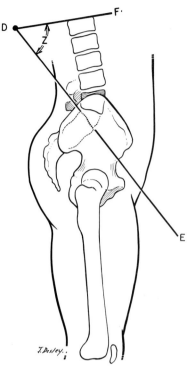

DE = PLANE OF SUPERIOR SURFACE OF S_I.
DF = PLANE OF SUPERIOR SURFACE OF L_I.
Z = ANGLE OF LUMBAR LORDOSIS.

FIGURE 18–7. Lumbar lordosis is measured as the angle between the plane of the superior surface of the first sacral segment and the plane of the superior surface of the first lumbar vertebra.

extension of the hip is not as great as when the patient stands erect. The average extension when a patient is lying prone or supine on a hard surface is 155 degrees (Fig. 18–11), whereas the average extension during relaxed standing is 170 degrees.[22] The extension of the hip when the patient is lying in bed varies from 135 to 150 degrees. The greater extension when standing is due to the greater extensor torque created by the weight of the torso centered slightly posterior to the hip joint. Patients who must remain in bed, even though they are positioned properly, will develop progressive hip flexion contractures unless they receive daily stretching of the hip flexors (Fig. 18–12).

KNEE. Tightness causing flexion of the knees develops in the hamstring and gastrocnemius muscles and the posterior capsule of the joint if the knees are not stretched to full extension by standing and walking each day. When a patient has a paretic or painful disability and habitually sits or lies with the knees flexed, contractures develop rapidly with progressive limitation of extension of

the knees. For arthritic patients or patients with neurological diseases, the placing of pillows under the knees results in the rapid development of contractures of the knees. The compressive force that must be exerted on the flexed knee during walking is considerably greater than the force exerted when the knee is extended, and, consequently, patients with arthritis in the knees have far less tolerance for standing and walking when there are flexion contractures than when the knees can extend fully (Fig. 18–13).

ANKLE. When a patient lies in bed without the support of a footboard or sits with the feet plantarflexed much of the time, progressive tightness develops in the muscles of the calf and may become great enough so that the sole of the foot cannot assume a position perpendicular to the long axis

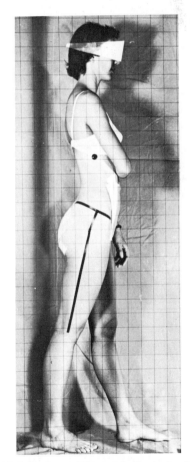

FIGURE 18–8. During walking, as the leg trails, the pelvis is tilted forward and the center of gravity of the head, arms, and trunk falls in front of the acetabulum. (From Kottke, F. J., and Kubicek, W. G.: Relationship of the tilt of the pelvis to stable posture. Arch. Phys. Med., 37:81–90, 1956.)

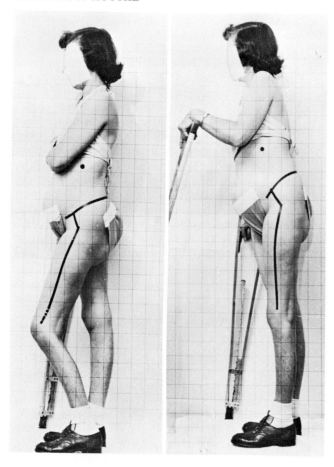

FIGURE 18–9. The combination of tightness of the flexor structures of the hip and weakness of the extensor muscles of the hip produces instability of both the hip and knee. During relaxed standing, the left thigh is flexed forward because tightness of the flexor ligaments and fascia prevents further extension of the left hip. The center of gravity is over the pelvis, but all weight is borne on the right lower extremity. If the left knee is forced into extension, the fixed flexion contracture of the left hip causes the pelvis to tilt forward and the center of gravity of the body is shifted ahead of the acetabulum. Since the extensor muscles of the hip are weak, the hip will collapse if anterior support is not provided. Attempts to center the weight of the body behind the acetabulum so that the hip becomes stable result in flexion of the knee because of the limitation of extension of the hip. Consequently, either the hip or the knee is always in a position of instability. (From Kottke, F. J., and Kubicek, W. G.: Relationship of the tilt of the pelvis to stable posture. Arch. Phys. Med., 37:81–90, 1956.)

of the tibia. Thus the patient cannot bear weight on the heel when standing. Even before this degree of tightness has been reached, tightness in the gastrocnemius increases stress on the longitudinal arch of the foot and the heads of the metatarsal bones when the patient walks. For patients who are chronically ill with painful or paretic disease, tightness in the triceps surae is accentuated by lack of a footboard on the bed, by lack of foot support when sitting, and by lying prone with the feet plantar-flexed.

Mobility Exercises to Maintain the Range of Motion

Twice daily all joints should be carried through the full range of motion three times. (See the normal ranges of motion in Chapter 2.) The patient should perform mobility exercises actively after having been taught the proper procedures. Exer-cises must be carried out with assistance to the patient if the patient is weak or has pain.

The greater the inflammation and pain, the more gentle the exercise must be. For cases of acute rheumatoid arthritis, passive motion should be carried out slowly and gently, with the patient completely relaxed. Joint inflammation requires more gentle motion than does muscular tightness. The therapist, nurse, or member of the family should gently move the part through the full range of free motion but not force motion or cause pain. The joint must be moved very slowly and gently. For patients with acute joint involvement it is highly desirable to have a skilled therapist carry out the passive motions. As the patient improves, the range can be increased slowly with gradual progression to active assisted exercise and then to active exercise. The use of improper exercise or overexercise may impede rather than help recovery in the acute stage. If motion is not maintained in the presence of inflammation, contractures occur rapidly and may become irreversible.

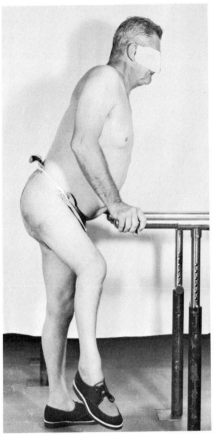

FIGURE 18–10. Typical postural deformity of flexion, abduction, and external rotation of the hip due to paresis and flexion contractures of the hip.

The therapists, nurses, or family should be taught any stretching procedures that are desired. Repeated examinations and supervision of the procedures are essential to ensure that the proper motions are obtained. The difference between properly supervised and unsupervised exercise is usually the same as the difference between adequate and inadequate care.

Stretching to Increase Range of Motion

When the stretching must be much more mild, a tight muscle can be stretched vigorously unless there is inflammation. For conditions such as poliomyelitis or Guillain-Barré syndrome, stretching should be past the point of pain, but there should be no residual pain when the stretching is discontinued. When performing manual stretching, hold for several seconds at the point of maximal stretch. This type of stretching should be done by a trained therapist. The therapist must use caution in cases of prolonged disuse, paralysis, or anesthesia, because osteoporosis may have occurred and vigorous stretching may cause fractures. In the presence of paralysis or hypesthesia, overstretching commonly occurs, causing bleeding into the disrupted connective tissue and subsequent heterotopic calcification and ossification. In quadriplegic patients, this is seen most frequently in the muscles around the hips and the flexors of the elbows.

Stretching of tight joints must be less vigorous than stretching of muscles. The motion should be slow and gentle with the patient completely relaxed, and it should stop short of the point that produces pain in the joint, although the patient may experience discomfort from stretch of the soft tissues. Inflamed joints tolerate vigorous stretching less well than joints that are not acutely inflamed. Edematous tissue is more likely to be torn than normal tissue, resulting in residual pain, swelling, and soreness. Inflammation in any joint may reduce the tensile strength of the capsule and collateral ligaments to as little as 50 per cent of the normal tensile strength.[18]

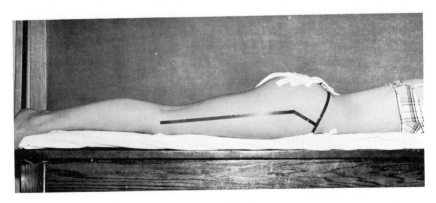

FIGURE 18–11. Normal hip extension when lying prone or supine on a flat surface is 10 to 20 degrees less than when standing.

FREDERIC J. KOTTKE

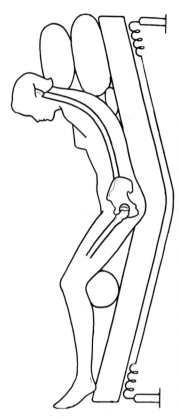

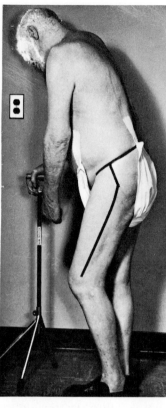

FIGURE 18–12. The prolonged bedfast position without maintenance of the normal range of motion results in a kyphosis of the spine and flexion contractures of the hips, knees, and ankles.

Certain principles apply to all techniques of stretching. The body segments on each side of the joint to be stretched must be properly stabilized so that the maneuver is under complete control. The force must be applied in the precise direction that produces tension in the appropriate connective tissues. Prolonged moderate stretching is more effective than momentary vigorous stretching; connective tissue shows the plastic property of "creeping" in response to prolonged tension, although it will resist a much greater momentary force. The plastic creeping of connective tissue under moderate stretch increases as the tissue temperature increases up to the maximal tolerated temperature, which is approximately 43° C (109.4° F) for tissues with normal circulation.[29] Therefore, thermotherapy to raise the temperature close to 43° C (109.4° F) during the period of stretching will increase the effectiveness of the treatment. At a temperature of 20 to 30° C (68.0° to 86.0° F), connective tissue requires about three times as much tensile force to effect a specified elongation as is necessary at 43° C (109.4° F).[10]

Stretching must be held within the limits of pain tolerance of the patient; during brief manual stretching, there may be pain when the stretch is applied, with relief of pain as soon as stretch ceases; prolonged stretching should remain within the patient's pain threshold to avoid tearing of blood vessels. Stretching should be repeated in less time than is required for connective tissue to "set" in a shortened position, daily or more often. Inflammation indicates decreased tensile strength of connective tissue, which must be stretched cautiously. Special procedures are used for prolonged stretching of joints that do not respond well to manual stretching (Fig. 18–14).

Hip Flexors. The patient, lying prone, is strapped snugly to a padded plinth by a strap run through C-clamps on either side of the hips and across the ischial tuberosities. A sling under the distal end of the thigh is attached by a rope through overhead pulleys to a weight that provides a constant tension. A stretching weight of 30 to 50 lb is added to the weight necessary to counterbalance the lower extremity. Only one hip is stretched at a time because it is not possible to immobilize the pelvis adequately to stretch both hip flexors simultaneously. The contralateral hip and knee are flexed, and the leg is supported on the seat of a chair or cushion of appropriate height. This stretch is maintained for 20 minutes each day.[16] It has

FIGURE 18–13. The compressive force, P, exerted on the flexed knee is a combination of the weight of the body and tension exerted by the quadriceps, M. If a patient weighing 150 pounds walks with the knee extended to 130 degrees, the calculated compressive force on the knee is:

$$\Sigma\, F_x = 0$$

$$P \cdot \frac{14}{33}\, M \cdot \frac{25}{42.6} = 0$$

$$P = 1.38M$$

$$\Sigma\, F_y = 0$$

$$150 + P \cdot \frac{30}{33} - M \cdot \frac{34.4}{42.6} = 0$$

$$150 + \frac{30}{33} \cdot 1.38M - \frac{34.4}{42.6}\, M = 0$$

$$M = 342 \text{ lb.}$$

$$P = 472 \text{ lb.}$$

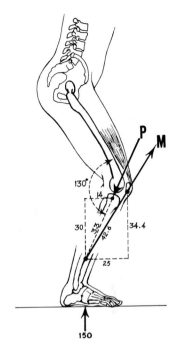

been found for conditions such as dermatomyositis, in which there is a relative decrease, if not a complete absence, of circulation through the stretched soft tissues, that the reduced circulation during stretching results in a decrease of the plastic elongation of the contractures. For patients with this condition, relieving the stretch for one minute in every five minutes allows a resumption of the circulation. It has been found that the plastic elongation of the tight connective tissue occurs

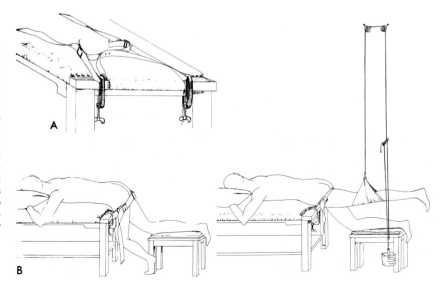

FIGURE 18–14. Counterbalanced stretching of the hip flexors. *A,* Two C-clamps fastened to the end of a padded table at hip width provide attachment for a double-ended stretching strap. *B,* The pelvis is immobilized by a strap fastened over the ischial tuberosities while the hips are flexed. A sling under the distal end of the thigh is attached by rope and overhead pulley to counterbalanced weights, which exert a continuous force on the hip flexors. Thirty to fifty pounds plus the weight counterbalancing the lower extremity are applied for 20 minutes.

more rapidly when such a schedule of intermittent stretching is used.

Knee Flexors. Contractures of the knees can be stretched by placing the patient prone on a firm surface with a pad under the knee and the leg extending unsupported. A 5- to 15-lb sandbag or weight is placed across the heel for 20 minutes (Fig. 18–15).

Alternatively, the patient sits with the knee extended, the heel supported at seat level, and the thigh and leg unsupported, and a sandbag weighing 10 to 15 lb is placed across the knee for 20 minutes.

Triceps Surae. The patient sits on an Elgin table or other apparatus to which an exercise boot with a toe extension may be attached. The foot is strapped to the exercise boot and 10 to 30 lb of tension is exerted at the end of the toe extension bar for 20 minutes (Fig. 18–16).

Alternatively, to dorsiflex the ankle, the patient stands at arm's length from a wall with the feet on a wedgeboard that elevates the front of the foot 20 degrees above the horizontal. The patient leans forward against the wall for one to five minutes, three to five times each day. This exercise is the most convenient to do at home. To be effective, the knees must be kept extended and the heels kept in contact with the floor. The same stretch may be obtained by placing the patient on a tilt table (Fig. 18–17).

Shoulders. Stretching of contractures in the soft tissues of the shoulder in the supine or upright position causes the head of the humerus to ride up under the acromion, pinching the intervening soft tissues and causing pain and inflammation. The pain produces spasm of the muscles of the rotator cuff, causing further compaction of the humerus against the acromion and preventing an effective stretching of the tight connective tissues. Codman[5] wrote a monograph on the treatment of restricted motion of the shoulder in which he inveighed against stretching in the supine or upright positions because of the adverse effects. Instead, he advocated dependent circumduction to allow gravity to distract the head of the humerus away from the acromion as the patient carried out active circumduction to the limits of the free range of motion. He pointed out that no special equipment was necessary. Instead, the patient bends forward at the hips so that the body is horizontal and the relaxed arm hangs dependent; then circumduction is performed in an increasing arc in both directions to stretch any tight connective tissues without compressing the head of the humerus against the acromion. At least $2/3$ of the range of motion of the shoulder is possible in this position, in which the weight of the dependent arm distracts the head of the humerus away from the acromion.

Hellebrandt and associates[12] compared the Codman position to the Chandler position, in which the patient lies prone or on the side with the arms hanging dependent through a suitable hole in a treatment table and a 2- to 5-lb weight hung on the wrist (Fig. 18–18). Electromyographic measurements of the activity of the muscles of the rotator cuff demonstrated greater relaxation of the muscles around the shoulder when the Chandler position was used than when the Codman position was assumed. A further advantage of the recum-

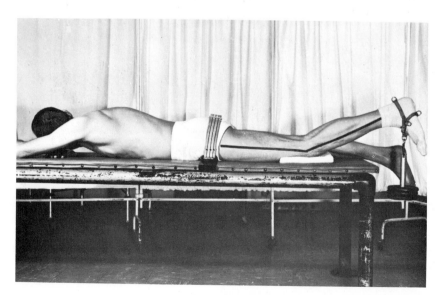

FIGURE 18–15. Prone stretching for the knee with a weight of 5 to 15 pounds applied at the heel.

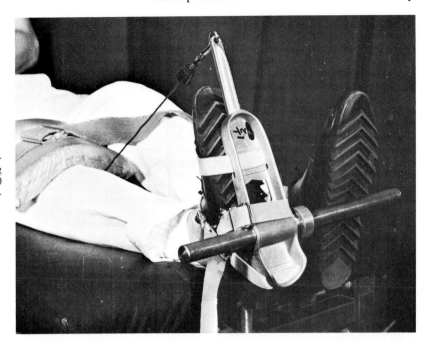

FIGURE 18–16. Stretching of the triceps surae on an exercise table using a toe extension boot. A weight of 10 to 30 pounds is applied for 20 minutes.

bent position is that it is more stable and secure and easier to maintain for older patients or patients with arthritis.

Elbows. Only active motion is used for mobilizing the elbow, because stretch applied through the long lever of the forearm to the relatively weak ginglymus joint results in overstretching and tearing of connective tissue, which increases the contracture rather than relieving it. It has been reported that mild, prolonged spring tension, which allows frequent motion but maintains tension during the intervals of relaxation, is effective to stretch flexion contractures of the elbows. Icing the elbow for 30 to 60 minutes after stretching has been found to decrease any edema resulting from the stretching.

Fingers. Stretching of the fingers in flexion and extension without first mobilizing the soft tissues around the joint is inadequate. The metacarpophalangeal joints have limited motion in other directions, including distraction, rotation, anteroposterior sliding, lateral sliding, and lateral bending as well as flexion and extension. The interphalangeal joints are capable of all of these motions except lateral bending.[21] General mobility of these joints must be reestablished by gentle manipulatory stretching before full flexion and full extension are possible. All motions are carried out gently a number of times daily. The connective tissue

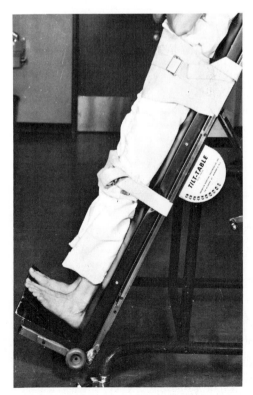

FIGURE 18–17. Prolonged stretching of the triceps surae using a tilt table and wedge board.

FREDERIC J. KOTTKE

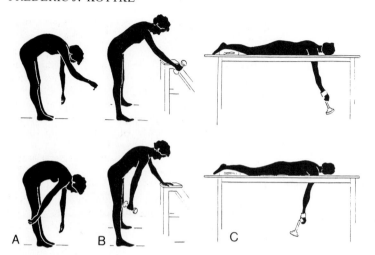

FIGURE 18–18. Three postures of dependent circumduction, *A,* Codman; *B,* Sperry, in which the patient holds a 5-pound weight in the hand; and *C,* Chandler, in which the patient is recumbent with a weight hanging on the wrist, are shown. The Chandler technique is the best, since it is associated with the greatest amount of muscular relaxation around the shoulder and, therefore, allows the greatest range of motion to stretch connective tissue. All three methods are superior to upright or supine postures, since traction from gravity prevents pinching of subacromial soft tissues. (From Hellebrandt, F. A., Houtz, S. J., Partridge, M. J., and Walters, C. E.: The Chandler table: Analysis of its rationale in the mobilization of the shoulder joint. Phys. Ther. Rev., 35:545–555, 1955, with permission of the American Physical Therapy Association.)

around the joints of the fingers tends to gel rapidly if there is no motion. Splinting devices that hold the hand in one position are not entirely effective because they do not provide the repetitive motion necessary to restore suppleness to the connective tissues around the joints. The joint capsules of immobilized hands quickly become edematous and sclerotic. Effective manipulation of fingers is difficult and is best carried out by a skilled therapist.

Continuous Passive Motion

It has been recognized for many years that lack of motion of joints and the surrounding soft tissues has the adverse effects discussed above. Normal mobility in loose connective tissue is neither regained nor maintained by infrequent motion.

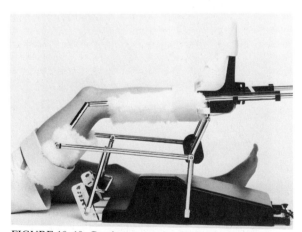

FIGURE 18–19. Continuous passive motion apparatus that can be adjusted to provide motion to the hip and knee at an adjustable rate and range. (Courtesy of Empi, Inc., St. Paul, Minnesota.)

When there is trauma or inflammation, with or without pain, frequent, nontraumatic and nonpainful motion is necessary to maintain and restore the pliability of the connective tissues. Over many years, there have been episodic preliminary reports of the benefits that may be obtained from using mechanical devices that provide continuous passive motion to the injured part.[31] Nutrition of cartilage in the diarthrodial joints is enhanced with acceleration of healing of defects.[26, 27] Deep venous thrombosis following surgery or trauma is diminished by using continuous passive motion prophylactically.[20] Adhesions and contractures are prevented.[7, 8, 9, 19] When continuous passive motion is applied precisely, slowly, and with appropriate range and force so that there is no overstretching or mechanical trauma, the range of motion can be restored again.[11]

Recently, a variety of mechanical devices have become available commercially to provide continuous passive motion to the various joints (Fig. 18–19). If these devices are properly fitted and adjusted for the correct range of motion, the correct force, and the correct speed of rotation of each joint being manipulated, they have the potential to be very beneficial. However, each machine is limited by its inflexibility. It must be set up and adjusted by a skilled kinesiologist who ascertains that orientation, force, and speed are correct. It must be checked frequently to assure that the proper performance is occurring. As the range of motion of the joint changes, the machine must be adjusted to adapt for that change. If these appropriate adjustments are made at the appropriate times, then it would appear that continuous passive motion should produce results superior to those of any regimen of intermittent motion. However, it must be cautioned that too forceful motion, too little or too great range, or too prolonged duration of an activity could produce detrimental results.

References

1. Becker, H., and Diegelmann, R. F.: The influence of tension on intrinsic tendon fibroplasia. Orthop. Rev., 13:153–159, 1984.
2. Becker, H., Orak, R., and Duponselle, E.: Early active motion following a beveled technique of flexor tendon repair; Report of fifty cases. J. Hand Surg., 4:454–460, 1979.
3. Buck, R. C.: Regeneration of tendon. J. Pathol. Bacteriol., 66:1–18, 1953.
4. Clayson, S. J., Newman, I. M., Debevec, D. F., Anger, R. W., Skowland, H. V., and Kottke, F.: Evaluation of mobility of hip and lumbar vertebrae of normal young women. Arch. Phys. Med. Rehabil., 43:1–8, 1962.
5. Codman, E. A.: The Shoulder. Rupture of the Supraspinatus Tendon and Other Lesions In and About the Subacromial Bursa. Boston, Thomas Todd Co., 1934.
6. Fernando, N. V. P., and Movat, H. Z.: Fibrillogenesis in regenerating tendon. Lab. Invest., 12:214–229, 1963.
7. Fronek, J., Frank, C., Amiel, D., Woo, S. L.-Y., Coutts, R. D., and Akeson, W. H.: The effects of intermittent passive motion (IPM) in the healing of a medial collateral ligament. (Abstract.) Proc. Orthop. Res. Soc., 8:31, 1983.
8. Gelberman, R. H., Amiel, D., Gonsolves, M., Woo, S. L.-Y., and Akeson, W. H.: The influence of protected passive mobilization on the healing of flexor tendons: A biochemical and microangiographic study. Hand, 13:120, 1981.
9. Gelberman, R. H., Woo, S. L.-Y., Lothringer, K., Akeson, W. H., and Amiel, D.: Effects of early intermittent passive mobilization on healing canine flexor tendons. J. Hand Surg., 7:170, 1982.
10. Gersten, J. W.: Effect of ultrasound on tendon extensibility. Am. J. Phys. Med., 34:362–369, 1955.
11. Greene, W. B.: Use of continuous passive slow motion in the postoperative rehabilitation of difficult pediatric knee and elbow problems. J. Pediatr. Orthop., 3:419–423, 1983.
12. Hellebrandt, F. A., Houtz, S. J., Partridge, M. J., and Walters, C. E.: The Chandler table: Analysis of its rationale in the mobilization of the shoulder joint. Phys. Ther. Rev., 35:545–555, 1955.
13. Jackson, D. S., Flickinger, D. B., and Dunphy, J. E.: Biochemical studies of connective tissue repair. Ann. N.Y. Acad. Sci., 86:943–947, 1960.
14. Kelton, I. W., and Wright, R. D.: The mechanism of easy standing by man. Aust. J. Exp. Biol. Med. Sci., 27:505–515, 1949.
15. Kottke, F. J., and Kubicek, W. G.: Relationship of the tilt of the pelvis to stable posture. Arch. Phys. Med., 37:81–90, 1956.
16. Kottke, F. J., Pauley, D. L., and Ptak, R. A.: The rationale for prolonged stretching for correction of shortening of connective tissue. Arch. Phys. Med. Rehabil., 47:345–352, 1966.
17. Lindstedt, S., and Prockop, D. J.: Isotopic studies on urinary hydroxyproline as evidence for rapidly catabolized forms of collagen in the young rat. J. Biol. Chem., 236:1399–1403, 1961.
18. Lippmann, R. K.: Arthropathy due to adjacent inflammation. J. Bone Joint Surg., 35A:967–979, 1953.
19. Long, M. L., Frank, C., Schacher, N. S., Dittrich, D., and Edwards, G. E.: The effects of motion on normal and healing ligaments. (Abstract.) Proc. Orthop. Res. Soc., 7:43, 1982.
20. Lynch, J. A., Baker, P. L., Polly, R. L., McCoy, M. T., Sund, K., and Roudybush, D.: Continuous passive motion: A prophylaxis for deep venous thrombosis following total knee replacement. American Academy of Orthopedic Surgeons, Atlanta, 1984.
21. Mennell, J.: The Science and Art of Joint Manipulation, Vol. I: The Extremities, 2nd Ed. Philadelphia, The Blakiston Co., 1949, pp. 51–69.
22. Mundale, M. O., Hislop, H. J., Rabideau, R. J., and Kottke, F. J.: Evaluation of extension of the hip. Arch. Phys. Med., 37:75–80, 1956.
23. Perkins, G.: Rest and movement. J. Bone Joint Surg., 25B:521–539, 1953.
24. Portnoy, H., and Morin, F.: Electromyographic study of the postural muscles in various positions and movements. Am. J. Physiol., 186:122–126, 1956.
25. Ross, R.: The fibroblast and wound repair. Biol. Rev. 43:51–96, 1968.
26. Salter, R. B., Minster, R. R., Clements, N., Bogooh, E., and Bell, R. S.: Continuous passive motion and the repair of full-thickness defects: A one year follow-up. Orthop. Trans., 6:266, 1982.
27. Salter, R. B., and Simmonds, D. F.: The effects of continuous passive motion on the healing of articular cartilage defects: An experimental investigation in rabbits. (Abstract.) J. Bone Joint Surg., 57:570, 1975.
28. Viljanto, J.: Biochemical basis of tensile strength in wound healing. An experimental study with viscose cellulose sponges in rats. Acta Chir. Scand. (Suppl.), 333:1–101, 1964.
29. Warren, C. J., Lehmann, J. F., and Koblanski, J. N.: Elongation of rat tail tendon: Effect of load and temperature. Arch. Phys. Med. Rehabil., 52:465–474, 1971.
30. Watson-Jones, R.: Fractures and Joint Injuries, Vol. I, 4th Ed. Baltimore, Williams & Wilkins Co., 1952, p. 5.
31. Zander, J. G. W.: The Apparatus for Medico-Mechanical Gymnastics and Their Use. Stockholm, P. A. Norstedt, 1984.

19

Therapeutic Exercise to Develop Neuromuscular Coordination

FREDERIC J. KOTTKE

The development of the ability to regulate multiple muscles simultaneously or in sequence to perform apparently simple or complex activities is the aspect of therapeutic exercise that is most difficult to understand. There has been continuing controversy regarding both the neurophysiological mechanisms involved and the functional process that is used to activate single or multiple muscles to perform a task. There is lack of agreement regarding what part of neuromuscular activity is voluntary, what part is based on automatic patterns, what part is purely the result of heredity, what part has to be learned, and when learning is necessary what the fundamentals of that process may be. This chapter attempts to deal with these issues.

As used in this chapter, *control* is defined as the ability to voluntarily activate one motor unit or a small number of motor units of a single muscle without activating any other muscle. Control has no capacity for selective inhibition of unwanted activity while the desired muscle is being excited. Therefore, isolated control can be demonstrated only in a relaxed subject when there is minimal activation of one pyramidal pathway producing one individual, weak, slow contraction. Control involves conscious and continuous awareness and intentional guidance of an activity. Strong contraction of a single muscle can occur in isolation only after a coordination engram has been developed that causes inhibition of all other muscles at the same time that motor units of the contracting muscle are being activated. *Coordination* is the

process that results in the activation of patterns of contraction of many motor units of multiple muscles with the appropriate forces, combinations, and sequences and with *simultaneous inhibition of all other muscles* in order to carry out the desired activity. Such patterns of multimuscular activity are automatized in that the individual component muscles are not under voluntary awareness or control as the activity is being performed. The development of automatic multimuscular patterns is dependent upon the development of *engram pathways* in the extrapyramidal system by training. Engrams are not inherent but can be trained to perfection only by the repetition of the correct pattern of muscular performance hundreds of thousands or millions of times. An engram represents the neurological organization of a preprogrammed pattern of muscular activity. Once an engram has been developed, each time it is excited it automatically produces the same pattern. In this automatic activity produced by an engram, not only must all of the involved muscles be excited in the correct sequence and at the right intensity but also all muscles not required for the activity must be inhibited if the pattern is to be produced smoothly with minimal expenditure of energy. The activities of the component muscles of a well-coordinated motion are automatic in that they are not consciously perceived or selected. Only the accomplishment of the activity is perceived.[28] Except for very light and unusual activity, most muscular activity occurs as the synchronized activation and inhibition of a number of muscle groups through the mechanism of excitation of reflexes rather than by the isolated contraction of a single prime mover. When exercise occurs against resistance, there is always cocontraction of synergists and stabilizers. The greater the resistance, the greater the spread of activity to produce cocontraction in more distant muscles, both ipsilateral and contralateral.[59] This spread of excitation must be inhibited by the engram before it reaches the anterior horn cells; otherwise the muscular response will be incoordination rather than precise coordination. In other words, the inhibitory capacity of the engram, derived from the inhibitory components of the spinal and supraspinal reflexes, is the sole basis for the limitation of motor unit activity to those muscles that actively participate in each motor pattern. This makes the basic neurological mechanism of coordination entirely different from the mechanism that produces individual muscle control.[45]

Because it is possible after engrams have been developed to select and activate sequences of preprogrammed patterns and at any time to superimpose on the preprogrammed pattern an additional controlled muscular activity to modify the response, it has been difficult to understand the difference between coordination and control. Most of our common activities are initiated by willing an automatic preprogrammed motor pattern (a coordination pattern) to occur. The pattern may be limited or extensive but occurs as it was preprogrammed by previous practice. In addition, an individual muscle can be activated, i.e., controlled, by directing attention to the sensations produced solely by that specific muscular action. When a muscular action is being voluntarily controlled, the neuromuscular process occurs more slowly than when the action is preprogrammed. Only one muscular action can be observed at a time. Attention may be switched from the control of one activity to the control of another only at the rate of two to three times per sec.[27, 34, 35, 66] In rapid, strong multimuscular activities, all components must be integrated into a timed sequence of interrelated responses, most of which are performed automatically. The goal of coordination training is to develop the ability to reproduce at will automatic multimuscular motor patterns that are faster, more precise, and stronger than those that can be produced when only voluntary control of each individual muscle is used (Fig. 19–1).

If a muscle is of major importance in performing a motion of a joint, it is called a prime mover or agonist. Other muscles that assist that motion are called synergists. Muscles that oppose the motion are called antagonists. Muscles of the same or adjacent joints that maintain position to allow the motion and are used synchronously with the prime mover are called stabilizers. Neuromuscular education, or control training, refers to the teaching of the discrete control of a prime mover of a motion under the direct consciousness of the patient. Coordination training refers to the training that develops preprogrammed automatic multimuscular patterns or engrams. "Control of coordination" is a frequently confusing and misused term that is employed to indicate the voluntary initiation and ending of a coordination engram. Since control and coordination are quite different mechanisms carried out by different parts of the brain, this term should not be used.

When a muscle is contracting against a load that is very light relative to the total voluntary strength of that muscle, it is possible to limit activity to that muscle voluntarily.[62] As the load becomes heavier, synergists as well as the prime mover begin to contract.[23] When the load becomes still heavier, the stabilizer muscles in the extremities and also in the trunk establish stability and balance in relation to gravity. With even heavier loading, antagonists and distant muscles that serve no useful purpose become active during the motion[13, 32, 59] because the amount of activity excited in the internuncial pool exceeds the capacity for selective inhibition. Practice of precisely coordinated activities at the highest possible intensity increases the capacity for selective inhibition, and because the selective inhibition increases, the capacity for coordination is increased. Prolonged activity causes fatigue of any muscle and increases the proportionate resistance that a constant load imposes on the available strength of the prime mover, thereby increasing incoordination with increasing fatigue.

Coordination Results from Engrams of Automated Movement

The development of coordination depends on repetition. When training for coordination is first carried out, the movement must be simple and the rate slow enough so that the person can consciously monitor all components of the activity. As the activity is repeated precisely many times, an engram is formed. The activity then can be performed with greater effort without the occurrence of errors in performance. The speed of performance can be

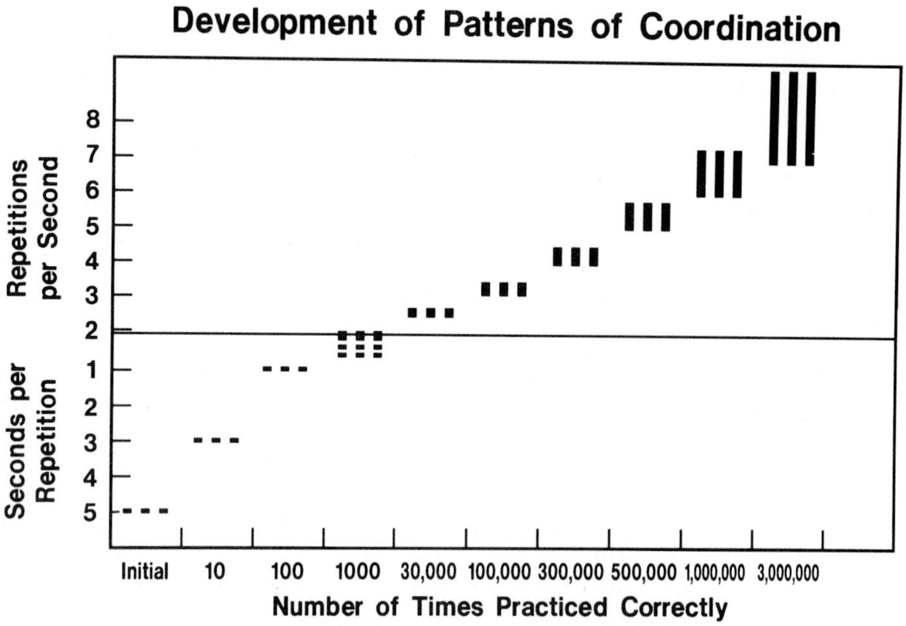

FREDERIC J. KOTTKE

Development of Patterns of Coordination

FIGURE 19–1. Conscious voluntary regulation of muscular contractions and automatic coordination of muscular activities have entirely different response times and require widely variable numbers of training repetitions before maximal performance is achieved. Conscious activation of the contraction of a muscle, as shown in the lower panel, may require a number of seconds to initiate if the activity is entirely new and unpracticed (naive). After relatively few repetitions (10 to 100), the response time decreases markedly, but the shortest response time under conscious volition is 300 to 500 milliseconds, with the longer time prevailing if continued conscious activation is required. Automatic coordination, shown above the horizontal line, not only can result in repetitions of muscular contraction two to four times as rapidly but also can regulate several muscles at the same time (as indicated by the relative height of the vertical bars when compared to the height of the block indicating contraction of a single muscle, shown in the lower panel). However, automatic coordination does not begin to develop until 30,000 to 50,000 correct repetitions have been practiced, and high levels of skillful coordination require millions of repetitions of correct practice.

increased. The conscious attention required for precise performance becomes less and inhibition reduces the spread of excitation to other neurons outside of the activity pattern. Eventually, the pattern can be carried on with little conscious perception of its individual components and is said to be automatic, or a preprogrammed engram.[45]

A high degree of coordination and speed does not develop until the activity pattern becomes so well developed through repeated practice that it does not require awareness of all phases of the activity. For example, a pianist when playing a piano does not need to think of the contraction of the individual muscles involved or even the individual placement of each finger, because the symbols on a page signify a whole pattern of responses, and cerebral awareness provides the initiation of an *automatized preprogrammed pattern* without need for conscious attention to the components of that activity. During motor activity, proprioceptive feedback provides both subconscious and conscious monitoring of whether or not the perform-

ance was successful rather than awareness of the precise activity of each muscle.

How the flow of nerve impulses becomes limited to specific neural pathways by repetition and how sensory feedback from a precisely performed activity becomes integrated by repetition into automatic patterns of activity have not been fully defined. Nevertheless, all skilled muscular activities are developed only in this way.* Repetition of activity with perceived sensory feedback to regulate performance is the basis for the development of motor skills in the infant and child. It is the mechanism by which highly skilled performance is perfected in the adult. Likewise, it is the basis for relearning coordination for the patient who has suffered injury to the neuromuscular system.

The components of skilled automatic performance are the following:

1. Volition: the ability to initiate the activity when it is wanted, to maintain it as long as desired,

---

*See references 17, 33, 45, 51, 54, and 58.

and to discontinue it at will. When an engram has been formed, volition can excite, maintain, and discontinue that engram, but the engram runs as it was preprogrammed.[51] Volition is used to select or modify the sequence of engrams and, therefore, to determine the order of the performance.

2. Perception: to tell whether or not the performance is occurring as desired. Coordinated activity is monitored primarily by sensory stimuli transmitted through proprioceptive pathways and reinforced by visual and tactile perception. A patient must have intact proprioception and intact subcortical centers for integrating proprioceptive impulses with motor impulses in order to achieve a high degree of coordination.[63] When there is damage to the proprioceptive pathways, visual monitoring must be substituted for proprioceptive monitoring, but the degree of coordination achieved is never as great as when the proprioceptive pathways are intact. Conscious awareness of the components of the activities being performed is only superficial. The monitoring of position and motion for skilled motor patterns is largely automatic through interaction between the cerebellum and the cerebral basal ganglia in conjunction with the precentral cortex. Perception is processed in the central nervous system more slowly than is performance and, therefore, results in retrospective recognition of error and a correction of subsequent performance.

3. Engram formation: the development of preprogrammed patterns of activity is the basis for coordination. Development of a motor engram is dependent upon the establishment of an internuncial network that programs each motor pattern. Repetition of each pattern many times at the maximal speed and force consistent with precision results in the development of a fast and forceful motor engram. Repetition involves the activation of nervous pathways to motor units that should be contracting at the same time that all other motor units are inhibited. *The only way by which automatic engrams can be developed is by voluntary repetition of the precise performance until the engram is formed.* From the limited data from research available at this time, it appears that 20,000 to 30,000 repetitions of precise performance of an activity pattern must be performed in order to begin to develop an engram[17, 57, 58] (see Fig. 19–1). The component units of a coordinated activity must be performed with precision several million times before peak performance is reached.[17]

Inhibition is the heart of coordination. The development of coordination results in greater preciseness of motion and greater economy of muscular effort because there is less extraneous muscular activity. This precision of motion depends upon active inhibition of all motor neurons other than those involved in the desired motion. *Inhibition of undesired activity is an essential part of the automatic regulation of coordination.* In one of his lectures, Karel Bobath used the metaphor, "Each motor engram is a pathway of excitation surrounded by a wall of inhibition." Precise coordination can be developed only to the extent that a person can train the inhibition of all undesired activity. Although inhibition is the heart of coordination, it cannot be trained directly but only by the execution of precise activity and by increasing the intensity of effort as precision can be maintained. There is no voluntarily controllable system by which inhibition can be imposed selectively on any anterior horn cell. As engrams develop, the capacity for inhibition also develops. Inhibition of undesired activity is more difficult to train than is the initiation of desired activity. The training of coordination results in the progressive development of selective inhibition during increasing effort. When the capacity for inhibition increases, voluntary effort can be increased to produce a stronger and faster specific motor activity, whereas neuronal excitation remains restricted to the desired neuromuscular pathways. Coordination of the most complex, most rapid and skillful, and most powerful contractions is an activity automatized by the extrapyramidal system rather than a voluntary activity controlled through the corticospinal pathway.

Training of Control of Individual Muscles

Conscious Control of a Muscle

The corticospinal pathway from the gamma-4 cortex has the ability to activate small groups of motoneurons of individual muscles under the direct attention of the individual. This is the only pathway for motor control in the nervous system that does not need training other than awareness of sensory-motor relationships. However, this pathway is limited to attending to one muscle or one motion at a time, and attention cannot be shifted more rapidly than two to three times per sec.[27, 35, 66] In addition, this is solely an excitatory pathway with no capacity for inhibition. It appears that this controllable pathway is used by the normal infant

FREDERIC J. KOTTKE

to augment or oppose reflex responses by imposing additional neural impulses to facilitate a muscular activity and, through this laborious mechanism, gradually to develop multimuscular coordination. It appears that the normally coordinated adult is able to modify multimuscular activity by imposing additional muscular activities, one by one, over the corticospinal pathway.

When a patient is unable to activate even the simple combinations of muscles to produce a coordinated contraction consistently without error, therapeutic exercise to teach coordination must be begun by teaching isolated control of the individual muscles under direct attention.

The patient must learn to control each muscle individually before its actions can be integrated into a coordination engram. Kenny[43] and Knapp[42] developed and described the clinical techniques for training control of individual prime movers. In the laboratory, Simard and Basmajian[62] showed that a similar technique could be used to teach control of individual motor units using electromyographic feedback. In 1960, Marinacci and Horance proposed the use of electromyography as a mechanism to provide specific feedback for retraining of precise muscular control.[47] Since that time, numerous studies have reported successfully augmented training of control of specific muscles without activation of antagonists by sensory feedback from an electromyograph monitoring the activity of the prime mover to be trained and the antagonists to be inhibited.[2, 3, 9, 10, 38]

Success has been reported, especially in the inhibition of activity of those muscles that should not participate in the motor pattern. Somewhat more recently, certain investigators have been more negative in their reports in a number of respects: (1) The results obtained have not been superior to those obtained by standard methods of muscle re-education if the patients have good proprioceptive sensation. (2) The prime movers may be trained to respond, but that response remains only a few per cent as strong as contractions of normal muscle and, therefore, does not contribute adequately to normal activities. (3) The effects of training do not persist when training is discontinued.[49, 50, 57]

Requirements for the Training of Control

The training of control of the individual prime mover muscles is an educational process requiring intense concentration and participation. The patient must be rational, old enough to comprehend and follow instructions, and able to learn, cooperate, and concentrate on the muscular training during the exercise period. The individual should be alert and emotionally calm. The patient should be allowed to have frequent short rest periods. As soon as the patient begins to tire or become inattentive, the training session should be discontinued.

The training exercise should be carried on in a quiet room so that the patient will not be distracted. The patient must be positioned to be relaxed, comfortable, and securely supported. A patient who is unsteady or insecure cannot concentrate on controlling the activity of an isolated muscle. If the patient has generalized weakness or a problem of balance, the body should be fully supported in the recumbent position. Patients with cerebral palsy may not relax fully when lying on a high or narrow table or when sitting in an erect position. They relax much better and, therefore, can concentrate on the task to be trained when lying on a mat on the floor.

The patient must have intact proprioceptors or teleceptors to monitor muscular activity. If proprioception is normal, the patient is taught while recumbent and relaxed and the emphasis is placed on proprioception, because proprioceptive sensation is more rapid and precise than other sensations.[5] If proprioception is impaired, the patient must be positioned in such a way that the activity can be watched in order to monitor it. Electromyography is a specific, strong sensory reinforcer and, therefore, facilitates learning. It can be used to augment impaired sensation, either to reinforce the activity of the prime mover or to suppress undesired activity of other muscles during the training of control;[9, 10] however, central neurophysiological processing of the conscious monitoring by electromyography is too slow to be utilized during the performance of a coordination engram at normal speed. Patients who have no mechanism available for perception of position or muscular activity cannot be taught precise control.

The patient must have a pain-free arc of motion of the joint across which the muscle is working. The sense of position and movement is derived primarily from joint receptors that are stimulated by motion of that joint.[33] A motion of approximately 10 degrees in a joint is adequate to initiate proprioceptive monitoring if that sensation is normal. In the presence of pain, inhibition of activity occurs and incoordination results. In addition, when pain is present, the patient learns to anticipate the pain and to restrict activity before motion produces pain. Usually, when pain may occur at both ends of the range of motion, neuromuscular education can be carried out if there is a pain-free arc of motion of about 30 degrees. This larger range affords the therapist adequate motion within the totally pain-free range in which to stimulate proprioceptive feedback.

During training, there must be competent direction from a trained therapist who provides clear-cut commands for precise performance and is alert to monitor and confirm that the correct performance is occurring. If there is any substitution or incoordination, the therapist must teach the patient how to limit the activity to the desired prime mover by decreasing the effort appropriately. This may require that the activity be an assisted motion with minimal voluntary effort. In addition, the therapist encourages the patient to be working continually at the maximal level of his or her ability.

Technique for the Training of Control of Individual Muscles

Verify That There Is a Lower Motor Neuron Pathway. For the hyporesponsive muscle that is not contracted by volition, the stretch reflex may be stimulated by a tendon tap or by rapidly repeated lengthening and relaxation to demonstrate that the lower motor neuron pathway is intact. A minimal reaction often can be observed best by palpation of the tendon of insertion. Multiple quick short stretches or vibration using an electric vibrator may be more effective to initiate the response than a single stretch. Vibrations at 200 Hz will saturate the discharge rate from Ia sensory endings of muscle spindles. Function of the lower motor neuron may also be verified by electromyography.

Verify the Upper Motor Neuron Pathway by Facilitation. For upper motor neuron diseases in which the stretch reflexes are readily elicited, the problem is to determine whether or not there is a trainable upper motor neuron pathway. It may be necessary to use one or more of the facilitation techniques to demonstrate that there is an upper motor neuron pathway over which volitional control of motor function may be transmitted.[11, 40, 44] When motor neurons cannot be activated by volition alone, facilitation is used to initiate and increase excitability of the upper motor neuron pathway before control training is begun. Facilitation techniques utilize overflow of nerve impulses from

one interneuronal pathway to another to reduce synaptic resistances and activate motor neurons not otherwise receiving threshold stimulation. Either reflex stimulation or mass cerebral discharge over multiple motor pathways may be used to activate inactive motor neurons.[24, 39] This type of facilitation can be used to demonstrate a potential pathway to a muscle. It is postulated that repeated activation of a motor neuron or motor pathway that has a high threshold in some way lowers that threshold.[39] Many of the specialized therapeutic exercises have focused on techniques for facilitation of voluntary function.[40, 53] If volition is insufficient to excite contraction of a prime mover, then facilitation is necessary to attempt to achieve that goal. The less effective the volitional excitation is, the greater must be the facilitation. As volitional excitation becomes more effective, the reflex facilitation can be decreased. After it is possible to produce a voluntary contraction of the prime mover, then reflex or mass proprioceptive neuromuscular facilitation must be withdrawn before training of control can be used as the basis for training coordination. The ability to produce activity in a muscle by facilitation techniques does not necessarily ensure that the neural pathway can be retrained to the level of useful performance. But since facilitation to activate voluntary muscular contraction followed by prolonged training to develop control and then coordination engrams is the only course available to regain useful function, a therapeutic trial is necessary.

Cutaneous Reinforcement of Excitation. Stimulation of the skin over the tendon of insertion and the belly of the muscle reflexly increases the sensitivity of the stretch reflex through the cutaneous-gamma reflex and facilitates the contraction of the muscle.[29, 42, 43] This stimulus is applied immediately before each command to contract the muscle. Stroking, tapping, cold, chemical irritants, or electrical stimulation of the skin over the muscle belly may be effective to increase the motor response.[60]

Teach Mental Awareness of Correct Function. Instruct the patient in the function of each muscle, indicating the origin and insertion of the muscle, the line of pull, and the action produced by the muscle. Demonstrate the action while the patient remains passive. Instruct the patient to think of the pull as coming from the insertion and moving in the direction of the shortening muscle to give the patient a concept of the sensations to be experienced as the muscle contracts and moves the body part. Stroke the skin over the insertion in the direction of pull and tell the patient to concen-

FREDERIC J. KOTTKE

trate on the sensation of motion occurring during this sensorially reinforced passive motion.

Train Perception of Contraction. The training of precise control of individual muscles is basically the training of awareness of the sensation produced by the isolated contraction of the prime mover so that it may be contracted independently from any other muscle. Control training or neuromuscular education begins with minimal effort against minimal resistance and is increased by small increments of intensity as the patient develops control.[42, 43] The specific sensations produced by the contraction of the prime mover are perceived only during very light effort because an isolated contraction of an individual muscle can be performed only when the muscle is contracting against a resistance that is small in relation to the total strength of that muscle. Greater effort, which would cause the spread of excitation to other motor neurons and result in the cocontraction of other muscles, should not be allowed. If such spread of excitation is allowed to occur, any stronger sensations produced by the contractions of stronger synergists and antagonists are perceived more readily than are sensations arising from the weakly contracting prime mover. The patient then learns to monitor the strong but incorrect motor activity and ignores the sensations arising from the lesser activity of the prime mover. Therefore, the patient does not learn to control the prime mover and it does not develop its potential strength and usefulness. If this type of incoordination is allowed during therapeutic exercise, a motor pattern is developed that does not include the paretic prime mover. The final result is an uncoordinated contraction of less than the potential strength.

When the muscle is weak in relation to the weight of the part, that weight constitutes a heavy resistance for the muscle and the effort to lift the part causes irradiation of impulses and incoordination. Therefore, control exercises are begun with maximal assistance so that the muscle contracts against minimal resistance, and the resistance is increased only as ability is developed to contract the prime mover without activating other muscles.

Sequence for Training Neuromuscular Control. For the training of control when there is an upper motor neuron lesion, it is necessary first to obtain relaxation of all muscles that show a reflex hypertonia. Then the patient must limit the intensity of effort to avoid exciting irradiation of impulses beyond the prime mover. Specific control of the prime mover or unit of contraction that is controllable is trained by performance of that motion with minimal effort and as much assistance as is necessary to produce motion through a range of 20 to 30 degrees. (1) The patient is instructed to think about the motion while that motion is carried out passively by the therapist in order that the patient may feel the sensations produced. The skin over the tendon of insertion is stroked in the direction of the motion just before the motion is carried out by the therapist, with the patient passive, to reinforce the sensation of the motion. Even this level of participation during which the patient is told only to think about the motion may result in cocontraction of other muscles as the patient tries to participate. If that is the case, the patient must be taught to diminish the effort so that overflow does not occur. (2) As the second step, after stimulating the skin over the tendon of insertion, the therapist carries out the motion while the patient assists only slightly by a minimal contraction of the prime mover. When the patient can limit the performance to the muscle or unit of motion being trained, the patient is allowed to increase participation gradually, and the assistance is decreased as the precision is maintained. (3) The patient produces increasingly stronger contractions as the therapist continues the technique of cutaneous stimulation followed by the desired movement. As the precise activity is carried on repeatedly, the patient learns how to control that prime mover without initiating other activity. The repetitions begin to form the correct engram of that single activity. (4) As the patient develops the ability to produce a stronger controlled contraction of the desired motion, the therapist gradually decreases assistance until the patient is producing the correct antigravity contraction.

Progression from one step to the next should be permitted only when the first step can be performed accurately without substitution or incoordination. At the beginning of training, the step being trained is carried out three to five times for each muscle or motion at each training session, depending upon the fatigability of the muscle. As the muscle gets stronger and endurance increases, the number of repetitions can be increased, but a short rest period must be allowed after each two to three attempted contractions to allow recovery time so that fatigue is avoided. Throughout control training, avoidance of substitution must be emphasized. Control of the individual muscles of a pattern should be achieved before more complex coordination training is attempted. Control of simple motions with inhibition of other activities represents the beginning of coordination.

Training of Multimuscular Coordination

Therapeutic exercise to train coordination has as its objective the development of a high level of coordination in the shortest possible time. The purpose of this training is to strengthen the selection and utilization of the best method of performance of each activity to be carried out. In order to accomplish this, the trainer must know each method to be used. This knowledge includes both the perceptual and the motor components of the coordinated performance. Then that method needs to be put into the patient's repertoire by the repetition of the correct pattern of performance.[17, 45]

For optimal learning of coordination, conditions should be set up in which each muscular pattern is consistently and successfully performed. A learning environment must be established in which the patient can concentrate on the task and can carry out the necessary activity correctly under direct perception (see Training of Control of Individual Muscles). To do this, the activity is broken down or *desynthesized into components that are simple enough to be performed correctly.* Desynthesis increases the consistency and frequency of correct performance and eliminates errors. The more complex the task to be learned, the more extensively it must be desynthesized to ensure that each sub-task can be correctly practiced. If a patient has such poor control that any simple subunits of coordination have not been developed, it is necessary to completely desynthesize the multimuscular movement and practice the contraction of the individual prime mover muscles. During training, it is necessary to keep the effort low by decreasing both the speed and the resistance against which the patient must perform, because as effort increases there is an increased spread of excitation to activate motor neurons that are not a part of the desired coordination pattern.

When the motor pattern is desynthesized to unit motor tasks that can be performed successfully, each task is trained by practicing it under voluntary control. The patient is instructed in the desired performance that is accompanied by sensory stimulation and passive movement. In the early stages of training, each step of the task must be observed and modified voluntarily by the patient. It is imperative to practice slowly because it is not possible for the patient to attend to more than one unit of function at any instant. It takes time for an individual to think through the sensations and muscular response of each untrained motion. An untrained activity requires a *minimum* of 500 msec per observation and response (see Fig. 19–1).

When the activity is strange or new, it may require several seconds for the patient to process the sensations generated by muscular contractions and relate them to the motion desired. At the same time, the patient must sort out conflicting sensory stimuli produced by contractions of other muscles and suppress that activity. Awareness of the sensations produced by this desired movement is reinforced. Whatever assistance is necessary to reduce the effort to the level at which precision is maintained is provided while the patient concentrates on the sensations produced by the activity. Fatigue occurs quickly during attempts to attend to precise or isolated contractions produced by voluntary control. As fatigue occurs, the ability of the patient to concentrate on the activity to be trained diminishes and, as a consequence, mistakes begin to occur. Therefore, the patient should have a short rest after each two or three repetitions to prevent cumulative fatigue. If the patient shows continuing fatigue or diminished control in spite of these short rests, that activity should be discontinued for that treatment session in order to avoid practice of an erroneous pattern.

As the patient develops the ability to produce a precise contraction with no evidence of cocontractions of other muscles, the patient may be allowed to exert more effort, always staying within the ability to maintain the pattern. At each step of the training, the therapist must be sure that the patient can perform independently and correctly before proceeding to a more advanced activity.

Repetition of the correct performance many times causes the formation of a coordination engram in the central nervous system (Fig. 19–2). The engram that is developed is determined by the pattern that is practiced. If the practice is imprecise, the engram will be imprecise. If errors are made during practice, the resulting engram will show frequent errors. Therefore, one should maintain precision at all times by keeping the task within the capacity of the patient to perform it correctly. Performance of an incorrect or variable pattern not only delays the development of the correct engram but also begins to introduce an incorrect engram, which then will have to be "unlearned." It requires a longer time to "unlearn" an incorrect pattern and establish a correct pattern than it does merely to establish a correct pattern when there is no interfering engram.

Repetition of precise activity is the only way by which engrams of skillful coordination are devel-

FREDERIC J. KOTTKE

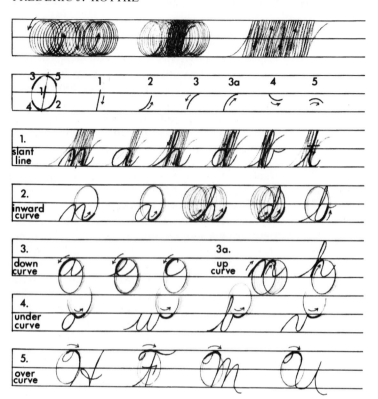

FIGURE 19–2. Repeated correct performance of simple components of a complex coordinated movement is the quickest way to develop the basic engrams, which then can be linked to practice more complex activities. Any guides that increase the awareness of correct performance or provide immediate comparison of correct performance hasten the development of coordination. As an example, in Palmer method writing, the practicing of the compact oval and vertical push-pull movements provides the pattern for the components of motions used when writing.

oped. The research that demonstrated the relationship between the number of repetitions performed and the level of skill in performance of an engram was reported by Crossman in 1959.[17] He showed that in the development of manual coordination required for an industrial task, a young adult with normal dexterity required three million repetitions of that act in order to develop maximal speed and skill (Fig. 19–3). In an investigation of other types of repetitive activities, it was found that a high level of coordination was not achieved until repetitions occurred a million or more times.[46]

Patients need to repeat the precise contraction of each movement unit many hundreds or even thousands of times each day if they are to develop precise and highly skillful engrams of that activity in as short a time as three years. However, less fast and less skillful engrams begin to appear much earlier when many fewer correct repetitions of a motor pattern have been performed. Crossman's data indicate improvement beyond the maximal capacity of voluntary control after 30,000 repetitions.[17] Rabbitt reported a significant shortening in reaction time after practicing 20,000 repetitions and still further improvement after 40,000 repetitions.[58] On the other hand, Prevo, Visser, and

Vogelaar reported that 10,000 repetitions of retraining of a motor pattern of a hemiplegic arm did not improve performance beyond that achieved by the learning of direct voluntary control.[57] From these admittedly limited data, it still may be concluded that little or no engram formation will occur until approximately 30,000 repetitions of a motor pattern have been performed, and the same number of repetitions will be necessary for each variation of each pattern in the patient's repertoire. It requires 1000 repetitions of an engram daily for three years to approximate one million repetitions. If only 100 repetitions are performed per day, it requires 30 years to accumulate one million repetitions. In our daily activities, commonly used patterns of coordination are repeated, or practiced, many thousands of times each day. For example, for each mile walked, each lower extremity takes at least 1000 steps and each upper extremity exhibits the reciprocal swing of the long spinal reflex with each step. Inadequate repetitions result in imperfect performances. Many of our daily activities have common component movements of the arms, legs, and trunk, and the practice of those components in one activity appears to have a carryover to other activities. However, any units of

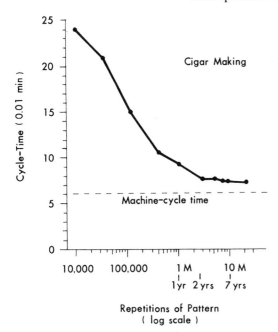

FIGURE 19–3. The development of skillful and automatic performance of a new task requires millions of repetitions to reach its peak, as demonstrated by the decrease of the unit performance time for this manual motor activity by newly employed normal young women. (From Kottke, F. J.: From reflex to skill: The training of coordination. Arch. Phys. Med. Rehabil., 61:551–561, 1980. Adapted from Crossman, E. R. F. W.: Theory of acquisition of speed-skill. Ergonomics, 2:153–166, 1959.)

activity that are specific to only one task must be practiced specifically to develop a coordination engram for that task.

As the patient develops the ability to produce the individual units of the engram easily and accurately, these are then linked into subtasks, each of which, in turn, is practiced as a unit until it, too, is automated as a larger engram of performance. As the individual movement units each become an engram unit through practice, the rate of performance for each of those units increases. However, when these engram units are linked together, at first that linkage must be made by conscious control, and that rate can be no faster than three per second. As practice of the linked pattern progresses, the linkage becomes a part of the new, bigger engram pattern, and the rate of performance then increases to four to six times per second or even faster (Fig. 19–4). Therefore, with each expansion of an engram or any change that requires the use of voluntary control, the rate of performance of that controlled component must be carried out no faster than two to three per second, and it is only as that consciously controlled

unit becomes a part of the engram through repetition that performance regains a faster speed. The necessity of slowing the rate of performance with each addition to a pattern and repeating the pattern with precision at that slow rate until the new more complex engram begins to form is frequently overlooked or ignored; and, as a result, errors creep into the performance and the patient ceases to make progress toward a precise, fast new engram. Because Kabat, Knott and Voss, Brunnstrom, and their followers were not concerned with the impairment of inhibition of muscles not participating in coordination patterns, they did not question the potentially detrimental effect of spread of excitation to many motor neurons outside of the coordination pattern each time that facilitation techniques were used. Therefore, in their therapeutic programs, precise performance of an activity was not an immediate requirement during therapeutic exercise. It was assumed that, if some performance developed, it could be shaped over time to the desired performance, just as occurs in the development of coordination by the growing child.

The engrams of the subtasks as they are perfected by practice are chained progressively until the full pattern can be performed precisely with speed and force. As these engrams of subtasks and, later, full engrams are developed, the conscious regulation becomes one of selecting the sequences in which these engrams will appear. If the patterned activity is such that sequences of engrams will appear many times, then through practice the entire sequence can be made into a continuous engram and run automatically.

The intensity of effort is increased during practice only within the range in which precise performance can be maintained. Increasing the speed, the force, or the complexity of an activity increases the intensity of effort that is required. Attention must be paid to each of these characteristics of performance, since excessive effort always leads to incoordination. Improvement in performance is achieved by gradually increasing the force, speed, and complexity of performance within the capacity to maintain precision. Performance improves only when practicing near the peak of ability. Performance should be encouraged at the highest level at which the patient can succeed. Repeated near-maximal practice is necessary to perfect and maintain fast and skillful coordination.

Although each test of maximal ability exceeds the peak of performance, practice should be carried on within the range in which every repetition, insofar as possible, is correct, since engrams de-

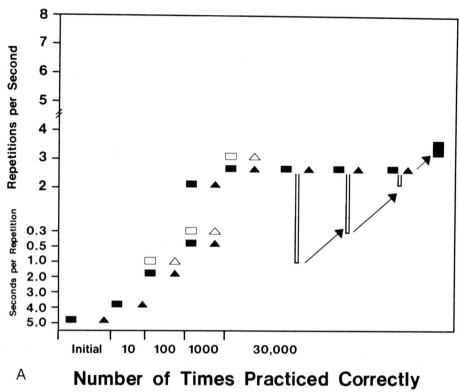

A **Number of Times Practiced Correctly**

FIGURE 19–4. *A,* Coordination develops progressively by practicing small units of activity under conscious control until an engram of each begins to form. The maximal rate of repetition under conscious control is two to three per second, with the slower rate quickly prevailing if the activity is continued for any period of time. The sequencing or linking of these controlled units of activity occurs at the same limited rate. After approximately 30,000 repetitions of practice, an engram of each unit of activity begins to form in the extrapyramidal system and the rate of performance begins to increase beyond the rate achievable by control through the pyramidal system. However, when these engram units are linked consciously, each linkage requires the response time of conscious control, i.e., 300 milliseconds, and that interval does not decrease until a sufficient number of repetitions have been practiced to make that linkage a part of the total engram.

velop only as the result of successful performance and nothing beneficial is accomplished by performing erroneously. Therapists, therefore, should try to avoid setting up practice situations in which there are errors in performance. Successful performance has a dual effect. Physiologically, it reinforces the strength of the engram and, psychologically, it rewards the patient so that he or she is more willing to continue to perform that activity.

The Role of Repetition in the Formation of Engrams

There is an interesting dichotomy of opinion that the usual activities of a normal child emerge as the result of genetic inheritance but that maximal performers of any neuromuscular act must train by practicing for years before they reach their peak skill. We usually overlook the fact that young children practice simple engrams many times each day for many months before they acquire the level of coordination necessary to begin to perform more complex activities. It requires many years of practice during play before the coordination of the child develops to the lowest level of the range of coordination found in normal adults (Fig. 19–5). Many activities are highly repetitive. Walking, a variety of forms of hand grasping, reaching, balancing—all are activities repeated thousands of times each day by all normal persons. Athletes, musicians, acrobats, and persons using finger dexterity in their occupations practice for years to perfect their skills. In recent years, it has become apparent that intense training of children in athletics or musical skills can shorten the time to reach the maximal level of performance; it is not a matter

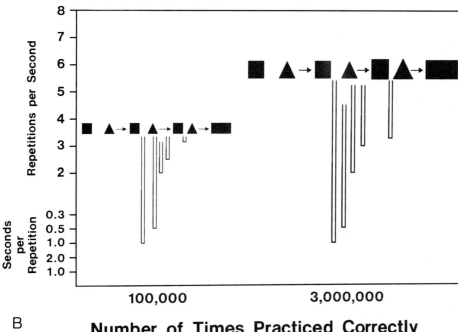

B

Number of Times Practiced Correctly

FIGURE 19–4 *Continued B,* Engrams develop their greatest rate of performance through practice at the maximal rate of correct performance for millions of times. This requires active inhibition of all muscles that should not contract as well as activation of the participating muscles in the correct sequence and with the correct intensity. Greater length and complexity of engrams are developed by the linking and chaining of subunit engrams, and then by practicing these longer units until all linkages have become a part of the engram. Initially, each linkage is a consciously controlled activity limited to the slow rate of performance of conscious control. Through practice, each link is integrated into the engram, and, as a result, the rate of performance is increased. Even when highly developed engrams are linked together, at first the duration of that linkage is no shorter than 300 to 500 milliseconds, and only after prolonged practice makes each linkage a part of the engram does the linkage speed up to the speed of the rest of the engram. The greater the number of repetitions of the sequences of engram units, as prolonged patterns, the more rapidly the linkages will become integrated component parts of the engram. In this way, a complex sequence of coordinated muscular activities is trained into the development of one highly skilled engram.

of maturation with age, but rather the achievement of millions of correct repetitions to perfect the necessary engrams.

Programs of therapeutic exercise to train coordination should provide for as many repetitions as possible of each activity each day, since engrams do not become well developed until hundreds of thousands of repetitions have been performed. Lack of sufficient repetitions has been a major flaw in much of the programming of therapeutic exercise for the training of coordination. In a single short period scheduled for coordination training each day, a child or adult with hyperreflexia may perform only a very few repetitions of each movement. Between therapies, many hours elapse during which correctly coordinated activity is not performed. Moreover, incoordinated activity may be allowed during the interval between therapies, whereas therapists focus on correct performance only during the few moments of the therapy. The

lack of understanding of the mechanism of formation of engrams of coordination results in the failure to provide enough practice to obtain adequately developed engrams and in the tolerance of incorrect performance, which develops incoordination. Such faulty scheduling of training guarantees that the result will be poor.

For the training of the handicapped person to be successful, therapeutic exercise needs to be organized similarly to the training of any skillful performer. Training schedules for those individuals provide for thousands of repetitions of specific activities each day. The level of practice is set and monitored so that, throughout the entire schedule, the performance is precise and exact. Before any performer can carry out the final complex pattern of coordination, the ability to carry out each of the simple component parts must be developed. Then each of these simple component parts, or subunits, must be practiced until each becomes a

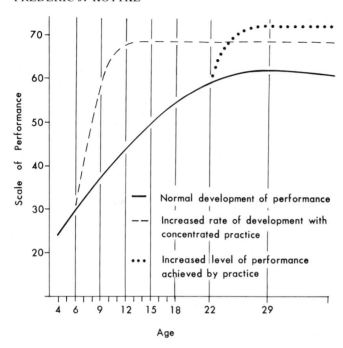

FIGURE 19–5. Under normal conditions coordination develops progressively through childhood and reaches its peak in the third decade. Concentrated training of a specific activity results in achievement of peak coordination for that activity at a much earlier age. Likewise, concentrated training of an activity in adulthood results in a significant increase in the peak performance of that activity. The number of correct repetitions in each situation rather than the length of time for their completion determines the level of coordination achieved. (From Kottke, F. J., Halpern, D., Easton, J. K. M., Ozel, A. T., and Burrill, C. A.: Training of coordination. Arch. Phys. Med. Rehabil., 59:567–572, 1978.)

precise engram. The subunit engrams are linked by control at that slower rate and practiced until that linkage becomes a part of the engram. Subunits and units are linked and chained in this way and, by practice, developed into precise engrams. We are only now beginning to recognize that maximal skill is not attained until an engram has been practiced millions of times. The task, then, in therapeutic exercise must be to establish conditions in which each day patients can perform many reproducible subunits of each of the coordination patterns to be trained. Practice is restricted to units of performance that can be controlled precisely. This requires that coordination training should begin by desynthesizing each coordination pattern into units, subunits, or even individual prime movers if more complex units cannot be controlled without cocontractions of any other muscles that should not be in that coordination pattern. Each of these precisely performable activities is practiced hundreds of times each day, increasing speed and force to the greatest limit possible while precision is maintained. Only in this way can the tens of thousands, hundreds of thousands, and even millions of repetitions of each pattern be carried out to develop a satisfactorily useful engram. Inspection of Crossman's data suggests that improvement in performance, indicating the development of a more skillful engram, begins to become evi-

dent only after a number of tens of thousands of repetitions (see Fig. 19–3).

The writings of Fay,[19] Kabat,[40] and Brunnstrom[11] indicate that for the retraining of adults after strokes and the training of children with cerebral palsy they considered the strengthening of the contractions of prime mover muscles of coordination to be the major consideration. None of these systems of therapy placed emphasis on the development of inhibition of opposing muscles in order that prime movers could function without muscular opposition. The focus of attention for those systems has been on increasing the excitation to the prime movers of each activity by volition transmitted over the corticospinal tract. Fay[19] considered spinal and supraspinal reflexes to be primitive pathways that had become obsolete in modern humans and to lie outside the corticospinal pathway for coordination. However, he recognized that in the presence of an upper motor neuron lesion in humans the initiation of specific reflexes could be used to unlock (block) the activity of other reflexes. When this was done repeatedly, together with initiation of desired reflex motor patterns, patients might regain progressive ability to produce useful motions with some degree of coordination. Kabat[39] likewise considered spinal reflexes to be obsolete and outside of the normal pathway of motor coordination but, in the presence of an upper motor lesion, to be available to facilitate weak cerebrospinal excitation that would activate the lower motor neuron. Moreover, he considered irradiation of excitation of cerebral origin and of reflex origin to be highly beneficial to develop a new pathway for motor control if it caused stronger contractions of the prime movers under consideration. Fay, Kabat, and Brunnstrom considered that prolonged repetition of muscle patterns activated in this way would strengthen the function of the voluntary cerebrospinal pathway until voluntary coordination was regained again. However, none of these investigators documented this phenomenon with a published series of cases.

Although great emphasis has been placed on specific methods for retraining coordination after stroke, several studies have been more than dubious about their effectiveness. Feldman, Rusk, and associates[20] compared a program of total rehabilitation that included therapeutic exercise for retraining coordination with a simultaneously conducted program in another institution in which therapy was limited to mobility exercises to establish and maintain normal range of motion and retraining in activities of daily living (ADLs). They found that the performance achieved by the two groups of patients was the same. Stern[64] treated one group of patients after stroke with mobilization and ADLs and to another group added proprioceptive facilitation training as determined to be necessary by each therapist. Stern did not observe any improvement as the result of the facilitation therapy.

The Bobaths first attracted wide attention in this country with their techniques for producing reflex inhibitory postures that were supposed to normalize the hypertonic reflexes.[7] It soon became apparent that these were not prolonged changes but were temporary changes of hyperreflexia. However, during the period of normoreflexia that followed the inhibitory maneuvers, the patients were able to participate in progressively more complex coordinated activities. Mrs. Bobath did develop excellent techniques for using reflex facilitation and inhibition to train antigravity posture and movement from lying to sitting to standing and walking by children with mild or moderate cerebral palsy.[6] Although she had no controls other than the changes in each child, the improvement of antigravity posture and ambulation was impressive for many children. No technique has been developed or asserted that produces great improvement of the coordination of the hands.

Factors Increasing Incoordination

A number of conditions increase incoordination. Strong effort to produce a contraction causes irradiation of impulses in the central nervous system from the pathway of a coordinated activity to other motorneurons. Constant repetition of an activity in combination with the same extraneous motion will incorporate that extraneous motion into the activity pattern and produce persistent incoordination. When a patient is insecure or fearful, there is a greater spread of excitation within the central system with activation of more motor neurons than those essential for an activity pattern. This results in a greater expenditure of effort, less precision of motion, and interference with the desired pattern of activity. If patients have to support themselves against gravity, if they are weak, or if they must overcome resistance that is great in relation to the strength of a muscle, incoordination will be increased. Excitement and strong emotions increase incoordination. Pain or increased sensory stimuli reaching the central nervous system increase irradiation from an activated pathway to other motor neurons. Fatigue increases incoordination, probably because of the inability of the inhibitory centers to restrict impulses from irradiating beyond the desired activity pathway.

Just as coordination is produced by repetition, it is lost through periods of inactivity. It is necessary to reteach coordination to muscles that have been inactive or paretic. The "alienation" or dropping of paretic muscles from an activity pattern occurs frequently. Only through specific training of control and coordination do these muscles again become incorporated as a part of the normal activity pattern.

Systems of Therapy

A comparison of the requirements for the training of coordination discussed above with the various systems of therapy that are being used throughout the United States at this time reveals that each of those systems concentrates on a limited range of the entire spectrum of need for training coordination. Each advocate of selected specified procedures of therapeutic exercise has concentrated on selected problems that must be resolved in the therapeutic program. Some methods such as those of Kabat,[39] Knott and Voss,[44]

FREDERIC J. KOTTKE

Rood,[60] and as quoted by Stockmeyer[65] and Brunnstrom[11] have concentrated on reflex or mass proprioceptive neuromuscular facilitation (PNF) to activate and attempt to strengthen voluntary control. For these methods, the assumption appears to be that as the voluntary activity becomes stronger there will be a fading of incoordination. The major limitation of each of these methods is that after facilitation has developed activation of prime mover muscles as a part of mass activity, there are no procedures in those methods focusing on the development of inhibition of undesired activity. Continued practice of reflex facilitation or mass PNF strengthens and perpetuates incoordination. In the only controlled study of PNF compared with treatment by restoring range of motion and training in ADLs, Stern found that the much greater time spent on PNF each day did not result in any greater functional improvement than occurred in the control group.[64] This is to be expected, because PNF increases diffuse activation (incoordination) but provides no training of inhibition to suppress overflow of excitation to muscles that should not participate in the muscular pattern so that precise coordination will develop. The only way by which inhibition of undesired activity can be developed is by prolonged practice of the desired patterns in order to develop coordination engrams. Therefore, systems of reflex facilitation must be followed by coordination training if mass patterns of activity are to be converted to useful coordination.

Phelps,[55] who developed one of the early programs for cerebral palsy in the United States, was eclectic in his approach to treatment. Many components of his treatment continue to be used. Among other contributions, he recognized that a patient who learned to relax completely showed less involuntary activity during relaxation than during activity. Therefore, patients were taught prolonged relaxation. However, Phelps did not distinguish between general relaxation on the one hand and inhibition of undesired muscular contraction during activity on the other. General relaxation alone does not train inhibition during activity.

Phelps recognized that repetition of a desired pattern of motion improved the performance of that pattern. He taught his patients to practice repetition of desired activities, with or without assistance, accompanied by songs or jingles each day. In effect, he was using repetition to develop engrams. His insistence on the continued practice of the same basic activities indicates his awareness of the need for many repetitions before coordination begins to develop.

Temple Fay recognized that the hierarchical organization of the nervous system imposed brain stem and forebrain controls on the reflex organization of the spinal cord to produce coordination.[18] He recognized that control of the basic reflexes was essential before more advanced coordination could be trained. He utilized reflex patterning and repetition as the means to begin to modify basic reflexes and referred to this as neurophysiological organization of the nervous system. Although Fay recognized that undesired reflex activity must be inhibited in any motor pattern, it is not clear to what extent he recognized the importance of training inhibition as the basis for the formation of correct engrams. It is evident that he did recognize that prolonged repetition through patterning was essential for the development of coordination engrams.[53]

Karel and Berta Bobath[6, 7] emphasized both the need for inhibition of hypertonia in patients with cerebral palsy prior to the beginning of training and the necessity for carrying out proper training in order to develop correct patterns of performance without overflow of activity to other muscles. They, like Fay, emphasize that training of posture progresses from simple activities to the more complex in a regular sequence and called this the neurodevelopmental sequence of therapy (Fig. 19–6). They utilize reflex facilitation to reinforce the motor patterns with which they are concerned, particularly in the postural activities.

Margaret Rood[60] and her students[65] have used a variety of reflex facilitatory methods to excite or inhibit motor activity. Rood, too, has focused her attention more on excitation of prime mover function than on the inhibition of the muscles producing incoordination.

The persons who have focused our attention on incoordination resulting from effort that causes the spread of muscular activity from prime movers to other muscles to an excessive degree were Kenny[43] and Knapp.[42] Their concepts grew out of their experience in the treatment of acute anterior poliomyelitis, quite a different disease from cerebral palsy. In poliomyelitis, when a prime mover is paralyzed, the uncoordinated overuse of other muscles because of the effort exerted to activate the paralyzed muscle is a predominant finding. In the early 1940s, it was presumed that the incoordination of poliomyelitis, and that of all other neurological diseases, was specific to that disease.

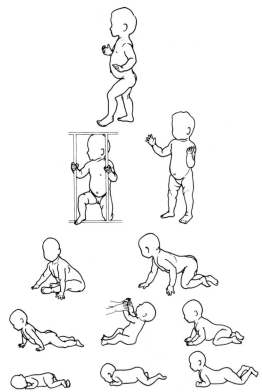

FIGURE 19–6. The development of antigravity posture shows a pyramidal contour from a broad base and low profile at birth to a progressively higher profile on a narrower base as coordination for balance and the ability to utilize and inhibit reflexes develop.

Gellhorn[23] was the first investigator to demonstrate that the incoordination of poliomyelitis was the overuse of synergists, stabilizers, and antagonists in the same typical pattern that occurred in normal individuals with increasing effort. This was the beginning of our understanding that the incoordination of motor activity is based on the normal reflex organization of the nervous system rather than being due to abnormal discharges from damaged neurons. The failure to recognize that incoordination is not a specific phenomenon peculiar to each disease but has a characteristic pattern in all diseases has delayed the development of our understanding regarding the mechanism of incoordination. Kenny and Knapp demonstrated that only when effort was decreased so that there was no irradiation of neuronal impulses to other pathways could a person produce an isolated contraction of a prime mover. *This is the basis for the training of control of the individual muscles.*

Hypothesis of Inheritance of Motor Coordination

The hypothesis that basic patterns of coordination are inherited as opposed to being learned through the development of engrams merits presentation here because it is the widely accepted doctrine.[15, 25, 48] Many of the early students of development observed that the basic patterns of posture and movement—sitting, standing, balancing, walking, running, reaching, grasping—all appeared in a uniform sequence and time during maturation, and they assumed that this uniformity was the result of genetic endowment. A logical extension of this concept, then, was that any reflex activity that interfered with the emergence of these automatic coordination patterns was an "abnormal" reflex rather than inadequate inhibition of a normal reflex. Coordination or automatic neuromuscular activity was assumed to develop in the normal child with age as the result of maturation of neurons and myelination of nerve pathways. Lapse of time rather than prolonged practice of each activity was considered to be the essential requirement for the development of coordination for those activities common to most people. In the young, lack of muscular strength and immaturity were assumed to be the factors limiting automatic coordination. Mass movement of multiple muscles was reported to precede the development of activity of individual muscles,[16] and from this, automatic coordination of multiple muscles was assumed to precede the development of control of individual muscles. It was deduced that multimuscular automatic coordination is inherent and only later does a person learn to control individual muscles by conscious practice. This concept is the converse of that of the progressive development from reflexes to control of the individual muscle to coordination of multiple muscles as the result of repetitive practice.[45] Part of the confusion may have resulted from equating mass reflex activity with multimuscular contractions which are coordinated. Coordination was viewed as being due solely to the excitation of the appropriate muscles, and little attention was paid to the need to inhibit those components of reflexes that did not contribute to the muscular patterns. Even mass reflex movements were shown by Windle[69] to develop in the fetus after the prior development of local reflexes. This reflex activity, either local or general, is far more rudimentary than the coordinated muscular activity with which we are concerned. However,

FREDERIC J. KOTTKE

normal infants and children in a normal environment develop motor patterns so easily and on such a regular schedule that genetic inheritance appeared adequate to explain development without invoking environment or experience.[12, 16, 25, 26] If these assumptions were accepted, it seemed quite logical also to assume that when brain damage arrested muscular performance at a low level, the impairment of function was imposed by loss of motor patterns genetically coded in the damaged neurons rather than resulting from lack of practice to develop coordination engrams.

It was only as the design of experiments changed to follow each patient and chronicle the patient's experiences and activities, rather than to evaluate performances of groups of infants at fixed ages of development, that genetic determinism appeared to be inadequate as a total explanation. Piaget[56] first, followed by others,[31, 61, 68] observed serial development of performance from the simple to the more complex as the result of many repetitions of each act. Environmental stimuli that encouraged the repetition of an activity speeded its development.[68] Prevention of activity severely delayed development.[52, 61]

Coordination Activities for the Hand and Upper Extremity

Prehension. The complex activities of pinch and grasp require multimuscular coordination for each digit. There is usually simultaneous movement of wrist, elbow, and shoulder to carry the hand to the desired place of activity. Prehension occurs most frequently as pinch, or precision grip between the thumb, index, and middle fingers like a three-jawed chuck (Fig. 19–7). Seventy per cent of prehensile activity is carried out by variants of this position. Power grasp, performed by approximating the four fingers toward the thenar eminence, is used in its various modifications for about 20 per cent of activities. Apposition of the thumb to the radial side of the index finger or to one fingertip occurs less frequently. Modifications of these basic patterns occur by varying the number of fingers in fingertip grasp; abducting, adducting, or rotating at the metacarpophalangeal joints; varying the position of terminal pad contact by the amount of interphalangeal flexion; or varying the degree of closure or the number of fingers involved in the power grip (Fig. 19–8). Each of these variants of position requires the development of a multimus-

cular coordination engram through prolonged practice in infancy and childhood.

The activities of the multiple muscles involved in the positioning or movement of even one finger exceed the supervisory capacity of totally voluntary observation and regulation. The development of preprogrammed engrams is essential for all finger activities, and, in the absence of these engrams, incoordination occurs even though each of the prime movers can be contracted voluntarily. This may be seen in the repeated reversal of consecutive joints of the fingers of the athetoid patient as grasp is attempted but muscles, other than the prime mover that is under immediate attention, deviate from the desired pattern. As the patient shifts attention consecutively from joint to joint, the joint receiving direct observation is brought under control, but other joints not being observed move out of position because automatic activation and inhibition are not imposed on the reflexes of the muscles that control them. These same patterns that are seen in the athetoid patient who is unable to develop engrams may be seen in the infant before engrams develop. In children or adults in whom the demands of performance exceed the engrams that have been developed, errors are more likely to result in the selection of the incorrect engram or incomplete inhibition of reflex activity. Moreover, because of lack of adequate inhibition, stronger stimuli will produce stronger reflex motor responses that will dominate the more weakly stimulated reflexes.

As might be expected, the most complex patterns are the most difficult to program and require the longest period of training. Finger-thumb prehension has far too many components and too many variations to be successfully controlled by volition through the single-channeled corticospinal tract in the absence of coordination engrams. The thumb, because of its mobility at the carpometacarpal joint, is the most mobile digit and by far the most difficult to learn to coordinate. It requires the coordinated contractions of multiple muscles to maintain one position or to move to another position. As a consequence, until the engrams of thumb coordination have developed, the thumb is a continual impediment to the use of the other fingers. Also each of the other fingers has metacarpophalangeal mobility in multiple planes: rotation, abduction-adduction, and flexion-extension. Each of these motions at each of these joints must be regulated by the appropriate contractions of the controlling muscles and inhibition of all other muscles for each of the possible variations of

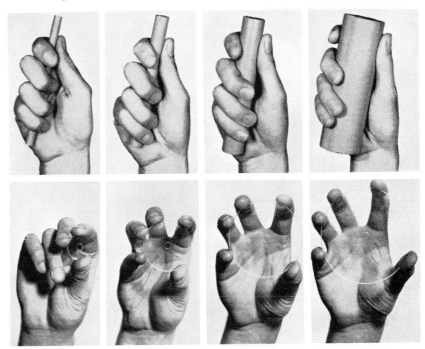

FIGURE 19–7. Prehension using the power grip or precision grip on objects of various sizes. (From Napier, J. R.: The prehensile movements of the human hand. J. Bone Joint Surg., 38B:902–913, 1956.)

prehension. Coordination of all of these potential patterns requires the formation of engrams developed only by prolonged practice. In particular, the untrained thumb persistently interferes with the use of the index and middle fingers. Athetoid children learn to avoid the interfering thumb by concentrating on the use of the fourth and fifth fingers for grasp—the so-called ulnar grasp. Ulnar grasp is not a more fundamental or primitive grasp but is the grasp that can be more successfully practiced to develop an engram because the patterns are not continually disrupted by uncontrolled motions of the thumb.

It is only after basic engrams form that useful function begins to emerge in the hand. When the activities of the normal individual without preprogrammed engrams are observed, i.e., the normal infant, as was done by White,[67] it is seen that the hand may be moved reflexly but not in a coordinated manner for the first three to four months.

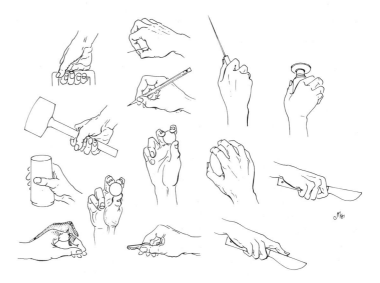

FIGURE 19–8. Although most prehensile motions are variants of the precision grip or the power grip, each position constitutes a separate engram.

FREDERIC J. KOTTKE

During that time, the infant may spend minutes at a time gazing at the motionless fisted hand (probably because he has no conception of how to initiate motion in the arm). At four months, there still is little prehension, and upper extremity activity is mainly swiping at an object in the visual field during which the hand may be fisted or open. It is only long after that and following practice each day throughout the waking period that the child develops crude one-handed, and later, bimanual grasp. Controlled thumb-to-index pinch does not begin to develop for about eight months, and three-finger pinch requires several more months of practice before rudimentary coordination is seen. Even then these activities are poorly programmed for integration into prehensile patterns. Two more years of daily practice are necessary before the child can integrate thumb position with arm motion and position in space to grasp a pencil and draw a simple vertical line (Fig. 19–9), and an additional 30 months of training are necessary before the child can copy a triangle. The purpose in focusing attention on this long period required for the training of a normal child in the use of the hand is to demonstrate that in every normal person the development of multimuscular engrams does not rely on merely the cognitive learning of the task to be performed but on millions of repetitions before muscular patterns become automatic and well coordinated.

The voluntary component of normal prehension consists of the selection of the engrams to be used and of modifying activity by shifting from one engram to another in relation to the shape and position of the object being manipulated. Skillful prehension develops slowly. The slow development of the drawing and writing skills of children that is extended into adulthood in the training time required for artists and architects is a good indication of the prolonged period of practice necessary before the fundamental multimuscular patterns of manual performance begin to develop. Tests of manual manipulation show that these skills increase in a linear fashion through youth and adolescence and do not peak until the third decade of life[8] (see Fig. 19–5).

For the patient with impaired coordination, if such a complex activity as precision grip is not desynthesized to the level that each controllable subunit can be practiced accurately under direct volition, then good coordination will never be developed. When there is damage to the extrapyramidal system so that cocontraction is difficult to coordinate and automatic inhibition is slow to

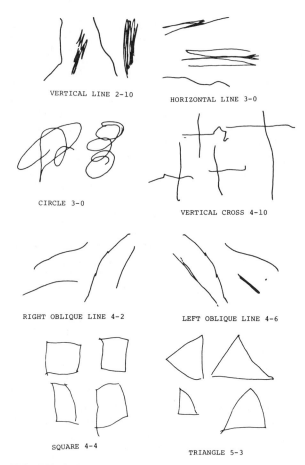

VERTICAL LINE 2-10

HORIZONTAL LINE 3-0

CIRCLE 3-0

VERTICAL CROSS 4-10

RIGHT OBLIQUE LINE 4-2

LEFT OBLIQUE LINE 4-6

SQUARE 4-4

TRIANGLE 5-3

FIGURE 19–9. It requires many months of manual activities before a child develops the ability to hold a pencil and successfully copy a figure on paper. The numerals indicate the age in years and months at which a child would be expected to perform increasingly difficult pencil-on-paper tasks on request. (From Beery, K. E.: Developmental Test of Visual-Motor Integration: Administration and Scoring Manual. Chicago, Follette Publishing Co., 1967.)

develop, it is essential to provide the environment and the practice routines that make the execution of performable motions possible in the correct patterns for thousands of times each day. How is this to be done? Specific programs with progressive sequences of activities to be practiced, from the simplest to the progressively more complex, need to be developed.

The first criterion for repeated performance is that the patient is willing to, or better, wants to perform. The reinforcing effect of a participating and observing therapist, parent, or friend is one way to augment this incentive. However, time each day for such participation is frequently limited. An activity that provides its own rewarding feedback so that the patient wishes to perform repeatedly is a second mechanism. Such rewarding activities should be readily available so that the patient can have the opportunity to practice at any time. Musical instruments, toys, typewriters, games, and construction crafts all come to mind as conventional self-rewarding activities. For most of these currently available modes of rewarding activity, participation can occur only when prehension is well advanced. The greatest unmet need at the present time is the development of the mechanical devices that link individual prime mover contractions or the contractions of simple subunits of coordinated muscular function to self-rewarding activities. In order to make these self-rewarding activities useful as independent training devices, it is essential that the device be constructed so that it responds only to the appropriate contraction of the engram subunit or unit to be trained and does not respond to any other substituted contraction. A variety of linking transducers needs to be developed to make it possible to initiate or carry out these self-rewarding activities by use of the subunit or unit engram that is to be trained. For example, it may be possible by a hinged hand splint, similar to the flexor-hinge splint for the metacarpophalangeal joints, to restrict activity to one simple agonist-antagonist pair and to use this motion to control a video game, an electronic organ, or another type of self-rewarding activity, so that for many minutes each day the patient gains pleasure from practicing that unit of prehension. Similarly adapted splints may allow the precise practice of subunits of function of the muscles of the thumb. As these subunits are mastered by the formation of engrams, the activities must be combined to activate other types of transducers, which requires linking of the subunits to perform a larger or more complex function. Variations of activities are necessary to prevent monotony and frustration, especially if the coordination of the patient is poor. Participation in multiple activities increases general coordination and aids in maintaining interests and attention.

At each step in chaining small engrams into larger ones, the activity must be performed more slowly than was necessary for the individual small engram in order to allow time for voluntary supervision of the linkage (see Fig. 19–4). As practice incorporates the linkage into the engram, the speed of performance can be increased again. When the coordination of the prehensile pattern has been developed to the force and speed that make the activity useful, it can be combined with arm motion in a wide variety of activities for both precision

grasp and palmar grasp.[37] In all of these activities, at each stage the patient should have the opportunity to practice the pattern with consistent accuracy. Each stage will need to be practiced tens of thousands of times before significant improvement is seen. Therefore, planned rewards and reinforcers of performance are essential to maintain interest in the activity.

In contrast to the emphasis on the need for prolonged, progressive training of prehension that has just been described, it should be pointed out that very many of the so-called adaptations for hand function are substitutes or holders that make prehension unnecessary. If the patient uses one of these substitutes, it dissuades the patient from attempting to use or improve prehension even though it may encourage the use of motions of the arm.

Transfer Motions of the Arm

The arm and forearm function like a retractable derrick carrying the hand as a prehensile organ. Motions of the shoulder, elbow, and wrist that carry the hand to the site of activity normally are automatic and not under specific attention. These automated motions of reaching, moving, and positioning the upper extremity develop through practice.[14] During coordinated motion, the traversing motion of the arm is fast, strong, and automatically guided by a preprogrammed engram (Fig. 19–10). Little attention needs to be paid to that automatic pattern. In the final approach, the positioning of the hand is under conscious visual and proprioceptive perception to ensure accuracy of positioning and is carried out more slowly and with less force. Athetoid patients who never have been able to practice precise patterns or children who have not yet developed automatic engrams show erratically unpredictable movements of both the traverse and the approach, since automated precise engrams have not been developed and the multimuscular demands of the traverse as well as the approach exceed the ability of the single-channeled corticospinal control system to monitor them (Fig. 19–11).

Maintenance of Balance

Coordination provides automatic postural balance and antigravity support as well as the integrated activities in the extremity. To grasp with

FREDERIC J. KOTTKE

UPPER EXTREMITY MOTION

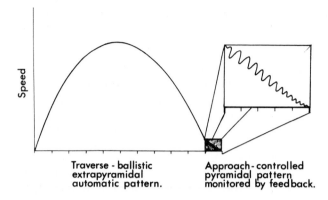

FIGURE 19–10. A reaching motion to a precise position consists of an automatic engram phase and an approach phase, which is guided by voluntary control to the target.

the hand, for example, prime mover responses provide motion and position for the fingers and thumb. Synergistic muscles contract with the prime movers to assist or modify those activities. Stabilizer cocontractions occur in the muscles of the wrist, elbow, and shoulder. Before this apparently primary activity can begin, a stable base must be established in relation to gravity by the properly coordinated contractions of the muscles that establish a stable posture for the body and head. To change the location of the hand requires motion produced by contraction of the muscles of the shoulder and elbow. As the arm moves, there must be postural adjustments to maintain balance. The effects of these muscular contractions must be monitored by sensory feedback from the joints, musculotendinous junctions, fascia, and skin to the central nervous system. The person remains unaware of most aspects of this complex performance

unless gross errors occur that require modification of the pattern. Even then the perception is of the achievement of the task rather than perception of the changes of contractions of individual muscles.

At each level of practice in the development of an engram, the ability to perform against a template or target positions for comparison increases the accuracy of performance and hastens learning. As the basic subunits are trained by matching performance against that template, the correct motor pattern emerges and, by practice, becomes an engram. Engrams developed more rapidly in this way can be combined progressively into more and more complex patterns of performance. A template allows more frequent and more precise comparisons than would occur otherwise so that the performance becomes more precise and the repetition of the correct pattern develops the engram more quickly. As an example of the use of a

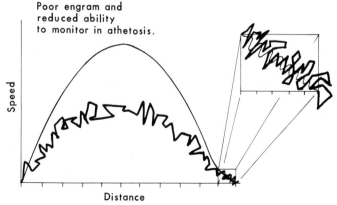

FIGURE 19–11. Children who have not yet developed coordination engrams or athetoid patients who are unable to do so show an erratic pattern of motion both in the traverse phase and in the approach phase of upper extremity motion.

guide to performance, the making of compact ovals or push-pull vertical lines in the Palmer method of penmanship provides a visual-spatial monitor of the motor activity as it occurs (see Fig. 19–2). The precision of or errors of performance can be recognized immediately. Comparison is available after each repetition. The spatial and temporal proximity of the template to the performance provides an excellent opportunity for comparison. As these basic components of the coordination engrams for writing develop, they can be selected and chained to form all of the components of the letters used in cursive writing. The development of similar types of templates or targets for other manual activities is necessary if precise coordination is to be developed rapidly.

Electromyographic feedback from the prime mover and synergists to be activated in contrast to the antagonists and other interfering muscles to be inhibited provides a close-linked means of monitoring a small number of muscles in simple patterns. Retrospective review of complex performances by video recording is of special value in recognizing undesired reflexes or other cocontractions that must be inhibited in order to obtain the coordination pattern desired. However, the greater the delay between performance and feedback, the less effective the monitor becomes.[67] In a similar way, repetitively retracing figures helps to develop visual-spatial-manual orientation as well as manual coordination. Spatial memory and orientation depend, at least in part, on the establishment of motor engrams in the extrapyramidal system.[21]

Occupational therapy can be used to develop varying degrees of strength and endurance at the same time that coordination is stressed. Occupational therapy is especially suited to the development of dexterity of the fingers and hand. The constructive aspects of occupational therapy aid in maintaining attention (Fig. 19–12). Similar training may also be carried on in a prevocational shop. Such activities should be designed to encourage the patient to work at the maximal rate of speed consistent with maximal precision. Modification of craft activities by incorporating artificial maneuvers or excessive resistance not only discourages the patient from prolonged participation but also interferes with the improvement of coordination.

Coordination Activities for the Lower Extremities. Ambulation training begins with the training of the basic engrams of balance and recovery of balance. Early training needs to be carried out by practicing units of these patterns that are simple enough so that the patient can perform each pat-

tern correctly. Selective external stabilization may need to be provided at each stage of the training so that antigravity support is secure and the patient can concentrate on voluntary activation of the assigned motor patterns without the distraction of other muscular activities required to maintain balance. This training should be initiated in infants who have not gained enough coordination to make balancing of the head possible by six months of age. With adequate support provided to secure trunk and lower extremity posture, neck control and balance are practiced until they become automatic.[30] Training of neck control is followed, in order of development, by training of independent trunk balance and motion, training of the upper extremities for protective extension and support to balance the trunk, hip balance and motion, knee balance and motion, and free standing.

For severely involved patients, the initial upright posture may be attained on a tilt table, where control of orthostatic blood pressure may be trained at the same time that progressive training of the engrams to ensure antigravity balance is begun (Fig. 19–13). As stable posture develops from the neck down, the patient can be transferred to an upright stander (Fig. 19–14) and later to the parallel bars.

The development of coordination adequate to provide stable balance and weight shifting and recovery are the necessary preludes to walking. Automatic engrams for control of motion of the joints at each level or suitable bracing to make muscular activity unnecessary is essential before the patient can learn standing balance and practice weight-shifting preparatory to walking. These patterns should be practiced as lead-up drills before walking is attempted. The ability to walk with crutches does not develop if the patient attempts to walk in the parallel bars or walker before he has gained the basic skills for maintaining balance while standing. Basic balance training is initiated while the patient is standing on both feet with balance provided by both hands, then shifting weight from one foot to the other and establishing balance with the weight supported fully on one lower extremity while the hands are used only to maintain balance. Training of balance in parallel bars provides excellent stability and security but also the opportunity for misuse by pulling or pushing forward or sideways on the bars, which cannot be done when using crutches or canes. Broad-base canes provide good stability but can be used only to push in the downward direction (Fig. 19–15). If balance is not attained before walking is initiated,

FREDERIC J. KOTTKE

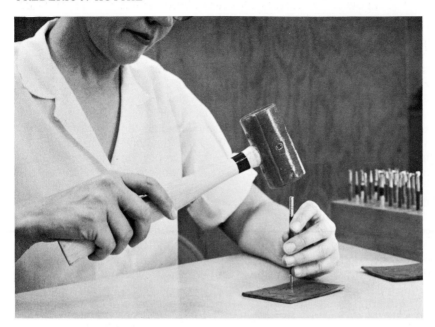

FIGURE 19–12. Leather stamping in occupational therapy requires the use of the power grip with the dominant hand and the precision grip with the nondominant hand.

the patient develops a lurching, falling gait that is unstable and fatiguing. Therefore, the ability to maintain balance throughout all phases of ambulation should be a fundamental component of the initial ambulation training. From full, broad, four-extremity support, the patient should practice balancing on a progressively smaller base until weight-bearing can be maintained on one foot with balance provided by only one hand. Weight shifting from one foot to the other should become easy, reliable, and rapid as practice develops motor engrams. Shifting of weight and balance forward one step, backward one step, and during turning from side to side also needs to be practiced until automatic. Practicing lead-up drills to appropriate music provides a pleasant mechanism for monitoring the rhythm and rate of performance of the drills. Daily calisthenics of foot shifting, hand shifting, simultaneous hand and foot shifting, stepping forward or backward, knee bending and straightening, all constitute basic engrams that are coordinated in the walking pattern.

Walking requires that balance be shifted and re-established with each step. Preservation of balance requires the automatic integration of the activities of the many muscles coordinating the motion, not only of the joints of the extremities but also of the trunk and neck at each step. As the base of support is widened by two crutches or two broad-base canes, there is decreased need for precision of balance, but engrams must be present that coor-dinate all four extremities and trunk (Fig. 19–15). Children under four years of age have not yet developed engrams adequate to coordinate reciprocal motion in all four extremities, which is necessary when walking in the parallel bars or when using crutches or canes. They learn to balance and walk much more readily by using a stable transverse bar on a push cart (Fig. 19–16) so that they need think only about the reciprocating motion of the two lower extremities. After they have developed their lower extremity engrams while pushing the cart, then they can begin training reciprocal motion of the upper extremities while using crutches.

Retraining Coordination for Proprioceptive or Cerebellar Dysfunction (Frenkel's Exercises). Frenkel's exercises are a series of exercises of increasing difficulty to improve proprioceptive control in the lower extremities.[22] These exercises begin with simple movements, with gravity eliminated, and gradually progress to more complicated movement patterns, utilizing simultaneous hip and knee motions carried on against gravity. They are especially useful when there is impairment of proprioception due to disorders in the central nervous system. Repeated practice helps to develop the usefulness of any proprioception that the patient has available. If the patient does not have adequate proprioception to monitor the movements during the training exercises, the patient must be positioned so that activity can be monitored by vision.

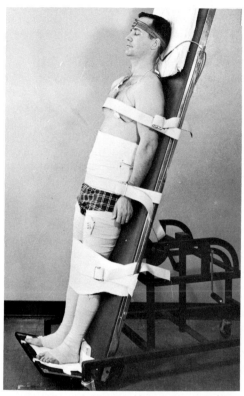

FIGURE 19–13. A tilt table may be used for stabilization of unstable joints of the lower extremities and trunk so that the patient can begin to practice controlled motion of the neck and upper trunk. At the same time the patient can develop cardiovascular tolerance to the upright position.

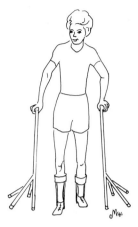

FIGURE 19–15. Canes that have a broad base enlarge the base of support during ambulation and decrease the precision of coordination that is necessary to balance and to walk.

The initial training exercise is conducted under the supervision of a therapist, and the emphasis is on slow, precise motion and positioning. To avoid fatigue, each exercise is performed not more than four times at each session. The first simple exercises should be accomplished adequately before progressing to the more difficult patterns. As the patient gains the ability to perform each exercise, the patient is instructed to perform it every three or four hours.

Exercises While Supine. The patient lies on a bed or plinth with a smooth surface along which the heels may slide easily. A caster shoe rolling on a large board positioned under the lower extremities may be used to make the activities easier by

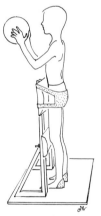

FIGURE 19–14. A standing frame provides postural stability from the floor up to the trunk so that neck, trunk, and upper extremity balance and coordination may be trained by practice. As coordination engrams develop in the upper segments, the support provided by the stander may be lowered progressively to require practice of coordination of the lower trunk, hips, and knees to prepare for free standing.

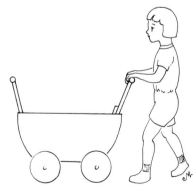

FIGURE 19–16. Until a child has developed engrams of coordination for all four extremities, the child has great difficulty in consciously monitoring two legs and two crutches while learning to walk. When holding a transverse bar attached to a weighted wagon the child needs to monitor only the reciprocal motion of the two lower extremities during walking. After the engrams for reciprocal motion in the lower extremities have developed, the child can consciously monitor the position of the two crutches as walking is practiced.

FREDERIC J. KOTTKE

reducing friction. The various motions to be practiced may be indicated by lines painted on the board. The head should be supported so that the patient can see the legs and feet.

1. Flex the hip and knee of one extremity, sliding the heel along in contact with the bed. Return to the original position. Repeat with the opposite extremity.

2. Flex as in exercise 1. Then abduct the flexed hip. Return to the flexed position and then to the original position.

3. Flex the hip and knee only halfway and then return to the extended position. Add abduction and adduction.

4. Flex one limb at the hip and knee, stopping at any point in flexion or extension on command.

5. Flex both lower extremities simultaneously and equally; add abduction, adduction, and extension.

6. Flex both lower extremities simultaneously to the halfway position; add abduction and adduction to half-flexed position. Extend. Stop in the pattern on command.

7. Flex one extremity at the hip and knee with the heel held 2 in above the bed. Return to the original position.

8. Flex as in exercise 7. Bring the heel to rest on the opposite patella. Successively add patterns so that the heel is touched to the middle of the shin, to the ankle, to the toes of the opposite foot, to the bed on either side of the knee, and to the bed on either side of the leg.

9. Flex as in exercise 7 and then touch the heel successively to the patella, shin, ankle, and toes. Reverse the pattern.

10. Flex as in exercise 7 and then on command touch the heel to the point indicated by the therapist.

11. Flex the hip and knee with the heel 2 in above the bed. Place the heel on the opposite patella and slowly slide it down the crest of the tibia to the ankle. Reverse.

12. Use the pattern in exercise 11, but slide the heel down the crest of the opposite tibia, over the ankle and foot to the toes. If the heel is to reach the toes, the opposite knee must be flexed slightly during this exercise. Stop in the pattern on command.

13. With malleoli and knees in apposition, flex both lower extremities simultaneously with the heels 2 in above the bed. Return to the original position. Stop in the pattern on command.

14. Perform reciprocal flexion and extension of the lower extremities with the heels touching the bed.

15. Perform reciprocal flexion and extension of the lower extremities with the heels 2 in above the bed.

16. Perform bilateral simultaneous flexion, abduction, adduction, and extension with the heels 2 in above the bed.

17. Place the heel precisely where the therapist indicates with the finger on the bed or the opposite extremity.

18. Follow with the toe the movement of the therapist's finger in any combination of lower extremity motion.

Exercises While Sitting

1. Practice maintaining correct sitting posture for two minutes in an armchair with the back supported and the feet flat on the floor. Repeat in a chair without arms. Repeat without back support.

2. Mark time to the counting of the therapist by raising only the heel from the floor. Progress to alternately lifting the entire foot and replacing it precisely in a marked position on the floor.

3. Make two cross marks on the floor with chalk. Alternately glide the foot over the marked cross; forward, backward, left and right.

4. Practice rising from and sitting on a chair to the therapist's counted cadence: (a) Flex the knees and draw the feet under the front edge of the seat. (b) Bend the trunk forward over the thighs. (c) Rise by extending the knees and hips and then straightening the trunk. (d) Bend the trunk forward slightly. (e) Flex the hips and knees to sit. (f) Straighten the trunk and sit back in the chair.

Exercises While Standing

1. Walking sideways. Balance is easier during sideward walking because the patient does not have to pivot over the toes or heels, which decreases the base of support. The exercise is performed to a counted cadence: (a) Shift the weight to the left foot. (b) Place the right foot 12 in to the right. (c) Shift the weight to the right foot. (d) Bring the left foot over to the right foot. The size of the step taken to the right or left may be varied.

2. Walk forward between two parallel lines 14 inches apart, placing the right foot just inside the right line and the left foot just inside the left line. Emphasize correct placment. Rest after 10 steps.

3. Walk forward placing each foot on a footprint traced on the floor. Footprints should be parallel and 2 inches lateral to the midline. Practice with quarter steps, half steps, three-quarter steps, and full steps.

4. Turning. (a) Raise the right toe and rotate the right foot outward, pivoting on the heel. (b)

Raise the left heel and pivot the left leg inward on the toes. (c) Bring the left foot up beside the right.

Exercises to Teach Relaxation. Anxiety produces a state of tension that causes increased activity in the central nervous system and affects many systems. The neuromuscular system responds by prolonged muscular contraction, causing discomfort in muscles and joints, neckache, and headache. As a result of the pain produced by prolonged muscular contraction, secondary reflex contractions also develop. The anxiety and tension of the patient are increased. Effective reversal of these secondary effects may be achieved by teaching the patient awareness of muscular tensions and how to control and inhibit them.[36]

Relaxation is taught in a quiet semidarkened room with the patient comfortably positioned on a treatment table or bed. A small pillow should be placed under the head, and another pillow should be placed under the knees to relax the hip and knee musculature. The feet should be supported so that the muscles in the legs can relax. Constricting garments should be loosened.

Breath control is taught by using prolonged slow breathing with proper diaphragmatic and abdominal coordination together with intercostal breathing. The patient is taught to exhale slowly through the mouth to emphasize awareness of breathing rate and breath control. As the patient gains control of breathing in the fully relaxed position, the patient then begins to practice breathing properly while sitting or standing.

Proprioceptive awareness of muscular contraction in the extremities is taught by having the patient flex and extend each joint in the extremity, feeling the difference between tightness and relaxation of the contracting muscles. Following a strong voluntary contraction, the patient is asked to relax and feel the difference between contraction and relaxation. Then progressively weaker contractions are alternated with complete inhibition of muscular activity so that the extremity becomes fully relaxed. Functional muscle groups at each joint are considered individually in the alternate tensing and relaxation activities so that the patient becomes fully aware of muscular activity in each region of the extremity. The patient should perceive the tenseness of the muscle rather than any tension, position, or motion of a joint. Jacobson[36] emphasized that persons could learn proprioceptive awareness of tension and then use it in almost any situation to relax from a state of tension.

Electromyographic monitoring by cutaneous or intramuscular electrodes may be used to indicate whether complete relaxation has occurred. This monitoring provides auditory reinforcement of perception of tension or relaxation and hastens learning. Dropping of the completely limp arm or leg is another method used to demonstrate the difference between partial contraction and relaxation. As the patient becomes aware of the sensations associated with a muscular contraction, the ability to initiate or inhibit that contraction is developed.[36]

The sequence of training is applied to all four extremities, to the shoulders by shrugging and relaxing the pectoral muscles, to the chest by tightening and relaxing the pectoral muscles, to the back by arching and relaxing, and to the facial muscles by contracting and relaxing the muscles about the mouth and eyes and on the forehead. For the tense patient, the training sessions may have to be repeated many times before the patient develops the proprioceptive awareness to know when the muscles have relaxed completely. Patients are instructed to practice this relaxation at home or at work when they become tense during the day or in the evening at bedtime if they have difficulty in relaxing before they go to sleep. When the patient is able to inhibit muscular contraction adequately in the various segments of the body while recumbent, the patient is taught to reproduce the same relaxation when sitting in a fully supporting arm chair and later when sitting in a straight chair. Training in relaxation is useful not only to relax and rest but also to enhance performance during skilled activities.

The patient should be instructed that selective muscular relaxation is possible at the same time that a person is thinking or carrying on an activity. It is not necessary for the mind "to become a perfect blank" or for the person to forego all activity in order to inhibit muscular tension. Even in the initial training period, the patient will soon observe that the muscles may be relaxed, even though the mind remains active. However, disturbing stimuli or ideas make relaxation more difficult. In spite of this, the patient can learn to relax the muscles to avoid prolonged muscular tension even during periods of active cerebration.

Through controlled relaxation, the individual learns to relax the muscles that do not need to be used for a specific activity and thereby decreases the energy used during ordinary activity. As a result, the individual is less fatigued by work. Selective relaxation of the unneeded muscles during activity allows the person to avoid the pain arising secondary to prolonged muscular tension.

FREDERIC J. KOTTKE

References

1. Armstrong, T. R.: Training for the production of memorized movement patterns. Technical Report No. 26. Human Performance Center. Ann Arbor, University of Michigan, 1970.
2. Baker, M., Regenos, E., Wolf, S. A., and Basmajian, J. V.: Developing strategies for biofeedback: Applications in neurologically handicapped patients. Phys. Ther., 57:402–408, 1977.
3. Basmajian, J. V., Gowland, C., Brandstater, M. E., Swanson, L., and Trotter, J.: EMG feedback treatment of upper limb in hemiplegic stroke patients: A pilot study. Arch. Phys. Med. Rehabil., 63:613–616 (Dec), 1982.
4. Beery, K. E.: Developmental test of visual-motor integration: Administration and scoring manual. Chicago, Follette Publishing Co., 1967.
5. Beevor, C.: Croonian Lectures on Muscular Movements. New York, Macmillan Co., 1903.
6. Bobath, K., and Bobath, B.: Cerebral palsy. In Pearson, P. H., and Williams, C. E. (Eds.): Physical Therapy Services in the Developmental Disabilities. Springfield, Ill. Charles C. Thomas, Publisher, 1972, pp. 31–175.
7. Bobath, K., and Bobath, B.: Treatment of cerebral palsy based on analysis of patient's motor behavior. Br. J. Phys. Med., 15:107–117, 1952.
8. Briggs, P. R., and Tellegen, A.: Development of the manual accuracy and speed test. Percept. Motor Skills (Monograph Suppl. 3) 32:923–943, 1971.
9. Brudny, J., Korein, J., Grynbaum, B. G., Belandres, P. V., and Gianutsos, J. G.: Helping hemiparetics to help themselves: Sensory feedback therapy. J. A. M. A., 241:814–818 (Feb 23), 1979.
10. Brudny, J., Korien, J., Levidow, L., Grynbaum, B. B., Lieberman, A., and Friedmann, L. W.: Sensory feedback therapy as a modality of treatment in central nervous system disorders of voluntary movement. Neurology, 24:925–932 (Oct) 1974.
11. Brunnstrom, S.: Movement Therapy in Hemiplegia. New York, Harper & Row, Publishers, 1970.
12. Bullock, T. H.: The origin of patterned nervous discharge. Behavior, 17:48–59, 1961.
13. Carey, J. R., Allison, J. D., and Mundale, M. O.: Electromyographic study of muscular overflow during precision grip. Phys. Ther., 63:505–512 (Apr), 1983.
14. Chyatte, S. B., and Birdsong, J. H.: Methods-time measurements in assessment of motor performance. Arch. Phys. Med. Rehabil., 53:38–44, 1972.
15. Coghill, G. E.: Anatomy and the Problem of Behavior. London, Cambridge University Press, 1929.
16. Coghill, G. E.: Flexor spasms and mass reflexes in relation to the autogenetic development of behavior. J. Comp. Neurol., 76:463–486, 1943.
17. Crossman, E. R. F. W.: Theory of acquisition of speed-skill. Ergonomics 2:153–166, 1959.
18. Fay, T.: The neurophysiologic aspects of therapy in cerebral palsy. Arch. Phys. Med. Rehabil., 29:327–334, 1948.
19. Fay, T.: The origin of human movement. Am. J. Psychiat., 3:644–652 (Mar), 1955.
20. Feldman, D. J., Lee, P. R., Unterecker, J., Lloyd, K., Rusk, H. A., and Toole, A.: A comparison of functionally orientated medical care and formal rehabilitation in the management of patients with hemiplegia due to cerebrovascular disease. J. Chronic Dis., 15:297–310 (Mar), 1962.
21. Flowers, K.: Lack of prediction in the motor behavior in parkinsonism. Brain, 101:35–52, 1978.
22. Frenkel, H. S.: The Treatment of Tabetic Ataxia. Translated and edited by Freyberger, L. Philadelphia, Blakiston's, 1902.
23. Gellhorn, E.: Patterns of muscular activity in man. Arch. Phys. Med. Rehabil., 28:568–574, 1947.
24. Gellhorn, E., Riggle, C. M., and Ballin, W. M.: Summation, inhibition and proprioceptive reinforcement under conditions of stimulation of the motor cortex and their influence on activities of single motor units. J. Cell Comp. Physiol., 43:405–414, 1954.
25. Gesell, A.: Maturation and infant behavior pattern. Psychol. Rev., 36:307–319, 1929.
26. Gesell, A., and Halvorson, H. M.: The development of thumb opposition in the human infant. J. Genet. Psychol., 48:339–361, 1936.
27. Glencross, D. J.: Control of skilled movements. Psychol. Bull., 84:14–29, 1977.
28. Granit, R.: The Purposive Brain. Cambridge, MIT Press, 1977.
29. Hagbarth, K. E.: Excitatory and inhibitory skin areas for flexor and extensor motoneurons. Acta Physiol. Scand., 26 (Suppl. 94):1–8, 1952.
30. Halpern, D., Kottke, F. J., Burrill, C. A., Fiterman, C., Popp, J., and Palmer, S.: Training of control of head posture in children with cerebral palsy. Develop. Med. Child. Neurol., 12:290–305, 1970.
31. Hein, A., and Held, R.: Dissociation of visual placing response into elicited and guided components. Science, 158:390–391, 1967.
32. Hellebrandt, F. A., and Waterland, J. C.: Expansion of motor patterning under exercise stress. Am. J. Phys. Med., 41:56–66, 1962.
33. Herman, R.: Electromyographic evidence of some control factors involved in the acquisition of skilled performance. Am. J. Phys. Med., 49:177–191, 1970.
34. Hick, W. E.: Reaction time for the amendment of a response. Q. J. Exp. Psychol., 1:175–179, 1949.
35. Holding, D. H., and Macrae, A. W.: Guidance, restriction and knowledge of results. Ergonomics 7:289–295, 1964.
36. Jacobson, E.: Progressive relaxation. Chicago, University of Chicago Press, 1938.
37. Jebsen, R. H., Taylor, N., Trieschmann, R. B., Trotter, M. J., and Howard, L. A.: An objective and standardized test of hand function. Arch. Phys. Med. Rehabil., 50:311–319, 1969.
38. Johnson, H. E., and Garton, W. H.: Muscle re-

education in hemiplegia by use of electromyographic device. Arch. Phys. Med. Rehabil., 54:320–323 (Jul), 1973.

39. Kabat, H.: Studies on neuromuscular dysfunction. XV. The role of central facilitation in restoration of motor function in paralysis. Arch. Phys. Med. Rehabil., 33:521–533, 1952.

40. Kabat, H.: Proprioceptive facilitation in therapeutic exercise. In Licht, S. (Ed.): Therapeutic Exercise, 2nd Ed. New Haven, Connecticut, Elizabeth Licht, Publisher, 1961.

41. Kelso, J. A. S., and Frekany, G. A.: Coding processes in preselected and constrained movements: Effect of vision. Acta Psychol., 42:145–161, 1978.

42. Knapp, M. E.: The contribution of Sister Elizabeth Kenny to the treatment of poliomyelitis. Arch. Phys. Med. Rehabil., 36:510–517, 1955.

43. Knapp, M. E.: Exercise for lower motor neuron lesions. In Basmajian, J. V. (Ed.): Therapeutic Exercise, 3rd Ed. Baltimore, Williams & Wilkins Co., 1978.

44. Knott, M., and Voss, D. E.: Proprioceptive Neuromuscular Facilitation: Patterns and Techniques. New York, Paul B. Hoeber, Inc., 1956.

45. Kottke, F. J.: From reflex to skill: The training of coordination. Arch. Phys. Med. Rehabil., 61:551–561, 1980.

46. Kottke, F. J., Halpern, D., Easton, J. K. M., Ozel, A. T., and Burrill, C. A.: Training of coordination. Arch. Phys. Med. Rehabil., 59:567–572, 1978.

47. Marinacci, A. A., and Horance, A.: Electromyogram in neuromuscular reeducation. Bull. Los Angeles Neurol. Soc., 25:57–71, 1960.

48. McGraw, M. B.: The Neuro-Muscular Maturation of the Human Infant. New York, Columbia University Press, 1945.

49. Mroczek, N., Halpern, D., and McHugh, R.: Electronic feedback and physical therapy for neuromuscular retraining in hemiplegia. Arch. Phys. Med. Rehabil., 59:258–267 (Jan), 1978.

50. Mulder, T., Hulstijn, W., and van der Meer, J.: EMG feedback and the restoration of motor control. Am. J. Phys. Med., 65:173–188 (Aug), 1986.

51. Neisser, V.: The limits of cognition. In Juszyk, P. W., and Klein, R. M. (Eds.): On the Nature of Thought: Essays in Honor of D. B. Hebb. Hillsdale, N. J., Laurence Erlbaum Associates, 1980.

52. Nissen, H. W., Chow, K. L., and Semmes, J.: Effects of restricted opportunity and manipulative experience on the behavior of the chimpanzee. Am. J. Psychol., 64:485–507, 1951.

53. Page, D.: Neuromuscular reflex therapy as an approach to patient care. Am. J. Phys. Med., 46;816–835, 1967.

54. Pascual-Leone, J.: Mathematical model for the transition role in Piaget's developmental stages. Acta Psychol., 63:301–345, 1970.

55. Phelps, W. M.: The role of physical therapy in cerebral palsy. In Illingworth, R. S. (Ed.): Recent Advances in Cerebral Palsy. Boston, Little, Brown and Co., 1958.

56. Piaget, J.: The origins of intelligence in children, 2nd Ed. Trans. by M. Cook. New York, International Universities Press, 1953.

57. Prevo, A. J. H., Visser, S. L., and Vogelaar, T. W.: Effect of EMG feedback on paretic muscles and abnormal cocontraction in the hemiplegic arm compared with conventional physical therapy. Scand. J. Rehabil. Med., 14:121–131, 1982.

58. Rabbitt, P. M. A.: Sequential reactions to holding. In Holding, D. H. (Ed.): Human Skills. Chichester, England, John Wiley and Sons, 1981, pp. 153–174.

59. Ramos, M. U., Mundale, M. O., Awad, E. A., Witsoe, D. A., Cole, T. M., Olson, M., and Kottke, F. J.: Cardiovascular effects of spread of excitation during prolonged isometric exercise. Arch. Phys. Med. Rehabil., 54:496–504, 1973.

60. Rood, M. S.: Neuromuscular mechanisms utilized in the treatment of neuromuscular dysfunction. Am. J. Occup. Ther., 10:220–225, 1956.

61. Schneirla, T. C.: Behavioral development and comparative psychology. Q. Rev. Biol., 41:283–302, 1966.

62. Simard, T. G., and Basmajian, J. V.: Methods in training conscious control of motor units. Arch. Phys. Med. Rehabil., 48:12–19, 1967.

63. Skoglund, S.: Anatomical and physiological studies of knee joint innervation in the cat. Acta Physiol. Scand., 36 (Suppl. 124):58, 1956.

64. Stern, P. H., McDowell, F., Miller, J. M., and Robinson, M.: Effects of facilitation exercise techniques in stroke rehabilitation. Arch. Phys. Med. Rehabil., 51:526–531 (Sep), 1970.

65. Stockmeyer, S. A.: Sensorimotor approach to treatment. In Pearson, P. H., and Williams, C. E. (Eds.): Physical Therapy Services in the Developmental Disabilities. Springfield, Ill., Charles C. Thomas, Publisher, 1972, pp. 186–222.

66. Vince, M. A.: Intermittence of control movements and psychological refractory period. Br. J. Psychol., 38:149–157, 1948.

67. White, B.: Experience and development of motor mechanisms. In Connelly, K. (Ed.): Mechanisms of Motor Skill Development. New York, Academic Press, 1970.

68. White, B. L., and Held, R.: Plasticity of sensorimotor development in the human infant. In Hellmuth, J. (Ed.): Exceptional Infant, Vol. 1. Seattle, Special Child Publications, 1967.

69. Windle, W. F.: Physiology of the Fetus: Origin and Extent of Function in Prenatal Life. Philadelphia, W. B. Saunders Company, 1940.

20

Therapeutic Exercise to Develop Strength and Endurance

BARBARA J. DE LATEUR
JUSTUS F. LEHMANN

Exercise vies with heat as the most commonly applied therapeutic modality. As with heat, virtually everyone applies this modality to himself or herself regardless of whether it is prescribed by a physician or carried out under the supervision of a therapist. Some degree of muscular effort is expended to move from one spot to another. Because of this universal employment of exercise, virtually everyone considers himself or herself to be to some degree knowledgeable if not actually expert on this topic. This familiarity has both advantages and disadvantages for one who would attempt to write scientifically about the topic. The advantage is the comfort and interest with which readers approach the topic. The disadvantage is the misuse, in common parlance, of technical terms. An example of the latter would be the common usage of the term *tone*. Advertisements for commercial exercise establishments often speak of "toning up your muscles," as though increase of tone were something that (1) results from an exercise program; (2) increases the firmness of muscle to palpation or increases the definition of muscle contours; and (3) somehow reflects the strength or endurance, or both, of the muscles. In point of fact, muscle tone is the resistance (tension) developed in a muscle as a result of passive stretch of a muscle. This is the technical definition of tone. It cannot be determined by palpation or inspection of the muscle. It has little or nothing to do with the voluntary strength of the muscle. Thus, in

order to use familiar terms in a precise way, some definitions would be useful.

Definitions

Force: A push or a pull. A force is equal to the mass of an object times the acceleration imparted to that object. F = m × a. Force is a vector quantity; that is to say, it has direction as well as magnitude. In the English system, a force may be expressed in pounds. In the meter-kilogram-second (MKS) system, force is expressed in newtons (N). A newton is that force that gives a mass of one kilogram an acceleration of one meter per second squared (1 meter per sec²). The term *kilopond* is also used. This is the force exerted by the mass of one kilogram on earth, i.e., the mass of one kilogram subjected to the acceleration of earth's gravity, or 9.81 meters per sec². A kilopond thus equals 9.81 newtons or about 10 N.

Mass: The amount of matter contained in an object. This is expressed as kilograms in the MKS system and as grams in the centimeter-gram-second (CGS) system. In the English system, mass is expressed as slugs. The slug, a unit no longer in common use, is the amount of matter contained in an object that exerts a force (weight) of 32 pounds on earth. Mass is a scalar quantity; that is, it has magnitude only, not direction.

Vector: A quantity that has both magnitude

and direction, such as force; an arrow whose length represents the magnitude and whose direction represents the direction of such a quantity.

Strength: The maximal force (actually torque; see definition later) that can be exerted by a muscle. This is subdivided into static and dynamic strength.

Static or Isometric Strength: The maximal force that can be exerted against an immovable or relatively immovable object. It is expressed as the maximal voluntary contraction or MVC. The term *isometric* refers to the fact that the overall length of the muscle stays essentially the same (although there is internal length change within the muscle, for example, to take up the slack in the series elastic elements). The kinesiological function of an isometric contraction is stabilization.

Dynamic Strength: Dynamic strength has many theoretically possible subdivisions, since a muscle may vary in its rate of lengthening or of shortening as well as in the amount of force (tension) developed at any given point from beginning to end of the arc described by the moving segment of the limb. For practical purposes the most commonly used terms are *isotonic* and *isokinetic strength*.

Isotonic: The term *isotonic* is, in most circumstances, a misnomer, since it implies that either the torque exerted by the muscle or even the internal tension of the muscle remains the same throughout the arc of movement of the limb. The achievement of either of these conditions is rare. For practical purposes, in the clinical literature isotonic has been equated with kinetic or dynamic and is often expressed in such definitions as the 1 repetition maximum or 10 repetition maximum.

One Repetition Maximum (1 RM): The highest weight that the subject can lift through the full range of motion one time only.

Ten Repetition Maximum (10 RM): The greatest weight that the subject can lift through the full range of motion 10 times only.

Shortening or Concentric Contraction: A muscle contraction in which the two ends of the muscle move toward each other. The kinesiological function of such a contraction is acceleration.

Lengthening or Eccentric Contraction: A muscle contraction in which the two ends of the muscle diverge; i.e., the muscle "plays out" its length. The kinesiological function of such a contraction is deceleration (shock absorption).

Rotatory Force: That component of the muscle tension that produces angular motion about the

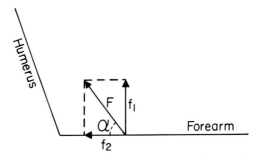

FIGURE 20–1. Resolution of muscle force (F) applied to the tendon into rotatory (f_1) and stabilizing (f_2) forces. The rotatory force acts at right angles to the lever: $f_1 = F \sin$ alpha; $f_2 = F \cos$ alpha. (From Brunnstrom, S.: Clinical Kinesiology, 2nd Ed. Philadelphia, F. A. Davis, 1966.)

joint. It is equal to the product of the total muscle tension applied to the tendon times the sine of the angle of application of the tendon (Fig. 20–1).

Stabilizing Force: That component of the total muscle force that approximates the two limb segments at the joint. It is equal to the muscle tension applied to the tendon times the cosine of the angle of application of the tendon (Fig. 20–1).

Torque (Moment of a Force): The effectiveness of a force in producing rotation about an axis. Torque is equal to the product of a force times the perpendicular distance from the site of application to the axis (Fig. 20–2).

Isokinetic Strength: The maximum torque that can be exerted against a pre-set rate-limiting device. This may be defined as the peak torque that occurs at any given velocity of contraction, regardless of the angle at which it occurs, or it may be defined as angle-specific.

Endurance: The ability to continue a specified task.

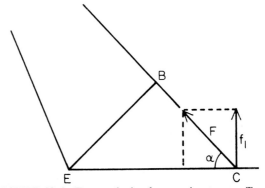

FIGURE 20–2. Two methods of computing torque. Torque equals $f_1 \times EC$ or $F \times EB$. (From Brunnstrom, S.: Clinical Kinesiology, 2nd Ed. Philadelphia, F. A. Davis, 1966.)

BARBARA J. DE LATEUR AND JUSTUS F. LEHMANN

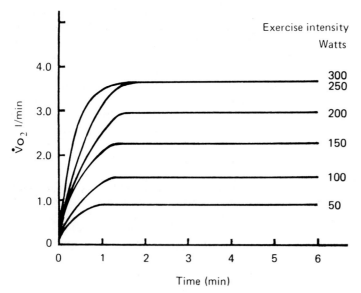

FIGURE 20–3. Relationship of oxygen uptake to various exercise intensities utilizing several muscle groups in reciprocal concentric contractions. There is no additional increase in oxygen uptake with further increase in exercise intensity (external work) once maximal oxygen uptake is reached. (From Soule, R. G.: Physiological response to physical exercise. *In* Knuttgen, H. G. [Ed.]: Neuromuscular Mechanisms for Therapeutic and Conditioning Exercise. Baltimore, University Park Press, 1976, pp. 79–96. Data from Saltin, B., and Åstrand, P. O.: Maximal oxygen uptake in athletes. J. Appl. Physiol., 23:353–358, 1967.)

Endurance Exercise: An exercise involving the reciprocal and dynamic use of several large groups of muscles. An exercise calling upon the ability of the cardiovascular-pulmonary system to deliver oxygen to such groups of muscles.

Fatigue: The decreased capacity of muscle to produce tension or shortening resulting from prior activity. Fatigue has both behavioral and measurable physiological components.

Maximal Aerobic Capacity: The maximal rate at which oxygen may be utilized (taken up) by the organism. The symbol for this is $\dot{V}O_2max$. (The dot over a symbol always indicates a rate.) This is determined as that rate of oxygen consumption that shows no further increase in spite of increasing mechanical work or rate of exercise performed by the subject (Fig. 20–3).

Work: Work is equal to the product of force times the distance through which the force is exerted. $W = F \times D$. Work may be expressed as newton-meters or kilopond-meters. In the older literature, the latter was expressed as kilogram-meters. Energy is expended in doing work; thus, units for work are often used as units for energy. One newton-meter = one joule (J) (see *Energy*, later).

Power: Power is the rate of performing work. It is equal to work divided by time. It is often expressed as watts or as kilopond-meters per minute (kpm per min). One watt = 1 J per sec = 6.12 kpm per min.

Energy: Energy is the product of power and the time that power is expended. The homeowner is accustomed to the energy unit of kilowatt-hours. Energy can also be expressed as kilopond-meters or as joules. One kpm = about 10 J. The biologic energy unit is the calorie (cal). One calorie = 4.2 J, and therefore one Kcal (ordinarily used to express the energy content of foodstuffs) = 4.2 K J.

Theoretical Considerations

Force-Velocity Relationships

The force-velocity relationship for mammalian muscle is described by this equation:

$$(P + a)V = b (P_O - P)$$

where V is the speed of shortening, P_O is the maximum isometric tension, P is the load, and a and b are constants.[35] There is an inverse relationship between the rate of shortening of a muscle and the tension that it can develop (Fig. 20–4).

Figure 20–4 shows an idealized force-velocity curve. The highest tensions are developed maximal contractions during externally forced lengthening of the muscle. The lowest tensions are developed with fast shortening contractions. The tension developed with an isometric contraction is shown at the inflection point of the curve. One may verify

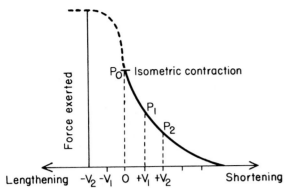

FIGURE 20–4. Force velocity curve of human muscle. Solid line: data obtained from elbow flexors of human subjects. At the time this curve was drawn, the dotted line was made by extrapolation. This portion of the curve has subsequently been confirmed experimentally (see Fig. 20–5). (From Brunnstrom, S.: Clinical Kinesiology, 2nd Ed. Philadelphia, F. A. Davis, 1966. Redrawn from Wilkie, D.: The relation between force and velocity in human muscle. J. Physiol., 110:249–280, 1950, and Abbott, B. C., Bigland, B., and Ritchie, J. M.: The physiological cost of negative work. J. Physiol., 117:380–390, 1952.)

this personally in a qualitative or roughly quantitative fashion by reflecting upon the fact that one can hold a weight that one cannot lift and that one can rapidly lower a weight that one cannot hold, much less lift. Such a relationship for maximal force of human elbow flexor muscles to velocity of contraction is expressed in Figure 20–5. This curve represents the performance of several human subjects at any given point in time. From Figures 20–4 and 20–5 one may infer the relationship between dynamic and static or isometric strength, but one

may not necessarily conclude that a dynamic training program will improve static strength performance or vice versa. One may anticipate that the general shape of these curves will stay the same regardless of a training program, and thus one may anticipate some degree of positive transference from one type of exercise program to the opposite type of performance, but one may not accurately predict, quantitatively, the degree of transfer.

The work of Seliger and co-workers has confirmed these relationships (Tables 20–1 and 20–2).[66] They determined the maximal voluntary forces produced upon a weightlifting rod by subjects changing from standing to squatting positions during a halfway knee bend. The rod was placed on a special stand and moved up and down at a constant speed of 8.5 meters per sec by a motor. They found that at an angle of 90 degrees, with a constant angle speed of flexion (17 degrees per sec) and with a maximal voluntary effort, the muscles exerted approximately three times greater force on a load during eccentric contractions than during concentric contractions. Muscle force exerted on a load during maximum isometric contraction at an angle of 90 degrees in the knee joint was greater than during maximum concentric contraction and lower than during eccentric contraction with the same angle.

The force-velocity relationships for concentric contractions have been confirmed by a number of authors with isokinetic tests.* A negative exponen-

---

*See references 9, 27, 41, 51, 57, 65, 69, and 72.

TABLE 20–1. Strength (Newtons) of Eccentric and Concentric Contractions of Lower Extremity Extensors at Different Angles of the Knee Joint of Normal Subjects Performing Knee Bends*

Angle	C. ECCENTRIC STRENGTH		C. CONCENTRIC STRENGTH		Statistical Significance†
	X̄	SD	X̄	SD	
70°	1800	820	459	106	0.01
80°	1899	857	543	189	0.01
90°	2101	735	737	252	0.01
100°	2221	576	866	347	0.01
110°	2229	551	996	370	0.01
120°	2157	530	1098	442	0.01
130°	2103	541	1229	521	0.01
140°	1971	524	1236	412	0.01
150°	1800	583	1125	339	0.01
160°	1321	578	918	365	0.05

*From Seliger, V., Dolejs, L., and Karas, V.: A dynamometric comparison of maximum eccentric, concentric and isometric contractions using EMG and energy expenditure measurements. Eur. J. Appl. Physiol., 45:235–244, 1980.

†Values of statistical significance were obtained by t test (for paired data).

BARBARA J. DE LATEUR AND JUSTUS F. LEHMANN

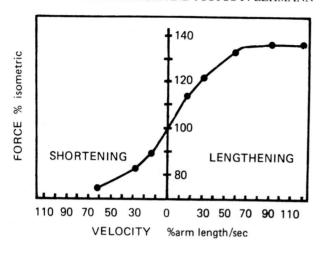

FIGURE 20–5. Relationship of maximal force of human elbow flexor muscles to velocity of contraction. Velocity on abscissa is designated as per cent of arm length per second. (From Knuttgen, H. G.: Development of muscular strength and endurance. *In* Knuttgen, H. G. [Ed.]: Neuromuscular Mechanisms for Therapeutic and Conditioning Exercises. Baltimore, University Park Press, 1976, pp. 97–118. Redrawn from Asmussen, E., Hansen, O., and Lammert, O.: The relation between isometric and dynamic muscle strength in man. Comm. Dan. Natl. Assoc. Inf. Paral., 20:11, 1965.)

tial model characterized the decline of strength as a function of increased isokinetic velocity of angular motion.[19] Fugl-Meyer and associates found close correlations between isokinetic and static peak torques (Table 20–3). However, as would be anticipated from the force-velocity curves, the static maxima were much greater than the torques at the various speeds of contraction and could be described by a negative exponential model between the maximal plantar flexion torque and isokinetic velocity of angular motion (Fig. 20–6).

The extent to which one may alter the form of such force-velocity or torque-velocity curves underlies the question of specificity of training; the latter is subsequently discussed in greater detail.

TABLE 20–2. Strength (in Newtons) of Lower Extremity Extensors of Normal Subjects Throughout a 7-Sec Isometric Contraction with the Knee Joint at a 90-Degree Angle*

CONTRACTION TIME (SECONDS)	STRENGTH	
	$\bar{X}$	SD
1	636	245
2	884	289
3	1027	329
4	1130	409
5	1146	415
6	1161	429
7	1143	438
1–7: average	1017	327

*From Seliger, V., Dolejs, L., and Karas, V.: A dynamometric comparison of maximum eccentric, concentric and isometric contractions using EMG and energy expenditure measurements. Eur. J. Appl. Physiol., 45:235–244, 1980.

Absolute Muscle Strength

It has long been known that the maximal force that a muscle may develop is related to the size of the muscle, i.e., to the physiological cross-sectional area of the muscle. The physiological cross-sectional area of a muscle is the combined cross section of all of its muscle fibers. Some muscles have long parallel fibers running through the belly of the muscle and the physiological cross section is the cross section of the muscle belly (Fig. 20–7). To calculate the physiological cross section of a pennate muscle, multiple sections perpendicular to the long axis of the muscle fibers must be made until all are included (Fig. 20–8). Some muscles in the body are particularly suited to speed of contraction by their anatomical configuration. Such muscles have long parallel fibers and are placed close to the axis of rotation of the joint. Other muscles are particularly well suited to the development of large forces but with relatively small distances covered by the distal portion of the limb. Such muscles insert relatively far from the axis of motion of the joint (Fig. 20–9). The absolute muscle strength, then, is in proportion to the physiological cross-sectional area and is generally considered to be about 3.6 kg per cm² of physiological cross-sectional area.[2, 74] This is a useful and probably essentially accurate concept, although some other factors may be involved. The work of Gordon suggested that performance of high-force tasks may be improved without gross hypertrophy.[26] Progressively increasing weights were attached to the backs of the experimental animals (rats), which were then made to climb poles. Their muscles showed no overall increase in weight, but the type II (fast twitch) muscles did show an

TABLE 20–3. Mean Maximum Isokinetic Plantar Flexion Torques for 135 Sedentary Northern Swedish Females and Males*†

			STAT. MAX.		90 DEGREES		180 DEGREES	
			Nm	± SD	Nm	± SD	Nm	± SD
AGE	SEX	n‡	R/L	R/L	R/L	R/L	R/L	R/L
20–29	F	15	80/87	17/16	46/55	12/11	24/29	6/8
	M	15	121/131	21/20	70/80	14/21	37/44	10/14
30–39	F	15	87/95	20/21	50/58	13/14	26/32	7/7
	M	15	126/133	19/18	74/80	12/16	37/41	9/11
40–49	F	15	74/82	15/14	41/47	11/13	18/22	7/9
	M	15	128/136	21/23	74/79	19/15	35/40	12/10
50–59	F	15	63/72	12/14	36/38	6/6	17/19	4/5
	M	15	114/118	18/14	66/74	10/13	30/36	7/11
60–65	F	9	54/60	10/13	29/33	8/7	13/14	4/7
	M	6	66/88	26/26	37/48	13/19	17/18	8/5

*From Fugl-Meyer, A. R., Gustafsson, L., and Burstedt, Y.: Isokinetic and static plantar flexion characteristics. Eur. J. Appl. Physiol., 45:221–234, 1980.

†Maximal torques measured for three different velocities of angular motion with the knee fully extended (0 degrees).

‡n: Number of subjects; Nm: Newton-meters; R: Right; L: Left.

increase in cross-sectional area. Certainly the ability to exert large brief forces relates both to muscle cross-sectional area and to motor unit recruitment patterns. In 1951, DeLorme and Watkins suggested that "the initial increase in strength on progressive resistance exercise occurs at a rate far greater than can be accounted for by morphological changes within the muscle. These initial rapid increments in strength noted in normal and disuse-atrophied muscles are, no doubt, due to motor learning. . . . It is impossible to say how much of the increase is due to morphological changes within the muscle or to motor learning."[16] Since that time, it has, indeed, become possible to tease apart the relative contribution of these two major determinants of increasing strength. Moritani and deVries make use of the fact that under carefully controlled conditions, the ratio of integrated electrical activity of muscle to the isometric force exerted by the elbow flexors is linear throughout the entire range of forces up to and including maximal voluntary contraction.[53] Figure 20–10A shows a theoretical possibility in which all strength (force) gain is due to neural factors, i.e., increased activation. Figure 20–10B shows a scheme in which all strength gained is due to hypertrophy. In this scheme, any given force requires less EMG activity. Moritani and deVries describe this as an improved electrical/force ratio or efficiency of electrical activity.* Figure 20–10C shows a scheme that allows evaluation of the percentage contributions of neural factors and muscular hypertrophy to the strength gain with training. The authors actually carried out such a study on the elbow flexors of seven young healthy males and eight such females who were subjected to an eight-week weight-training program. Figure 20–11 displays the electrical activity ratios obtained. This indicates that the strength increases of the first two weeks were almost entirely due to neural factors and the strength gains of subsequent weeks were mostly due to muscular hypertrophy. Comparison of Figures 20–11A and B may explain conflicting data in the literature regarding cross-training. Unless the untrained limb is heavily involved in stabilization, the improvement in strength sometimes found in the unexercised limb may be due to neural factors.

Milner-Brown and colleagues[50] found elevated synchronization ratios in weightlifters. The synchronization ratio reflects the extent to which the motor units fire simultaneously (Fig. 20–12). Such

*Ordinarily efficiency is expressed as the ratio of mechanical output to input. In that case it would be expressed as force over electrical activity. The authors have expressed this as electrical activity over force, the opposite of the custom, but it is clear that the meaning is the same.

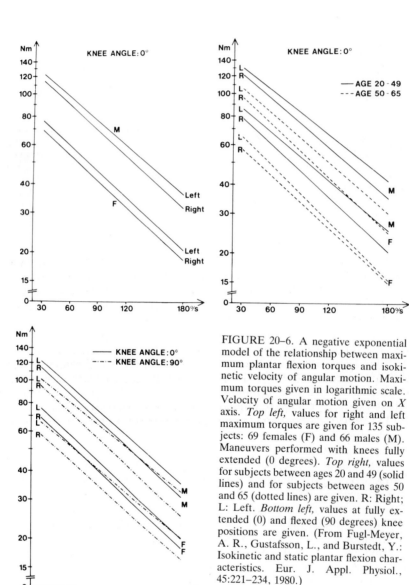

FIGURE 20–6. A negative exponential model of the relationship between maximum plantar flexion torques and isokinetic velocity of angular motion. Maximum torques given in logarithmic scale. Velocity of angular motion given on *X* axis. *Top left,* values for right and left maximum torques are given for 135 subjects: 69 females (F) and 66 males (M). Maneuvers performed with knees fully extended (0 degrees). *Top right,* values for subjects between ages 20 and 49 (solid lines) and for subjects between ages 50 and 65 (dotted lines) are given. R: Right; L: Left. *Bottom left,* values at fully extended (0) and flexed (90 degrees) knee positions are given. (From Fugl-Meyer, A. R., Gustafsson, L., and Burstedt, Y.: Isokinetic and static plantar flexion characteristics. Eur. J. Appl. Physiol., 45:221–234, 1980.)

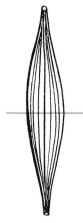

FIGURE 20–7. Parallel arrangement of muscle fibers. Physiological cross section is equal to cross section of muscle belly. (From Brunnstrom, S.: Clinical Kinesiology, 2nd Ed. Philadelphia, F. A. Davis, 1966.)

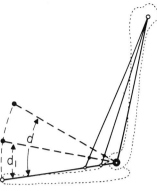

FIGURE 20–9. Relation of tendon lever arm to speed and force. If the lever arm is a short distance from the center of motion, there is greater excursion per unit of contraction but low force at the distal end of the lever. If the tendon is inserted at a greater distance from the center of motion, there is less excursion per unit of contraction but greater force at the distal end of the lever. (Redrawn from Steindler, A.: Kinesiology of the Human Body. Springfield, Ill., Charles C. Thomas, Publisher, 1955.)

synchronization occurs randomly at high levels of recruitment (Fig. 20–13). However, a greater incidence of simultaneous firing than normal, i.e., elevated synchronization ratios, occurs in weightlifters or in subjects, such as bus drivers, whose occupation requires frequent exertion of large,

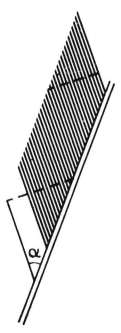

FIGURE 20–8. In pennate muscle, the physiological cross section is determined by multiple sections at right angles to the fibers until all are included. (From Brunnstrom, S.: Clinical Kinesiology, 2nd Ed. Philadelphia, F. A. Davis, 1966.)

brief forces (Fig. 20–14). The authors found that a high-force training program altered synchronization ratios in previously untrained subjects. A 20 per cent increase in maximal isometric force (MVC) was associated with a doubling of the synchronization ratio. After a further period of six weeks of no exercise, the synchronization ratio declined but not to control levels. The extent to which this occurs with prolonged, low-force, static or dynamic training is not known at present.

Intensity and Endurance Relationships

The extent to which muscle endurance is related to muscle strength and the specificity of exercise programs designed to improve one or the other are subjects of controversy. Within limits, strength or the intensity of activity and endurance at that activity are mathematically related. Figure 20–15, *left,* shows the relationship of endurance as total contractions of repeated flexion of the third digit to the effective force of contraction. Figure 20–15, *right,* shows the relationship of endurance (as minutes to fatigue) of cycle exercise to external power production. In both figures, the intercept with the abscissa represents the exercise intensity for which the maneuver could be performed only once; this would, therefore, define the strength of concentric contraction. Also, in both figures, endurance could be specified as either the total number of contractions or minutes to fatigue. The shape of the curve, then, represents the endurance at any given intensity level. It should be noted that the curves have a very similar shape in spite of the

BARBARA J. DE LATEUR AND JUSTUS F. LEHMANN

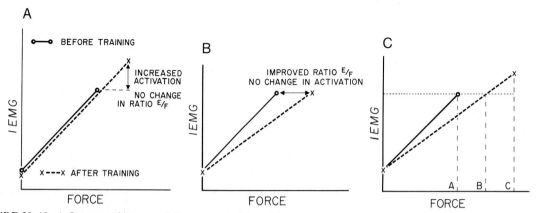

FIGURE 20–10. *A*, Increase of integrated electromyographic activity plotted against force of contraction as an index of strength due to neural factors gained during training. *B*, Strength gained due to hypertrophy when neural activity is maintained constant. *C*, Schema for evaluation of per cent contributions of neural factors (NF) versus muscular hypertrophy (MH) to the gain of strength through progressive resistance exercise based upon efficiency of electrical activity (EEA). Strength increase per cent (MH) = (B − A)/(C − A) × 100. Strength increase per cent (NF) = (C − B)/(C − A) × 100. (Redrawn from Moritani, T., and de Vries, H. K.: Neural factors versus hypertrophy in the time course of muscle strength gain. Am. J. Phys. Med., 58:115–130, 1979.)

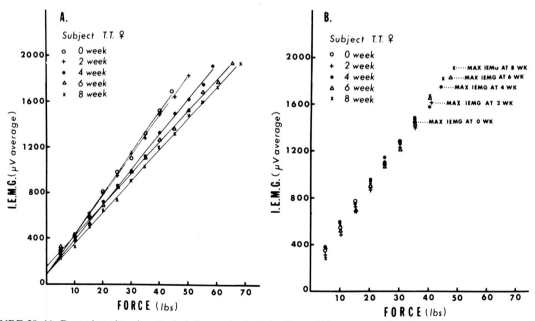

FIGURE 20–11. Data plotted to show typical changes in the trained arm (*A*) as compared to the untrained arm (*B*). Both arms gained in strength but only the trained arm showed significant changes in the E/F ratio (hypertrophy). (From Moritani, T., and de Vries, H. K.: Neural factors versus hypertrophy in the time course of muscle strength gain. Am. J. Phys. Med., 58:115–130, 1979.)

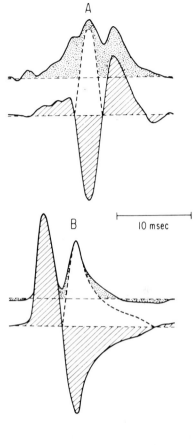

FIGURE 20–12. Average responses of 500 sweeps obtained before and after rectification of the surface EMG were used to determine the degree of synchronization. Each sweep was triggered by an impulse from a single motor unit recorded by a needle in the first dorsal interosseous muscle of (A) a weightlifter and (B) a control subject. The lower horizontal lines in each part indicate the zero voltage level and the upper horizontal lines the mean rectified surface EMG, which gives a measure of the total electrical activity in the muscle. Note that there is a substantial rise in the activity near the time of the impulses from the single motor unit in the weightlifter (dotted area), but not in the control subject. This indicates that the impulses of this unit were grouped or synchronized with those of other motor units in the muscle. The surface EMG was delayed electronically 5 or 10 msec to show the full time course of this synchronization. The only peaks observed for the control subject were those expected from the unrectified average, which represents the contribution of the single unit to the surface EMG (diagonal lines). As a measure of synchronization, Milner-Brown et al. computed the ratio of the dotted area to the diagonally hatched area for a number of motor units. Any dotted area that fell below the mean rectified level was subtracted from that which exceeded this level. (From Milner-Brown, H. S., Stein, R. B., and Lee, R. G.: Synchronization of human motor units: Possible role of exercise and supraspinal reflexes. E. E. G. Clin. Neurophysiol., 38:245–254, 1975.)

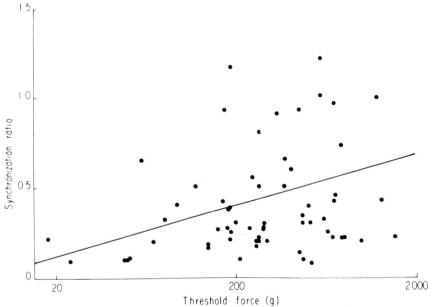

FIGURE 20–13. Synchronization ratios for different motor units in seven weightlifters as a function of the overall force in the muscle required to recruit a given unit to fire continuously (threshold force). There is a weak trend, indicated by the computed best-fitting straight line, for the higher threshold units to have larger synchronization ratios (linear correlation coefficient = 0.34). (From Milner-Brown, H. S., Stein, R. B., and Lee, R. G.: Synchronization of human motor units: Possible roles of exercise and supraspinal reflexes. E. E. G. Clin. Neurophysiol., 38:245–254, 1975.)

BARBARA J. DE LATEUR AND JUSTUS F. LEHMANN

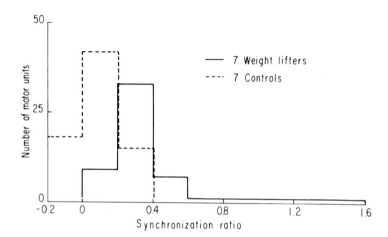

FIGURE 20–14. Synchronization ratios computed as shown in Figure 20–13 for a number of motor units from weightlifters and controls. A value greater than 0.2 was assumed to represent a significant degree of synchronization. These values were rarely observed in control subjects, but were generally found in weightlifters. (From Milner-Brown, H. S., Stein, R. B., and Lee, R. G.: Synchronization of human motor units: Possible roles of exercise and supraspinal reflexes. E. E. G. Clin. Neurophysiol., 38:245–254, 1975.)

FIGURE 20–15. *Left panel*, Relationship of endurance (as total contractions) of repeated flexion of third digit to effective force of contraction. *Right panel*, Relationship of endurance (as minutes to fatigue) of cycle ergometer exercise to external power production. In both panels, the intercept with the abscissa represents the exercise intensity for which the maneuver could be performed only once (and, therefore, the strength of the concentric movement). In both panels, endurance could be presented as either total contractions or minutes to fatigue and, as the contraction rate and velocity are designated, either abscissa could be designated as force (per individual repetition) or power (work per unit time). (From Knuttgen, H. G.: Development of muscular strength and endurance. *In* Knuttgen, H. G. [Ed.]: Neuromuscular Mechanisms for Therapeutic and Conditioning Exercises. Baltimore, University Park Press, 1976, pp. 97–118.)

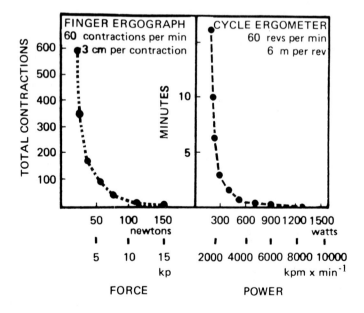

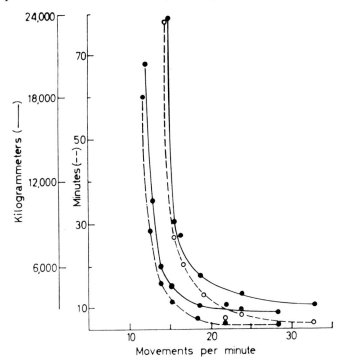

FIGURE 20–16. Endurance and intensity of work. Arm ergograph. Movements per minute plotted against duration of work and total amount of work performed. (From Monod, H., and Scherrer, J.: Capacité de travail statique d'un group musculaire synergique chez l'homme. C. R. Soc. Biol., 151:1358–1362, 1957.)

fact that the ergograph requires the use of one muscle group and the cycle ergometer requires the reciprocal use of several large muscle groups. Figure 20–16 shows the relationships of intensity of work, in kilogram-meters, to the duration of work and the amount of work performed.[52] Figure 20–17 shows the maximal holding time as a function of force. It can be seen that there is a tight mathematical relationship over a large number of observations with various muscle groups in subjects of both sexes.[58] This may be described as a hyperbolic curve with ends asymptotically approaching

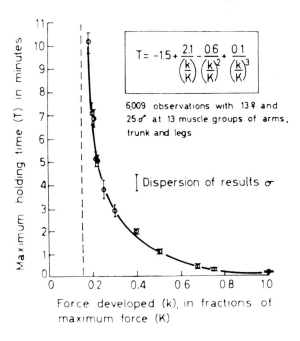

$$T = -1.5 + \frac{2.1}{\left(\frac{k}{K}\right)} - \frac{0.6}{\left(\frac{k}{K}\right)^2} + \frac{0.1}{\left(\frac{k}{K}\right)^3}$$

6,009 observations with 13 ♀ and 25 ♂ at 13 muscle groups of arms, trunk and legs

Dispersion of results σ

FIGURE 20–17. Endurance and intensity of work. Static work: tension at fractions of maximal strength. (From Simonson, E.: Recovery and fatigue. In Simonson, E. [Ed.]: Physiology of Work Capacity and Fatigue. Springfield, Ill., Charles C. Thomas, Publisher, 1971, pp. 440–458. Redrawn from Rohmert, W.: Ermittlung von Erholungspausen für statische Arbeit des Menschen. Int. Z Angew. Physiol., 18:123–164, 1960.)

BARBARA J. DE LATEUR AND JUSTUS F. LEHMANN

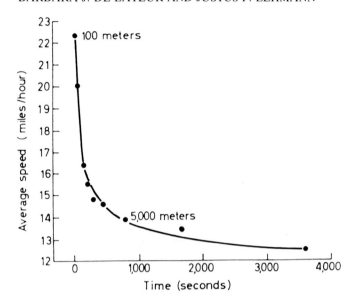

FIGURE 20–18. Intensity of work versus endurance for world record runs. (From Simonson, E.: Recovery and fatigue. *In* Simonson, E. [Ed.]: Physiology of Work Capacity and Fatigue. Springfield, Ill., Charles C. Thomas, Publisher, 1971, pp. 440–458, plotted from Lloyd, B. B.: World running records at maximal performances. Circ. Res., 20 and 21 [Suppl 1]: 1, 1967.)

the ordinate and abscissa. It should also be noted that this experiment has not been carried out below 20 per cent of the maximal isometric force. Hill calculated that below 15 per cent of the maximal isometric force an isometric contraction may be sustained indefinitely, since the rate at which the circulatory system can carry away the heat equals or exceeds the rate at which heat is generated.[34] This calculation does not take into consideration the rate of consumption and regeneration of metabolic substrate, however.

The average speed in miles per hour has been plotted against the time, in seconds, of world record runners[46] (Fig. 20–18). It is of some interest to note that even for a very different type of exercise, the acute intensity-endurance relationships remain the same, i.e., have a similar hyperbolic curve.

Knuttgen suggests the physiological significance of the curves in Figure 20–15.[42] (His comments would also apply to Figures 20–16 and 20–17.) The intercept with the abscissa, i.e., the one repetition maximum or strength, is determined by the physiological cross-sectional area of the muscles involved. To the author's comment one may add that the ability to synchronize may also have an influence upon the intercept with the abscissa or one repetition maximum. Knuttgen states that the horizontal portion of the curve is determined predominantly by the capacity of the anaerobic energy release process. The vertical portion of the curve is determined by the aerobic energy release capac-

ity as dominated by the delivery of oxygen to the muscles by the circulatory system. The portion of greatest curvilinearity is related to a combination of aerobic and anaerobic power capacities. At the very high force levels at which contractions can be repeated up to 10 times, Knuttgen suggests that depletion of high-energy phosphate at the sites of contractile activity may be the limiting factor. Dissociation between integrated electromyographic activity and force in a sustained isometric contraction suggests that it is not failure of nerve impulses or failure of the spread of excitation of the muscle membrane (Fig. 20–19).

Infante and associates demonstrated *in vitro* that when adenosine triphosphate (ATP) resynthesis is blocked by 1-fluoro-2, 4 dinitrobenzene, frog sartorius muscle can produce only three near-maximal contractions in response to electrical stimulation before the ability of the muscle to contract is definitely reduced.[37] Mundale reported that during maximal voluntary isometric contractions of handgrip in humans, maximal tension could not be maintained more than one sec[55, 56] (Fig. 20–20). Anaerobic restoration of ATP occurs more slowly than breakdown during maximal metabolic activity of muscle, resulting in a progressive decrease in muscular contractile capacity with increasing duration of activity due to the progressively diminishing supply of ATP to fuel the actin-myosin interaction in the sarcomeres. Keul, Doll, and Keppler report the relative availability of energy-supplying substrates to restore ATP during early activity.[39]

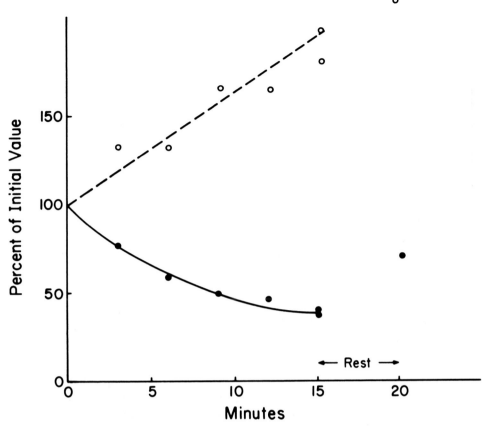

FIGURE 20–19. Effect of intense dynamic work on the maximal isometric force of the muscle and on the integrated global EMG. Triceps, recording by surface electrodes during work to exhaustion lasting 15.1 minutes. Every three minutes the subject performed a maximal isometric contraction, whose force (in a continuous line) and integrated electrical activity (in an interrupted line) are measured. Note how the electrical activity increases again during the phase of relaxation. (From Scherrer, J., and Bourguignon, A.: Changes in the electromyogram produced by fatigue in man. Am. J. Phys. Med., 38:148–158, 1959.)

FIGURE 20–20. Maximal tension can be maintained during a voluntary maximal contraction of hand grip for less than one sec before evidence of fatigue appears as the available supply of ATP is exhausted. Fatigue (unavailability of ATP) increases in proportion to the intensity of activity but can be demonstrated following 10 min of intermittent contractions at 5 per cent of maximal. (From Mundale, M. O.: The relationship of intermittent isometric exercise to fatigue of hand grip. Arch. Phys. Med. Rehabil., 51:532–539, 1970.)

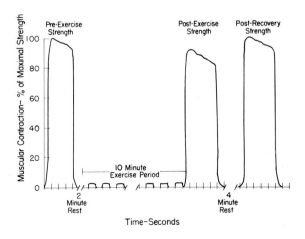

BARBARA J. DE LATEUR AND JUSTUS F. LEHMANN

Energy Sources in Relation to Duration of Contraction

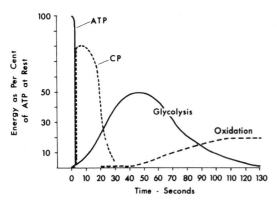

FIGURE 20–21. Muscular metabolism available from the various substrates participating in supplying energy during the first two min of an attempted maximal contraction. The relative contribution of each substrate at any moment is indicated. The intensity of metabolic activity over the two-minute period is adjusted to the change of the isometric tension produced during a sustained voluntary maximal contraction.[54, 56] (Redrawn from Keul, J., Doll, E., and Keppler, D.: Energy Metabolism of Human Muscle. Medicine and Sport, Vol. 7. Baltimore, University Park Press, 1972.)

The stored ATP at rest is sufficient for only three to four sec of contraction. Creatine phosphate–splitting can maintain ATP at a somewhat reduced rate of activity for approximately 20 sec. During this time, glycolytic metabolism increases to peak at approximately 40 to 50 sec and then begins to fall. Oxidative metabolism rises slowly so that by 90 sec the major contribution to the metabolic rate is oxidation. After three to four minutes of constant exercise, a person reaches a metabolic steady state or a constant rate of consumption of oxygen. Figure 20–21 presents the relative contributions of the various energy-supplying substrates to total energy utilization during maximal metabolism at any instant in the first two min of activity. These values were calculated by Keul, Doll, and Keppler[39] and adapted by Kottke and Mundale[44] according to the decreasing intensity of maximal voluntary isometric tension that occurs during that time. Glycolytic metabolism can restore ATP at approximately 30 to 50 per cent of the maximal rate of muscular metabolism, whereas oxidative metabolism can produce ATP only at a rate of approximately 10 to 20 per cent of maximal muscular metabolism. To what extent the various kinds of training exercises cause shifts in these relative rates of metabolic activity has yet to be established.

It must be emphasized that these relative contributions to metabolism apply to attempts at sustained, maximal, isometric contraction.

The limit of the mechanism of oxidative phosphorylation (Krebs' cycle and electron transport system) to resynthesize ATP determines the exercise rate for the first five min, after which oxygen delivery becomes the decisive factor. Knuttgen[42] suggests that for exercise intensities that can be maintained for extended periods (one to two hours), depletion of glycogen stored in the muscle cells becomes the most likely limiting factor. Since the uptake rate of glucose from the blood is limited, depletion of the glycogen curtails both glycolytic phosphorylation and the availability of carbohydrate-provided substrate (pyruvate) for the Krebs' cycle. It should be noted that the aerobic capacity of the total individual is of great importance in the ergometer exercise but of little or no importance in the finger ergograph exercise.

The following studies shed further light on the relationship between strength and endurance. It is generally conceded that there is a significant positive correlation between maximal dynamic strength and absolute dynamic endurance.[67] Evidence is also available that this holds true of the relationship between maximum static strength and absolute static endurance.[73] These relationships are demonstrated in Figures 20–15 to 20–17. An example may serve to illustrate this relationship: If one's maximal isotonic strength of the biceps is 20 lb, the individual will be able to lift this weight (by definition) for only one repetition. In contrast, if one's maximal isotonic strength is 40 lb, the individual will be able to carry out the contraction at the 20-lb load for many more repetitions. By the same token, the tight mathematical relationship (with little scatter) suggests that greater strength does not improve one's *relative* endurance. Thus, no matter how strong one is, 100 per cent of MVC is 100 per cent, and this will fall on the intercept with the abscissa. Barnes has studied the relationship between maximal isokinetic strength and isokinetic endurance[4] (Table 20–4). When isokinetic endurance is defined as the number of repetitions performed at any given percentage of maximal isokinetic strength (i.e., relative isokinetic endurance), there is a nonsignificant correlation between strength and endurance (Table 20–5). However, when maximal isokinetic strength was correlated with absolute endurance, defined as the total ft-lb of work done at any given percentage of maximal strength, the correlation coefficients were both positive and significant. This is a measure of ab-

TABLE 20–4. Comparison During Isokinetic Exercise of Maximal Isokinetic Strength, Relative Isokinetic Endurance, and Absolute Endurance or Ability to Perform Work*

VARIABLE	X̄	SD
Peak torque, ft-lb	113.65	29.19
Repetitions > 90% peak torque†	5.88	3.46
Repetitions > 75% peak torque†	15.29	4.88
Work > 90% peak torque, ft-lbs	638.82	440.95
Work > 75% peak torque, ft-lbs	1536.55	670.83

*From Barnes, W. S.: The relationship between maximal isokinetic strength and isokinetic endurance. Res. Q., 51:714–717, 1980.

†Repetitions at 90% or 75% of peak torque represent relative endurance. Work performed at 90% or 75% of peak torque represents absolute endurance.

solute endurance. Barnes' findings support the concept that the work output of high-strength individuals is greater than that of low-strength individuals. In summary, there is no evidence that relative endurance increases as strength increases. However, there is a strong positive correlation between strength and absolute endurance or ability to perform work. As Barnes[4] cautions, this positive correlation between maximal strength and absolute endurance accounts for only approximately 10 to 20 per cent of the observed variance, and a major portion of endurance cannot be accounted for by strength alone. Other factors such as inherent differences in muscle fiber type, myoglobin stores, and enzymatic profiles, as well as the elusive factor of motivation, may contribute to any individual's endurance capacity.

Length-Tension Relationships

If a relaxed (nonstimulated) muscle is detached from its insertion and gradually stretched, a passive length–tension relationship can be determined

TABLE 20–5. Comparison of Correlations of Isokinetic Strength with Relative Isokinetic Endurance and with Absolute Endurance to Do Work*

ENDURANCE PARAMETER VERSUS	STRENGTH "R"
Repetitions > 90% peak torque	− 0.03
Repetitions > 75% peak torque	0.04
Work > 90% peak torque	0.36†
Work > 75% peak torque	0.27‡

*From Barnes, W. S.: The relationship between maximal isokinetic strength and isokinetic endurance. Res. Q., 51:714–717, 1980.

†$p < 0.01$.

‡$p < 0.05$.

(Fig. 20–22). The length at which the passive tension begins to exceed zero is defined as the resting length. If the length-tension relationships are again measured, but this time at each new length, a tetanizing volley of electrical stimuli is delivered to the motor nerve and a new curve will be determined (Fig. 20–22; this figure is also referred to as the Blix diagram). The total tension at any point will be the sum of the active tension and passive tension. At all lengths below the resting length, the passive tension is, by definition, zero, and therefore, at those lengths the total tension will be equal to the active tension. At all lengths beyond the resting length, the active tension is determined by subtracting the passive tension from the total tension. Thus, it can be seen that the greatest active tension is developed at the resting length and the greatest total tension is developed at or slightly longer than the resting length. Kidd and Brodie have suggested the superimposition of the force-velocity and active length-tension diagram to illustrate the concept that at any given velocity of lengthening or shortening, there is a length-tension relationship as the muscle passes through various lengths.[40] The classic

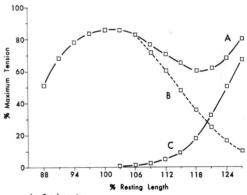

Length – Tension Diagrams of Total and Passive Tension

A - Total tension
B - Tension due to active contraction
C - Passive tension due to stretch

FIGURE 20–22. Length-tension diagram for passive stretch of an unstimulated muscle is shown in lower Curve C. Curve A, showing total isometric tension when the muscle was stimulated at various lengths from maximal stretch through moderate shortening, represents the summation of active contraction plus passive tension due to the stretch. Active tension due solely to muscular contraction is obtained by subtracting passive tension, C, from total tension, A, and is represented by Curve B. Normal resting length is 100 per cent. (Redrawn from Schottelius, B. A., and Senay, L. C.: Effect of stimulation-length sequence on shape of length-tension diagram. Am. J. Physiol., 186:127–130, 1956.)

BARBARA J. DE LATEUR AND JUSTUS F. LEHMANN

length-tension relationship, as shown in the previous figures, is an isometric one. Thus, theoretically there would be a whole family of length-tension curves, one for each contraction velocity.

Leverage Effect

The influence of the mechanical factor of leverage, deriving from tendon location and angle of insertion, upon torque when the force of the muscle is maintained constant varies with the sine of the angle of insertion. Figure 20–23 shows leverage curves for the elbow flexors. These are not torque curves but represent the mechanical factors contributing to torque.

Torque

As defined earlier, muscle torque represents the effectiveness of a muscle's force in producing ro-

tation about a joint. It is the net effect of the physiological and mechanical factors. These factors do not have an equal effect at all joints. In one, the mechanical effect may be more important, whereas in another, the physiological effect of length-tension relationships has greater impact upon the net torque. Figures 20–24 to 20–26 show several examples of isometric torque curves. For pronation and supination of the forearm and for flexion and extension of the shoulder, the physiological factor of the length-tension relationship predominates, with greater tension developed at longer lengths. For elbow flexion, there is an interaction between the two factors—physiological and mechanical. The angle of insertion of the biceps and brachialis muscle (mechanical factor) is very favorable at 90 degrees. It remains favorable at 100 to 120 degrees, but this factor is overshadowed by the physiological factor of very short muscle length.

The Cybex II dynamometer (for description, see *Equipment*) permits the measurement of torque curves throughout the range of motion and at various contraction speeds. Figure 20–27 shows examples of such measurements on the author's right quadriceps and hamstrings at the maximal torque possible at each angle from 90 degrees to 0 degrees of flexion at three contraction velocities. The angle of peak torque shifts with the increasing velocity of contraction. New equipment, currently or soon to become available, permits the extension of the torque measurement curves to the eccentric (lengthening) portion.

Muscle Fiber Types[36]

That there might be some specialization of muscle fibers has been known at least since the "dark meat" and "white meat" of fowl were observed. Attempts have been made on the basis of various muscle characteristics to classify muscles, but in humans muscle is a mosaic and not easily distinguishable on the basis of color. Attempts have been made to classify muscle types on the basis of oxidative or glycolytic capability, but the metabolic capacity of muscle is highly influenced by the state of activity and training and, therefore, is not a stable characteristic. Figure 20–28 shows the contraction-relaxation curves for fast twitch and slow twitch mammalian skeletal muscles. The slow twitch muscle is also known as type I, and the fast twitch muscle is known as type II. Under ordinary circumstances, these fiber types are extremely stable. They are under control of the nerve supply. Figure 20–29 gives a diagrammatic illustration of the influence of the innervation pattern.[28, 29, 61, 62]

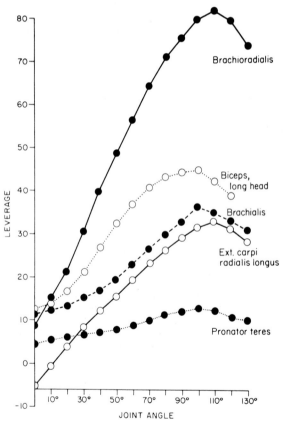

FIGURE 20–23. Leverage curves of elbow flexors. Zero degrees—elbow extended. (From Brunnstrom, S.: Clinical Kinesiology, 2nd Ed. Philadelphia, F. A. Davis, 1966; redrawn from Braune, W., and Fischer, O.: Die Rotationsmomente der Beugemuskeln am Ellbogengelenk des Menschen. Abhandlungen der Königlich Sächsischen Gesellschaft der Wissenschaften, 26:243–310, 1890.) Leverage is effective lever arm length: $l_f \cdot \sin \alpha$, where l_f is the distance from the joint axis to the site of application of the tendon of insertion and α is the angle of insertion of the tendon at that joint angle.

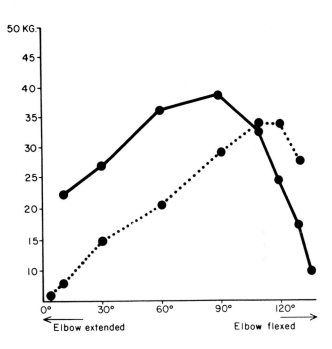

FIGURE 20–24. Torque curves for flexion and extension of right elbow, from determinations on four male subjects. Solid curve: elbow flexion curve; dotted curve: elbow extension. (From Brunnstrom, S.: Clinical Kinesiology, 2nd Ed. Philadelphia, F. A. Davis, 1966; redrawn from Bethe, A., and Franke, F.: Beiträge zum Problem der willkürlich beweglichen Armprothesen. IV. Die Kraftkurven der indirekten natürlichen Energiequellen. Münch. Med. Wochenschr., 66:201–205, 1919.)

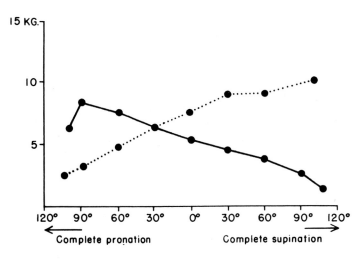

FIGURE 20–25. Torque curves for pronation and supination of right elbow, derived from determinations on four male subjects. Elbow at 90 degrees of flexion. Solid curve: supination. Dotted curve: pronation. Zero: thumb upward. (From Brunnstrom, S.: Clinical Kinesiology, 2nd Ed. Philadelphia, F. A. Davis, 1966; redrawn from Bethe, A., and Franke, F.: Beiträge zum Problem der willkürlich beweglichen Armprothesen. IV. Die Kraftkurven der indirekten natürlichen Energiequellen. Münch. Med. Wochenschr., 66:201–205, 1919.)

BARBARA J. DE LATEUR AND JUSTUS F. LEHMANN

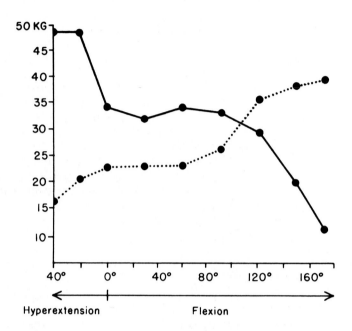

FIGURE 20–26. Torque curves for flexion and extension of right shoulder, derived from determinations on four male subjects. Solid curve: flexion. Dotted curve: extension. (From Brunnstrom, S.: Clinical Kinesiology, 2nd Ed. Philadelphia, F. A. Davis, 1966; redrawn from Bethe, A., and Franke, F.: Beiträge zum Problem der willkürlich beweglichen Armprothesen. IV. Die Kraftkurven der indirekten natürlichen Energiequellen. Münch. Med. Wochenschr., 66:201–205, 1919.)

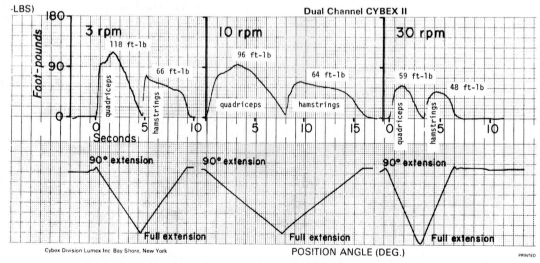

FIGURE 20–27. Torque curves of quadriceps and hamstrings throughout 90 degree range of motion and at various speeds. Note the greater strength of the quadriceps versus the hamstrings. With the subject seated, gravity hinders the quadriceps and helps the hamstrings progressively more at higher speeds.

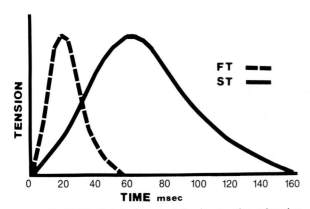

FIGURE 20–28. Twitch characteristics (contraction relaxation curves) of slow twitch (type I) and fast twitch (type II) muscles. (From Ianuzzo, C. D.: The cellular composition of human skeletal muscle. *In* Knuttgen, H. G. [Ed.]: Neuromuscular Mechanisms for Therapeutic and Conditioning Exercise. Baltimore, University Park Press, 1976, pp. 31–53.)

Cross-innervated muscles originally having fast twitch properties and low oxidative capacity take on slow twitch characteristics and an increased oxidative capacity, whereas the inverse occurs in slow twitch muscles experimentally innervated with nerves from fast muscles. In addition, the changes in the metabolic apparatus are accompanied by corresponding changes in the density of the capillaries surrounding the fibers. It has been shown that the fast twitch muscles and slow twitch muscles have their own force-velocity relationships. The general shape of the curve is the same, but there

are quantitative differences, with the rate of shortening being greater for fast twitch muscles than for slow twitch muscles with the same relative load. It should be noted, however, that the length-tension relationships of slow and fast muscles are similar when the amount of force developed is expressed per unit of cross-sectional area.[10, 75] One metabolic characteristic that is relatively stable is the reaction, with supravital stain, for myofibrillar adenosine triphosphatase (ATPase). When the section of muscle is pre-incubated at pH of 9.4 (or, more recently, at pH 10.2), the type II fibers (fast twitch) will stain darkly for myofibrillar ATPase. After this technique has been used for identifying the fiber types, these muscle fibers may then be stained, on adjacent serial sections, for other enzymes reflecting other metabolic capabilities. For example, Figure 20–30 shows adjacent serial sections from human muscle. On the left, the section had been stained for myofibrillar ATPase. The darkly staining fibers are the type II or fast twitch fibers. The light fibers are the type I or slow twitch fibers. The adjacent section, shown on the right, has been stained for NADH-tetrazolium reductase (NADH-TR), which reflects aerobic capability of the fibers. The slow twitch fibers are thus shown to be high in aerobic capacity. Qualitative or roughly quantitative changes resulting from training programs could be demonstrated by such stains as NADH-TR on repeated biopsy. Such techniques have been used in recent years to study fiber typing

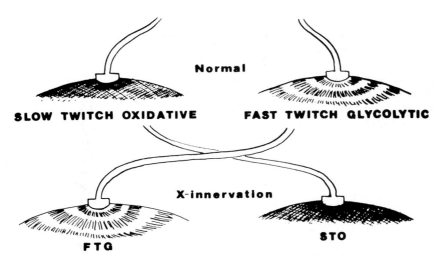

FIGURE 20–29. Cross-innervated muscles take on twitch characteristics and metabolic properties dependent on their innervation and become like the muscles of the opposite type. (From Ianuzzo, C. D.: The cellular composition of human skeletal muscle. *In* Knuttgen, H. G. [Ed.]: Neuromuscular Mechanisms for Therapeutic and Conditioning Exercise. Baltimore, University Park Press, 1976, pp. 31–53.)

BARBARA J. DE LATEUR AND JUSTUS F. LEHMANN

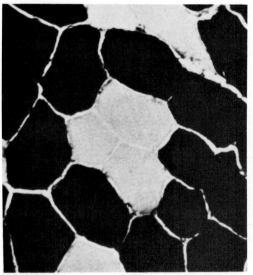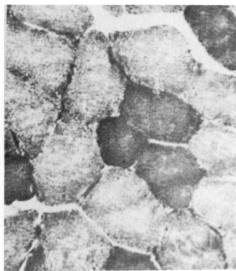

FIGURE 20–30. Histochemical micrograph illustrating the fast twitch and slow twitch muscle fibers in human skeletal muscle. The micrograph on the left has been stained for myofibrillar ATPase. The light and dark stained cells are slow twitch and fast twitch fibers, respectively. The micrograph at the right is from a serial section of the muscle and has been stained for NADH-TR, which indicates the aerobic potential of the fibers. These micrographs illustrate that in human skeletal muscle slow twitch fibers have a relatively high aerobic capacity, whereas FT fibers have a low capacity. (From Ianuzzo, C. D.: The cellular composition of human skeletal muscle. *In* Knuttgen, H. G. [Ed.]: Neuromuscular Mechanisms for Therapeutic Conditioning Exercise. Baltimore, University Park Press, 1976, pp. 31–53.)

and responses to training in athletes in various sports. It should be emphasized that the aerobic and glycolytic capabilities as well as glycogen content of muscle change, but the twitch characteristics and the myofibrillar ATPase staining remain stable. Such histochemical techniques may be supplemented by purely chemical techniques that are more quantitative but do not distinguish between fiber types. The change in enzyme activity reflects an average of both fiber types taken in the biopsy and does not distinguish the changes that may occur predominantly in slow twitch muscle fibers or fast twitch muscle fibers. One may also count percentages of fibers and look at the areas of individual slow twitch fibers and fast twitch fibers (i.e., the absolute area of each), as well as the ratio of slow twitch fiber areas to fast twitch fiber areas before and after training. Finally, the recruitment patterns of muscle fibers may be studied in acute experiments by repetitive biopsies during the course of various types of strenuous activity. The pattern of glycogen depletion in the fiber types may thus be followed at intervals throughout the activity.

In addition to the two basic types of muscle fibers, i.e., type I slow oxidative (SO) and type II fast glycolytic (FG), evidence is accumulating that in humans there is at least one additional type, i.e., fast oxidative glycolytic (FOG), a subtype of the type II fiber. Table 20–6 summarizes the properties of these three muscle types. To this table, one may add the recruitment level. The slow oxidative fibers are in motor units that have a low threshold, are recruited earlier, and, therefore, contract more frequently.

Motor Unit Recruitment Patterns and the Size Principle

Evidence supports the size principle enunciated by Henneman.[31] There are variations in size of the motor unit and its component parts, including the soma of the neuron as well as the number and cross-sectional area of the muscle fibers innervated. The smaller units are type I (slow oxidative), which have a low threshold of recruitment and generate low forces. The size principle is followed electromyographically. The electromyographer will observe that the earliest recruited motor units have smaller electrical potentials (amplitude) than units that recruit later. Although with biofeedback one can vary the order of recruitment of units of approximately the same amplitude, one cannot recruit a larger unit without first recruiting the relatively smaller one. The size principle is followed in the generation of mechanical force as

TABLE 20–6. A Characterization of Skeletal Muscle Fibers Based upon Their Metabolic and Mechanical Properties

	MUSCLE FIBER CHARACTERISTICS		
	Slow Oxidative	**Fast Glycolytic**	**Fast Oxidative Glycolytic**
Major source of ATP	Oxidative phosphorylation	Glycolysis	Oxidative phosphorylation
Mitochondria	Numerous	Few	Numerous
Myoglobin content	High	Low	High
Capillarity	Dense	Sparse	Dense
Muscle color	Red	White	Red
Glycogen content	Low	High	Intermediate
Glycolytic enzyme activity	Low	High	Intermediate
Myosin ATPase activity	Low	High	High
Speed of contraction	Slow	Fast	Fast
Rate of fatigue	Slow	Fast	Intermediate
Muscle fiber diameter	Small	Large	Intermediate

*From Kidd, G., and Brodie, P.: The motor unit: A review. Physiotherapy, 66:146–152, 1980.

well. The force generated by each motor unit varies linearly with recruitment order, so that the motor unit recruited earliest generates the least force.[50] These low-force units are recruited early, fire regularly, and are relatively fatigue-resistant. The term *tonic* is often used to refer to these units (see the next paragraph). The type II units, recruited later and exerting higher force, fire irregularly in bursts and fatigue relatively rapidly, although the subtype of fast oxidative glycolytic has an intermediate aerobic capacity and fatigues less rapidly while still retaining a rapid rate of contraction.

Maton, studying single motor units in the biceps of 15 normal subjects, found that a motor unit that does not discharge for a given level of static force will discharge during the following dynamic work and can also be recruited for a higher level of static force.[49] Thus, any given motor unit activity is dependent on the level of external force in keeping with the previous force-velocity relationships. Since higher levels of force are developed with isometric contractions, a higher level of static force is required to recruit a motor unit that would be recruited with dynamic work at the same force. Thus, the author points out that the qualifications *tonic* and *phasic* characterize the motor unit twitches and do not imply any static-dynamic differentiation. In further support of this concept, Desmedt and Godaux found that during ballistic (very rapid or steep ramp) contractions, higher order units, including type II, are recruited at lower force levels than during slow contractions.[17]

The work of Moritani and deVries reported earlier in the chapter suggested that the rapid increase in strength seen in the first two weeks of an isometric program was largely due to neural factors, i.e., increased activation of motor units, and the subsequent improvement of strength was due more to hypertrophy. That a similar pattern may be seen with heavy resistance (isotonic) exercise is shown in a study by Lüthi and associates,[47] using a very different methodology, i.e., computed tomography (CT) measurements of cross-sectional areas of the thigh. Figure 20–31 shows that force and cross-sectional area change in the same direction but that the increase in cross-sectional area is much steeper between weeks three and six.

Fatigue

Fatigue is any decrement in performance due to previous activity. True fatigue may not always be easy to determine. Fatigue may be operationally defined as the inability or unwillingness to carry out the assigned task in the assigned manner, under the specific conditions of reinforcement in effect and known to the subject, as the result of prior activity. This is, in essence, a behavioral definition. However, it would be desirable to have a definition of a physiological endpoint of fatigue. In at least two circumstances, such a definite biological endpoint is available. One is the maximum aerobic capacity. As defined, this is the rate of oxygen consumption ($\dot{V}O_2$), which does not increase in spite of increased performance of external work. Thus defined, this is the $\dot{V}O_2$max, which is illus-

BARBARA J. DE LATEUR AND JUSTUS F. LEHMANN

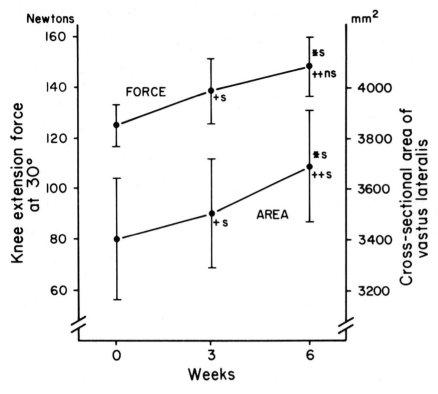

FIGURE 20–31. Force production as measured on the Cybex II apparatus and increase of muscle cross-sectional area as estimated from computed tomography before and after three and six weeks of strength training (means ± SD; s = significant; ns = not significant; + = 0–3 weeks; + + = 3–6 weeks; * = 0–6 weeks). (Lüthi, J. M., Howald, H., Claassen, H., Rösler, K., Vock, P., and Hoppeler, H.: Structural changes in skeletal muscle tissue with heavy resistance exercise. Int. J. Sports Med., 7:123–127, 1986.)

trated in Figure 20–3. This idealized figure shows that at all exercise intensities below 250 watts, the subject goes to a new rate of oxygen consumption. However, when the subject jumps from 250 watts to 300 watts, no increase in the rate of oxygen consumption occurs in spite of an increase in exercise intensity and external work performed. This additional 50 watts of external work is being carried out anaerobically, and fatigue will quickly result in failure to continue working at that intensity. Another situation in which a good physiological endpoint for fatigue may be determined is one in which the subject exerts a maximal isometric contraction (MVC) and the integrated electrical activity of the muscle is measured. Figure 20–19 shows the effect of intense dynamic work on maximal isometric force and on the integrated surface EMG. The fact that the integrated electrical activity *is increasing* at the time that the mechanical force is decreasing ensures that the subject is putting out a full effort but that fatigue is occurring in spite of the effort. There are concomitants of fatigue in other situations, but the endpoint is not so clear cut.

Response to Training

Are Athletes Born or Made?

Marked differences between athletes participating in different types of sports can be detected by the casual observer or the devotee of sport and in greater detail by the scientist in the human performance laboratory. The weightlifter is heavy and extremely strong. The distance runner is slight of build with very little body fat and relatively low strength but has the ability to continue running literally for hours. Definite but more subtle changes are observed between the sprinter and the distance runner. Differences in local metabolic capacity of the muscle as well as differences in fiber type have been determined by large-needle biopsy.[5] Gollnick sampled the upper and lower extremity muscles of athletes participating in various sports.[21] A total of 74 trained and untrained men were studied. The quantitative chemical studies that were carried out include succinate dehydrogenase (SDH) and phosphofructokinase (PFK), representing, respectively, the oxidative and glycolytic capabilities of the muscle sample as a whole, without distinction between the fiber types. Histochemical studies included myosin adenosine triphosphatase (ATPase) for fiber-typing, as well as NADH-TR and alpha-glycerophosphate dehydrogenase for estimating (semiquantitatively only) relative (type I versus type II) oxidative and glycolytic capabilities. The distribution of glycogen was estimated (in serial sections) from the periodic acid–Schiff (PAS) reaction. Standard photographs were made so that planimetry could be used for fiber areas. In addition, each subject's maximal aerobic capacity ($\dot{V}O_2$max) was determined while the subject was either running on a treadmill or pedaling a bicycle. Whereas only minor differences existed for PFK (glycolytic capacity), remarkable differences were found in local muscle oxidative capacity (SDH) and in $\dot{V}O_2$max. The SDH and $\dot{V}O_2$max of the weightlifters were no greater than those of the untrained men; in fact, they were slightly less. The endurance-trained athletes had much higher $\dot{V}O_2$max and local muscle SDH activity than the untrained or the weightlifters. Of particular interest is the selective effect upon the muscles used predominantly in the sport. For instance, in the group of bicyclists the SDH activity of the vastus lateralis (11.0 ± 1.0 µmole per g min) was much greater than that of the deltoid (6.1 ± 0.2), whereas in canoeists, the SDH activity of the deltoid (7.9 ± 0.6) was much higher than that of the vastus lateralis (5.8 ± 0.9). Table 20–7 shows the fiber sizes, populations, and contribution to muscle area of several individual subjects. It can be seen that in the untrained athletes, the weightlifters, and the sprinter, the slow twitch fibers (type I) occupied a relatively small percentage of the muscle fiber area ($21.9 - 30.0$ per cent), whereas in the endurance-trained athletes, the slow twitch fibers occupied as much as 84 per cent of the area. This study examined the state of the athletes at the time of the test and did not constitute a before-and-after experiment. It might be argued that very early in their athletic careers these athletes found that they were able to compete much more effectively in one type of sport than in another and,

TABLE 20–7. Relationship of Exercise Training of Upper and Lower Extremity Muscles to Fiber Diameters, Total Cross-Sectional Areas, and Percentages of Slow Twitch and Fast Twitch Muscle Fibers*

SUBJECT	SAMPLE SITE (ARM OR LEG)		FIBER DIAMETER, µ		AREA, µ³		ST FIBERS	% AREA ST FIBERS
			Slow Twitch	Fast Twitch	Slow Twitch	Fast Twitch		
PG	L	Untrained	75.2 ± 2.9	85.8 ± 2.0	4567.5 ± 343.2	5843.0 ± 273.9	34.0	28.7
CS	L	Untrained	80.3 ± 3.3	93.2 ± 2.2	5234.5 ± 440.3	6902.0 ± 329.9	30.0	24.5
MKS	L	Untrained	63.4 ± 2.4	67.7 ± 2.4	3057.5 ± 273.6	3683.0 ± 250.0	34.0	30.0
GK	A	Untrained	63.6 ± 2.0	67.3 ± 1.7	3234.0 ± 181.2	3594.0 ± 177.8	48.3	45.7
			72.2 ± 3.5	75.0 ± 1.4	4275.0 ± 382.1	4445.0 ± 169.1	48.6	47.6
NP	L	Sprinter	79.5 ± 2.6	89.4 ± 2.1	5060.5 ± 314.0	6336.5 ± 284.2	26.0	21.9
DM	L	Distance runner	67.1 ± 1.7	58.0 ± 1.3	3581.1 ± 186.2	2668.0 ± 122.0	75.0	80.1
DS	L	Distance runner	85.1 ± 3.5	105.2 ± 2.5	5858.0 ± 445.8	8776.1 ± 408.2	70.0	50.9
DF	L	Middle-distance runner	95.5 ± 3.2	87.9 ± 3.4	7307.8 ± 499.6	6235.0 ± 448.2	55.0	58.9
RP	L	Middle-distance runner	59.2 ± 2.7	71.6 ± 2.5	2856.5 ± 231.8	4118.0 ± 295.9	47.0	38.1
BA	L	Former weightlifter	107.1 ± 3.8	108.9 ± 3.4	9199.1 ± 656.7	9482.9 ± 666.9	24.0	23.5
MH	L	Weightlifter	85.6 ± 4.9	110.8 ± 3.0	6035.6 ± 629.4	9758.1 ± 516.6	25.3	23.5
	A		83.5 ± 2.4	105.0 ± 3.3	5553.5 ± 303.8	8917.2 ± 543.1	48.4	36.9
JR	A	Bicyclist	83.1 ± 1.4	96.2 ± 1.9	5467.0 ± 187.9	7337.0 ± 273.7	52.1	48.6
	L		104.6 ± 2.3	112.2 ± 2.2	8651.5 ± 763.9	9446.6 ± 401.5	51.3	44.0
BL	A	Canoeist	101.9 ± 2.6	102.9 ± 2.3	8244.0 ± 570.3	8391.0 ± 361.9	57.9	74.6
	L		90.5 ± 2.7	80.3 ± 1.5	6544.0 ± 387.5	5100.0 ± 190.1	69.9	57.5
SH	A	Swimmer	88.0 ± 1.7	91.0 ± 2.4	6124.0 ± 233.9	6552.0 ± 263.2	85.3	84.4
	L		79.0 ± 2.0	93.6 ± 1.9	4954.0 ± 237.6	6928.0 ± 266.9	79.7	73.7

*From Gollnick, P. D., Armstrong, R. B., Saubert, C. W., IV, Piehl, K., and Saltin, B.: Enzyme activity and fiber composition in skeletal muscle of untrained and trained men. J. Appl. Physiol., 33:312–319, 1972.

BARBARA J. DE LATEUR AND JUSTUS F. LEHMANN

thus, because of positive reinforcement, selected the sport at which they were successful. However, there is some suggestion that the changes seen in their muscles were, at least to some extent, the result of training, because one would anticipate genetically a more or less constant ratio of slow twitch to fast twitch fibers in the upper and lower extremities. (This is not to say that one expects the *same* ratio of slow twitch to fast twitch fibers in the deltoid and in the vastus lateralis; however, if the ratio of slow twitch to fast twitch fibers is X in the deltoid and Y in the vastus lateralis in one subject, and if the ratio of slow twitch to fast twitch fibers in the deltoid is A and the ratio of slow twitch to fast twitch fibers in the vastus is B in another subject, then, if differential usage (training) has no effect, one might expect X/Y to equal A/B.) However, those athletes who used the upper or the lower extremity more in a specific sport had enhancement of the metabolic capability and a larger per cent area of the slow twitch fibers in the muscles used.

Gollnick also carried out a five-month training program with biopsy studies before and after training.[20] The training program consisted of pedaling a bicycle ergometer one hour per day for four days a week at a load requiring 75 to 90 per cent of maximal aerobic power. The subsequent biopsies showed an increase in the ratio of the areas of slow twitch to fast twitch fibers from 0.82 to 1.11 ($p \leq 0.01$). Oxidative capacity increased in both fiber types; anaerobic capacity increased only in the fast twitch fibers. This study indicates the possibility of great enhancement of local muscle metabolic capability, particularly oxidative capacity, with endurance training and strongly supports the notion of some degree of specificity of training.

In studies with human subjects, fiber number does not appear to increase. However, in an animal study, Gonyea and co-workers[25] were able to excise and tease apart the fibers of an entire muscle using nitric acid digestion and they found a small but significant increase in the number of fibers in response to unilateral exercise. The fact that they found a significant increase means either that the animals had been born with more fibers on one side than on the other or that there was an actual increase in fiber number in response to exercise.

Regarding the question of whether athletes are born or made, it appears that the genotype sets the rather wide limits, with the actual performance capability determined by the extent and type of training.

Further Studies on the Specificity of Training

Transferability is the converse of specificity of training. It is of considerable interest to anyone who must prescribe exercise programs to know to what extent training acquired under one set of circumstances transfers to performance under another set of circumstances. The DeLorme axiom states that "high-power (high-force), low-repetition exercises build strength; low-power, high-repetition exercises build endurance" and that "each of these types of exercise is wholly distinct and wholly incapable of producing the results obtained by the other."[15] In the extreme case, it seems clear that the DeLorme axiom must be correct, but there is also reason to think that there may be a rather large middle ground where, under certain conditions, the DeLorme axiom may not apply. De Lateur and co-authors utilized a double-shift, transfer-of-training design to assess this axiom with the intensity range of 40 to 100 per cent of maximal.[12] Healthy young adult males were randomly assigned to one of four groups, two of which trained to fatigue on the high weight of 55 lb and two of which trained on the relatively low weight of 26 lb. The task was identical except for the amount of weight used. Subjects were seated in standard wooden chairs. To the metronome beat of 52 per min, the knee was extended on the count of one, held in full extension through the count of six, lowered on seven, and raised again on one. Subjects were paid a small amount per repetition. Each session yielded a score. Thus training and testing were one and the same. At the completion of 15 sessions, one of the high-weight–trained groups shifted to the low-weight condition, and one of the low-weight–trained groups shifted to the high-weight condition and all continued for four more sessions. Results are shown in Figure 20–32. The transference was complete. In addition, when, in a fifth test session, all four groups were tested on a common power test (maximum work performed per unit time), the group averages were identical.

The task in the above-described study was qualitatively identical; only the amount of weight (and thus the repetitions needed to achieve fatigue) was different. The author carried out a subsequent study to assess the amount of transference of isotonic training to isometric performance and vice versa.[14] Healthy young adult males were randomly assigned to one of four groups, two isometric and two isotonic. The weight attached to the foot was

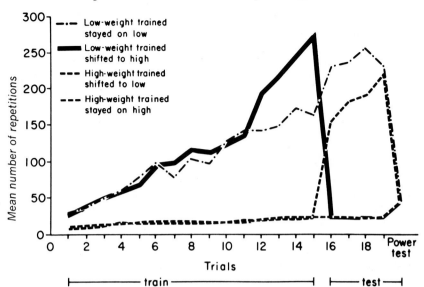

FIGURE 20–32. Mean scores for each of the four groups for each of 15 training trials and each of 4 test trials. The mean score for each of the four groups on the power test is also shown. (From de Lateur, B. J., Lehmann, J. F., and Fordyce, W. E.: A test of the DeLorme axiom. Arch. Phys. Med. Rehabil., 49:245–248, 1968.)

the same for all, 50 lb. The tasks were pure, i.e., no lifting or lowering for the isometric group and no holding of the knee in extension for the isotonic group. Subjects were again encouraged to continue to the point of muscle fatigue by being paid per second of holding time for the isometric group and per repetition for the isotonic group (Fig. 20–33). At the completion of 29 sessions, one isometric-trained group shifted to the isotonic condition and one isotonic-trained group shifted to the isometric condition, and all continued for five more sessions. In contrast to the DeLorme axiom study, there was very little transfer of training: subjects did much better on the task on which they had been trained.

Gollnick and co-workers used the biopsy technique to study the patterns of glycogen depletion in bicycling exercise of work intensities ranging from 30 to 150 per cent of $\dot{V}O_2$max.[24] They found that the slow twitch, high oxidative fibers were the first to lose glycogen at all workloads below 100 per cent of $\dot{V}O_2$max, but that as work continued the fast twitch fibers also became depleted of glycogen. At workloads exceeding maximal aerobic power, both fiber types lost glycogen. They concluded that there was primary reliance upon slow twitch fibers during submaximal endurance exercise, with recruitment of fast twitch fibers after slow twitch fibers were depleted of glycogen; during exertion requiring energy expenditure greater

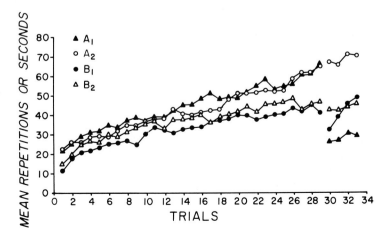

FIGURE 20–33. Results of the isotonic-isometric comparison. Groups A_1 and A_2 were isotonically trained. Groups B_1 and B_2 were isometrically trained. Group A_1 shifted to the isometric task on day 30. Group B_1 shifted to the isotonic task on day 30. (From de Lateur, B. J., Lehmann, J., Stonebridge, J., and Warren, C. G.: Isotonic vs. isometric exercises: A double-shift, transfer-of-training study. Arch. Phys. Med. Rehabil., 53:212–217, 1972.)

BARBARA J. DE LATEUR AND JUSTUS F. LEHMANN

than maximal aerobic power, both fiber types were continuously involved in the task.

Gollnick and associates also studied glycogen depletion patterns in the vastus lateralis muscles of six healthy males who carried out isometric contractions of various intensities related to their MVC.[23] In all experiments, a selective glycogen depletion was observed. Instead of any gradation of depletion, there was a reversal of depletion patterns above and below the critical tension of 20 per cent of MVC. Below 20 per cent, there was depletion of the slow twitch fibers; above 20 per cent, the fast twitch fibers were depleted. Even at 30 min of isometric contractions below 20 per cent of MVC, the type II fibers were not depleted of their glycogen. However, other studies[22] indicate that, in cycle ergometry, only 10 to 20 per cent of MVC is used in pedaling. If this work is continued to the point of exhaustion, type II fibers are also depleted of their glycogen.

The studies noted above collectively suggest that, for qualitatively identical tasks, comparable results from training in the range of 30 to 100 per cent MVC may be obtained as long as the task is carried to the point of fatigue (but it is much more difficult to reach true muscle fatigue with the lower weights; boredom is the more likely reason for cessation of the activity). For qualitatively different tasks, or for extreme quantitative differences, the best training is that task itself.

Newer dynamometric equipment has facilitated the study of the specificity of velocity of contraction in training, i.e., the extent to which it is possible to change the shape of the force-velocity curves by selective training. Moffroid and Whipple compared the results of six weeks of training on a slow (6 rpm) maximal task versus a fast (18 rpm) maximal task.[51] The outcome is shown in Figures 20–34 and 20–35. This study suggested that training at the higher rpms transferred to the lowered velocities, but that training at the lower rpms had little or no transference to the higher velocities. However, de Lateur and associates[11] addressed the problem of motivation on an isokinetic device by paying subjects per foot pound of torque in training and in testing for each quadriceps contraction. This reinforcement schedule thus encouraged the maximal production of torque in training as well as in testing. The subjects who trained at 6 rpm and who trained more forcefully, because of force-velocity relationships, had significantly greater increases in torque throughout the force-velocity curve than did those who trained at 18 rpm. This outcome suggests that the critical variable in the development of strength is the force exerted by the muscle in training.

Having little or no positive transfer from training to a desired performance task is certainly inefficient and undesirable. It is possible, however, that an even more undesirable outcome may occur, i.e., negative transference or interference. Such an outcome was found by Kennedy and co-workers, who randomly assigned six distance runners to experimental and control groups whose training during running differed only in that the experimental subjects wore weighted wristlets, anklets, and belts. In pre- and post-training measurements it was found that the energy cost of a low-intensity

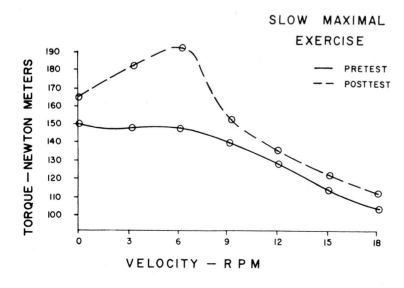

FIGURE 20–34. Peak torques of quadriceps plotted against velocity of contraction before (solid line) and after (dotted line) a maximal exercise regime at 6 RPM. (From Moffroid, M. T., and Whipple, R. H.: Specificity of speed of exercise. Phys. Ther., 50:1692–1700, 1970.)

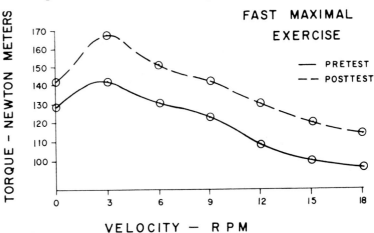

FIGURE 20–35. Peak torques of the quadriceps plotted against velocity of contraction before (solid line) and after (dotted line) a maximal exercise regime at 18 RPM. (From Moffroid, M. T., and Whipple, R. H.: Specificity of speed of exercise. Phys. Ther., 50:1692–1700, 1970.)

run (9.7 km per hr at 0 per cent grade with weights removed) was *increased,* and an unexpected shift toward greater anaerobic metabolism was observed.[38]

Hickson carried out a study designed to determine how individuals respond to a combination of strength and endurance training as compared with the adaptations produced by either strength or endurance training separately. The endurance training referred to is not isolated muscle endurance but aerobic training. The strength training program (group S) consisted of lower extremity weight training 5 days per week for 10 weeks. The endurance training program (group E) consisted of cycle ergometer work for 6 days per week for 10 weeks or at least 30 min of continuous running (cycling and running on alternate days). Groups S and E performed both programs at the same intensities, and with at least two hours' rest between the two programs. Results are displayed in Figures 20–36 and 20–37. Based upon this outcome, Hickson suggests that at the upper limits in the development of strength, aerobic training inhibits or interferes with further increases in strength.[33] Caution must be exercised in drawing conclusions

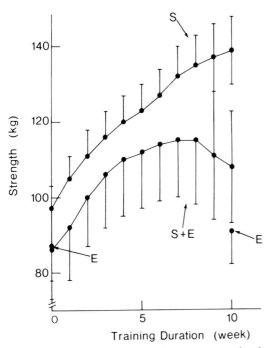

FIGURE 20–36. Strength changes in response to the three types of training. Measurements were made on a weekly basis in the strength (S) and strength and endurance (S and E) groups. The endurance (E) group was tested before and after 10 weeks of training. (From Hickson, R. C.: Interference of strength development by simultaneously training for strength and endurance. Eur. J. Appl. Physiol., 45:255–263, 1980.)

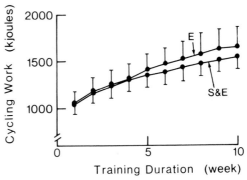

FIGURE 20–37. Increases in average total bicycle work per week during the 10 weeks of training in the endurance (E) and strength and endurance (S and E) groups. (From Hickson, R. C.: Interference of strength development by simultaneously training for strength and endurance. Eur. J. Appl. Physiol., 45:255–263, 1980.)

BARBARA J. DE LATEUR AND JUSTUS F. LEHMANN

because the subjects in Hickson's study were allowed to volunteer for the groups rather than be randomly assigned. If the conclusion holds up with further study, it will support the notion of making the training as close to the performance task as possible.

Thus, one may say that for qualitatively identical or very similar exercises, there is a high degree of transfer of training for tasks ranging between 40 and 100 per cent of muscle contractile power (and perhaps between as wide a range as 20 to 100 per cent). This is true as long as the task performed (at whatever relative level) is carried to the point of fatigue, as previously operationally defined. In contrast, for qualitatively dissimilar tasks, or in the case of extreme quantitative differences, the best training for a task is that task itself.

Relative Roles of Mechanical Work
Versus Fatigue

The results of the DeLorme axiom study showed no difference in ultimate performance ability between low-weight–trained (about 40 per cent

MVC) and high-weight–trained (about 85 to 100 per cent MVC) groups, as long as all subjects worked to fatigue in training. However, the low-weight–trained group required far more mechanical work and time to reach muscle fatigue. This suggested, but was not critically designed to show, that muscle fatigue was of greater importance in training than the amount of mechanical work performed. De Lateur and associates[13] carried out a two-phase, double-shift transfer-of-training study specifically designed to determine the relative importance of these two factors. In phase I, mechanical work was kept the same between right and left quadriceps, but one side, randomly determined, was subjected to more fatigue than the other. Subjects were paid for the number of repetitions (of complete cycles) performed by the fatigued side. The repetitions done on the nonfatigued side had to match the number of repetitions done on the fatigued side, but did so with one or more cycles of rest. Both sides lifted a 45-lb weight. The scheme for phase I and its five subsections is shown

	Seconds/Cycle	Nonrested Quad, Verbal Count	Rested Quad, Cycles Work/ Cycles Rest	Rested Quad, Verbal Count
Phase I	7	"up/2/3/4/5/6/ down"	1/1	"up/2/3/4/5/6/ down/rest/2/3/ 4/5/6/ready"
	6	"up/2/3/4/5/down"	1/2	"up/2/3/4/5/down/ rest/2/3/4/5/6/7/ 8/9/10/11/ready"
	5	"up/2/3/4/down"	1/3	"up/2/3/4/down/ rest/2/3/4/5/6/ 7/8/9/10/11/12/ 13/14/ready"
	4	"up/2/3/down"	1/4	"up/2/3/down/ rest/2/3/4/5/6/ 7/8/9/10/11/12/13/ 14/15/ready"
	3	"up/2/down"	1/5	"up/2/down/rest/ 2/3/4/5/6/7/8/9/ 10/11/12/13/14/ ready"
Phase II	7	"up/2/3/4/5/6/ down"	1/1	"up/2/3/4/5/6/ down/rest/2/3/4/ 5/6/ready"

FIGURE 20–38. The chart presents the number of seconds per cycle, the number of cycles of rest per cycle of work, and verbal counts for each leg under nonrested and rested conditions in Phase 1 and Phase 2. (From de Lateur, B. J., Lehmann, J. F., and Giaconi, R.: Mechanical work and fatigue: Their roles in the development of muscle work capacity. Arch. Phys. Med. Rehabil., 57:319–324, 1976.)

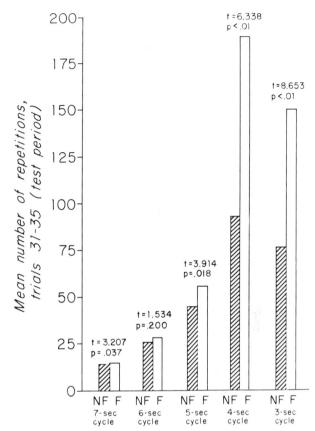

FIGURE 20–39. Comparison of exercise performance at days 31 to 35 of nonfatigued versus fatigued quadriceps exercised according to schedule of Phase 1. Both muscles performed the same amount of work each day during the first 30 days of training. NF = Nonfatigued quadriceps. F = Quadriceps exercised to fatigue. (From de Lateur, B. J., Lehmann, J. F., and Giaconi, R.: Mechanical work and fatigue: Their roles in the development of muscle work capacity. Arch. Phys. Med. Rehabil., 57:319–324, 1976.)

in Figure 20–38. The results are summarized in Figure 20–39. They may be interpreted as showing that more rest and less fatigue during training result in poorer performance in the test period. In phase II with a new set of subjects, both sides were exercised to fatigue during training, but one side, randomly determined, did so with a rest cycle between duty cycles and one side did so without a rest between duty cycles (see Fig. 20–38). Thus the side with a rest cycle did far more mechanical work than the side without the rest cycle in the process of continuing to fatigue bilaterally. The results are shown in Figure 20–40. The side that did more mechanical work did better in the test period, but not in proportion to the amount of time spent in training. For example, group one performed 91 per cent better than group two in the test period, in which both sides exercised to fatigue with a rest cycle between duty cycles, but spent 567 per cent more time in training. Comparing groups three and four in the test period, in which both sides exercised to fatigue without a rest cycle between duty cycles, one sees that group three, which trained with a rest cycle and thus had

more mechanical work, did 21 per cent better than group four, which trained without a rest cycle but spent 917 per cent more time in training. Thus, it may be said that if time and willingness to spend it in training are not a limiting factor, pacing oneself to fatigue may be somewhat more *effective*, but continuing to fatigue without a rest cycle is much more *efficient*.[13]

Rate of Improvement and Rate of Loss

How much exercise provides optimal training and the fastest increases in strength or work capacity, or both? The previously reported studies suggest that within wide limits, and provided there is no joint disease or tendinitis, the more exercise the better. Figure 20–41 shows that the time to reach the asymptote of limiting strength was less with heavier and more frequent isometric training.[54] Depending upon the previous state of training, Müller states that, with maximal exercise, the rate of increase may be 12 per cent per week. Rate of loss of strength, in the absence of any contraction of a muscle, is about 5 per cent per day (Fig. 20–42).

MacDougall and co-workers give somewhat dif-

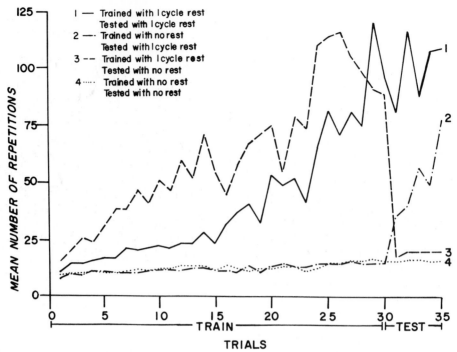

FIGURE 20–40. Comparison of exercise performance during training of quadriceps muscles with and without rest periods and during double-shift testing at days 31 to 35. Both rested and nonrested muscles were exercised to fatigue each day. (From de Lateur, B. J., Lehmann, J. F., and Giaconi, R.: Mechanical work and fatigue: Their roles in the development of muscle work capacity. Arch. Phys. Med. Rehabil., 57:319–324, 1976.)

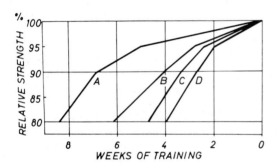

FIGURE 20–41. Weeks needed to reach limiting strength from an initial relative strength of 80 per cent: *A*, by submaximal training (one daily contraction at 65 per cent of maximum for one sec); *B*, by standard training (one daily maximal contraction for one sec); *C*, by one daily maximal contraction for 6 sec; *D*, by multiple daily maximal contractions totaling 30 sec in duration. (From Müller, E. A.: Influence of training and of inactivity on muscle strength. Arch. Phys. Med. Rehabil., 51:449–463, 1970.)

FIGURE 20–42. Observed decrease of strength per day of biceps of normal men when the arm was immobilized in a cast. (From Müller, E. A.: Influence of training and of inactivity on muscle strength. Arch. Phys. Med. Rehabil., 51:449–463, 1970.)

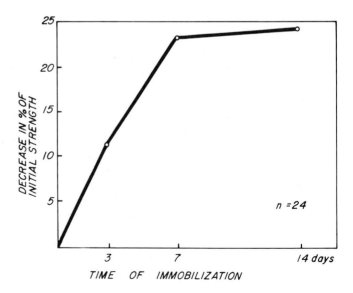

510

ferent figures.[48] Following five to six months of heavy resistance training, increase of strength had averaged 5 per cent per week; after five to six weeks of immobilization in a cast, strength had decreased an average of 8 per cent per week. These apparent discrepancies between Müller and MacDougall can be reconciled if one recalls that the greatest increases with training and losses with immobilization occur early in the course of the process, with subsequent leveling off. Moreover, isometric exercise within a cast against the resistance provided by the cast may retard the rate of loss of strength.

The work of Komi,[43] utilizing combined concentric and eccentric training, shows the time course of size changes in fast and slow twitch muscle fibers with training and detraining. It should be noted that, with 16 weeks of training, the greatest increases in fiber size were in the last half of the training process, i.e., the last eight weeks. In contrast, rapid changes occurred, particularly in the fast twitch muscles, in the first eight weeks of detraining.

Isometric Programs

Brief isometric programs, as described by Hettinger and Müller[32] and others,[45, 59] have as advantages the fact that they can be done virtually anywhere, require no special equipment (using antagonistic muscles, for example, as resistance), consume very little time, and are highly effective in increasing isometric strength. However, since most activities in physical restoration and sports require some dynamic contractions (some of them quite rapid), it would be unwise to confine training only to isometric programs.

Equipment

Although exercise programs may be carried out with no special equipment at all, using only the force of gravity and the resistance of one's opposing muscles or ligaments, or both, a wealth of equipment, ranging from simple to complex and from inexpensive to expensive, has become available.

In 1945, DeLorme described a technique of progressive resistive exercise that makes readily apparent use of the overload principle by literally increasing the load on the muscle.[15] (There are various ways to formulate the overload principle, some narrower and some broader. Very broadly, the overload principle holds that muscle perform-

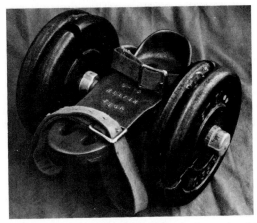

FIGURE 20–43. Quadriceps boot with crossbar and weights.

ance cannot be improved unless the muscle is taxed beyond usual daily activity.) The distal part of the extremity moved by the muscle or muscle group to be trained is weighted in one of several ways. A typical method for the quadriceps muscle involves the application of a quadriceps boot, sometimes called a DeLorme boot, which is an iron boot (or full sole plate) with a crossbar, iron weights of various sizes, collars and screws to hold weights on, and leather straps. Figure 20–43 shows a quadriceps boot. At the beginning, and once a week thereafter, the 10 repetition maximum is determined. The daily program, then, consists of 10 repetitions (each repetition consisting of full extension of the knee of the seated subject) at each of several percentages of the 10 RM. A typical session would consist of 10 repetitions at 50 per cent, 10 at 75 per cent, and 10 at 100 per cent of the 10 RM. As strength increases, the 10 RM increases, and therefore the load is also increased.

It often happens that, because of the previous repetitions at 50 per cent and 75 per cent of the 10 RM, the subject is unable to carry out 10 repetitions at 100 per cent 10 RM. For this reason, Zinovieff and associates described a method that has been dubbed the Oxford technique.[77] All aspects are the same as the DeLorme technique except that, during the exercise session, instead of starting with the lower weights and adding weight to reach 100 per cent of the 10 RM, the subject starts at 100 per cent and subsequently does 10 repetitions at 75 per cent and 10 repetitions at 50 per cent. In this way, the subject is less fatigued and is able to complete all of the prescribed repetitions. The results of the study of mechanical work versus fatigue would suggest that less fatigue

BARBARA J. DE LATEUR AND JUSTUS F. LEHMANN

is a training disadvantage rather than an advantage, but the critical transfer-of-training study of the Oxford technique versus the DeLorme technique remains to be done.

The Oxford and DeLorme techniques are highly effective, time-tested methods of strengthening muscle, but both have actual or potential disadvantages. One such disadvantage is that they are time-consuming, with the need to remove the collars from the bars in order to add or subtract weights and then replace the collars and tighten the screws. The problem of time consumption was even greater with earlier forms of the DeLorme technique, which involved 90 to 100 repetitions, 10 each at 10 per cent of the 10 RM, 30 per cent, 40 per cent, and so on, to 100 per cent of the 10 RM.[16] This time consumption is expensive in the use of therapist and patient time and is multiplied by the number of muscle groups studied. Another potential disadvantage of these techniques, applied to the seated subject attempting to strengthen the quadriceps muscle, is that the force required to extend the knee in the early part of the range (e.g., between 90 and 80 degrees of flexion) is relatively small and becomes greater as the knee approaches full extension. (This illustrates the fact that most dynamic exercises are not correctly called isotonic.) This a purely mechanical factor and is quite distinct from the angle at which the muscle is *able* to exert maximal torque. To the extent that training is joint-angle specific, then the quadriceps will be undertrained in the early part of the range.

Several approaches have been made to the problems of time consumption and uniformity of training. One approach, used by the authors of this chapter and others at the University of Washington hospitals, is to find a weight that the patient can lift three to five times and thereafter count repetitions to fatigue. So that the repetitions are a reliable measure of performance, they should be done to a metronome, raising the weighted limb on one beat and lowering it smoothly on the next. After the session in which the patient reaches 30 repetitions, the weight is increased substantially, so that the patient reverts to the three to five RM range. Thus, the weight needs to be changed only once every several sessions instead of several times per session. Graphing repetitions is an easy way to record and reinforce progress in performance. This method helps reduce time consumption considerably but does nothing about the problem of angle specificity during training.

Ankle and wrist cuff weights with Velcro clo-

sures can help with both problems to some extent. Whether used with the progressive resistive exercise technique of DeLorme, with the Oxford technique, or with the authors' technique, they will save time because of their rapidity of donning and doffing. They can help with the problem of undertraining of the early part of the range if the patient will add one set of repetitions in a different body position. For example, for the second set of quadriceps exercises, the patient could be supine, flex the hip 90 degrees, and take the weighted ankle from full knee flexion to full knee extension. This multiple-position exercise, however, increases the problem of time consumption while helping with the problem of angle of training. Also, the maximal weight of the cuff is limited to about 20 lb.

Another method to conserve time can be derived from the work of Hellebrandt, who showed that muscular performance could be improved by increasing the *rate* of training (rate of contraction) while keeping the load constant.[30] Thus, for example, a weight could be chosen that the patient

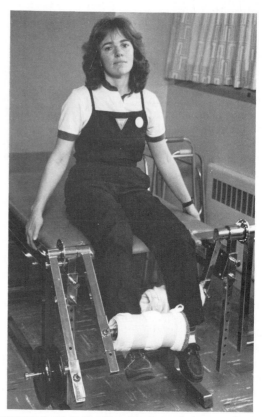

FIGURE 20–44. N-K table with the angle between load and lower arm set at 0 degrees.

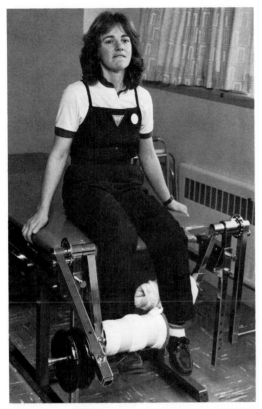

FIGURE 20–45. N-K table with the angle between load and lever arm set at 45 degrees.

can lift 10 to 20 times at the lowest metronome setting (raise on one beat; lower the weighted limb smoothly on the next beat). Thereafter, the load (weight) is kept the same, but each day the metronome setting is increased one notch. The patient carries out repetitions at this new *rate* to fatigue or 20 repetitions, whichever is less. The problem of time is not only controlled but gets a bit better each day. To the authors' knowledge, such a program is not widely used, but has much to recommend it, the chief drawback being the possible annoyance of the tick-tock of the metronome.

The N-K table (Fig. 20–44) is a piece of equipment found in many physical therapy departments. It can help with time consumption and angle problems to a limited extent. Weights can be added and removed rapidly since a collar does not have to be used. Also, changing the angle between the load arm and lever arm (Fig. 20–45) will vary the angle of maximum load on the muscle. It will not, however, be a uniform load throughout the range.

The load *can* be kept uniform throughout the range by the use of pulleys or special cams. On the Elgin table, the load on the hip extensor (Fig. 20–46) or adductors (Fig. 20–47) is maintained nearly constant throughout their range. The single fixed pulley offers no mechanical (force) advantage, but does redirect the angle of pull. Thus, with a single fixed pulley, if a 10-lb weight is used, it requires a 10-lb force to lift or lower it at any point in the range.

At this point, it should be recalled that the torque that can be exerted at any point throughout the range of motion is the net effect of the length-tension relationships and such mechanical factors as angle of application of the tendon of insertion, which vary independently. Figures 20–24 to 20–27 show variability of torque throughout the range for several muscle groups. Since the training effect upon a muscle depends not only upon load but upon the relationship of that load to the muscle's position of maximal voluntary contraction, a *constant* load will have a *variable* effect at different points in the range, having least effect where the muscle is capable of exerting the greatest torque. This complicates the angle-specificity problem further.

This angle-specificity problem is also addressed very well by the Cybex Extremity Testing System, which limits the angular velocity of contraction (rpm; degrees per sec; radians per sec) to some pre-set rate that cannot be exceeded, no matter how forcefully the subject pushes against the lever arm. The device thus provides accommodating resistance that matches anything the muscle can produce (large or small) throughout the range.

The Nautilus system, so named because of somewhat fanciful resemblance of its special cam to a cross section of the sea creature of that name, thoughtfully addresses the problem of uniformity of load throughout the range (Figs. 20–48 and 20–49). Because of the variation of torque that the muscle can exert in various portions of the range, a constant load will not provide uniform stress to the muscle and, therefore, presumably not provide uniform training. The Nautilus equipment is responsive to this problem. The special cam varies the resistance to match the torque curve of each muscle group. Thus, variable resistance is used to provide uniformity of training throughout the range of motion. Because the resistance so closely matches the angle-specific torque capabilities of the muscle, the resistance subjectively seems uniform throughout the range. The Nautilus training program emphasizes slow, very forceful concentric and eccentric contractions, i.e., just to the right

BARBARA J. DE LATEUR AND JUSTUS F. LEHMANN

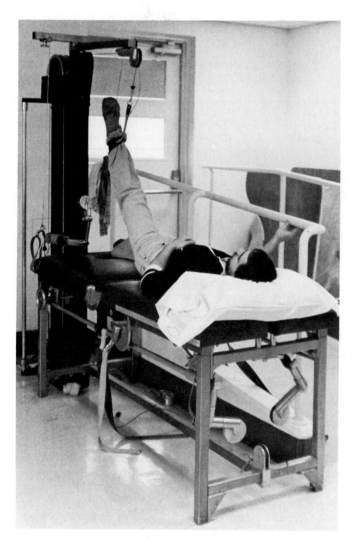

FIGURE 20–46. Exercising hip extension on an Elgin table.

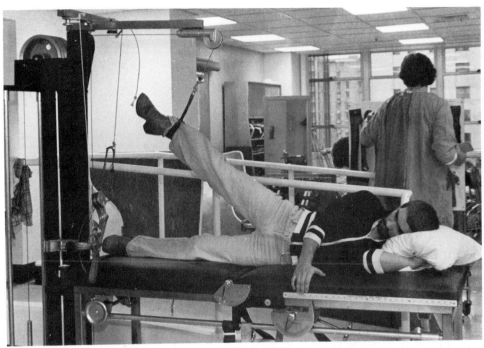

FIGURE 20–47. Exercising hip adduction on an Elgin table.

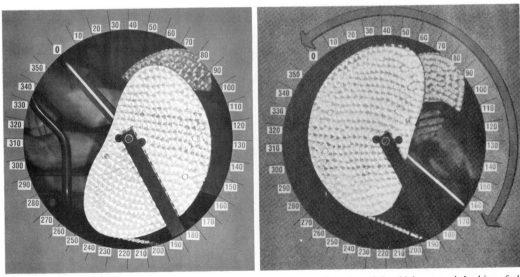

FIGURE 20–48. The Nautilus hip and back machine cam, providing range of motion of the thighs around the hips of about 160 degrees. (Photograph courtesy of Nautilus.)

BARBARA J. DE LATEUR AND JUSTUS F. LEHMANN

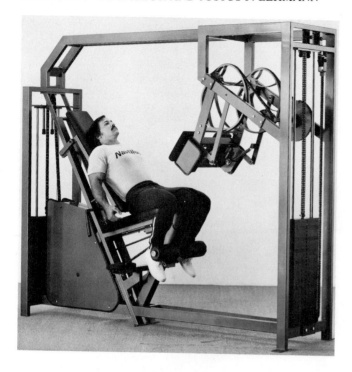

FIGURE 20–49. Nautilus compound leg machine, showing a subject performing a quadriceps extension. The upper portion of the apparatus is used to perform a compound leg press. (Photograph courtesy of Nautilus.)

and to the left of isometrics on the force-velocity curve. Cost of purchase and space required increase with the variety of Nautilus machines desired. At the time of this writing, the machines are more widely used in athletic departments or free-standing Nautilus programs than in hospital physical therapy departments.

The Cybex Extremity Testing System also addresses another problem, i.e., the specificity of rate of training. It was previously pointed out that force of contraction is dependent both on muscular hypertrophy and upon neural factors, such as patterns of recruitment. Evidence was presented that the force-velocity curves can be altered to some extent and thus, if the task for which one is training requires quick movement, it would be wise to do at least some of the training at the higher rpm. The flexibility of this system allows the user to vary the program in many ways. The individual can, for example, begin training at slow rpm's and gradually increase the rate without the annoyance of the metronome accompanying Hellebrandt's and the authors' systems. (In the authors' system, the metronome is desirable, but not essential in clinical application. For the Hellebrandt system, the metronome is necessary even in the clinic. The metronome would be essential for both systems for the precision required in research.) In contrast

to any other system, the Cybex Extremity Testing System has the advantage that it automatically accommodates to any torque the muscle can produce at any rate of contraction. Also, the one system can be adapted to the various large muscle groups of the limbs. Immediate feedback and a permanent record of progress on moving graph paper may be obtained.

It may be noted that the proponents of the Nautilus and the Cybex systems use the same basis, force-velocity curves, to support the use of their respective systems, i.e., low-velocity, high-force training versus high-velocity, lower-force training. Rather than viewing one system as superior to another, it may be wise to emphasize training specificity and to make the training as close as possible to the task one will be performing.

Other isokinetic systems have become available and would include LIDO Active and Digital systems (Loredan Biomedical, Inc., P.O. Box 1154, Davis, CA 95617); Kin-Com (Chattecx Corporation, P.O. Box 4287, Chattanooga, TN 37405); Biodex Multi-Joint System (Biodex Corporation, P. O. Drawer S, Shirley, NY 11967); and Merac (Universal Subsidiary of Kidde, Inc., P.O. Box 1270, Cedar Rapids, IA 52406). The first three systems allow eccentric as well as concentric contractions.

Aerobic Equipment and Physical Disability

As has previously been mentioned, strength and local muscle endurance have been shown to be mathematically related over as large a range as 20 to 100 per cent of maximal contraction ability. However, improving the aerobic capacity of the individual requires prolonged low-level (left-hand portion of curve in Figure 20–16) reciprocal use of multiple muscle groups. There are many options (jogging, cycling, use of the cycle ergometer, and so on) for able-bodied persons, but options for establishing a quantitative aerobic program for persons with lower-extremity physical disabilities, such as paraplegia, are more limited. A useful piece of equipment for persons with such disabilities is the Monark Rehab Trainer (Model No. 881) (Fig. 20–50). This is a true ergometer, permitting quantification of work intensity (power) and total amount of external work accomplished and calories consumed. Programs with such equipment can be varied widely, but to improve aerobic capacity, a low enough intensity should be selected so that the individual can continue for 20 to 30 min (less than 20 min may have insufficient training effect; more than 30 min may be impractical owing to boredom and the expense of patient and therapist time). With improvement in training, the intensity can be increased.

ACKNOWLEDGMENT

This chapter is in part based on research supported by Research Grant #G00830076 from the National Institute on Disability and Rehabilitation Research, Department of Education, Washington, D.C., 20202.

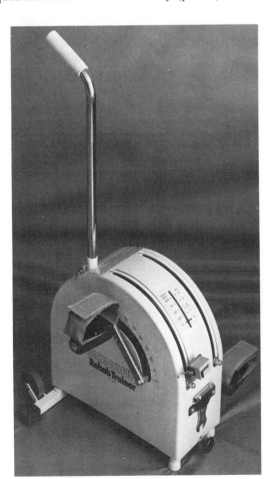

FIGURE 20–50. Rehab trainer.

References

1. Abbott, B. C., Bigland, B., and Ritchie, J. M.: The physiological cost of negative work. J. Physiol., 117:380–390, 1952.
2. Arkin, A. M.: Absolute muscle power: The internal kinesiology of muscle. Master of Science thesis, Department of Orthopedic Surgery, State University of Iowa, 1939.
3. Asmussen, E., Hansen, O., and Lammert, O.: The relation between isometric and dynamic muscle strength in man. Commun. Danish Nat. Assoc. Inf. Paral., 20:3–11, 1965.
4. Barnes, W. S.: The relationship between maximum isokinetic strength and isokinetic endurance. Res. Q., 51:714–717, 1980.
5. Bergström, J.: Muscle electrolytes in man. Scand. J. Clin. Lab. Invest., 14 [suppl 68]:11–13, 1962.
6. Bethe, A., and Franke, F.: Beiträge zum Problem der willkürlich beweglichen Armprothesen. IV. Die Kraftkurven der indirekten natürlichen Energiequellen. Münch. Med. Wochenschr., 66:201–205, 1919.
7. Braune, W., and Fischer, O.: Die Rotationsmomente der Beugemuskeln am Ellbogengelenk des Menschen. Abhandlungen der Königlich Sächsischen Gesellschaft der Wissenschaften, 26:243–310, 1890.
8. Brunnstrom, S.: Clinical Kinesiology, 2nd Ed. Philadelphia, F. A. Davis, 1966.
9. Caiozzo, V. J., Perrine, J. J., and Edgerton, V. R.: Training-induced alterations of the in vivo force-velocity relationship of human muscle. J. Appl. Physiol., 51:750–754, 1981.
10. Close, R. I.: Dynamic properties of mammalian skeletal muscles. Physiol. Rev., 52:129–197, 1972.
11. de Lateur, B. J., Alquist, A. D., Giaconi, R. M., and Esselman, P. C.: Specificity of velocity of train-

BARBARA J. DE LATEUR AND JUSTUS F. LEHMANN

ing: Unexpected outcome. Arch. Phys. Med. Rehabil., 67:643, 1986.

12. de Lateur, B. J., Lehmann, J. F., and Fordyce, W. E.: A test of the DeLorme axiom. Arch. Phys. Med. Rehabil., 49:245–248, 1968.

13. de Lateur, B. J., Lehmann, J. F., and Giaconi, R.: Mechanical work and fatigue: Their roles in the development of muscle work capacity. Arch. Phys. Med. Rehabil., 57:319–324, 1976.

14. de Lateur, B., Lehmann, J., Stonebridge, J., and Warren, C. G.: Isotonic versus isometric exercise: A double-shift transfer-of-training study. Arch. Phys. Med. Rehabil., 53:212–217, 1972.

15. DeLorme, T. L.: Restoration of muscle power by heavy-resistance exercises. J. Bone. Joint. Surg. 27A:645–667, 1945.

16. DeLorme, T. L., and Watkins, A. L.: Progressive Resistance Exercise. East Norwalk, CT, Appleton-Century-Crofts, 1951.

17. Desmedt, J. E., and Godaux, E.: Ballistic contractions in man: Characteristic recruitment pattern of single motor units of the tibialis anterior muscle. J. Physiol., 264:673–693, 1977.

18. Engel, W. K.: Selective and nonselective susceptibility of muscle fiber types. Arch. Neurol., 22:97–117, 1970.

19. Fugl-Meyer, A. R., Gustafsson, L., and Burstedt, Y.: Isokinetic and static plantar flexion characteristics. Eur. J. Appl. Physiol., 45:221–234, 1980.

20. Gollnick, P. D., Armstrong, R. B., Saltin, B., Saubert, C. W., IV, Sembrowich, W. L., and Shepherd, R. E.: Effect of training on enzyme activity and fiber composition of human skeletal muscle. J. Appl. Physiol., 34:107–111, 1973.

21. Gollnick, P. D., Armstrong, R. B., Saubert, C. W., IV, Piehl, K., and Saltin, B.: Enzyme activity and fiber composition in skeletal muscle of untrained and trained men. J. Appl. Physiol., 33:312–319, 1972.

22. Gollnick, P. D., Armstrong, R. B., Saubert, C. W., IV, Sembrowich, W. L., Shepherd, R. E., and Saltin, B.: Glycogen depletion patterns in human skeletal muscle fibers during prolonged work. Pflügers Arch., 344:1–12, 1973.

23. Gollnick, P. D., Karlsson, J., Piehl, K., and Saltin, B.: Selective glycogen depletion in skeletal muscle fibres of man following sustained contractions. J. Physiol., 241:59–67, 1974.

24. Gollnick, P. D., Piehl, K., and Saltin, B.: Selective glycogen depletion pattern in human muscle fibres after exercise of varying intensity and at varying pedalling rates. J. Physiol., 241:45–57, 1974.

25. Gonyea, W. J., Sale, D. G., Gonyea, F. B., and Mikesky, A.: Exercise induced increases in muscle fiber number. Eur. J. Appl. Physiol., 55:137–141, 1986.

26. Gordon, E. E., Kowalski, K., and Fritts, M.: Protein changes in quadriceps muscle of rat with repetitive exercises. Arch. Phys. Med. Rehabil., 48:296–303, 1967.

27. Gregor, R. J., Edgerton, V. R., Perrine, J. J., Campion, D. S., and DeBus, C.: Torque-velocity relationships and muscle fiber composition in elite female athletes. J. Appl. Physiol., 47:388–392, 1979.

28. Guth, L.: "Trophic" influences of nerve on muscle. Physiol. Rev., 48:645–687, 1968.

29. Guth, L., Samaha, F. J., and Albers, R. W.: The neural regulation of some phenotypic differences between the fiber types of mammalian skeletal muscle. Exp. Neurol., 26:126–135, 1970.

30. Hellebrandt, F. A., and Houtz, S. J.: Methods of muscle training: The influence of pacing. Phys. Ther. Rev., 38:319–322, 1958.

31. Henneman, E.: Peripheral mechanisms involved in the control of muscle. In Mountcastle, V. B. (Ed.), Medical Physiology, 13th Ed. St. Louis, C. V. Mosby, 1974.

32. Hettinger, T., and Müller, E. A.: Muskelleistung und Muskeltraining. Arbeitsphysiol., 15:111–126, 1953.

33. Hickson, R. C.: Interference of strength development by simultaneously training for strength and endurance. Eur. J. Appl. Physiol., 45:255–263, 1980.

34. Hill, A. V.: The dynamic constants of human muscle. Proc. R. Soc., 128B:263–274, 1940.

35. Hill, A. V.: The heat of shortening and the dynamic constants of muscle. Proc. R. Soc., 126B:135–195, 1938.

36. Ianuzzo, C. D.: The cellular composition of human skeletal muscle. In Knuttgen, H. G. (Ed.): Neuromuscular Mechanisms for Therapeutic and Conditioning Exercise. Baltimore, MD, University Park Press, 1976.

37. Infante, A. A., Klaupiks, D., and Davies, R. E.: Length, tension and metabolism during short isometric contractions of frog sartorius muscles. Biochim. Biophys. Acta, 88:215–217, 1964.

38. Kennedy, C., Van Huss, W. D., and Heusner, W. W.: Reversal of the energy metabolism responses to endurance training by weight loading. Percept. Mot. Skills, 39:847–852, 1974.

39. Keul, J., Doll, E., and Keppler, D.: Energy stores of the muscle cell and anaerobic energy supply. Med. Sport. 7:19–51, 1972.

40. Kidd, G., and Brodie, P.: The motor unit: A review. Physiother., 66:146–152, 1980.

41. Knapik, J. J., and Ramos, M. U.: Isokinetic and isometric torque relationships in the human body. Arch. Phys. Med. Rehabil., 61:64–67, 1980.

42. Knuttgen, H. G.: Development of muscular strength and endurance. In Knuttgen, H. G. (Ed.): Neuromuscular Mechanisms for Therapeutic and Conditioning Exercise. Baltimore, MD, University Park Press, 1976.

43. Komi, P. V.: Training of muscle strength and power:

Interaction of neuromotoric, hypertrophic, and mechanical factors. Int. J. Sports Med., 7[suppl]:10–15, 1986.

44. Kottke, F. J., and Mundale, M. O.: Personal communication.

45. Liberson, W. T.: Further studies of brief isometric exercises. Arch. Phys. Med. Rehabil., 40:330–336, 1957.

46. Lloyd, B. B.: World running records as maximal performances. Circ. Res. 20,21 [suppl 1]:I-218–I-226, 1967.

47. Lüthi, J. M., Howald, H., Claassen, H., Rösler, K., Vock, P., and Hoppeler, H.: Structural changes in skeletal muscle tissue with heavy resistance exercise. Int. J. Sports Med., 7:123–127, 1986.

48. MacDougall, J. D., Elder, G. C. B., Sale, D. G., Moroz, J. R., and Sutton, J. R.: Effects of strength training and immobilization on human muscle fibres. Eur. J. Appl. Physiol., 43:25–34, 1980.

49. Maton, B.: Fast and slow motor units: Their recruitment for tonic and phasic contraction in normal man. Eur. J. Appl. Physiol., 43:45–55, 1980.

50. Milner-Brown, H. S., Stein, R. B., and Lee, R. G.: Synchronization of human motor units: Possible roles of exercise and supraspinal reflexes. Electroenceph. Clin. Neurophysiol., 38:245–254, 1975.

51. Moffroid, M. T., and Whipple, R. H.: Specificity of speed of exercise. Phys. Ther., 50:1692–1700, 1970.

52. Monod, H., and Scherrer, J.: Capacité de travail statique d'un groupe musculaire synergique chez l'Homme. C. R. Soc. Biol., 151:1358–1362, 1957; cited in Simonson, E. (Ed.): Physiology of Work Capacity and Fatigue. Springfield, IL, Charles C. Thomas, 1971.

53. Moritani, T., and deVries, H. A.: Neural factors versus hypertrophy in the time course of muscle strength gain. Am. J. Phys. Med., 58:115–130, 1979.

54. Müller, E. A.: Influence of training and of inactivity on muscle strength. Arch. Phys. Med. Rehabil., 51:449–462, 1970.

55. Mundale, M. O.: The relationship of intermittent isometric exercise to fatigue of hand grip. Arch. Phys. Med. Rehabil., 51:532–539, 1970.

56. Mundale, M. O.: A study of the relationship of endurance during isometric exercise to strength of isometric contraction of the muscles of hand grip. Master of Science thesis, University of Minnesota, 1964.

57. Perrine, J. J., and Edgerton, V. R.: Muscle force-velocity and power-velocity relationships under isokinetic loading. Med. Sci. Sports, 10:159–166, 1978.

58. Rohmert, W.: Ermittlung von Erholungspausen für statistische Arbeit des Menschen. Int. Z. angew. Physiol. einschl. Arbeitsphysiol., 18:123–164, 1960; cited in Simonson, E. (Ed.): Physiology of Work Capacity and Fatigue. Springfield, IL, Charles C. Thomas, 1971.

59. Rose, D. L., Radzyminski, S. F., and Beatty, R. R.: Effect of brief maximal exercise on the strength of the quadriceps femoris. Arch. Phys. Med. Rehabil., 38:157–164, 1957.

60. Saltin, B., and Åstrand, P-O.: Maximal oxygen uptake in athletes. J. Appl. Physiol., 23:353–358, 1967.

61. Samaha, F. J., Guth, L., and Albers, R. W.: Differences between slow and fast muscle myosin. J. Biol. Chem., 245:219–224, 1970.

62. Samaha, F. J., Guth, L., and Albers, R. W.: The neural regulation of gene expression in the muscle cell. Exp. Neurol., 27:276–282, 1970.

63. Scherrer, J., and Bourguignon, A.: Changes in the electromyogram produced by fatigue in man. Am. J. Phys. Med., 38:148–158, 1959.

64. Schottelius, B. A., and Senay, L. C., Jr: Effect of stimulation-length sequence on shape of length-tension diagram. Am. J. Physiol., 186:127–130, 1956.

65. Scudder, G. N.: Torque curves produced at the knee during isometric and isokinetic exercise. Arch. Phys. Med. Rehabil., 61:68–73, 1980.

66. Seliger, V., Dolejs, L., and Karas, V.: A dynamometric comparison of maximum eccentric, concentric and isometric contractions using EMG and energy expenditure measurements. Eur. J. Appl. Physiol., 45:235–244, 1980.

67. Shaver, L. G.: Maximum dynamic strength, relative dynamic endurance, and their relationships. Res. Q., 42:460–465, 1971.

68. Simonson, E.: Recovery and fatigue. In Simonson, E. (Ed.): Physiology of Work Capacity and Fatigue. Springfield, IL, Charles C. Thomas, 1971.

69. Smith, M. J., and Melton, P.: Isokinetic versus isotonic variable-resistance training. Am. J. Sports Med., 9:275–279, 1981.

70. Soule, R. G.: Physiological response to physical exercise. In Knuttgen, H. G. (Ed.): Neuromuscular Mechanisms for Therapeutic and Conditioning Exercise. Baltimore, MD, University Park Press, 1976.

71. Steindler, A.: Kinesiology of the Human Body. Springfield, IL, Charles C. Thomas, 1955.

72. Thorstensson, A., Grimby, G., and Karlsson, J.: Force-velocity relations and fiber composition in human knee extensor muscles. J. Appl. Physiol., 40:12–16, 1976.

73. Tuttle, W. W., Janney, C. D., and Thompson, C. W.: Relation of maximum grip strength to grip strength endurance. J. Appl. Physiol., 2:663–670, 1950.

74. Von Recklinghausen, H.: Gliedermechanik und Lähmungsprothesen. New York, Springer, 1920.

75. Wells, J. B.: Comparison of mechanical properties between slow and fast mammalian muscles. J. Physiol., 178:252–269, 1965.

76. Wilkie, D. R.: The relation between force and velocity in human muscle. J. Physiol., 110:249–280, 1950.

77. Zinovieff, A. N.: Heavy-resistance exercises: The "Oxford" technique. Br. J. Phys. Med., 14:129–132, 1951.

21

Bed Positioning

PAUL M. ELLWOOD, JR.

The prevention and treatment of contractures and decubiti through an effective bed positioning program is contingent upon proper equipment, a well-trained and well-motivated nursing staff, and appropriate physician's orders.

The Positioning Prescription

The positioning prescription should identify the equipment specifically needed for the positioning program, positions to be used, motions and positions to be avoided, and frequency of turning. In addition, it is important to recognize that the patient should assume increasing responsibility for the positioning program. If they are able, the patients should remind the staff when they need to be turned, know where positioning equipment is kept, actually assist in changing positions, and ultimately assume full responsibility.

The Equipment for Effective Bed Positioning

High-Low Bed. The use of beds that are adjustable to high (30 inches including the mattress) and low (20 inches including the mattress) positions is recommended. With the bed in the high position, more comfortable and efficient nursing care and range of motion exercises can be carried out. In the low position, the bed can be set at the ideal height for wheelchair transfers or crutch-walking.

Bed Boards. A ¾-inch plywood bed board equal in size to the spring frame is bolted between the spring and mattress (Fig. 21–1). Jointed (Gatch) features can be retained by breaking the continuity of the board at the hinge points. Some hospital beds now have a metal panel that substitutes for springs and provides excellent mattress support. Also available are slatted bed boards, which have the advantage of flexibility.

Mattresses. Firmness and durability are sought in mattress selection. Uniform firm support is obtained through a foam rubber mattress. A 4-inch foam rubber mattress made of 34-lb compression ratio material is the firmest available. Urethane foam of the same compression ratio is still undergoing evaluation for rehabilitation uses. The firm support provided by bed board and mattress is especially valuable in preventing hip flexion contractures.

Footboards. Heel cord contractures are prevented by the use of a footboard. It has been suggested, but not proved, that the footboard provides a valuable source of sensory input to the plantar surface of the feet so that the desirable extensor reflex dominance is maintained and the neuron networks normally involved in the standing position are activated. The board should be ½-inch thick and sufficiently high to keep the bedclothes from contact with the toes. To prevent decubiti over the posterior calcaneus and to facilitate prone positioning without knee flexion, the board is blocked 4 inches away from the end of the mattress (Fig. 21–2).

Short Side Rails. Side rails are used for safety, moving about, coming to a sitting position, and transferring in and out of bed (Fig. 21–3). Commercial short side rails are 33 inches long and should extend 11 inches above the level of the mattress. For most patients, the rails are attached only to the head end of the bed. If side rails are not required for protection, a single short rail is

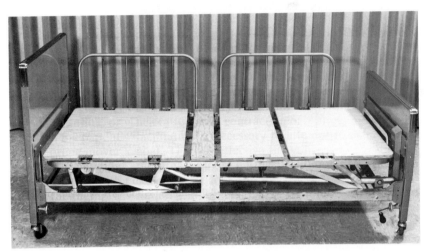

FIGURE 21–1. Three-quarter-inch plywood bed board.

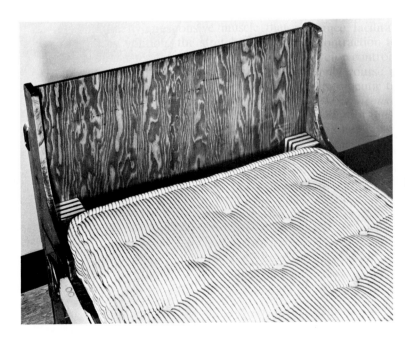

FIGURE 21–2. Footboard.

PAUL M. ELLWOOD, JR.

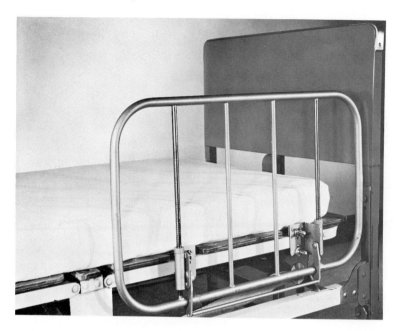

FIGURE 21–3. Short side rail.

attached at the head end of the bed on the stronger side to which the patient transfers.

Overhead Trapezes. Trapezes are rarely necessary to facilitate moving about in bed or for upper extremity exercise. In making unassisted transfers, they are not as useful as short side rails. They do simplify nursing care of very large patients or those in casts.

Positioning Frames (Foster, Stryker, and Others). When immobility of the spine is required, a bed consisting of canvas stretched on anterior and posterior frames that can be rotated along their long axes is used. Footboards for frames are often available and should be used. The narrow metal-rimmed canvas surface of the frame can be satisfactorily padded with 1-inch foam rubber covered with plastic. The foam rubber for the trunk section of the prone unit should be wider than the metal frame to protect the shoulders from pressure when the patient's arms are dropped downward for eating or reading. The foam rubber of the lower extremity section of the prone unit should be slightly longer than the canvas frame to protect the front of the patient's ankles. The foam rubber pieces of the supine section should cover the canvas to protect the patient's sacral area when using the bedpan. Armboards are available for positioning the upper extremities of the quadriplegic patient.

Powered Rotating Frames. Electrically powered frames that rotate along their short axes can be used to substitute for both canvas frames and standing beds. They permit more comfortable positioning and changes in position by the patient or a single staff member by the operation of remote control switches. They are costly, however, and because of their complexity are more subject to mechanical failure.

Standing Beds. Electrically or manually controlled beds to elevate patients to the upright position are thought to aid in the reduction of osteoporosis and renal calculi, the maintenance of vascular tone (thus preventing postural hypotension), the preservation of morale, and the shifting of weight-bearing to relieve pressure in other areas. Postural hypotension due to pooling in splanchnic and lower extremity veins is prevented in part by the use of scultetus binders and by wrapping the legs with 6-inch elastic bandages. Blood pressure should be taken at frequent intervals by the attendant. No patient on a standing bed should be left unattended. Many patients cannot attain the upright position on the first occasion on the standing bed. A useful routine is to begin at 30 degrees for 30 minutes. When this is readily tolerated, increase by 5- to 10-degree increments. Binders and bandages are progressively eliminated after the patient attains 80 degrees.

Small Positioning Devices. Most quadriplegic patients will require two trochanter rolls, two

TABLE 21–1. Some Common Deforming Forces

FORCE	RESULTANT DEFORMITY	METHOD OF PREVENTION
Gravity	Sagging mattress and springs + gravity = hip flexion contractures	Firm mattress plus bed board, prone position, prone cart
Shape of the extremity surface	Configuration of the ankle and foot + gravity = external rotation of the lower extremity and a tight gastrocnemius	A trochanter roll and footboard
Muscular imbalance	High above-knee amputation + strong hip abductors = hip abduction contracture	Prone position with leg adducted and internally rotated
Spasticity	Paraplegia + flexor spasticity = hip and knee flexion contractures	Prone position, buttocks and knees strapped in extension, prone cart, knee lockers during gait-training

shoulder rolls, three hand rolls, two small pillows, six large pillows, 6-inch-wide canvas straps, and, in the presence of lower extremity abduction spasticity, a 6-inch-wide canvas strap lined with soft leather. The application of these devices is described later in this chapter.

The Positioning Program

Positioning instructions and turning schedules are based on individual patient needs, but certain generalizations can be made about most disabilities that are associated with muscle weakness or joint deformity. In some institutions that serve large numbers of the chronically disabled, it has been found desirable to establish a set of positioning procedures for hemiplegia, quadriplegia, and paraplegia. The physician's order then may specify variations from the routine positioning procedure, positions to be avoided, and areas to be kept immobilized. Positions are prescribed to overcome certain natural and pathological forces, to provide a variety of joint positions for maintaining joint range, and to place the extremity in a more functional position (Table 21–1).

The Supine Position

Lower Extremities. The feet are positioned with the entire plantar surface firmly against the footboard. Contact with the posterior heel is avoided by placing it in the space between the mattress and the footboard that has been created by 4-inch-thick blocks. The legs are placed in a neutral position with the toes pointed toward the ceiling (Fig. 21–4). This position is maintained by friction of the feet against the footboard and a cloth roll placed under the greater trochanter (trochanter roll).

The knee and hips are positioned in extension (Fig. 21–5). Perhaps the most critical element of

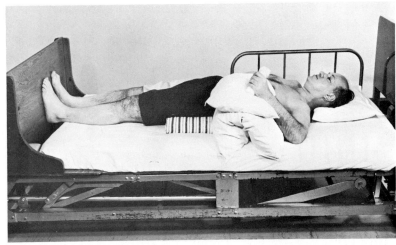

FIGURE 21–4. Routine positioning of lower extremities, plus one possible arm position.

PAUL M. ELLWOOD, JR.

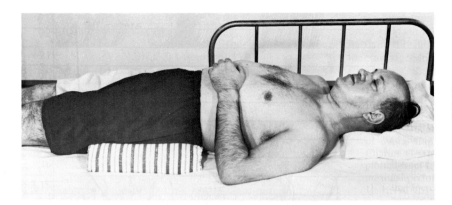

FIGURE 21–5. Use of trochanter roll in positioning of lower extremities.

the lower extremity positioning program is the prevention of hip and knee flexion contractures. Hip flexion contractures in the presence of lower extremity weakness are the principal deterrents to ambulation for patients with hemiplegia, paraplegia, and above-knee amputations. Stance phase stability of the knee and hip joints requires full extension so that gravitational forces are applied against ligaments and the normal configuration of the joint rather than requiring muscle power.

Upper Extremities. Nurses should be cautioned to position only within the painless or nonresistive range of motion. Spasticity must, however, be differentiated from other forms of resistance to joint motion.

POSITION 1. The shoulder is abducted to 90 degrees and slightly internally rotated, the elbow is at 90 degrees, and the forearm is partially pronated (Fig. 21–6).

POSITION 2. The shoulder is abducted to 90 degrees or more and externally rotated to the greatest degree compatible with comfort. The elbow is flexed at 90 degrees, and the forearm is pronated (Fig. 21–7).

POSITION 3. The shoulder is in slight abduction, the elbow extended, and the forearm supinated (Fig. 21–8).

Wrist and Hand

POSITION 1. The wrist is extended, the fingers are partially flexed at the interphalangeal and metacarpophalangeal joints, and the thumb is abducted, opposed, and slightly flexed at the interphalangeal joint (Fig. 21–9). Maintenance of these positions is facilitated by the use of a hand roll (Fig. 21–10).

POSITION 2. This position is similar to position 1 except that the fingers are extended at the

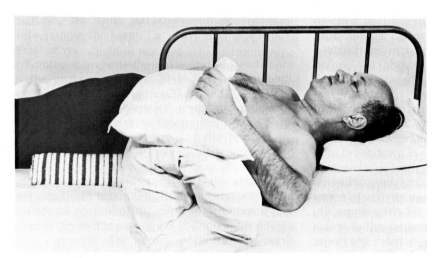

FIGURE 21–6. Positioning of the upper extremities, position 1.

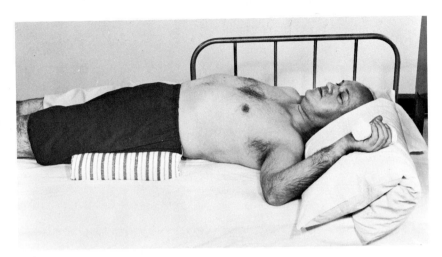

FIGURE 21–7. Positioning of the upper extremities, position 2.

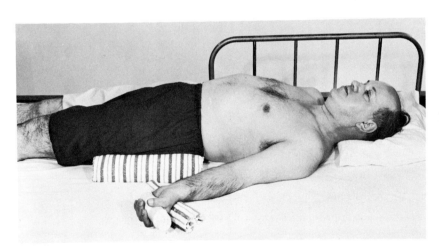

FIGURE 21–8. Positioning of the upper extremities, position 3.

FIG. 21–9 FIG. 21–10

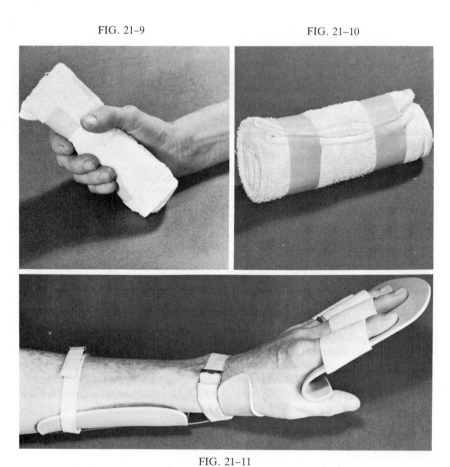

FIG. 21–11

FIGURE 21–9. Positioning of the wrist and hand, position 1.

FIGURE 21–10. Hand roll for use in wrist and hand positioning.

FIGURE 21–11. Palmar positioning splint for use in wrist and hand positioning, position 2.

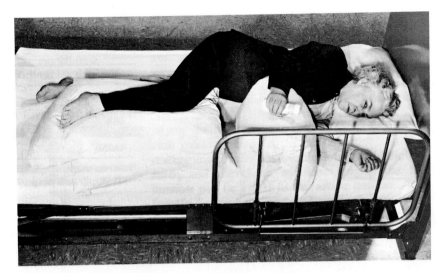

FIGURE 21-12. Side-lying position.

interphalangeal and metacarpophalangeal joints. A palmar positioning splint can be used to maintain this position (Fig. 21-11). The positioning program for the wrist and fingers should be particularly directed to *maintenance of joint motion of the wrist* from neutral to a fully extended position, *a full range of motion in the metacarpophalangeal joints,* flexion of the interphalangeal joints, and opposition of the thumb. To obtain tenodesis grasp in the quadriplegic patient who retains wrist extensor function, arthrodesis of thumb joints and interphalangeal joints to form a three-jawed chuck may be sought.

Side-Lying Position

Hemiplegic patients are most comfortable lying on their uninvolved side. Paraplegics and quadriplegics should be positioned on either side when they can tolerate it. The top leg is placed in a position of flexion at the hip and knee. Through use of pillows, contact with the under leg is avoided. The inner (bottom) arm is externally rotated and partially extended. The outer (top) arm is kept away from the patient's chest (Fig. 21-12).

The Prone Position

The prone position is ordered when pulmonary, cardiac, and skeletal status permit. Many patients do not tolerate it well at first. It is highly advantageous in maintaining full extension of the hips and relieving pressure over vulnerable posterior bony prominences that so commonly are sites of decubiti. The prone position also has its vulnerable points, such as the skin over the sternum, the iliac spines, the patella, and the dorsum of the foot. These areas should be inspected frequently. Foam rubber can be used above and below the contact points when pressure is producing focal ischemia. Synthetic fibers or sheepskin are also useful to protect the bony prominences. Narrow doughnut-shaped devices should *not* be used. They actually inhibit circulation to ischemic areas.

The prone position (Fig. 21-13) is simply one of good alignment with hips and knees extended. Toes should not be allowed to touch the footboard. The feet can be elevated slightly using a trochanter roll under the anterior ankle.

The arm is abducted slightly, extended at the elbow, and extended and supinated at the wrist. Finger flexion and wrist extension are achieved through the use of a hand roll. Shoulder rolls are placed lengthwise under each shoulder.

Frequency of Turning

Turning the patient every two hours is usually a safe routine to follow until the patient's skin sen-

PAUL M. ELLWOOD, JR.

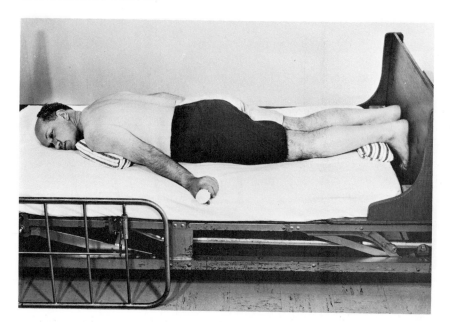

FIGURE 21–13. Prone position.

sitivity and tolerance of the positions have been determined. It may be necessary to decrease the amount of time spent in certain positions, or it may be found that time in other positions can be increased to two and a half or three hours. Generally it is best to order the more prolonged positioning periods for the night hours, thus lessening the amount of turning at night and enabling the patient to sleep more satisfactorily. More frequent turning will automatically be needed during the day to allow the desired positions for the patient's daily activities. Nursing staff should be encouraged to set up a definite schedule so that the patient will be in a proper position for activities (such as supine for physical therapy).

The physician should frequently check the skin in vulnerable areas to make certain that no decubiti are developing and to emphasize to the attending staff the importance of a proper turning schedule. Increased activities in the use of various appliances should call attention to new possible areas of ischemic ulceration. The patient who is spending a great deal of time in a wheelchair should have particularly close observation for possible ischemia in the region of the ischial tuberosities.

References

1. Coles, C. H., and Bergstrom, D. A.: Bed Positioning Procedures. Minneapolis, American Rehabilitation Foundation, 1969.
2. Elson, R.: Practical Management of Spinal Injuries for Nurses. Baltimore, Williams & Wilkins, 1965.
3. Hicks, D., Scarlisi, S., Woody, F., and Skinner, B.: Increasing upper extremity function. Am. J. Nurs., 64:69–73, 1964.
4. Hirshberg, G., Lewis, L., and Thomas, D.: Rehabilitation: A Manual for the Care of the Disabled and Elderly. Philadelphia, J. B. Lippincott, 1964.
5. Kosiak, M.: Etiology and pathology of ischemic ulcers. Arch. Phys. Med., 40:62–69, 1959.
6. Kosiak, M.: Etiology of decubitus ulcers. Arch. Phys. Med., 42:19–29, 1961.
7. Larson, C., and Gould, M.: Orthopedic Nursing. St. Louis, C. V. Mosby, 1970.
8. Strike Back at Stroke. U.S. Department of Health, Education and Welfare, Public Health Service Publication No. 596. U.S. Government Printing Office, Washington, DC 20201, 1960.
9. Sverdlik, S. S., and Chantraine, A.: A spongy cushion over hypersensitive areas of the skin to increase threshold to pain. Arch. Phys. Med., 45:430–432, 1964.

22
Transfers—Method, Equipment, and Preparation

PAUL M. ELLWOOD, JR.

A transfer is a pattern of movements by which the patient moves from one surface to another. This chapter is limited to a discussion of transfers to and from wheelchairs, since these are the earliest and most common types of transfer for the patient with neuromuscular disability. The ingredients of safe and efficient transfers are a combination of physical and perceptual capacities, proper equipment, and techniques that are suited to the patient's abilities. Firm, stable surfaces for the patient to move to and from are required for all transfers. It is also necessary that the patient have the ability to learn motor skills.

Assisted Transfers

Techniques for assisted transfers are not demonstrated in this chapter. However, assistance by another person for physical support and reinforcement of learning may be required during early learning, or permanently for more severely disabled patients. In an assisted transfer, the same general techniques are used, with the assistant compensating for the patient's inabilities. Providing support at the waist with a transfer belt assures a good grip on the patient without restricting the patient's use of the arms (Fig. 22–1).

Standing Transfers

Physical Requirements. The unassisted standing transfer requires good sitting balance without postural hypotension; the ability to maintain the hip and knee in a position of extension by means of voluntary muscle contraction, long leg braces, or extensor spasticity; reasonably strong shoulder depressors and adductors, elbow flexors and extensors; and, preferably, hand and wrist function on one side.

Preparing the Patient for Standing Transfers. Activities helpful in preparation for standing transfers are sitting on the edge of the bed without making a transfer; daily use of the standing bed, followed by actual standing at the parallel bar and practice in locking the knee; exercises designed to strengthen hip and knee extensors, shoulder depressors and adductors, and elbow and wrist extensors on the normal side; and mat work and bed activities to improve the ability to roll, balance, and shift weight.

Teaching Transfers. The process of teaching the patient to make a transfer with assistance is begun as soon as the patient is able to balance in the sitting position. Patients should be taught in short sequences, and they should master each step before proceeding to the next. Even patients with no verbal language can be taught to transfer by repetition and demonstration. Visual motor-perceptual defects may prevent motor learning.

Technique. Most transfers are made toward the more normal or stronger side, regardless of the cause of the disability. This text uses as an example a hemiplegic patient, but the principles set forth apply to any patient who can attain a stable standing position during the course of the transfer.

529

PAUL M. ELLWOOD, JR.

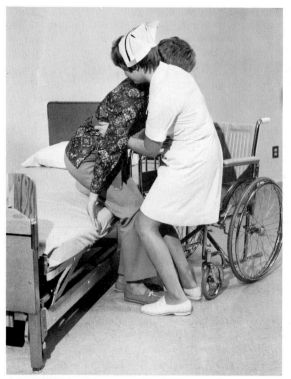

FIGURE 22–1. Using a belt around the patient's waist, the nurse assists her in a standing transfer.

Bed to Wheelchair Transfer

Equipment. The necessary equipment includes a stable bed approximately the same height as the wheelchair (a short side rail attached at the head end of the bed is optional) and a wheelchair with brakes and detachable footrests. For the hemiplegic patient, the footrest on the normal side should be removed.

Layout. The wheelchair is on the patient's normal side; it is slightly angled toward the foot of the bed for the transfer out of bed (Fig. 22–2) and toward the head of the bed for the transfer into bed. The footrest adjacent to the bed is removed or swung aside.

Coming to a Sitting Position. The patient begins the sequence lying in the center of the bed. With her normal hand, she picks up her involved arm at the wrist and places the forearm across her abdomen (Fig. 22–3).

The patient places her normal foot under the knee of her involved leg and slides her foot down the leg to her ankle. She then partly flexes and lifts her involved leg with her normal foot and leg.

Keeping the same foot-support position, she grasps the side rail with her normal hand and, rolling her legs toward her normal side, turns onto her side (Fig. 22–4).

Then, as she moves her legs over the edge of the bed, the patient grasps and pulls on the side rail and swings herself to a sitting position (Fig. 22–5). She makes full use of gravity and momentum by performing these motions in one unit. She then uncrosses her feet and places them firmly on the floor to maintain balance.

Coming to a Standing Position and Completing the Transfer. From her sitting position at the edge of the bed, the patient locks the brakes on both sides of the wheelchair, locking the rear brake first. By leaning her trunk forward and pushing down at the same time with her normal hand and foot, she moves forward toward the edge of the bed. She then flexes her normal knee more than 90 degrees and moves her normal foot slightly behind the involved foot so that her feet will be free to pivot. Grasping the side rail (or the middle of the farther armrest of the wheelchair if balance is poor), the patient is now in a position for standing (Fig. 22–6).

She moves her trunk forward, pushes down with her normal arm, and, bearing most of her weight on the normal leg, comes to a standing position (Fig. 22–7).

She moves her hand to the middle of the far arm of the wheelchair and pivots on her feet, bringing herself into a position to sit down (Fig. 22–8). After sitting down in the chair, she adjusts her sitting position, unlocks the brakes, lifts her involved foot with her normal foot, and backs the wheelchair away from the bed. Finally the patient swings the footrest into position and, lifting her involved leg with her normal hand, places her foot on the footrest.

Standing Transfer from Wheelchair to Low Bed

Again, the transfer is made toward the normal side. The wheelchair faces the head of the bed (Fig. 22–9). After locking the brakes and taking her involved foot off the footrest, the patient swings the footrest out of the way. By leaning forward and pushing down, she moves forward toward the edge of the wheelchair until her feet are under her and her normal foot is slightly behind the involved foot. Holding onto the wheelchair

Text continued on page 535

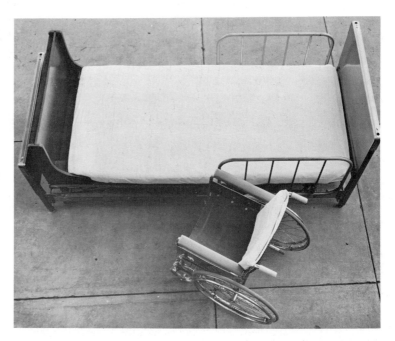

FIGURE 22–2. Position of the wheelchair for the standing transfer out of bed.

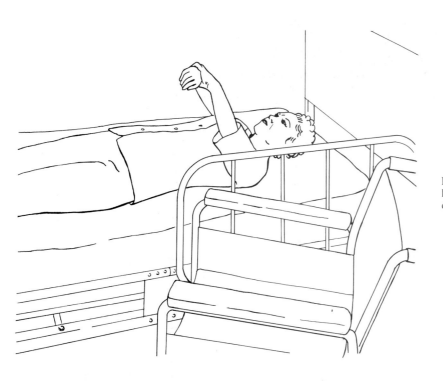

FIGURE 22–3. The patient moves her involved arm in preparation for coming to a sitting position.

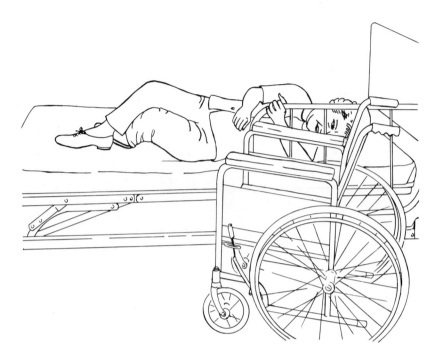

FIGURE 22–4. She moves her involved foot and leg, grasps the side rail, and turns onto her normal side.

FIGURE 22–5. She swings into a sitting position.

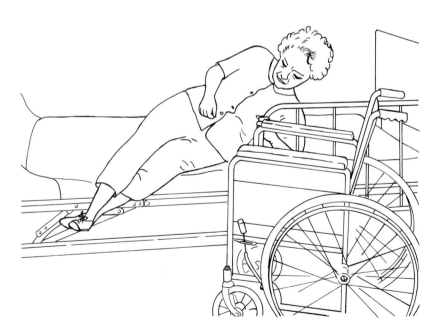

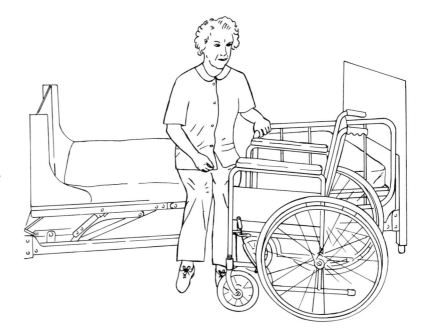

FIGURE 22–6. Grasping the side rail, the patient prepares to stand.

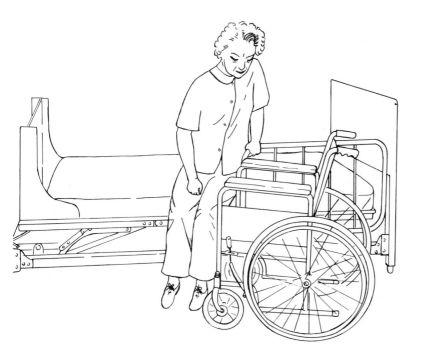

FIGURE 22–7. The patient comes to a standing position.

PAUL M. ELLWOOD, JR.

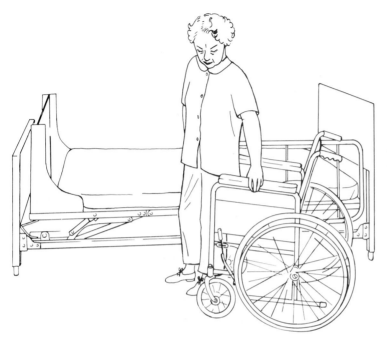

FIGURE 22–8. Grasping the far arm of the wheelchair, she pivots, and prepares to sit down.

FIGURE 22–9. Position of the wheelchair for the standing transfer from chair to bed.

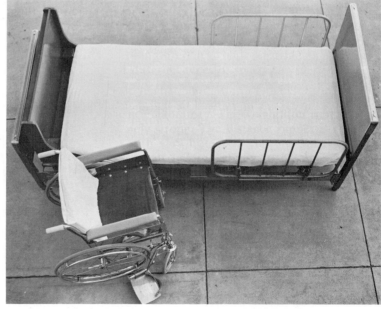

armrest (or the side rail), the patient moves her trunk forward and, bearing her weight on her normal leg and arm, comes to a standing position. After standing erect, she moves her hand to the side rail and pivots on her feet, bringing herself into a position to sit on the bed. Seated on the edge of the bed, she moves the wheelchair away so that she can swing her legs onto the bed and lie down.

Standing Transfer from Wheelchair to Toilet

A special requirement for an unassisted toilet transfer is that the patient be able to manage clothing.

Equipment. Preferably, the toilet seat is mounted 20 inches from the floor. Raised seats that can be fastened securely to the toilet bowl are available from hospital supply companies (Fig. 22–

10). The placement of a handrail generally depends on the position of the toilet in relationship to the side walls of the bathroom. The rail should be on the same side as the normal extremities when the patient is seated on the toilet. It is mounted on the wall at a 45-degree angle with the lower part of the bar placed 2 inches behind the leading edge of the toilet (Fig. 22–11). The length of the bar may vary from 15 to 35 inches. If for any reason the handrail cannot be attached to the wall beside the toilet, a right-angle rail may be bolted on the floor and wall (Fig. 22–12). The right-angle rail should extend 6 inches in front of the leading edge of the toilet.

Layout. The chair is angled with the patient's normal side adjacent to the toilet.

Transfer Procedure. After locking the brakes and removing her foot from the footrest, the patient swings the footrest out to the side (the clothing may be loosened at this time). Pushing down on the armrest with her normal hand, she moves forward in the chair, leans forward (Fig.

FIG. 22–10

FIG. 22–11

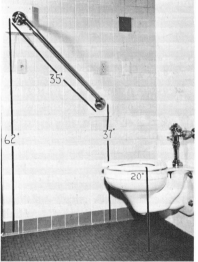

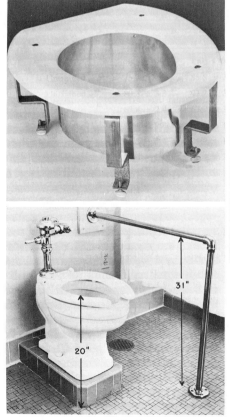

FIG. 22–12

FIGURE 22–10. A raised toilet seat attached to the toilet bowl facilitates transfer.

FIGURE 22–11. Position of the 45-degree-angle handrail at the toilet for transfers.

FIGURE 22–12. Position of the right-angle handrail at the toilet.

PAUL M. ELLWOOD, JR.

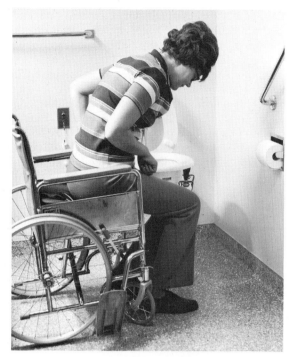

FIGURE 22–13. The patient has locked her wheelchair brakes, swung the footrest out of the way, and moved to the edge of the chair.

22–13), bearing most of her weight on her normal leg, and rises from the chair. Most of her lifting power should come from her normal leg. When standing, she uses the handrail to keep her balance and pivots on her feet until she is standing in front of the toilet (Fig. 22–14). Clothing is lowered and she sits down on the toilet.

To transfer from the toilet to the wheelchair, she reverses the procedure.

Bathtub Transfer

Getting in and out of the bathtub can be one of the most dangerous procedures for the patient and should always be supervised. Unlike most transfers, which should be made toward the patient's normal side, a tub transfer may be made toward either side, whichever is easiest for the patient.

Layout. A firm wooden chair should be placed beside the tub and another in the tub. These are used until the patient gains enough strength and confidence in his or her ability to transfer to a 9-inch or 5-inch stool or to the bottom of the tub. The legs of the chair placed in the tub should be shortened so that the seats of both chairs are the

same height as the edge of the tub. Rubber tips attached to the bottom of the chair legs on the shorter chair protect the tub and prevent the chair from slipping. A shampoo hose is attached to the faucet. Safety tread tape is used in addition to a bath mat. The bath mat covers the rough surface of the tape, and the tape keeps the mat from moving.

Transfer Technique. Pushing down on the chair seat with her normal hand, and on the floor with her normal leg, the patient moves to the edge of the chair and onto the edge of the tub. Then she picks up her involved leg with her normal hand and places it in the tub (Fig. 22–15).

Again pushing down with her normal arm and leg and using the wall handrail for support, she slides onto the chair in the tub (Fig. 22–16). She then lifts her normal leg into the tub.

Sitting Transfers

There are three basic types of sitting transfers: a lateral sliding transfer requiring the use of a

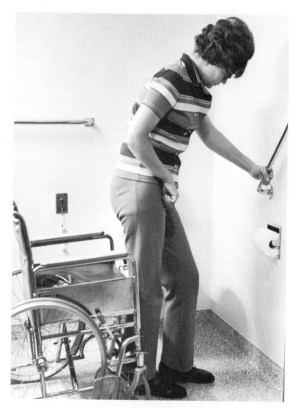

FIGURE 22–14. She pushes on the armrest to stand and reaches to the wall rail for support while turning and sitting down.

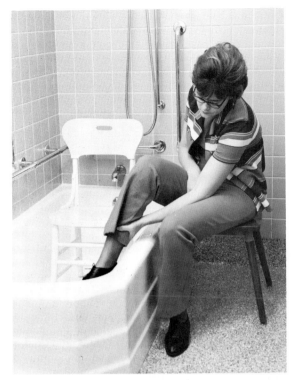

FIGURE 22–15. The patient places her involved leg in the tub.

stretching. For quadriplegic patients with weak triceps, training in locking the elbow is also included.

Bed to Wheelchair: Lateral Transfer Using a Sliding Board

Physical Requirements. Good sitting balance and arms powerful enough to lift the hips from the bed (strong shoulder depressors and adductors and elbow and wrist extensors) are necessary. This transfer is seldom accomplished unassisted by patients with lesions above the seventh cervical vertebra. Unusual quadriplegics with lesions at the fifth to sixth cervical segments who have weak triceps can use their biceps to lock their elbows in hyperextension sufficiently well to accomplish a sliding board transfer without assistance.

Equipment. A stable bed approximately the same height as the seat of the wheelchair; a wheelchair equipped with brakes, swinging detachable footrests, and detachable armrests; and a sliding board are needed.

Layout. The wheelchair is placed next to the bed and facing the head or foot of the bed at a

sliding board to bridge the space between the two surfaces; an anterior-posterior sliding transfer; and a lateral transfer without a sliding board.

In the sitting transfers described in this section, paraplegic patients are used as examples. The transfer techniques apply unmodified to patients with other lower extremity disabilities (e.g., double amputees). If upper extremity weakness is present, the assistance of another person may be required for the transfer. The type of transfer used depends on the patient's ability and the specific situation.

Preparing the Patient for Sitting Transfers. The following activities are valuable in preparation for sliding and swinging transfers: daily use of the standing bed, leading to the ability to stand at 80 degrees without postural hypotension; training in coming to a sitting position and sitting on the edge of the bed without making a transfer (transfer training is begun when the patient can balance in sitting position); progressive resistive exercises designed to strengthen shoulder depressors and adductors, elbow flexors and extensors, and wrist extensors and flexors; intensive mat work in the long sitting position to improve the ability to roll and balance and to elevate the hips; and hamstring

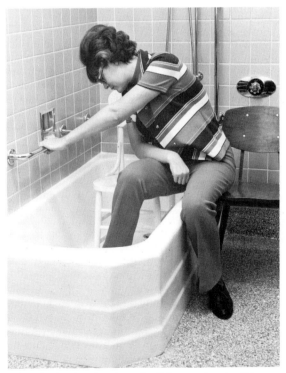

FIGURE 22–16. Using the wall rail for support, she slides onto the tub chair. She then moves her normal leg into the tub.

PAUL M. ELLWOOD, JR.

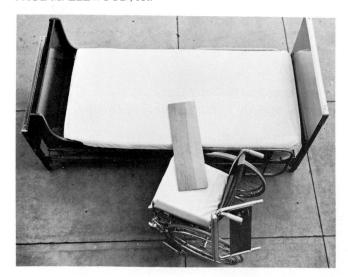

FIGURE 22–17. Position of the wheelchair and sliding board for a lateral sliding transfer.

slight angle. The principle of transfer toward the stronger side applies here also. The armrest is removed from the side next to the bed and is hung on the back of the chair. After the patient is sitting, the sliding board is placed between the chair and the bed (Fig. 22–17).

Coming to a Sitting Position. Paraplegics in the early stages of training and some quadriplegics attain sitting positions in a manner similar to the hemiplegic; i.e., after the patient rolls onto the side, the legs are brought independently or with assistance over the side of the bed. For more advanced patients, particularly those with good sitting balance and loose hamstrings, the following procedure can be used in coming to a sitting position.

The patient raises her head and bends it forward, then places her hands on the bed beside her hips, palms down, elbows flexed. She raises her shoulders by pushing down on her forearms and gradually "walking" her forearms backward (Fig. 22–18).

She transmits her weight to her right forearm and flexes her head to the right as she quickly straightens her left elbow. Keeping her left elbow in this locked position, she shifts her weight to her left arm and straightens her right elbow (Fig. 22–19).

To come to an upright sitting position, she must "walk" her hands forward one at a time until her trunk is forward. She must keep her head and shoulders slightly forward to maintain her balance and to keep from falling backward (Fig. 22–20).

She performs lateral and anterior-posterior movements by using her upper extremities to push against the bed to raise her hips off the bed, moving the desired direction while her hips are raised. She uses her fist rather than the palm of her hand for added height.

Transfer to the Chair. The patient reaches a sitting position on the side of the bed by moving her legs with her hands. She moves toward the edge of the bed, turning herself so that her knees are away from the wheelchair and her hips are toward the wheelchair (Fig. 22–21). As she turns, she must adjust her feet with her hands to bring them directly under her.

The patient leans over onto her right forearm, raising her left buttock off the bed enough to place one end of the sliding board under her (Fig. 22–22). Two corners of the board must rest securely on the bed and two corners must rest on the wheelchair seat, or the board may slip or break.

Using her upper extremities for balance and movement, the patient carefully moves laterally across the sliding board into the wheelchair (Fig. 22–23). She then leans over onto her left forearm to raise her buttock off the board and removes the sliding board.

She replaces the armrest on the wheelchair and swings the left footrest into place. After placing her left foot on the footrest, she unlocks the brakes and moves away from the bed. Finally she swings the right footrest into place and places her right foot on the footrest. When the patient becomes adept at using the sliding board, she may be able

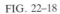

FIG. 22–18

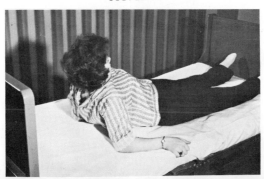

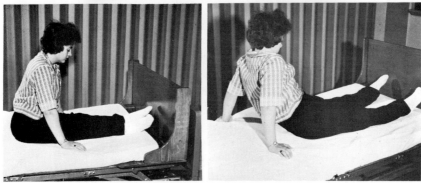

FIG. 22–19   FIG. 22–20

FIGURE 22–18. To come to a sitting position, the patient raises her shoulders by pushing down on her forearms and gradually moving them backward.

FIGURE 22–19. She straightens her elbows, one at a time.

FIGURE 22–20. She "walks" her hands forward one at a time until her trunk is forward and she has reached an upright sitting position.

FIG. 22–21  FIG. 22–23

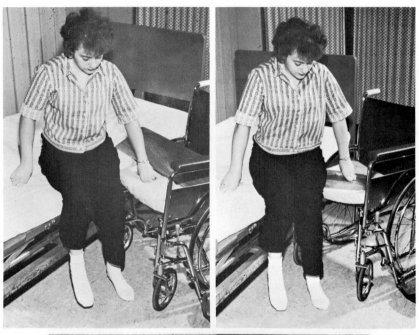

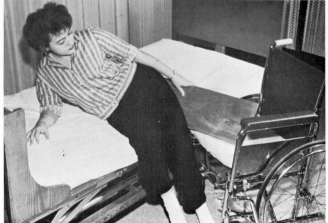

FIG. 22–22

FIGURE 22–21. She moves her legs over the side of the bed with her arms and slides to the edge of the bed in position for the sliding transfer to the wheelchair.

FIGURE 22–22. Leaning on her right forearm, the patient places one end of the sliding board under her.

FIGURE 22–23. She moves across the sliding board to the wheelchair.

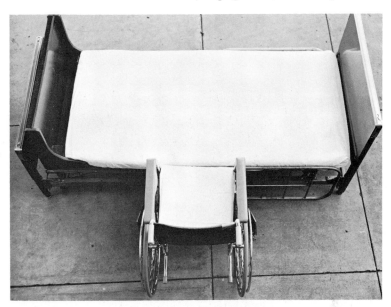

FIGURE 22–24. Position of the wheelchair for the anterior-posterior sliding transfer.

to progress to transferring without it. The movement would then be performed by using her upper extremities to boost her hips short distances rather than by sliding.

Bed to Wheelchair: Anterior-Posterior Sliding Transfer

Physical Requirements. This transfer requires loose hamstrings and slightly more strength, particularly in the elbow extensors, and better balance than for the lateral transfer.

Equipment. A bed that can be immobilized and set at approximately the same height as the wheelchair is needed.

Layout. The wheelchair is braked and placed with the front of the seat directly against the bed, and the footrests are swung aside (Fig. 22–24).

Transfer Techniques. During the entire transfer, the patient keeps her head and shoulders slightly forward to maintain her balance and prevent her from falling backward. She moves her legs to the side of the bed away from the wheelchair by moving one leg at a time with her hands.

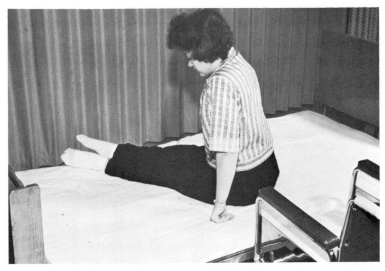

FIGURE 22–25. The patient pushes with her fists to move into position for the anterior-posterior transfer.

PAUL M. ELLWOOD, JR.

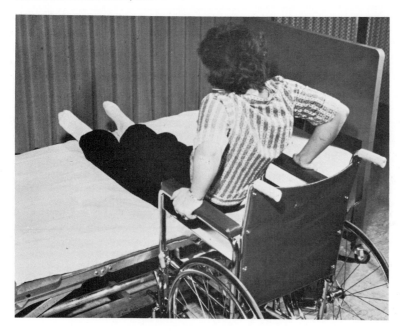

FIGURE 22–26. Grasping the middle of the wheelchair armrests, she lifts herself into the chair.

By pushing with her fists, the patient moves sideways and backward, moving each leg and hip alternately to bring her hips close to the wheelchair (Fig. 22–25).

When the patient is near the edge of the bed, she reaches behind her, places her hands on the middle of the wheelchair armrests, and lifts herself gently back into the wheelchair (Fig. 22–26). It is for this stage of the maneuver that strength in the elbow extensors is essential.

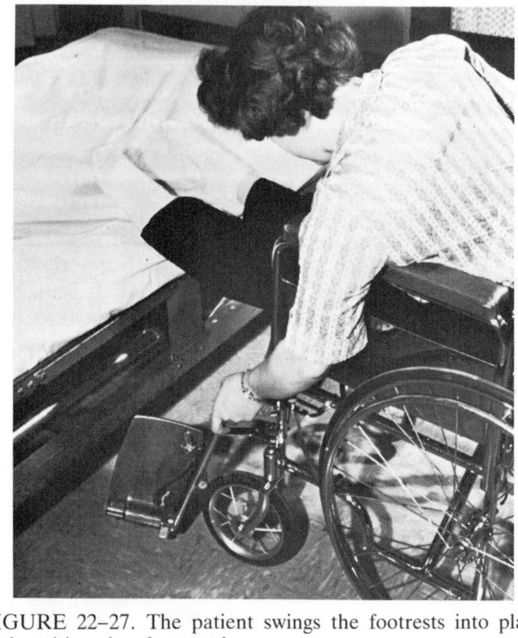

She moves the chair away from the bed until only her heels are resting on the edge of the bed. She locks her brakes; then, using the armrests for support, the patient leans to each side to swing the footrests into place (Fig. 22–27) and carefully places her feet on the footrests, watching to see that they are properly positioned. To get back into bed, she reverses the procedure.

Sitting Toilet Transfers

Equipment. It is recommended that the toilet seat be approximately the same height as the wheelchair seat. In a rehabilitation center where many patients need a higher toilet, the fixture may be installed at a height of 20 inches. When a standard toilet seat 16 inches high is the only one available, a securely fastened raised toilet seat may be used (see Fig. 22–10).

Layout. Depending on the space in the bathroom, the patient should position the wheelchair parallel or at an angle to the toilet. If space does not permit the use of the wheelchair in the bathroom, an ordinary sturdy wooden straight-back chair with small casters or gliders may be used instead of the wheelchair, provided the patient has

FIGURE 22–27. The patient swings the footrests into place and positions her feet on them.

sufficient balance to manage a chair without the support of armrests.

Transfer Technique. The patient lifts his feet off the footrests, places them on the floor one at a time, and swings the footrests out of the way. Next, he moves the chair until his knee is as close as possible to the toilet. He locks the wheelchair brakes (Fig. 22–28).

He shifts his hips so that he is sitting sideways on the chair and moves his legs so that his knees are away from the toilet (Fig. 22–29). He unlocks the brakes and moves the wheelchair as close as possible to the toilet. Then he relocks the brakes (Fig. 22–30). This final moving of the wheelchair is an important clue to a good transfer; it eliminates the space between the wheelchair seat and the toilet seat, thus reducing the distance the patient must cross. At this point, while he still has the support of the wheelchair armrests, the patient loosens his trousers and, by leaning from side to side, gradually works them under his buttocks to about midthigh.

Next he removes the armrest and places it on the back of the chair so that it will be within easy reach. He places one hand on the opposite side of the toilet seat and the other hand on the wheelchair seat. He uses his upper extremities to raise his hips and move toward the toilet (Fig. 22–31).

Several moves may be needed to complete the transfer. When the transfer procedure is com-

FIG. 22–28   FIG. 22–29

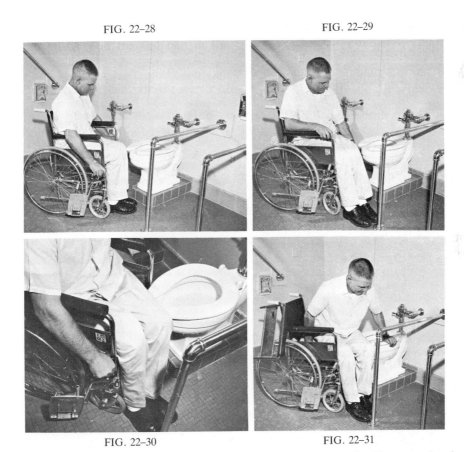

FIG. 22–30   FIG. 22–31

FIGURE 22–28. For the lateral transfer to the toilet, the patient swings the footrests to the side, moves the wheelchair so that his knee is close to the toilet, and locks the brakes.

FIGURE 22–29. The patient moves so that he is sitting sideways on the wheelchair.

FIGURE 22–30. He unlocks the brakes and moves the wheelchair as close as possible to the toilet. Then he relocks the brakes.

FIGURE 22–31. Removing the armrest and placing one hand on the opposite side of the toilet seat, the patient lifts himself to the toilet seat.

PAUL M. ELLWOOD, JR.

pleted, the patient must position his lower extremities.

Tub Transfers

Caution: When the patient has lost sensation to pain and temperature, the water temperature must be checked.

Equipment and Layout. See the bathtub transfer on page 536.

Transfer Technique. The patient transfers from a wheelchair to a straight chair next to the tub. He then straightens his knees and directs his feet toward the end of the tub so that his legs will move forward as he lowers himself into the tub. This is essential to a safe and efficient transfer. The patient positions his hands on the seat of the chair and on the handrail. Sometimes the edge of the tub may be used instead of a rail. Keeping his head and upper trunk forward, he gently lowers his body into the tub (Fig. 22–32). Gradual flexion of the elbows gives better control.

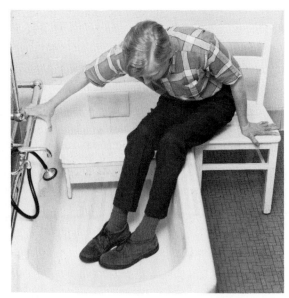

FIGURE 22–32. After placing his feet in the bathtub, the patient, using the handrail and the seat of the chair, lowers himself to a stool in the tub.

Bed to Wheelchair: Lateral Sitting Transfer Without Sliding Board

Physical Requirements. This transfer method can be used only by paraplegics with exceptionally good shoulder depressors and abductors as well as good balance. The patient must have the ability to lift the buttocks off the bed and to move from the bed to the wheelchair in one motion. Male paraplegics who develop very strong upper extremities may even be able to transfer to different levels with ease.

Layout. The wheelchair is set at a 45-degree angle next to the bed. For close placement, the footrests are swung aside. Very strong patients find this maneuver unnecessary.

Transfer Techniques. The patient comes to a sitting position on the side of the bed. She turns so that her knees are away from the wheelchair and her hips are directed toward the wheelchair. She adjusts her legs to bring her feet directly under her. She moves her hand to the middle of the farther armrest. By pushing down with her upper extremities, she raises herself off the bed and swings in one motion to the wheelchair (Fig. 22–33). She turns her trunk as she lowers herself into the chair.

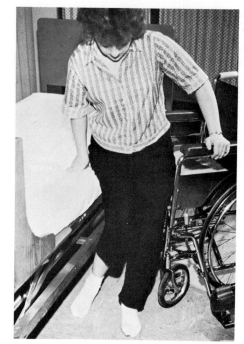

FIGURE 22–33. The patient pushes up on her arms to lift her buttocks from the bed to the wheelchair.

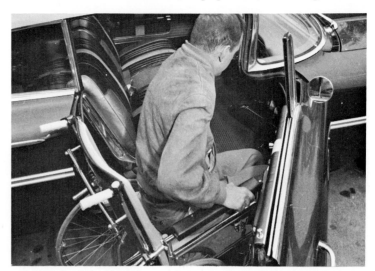

FIGURE 22–34. Position of the wheelchair for transfer to the car.

Car Transfers

Physical Requirements. This is an advanced transfer and can be accomplished unassisted only by patients with strong upper extremities.

Transfer Techniques. There are several methods by which patients can make a car transfer. Patients wearing long leg braces or who have sufficient extensor spasticity or one strong leg may be able to perform a standing transfer in which they stand, pivot and sit on the edge of the car seat. If the windows are rolled down, the window opening can be grasped for support during the transfer.

If the car door opens wide enough, the wheelchair can be placed directly facing the seat of the car. The patient's legs can be placed on the seat of the car and the patient can then slide forward into the car. This method is exactly the same as the one described for the anterior-posterior transfer from the wheelchair to the bed. A wide sliding board facilitates this transfer, particularly for the bilateral lower extremity amputee with prostheses.

The wheelchair can be placed at an angle to the car and the patient may be able to perform a swinging transfer, moving to the side (Figs. 22–34 and 22–35). This again is the same procedure that is so frequently used for bed or chair transfers except that there is a wider space between the wheelchair seat and the car seat. If the patient does not have sufficient strength to bridge this gap,

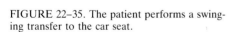

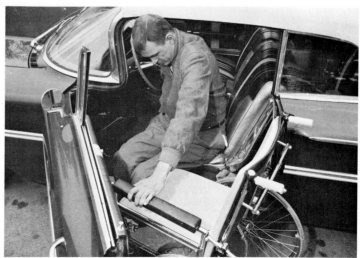

FIGURE 22–35. The patient performs a swinging transfer to the car seat.

PAUL M. ELLWOOD, JR.

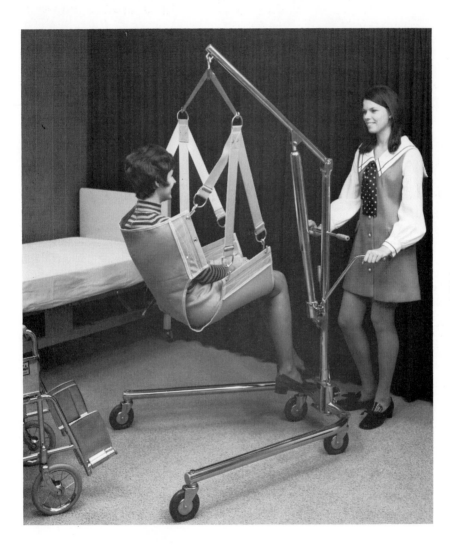

FIGURE 22–36. Mechanical lift for assistance in transfer. (Courtesy of Ted Hoyer & Company.)

a sliding board 28 to 34 inches long may be used. A completely independent transfer includes the ability to bring the wheelchair into the car after the transfer has been made and to remove the wheelchair before transferring out of the car.

For patients who cannot accomplish a transfer without extensive assistance, the various hydraulic or mechanical lifts have been found to be very effective (Fig. 22–36). A properly trained small woman, using these devices, can successfully lift and transfer a man more than twice her size. Family members or attendants should be trained to use such equipment if excessive lifting is required to assist a transfer. The rehabilitation center should have lifts available for training demonstrations.

ACKNOWLEDGEMENT

The author is indebted to the staff of Sister Kenny Institute for the preparation of photographs and drawings used in this chapter.

References

1. Audiovisual Aids Utilized in Teaching Rehabilitation Nursing. New York, Educational Services Division, American Journal of Nursing, Company, 1970.
2. Flaherty, P., and Jurkovich, S.: Transfers for Patients with Acute and Chronic Conditions. Minneapolis, American Rehabilitation Foundation, 1970.
3. Fowles, B. H.: Syllabus of Rehabilitation Methods and Techniques. Cleveland, Stratford Press Company, 1963.
4. Lawton, E. B.: Activities of Daily Living for Physical Rehabilitation. New York, McGraw-Hill Book Company, 1963, Chapter 3.
5. Narrow, B. W.: A hydraulic patient lifter. Am. J. Nurs., 60:1273–1275, 1960.
6. Rusk, H. A.: Rehabilitation Medicine, 2nd Ed. St. Louis, C. V. Mosby, 1964, Chapter 6.

23

Wheelchair Prescription

CATHERINE W. BRITELL

The achievement of optimal independent personal mobility is a vital step in the rehabilitation of the physically disabled individual. For a person unable to achieve and sustain a safe, comfortable, and energy-efficient gait, the proper wheelchair will afford necessary access to the social, educational, vocational, and recreational opportunities that compose a productive and rewarding life style.

Historically, the wheelchair has been associated with "invalidism." President Franklin D. Roosevelt, one of the world's most famous and successful wheelchair users, valued independent mobility and had a kitchen chair adapted to provide some measure of function in this respect (Fig. 23–1). Yet, he was reluctant to be seen or photographed in the wheelchair, fearing that this might give the impression of a certain weakness or ineptitude. This attitude prevailed for many years, and thus it has been only very recently that wheelchairs have been available to provide maximum function to meet the wide variety of user needs.

The goals of wheelchair prescription are as follows.

Maximization of Efficient Independent Mobility. The user should be able to move easily through the environment with acceptable energy expenditure and a minimum of assistance throughout the day.

Prevention/Minimization of Deformity or Injury. The user must be positioned and cushioned in such a manner as to prevent skin sores, contractures, joint deformities, or injuries to the extremities.

Maximization of Independent Functioning. The wheelchair must provide stable positioning and minimization of abnormal tone or movement so that functional head and extremity use can be

optimized and so that access to other adaptive devices is provided.

Projection of a Healthy, Vital, Attractive "Body Image." A wheelchair becomes a part of the disabled user's habitus. Therefore, its appearance should be as pleasing and attractive as possible.

Minimization of Short-term and Long-term Equipment Cost. Purchase, repair, maintenance, and replacement costs must be considered, and the least expensive alternative that is functionally and aesthetically appropriate should be considered, with particular attention to durability and repair and replacement cost.

Choice of a wheelchair will be determined by the user's size, weight, type and intensity of activity, and level of disability. Wheelchair prescription should be carried out by the rehabilitation team in an interdisciplinary manner as dictated by the complexity of the patient's needs. The physical or occupational therapist will often perform the major part of the evaluation and determination of specifications, with input from the physician, nurse, vocational rehabilitation specialist, and social worker, as appropriate. Because physicians must take overall responsibility for the wheelchair prescription, it is imperative that they understand the functions, mechanics, aesthetics, and economics of wheelchairs.

Manual Wheelchair Components

Modern manual wheelchair design takes advantage of a number of improvements in understanding of wheelchair mechanics and availability of materials. These improvements are ongoing, and

548

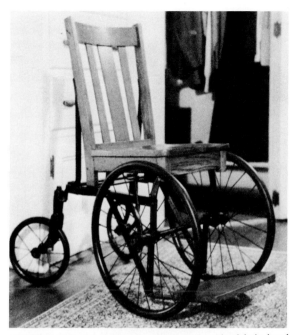

FIGURE 23–1. Franklin Delano Roosevelt's wheelchair, hand-made from a kitchen chair, provided an important measure of mobility during his everyday work. (Photograph courtesy of FDR Library.)

therefore it is important for the prescriber to keep abreast of changes in available materials and designs. Various components of a typical manual wheelchair are illustrated in Figure 23–2. The following considerations are important when choosing among the various options available.

Frame and Axle

There are a number of options for frame characteristics. Frame material may significantly determine both the durability and weight of the wheelchair. Weight is relatively unimportant in propulsion efficiency (a 5- or 10-lb difference is insignificant when the combined chair/user weight exceeds 200 lb). However, a lighter chair may be significantly easier to load into a vehicle. Frames that fold are easier to transport and store, whereas rigid frames often afford more stability to active users. Some newer frames that fold have a locking system to improve rigidity and maintain alignment. These are preferable for the active and highly mobile user. Many of the newer frames afford flexibility in the placement of the rear wheels by

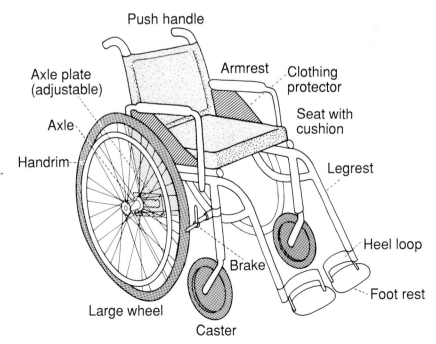

FIGURE 23–2. Typical wheelchair components.

CATHERINE W. BRITELL

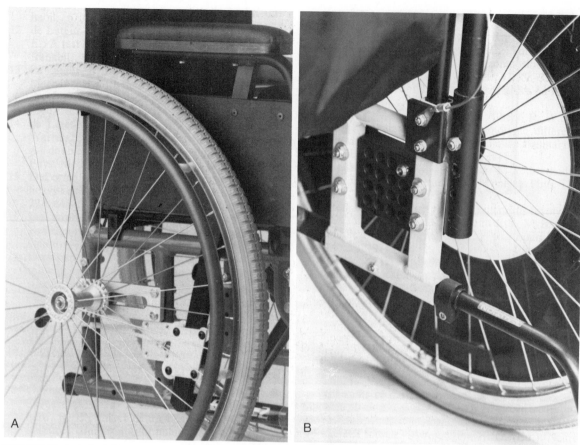

FIGURE 23–3. Adjustable axle plates. Position of the rear wheel can be changed by moving the axle plate vertically or the axle horizontally (*A*), or by providing a stationary axle plate with multiple holes (*B*).

means of an adjustable axle plate (Fig. 23–3). This allows modification of the wheelchair during the course of rehabilitation and makes adjustments possible that will significantly improve propulsion efficiency for most active wheelchair users.

Wheels and Tires

Wheel size affects overall height, rolling ease, transfer in and out of the chair, and upper extremity mechanics of pushing and is fairly standard in most general-purpose chairs. Solid, smooth tires generally work better on smooth, hard indoor surfaces (such as in a nursing home), whereas treaded pneumatic tires will give a smoother ride and easier maneuvering on rough terrain or wet or icy surfaces. Flat tires can be minimized by thorn-resistant tubes or by the addition of a latex gel,

which takes the place of the air but adds considerable weight.

Handrims, Wheel Locks, Grade Aids

Handrims may vary in size from a very small rim used in racing to a large rim used to maximize maneuverability and power. They may be modified to improve gripping by adding a coating, by increasing tube size, by changing the shape, or by adding rim projections.

Almost all users require wheel locks (Fig. 23–4). Handles must be positioned to provide easy access but not to interfere with wheelchair propulsion. For a very active user with a particularly long pushing stroke, it is sometimes helpful to position brakes lower down on the frame (Fig. 23–4*B*) to

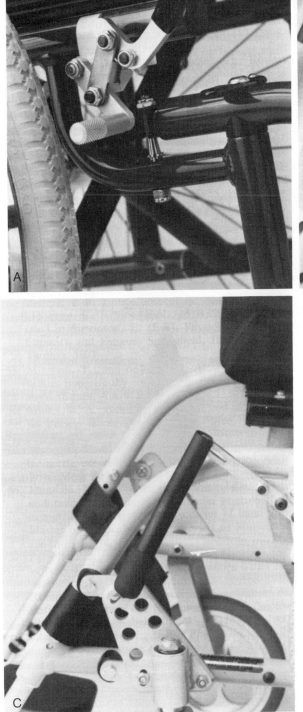

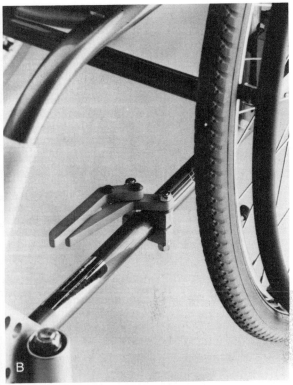

FIGURE 23–4. Wheel locks. Standard wheel locks (*A*) provide a solid stationary base. Lowered locks (*B*) may be useful for the very active individual. Extension handles (*C*) may be added as needed. (Photographs courtesy of Motion Designs, Inc.)

CATHERINE W. BRITELL

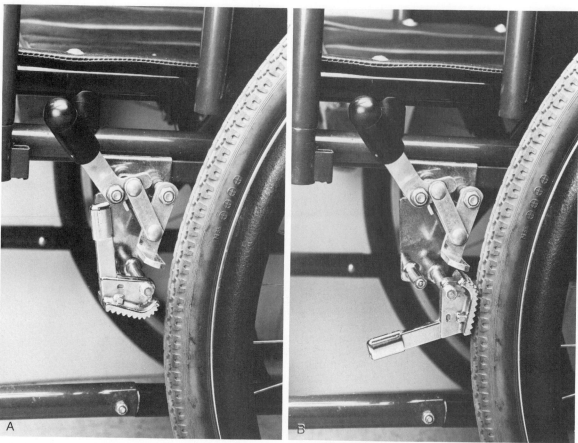

FIGURE 23–5. Grade aids. In the disengaged position (*A*), there is free backward and forward motion. When grade aids are engaged (*B*), backward motion is prevented.

prevent injury to the thumbs and fingers. Brake extension handles (Fig. 23–4*C*) may be needed by those with upper extremity dysfunction.

Grade aids (Fig. 23–5) are useful for those who have difficulty maintaining momentum on inclines, such as elderly individuals, those with quadriplegia, or users who have generalized weakness. These are simple, spring-loaded teeth that allow the chair to move forward only, and can be selectively activated while going uphill.

Casters

Casters are most often on the front of the chair. In general, a caster that is hard and of small diameter affords the best turning characteristics (as necessary for basketball or tennis). On the other hand, this kind of caster will get stuck on uneven terrain or soft ground, and so a larger pneumatic caster has greater utility outdoors. Many chairs allow casters to be interchanged easily, so that the user may use different casters for different situations (Fig. 23–6). Caster placement toward the rear of the chair will decrease turning radius, but will increase the tendency of the chair to tip forward. Caster "flutter" is a bothersome problem encountered by active users. It is noisy and affects the smoothness of the ride and straight tracking. This can be reduced by grooved casters or by increased damping of rotation of the casters. Caster locks are necessary when a patient requires absolute stability of the chair for transfers (such as a high paraplegic or quadriplegic). They are standard on most general-purpose chairs, but must sometimes be ordered specifically.

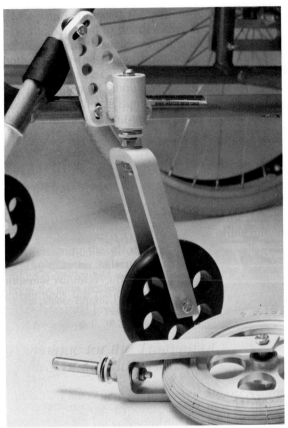

FIGURE 23–6. Interchangeable casters. The large pneumatic caster will allow easier wheeling on soft surfaces or rough terrain, whereas the hard nylon caster will provide quicker turning on hard, smooth surfaces. (Photograph courtesy of Motion Designs, Inc.)

Seat and Back Type

Most folding wheelchair seats and backs are sling-type, made of a flexible fabric. For a user with poor muscle control, spasticity, or a tendency toward deformity, it is difficult to attain adequate posture unless a solid seat, back, or both are substituted. These may be hinged to maintain folding ability, and add little to the weight of the chair. For example, if there is a tendency toward internal rotation and adduction of the lower extremities, a solid seat or seat insert is necessary to provide a base for pelvis and thigh positioning to correct this.

The problem of back support has historically been poorly addressed by wheelchair back design. In order to distribute the weight optimally over the thigh and ischial areas, proper lumbar support is especially necessary. Without lumbar support, there is a tendency to develop a sacral sitting posture (Fig. 23–7A), which can result in sacral and ischial pressure sores, increased thoracic kyphosis, and neck and upper back muscle strain. Adding a more stable seating surface and proper lumbar support (Fig. 23–7B) will significantly improve seated posture. Not only does this shift the seating weight off of bony prominences, but the thorax, head, and neck also come into better balance, reducing neck and upper back strain and improving respiratory function.

Back height should be low enough to avoid pushing the scapulae and shoulders forward, but high enough to provide proper back support. A common error is providing too low a back in order to achieve a "sporty" look. When the back is too low, it causes excessive pressure at its upper edge, and wheeling efficiency is decreased owing to poor stabilization of the shoulder girdle. A general rule of thumb is that for patients with abnormal trunk control above T 8–10 but with good head control, the back should come up to within 2 inches of the lower edge of the scapulae.

Push handles may be optional on the back. Some users favor being without these because of cosmetic factors and the desire to project an image of independence. Others find them useful for hanging backpacks, for stabilizing themselves for reaching, or as a means of having others push the chair.

Armrests

For many users, armrests can aid significantly in transfers and weight shifts, and they can reduce ischial pressure by carrying the weight of the arms and maintaining trunk balance. Armrests may be removable or fixed, and they may be adjustable. For most users with significant lower extremity dysfunction, removable armrests will make transfers easier. Various manufacturers offer different sets of options for arm support. At this time there is no standard selection available in all chairs; therefore, it will be necessary for the clinician to choose the particular one that best meets the user's needs of size, shape, stability, adjustability, and cosmesis. If a splint, custom arm trough, balanced orthosis, or lapboard is needed, this should be taken into account when choosing the armrest. In addition, the total width of the chair may be decreased by using wraparound armrests, if this option is indicated by the user's environment.

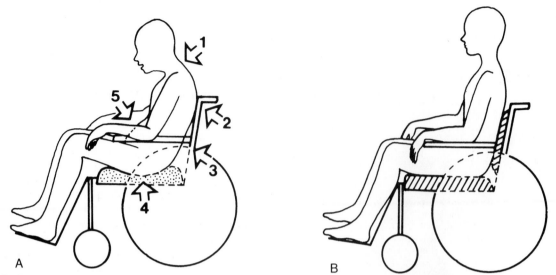

FIGURE 23–7. Lumbar and seat support. Poor lumbar and seat support (*A*) allows a sacral sitting posture, resulting in (1) neck and upper back strain, (2) excessive scapular pressure, (3) overstretching of lumbar extensors, (4) excessive sacral pressure, and (5) poor ventilation. Proper seat and lumbar support (*B*) greatly improves function and cosmesis.

Foot and Leg Support

Leg supports and footrests afford protection, proper positioning, and maximal balance and weight-bearing for the limbs. Footrests should be high enough so that the foot is supported sufficiently to maintain circulation in the lower extremity, but not so high as to shift the weight of the legs backward into the ischial tuberosities and sacrum. If significant spasticity is present, a large foot plate with a foot restraint system may be necessary. Foot plates that afford protection to the feet may be necessary if the feet are not clearly visible to the user, or if wheelchair control is imprecise. Calf support is seldom necessary if the feet and heels are well supported; however, calf pads can be added if the legs must occasionally be elevated. Swing-away, detachable footrests are necessary to facilitate transfers for many individuals. Close attention must be paid to whether the release mechanisms available on a particular model of chair can be managed independently by the user with impaired hand function.

Upholstery

Upholstery should be impervious to body secretions, be easily cleanable, and not stretch. For a person who spends significant time in a wheelchair, color and general appearance are of great importance. The user should be encouraged to choose colors and styles, since this is much like a piece of clothing and should be pleasing to the user.

Wheelchair Measurement

In prescribing a wheelchair, it is necessary to specify (1) seat width, (2) seat height, (3) seat depth, (4) back height, and (5) armrest height (Fig. 23–8). When measuring seat height, it is important to take into account the thickness of the compressed cushion. Other size considerations include overall width of the chair, overall height of the wheelchair-seated user, and distance from the lap to the floor. Minor adjustments can sometimes be made in the configuration of the chair to accommodate the seated individual within a limited space. These may include using wraparound armrests to make the chair up to 1 inch narrower, or a narrowing device that can temporarily narrow a folding chair to allow the user to traverse a narrow doorway.

In prescribing a manual wheelchair, one will often find that each manufacturer offers an array of options that may be unique. Therefore, the choice of manufacturer should be made after de-

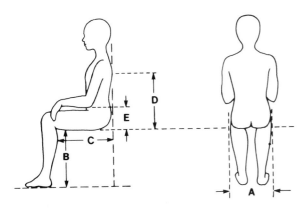

FIGURE 23–8. Wheelchair measurement.
Seat width: 1 inch wider than the width of the widest part of the buttocks (*A*).
Seat height: 2 inches higher than the distance from the bottom of the heel to the popliteal area (*B*).
Seat depth: 1 to 2 inches longer than the distance from the popliteal area to the back of the buttocks (*C*).
Back height: 2 inches less (may vary) than the distance from the bottom of the scapulae to the sitting surface (*D*).
Armrest height: Distance from bottom of buttocks to elbow (*E*).

termining the best wheelchair characteristics for the patient in a generic fashion. The cost of a manual wheelchair is often dependent on how unusual the prescription is and thus how many components must be custom-made or assembled. Therefore, the prescriber should make certain that an unusual custom specification will significantly enhance the utility of the chair before prescribing it.

Minimizing the Energy Requirements of Manual Wheelchair Use

A wheelchair's performance is generally considered to be inversely proportional to the energy required to propel it. Factors affecting this include the following.

Rolling Resistance

Rolling resistance is affected mainly by tire material, wheel diameter, bearings, and wheel alignment. The softer the tires, the more deformity and resistance to wheeling will occur on a flat surface.

Malalignment of the wheels by 1 degree can increase rolling resistance by five times.[3, 12] The weight of the wheelchair is relatively unimportant in affecting rolling resistance, since it is relatively small in comparison to the weight of the user.

Control and Maneuverability

As a chair becomes easier to control, the associated energy cost decreases. Generally, the closer the center of gravity of the user to the axis of the rear wheels, the better the control achieved. For example, when a person is wheeling on a sidehill, perpendicular to the slope of the terrain, there is a tendency for the wheelchair to turn downhill. The energy cost of wheeling on a 2-degree side slope is approximately twice that of wheeling on the level, due to this downhill turning tendency.[5] This can be minimized by placing the rear wheels forward, more directly under the user. Forward placement of the rear wheels also makes turning

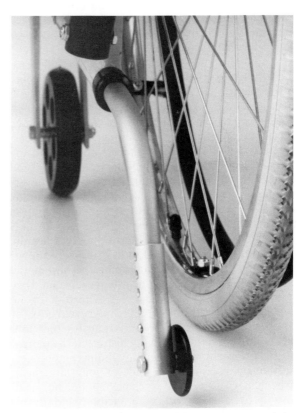

FIGURE 23–9. Anti-tip device will discourage backward tipping for the individual with impairment of trunk control. (Photograph courtesy of Motion Designs, Inc.)

CATHERINE W. BRITELL

easier and makes weight shift for negotiation of curbs ("wheelies") possible. On the other hand, static stability (resistance to tipping over backward) is decreased when the rear wheel is moved forward and must be considered, particularly when the user is elderly or has poor balance. In such a case, anti-tip devices (Fig. 23–9) should be tried before shifting the center of gravity forward, since the elderly or severely disabled individual can often benefit most from decreasing the energy cost of wheeling.

Wheelchair/User Interaction

The process of wheeling a wheelchair with the upper extremities is a complex one consisting of (1) positioning of the arms for maximal power stroke, (2) grasping the propulsion rim, (3) pushing down and forward through the propulsion arc, and (4) releasing the propulsion rim. By minimizing the energy required to reposition the extremities after the power stroke, propulsion efficiency can be greatly enhanced. For example, moving the seat as little as 1 inch back and upward may increase efficiency by as much as 50 per cent.[4] A user with unusually long or short arms may need additional modifications to maximize efficiency of extremity dynamics.

In general, the energy necessary to achieve mobility will determine the speed of travel, the range of the user within the environment, and the accessibility of various parts of the environment to the user. For example, normal wheelchair propulsion on flat, hard surfaces requires an energy expenditure of 0.46 kcal/kg km.[16] The addition of carpeting to the surface nearly doubles energy consumption per distance traveled.[11] Negotiating a standard (1-inch rise per foot) ramp requires 8 to 10 times the energy as does flat, smooth surface wheeling.[10] Although these requirements may be within the capabilities of the young, healthy paraplegic, they may be beyond those of the elderly person or one who has upper extremity deformity, weakness, or spasticity. Therefore, it is important for the clinician to take a careful mobility history. If the patient is limited in any way by energy requirements (i.e., avoids ramps, rough ground, or long stretches), wheelchair propulsion efficiency should be maximized by analysis of these factors, and if this continues to be a problem, some type of power-assisted mobility should be considered.

Electrically Powered Wheelchairs

For an individual who cannot achieve energy-efficient mobility in a manual wheelchair, an externally powered chair is usually necessary. Powered mobility may be a major determinant of self-esteem and may significantly enhance socializing, learning ability, and overall rehabilitation potential in both children and adults.[6, 13] Prescription of powered wheelchairs has the same overall goals as for manual chairs; however, their components must be considered in a different way. Components of a powered wheelchair prescription include the following.

The Wheelchair Power Base

Power bases are generally of two types: those with direct-drive motors and four small balloon tires (Fig. 23–10A), and those with belt-drive power linkages and a large rear hard rubber tire and small front pneumatic casters (Fig. 23–10B). The direct-drive power bases are generally more durable and more able to traverse rough terrain, whereas the belt-driven bases can often attain higher speeds and provide more stability, which is sometimes very important to those with high-level disabilities. A feature that is available on either type and can greatly assist the user with marginal or slowly responsive control is a "high brake bias," which brakes the chair when no control input is received. Major manufacturers who supply these power bases provide excellent product support and a complete selection of other components; therefore, choice of the power base can be made entirely on planned use and user preference.

Independent Maintenance of Posture, Trunk, and Limb Support

Often an individual who requires an electric wheelchair will also require some special consideration as to seating, back and limb support, and dynamic positioning. There is generally little indication for a sling seat and back for these individuals. A solid seat insert will allow management of spasticity and limb positioning as well as provide a level, stable base for the appropriate cushion, as

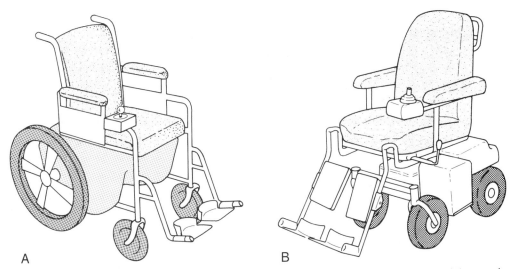

FIGURE 23–10. Electrically powered wheelchairs are available with belt-driven (*A*) or direct-drive (*B*) power bases.

discussed later in this chapter. A solid back will allow proper lumbar support as well as management of trunk stability with a minimum of restriction of motion. It is generally better to provide trunk support with lateral thoracic pads than by strapping the user into the chair, because the greater freedom of movement may allow the user to do weight shifts, and also respiration will not be restricted. A person who requires an electric wheelchair often has some limitations in the ability to perform adequate pressure relief. This individual seldom can perform a standard wheelchair pushup, and must therefore shift weight by leaning forward or to the side in order to shift pressure over the sitting area. If trunk stability or control is not adequate to carry this out, a reclining back is necessary. This can be manual or electrically powered. The powered system provides a greater degree of independence; however, it is quite costly and requires significant maintenance and repair. When there is need for a reclining wheelchair, it is also necessary to keep in mind the necessity of head, arm, and leg support in the reclining as well as in the sitting position.

Because of the rotation of the pelvis about the femur when changing between the supine and sitting positions, there is a relative lengthening of the posterior aspect of the body in the sitting position. This may cause significant shear on the sitting and back surfaces when changing between these two positions. The result of this shear is malpositioning of the user when coming to the seated position, and also a much greater tendency toward skin breakdown.

This shearing may be minimized in a number of ways: sliding the seat, sliding the back, or maintaining the seat and back at 90 degrees at all times with the "tilt-back" system. The "tilt-back" system provides the best shear protection; however, it is unstable for large individuals, it adds significant seated height to the user, and it is not adequate for those users who must occasionally straighten out the body (i.e., in order to empty the bladder). Recently, a spring-equipped power recline system that reclines at either a 90-degree angle or flat has been developed that shows promise in improving function while minimizing shear.

Selection of Optimal Primary and Secondary Controllers

The *primary control* of a wheelchair, that of direction, speed, and braking, may be in one of three modes: proportional control, multiple-switch control, or single-switch sequential scanning. Proportional control, most often using a joystick, provides the fastest, most efficient, and most precise control method. The joystick may be controlled by the hand, foot, chin, or any other site that can move independently in four directions and maintain a position in space. The joystick may be secured to the wheelchair or to the user's body. When using a joystick, a less axial (farther away from the center of the body) control site will provide better control on rough terrain. A switch array, such as a slot switch or a series of sip-and-puff switches, can adequately control a wheelchair in many settings; however, this method will slow the user considerably. A scanning system, although very useful for secondary controls, is seldom useful in controlling the motion of a wheelchair, since the time necessary for scanning is too long to provide safe control at any but the most excruciatingly slow speeds. The technology for voice-actuated control is readily available, and it is expected that this will be effectively applied to wheelchair control in the near future. Depending on the user, voice-actuated control will have approximately the same efficiency as a switch array.

The *secondary controls* include the on-off switch, gear selection, and selection of other modalities controlled, which may include reclining controls, call signals, or interfaces with communication devices, environmental control systems, or personal computers. These must be specifically fitted to the patient's needs and abilities as well as anticipated future needs. In general, these controls should be as simple, unobtrusive, and inexpensive as possible; yet at the same time the user may benefit from a capability for expansion as he or she becomes more proficient at controlling devices. When prescribing a complex wheelchair-based control system, it is imperative that the physical and occupational therapist, speech pathologist, patient, family, and physician—and, if necessary, the rehabilitation engineer, psychologist, social worker, and teacher—work closely together to ensure that the optimal system is prescribed. If the rehabilitation team involved with a patient is unfamiliar or inexperienced with high-level control systems, it is often cost-effective to obtain the services of a consulting occupational therapist or rehabilitation engineer who has special expertise with these systems.

Transportation of the electrically powered wheelchair poses a number of issues. These chairs are very heavy and generally do not fold easily; therefore, it is usually necessary to transport them in a wheelchair lift–equipped van or bus. In rare instances, the user can be transferred to a station wagon seat, and the partially disassembled chair can be stowed in the rear; however, this is not feasible unless the attendant has unusual strength and dexterity, and it is also quite time-consuming. Dependent wheelchair access to the outdoor environment is also complicated by the use of an electrically powered chair. Whereas the attendant or family member can readily get the user up a high curb or single step in a manual chair, the combined weight of the user and the electric chair often precludes this. Therefore, community mobility must be carefully addressed when prescribing an electric wheelchair.

Electric Carts and Add-On Power Devices

A number of three-wheeled and four-wheeled electric carts are marketed to improve mobility for the disabled individual (Fig. 23–11). These are sometimes of benefit to the user who has good trunk and limb control but for whom mobility is limited as a result of cardiac or pulmonary dysfunction, arthritis, or other conditions that compromise stamina. These devices are seldom adequate for an individual who has significant neuromuscular dysfunction or who requires a

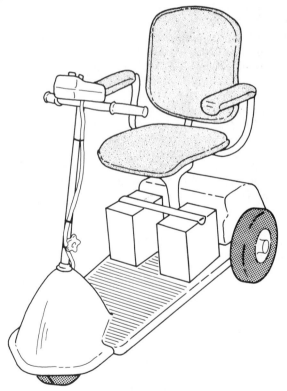

FIGURE 23–11. The electric cart may be useful for those with good neuromuscular control who have cardiopulmonary or orthopedic limitations.

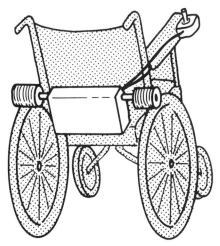

FIGURE 23–12. The add-on unit may be useful for the person who requires occasional powered assistance for ramps and rough terrain, or whose mobility range is small.

wheelchair at all times, since they may be difficult to transfer into, sometimes do not work well at tables or in small spaces, and provide poor trunk and limb support. Many electric carts can be disassembled for transport in an auto trunk. This makes them useful for increasing outdoor mobility.

The add-on unit (Fig. 23–12) consists of a battery pack and two motors that attach to the manual wheelchair frame and drive the wheels by friction on the existing tires. This device is almost always less than optimal in providing dependable mobility, but it can be folded and stowed in an auto trunk and also is much less expensive to purchase than an integrally powered chair. Because of the limited power supply, its major use is for those who are not very active but who would otherwise require assistance with ramps and rough ground.

Wheelchair Cushions and Seating Systems

Selection of the appropriate cushion and seating must take into account the following factors:
1. Stability of support for upper extremity function.
2. Pressure distribution.
3. Maintenance of posture to prevent deformity.
4. Weight.
5. Cleansability and durability.

Pressure relief and distribution is an especially important consideration in asensory individuals and the elderly[1] as well as those who, for reasons of physical inability or cognitive deficits, must sit still in the chair for long periods of time. Of course, no cushion will successfully prevent pressure sores without an adequate system of weight shifting. If the user cannot do this independently, a reclining chair or assistance in doing this will be necessary. Using commercially available sensors, it is possible to measure seated pressures under the ischial tuberosities and coccyx. In general, ischial pressures should not exceed 50 mm Hg, and pressures under the coccyx should be less than 20 mm Hg.[9, 14] The lower surface of the thigh can tolerate relatively high pressure, up to 100 mm Hg. A functional way to assess the adequacy of a cushion in providing pressure relief for an individual is to carefully monitor the skin for redness after sitting trials on the cushion, starting at 15 minutes, and lengthening sitting time to four hours in 15-minute intervals, with the user's customary weight-shift routine in effect.[18]

Table 23–1 illustrates a number of available cushions and outlines their salient characteristics. Every effort should be made to control the position of the spine and lower extremities by use of the appropriate cushion components, rather than adding on belts, restraints, and leg separators. In the case of severe spasticity and resultant deformity, a special modular or custom-molded seating system[2, 15] may be necessary to provide proper positioning and pressure relief while preventing further deformity.

Specific Prescription Considerations

The following examples illustrate the principles outlined in the preceding in the context of specific disabilities. It is important to keep in mind that each user is unique, and that there is no "standard" wheelchair prescription for a particular type of disability.

Hemiplegia

The user is a 72-year-old retired executive weighing 126 pounds with severe spastic right hemiplegia who walks short distances slowly with ankle-foot orthosis (AFO) and quad cane, and transfers independently. He lives with his 71-year-old wife, and enjoys visiting his children in New York, Seattle, and Chicago. His favorite activities include attending sports events, sightseeing, wheelchair bowling, and tending his raised flower and vegetable plots.

CATHERINE W. BRITELL

TABLE 23–1. Characteristics of Commonly Used Wheelchair Cushions

CUSHION TYPE	Pressure relief	Seating stability	Heat dissipation	Cleanability	Durability	Cost
Contoured foam with gel insert	GOOD	GOOD TO EXCELLENT	FAIR TO GOOD	EXCELLENT	GOOD TO EXCELLENT	HIGH
Air-filled villous	EXCELLENT	POOR TO FAIR	GOOD TO EXCELLENT	EXCELLENT	FAIR TO GOOD	HIGH
Gel-filled	GOOD	FAIR TO GOOD	EXCELLENT	EXCELLENT	FAIR	MODERATE TO HIGH
Coated contoured foam	FAIR TO GOOD	EXCELLENT	FAIR TO POOR	EXCELLENT	EXCELLENT	MODERATE TO HIGH
Foam	FAIR TO GOOD	GOOD	FAIR	POOR	FAIR TO GOOD	LOW TO MODERATE
Air-filled	FAIR	GOOD TO EXCELLENT	FAIR TO GOOD	EXCELLENT	GOOD	LOW

The proper cushion for the patient is dictated by which features are most desirable for that individual.

This active man will require a lightweight folding chair with an aluminum frame that his wife can load into the trunk of their sedan. Quick-disconnect axles will provide easier loading and storage for their frequent car and plane trips. Because he propels the chair with his left arm and foot, the seat height should be low enough to provide good traction on the floor without sliding forward in the seat. The wheels should have spokes to reduce their weight. Rear tires should be pneumatic, with smooth tread. Casters should be large-sized and pneumatic, to minimize "sticking" on rough surfaces. Brakes should be high, with an extension on the right. Push rims may be plastic-coated to improve gripping. The back is of standard height with push handles, and the removable armrests should have clothing protectors. The upholstery should be a washable, lightweight fabric. Detachable, swing-away footrests should provide good support for the right foot. The cushion should be light in weight. Four-inch foam will usually suffice. If there is significant adductor spasm of the right thigh in the seated position, a removable solid seat insert and contoured foam cushion may be needed.

Paraplegia

The user is a 28-year-old aircraft engineer with T 7 paraplegia who enjoys outdoor activities and recreational basketball, and who competes nationally in wheelchair track and road-racing events.

The chair must be durable, and therefore the frame should be of titanium or stainless steel and should provide a high degree of rigidity. Axle and caster position should be widely adjustable, and mag wheels with quick-disconnect axles will provide the greatest durability and portability. Tires should be pneumatic and treaded, and push rim type should be the preference of the user. Casters should be easily interchangeable and should lock, and the chair should be provided with one set of large pneumatic casters for everyday use, and a set of small nylon casters for his occasional recreational basketball. This chair will not be adequate for competitive racing. (The user will require a chair that is specifically designed for this purpose.) Brake type and grade aids should be the user's preference. Footrests should be detachable and swing-away, and should provide adequate heel support. Armrests should be adjustable and removable, and back height adjustable. Upholstery

should be the choice of the user. The cushion should also be the choice of the user, with emphasis on maintenance of good posture and adequate pressure distribution. Contoured foam with or without a gel insert is often a good choice. A lumbar support may be useful in maintaining posture and reducing upper back strain.

High Quadriplegia

The user is a 24-year-old single law student with C 5 quadriplegia. She lives on the university campus and has two hours' attendant care in the morning and one hour at night. She uses public transportation and her wheelchair for community mobility, and enjoys the theater, ballet, watching sports events, and chess playing.

A durable direct-drive power base with automatic braking and four medium-sized semi-pneumatic tires will be the best choice for mobility about the campus. Since she cannot do independent weight shifts, she will require a no-shear integrated power recline system. The wheelchair controller is a hand-operated joystick that doubles as an environmental control interface. A special lapboard holds her tape recorder and portable computer, which are indispensable as she prepares for her law career. She may require a villous pneumatic cushion for pressure relief; however, she may get better stability and positioning from a contoured foam cushion with a gel insert.

Cerebral Palsy

The user is a 4-year-old boy with spastic quadriparesis. He is sociable and communicative, although he has no speech. His head control is fair, but he cannot sit unsupported. He has severe muscle imbalance in his trunk and limbs with moderate deformity, making positioning difficult. He is beginning to master control of switches for mechanical toys with his hands and is working on self-feeding. He delights in being pushed along while his mother goes jogging, enjoys car rides, and likes to play with a small electronic musical keyboard.

Proper positioning will be the key to controlling tone and maximizing independence for this child. This may start with a vacuum-formed custom seat insert, which can fit into a wheelchair-stroller, car seat, or highchair frame. As he becomes more able

CATHERINE W. BRITELL

to manipulate switches, he may soon be ready for a power base with augmentive communication device and environmental control/computer interface.

Pulmonary Disease

The user is a 68-year-old widow who lives in an Arizona retirement community. She has severe chronic obstructive pulmonary disease, which makes her dependent on oxygen and on a number of medications, including steroids. She has severe osteoporosis and multiple thoracic compression fractures, with resultant severe thoracic kyphosis. She walks very short distances, using a wheeled walker with a bracket for her oxygen concentrator. She has excellent balance and judgment; she enjoys meeting her friends for meals in the community dining room and taking part in quilting bees, bridge tournaments, and her needlework club in the recreation hall.

Powered mobility is essential to this lady's quality of life. Because her neuromuscular function is essentially normal, she should be able to handle an electric scooter. If terrain is smooth, a three-wheeled vehicle will suffice; a four-wheeled scooter will provide greater stability over rough ground. She will require a bracket for her oxygen concentrator. Because she is involved in many activities that require her to sit at a table, a swivel seat with power height adjustment may be quite useful.

Wheelchairs for Institutionalized Individuals

When an elderly or disabled individual is confined to an institution as a residential alternative, it is imperative that he or she be able to have a wheelchair that serves the two essential functions of optimal mobility and safe, comfortable seating. If this is not the case, the result will often be lowered self-confidence and self-esteem, dysphoria, and a poor quality of life. Each individual who must sit in a wheelchair for any reason should be evaluated by a rehabilitation professional trained and skilled in this area. The optimal chair should then be provided, taking into account the principles outlined in this chapter.

Conclusion

Wheelchair prescription is an important function of the professional rehabilitation team, with medical, mechanical, psychosocial, and rehabilitative considerations all being relevant to proper selection and fitting. The proper wheelchair can make a profound difference in the quality of life for a disabled user when the basic factors of support, mobility, comfort, and cosmesis are optimally addressed.

ACKNOWLEDGMENT

The author would like to thank Mrs. Dale Leuthold for providing the original drawings.

References

1. Bennett, L.: Skin stress and blood flow in sitting paraplegic patients. Arch. Phys. Med. Rehabil., 65:186–190, 1984.
2. Bergen, A. F., and Colangelo, C.: Positioning the Client with Central Nervous System Deficits: The Wheelchair and Other Adapted Equipment, 2nd Ed. Valhalla, NY, Valhalla Rehabilitation Publ. Ltd., 1985.
3. Brubaker, C. E.: Wheelchair prescription: An analysis of factors that affect mobility and performance. J. Rehabil. Res. Dev., 23:19–26, 1986.
4. Brubaker, C. E., McLaurin, C. A., and McClay, I. S.: A pulmonary analysis of limb geometry and EMG activity for five seat positions. Proc. VIII Conf. Rehabil. Tech., RESNA, 1985, pp. 350–351.
5. Brubaker, C. E., McLaurin, C. A., and McClay, I. S.: Effects of side slope on wheelchair performance. J. Rehabil. Res. Dev., 23:55–57, 1986.
6. Butler, C., Okamato, G. A., and McKay, T. M.: Motorized wheelchair driving by disabled children. Arch. Phys. Med. Rehabil., 65:95–97, 1984.
7. DeLisa, J. A., and Greenberg, S.: Wheelchair prescription guidelines. Am. Fam. Physician, 25:145–150, 1982.
8. Fergusen-Pell, M. W., Wilkie, J. C., Reswick, J. B., and Burbend, J. C.: Pressure sore prevention for the wheelchair-bound spinal cord injured patient. Paraplegia, 18:42–51, 1983.
9. Fisher, S. V., and Patterson, R.: Long-term pressure recordings under the ischial tuberosities of tetraplegics. Paraplegia, 21:99–106, 1983.
10. Glaser, R. M., Barr, S. A., Lauback, C. C., Sawka, M. N., and Suryaprasad, A. S.: Relative stresses of wheelchair activity. Hum. Factors, 22:177–181, 1980.

11. Glaser, R. M., Sawka, M. N., Welde, S. W., Woodrow, B. K., and Suryaprasad, A. S.: Energy cost and cardiopulmonary responses for wheelchair locomotion and walking on tile and on carpet. Paraplegia, 19:220–226, 1981.

12. Kauzlarich, J. J., and Thacker, J. G.: Wheelchair tire rolling resistance and fatigue. J. Rehabil. Res. Dev., 22:25–41, 1985.

13. Nauman, S., Walder, S., Snell, E., and Milner, M.: A powered mobility for two to five year olds with neuromuscular disorder. Proc. V Ann. Conf. Rehabil. Engineering, RESNA, 1982.

14. Perkash, I., O'Neill, H., Politi-Meeks, D., and Beet, S. C. L.: Development and evaluation of a universal contoured cushion. Paraplegia, 22:358–365, 1984.

15. Trefler, E., Tooms, R. R., and Hobson, D.: Seating for cerebral-palsied children. Inter-Clinic Information Bull., 17:1–8, 1978.

16. Waters, R. L., and Lunsford, B. R.: Energy cost of paraplegic locomotion. J. Bone Joint Surg., 67A:1245–1250, 1985.

17. Wilson, A. B.: Wheelchairs: A Prescription Guide. Charlottesville, VA, Rehabilitation Press, 1986.

18. Zacharkow, D.: Wheelchair Posture and Pressure Sores. New York, Charles C Thomas, 1984.

24

Training for Functional Independence

LOREN R. LESLIE

The effectiveness of any program of medical intervention is determined by its therapeutic outcome. If possible, quantitative criteria should be used to measure outcome. Examples of rehabilitation outcome measurements are changes in muscle strength and endurance; degrees of range of motion; and levels of independence of physical function, referred to as self-care activities or activities of daily living (ADLs). This chapter presents a review of the basic principles involved in making a physically handicapped patient independent in the performance of those activities of daily living as well as some of the systems utilized to measure ADL rehabilitation outcome.

The activities that must be performed to achieve functional independence may be classified as mobility activities, hygiene, eating, dressing, and bowel and bladder control. Mobility activities include bed position, transfers, wheelchair mobility, and ambulation. Most programs for training physically handicapped patients to become independent in the activities of daily living are adapted from the original work of George G. Deaver and Mary Eleanor Brown at the Institute for the Crippled and Disabled, New York City.[1]

Any activity that must be performed is analyzed by breaking it down into its simplest components, and exercises or therapies are selected that will increase the ability of the patients to perform each component motion until they can perform the total activity.[2, 3] In addition, many of the activities of daily living can be performed with a variety of mechanical aids and assistive devices.[4-7] It is often necessary for the patients to use assistive devices and aids early in the rehabilitation program; however, when they have developed some flexibility, strength, and endurance, less equipment may be required.

Mobility Activities

Bed Mobility. The handicapped patient should be trained to shift about in bed, turn in both directions, sit erect in the long and short sitting positions, and reach objects on a bedside table. To facilitate bed mobility, the bed should have a ¾-inch plywood board under a firm flat mattress. A footboard should extend 4 inches from the lower end of the mattress, and the bed should have a half-length side rail to provide protection against falling and a handgrip for turning and positioning.

Patients with good arm strength may be able to push up to the erect sitting position. The side rail also may be used to pull themselves erect. Overhead trapeze bars enable patients to pull up to a sitting position and to transfer to a wheelchair beside the bed (Fig. 24–1).

Wheelchair Mobility. Wheelchair mobility includes transfers to and from the wheelchair, operation of the wheelchair, and sitting tolerance. The ability to transfer requires adequate strength to lift or shift the weight of the body, balance, and coordination. There are numerous methods of transfer.[8] The method of transfer selected should be the most convenient one in relation to the patient's residual abilities. To improve the ability to transfer, exercises are directed particularly to the muscles for shoulder depression, elbow extension, hand grip, hip extension, and knee extension.

564

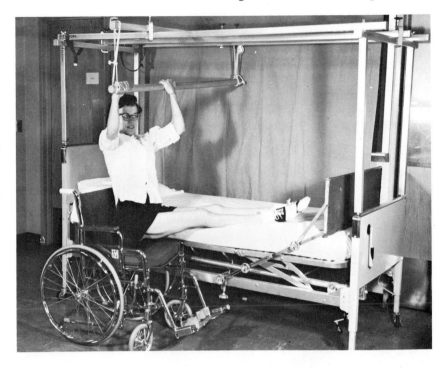

FIGURE 24–1. Transfer from bed to wheelchair by a paraplegic patient using a 4-foot trapeze bar. The long bar makes lateral transfers less difficult for any patient who has good strength in the upper extremities.

For the patient with hemiplegia or generalized weakness who has head and trunk balance, the pivot transfer can be performed independently or with the assistance of one person with little effort (Fig. 24–2). This is probably the most frequently used transfer when assistance is available. The nurse or therapist prevents buckling of the patient's knees with his or her knee and, by supporting the hips, assists the patient to stand and balance. The patient may then be pivoted to change directions. This transfer is stable and safe. Its relatively low energy requirement permits the movement of a large patient and decreases the risk of a back injury by the attendant.

For the patient who has lower extremity paraplegia, transfer to and from the bed by use of a trapeze bar is convenient (Fig. 24–1). The bed should be at the same height as the seat of the wheelchair. If the arm of the wheelchair is removable, the patient can transfer horizontally without having to lift the body vertically. Wheelchairs with detachable footrests can be wheeled close to the bed so that the distance for transfer is minimal. The transfer method that requires the least strength utilizes a transfer board or sliding board along which the patient slides from the bed, toilet, or chair to the wheelchair.

Wheelchair mobility requires more than the ability of the patients to propel themselves with the upper extremities. It is imperative that they are able to lock both wheels and adjust the footrests. In addition, the patient should be able to remove and replace the removable armrests as applicable. Use of the uninvolved lower extremities may assist in propelling the chair in a straight line or in turning the chair in either direction.

The disabled person who has reduced sensation or lacks the ability to shift weight is in danger of developing tissue damage as a result of ischemic necrosis. Normally, people shift position frequently enough that ischemia is not a problem. If the pressure produced by the weight of the body on a given surface exceeds capillary pressure for more than 30 minutes, ischemic damage begins to occur in that area.[9] Usually this pressure is greatest beneath the bony prominences of the ischial tuberosities and the greater trochanters. In addition to shifting weight for a few seconds every 10 minutes, persons with sensory loss should have a seat cushion in the wheelchair to distribute the sitting pressure more evenly. Sitting time and wheelchair mobility may be limited to the time during which the patient can sit without evidence of injury to the skin.

LOREN R. LESLIE

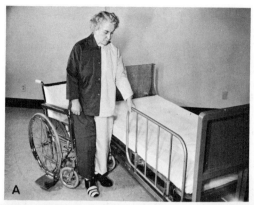

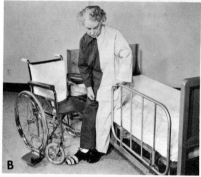

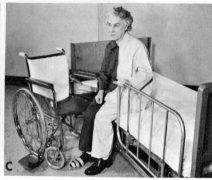

FIGURE 24–2. Sequence for independent transfer by a hemiplegic patient from a wheelchair to bed. The patient approaches the bed, locks the chair, and swings the footrest out of the way. She moves forward toward the edge of the chair seat and, grasping the arm rest, leans forward and pushes herself erect. After she is standing erect she grasps the side rail of the bed, pivots on her feet and lowers herself to sit on the bed. (From A Handbook of Rehabilitative Nursing Techniques in Hemiplegia. Minneapolis, Kenny Rehabilitation Institute, 1964.)

Ambulation. Ambulation training is dealt with elsewhere in this text; however, it should be noted that successful ambulation as a functional mobility activity requires that the patient be able to transfer from sitting to standing independently and to utilize ambulation aids such as crutches, canes, or appliances with ease.

The degree of functional independence determines the extent of ambulatory proficiency required both in complexity and in endurance of effort. Ambulation for short distances on level, smooth surfaces may be entirely satisfactory for the patient who is homebound or limited to an institutional domicile. For most patients, however, ambulatory mobility must also include the ability to climb stairs, curbs, and inclines as well as to walk on uneven surfaces or textures. Training in walking in a variety of environmental conditions and in the use of private and public transportation is an integral part of achieving functional independence in mobility.

Dressing

Patients should be evaluated for their ability to put on and take off the usual types of clothing.

Most dressing ADLs can be accomplished using one-handed techniques, although limitations of range of motion may make it difficult to put the arms through sleeves or slip clothing of usual design over the feet. Impairment of hand and finger coordination may interfere with buttoning, lacing, tying, and other small motions. By far the easiest adaptation today is the substitution of Velcro for other types of closures for all clothing including shoes. Otherwise, the use of assistive devices such as buttonhooks, long-handled reachers, and shoehorns often enables patients to dress themselves independently. Frequently, minor adaptations in the design of clothing, such as the relocation of buttons, hooks, or zippers or the substitution of elastic or Velcro closures, make dressing easier.[10] Recently, specially designed clothing for the handicapped has become available commercially.

Hygiene

The usual hygiene activities of washing, brushing teeth, shaving or applying make-up, combing hair, and using a handkerchief may require adapted equipment so that the patient can hold, control,

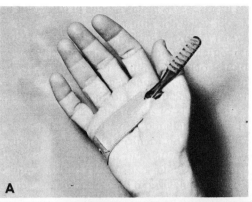

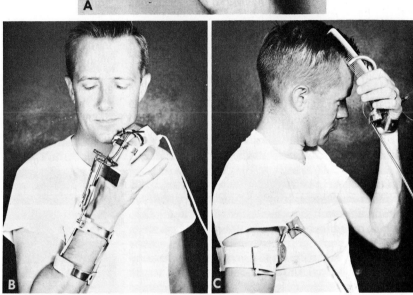

FIGURE 24–3. *A,* Cuff with pocket to hold the handle of a toothbrush. *B,* Finger flexion splint activated by wrist extension to hold a razor or other equipment for daily self-care. *C,* Robin-Aid splint hook attached to the hand for prehensile activities. The hook is closed by elastic bands and opened by abduction of the opposite arm.

or reach. Limitation of arm mobility or of grasp interferes with the performance of these activities. If the grasp is inadequate but the arm can be controlled, a holding device for such articles as a toothbrush, comb, or razor allows independence. Such a device may vary from a simple cuff to an elaborate splint or powered orthosis (Fig. 24–3). If the muscles of the shoulder or elbow are weak or incoordinated, a counterbalanced deltoid aid greatly increases the sphere of useful motion of the upper extremity (Fig. 24–4). Motorized equipment such as electric razors or toothbrushes also makes self-care easier for the patient with severe physical impairment. Bathing in a tub or shower requires the ability to transfer. A stool in the tub or shower may make independent transfers easier, and it should have nonskid mats or adhesive on the bottom for safety.

Bowel and Bladder Control

The establishment of bowel and bladder continence is needed to prevent perineal and sacral irritation. Urinary control may be achieved by an indwelling catheter; however, it is desirable to achieve a catheter-free status because of the multiple hazards of prolonged catheterization.[11] The use of condom catheter drainage or intermittent catheterization may be a part of the patient's self-care training. Bladder training is described in detail in Chapter 38.

Bowel control is somewhat easier to manage than bladder control. If normal bowel function cannot be restored, management of the bowel should prevent fecal incontinence, diarrhea, impaction, and irregularity.[12] Optimal function is established by developing regular bowel habits.

LOREN R. LESLIE

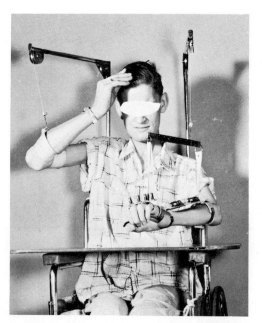

FIGURE 24–4. A counterbalanced deltoid aid allows flexion, abduction, and adduction of the shoulder with minimal muscular strength.

The gastrocolic reflex may enable the patient to attempt a bowel movement on a toilet or commode. This reflex occurs 20 to 40 minutes after a meal. The same postprandial period should be used every day if the patient's schedule of activities permits. Adequate time without emotional stress must be allowed so that the patient can relax, adequate peristalsis can occur, and the bowel can be emptied.

Other stimulation of colonic peristalsis may be used. Stimulation of the anorectal reflex by gently dilating the anal sphincter with a gloved finger or by the use of a glycerin suppository is an effective means of initiating defecation. Irritation of the rectum by irritant suppositories, cathartics, or enemas should be avoided. Usually bulk-forming agents such as Colace or Senokot will suffice to maintain stool consistency and intestinal peristalsis. If an atonic bowel does require a stimulus, Dulcolax suppositories or tablets are preferred, although milk of magnesia, tap water, or Fleet enemas may be used to initiate peristalsis. The least irritating procedure that is effective should be used.

Fecal incontinence is controlled best by dietary management. In the absence of an infectious gastroenteritis, just decreasing condiments or roughage in food or adding such foods as cheese, apple-

sauce, or tea may be adequate to solve the problem. Pectin, kaolin, or Metamucil may decrease intestinal motility. On occasion, anticholinergic drugs may be necessary, but the use of opium preparations is unsatisfactory.

The optimal position for defecation is the squat; therefore, the use of a commode or toilet is preferable to the bedpan or chucks. In addition to increased comfort, the commode requires less energy than the bedpan.[13] Suitable handrails in the bathroom assist the patient in toilet transfers and in minimizing the danger of a fall.

Eating

Physically disabled patients may be unable to feed themselves adequately because of loss of grasp, range of motion, or coordination. A holding device may be necessary for the knife, spoon, or cup. Adapted utensils are helpful (Fig. 24–5). If mobility or coordination of the upper extremities is limited, devices such as a Warm Springs feeder (Fig. 24–6), rocker feeder, or balanced forearm orthosis may be required.

Care should be taken in the placement of food on the plate or eating surface, especially if there is a visual field deficit. Difficulty in swallowing requires the appropriate selection of food consistency. Aspiration of liquid substances may occur in patients with bulbar paresis. Evaluation of the swallowing mechanisms should be a part of an ADL evaluation.

The oral ingestion of substances other than food, such as medications, is a part of functional independence training. Self-medication programs on the rehabilitation ward address the competence of the patient in the self-administration of prescribed drugs.

Rehabilitation ADL Measurement

Because self-care and ADL proficiency represent rehabilitation process outcomes and in addition are quantifiable, self-care rating systems are often used as indicators of rehabilitation effectiveness and program efficiency. Numerous assessment methods have appeared in rehabilitation literature, including the Barthel Index,[14] Pulses,[15] and Kenny Self Care Scale.[16] Combinations of these and other scales have been adapted to meet individual insti-

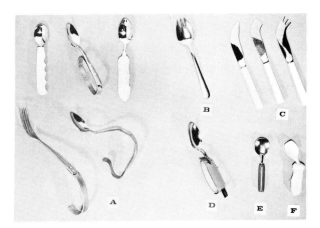

FIGURE 24–5. Adapted eating utensils for patients with impairment of grasp or reach.

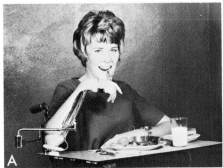

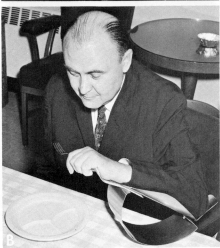

FIGURE 24–6. *A,* A balanced forearm orthosis mounted on the arm of a chair allows the patient to substitute shoulder depression for shoulder flexion and pivot the hand to the mouth during eating. This orthosis assists the function of weak shoulder flexors, adductors and abductors and weak elbow flexors. *B,* A forearm rocker feeder orthosis aids in the elevation of the hand during eating.

tution or program needs, or to form the basis for the functional component of a more comprehensive patient profile system.[17]

The importance of measuring functional outcome is emphasized by accreditation bodies such as the Commission on Accreditation of Rehabilitation Facilities (CARF) as a part of required program evaluation systems. Utilization review and third-party payers such as Medicare often employ functional scales for documentation of rehabilitation effectiveness in the monitoring of health care services.

It is important to recognize, however, that rehabilitation for self-care and functional independence is more than an intra-institutional exercise or a basis for documentation of rehabilitation program effectiveness. The ultimate outcome of training for functional independence is the use of this knowledge and techniques by patients in their home or post-discharge domicile. ADL training must be practical for daily use in order to be accepted by the patients and their families. For example, the time required by patients to dress or feed themselves may be excessive, resulting in family members or attendant staff providing assistance to expedite the process. If possible, these problems should be determined before the patient is discharged from the rehabilitation training program. Trial weekends at home or live-in facilities at the rehabilitation center should be utilized to assist families in learning to supervise the patient's self-care activities and to help determine the level of proficiency needed to function in the home environment. Home-bound health care or home nursing visits both before and after discharge are

LOREN R. LESLIE

also useful to monitor self-care proficiency and to reinforce the patients and their families in accomplishing a level of optimal functional independence.

References

1. Deaver, G. G., and Brown, M. E.: Physical Demands of Daily Life. New York, Institute for the Crippled and Disabled, 1945.
2. Lawton, E. B.: Activities of Daily Living for Physical Rehabilitation. New York, McGraw-Hill Book Company, 1963.
3. Rusk, H. A., and Taylor, E. J.: Living With a Disability. Garden City, NY, The Blakiston Company, 1953.
4. Self-Help Devices for Rehabilitation: Part I. New York University-Bellevue Medical Center Institute of Physical Medicine and Rehabilitation. Dubuque, IA, Wm. C. Brown Company, Publishers, 1958.
5. Self-Help Devices for Rehabilitation: Part II. New York University-Bellevue Medical Center Institute of Physical Medicine and Rehabilitation. Dubuque, IA, Wm. C. Brown Company, Publishers, 1965.
6. Goldsmith, S.: Designing for the Disabled, 2nd Ed. New York, McGraw-Hill Book Company, 1967.
7. Rosenberg, C.: Assistive Devices for the Handicapped. Minneapolis, American Rehabilitation Foundation, 1968.
8. A Handbook of Rehabilitative Nursing Techniques in Hemiplegia. Minneapolis, Kenny Rehabilitation Institute, 1964.
9. Kosiak, M.: Etiology of decubitus ulcers. Arch. Phys. Med., 42:19–29, 1961.
10. Kernaleguen, A.: Clothing for the handicapped. Physiother. Can., 30:135–138, 1978.
11. Price, M., Tobin, J. A., Reiser, M., Olson, M. E., Kubicek, W. G., Kottke, F. J., and Boen, J.: Renal function in patients with spinal cord injuries. Arch. Phys. Med., 47:406–411, 1966.
12. Mead, S.: A bowel training program in a rehabilitation center. Arch. Phys. Med., 37:210–213, 1956.
13. Benton, J. G., Brown, H., and Rusk, H. A.: Energy expended by patients on the bedpan and bedside commode. J.A.M.A., 144:1443–1447, 1950.
14. Mahoney, F. I., and Barthel, D. W.: Functional evaluation: Barthel index. Md. State Med. J., 14:61–65, 1965.
15. Moskowitz, E., and McCann, C. B.: Classification of disability in chronically ill and aging. J. Chronic Dis., 5:342–346, 1957.
16. Schoening, H. A., Anderegg, L., Bergstrom, D., Fonda, M., Steinkie, N., and Ulrich, P.: Numerical scoring of self-care status of patients. Arch. Phys. Med., 46:689–697, 1965.
17. Granger, C. V., and Gresham, G. E.: Functional Assessment in Rehabilitation Medicine. Baltimore, Williams & Wilkins, 1984.

25 Training in Homemaking Activities

LOREN R. LESLIE

Homemaking is probably the oldest vocation in history. In 1954, the Federal Rehabilitation Law was interpreted to include homemakers. Even earlier, in 1943, federal rehabilitation programs were included in the Social Security Law, and in 1946 homemaking was declared a vocation by the Vocational Rehabilitation Administration.[1]

Homemakers constitute the largest group among the disabled. One survey[2] pointed out that there were 1,875,000 women with arthritis, 4,000,000 women with cardiovascular disease, 175,000 women with active or arrested tuberculosis, 650,000 women with hemiplegia, and 800,000 women with orthopedic disabilities. The last group runs the gamut from tetraplegia to osteoarthritis of the hip. The total number of physically handicapped homemakers is now well over 10,000,000.

The disabled woman is not the only one who can benefit from training in homemaking. Men with physical impairment often must assume homemaking roles in order to allow other members of the family to work outside the home (Fig. 25–1). Men and women with a chronic illness are often relegated to a condition of complete dependency. Their potential for independence through training has never been realized. Children and young people with handicaps are certainly candidates for training. Development of homemaking skills may contribute to development of self-confidence and initiative.

It would be difficult to calculate the economic consequences of homemaking disability considering the diversity of tasks that a homemaker performs. Household management impacts not only on housekeeping but also on the emotional well-being of the individual and the family unit; therefore, the rehabilitation process must address much more than the development of work skills alone.

Homemaking activities—whether carried out by men, by women, or by children—contribute to the welfare of the family and to its economic productiveness and well-being. Homemaking itself is a composite of physical tasks, managerial functions, spirit, and emotional climate that holds the family or personality together and fosters development. The scope of activities related to homemaking includes the following:

1. Care of self.
2. Feeding the family.
3. Marketing and shopping.
4. Clothing the family.
5. Housing and maintenance.
6. Family relations.
7. Education and recreation.
8. Community participation.

Organization of a Training Program

Training may be arranged as a community service, as part of a hospital service, or, when possible, as a combination of the two.[2]

There are many agencies and facilities in most communities with an interest in homemaking. In planning the program, one should consider the local medical society, physical and occupational therapists, visiting or public health nurses, social

LOREN R. LESLIE

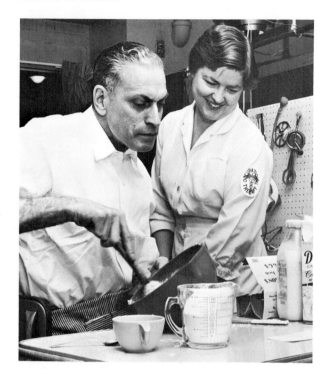

FIGURE 25–1. Men sometimes need homemaker training. (Connecticut Society for Crippled Children and Adults.) (From U.S. Department of Health, Education and Welfare, Vocational Rehabilitation Administration: Rehabilitation of the Physically Handicapped in Homemaking Activities, 1963.)

workers, voluntary agencies such as the National Society for Crippled Children and Adults, homemaker services in welfare departments or family service groups, home economists, dietitians, architects, designers, builders, and industrial engineers. Physiatrists and other physicians, such as orthopedic surgeons, neurologists, and cardiologists, should be encouraged to help in the planning.

The ideal training program should be based in a rehabilitation center or in a hospital with a department of physical medicine and rehabilitation and should begin when the homemaker is in the hospital.[3] Here the team concerned with the patient's rehabilitation can plan homemaking as an integral part of the general rehabilitation program. In addition, after discharge, the team can serve as a liaison to arrange continued training and follow-up. If the patient lives too far away from the rehabilitation facility, agencies in the patient's community can be alerted to his or her needs after return to the home.

The team may include all professional personnel in a department of physical medicine and rehabilitation. People most concerned are the physician (preferably a physiatrist), who directs training; the social worker, who acquaints the patient's family with the patient's particular needs and maintains the link with the physician, evaluates the possibilities for adaptations in the home, and helps in the purchase or procurement of special aids or devices; the physical therapist, who helps evaluate the patient's proficiency in activities of daily living and plans a conditioning program to maintain physical fitness; and the occupational therapist, who instructs in household management and the use of adaptive devices. Most often the actual home evaluation is carried out by a physical or occupational therapist who collaborates with the social worker. When the patient is a client of an outside agency, coordination of the rehabilitative program may be directed by a rehabilitation counselor. A very useful addition to the team is the home consultant or home economist who is trained in many areas of homemaking and whose skills are too often overlooked by the other members of the rehabilitation team. Duties of team members should complement each other.

Evaluation Content

The goal of homemaker training is efficient resettlement of the patient in the place of work—the home. Evaluation should anticipate

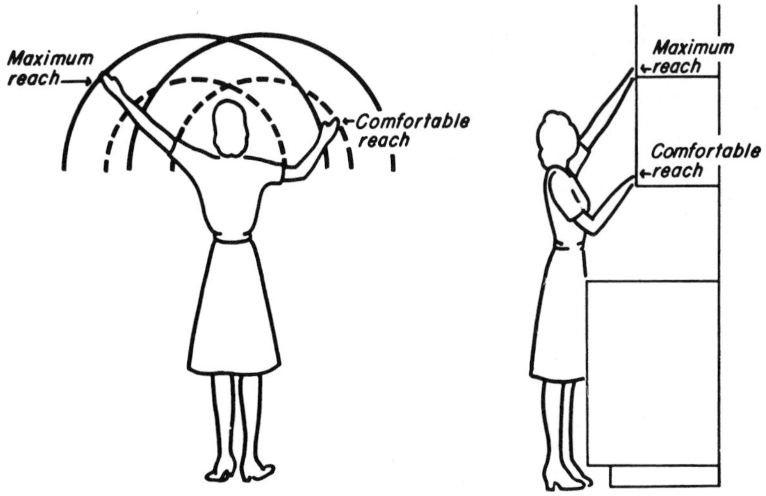

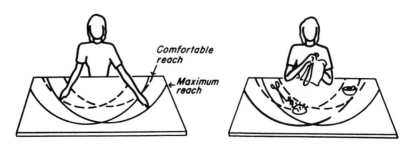

FIGURE 25–2. Determining vertical reaching areas. (From Rusk, H. A., et al.: A Manual for Training the Disabled Homemaker. Rehabilitation Monograph VIII, 2nd Ed. New York, The Institute of Physical Medicine and Rehabilitation, New York University Medical Center, 1961.)

problems or difficulties that the patient will encounter in the home. Domestic activities involve consideration of the following.[4]

Range of Reach. One should consider the maximal reach required, both in a vertical and in a horizontal direction. Prescriptions of tools for reaching, allocation of equipment, and arrangement of working surfaces depend on these measurements (Figs. 25–2 and 25–3). Conditions that limit range of reach are those requiring that work be done sitting down, such as paraplegia, and those severely limiting motion, such as crippling rheumatoid arthritis.

Movement from One Place to Another. A homemaker may walk as much as 25 km during a day's work. Cardiac patients, those limited to wheelchairs, and those requiring the use of canes, crutches, or leg braces are obviously limited.

Manual Activities. Patients with impaired use of hand or arm because of weakness, incoordination, or amputation may suffer limitations. It is this group that will call upon all the ingenuity the occupational therapist can muster.

Energy Consumption. Patients with cardiorespiratory diseases will usually find this the chief limiting factor. Bedmaking, ironing, or washing up requires the same rate of energy expenditure as housepainting, cabinetmaking, or plastering—3 to 4.5 calories per minute. Passmore and Durnin[5] describe the energy costs of many common household activities.

Safety. Lack of coordination, of sensation, and of spatial orientation may prove dangerous when one handles hot or sharp objects. The danger of falling because of vertigo, loss of consciousness, syncopal attacks, or epilepsy must be guarded against. It is in this group that one should consider elimination of certain household tasks altogether.

Communication. Contact with the outside world through the telephone or directly in such activities as shopping is difficult for patients with language difficulty. The aphasic patient is an example of this problem.

Almost all rehabilitation centers and physical medicine and rehabilitation services in general hospitals have a training kitchen facility. In addi-

FIGURE 25–3. Determining horizontal reach areas. (From Rusk, H. A., et al.: A Manual for Training the Disabled Homemaker. Rehabilitation Monograph VIII, 2nd Ed. New York, The Institute of Physical Medicine and Rehabilitation, New York University Medical Center, 1961.)

LOREN R. LESLIE

tion, bathroom and bed and sitting room training areas are often standard equipment. In such facilities, patients' skills in cleaning activities, meal preparation, meal service, laundry tasks, sewing, heavy household duties, marketing, child care, and special tasks may be thoroughly evaluated and plans made for adaptation in the home. Forms on which careful records are kept are an essential part of the training program. Accurate assessment of progress or changes in technique cannot be made any other way. Evaluation of skills in activities of daily living, such as bed to wheelchair transfer, walking, climbing, traveling, hand dressing, eating, and toilet activities, cannot be excluded from the program. Training in these areas must go on concomitantly with training in homemaking.

All members of the rehabilitation team try to help the homemaker to help herself. The primary therapeutic goal is work simplification—a scientific process of improving job method and adapting mechanical facilities to fit the physiological capacity of the worker. We may add two more: improved physical fitness—increased capacity for work—and improvement in psychological motivation so that the patient is encouraged to become proficient.

Principles of Work Simplification or Economy of Motion

Work simplification is of primary concern in homemaking training. The following outline is an excellent working guide.[2]

1. Whenever the condition allows, use both hands in opposite and symmetrical motions while working.

2. Lay out work areas within normal reach. Arrange supplies in a semicircle.

3. Slide—do not lift and carry. Use a table with wheels when moving from one work area to another.

4. Use fixed work stations. Have a special place to do each job so that supplies and equipment may be kept ready for immediate use.

5. Use the smallest number of work elements. Select equipment that may be used for more than one job; eliminate unnecessary motions.

6. Avoid the work of holding. Use utensils that rest firmly and are secured by suction cups or clamps. This will free hands for work.

7. Let gravity work. Examples are a laundry chute, refuse chute, and gravity-feed flour bin.

8. Position tools in advance. Store them so that they are placed in position for immediate grasping and use. For example, hang measuring cup and spoons separately within sight.

9. Position machine controls and switches within easy reach. Household appliances should be chosen on the basis of ease of operation.

10. Sit to work whenever possible. Use a comfortable chair and adjust work-place height to the chair. Or use an adjustable stool or chair.

11. Use a correct work-place height. The height should be right for the homemaker and the job. There are no standard heights. Morant[6] points out that the dimensions of a work space suitable for persons of normal size may differ appreciably from the best that can be found to accommodate workers of all sizes and that in a work space, a change of even ½ inch may make an appreciable difference in the ease of operation and comfort of a considerable proportion of workers.

12. Good conditions are important—good light and ventilation, comfortable clothing, and ambient temperature.

Rules of work simplification are not enough. The patient must learn to manage herself and her needs before she can manage homemaking activities and her family. She must become proficient in her activities of daily living.[7] She must begin to think like an industrial engineer. Is her strength adequate for certain jobs? What is her need for rest periods? What is the best time of day for the performance of certain duties? Ought she to plan some jobs as a daily chore, a weekly chore, or even a monthly chore? In what quantities ought food to be prepared? It is these and countless other questions that the homemaker tries to answer as she becomes more skillful in her job.

Assistive Devices, and Selection and Adaptation of Household Equipment

Tasks should be attempted without special aids. If it is decided that the homemaker will continue certain activities that require them, then plans can be made for the adaptation of a special aid or device. It would be unwise to plan for aids if the homemaker is not going to carry out activities for which the aids are designed.

Before planning to make a device, determine whether it is already available commercially. Often aids can be purchased more cheaply than they

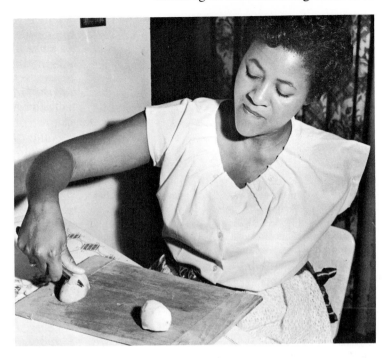

FIGURE 25–4. A spike on a board simplifies potato peeling. (J. A. Manter, University of Connecticut.) (From U.S. Department of Health, Education and Welfare, Vocational Rehabilitation Administration: Rehabilitation of the Physically Handicapped in Homemaking Activities, 1963.)

could be made. Basic considerations in the selection of devices are as follows:[8]

1. Use ordinary tools when they can be managed. Some homemakers hesitate to use tools that are obviously designed for the handicapped.

2. Homemakers are more likely to use assistive devices if they have a part in their selection.

3. Choose simple tools, and before their purchase or fabrication, consider the complications involved in taking them apart, keeping them clean, and finding a place to store them.

4. Consider an assistive device as temporary if that is possible. Change it as the homemaker acquires new skills.

Self-help devices or aids for the homemaker are used for stabilizing and holding objects (Figs. 25–4 and 25–5) or for extending reach and mobility (Fig. 25–6). In addition, one-handed aids and remote control devices (Fig. 25–7) may be useful in patients with limited upper extremity function.

Selection of proper appliances also can be of immense help to the homemaker. Care should be taken to see that all machines and appliances have openings and controls that can be reached and operated easily. It is also important that such appliances are placed in a convenient location. The designs of small household appliances and their use are discussed by Klinger.[19] In general, it can

be said that for the limited homemaker, front-opening equipment is better than top-opening equipment and that doors hinged on the side are best. A piece of equipment, such as a refrigerator, should not be purchased until the needs of the homemaker are clearly understood. Gas and electric utility companies can give very helpful advice.

Remodeling and Rearrangement of Home Facilities

In recent years there has been a great deal of emphasis on remodeling and rearrangement of home facilities, particularly kitchens. This work has emphasized space requirements for maneuvering a wheelchair, for vertical and horizontal reaches of the homemaker, for comfortable working heights, for necessary clearances of work areas, and for arrangement of the various centers such as sink center, range center, and mix center. Three basic kitchen arrangements, the U, the L, and the corridor, have been thoroughly worked out. There are advantages and disadvantages to each. Which one is best for a particular homemaker depends on the disability. However, the arrangement of the

LOREN R. LESLIE

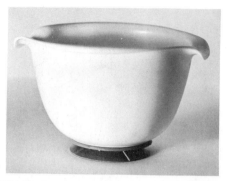

FIGURE 25–5. Suction bowlholder. (From Steinke, N., and Erickson, P.: Homemaking Aids for the Disabled. Minneapolis, Kenny Rehabilitation Institute, 1963.)

refrigerator, stove, and kitchen sink should form a work triangle. Most trips are made from the sink to the refrigerator and then to the stove.

The work center should have a definite and fixed place for all tools, utensils, and materials. This equipment should be located to permit a sequence of motion. Examples include the storage in the sink area of utensils that are first used with water, including all top-of-range utensils except skillets and pan covers. In the range area should be located utensils first used with heat, including covers to all utensils.

A logical extension of kitchen planning is the design of complete dwellings for the disabled. Obviously the limitations here are chiefly economic. In spite of these drawbacks, several approaches to housing for the disabled have been made. Design of dwellings for the disabled who require wheelchairs has been extensively discussed in two communications from the Testing and Observation Institute at Hellerup, Denmark,[9, 10] and in a recent publication by Laurie.[11]

At a conference of the International Society for Rehabilitation of the Disabled, the following criteria were stressed:[12]

1. The dwelling must allow the individual, whatever the handicap, to move about with maximal convenience and minimal effort.

2. The disabled person must be able to use all the facilities, not just the kitchen.

3. The dwelling must have maximal ease of communication with the outside world.

4. The house must have an adequate heating system.

5. Everything in the house must be planned for maximal serviceability and ease of maintenance.

6. The house must be usable regardless of the type of disability. It must never be planned for one disability only.

7. The price of every single component must be reduced to the absolute minimum.

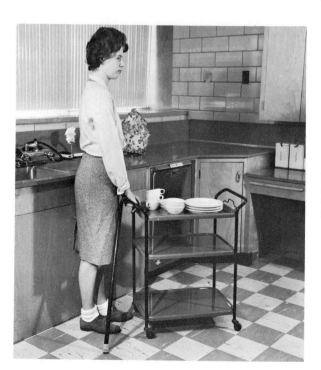

FIGURE 25–6. Wheeled utility table. The patient hangs her cane on the table rail and uses the table for support as she wheels it from place to place. (Courtesy of Kenny Rehabilitation Institute.)

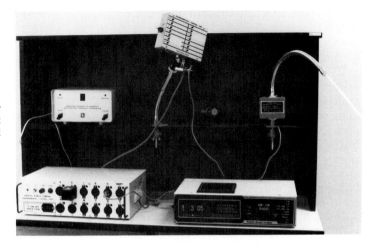

FIGURE 25–7. Environmental control unit. By sipping or puffing into the mouthpiece the patient activates this device, which can remotely control appliances, lights, and communication aids.

Planning the home for a disabled person requires accurate information concerning the physical limitations imposed by the disability or illness and the actual space available in the house. A planning consultant can save time and money. Any new construction or remodeling of a home for the disabled should include the following dimensions:

1. Walkways and halls should be at least 3 feet wide.

2. Doorways should be a minimum of 32 inches in width to accommodate the average wheelchair or some motorized chairs, which may be 2 feet 5 inches in width.

3. Ramp slopes are recommended at no more than 8.3 per cent, or a 1-foot rise in 12 feet.

4. Wall outlets should be no less than 16 inches from the floor.

5. Optimal table height for pull-out tables is 24 inches. If knee room is needed to accommodate a wheelchair, the height should be 30 inches, and for working while standing, 32 to 37 inches.

6. Sink heights should be 21 to 36 inches.

7. Toilet heights should be 15 to 23 inches.

8. An area of 15 square feet is required for wheelchair accommodation in a bathroom.

More detailed specifications are described in the publication by Laurie,[11] which also includes references to other resource materials about adaptations, techniques, and remodeling plans.

Child Care

Child care may be a particular problem for the disabled homemaker. It is important for her to develop a sense of discipline and responsibility in her children. Dressing the young child may be especially difficult for the handicapped mother. May and co-workers[8] have made some very practical suggestions concerning clothes for pre-school children that make dressing much easier.

It may happen on occasion that a handicapped homemaker has handicapped children. In such cases good work habits and a sense of pride in accomplishment are invaluable. This is an excellent way to encourage independence.

All children, whether handicapped or not, work much better under established rules and regulation. Disciplinary problems arise more often when there are no standards and when the child is not made responsible. Wall[13] points out that the desire to be helpful and independent is often at its height when the child is four years old. Instead of making the child more dependent, the mother should give the child the opportunity to develop into a cooperative member of the family.

A mother who teaches her children to be independent early, whether they are handicapped or not, will make time available for her own needs—needs for rest, for cultural enrichment, and for other tasks not related to child care.

Nutrition and Exercise

During her training in the hospital or rehabilitation center, the disabled homemaker should learn the principles of sound nutrition. This is of importance not only for herself but also for her family. Since mixes, canned, frozen, and dehy-

LOREN R. LESLIE

drated foods may be sources of work simplification, it is imperative that the homemaker learn to incorporate them in a balanced diet. The hospital dietitian has a very helpful role to play here.

It is probably true, however, that the homemaker will suffer far more often from overnutrition than from malnutrition. Because disability may limit markedly the homemaker's opportunity to perform tasks that require intense, prolonged physical effort, she will tend to eat more than she needs. The result is obesity, which in turn will increase the cost of work.[14] An occasional patient, however, who is taking large doses of medication, or of several medications, may have little or no appetite. The goal in this instance is to control medications and encourage sound nutritional habits.

The recommendation for daily periods of cardiorespiratory and muscular exercise may appear contradictory after we have stressed work simplification and efficiency. On the contrary, short periods of relatively intense graded exercise are the basis of physical fitness and will increase the homemaker's ability to perform useful work. Some activity aside from the fixed duties of homemaking is also necessary to maintain flexibility and optimal range of motion of joints. An exercise program may be contraindicated in the case of a patient with severe cardiopulmonary disease.

Psychology of Disability and Family Relationships

The handicapped homemaker has fears and anxieties that those who are well can only dimly perceive. She must learn to accept the difference in her appearance and she must finally adjust her life to a central fact—disability is permanent and the most fervent wishing will not make it disappear. She is perturbed by doubts concerning her abilities, her role as a wife and sexual partner, and the way her children may respond to her altered appearance. Litman,[15] in a study of 100 patients undergoing treatment in rehabilitation centers, has emphasized the importance of family support in the rehabilitation process.

If we are to help the homemaker achieve successful resettlement in her home, the family must be encouraged to take an active part in the training. Frequent visits to the hospital by family members help the patient, but also allow them to see the patient at work, to discover what she can do,

and to learn techniques of treatment that will be carried out at home.[16] Members of the rehabilitation team must learn to wait, to be patient, and to understand that the patient's adjustment is a dynamic, constantly changing process.[17]

Accounts of the trials and tribulations of disabled homemakers demonstrate that there are certain common factors in successful rehabilitation. They are courage, determination to succeed, family support, ability to change work habits and techniques, and intelligent use of available facilities.

The successful rehabilitation process is demonstrated in the words of a handicapped homemaker:

I am happy and thankful to do my own housework. I love to cook and wash and iron. It just is a thrill for me knowing I've done it myself, to see my clothes sparkling white and ironed smoothly, to see my family nicely dressed, and to see my husband's and son's eyes and hear their comments of pleasure as they enjoy their food.[11]

Home Care and Homemaker Services

These subjects have some relation to training in homemaking and deserve definition. Home care is the provision of health care and supportive services to the sick or disabled person in his or her place of residence. It may be provided in a diversity of patterns or organization and service running the gamut from nursing service under a physician's direction to a program that is centrally administered and that, through coordinated planning, evaluation, and follow-up procedures, provides physician-directed medical, nursing, social, and related services to selected patients at home. A logical link between the homemaker and the hospital would be a hospital extension service. Under titles XVIII and XIX of the Social Security Act (Medicare and Medicaid), home health care visits were included in a federal program of health insurance. Medicare benefits are limited to skilled nursing care or other therapeutic services prescribed by a physician and provided by an approved home health agency. This does not include homemaking services. Medicaid home health care benefits differ from Medicare in that eligibility for home health care for persons entitled to public assistance and Supplemental Security Income (SSI) is not related to the requirements for skilled care. Medicaid services may include home health aid services, medical equipment, and appliances. A new title XX enacted in 1974 called for states to provide for health support services to meet the needs of children, the aged, the mentally retarded, the blind, the emotionally disturbed, and the physically handicapped. These services include those related to the management and maintenance of the home.[11]

Homemaker services are services offered to families disrupted by death, illness, or accident. A homemaker in this frame of reference is a trained housekeeper and cook who has skill in handling children. Such services are provided by many welfare and family agencies.[18] Home health aides have been added to homemaker services. Their function is to help improve the patient's level of independence by helping in the carrying out of instructions left by the occupational therapist, physical therapist, physician, or other supervisor. The nutritionist or dietitian may offer useful services through consultation to staffs of home health agencies, membership on a professional advisory committee, and teaching programs for home health aides. Such services may be extremely helpful to individuals whose disability is so severe that independent function will never be possible.

References

1. Switzer, M. D.: Foreword. *In* Rehabilitation of the Physically Handicapped in Homemaking Activities. Proceedings of a workshop. Highland Park, IL, January 27–30, 1963. U. S. Department of Health, Education and Welfare, Vocational Rehabilitation Administration.
2. Rusk, H. A., Kristeller, E. L., Judson, J. S., Hung, G. M., and Zimmerman, M. E.: Introductions. *In* A Manual for Training the Disabled Homemaker. Rehabilitation Monograph VIII, 2nd Ed. New York, The Institute of Physical Medicine and Rehabilitation, New York University Medical Center, 1961.
3. May, E. E.: Suggestions for the rehabilitation of the physically handicapped homemaker. Am. J. Occup. Ther., 8: Part I, 1962.
4. Petrie, A.: Rehabilitation of the housewife. Occup. Ther., 27:19, 1964.
5. Passmore, R., and Durnin, J. V. G. A.: Human energy expenditure. Phys. Rev., 35:801, 1955.
6. Morant, G. M.: Body sizes and work spaces. *In* Symposium on Human Factors in Equipment Design. The Ergonomics Research Society. Proceedings, Vol. 2, edited by W. F. Floyd and A. T. Welford. London, H. K. Lewis & Co., Ltd., 1954.
7. Mossman, P. L.: A Problem Oriented Approach to Stroke Rehabilitation. Springfield, IL, Charles C Thomas, Publisher, 1976.
8. May, E. E., Waggoner, N. R., and Boettke, E. M.: Homemaking for the Handicapped. New York, Dodd, Mead, and Company, 1966.
9. Leschly, V., Exner, I., and Exner, J.: General Lives in Designs of Dwellings for Handicapped Confined to Wheelchairs. Part I. Communications from the Testing and Observation Institute of the Danish National Association for Infantile Paralysis, No. 6. Hellerup, Denmark, 1960.
10. Leschly, V., Kjaer, A., and Kjaer, B.: General Lives in Designs of Dwellings for Handicapped Confined to Wheelchairs. Part 2. Communications from the Testing and Observation Institute of the Danish National Association for Infantile Paralysis, No. 6. Hellerup, Denmark, 1960.
11. Laurie, G.: Housing and Home Services for the Disabled. Hagerstown, MD, Harper and Row, 1977.
12. Planning of Dwellings. *In* ISRD Conference, The Physically Disabled and Their Environment, Stockholm, October 12–18, 1961. New York, International Society for the Rehabilitation of the Disabled, 1962.
13. Wall, J. S.: Play Experiences Handicapped Mothers May Share with Young Children. Storrs, CT, University of Connecticut, School of Home Economics, 1961.
14. Gordon, E. E.: Development of the Applied Sciences to the Handicapped Homemaker. *In* Rehabilitation of the Physically Handicapped in Homemaking Activities. Proceedings of a workshop. Highland Park, IL, January 27–30, 1963. U. S. Department of Health, Education and Welfare, Vocational Rehabilitation Administration.
15. Litman, T. J.: An analysis of the sociologic factors affecting the rehabilitation of the physically handicapped. Arch. Phys. Med., 45:9, 1964.
16. Peszczynski, M., Fowles, B. II, and Mohan, S. P.: Function of home evaluations in discharging rehabilitated severely disabled from the hospital. Arch. Phys. Med. Rehabil., 43:109, 1961.
17. Christopherson, V. A.: The patient and the family. Rehabil. Lit., 23:34, 1962.
18. Homemaker Services in Public Welfare. U. S. Department of Health, Education and Welfare, Welfare Administration, April 1964.
19. Klinger, J. L.: Mealtime Manual for People with Disabilities and the Aging, 2nd Ed. New York, Institute of Physical Medicine, 1978.
20. Steinke, N., and Erickson, P.: Homemaking Aids for the Disabled. Minneapolis, Kenny Rehabilitation Institute, 1963.
21. Zmola, G. M.: You Can Do Family Laundry with Hand Limitations. Storrs, CT, University of Connecticut, School of Home Economics, 1959.

26

Upper Extremity Orthotics

LEONARD F. BENDER

Functional Anatomy

The shoulder-elbow-wrist-hand unit is a remarkable evolutionary development modified as humans arose and walked on their hind legs. The front legs developed the capacity for prehension and the mobility necessary to place the hand in an infinite number of positions.

The shoulder girdle is composed of seven joints: the costovertebral, costosternal, sternoclavicular, scapulocostal, acromioclavicular, suprahumeral, and glenohumeral.[1] Moving synchronously, these joints provide great mobility but only minimally essential stability. The glenohumeral joint is commonly referred to as the shoulder joint, in contrast to the group of joints that make up the shoulder girdle. Movements of the glenohumeral joint are controlled by two groups of muscles: (1) large muscles originating on the thorax and inserting on the humerus plus the deltoid, and (2) smaller muscles that arise on the scapula and insert through the rotator cuff on the humeral head and neck. The combined action of the short rotator muscles (supraspinatus, infraspinatus, teres minor, and subscapularis) pulls the humeral head into the glenoid fossa and fixes it there, depresses and rotates the head of the humerus, and, coupled with the deltoid muscle, assists in abduction of the arm through a rotatory force couple.[2] The short rotators receive their innervation primarily from the fifth and sixth cervical nerve roots through nerves that branch off the upper trunk and the posterior and lateral cords of the brachial plexus; they are spared in most cervical spinal cord injuries but are variously involved in injuries of the brachial plexus.

Elbow, forearm, and wrist motions combine to produce shortening and lengthening of the support system of the hand and rotation of the hand through 180 degrees from full pronation to extreme supination. Like a universal joint, these joints, in conjunction with the shoulder girdle, provide accurate and extensive positioning of the hand. Elbow flexor muscles are largely supplied by the fifth and sixth cervical nerve roots through the musculocutaneous nerve; extensors are innervated by the sixth and seventh cervical nerve roots in the radial nerve.

The forearm anchors most of the muscles that flex, extend, and rotate the wrist and also provide power grip and metacarpophalangeal extension, whereas the muscles responsible for many fine functions of the fingers are located in the hand. The intrinsic muscles of the hand are supplied by the eighth cervical and the first thoracic nerve roots, whereas the muscles of the forearm receive innervation from all nerve roots of the brachial plexus.

Individual muscles for the thumb and little finger (fifth digit) make these two digits uniquely mobile and useful. The first, second, and third digits are often used as a three-jaw chuck to grasp small objects. Napier has described this position as "precision grip."[3] It may be accomplished through fingertip, lateral, or palmar pinch. "Power grip" involves holding an object between flexed fingers and the opposed thumb. The same tool may be handled by either precision grip or power grip; it is the nature of the task, not the shape of the tool, that dictates which posture is employed. This difference must be carefully considered when prescribing orthoses or recommending surgery.

Forces

Orthotic devices apply forces to the braced extremity. Therefore, it is important to recognize and attempt to understand the role of force in producing motion and desired activities.

A force can be described according to its magnitude, direction, and point of application.[4] All movement is either rotation, translation, or a combination of the two. Rotation is angular motion, and translation is motion without change in angular orientation. Torque is the strength of a rotating tendency. The effectiveness of a force in causing joint motion depends both on its point of application or distance from the axis of rotation and on its magnitude. Moving the origin or insertion of a muscle to a different location may either decrease or increase the effectiveness of that muscle.

Levers can be used to amplify forces, and examples of all types of levers can be found in the musculoskeletal system. When applying force through orthoses, the principles of leverage and forces must be utilized to achieve optimal results.

Purposes of Orthoses

Orthoses are used to (1) assist, (2) resist, (3) align, and (4) simulate function of part of the body. Orthoses that assist movement generally incorporate a method of storing energy and releasing it at a desired time; springs, rubber bands, compressed gas, and electricity may be used. They may also transfer muscle power from an accustomed use to a new one, as in balanced forearm orthoses or flexor-hinge hand orthoses.

Occasionally, movements of the body need to be reduced; orthoses may rigidly support a bone fracture or an area of instability or weakness. Orthoses may restrict or resist movement by adding friction to orthotic joint motion or by using stops.

Alignment of joints damaged by arthritis or of a spine curved abnormally may be achieved through orthoses; such devices may reduce or possibly prevent deformity.

Certain surgical procedures may also achieve results similar to those produced by orthoses; in some instances, an orthotic device may be used to simulate the result of proposed surgery.

Classification of Orthoses

The confusing terminology used to describe braces, splints, calipers, appliances, and aids has included eponyms, descriptive phrases, and non-standardized terms. In 1971, the American Orthotic and Prosthetic Association urged the Committee on Prosthetic-Orthotic Education of the National Academy of Sciences to develop a standardized nomenclature. By mid-1972, a new terminology was developed and put into use[5]; in it all exoskeletal devices are called orthoses and they are described (1) by the joints they encompass, (2) by abbreviating each joint name to one letter, and (3) by using combinations of symbols to indicate the desired control of the designated function.

Orthoses may be made out of thin metal, heat-moldable plastic, polyurethane foam, epoxy resins, or plaster. The shorter the period of time one proposes using the device, the less durably it need be constructed. Thus, if one wishes to rest an inflamed joint for a few days, it is quite likely that a suitable orthosis can be constructed of plaster or heat-moldable plastic by the physician or by a therapist. But when use of the device for an extended period of time is anticipated, it will be cheaper and better to use metal, plastic, or epoxy resins and to have the device constructed by an orthotist.

Types of Orthoses

A convenient way to describe orthoses is to divide them into static positioning devices and functional ones.

Static Orthoses

SHOULDER STATIC DEVICES

The airplane splint is a classic example of a static positioning device applied to the shoulder. It holds the arm in approximately 90 degrees of abduction and permits no glenohumeral motion. It is held to the chest wall by straps or elastic bandages and is made of metal or plaster. Previously thought to be the best way to manage perinatal injury of the brachial plexus, it is no longer recommended for this purpose because it may contribute to the high-riding shoulder girdle frequently seen in Erb's palsy.[6] However, it is the orthosis of choice for burns of the axilla.

ELBOW STATIC DEVICES

Static positioning orthoses are used at the elbow primarily to hold a damaged, unstable joint in alignment. By adding straps or turnbuckles, force

LEONARD F. BENDER

may be applied to gently gain a desired increase in range of motion or to prevent an anticipated contracture after burns of the elbow.

WRIST STATIC DEVICES

At the wrist, static orthoses are commonly used to provide immobilization. In a case of neurapraxia of the radial nerve with a good prognosis for quick recovery, a plaster cock-up splint that holds the hand in 15 degrees of dorsiflexion at the wrist and prevents wrist motion may suffice. If a long period of recovery is anticipated, a functional device would be more appropriate.

In rheumatoid arthritis, a plastic or metal orthosis can be applied to the volar surface of the forearm and the wrist and is held in place by three straps over the styloid processes of the radius and ulna, the metacarpals, and the mid-forearm.[7] When correctly applied, this device can help prevent or correct subluxation of the carpal bones volarly on the radius and ulnar deviation of the hand at the wrist.

Spiral orthoses also can stabilize the wrist by wrapping a metal or plastic strap from the palm to the mid-forearm in 1½ turns (Fig. 26–1).

STATIC HAND ORTHOSES

Static hand orthoses vary considerably in design according to their purpose. They may be used to immobilize finger joints or to increase function by holding digits in a more favorable position.

Burns of the dorsum of the hand are appropriately splinted by holding the fingers on a platform with the interphalangeal joints extended, the metacarpophalangeal joints fully flexed, the thumb abducted, and the wrist slightly dorsiflexed.[8]

When the metacarpophalangeal joints are acutely inflamed, as in rheumatoid arthritis, these

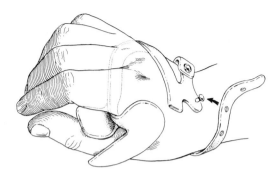

FIGURE 26–2. A simple or basic hand orthosis made from steel and held on by a Plastisol strap. A large C bar is attached to hold the thumb abducted.

joints should be supported in a neutral position with a volar platform extending to the flexor crease of the proximal interphalangeal joint. This support is most easily provided through heat-moldable plastic splints that extend either to or across the wrist on the volar surface and have a lip on the ulnar border high enough to prevent ulnar deviation of the fingers and a dorsal strap just behind the head of the metacarpals to reduce volar subluxation of the phalanges.

As one considers different ways to increase function in a weak or partially paralyzed hand, there appear to be two basic classes of orthoses that may be used: the simple hand orthosis and some type of flexor-hinge hand orthosis.

The simple hand orthosis is a device that consists of a metal or plastic band that runs either over the dorsum of the hand from the thumb web to the volar surface of the fourth metacarpal or volarly from the dorsal surface of the second metacarpal across the palm to the dorsal surface of the fourth metacarpal (Fig. 26–2). Each orthosis is held on the hand and prevented from sliding off by a strap around the volar surface of the wrist. A small, rolled bar protrudes between the first and second metacarpals to prevent the orthosis from migrating proximally. If this bar is enlarged to form a letter C, it can be used to hold the thumb abducted from the palm. An extension of the basic orthosis over the first metacarpal will hold the thumb in a position of opposition. If the thumb is flail, it can be held in a pair of rings with a bar connecting them to the simple hand orthosis. A bar set dorsally over the proximal phalanges will prevent hyperextension of the metacarpophalangeal joints, yet this "lumbrical" bar will permit the long finger extensors to act to extend the interphalangeal joints (Fig. 26–3).

Other units that may be added to a simple hand

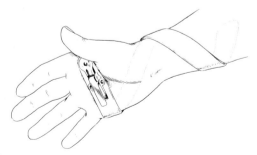

FIGURE 26–1. A spiral wrist orthosis with a spring-loaded clip on the palmar extension can be used to stabilize the wrist and to provide an attachment for writing and eating and other assistive devices.

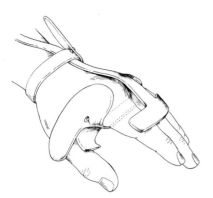

FIGURE 26–3. A wrist-hand orthosis with a metacarpophalangeal extension stop; this "lumbrical" bar can be used to enhance extension of the interphalangeal joints by the long finger extensor muscles in an ulnar nerve lesion.

orthosis utilize springs or movable parts and will be considered under the heading *Functional Orthoses*.

STATIC FINGER ORTHOSES

Static finger orthoses can stabilize individual interphalangeal joints or combinations of interphalangeal joints. They are usually constructed of stainless steel in the form of complete or partial rings fastened together with narrow metal bars. They may also be spirals similar to those used across the wrist. An unstable interphalangeal joint can be prevented from hyperextending and can be made stable with one of these devices (Fig. 26–4).

Functional Orthoses

Instead of immobilizing a joint or restraining its motion as static orthoses do, a functional orthosis

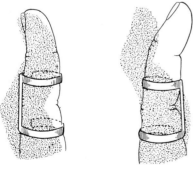

FIGURE 26–4. Static finger orthoses. The one on the left prevents fixed flexion of the proximal interphalangeal joint as is seen in a "boutonnière" deformity; the one to the right prevents hyperextension of the proximal interphalangeal joint, as may be seen in a "swan-neck" deformity.

improves function through the use of levers, pulleys, movable joints, and external power storage devices such as springs, rubber bands, batteries, and tanks of compressed gas.

FUNCTIONAL SHOULDER ORTHOSES

Functional orthoses to improve shoulder actions have not proved generally useful or successful. Several orthoses that were supported on the iliac crest and had uprights that extended to the axilla or laterally around the shoulder were designed and refined in the decades between 1950 and 1970.[9] They were relatively complex exoskeletal systems and have been discarded because they were cumbersome and difficult to fit and provided only limited additional function.

FUNCTIONAL ELBOW ORTHOSES

Functional orthoses can be constructed for weakness or instability of the elbow. The customary device has some type of pivot hinge aligned with the axis of the elbow joint, and stability is provided by cuffs above and below the elbow. Rubber bands, springs, or compressed gas may be used to assist either flexion or extension; generally, extension can be achieved through the pull of gravity and only flexion need be assisted. When elbow flexion muscle strength is less than antigravity and an elbow flexion assist is utilized, the orthosis must also incorporate a locking mechanism at the elbow to maintain a practical functional position for carrying loads. Elbow flexion assist may also be provided through a Bowden cable, which has the cable housing attached to a cuff around the arm while the cable extends through it from a figure eight harness around the shoulders to that portion of the orthosis that is below the elbow. Tension on the cable will flex the elbow, and an elbow-locking mechanism operated by scapular elevation will permit a choice of several stable positions of the elbow. A hollow tube of polyurethane foam can be used to provide moderate stability, to permit active elbow flexion, and to give elbow extension assist. Compressed foam seeks to return to its original shape; hence, elbow flexion compresses the foam, which returns to the straight contour when released. For ease of donning and doffing, the tube is slit and tapered down the side and uses Velcro fasteners (Fig. 26–5).

BALANCED FOREARM ORTHOSES

Perhaps the most useful device to assist both elbow and shoulder function, in the presence of

LEONARD F. BENDER

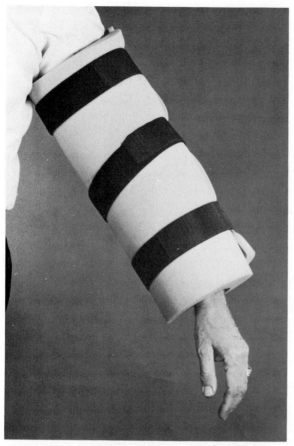

FIGURE 26–5. Polyfoam orthosis to assist elbow extension.

level of the iliac crest. It consists of a trough in which the proximal portion of the forearm rests; a pivot and linkage system underneath the trough can be adjusted and preset so that the patient can learn to produce motion at both the elbow and to a lesser extent the shoulder, with small motions of the trunk or shoulder girdle (Fig. 26–6).

FUNCTIONAL WRIST ORTHOSES

Functional wrist orthoses are rarely used without hand orthoses. If it is necessary to assist wrist extension only, it can be done by a volar plastic or metal trough on the forearm attached with Velcro straps around the dorsum of the forearm. Pivot hinges at the side of the wrist must be attached to the forearm piece and to a palmar bar. Springs or rubber bands attached to short dorsal uprights on either side of the wrist hinge can be adjusted to give assistance to wrist extension.

A group of devices known as wrist-driven, flexor-hinge hand splints have been developed and will be discussed under *Functional Hand Orthoses*, since they use wrist power to provide finger function, especially prehension.

FUNCTIONAL HAND ORTHOSES

Functional hand orthoses can be constructed by using a simple hand orthosis as a foundation and adding one or more special assistive devices.

A swivel thumb is a half-ring clip around the proximal phalanx of the thumb whose arm pivots from a point near the head of the second metacarpal to permit the thumb to swing in a fixed arc toward opposition from extension and abduction. The rigid pivot arm can be replaced with a spring wire, and the thumb then not only can pivot but

profound weakness in the upper extremity, is the balanced forearm orthosis. This can be mounted on a wheelchair, on a table or working surface, or occasionally on a belt around the person at the

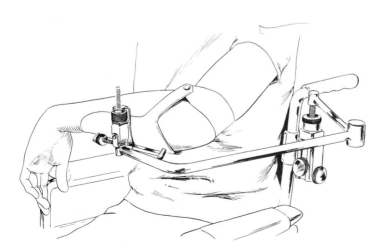

FIGURE 26–6. A balanced forearm orthosis mounted on a wheelchair. The patient's forearm rests in a trough. The pivot point of the trough and the position of the two movable arms must be carefully adjusted to achieve maximum range of hand placement in a patient with severe proximal weakness.

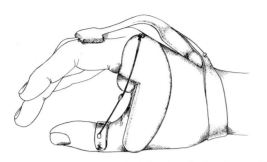

FIGURE 26–7. A spring swivel thumb assist has been added to a simple hand orthosis with a metacarpophalangeal extension stop. The thumb assist permits the thumb to be actively adducted, and the spring will assist abduction. The thumb can also pivot across the palm toward the fifth digit.

also can voluntarily be brought into adduction; abduction is assisted by the spring (Fig. 26–7).

A first dorsal interosseus assist also attaches near the head of the second metacarpal and utilizes a spring wire and a plastic ring to pull the index finger into abduction; the plastic ring may be placed over either the proximal or the middle phalanx.

A thumb interphalangeal joint extension assist is similar to a first dorsal interosseus assist but is attached near the head of the first metacarpal and exerts its pull on the distal phalanx of the thumb.

Interphalangeal extension assist in the absence of hand intrinsic muscles and long finger extensors can be achieved by mounting a "banjo"-shaped device on the hand orthosis and pulling on the distal phalanges through plastic rings attached to

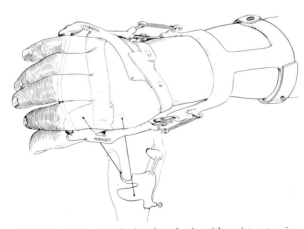

FIGURE 26–8. A wrist-hand orthosis with wrist extension assist and metacarpophalangeal extension assist. The wrist extension assist is provided by rubber bands dorsal to the axis of wrist motion; metacarpophalangeal extension assist comes from coiled springs that support a volarly placed "lumbrical" bar. This orthosis is designed for use in radial nerve paralysis.

rubber bands that are fastened to the crossbar of the "banjo." Unfortunately, the device is cumbersome and the assisting force cannot be constant, since the rubber band tension increases with stretch.

Metacarpophalangeal extension assist no longer requires a "banjo." It can be accomplished by a bar similar in contour to a lumbrical bar but placed on the volar surface of the proximal phalanges with stiff coil springs holding each end of the bar to the hand orthosis. The springs must be placed to push the proximal phalanges into extension at the metacarpophalangeal joint and to permit full range of finger flexion (Fig. 26–8).

FLEXOR-HINGE HAND ORTHOSES

Hand orthoses with various attachments described in the preceding work well in isolated and mild to moderate weaknesses or abnormal functions of the hand. However, when paralysis or weakness is widespread or severe, it may be advisable to use an orthosis built on the flexor-hinge hand principle. This principle permits only metacarpophalangeal motion, stabilizes the interphalangeal joints of digits two and three and both the interphalangeal and metacarpophalangeal joints of the thumb, creates a three-jaw chuck prehension, and may utilize several different power-assist sources. A hand with unstable metacarpophalangeal joints, such as is seen in rheumatoid arthritis, may need only the alignment provided by a finger-driven flexor-hinge hand orthosis. The intact muscles are used to flex and extend the metacarpophalangeal joints, and the orthosis guides the fingers in the desired path of movement.

In cervical spinal cord injuries in which no muscles to flex or extend the fingers remain innervated, but the extensor carpi radialis muscle is intact, a wrist-driven flexor-hinge hand orthosis can be used. This device has a parallelogram of metal bars that transforms wrist extension and flexion into finger flexion and extension. Usually, the top bar of the parallelogram is adjustable in length so prehension can be accomplished in several different positions of wrist flexion or extension. Instead of being a hand orthosis, it is a wrist-hand orthosis with a cuff or trough on the forearm (Fig. 26–9).

A variation of the wrist-driven flexor-hinge hand orthosis has been developed. A one-piece molded dorsal cover for the three phalanges each of the second and third digits is adjustably attached by a cord to a wrist cuff (Fig. 26–10). A hand orthosis

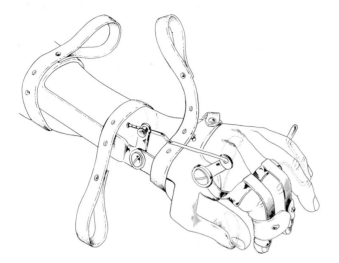

FIGURE 26–9. A wrist-driven flexor-hinge wrist-hand orthosis is operated by the power of wrist extension and is used in spinal cord injuries where no active finger function remains but wrist extension, elbow flexion, and shoulder motions are all at least antigravity strength. The top bar of the parallelogram at the wrist is adjustable in length so that prehension can be accomplished in different wrist positions.

with a thumb post holds the thumb in a stable position. Again, wrist extension causes finger flexion. The device is less bulky and somewhat less stable than the metal wrist-driven flexor-hinge hand orthosis with parallelogram bars but is used primarily as a testing and training device.

Another newer variation of the wrist-driven flexor-hinge hand orthosis is the Key Grip or Lateral Pinch Orthosis. In this device, developed at Burke Rehabilitation Center, a wrist-driven orthosis holds the index finger stabilized at the metacarpophalangeal and interphalangeal joints in a position of partial flexion and then pulls the thumb into flexion by a Bowden cable attached volarly at the wrist and to the plastic thumb post. This creates a lateral pinch type of grip that is preferred by some persons with severe paralysis of the hand.

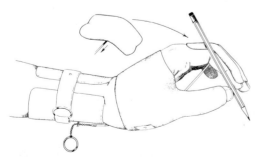

FIGURE 26–10. A three-piece wrist-hand orthosis is simpler, lighter, and less expensive than a wrist-driven flexor-hinge wrist-hand orthosis, yet it provides similar function.

When both the hand and the forearm muscles are paralyzed, a cable-driven or motor-driven flexor-hinge hand orthosis may be utilized. A Bowden cable can be attached to a figure eight harness similar to that used to operate the terminal device of an upper extremity prosthesis. Scapular abduction or humeral flexion will operate the orthosis. To provide prehension for an extended period of time without constant tension on the control cable, a clutch-locking device or spring-assisted prehension and a tension-relief control must be included. The development of small electrical motors has made it possible to open and close a flexor-hinge hand orthosis electrically. Myoelectrical control may be used, but the current state of the art leaves much to be desired. Reliable, implantable electrodes for controlled voltages are still in the developmental stage. Surface electrodes are not consistent or reliable from day to day; it is difficult to place them accurately daily, and varying skin impedance requires resetting the amplifier gain. Instead of myoelectrical control, one can use on-off switches of many designs; generally, it is difficult to place them in a position where they can be utilized over extended periods of time. Often, these switches are attached to the wheelchair and operated by head motion or scapular motion; this correct relationship between the person and the switch is difficult to maintain.

MOUTHSTICKS

A few devices have been developed that consist of a lightweight but strong metal tube or rod

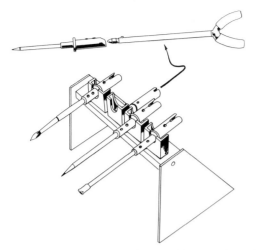

FIGURE 26–11. A mouthstick is grasped between the patient's teeth and can be inserted into a choice of several devices that hold a pencil, a paint brush, a pen, or a typing stick.

attached to a mouthpiece and capable of holding simple tools like a pencil, pen, or paintbrush. The rod is usually about 12 inches long, permitting the person to see what he or she is drawing or painting (Fig. 26–11). The mouthpiece should be carefully constructed by a dentist so that an accurate impression of the teeth or gums is made and the mouthpiece constructed to the same contour. If simple half-rings or flat pieces are used, damage to the teeth is likely to result.

Environmental Control Systems

Electrical devices are available that control a selection of a variety of outputs from one of a number of possible input mechanisms. They were developed to permit persons who have limited or no use of the extremities to turn on and off a small number of electrical devices that can be plugged into the master control box. In one such device, 10 different electrical appliances can be operated. The handicapped person can select one of several control mechanisms: a sip-and-puff switch, a joystick switch, a manual rocker switch, and a toggle switch. Whichever switch works best for the person can be selected and attached to the control system. A small box on which scanning lights move from the name of one object to the next at a controllable rate is placed in a position where the handicapped person can see it. Each actuation of the control mechanism orders the scanning device to begin scanning or to stop at the desired point. When it

stops at the desired point, a different mode of operation of the control switch turns on the device connected to that particular circuit; it may be a radio, an electrical door controller, an electrical window shade controller, a lamp, a television set, or a telephone. Any small device that can be operated electrically can be controlled by the environmental control system (Fig. 26–12). In the case of a television set, there is a separate position on the scanning box for changing channels after the set is turned on. The telephone requires a special dialing device that performs the dialing function electronically and utilizes a speaker-phone so that no hands are needed.

Inexpensive environmental control systems are available that do not require that the device to be activated be plugged into the controller. The controller may operate up to 16 separate devices by sending electronic signals to modules anywhere in the house. The modules plug into wall outlets; the devices plug into the modules.

Evaluation for an Orthosis

Analysis of Handicap

What does the physician need to know about the patient in order to prescribe an orthosis for the upper limb? First, the history of the present problem and information about any other conditions that may influence the ability of the patient to use an orthosis form the basic information base. Evaluation of the impaired upper extremity includes accurate assessment of

1. Range of motion of all joints in the extremity.
2. Muscle strength.
3. Sensation.
4. Adequacy of skin coverage.
5. Pain.
6. Vocational and avocational needs.

From a general standpoint, it is important to try to estimate the patient's tolerance for devices and the degree of mobility. Some people simply do not have the patience or motivation to use complicated devices, such as a myoelectrically controlled, motor-powered orthosis, and they would best be provided with a simpler device to achieve more limited function. Persons who are mobile in a wheelchair may need a different hand orthosis from those who walk because they must propel the wheelchair and the orthosis must not interfere with their mobility.

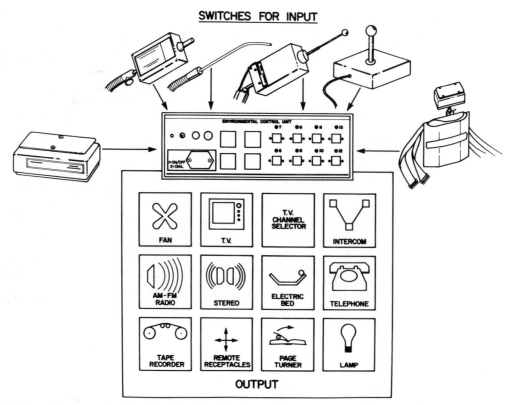

FIGURE 26–12. A diagrammatic representation of an environmental control unit. Any one of six different types of input switches can be used to control many different electrical appliances. The most appropriate switch is selected and attached to the control system. A small box contains scanning lights that move from the name or symbol of one device to the next at a controllable rate. Actuating the input switch starts the device scanning. When the desired appliance is reached by the scan, the input switch can be used to stop scanning and to actuate the appliance.

Prescription of Orthoses

The requirements of the patient must be established and the purpose of the device carefully delineated. The proposed device must be comfortable, provide adequate cosmesis, fill a real need, and be relatively inexpensive and lightweight. The many devices previously described are available, either through prefabricated kits or directly from an orthotist. A full range of sizes of both flat precut blanks and partially assembled devices is available for many hand and wrist orthoses. The use of these kits often saves time, effort, and money (Fig. 26–13).

Conditions Requiring Orthoses

The specific conditions that most frequently call for a prescription of orthotic devices include lower motor neuron lesions at any level from the spinal nerve root to the terminal branches of a peripheral nerve; upper motor neuron lesions, particularly those in the spinal cord and cerebral cortex; burns; and arthritis. The orthoses for these various conditions differ greatly, but all are based on the principles of providing immobilization, improved alignment, or assisted or resisted function.

Lower Motor Neuron Lesions

Complete interruption of the brachial plexus, either by avulsion of all the motor and sensory roots of the plexus or by severance of the entire plexus, as is sometimes seen in motorcycle accidents and gunshot wounds, cannot be helped by currently available orthoses. Absence of motor power at the shoulder, elbow, wrist, and hand requires such a complicated, motor-powered, com-

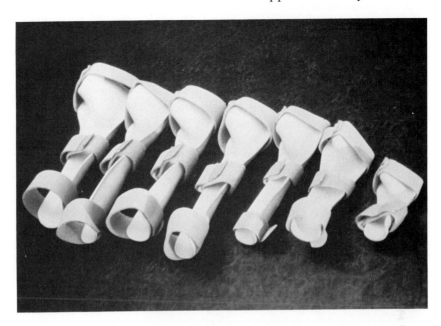

FIGURE 26–13. Prefabricated wrist-hand orthoses in a range of sizes incorporating a hand anatomical cone.

puter-controlled orthosis that it is impractical, and such a device is still experimental.[10] Upper brachial plexus (Erb's) palsy is now managed without splinting,[6] although there are probably still some advocates of airplane orthoses to hold the arm abducted and externally rotated.

Musculocutaneous nerve lesions may cause sufficient weakness of elbow flexion that an elbow flexion-assist orthosis is desired.

Ulnar nerve lesions in the distal forearm are best treated with a hand orthosis with "lumbrical bar." This permits the long finger extensor muscles to extend the interphalangeal as well as the metacarpophalangeal joints. To enhance pinch, a first dorsal interosseus assist may be added. Ulnar nerve lesions above the elbow create an imbalance of wrist flexor pull but seldom require a wrist extension of the hand orthosis.

Median nerve lesions at the wrist create loss of active thumb abduction and opposition; they can be treated with a hand orthosis with spring-swivel thumb assist. Since the thumb adductor still functions, it is not advisable to use a swivel thumb with rigid post. Median nerve lesions above the elbow create a serious problem by paralyzing thumb flexion, abduction, and opposition as well as radial wrist flexion and all finger flexion, except for those fingers supplied by the ulnar innervated portion of the flexor digitorum profundus muscle. Precision grip is lost; power grip is weakened significantly. A wrist-driven flexor-hinge hand orthosis can be utilized, but the patient may prefer no device, since lateral prehension is still possible through muscles innervated by the ulnar nerve.

Radial nerve lesions above the elbow cause paralysis of the wrist, thumb, and finger extensors. The least cumbersome, most functional device is a wrist-hand orthosis with side wrist pivot hinges, wrist dorsiflexion assist, a spring-loaded "volar lumbrical bar" to assist metacarpophalangeal extension, and a thumb interphalangeal stabilizer.[11]

Lesions of two or more peripheral nerves simultaneously or partial lesions of one or more nerves require a careful evaluation of the functional loss so that the correct device can be prescribed.

Upper Motor Neuron Lesions

Transection of the cervical spinal cord with paralysis below the level of the damage creates a myotomal type of sparing. The upper extremity is supplied by the fourth through eighth cervical roots and the first thoracic; since the interossei, lumbricals, and thenar and hypothenar muscles are largely supplied by the eighth cervical and first thoracic roots, they will be paralyzed in a lesion that spares the seventh cervical roots and above. Function may be improved in this case by a hand orthosis with "lumbrical bar" and thumb post, but most persons with this lesion seem to prefer to wear no device. Persons with sparing of the sixth cervical roots benefit from some type of wrist-driven flexor-hinge hand orthosis. Any of those previously described may be utilized. A spontaneous finger flexor tenodesis will usually develop if judicious physical therapy does not overstretch the long finger flexors, and the person will then be nearly as functional without a device as with it.

Sparing at the fifth cervical root level leaves the forearm and hand muscles paralyzed plus loss of elbow extension and weakened elbow flexion. Limited function can be obtained from a palmar band with clip, which can hold many small utensils or writing instruments. A spiral wrist orthosis can stabilize the wrist to enhance function of devices held in a palmar band. The spiral wrist orthosis may also be adapted to hold utensils and devices. A motor- or cable-driven flexor-hinge hand orthosis can provide prehension and stability at the wrist. Since persons with this level of spinal cord

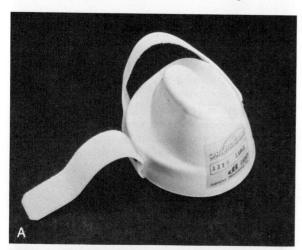

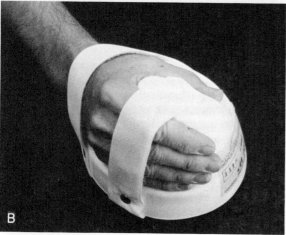

FIGURE 26–14. *A* and *B*, Prefabricated hand orthosis with anatomical cone for hand positioning.

injury usually have an electric wheelchair, a source of electricity is readily available and a motor-driven device becomes reasonably practical.

Cervical spinal cord injuries with sparing only of C4 and above leave the arm, forearm, and hand paralyzed, and there remains only weak shoulder function. A balanced forearm orthosis can usually provide hand placement, and those devices used at the C5 level will provide hand function.

Environmental control systems that permit the handicapped person to operate a number of electrically powered devices are available with a variety of control switches that interface the handicapped person to the system. They may be very useful in high-level cervical spinal cord injuries.

Devices held in the mouth, either between the teeth or between the gums, can be used to operate devices such as an electric typewriter, control switches, and environmental control systems and may also be used for writing and drawing.

Cerebral damage resulting in hemiparesis is often accompanied by distal edema and a spastic, fisted hand. An anatomical hand cone of prefabricated molded plastic may be helpful; it is available also as a wrist-hand cone (Fig. 26–14). To reduce hand edema, the forearm may be placed on an inclined slope of a contoured polyurethane foam block.

Burns

When burns damage the full thickness of the skin, contractures can be expected to develop. The resultant deformities may be minimized by using static or functional orthoses early in the course of treatment.

Burns of the axilla are best treated by holding the arm abducted, especially after grafting. A padded metal or plastic orthosis that can be sterilized should be adjusted to hold the arm in maximum obtainable abduction. The orthosis may be needed for four weeks or more.

When the antecubital fossa is burned, the impending elbow flexion contracture can be minimized by using a padded metal trough to hold the elbow extended until the skin has healed.

Burns of the hands frequently involve the dorsum, since the hand may be used to shield the face. The resulting deformity of hyperextension of the metacarpophalangeal joints and flexion of the interphalangeal joints can be counteracted by a static, volar, wrist-hand orthosis that holds the wrist 10 degrees dorsiflexed, metacarpophalangeal joints fully flexed, and interphalangeal joints extended.[12] Later, a hand orthosis with rubber band metacarpophalangeal flexion assist and interphalangeal extension assist may be needed to improve motion. If the palm is burned, immobilization by a static dorsal orthosis will be needed for at least four weeks.

Arthritis

When rheumatoid arthritis involves the joints of the hand and wrist, various orthoses may be utilized. According to the theory of Smith and colleagues,[13] the pull of the flexor digitorum sublimis and profundus tendons at the metacarpophalangeal joint is largely responsible for the deformity of volar subluxation and ulnar drift and dislocation at the metacarpophalangeal joints. Based on this theory, immobilization of the metacarpophalangeal joints of the second through fifth digits, when those joints are acutely inflamed and swollen, has been instituted, and a heat-moldable plastic orthosis that extends to the proximal interphalangeal joints of those digits on the volar surface and crosses the wrist to the mid-forearm has been designed. This orthosis must be carefully contoured to provide support at the base of the proximal phalanges and to create a shear force in the dorsal direction by pressing down upon the head of the metacarpals with a padded Dacron strap. Similarly, a strap over the styloid processes with pressure from the orthosis against the carpal bones from the volar aspect will reduce the tendency to volar subluxation at that joint. By preventing ulnar deviation of the hand on the wrist and of the fifth digit on the hand, the tendency to ulnar dislocation will be reduced (Fig. 26–15).

When only the wrist is acutely involved, the volar orthosis need extend only to the head of the

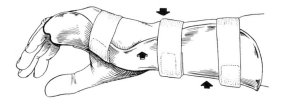

FIGURE 26–15. A plastic wrist-hand orthosis for use in rheumatoid arthritis. Carefully contoured, it extends to the proximal interphalangeal joints of the fingers to support the metacarpophalangeal joints and the wrist joints. It is designed to reduce deforming forces that contribute to ulnar deviation and volar subluxation at the wrist and fingers.

metacarpals rather than to the proximal interphalangeal joint. A static wrist-hand orthosis then is carefully contoured to reduce the volar subluxation tendency of the carpal bones on the radius.

If only the proximal interphalangeal joints are acutely involved and are developing either "boutonnière" or "swan neck" deformities, the joint can be immobilized by using static interphalangeal joint orthoses.

When acute involvement of joints of the wrist and fingers is no longer present, but the collateral ligaments of the joints have stretched or deteriorated, it is possible to provide alignment to finger motion by using a finger-driven flexor-hinge hand splint. Some persons may prefer to use no orthosis at this stage of the disease.

Training the Patient to Use an Orthosis

The simpler positioning and functional splints require little or no training in their application and removal. However, modification of techniques of performing activities of daily living may be necessary and should be undertaken by the therapist most skilled in this area. The more complicated orthoses utilizing external power and the balanced forearm orthosis require hours of careful adjustment and training to maximize their usage.

Patient Acceptance of Orthoses

It is essential that the orthosis be comfortable, cosmetic, complementary, and cheap as well as being easy to put on and take off and to repair. Pre-prescription thought and discussion with the patient as well as the orthotist may save considerable time and effort. The patient must have the same goals and expectations for the orthosis that the physician and orthotist have. Effective communication among patient, physician, and orthotist will develop the best orthotic solution by specifying acceptable criteria to achieve their common goal.

An ugly but functional orthosis may be rejected by a patient who values appearance over function. A complicated orthosis may exceed the patient's gadget tolerance. If the device cannot easily be put on and removed, it may remain in the drawer. If the device provides improved function desired by the patient or decreased pain, the patient will ordinarily wear it as instructed. However, if the device impairs function and creates pain or discomfort, it may well be discarded. When patients with rheumatoid arthritis understand the necessity to protect joints, they, too, will wear the devices, and they soon find that they are more comfortable. The extremely complicated devices with myoelectrical controls must be carefully prescribed and must provide increased function without undue technical problems. They are the ones most likely to be rejected because the improved function they provide may be only marginal.

References

1. Cailliet, R.: Shoulder Pain. Philadelphia, F. A. Davis, 1966.
2. Inman, V. T., Saunders, J. B. de C. M., and Abbott, L. C.: Observations on functions of shoulder joint. J. Bone Surg., 26A:1, 1944.
3. Napier, J.: The evolution of the hand. Sci. Am., 207:1–8, 1962.
4. Smith, E. M., and Juvinall, R. C.: Mechanics of bracing. In Licht, S. (Ed.): Orthotics, Etcetera. Baltimore, Waverly Press, 1966.
5. American Orthotics and Prosthetics Association Almanac, March 1973, p. 11.
6. Johnson, E. W., Alexander, M. A., and Koenig, W. C.: Infantile Erb's palsy (Smellie's palsy). Arch. Phys. Med. Rehabil., 58:175, 1977.
7. Smith, E. M., Juvinall, R. C., Bender, L. F., and Pearson, J. R.: Flexor forces and rheumatoid metacarpophalangeal deformity. J.A.M.A., 198:130–134, 1966.
8. Koepke, G. H., and Feller, I.: Physical measures for the prevention and treatment of deformities following burns. J.A.M.A., 199:791–793, 1967.
9. Anderson, M.: Functional Bracing of the Extremities. Springfield, IL, Charles C Thomas, Publisher, 1958.
10. Long, C.: Upper limb bracing. In Licht, S. (Ed.): Orthotics, Etcetera. Baltimore, Waverly Press, 1966.
11. Bender, L. F.: Prevention of deformities through orthotics. J.A.M.A., 183:946–948, 1963.
12. Koepke, G. H., Feallock, B., and Feller, I.: Splinting the severely burned hand. Am. J. Occup. Ther., 17:147–150, 1963.
13. Smith, E. M., Juvinall, R. C., Bender, L. F., and Pearson, J. R.: Role of the finger flexors in rheumatoid deformities of the metacarpophalangeal joints. Arthritis Rheum., 7:467–480, 1964.

27 Spinal Orthoses

STEVEN V. FISHER

As with any proper prescription, a spinal orthosis cannot be adequately prescribed without proper understanding of the anatomy, kinesiology, biomechanics, and pathophysiology of the disorder being treated.

The prescribing physician must be knowledgeable concerning the positive and negative effects of a spinal orthosis for a particular pathological condition. At times, an accurate assessment of the pathophysiology and faulty biomechanics of the spine is difficult, making the proper prescription of an orthotic device an analytical problem. It is beyond the scope of this chapter to deal in sufficient detail with the anatomy, kinesiology, and disease conditions of the spine to allow a reader to become expert in the prescription of spinal orthoses. The basic principles of spinal bracing will be reviewed, and some of the common spinal orthoses will be discussed. The reader is referred to other sources for more detail.[1–4] Scoliosis bracing will not be considered.

Spinal bracing is used to decrease pain, to protect against further injury, to assist weak muscles, and to prevent or help correct a deformity.[4] These objectives are gained through the biomechanical effects of (1) trunk support, (2) motion control, and (3) spinal realignment.[3] When dealing with the cervical spine, an additional biomechanical effect is partial weight transfer of the head to the trunk when the patient is upright.

The negative effects of spinal orthoses must also be considered. Muscle atrophy and weakness may result from the use of spinal orthotics by reducing the amount of muscular activity needed to maintain trunk support. This problem can be partially avoided by an isometric exercise program. Control of the motion of an orthosis can promote contrac-

ture in the immobilized area. Psychological dependence on an orthosis[3] and increases in energy expenditure while ambulating with a spinal orthosis have been documented.[5]

Ralston found that when subjects walked at a comfortable speed while immobilized in a posterior plastic shell, a 10 per cent increase in oxygen consumption resulted. This factor must be taken into consideration when fitting a debilitated patient. Since axial rotation is necessary between the pelvis and shoulders during ambulation, not only is the energy consumption of ambulating increased, but there may be an increased motion at the unrestrained segments rostral and caudal to the orthosis.[3]

Nomenclature for spinal orthotics is confusing. Eponyms are commonly used for spinal orthotics, and the standardized nomenclature given orthotic devices omits sufficient detail. Therefore, a sketch of each orthosis discussed is shown. Orthotic devices are grouped according to level of the spine to which they are applied, and the most common general types are shown. For further discussion of other spinal orthoses, detailed references are available.[2, 4]

Cervical Orthoses (CO)

General Considerations

The cervical spine provides the greatest range of motion of the entire spinal column in extent, direction, and variation of motion.[6] Cervical orthotic devices are often used in the treatment of neck disorders of both traumatic and nontraumatic causation. Such orthoses are used to provide support and protection as well as to limit range of motion. In general, cervical orthotic devices are most effective in limiting flexion and extension. With even the most effective cervical orthosis, lateral bending can be limited only to approximately 50 per cent of normal motion and rotation to 20 per cent of normal. Sagittal plane motion is better restricted, although the reported effect of the orthotic devices varies somewhat depending on the literature cited.[7–10]

Although the orthotic device must fit precisely, it should not be fitted so tightly that the pressure exerted by the orthotic device on the patient exceeds a capillary pressure of 20 to 30 mm Hg. If this does occur, the patient experiences ischemic pain. The patient will attempt to change posture in the orthosis to provide comfort. If the orthosis is too tight, however, the patient will either loosen the orthotic device or reject it altogether. It has been shown that fitting a cervical orthotic device to within capillary pressure does not decrease the effectiveness of the orthosis as compared with the usual manner of fitting.[11]

Types of Orthoses

COLLARS

Cervical orthoses are of several basic design types. The first type to be considered is the collar made out of foam, which can be a firm Plastizote material or a more rigid polyethylene. The foams may vary in their thickness or firmness. The hard collars (polyethylene) may have occipital and mandibular projections for added support. The collars are applied in a circular manner about the neck.

The effectiveness of the collars is limited. The soft cervical collar provides its restriction of motion more through a sensory feedback and a reminder to limit head and neck motion than through actual mechanical restriction of motion (Fig. 27–1).[7] A firmer cervical collar made out of a Plastizote material with anterior and posterior plastic rigid supports (Philadelphia collar) limits the anterior-posterior cervical motion to approximately 30 per cent of normal (Fig. 27–2).[7, 8] This support allows 43 per cent of normal rotation and 67 per cent of lateral bending.[7] The firmer polyethylene collar with a mandibular and occipital piece demonstrates similar effectiveness in limiting anterior-posterior neck motion.[8] This collar, however, can be quite uncomfortable because it rests over the clavicles (Fig. 27–3).

RIGID SUPPORTS

A more rigid type of orthosis fabricated with metal uprights can be classified as a "poster" appliance. The four-post orthotic device (Fig. 27–4) consists of a chin and occipital piece connected with four uprights to a sternal and posterior thoracic plate.[4] The four posts are easily adjusted. This orthosis has been reported to allow sagittal

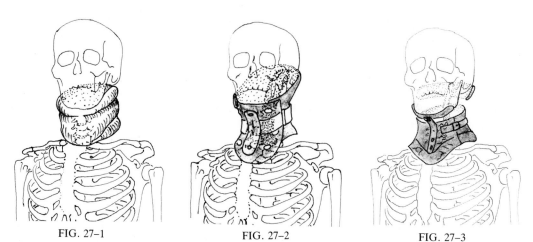

FIG. 27–1   FIG. 27–2   FIG. 27–3

FIGURE 27–1. Foam soft collar.

FIGURE 27–2. Firm Plastizote (Philadelphia) collar.

FIGURE 27–3. Polyethylene rigid collar with mandibular and occipital supports.

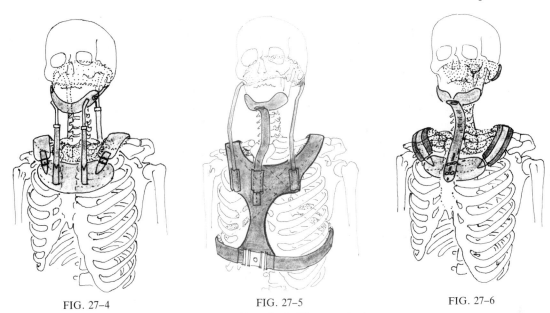

FIG. 27–4   FIG. 27–5   FIG. 27–6

FIGURE 27–4. Four-post adjustable orthosis (Thomas collar).

FIGURE 27–5. Sternal-occipital-mandibular immobilizer (SOMI) orthosis.

FIGURE 27–6. Two-post adjustable orthosis with mandibular and occipital supports.

motion of 5 per cent[8] to 21 per cent[7] of normal, rotation of 27 per cent of normal, and lateral bending of 46 per cent of normal.[7]

The SOMI (sternal-occipital-mandibular immobilizer) (Fig. 27–5) is another type of "poster" appliance. This support has one strip of metal running anteriorly to hold the chin piece and two rigid metal rods running posteriorly to hold the occipital piece. The device is easily applied with the patient supine in the case of spinal cord injury and requires very little patient movement by the orthotist in its application and fitting. It is a comfortable orthosis and is very lightweight. The SOMI has been reported to allow 13 per cent[8] to 27 per cent[7] of normal sagittal motion, 34 per cent of rotation, and 66 per cent of lateral bending.[7] Both orthotic devices are quite effective in limiting cervical range of motion.

Other "poster" type appliances exist, for example, the two-post (Fig. 27–6), and are probably as effective as the four-post or the SOMI mentioned before, but they may provide less lateral stability. Johnson and co-workers[7] developed a cervicothoracic (CTO) four-post brace that extended farther down the trunk and appeared to be more effective than the SOMI or four-post in limiting overall sagittal plane movement. The Jewett J-21 brace (Fig. 27–7) is a two-post CTO that extends well down the thorax, with rigid metal bands from the sternal pad across the shoulders and down the back to the lower thoracic band. This brace is more difficult for the orthotist to apply to the patient in a supine position. A "Peterson" is a similar cervicothoracic (CTO) two-post device but has enlarged mandibular and occipital supports and a forehead strap (Fig. 27–8). It is doubtful that the additional support offered, compared with the SOMI, warrants its prescription, especially in view of its difficulty in fitting and pressure problems on the skin in the supine spinal cord injury patient.

Another type of cervical orthotic device could be classified as a custom-molded, total contact, chin-occipital-sternal-thoracic orthosis of the Minerva type (Fig. 27–9). This orthosis, if fabricated properly, would seem to control more lateral and rotatory movement of the cervical spine than the "poster" type orthosis. A formal study of its effectiveness has not been published. As with any orthosis, the fabrication technique for this appliance is crucial to its success in limiting cervical range of motion. If more control of the cervical spine is required, rather than tightening an orthosis

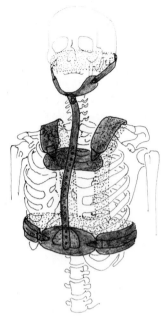

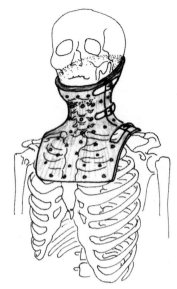

FIGURE 27–9. Molded "Minerva" cervical orthosis.

FIGURE 27–7. Jewett J-21 two-post cervical orthosis with thoracic extension.

to unbearable limits, a rigid jacket made out of either plaster or polyethylene with a halo attached to the skull becomes necessary (Fig. 27–10).

Johnson and associates have reported on the effectiveness of the halo vest on normal individuals and found that it allowed almost no motion overall in the cervical spine; however, at an individual vertebral level, the spine appeared to "snake" with flexion at one level and extension at the next. This "snaking" motion illustrates that not even the halo eliminates all spine motion. They suggested an intimate fit of the chest portion of the halo.[12]

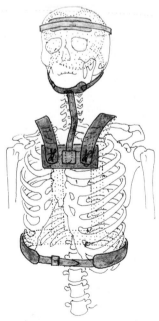

FIGURE 27–8. Peterson cervical orthosis with thoracic extension.

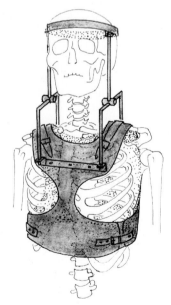

FIGURE 27–10. Halo-type cervical orthosis attached to a polyethylene jacket.

Koch and Nickel studied quadriplegics in halo vests and found the overall average sagittal movement in a halo vest was reduced to 31 per cent of normal, and they concluded that the absolute motion in a halo vest has been underestimated. They consider that insufficient support is achieved from the sternum and thorax, and suggest an intimate molded body vest.[13]

Many of the newer halo devices on the market, however, emphasize less vest and more fixation onto a sternal and a midline posterior thoracic plate, eliminating the classic vest. If these new halo orthoses do immobilize the patient well enough as documented in each individual patient case, they have a significant advantage in the rehabilitation of the quadriplegic because of their lighter weight, the ability to perform full arm range of motion, and the ability to fully examine insensate skin.

Forces on the halo vest, as measured by strain gauges, suggest that vest distortion occurs from changes in body position and with direct pushing of the lower abdomen, the arms, and the shoulders with body movement. Changing the vest design may greatly improve effectiveness of the halo device in limiting cervical range of motion.[14]

Thoracolumbosacral Orthoses

Lumbosacral and thoracolumbosacral orthoses are prescribed more frequently than cervical orthoses, and there are more numerous variations of the designs for each type. This chapter will concentrate on the most commonly prescribed orthotic devices[15] and the representative types of design and material.

General Considerations

The work of Norton and Brown[16] was the first and still remains one of the most important articles dealing with the effectiveness of back braces. Some of the findings are pertinent to this discussion. Orthoses vary widely in their effectiveness in controlling the lower lumbar intervertebral levels. This variability of orthotic effectiveness probably relates to an individual's lumbar flexion pattern.

All spinal devices employ three-point pressure, and the effectiveness of each orthotic device in the production of controlling forces varies considerably. Orthotic devices that are well fixed to the chest but inadequately fixed to the pelvis produce a concentration of forces in the upper lumbar and thoracolumbar region as the trunk flexes. This leaves the lumbosacral segments unsupported. This was particularly noted in braces of the Taylor-type construction. In contrast, the chairback brace that has short supports tends to pull away from the body much less. In this way, the supportive force offered by the orthotic device is maintained in the lumbosacral area.[16]

No brace actually immobilizes; it only tends to limit interspinous motion. No orthotic device can totally control the sagittal or axial lumbosacral motion.[16, 17] Therefore, if an orthotic device is to be effective, it must supply sufficient localized pressure over bony prominences to cause enough discomfort to remind the patient wearing the orthosis to change or maintain posture in the orthotic device.

Morris and associates[18] wrote that increased abdominal pressure decreases the net force applied to the spine when attempting to lift a weight from the floor. They believed that one of the major functions of a lumbar support, including corsets and rigid braces, was abdominal compression. The resultant increased intra-abdominal pressure thereby created a semirigid cylinder surrounding the spinal column capable of relieving some of the imposed stresses on the vertebral column itself.[19] Nachemson and co-workers more recently noted, however, that no lumbosacral orthosis raised intragastric pressure significantly.[20] Intra-abdominal pressure will increase only with closure of the glottis during muscular activity. The lumbosacral support, when tightened within patient tolerance, decreases the intradiskal pressure at the lumbar spine by approximately 30 per cent.[21] In a later work, Nachemson demonstrated a reduction in disk pressure values in about two thirds of the exercises and an increased pressure in the remaining third when a lumbosacral orthosis is worn.[20]

At rest, both the chairback brace and the lumbosacral corset either decrease or have no effect on the electrical activity of back muscles in the majority of subjects.[18] Nachemson, however, found no consistent trends in myoelectrical activity when four normal volunteers performed six tasks while using lumbosacral orthoses. Erector spine myoelectrical activity was sometimes reduced by about one third, although it was at times also increased by that amount.[20] Lantz and Schultz similarly found inconsistent changes in the myoelectrical activity when normal volunteers wore spinal orthoses. Some of the increased activity was thought to be due to antagonistic muscle activity. It is thought, but not verified experimentally, that low back pain patients wearing an orthosis daily relax into the brace and perhaps reduce antagonistic muscle activity.[22] When the subjects walk at their comfortable walking speed, neither support has any effect on electrical muscular activity. However, when subjects wearing the chairback brace walk at a fast pace, the muscle activity increases in comparison with the activity of that muscle when no support is worn. It is thought that the greater electrical activity recorded in subjects walking rapidly while wearing the chairback brace reflects the increase in muscular exertion of the back muscles in attempting to overcome immobilization of the chairback brace.[23] Persons with back pain usually do not walk fast, and the significance of this electrical activity is uncertain.

It would seem that the effectiveness of an orthosis results from a combination of trunk support as well as gross and intersegmental motion restriction. The motion control that is created by the orthotic devices might very well be more on the basis of painful stimuli to the subjects wearing the brace, reminding them to correct their position, than by the actual three-point support system. Spinal realignment would be a very difficult task for an external support to perform passively. Active muscle realignment with the orthotic device seems necessary.

Types of Orthoses

These appliances can be classified as corsets, rigid braces, hyperextension braces, and jackets. All spinal orthoses with the exception of hyperextension braces give abdominal support. The ability of these devices to restrict motion has not been measured with as great detail as for the cervical orthoses, so that the evaluation of effectiveness is more subjective.

CORSETS

The most commonly prescribed lumbosacral support is the lumbosacral corset, which is prescribed approximately 44 per cent of the time.[15] In general, a corset is made of canvas with rigid back steels. There is adjustable side or back lacing. A corset is a stock item and can be fitted by a corseteer without difficulty. The corset can be lumbosacral (LS) or thoracolumbosacral (TLS) in nature. The

steels can be either rigid or semirigid. Fidler[24] and Lantz[25] found even the corset significantly reduced spinal motion by as much as two thirds. However, the steels serve to give a little support and to supply painful stimuli if the patient leans against the stays, especially the lateral ones. Therefore, the corset not only gives some support but reminds the patient to maintain adequate posture.

RIGID BRACES

Lumbosacral Orthoses (LSO). Of the rigid braces, the chairback brace is the most popular.[12] The chairback brace consists of two paraspinal uprights and two uprights in the mid-axillary line (Fig. 27–11). It may have an anterior corset or apron front with side lacing and is designed to control flexion-extension and lateral motion (Fig. 27–12).

Another lumbosacral orthosis commonly prescribed is the William's back brace, which is used primarily to control extension and lordosis, and to give some lateral control (Fig. 27–13). It is a specialized orthosis in that it allows free flexion but limits extension and uses a lever action and abdominal support to reduce lumbar lordosis.

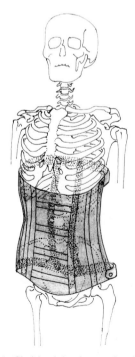

FIGURE 27–11. Chairback lumbosacral orthosis with attached abdominal apron closed by Velcro straps.

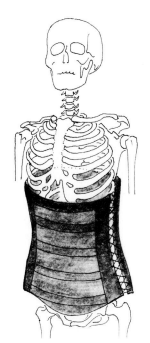

FIGURE 27–12. Chairback lumbosacral orthosis with side-lacing attachment of abdominal apron.

Thoracolumbosacral Orthoses (TLSO). There are two major types of thoracolumbosacral orthoses. The more common is the Taylor orthosis, which is constructed to restrict flexion and extension (Fig. 27–14). However, as mentioned earlier, this type of orthosis is ineffective for limiting the lumbar spine motion.[16] The Taylor orthosis limits thoracic motion only if the axillary straps are tightened to a point of discomfort. Therefore, when the patient loosens the straps because of discomfort, the orthosis becomes ineffective. This orthosis, therefore, seems to be a poor choice for thoracolumbosacral immobilization. The chairback brace with cowhorn or sternal pad attachments (Fig. 27–15), which transmits pressure through the sternum and ribs directly to the spine, provides better lumbosacral and thoracic immobilization than a brace by which force is transmitted through the pectoral girdle, which is attached to the spinal axis only by muscles and the sternoclavicular joints.

Molded jackets are made either of plaster of Paris or of a thermoplastic to conform to the contours of the body (Fig. 27–16). If made properly, they become a nearly total contact type of orthotic device. Therefore, the pressure distribution is more uniform and more support is afforded. Fidler[24] and Lantz[25] verified the expected: the molded TLSO restricts spinal movement better than does a corset or chairback brace. A spica attachment to the molded TLSO not unexpectedly was best at restricting movement, presumably by partially immobilizing the pelvis. These jackets are used frequently for patients with spinal fractures or scoliosis to allow early mobilization and rehabilitation. They also may be of value when there are metastases in vertebrae to provide support and control pain. Donning and doffing the molded jacket is more difficult than with other orthoses.

The hyperextension orthosis differs from other devices because it does not have an abdominal apron and does not give abdominal support; it functions to give a hyperextension moment (Fig. 27–17). This hyperextension brace applies three-point pressure over the sternum and the hypogastrium anteriorly and over the upper lumbar spine posteriorly. This orthosis is used to permit the upright position, especially to prevent flexion after a compression fracture of a vertebral body. It is not recommended, however, to manage compression fractures in osteoporotic elderly patients because it may place excessive hyperextension forces on lower lumbar vertebrae, which can induce posterior element fractures or exacerbate a degenerative arthritic condition.

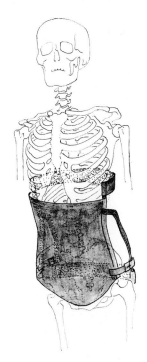

FIGURE 27–13. William's hyperextension lumbosacral orthosis.

STEVEN V. FISHER

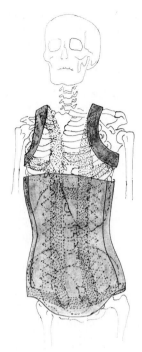

FIGURE 27–14. The Taylor thoracolumbosacral brace is too frequently prescribed and usually ineffective.

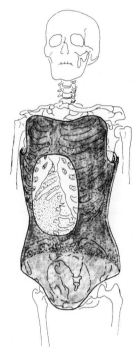

FIGURE 27–16. The molded jacket, when properly fitted, provides total contact support.

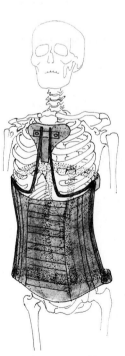

FIGURE 27–15. Chairback brace with sternal pad transmitting bony support to the thoracic spine.

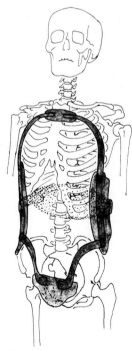

FIGURE 27–17. The hyperextension orthosis restricts spinal flexion by anterior pressure over the sternum and hypogastrium, and posterior pressure across the upper lumbar and lower thoracic region.

It should be stressed that orthotic devices only partially limit rather than immobilize the spine. Spinal orthoses should be considered to be temporary devices. At the same time that the orthotic device is prescribed, a rehabilitation treatment plan should be outlined to attempt to rid the patient of the need for the device in the future.

References

1. McCollough, N. C. III: Biomechanical analysis of the spine. *In* Atlas of Orthotics: Biomechanical Principles and Application. American Academy of Orthopedic Surgeons. St. Louis, C. V. Mosby, 1975.
2. Berger, N., and Lusskin, R.: Orthotic components and systems. *In* Atlas of Orthotics: Biomechanical Principles and Application. American Academy of Orthopedic Surgeons. St. Louis, C. V. Mosby, 1975.
3. Lusskin, R., and Berger, N.: Prescription principles. *In* Atlas of Orthotics: Biomechanical Principles and Application. American Academy of Orthopedic Surgeons. St. Louis, C. V. Mosby, 1975.
4. Lucas, B. D.: Spinal orthotics for pain and instability. *In* Redford, J. B. (Ed.): Orthotics, Etcetera. Baltimore, Williams & Wilkins, 1980, pp. 123–152.
5. Ralston, H. J.: Effects of immobilization of various body segments on energy cost of human locomotion. Proceedings of Second International Congress on Ergonomics, Dortmund, 1964. Ergonomics [Suppl.], 1965, pp. 53–60.
6. Calliet, R.: Neck and Arm Pain. Philadelphia, F. A. Davis, 1964.
7. Johnson, R. M., Hart, D., Simmons, E. F., Ramsby, G. R., and Southwick, N. O.: Cervical orthoses. J. Bone Joint Surg., 59A:332–339, 1977.
8. Fisher, S. V., Bowar, J. F., Awad, E. A., and Gullickson, G.: Cervical orthoses effect on cervical spine motion: Roentgenographic and goniometric method of study. Arch. Phys. Med. Rehabil., 58:109–115, 1977.
9. Colachis, S. C. Jr., Strohm, B. R., and Ganter, E. L.: Cervical spine motion in normal women: Radiographic study of effect of cervical collars. Arch. Phys. Med. Rehabil., 46:753–760, 1965.
10. Hartman, J. T., Palumbo, F., and Hill, B. J.: Cineradiography of braced normal cervical spine: Comparative study of five commonly used cervical orthoses. Clin. Orthop., 109:97–102, 1975.
11. Fisher, S. V.: Proper fitting of the cervical orthoses. Arch. Phys. Med. Rehabil., 59:505–507, 1978.
12. Johnson, A. M., Owen, J. R., Hart, D. L., and Callahan, R. A.: Cervical orthoses, a guide to their selection and use. Clin. Orthop. Rel. Res., 154:34–45, 1981.
13. Koch, R. A., and Nickel, V. L.: The halo vest, an evaluation of motion and forces across the neck. Spine, 3:103–107, 1978.
14. Walker, P. S., Lamser, D., Hussey, W., Rossier, A. B., Farberov, A., and Dietz, J.: Forces in the halo vest apparatus. Spine, 9:773–777, 1984.
15. Perry, J.: The use of external support in the treatment of low back pain. J. Bone Joint Surg., 52A:1440–1442, 1970.
16. Norton, P. L., and Brown, T.: The immobilization efficiency of back braces, their effect on the posture and motion of the lumbosacral spine. J. Bone Joint Surg., 39A:111–139, 1957.
17. Lumsden, R. M., and Morris, J. M.: An in vivo study of axial rotation and immobilization at the lumbosacral joint. J. Bone Joint Surg., 50A:1591–1602, 1968.
18. Morris, J. M., Lucas, D. B., and Bresler, B.: Role of the trunk in stability of the spine. J. Bone Joint Surg., 43A:327–351, 1961.
19. Morris, J. M.: Low back bracing. Clin. Orthop., 102:126–132, 1974.
20. Nachemson, A., Schultz, A., and Andersson, G.: Mechanical effectiveness studies of lumbar spine orthoses. Scand. J. Rehabil. Med. [Suppl.], 9:139–149, 1983.
21. Nachemson, A., and Morris, J. M.: In vivo measurements of intradiscal pressure: Discometry, a method for the determination of pressure in the lower lumbar discs. J. Bone Joint Surg., 46A:1077–1092, 1964.
22. Lantz, S. A., and Schultz, A. B.: Lumbar spine orthosis wearing. II. Effect on trunk muscle myoelectric activity. Spine, 11:838–842, 1986.
23. Walters, R. L., and Morris, J. M.: Effect of spinal supports on the electrical activity of muscles of the trunk. J. Bone Joint Surg., 52A:51–60, 1970.
24. Fidler, M. W., and Plasmans, C. M. T.: The effect of four types of support on the segmental mobility of the lumbosacral spine. J. Bone Joint Surg., 65A:943–947, 1983.
25. Lantz, S. A., and Schultz, A. B.: Lumbar spine orthosis wearing. I. Restriction of gross body motions. Spine, 11:838–842, 1986.

28

Lower Extremity Orthotics

JUSTUS F. LEHMANN
BARBARA J. DE LATEUR

Historically, design features for lower extremity orthotics have changed slowly. In recent years, however, two factors have led to a rapid increase in the number of changes, i.e., the application of engineering skills to orthotic design and the introduction and widespread availability of plastic materials suitable for use in these orthoses. As a result, not only are there many more designs from which to choose, but they are also constantly changing. Therefore, guidelines for evaluation of patients and selection of the appropriate orthosis assume an even greater importance than in the past. An understanding of the functional biomechanical principles used in orthotic design provides the foundation for these guidelines and simplifies the approach to the patient.[1] Also, new developments in electrophysiological bracing have been of greater interest recently.

Orthoses for Skeletal and Joint Insufficiency

The design of these orthoses provides for adequate bone and joint alignment and allows quantifiable limits of lower extremity weight-bearing through the skeletal system.

Ischial Weight-Bearing Orthoses

Orthotic Components. These orthoses are designed to transmit force from the ischium to the orthosis and through the orthosis to the ground.

The components consist of standard stainless steel bar stock for the uprights connected at the bottom by a stirrup, which is often riveted to a steel sole plate extending to the metatarsal head area. A rocker or patten bottom[2] may be added. The most common design of the weight-bearing area used is a quadrilateral cuff of the same configuration as the quadrilateral socket of the prosthesis for an above-knee amputee.[3–7] The ischial (Thomas) ring[8] is no longer used as a standard design.

Biomechanical Function. The amount of reduction of force transmission through the skeletal system depends on several elements in the orthotic design, such as the configuration of the ischial weight-bearing area, the use of a locked or free knee joint, the design of the ankle joint, the sole plate, and the addition of a rocker or patten bottom. Training of the patient in the proper use of the orthosis also has a major effect on reliable weight-bearing relief.

The use of the rigid quadrilateral cuff (Fig. 28–1) markedly improved the weight-bearing function of the orthosis, which, in general, is maximal during heel strike and drops off significantly during the push off phase. However, if the patient is trained to avoid active push off, which loads the skeletal system, weight-bearing of the orthosis during the latter part of the stance is greatly improved. Also, the patient should be instructed in the appropriate utilization of the ischial seat of the orthosis, i.e., weight-bearing with the ischium on the seat.[9, 10] In addition, the greater the clearance between heel and shoe provided during fitting, the greater the reliability of weight-bearing through the orthosis. A minimum of ⅜ in heel clearance

602

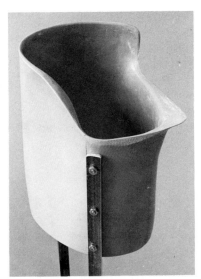

FIGURE 28–1. Rigid, quadrilateral cuff for ischial weight-bearing orthoses. (From Lehmann, J. F., Warren, C. G., de Lateur, B. J., Simons, B. C., and Kirkpatrick, G.: Biomechanical evaluation of axial loading in ischial weight bearing braces of various designs. Arch. Phys. Med. Rehabil., 51:331–337, 1970.)

of the hip joint, since not all forces are transmitted through the ischial seat and, therefore, do not all bypass the hip joint. Actual measurements with an instrumental ischial seat show that only approximately 40 per cent of the force is transmitted through it:[10] the rest apparently passes from the quadrilateral cuff through the soft tissue mass of the thigh into the skeletal structure. Therefore, canes or crutches should be used to protect the hip joint.

The Thomas ring may be considered obsolete as a component of a weight-bearing orthosis. Because of the small contact area between the ischium and the ring,[8] discomfort is frequently produced, causing patients to loosen the thigh lacer to obtain relief. The ischium then drops into the ring and the weight-bearing function is lost.[10]

In general, the weight-bearing function of an ischial weight-bearing orthosis depends on design and training as follows:

1. The orthosis with a locked knee and a patten bottom produces 100 per cent weight-bearing through the orthosis.

2. The orthosis with a locked knee, fixed ankle, rocker bottom, and training produces weight-bearing through the orthosis at 90 per cent or more of body weight (Fig. 28–2).

3. The orthosis with a locked knee and a fixed ankle, with training, produces weight-bearing

as measured in mid-stance should be provided, and occasionally a greater amount may be desirable.

The ischial weight-bearing orthosis with a quadrilateral cuff does not provide complete protection

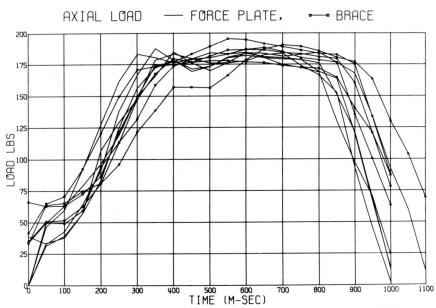

FIGURE 28–2. Axial loads developed on force plate and in uprights of a brace with fixed ankle, fixed knee, quadrilateral shell, and rocker bottom during five stance phases. (From Lehmann, J. F., Warren, C. G., de Lateur, B. J., Simons, B. C., and Kirkpatrick, G.: Biomechanical evaluation of axial loading in ischial weight-bearing braces of various designs. Arch. Phys. Med. Rehabil., 51:331–337, 1970.)

JUSTUS F. LEHMANN AND BARBARA J. DE LATEUR

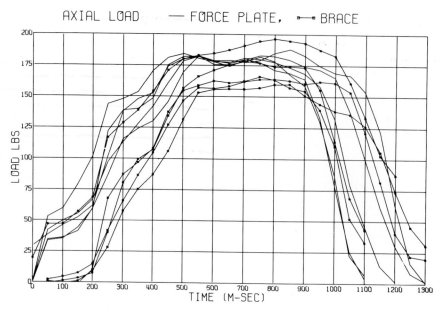

FIGURE 28–3. Axial loads developed on force plate and in uprights of a fixed ankle, fixed knee brace with a volunteer attempting active dorsiflexion to avoid push-off during five stance phases. (From Lehmann, J. F., Warren, C. G., de Lateur, B. J., Simons, B. C., and Kirkpatrick, G.: Biomechanical evaluation of axial loading in ischial weight-bearing braces of various designs. Arch. Phys. Med. Rehabil., 51:331–337, 1970.)

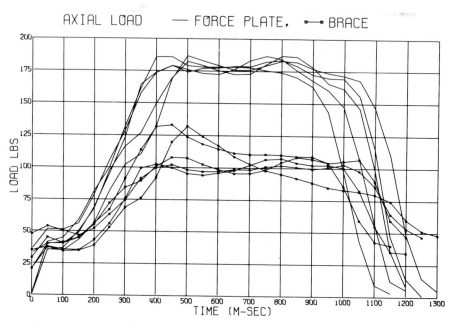

FIGURE 28–4. Axial loads developed on force plate and in uprights of a brace with fixed ankle, fixed knee, and quadrilateral shell during five stance phases. (From Lehmann, J. F., Warren, C. G., de Lateur, B. J., Simon, B. C., and Kirkpatrick, G.: Biomechanical evaluation of axial loading in ischial weight bearing braces of various designs. Arch. Phys. Med. Rehabil., 51:331–337, 1970.)

through the orthosis at approximately 86 per cent of body weight (Fig. 28–3).

4. The orthosis with a locked knee and a fixed ankle, without training, produces weight-bearing through the orthosis at 50 per cent of body weight with little variation (Fig. 28–4).

5. The orthosis with a locked knee and a free ankle joint, with training, produces 50 per cent or more variable weight-bearing through the orthosis throughout the stance phase.

6. The orthosis with a locked knee and a free ankle joint, without training, produces 50 per cent or more weight-bearing through the orthosis only during heel strike.

Patellar Tendon–Bearing Orthoses

Orthotic Components. The most important advance in the design of this orthosis is the use of a patellar tendon–bearing cuff of the same design as the patellar tendon–bearing socket of the below-knee prosthesis for amputees. It is designed to transmit the majority of the force from the knee through the patellar tendon area into the cuff, and from there through the upright and shoe to the ground. A rocker bottom can also be fitted to the shoe, as in the ischial weight-bearing orthosis. For ease of donning and doffing, the patellar tendon-bearing cuff is bivalved and must be closed by rigid ski boot–type buckles to avoid the yielding found with soft leather or Velcro, which decreases the weight-bearing function of the orthosis (Fig. 28–5).[11–14] To make effective use of the patellar tendon–bearing area, the cuff should be flexed to approximately 10 degrees in relation to the uprights. If a fixed ankle joint is used, the stop should be adjusted to 7 degrees dorsiflexion from the 90-degree neutral position.[15]

Biomechanical Function. The weight-bearing function of the orthosis depends on whether the design uses a locked ankle joint with a sole plate, a free ankle, or a rocker bottom as well as the amount of heel clearance. In addition, training has a significant influence, and the patient should be taught to avoid active push off, which would load the skeletal system. The patient should also be shown how to maximally use the weight-bearing area of the patellar tendon–bearing cuff.

The weight-bearing function of the patellar tendon–bearing orthoses of various designs can be summarized as:

1. If a free or cable ankle joint is used with ⅜

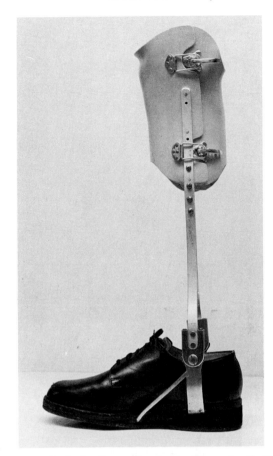

FIGURE 28–5. Patellar tendon–bearing brace for limiting weight-bearing, incorporating bivalved patellar tendon bearing cuff closed by skin boot buckles, standard uprights, double-stopped ankle joint, and sole plate extending to the metatarsal head area.

in heel clearance, the weight-bearing function of the orthosis during the heel strike phase is limited to approximately 42 to 44 per cent of the total force transmitted to the ground (Fig. 28–6). During the push off phase, there is a marked drop-off to no weight-bearing. However, with training, the weight-bearing function can be improved by avoiding active push off.

2. If a fixed ankle is used with heel clearance of ⅜ in but no training is given, approximately 40 per cent of the total force transmitted to the ground is borne by the orthosis with a drop-off to approximately 30 per cent during the push off phase (Fig. 28–7).

3. In the same design, using a fixed ankle and an increased heel clearance of 1 in and training, more than 70 per cent of the weight is borne by

JUSTUS F. LEHMANN AND BARBARA J. DE LATEUR

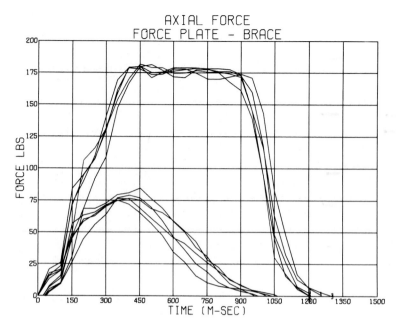

AXIAL FORCE
FORCE PLATE - BRACE

PTB BRACE   CABLE   ANKLE

SHELL — SHORT   10°   HEEL   CLEARANCE — 3/8"

FIGURE 28–6. Patellar tendon–bearing, cable ankle joint, short shell at 10 degrees flexion, heel clearance ⅜ inch. Upper curves force plate force, lower curves brace forces. (From Lehmann, J. F., Warren, C. G., Pemberton, D. R., Simons, B. C., and de Lateur, B. J.: Load bearing function of patellar tendon bearing braces of various designs. Arch. Phys. Med Rehabil., 52:367–370, 1971.)

the orthosis, with a drop of 50 to 60 per cent during the push off phase (Fig. 28–8).

4. With a fixed ankle and 1 in heel clearance, the weight-bearing during push off can be further improved by adding a rocker bottom. This makes the patient unstable in order to prevent active push off and also increases difficulty in ambulation.

Weight-bearing during the heel strike phase is not likely to be improved beyond 70 per cent.

According to Davis and associates,[14] the indications for the use of patellar tendon–bearing orthoses on a short-term basis are

1. Healing of os calcis fractures.
2. Postoperative fusions about the ankle.

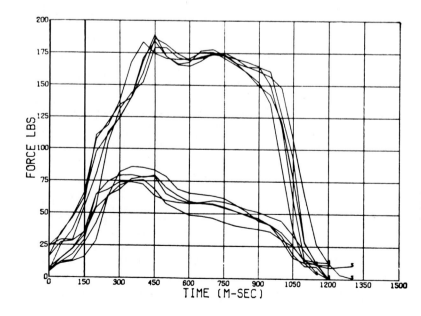

FIGURE 28–7. Patellar tendon–bearing brace with rigid closure, short shell at 10 degrees, fixed ankle at 7 degrees, heel clearance ⅜ inch. Upper curves force plate force, lower curves brace forces. (From Lehmann, J. F., Warren, C. G., Pemberton, D. R., Simons, B. C., and de Lateur, B. J.: Load bearing function of patellar tendon bearing braces of various designs. Arch. Phys. Med. Rehabil., 52:367–370, 1971.)

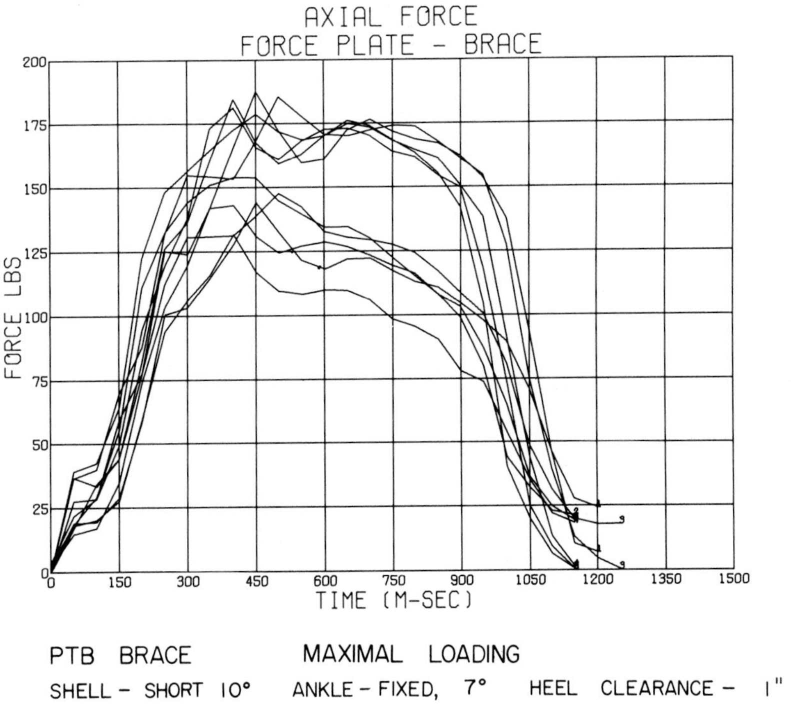

FIGURE 28–8. Patellar tendon–bearing brace used with training, short shell at 10 degrees, fixed ankle at 7 degrees, flexion, heel clearance 1 in. Upper curves, force plate force; lower curves, brace forces. (From Lehmann, J. F., Warren, C. G., Pemberton, D. R., Simons, B. C., and de Lateur, B. J.: Load bearing function of patellar tendon bearing braces of various designs. Arch. Phys. Med. Rehabil., 52:367–370, 1971.)

3. Painful conditions of the heel that have been refractory to conservative management and for which surgery is contraindicated.

The orthosis is recommended for long-term use in the following conditions:

1. Delayed unions or nonunions of fractures and fusions.

2. Avascular necrosis of the talar body.

3. Degenerative arthritis of the subtalar or ankle joint.

4. Osteomyelitis of the os calcis.

5. Sciatic nerve injury with secondary anesthesia involving the sole of the foot.

6. Chronic dermatological problems, such as diabetic ulceration.

7. Other chronic and painful conditions of the foot that are not amenable to surgery.

Davis identified as contraindications conditions of the skin and peripheral circulation such that pressure about the patellar tendon and popliteal regions cannot be tolerated.

Fracture Cast Bracing

Casts with patellar tendon or ischial weight-bearing designs have been successfully used in the treatment of lower extremity fractures.[16] The bio-mechanics of the weight-bearing function are the same as those in the weight-bearing orthoses described. In addition, however, the cast or the plastic materials used to encase the limb or a portion of it must maintain bone alignment. Sarmiento suggested that the fluid column of the soft tissue when completely encased may add to the weight-bearing function.[17] This requires further investigation, since no significant difference in the amount of weight-bearing was found between the patellar tendon–bearing orthosis that tightly encased the entire leg to the ankle and an orthosis with a short patellar tendon–bearing cuff.[16] The use of these orthoses in the management of fractures has been advantageous when compared to the traditional methods of treatment, since the period of immobilization is reduced, and even fractures with delayed union or nonunion frequently heal well. Nickel and co-workers described 102 femoral fractures treated with ischial weight-bearing fracture cast orthoses as healing after traction in an average of 12 weeks.[4-6] Similarly, Sarmiento used patellar tendon–bearing orthoses in 382 patients with tibial fractures and reported an average healing time of 14.5 weeks.[18] No significant shortening of the limbs associated with this treatment was observed, and fractures with delayed union or nonunion responded well. It is likely that these orthoses are effective because they maintain bone alignment and limit weight-bearing through the fracture site to a tolerable level, which promotes bone healing while simultaneously allowing early ambulation.

Weight-Bearing Orthoses to Maintain and Correct Joint Alignment

In cases of joint disease such as rheumatoid arthritis, it may be desirable not only to limit weight-bearing but also to support joint alignment. Orthoses used for this purpose are of the same design as the ischial and patellar tendon weight-bearing orthoses; however, they are modified to maintain joint alignment and stability. They may also be used without the weight-bearing features. Clinically, the major problems that can be treated with these types of orthoses occur at the level of the knee joint, as in rheumatoid arthritis where destruction and loosening of the medial collateral ligaments lead to valgus deformity. Orthoses can be designed to counteract the bending moment that forces the knee into valgus position. This is therapeutically significant, since the center of rotation for medial deviation of the knee is moved medial to the extension of the ground reactive force line, thus creating a moment arm that bends the knee further medially into valgus. Consequently, the more the knee is deformed, the greater the moment arm, and, therefore, the greater the deforming force. This is an accelerating process that can be prevented by the proper use of orthoses. The corrective force must be applied medial to the knee and countered by two forces, one applied to the limb above the knee and one below. The corrective force may be applied by a pressure pad to the medial side, but it is better if a form-fitting plastic shell is added that extends from below to just above the knee level (supracondylar extension). Thigh position can be better controlled by substituting a plastic, form-fitting shell for the standard thigh bands (Fig. 28–9).[19–21] The plastic shell, both above and below the knee, must be manufactured from an accurate plaster cast made when the limb is in its optimally correct position. When the orthosis allows free knee flexion and extension, it is important to align the center of rotation of the brace axis as accurately as possible to coincide with the location of the anatomical knee axis. Otherwise, the force generated by the relative motion of the orthosis and

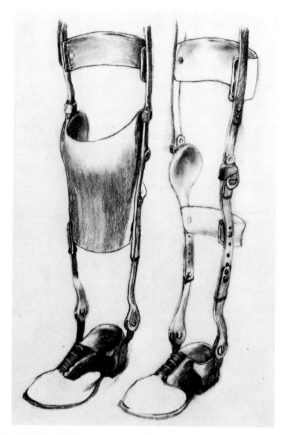

FIGURE 28–9. Braces with standard medial knee support (R) and pretibial shell (L).

limb may further injure the diseased joint and make the wearing of the orthosis uncomfortable. Since single axis knee joints are used for the most part and since the location of the instantaneous center of rotation of the anatomical knee changes with motion,[22] special attention must be given to optimal alignment. A commonly used method for aligning the orthotic knee joint with the anatomical joint axis is as follows:

1. Locate the maximum bone prominence of the medial femoral condyle.

2. Draw a line horizontally at the mid-patellar level and subdivide it into three equal parts.

3. The axis is located at the junction of the middle and posterior third (Fig. 28–10).

To check the alignment of the knee axis with the completed orthosis, the following points should be observed:

1. When the patient sits down, there should be no relative motion between the orthosis and the limb.

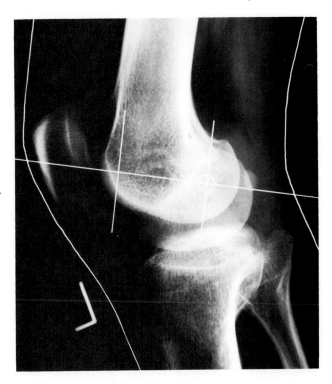

FIGURE 28–10. Location of knee axis.

2. If the axis of the orthosis is too high, the lower thigh band digs into the thigh.

3. If it is too low, the calf band bites into the calf.[23]

In their evaluation of single and double upright orthoses for patients with rheumatoid arthritis and valgus deformity at the knee, Smith and associates[20] found:

1. The use of a single upright is limited to conditions requiring a corrective force of 18 to 20 lb.

2. Either the single or double upright orthosis could be worn only if flexion contracture at the knee was less than 15 to 20 degrees. They found that of 50 patients thus fitted, 38 patients wore their orthoses successfully for 7 to 48 months.

In order to correct the valgus, a padded dial over the medial side of the knee that was attached to the brace kept the knee in alignment. In the single upright orthosis, this was attached to a medial bar that was, in turn, attached to the lateral full upright. In the bilateral upright orthosis, it was attached directly to the medial upright.

Knee extensor weakness or muscle imbalance, which may be caused by an absence of sensory feedback as in tabes dorsalis, may produce a genu recurvatum. In cases with muscle weakness, the patient stabilizes the knee against the posterior capsule and extension check ligaments by manipulating the ground reactive force line so that it falls in front of the knee, creating an extension moment. Thus, the knee is locked in extension. The posterior capsule is weak and will gradually yield. A "back knee" can be produced by a tight gastrocnemius, soleus, or other bone abnormalities fixing the foot in equinus, thereby creating an excessive extension moment at the knee, especially during the latter part of the stance. In addition to standard medical or surgical care, or both, and an appropriate physical therapy program, orthoses are prescribed for this condition. In mild genu recurvatum, often seen as a knee control problem in the early phase of recovery after the onset of hemiplegia, an ankle-foot orthosis with plantar and dorsiflexion stops and sole plate can be used as a training device. The ankle is set in some dorsiflexion. As the patient rocks over the heel from heel strike to foot flat, the contact point with the ground is at the posterior edge of the heel, with the extension of the ground reactive force falling behind the knee joint, creating a bending moment; whereas during the push off phase, the adjustment of the ankle reduces the extension moment at the knee. It may be advisable in some cases to remove

JUSTUS F. LEHMANN AND BARBARA J. DE LATEUR

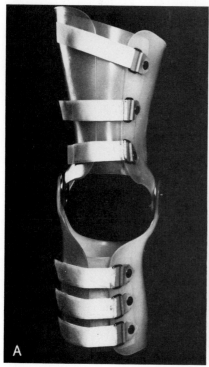 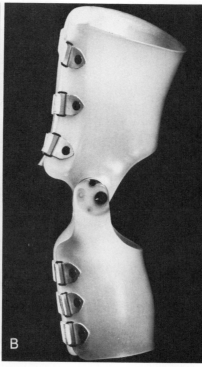

FIGURE 28–11. Anterior *(A)* and medial *(B)* views of the genucentric knee orthosis. (From Foster, R., and Milani, J.: The genucentric knee orthosis—a new concept. Orthot. Prosthet., 33:31–44, 1979.)

the dorsiflexion stop, but the patient must have enough voluntary control to keep the knee from buckling. The biomechanical details are discussed in the section on ankle-foot orthoses for paralysis and paresis.

Most commonly, genu recurvatum is treated with a knee-ankle-foot orthosis positioning the knee in slight flexion. The posterior capsule and check ligaments may tighten enough so that the patient might not have to wear the orthosis permanently. To achieve proper knee position, the upper thigh band should be relatively deep and the lower thigh bands relatively shallow. Thus, according to Bennett,[23] the knee is put in a flexed position. Better control can be achieved with a rigid plastic cuff instead of thigh bands, supplemented by a plastic posterior shell below the knee instead of a calf band.[24]

The knee cage is a relatively short orthosis extending from the area just above the knee to the area just below the knee. It has rigid cross connections or bands between the orthotic uprights posteriorly and two counter forces applied by elastic straps just above and below the knee. More recently, plastics have been used to improve this design,[25] although none of them has been totally satisfactory, some tending to slide off the leg. The

hinged knee cage and the double anterior loop knee orthosis[25, 26] are some of the commonly used modifications of the knee cage. Also, plastic orthoses have been advocated.[25, 26] The genucentric knee orthosis, as shown in Figure 28–11, accommodates the axis of rotation to the instantaneous center of rotation of the knee as it moves through flexion and extension.[74, 75] It also prevents sliding of the orthosis up or down the leg because of the shape of the plastic above and below the knee. Also, hyperextension of the knee can be stopped.

The Toronto abduction orthosis for Legg-Perthes disease is a specialized orthosis for the hip joint.[27, 86] This orthosis allows ambulation and knee and hip flexion while maintaining the hip at 45 degrees abduction and 18 degrees internal rotation. An angle of 90 degrees is maintained at all times between the legs. The treatment rationale is that the femoral head will re-form if weight-bearing is allowed only in the abducted position.

Orthoses for Weakness of the Lower Extremity

These orthoses are used in cases of paralysis and paresis from upper and lower motor neuron disease or in cases of weakness from muscle pathology. They also prevent the development of deformities.

Ankle-Foot Orthoses

These are by far the most commonly used orthoses, and the most important reasons for prescribing them are that they provide (1) mediolateral stability at the ankle during the stance phase to prevent inadvertent twisting of the ankle; (2) toe pickup during the swing phase to prevent dragging of the toe, stumbling, and falling; and (3) push off simulation during the latter part of the stance phase, thus approximating more normal gait and reducing energy expenditure.[76] They may also be used to prevent the development of deformities.

The criteria listed above take into consideration the fact that many patients may be able to ambulate without an orthosis; however, they cannot do so safely because they may frequently fall, stumble, or twist an ankle. Thus the orthoses are prescribed in those cases to provide safety of ambulation. All ankle-foot orthoses inevitably have a significant influence on knee stability.

The biomechanical function of different ankle-foot orthoses may be the same irrespective of materials and components used in their construction. This function can be demonstrated in the conventional metal double upright orthosis. This orthosis is attached to a firm Blücher[28] type shoe for ease of donning and doffing. Most commonly used is a stirrup, i.e., a steel plate bent in a U shape that is incorporated into the shoe. The upper ends form part of the ankle joints. A rigid steel sole plate is often riveted to the stirrup, extending into the sole of the shoe just short of the metatarsal head area. Designs such as the split stirrup with flat channels or stirrups that accommodate round calipers for attachments of the uprights allow the detachment of the uprights from the stirrup but have major disadvantages. In the split stirrup, the uprights may slip out inadvertently because of dirt and corrosion in the channels, and they may be difficult to remove. The round calipers eliminate the ankle joint and, therefore, the axis of motion is coincident with the instep rather than the anatomical ankle axis. Pistoning of the brace against the limb is thus inevitable, but this is less of a problem with children because of the short distance between the instep and ankle. The conventional ankle joint allows motion only on one plane, i.e., dorsiflexion or plantar flexion. The so-called free ankle does not significantly limit motion in either direction, and in order to prevent footdrop, a plantar flexion or posterior stop may be added (Fig. 28–12). A steel pin is inserted into the channel that rests against the posterior flange of the stirrup, stopping plantar flexion. The angle at which this occurs is determined by a set screw. A

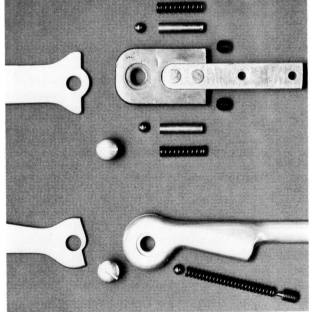

FIGURE 28–12. Double-stopped Becker ankle joint with pin and spring stops *(top)*; single-stopped Klenzak ankle joint with spring assist *(bottom)*.

spring inserted into the same channel will also counteract plantar flexion somewhat and is called a lift assist. A double-stopped ankle joint adds a similarly constructed dorsiflexion or anterior stop (Fig. 28–12) that, to be fully effective, is usually combined with a steel sole plate or a long flange stirrup extending to the metatarsal heads. The uprights consist of stainless steel bar stock or, for a lighter weight, are made of aluminum. They are posteriorly connected at the top of a rigid, padded calf band with an anterior soft closure.

The biomechanical function of the standard double-upright orthosis is as follows:

1. Mediolateral stability: This orthosis, when attached to a firm shoe, provides satisfactory mediolateral stability; however, in those patients with significant spasticity, such as stroke patients who tend to invert the foot, this is not the case. In such situations, a T-strap attached to the outside of the shoe covering the lateral malleolus and cinched around the medial upright can be added. When cinched, the lateral malleolus is pushed medially, thus correcting the varus (inversion) position. The valgus position, when there is a tendency toward eversion, can be corrected by attaching the T-strap to cover the medial malleolus and cinching it around the lateral upright (Fig. 28–13).

2. Ankle and knee stability: The plantar flexion stop at the ankle joint is a substitute for weak foot dorsiflexors, thus preventing toe drag and stumbling during the swing phase. In moderate to severe spasticity, a firm pin stop may be required to prevent a lapse into the equinus position; however, in flaccid paralysis or mild spasticity, a spring assist may be adequate.

Knee stability is also significantly influenced by the type of stop used. With a pin stop, the patient rocks over the posterior portion of the heel rather than letting the foot down slowly from heel strike to foot flat through a contraction of the foot dorsiflexors. As a result, the ground reactive force is extended behind the knee joint (Fig. 28–14) with the moment arm (perpendicular distance from knee axis to force line) posterior to the knee, creating a bending moment at the knee greater than that produced by the normal lengthening contraction of the foot dorsiflexors. This bending moment must be overcome by knee extensor musculature. It is essential for the orthotic design to minimize this bending moment, since in many cases of significant weakness around the ankle, the muscles that extend the knee are also affected. Therefore, during the swing phase, only the minimal force necessary to pick up the toe should be used.

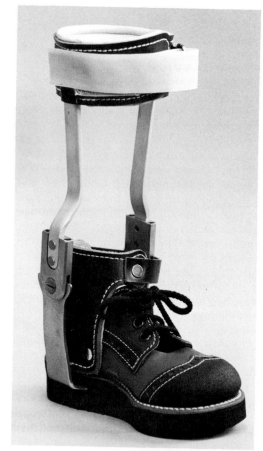

FIGURE 28–13. Inside T-strap correcting valgus position.

This would reduce the bending moment at the knee because the resistance to plantar flexion is less. A spring assist, if adequate, should be used rather than the rigid pin stop.

The influence of the adjustment of the plantar flexion pin stop on the knee moment in a case of peroneal paralysis is shown in Figure 28–15.[77] With the posterior stop adjusted in five degrees dorsiflexion, the duration and magnitude of the knee flexion moment is exaggerated as compared with normal flexion. If adjusted in five degrees plantar flexion, the duration and magnitude of this bending moment is less. Also, the spring-assisted dorsiflexion produced less flexion moment than the posterior pin stop but was adequate for picking up the toe in flaccid paralysis. The gait events, especially the timing of heel strike and toe strike, approached normal both with the posterior plantar flexion pin stop and with the spring stop (Fig. 28–16).

There is a direct trade-off—the more dorsiflexion provided by the pin stop at the ankle, the

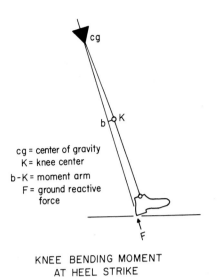

cg = center of gravity
K = knee center
b-K = moment arm
F = ground reactive
force

KNEE BENDING MOMENT
AT HEEL STRIKE

FIGURE 28–14. Knee-bending moment at heel strike (on photo). (From Lehmann, J. F.: The biomechanics of ankle foot orthoses: Prescription and design. Arch. Phys. Med. Rehabil., 60:200–207, 1979.)

provides an almost normal forward movement of the vertical force moment arm with respect to the ankle (center of pressure). The adjustment in five degrees dorsiflexion is not as close to normal (Fig. 28–17). Correspondingly, the total ankle moments (due to shear and vertical loading) are restored close to normal by the anterior stop in five degrees plantar flexion (Fig. 28–18). As a result, the forward movement of the pelvis during push off is normal (Fig. 28–19), with the heel rising and the foot pivoting over the forefoot. The step length on the opposite side is restored. The bending and extension moments at the knee are virtually returned to normal (Fig. 28–20), whereas the adjustment of the anterior stop in five degrees dorsiflexion only partially restores the described parameters to normal. If a spring is used as a dorsiflexion stop, it is not strong enough to withstand the ankle moment created and therefore the brace is not able to assist push off.[79] If the dorsiflexion stop is adjusted toward too much plantar flexion, creating too much of an extension moment at the knee, genu recurvatum may develop.

better the toe clearance during the swing phase but the greater the bending moment at the knee at heel strike that the patient must overcome through voluntary muscle effort. Conversely, the more plantar flexion provided, the more toe drag during swing phase but the less bending moment at the knee at heel strike. Also, the greater the force with which plantar flexion is stopped (greater force in the pin than in the spring), the greater the bending moment during heel strike phase. *Conclusion*: A posterior stop should be used that provides only the minimal necessary force to pick up the toe during the swing phase. The stop should be engaged to provide adequate toe clearance during the swing, but there should be no more adjustment in dorsiflexion than is needed for toe clearance to avoid the excessive bending moment during the heel strike phase.

3. When the anterior, dorsiflexion stop is combined with a sole plate extending to the metatarsal head area, the center of gravity of the body moves forward, the heel rises, the shoe pivots over the end of the sole plate, and push off is simulated. Consequently, the lowest point of the center of gravity pathway is elevated during the phase of double support; i.e., there is a reduction in the total amplitude of the center of gravity pathway. In the case of tibial paralysis, with no gastrocnemius and soleus function,[78] the anterior dorsiflexion stop adjusted in five degrees plantar flexion

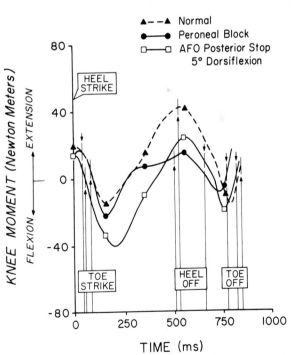

FIGURE 28–15. Knee moment versus time. Curves represent the mean of six trials of one subject. (From Lehmann, J. F., Condon, S. M., de Lateur, B. J., and Price, R.: Gait abnormalities in peroneal nerve paralysis and their corrections by orthoses: A biomechanical study. Arch. Phys. Med. Rehabil., 67:380–386, 1986.)

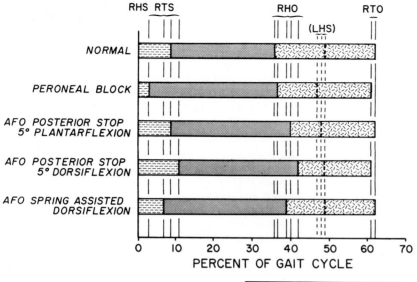

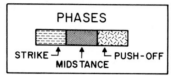

FIGURE 28–16. Mean timing of gait events for six subjects. Gait events are denoted as follows: right heel strike (RHS), right toe strike (RTS), right heel off (RHO), right toe off (RTO), and left heel strike (LHS). (From Lehmann, J. F., Condon, S. M., de Lateur, B. J., and Price, R.: Gait abnormalities in peroneal nerve paralysis and their corrections by orthoses: A biomechanical study. Arch. Phys. Med. Rehabil., 67:380–386, 1986.)

FIGURE 28–17. Vertical force moment arm with respect to the ankle versus time. Curves represent the mean of six trials of one subject. (From Lehmann, J. F., Condon, S. M., de Lateur, B. J., and Smith, J. C.: Ankle-foot orthoses: Effect on gait abnormalities in tibial nerve paralysis. Arch. Phys. Med. Rehabil., 66:212–218, 1985.)

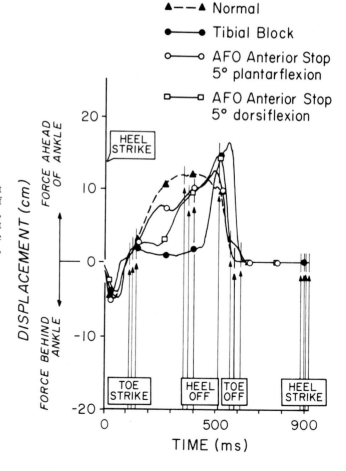

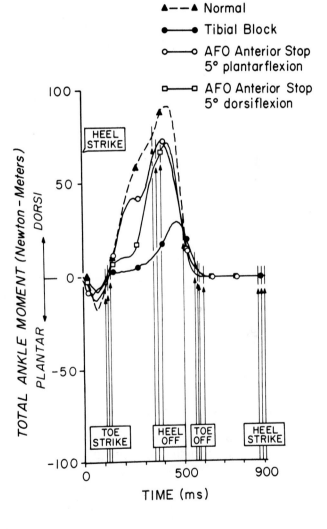

FIGURE 28–18. Total ankle moment versus time. Curves represent the mean of six trials of one subject. (From Lehmann, J. F., Condon, S. M., de Lateur, B. J., and Smith, J. C.: Ankle-foot orthoses: Effect on gait abnormalities in tibial nerve paralysis. Arch. Phys. Med. Rehabil., 66:212–218, 1985.)

JUSTUS F. LEHMANN AND BARBARA J. DE LATEUR

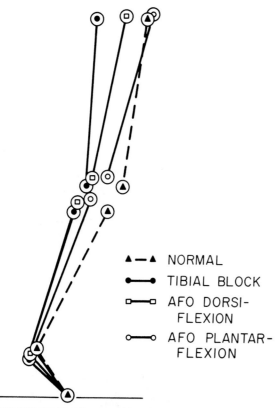

▲–▲ NORMAL

●–● TIBIAL BLOCK

□–□ AFO DORSI-
        FLEXION

○–○ AFO PLANTAR-
        FLEXION

FIGURE 28–19. Mean position of right lower limb at the time of LHS. Stick figures represent the means of six trials of one subject. Circles represent markers placed on the greater trochanter, lateral epicondyle, fibular head, lateral malleolus, and fifth metatarsal head. (From Lehmann, J. F., Condon, S. M., de Lateur, B. J., and Smith, J. C.: Ankle-foot orthoses: Effect on gait abnormalities in tibial nerve paralysis. Arch. Phys. Med. Rehabil., 66:212–218, 1985.)

The dorsiflexion stop, in combination with the sole plate, has a profound effect on knee stability. In gastrocnemius-soleus paralysis, the knee is subjected to a major bending moment that requires considerable muscular effort to keep it from buckling. This bending moment can be restored to normal by adjustment of the stop in five degrees plantar flexion and can be improved but not to normal with adjustment in five degrees dorsiflexion (Fig. 28–20). Also, the ground reactive force line moves in front of the knee, creating a moment arm extending and stabilizing the knee (Fig. 28–21). Conclusion: The dorsiflexion stop in combination with a sole plate is a substitute for the plantar flexion musculature, the gastrocnemius, and the soleus. For a double-stopped ankle joint, there is a trade-off between toe pickup and knee

stability in that the more toe pickup or dorsiflexion of the ankle needed to clear the ground adequately during the swing phase, the more knee instability is produced by the plantar flexion stop during the heel strike phase, and the less knee stability and push off simulation can be gained from the dorsiflexion stop, and vice versa.

If significant spasticity forces the foot into the equinus position during the swing phase, a solid posterior plantar flexion pin stop is needed to prevent the toe from dragging. If, at the same time, the adjustment of the stop, i.e., the angle at which it becomes effective, is such that the knee buckles during the heel strike phase, the bending moment can be changed. This is accomplished by moving the location of the ground reactive force forward (Fig. 28–22),[29] either by cutting off part of the heel of the shoe at a 45-degree angle or by inserting a cushion wedge into the heel.[30]

USE OF BIOMECHANICAL PRINCIPLES IN EVALUATION OF ORTHOSES

With an understanding of the biomechanical function of the orthotic components, selection of the design that best corresponds to a patient's needs is greatly simplified. This is especially important in view of the many recent orthotic designs and modifications using new materials such as plastics, and it can be anticipated that there will continue to be a fairly rapid increase in modifications of existing designs, design changes, and materials used.

When prescribing an orthosis, it is of primary importance to determine the patient's need for mediolateral stability at the ankle, toe pickup, knee stability, and simulated push off. A gross assessment of the forces required, especially for toe pickup, is desirable. With this in mind, several examples of the application of biomechanical principles are as follows:

Orthosis with Single Metal Upright and Posterior Plantar Flexion Stop (Fig. 28–23). It is obvious that this orthosis does not provide as much mediolateral stability as a double upright orthosis, but the medial malleolus of the opposite leg is less likely to be bumped because of the absence of a medial upright. The plastic laminated shoe insert allows shoes to be changed, and, if an anterior dorsiflexion stop is added, the insert would also serve as an equivalent to the sole plate for push off. This design could be used as a toe pickup orthosis, but the patient using it should not have

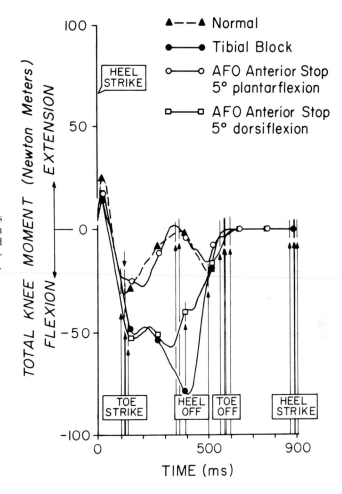

FIGURE 28–20. Total knee moment versus time. Curves represent the mean of six trials of one subject. (From Lehmann, J. F., Condon, S. M., de Lateur, B. J., and Smith, J. C.: Ankle-foot orthoses: Effect on gait abnormalities in tibial nerve paralysis. Arch. Phys. Med. Rehabil., 66:212–218, 1985.)

JUSTUS F. LEHMANN AND BARBARA J. DE LATEUR

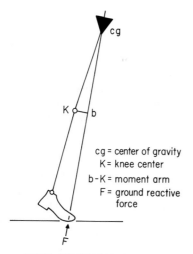

cg = center of gravity
K = knee center
b-K = moment arm
F = ground reactive force

KNEE EXTENSION MOMENT
DURING PUSH OFF

FIGURE 28–21. Knee extension moment during push off. (From Lehmann, J. F.: The biomechanics of ankle foot orthoses: Prescription and design. Arch. Phys. Med. Rehabil., 60:200–207, 1979.)

much spasticity driving the foot into an equinovarus position.

Teufel Orthosis (Fig. 28–24).[1, 31, 32] This orthosis is a stock item that is available in different sizes. As can be seen from its appearance, it provides

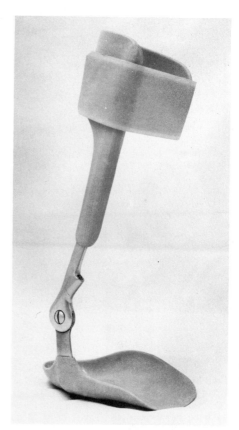

FIGURE 28–23. Orthosis with single upright and posterior plantar flexion stop.

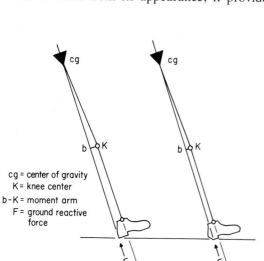

cg = center of gravity
K = knee center
b-K = moment arm
F = ground reactive force

REDUCTION OF KNEE BENDING MOMENT
DURING HEEL STRIKE PHASE BY HEEL CUTOFF

FIGURE 28–22. Reduction of knee bending moment during heel strike by heel cutoff. (From Lehmann, J. F.: The biomechanics of ankle foot orthosis: Prescription and design. Arch. Phys. Med. Rehabil., 60:200–207, 1979.)

limited mediolateral stability. It is effective in patients needing a moderate amount of force for toe pickup, but it provides little additional knee stability during the latter part of the stance. It is fairly rigid in resisting plantar flexion when stressed manually but yields easily when the same amount of force is applied to push it into dorsiflexion. Because the orthosis acts as a posterior leaf spring allowing dorsiflexion, the center of rotation in the orthosis differs from the location of the anatomical axis of the ankle, resulting in some relative motion between the orthosis and the limb, a problem in some patients.

Seattle Orthosis (Fig. 28–25). This orthosis is manufactured by lamination over a positive mold taken from a cast and was the first plastic orthosis described in the literature.[33, 34] The orthosis is rigid and encases the ankle, thereby providing the biomechanical equivalent of an anterior and posterior pin stop with a sole plate extending to the metatarsal head area. It provides maximal mediolateral

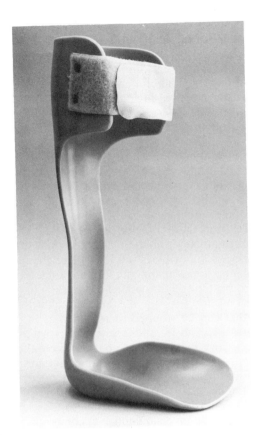

FIGURE 28–24. Teufel orthosis.

In order to achieve the same ankle rigidity in the polypropylene ankle-foot orthosis as found in the laminated orthosis, a thicker sheet of plastic or, as Fillauer[80] has suggested, carbon composite inserts at the level of the ankle can be used. Since these inserts have beveled edges, they allow the thermoplastic to lock the insert in place during the vacuum-forming process (Fig. 28–27). A variant of the Seattle orthosis, which wraps around the entire circumference of leg and ankle but uses rather thin thermoplastic, has been proposed by Gans and associates for use in children with cerebral palsy, myelomeningocele, and muscular dystrophy.[81]

TIRR Orthosis (Engen) (Fig. 28–26). Polypropylene is used in the manufacture of this orthosis, which was designed by Engen.[31, 32] It is corrugated posteriorly for greater strength. The orthosis resists mild to moderate forces pushing it into plantar flexion, depending on thickness of plastic and trim line; however, there is very little resistance to being pushed into dorsiflexion. Depending on the trim line, limited mediolateral stability is provided. Therefore, since the orthosis gives little additional knee stability during push off or the latter part of the stance phase, its primary use is to provide toe pickup during the swing phase for patients with flaccid paralysis or mild spasticity.

stability, but since knee stability is dependent on the degree of plantar flexion or dorsiflexion at which the foot is fixed, casting at the correct angle of the ankle is of critical importance, and heel and sole height of the shoe must be taken into consideration when casting. Consequently, shoes can be changed only if heel and sole height are the same as those of the shoes used for casting. A cushion wedge[34] or cutoff heel can be used to reduce the bending moment at the knee during heel strike. The anterior portion of the orthosis can be slightly trimmed back to reduce the extension moment at the knee, if desired.

The staff at Rancho Los Amigos have modified the design of this orthosis using plastics such as polypropylene (Fig. 28–26).[31] The cost of manufacture is thus reduced, since vacuum-forming techniques can be used with these plastics. The biomechanical function of this orthosis is basically the same as that of the Seattle orthosis; however, it is somewhat less rigid, depending on the thickness of the plastic used and the trim lines.

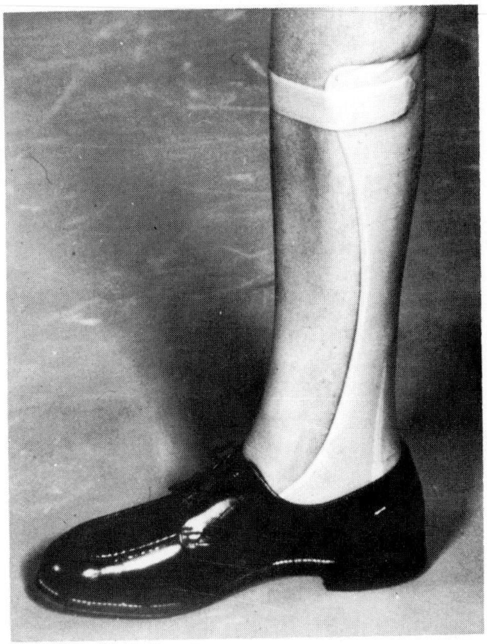

FIGURE 28–25. Seattle orthosis. (From Lehmann, J. F.: The biomechanics of ankle foot orthoses: Prescription and design. Arch. Phys. Med. Rehabil., 60:200–207, 1979.)

JUSTUS F. LEHMANN AND BARBARA J. DE LATEUR

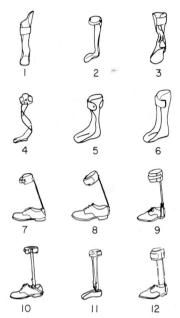

FIGURE 28–26. Small selection of recent orthotic designs:
  1. Plastic solid ankle.
  2. Teufel.
  3. Texas Institute of Rehabilitation Research (Engen).
  4. Institute of Rehabilitation Medicine Spiral.
  5. Rancho Los Amigos.
  6. Seattle.
  7. Veterans Administration Prosthetics Center Shoe-Clasp.
  8. Army Medical Branch Research Laboratory Posterior Bar.
  9. VAPC Single Side Band.
 10. University of California Biomechanics Laboratory Dual Axis.
 11. New York University.
 12. AMBRL—Double Upright.

VAPC Shoe Clasp Orthosis (Fig. 28–28).[1, 31, 35] This orthosis is a plastic leaf spring orthosis with its main advantage being that it is ready made and requires only a firm shoe for application. It can be attached to the heel counter of a shoe by a clasp and loosely to a calf band to absorb the relative motion of the orthosis against the limb. Although the center of rotation of the ankle and the orthosis are in different locations, pistoning of the plastic bar within the calf band is possible. Although readily available and easily applied, this orthosis provides only moderate force for toe pickup and no significant mediolateral stability, and it collapses readily into maximal dorsiflexion even in the absence of stress, thus contributing no additional knee stability (Fig. 28–28).

Spring Wire Orthosis.[36, 37] This orthosis provides only a moderate spring foot dorsiflexor assist for toe pickup. It resists dorsiflexion at push off in the

same proportion, but the force is not strong enough to produce any significant push off simulation. Because it allows plantar flexion at heel strike with little resistance, a buckling moment at the knee is minimized. Mediolateral ankle stability is limited, and plastic orthoses are now frequently used instead of this orthosis.

University of California at Berkeley Dual Ankle Orthosis.[38] This is just one example of special orthoses designed for unusual conditions and, like the others in this group, is applicable to only a few patients. In developing this orthotic design, Inman and associates[39, 40] determined that the axis of inversion and eversion of the subtalar joint is 42 degrees from the horizontal plane and 23 degrees from the midline of the foot. With this information as the basis, an orthosis was designed with an axis for plantar flexion and dorsiflexion and an axis located posteriorly at the heel of the shoe to allow inversion and eversion. A standard ankle joint is used that can be stopped or modified as in other orthoses. However, the use of this orthosis is limited, since it can seldom be used where there is weakness of the anterior leg musculature. The necessity for toe pickup requiring a stopped ankle joint implies that the foot dorsiflexors are either nonfunctioning or weak. Since these muscles are also part of the inversion and eversion group, most patients are unable to use this orthosis with its additional freedom to invert and evert, since they need mediolateral stability at the ankle.

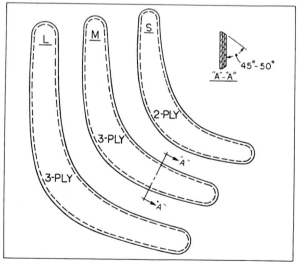

FIGURE 28–27. Patterns used for carbon composite inserts. Note the beveled edges that allow the thermoplastic to lock in the insert during the vacuum-forming process. (From Fillauer, C.: A new ankle-foot orthosis with a moldable carbon composite insert. Orthot. Prosthet. 35:13–16, 1981.)

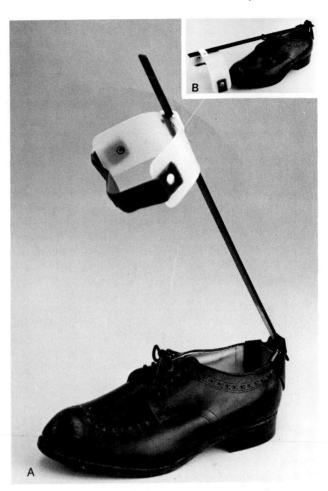

FIGURE 28–28. *A*, VAPC shoe clasp orthosis. *B*, No resistance to dorsiflexion.

Only a few of the available orthoses have been discussed or illustrated in Figure 28–26, but this relatively small number demonstrates the value of understanding and using the basic biomechanical principles when prescribing orthoses. This understanding not only allows more individualization in prescribing orthoses but also eliminates the need for rote memorization of their indications and contraindications.

In addition to the biomechanical principles discussed, another important consideration in prescription should be whether or not the orthotic design increases functional ambulation capability and decreases energy expenditure. As shown in Table 28–1, hemiplegic ambulation is slow and therefore the rate of energy consumption is not greatly increased, but the efficiency, as measured in calories per meter walked per kilograms of body weight, is very poor. A comparison between normal subjects and hemiplegic patients walking without an orthosis, with the Seattle orthosis, and with a double upright ankle-foot orthosis with anterior and posterior pin stops and sole plate showed the following:

1. Oxygen consumption was lowest in normal subjects for any given walking speed and highest in hemiplegics walking without an orthosis. When walking with an orthosis, oxygen consumption was reduced but was still considerably higher than that of normal subjects.

2. There was no difference in oxygen consumption at various speeds with patients using the Seattle or the double upright ankle-foot orthosis.

3. The use of either the Seattle or double upright ankle-foot orthosis increased the comfortable walking speed, i.e., that walking speed at which the minimum amount of energy is required to cover a given distance. The use of either of these

JUSTUS F. LEHMANN AND BARBARA J. DE LATEUR

TABLE 28–1. Hemiplegic Ambulation*

RESEARCHER, DATE, AND REFERENCE NO.	N	TYPE OF DISABILITY AND APPLIANCES	SPEED (M/MIN)	ENERGY EXPENDITURE	
				kcal/min/kg	kcal × 10⁻³/m/kg
Bard, 1963†	15	Hemiplegics	41‖	0.044§	1.06
Corcoran, 1970	15	Hemiplegics - no brace	42‖	0.062	1.49‡
Corcoran, 1970	15	Hemiplegics with plastic brace	49‖	0.067	1.37‡
Corcoran, 1970	15	Hemiplegics with metal base	49‖	0.067	1.37‡

*From Fisher, S. D., and Gullickson, G.: Energy cost of ambulation in health and disability: A literature review. Arch. Phys. Med. Rehabil., 59:124–133, 1978, p. 130.

†Bard, B.: Energy expenditure of hemiplegic subjects during walking. Arch. Phys. Med. Rehabil., 44:368–370, 1963.

‡Calculated knowing kcal/min and m/min.

§Calculated knowing kcal/meter and m/min.

‖Speed chosen by the subjects.

orthoses also increased the maximum walking speed when compared with the same patient walking without the orthosis. In these respects, there was no difference between the two types of orthoses used (Fig. 28–29).[41, 42]

4. Most important, however, whereas the patients walked safely with either of the orthoses, they had to be closely guarded against falls when walking without an orthosis.

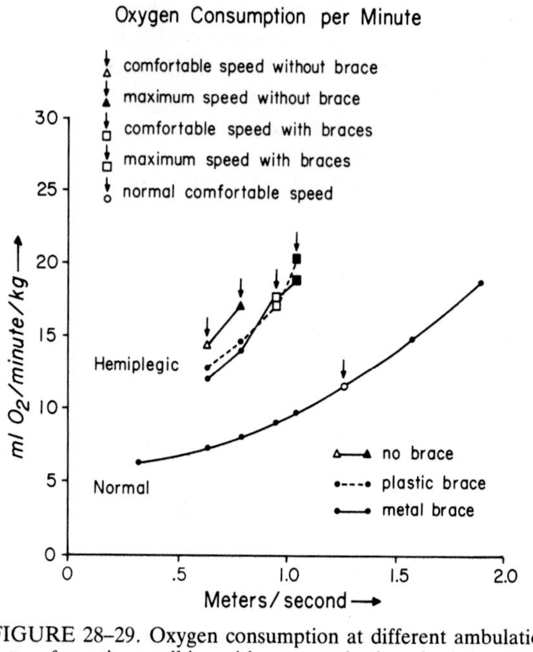

FIGURE 28–29. Oxygen consumption at different ambulation rates of a patient walking without an orthosis and using a plastic laminated ankle-foot orthosis and using an ankle-foot orthosis with double metal uprights, anterior and posterior stops, and a sole plate extending to the metatarsal head area. (From Lehmann, J. F.: The biomechanics of ankle foot orthosis: Prescription and design. Arch. Phys. Med. Rehabil., 60:200–207, 1979. Redrawn from Corcoran.[41, 42])

In summary, proper bracing increases functional ambulation while decreasing energy consumption and provides a greater degree of safety for the patient. Second, even though the materials used and the appearance of orthoses are different, results are quantifiably similar, provided the same biomechanical design is used in the orthoses. Third, minor differences in the weight of the orthoses are not as important in determining energy consumption as biomechanical function and its influence on the center of gravity pathway.

USE OF BIOMECHANICAL PRINCIPLES IN CHECKING ORTHOSES

After fitting the patient, it is most important to check the orthosis to determine whether it fulfills its intended functions. This checking procedure can be divided into several parts:

1. The simple fit of the orthosis should be checked in a static situation. There should be no pressure areas or areas where the orthosis may produce abrasions. With the metal double upright orthosis, common problem areas include the impingement of the peroneal nerve as it passes around the fibular neck by the calf band and where the uprights touch the malleoli. The patient with a plastic orthosis should be managed in the same way as an amputee with a new prosthetic socket. Initially, frequent checks for pressure areas are necessary, and redness should fade after a short period of time. Skin intolerance must be built up by gradually increasing wear.

2. The dynamic checkout is very important. While the patient is standing, the sole and heel of the shoe should be flat on the floor. While walking, the patient should be closely observed for potential knee instability during the heel strike phase from

heel strike to foot flat. This relates to the function of the plantar flexion or posterior stop of the orthosis or its equivalent. If, during the push off phase, a tendency toward back knee is noted, this can be related to the anterior dorsiflexion stop and the length of the sole plate. During the entire swing phase, a determination should be made as to adequacy of toe clearance and, if a dorsiflexion spring assist is used, it should be observed for sufficient toe clearance.

3. The ankle should also be closely observed for possible movement. If the orthosis does allow movement, the axis of the ankle joint for plantar flexion and dorsiflexion should be aligned to coincide as closely as possible with the location of the anatomical joint axis. It was determined by Inman and associates[39] that this axis can be approximated by connecting the tips of the medial and lateral malleoli. This alignment prevents forces from developing between the orthosis and the limb. A special problem is present in plastic or posterior spring orthoses where the center of rotation in the orthosis differs from that of the ankle joint.

Knee-Ankle-Foot Orthoses (KAFOs)

As in the ankle-foot orthoses, an understanding of the biomechanical function of these orthoses will allow their prescription and modification to meet the specific needs of a particular patient. New approaches to design have recently been introduced, and their advantages and disadvantages over the standard double upright metal orthosis can be best understood in terms of their biomechanical function. KAFOs are usually needed by patients who not only have weakness around the foot and ankle but also are unable to stabilize the knee securely during the weight-bearing phase of the gait cycle. Weakness of this type may be caused by upper or lower motor neuron lesions. A severe disability commonly managed with these orthoses is spinal cord injury, including conus and cauda equina lesions. The orthoses may be used for functional ambulation or for ambulation as exercise. Patients with spinal cord injury usually use a swing-to or swing-through gait and become functional ambulators only at lesion levels below T10,[43, 44] their functional ambulation ability depending on age, strength, and coordination.

The KAFO should provide the following biomechanical functions during the stance phase:

1. Mediolateral stability at the ankle.

2. Knee stability in cases where the ankle-foot orthosis is not adequate to control the knee.

3. Push off simulation during the latter part of the stance phase if the orthosis is equipped with an anterior dorsiflexion stop and a rigid sole plate extending to the metatarsal head area.

During the swing phase the posterior plantar flexion stop should ensure toe clearance.

Thus, the basic difference between the ankle-foot and knee-ankle orthoses is the stabilization of the knee by the knee-ankle orthosis. This is achieved by three force applications, one stabilizing force applied in front to keep the knee from buckling under weight-bearing and two counterforces applied at the upper part posteriorly and at shoe level to keep the limb from moving. The components used to achieve such biomechanical function in the standard metal double upright orthosis, i.e., shoes, stirrups, ankle joints, calf bands, and uprights, are the same as those in the ankle-foot orthosis. Commonly available knee joint designs are a free knee, a knee joint with a drop or ring lock, and a bail or Swiss lock (Fig. 28–30). At the top of the orthosis the two uprights are connected by a posterior, rigid, padded upper thigh band with anterior soft closure. This band should clear the ischium by approximately 1½ inches. Usually a lower thigh band with a soft front closure is also used. Knee stabilization is provided by a number of different devices, six common versions of which are shown in Figure 28–31.[45]

A pelvic band is sometimes used in conjunction with the knee-ankle orthosis.[46] The pelvic band is a padded, rigid steel band worn posteriorly and laterally that fits between the greater trochanter and the iliac crest. A soft front closure is used. The pelvic band is connected to the lateral uprights of the knee-ankle orthosis by a hip joint that may be locked, for instance, by a drop lock. Most hip joints of this type allow only flexion and extension movements.

Through an analysis of the function of the KAFO, a determination can be made of the basic principles necessary for understanding the function of the orthosis. These principles are as follows:

1. Force applications should be well within tolerance limits, particularly in patients with anesthetic skin.

2. Forces should be distributed over tolerant areas of the tissues.

3. Unnecessary shear stresses that may loosen ligaments of the knee should be avoided.

4. Energy consumption required for walking should be kept to a minimum.

JUSTUS F. LEHMANN AND BARBARA J. DE LATEUR

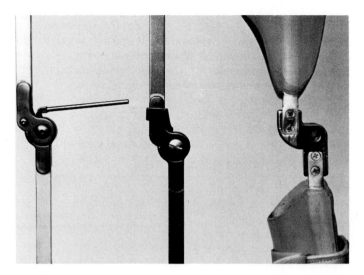

FIGURE 28–30. Swiss or bail lock, drop lock, and free knee off set.

5. The orthosis should allow ease of donning, doffing, and transfer activities.

When the forces between the upper thigh band and thigh were measured, no differences were found in the various designs applying the knee-stabilizing force.[45] However, significant differences were found in the amount of total stabilizing force required to counteract a given bending moment at the knee. The highest force was required when the lower thigh band and calf band were used together to stabilize the knee (Fig. 28–32). From these experiments it can be concluded that the knee-stabilizing force can be kept to a minimum if it is applied close to the center of the knee, since this provides a better leverage to counteract the bending moment at the knee. In addition, the more flexion allowed at the knee, the greater the bending moment during the weight-bearing phase of the stance. Therefore, it is essential that the orthosis be designed to keep the knee straight in the orthosis, thus reducing the required stabilizing force. It is equally important for an orthosis so designed to be correctly applied and the straps cinched evenly and tightly enough to prevent any bending during weight-bearing (Fig. 28–33).

If one looks at the forces per strap that approx-

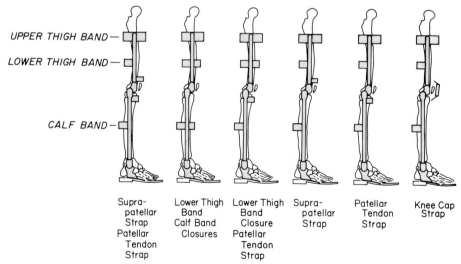

FIGURE 28–31. Six common orthotic configurations. (From Lehmann, J. F., and Warren, C. G.: Restraining forces in various designs of knee ankle orthoses: Their placement and effect on anatomical knee joint. Arch. Phys. Med. Rehabil., 57:430–437, 1976.)

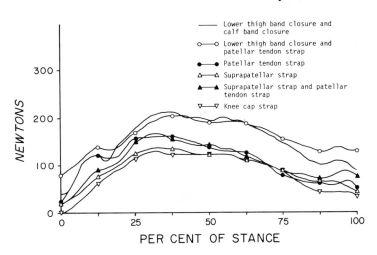

FIGURE 28–32. Total force required to stabilize the knee in the same patient using the six orthoses. (From Lehmann, J. F., and Warren, C. G.: Restraining forces in various designs of knee ankle orthoses: Their placement and effect on anatomical knee joint. Arch. Phys. Med. Rehabil., 57:430–437, 1976.)

imately represent the force per unit of surface area of tissue, one finds very significant differences (Fig. 28–34). The lowest force per strap was found when the forces were applied close to the center of the knee and distributed over two straps, such as the patellar tendon and suprapatellar straps. These straps have the additional advantage of being applied to areas very tolerant of pressure, i.e., the patellar tendon and the musculature above the patella. Single straps can be safely used only if they are large enough to distribute the forces over a large area and especially if applied to tolerant areas such as the patellar tendon.

The forces required to counteract the knee bending moment by the application of stabilizing straps are biologically significant. The range of these forces was measured and found to be from 100 to 170 newtons during paraplegic ambulation using a swing-through gait. For the calculation of pressure, a variable contact area between tissue and the

straps or bands was assumed. Depending on the width of the area of interaction between the band and the tissues, these pressures were on the order of magnitude of 10 newtons per sq cm or 750 mm Hg. In a poorly fitting orthosis, the patient's ischium may be sitting on the edge of the upper posterior thigh band. The force interaction between the ischial area and the band was measured by determining the bending moment created in the orthosis uprights below the band. The forces in swing-through ambulation ranged from 3 to 5 newtons. If one calculates the pressure for interaction between the tissue and various widths of the edge of the posterior thigh band, it is on the order of magnitude of 25 newtons per sq cm or 1875 mm Hg (Fig. 28–35). These are significant and potentially destructive forces and, therefore, should be kept to a minimum in an optimal orthotic design. Even then they occlude the blood flow; however, this occurs during ambulation only in the stance

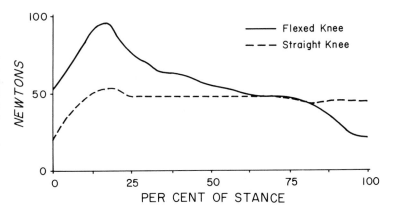

FIGURE 28–33. Comparison of total stabilizing force required with the knee maintained as straight as possible and flexed at 12 degrees. (From Lehmann, J. F., and Warren, C. G.: Restraining forces in various designs of knee ankle orthoses: Their placement and effect on anatomical knee joint. Arch. Phys. Med. Rehabil., 57:430–437, 1976.)

JUSTUS F. LEHMANN AND BARBARA J. DE LATEUR

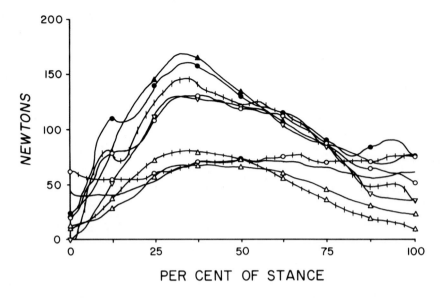

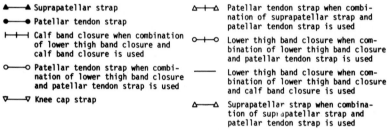

Suprapatellar strap

Patellar tendon strap

Calf band closure when combination of lower thigh band closure and calf band closure is used

Patellar tendon strap when combination of lower thigh band closure and patellar tendon strap is used

Knee cap strap

Patellar tendon strap when combination of suprapatellar strap and patellar tendon strap is used

Lower thigh band closure when combination of lower thigh band closure and patellar tendon strap is used

Lower thigh band closure when combination of lower thigh band closure and calf band closure is used

Suprapatellar strap when combination of suprapatellar strap and patellar tendon strap is used

FIGURE 28–34. Forces on each of the individual strap closures stabilizing the knee in the same patient using the six orthoses. (From Lehmann, J. F., and Warren, C. G.: Restraining forces in various designs of knee ankle orthoses: Their placement and effect on anatomical knee joint. Arch. Phys. Med. Rehabil., 57:430–437, 1976.)

FIGURE 28–35. Possible distribution of pressure calculated assuming a variable contact area on the superior edge of the upper thigh band. (From Lehmann, J. F., and Warren, C. G.: Restraining forces in various designs of knee ankle orthoses: Their placement and effect on anatomical knee joint. Arch. Phys. Med. Rehabil., 57:430–437, 1976.)

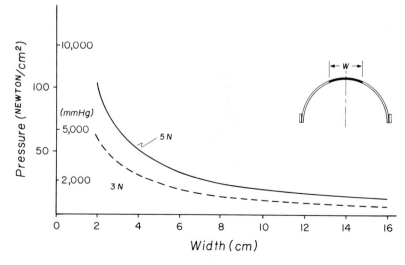

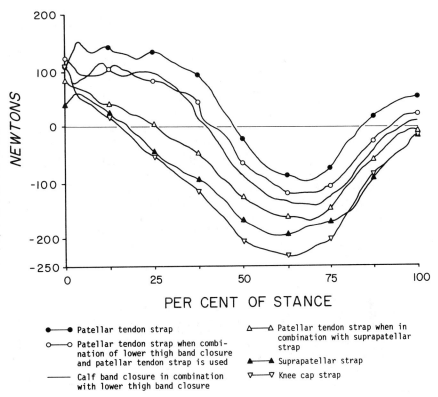

FIGURE 28–36. Anatomical knee shear showing force interaction between femur and tibia. Positive values indicate the femur shearing forward on the tibia; negative values indicate the femur shearing backward on the tibia. (From Lehmann, J. F., and Warren, C. G.: Restraining forces in various designs of knee ankle orthoses: Their placement and effect on anatomical knee joint. Arch. Phys. Med. Rehabil., 57:430–437, 1976.)

●——● Patellar tendon strap

○——○ Patellar tendon strap when combination of lower thigh band closure and patellar tendon strap is used

——— Calf band closure in combination with lower thigh band closure

△——△ Patellar tendon strap when in combination with suprapatellar strap

▲——▲ Suprapatellar strap

▽——▽ Knee cap strap

phase and, therefore, this temporary interruption of capillary flow is tolerated. However, tolerance may be exceeded if straps are used over less tolerant areas such as bone prominences.

Anatomically, knee shear varied greatly with the type of knee-stabilizing force applied (Fig. 28–36). In all cases, the initial shear during heel strike was positive, i.e., the femur sheared forward on the tibia. During the latter part of the stance or push off, it sheared backward on the tibia; i.e., a negative shear was recorded. Two types of curves were obtained with the different orthotic designs, one with relatively even distribution of duration and amplitude between positive and negative shear, the other with a minimum positive shear during the heel strike phase and a maximum amplitude and duration of negative shear during the latter part of the stance, with total shear amplitude negative and greater than in the other types of curves. It can be assumed that the latter distribution of shear would be destructive to knee ligaments, especially if the patients are vigorous ambulators. The result is usually a back knee or genu recurvatum. The explanation for this difference and the types of shear curves during the push off phase are shown in Figures 28–37 and 28–38.

If the force is applied by a patellar tendon strap (Fig. 28–37), the shear transmitted to the knee ligaments is reduced considerably, thereby decreasing the chance of loosening them. The explanation for this reduction in shear is as follows:

1. The shear measured in the orthosis is in an anterior direction, whereas the shear against the floor is in a posterior direction.

2. Shear transmitted through the skeletal system equals floor shear minus the shear measured in the orthosis.

3. Since these shear forces are vectors, the shear in the orthosis is added to the floor shear in the opposite direction. The shear in the skeletal system is, therefore, large and posterior.

4. This large amount of shear is transmitted up the skeletal leg column until another force is applied, in this case by the patellar tendon strap.

However, when the strap is applied above the knee, the total shear force is transmitted across the knee and might very well stretch the ligaments (Fig. 28–38). With this application of force, the shear force generated in the leg column is not reduced until it meets another force about the knee.

If the strap is applied below the knee, the

JUSTUS F. LEHMANN AND BARBARA J. DE LATEUR

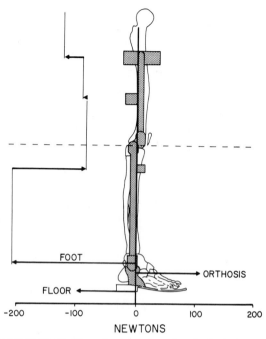

FIGURE 28–37. Shear in the limb and orthosis during push off, the stabilizing force below the knee. (From Lehmann, J. F., and Warren, C. G.: Restraining forces in various designs of knee ankle orthoses: Their placement and effect on anatomical knee joint. Arch. Phys. Med. Rehabil., 57:430–437, 1976.)

positive shear phase is enhanced, providing a more even distribution between positive and negative shear through the stance phase (Fig. 28–39). If, on the other hand, the stabilizing strap is applied above the knee, only a minimum amount of positive shear is transmitted through the knee during heel strike, producing an even distribution between positive and negative shear (Fig. 28–40).

Efforts have been made to reduce the weight of the orthoses by eliminating unnecessary structural components, thus making them more functional and easier to don and doff. The Craig-Scott orthosis[47–49] was specifically designed for this purpose for paraplegic patients. This orthosis eliminates the lower thigh band and calf bands, retains the bail lock at the knee, and applies a stabilizing force to the knee through an anterior pre-tibial rigid piece that may either be hinged and locked into position or permanently attached to the uprights. As in the conventional designs, a double pin–stopped ankle joint with a sole plate at the metatarsal head area is used. When this orthosis was evaluated (Fig. 28–41),[49] it was found that the total force required to stabilize the knee is small, since the force is applied near the center of the knee. If the forces applied by the pre-tibial piece are compared with forces applied by straps used in the other configurations, they are found to be relatively high, since only one strap is used for stabilization. In spite of careful fitting and padding, the original design of the shin piece applies too much force over the tibia so that functional ambulators suffer skin abrasions or unduly prolonged reddening after wearing the orthosis. This can be eliminated by widening the shin piece, manufacturing it from a plaster cast mold to make it form-fitting, and extending the area of maximal pressure to the patellar tendon area. The shear forces were relatively small and well distributed in this orthosis, since the knee-stabilizing force was applied below the knee (Fig. 28–42). When the rigidity of the orthosis with reduction of rigid cross connections between the uprights was tested, it was found that mediolateral displacement and rotation at the upper thigh band level and posterior displacement at the knee level were minimal and temporary in the standard configuration of this orthosis. Only when all rigid cross connections, including the bail, were removed between the upper thigh band and the

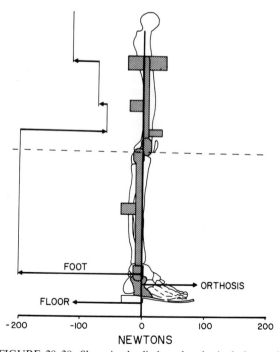

FIGURE 28–38. Shear in the limb and orthosis during push off, the stabilizing force above the knee. (From Lehmann, J. F., and Warren, C. G.: Restraining forces in various designs of knee ankle orthoses: Their placement and effect on anatomical knee joint. Arch. Phys. Med. Rehabil., 57:430–437, 1976.)

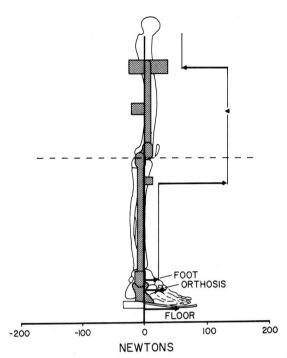

FIGURE 28–39. Shear distribution in limb and orthosis at heel strike with stabilizing force below the knee. (From Lehmann, J. F., and Warren, C. G.: Restraining effects in various designs of knee ankle orthoses: Their placement and effect on anatomical knee joint. Arch. Phys. Med. Rehabil., 57:430–437, 1976.)

at the lowest point of the center of gravity pathway curve. This is the result of the dorsiflexion stop and the sole plate. The shoe and foot pivot over the end of the sole plate at this time. If the ankle joint allows free dorsiflexion, the sole of the shoe stays flat on the floor and the center of gravity at this point is at a lower elevation from the floor than in the orthosis equipped with a dorsiflexion stop and sole plate. As a result, the patient must lift the limb higher to clear the ground during the swing phase (Table 28–2). During the lift phase, the actual difference in mechanical work between patients wearing these two designs of orthoses can be determined by multiplying the center of gravity displacement by the force exerted against the ground through the crutches. The latter can be measured through the use of a force plate. It was found[51] that the mechanical work was reduced by an average of 34 per cent. Since energy is also consumed when mechanical work is not done—i.e., for balance, shock absorption, deceleration—oxygen consumption was also measured (Table 28–3). The total energy consumption thus measured was reduced by the addition of the

stirrup below did the orthosis significantly deform under load conditions comparable to those measured in paraplegic ambulation. Thus, the Craig-Scott orthosis with a bail for the knee lock and an anterior rigid pre-tibial shell should have adequate structural rigidity.

The ability to functionally ambulate, especially for paraplegic patients, depends largely on the amount of oxygen consumed.[50] With a KAFO, the amount of energy consumption during ambulation primarily depends on the influence of the design on the center of gravity pathway. The six conventional orthoses (see Fig. 28–31) share with the Craig-Scott design the double pin–stopped ankle joint used in conjunction with a rigid steel sole plate extending to the metatarsal head area, which provides a simulated push off. Another common design uses a single joint with a posterior plantar flexion stop to provide toe clearance during the swing phase but allows free dorsiflexion. As a paraplegic patient using a swing-through gait with crutches leans forward on the crutches, the heel rises and the center of gravity pathway is maintained at a relatively high elevation from the floor

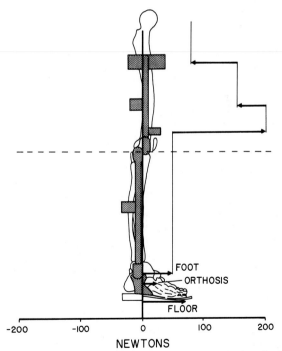

FIGURE 28–40. Shear distribution in limb and orthosis at heel strike with stabilizing force above the knee. (From Lehmann, J. F., and Warren, C. G.: Restraining forces in various designs of knee ankle orthoses: Their placement and effect on anatomical knee joint. Arch. Phys. Med. Rehabil., 57:430–437, 1976.)

JUSTUS F. LEHMANN AND BARBARA J. DE LATEUR

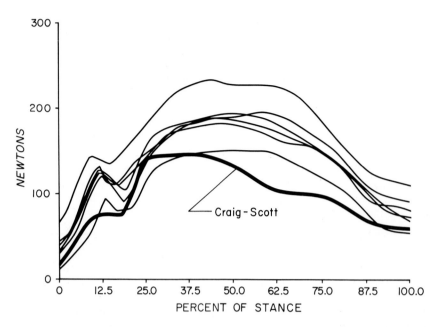

FIGURE 28–41. Total stabilizing force on the knee as compared with six other configurations. (From Lehmann, J. F.: Lower limb orthotics. *In* Redford, J. B. [Ed.]: Orthotics Etcetera, 2nd Ed. Baltimore, Williams & Wilkins Co., 1980, p. 320.)

dorsiflexion stop and the sole plate. It is also interesting to note that the greatest amount of energy consumed when the dorsiflexion stop and sole plate were used occurred during ambulation or in the first part of the rest period. However, with free ankle dorsiflexion, this occurred late in the rest period, which suggests that these patients incurred an oxygen debt to a degree that would limit ambulation with this type of orthosis to walking for exercise purposes only. The same patients equipped with a dorsiflexion stop and sole plate could ambulate for greater distances and longer periods of time and would thus be more likely to become functional ambulators. These findings on energy expenditure comparing the Craig-Scott orthosis with a single-stopped orthosis, which limits

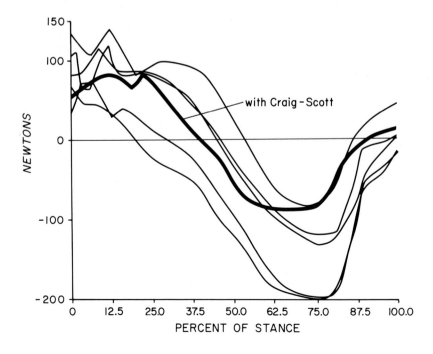

FIGURE 28–42. Anatomical knee shear as compared with six other configurations.

TABLE 28–2. Comparison of Vertical Lift of Center of Gravity Area*

PATIENT NO.	SEX	LEVEL OF LESION	(n = 10) POSTERIOR STOP	(n = 10) POST. AND ANTERIOR STOP	t VALUE (p†)
1	F	T12	13.2	9.0	5.998 (0.0001)
2	F	T7-T8	12.0	6.85	6.414 (0.0006)
3	M	L2-L3	21.6	13.3	5.534 (0.00002)

*From Lehmann, J. F., de Lateur, B. J., Warren, C. G., Simons, B. C., and Guy, A. W.: Biomechanical evaluation of braces for paraplegics. Arch. Phys. Med. Rehabil., 50:179–188, 1969.

†p = probability.

plantar flexion and allows dorsiflexion, were confirmed by Merkel and co-workers.[82] Also, the double-stopped ankle joint with a sole plate provides a platform over which the patient can balance and, therefore, the standing balance without handholds or crutches was significantly increased with the use of this orthotic design.

Energy cost seems to be one of the major limitations on paraplegic ambulation. It is for this reason that Long and Lawton[43] believed that paraplegics with lesions at levels T10 and above would not become functional ambulators, a finding confirmed by Rosman and Spira.[52] They found that paraplegics with lesions at levels T1 through T6 did not use their orthoses. A few paraplegics with lesions at T7 to T11 used their orthoses primarily for exercise purposes, whereas the functional ambulators usually had lesion levels at T12 or below. Patients with lesions at levels L2 to L5 are especially likely to become functional ambulators. Clinkingbeard's[50, 53–55] group, in a study of para-

plegics, found that the energy required for ambulation ranged from 2.32 to 9.05 kcal $\times 10^{-3}$ per m per kg. This represents a 3- to 10-fold increase when compared with normal subjects.

It is not so much the mechanical ability to walk with normal speed that limits ambulation using a swing-through gait with bilateral KAFOs. Rather, it is the high metabolic demand that limits endurance at any practical walking speed, especially since the work has to be done by the small muscle groups of the upper extremity as compared with the large musculature of the legs in the normal individual (Table 28–4).[83, 84] The high metabolic demand may also be associated with a high heart rate because of reduced venous return to the heart resulting from pooling of blood in the lower extremities.[85] The data available on functional electrical stimulation (FES) for paraplegic ambulation, with about 8.0×10^{-3} kcal per m per kg,[86] still show the excessive metabolic demand with decreased efficiency, yet the fact that a larger group

TABLE 28–3. Comparison of Energy Consumption of Patient Ambulating with Each Brace*

INTERVALS OF O₂ CONSUMPTION	POSTERIOR ANKLE STOP		POSTERIOR AND ANTERIOR ANKLE STOP	
	Run 1	Run 3	Run 2	Run 4
Rest 1 min	0.42 l	0.44 l	0.67 l	0.66 l
Ambulation 200 feet	2.48 l	2.49 l	2.56 l	2.04 l
Min 1 and 2 rest	1.56 l	1.58 l	1.82 l	2.22 l
Min 3 and 4 rest	3.35 l	3.38 l	1.01 l	0.95 l
Total O₂ consumed†	7.39 l	7.45 l	5.39 l	5.21 l
Total caloric† equivalent	36.95 cal	37.25 cal	26.95 cal	26.05 cal
Ambulation time	1 min, 11 sec	1 min, 19 sec	1 min, 13 sec	1 min, 17 sec

*From Lehmann, J. F., de Lateur, B. J., Warren, C. G., Simons, B. C., and Guy, A. W.: Biomechanical evaluation of braces for paraplegics. Arch. Phys. Med. Rehabil., 50:179–188, 1969.

†Prerun rest not included in totals.

JUSTUS F. LEHMANN AND BARBARA J. DE LATEUR

TABLE 28–4. Paraplegic Ambulation*

RESEARCHER, DATE, AND REFERENCE NO.	N	TYPE OF DISABILITY AND APPLIANCES	SPEED (M/MIN)	ENERGY EXPENDITURE	
				kcal/min/kg	kcal × 10⁻³/m/kg
Clinkingbeard, 1964[53]	4	Thoracic paraplegics	4	0.043	9.05
Clinkingbeard, 1964[53]	3	Lumbar paraplegics	20	0.048	2.37
Gordon, 1956[54, 55]	3	Thoracic paraplegics	27	0.090	2.44
Gordon, 1956[54, 55]	10	All paraplegics	27	0.086	2.32

*From Fisher, S. D., and Gullickson, G.: Energy cost of ambulation in health and disability: A literature review. Arch. Phys. Med. Rehabil., 59:124–133, 1978, p. 130. Original data reanalyzed.

of muscles is used as compared with the brace ambulation may improve endurance somewhat. No clear evidence in this respect is available. On the other hand, the slowness of the gait with FES[87] using a reciprocating gait pattern does not seem to compare well with brace ambulation.

Waters and Miller[88] stated, "Even those patients, who are physiologically capable of sustaining the intense physical effort of a swing-through gait for a sustained time period to travel longer distances, find tachypnea, tachycardia, and hidrosis unacceptable for routine activities of daily living."

In spite of these serious metabolic limitations of ambulation, the prescription of orthoses and the training of the patient to use orthoses in ambulation are still frequently useful. The need for ambulation with braces and crutches should be evaluated in the light of the demand placed upon the patient by the environment. Even if the patient would not be able to use sustained ambulation at a practical speed for daily activities and has to primarily rely on the wheelchair, the capability of walking with braces may be essential in other situations. For instance, the patient may have to walk only a short distance to have access to a job site or to the bathroom facilities at the site of work. In this situation, the ability to walk may make the difference between employment and unemployment. At lower levels of capability, the ambulation could be used in homemade parallel bars as an exercise program to stretch hip flexors, knee flexors, and the gastrocnemius and soleus muscles and maintain strength in the upper extremities. In short, therapeutically, one should match the patient's capability with essential demands placed upon the patient by the environment and correspondingly decide whether braces should be prescribed. Consistent with this concept, Merkel and associates[89] stated, "Our data do not support the concept of denying, on the basis of the level of lesion alone, young, otherwise healthy, well-motivated patients with thoracic paraplegia the

opportunity of using Scott-Craig orthoses to supplement wheelchair mobility and activities of daily living."

In contrast to ambulation with braces and crutches or FES, wheelchair ambulation does not have the same metabolic and cardiovascular limitations. Ambulation in the wheelchair at comparable speeds is as efficient and requires energy as much as or less than normal walking.[50, 90] However, there is a significant difference in the energy requirements, depending on the surface of the ground.[91]

Orthotic design features should make donning and doffing easy, and the time required for this purpose was used as a measure of the difficulty encountered. When the Craig-Scott orthosis was compared with the standard double upright orthosis using the patellar tendon–suprapatellar strap combination, the average donning time was 111 sec for the Craig-Scott orthosis and 153 sec for the standard orthosis. The doffing time for the former was 28 sec and for the latter 33 sec. However, on evaluation of the Craig-Scott orthosis, it was noted that it slid off the thigh when the patient sat because the posterior calf band normally restraining the orthosis was missing. This could be readily corrected by a posterior soft closure below the knee, which, however, added four seconds to the doffing time.[49] It can, therefore, be concluded that one posterior connection between the uprights below the knee is essential to stabilize the orthosis on the limb when the patient sits. There was no difference between the standard orthosis and the Craig-Scott design in transfer activities. Also, standing balance was identical, since these two types of orthoses are the same from the ankle joint down.

The necessity for a pelvic band is somewhat controversial. Although a pelvic band designed with a lockable hip joint is frequently used for stabilizing the hips, patients can be quite stable when using a swing-through and swing-to gait without such a band. With crutches in front, the forces of gravity pull the hips into extension to provide stability, and hyperextension is checked by extremely strong ligaments. Following swing-through, the patient is stable with the crutches behind the body. If the patient's trunk is arched, the center of gravity force line falls behind the hip joints into an area of support between the legs and crutches. The hips are again locked by the extension moment created by the force line falling behind the hip axis of flexion extension. In this manner, patients can ambulate effectively without being encumbered by a pelvic band.

The literature suggests that excessive lumbar excursion is reduced by the use of a pelvic band and that it controls the forward swing of the legs, especially in cases of uneven spasticity. An experiment was developed to test this suggestion by applying an electrogoniometer to the backs of paraplegic patients in order to estimate the maximal excursion of the lumbar spine throughout the gait cycle.[56] The results showed that while the hips were somewhat limited by the pelvic band, lumbar excursion was significantly increased as the lumbar spine compensated for lack of mobility at the hips. The use of the pelvic band resulted in a significant reduction of mean stride length and an increase in the center of gravity pathway amplitude (Table 28–5). Without the pelvic band, the patient walked with a lower center of gravity pathway amplitude (Table 28–5), and mobility at the hips allowed the patient to clear the ground more easily during the swing phase.

The inference can be made from these measurements that energy consumption will be greater when the orthosis includes a pelvic band. Also, donning and doffing times were found to be longer with this device than with others. If the patient had some spasticity, it was found that standing balance was slightly improved. However, all patients tested learned to overcome their initial difficulties when using orthoses without pelvic bands

and chose permanent orthoses without the band even though forward leg swing might be better controlled with the pelvic band. Therefore, in most cases of paraplegia, pelvic bands are probably unnecessary, although they may be useful in some exceptional cases of spasticity.[56]

In summary, the following biomechanical principles apply to the design and fitting of all KAFOs:
1. Mediolateral stability of ankle and toe pickup during the swing phase is provided in the same fashion as in the ankle-foot orthosis. In addition, knee stability is provided during the stance phase and simulated push off.
2. To reduce the possibility of excessive forces being applied to the knee by bands or straps, the following should be observed:
   a. The orthosis should be designed and applied with the knee straight to reduce the bending moment at the knee.
   b. Any stabilizing straps should be applied close to the center of the knee to reduce the force required to counteract a bending moment at the knee.
   c. The straps or bands stabilizing the knee should distribute the required force over a large and also tolerant area, such as the patellar tendon and suprapatellar areas.
   d. To reduce the shear on the knee ligaments, a major portion of the total knee-stabilizing force should be applied below the knee.
3. An anterior dorsiflexion stop combined with a sole plate extending to the metatarsal head area simulates push off with a decreased center of gravity pathway and amplitude and a significant reduction of energy consumption.
4. The rigid platform provided by a double pin–stopped ankle joint combined with a sole plate provides better standing balance with the hands free.
5. Reduction of structural components in the standard double upright orthosis and its modifications (Craig-Scott orthosis) is possible, but to

TABLE 28–5. Lumbar Excursion, Stride Length, and Center of Gravity Amplitude With and Without Pelvic Band*

	WITH PELVIC BAND	WITHOUT PELVIC BAND	WILCOXON TEST†
Mean maximum range of lumbar excursion (degrees)	29.0	26.8	$p < 0.05$
Mean stride length	0.96 m	1.03 m	$p < 0.05$
Mean center of gravity amplitude	10.8 cm	8.7 cm	$p < 0.05$

*From Warren, C. G., Lehmann, J. F., and de Lateur, B. J.: Pelvic band use in orthotics for adult paraplegic patients. Arch. Phys. Med. Rehabil., 56:221–223, 1975.
†Matched-pairs signed-ranks test.

JUSTUS F. LEHMANN AND BARBARA J. DE LATEUR

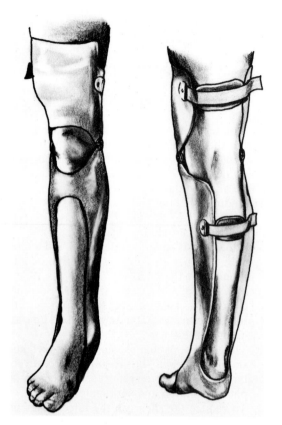

FIGURE 28–43. Design developed by Lehneis. For further discussion, see references 57 and 58.

maintain structural stability, at least one rigid cross connection, which can be the bail at the knee lock, should be built into the orthosis between the rigid posterior upper thigh band and the stirrup below. To restrain the orthosis from sliding off the leg when sitting, a strap or band applied posteriorly below the knee is necessary.

6. Pelvic bands are needed only in exceptional cases to control rotation or adduction of the legs in adults. The pelvic band combined with a hip lock reduces stride length, increases center of gravity amplitude, and makes donning, doffing, and transfers more difficult.

With the understanding of the basic principles of orthotic design, it is relatively easy to examine new designs and identify their functions. To illustrate this idea, the following can be determined by examining a design developed by Lehneis (Fig. 28–43):[57, 58]

1. Knee-stabilizing force is applied in the suprapatellar and patellar tendon areas.

2. A rigid ankle is used that is functionally equivalent to an anterior and posterior stop with sole plate extending to the metatarsal head area.

3. The malleoli are encased to provide maximum mediolateral stability.

4. A posterior soft closure prevents the orthosis from sliding off the thigh when sitting.

5. The upper closure is equivalent to the posterior thigh band.

ParaWalker (Hip Guidance Orthosis) and Reciprocating Gait Orthosis

Recently, bracing of the hip has been proposed for specific conditions. Major and colleagues[92] and Butler and associates[93] braced the hip with a ball bearing hip joint that allowed limited hip flexion through provision of a stop. Free motion in extension was available. Extension could be restricted in a similar fashion by a stop. This joint is incorporated into a body brace with the KAFO. The orthosis also includes a shoe rocker for lateral rocking. The hip motion is guided in the flexion-extension plane, and abduction and adduction are controlled (Fig. 28–44).[92, 94–96] Flexion motion in this orthosis is initiated by gravity through trunk motion and checked by the stop. The authors proposed this orthosis for patients with an L2 lesion and complete flaccidity of the lower extremities. Rose and associates[96] evaluated the use of this orthosis in children with spina bifida. In a series of 27 children ranging in age from 5 years 8 months to 15 years 7 months, 17 were totally flail, 7 were flail in one leg, and the remaining 7 had some power in both hips. Thirteen patients improved in ambulation with the orthosis. Nene and Major[97] conducted force plate studies with nine adult complete paraplegics who had lesions at the thoracic level. They found that each patient had to apply extra stabilizing forces through the crutches for safe walking. These forces are attributed to an increased crutch force applied to prevent lateral deformation of the orthoses in stance phase. Consequently, alternative methods of compensating for the lack of structural rigidity by means of a hybrid system incorporating both the mechanical orthosis and electrical stimulation of selected muscle groups need to be investigated.[98]

Fillauer[8] has proposed the development of a reciprocating gait orthosis (Fig. 28–45). This orthosis also incorporates a special hip joint that

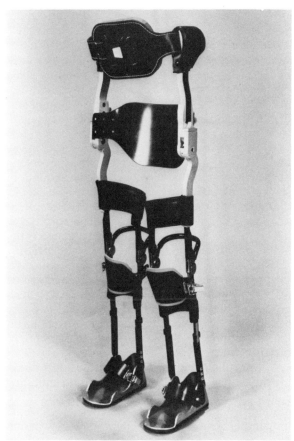

FIGURE 28–44. The ParaWalker. (Photograph courtesy of ORLAU Publishing, used by permission.)

transfers forces from one hip to the other via one or two Bowden cables. The pelvic band design covers the gluteal and sacral areas and includes a thoracic extension, featuring a closure with Velcro bands. The basic concept of the design is that flexion force on one hip can be transferred to an extension force on the other hip, or vice versa. Either flexion or extension is possible in a reciprocal pattern. This design, therefore, is most appropriate for special cases.[99] Special locks for hip and knee are available.[100] Unpublished data obtained by Merritt[101, 102] showed that the reciprocating gait orthosis using a reciprocating gait pattern required more calories per meter walked per kilogram body weight than did the standard Craig-Scott orthosis. On the other hand, if a swing-through gait pattern was used, the energy consumption was the same. The reciprocating gait pattern was also slow as compared with the swing-through gait. To enhance the usefulness of this

orthosis, Solomonow and co-workers[103] suggested using it with functional electrical stimulation of the quadriceps simultaneously with the contralateral gluteus maximus muscle or using implanted electrodes to stimulate the iliopsoas muscle directly for hip flexion. The utility of the reciprocating gait orthosis as compared with standard KAFOs remains to be assessed.

Pneumatic Orthosis

Pneumatic orthoses were introduced in this country for paraplegics by Silber and associates and were tested by Ragnarsson.[59, 60] Inflatable tubes in front and back provide rigidity when properly

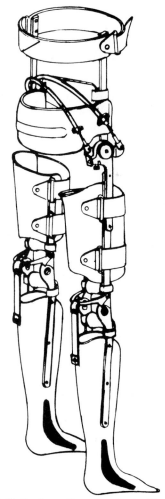

FIGURE 28–45. Reciprocating gait orthosis. (Photograph courtesy of Durr-Fillauer Medical, Inc., used by permission.)

JUSTUS F. LEHMANN AND BARBARA J. DE LATEUR

inflated. Deflation allows bending at hips and knees for sitting. The long version of the orthosis covers the hips and a portion of the trunk. This pneumatic orthosis has approximately the same length as a standard double upright metal orthosis. Toe pickup during the swing phase is provided by a pickup strap, and mediolateral stability at the ankle by wearing high-top boots. On evaluation of these orthoses, it was found that[61]

1. Much better mediolateral stability of the ankle and simulated pushoff could be produced by using the orthosis in combination with a plastic ankle-foot orthosis of the Seattle or Rancho type as an insert. Only with this ankle-foot orthosis were our patients able to use the short orthosis effectively.

2. The center of gravity pathway amplitude was definitely greater when the patients used pneumatic orthoses rather than the standard double upright orthosis. The greatest amplitude was found with the short pneumatic orthosis even when used in combination with the ankle-foot orthosis. An equally large amplitude of the center of gravity pathway was observed when the patients wore the long pneumatic orthosis without the ankle-foot orthosis followed by the long pneumatic orthosis, using it in combination with the ankle-foot orthosis. The least amplitude was produced with the patients walking with the standard double upright orthosis with anterior and posterior stops and a sole plate extending to the metatarsal head area. These larger amplitudes in the pneumatic orthosis were the result of the angular motion at the knee under the impact of heel strike as well as some movement at the ankle even when used with the plastic ankle-foot orthosis. The ankle motion was maximal if the orthosis was used without the ankle-foot orthosis as an insert.

3. When the metabolic requirements were measured, it was surprising that the long pneumatic orthosis required the least oxygen consumption in spite of the center of gravity amplitude being larger than that observed in the standard double upright orthosis. The difference was significant at the $p \leq 0.05$ level (Fig. 28–46). The only explanation is the better stabilization of hip and trunk by the orthosis, resulting in less voluntary effort being required by the patient.[104] Even when using the long pneumatic orthosis without the ankle-foot orthosis, which produced the largest center of gravity pathway amplitude, the oxygen consumption was equal to that of patients using the standard double upright orthosis.

4. Functional ambulation was evaluated by having the patients walk at a prescribed rate until they could no longer maintain that speed. Distances are plotted in Figure 28–47. At slow walking speeds, i.e., those below 70 m per min, patients wearing

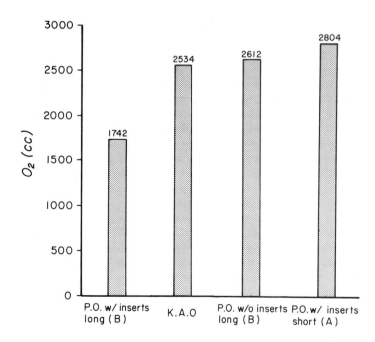

FIGURE 28–46. Total oxygen consumption while a T-12 paraplegic ambulated 300 meters with different orthoses. Average of 6 runs with each orthosis. PO = pneumatic orthosis, KAO = standard double upright knee ankle orthosis (From Lehmann, J. F., Stonebridge, J. B., and de Lateur, B. J.: Pneumatic and standard double upright orthoses: Comparison of their biomechanical function in three patients with spinal cord injuries. Arch. Phys. Med. Rehabil., 58:72–80, 1977.)

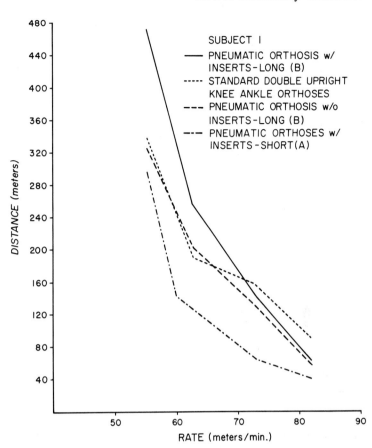

FIGURE 28–47. Maximum distance traveled by a T-12 paraplegic ambulating at various speeds while wearing different orthoses. (From Lehmann, J. F., Stonebridge, J. B., and de Lateur, B. J.: Pneumatic and standard double upright orthoses: Comparison of their biomechanical function in three patients with spinal cord injuries. Arch. Phys. Med. Rehabil., 58:72–80, 1977.)

the long pneumatic orthosis with the ankle-foot orthosis as an insert could walk greater distances at the various speeds than those with other orthoses. This performance was closely followed by the use of the standard double upright metal orthosis. At higher speeds, the pneumatic orthoses were more likely to buckle at the knee with the increased impact of heel strike. This increased the center of gravity amplitude significantly, rendering the pneumatic orthoses less efficient. The angular change at the knee increased from 4 degrees at 55 m per min to 10 degrees at 75 m per min. The center of gravity amplitude changed from 10.81 cm to 25.72 cm.

5. For marginal ambulators and for ambulators who walk for exercise purposes only, the long pneumatic orthosis with the ankle-foot orthosis may be most effective. However, it was found that even paraplegic patients with good use of the arms had difficulties in correctly donning and doffing the garment. The inflation mechanism is, at the very least, cumbersome because it depends on availability of compressed gas cans or an electrical outlet for a pump.[61]

6. For early mobilization of recent paraplegics, the long pneumatic orthosis compresses the abdomen and legs, as pointed out by Silber, and reduces the likelihood of orthostatic hypotension.

7. The short pneumatic orthosis has none of the advantages of the long pneumatic orthosis, but most of its disadvantages.

Since the garment is available as a shelf item in different sizes and can be adjusted to individual patients, it may be used for the initial phase of mobilization of paraplegic patients. An additional benefit to the patient is the reduction of cost, since the orthosis can be reused by subsequent patients. For marginal ambulators or those who ambulate for exercise purposes only, the long pneumatic orthosis may be the choice in exceptional cases. For functional ambulation, however, the standard double upright metal orthosis is preferred.

JUSTUS F. LEHMANN AND BARBARA J. DE LATEUR

Orthoses Using Electrical Stimulation

The concept of FES was introduced by Liberson and co-workers,[62] and it is used primarily to control footdrop during the swing phase in hemiplegic patients. The theory upon which its use is based is the survival of the lower motor neuron, including the axon in upper motor neuron lesions; therefore, a contraction of the muscles innervated by the peripheral nerve can be induced by electrical stimulation of this nerve, although stimulation must be properly phased to obtain a functional result.[63, 105]

There are two types of electrical stimulators available, one using external stimulation of the peroneal nerve through the skin, the other using an implanted electrode that is applied surgically to the nerve. Common to both applicators is a miniature electrical stimulator producing currents between 20 and 300 μsec of pulse duration with a repetition of 24 to 100 Hz, current intensities between 90 and 200 mA, and voltages between 50 and 120 V.[106]

In using an external stimulator, the power pack is worn on a waist belt, and the skin electrode is applied to the peroneal nerve below the fibular head, with the inactive electrode applied to the leg below. The stimulator is activated by a switch incorporated in the shoe that turns on the stimulator when the heel leaves the ground and turns off the stimulator on heel strike.[65]

When an implanted electrode is used, it must be surgically placed directly on the nerve with a flexible wire lead connected to a subcutaneously implanted receiver located over the anteromedial aspect of the thigh. The power pack for the stimulator and transmitter is worn at the waist, and the transmitter is connected to an antenna located on the surface of the skin over the implanted receiver. Phasing of the stimulation is controlled by a heel switch with a transmitter incorporated into the shoe, its signal being received by the receiver section of the stimulator-transmitter assembly at the waist (Fig. 28–48).[63]

According to Waters, conduction velocity of the nerve is not significantly affected by the stimulation.[66] Fuhrer found that repetitive stimulation slightly decreased skin impedance and slightly increased current levels.[67]

Both the external and implanted stimulators have been applied to hemiplegic patients with the ability to walk without an orthosis.[107] However, certain criteria have been developed in various

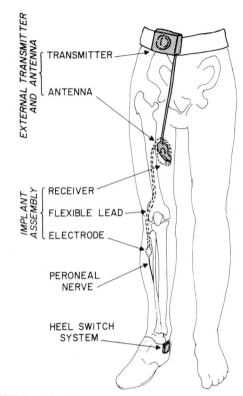

FIGURE 28–48. Relative location of neuromuscular assist equipment on a patient with right side hemiplegia. (From Lehmann, J. F.: Lower limb orthotics. *In* Redford, J. B. [Ed.]: Orthotics Etcetera, 2nd Ed. Baltimore, Williams & Wilkins Co., 1980, p. 320. Redrawn from Waters et al.[68])

studies for the use of these types of functional orthoses. The following is a brief summary of the findings of these studies:

1. Waters and associates felt that it was necessary for the patient to be able to walk more rapidly than 25 m per min without an orthosis, that the patient should have good balance, and that the major gait problem should be footdrop, which could also be corrected by an ankle-foot orthosis.[68] Proprioception should also be intact, and, during the stance phase, the patient's ankle should not be plantar flexed more than 10 degrees.

2. In addition, Takebe and co-workers stated that the patient should be able to apply the electrodes manually without difficulty if the external stimulator is used and should also be able to tolerate the discomfort caused by stimulation.[65]

3. Liberson suggested that an increase in strength of foot dorsiflexors could be attributed to this therapy and that on a long-term basis it would be helpful in re-educating the patient's muscles,

even without continued use of the electrophysiological orthosis.[62] Also, Van Griethuysen and colleagues[108] suggested that in some patients, the FES may successfully improve the gait pattern through re-education.

4. Rather than stimulating the peroneal nerve, Lee and Johnston applied a train of electrical pulses to a single skin area to induce a flexion reflex in order to effect an improvement in gait pattern during the swing phase.[69]

5. Dimitrijevic and associates claim that a reciprocal inhibition of the triceps surae results from stimulation of the foot dorsiflexors, and, therefore, they conclude that the electrophysiological orthosis prevents undesirable ankle clonus.[70]

The principle used in these electrophysiological orthoses has been applied to major hip and thigh muscle groups in patients with spinal cord injuries.[7] Kralj and associates[109, 110] and Cybulski and associates[111] investigated FES for spinal cord injuries. This procedure has been investigated as a tool for muscle strengthening,* for maintaining standing posture,[117] and for ambulation.[117-119] Braun and associates[120] used FES for standing and walking in four paraplegic patients. A good standing position was achieved by stimulation of the quadriceps muscle supplemented by stimulation of the gluteus maximus and the gluteus medius muscles. Gait was initiated by activation of the flexion reflex in a single stimulation of the shank and by tilting the trunk. Difficulties were encountered due to uncontrolled strong adduction of the legs. External support such as parallel bars, walkers, or crutches was needed. The stimuli were rectangular, 0.3 msec in duration and up to 120 V with a current intensity of 200 mA, and with a frequency of 24 Hz. Similarly, Bajd and co-workers[118] used four channels of electrical stimulation to produce a reciprocal gait pattern. During the phase of double support, knee extensor musculature was stimulated bilaterally for support. The transition from double stance to swing phase was controlled by hand switches placed in the handles of the walking frame or crutches. It was achieved through electrical stimulation of afferent nerves eliciting a synergistic flexor muscle response.

In studies by Marsolais and Kobetic,[121, 122] 3 of 11 subjects with spinal cord injury found the regimen of exercise and testing as part of FES for ambulation purposes too time-consuming. Another subject was unable to bring the strength of the quadriceps to an adequate level for FES and am-

*See references 84, 112, 113, 114, 115, and 116.

bulation. Nine subjects achieved the ability to stand, seven were able to walk in parallel bars, and six were able to walk using a reciprocal or rolling walker. The speed of walking with the assistance of FES among the subjects ranged from 12 to 48 m per min.

Isakov and colleagues[86] noted that the effort invested during ambulation by means of FES was too exhausting and felt that the use of FES would be advisable only in young subjects. In two patients, the values in terms of oxygen uptake in milliliters per minute during ambulation were 812 and 1381, with a velocity of 8.31 m per min and 11.15 m per min, respectively. The efficiencies, as measured in milliliters per kilogram of body weight per meter walked, were 1.53 and 1.65, respectively. These values can be recalculated and are approximately 8 kcal per kg body wt per m walked, which contrasted with normal values of about 0.8 kcal per kg body wt per m walked,[50] thus representing a very marked decrease in efficiency. According to the authors, it must also be realized that these patients probably were very limited ambulators using KAFOs, producing a low energy efficiency of walking.

Most recently, Marsolais and Edwards[123] reviewed the energy cost of walking and standing with FES and KAFOs with rigid ankle joints. Patients walked with FES using reciprocal gait and a rolling walker. With the KAFOs a swing-to gait pattern was used. Table 28–6 shows the energy cost of ambulation of the patients walking with neuromuscular stimulation. It should be noted that the rate of energy consumption with an average of 0.095 ± 0.005 kcal per kg per min is increased over the normal values as compiled by Fisher (Table 28–7).[50] The walking speed, which ranged from 6.6 m per min to 33.6 m per min, was markedly reduced from normal. The increase of energy expenditure in terms of kcal $\times 10^{-3}$ per kg body wt per m walked was on average 8.42 with FES, with a minimal value of 2.77 and a maximal value of 13.40. This represents a much higher value, that is, a greater decrease in efficiency for paraplegic walking compared with comparable data from the literature reviewed by Fisher. It also should be noted that subjects 1 and 2 in Table 28–6 were able to walk distances greater than 200 m at rates of 18 m per min or more with FES, whereas subject 3 was unable to walk at speeds of 18 m per min. Subjects 1 and 2 also walked at comparable speeds for unlimited distances using KAFOs. Marsolais and Edwards also found a somewhat increased heart rate with FES as compared with

JUSTUS F. LEHMANN AND BARBARA J. DE LATEUR

TABLE 28–6. Energy Costs of Ambulation with Functional Neuromuscular Stimulation*

SUBJECT	TRIAL	DISTANCE (m)	SPEED (m/sec)	O$_2$ CONSUMPTION (l/min)	ENERGY EXPENDITURE (kcal/kg/min)	(kcal/kg/m)	O$_2$ DEBT (l)
1	1	58.5	0.32	1.36	0.089	4.74×10^{-3}	1.89
1	2	30.5	0.35	1.43	0.094	4.43×10^{-3}	1.62
1	3	29.6	0.17	1.57	0.099	9.84×10^{-3}	2.30
1	4	30.5	0.39	1.42	0.094	4.05×10^{-3}	1.33
1†	5	28.7	0.11	1.38	0.091	13.40×10^{-3}	1.62
2	1	58.5	0.16	1.64	0.103	10.98×10^{-3}	1.59
2	2	30.2	0.15	1.39	0.088	9.53×10^{-3}	1.73
2	3	39.6	0.13	1.52	0.101	13.13×10^{-3}	1.79
2	4	30.5	0.16	1.49	0.099	10.13×10^{-3}	1.59
2†	5	30.2	0.16	1.46	0.093	9.66×10^{-3}	1.80
3	1	58.5	0.56	1.48	0.093	2.77×10^{-3}	2.90
			$\bar{x} = 0.24$ m/sec		$\bar{x} = 0.095$, SD $= 0.005$		

*From Marsolais, E. B., and Edwards, B. G.: Energy costs of walking and standing with functional neuromuscular stimulation and long leg braces. Arch. Phys. Med. Rehabil., 69:243–249, 1988.
†No hamstrings or gluteals; Subject 1: $\bar{x} = 0.093$, SD $= 0.003$; Subject 2; $\bar{x} = 0.097$, SD $= 0.007$.

KAFOs. This paper, which essentially points out the slow speed of ambulation with FES, shows that FES has the same problem as the KAFOs with high metabolic rate and low efficiency of ambulation at speeds the paraplegics were able to deliver (Fig. 28–49). However, it was also pointed out that with FES both the muscle mass of the arm and some of the muscles in the lower extremities are used, which may decrease the likelihood of going into the aerobic phase of the metabolism.

On the other hand, one also has to consider the vascular adjustments. It is well known, for instance, that FES in bicycle ergometry may produce orthostatic hypotension and, sometimes, at higher levels of cord lesions, autonomic dysreflexia.

It is not so much the mechanical ability to walk with normal speed that limits the ambulation with bilateral KAFOs. Rather, it is the high metabolic demand that limits endurance at any practical walking speed, especially since the work has to be

TABLE 28–7. Normal Ambulation*

RESEARCHER, DATE, AND REFERENCE NO.	N	TYPE OF DISABILITY AND APPLIANCES	SPEED (M/MIN)	ENERGY EXPENDITURE kcal/min/kg	kcal $\times 10^{-3}$/m/kg
McDonald, 1961	583	Normals (F)	80	0.067‡	0.83
		Normals (M)	80	0.061‡	0.76
Ralston, 1958	19	Normals (M & F)	74§	0.058‡	0.78
Corcoran, 1970	32	Normals (M & F)	83§‖	0.063‡	0.76
Waters, 1976	25	Normals (M & F)	82‖	0.063‡	0.77
Ganguli, 1973	16	Normals (M)	50¶	0.044	0.088†
Bobbert, 1960	2	Normals (M)	81¶	0.063**	0.079†
Pelzer, 1969	?	Normal (?)	80††	0.043††	0.57

*From Fisher, S. D., and Gullickson, G.: Energy cost of ambulation in health and disability: A literature review. Arch. Phys. Med. Rehabil., 59:124–133, 1978.
†Calculated knowing kcal/min and m/min.
‡Calculated knowing kcal/meter and m/min.
§Most efficient speed of ambulation.
‖Speed chosen by the subjects.
¶Speed chosen by the researcher (the only speed or a representative speed).
**Calculation from author's equation and/or percentage figure.
††Approximated from a graph.

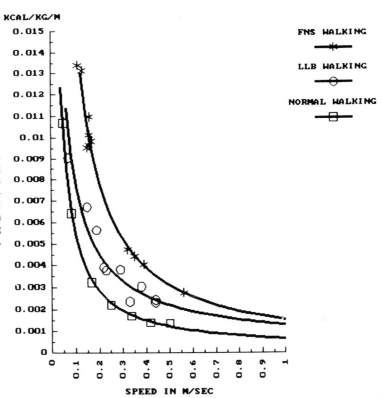

FIGURE 28–49. Energy efficiency of para- plegic persons walking with FNS (functional neuromuscular stimulation) and with LLB (long leg braces) compared with normal walk- ing. (Marsolais, E. B., and Edwards, B. G.: Energy costs of walking and standing with functional neuromuscular stimulation and long leg braces. Arch. Phys. Med. Rehabil., 69:243–249, 1988.)

done by the small muscle groups of the upper extremity as compared with the large musculature of the legs in the normal subject. In this respect, the data available on FES for paraplegic ambula- tion still show the excessive metabolic demand with decreased efficiency, yet the fact that a larger group of muscles is used as compared with the brace ambulation may improve endurance some- what. No clear evidence in this respect is available. The slowness[87] of the gait with FES does not seem to compare well with brace ambulation. Again, not enough data are available for a final evaluation.

The combination of orthotic devices with FES of critical muscle groups is currently being devel- oped.[103, 124] Solomonow and associates[103] used a Louisiana State University (LSU) reciprocating gait orthosis in combination with stimulation of the quadriceps muscle with the contralateral glu- teus maximus muscle. For more powerful hip flex- ion, an electrode implanted in the iliopsoas muscle was used. Also, attempts are being made to de- velop externally powered orthotic devices.[125]

In summary, FES is promising as a standard therapeutic procedure, especially if the system is simplified, reducing the difficulties encountered

with stimulation through the skin and reducing the problems with implanted electrodes. Marsolais and Kobetic[126] implanted fine wire electrodes into the motor points. Of 1025 implantations in six patients over a period of 38 months, 35 per cent failed within the first four months. More than 75 per cent of those early failures resulted from electrode movement. The use of stimulation of a limited key muscle group in combination with bracing seems to be especially promising in its practicality and in its capacity to make the patient more functional. At this point, the FES used for walking has the same problems of high energy requirement and low energy efficiency as the use of bilateral KAFOs with a swing-through gait pattern. The metabolic requirements limit endurance and distance of walk- ing. The speed of walking, however, seems to be more limited mechanically with FES than with the use of bilateral KAFOs.

Summary

An understanding of the biomechanical function of orthoses can markedly improve the prescribing

JUSTUS F. LEHMANN AND BARBARA J. DE LATEUR

physician's ability to select the most effective orthosis for each patient's needs. It has also led to better and more varied orthotic designs as well as to the development of new materials to be used in those designs. Patient acceptance has been enhanced because of the higher cosmetic value of many of the new orthoses, although patient acceptance through improved cosmesis should never be gained at the expense of psychological treatment of the patient's problem. It should also be noted that prescription of an orthosis should always be an integral part of a comprehensive treatment program and should not be considered in isolation from other treatment strategies. The best results can be obtained only when other possibilities such as drugs or motor point blocks are also considered and a comprehensive treatment program is developed that best suits the particular patient. If an orthosis is a part of the treatment program, then the biomechanical principles discussed in this chapter can be very helpful in the selection and ultimate effectiveness of that orthosis.

Acknowledgment

This chapter is based in part on research supported by Research Grant #G00830076 from the National Institute on Disability and Rehabilitation Research, Department of Education, Washington, D.C. 20202

References

1. Lehmann, J. F.: The biomechanics of ankle foot orthoses: Prescription and design. Arch. Phys. Med. Rehabil., 60:200–207, 1979.
2. Lehmann, J. F.: Lower limb orthotics. In Redford, J. B. (Ed.): Orthotics Etcetera, 3rd Ed. Baltimore, Williams & Wilkins Co., 1986, pp. 331–332.
3. Russek, A., and Eschen, F.: Ischial weight bearing brace with quadrilateral wood top—preliminary report. Orthop. Prosthet. Appl. J., 12:31–35, 1958.
4. Nickel, V. L., and Mooney, V.: The application of lower extremity orthotics to weight bearing relief. Final narrative report. Rancho Los Amigos Hospital, Downey, California.
5. Lesin, B. E., Mooney, V., and Ashby, M. E.: Cast bracing for fractures of the femur. J. Bone Joint Surg., 59A:917–923, 1977.
6. Mooney, V., Nickel, V. L., Harvey, J. P., and Snelson, R.: Cast brace treatment for fractures for the distal part of the femur. A prospective controlled study of one hundred and fifty three patients. J. Bone Joint Surg., 52A:1563–1578, 1970.
7. Grynbaum, B. B., Sokolow, J., and Fleischman, E. P.: An adjustable ischial weight bearing brace for early ambulation in lower extremity fractures. Arch. Phys. Med. Rehabil., 54:566–568, 1973.
8. American Academy of Orthopedic Surgeons: Orthopedic Appliances Atlas, Vol. 1. Ann Arbor, Mich., J. Edwards, 1952, pp. 398–399.
9. Warren, C. G., and Lehmann, J. F.: Effect of training on the use of weight bearing orthoses. Phys. Ther., 55:487–492, 1975.
10. Lehmann, J. F., Warren, C. G., de Lateur, B. J., Simons, B. C., and Kirkpatrick, G.: Biomechanical evaluation of axial loading in ischial weight bearing braces of various designs. Arch. Phys. Med. Rehabil., 51:331–337, 1970.
11. McIlmurray, W. J., and Greenbaum, W.: A below knee weight bearing brace. Orthop. Prosthet. Appliance J., 12:81–82, 1958.
12. Nitschke, R. O., and Marschall, K.: The PTS knee brace. Orthop. Prosthet., 22:46–51, 1968.
13. Lehmann, J. F., de Lateur, B. J., Warren, C. G., and Simons, B. C.: Trends in lower extremity bracing. Arch. Phys. Med. Rehabil., 51:338–353, 1970.
14. Davis, F. J., Fry, L. R., Lippert, F. G., Simons, B. C., and Remington, J.: The patellar tendon bearing brace: Report of 16 patients. J. Trauma, 14:216–221, 1974.
15. Lehmann, J. F., Warren, C. G., Pemberton, D. R., Simons, B. C., and de Lateur, B. J.: Load bearing function of patellar tendon bearing braces of various designs. Arch. Phys. Med. Rehabil., 52:367–370, 1971.
16. Sarmiento, A., and Sinclair, W. F.: Application of prosthetics-orthotics principles to treatment of fractures. Artif. Limbs, 11:28–32, 1967.
17. Sarmiento, A.: A functional below-the-knee cast for tibial fractures. J. Bone Joint Surg., 49:855–875, 1967.
18. Sarmiento, A.: A functional below the knee brace for tibial fractures. A report of its use in 135 cases. J. Bone Joint Surg., 52:295–311, 1970.
19. American Academy of Orthopedic Surgeons: Atlas of Orthotics, 2nd Ed. St. Louis, The C. V. Mosby Co., 1975, p. 209.
20. Smith, E. M., Juvinall, R. C., Corell, E. B., and Nyboer, V. J.: Bracing the unstable arthritis knee. Arch. Phys. Med. Rehabil., 51:28, 36, 1970.
21. Heizer, D.: Bracing design for knee joint instability. In Perry, J., and Hislop, H. (Eds.): Principles of Lower Extremity Bracing. New York, American Physical Therapy Association, 1967.
22. Frankel, V. H., and Burstein, A. H.: Orthopedic Biomechanics. Philadelphia, Lea & Febiger, 1970.
23. Bennett, R. J.: Orthotics for function. Part I: Prescription. Phys. Ther. Rev., 36:1–25, 1956.
24. Simons, B. C., C. P. O.: Personal communication.
25. Lehneis, H. R.: New developments in lower-limb

orthotics through bioengineering. Arch. Phys. Med. Rehabil., 53:303–310, 1972.

26. American Academy of Orthopedic Surgeons: Atlas of Orthotics, 2nd Ed. St. Louis, The C. V. Mosby Co., 1975, pp. 216–219.

27. Fifth Workshop Panel on Lower Extremity Orthotics. Subcommittee on Design and Development, Committee on Prosthetics Research and Development. Division of Engineering, National Research Council, National Academy of Sciences, National Academy of Engineering. Atlanta Ga., April 3–4, 1968, p. 17.

28. Kamenetz, H. L.: Eponymic orthoses. In Redford, J. B. (Ed.): Orthotics Etcetera, 3rd Ed. Baltimore, Williams & Wilkins Co., 1986, p. 747.

29. Lehmann, J. F., Warren, C. G., and de Lateur, B. J.: A biomechanical evaluation of knee stability in below knee braces. Arch. Phys. Med. Rehabil., 51:687–695, 1970.

30. McIlmurray, W., and Greenbaum, W.: The application of SACH foot principles to orthotics. Orthop. Prosthet. Appl. J., 13:37–40, 1959.

31. Rubin, G., and Dixon, M.: The modern ankle foot orthoses (AFO's). Bull. Prosthet. Res., Spring:20–40, 1973.

32. Stills, M.: Thermoformed ankle foot orthoses. Orthop. Prosthet., 29:41–51, 1975.

33. Jebsen, R. H., Simons, B. C., and Corcoran, P. J.: Experimental short leg brace fabrication. Arch. Phys. Med. Rehabil., 49:108–109, 1968.

34. Simons, B. C., Jebsen, R. H., and Wildman, L. E.: Plastic short leg brace fabrication. Orthop. Prosthet. Appl. J., 21:215–218, 1967.

35. Siegel, I. M.: Plastic-molded knee-ankle-foot orthoses in the treatment of Duchenne muscular dystrophy. Arch. Phys. Med. Rehabil., 56:322, 1975.

36. Heizer, D.: Short-leg brace design for hemiplegia. In Perry, J., and Hislop, H. (Eds.): Principles of Lower Extremity Bracing. New York, American Physical Therapy Association, 1967.

37. American Academy of Orthopedic Surgeons: Atlas of Orthotics, 2nd Ed. St. Louis, The C. V. Mosby Co., 1975, p. 209.

38. LeBlanc, M.: A clinical evaluation of four lower limb orthoses. Orthop. Prosthet., 26:27–43, 1972.

39. Inman, V. T.: The Joints of the Ankle. Baltimore, Williams & Wilkins Co., 1976.

40. Inman, V. T.: UC-BL dual axis ankle control system and UC-BL shoe insert. Bull. Prosthet. Res., Spring:130–145, 1969.

41. Corcoran, P. J.: Evaluation of a plastic short leg brace. M. Sc. Thesis, University of Washington, Seattle, 1968.

42. Corcoran, P. J., Jebsen, R. H., Brengelmann, G. L., and Simons, B. C.: Effects of plastic and metal leg braces on speed and energy cost of hemiparetic ambulation. Arch. Phys. Med. Rehabil., 51:69–77, 1970.

43. Long, G., and Lawton, E. B.: Functional significance of spinal cord lesion level. Arch. Phys. Med. Rehabil., 36:249–255, 1955.

44. Stauffer, E. S.: Symposium on spinal cord injuries. Clin. Orthop., 112:1–165, 1975.

45. Lehmann, J. F., and Warren, C. G.: Restraining forces in various designs of knee ankle orthoses: Their placement and effect on anatomical knee joint. Arch. Phys. Med. Rehabil., 57:430–437, 1976.

46. American Academy of Orthopedic Surgeons: Atlas of Orthotics, 2nd Ed. St. Louis, The C. V. Mosby Co., 1975, p. 232.

47. Hahn, H.: Lower extremity bracing in paraplegics with usage followup. Paraplegia, 8:147–153, 1969.

48. Scott, B. A.: Engineering principles and fabrication techniques for Scott-Craig: Long leg brace for paraplegics. Orthop. Prosthet., 28:14–19, 1974.

49. Lehmann, J. F., Warren, C. G., Hertling, D., McGee, M., and Simons, B. C.: Craig Scott orthosis: A biomechanical and functional evaluation. Arch. Phys. Med. Rehabil., 57:438–442, 1976.

50. Fisher, S. D., and Gullickson, G.: Energy cost of ambulation in health and disability: A literature review. Arch. Phys. Med. Rehabil., 59:124–133, 1978.

51. Lehmann, J. F., de Lateur, B. J., Warren, C. G., Simons, B. C., and Guy, A. W.: Biomechanical evaluation of braces for paraplegics. Arch. Phys. Med. Rehabil., 50:179–188, 1969.

52. Rosman, N., and Spira, E.: Paraplegic use of walking braces: Survey. Arch. Phys. Med. Rehabil., 55:310–314, 1974.

53. Clinkingbeard, J. R., Gersten, J. W., and Hoehn, D.: Energy cost of ambulation in the traumatic paraplegic. Am. J. Phys. Med., 43:157–165, 1964.

54. Gordon, E. E.: Physiological approach to ambulation in paraplegia. J.A.M.A., 161:686–688, 1956.

55. Gordon, E. E., and Vanderwalde, H.: Energy requirements in paraplegic ambulation. Arch. Phys. Med. Rehabil., 37:276–285, 1956.

56. Warren, C. G., Lehmann, J. F., and de Lateur, B. J.: Pelvic band use in orthotics for adult paraplegic patients. Arch. Phys. Med. Rehabil., 56:221–223, 1975.

57. American Academy of Orthopedic Surgeons: Atlas of Orthotics, 2nd Ed. St. Louis, The C. V. Mosby Co., 1975, p. 226.

58. Casson, J.: Advanced designs of plastic lower orthoses. Orthop. Prosthet., 26:24–30, 1972.

59. Silber, M., Chung, T. S., Varghese, G., Hinterbuchner, C., Bailey, M., and Hivry, N.: Pneumatic orthosis: Pilot study. Arch. Phys. Med. Rehabil., 56:27–32, 1975.

60. Ragnarsson, K. T., Sell, G. H., McGarrity, M., and Offir, R.: Pneumatic orthosis for paraplegic patients: Functional evaluation and prescription consideration. Arch. Phys. Med. Rehabil., 56:479–483, 1975.

61. Lehmann, J. F., Stonebridge, J. B., and de Lateur, B. J.: Pneumatic and standard double upright orthoses: comparison of their biomechanical function in three patients with spinal cord injuries. Arch. Phys. Med. Rehabil., 58:72–80, 1977.

62. Liberson, W. T., Holmquest, H. F., Scott, D., and Dow, M.: Functional electrotherapy: Stimulation of the peroneal nerve synchronized with the swing phase of the gait of hemiplegic patients. Arch. Phys. Med. Rehabil., 42:101–105, 1961.

63. Gracanin, F., and Trnkoczy, A.: Optimal stimulus parameters for minimum pain in the chronic stimulation of innervated muscle. Arch. Phys. Med. Rehabil., 56:243–249, 1975.

64. Post, B. S., Foster, S., Rosner, H., and Benton, J. G.: Use of functional electrotherapy in neuromuscular diseases. N.Y. State J. Med., 63:1808–1811, 1963.

65. Takebe, K., Kukulka, C., Narayan, M. G., Milner, M., and Basmajian, J. V.: Peroneal nerve stimulator in rehabilitation of hemiplegic patients. Arch. Phys. Med. Rehabil., 56:237–240, 1975.

66. Waters, R. L., McNeal, D. R., and Tasto, J.: Peroneal nerve conduction velocity after chronic electrical stimulation. Arch. Phys. Med. Rehabil., 46:240–241, 1975.

67. Fuhrer, M. J., and Yegge, B.: Effects of skin impedance changes accompanying functional electrical stimulation of the peroneal nerve. Arch. Phys. Med. Rehabil., 53:276–281, 1972.

68. Waters, R. L., McNeal, D., and Perry, J.: Experimental correction of foot drop by electrical stimulation of the peroneal nerve. J. Bone Joint Surg., 57A:1047–1054, 1975.

69. Lee, K. H., and Johnston, R.: Electrically induced flexion reflex in gait training of hemiplegic patients: Induction of the reflex. Arch. Phys. Med. Rehabil., 57:311–314, 1976.

70. Dimitrijevic, M. R., Gracanin, F., Prevec, T., and Trontelj, J.: Electronic control of paralysed extremities. Biomed. Eng., 3:8–14, 1968.

71. Varken, E., and Jeglic, A.: Application of an implantable stimulator in the rehabilitation of the paraplegic patient. Int. Surg., 61:335–339, 1976.

72. Burke, J. F., Pocock, G. S., and Wallis, W. D.: Electrophysiological bracing in peripheral nerve lesions. J. Am. Phys. Ther. Assoc., 43:501–504, 1963.

73. Merletti, R., Acimovic, R., Grobelnik, S., and Cvilak, G.: Electrophysiological orthosis for the upper extremity in hemiplegia: Feasibility study. Arch. Phys. Med. Rehabil., 56:507–513, 1975.

74. Foster, R., and Milani, J.: The genucentric knee orthosis—a new concept. Orthot. Prosthet., 33:31–44, 1979.

75. Walker, P. S.: Knee orthoses. Phys. Med. Rehabil.: State Art Rev., 1:83–94, 1987.

76. Halar, E., and Cardenas, D.: Ankle-foot orthoses: Clinical implications. Phys. Med. Rehabil.: State Art. Rev., 1:45–66, 1987.

77. Lehmann, J. F., Condon, S. M., de Lateur, B. J., and Price, R.: Gait abnormalities in peroneal nerve paralysis and their correction by orthoses: A biomechanical study. Arch. Phys. Med. Rehabil., 67:380–386, 1986.

78. Lehmann, J. F., Condon, S. M., de Lateur, B. J., and Smith, J. C.: Ankle-foot orthoses: Effect on gait abnormalities in tibial nerve paralysis. Arch. Phys. Med. Rehabil., 66:212–218, 1985.

79. Lehmann, J. F., Ko, M. J., and de Lateur, B. J.: Double-stopped ankle-foot orthosis in flaccid peroneal and tibial paralysis: evaluation of function. Arch. Phys. Med. Rehabil., 61:536–541, 1980.

80. Fillauer, C.: A new ankle-foot orthosis with a moldable carbon composite insert. Orthot. Prosthet., 35:13–16, 1981.

81. Gans, B. M., Erickson, G., and Simons, D.: Below-knee orthosis: A wrap-around design for ankle-foot control. Arch. Phys. Med. Rehabil., 60:78–80, 1979.

82. Merkel, K. D., Miller, N. E., Westbrook, P. R., and Merritt, J. L.: Energy expenditure of paraplegic patients standing and walking with two knee-ankle-foot orthoses. Arch. Phys. Med. Rehabil., 65:121–124, 1984.

83. Cerny, K., Waters, R., Hislop, H., and Perry, J.: Walking and wheelchair energetics in persons with paraplegia. Phys. Ther., 60:1133–1139, 1980.

84. Huang, C.-T., Kuhlemeier, K. V., Moore, N. B., and Fine, P. R.: Energy cost of ambulation in paraplegic patients using Craig-Scott braces. Arch. Phys. Med. Rehabil., 60:595–600, 1979.

85. Chantraine, A., Crielaard, J. M., Onkelinx, A., and Pirnay, F.: Energy expenditure of ambulation in paraplegics: Effects of long term use of bracing. Paraplegia 22:173–181, 1984.

86. Isakov, E., Mizrahi, J., Graupe, D., Becker, E., and Najenson, T.: Energy cost and physiological reactions to effort during activation of paraplegics by functional electrical stimulation. Scand. J. Rehabil. Med. (Suppl.), 12:102–107, 1985.

87. Mizrahi, J., Braun, Z., Najenson, T., and Graupe, D.: Quantitative weight-bearing and gait evaluation of paraplegics using functional electrical stimulation. Med. Biol. Eng. Comput. 23:101–107, 1985.

88. Waters, R. L., and Miller, L.: A physiologic rationale for orthotic prescription in paraplegia. Clin. Prosthet. Orthot., 11:66–73, 1987.

89. Merkel, K. D., Miller, N. E., and Merritt, J. L.: Energy expenditure in patients with low-, mid- or high-thoracic paraplegia using Scott-Craig knee-ankle-foot orthoses. Mayo Clin. Proc., 60:165–168, 1985.

90. Hildebrandt, G., Voigt, E.-D., Bahn, D., Berendes, B., and Kroger, J.: Energy costs of propelling wheelchair at various speeds: Cardiac response and effect on steering accuracy. Arch. Phys. Med. Rehabil., 51:131–136, 1970.

91. Glaser, R. M., and Collins, S. R.: Validity of

power output estimation for wheelchair locomotion. Am. J. Phys. Med., 60:180–189, 1981.

92. Major, R. E., Stallard, J., and Rose, G. K.: The dynamics of walking using the hip guidance orthosis (hgo) with crutches. Prosthet. Orthot. Int., 5:19–22, 1981.

93. Butler, P. B., Major, R. E., and Patrick, J. H.: The technique of reciprocal walking using the hip guidance orthosis (hgo) with crutches. Prosthet. Orthot. Int., 8:33–38, 1984.

94. Rose, G. K.: The principles and practice of hip guidance articulations. Prosthet. Orthot. Int., 3:37–43, 1979.

95. Rose, G. K., Sankarankutty, M., and Stallard, J.: A clinical review of the orthotic treatment of myelomeningocele patients. J. Bone Joint Surg. [B], 65:242–246, 1983.

96. Rose, G. K., Stallard, J., and Sankarankutty, M.: Clinical evaluation of spina bifida patients using hip guidance orthosis. Dev. Med. Child. Neurol., 23:30–40, 1981.

97. Nene, A. V., and Major, R. E.: Dynamics of reciprocal gait of adult paraplegics using the ParaWalker (Hip Guidance Orthosis). Prosthet. Orthot. Int., 11:124–127, 1987.

98. Patrick, J. H., and McClelland, M. R.: Low energy reciprocal walking for the adult paraplegic. Paraplegia, 23:113–117, 1985.

99. Yngve, D. A., Douglas, R., and Roberts, J. M.: The reciprocating gait orthosis in myelomeningocele. J. Pediatr. Orthop., 4:304–310, 1984.

100. Douglas, R., and Solomonow, M.: The LSU reciprocating gait orthosis. J. Rehabil. Res. Dev., 25:57–58, 1987.

101. Merritt, J. L.: Personal communication.

102. Merritt, J. L.: Knee-ankle-foot orthotics: Long leg braces and their practical applications. Phys. Med. Rehabil.: State Art. Rev., 1:67–82, 1987.

103. Solomonow, M., Douglas, R., King, A., and Shoji, H.: Development of an improved walking system for paraplegics with FES adjunct to the LSU reciprocating gait orthosis. J. Rehabil. Res. Dev., 25:235, 1987.

104. Strachan, R. K., Cook, J., Wilkie, W., and Kennedy, N. S. J.: An evaluation of pneumatic orthoses in thoracic paraplegia. Paraplegia 23:295–305, 1985.

105. Stanic, U., Acimovic-Janezic, R., Gros, N., Trnkoczy, A., Bajd, T., and Kljajic, M.: Multichannel electrical stimulation for correction of hemiplegic gait. Scand. J. Rehabil. Med., 10:75–92, 1978.

106. Braun, Z., Mizrahi, J., Najenson, T., and Graupe, D.: Activation of paraplegic patients by functional electrical stimulation: Training and biomechanical evaluation. Scand. J. Rehabil. Med. (Suppl.), 12:93–101, 1985.

107. Brandell, B. R.: The study and correction of human gait by electrical stimulation. Am. Surg., 52:257–263, 1986.

108. Van Griethuysen, C. M., Paul, J. P., Andrews, B. J., and Nicol, A. C.: Biomechanics of functional electrical stimulation. Prosthet. Orthot. Int., 6:152–156, 1982.

109. Kralj, A., Plevnik, S., Ugrinovski, S., and Acimovic-Janezic, R.: Report, April 1, 1979, to March 31, 1981, of Rehabilitation Engineering Center, Univerza v Ljubljani, Fakulteta za Elektrotehniko, 61001 Ljubljana, Trzaska 25, Yugoslavia. Bull. Prosthet. Res. (BPR 10–35), 18:229–234, 1981.

110. Kralj, A., Turk, R., and Bajd, T.: FES of spinal-cord-injured patients. Bull. Prosthet. Res. (BPR 10–37), 19:105, 1982.

111. Cybulski, G. R., Penn, R. D., and Jaeger, R. J.: Lower extremity functional neuromuscular stimulation in cases of spinal cord injury. Neurosurgery 15:132–146, 1984.

112. Kralj, A., and Grobelnik, S.: Functional electrical stimulation—a new hope for paraplegic patients. Bull. Prosthet. Res. (BPR 10–20):75–102, 1973.

113. Kralj, A., Bajd, T., Turk, R., Krajnik, J., and Benko, H.: Gait restoration in paraplegic patients: A feasibility demonstration using multichannel surface electrode FES. J. Rehabil. Res. Dev. (BPR 10–38), 20:3–20, 1983.

114. Kralj, A., Bajd, T., and Turk, R.: Electrical stimulation providing functional use of paraplegic patient muscles. Med. Prog. Technol., 7:3–9, 1980.

115. Arnold, P. B., McVey, P., Farrell, W., and Deurloo, T.: Functional electrical stimulation at Newington Children's Hospital. Arch. Phys. Med. Rehabil., 68:662, 1987.

116. Spielholz, N. I., Axen, K., Pollack, S., Haas, F., and Ragnarsson, K.: Effect of an FES bicycle exercise program on velocity of shortening of quadriceps muscles in spinal cord injured people. Arch. Phys. Med. Rehabil., 68:662, 1987.

117. Bajd, T., Kralj, A., and Turk, R.: Standing-up of a healthy subject and a paraplegic patient. J. Biomech., 15:1–10, 1982.

118. Bajd, T., Kralj, A., Turk, R., Benko, H., and Sega, J.: The use of a four-channel electrical stimulator as an ambulatory aid for paraplegic patients. Phys. Ther., 63:1116–1120, 1983.

119. Turk, R., and Obreza, P.: Functional electrical stimulation as an orthotic means for the rehabilitation of paraplegic patients. Paraplegia, 23:344–348, 1985.

120. Braun, Z., Mizrahi, J., Najenson, T., and Graupe, D.: Activation of paraplegic patients by functional electrical stimulation: Training and biomechanical evaluation. Scand. J. Rehabil. Med. (Suppl.), 12:93–101, 1985.

121. Marsolais, E. B., and Kobetic, R.: Functional electrical stimulation for walking in paraplegia. J. Bone Joint Surg. [A], 69:728–733, 1987.

122. Marsolais, E. B., and Kobetic, R.: Functional walking in paralyzed patients by means of electrical stimulation. Clin. Orthop., 175:30–36, 1983.

123. Marsolais, E. B., and Edwards, B. G.: Energy costs of walking and standing with functional neuromuscular stimulation and long leg braces. Arch. Phys. Med. Rehabil., 69:243–249, 1988.

124. McClelland, M., Andrews, B. J., Patrick, J. H., Freeman, P. A., and El Masri, W. S.: Augmentation of the Oswestry Parawalker orthosis by means of surface electrical stimulation: gait analysis of three patients. Paraplegia, 25:32–38, 1987.

125. Miyamoto, H., Sakurai, Y., Shimazaki, Y., and Tokimura, K.: Development of a powered orthosis for lower limbs. J. Rehabil. Res. Dev., 25:60, 1987.

126. Marsolais, E. B., and Kobetic, R.: Implantation techniques and experience with percutaneous intramuscular electrodes in the lower extremities. J. Rehabil. Res. Devel., 23:1–8, 1986.

29

Prescription Writing in Physical Medicine and Rehabilitation

GORDON M. MARTIN   GAIL L. GAMBLE

The ability to formulate a concise yet thorough prescription is a hallmark of the well-trained physiatrist. Written prescriptions allow the physician to plan, specify, and correlate various techniques and procedures into a suitable, realistic program designed to improve or develop a patient's physical function. The prescription may be a simple one for short-term treatment, or it may provide a complex program that changes over a prolonged period for the severely and chronically disabled patient. In any case, the prescription must be concise, legible, specific, and individualized. The appropriateness of the prescription and, therefore, of the therapy depends on the physician's skill and interest in the area of physical medicine and rehabilitation, on the physician's ability to communicate well with therapists, and on the physician's knack for keeping patients motivated and cooperative.

Goals

Several important goals must be taken into consideration in writing a prescription in physical medicine and rehabilitation. The prescription guides the therapist in the basic objectives of the treatment program. The prescription is designed to enhance and clarify communication between the physician and other members of the rehabilitation team and prevents misunderstandings that might affect patient care. Also it provides a record of the treatment prescribed and administered by all rehabilitation personnel. Such records are valuable for use in the future care of a patient. Finally,

accurate and detailed information serves to protect both the physician and the therapist in case of medicolegal problems in insurance or compensation cases.

The Physician As Prescriber

Certain qualifications are expected of the person prescribing physical therapy and other rehabilitative procedures. At present, in most states, only a licensed physician may write such prescriptions. (However, the physician need not always have had special training in rehabilitation medicine.) In some states, physical and occupational therapists are allowed, by law, to evaluate and prescribe programs independent of physicians. When such is the case, it is important that the physician care giver, who has knowledge of the patient's medical situation, maintain an open dialogue with the therapist.

A physician's evaluation establishes an adequate working diagnosis based on the patient's history, physical findings, x-ray studies, and laboratory values. When physicians are prescribing, they should have a basic knowledge of the physiological, biomechanical, and psychological effects of the treatments prescribed. They should know the indications for these treatments, along with any contraindications and limitations. They should also be aware of the training, special expertise, and possible limitations in the experience of the therapists involved.

647

GORDON M. MARTIN AND GAIL L. GAMBLE

Patient Considerations in Treatment Selection

As stated above, an accurate assessment of the clinical problem is imperative, but other factors affecting the patient's status also need to be considered. The patient's present physical status, mental capacity, and physical endurance may preclude an aggressive treatment program. The time constraints of patients, who may be involved in other medical evaluations, or outpatients, who have a busy work schedule, may limit what can realistically be prescribed. Many health care insurance programs place restrictions on therapy and equipment, and these issues should be considered so that the patient's prescription should also be assessed within the context of the patient's goals for an adequate quality of life. The patient's ability to achieve the desired functional level, the availability of community resources, and the family's energy and limitations must be considered in trying to establish a realistic program.

Essentials of a Good Prescription

The written prescription for physical medicine and rehabilitation should become a permanent part of the patient's medical record in the hospital or office setting. A diagnosis, whether tentative or final, is an integral part of any physiatric evaluation and should be recorded and communicated to the referring physician and the members of the rehabilitation team.

Initially, a summary of the patient's history and physical examination will provide pertinent information for the therapists and the referring physician. Because the full clinical history is often not available at the time of individual treatment sessions, enough information must be recorded to allow accurate interpretation and appropriate patient care by the therapists. Statements such as "see record" or "see history" are generally useless to those who are caring for the patient. Measurements of range of motion and muscle strength, which are recorded with the original prescription, provide baselines for evaluation of the patient's progress.

Each body area that is designated for treatment should be listed specifically. Modalities should be indicated with special notations regarding a particular prescribed technique. Guidance as to frequency of therapy sessions during an initial trial of a modality is helpful. Requesting a specific date for a follow-up visit is an integral part of any prescription. The status of the condition being treated usually changes during the course of therapy, and the treatment plan and prescription will, therefore, require frequent updating and modification.

Special instructions or cautions should be clearly indicated. The presence of unstable angina, confusion or dementia, diabetes, or a convulsive disorder should be clearly indicated so that the therapist can observe the necessary precautions. The need for precautions against infectious diseases should be clearly identified, and standardized procedures should be followed.

Written instruction sheets for home care are very helpful, particularly when only a few supervised treatments are possible, and should be included as part of the prescription. The technical details of the instructions are taught during several therapy sessions. Printed or written instructions given to the patient serve as reminders of what to do, but exactly how it is to be done can only be learned by actually doing it under the close supervision of a competent instructor.

The record sheet should include dates of treatment, names of therapists treating the patient, progress notes by physicians and therapists, and an assessment of the patient's condition at the time of dismissal with final recommendations. (See the sample prescriptions at the end of this chapter.)

Common Errors

A faulty prescription is usually due to an inadequate evaluation, perhaps with inappropriate selection of therapies. At a time when efficient use of health care resources is mandated, the prescriber must justify therapeutic goals for any condition treated. Whether or not the patient and the patient's condition are amenable to treatment and whether or not the treatment has proved worthwhile should be constant questions in assessment. If treatment is delayed (perhaps postoperatively) or, occasionally, if it is started too early (before medical stability has been established), the chances of optimal benefit may be compromised.

The use of "shotgun" orders—listing a menu of modalities and exercises such as prescribing a full multijoint program for an arthritic patient when only one joint is affected—is to be avoided. The patient may miss the primary goal of the treatment if he or she is confused by an unnecessarily complex program. The orders should be specific enough to provide the guidance intended yet not so regimented as to restrict the initiative of the therapist and interaction among members of the rehabilitation team during the course of treatment. The use of routine orders is a gross misuse of the privilege of prescription writing in physical medicine and rehabilitation and is a disservice to the evaluator and the patient alike. The physician is not using his or her skills of evaluation, problem assessment, program development, and problem resolution to full potential unless an individualized total plan is formulated.

Inadequate or delayed follow-up and rechecking by the physician is a common pitfall that may unnecessarily prolong treatment in some cases. The physician should closely follow the patient's progress and "graduate" the patient to a home program when appropriate relief has been achieved or the necessary skills have been learned. Additionally, third-party payers cease reimbursement for therapy received after the patient's progress has stabilized and little change in a patient's condition is being documented.

Prescriptions for Physical Therapy

A constant relationship between the physician and the physical therapist is an essential part of the rehabilitation prescription. The specific orders for physical therapy are not limited to one modality but involve a gamut of therapies intended to build a sense of comfort and security for patients as they proceed through the rehabilitation process. The primary goals of these elements of the prescription are, of course, to relieve pain and restore function.

Prescriptions for Pain Relief

The initial orders of the prescription are usually directed at relief of pain, which will enhance patient acceptance of the therapeutic exercise that will follow.

Heat. Multiple thermal modalities are utilized to relieve pain through muscle relaxation.[1] The source of heat to be used (such as superficial heat, ultrasound, and diathermy) should be specified. The specific location or problem area should also be described. The physician should be cautious about prescribing heat for the unreliable, severely debilitated, or insensate patient. One must also remember that each modality has an individual set of precautions for its use (see Chapter 13).

Hydrotherapy continues to be a dependable therapeutic resource. It may prove useful when the part to be treated is not amenable to other forms of systemic or superficial heat or when assistive and supportive exercise is indicated. The temperature of the water should be indicated, taking into consideration the patient's tolerance, age, and debility. The prescription should indicate whether hydrotherapy is to be used for underwater exercises, thermotherapy, or for cleansing of an open wound, which requires the use of tank-cleaning techniques and necessary precautions against the spread of infection.

Massage. In the prescription for therapeutic massage, the type or types of massage should be specified, such as stroking and kneading, which are usually combined; friction massage; or decongestive massage, which may be indicated for specific areas. Other types of manual massage or mechanical massage devices are infrequently prescribed.

Specifications should indicate whether the massage is to be deep or light and sedative (most common) or stimulating. The need to avoid recent surgical incisions or varicosities during massage should be noted. The parts to be massaged should be specifically listed (patients have a tendency to ask therapists to massage more extensive areas). Therapeutic manual massage is time consuming and, therefore, expensive and should not be prescribed indiscriminately (see Chapter 17).

Electrical Stimulation. Electrical stimulation in various forms is often used to achieve relief of pain. The sources and availability of these stimulators are growing, and the physician should be familiar with the units most often used. In addition to noting the specifics of the problem when writing a prescription, one must consider whether or not treatment is to be used in a rehabilitation department or at home. Some modalities (inferential current and neuroprobe) are designed for office use only. The more conventional transcutaneous electrical nerve stimulators are portable and are suitable for home use. One must also be aware of the different current options available (see Chapter 15) and guide the patient and therapist appropriately. The prescription should always be recorded as an initial trial of two to four days, because patients may find initial relief of pain with the approach but then, with accommodation, obtain little relief thereafter. (For the same reason the prescription should indicate initial rental of necessary equipment for one to three months with an option for purchase.) The physician should request follow-up and appropriately document the patient's pain relief on a numerical scale; such documentation is being demanded regularly from third-party payers.

Prescriptions for Restoration of Function

The physical therapist traditionally is thought of as a teacher of specific exercise functions and as a monitor of increasing strength. As with other areas of rehabilitation, the role and experience of therapists have increased, and their skills should be kept in mind when addressing the physical therapy prescription.

Therapeutic Exercise. The prescription for therapeutic exercise is generally the most complex and difficult part of the prescription for physical therapy. (For appropriate definitions regarding types of exercises, please see Chapters 18, 19, and 20.) For a patient with significant loss of motor function, a graduated program progressing through multiple levels of therapeutic exercise would be appropriate. To avoid contracture, the prescription would initially request only active or assistive range of motion exercises. As motor function returns, muscle re-education exercises would be appropriate, in which techniques would be employed to isolate function and then retrain individual muscle groups. The prescription would then progress to muscle-strengthening exercises, providing resistance against the desired groups. Multiple factors must be considered at each step (such as patient debility, cardiovascular status, and musculoskeletal stability), as each type of exercise is chosen for a particular problem.

Relaxation Therapy. The principles of relaxation and the appropriate exercises are prescribed for patients who exhibit persistent muscle guarding and spasms with organic hypertonicity, as well as those with tension states. Relaxation therapy has become an important area of therapeutic exercise, and a therapist's skills are very helpful. Many therapists have developed expertise in the use of electromyographic biofeedback as a technique to enable the patient to master appropriate muscle relaxation; the prescription should utilize these techniques when available. Many other forms of exercise may be requested for other types of problems, such as coordination exercises for the patient

with cerebellar dysfunction or severe sensory impairment.

Again, electrical stimulation is a rapidly developing modality in physical therapy and should be considered for various forms of muscle and nerve stimulation and muscle re-education. It is being used with some success for re-education of hemiparetic limbs, post-tendon transfer, and nerve injury. The physician should be familiar with the skills of the therapist and the technology available and prescribe accordingly.

In writing the physical therapy prescription, the physician should also recognize the expanding use of exercise equipment, particularly in the area of sports medicine and back rehabilitation. The physician should be familiar with the available equipment and request the use of a particular system (Cybex, Kinetron, and so on) that documents strength or range of motion for use in retraining.

Ambulation. Training of and assistance with ambulation are often important parts of physical therapy. The need for a cane, a German or axillary crutch, a walker, braces, or other special assistive devices should be determined by the physician, therapist, and patient as the patient's condition changes over time.

Preliminary strengthening exercises may be needed and should be included in the prescription. Preparatory to walking on crutches, progressive resistive exercises for latissimus dorsi, triceps, and biceps muscles may be indicated, along with those for quadriceps and hip extensors and abductors. Mat exercises, crawling, rolling, sitting balance, transfers, or tilt-table procedures may precede ambulation for some patients (for example, paraplegics). Parallel bars may be prescribed for balance and security for patients who are learning specific patterns of gait. Practice on curbs and steps and car transfers are important after a stable gait on a level surface has been attained (see Chapters 4, 22).

The physical therapist is very helpful when fitting of equipment, particularly a wheelchair, is required. Many components must be considered in an individual wheelchair prescription, including goals for use, patient height and girth, functional capabilities of the upper and lower extremities, ability for transfer, and other factors (see Chapter 23). The therapist and the patient should work together to arrive at the correct chair width and height and other features to allow optimal function. The prescription must specifically reflect these considerations when the wheelchair is ordered. For some patients, selection of a motorized wheelchair with basic or specially adapted controls must be considered.

Last, when appropriate, the prescription should reflect the integral role of physical therapy in such areas as chronic pain management, with appropriate use of group therapy and endurance training, cardiac retraining after myocardial infarction, and respiratory management, particularly if the patient has been in the intensive care unit. The physical therapist is trained in these areas of health care, and the prescription should include therapy programs for patients with such problems.

Prescriptions for Occupational Therapy

The field of occupational therapy has expanded in scope and depth in recent years, and the potential contributions from this field are many.[2] Occupational therapy should be considered in detail when a physiatric prescription is developed. The physician's initial assessment and written summary can be the same as for physical therapy except that more detail in functional activity should be recorded. The diagnosis is, of course, included. The present physical status and endurance level of the patient should be noted, along with any cognitive deficits and emotional or psychological factors. Depending on the stamina of the patient, a recommendation may be made as to whether therapy should be started at the bedside or in the department.

The occupational therapist has traditionally offered a functional approach to the patient's therapy. Special functional assessments of the upper extremities, sensory evaluations, and cognitive assessment may be requested. The functional level of the patient is established before therapy begins.

Training of the patient in functional independence in the performance of the activities of daily living is an integral role for the occupational therapist and should be requested in many situations. Motor strength, coordination skills, and appropriate planning are retaught within this context. The assessment for the need for adaptive equipment can also be requested as part of the retraining process in this area.

Occupational therapists play a significant role in the rehabilitation of the brain-injured adult. The physiatric prescription may call on occupational therapy skills at a variety of levels. Initially, cognitive stimulation and orientation skills may be appropriate for the near-comatose patient. Cogni-

tive and perceptual testing and retraining may be requested when the patient becomes more alert, along with re-education and strengthening of a hemiparetic upper limb. Orders for upper extremity splinting may be helpful for appropriate positioning. As the patient progresses, cognitive therapy by means of computer software programs may be suggested, if such equipment is available.

Significantly, the occupational therapist may be called on in the assessment of dysphagia,[3] including assisting with videofluoroscopy in the diagnosis of a swallowing difficulty. Re-education in swallowing may be a vital component of the physiatric prescription in the brain-injured patient, and it is often overlooked in the more acute management of the patient with this condition.

Hand and upper extremity rehabilitation are included in occupational therapy training and should be reflected in the physiatric prescription. Intricate re-education following tendon reconstruction may be requested; specific static and dynamic splinting may be outlined. Edema control measures, including pressure garments, massage, or positioning, are to be considered in many patients with upper extremity dysfunction from trauma, fracture, or burn injury.

Occupational therapy orders are also often pertinent as part of the physiatric program for chronic pain management, psychiatric rehabilitation, cardiac rehabilitation, and so on. Accordingly, the physiatrist should be well versed in the use of these resources.

Prescriptions for Recreational Therapy

Recreational therapy has developed significantly in recent years and a representative from this discipline should be on the rehabilitation team. The physiatrist should be familiar with the skills and programs available and should utilize these resources when appropriate when writing the physical medicine prescription.[4]

In the early 1980s, the National Therapeutic Recreation Society adopted a position statement declaring that "the purpose of recreation therapy is to facilitate the development, maintenance, and expression of an appropriate leisure lifestyle for individuals with physical, mental, emotional, or social limitations."[4] Services include specific therapy, leisure education, and the opportunity to participate in recreational activities.

The prescription should reflect specific goals for

treatment. In the hospital setting, the physician may want to emphasize one-handed leisure skills for the patient with newly acquired hemiplegia or coordination skills for the patient who is recovering use of an upper extremity. The introduction of leisure activities that can be performed from a sitting position will be appropriate for a newly chairbound patient. Community reintegration for the newly disabled patient is a vital part of the rehabilitation process, and a comprehensive recreational therapy department will be the cornerstone for progressive activities in this area. As outpatient rehabilitation programs grow, the patients' needs for recreational therapy will become an increasingly vital part of the physiatric therapeutic prescription, resulting in coordination of specific recreational activities within the community.

Other Areas of Consideration

The rehabilitation prescription should not be limited to suggestions for physical and occupational therapies. Other areas often have to be considered, and many of these are discussed in great detail in other chapters of this text. Specifically, the physiatrist should be able to assess the need for gait aids for ambulation, exercise equipment, and wheelchairs and to recommend the proper equipment when appropriate. The technological improvements and available options for equipment, particularly wheelchairs, have exploded in recent years, and physiatrists must keep abreast of these new developments so that they may provide their patients with the most useful equipment available. If new or specific options are ordered, these must be specified within the context of the individual patient's needs, since insurance carriers are reluctant to reimburse for expensive equipment without specific justification.

A physician's prescription is generally required to authorize reimbursement for pressure garments used in peripheral vascular disease or chronic edema or as part of burn rehabilitation. The industry of pressure garment fabrication has expanded to the extent that the physiatrist must have detailed knowledge of the various materials available in terms of therapeutic pressure, ease of donning, and custom modifications that are possible.

Orthotic devices should be considered in the physiatric evaluation and may be an important component of the rehabilitation prescription (see Chapters 26, 27, 28). Discussion with the patient, therapist, and orthotist may be necessary for obtaining the optimal appliance for an individual condition. Follow-up is mandatory when an orthosis has been ordered in order to ensure a proper fit (especially in the patient with decreased sensation) and to enhance patient compliance.

Assessment for prosthetic fitting and care is another important area in the comprehensive consideration of the physiatric prescription (see Chapters 48, 49). Many other factors to be considered are beyond the scope of this chapter, but accurate prescription writing reflects the importance of the ongoing relationship between the patient and the rehabilitation team and the changing needs of the patient over time.

Conclusion

The physician, as the coordinator of the patient's comprehensive rehabilitation program, needs to maintain communication with all members of the rehabilitation team, including a psychologist, speech therapist, and social worker. In both hospital and outpatient settings, the physician may see the need for another professional's involvement. The effective rehabilitation prescription is the product of an evaluation that involves all members of the health care team.

Sample Prescriptions

These sample prescriptions illustrate some of the principles that have been discussed. They are not to be considered as standard or routine prescriptions or necessarily ideal prescriptions for patients with the condition listed. Each prescription must be individualized and then modified as changing status indicates need for variations and progression.

Prescription Writing in Physical Medicine and Rehabilitation

Chronic Postmastectomy Lymphedema (Right)

TREATMENT	SPECIFICATIONS
Patient education	Anti-edema principles (with elevation) Instruct one-handed Ace wrap from hand to axilla; wrap continually during day
Volume	Measure arm volumes before first treatment and at end of one week
Compression pump	Full arm pneumatic compression pump at 50 to 60 mm Hg for 45 to 50 minutes
Massage	Decongestive massage of digits, hand, forearm, 5 to 10 minutes
Exercise	Overhead isometric hand and wrist strengthening exercises Isometric shoulder group strengthening exercises
Occupational therapy	Coban wrapping of digits and hand for 10 minutes, 4 times per day Right upper extremity protection principles Activities of daily living

Frequency: Treat twice daily for one week. Detailed home instructions.
Follow-up: At the end of one week, if reduced volume is maintained, prescribe a pressure garment.

Adhesive Capsulitis, Right Shoulder

TREATMENT	MINUTES	SPECIFICATIONS
Ultrasound	10	To right shoulder
Massage	5 to 10	Deep sedative to right shoulder
Exercise	10 to 15	Active and assistive for the right shoulder Moderate stretch Wall ladder Overhead pulley Shoulder wheel Codman's exercise with 5-lb sandbag.

Treat daily. Physician needs to recheck after five treatments.
Instruct: Infrared lamp, 30 min daily.
Active exercises and pulley and ladder assistive exercises, two times daily at home.

Chronic Left L5 to S1 Radiculopathy (For Static and Night Pain Two Years After Lumbar Laminectomy)

TREATMENT	MINUTES	SPECIFICATIONS
Transcutaneous electrical nerve stimulators	30	Trial treatment with two electrodes over the left lumbar paraspinal area Two electrodes over the sciatic nerve, the thigh, and the popliteal area (place one on the common peroneal, one at the sciatic notch) Evaluate combinations of intensity and frequencies Have patient stand during trial

Treat two times daily for two or three days.
Provide stimulator on loan for overnight use, if feasible.
Physician to recheck after four treatments.

GORDON M. MARTIN AND GAIL L. GAMBLE

Left Hemiplegia (Onset on January 26)

DATE	TREATMENT	TIME, MINUTES	SPECIFICATIONS
2–1	Passive exercise	10	Left upper and lower extremities through normal range, three to four times each joint (remove footdrop splint for treatment)
2–7	Re-education and coordination exercise	20	Left upper and lower extremities
	Active exercise		Normal range, right upper and lower extremities (avoid fatigue; encourage use of normal extremities for activities of daily living)
2–16	Active and assistive exercise		Left shoulder and elbow Left hip and knee Powder board with assistance for hip and knee flexion and extension, and hip abduction and adduction
	Resistive exercise		Right quadriceps—isometric (mild), 30 contractions daily—10 each of ½, ¾, and full 10 repetitions maximum
2–18	Gait training	Twice a day (b.i.d.)	Parallel bars with knee splint and foot support Sling left arm 1. Standing balance 2. Walking
2–22	Gait training	b.i.d.	Start on glider cane with assistance (cane in right hand)
3–2	Gait training	b.i.d.	Walk with regular cane and ankle-foot orthosis
3–6	Gait training	b.i.d.	Climb stairs, ramp Getting in and out of chairs Getting in and out of car
2–3	Occupational therapy (OT)		Orientation assessment Begin perceptual assessment Passive range of motion of left upper extremity Proper position to avoid edema; Jobst's glove
2–8	OT		Activities to increase function of left upper extremity Re-education for neglect of paretic side
2–10	OT		Start assessment of patient's performance of activities of daily living and begin training Recommend adaptive equipment as necessary
2–22	OT		Start home assessment for necessary modification and progressive program instruction

2–1	Treat once daily in patient's room. Physician check every three to four days.
2–7	Treat in physical medicine and rehabilitation department twice daily.
3–4	Instruct in normal range of motion exercises for home use.

Prescription Writing in Physical Medicine and Rehabilitation

Rheumatoid Arthritis (for Involvement of Hands, Elbows, Shoulders, Knees, and Feet)

TREATMENT	MINUTES	SPECIFICATIONS
Radiant heat	30	To elbows, wrists, knees (alternate with hydrotherapy)
Hydrotherapy	30, three times weekly	Hubbard tank—water temperature 38.9° C (102° F) with active assistive underwater exercise of shoulders, elbows, and knees
	30	Contrast baths, hands, and feet; once for instruction
Massage	20	Deep stroking and kneading to hands, shoulders, knees
Exercise	10	Active and assistive, work toward normal range in joints mentioned above
		Resistive isometric with 5-lb sandbag. Later progressive resistive exercise program for quadriceps
		Posture correction and principles to stand, to sit, and to lie
Gait		Supervise walking of short distances, getting in and out of chair, stair climbing
Occupational therapy	Treat daily for two weeks	Energy conservation
		Resting hand splints
		Hand use and protective principles
		Assessment of activities of daily living
		Adaptive equipment for hand function and activities of daily living

Treat daily for two weeks
Instruct: Daily contrast baths at home, water temperature 43.3° C (111° F) and 18.3° C (65° F) for hands and feet.
　　　　Warm tub bath twice a week, water temperature 102° F (39.9° C), 20 minutes.
　　　　Home exercise program: active and progressive resistive

References

Griffin, J. E., and Karselis, T. C.: Physical Agents for Physical Therapists. 2nd Ed. Springfield, IL, Charles C. Thomas, 1982.

Logemann, J. A.: Evaluation and Treatment of Swallowing Disorders. San Diego, College-Hill Press, Inc., 1983.

Pedretti, L. W.: Occupational Therapy: Practice Skills for Physical Dysfunction. St. Louis, C. V. Mosby Company, 1985.

Peterson, C. A., and Gunn, S. L.: Therapeutic Recreation Program Design: Principles and Procedures. Englewood Cliffs, NJ, Prentice-Hall, Inc., 1984.

30
Rehabilitation of Patients with Completed Stroke

THOMAS P. ANDERSON

Stroke is usually defined as a cerebrovascular accident. However, when the term is used in this broad sense, it also includes transient ischemic attacks, which some writers believe comprise 60 to 75 per cent of all strokes.[37] Because these transient ischemic attacks, by definition, result in complete recovery, they are not included in discussions about rehabilitation for stroke. This is the reason for using the term *completed stroke* when rehabilitation is discussed. In this chapter, when general references are made to completed stroke, it usually means the stereotypical completed stroke involving the middle cerebral artery. When it does not mean this, it is designated that the anterior cerebral artery or posterior cerebral artery or vertebral arteries are involved. Certainly not all completed strokes should be lumped together and considered to be the same, since they vary so widely in their manifestations (Table 30–1) and, hence, in their evaluation and management.[12] For example, brain stem strokes are significantly different in their manifestations and management from middle cerebral artery strokes.

Many of the principles in the rehabilitation of completed stroke apply to the hemiparesis resulting from traumatic brain damage, but there are sufficient differences so that generalizations for completed stroke should not be made for post-traumatic hemiplegia. Before a patient with completed stroke is evaluated for rehabilitation training, the professional should ask the question, "Is this stroke?" The differential diagnosis of completed stroke[38] is extensive, and with the new diagnostic procedures of various types of brain scans and magnetic resonance imaging, one may be able to determine not only whether this patient

TABLE 30–1. Common Syndromes Occurring After Cerebral Vascular Accidents

Disturbance of consciousness
Mental confusion
Paralysis, paresis
Motor
Sensory
Spasticity
Incoordination
Dyspraxia
Anosognosia
Visual field deficits
Cognitive dysfunction
Perseveration
Impaired judgment and planning
Impulsivity
Ataxia
Communication disorders
Language (aphasia)
Speech production (dysarthria, dyspraxia, dysphonia)
Emotional lability

has a completed stroke but also the probable mechanism of the stroke, i.e., thrombosis, embolus, or hemorrhage. Furthermore, it is rare that one treats a patient with completed stroke as the only problem. There are usually concomitant disorders, such as hypertension, cardiac failure, angina, diabetes mellitus, peripheral vascular disease, and more.

Recovery

It should be kept in mind that there are two types of improvement that occur in completed

656

stroke: neurological recovery and improvements in functional abilities or performance. Neurological recovery depends on the mechanism of the stroke and the location of the lesion, so that no one generalization about neurological recovery is applicable to an individual case. However, it is generally agreed that 90 per cent of the neurological recovery has occurred by the end of three months following onset of the stroke, with the exception of some hemorrhagic-type strokes that may continue to show some slow neurological recovery for a longer period.

The improvement in function depends upon the environment in which the patient with completed stroke is placed and how much training and motivation there is for the patient to learn to become independent again in self-care and mobility. It is still not proved that the early initiation of rehabilitation treatment, particularly some of the facilitation techniques, can influence a greater return of neurological function. However, there are other justifications for beginning rehabilitation early in the course of completed stroke, e.g., to prevent avoidable complications such as depression. Several studies[4, 31] for developing predictive factors to determine which patients are good candidates for stroke rehabilitation and which are not concluded that there is no single predictive finding in early evaluation of the stroke patient that will indicate what the long-term outcome will be. However, some conditions are often associated with unfavorable outcomes,[19] such as marked concomitant disease, bilateral brain damage, dementia, persistent neglect, bowel and bladder incontinence lasting more than three to four weeks, gross perceptual deficits, flaccid paralysis lasting more than two months, severe dysphasia, prolonged bed rest, clinical depression, and a long interval between onset and initiation of rehabilitation. The influence of age on the outcome of stroke rehabilitation has not been clarified by recent reports. One study reported no significant differences in ambulation and self-care among stroke patients in four age groups. One study by Wade and co-workers[54] found age had little influence on the severity of stroke, the deficits seen initially, or the functional ability six months later. However, in a second study reported two years later, the same author found that not only did older patients appear to have more functional loss but also appeared not to recover as well as younger patients both socially and in terms of function in the activities of daily living. The interpretation of incidence is difficult because the older group, primarily women, had a greater incidence of pre-stroke impairment, and a large proportion were living alone so that they may have had an inadequate environmental support system.

Should the Patient with Completed Stroke Have Rehabilitation?

The old myth that the survival of patients with completed stroke is not sufficiently long to justify the great expense and effort of rehabilitation has been disproved by recent studies,[3, 5, 36] which show that at least 50 per cent of the survivors lived for 7 1/2 years or longer. A study has recently been completed comparing the long-term outcomes of those stroke patients who had rehabilitation with those who did not.[6] It showed that those who had rehabilitation had better long-term outcomes. There has also been some confusion about what rehabilitation is and where it should be done,[57] that is, in a nursing home versus a rehabilitation center. Stroke rehabilitation that is carried out in a comprehensive manner in a large rehabilitation center moves the stroke patient from a low level of functioning to a higher level in a relatively short period of time, whereas the activities in physical therapy, occupational therapy, and other therapies in extended care facilities, community hospitals, and nursing homes could often be labeled maintenance rehabilitation, which is carried out to prevent the deterioration of function in the patient but does not actually aid the patient to rapidly progress from a low level to a high level of function. Furthermore, studies are being considered that measure the costs and benefits or the cost effectiveness* of stroke rehabilitation.[32] Many comprehensive rehabilitation centers have reported a reduction in the length of stay for stroke rehabilitation patients in recent years. Some outcome studies have shown that the gains during rehabilitation are maintained for as long as several years thereafter.[3, 5, 6] If the patient survives 22 months or longer after rehabilitation for completed stroke, there is a lessening of costs.[32] Reports have appeared about the ineffectiveness of stroke re-

---

*The term *cost/benefit analysis* usually refers to a comprehensive inclusion of all costs, direct and indirect, as well as all benefits, direct and indirect, whereas *cost effectiveness* usually refers only to the more direct costs and benefits. See Table 30–2 for examples.

THOMAS P. ANDERSON

habilitation in which there was no distinction made between the type of rehabilitation care provided in a small community hospital[57] and another hospital in which patients were admitted to a large comprehensive rehabilitation center 40 days (on the average) after the onset of the stroke.[20] Most stroke rehabilitation programs are completed by patients before the end of 40 days after the onset of the condition. In carrying out cost benefit studies of stroke rehabilitation, it has been recognized that not just financial benefits but all benefits should be considered, such as those contributing to the quality of life of the patient (Table 30–2).

Referral to a Rehabilitation Center?

Which patients with completed stroke should be referred to a rehabilitation center? Attitudes about this question have changed in recent years. It was formerly felt that there were such a great number of patients with completed stroke and so few comprehensive rehabilitation centers and such difficulty in transportation that the majority of stroke patients had no access to rehabilitation centers. However, now it is rare that any patient in southern Canada or the United States is more than a few hours' drive from a comprehensive rehabilitation center. Because there is such a wide variation in patients with completed stroke and their evaluations are so complex, the stroke patient should go to a rehabilitation center in order to have an individually designed rehabilitation program. After

TABLE 30–2. Examples of Direct and Indirect Costs and Benefits of Stroke Rehabilitation

Direct Costs
  Hospital bills
  Doctors' bills

Indirect Costs
  Modification of home
  Special transportation
  Time lost from employment by family member

Direct Benefits
  Improved functions
  Improved performance
  Less dependency
  Employment

Indirect Benefits
  Improved quality of life
  Greater socializing
  Greater community involvement

the principal aspects of stroke rehabilitation training have taken place in a rehabilitation center, some of the long-term aspects of rehabilitation training, e.g., speech therapy, may be done in the home community.

When Should a Patient with Completed Stroke Be Referred to a Rehabilitation Center?

Generally, some principles of rehabilitation can be implemented on the first or second day after the onset of stroke. Usually, as soon as the stroke has stabilized, when the patient shows no further progression of neurological deficits, it is desirable to move the patient to a rehabilitation service or ward, provided the patient can meet a few simple criteria such as having a level of consciousness that permits him or her to follow two-step or, preferably, three-step directions. Also, can the patient remember and apply today what he learned yesterday? If both of these criteria can be fulfilled, then it is not too early to transfer the patient with completed stroke for rehabilitation training.

In planning the organization of this chapter, it was decided that using the approach taken by each of the rehabilitation disciplines to the patient with completed stroke was not as appropriate as a problem-oriented approach to stroke rehabilitation. Instead of having one section of the chapter on evaluation of the stroke patient and another on management, the evaluation and management will be discussed for each problem that is presented.

Rehabilitation During the Acute Phase of Stroke

How soon after the onset of stroke should rehabilitation begin? Some rehabilitation procedures should begin on the first day, particularly those aimed at preventing the development of complications. How long does the acute stroke patient have to remain in bed or in a chair? In the past there has been a tendency to leave stroke patients in bed much too long for fear of making the stroke progress if the patient starts sitting up too soon. However, the practice of having stroke patients sit up early has proved this myth to be untrue. Most authorities agree that the stroke patient can start sitting up in bed, and even in a chair beside the bed, just as soon as the stroke has stabilized. There has been some difficulty in determining when the stroke has stabilized or has been completed. Some physicians feel that the stage of stabilized stroke has been reached when there has been no further evidence of progression of neurological deficits for 48 hours.[7]

Enlightened rehabilitation practices applied early to the patient with completed stroke have made it apparent that many aspects of stroke that were formerly considered part of the natural history of completed stroke have, in reality, been complications that are preventable and avoidable. A recent report[26] indicates that the early intervention of rehabilitation after stroke or head injury shortens hospital stay. Patients admitted to a rehabilitation program 35 days after onset required twice as much acute rehabilitation as patients admitted earlier.[18]

Preventable Complications

Intellectual Regression. Probably the most common complication in completed stroke is intellectual regression due to sensory deprivation. Also, some complications are enhanced by prolonged sensory deprivation, such as depression, short attention span, and poor motivation. There has been a tendency in the past to isolate the stroke patient during the acute phase to a quiet, dark room, disturbing the patient as infrequently as possible. The patient sometimes is placed in a bed so that little, if any, stimulation is provided by the environment: when the patient lies flat, only the ceiling is seen and when lying on the one side, the patient is able to see only a blank wall. Although nursing personnel and physicians are briefly present on rounds, they sometimes have a tendency to speak of the patient in the third person, even in the patient's presence. Without external stimulation from the environment, even the most well-integrated personality tends to deteriorate rapidly. For example, astronauts who were placed in dark, quiet tanks began to hallucinate within an average of 14 hours. It is true that some stroke patients have short attention spans at first and fatigue easily and quickly. Consequently, the environmental stimulation has to be provided in brief intervals.

Depression. If sensory deprivation is prolonged, the patient soon develops depression along with the intellectual deterioration. There is then a tendency to blame depression on brain damage rather than on the environmental situation. More is discussed about depression later in this chapter.

Physical Deterioration. With intellectual regression, depression, and physical disability, the patient becomes increasingly dependent on the nursing personnel. Dependency frequently leads to resentment, and, hence, the patient becomes an increasing problem in nursing care. When this withdrawal, apathy, and depression are allowed to persist, it does not take long before a physical breakdown begins to develop. Decubitus ulcer occurs, particularly if the patient has some sensory deficits on the involved side or has been under the influence of heavy sedation or analgesia. Until the patient has learned to use the less affected side in changing position in bed, it should be part of the standard nursing care procedures to change the patient's position frequently.

Contractures. Probably the second most common complication of completed stroke is the development of contractures, a complication that is generally avoidable. The presence of contractures has many effects on the stroke patient other than just the loss of motion. For example, when the contractures are permitted to progress, they soon become painful. The presence of contractures often enhances the amount of spasticity and can greatly interfere with ambulation. The two principal procedures that are used to prevent the development of contractures can be accomplished by nursing personnel. These are (1) proper positioning of the more affected limbs in bed and when the patient is sitting and (2) range of motion exercises to maintain full range of motion. Excellent inexpensive monographs are available for nursing personnel who are not familiar with proper positioning of the more affected limbs of the stroke patient.[42] The majority of nursing personnel have been well instructed in performing passive range-of-motion exercises to prevent contractures, even though sometimes these exercises may also be carried out by the physical therapist. It is the physician's duty to see that these exercises are ordered to be carried out routinely, on a daily basis by nursing personnel. It should be pointed out that a distinction should be made between passive range-of-motion exercises that are performed by nursing personnel to *prevent* contractures and the stretching exercises for *correction* of contractures; the latter are usually performed by trained physical therapists.

Bladder Incontinence. After the onset of stroke, the presence of urinary incontinence may be due to confusion, to a communication disorder, or to the presence of a flaccid, distended bladder with a type of incontinence involving dribbling overflow.

THOMAS P. ANDERSON

If the involved extremities are flaccid and an altered level of consciousness is noted, it is reasonable to assume that a situation has occurred in which catheter drainage is indicated. Later, the neurological effect on bladder function may change as peripheral reflexes return and perhaps some spasticity appears and the incontinence changes to an inability to inhibit the detrusor reflex. When the filling bladder begins to contract, the patient cannot postpone this urgency volitionally and incontinence results. In evaluating bladder dysfunction, three aspects of voiding have to be evaluated and considered,[40] namely, bladder filling, the detrusor activity for emptying the bladder, and the external sphincter relaxation that permits the flow of urine. In addition, an impairment of urine flow may be caused by a mechanical obstruction such as an enlarged prostate or a scarred urethra. By asking the nursing service to initiate a total bladder training program, urinary dysfunction can often be accommodated without the demoralizing effect of incontinence but still avoiding the use of an indwelling catheter.

Urinary Sepsis. The period of urinary incontinence in many stroke patients does not last very long, and in many male patients, frequent changes of bed linen may be avoided by simply keeping a urinal in place, by using an external catheter to avoid bed wetting, or by simply arousing the patient at frequent intervals and offering the bedpan or urinal. Unfortunately, it is much easier to take care of the patient by using an indwelling catheter. The tendency is to leave the catheter in much too long. The longer the catheter, which acts as a foreign body, stays in the bladder, the greater the likelihood of urinary sepsis. It is rare to hear of a trial in which the stroke patient is taken off the catheter unsuccessful because it was tried too early.

Bowel Dysfunction. Even with severe brain damage, intestinal peristalsis continues so that fecal material arrives at the rectum automatically without volition of the patient. When this happens, if the stroke patient is unable to inhibit the urge or reflex to defecate, fecal incontinence occurs. This type of incontinence is often accompanied by urinary incontinence and is seen more commonly and more extensively in cases in which the brain damage is more extensive or even bilateral. However, even in those cases of bowel incontinence associated with severe brain damage, bowel incontinence can often be avoided by the initiation of an effective bowel program by the nursing service. Such a program has to take many factors into consideration, such as the patient's previous habits

of timing of bowel movements, diet, food intake, and amount of physical activity. Even though the patient may not be able to request a bedpan or commode, an individualized bowel program may take care of emptying the rectum at a regular, natural time so that accidents are avoided at other times of the day. This training by the nursing service, sometimes called bowel training of the stroke patient, plays a large role in helping to relieve depression by avoiding incontinence.

Deep Vein Thrombosis

Although not always preventable, deep vein thrombosis can be successfully detected early in high-risk stroke patients by impedance plethysmography, thus leading to prompt medical management, reduction of morbidity and mortality, and improved rehabilitation outcome.[28]

Motor Aspects

Paralysis and Weakness

Many people, when hearing the word *stroke*, think first of paralysis or weakness as the most outstanding characteristic of completed stroke. Hence, they tend not to realize that this process or weakness may not be the most disabling factor to the patient with completed stroke. In evaluating the extent and amount of paralysis or weakness, or both, manual muscle testing is of limited value because the response of individual muscle groups to testing depends upon a wide variety of factors, such as spasticity, incoordination, apraxia, uninhibited reflexes, relationship to gravity, and posture. It may take a considerable time before a full appreciation can be developed of how much motor function has been retained or regained. Often, additional motor function can be demonstrated in the more affected lower extremity when the patient is supported in the standing position than when examined while lying supine.

A new study of stroke patients with significant loss of motor function[48] compared with those without revealed they had a highly significant difference in problem-solving, spatial neglect, communication, and postural function. It was concluded that the significant loss in motor function had a negative prognostic effect on functional outcome, length of stay in the hospital, and survival.

Spasticity

During the recovery phase, the limbs affected by the stroke progress from a state of flaccidity to increased stretch reflexes (spasticity) as exhibited by increased deep tendon reflexes, clonus, and clasp-knife reaction to flexor and extensor synergies and finally to return of voluntary motor function. This general pattern of recovery may cease to progress at any phase. Hence, spasticity cannot always be considered to herald return of voluntary motor function. For an excellent, yet brief, explanation of the neurophysiological basis of spasticity, see Chapter 3 in *Mossman's Problem Oriented Approach to Stroke Rehabilitation*.[40] Some spasticity may be useful to the patient, particularly for standing and walking. In dealing with spasticity in the stroke patient, the professional should ask the question: "How disabling is it?"

A wide variety of pharmacological and surgical approaches to spasticity are available. These tend to dominate consideration before these questions are asked: "Had the spasticity been about the same for a long period of time and only recently become sufficiently worse to produce an increase in disabling effects? If so, what has occurred that might be enhancing the spasticity?" Factors that are well known for enhancing spasticity include the presence of contractures, anxiety, extremes of heat or cold, or any ordinarily painful condition, such as an ingrown toenail, an infection, or a decubitus ulcer. An attempt should be made to eliminate or diminish these factors before any pharmacological or surgical approach to treating the spasticity is tried (see Chapter 11).

The use of both heat and cold has been noted to have some temporary effect on reducing the amount of spasticity in some stroke patients. Sometimes this permits a brief period in which the patient can better practice certain exercises or neurophysiological retraining. Probably the most well-publicized approach to spasticity is through drugs. There are several classes of drugs that have different sites of action. Although some of them have proved to reduce measurably the amount of spasticity, when patients who have tried them are given the option of continuing or going without the antispasmodic, many give up the drug treatment and tolerate the increased spasticity because they do not like the drug's side effects. Because most of the drugs used for spasticity also have some effect on the functioning of the central nervous system, particularly alertness, stroke patients tend to find these side effects more undesirable

than the more pronounced spasticity. A long-term follow-up study is needed to determine how many patients continue taking drugs for spasticity over a long period of time.

The use of phenol blocks,[24] either for neurolysis of a main nerve trunk or intramuscularly for a few selective motor units, has been quite effective in reducing the amount of spasticity. These effects are not permanent but can be repeated when the spasticity increases again. Following such procedures, some patients have had a complication of discomfort in the blocked muscle for two to three days. Early initiation of daily range-of-motion exercises to lower and upper extremity joints, both during the phase of acute hospitalization and during rehabilitation, has decreased the occurrence of connective tissue contractures. Surgical lengthening of tendons of the spastic muscles is rarely done anymore.

Incoordination

Incoordination in patients with completed stroke may be associated with spasticity or may be due to involvement of the cerebellum or cerebellar tracts. For evaluation and management of the latter, see the section on brain stem involvement. For incoordination associated with spasticity, see the later section on management.

Dyspraxia

In stroke patients, dyspraxia is a disorder of voluntary movement wherein the individual cannot initiate a willed or planned purposeful movement or activity despite the presence of adequate strength, sensation, coordination, and comprehension. A wide variety of types of dyspraxia have been described in stroke patients, such as oral-verbal dyspraxia, constructional apraxia, dressing apraxia, ideational apraxia, and motor dyspraxia. It is the motor, or kinetic, dyspraxia that is most commonly encountered in stroke patients. A common example of motor dyspraxia is exhibited by the patient who can perform a movement spontaneously quite accurately but when requested to perform this same act so that the movement must be planned, the patient is then unable to initiate the movement. Once the patient is given some assistance to initiate the movement, the patient can then go ahead and complete it, often with good coordination or dexterity. This phenomenon has a definite neurological basis, although it often resembles a problem in attitude, cooperation, comprehension, awareness, or motivation. Once the problem is recognized, it can be dealt with in rehabilitation training by giving the patient assistance for starting a complex performance that the patient completes successfully. The prognosis is good for overcoming most types of dyspraxia if consistent training is pursued. This is true even for oral dyspraxia and oral-verbal dyspraxia, which will be further discussed in the section on communication disorders.

Management of Motor Dysfunction

It is not difficult for the physician to write an adequate prescription for physical therapy, even for the patient with a paretic limb that continues to progress in neurological recovery. The order can be written: "Re-education, including neurophysiological techniques, for all muscle groups in the extremity; progressing each group as improvement occurs to active assistive, active, active against gravity, and finally resistive exercise." This will permit the physical therapist to allow the patient to progress as neuromuscular functioning improves without having to have the physical therapy prescription rewritten at frequent intervals. The problem that is still quite controversial is the selection of neurophysiological techniques to use for this returning function. Two studies reported help in this dilemma. One study found that, with the single exception of self-feeding, no significant statistical differences in skill level were found between two groups of stroke patients—one group received traditional functional retraining (integrated behavioral technique) whereas the other group received neuromuscular retraining (Bobath technique). The other study[11] reported that there was no statistically significant superiority of either type of physical therapy program for stroke. Fields has developed electromyographically triggered electrical muscle stimulation for treating stroke.[21] He reports that the technique is designed to directly intervene in the dynamics of sensorimotor control, reinstating proprioceptive feedback that is time-locked to attempts at muscular movement.

Some people are under the incorrect impression that these neurophysiological techniques are designed to overcome pathological reflexes, but Kottke[29] points out that, rather than pathological reflexes, in stroke patients there are specific spinal and supraspinal reflexes that vary only in intensity or extent of response as the result of diminution or loss of inhibition because of damage to the higher centers. Kottke further points out that to train a normal adult to the peak of coordination in a specific activity, the activity must be performed with maximal skill for hundreds of thousands, possibly millions, of repetitions. Just as coordination is developed by frequent and multiple repetitions, it is lost progressively over time with inactivity. Therefore, the therapeutic program should be adjusted to ensure that coordination activities are repeated at frequent intervals throughout each day and continued until a functional level of activity is achieved. In the treatment of stroke, Kottke divides the neurophysiological techniques into four phases, depending on the state of neuromuscular function of the patient: (1) activation of nonresponsive muscles, (2) reinforcement of feedback, (3) inhibition of muscles not in a coordinated engram, and (4) improving performance of the engram. Instead of recommending any one of the many detailed techniques of treatment, he recommends that techniques be used that are appropriate for the state of neuromuscular function of the muscle group or limb in that individual patient that seem to be the most effective.

One of the difficulties in using these neurophysiological methods of treatment of stroke patients is that they have to be carried out over a long period of time, with many repetitions. In the short period of time that stroke rehabilitation usually takes place on an inpatient basis, there has been insufficient time to note much significant change in the patient's performance with these methods.[49] Ideally, those stroke patients who show a good early response to such training should have the opportunity to continue the training on an outpatient basis over a long period of time.

Sensory Deficits

Because the patient may not complain of sensory deficits, their importance in causing disability in the hemiplegic patient tends to be overlooked by rehabilitation professionals. This is particularly true in the upper extremity that has good return of voluntary motor functioning but that is not utilized by the patient because of the persistent sensory deficits. This patient is accused of poor motivation or emotional overreaction for not using the upper extremity more. The types of sensory modalities involved in completed stroke in the order of importance of the disabilities they produce are proprioception, tactile sensation, vibration, pain, and temperature.

In some hemiplegics who have some sensory impairment but not complete sensory paralysis of the more involved limbs, there is a tendency to recognize all stimuli as pain. This is probably most pronounced in partial lesions in the thalamus. Such a situation makes carrying out range-of-motion exercises for prevention of contractures difficult because all light touch and movement of the involved extremities are recognized by the patient as pain. One of the ways this problem can be lessened is that the therapist, recognizing that the patient's sensation has the ability to adapt, does not change tactile sensations once the extremity is grasped for conducting the passive movements. After a few minutes, the patient's reaction of pain to the tactile sensation of having the limb held by the therapist will adapt. Then when the therapist performs the movements at the same rate of speed without sudden stops and starts, the amount of pain recognized by the patient from the movement will be lessened. In addition, the therapist needs to repeatedly reassure the patient that what is being done is not actually painful but is just being misperceived.

The level of the lesion has considerable effect on the sensory deficit. Lesions of the ascending sensory tracts in the brain stem may produce sensory loss of the entire extremity, whereas higher lesions in the internal capsule or cortex tend to produce a loss of sensation that is greater distally than proximally. The ventral nucleus of the thalamus may be affected, particularly following interruption of the posterior cerebral artery circulation. This is the level for the first appreciation of primary sensations of touch, temperature, pain, vibration, and some cruder aspects of proprioception. Projections from the ventral nucleus of the thalamus to the parietal cortex pass through the posterior limb of the internal capsule, which is a frequent site of damage in strokes involving the internal carotid or middle cerebral artery circulation. The sensory projections are commonly involved in conjunction with the descending motor tracts that pass more anteriorly in the internal capsule, giving rise to associated hemiplegia and sensory losses. It is the area of the parietal cortex in which the crude sensations that were initially perceived by the thalamus undergo fine discrimination. Because the fibers within the internal capsule are more closely concentrated than the more diffused projections in the cortex, a lesion of equal size produces greater damage within the internal capsule than one in the cortex.

In cortical sensory lesions impairing proprioception from the knee down, the lower extremity can function adequately with a gross motor pattern for walking. Useful distal function in the upper extremity requires not only fine motor coordination for prehension but also sensory sophistication of a high order of complexity. Hence, when cortical proprioception is involved, there is a poorer prognosis for regaining useful function in the upper extremity than in the lower extremity. However, occupational therapists have found that teaching the patient to use visual monitoring of hand activity can help compensate for the impaired proprioception. Other cortical functions for sensation that can be tested are localization and discrimination of stimuli by tests of two-point discrimination, sensory extinction, stereognosis, and graphesthesia. After time is allowed for spontaneous recovery, the stroke patient who performs well on these tests of cortical functioning has a much better prognosis for use of the involved extremity in vocational rehabilitation.

Studies have shown that some stroke patients with impairment of sensation do recover part of the impaired sensation, usually within the first or second month.[51] The number of patients experiencing recovery of sensory function varied, depending on the types of sensation that were involved. Generally, one half to two thirds of the patients experienced some improvement in sensory deficits. Those patients with no sensory deficits had a much shorter period of initial hospitalization. Those that achieved no recovery had a still longer period of hospitalization than those with some recovery. It is still questionable whether retraining can help patients with impaired, but not absent, sensation to improve their recognition of these sensations for practical clinical purposes.

Anosognosia is a term coined by Babinski, but the meaning and cause of the condition are still not well understood. Generally, the term applies to a condition in some patients with left hemiparesis or hemiplegia who do not recognize their left extremities as their own or who do not recognize the disabilities in those extremities. Friedlander[23] has pointed out that there are three theoretical mechanisms underlying anosognosia: (1) a defect in morphosynthesis, (2) a defect of body concept, and (3) a maladaptation to illness in a personality that premorbidly denied illness. Whatever the defect, the phenomenon of anosognosia significantly impedes rehabilitation training.

THOMAS P. ANDERSON

Visual Field Deficits

Vascular lesions of the brain can cause interference with vision if they occur anywhere along the visual pathways but occur more often in circulatory embarrassment in the territory of the middle cerebral artery and less commonly in the area of distribution of the posterior cerebral artery. The effect on vision may be complete ablation, so that it is referred to as a field cut (Fig. 30–1), or it may be partial. Since it is so difficult to distinguish between these two effects early after the onset of stroke, it is probably preferable to label such lesions as visual field deficits. The pattern of involvement can vary from one quarter, one half, or three quarters of a visual field. It may involve the same amount of the visual field of each eye, which is the most common type of deficit. These deficits in visual field should not be called problems in perception or perceptual deficits. The term *perceptual* relates to right hemisphere function.

Visual field impairments are often not recognized and appreciated by the rehabilitation staff early after onset of stroke, but becoming aware of these problems allows the staff to help avoid a lot of frustration for the patient. For example, when the patient is learning self-feeding techniques, the staff learns to place the food in the area of the patient's functioning field of vision, avoiding the side on which the deficit is located. Some patients with these problems can learn to compensate for the visual field deficit. Some either learn to compensate very well so that the problem no longer appears to exist, or perhaps they actually recover and regain visual functioning. One of the greatest problems in teaching such patients to compensate for the visual deficit is the patient's tendency to deny that such a visual impairment exists. This denial should not be confused with another condition called visual field neglect, in which the patient when tested by perimeter examination has a full field of vision but tends to ignore and neglect visual stimuli coming from the involved side. Often this type of extinction, or perceptual rivalry, is encountered in other areas of sensory perception, such as double simultaneous stimulation and kinesthetic perception. In Britain, the Rivermead Behavioral Inattention Test[60] has been developed, which appears to be a valid and reliable test of visual-spatial neglect and one which is likely to provide more information about everyday problems of the patient with stroke than existing measures of evaluation of neglect.

Hearing Deficits

Although there are no well-recognized specific deficits in hearing ability that are caused by stroke, the impairment of hearing in stroke patients is quite common. It is usually assumed that the hearing loss was present prior to the stroke. The rehabilitation staff should suspect possible hearing difficulties in the older stroke patient. Audiometric examination is quite useful to the staff in knowing how to communicate with the stroke patient.

Cognitive and Other Dysfunctions

Differences Between Right and Left Hemisphere Involvement

Generally it is recognized that the left hemisphere controls the right side of the body and is the dominant one for communication ability, whereas the right hemisphere controls the left side of the body and various integrative factors in cognition and intellectual functioning. However, it is erroneous to think that all stroke patients have

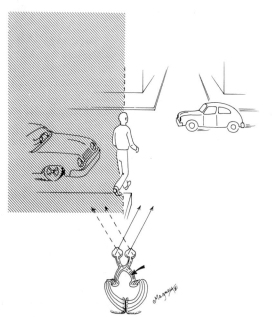

FIGURE 30–1. Example of visual field deficit on the left. The individual does not respond to the visual stimuli of the approaching auto on his left owing to a lesion in the optic radiation at the point of the arrow.

only one side of the body involved. Even though the lesion may be in one side of the brain, the effects on brain function are often bilateral so that we should say that one side is "the more involved" and the other side is "less involved," rather than saying that the patient is left hemiparetic or right hemiparetic. It is also generally recognized that the intelligence quotient is made up of an average of the verbal IQ, which mainly represents left hemisphere function, and the performance IQ, which mainly represents right hemisphere function. The effects of left hemisphere lesions on communication will be dealt with under communication disorders later in this chapter.

Right Hemisphere Dysfunction

The right parietal lobe in the majority of people, including most left-handed people, provides the ability to correctly organize stimuli into concepts, which is termed *morphosynthesis*. Interference in this functioning is often termed a *perceptual disorder*. However, because of the ambiguity of this term, such as applying it to visual field disorders, it is probably preferable to refer to dysfunctions of the right parietal lobe more specifically with terms such as *visual-spatial* and *visual-motor disorders*. These are seen in stroke patients most often as difficulties in the performance of activities of daily living in which they seem impaired in making the right spatial analysis of problems they encounter. A classic example is the patient who easily recognizes that something is wrong with his or her shirt yet cannot recognize that one sleeve is turned wrong side out.

Some studies of rehabilitation of stroke patients have shown that patients with right hemisphere damage that produces this type of deficit are slower in learning activities of daily living than those patients with left hemisphere involvement. However, other studies[4, 31] show that there is no difference between right and left hemisphere involvement. Perhaps this variation occurred owing to differences in the number of nonverbal cues given in instructing the patient in the training in activities of daily living. There appears to be no correlation of visual-spatial and visual-motor dysfunctions with the amount of motor impairment in the left limb. Generally all patients who have had right hemisphere involvement should not be permitted to drive an automobile again until they have passed special testing for visual-spatial and visual-motor

functioning as well as for visual field neglect and other types of deficits.

Psychometric Testing

One of the most widely used tests of right parietal lobe functioning is the Bender-Gestalt Visual Motor Test. It consists of asking the patient to copy on paper meaningless geometric designs and dots. This is a cross-cultural test that can detect spatial distortions, separations, and errors in orientation or rotation. It may also demonstrate unilateral visual field neglect. The Gram Kendall Memory for Design Test and Sequin Formboard require perception of visual-spatial relationships and discrimination of the test object by the patient. The Wechsler Adult Intelligence Scale has a variety of assembly and completion tasks involving varying levels of visual-spatial reasoning, analysis, and manipulation of relationships as well as higher cognitive visual-spatial reasoning. The scores in the performance part of this test are often low in patients with right hemisphere involvement, whereas their verbal IQ may remain quite high, similar to the premorbid level. These tests have not proved to be useful in their predictive value[4, 31] as had been hoped by an earlier study.

Other Dysfunctions

Perseveration is a repetitive and involuntary motor or verbal response that possibly was appropriate to a first stimulus but continues to be repeated even after the first stimulus has been removed and other new stimuli or instructions have been introduced. It is found in people with a wide variety of brain damage. It usually is associated with severity of involvement or is indicative of recent involvement, since it often gradually subsides as neurological recovery takes place.

Some patients with brain damage also exhibit a quality of behavior called impulsivity. This is most often encountered in patients who begin an action before they completely process what the full scope of the action will be. For example, they begin following instructions before the instructions have been completed. Patients exhibiting impulsivity seem to be unable to withhold a response and make a judgment about which alternatives and course of action would be most appropriate. They act with a quick motor response without taking time to consider its appropriateness or its effects.

Another characteristic of brain damage that interferes with the rehabilitation process is impaired judgment and impaired planning and foresight. This can be easily tested and demonstrated by asking the patient to perform on Porteus mazes. Clinically, this problem often becomes manifest when patients are undergoing homemaking evaluation in which they exhibit poor judgment or inability to plan or execute preparation of a meal. These dysfunctions tend to be most noticeable immediately after the onset of the stroke and gradually diminish with time. Often the dysfunctions completely disappear or recur only with marked fatigue. Since they tend to resolve spontaneously, either rapidly or gradually, it has been difficult to study training programs that might lead to a better resolution or a more rapid resolution of the problem.

Mobility

During the Acute Phase

Some patients with stroke view themselves at first as totally paralyzed instead of paralyzed on just one side of the body. They feel totally helpless. One of the first steps in overcoming this feeling is helping them learn to use the less involved arm and leg to move themselves in bed. Because the dangers of having the stroke patient sit up early have been exaggerated in the past, one should consider rolling up the head of the bed quite early, particularly while the patient is awake. When this is tolerated well, the patient can learn to come to a sitting position on the edge of the bed. The patient rolls to his less involved side and then uses the less involved lower extremity under the involved one to guide it over the edge of the bed and uses the less involved arm to push up to the sitting position. These techniques are well described and illustrated in a monograph on nursing procedures for stroke patients published by the Elizabeth Kenny Institute.[42]

Common to nearly all patients with completed stroke is the difficulty in maintaining sitting balance and, of course, standing balance. This problem is not necessarily related to which hemisphere is involved but rather is related to the need to learn to develop new reflexes for maintaining balance. There are three major determinants for maintaining balance in the normal individual: vision, proprioception, and labyrinthine function. Generally, at least two of these three factors should be oper-

ating. If the patient has been left for a long time in bed, transient hypotension due to the sudden change in posture may cause cerebral vascular insufficiency with transient vertigo. Undoubtedly visual-spatial and visual-motor dysfunctions could also interfere with maintenance of balance.

Another factor is the sense of verticality in the hemiplegic patient (Fig. 30–2). Special tests have been developed for measuring this sensation, such as the Rod and Frame Test. Most studies[16] reveal that early after onset nearly all hemiplegic patients show some impairment of performance in ascertaining the vertical position of the test rod. Not all of the studies[13] agree that right hemiplegic patients perform this test better than left hemiplegic patients. Fortunately, the sense of verticality and particularly the sense of balance can be relearned. It is rare that these problems persist for a long period of time if the stroke patient has been given an adequate trial of relearning sitting balance while using visual input as well as proprioceptive input from the less involved upper extremity, and then relearning standing balance.

Transfers and Wheelchairs

Getting out of bed, particularly when the patient has learned to do so by himself or herself, is probably more significant to the stroke patient than any other factor in overcoming the feeling of still being a sick patient; it signifies that the individual is learning to become a person again instead of a patient. For the hemiplegic or hemiparetic patient, there is a definite method to be used (see

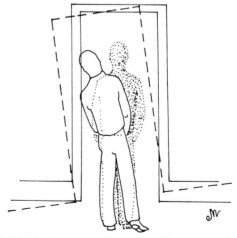

FIGURE 30–2. Illustration of a person with an impaired sense of verticality.

Chapter 22), even when the patient needs assistance or direction, so that eventually using this same procedure the patient can learn to perform the transfer without assistance. Detailed instructions of a step-by-step procedure of transfer training are well outlined in the Elizabeth Kenny Institute publication on stroke.[42] Each time a transfer is performed with assistance, training should be given so that eventually the patient will learn to do it independently.

For the stroke patient, an important aspect of getting up in a wheelchair is to be able to propel the wheelchair independently. It is not necessary to have an expensive one-hand-driven wheelchair. If the patient has one functioning upper extremity and a functioning lower extremity, the patient can quickly learn how to use that foot and hand together to propel the wheelchair forward and to turn and guide the chair (see Chapter 23). Even patients with visual-spatial and visual-motor dysfunctions associated with right hemisphere damage can learn to use a wheelchair by practicing to get themselves around the building independently.

Ambulation

For ambulation, the patient with completed stroke should possess the following:

1. The ability to follow instructions, preferably three-step directions. Even though the patient may have marked impairment in comprehension of verbal instructions, he or she may be able to learn readily from nonverbal directions such as demonstrations.

2. The ability to maintain standing balance, which can be evaluated when the patient is transferring.

3. The absence of contractures in hip and knee flexors and heel cord.

4. Adequate return of voluntary motor function to stabilize the hip, the knee, and the ankle on the involved side. For the patient with completed stroke to learn to walk again, return of voluntary motor function is necessary in only one muscle group—the hip extensors. These muscles not only stabilize the hip in extension but also help stabilize the knee in extension by pulling backward on the femur. Lateral stabilization of the hip that is impaired by weakness or paralysis of the hip abductors can be compensated for by placing the opposite (less involved) hand on a stable object such as a cane. For paralysis or weakness of foot and ankle muscles, an ankle-foot orthosis not only can help

keep the forefoot up but also can aid medial and lateral stability of the ankle. If the ankle-foot orthosis resists dorsiflexion beyond 90 degrees, it can also help to stabilize the knee to keep it from flexing during stance. It is rare that a patient with hemiparesis needs a long leg brace. In evaluating the patient to determine how much return of voluntary motor function is present, manual muscle testing while the patient is lying supine can be misleading. Often the stimulus of being in the upright standing position and attempting to bear weight on the more involved lower extremity demonstrates more voluntary motor function than is apparent when the patient is lying supine.

5. An intact sense of position in the more involved lower extremity. This is not an absolute requisite because patients with impaired proprioception can learn to walk again by using the lower extremity in which sensory function is still intact.

Progression of Gait Training

Olney and associates[41] classified three major types of gait disturbances in stroke patients and concluded that each would require a different approach to gait training. After studying 25 patients, Wall and Turnbull[57] concluded that it is not possible to design a single gait re-education program for all residual stroke patients; rather, the training prescribed must address the unique deficiencies of each patient.

For successful gait training of the patient with completed stroke, a well-trained physical therapist is most helpful, if not essential. The patient first learns balance by holding onto a bar or other stable support while standing. When balance is beginning to be reliable, the patient learns to shift full weight onto the more affected lower extremity. Once this is feasible, the patient can begin performing gait drills by standing in place, shifting the weight from one lower extremity to the other. When this procedure appears to be going well, with the hip, knee, and ankle well stabilized, actual walking at the bar can begin, with the aim of developing an optimal reciprocal pattern of gait. Once a good reciprocal pattern at the bar has been achieved, the patient progresses to using a four-point cane. A crutch at this point is not desirable because, with a crutch, the patient can easily develop a habit of leaning away from the more involved lower extremity, thereby not placing full weight on it, which will make the later progression to a cane difficult. When the patient is doing well

THOMAS P. ANDERSON

with a four-point cane and appears to have confidence, an attempt can be made to use a single-ended cane. Gait training is not completed, however, until the patient has learned to negotiate stairs and ramps. For the patient with right hemisphere involvement that has produced some spatial and visual-motor impairment, the patient may have difficulty remembering which foot to use first when going up or down stairs. However, this can sometimes be helped if the patient has good verbal functioning. The patient can learn to negotiate stairs through conscious effort with the aid of verbal cues, such as the little mnemonic device, "up with the good foot, down with the bad."

Factors Interfering with Ambulation

Paralysis and Weakness. Since antigravity strength in the hip extensors on the more involved side is the only motor function required for walking, paralysis and weakness play little role in the interference with gait training.

Spasticity. This is undoubtedly the most common disabling factor in gait training. When this occurs, first a search should be made for factors that may be enhancing the spasticity, such as pain, contracture, ataxia, fear, and anxiety. For many stroke patients, spasticity that interferes with walking is most marked in the plantar flexors. This can often be adequately controlled with the use of an ankle-foot orthosis (see Chapter 28 on *Lower Extremity Orthotics*). If the spasticity is rather marked, the Klenzak brace seems to be more effective than the posterior molded plastic splint. It should be pointed out that there is no truth in the persistent myth that spring action braces enhance spasticity.[35] An outside T-strap on a Klenzak brace may help lessen the problem of spastic invertors pulling the foot over medially so that the patient has a tendency to walk on the outer edge of the foot. Intramuscular neurolysis may also be used to reduce the amount of spasticity.[24] A pharmacologic approach to spasticity in patients with completed stroke often adds a burden of central nervous system depression. Drugs should be considered only when all the above measures have been tried and yet the spasticity is still interfering with the patient's attempt at walking.

Common Pitfalls in Gait Training for Stroke Patients[8]

Some physical therapists who are eager to make the patient feel that progress is occurring in am-

bulation have a tendency to start the patient walking at a bar before adequately learning to shift the full weight onto the more involved lower extremity. This leads to the development of a gait pattern that will make it very difficult for the patient ever to progress to using a cane. There is also a tendency for both the therapist and the patient to want to complete training at the bar too soon, before a good pattern is established, thereby initiating a persistently poor gait pattern. Then, once the patient has graduated from the bar and is walking well with a four-point cane, there is a tendency to move the patient to a single-ended cane too soon. In fact, the single-ended cane should not be used until the therapist notices no differences in the patient's gait pattern whether the patient uses a four-point cane or a single-ended cane. For those patients with dyspraxia, a physical therapist has to learn to refrain from giving instructions for each movement in sequence but instead allow the patient to move ahead automatically as feasible.

Activities of Daily Living

One-Handed Methods

The reader is referred to Chapter 24 on activities of daily living. For all the listed activities, methods have been worked out for one-handed performance. For specific written guides to be used for stroke patients in the performance of self-care and other activities of daily living, the Sister Elizabeth Kenny publications[43] are excellent guides with good illustrations. For most patients with completed stroke, the difficulties involved in learning activities of daily living are less commonly due to physical factors, such as weakness and one handedness or to communication factors, but more often are due to problems such as poor sitting balance, a visual field defect, and visual-spatial and visual-motor dysfunctions.

Self-Care

Training in self-care by nursing personnel should begin early while the patient is still in bed. Even then, the patient can begin learning to use the less involved extremities for turning in bed and self-feeding, and can start to perform some aspects of personal hygiene, to bathe, and eventually to learn to come to a sitting position on the edge of the bed without assistance. When sitting balance has been achieved, then the patient can start to learn to dress and also to transfer to a bedside commode or toilet. Finally when the patient has achieved standing balance and the ability to transfer to and from a toilet independently, the patient still needs to learn to rearrange clothing in a standing position before and after using the toilet.

Homemaking

It should not be assumed that mainly female patients with completed stroke are interested in evaluation and training in homemaking. Almost as many males are interested in including this in their rehabilitation training. Often this evaluation and training are postponed until shortly before discharge from the comprehensive inpatient rehabilitation period so that the patient may have attained maximal potential in mobility and communication. Better recommendations for what the patient is able and not able to do at home can then be made. Although most of this evaluation is done by the occupational therapist, the entire team contributes to the assessment of some aspects of the evaluation. For example, the physical therapist reports on whether the patient should work from a wheelchair or from a standing position, whether transfers are performed safely, and whether transfer to a stool in the kitchen is practical. The social worker reports on the family's general attitude toward the patient's return home, what their expectations are, and if the patient will be expected to resume a full or limited homemaking role. The occupational therapist reports on factors such as the degree of function that remains in the more involved upper extremity, whether it can be used in a helping way or a stabilizing way, whether there is a visual field deficit, whether the patient has learned to compensate for the deficit and whether visual-spatial and visual-motor problems affect the patient's ability. The speech pathologist recommends what communication methods should be used with the patient during the homemaker's evaluation, and the psychologist may report from results of psychometric testing about the patient's judgment and reliability. The homemaking evaluation itself gives a great deal of information about judgment, reliability, and ability to plan ahead.

When the final report of this evaluation is made, recommendations are given about which activities will need no help, some help, much help, or complete help. Some of the other problems that affect the outcome of the homemaking evaluation are perseveration, impulsivity, ataxia, unreliability, and poor tolerance of frustration. After the evaluation of homemaking abilities has been completed, the homemaking training often focuses on factors such as work simplification in the patient's home, organization of the work areas there, and the determination of the patient's reaching ranges.

Other Activities

Consideration should be given to how the patient functions not only in the home but also outside the home, and how the patient is able to negotiate certain types of architectural barriers, use public transportation, go shopping, and drive an automobile. For driving an automobile, special consideration should be given to factors such as slowed reaction time, visual field neglect, and visual-spatial dysfunction, which are usually not demonstrated in the average medical or driving evaluation for reissuing a driver's license.

Upper Extremity Problems

Neurological Recovery

In the typical middle cerebral artery stroke, the upper extremity is usually more involved than the lower extremity, and recovery is usually not as complete. With the exception of those patients whose stroke involved the anterior cerebral artery, the pattern of long-term return of motor function is usually more proximal, with the distal functioning in the fingers being the last to return. Stroke patients who regained full recovery of motor function in the upper extremity exhibited the onset of this return of function within the first two weeks of the onset of the stroke, and always within the first month.[9] Most subjects achieved full active movement within the first month, and all of them recovered function by the third month. A recent study[55] reported that statistically significant improvement in arm function is seen only in the first three months following the onset of stroke. If the patient has had no return of voluntary motor function in the hand six months after the onset of the stroke, the prognosis for any return of useful function in that hand is poor. Carroll[17] found that if there was no return of voluntary motor function within the first week, it was unlikely the patient would regain full use of the hemiplegic upper

THOMAS P. ANDERSON

extremity. There are other differences between the upper extremity and lower extremity on the involved side. For the lower extremity to be useful in ambulation, it requires only minimal return of voluntary motor function of the hip extensor for that extremity to serve as a pillar for weight bearing. For the upper extremity to be useful, there has to be almost complete return of voluntary motor and sensory function to provide fine coordination and finger dexterity. It is always difficult to know even with knowledge of these statistical studies[9, 17] about return of function (Table 30–3), when to start training the nondominant hand to become the dominant one after a completed stroke. In the treatment of the upper extremity, therapists often incorporate the use of bilateral activities in the hope that movement might more readily return in the involved dominant upper extremity. However, it has been pointed out[25] that the function in the unaffected nondominant hand may be less efficient and inferior to the paretic dominant hand's capability when it functions separately. There is still considerable question about whether specialized neurophysiological techniques utilizing synergies and facilitation produce a significant improvement in the paretic hand. Stern and co-workers[49] indicated that the specialized facilitation techniques have no better results than a traditional approach in teaching self-care techniques to the stroke patient. Others point out that for new patterns of motion to become effective and useful they have to be repeated many times over a long period of time. Hence, the short period of three to four weeks that a stroke patient is in traditional inpatient rehabilitation is not long enough to show effective results. It would appear that before the value of these specialized neurophysiological techniques can be assessed, a group of patients would have to experience a long period of training as outpatients.

TABLE 30–3. Time After Onset Until Initial Voluntary Motion in Upper Extremity (Months)*

	1	2	3	4	>4
Patients recovering full motion	39	0	0	0	0
Patients recovering partial motion	17	5	5	1	0

*Used with permission from Bard, G., and Hirschberg, G. G.: Recovery of voluntary motion in the upper extremity following hemiplegia. Arch. Phys. Med. Rehabil., 46:567–572, 1965.

Painful Shoulder

In those patients with completed stroke who have a subluxation of the shoulder on the more involved side, the tendency is always to blame the shoulder pain on the subluxation. However, many subluxed shoulders are not painful. What tends to be overlooked is a painful contracture of the shoulder that is also present. To give such a patient a sling without also adding stretching exercises to correct the contractures will fail to relieve the pain. Although no comparative studies are known to have been reported, it is the clinical impression that the incidence of painful contractures is much less today than two or three decades ago when daily range-of-motion exercises were not as common and routine as they are at present. The number of patients with hemiparesis who exhibit a fully developed reflex sympathetic dystrophy involving the hand and shoulder also seems much less in recent years. Bohannon and colleagues[14] studied hemiplegic patients and found that range of external rotation was considered the factor related most significantly to shoulder pain, whereas Van Ouwenaller and associates,[52] who looked at spasticity in association with shoulder pain in hemiplegia, did not even mention checking the range of motion in the shoulder. Another study[30] reported that a lesion of the suprascapular nerve is not responsible for the painful contracted shoulder of a hemiplegic patient, although such a lesion may coexist incidentally. When early signs of reflex dystrophy associated with vasoconstriction are detected, the vicious circle can usually be rapidly reversed through the use of simple measures such as heat, gentle stretching exercises to regain full pain-free motions in the shoulder, oral analgesic agent, contrast baths for the hand and arm, and other similar measures to counteract the pain and vasoconstriction. If these are used frequently and vigorously before structural changes have begun to develop, it is seldom necessary to use more drastic measures for the reflex dystrophy such as stellate ganglion blocks. Even so, reflex sympathetic dystrophy frequently contributes to a chronic painful shoulder after a stroke, and the treatment measures mentioned above should not be neglected when there are no signs of sympathetic hyperactivity.

The upper extremity with a subluxed shoulder can be supported by a sling. There are many types of slings (Fig. 30–3). The type most commonly used is the one that places most of the weight-

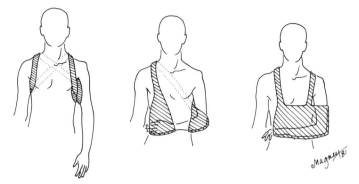

FIGURE 30–3. Some types of arm slings. From left to right: Bobath, common hemiplegic, Breuer-Kauper.

bearing on the back of the neck. The other types of slings are more difficult to put on by the patients with visual-spatial and visual-motor difficulties. Basmajian[10] has pointed out that it is the downward droop of the glenoid fossa, which becomes less vertical, that enhances the subluxation of the shoulder (Fig. 30–4). Hence, he recommends retraining the upper trapezius muscle to perform its function better in keeping the shoulder elevated in its normal position and thus preventing the downward droop and resulting subluxation.

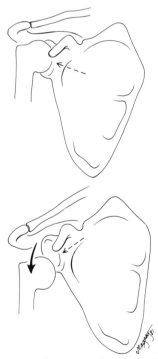

FIGURE 30–4. Basmajian's principle. *Lower,* Drooping of the shoulder in some hemiplegics permits subluxation out of the downward tilted glenoid fossa (dotted arrow). *Upper,* Normally positioned shoulder prevents subluxation because the humeral head cannot displace laterally out of the upward-tilted glenoid fossa (dotted arrow).

The Hand and the Wrist

Probably the most common problem in the paralytic or paretic hand and wrist is the development of contracture, usually in the flexors. Some patients who have accepted the fact that the paralysis of the hand is going to be permanent wonder why they should bother with continuing with the range-of-motion exercises. Unfortunately, contractures can become painful, and even if they are not painful, the presence of a contracture enhances spasticity in the upper extremity and then also indirectly in the lower extremity, which may in turn interfere with walking. If the patient and family understand this relationship, they do a better job of preventing contractures in the paralyzed, useless upper extremity.

The use of a pancake resting splint (Fig. 30–5) at night, as well as the daily routine of stretching exercises, can be helpful in preventing the development of contractures of the finger flexors. The patient who has some return of voluntary motor function in the upper extremity but spasticity in the more dominant flexors and thus tends to keep the hand and wrist in a flexed position would do well to use a dorsal cock-up splint for the hand to keep the hand and wrist in a better position of function and to prevent the spasticity in the flexors from dominating the posture of the hand (Fig. 30–6).

Dependent edema of the hand, sometimes ex-

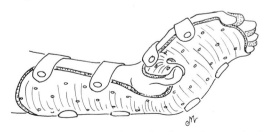

FIGURE 30–5. Pancake (resting) splint for hand and wrist.

THOMAS P. ANDERSON

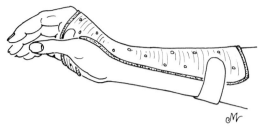

FIGURE 30–6. Dorsal cock-up splint.

tending up into the arm, occurs in hemiplegia, particularly when there is little, if any, voluntary motor function in the upper extremity. The pumping mechanism for helping the venous and lymphatic flow in the arm is impaired. When the dependent edema begins to accumulate, it is preferable to provide the patient with other means of keeping the extremity elevated rather than putting it in a sling against the patient's chest. It is more desirable to use a forearm tray on the patient's wheelchair with the hand end elevated. While the patient is lying down, the involved upper extremity can be elevated on pillows. The use of the sling can be limited to times when the patient is walking.

Communication Disorders

Confusion of Terms

Communication may be affected by a language disorder, an impairment of speech production, or both. It is important to determine in which of these ways communication is affected, because impaired communication is very frustrating to the stroke patient and also because professionals dealing with the patient and the family will better understand how to communicate with the patient. There still tends to be an old persisting custom of referring to all communication disorders collectively as aphasia. Aphasia refers specifically to language problems and not to speech production problems.

Aphasia

Aphasia can be defined as an acquired impairment of verbal language behavior at the linguistic level caused by brain damage to the dominant cerebral hemisphere (usually the left).[44] It ordinarily affects all language areas to some degree, such as understanding the speech of others, speaking, reading, writing, and arithmetic, but may involve principally verbal expression or principally comprehension. The term *aphasia* does not apply to language disorder associated with primary sensory deficits (for example, deafness), mental deficiency, psychiatric problems, or neuromuscular involvement of the speech mechanism. The majority of stroke patients with aphasic communication disorders have difficulty with both input (auditory comprehension and reading) and output (speaking and writing). Usually their impairment is more marked in one area than in another. Hence, it is inappropriate to use specific labels such as *receptive aphasia, expressive aphasia,* and *mixed aphasia.* Terms sometimes used that relate to impairment of verbal expression are determined according to the classification used. Schuell and her colleagues[47] have designated five groups. Wepman and Jones[59] have a different type of classification: (1) syntactic aphasia, (2) semantic aphasia, (3) jargon aphasia, and (4) global aphasia. Aphasias can also be classified according to the anatomical localization of the lesion, such as Broca's aphasia and Wernicke's aphasia. Probably the most commonly used terms by speech pathologists are listed in Table 30–4, showing the distinguishing features in fluency, ability to repeat, and comprehension.

It is difficult to ascertain quickly what the patient's specific problems are in aphasia. Sometimes evaluation must be continued over many visits before the speech pathologist can adequately determine the types of aphasia and advise the other members of the rehabilitation team as to how they should attempt to communicate with the patient. In a rehabilitation team, most of the other members of the team may actually be performing more speech therapy than the speech pathologist, but the speech pathologist serves as the team's expert. The methods used may vary considerably as the rehabilitation process progresses and the patient makes some improvement.

Because categorization of the type of aphasia is not easy and takes time, it is difficult for the speech pathologist to state early what the prognosis for regaining language function is, unless the patient happens to have severe global aphasia. If the patient is classified according to Schuell's groupings, the group that the patient is placed in has a hierarchy of prognosis, the poorest being for group five, i.e., irreversible aphasia syndrome, which is virtually complete loss of language skills. In patients with severely involved aphasia, the principal early benefits of speech therapy are the supportive care given to the patient by the speech pathologist.[45] Most speech pathologists agree that spontaneous recovery of speech is probably not finished

TABLE 30–4. Distinguishing Features of Major Forms of Aphasia*

	FLUENCY	ABILITY TO REPEAT	COMPREHENSION
Broca's aphasia	Nonfluent	↓	+
Transcortical motor aphasia	Nonfluent	+	+
Global aphasia	Nonfluent	↓	↓
Wernicke's aphasia	Fluent	↓	↓
Transcortical sensory aphasia	Fluent	+	↓
Conduction aphasia	Fluent	↓	+

* ↓ , impaired.
+ , relatively intact.

until the end of the first three months. Following that time, as the patient reaches a plateau in functional improvement with speech therapy and makes no progress for two or three weeks, speech therapy may be discontinued for a while or limited to a few drills that can be performed at home with a periodic follow-up. However, in most cases patients do show progress with speech therapy, and it is feasible for the patient to continue speech therapy on an outpatient basis[46] (Fig. 30–7). This may continue for a long period of time, from 12 to 24 months. It is important to include the evaluation by a speech pathologist for those patients with completed stroke who have a communication disorder.

With neurologists, psychologists, and linguists working together in the study of aphasia, practical benefits in the treatment for aphasic patients should result, such as the development of theory-based aphasia test batteries and a new approach to aphasia therapy. A new national organization, the National Aphasia Association, which was

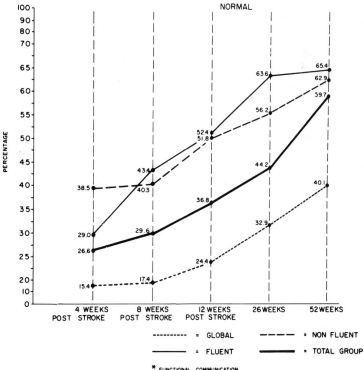

FIGURE 30–7. Functional Communication Profile Overall Scores (based on median scores by groups). (Included with permission of Sarno and Levita in STROKE, 10:633–670, 1979, by permission of the American Heart Association, Inc.)

founded in 1987, has been formed to help with the long-term needs of aphasic persons and their families.

Other Language Impairments in Stroke

Not all language impairments in stroke are due to involvement of specific speech areas in the left hemisphere. There may be confusion in language related to generalized reduced cognitive functioning. The patient with involvement of the right hemisphere may have impairment in language (particularly reading) due to visual-spatial and visual-motor impairment. In performing written arithmetic and reading the patient finds it difficult to follow the line across the page and to shift down from one line to the next. The speech pathologist can evaluate whether the patient is reliable in keeping a checkbook and whether, even though single words or sentences can be read that are single lines, the patient cannot read an entire paragraph and control the eyes to read it in the proper sequence to ascertain the meaning. Even for these disorders, there are some aspects of speech therapy that can be helpful, such as using a red line down the left margin of the page if the patient is having difficulty making the eyes track back far enough to the left. Also, if the patient has difficulty following a single line across the page in a paragraph, sometimes a piece of paper with a single line cut out, restricting visibility to one line at a time, will help.

Disorders of Speech Production

Dyspraxia. Dyspraxia in speech production is similar to dyspraxia in other kinds of motor function. It is an impairment of the ability of the patient to initiate simple voluntary motor acts. When the patient has difficulty in initiating voluntary motor function of the tongue and lips or cannot touch the tongue from one corner of the mouth to the other as directed or demonstrated, this condition is referred to as oral dyspraxia. On the other hand, some patients are able to move their tongue and lips on command or imitate tongue and lip movements of others but cannot initiate speech when asked to, even though they are capable of automatic speech that is quite clear and distinct. This is called oral-verbal dyspraxia. Sometimes patients with this condition need only a slight clue to get them started, such as making the first sound of a word. Unless the dyspraxia is severe, the prognosis is usually much better than the more severe forms of aphasia. However, it is not unusual for patients who have aphasia also to have some dyspraxia. It may take the speech pathologist working with the patient some time to be able to determine that both of these disorders are present. Hence, it is of great importance to have stroke patients with a confusing communication disorder evaluated by a speech pathologist who can advise others on the types of communication disorders present and on how to deal with the patient. For example, they can advise whether to try to guess the word that the patient is searching for, or to wait and give the patient time to find the word, or to give a clue by giving the first sound of the word that the patient is having difficulty initiating.

Dysarthria and Dysphonia. Other disorders of speech production are those associated with muscular weakness. Facial weakness on one side can be a cause of slurred speech referred to as dysarthria. Brain stem strokes may produce sufficient weakness in the laryngeal area to cause dysphonia or aphonia and render the patient speechless. Sometimes aphonic patients are mistakenly called aphasic and are even assumed to have no auditory comprehension, when actually their only problem is difficulty in speech production. Of course, patients with dysarthria and dysphonia can communicate by writing, which is ordinarily unimpaired, but they have to perform this act with their dominant hand.

Emotional Response and Personality Aspects of Completed Stroke

In addition to the effects of brain damage on cognitive functioning and personality, the patient with recent onset of completed stroke reacts to the newly acquired disability in a manner similar to those with other types of new disability. These reactions can usually be categorized in order of occurrence and frequency as denial, depression, anxiety, and hostility.

There tends to be confusion regarding patients with brain damage who have the phenomenon of anosognosia, those who ignore the extremities on the involved side, and those who display the emotional response termed denial. Most feel that these are two separate phenomena, the anosognosia being neurological[23] and the denial being emotional.[22] They discourage the use of the term *anatomical denial* to substitute for the term anosognosia. Generally, denial is seen as a protective mechanism to allow the patient to prepare to accept the reality of the loss and thereby perhaps avoid a sudden profound depression.[40] Furthermore, most patients who experience completed stroke know of some stroke patients who had remarkable recoveries. They like to cling to the idea that the neurological deficits they have experienced may be only temporary.

Depression has been considered by some to be part of the natural history of stroke. They maintain that all patients with significant deficits in completed stroke are bound to experience considerable depression simply because brain damage itself causes depression. However, some of the depression may be preventable, particularly that associated with intellectual deterioration due to environmental deprivation originating from isolation. A double-blind study of post-stroke depression[33] showed significantly better improvement in patients with nortriptyline than in a similar group of placebo-treated patients. Emotional lability associated with brain damage is sometimes confused with depression. The patient loses some of the inhibitory control over the expression of emotions, especially crying. This occurs with the slightest provocation but tends also to subside quickly. It often is much more easily tolerated by the patient and the family, particularly if the patient is male, if it is explained to them that this occurrence does not indicate a weakness of character or that the patient is losing control of mental faculties and that usually it is not a permanent condition. Emotional lability gradually subsides, lasting rarely past the first year after onset of the stroke.

Nearly all patients with completed stroke have very easy fatigability. Some of these patients, when placed in an environment or situation in which they feel obligated to remain active for longer periods of time than they feel like doing, will experience cumulative fatigue that can sometimes give the impression of a depressive state. During the early rehabilitation phase, it is well for a patient to have rest periods between appointments at various therapies. Generally, for most stroke patients, one of the most effective ways of counteracting depression is promoting a sense of progress and improvement. This can happen in rehabilitation, even when no further spontaneous return of neurological function occurs, if the therapist makes sure that the patient ends the daily periods of training with a performance the patient has learned to do well and provides positive verbal feedback to the patient for this successful performance.

It has been observed that premorbid personality traits of the patient appear to be exaggerated following completed stroke.[2] If the patient tended to be impulsive premorbidly, he or she tends to be even more impulsive after the stroke. For help in relieving both anxiety and depression reactions to stroke, counseling is certainly in order,[22] but nothing may be as helpful to the patient as seeing that he or she is making progress, improving functional abilities, and becoming less dependent. The professional staff working with the stroke patient who expresses hostility toward them should realize that sometimes this is a defense mechanism that shields the patient from acute guilt feelings and feeling responsible for the stroke. Rather, the patient transfers the responsibility to the health care profession. This may be a way of reducing the overwhelming emotional impact of the stroke.

Because there is a wide variation among people in all age groups in the amount of sexual activity they have, it cannot be assumed that sexuality is not important to the stroke patient; instead, this subject should be explored.[15] For those patients who are concerned, specific counseling should be sought. One study[39] reported that the most common factor identified as causing decline of sexual activity of stroke patients was the fear that having sex might adversely affect blood pressure and cause another stroke. The majority of stroke patients can continue to function sexually from a physical standpoint but need guidance and understanding from health professionals as well as their partners about readaptations that may need to be made.

Brain Stem Involvement

One should be cautious in applying generalizations to an individual patient. Each patient should be evaluated and treated individually. This is certainly true for patients with involvement of the brain stem because it contains both the ascending and descending tracts as well as cranial nerve nuclei. Damage within this area can produce a wide variety of symptoms. An impairment of the vertebral vascular system in the brain stem can produce a crossed hemiplegia or quadriplegia as well as a variety of signs of cranial nerve, cerebel-

THOMAS P. ANDERSON

lar, and sensory tract involvement. (See the section on dysarthria and dysphonia.) The patients with resulting ataxia may have normal motor strength but may be quite disabled by the ataxia. There are specific types of coordination exercises for both upper and lower extremities that help the patient regain control of coordination and reduce the amount of ataxia. However, this type of training must continue for a long period of time to produce significant clinical results that are observable in walking ability or in activities of daily living.

The speech pathologist can be of great help to patients who have brain stem involvement, not only to those who have difficulty in phonation but also to those who have difficulty in swallowing. Sometimes by experimentation, the speech pathologist, occupational therapist, and a nurse all working as a special team in the treatment of swallowing disorders can find ways to enhance the swallowing mechanism so that the patient does not have to continue nasogastric tube feeding for a long period or have a gastrostomy performed.

In a study[27] of 38 patients with a cerebrovascular accident who exhibited a variety of physiological disturbances in swallowing, the disturbances usually occurred in various combinations rather than as isolated disorders. A delayed swallowing reflex was the most frequent disorder. In another report,[53] seven consecutive patients who had lost the ability to swallow saliva or ingested food following a cerebrovascular accident were taught to eat again by instructing and drilling them in sucking, the elevation of the larynx, and the coordination of those functions.

Vocational Aspects

There has been a tendency in the past for patients who have completed stroke to be considered fit only for retirement, even though some of them may be considerably younger than retirement age. Part of this may be due to an attitude of the public of reluctance to hire or rehire a patient who has obvious hemiparesis. However, recent outcome studies[3, 5, 6] have made it clear that a larger percentage of patients with completed stroke are capable of some type of employment than had been assumed earlier. At the University of Minnesota, a special long-term outcome study[5] of younger stroke patients was made because it was felt that vocational aspects may have been neglected. In these patients, 54 per cent had returned to their usual daily activities, ranging from being employed full time or part time to being a full-time or part-time homemaker. In another study at the University of Minnesota,[3] only 53 per cent of post-rehabilitation stroke patients at all ages were unemployed at the time of follow-up. Hence the old attitude that most stroke patients are too old or too impaired to be able to return to employment has been proved to be erroneous. Vocational rehabilitation replacement should be considered for all those patients with completed stroke who are under retirement age, if this is feasible.

References

1. Adler, M. K., et al.: Stroke rehabilitation—is age a determinant? J. Am. Geriatr. Soc., 28:499–503, 1980.
2. Allison, R.: The Senile Brain. London, Edw. Arnold, Ltd., 1962.
3. Anderson, E., Anderson, T. P., and Kottke, F. J.: Stroke rehabilitation: Maintenance of achieved gains. Arch. Phys. Med. Rehabil., 58:345–352, 1977.
4. Anderson, T. P., et al.: Predictive factors in stroke rehabilitation. Arch. Phys. Med. Rehabil., 55:545–553, 1974.
5. Anderson, T. P., et al.: Stroke rehabilitation: Evaluation of its quality by assessing patient outcomes. Arch. Phys. Med. Rehabil., 59:170–175, 1978.
6. Anderson, T. P., et al.: Quality of care of stroke without rehabilitation. Arch. Phys. Med. Rehabil., 60:103–107, 1979.
7. Anderson, T. P.: Management of completed stroke. J. Okla. State Med. Assoc., 63:403–411, 1970.
8. Anderson, T. P., and Kottke, F. J.: Stroke rehabilitation: A reconsideration of some common attitudes. Arch. Phys. Med. Rehabil., 58:175–181, 1978.
9. Bard, G., and Hirschberg, G. G.: Recovery of voluntary motion in upper extremity following hemiplegia. Arch. Phys. Med. Rehabil., 46:567–572, 1965.
10. Basmajian, J. V.: Muscles Alive: Their Functions Revealed by Electromyography. Baltimore, Williams & Wilkins, 1967.
11. Basmajian, J. V., et al.: Stroke treatment: Comparison of integrated behavioral-physical therapy versus traditional physical therapy programs. Arch. Phys. Med. Rehabil., 68:267–272, 1987.
12. Basmajian, J. V., and Gowland, C. A.: The many hidden faces of stroke: A call for action. Arch. Phys. Med. Rehabil., 68:319, 1987.
13. Birch, H. G., et al.: Perception in hemiplegia: I. Judgement of vertical and horizontal. Arch. Phys. Med. Rehabil., 41:19–27, 1960.
14. Bohannon, R. W., et al.: Shoulder pain in hemiplegia: Statistical relationship with five variables. Arch. Phys. Med. Rehabil., 67:514, 1986.

15. Bray, G. P., et al.: Sexual functioning in stroke survivors. Arch. Phys. Med. Rehabil., 62:286–288, 1981.

16. Bruell, J. H., et al.: Perception of verticality in hemiplegia: Patients in relation to rehabilitation. Clin. Orthop., 12:124–130, 1958.

17. Carroll, D.: Hand function in hemiplegia. J. Chronic Dis., 18:493–500, 1965.

18. Cope, D. N., and Hall, K.: Head injury rehabilitation: Benefit of early intervention. Arch. Phys. Med. Rehabil., 63:433–437, 1982.

19. Delisa, J. A., et al.: Stroke rehabilitation, Part I. Cognitive deficits and prediction of outcome. Am. Fam. Pract., 26:207–214, Nov. 1982.

20. Feigenson, J. S., et al.: A comparison of outcome and cost for stroke patients treated in academic and community hospital centers. J.A.M.A., 240:1878–1880, 1978.

21. Fields, R. W.: Electromyographically triggered electric muscle stimulation for chronic hemiplegia. Arch. Phys. Med. Rehabil., 68:407–414, 1987.

22. Fisher, S. H.: Psychiatric considerations of cerebral vascular disease. Am. J. Cardiol., 7:379–385, 1961.

23. Friedlander, W. J.: Anosognosia and perception. Am. J. Phys. Med., 46:1394–1408, 1967.

24. Halpern, D., and Meelhuysen, F. E.: Duration of relaxation after intramuscular neurolysis with phenol. J.A.M.A., 200:1152–1154, 1967.

25. Hausmanouva-Petrusewicz, I.: Interaction in simultaneous motor functions. A.M.A. Arch. Neurol. Psychiatr., 81:173–181, 1959.

26. Hayes, S. H., and Carroll, S. R.: Early intervention care in the acute stroke patient. Arch. Phys. Med. Rehabil., 67:319–321, 1986.

27. Heimlich, H. J.: Rehabilitation of swallowing after stroke. Ann. Otol. Rhinol. Laryngol., 92:357, 1983.

28. Izzo, K. L., and Aquino, E.: Deep venous thrombosis in high risk hemiplegic patients: Detection by impedance plethysmography. Arch. Phys. Med. Rehabil., 67:799, 1986.

29. Kottke, F. J.: Neurophysiologic therapy for stroke. In Licht, S.: Stroke and Its Rehabilitation. New Haven, Conn., Elizabeth Licht, 1975.

30. Lee, K. H., and Khunadorn, F.: Painful shoulder in hemiplegic patients: A study of the suprascapular nerve. Arch. Phys. Med. Rehabil., 57:818, 1986.

31. Lehmann, J. F., et al.: Stroke rehabilitation: Outcome and prediction. Arch. Phys. Med. Rehabil., 56:383–389, 1975.

32. Lehmann, J. F., et al.: Stroke: Does rehabilitation affect outcome? Arch. Phys. Med. Rehabil., 56:375–382, 1975.

33. Lipsey, J. R., et al.: Nortriptyline treatment of post-stroke depression: A double-blind study. Lancet, 1(8372):303, 1984.

34. Lord, J. P., and Hall, K.: Neuromuscular reeducation versus traditional programs for stroke rehabilitation. Arch. Phys. Med. Rehabil., 67:88, 1986.

35. Machek, O.: Is elastic bracing contraindicated in spastics? Arch. Phys. Med. Rehabil., 39:245–246, 1958.

36. Matsumoto, N., et al.: Natural history of stroke in Rochester, Minnesota, 1955 through 1969: Extension of previous study 1945 through 1954. Stroke, 4:20–29, 1973.

37. McHenry, L. C., et al.: Essentials of stroke diagnosis and management. Philadelphia, Smith, Kline and French, 1973.

38. McHenry, L. C., and Jaffee, M. E.: Cerebrovascular disease, Part I. G.P., 37:88, 1968.

39. Monga, T. N., et al.: Sexual dysfunction in stroke patients. Arch. Phys. Med. Rehabil., 67:19, 1986.

40. Mossman, P. L.: A Problem Oriented Approach to Stroke Rehabilitation. Springfield, Ill., Charles C Thomas, Publisher, 1976.

41. Olney, S. J., et al.: Mechanical energy of walking of stroke patients. Arch. Phys. Med. Rehabil., 67:92–98, 1986.

42. Rehabilitation Nursing Techniques—1: Bed Positioning and Transfer Procedures for the Hemiplegic. Minneapolis, Kenny Rehabilitation Institute, 1962.

43. Rehabilitation Nursing Techniques—4: Selfcare and Homemaking for the Hemiplegic. Minneapolis, Kenny Rehabilitation Institute, 1962.

44. Sarno, M. T.: Disorders of communication. In Licht, S.: Stroke and Its Rehabilitation. New Haven, Conn., Elizabeth Licht, 1975.

45. Sarno, M. T., Silverman, E., and Sands, E.: Speech therapy and language recovery in severe aphasia. J. Speech Hear. Res., 13:607, 1970.

46. Sarno, M. T., and Levita, E.: Recovery in treated aphasia in the first year post-stroke. Stroke, 10:663–670, 1979.

47. Schuell, H. M., et al.: Aphasia in Adults. Diagnosis, Prognosis and Treatment. New York, Hoeber, 1964.

48. Smith, D. L., et al.: Motor function after stroke. Age Ageing, 14:46–48, 1985.

49. Stern, P., et al.: Effects of facilitation exercise techniques in stroke rehabilitation. Arch. Phys. Med. Rehabil., 51:526–531, 1970.

50. Taylor, M., et al.: Perceptual training in patients with left hemiplegia. Arch. Phys. Med. Rehabil., 52:163–169, 1971.

51. Van Buskirk, C., and Webster, D.: Prognostic value of sensory defects in rehabilitation of hemiplegics. Neurology, 5:407–411, 1955.

52. Van Ouwenaller, C., et al.: Painful shoulder in hemiplegia. Arch. Phys. Med. Rehabil., 67:23, 1986.

53. Veis, S. L., and Logemann, J. A.: Swallowing disorders in persons with cerebrovascular accident. Arch. Phys. Med. Rehabil., 66:372–375, 1985.

54. Wade, D. T., et al.: Stroke: The influence of age upon outcome. Age and Ageing, 13:357–362, 1984.

55. Wade, R. L., et al.: The hemiplegic arm after stroke: Measurement and recovery. Neurol. Neurosurg. Psychiatr., 46:521–524, 1983.

56. Wade, D. T., and Hewer, R. L.: Stroke: Associations with age, sex, and side of weakness. Arch. Phys. Med. Rehabil., 67:540, 1986.

THOMAS P. ANDERSON

57. Wall, J. C., and Turnbull, G. I.: Gait asymmetries in residual hemiplegia. Arch. Phys. Med. Rehabil., 67:550, 1986.
58. Waylonis, G. W., et al: Stroke rehabilitation in a mid-western county. Arch. Phys. Med. Rehabil., 54:151–155, 1973.
59. Wepman, J. M., and Jones, L. V.: Five aphasias. A commentary on aphasia as a regressive linguistic phenomenon. *In* Rioch, D. M., and Weinstein, E. A.: Disorders of Communication. Baltimore, Williams & Wilkins Co., 1964.
60. Wilson, B., et al.: Development of a behavioral test of visuospatial neglect. Arch. Phys. Med. Rehabil., 68:98–102, Feb 1987.

31

Rehabilitation in Arthritis and Allied Conditions

ROBERT L. SWEZEY

Physiatrists are frequently called on to assess and treat acute rheumatological and related musculoskeletal problems. Frequently, they serve as the primary diagnostician and manager to patients with degenerative joint disease and soft tissue rheumatism, as well as related diskogenic disorders. They are therefore called on to identify and distinguish systemic, inflammatory, and metabolic disorders that affect the joints and soft tissues, and physiatrists may play a primary or adjunctive role in the management of these conditions. Therefore, the physiatrist must be equipped to diagnose and understand the significance of various diagnostic categories of rheumatic diseases and to perceive when additional diagnostic clarification may be required in those patients referred for adjunctive therapies.

There are four major categories of rheumatological disorders to be considered: degenerative joint diseases, rheumatoid arthritis and related inflammatory processes, metabolic disorders affecting joints, and periarticular conditions. As is invariably the case in medical diagnosis, a careful history and physical examination are essential for an accurate diagnosis. A careful searching for clues of relevant systemic disease, such as a history of sun sensitivity, neuritis, urethritis, syphilis, exposure to hepatitis, and passage of a kidney stone, as well as familial predispositions, may alert the clinician to select those diagnostic measures most likely to lead to a correct diagnosis.

From a musculoskeletal disease standpoint, the clinician must first determine if the joint is indeed involved. Circumferential tenderness around the joint is highly indicative of an intra-articular process. In degenerative joint disease only one surface of the joint may be tender, but this is rarely the case in an inflammatory disorder. Restriction of joint motion, swelling, redness, and heat all point to intra-articular inflammatory disease. The clinician must then determine whether more than one joint is involved. Here, again, careful palpation of all symptomatic joint margins may elicit evidence of more than one affected joint and lead to the appropriate polyarticular diagnostic category.

Table 31–1 outlines the major diagnostic considerations when one is confronted with a true monarticular arthritis. In a monarticular arthritis, the most important decision to be made is whether infection is present. Synovial fluid aspiration is therefore essential; even if it is questionable whether synovial fluid has been obtained, a culture should be made from serum or blood from the aspirating needle.[1] Table 31–2 indicates various diagnoses that can be sorted out by an analysis of the synovial fluid. An elevated synovial fluid leukocyte count with a high percentage of polymorphonuclear leukocytes suggests infection; an analysis for crystals using polarizing light with a red compensating filter is invaluable in identifying sodium urate or calcium pyrophosphate crystals. A low serum complement is suggestive of rheumatoid arthritis or lupus, and an elevated serum complement is suggestive of Reiter's syndrome. A depression of the synovial fluid sugar may be seen in a number of inflammatory disorders but is suggestive of infection. Less specific indicators of inflammation are an elevated synovial fluid protein and reduced synovial fluid mucin viscosity.

If the disorder is polyarticular, then a much wider range of diagnostic considerations must be entertained. Table 31–3 outlines many of those

ROBERT L. SWEZEY

TABLE 31–1. Diagnostic Considerations in Monarticular Arthritis

TRANSIENT (<2 WEEKS)	ACUTE	SUBACUTE-CHRONIC
Initial phase of polyarthritis	Infection—septic	Infection—granuloma, TB
Palindromic rheumatism	Gout/pseudogout	Gout/pseudogout
Intermittent hydroarthrosis	Rheumatoid and variants	Rheumatoid and variants
Acute periarthritis	Trauma	Osteoarthritis
		Tumor
		Neuropathic (Charcot)
		Chronic Periarthritis

TABLE 31–2. Major Categorizations by Synovial Fluid Analysis

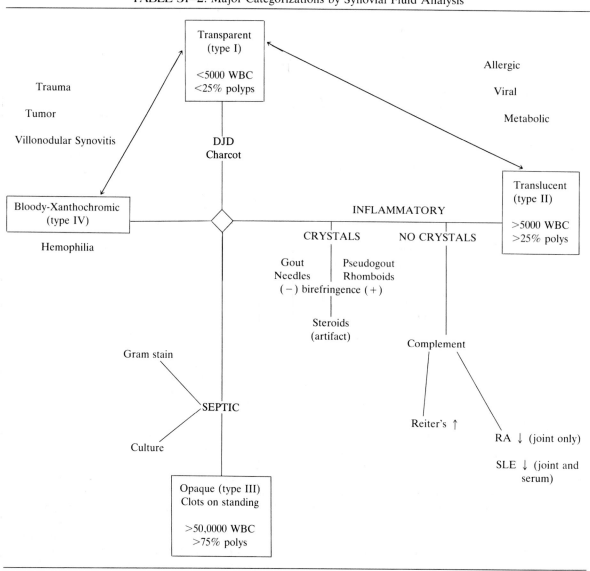

TABLE 31–3. Differential Diagnosis of Polyarthritis

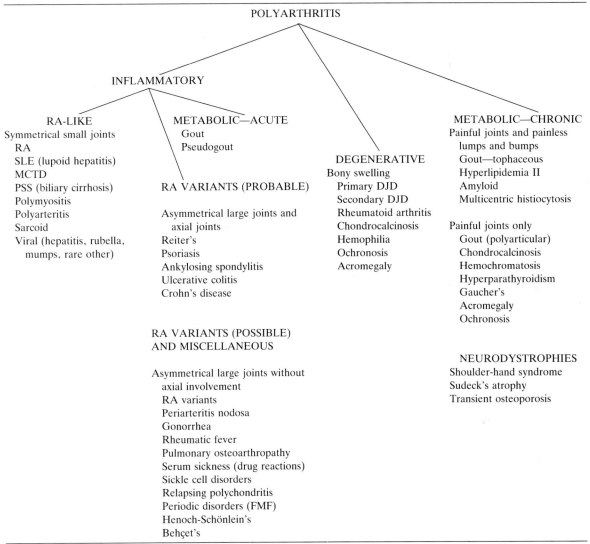

POLYARTHRITIS

INFLAMMATORY

RA-LIKE
Symmetrical small joints
RA
SLE (lupoid hepatitis)
MCTD
PSS (biliary cirrhosis)
Polymyositis
Polyarteritis
Sarcoid
Viral (hepatitis, rubella,
  mumps, rare other)

METABOLIC—ACUTE
  Gout
  Pseudogout

RA VARIANTS (PROBABLE)

Asymmetrical large joints and
  axial joints
Reiter's
Psoriasis
Ankylosing spondylitis
Ulcerative colitis
Crohn's disease

**RA VARIANTS (POSSIBLE)
AND MISCELLANEOUS**

Asymmetrical large joints without
  axial involvement
RA variants
Periarteritis nodosa
Gonorrhea
Rheumatic fever
Pulmonary osteoarthropathy
Serum sickness (drug reactions)
Sickle cell disorders
Relapsing polychondritis
Periodic disorders (FMF)
Henoch-Schönlein's
Behçet's

DEGENERATIVE
Bony swelling
Primary DJD
Secondary DJD
Rheumatoid arthritis
Chondrocalcinosis
Hemophilia
Ochronosis
Acromegaly

METABOLIC—CHRONIC
Painful joints and painless
  lumps and bumps
Gout—tophaceous
Hyperlipidemia II
Amyloid
Multicentric histiocytosis

Painful joints only
Gout (polyarticular)
Chondrocalcinosis
Hemochromatosis
Hyperparathyroidism
Gaucher's
Acromegaly
Ochronosis

NEURODYSTROPHIES
Shoulder-hand syndrome
Sudeck's atrophy
Transient osteoporosis

considerations and characterizes them further into the rheumatoid-like inflammatory disorders, the degenerative disorders, and acute and chronic metabolic disorders. In Table 31–4 the various diagnostic considerations that can be brought forward from the laboratory are outlined. Table 31–5 delineates those clues that can be obtained from x-ray examination of joints in addition to the affected joint or joints in question. Specific radiographic features that are often diagnostic are outlined in Table 31–6, and Table 31–7 lists supplementary nonarticular radiographic examinations that may be of great importance in establishing the final rheumatological diagnosis.

The various diagnostic laboratory and x-ray procedures accompanied by appropriate joint or other tissue biopsy will usually lead to the correct diagnosis, but only if the clinician has carefully performed the initial clinical evaluations. In making an assignment, there are *certain features that must be kept in mind if an accurate assessment of the clinical findings is to be made.* Whenever an apparently normal range-of-joint mobility is found where one has reason to suspect an abnormality, hypermobility on the *opposite side should be sought.* Bilateral *elbow joint contractures* are often telltale indicators of current or previous rheumatoid disease. They may, however, represent con-

TABLE 31–4. Laboratory Determinations of Diagnostic Help*

LABORATORY TEST	HELPFUL IN FOLLOWING CONDITIONS
Initial Survey	
Antinuclear antibodies or ANA	JRA (chronic iritis), MCTD, PSS, SLE, anti-ds DNA (SLE)
Complete blood count	Anemia, infection, leukemia, leukopenia (Felty's syndrome), sickle cell disorders, SLE
Culture, blood	Sepsis, SBE
Culture, special site (mouth, anus)	Gonorrhea, sepsis
Rheumatoid factor (latex)	RA (falsely positive in chronic inflammation, leprosy, liver disease, SBE, syphilis)
Sedimentation rate	Inflammatory disorders, PMR (high)
SMA 12	
Alkaline phosphatase	Acromegaly, biliary cirrhosis, fracture, Paget's disease
Calcium, inorganic phosphorus	Hyperparathyroidism, sarcoidosis, vitamin D intoxication
Cholesterol	Type II hyperlipidemia
Glucose	Charcot joint disease, diabetes mellitus
Lactic acid dehydrogenase (LDH), aspartate aminotransferase (AST)	Hepatitis with arthritis, polymyositis
Total bilirubin	Biliary cirrhosis, hepatitis
Urea nitrogen	Vasculitis with renal disease
Uric acid	Gout
Urinalysis, routine	Amyloidosis, metabolic disease, renal calculus, systemic vasculitis
Augmented Survey	
Antistreptolysin-O (ASO) titer	Rheumatic fever
Creatine phosphokinase, aldolase	Polymyositis
Deoxyribonucleic acid (DNA), extractable nuclear antigen (ENA)	SLE, MCTD, anticentromere (PSS, CREST)
Hemoglobin electrophoresis	Sickle cell disorders
Heterophile agglutinins	Infectious mononucleosis
HLA B27	Ankylosing spondylitis, RA variants, Reiter's syndrome
Protein electrophoresis	Agammaglobulinemia, multiple myeloma, sarcoidosis, Sjögren's syndrome, SLE
Serum amylase, lipase	Arthritis in pancreatic disease
Serum complement	Polyarteritis, serum sickness, SLE (reduced)
Triiodothyronine (T3), thyroxine (T4)	Arthralgia, hyper- or hypothyroidism, myopathy
VDRL (Venereal Disease Research Laboratories)	Charcot joint disease, secondary syphilis, SLE (biologic false-positive)
Supplemental Survey	
Anticytoplasmic antibodies	Anti-Ro (SS-A) primary Sjögren's
Coagulation profile	Clotting disorders
Cryoglobulin, immunoglobulins	Lymphomatous disorders, serum protein abnormalities
Serum iron (transferrin)	Hemochromatosis, iron deficiency

*Table adapted from Rehabilitation in joint and connective tissue disorders. *In* Medical Knowledge Self-Assessment Program in Physical Medicine and Rehabilitation Syllabus. Chicago, American Academy of Physical Medicine and Rehabilitation, 1977, p. G6. Reprinted with permission from the publisher.

CREST, a mild PSS variant; JRA, juvenile rheumatoid arthritis; LE, lupus erythematosus; MCTD, mixed connective tissue disease; PMR, polymyalgia rheumatica; PSS, progressive systemic sclerosis; RA, rheumatoid arthritis; SBE, subacute bacterial endocarditis; SLE, systemic lupus erythematosus; SMA 12, sequential multiple analysis (12 tests).

TABLE 31–5. X-Ray Survey

Hands (posterior-anterior)	Osteoarthritis, rheumatoid arthritis, sarcoid, chondrocalcinosis (calcification of the triangular cartilage in wrist)
Chest (posterior-anterior and lateral)	Tuberculosis, sarcoid and other granuloma, pneumonitis and pleuritis with collagen vascular disease, malignancy, erythema nodosoum, osteoporosis, compression fractures
Cervical spine (lateral in mild flexion)	C 1–C 2, subluxation in rheumatoid arthritis C 2–C 3, fusion in juvenile rheumatoid arthritis C 4–C 7, fusion in ankylosing spondylitis, osteophytes in degenerative joint disease of cervical spine;
Pelvis (anterior-posterior)	Sacroiliac joint disease in ankylosing spondylitis, hip joint disease, and calcification of symphysis in chondrocalcinosis
Knee (standing anterior-posterior)	Degenerative joint disease, rheumatoid arthritis, Charcot (or neuropathic) arthritis, and chondrocalcinosis of menisci

genital abnormalities, and this can usually be established by asking the patient. Congenital flexion contractures of the proximal interphalangeal (PIP) joints of the fifth fingers are particularly common. Restricted flexion of the distal interphalangeal (DIP) joints to 45 degrees found in multiple joints or in symmetrical joints is usually a congenital variation. A normal PIP joint should flex beyond 90 degrees to approximately 110 to 120 degrees. A *subluxation of a small joint is detected by the sensation of a distinct ledge,* rather than an indented cleft (a bayonet configuration) at the adjacent joint margins. Most patients over the age of 50 years have restriction of internal rotation of both hips. If restriction of mobility of the hip joints is asymmetrical or all planes of motion are restricted and painful, then hip joint involvement is highly suspect. Restrictions of joint mobility may be very difficult to assess in the presence of severe pain, and one should not assume a contracture where reflex muscle spasm may be restricting joint motion. Pain also alters the response on muscle testing. In the presence of joint disease, the joint should be placed and supported to minimize pain and then the muscle in question tested isometrically. If care is taken to avoid pain, one will get a "normal" response to manual tests performed in this manner unless true neuropathic or myopathic disease or muscle-tendon rupture is present.[2, 3]

Diagnostic and Therapeutic Considerations in Joint Diseases

Just as certain features of various joint disorders help characterize them diagnostically, the pathophysiological features of the joint disorder, its natural history, the location of the joints that are affected, the severity of the joint involvements, and the customary response to treatment of the joint disorder in question will all help determine the ordering of specific therapeutic interventions.

Osteoarthritis (Degenerative Joint Disease)

Although osteoarthritis is relatively rare in young adults, it can be predictably diagnosed in association with the inevitable disk degeneration of the spine in all patients over the age of 50 years. The problem is whether roentgenographic confirmation of osteoarthritis can be correlated with clinical symptoms. Obviously this is not true in the case of spinal diskogenic disease in the geriatric population, but *most patients with radiographic evidence of osteoarthritis in other axial or peripheral joints will either have or give a history of having had symptoms.*

Osteoarthritis is a disorder in which bony proliferation at the joint margins and subchondral bone is a consequence of deterioration in the articular cartilage. The earliest changes in osteoarthritis are a depolymerization of the glycoprotein ground substance surrounding the chondrocytes, and this is subsequently associated with fissuring of the overlying cartilage surface, wearing away of the cartilage surface, and bony proliferations that may lead to juxta-articular bony cyst formation with ultimate collapse of these cysts and derangements of joint surfaces.[4] The synovial fluid that nourishes the cartilage and lubricates the joint surfaces does not appear to be at fault as a lubricant, and the exact mechanism whereby the cartilage deteriorates cannot always be ascertained.[5–7]

In those disorders in which the osteoarthritis is secondary to a previous trauma or inflammation,

TABLE 31–6. Disorders for Which X-Ray Examination is Often Diagnostic

BONE AND JOINT	Osteophyte	Sclerosis	Free Joint Ossicles	Joint Narrowing	Bone Proliferation	Periosteal Proliferation	Bone Resorption	Joint Margin Erosion	Bony Cysts	Osteoporosis	Cartilage Calcification	Extra-Articular Calcification	Subluxation	Bony Ankylosis	
Osteoarthritis (DJD)	X	X	X	X	X										Asymmetrical joint narrowing; findings of DJD are common in gout, chondrocalcinosis, trauma, osteochondromatosis
Neuropathic (Charcot)	X	X	X	X	X	X	X		X		X	X	X		Highly variable findings with large effusions characteristically observed
Ochronosis	X	X	X	X	X			X	X		X				Disk calcifications and severe generalized DJD
Acromegaly	X	X			X										Tufting of terminal phalanges due to bone growth; widening of joint spaces due to cartilage growth
Rheumatoid (RA)				X		X	X	X	X	X			X	X	Diffuse cartilage loss (joint narrowing), marginal erosions of MCP and MTP joints
Juvenile RA				X	X	X	X	X	X	X			X	X	Hypoplastic mandible, irregular epiphyseal closures; fusion of C 2–C 3 or C –3–C 4
Psoriasis				X	X	X	X	X		X			X	X	Destructive widening of DIP joints
Septic Arthritis				X	X	X	X	X		X					Soft tissue changes are seen only for 2 to 3 weeks
Hyperparathyroidism						X	X		X	X	X				Resorption of radial aspect of middle phalanges and of distal clavicles
Paget's		X			X										Secondary DJD is common
Aseptic necrosis		X	X			X				X					Cartilage loss and secondary DJD come late; bone scan is more sensitive; MRI is most sensitive

Disorder	Comments
Tophaceous gout	Calcification of tophus
Chondrocalcinosis	May occur coincidentally in other diseases
Calcific periarthritis	Calcifications may be transient
Scleroderma (PSS)	Subcutaneous calcifications, resorption of distal phalanges is typical
Reiter's	When periosteal thickening or bone proliferation on the anterior calcaneus is present
Pulmonary osteoarthritis	Distal ends of long bone ± clubbing
Sarcoid	Usually x-ray study is of no assistance
Ankylosing spondylitis (AS)	These findings apply to sacroiliac joints and axial joints; CT is more sensitive
Osteochondromatosis	Single to multiple

DISORDERS FOR WHICH X-RAY EXAMINATION OFTEN SUGGESTS THE DIAGNOSIS

Disorder	Comments
Amyloidosis	Large soft tissue shoulder masses are rare but distinctive
Chronic SLE	MCP and PIP subluxations without erosions are suggestive
Hemochromatosis	Erosions of index and middle MCP joints
Lymphomas	
Multicentric reticulohistiocytosis	Can be confused with RA, psoriasis, gout

685

ROBERT L. SWEZEY

TABLE 31–7. Radiographs Often Helpful in Diagnosing Extra-Articular Manifestations

Barium swallow	Polymyositis and progressive systemic sclerosis (PSS)
Dental films	Resorption of lamina dura in hyperparathyroidism and PSS
Upper GI	Duodenal widening in progressive systemic sclerosis
Small bowel follow-through	Crohn's disease
Barium enema	Ulcerative colitis, wide-mouth diverticuli in PSS
Chest film	Granuloma, infection, TB, sarcoid, Wegener's granulomatosis, rheumatoid arthritis, progressive systemic sclerosis, SLE, periarteritis nodosa, malignancy
Abdominal arteriogram	Polyarteritis (aneurysms)
Bone scan	Malignant disorders or osteomyelitis
MRI	Aseptic necrosis, loose bodies, torn menisci, metastasis

the basis for the particular cartilage deterioration is apparent. In the so-called primary osteoarthritis, a genetic factor is clearly operative, but the biochemical nature of the defect that renders the cartilage susceptible to deterioration has not yet been identified. Primary osteoarthritis is characterized by its dominant genetic inheritance pattern, which is fully expressed in females after the menopause and less often expressed in the male siblings. Characteristically it affects the distal interphalangeal joints and the carpometacarpal joint of the thumbs. The distal interphalangeal joint involvement creates bony prominences on the dorsal surface, originally described by Heberden, and similar subsequent involvement of the proximal interphalangeal joints is called Bouchard's nodes. Patients with severe primary generalized osteoarthritis may also have involvement of the knees, much less commonly the hips, and occasionally the small joints in the toes in addition to the first metatarsophalangeal (MTP) joint.[7] Acromioclavicular joints may be affected, and only rarely are the glenohumeral joints involved. Generally the elbows and ankles are spared. The wrists, however, are occasionally involved in the joints between the navicular and lunate and navicular and greater multangular.

There are two distinctive features of primary osteoarthritis that merit comment. Although the typical development of Heberden's nodes is minimally symptomatic or asymptomatic, on occasion the onset can be fairly acute and accompanied by a cystic erythematous mass overlying the DIP joint, which is red and extremely tender. The mass, which may persist for months, consists of a mucinous cyst that communicates with the joint. Local steroid injections and rest or splinting will usually relieve the acute symptoms. Less commonly the distal interphalangeal and occasionally proximal interphalangeal joint involvement is characterized by an aggressive, erosive, destructive process that pathologically is manifested by an acute inflammatory reaction and that leads to marked destruction and derangement of the affected DIP and PIP joints, the so-called erosive osteoarthritis. Synovectomy and surgical stabilization of the affected joints may occasionally be necessary to preserve function in such cases.[8]

The *most disabling problem in the hand in association with primary osteoarthritis* is *the involvement of the first carpometacarpal joint.* Atrophy of the overlying thenar musculature and inhibition of normal joint use lead to an adductor contracture with impairment of grasp and pinch. Splinting to stabilize this joint in addition to occasional use of local steroid injections with gentle stretching of the adductor musculature between the thumb and index metacarpals can help preserve mobility (Fig. 31–1). Excision of the greater multangular or joint replacement and occasionally fusion of the carpometacarpal joint are sometimes necessary to relieve pain and preserve function. As is generally true in the management of osteoarthritis when avoidance of joint stress, stabilization, and the use of occasional local steroid injections are insufficient, local heat, salicylates, and occasional use of other analgesics or nonsteroidal anti-inflammatory drugs may be helpful in management of the specific joint problem.

Osteoarthritis of the hip is an insidious problem of middle and late adult life that typically manifests itself with pain in the groin, as well as in the buttock and lateral thigh. Congenital shortening of the leg on the affected side, pathological change of the opposite knee, a childhood slipped capital femoral epiphysis, and osteochondritis are common predisposing factors in addition to previous inflammatory arthritis or trauma.[7] Nevertheless, for most patients who develop osteoarthritis of the hip, the cause is not easily ascertained. Pain in the buttock area is often attributed to the hip when in fact it may be due to lumbar diskogenic disease. Pain in the upper lateral thigh may be due to trochanteric bursitis, which is commonly seen in

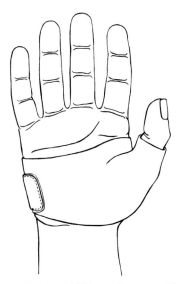

FIGURE 31–1. Plastic stabilizing splint to restrict motion of the carpometacarpal and metacarpophalangeal joints of the thumb. This splint allows full interphalangeal flexion. The distal palmar edge of the splint is proximal to the distal palmar crease so as not to restrict MCP flexion of the fingers. (From Swezey, R. L.: Arthritis: Rational Therapy in Rehabilitation. Philadelphia, W. B. Saunders Company, 1978.)

association with osteoarthritis of the hip, but it may also be an unrelated problem. In addition to pharmacological measures, which again include salicylates, mild analgesics, nonsteroidal anti-inflammatory drugs, and a trial of local steroid injections, the rehabilitative management consists of relief of weight-bearing stresses by the use of a cane or crutches, early stretching of the tight hip musculature to maintain good mobility and joint surface apposition for optimal joint nutrition, and strengthening of the hip musculature.[9] Activities that cause undue stress, including jogging and hiking, are best avoided. In all overweight patients with arthritis in weight-bearing joints, weight reduction is an important factor. Bicycling may be tolerated if there is little inflammatory reaction in the hip. Swimming is the optimal overall exercise, both for mobilizing the hip and strengthening the musculature and for its general conditioning effect on patients whose athletic activities are otherwise circumscribed. When pain cannot be well controlled with these regimens and particularly when pain consistently disturbs rest at night or functional activities are greatly limited, surgical therapy is indicated.[10, 11]

Osteoarthritis of the knee is frequently a result of damage secondary to meniscal injury and other trauma. Patellofemoral compartment degeneration (chondromalacia of the patella) is a disorder that affects young people and is the exception to the usual pattern of medial tibiofemoral joint disease with narrowing of the tibiofemoral compartment and early proliferation of osteophytes on the opposing medial tibial and femoral borders.[12] People with genu varus deformities carry the bulk of their weight-bearing stresses in the medial compartment and are predisposed to osteoarthritis in that area, as opposed to those with valgus angulation of the knee joint, who are predisposed to lateral tibiofemoral joint disease.

The treatment of osteoarthritis of the knee includes the same drug and local steroid considerations previously described for the hip, as well as the recommendations for avoidance of weight-bearing stress. In all disorders of joints, as is particularly obvious in the knee, atrophy of the related musculature occurs as a consequence of the reduction in active use of the affected joint. Quadriceps strengthening and instruction in body mechanics to avoid unnecessary knee stress that may occur when arising from chairs or toilet stools that are too low are key features in successful management. Isometric strengthening of the quadriceps musculature should be initiated in a regimen consisting of six seconds of quadriceps strengthening twice daily (Fig. 31–2). The exercise should be performed in a position of maximum comfort, which is usually in extension for the patient with osteoarthritis of the knee, and particularly for those patients with patello-femoral compartment disease. There is no established basis for the additional use of isotonic or isokinetic exercise, although these may be added if desired, but only when pain permits (see *Exercise Therapy*).[13]

Flexion contractures in osteoarthritic knees are usually minimal, and apparent contractures in more advanced cases may be a consequence of bone obstruction; therefore, range-of-motion exercises may not be required in many cases of osteoarthritis of the knee.

Attention to leg length discrepancies should be given, and at least a 50 per cent compensation in the height of the shortened extremity should be made. For both the hip and the knee, good supporting footwear is essential to minimize joint stress. A shock-absorbing sole is useful; however, the sole should not be made of a crepe so soft that it creates an unstable gait because of excessive yielding at heel strike. A maximum heel height of 1 inch is recommended for any patient with osteoarthritis of the knee, and this is particularly important in patients with patellofemoral joint

ROBERT L. SWEZEY

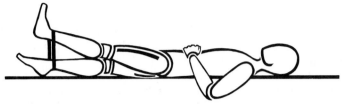

FIGURE 31–2. Isometric counterresistance exercise of quadriceps vs. contralateral gluteal and hamstring muscles using an elastic band or belt looped over both ankles. (From Swezey, R. L.: Arthritis: Rational Therapy in Rehabilitation. Philadelphia, W. B. Saunders Company, 1978.)

compartment disease, for which a negative heel may actually be preferred.

When conservative measures have failed to provide sufficient pain relief or restoration of function, surgical procedures must be considered. The success rate of the numerous variations on total knee replacement does not approach that of the total hip procedures.[10, 11, 14, 15] The postoperative management is difficult because of pain and because more cooperation on the part of the patient is required during the postoperative period to restore mobility and function.

Osteoarthritis of the foot and ankle. The ankle is essentially spared by osteoarthritic disorders except as a consequence of trauma or secondary to another disease process such as rheumatoid arthritis. The management of these problems includes the usual pharmacological and local steroid therapy considerations, avoidance of weight-bearing stresses, and use of appropriate supporting footwear. Supportive footwear may include a high-top shoe, a rigid shank, a cushion heel, a rocker sole, or a supportive leg-hindfoot orthosis.[16] In those patients in whom distress is not being controlled by these measures, a below-knee weight-bearing brace or surgical therapy must be considered.[17] *Osteoarthritic changes in the proximal tarsal joints* are not uncommon; the bony prominences protruding from the dorsal surfaces of these joints are common and sometimes symptomatic. Therapeutic considerations include good supporting footwear with multiple lacings to give a supporting corset effect to the proximal tarsal joints.

The most common problems in the forefoot are those that affect the great toe. Hallux valgus and secondary osteoarthritis of the first MTP joint and/or IP joint are common disabling disorders. Appropriate shoewear with adequate room in the forefoot and a rigid sole with the roll-over or rocker feature or an orthosis providing similar features to minimize stress in the joints is helpful.[17] Local steroid injections are occasionally of value in relieving acute symptoms. Surgical therapy to improve cosmesis is useful and can be helpful in relieving pain in refractory cases. The status of prosthetic arthroplasties of the MTP joint is not established, but this may hold promise to achieve not only improved cosmesis and pain relief, but also improved toe-off function during ambulation.

Soft Tissue Rheumatism (Bursitis and Fibrositis)

If, until the recent advent of reconstructive surgery, osteoarthritis has been the stepchild of rheumatology, then the soft tissue disorders have been the orphans. Musculoskeletal complaints attributable to soft tissue rheumatism probably account for the vast majority of rheumatological disorders. Because the complaints are often mild and accepted as part of the natural course of events, and because many of the problems are self-limited and the justification for surgical intervention is almost nil, there has been relatively little interest in defining the nature of these problems and in developing rational approaches to their management. Perhaps the major deterrent to careful assessment of these disorders is the lack of "objective" findings such as laboratory or x-ray confirmation of a diagnosis. Calcium deposits in tendons and bursae may be found on occasion, and they may or may not correlate with the clinical condition in question. Clinicians are left with their fingertips and thumbs and their knowledge of anatomy and kinesiology to locate the source of the patient's complaint. Having done so, they must presume more knowledge than they can confirm in establishing the diagnosis; e.g., is the painful shoulder due to a rotator cuff tendinitis, a bicipital tendinitis, a subacromial bursitis, a referred cervical myalgia, an idiopathic adhesive capsulitis, or a true arthritis? The examiner's knowledge and hands, and the lack of supporting evidence for other conditions, allow a diagnosis to be made—i.e., bicipital tendinitis. Who can refute it?

There are, in fact, a number of disorders that are commonly seen and for which either definitive or presumptive diagnoses of soft tissue rheumatism can be made.[18] In general, one can say that *the management of soft tissue disorders* will depend on their severity and chronicity. Treatments will consist variably of the use of cold applications in acute processes; warm compresses in more chronic processes; diathermy for diffuse chronic processes, and ultrasound for focal chronic processes; rest of the part, which may include immobilization by sling or splint in the more acute disorders and functional splinting in more quiescent disorders; and adjunctive therapy consisting of analgesics and non-steroidal anti-inflammatory drugs, depending on the severity of the process.[19] By and large, *those focal disorders* of ligaments, tendons, or bursae (see muscle trigger points) *that are either very severe* or *very persistent,* e.g., lasting more than three or four weeks, are most expeditiously treated by the use of a local steroid injection consisting of approximately 2.5 mg of triamcinolone in 1 to 2 ml of 1 per cent lidocaine, followed by range of motion exercises to increase mobility if mobility of the affected joint area has been lost, and then isometric exercises of the affected related musculature. Isometric exercises are first performed in a restricted range and, when tolerated, at the extremes of joint range with or without the addition of isokinetic exercise. Instruction in body mechanics is essential to help avoid the stresses that predispose to the problem.

Fibrositis Syndrome. The most elusive disorder of the various conditions that can be categorized under soft tissue rheumatism is the fibrositis syndrome. It consists of local and focal areas of muscle tenderness *(trigger points)* and soft tissue enthesis and bursae (tender points), usually limited to the region of the axial skeleton extending over the shoulder and hip areas and out onto the trunk.[20] Occasionally ramifications of this disorder will be felt in so-called tender areas as far as the ankle, and not uncommonly in the posterior calf in either of the heads of the gastrocnemius muscle or at the musculotendinous juncture of the soleus muscle.[21–23] The term *fibrositis* is undoubtedly a misnomer, because cellular inflammation has not been observed.[24] The basic pathological change appears to be the development of hyperirritable and usually anatomically predictable so-called trigger points of muscle spasm, usually as a consequence of pain referral from axial skeletal or, less commonly, large proximal joint derangements.[21–24] Pathologically, whereas inflammation is lacking, an in-

creased intracellular amorphous deposit with increased numbers of mast cells, platelets, and giant intracellular myofilaments has been observed.[24] Electromyographical abnormalities have been inconsistent, but short-duration high-pitched motor unit potentials have been noted by several observers when a needle electrode is inserted into the trigger point. There has been no evidence of consistent motor unit firing nor evidence of muscle spasm *per se* by electromyographical criteria.[19, 25] A recent report indicates a disturbance of normal delta wave sleep patterns in patients with the fibrositis syndrome with reduction in symptoms as a consequence of chlorpromazine therapy used to induce normal sleep patterns.[21] From a clinical standpoint a fibrositic syndrome may therefore occur as a primary disorder, perhaps related to sleep disturbance, and as a secondary disorder related to a variety of focal or general inflammatory and degenerative joint disorders. The recognition of the primary fibrositic syndrome is important in that many of these patients who are tense, worried, and particularly fearful that they are developing a severe arthritic disease are greatly benefited by the reassurance that this is not the case. These patients are susceptible to cold and drafts. Fatigue and nervous tension aggravate their symptoms. They should be cautioned against exposing themselves to these stresses, but at the same time it should be pointed out that the only danger is temporarily increased pain and discomfort, and not a progressive crippling joint problem.

Mechanical stresses from inappropriate body mechanics during activities or during sedentary occupations should be avoided. Typically, it is suggested to patients that they obtain a firm mattress or place a board under the mattress and that they obtain proper seating and lighting as well as needed spectacles for reading purposes or television viewing. Instructions are given in general warm-up and conditioning exercises to maintain body mobility and conditioning so that unaccustomed activities are less apt to precipitate fibrositic stresses. When symptoms are persistent, the local trigger points can be treated with ice massage, fluorimethane spray and stretch techniques, kneading massage, local heat, local electrical stimulation, and local ultrasound, in addition to mild analgesics such as aspirin or acetaminophen.[19, 26, 28] Local 1 per cent lidocaine injections are often helpful in the management of severe or refractory "trigger" points. Note that since the trigger points are apparently areas of reflex muscular irritability rather than inflammation, the addition of steroids to

ROBERT L. SWEZEY

injection therapy offers no additional advantage and may produce unneeded irritation at the injection site.

The fact that tension, fatigue, and psychological stresses exacerbate this problem does not make it a psychogenic rheumatism *per se*, but psychological and social counseling may be of additional benefit in many of these patients, and low dosages of antidepressant drugs are often helpful.[20] When the fibrositic nodules occur secondary to other disorders such as lumbar or cervical diskogenic disease, appropriate therapy directed to these problems, in addition to the local therapy to the reflex trigger points, may facilitate the total management.

Some of the *common locations for trigger points* in muscles are the origins and insertion of the upper trapezii at the base of the skull and just superior to the superior medial angle of the scapulae along the lower third of the medial angle of the scapulae and the rhomboid, in the paracervical musculature, at the lateral edge of the quadratus lumborum, at the origin of the erector spinae just medial to the posterior superior iliac spine, in the gluteus medius origin just below the iliac crest, and in the areas overlying the sciatic outlet, the subgluteus medius, and subgluteus maximus bursae.[22, 23, 27, 28] Less commonly they can be found in the scalenes, infraspinati, anterior tibials, gastrocnemii, and soleus muscles.[22, 23, 27, 28]

Often confused with these focal trigger points are fibrofatty nodules that may range in number from one to many and that are typically located in the region of the posterior superior iliac spines.[29] These are benign and in this author's experience rarely a cause of symptoms. Severe and diffuse stiffness, aching, and "fibrositic" symptoms are characteristic of polymyalgia rheumatica and accompany rheumatoid arthritis, ankylosing spondylitis, hypothyroidism, and viral infections.

Focal Syndromes

Tendinitis and bursitis occur as a consequence of repeated low-grade irritation due to unaccustomed or excessively strenuous activity in otherwise normal structures or as a result of such activity that is poorly tolerated in abnormal structures. Typical examples are trochanteric bursitis associated with hip joint disease or anserine bursitis in association with osteoarthritis of the knees. Calcific deposits (calcium hydroxyapatite crystals) in tendinous areas, most notably the rotator cuff tendon, may be extruded into adjacent bursae and produce an acute crystal-induced bursitis.[30] This is often an extremely painful disorder, such that the patient suffers agonizing pain even at rest and will not accept the best-intended examination. X-ray documentation of this diagnosis may or may not be made because of the edema associated with the inflammatory reaction and the diffusion of the extruded calcium hydroxyapatite crystals into the swollen bursal area may obscure calcium deposits. Calcium hydroxyapatite crystals associated with tendinitis may also occasionally be seen in the region of the trochanteric bursa and rarely in the region of the short thumb extensor tendon in association with de Quervain's disease.

There is a disorder, acute calcific periarthritis, in which calcific deposits recur variously, most commonly in the region of the extensor carpi ulnaris at the wrist and in and around the small joints of the hands.[31] Although usually idiopathic, it may rarely be seen in association with either hyperparathyroidism or as a complication of chronic kidney disease, in particular renal dialysis.[32]

Acute bursitis, with or without local crystal extrusions, is treated with analgesic medication, cold or ice applications, immobilization, and nonsteroidal anti-inflammatory agents.[30] If a prompt response is not seen, short-term oral steroids (if not otherwise contraindicated) such as prednisone in a dose of 0.5 mg/kg for three or four days will usually provide relief. Local steroid injections are equally beneficial, but when the pain is extremely severe, the patient may not accept this procedure. When symptoms have abated sufficiently, first gentle range-of-motion exercises followed later by active stretching to restore loss of mobility and finally isometric exercises to regain strength should be instituted.

A *rule of thumb in the management of all painful joint disorders* is to *restore mobility as a first priority* rather than risk exacerbation of symptoms in a strengthening regimen that might lead ultimately to aggravation of the joint problem and loss of motion and function. It should also be mentioned that local corticosteroid injections into tendons can cause collagen necrosis, and a steroid should never be forced from the syringe but rather should flow freely into the tendon sheath or bursal space during the injection. Excessive use of a damaged tendon made possible by pain relief from steroid injection may predispose a tendon to rupture. The patient should be instructed to avoid excessive use of tendinous structures following injections for a period of four weeks.

There are several bursal areas in addition to the subacromial bursa that merit comment. The *olecranon bursa* may swell as a consequence of rheumatoid arthritis, often with associated subcutaneous nodule formation, and it may also become swollen without severe pain in patients with gout. Where there is no adequate explanation for the olecranon bursal swelling, the bursa should be aspirated and a synovial fluid analysis made. There are two bursae that are consistently present around the hip: the *subgluteus medius bursa*, which lies deep to the insertion of the gluteus medius muscle at the superior angle of the greater trochanter, and the *subgluteus maximus bursa*, which lies beneath the muscle at the inferior lateral edge of the greater trochanter near the insertion of the gluteus maximus into the fascia lata. These bursae become irritated in association with mechanical stresses about the hip joint secondary to arthritis of the hip, leg length discrepancies associated with contractures of the muscles attaching to the fascia lata (the fascia lata syndrome), or static or dynamic postural stresses in association with low back pain.[33] In many instances in which lumbar diskogenic disease is present and pain is referred, trochanteric bursal irritation can be confused with radiculitis because of its referral into the lateral thigh. It is difficult, if not impossible, to determine whether the focal tenderness found in the trochanteric bursal locations is secondary to muscle trigger points or to bursal involvement *per se*, but in this author's experience, in contrast with muscle trigger points, local steroid injections have proved to be far more effective than any other therapeutic intervention regardless of whether the hip joint or a lumbar disk disease was the inciting factor.

When the bursitis is severe, cold compresses are useful; when the bursitis has largely subsided, gentle mobilizing exercises are performed, initially with the patient supine with the knees flexed and feet flat, and then both legs rotated to the side opposite that of the affected bursa in a manner to cause a mild stretch but to avoid exacerbating pain. When the contralateral knee can be rotated to touch the floor, then a more advanced pelvis and hip rotation exercise can be instituted (Fig. 31–3).

The *anserine bursa* lies on the anterior medial surface of the tibia about 2 to 3 cm below the tibial plateau. It separates the junction of the sartorius, gracilis, and semi-tendinosus muscles from the tibia. Irritation of this bursa occurs in association with osteoarthritis of the knee and the mechanical stresses that accompany varus deformity.[34] Treat-

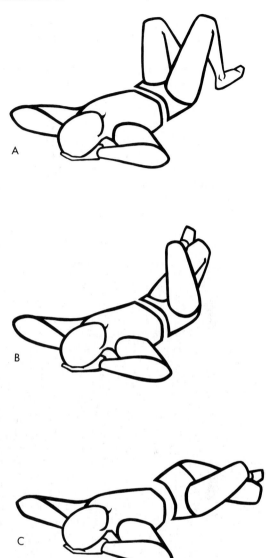

FIGURE 31–3. Active assisted stretch of external rotary components of hip and lumbosacral fascia. (From Swezey, R. L.: Arthritis: Rational Therapy in Rehabilitation. Philadelphia, W. B. Saunders Company, 1978.)

ment directed toward relieving irritation in the knee, improving the quadriceps function, and stabilizing the knee with an elastic knee support and the use of a cane or crutches all may be beneficial. Local steroid injections are very useful in obtaining prompt relief and may obviate the need for more aggressive therapy to the knee joint *per se*. As in all chronic conditions, analgesics and nonsteroidal anti-inflammatory drugs may be of additional benefit. In addition to the anserine bursa, there are bursae located between the skin and the pa-

ROBERT L. SWEZEY

tella—the so-called prepatellar bursa, the suprapatellar bursa or pouch, which is actually a part of the knee joint itself, and the small bursae lying between the medial or lateral collateral ligaments and the joint margins.[35] These small bursae can become highly irritated in patients with osteoarthritis of the knee and will respond to measures outlined for the anserine bursa.

There are several other bursae that much less commonly cause symptoms. The ischiogluteal bursa, when irritated, can be a source of pain on sitting (Weaver's bottom). Hyperflexion of the thigh performed with the knee flexed to eliminate sciatic stretch will cause exquisite tenderness over the ischial tuberosity. Just proximal to the ischiogluteal bursa is the obturator internus bursa, which is a frequent source of buttock pain. Modification of patients' activities and the use of padded seating, as well as the general therapeutic principles previously described, are recommended. There are bursae lying superficial to and deep to the Achilles tendon that can be irritated. These may be affected in association with ankylosing spondylitis, and indeed this disorder would be suspected when bursitis in this area is observed. In addition to the usual therapeutic consideration, the use of a cushioned and raised heel to minimize stretch on the Achilles tendon may increase comfort and minimize recurrences.

Tendinitis

The hypermobility of the glenohumeral joint may predispose it to the stresses that make tendinitis and bursitis so common in this joint area. Except in those cases in which aspiration of the subacromial-deltoid bursa reveals synovial fluid and calcium hydroxyapatite crystals, there is really no sure way to distinguish between subacromial bursitis, rotator cuff tendinitis, and biceps tendinitis. Calcification in the rotator cuff tendon may suggest that a tendinitis exists, but does not prove its cause in the patient's shoulder complaint. The clinician can palpate the anterior capsule of the glenohumeral joint just lateral to the coracoid process, and the findings of an accentuation of tenderness in this area suggest intra-articular glenohumeral joint disease. By the same token, palpation over the acromioclavicular joint may localize a diagnosis to that area. One is left with palpation in most instances to arbitrarily distinguish between biceps tendinitis and rotator cuff tendinitis. With the arm in the anatomical position, the biceps tendon passes anteriorly over the humerus, and local tenderness in that area as opposed to tenderness over the greater tuberosity is the usual basis for distinguishing these two disorders. A positive Yergason's sign—shoulder pain elicited by resisting supination and external rotation of the forearm while the upper arm is kept adducted and fixed alongside the trunk—adds strong support to the diagnosis of biceps tendinitis.[30] As a practical matter, one uses palpation to attempt to localize the seat of the pathological change and then is guided clinically by what is found. If rotator cuff tendinitis or biceps tendinitis is suspected, local measures depending on the severity of the problem are used for pain relief, and stress of the affected area is avoided. By and large, the use of diathermy and ultrasound or other modalities is not as effective as local steroid injections in obtaining prompt subsidence of pain. Friction massage is often useful in relieving pain, and steroid phonophoresis has its advocates.[37, 38] The use of local cold or heat and occasionally transcutaneous nerve stimulation may facilitate joint mobilization. Because of the propensity of the glenohumeral joint to undergo contracture, early and prompt attention is directed toward mobilizing exercises beginning with pendulum (Codman's) exercises (Fig. 31–4) in the more acute cases, and progressing through reciprocal pulleys and wand exercises to attempt to restore full mobility if possible when pain has subsided (Figs. 31–5 and 31–6). When pain is under sufficient control that resistive exercises can be commenced, isometric exercises first to the deltoid and then to the external and internal rotators are taught. These should be performed in the com-

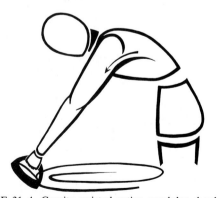

FIGURE 31–4. Gravity-assisted active pendular shoulder exercise to increase range of motion. There is better relaxation if the patient lies prone with the arm hanging over the side of the plinth and a 5-pound weight is suspended from the wrist. (From Swezey, R. L.: Arthritis: Rational Therapy in Rehabilitation. Philadelphia, W. B. Saunders Company, 1978.)

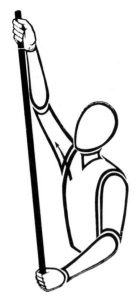

FIGURE 31–5. Shoulder mobility exercises using a wand to provide active assistance from the opposite upper extremity. (From Swezey, R. L.: Arthritis: Rational Therapy in Rehabilitation. Philadelphia, W. B. Saunders Company, 1978.)

fortable range of motion of the shoulder in order to obtain forceful contractions and to avoid exacerbating the painful shoulder disorder itself. Exercises to increase mobility of the shoulder should focus first on restoration of flexion and then on external and internal rotation.[36] When these are restored, abduction is usually restored as well; if not, it can be more easily accomplished at the time that the other motions have returned toward normal and pain has abated. To attempt to achieve

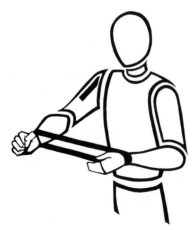

FIGURE 31–6. Isometric bilateral shoulder abduction and external rotation resistance exercise using a belt around the wrists. (From Swezey, R. L.: Arthritis: Rational Therapy in Rehabilitation. Philadelphia, W. B. Saunders Company, 1978.)

abduction, particularly with the hand pronated, is to risk impingement of the greater tuberosity on the coracoacromial ligament and exacerbation of pain and prolongation rather than amelioration of the shoulder problem.

Lateral and Medial Epicondylitis ("Tennis" and "Golfer's" Elbows). Epicondylitis is a strain of the tendinous insertions of the finger and wrist extensors (lateral epicondylitis) or flexors (medial epicondylitis) and occurs as a consequence of repetitive or forceful actions by these muscle groups either in work or in recreational activities. "Tennis elbow" can occur in various hand activities such as wood chopping, hammering, and nut grinding, and the same applies to medial epicondylitis. Management of these problems consists of rest of the affected extremity, avoidance of stress (handshaking by politicians and ministers is a notorious offender), use of mild analgesics and cold or warm compresses, depending on the severity of the disorder and the effectiveness of these modalities.[39, 40] Local ultrasound can be tried, but this has not often proved to be effective in this author's experience, and local steroid injections are generally the most effective way to restore pain-free functional activities.[41] To ensure that function can be restored, reconditioning of the affected musculature by graded isometric and isotonic exercises is recommended when pain permits.[36] Wearing a forearm strap measuring approximately 1½ inches in diameter over the bulky muscular area approximately 4 to 5 cm distal to the cubital fossa helps minimize stress at the insertion of the muscle groups on the epicondyles. Caution should be taken in injecting steriods in the region of the medial epicondyle to assure that the ulnar nerve is avoided.

Flexor Tenosynovitis (Trigger Fingers). Tenosynovitis can affect any of the fingers and thumb and cause irritation or crepitation. Most commonly and dramatically, the patient's attention is drawn to this problem by a tendency for a finger or fingers to become "stuck" after forceful flexion and for them to become "unstuck," "triggered," in a jerking and often very painful fashion by forcible extension of the affected joint. Tenosynovitis can occur as a manifestation of a systemic disorder, but most often it is idiopathic or a consequence of unusual hand stress. Palpation of the tendon area at the metacarpophalangeal (MCP) joint will usually elicit tenderness and crepitation and often a sense of a nodular thickening under the examining finger. Similar findings are less commonly observed at the IP joint on its palmar surface. Specific

ROBERT L. SWEZEY

therapeutic interventions for these problems include modification of tools with built-up handles to avoid joint stress and other work modification measures. The use of a simple elastic splint designed to permit partial but not full flexion of the finger may relieve symptoms and expedite subsidence of these problems.[42] In persistent or very painful cases, local steroid injections into the tendon sheath are usually beneficial. Rarely surgical release of tendinous constraints or synovectomy is required.

De Quervain's Disease (Stenosing Tenosynovitis of the Long Thumb Adductor and Short Thumb Extensor Tendons). Pain in the region of the thumb may be difficult to localize. Osteoarthritis of the first MCP joint or carpometacarpal joint is commonly a cause of thumb pain in the older age group in the absence of other associated arthritic disorders. IP joint involvement is also a possible source of thumb pain, as is the carpal tunnel syndrome and flexor tenosynovitis. As common as any of these disorders is de Quervain's disease. Careful examination will usually reveal tenderness along the lateral aspect of the radial styloid, frequently extending into the area just volar to the anatomical snuff box. There may be mild swelling over the radial styloid extending somewhat proximally and dorsally. On occasion evidence of calcification in the tendon or tendon sheath can be noted on x-ray examinations. The tenderness along the radial styloid as opposed to articular or other tendon areas is crucial to the diagnosis. Finkelstein's test (sign) consists of putting the affected tendons on stretch by placing the thumb across the palm of the hand, grasping it with the fingers, and then ulnar-cocking the hand.[43] This can cause exquisite pain in the region of the radial styloid at the point of stenosis of the affected tendons. Care must be taken to first test the unaffected side because this test can cause mild to moderate discomfort in apparently normal patients. Therapy consists of avoidance of stress, mild analgesics, and local steroid injections. The use of a splint to stabilize the base of the thumb while permitting full flexion of the IP joint is very useful in restoring function and relieving pain (see Fig. 31–1). Surgical release of the stenosed tendon sheath is rarely necessary.[43, 44]

Peroneal Tenosynovitis. Tenosynovitis affecting these tendons as they pass behind the lateral malleolus is usually seen in association with other foot disorders, most notably marked pes planus or spasticity of the foot secondary to upper motor neuron lesions. Tenderness, swelling, and heat are frequently noted. Correction of the predisposing factors, ice or heat, analgesics, nonsteroidal anti-inflammatory drugs, and local injections are used depending on the severity and persistence of the problem.

Morton's Neuroma or Neuralgia. Although not properly a tendinitis or bursitis or even an arthritis, pain in the ball of the foot that may be burning and quite disabling is so commonly confused with an arthritic or related disorder that a Morton's neuralgia is appropriate to consider here. The junction of the medial and lateral plantar nerves of the foot in the area underlying or plantar to the intermetatarsal ligament between the third and fourth or less commonly the second and third distal metatarsal heads places the thickened nerve (rarely an actual neuroma) in jeopardy from compression due to tight shoes or high heels.[45] This is particularly true in the foot that is beginning to spread with increased age or in disorders associated with edema formation. The diagnosis is suspected by palpation of the exquisite tenderness between the third and fourth metatarsal heads and usually occurs in the absence of local callus formation or marked tenderness in the adjacent joints. A local injection of 1 per cent lidocaine into the tender area will usually cause a prompt subsidence of tenderness. Symptoms can be relieved by wearing appropriate footwear with restricted heel height, metatarsal pads, and ample room for the forefoot structures. Local steroid injections into the irritated area will often give lasting relief; however, the problem tends to recur if appropriate shoe modifications cannot be made, and surgical excision is sometimes necessary.[45] Following surgery, the patient should be advised and encouraged to continue to wear appropriate footwear to avoid recurrences.

Morton's neuroma is a true nerve entrapment syndrome but one that is *not* diagnosable by nerve conduction studies. The most common disorder in this category is the carpal tunnel syndrome. This, along with the relatively infrequent tarsal tunnel syndrome, lateral femoral cutaneous nerve entrapment, and others as well, is discussed in Chapter 4.

Ganglions. Related to tendon degeneration, these mucus-containing cystic masses may occur in a number of locations, most commonly around the wrist and less commonly about the fingers, over the dorsum of the foot, and around the ankle. They may be associated with a localized tenosynovitis or may be asymptomatic and present merely as a very firm mass that moves with tendon motion and sometimes disappears in certain positions of the wrist or hand, only to reappear when the position is changed. If the margins of the suspected ganglion on the dorsal surface of the wrist are not well defined and rather tend to blur, a tenosynovitis related to a systemic process should be seriously considered, most notably rheumatoid arthritis and its related disorders. Avoidance of stressful activities or movements in painful cases is helpful, as is splinting. Ganglia may subside spontaneously and when they are asymptomatic usually do not require treatment. Those that are painful will usually respond to local steroid injections. Surgical excision may be required in some instances, but again there is a tendency for the lesions to recur after apparently successful surgery.[46]

Dupuytren's Contracture. This consists of a painless nodular thickening of the palmar fascia, which usually originates in the region overlying the palmar surface of the third or fourth metacarpophalangeal joints. A progressive proliferation of this fascial tissue may lead to a gradual contracture of all of the fingers into the palm.[47] The plantar fascia is similarly affected in some cases.[47] This process is frequently seen in association with the late stages of the shoulder-hand syndrome.[30] Attempts to prevent progression of the contracture by daily metacarpophalangeal stretching exercise or splinting can be tried. There is no established treatment to arrest the process, but surgical release of the tissue causing the contracture can restore function. Postsurgical recurrences are common.[47]

Rheumatoid Arthritis

The most dramatic and usually the most devastating of the arthritides is rheumatoid arthritis. Unlike the descriptive "ovia" in synovia, which alludes to the egg white–like mucinous characteristic of synovial fluid, the "oid" in rheumatoid deliberately obfuscates all those disorders that are similar to, but can be separated from, rheumatic fever. It follows, therefore, that under the umbrella of the term *rheumatoid arthritis* one can find a wide variety of joint and systemic manifestations, a wide variety of clinical presentations, a wide variety of clinical courses, a wide variety of numbers and locations of joints affected, and a wide variety of responses to therapy or indeed to the absence of therapy. Therefore, it is clearly beyond the scope of this chapter to attempt to delineate all of the clinical, pathological, and therapeutic ramifications that might occur under the diagnostic rubric of rheumatoid arthritis. One has only to witness the recent fragmentation of juvenile rheumatoid arthritis (JRA) into at least three subgroups—systemic onset disease (Still's disease), polyarticular disease, and pauciarticular disease—and its further differentiation into subsets of rheumatoid factor–positive and rheumatoid factor–negative polyarthritis and pauciarticular arthritis associated with chronic iridocyclitis with and without sacroiliitis.[48] These types of JRA are further distinguished from rheumatic fever, juvenile ankylosing spondylitis, lupus erythematosus, rheumatoid variants, and dermatomyositis.[48] Advances in the techniques for tissue typing play a major role in ability to distinguish a number of apparently similar disorders that are currently classified as rheumatoid arthritis.[49–52] It is too early to determine whether most of these disorders are indeed similar in etiology (witness the broad spectrum of manifestations of syphilis) or whether indeed genetic factors primarily affecting the immune control mechanisms are the determinants of individual responses to a variety of pathogenetic factors.[50–53] An example of the latter is the susceptibility of those persons who carry the HLA B27 tissue antigen to the development of Reiter's syndrome as a consequence of infections with Salmonella, Shigella, and Yersinia organisms.[49]

At the time of this writing the explosion of information relating to the immunological aspects of rheumatoid arthritis and related disorders still permits only a glimpse at the basic mechanisms and only a hint as to how different immunological responses in clinically similar disorders come about and how they operate. The recent association of HLA Dw-4 with rheumatoid arthritis caused a reexamination of genetic factors in rheumatoid disease.[51, 54] It is now known that rheumatoid factors not only may exist in the IgM class, but also are found in the IgG and IgA immunoglobulin classes and create complexes of various affinities and sizes, and therefore sensitivities to detection by classic rheumatoid factor analyses.[55, 56] The importance of rheumatoid factor complex binding with synovial fluid complement in the genesis of the inflammatory reaction of a rheumatoid joint is well documented, and the association with circulating immune complexes and the more virulent systemic complications of rheumatoid arthritis and vasculitis has also been demonstrated.[55] The demonstration of synovial plasma cell production of IgG rheumatoid factors and their relationship to synovial fluid IgG rheumatoid factor complexes has also been established.[55] The role of the T cell, which is the predominant cell in both the synovial fluid and

ROBERT L. SWEZEY

peripheral blood, as a significant factor in the pathogenesis of rheumatoid arthritis is dramatically illustrated by the remissions in rheumatoid arthritis demonstrated through thoracic duct drainage of circulating T lymphocytes. The interactions between local tissue antigens (including collagen), T lymphocytes, B lymphocytes, plasma cells, rheumatoid factor production, immune complex formation, and release of lymphokines from activated T cells and lysosomal enzymes from activated leukocytes and macrophages are all significant parts of a complex web of events. These events, partially determined by genetic susceptibilities and to an indeterminant degree by environmental factors, coalesce in the ultimate manifestations of rheumatoid joint disease and determine the presence or absence of systemic complications.[52, 55]

Whatever the mechanisms, the ultimate effect is that rheumatoid arthritis is usually manifested as a disorder that symmetrically involves the small joints of the hands and feet. Characteristically, to the exclusion of most noninflammatory disorders, it affects the MCP joints, and almost as frequently the PIP joints, wrists, elbows, shoulders, knees, ankles, and proximal tarsal and metatarsal phalangeal joints. Less commonly, the temporomandibular joints, the cervical spine, and the hips are affected. The pathological joint change consists of a chronic granulomatous process that is associated with proliferation of the synovial lining, overgrowth of articular surfaces by a pannus of this proliferating granulomatous synovial tissue, an undermining of the joint margins, and a destruction of the overlying cartilage. Penetration of the proliferating synovia into the subchondral bone leads to cyst formation and, in more severe cases, to complete destruction of the articular surfaces with fibrous or, more rarely, bony ankylosis.[55]

As in all things in nature, the symmetry of the joint involvement is never perfect, nor is the intensity of the inflammatory reaction consistent in the various joints that may be affected. The disorder may be monocyclic, characterized by a generalized flare, which may be either insidious or acute in onset and which may last a period of months and then remit. It may be cyclical, with one to several joints involved for durations as short as a few days to as long as years and with joints variously involved such that one PIP joint may undergo severe destructive changes and an indolent inflammation may persist in a knee, while other joints may be variously affected acutely or not affected at all. The lack of predictability of the course of the disease makes generalizations about its treatment extremely complex and assessment of the results of therapy equally confusing. In general, those patients who develop early destructive changes manifested by x-ray examination require more aggressive therapy in order to control and contain the disease. The presence of high-titer rheumatoid factor, rheumatoid nodules, or antinuclear antibodies in patients with rheumatoid arthritis is usually associated with more severe arthritic disease than in those cases in which these serological manifestations are lacking.[57]

Patients with rheumatoid arthritis and rheumatoid factor (usually high-titer) commonly develop subcutaneous granulomatous nodules at points of pressure, most notably in the region of the olecranon bursa; similar granulomatous lesions can be seen in the lung, heart, sclerae, and even the meninges. The presence of severe necrotizing vasculitis, which is a rare complication of rheumatoid arthritis, may be manifest by small or large areas of gangrene and peripheral neuropathies, the most characteristic pattern of which is the so-called mononeuritis multiplex—a series or cluster of unrelated sensory or motor neuropathies secondary to vasculitis. These complications are related to circulating immune complex formation and their deposition into the endothelia of small and large arteries. The use of high dosages of steroids and immunosuppressive therapy may be lifesaving in such cases.[55]

The systemic nature of rheumatoid arthritis is typically more subtle and associated with weight loss, low-grade fever, severe generalized stiffness, depression, and less commonly generalized lymphadenopathy, pleuritis, pericarditis, and sicca (Sjögren's) syndrome. This last syndrome is characterized by lacrimal and salivary involvement with dry eyes and dry mouth, as well as, in severe cases, dryness of other mucus-secreting tissue surfaces.[58] Gamma globulins, antinuclear antibodies, and rheumatoid factor are commonly found in high titers. Sjögren's syndrome can occur in association with other connective tissue diseases and as a primary disease. It may be associated with the development of lymphomas.[58] Felty's syndrome is another rare complication of severe rheumatoid arthritis associated with neutropenia, anemia, hepatosplenomegaly, and in many cases susceptibility to infection. Disturbances in hematopoiesis and antileukocyte antibodies leading to impaired phagocytosis and enhanced removal of polymorphonuclear leukocytes in the circulation by margination and splenic sequestration are important factors in this disorder. In Felty's syndrome, the indications for splenectomy are still not firmly established; the role of gold therapy has some credibility; the status of lithium carbonate in stimulating granulopoietic activity is currently being investigated.[55, 59]

In the management of rheumatoid arthritis, it is important to recognize the role of a number of drugs that, among other things, inhibit prostaglandin synthetase activity. These include aspirin in the dose of approximately 4 gm daily and a rapidly expanding number of nonsteroidal anti-inflammatory drugs that have superseded phenylbutazone, because of its various toxicities, and indomethacin, because of its poor tolerance and requirement for high-dosage therapy for suppression of rheumatoid arthritis.[60] These now include ibuprofen, naproxen, and phenoprofen in the phenylalkanoic acid group; tolmetin sodium, which is related to indomethacin, in the pyrrole group; and Sulindac, a fluoridated indole, or sulfone.[60, 61] These drugs and some more recent additions have in common a prostaglandin synthetase–inhibiting effect and share to a greater or lesser extent the side effects of gastrointestinal irritation, central nervous system disturbance, dermatitis, tendency to salt retention, and, according to occasional reports, bone marrow suppression.[60] In general they are all as effective as high-dose salicylates and, with the exception of choline magnesium trisalicylate and salsalate, have fewer side effects, and in particular cause less gastrointestinal bleeding than aspirin. There are many potential hazards when two or more drugs are prescribed simultaneously, and this is true of many antirheumatic drug combinations.[62, 63] At this time it is not possible to predict which of these drugs will be effective or tolerated in any given patient. A trial of each in turn in full dosages for a period of at least two weeks is recommended in the event that a month's trial of full-dose salicylates has already proved ineffective in controlling inflammatory manifestations of rheumatoid arthritis and its related and variant disorders.[60, 61]

When nonsteroidal anti-inflammatory drugs have proved inadequate or where the aggressive and destructive nature of the ongoing rheumatoid disease is of sufficient severity, an agent that will better control the basic disease process is required. The three agents most widely used for this purpose are gold compounds (gold thiomalate and gold thiosulfate), D-penicillamine, and antimalarials (hydroxychloroquine). The mechanism of action of these agents has not been established, but the efficacy of both gold and penicillamine has been confirmed.[64, 65] Both gold and penicillamine have

serious side effects, most notably bone marrow suppression and renal insufficiency, and require close observation of the patient for these as well as other manifestations of drug toxicity. Both agents require two to six months for an effect to be determined and require long-term maintenance therapy. The role of hydroxychloroquine is more controversial; both because its efficacy is less firmly established and because of the potential for an irreversible retinopathy, many clinicians have been reluctant to use the agent.[66] Nonetheless, hydroxychloroquine, which also requires two to four months for its effect to be established, continues to have a role in the management of rheumatoid arthritis. Sulfasalazine, long used in the treatment of Crohn's disease, has recently secured a role alongside gold as a rheumatoid arthritis–remitting drug.[67] Two immunosuppressive drugs, methotrexate and azathioprine, are now approved for use in rheumatoid arthritis.[55, 68] Both of these drugs have demonstrated their capability of suppressing rheumatoid arthritis. Both drugs have a wide spectrum of toxic side effects, and the emergence of carcinoma in patients treated with azathioprine is the most alarming of these.[55] The most heroic of all treatments, total lymphoid irradiation, has not been shown to be more effective than drug therapy.[69]

Systemic steroid therapy is occasionally required for suppression of symptoms in patients with otherwise uncontrollable rheumatoid arthritis. The prednisone dose should be kept below 7.5 mg to minimize (but certainly not avoid) the disastrous consequences of iatrogenic Cushing's disease.[70] Local steroid injection into affected joints and tendon sheaths is a major adjunctive therapy in the management of rheumatoid arthritis and related disorders.[71, 72] Large joint injections of approximately 20 to 30 mg of prednisone or its equivalent and small joint injections of doses ranging variously from 2.5 mg for an interphalangeal joint to 10 to 15 mg for an intercarpal or wrist injection and 2 to 10 mg for a tendon sheath injection are efficacious.[71, 72] The risk of tendon rupture and joint destruction from repeated injections or excessive use of recently injected joints is recognized; however, one must weigh the risk of the destructive rheumatoid process versus its amelioration and suppression by steroids against the inherent joint- and tendon-damaging properties of the local steroids per se.[73, 74] At this time it is very difficult to determine with precision exactly what that trade-off is in any given case. The usual recommendation of not more than three or four injections per joint per year would certainly avoid any serious problems; however, more frequent injections, particularly in non–weight-bearing joints such as the shoulder, may be required to assist in maintaining mobility and compliance in an exercise regimen designed to prevent progression of contracture or reverse joint contracture.[75] In the author's experience, injections given as frequently as every two weeks for a series of three injections into a shoulder may safely be administered during a concomitant course of intensive therapy designed to overcome contracture. One must bear in mind that there are individual cases in which the risk of the destructive effects of repeated intrasynovial injections administered to maintain joint function is justified when weighed against the equally destructive surgical alternative—which may not be accepted by the patient.

Basic Principles of Joint Therapy in Inflammatory Joint Disease

Repetitive joint movement and in fact any joint activity not specifically performed in a therapeutic context will create undesirable joint stress and tend to aggravate an inflammatory joint disorder. In addition to the pharmacological efforts to suppress joint inflammation, patients should be cautioned to avoid both physical and mental exhaustion, and rest should be prescribed sufficient to ensure that both general fatigue and local joint fatigue and discomfort are kept at a minimum. This usually requires eight hours of bed rest at night and at least an hour nap in the day for patients with very active generalized rheumatoid and related joint diseases.

Splinting of affected joints during the acute phase of the disorder should be designed to maintain optimal functional position and insofar as possible permit functional activities to take place.[76] Although immobilization of arthritic joints for three to four weeks has been shown to ameliorate the inflammatory process in the splinted joints without significant risk of contracture, this degree of immobilization is warranted only for short periods of time in patients with a very severe acute form of inflammatory joint disease prior to control by pharmacological means.[76] There are two splints of particular value in this regard: one is a static working wrist splint designed to stabilize the inflamed wrist (which can be extended to include

partial stabilization of the MP joints), and the other is a posterior molded leg splint to stabilize the knee or ankle.[76]

The patients should be carefully instructed in body mechanics and joint protection and pacing of their activities to minimize joint stress and maximize postural patterns that will best preserve joint function.[77] A firm mattress, the use of built-up handles for grasp, avoidance of a pillow under the knee to prevent hip and knee and ankle contractures, and prone positioning during rest to minimize hip flexion contracture are some of the basic considerations in this regard. The use of raised toilet seats, raised chairs, and raised beds to facilitate transfer are protective of lower extremity joints and also minimize stress on upper extremities—in particular the hands, which might be required to assist in transfer.[77]

The use of modalities as specific curative treatments for joint diseases has no established value. Generally moist heat administered as a compress or by tub, shower, or pool is effective in providing pain relief, and this is particularly useful just prior to any exercise therapy.[78] In many patients, cold compresses are equally or more effective in relieving joint discomfort.[79]

Patients with rheumatoid arthritis and related diseases suffer not only from painful joints but also from the indignities that loss of function and the visible alterations in their bodies impose. "Psychic rest" may require social counseling, psychological counseling, sexual counseling, psychiatric counseling, or pharmacological intervention, as well as patient and family education. Patients and their families must learn the nature of the disease, the specifics of the regimens for drugs, exercise, and other therapeutic modalities, and the optimal ways for compliance with these regimens.[80]

The coordination of the health professionals and integration of their effort into a teamlike configuration to optimize the potential beneficial effects to the patient and his or her family require that each health professional be highly skilled in his or her profession and both trained and experienced in the management of the various rheumatic diseases. The various disciplines must cooperate and collaborate and must often, therefore, subordinate some of their own areas of interest or expertise in the conduct of the patient's treatment program. Unfortunately the ideal configuration of such highly experienced health care professionals working with arthritis patients in a smooth and efficient manner is rarely achieved because of the lack of such trained personnel and because of the bureaucratic barriers that exist or are all too often created to interfere with coordinated rehabilitative team therapies.[81, 82]

EXERCISE THERAPY

Strengthening. Since repeated and stressful joint motion will aggravate an inflammatory joint disorder, it is essential that these movements be kept to a minimum during therapeutic exercise. From the standpoint of strengthening the musculature that activates an affected arthritic joint (a task that is essential if sufficient strength is to be available for the joint to perform its essential functional tasks in a smooth and coordinated fashion), one must design the exercises to strengthen those muscles in a manner that minimizes joint irritation and pain. If one provokes pain, forceful muscular contractions will be inhibited and the stimulus required for muscle strengthening may not be achieved.[83]

What is required of the musculature related to an arthritic joint is that it perform brief dynamic or static holding activities essential to basic functions, such as lifting a cup of tea, arising from or sitting down onto a chair, walking across the room, and dressing. These are basically "weight-lifting" functions associated with type II (glycolytic, anaerobic) muscle fiber activity that is capable of brief, forceful, resistive contractions.[84] These fibers are strengthened preferentially by isometric contractions. This is fortunate because one can position the affected arthritic joint in the least painful posture (usually in mid-joint range, with all aspects of the joint capsule under minimal stretch), and then a brief maximum contraction can be performed isometrically.[83] The basic principles of brief isometric exercises are discussed elsewhere, but their efficacy in the face of inflammatory joint disease has also been shown.[83, 85-87] A six-second maximum contraction twice daily (with the patient instructed to count out loud while forcibly exhaling to avoid a Valsalva stress) is prescribed for each muscle group unless contraindicated by cardiovascular considerations.[83] The use of an elastic belt or rubber loop made of dental dam or tire inner tube or of a partially inflated beach ball is a practical way to provide proprioceptive feedback as the extremity is "isometrically" contracting against a barely yielding resistance[83] (see Figs. 31-2 and 31-7).

The isometric exercise regimen can help to provide useful coordinated functional movements with joints protected from adverse stress during the exercise program. With subsidence in the joint

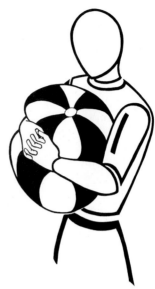

FIGURE 31-7. Isometric exercise to strengthen biceps brachii bilaterally using beachball resistance. (From Swezey, R. L.: Arthritis: Rational Therapy in Rehabilitation. Philadelphia, W. B. Saunders Company, 1978.)

disease, isotonic activities and exercise can be incorporated into the overall patient management program. However, whereas isotonic *functional activities* may not be avoidable (e.g., the secretary may have to type), isotonic and isokinetic *exercise* has not been shown to have any specific added value in the management of inflammatory joint disease. Nonetheless, when the patient's general condition improves, a desire for overall physical exercise beyond that which is incurred in daily activities and aerobic conditioning is frequently expressed. Swimming and water activities are usually the most suitable exercise for such purposes because the buoyancy (and warmth) of water minimizes joint stress. Exercycles, walking, yoga, and weight work can be suitably modified for conditioning purposes to avoid exacerbating joint problems in many cases.[88]

Stretching. The basic principles of avoidance of joint irritation by repeated movement or stressful actions apply to stretching as well as to strengthening exercise.[83] In general, the nature of the exercise will depend on the acuteness of the joint process. When joint inflammation is severe and pain is great, the goal of therapy is to minimize further loss of joint movement. As the severity of the inflammation decreases, restoration of joint mobility or preservation of joint movement becomes the objective. Once a joint has become subluxed or dislocated, no exercise will restore alignment; but if the malalignment is due to contracture alone, then there is a reasonable expectation of restoration of joint mobility, provided the articular surfaces are not excessively damaged or deranged. Therapeutic exercise in all patients with inflammatory joint disease should be performed when the patient is at his or her best. This usually means sometime in the mid-morning when the characteristic morning stiffness has subsided. The use of moist heat or cold (as preferred by the patient) to minimize joint discomfort and, if need be, supplementary analgesics may be prescribed to be effective at the time of the exercise regimen.[83]

In the very acute phase of joint inflammation, active and gently assisted exercises with one to three gentle repetitions once or twice daily is usually all that will be tolerated in the effort to preserve joint mobility. At this state, splinting and posture-corrective measures are used to maintain functional position of joints.[76, 77] As inflammation subsides and the goal is increase of joint motion, the patient is instructed to repeat the specific exercise three to five times with the initial repetitions being in essence a "warm-up" and the final two or three repetitions the actual stretching exercise just into the range of pain. The rule of thumb is that no exercise, strengthening or stretching, should cause severe pain at the time the exercise is performed, nor should it cause pain lasting more than two hours, nor should it be associated with either increased joint inflammation or excessive pain on the day following the exercise regimen.[83]

When inflammation is only moderate, the exercise regimen to increase mobility where contractures have occurred can be performed three to four times daily. In those joints for which the goal is maintenance of motion, once-daily exercise should suffice. It should be borne in mind that the patient's compliance with an exercise regimen that is painful, time-consuming, and fatiguing and that requires repetitive performances will be markedly attenuated as the complexity, frequency, and pain of these regimens are increased. The goals of exercise therapy should be precisely defined, and once they are achieved, they should be revised so that either a new goal requiring additional exercise is prescribed and the previous exercise is discontinued or the regimen is altered according to the newly perceived needs and realities. It must be remembered that patients with inflammatory joint disease tend to have a variable course in terms of the overall disease and in terms of the problems relating to any given joint at any given time. This is particularly true as new medical treatments are implemented during the course of the joint disorder.

Key Joint Problems in Rheumatoid and Related Arthritides

Temporomandibular Joint. The temporomandibular (TM) joint is occasionally the source of significant trouble to patients with rheumatoid arthritis. Transient pain is not uncommon, but on occasion a destructive process involving one or both of the temporomandibular joints can cause severe disability. Mandibular contracture, loss of inter-incisor separation or lateral translation in mastication, and even mandibular resorption may be noted; however, the chief problem is pain on mastication. Persistent transient inflammatory reactions not ameliorated by a soft diet and local heat can often be relieved by local steroid injections into the TM joint with due care that the facial nerve is avoided. Arthroplasties and joint replacement are occasionally necessitated by severe TM joint pain and malfunction.[89] Mandibular hypoplasia is a sequela in some cases of JRA and may require mandibular reconstruction.

Cervical Spine. Subluxation of C 1 on C 2 may rarely lead to severe upper and lower neuron complications and death. Painful C 1–C 2 subluxations without neurological deficit are best treated with a soft or plastic collar fitted to minimize hyperflexion of the cervical spine.[90] All patients with cervical spine involvement should be cautioned to avoid excessive neck manipulation in a dental chair, under anesthesia, during x-ray procedures, or in therapy.[91] Even in cases in which neurological manifestations have occurred, the use of these collars and instruction in appropriate body mechanics may suffice.[90] When the atlas is sufficiently eroded to allow penetration of the odontoid process into the foramen magnum, the risk of catastrophic neurological damage due to spinal cord compression is great, and surgical intervention may be mandatory. Mid- or lower cervical instability and subluxation secondary to rheumatoid disease is also a common complication and may lead to spinal cord compression.[90] All of these complications tend to be more prevalent in patients on long-term steroid therapy, which may reflect both a complication of steroid therapy and a selection of more severely involved patients. When neurological signs and symptoms cannot be stabilized with the use of cervical immobilization, which in the case of the lower cervical spine is best effected by a Philadelphia collar or SOMI brace, surgical stabilization may be required.[76, 90] Unfortunately, the poor quality of bone in patients with these complications may militate against a successful stabilization procedure.

Shoulders. Both the acromioclavicular joint and the glenohumeral joint are commonly involved. Swelling of the glenohumeral joint is often difficult to detect. Contractures of the glenohumeral joint capsule occur early; these should be avoided when possible, and an attempt to reverse them should be made as soon as they are detected. A progressive exercise program may commence, with pendulum (Codman's) exercises, progress to reciprocal pulleys, finger-wall "walking," and "wand" exercises, accompanied in the last instance by isometric exercises to the deltoid and internal and external rotators (see Figs. 31–5 and 31–6).[36] Local steroid injections may permit more rapid restoration of shoulder motion. Patients should be instructed to avoid excessive reaching, repetitive overhead activities, and movements such as mopping, sweeping, and the like. When these are unavoidable, the use of long-handled, lightweight tools or power tools and an arrangement of household supplies to avoid unnecessary stretching or the use of reachers where appropriate should be instituted. The status of total shoulder arthroplasties remains to be determined.[92, 93]

Elbow. Elbow contractures are common in rheumatoid arthritis and occur with pain or minimal effusions in the elbow joint. The use of local steroids to minimize swelling and inflammation while accompanied by extension exercises tends to minimize the problem and help reverse early contractures. Fixed contractures in extension are extremely difficult to overcome, and attention should be directed at preventing loss of flexion because of the severe functional embarrassment in self-care activities that this loss of range of motion can impose—particularly in patients with rheumatoid arthritis, whose shoulder and wrist mobility are often impaired as well. Flexion exercises, active and assisted, should be designed to maintain mobility and increase mobility where loss of range is detected. Pronation and supination of the elbow and wrist, particularly of the wrist, require range-of-motion exercise to preserve mobility.[94] Platform crutches facilitate crutch-walking in patients with wrist and elbow involvement. Synovectomy combined with radial head resection is a useful procedure for pain relief but creates difficulties for some crutch users.[95, 96] Considerable experimentation in total elbow prostheses is being done, but no entirely satisfactory resolution of the problems has been forthcoming as yet.[97, 98]

Wrist. In contrast to most other joints affected in rheumatoid arthritis, the intercarpal joints have a tendency to undergo bony fusion. This may bridge the radiocarpal joint space or be associated with subluxations in that same area. When the wrist is affected, a static working wrist splint may be employed to minimize joint irritation during function (Fig. 31–8). This should be accompanied by twice-daily wrist range-of-motion exercises to minimize loss of mobility. Chronic wrist pain may require surgical intervention. Wrist synovectomy with removal of severely eroded ulnar styloids (the Darrach procedure) may permit restoration of useful function. Temporary fixation to permit a fibrous ankylosis or a bony fusion may be necessary to stabilize the wrist. Replacement arthroplasties are gaining acceptance as a method to preserve mobility and stability and relieve wrist pain.[99–101]

A breakdown in the integrity of the carpal joint and tendon sheaths and resultant communication with the intercarpal and radiocarpal joints and the overlying extensor and underlying flexor tendons is common in rheumatoid arthritis and can be associated with tenosynovitis. Rupture of the extensor tendons is very commonly associated with tenosynovitis and a prominent dorsally subluxed distal ulnar head and ulnar styloid erosions. Prompt surgical intervention when a tendon rupture is detected should be made in order to minimize the extent of surgery and further loss of function in adjacent fingers.

Hands. The selection of the metacarpophalangeal joint as a primary locus of rheumatoid arthritis leads to a weakening of the joint-supporting structures, contractures of the interosseous musculature, and, as a consequence of the stresses imposed by normal hand activities, the characteristic ulnar deviation and swan neck deformities.[102] Splinting to stabilize the MCP joints accompanied with exercises designed to stretch the interossei may help prevent these deformities, but this has not been established.[76]

Subluxation of the lateral slips of the extensor tendons volarly in association with attenuation or rupture of the central slip at its attachment on the dorsum of the base of the middle phalanx leads to PIP contracture and the boutonnière deformity.[102] The intact extensor tendon attachment to the dorsum of the base of the distal phalanx tends to

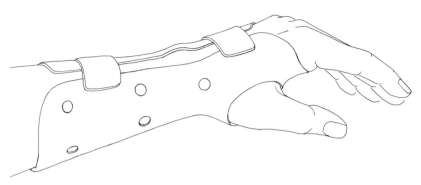

FIGURE 31–8. Static wrist stabilizing (working) splint. This splint is a custom-molded thermolabile plastic splint. It extends from distally just proximal to the distal palmar crease to the proximal one third of the forearm. There is a wide aperture for thumb clearance. It is useful in arthritis of the wrist and to prevent hyperflexion and hyperextension of the wrist in the carpal tunnel syndrome. (From Swezey, R. L.: Arthritis: Rational Therapy in Rehabilitation. Philadelphia, W. B. Saunders Company, 1978.)

maintain the DIP joint in hyperextension.[102] This can lead to a loss of effective apposition during pinch unless range of motion to the DIP joint is prescribed for maintenance of the DIP joint's mobility or to overcome an incipient contracture. It is doubtful that any exercise can prevent the PIP contractures that occur with the boutonnière deformity; however, the use of local steroid injection into the joint may minimize the inflammatory process and the progression of the PIP lesions, particularly when systemic antirheumatic disease therapy can be anticipated to ultimately control the disease. Splinting to stabilize the thumb CMC, MCP, and IP joints can reduce pain and improve function.[76]

The role of synovectomy, either chemical or surgical, in the management of rheumatoid joints in the hand or elsewhere remains controversial.[103–105, 107] Joint arthroplasties of the MCP joints have been shown to improve cosmesis and relieve pain, but cannot be relied on to improve function.[106] Surgical treatment of the PIP joints is less predictable in its outcome with the exceptions of stabilizing procedures designed to improve function. Arthroplasties to stabilize the CMC joint in the thumb, replacement of the trapezium or stabilization of the thumb IP joint, and replacement of the MCP joint in the thumb are useful in selected cases.[103, 107]

Hip. Progressive destructive changes in the hip are not uncommon in rheumatoid arthritis and are even more common in rheumatoid variant disease. Exercises to maintain mobility, posture corrections to minimize hip flexion contractures, and strengthening by isometric contractions of the hip musculature can be helpful in preventing progressive weakness and irreversible deformity.[108] Swimming and pool therapy are very useful. Relief of weight-bearing stresses by crutch or cane is often required. Raised toilet seats and elevated seating minimize stress during transfer. Reachers and special dressing devices, such as stocking putter-on-ers and long-handled shoe horns, can facilitate function.

Fortunately, when satisfactory control cannot be achieved by conservative means, a total hip prosthesis offers an excellent functional solution to the pain of progressive inflammatory hip disease.[109] Long-term experience is lacking in the use of these prostheses in young patients, but their use in middle-aged and older patients appears safe and represents a major achievement in the management of arthritic disorders.[109] The rheumatoid arthritis patient has the advantage of being generally less active than the patient who has osteoarthritis and hip involvement and hence tends to have less risk of abusing the replaced joint and stressing the prosthesis.

Knee. The knee is commonly involved in rheumatoid arthritis. Inflammation of the knee leads to rapid quadriceps atrophy and weakness, which minimize the joint protective action of the key muscle for this crucial weight-bearing joint. Possibly as a result of the quadriceps inhibition, pain, and resultant weakness, patients with rheumatoid arthritis tend to externally rotate the hip, pronate the foot, and stabilize the knee by leaning into the medial collateral ligament rather than relying on the quadriceps to support the knee in its unstable flexed position during weight-bearing. Whatever the mechanism, medial collateral ligament overstretching and valgus deformity are the usual late manifestations of rheumatoid knee involvement.

Effusions of the knee, unless accompanied by a lax or overstretched capsule, restrict knee movement particularly in extension and predispose the knee to flexion contractures. The use of a pillow under the knee for support and comfort tends to further aggravate this problem and must be avoided. Stabilization of the knees with a posterior removable splint to maintain position at rest during the acute phases is therefore extremely important and should be combined with aspiration or local steroid injections when knee effusions preclude full extension.

Relief of weight-bearing stresses by crutches or canes is useful. In patients with very unstable knees, a long-leg, plastic-metal orthosis can provide stability and pain relief, but long-leg orthoses are not well accepted by most patients. The use of an elastic knee support with or without metal side hinges is sometimes helpful in relieving pain even though it provides little actual stabilization for the knee.

Quadriceps isometric exercises with the knee in partial flexion can be initiated as soon as pain permits. Range-of-motion exercises should be performed with assistance twice daily in acute stages, and more frequently if a contracture persists and exercise is tolerated. Traction and serial casting can be helpful in overcoming contractures.[19, 76] Synovectomy of the knee, preferably by arthroscopy,[110] may buy time and pain relief if performed at a time before severe destructive changes have occurred.[103-105, 111, 112] In those patients with marked loss of joint cartilage and destructive changes with uncontrolled active painful synovitis, a joint replacement prosthesis will be required.[113] It should be noted, however, that in those patients in whom the disease can be well controlled by antirheumatic drugs, the x-ray appearance alone should not dictate the decision for surgical treatment.

A complication of rheumatoid arthritis and variant disease in the knee is the rupture of a popliteal cyst that may form as a posterior extension of the knee joint in the presence of inflammatory joint disease. This can result in pain in the calf and swelling in the leg, and is frequently confused with thrombophlebitis.[114] Ultrasound and MRI studies can detect posterior effusions, and arthrography can document synovial rupture.[115, 116] A local steroid injection into the knee will usually cause a rapid subsidence of the inflammatory reaction in the calf, and this should be followed with one to three days of elevation and warm compresses to reduce the swelling and irritation in the leg.

Ankle and Hindfoot. The ankle is commonly involved in rheumatoid arthritis and in variant disease. With or without destructive changes in the articular surface, significant problems with ambulation are common. Relief of weight-bearing forces with crutches or a cane should be attempted. Stress on the foot itself during gait can be partially relieved by the use of a Sach heel and rocker sole, and in more severe cases this shoe modification can be attached to a below-knee weight-bearing brace to partially relieve some of the load on the ankle joint.[17] A recently developed ankle-hindfoot orthosis appears to be a useful bracing alternative.[16] Local steroid injections are often beneficial.

Synovectomy is rarely useful in recalcitrant cases in which severe destructive changes have not yet occurred, and the role of total ankle replacement is gaining acceptance over arthrodesis in severe chronic ankle problems.[103] Caution in making a recommendation for ankle surgery should be exercised because very often both the ankle and the proximal tarsal joints are involved. The latter may be a source of more discomfort than the ankle, in which case the results of ankle surgery may be disappointing indeed.[117]

Rheumatoid involvement of the *proximal tarsal joints* may affect any or all of these joints and is occasionally associated with bony ankylosis similar to that seen in the wrist. Selected local steroid injections can be helpful. The use of shoe modifications and bracing as described for the ankle are also of value. The shoe selected for the patient with proximal tarsal involvement should be a Blucher model with a steel shank and multiple lacings such that when it is properly laced, a corset-like effect can be achieved to help stabilize the proximal tarsal joints.

The *subtalar joint* is commonly involved in rheumatoid arthritis. Inflammation of the bursae surrounding the insertion of the *Achilles tendon* with or without associated rheumatoid nodule formation is not uncommon. Pain at the insertion of the plantar fascia on the anterior surface of the calcaneus as well as at the insertion of the Achilles tendon posteriorly is commonly seen in rheumatoid variant diseases. The use of a Sach heel, as well as a cushioned inner heel, is helpful in relieving stress on the hindfoot structures during heel strike and weight-bearing. Occasionally undermining and filling the heel with soft foam for further relief is of value. A raised heel can reduce stress in cases of Achilles tendinitis. Cane, crutches, and below-knee weight-bearing braces may be required. Again, local steroid injections may be useful in relieving persistent symptoms.

Forefoot. Characteristic rheumatoid involvement of the metatarsophalangeal joints leads to secondary muscle contractures and a kaleidoscope of deformities that most commonly include hallux valgus, hyperextension of the MTP joints with hyperflexion of the PIP joints, and a bunionette deformity of the fifth toe. Compounding these so-called hammer toe and bunion deformities are the hard callosities that occur on the dorsal surface of the PIP joints, on the lateral surfaces of the first and fifth toes, and under the depressed metatarsal heads. The metatarsophalangeal joints can be further traumatized as their protective fat pads are pulled distally by the toe contractures.

The use of a shoe with a rigid shank to provide stability, a metatarsal pad to relieve the weight-bearing stress on the metatarsophalangeal joints with ample width to allow room for the splayed toes medially and laterally, and ample (extra depth) depth of the toe box to allow for the cocked-up deformities of the PIP joints will help minimize pain on walking. The soles should be cushioned, and a crepe or rippled sole is helpful; however, a sole that is too soft can create instability beneath the foot during ambulation. Metatarsal bars can be placed on the outside of the shoe and perform the same service as a metatarsal pad. They have the advantage of not altering the volume on the inside of the shoe in which the foot must be contained, but they have the disadvantage that they may cause the patient to trip over slight defects in the pavement. The rheumatoid foot generally tends to undergo pronation due to stretching of lax proximal tarsal and subtalar ligaments. Good supporting footwear, therefore, is essential to minimize these deforming forces, and a molded insole should be provided to maintain the foot such that the longitudinal arch is held stable in its most comfortable position. Attempts to correct the depressed longitudinal arch usually result in pain on ambulation, and there is no evidence that they are successful. When attempts to relieve pain by shoe correction and pharmacological therapy fail or when the patient rejects on cosmetic grounds shoes designed to accommodate and support the arthritic foot, then surgical treatment is advisable. Resection of metatarsal heads or the bases of the phalanges can be anticipated to provide excellent pain relief as a consequence of functional gait and a more varied choice of footwear to the patient.[113] The status of prosthetic implants in the first MTP joint as well as other joints in the forefoot is not yet clear.[113]

Rheumatoid Arthritis Variants

Ankylosing Spondylitis. Ninety per cent of patients with ankylosing spondylitis are HLA B27–positive.[53, 118] This disorder characteristically affects young men with variable pain in the low back and buttocks, and often progresses to involve the dorsal and cervical spine and may originate initially in any of these areas. Sacroiliitis is the hallmark of this disorder, and varying progression of bony proliferation leading to fusion between the vertebral bodies and loss of spinal mobility is a distinctive feature.[119] It has recently been shown that whereas the clinical manifestations of the full-blown picture of ankylosing spondylitis are relatively rarely seen in women, the disorder in a mild form probably occurs as often in women as in men when assessed on the basis of HLA B27 antigen positivity, back complaints, and sacroiliitis.[120]

The joints that are characteristically affected are those of the axial skeleton, which include the temporomandibular, the acromioclavicular, and the sternoclavicular joints, as well as the rib articulations. A loss of chest expansion is a characteristic clinical sign, as is early loss of lumbar flexion and atrophy of the lumbar paraspinal musculature. Iritis can lead to loss of vision, aortitis can necessitate aortic valve replacement, apical pulmonary infiltration may be associated with loss of pulmonary function, and amyloidosis, a rare complication, may lead to renal failure.

The characteristic pathological feature of this disorder is enthesitis (an inflammation of ligamentous and tendinous insertions).[121] Focal areas of pain in these locations may be very troublesome, and this is particularly true of the insertion of the Achilles tendon into the plantar fascia with the accompanying heel pain that may be a severe disabling complication of this disorder.

Hip joint involvement occurs in about 20 per cent of patients and may lead to severe disability because of the concomitant loss of motion in the spine. Further, surgical procedures such as total hip operations have a higher incidence of failure than does surgery for other disorders because of the tendency for heterotopic bone deposition and ankylosis to occur following hip surgery.[109, 122]

Pharmacological treatment consists of the use of nonsteroidal anti-inflammatory drugs. Patients with ankylosing spondylitis often will respond to lower dosages than are usually effective in other conditions (e.g., indomethacin, 25 mg two to three times daily may suffice to ameliorate severe spondylitic back and neck pain).

Rehabilitative Therapy. *Exercise* to maintain position and pulmonary expansion, as well as postural corrective measures, is the mainstay of rehabilitation therapy. Bracing to prevent kyphosis is of doubtful value. The patient should be instructed to use a firm mattress and a minimal pillow (or a Jackson pillow, which allows lateral cervical support in the side-lying position but does not cause cervical flexion in the supine position). *Prone positioning* for periods of at least one hour daily during the active phase of the disease and in patients with hip joint involvement is stressed.

EXERCISES. Early morning warm-ups should be prescribed to facilitate daily activities. This consists of having the patient assume the "all-fours" position (on the hands and knees in bed), rock back onto the heels, rock forward onto the shoulders, alternately stretch one arm and the opposite leg, and indeed to crawl when necessary to facilitate mobility. An excellent illustrated booklet detailing exercise therapy for ankylosing spondylitis is now available.[123] Neck and back extension exercises can be initiated from the "all-fours" position. Both upper extremities and the upper back and neck are then extended against gravity as far as possible, and this stretch is held for a count of three. This exercise can be repeated three to five times and the holding phase continued to the point of fatigue to encourage strengthening of the erector spinae musculature. The patient can be more vigorously exercised in the prone position with a pillow placed under the upper abdomen and lower thorax. Alternating arm and leg extension is then followed by simultaneous upper extremity extension and simultaneous lower extremity extension, and then both upper and lower extremity and neck extension stretches with isometric holding at the extreme of the stretch to increase strength in the extensor muscles. Range of motion of the cervical spine consists of gentle flexion-extension, rotation, and lateral flexion movements in a series of three to five repetitions.[83] Neck extension and posture can be reinforced by having the patient attempt to place the occiput against a wall or door and slide up and down doing partial knee bends.[83] Rotation of the thoracic spine is best performed with the patient straddling a chair and twisting, first to one side and then to the other. This is done at least once daily for maintenance, and two to three times daily during the early phase of the disease, where evidence for loss of mobility is found. If patients with ankylosing spondylitis are kept under observation, the need for continuing exercise in each area can be assessed and the exercise regimen reduced to its essentials. Progress can be gauged by the ability of the patient to touch the floor, by measurements of chest expansion, by measurements of the occiput-to-wall distance while standing, and by the Schober test, a measurement of the lumbosacral vertebral interspinous lengthening during lumbar flexion.

In those patients in whom a relentless deformity and pain are not responsive to nonsteroidal antiinflammatory drugs, the use of x-ray therapy should be considered; however, the late complications of acute myelogenous leukemia following x-ray therapy should be heavily weighed in considering this modality. A vertebral osteotomy can be performed to correct spinal alignment when severe flexion deformity has not been preventable or has already occurred. The failed total hip operation in patients with ankylosing spondylitis may be salvaged to the extent that mobility at the expense of instability can be restored by a Girdlestone procedure that consists of amputation of the femoral head and neck.[124]

The peripheral joints most commonly involved outside of the axial skeleton are the knees and ankles. The small joints in the hands and feet as well as wrists and elbows may also be involved, but generally the synovitis that occurs is less damaging to peripheral joints than to the axial and spinal joints, and is less destructive in the majority of cases than that seen in rheumatoid arthritis.[119] Treatment of peripheral joint involvement from a physiatric standpoint is essentially that of rheumatoid arthritis. From a pharmacological standpoint, local steroid therapy and systemic nonsteroidal anti-inflammatory drugs are the only agents effective in this disorder, and drugs such as antimalarials, D-penicillamine, and gold compounds are not indicated, although sulfasalazine is being evaluated currently.

Reiter's Syndrome

Reiter's syndrome is another disorder in which the HLA B27 antigen occurs in 90 per cent of cases.[118] This is also typically a disease of young males characterized by arthritis, usually asymmetrical and typically in weight-bearing joints, conjunctivitis or iritis, and a nonspecific urethritis.[125] Balanitis, a painless stomatitis, diarrhea, and an acute pustular psoriasis are very commonly associated.[125] About one third of the patients develop features of ankylosing spondylitis. Synovial fluid analysis typically reveals an elevated synovial fluid complement.[125]

Patients are managed with nonsteroidal anti-inflammatory drugs, although the response is usually incomplete. The attacks tend to be self-limiting, lasting two to four months with a recurrence rate of 15 per cent per year.[125] In some patients the development of a severe generalized psoriasis, ankylosing spondylitis, persistent hindfoot and heel pain, or systemic complications may result in considerable disability.[125] The physiatric management is as described under *Ankylosing Spondylitis* and *Rheumatoid Arthritis*.

Psoriatic Arthritis

Psoriatic arthritis in the majority of cases is essentially indistinguishable from rheumatoid arthritis except that rheumatoid factor and nodules are not present.[126] Skin lesions usually antedate the arthritis, and exacerbations and remissions of psoriatic arthritis are poorly correlated with the course of the skin lesions.[126] The presence of HLA B27 antigen is highly correlated with the development of spondylitic manifestations in those patients with psoriasis. The HLA B13 and B17 antigens have been associated with HLA B27–negative patients with psoriasis and peripheral arthritis.[127] Distinctive features of psoriatic arthritis include seronegativity, distal interphalangeal joint involvement, periosteal proliferation, and the association of nail fissuring, pitting, or undermining keratosis. Occasionally (as in Reiter's syndrome as well) the arthritis may affect predominantly one digit, causing an inflammatory dactylitis with considerable overlying soft tissue inflammation—the so-called "sausage" digit. Severe osteolysis at the opposing articular surfaces may occur in peripheral and occasionally in proximal joints. A tendency to bony fusion may typically be seen in severe cases of psoriatic arthritis. These latter manifestations are more likely to occur in patients with generalized psoriatic erythroderma. The severe resorptive arthropathy in which the loss of bone-stock and joint surface is so extensive that the skin overlying the fingers or wrists may fold upon itself—the so-called main en lorgnette syndrome—may occur in a variety of arthritic conditions but most typically occurs in psoriatic and rheumatoid arthritis.[128]

The physiatric treatment of psoriasis is that of rheumatoid arthritis. The pharmacological therapy at this time does not include penicillamine or hydroxychloroquine. Hydroxychloroquine has been shown to exacerbate psoriasis.[126] Gold therapy is being re-evaluated at this time, and in severe cases immunosuppressive therapy, particularly methotrexate, may be required for control of the disease.[129] Steroids are occasionally necessary for control of the joint disease and they also ameliorate the skin manifestations. Local skin therapy, including topical steroids and various modifications of the Goeckerman regimen, may alleviate the skin manifestations but do not seem to alter the course of the joint disease.[130]

Arthritis and Colitis

The HLA B27 antigen has again helped us to understand the association between chronic inflammatory disorders of the gastrointestinal tract and ankylosing spondylitis.[118] Patients with ulcerative colitis or Crohn's disease may develop erythema nodosum with transient arthritis; episodes of usually symmetrical, nondestructive large joint synovitis, which may persist for weeks or months and subside; and localized sacroiliac disease or full-blown ankylosing spondylitis.[131] The course of the ankylosing spondylitis, once initiated, is independent of the activity of the bowel disease.[131] The use of nonsteroidal anti-inflammatory drugs in these patients requires some caution because of the possibility of exacerbating the diarrheal disorder. Sulfasalazine appears to be beneficial in patients with ankylosing spondylitis with and without inflammatory bowel disease.

Systemic Lupus Erythematosus (SLE) and Related Disorders

There are several rheumatic diseases that in some instances resemble each other so closely that they cannot be distinguished with confidence. Some of these disorders may on occasion so closely resemble rheumatoid arthritis in their articular manifestations that terms such as *cross-over disease* or *overlap syndromes* are applied. As refinements in immunological, pathological, and clinical observations multiply, the criteria for distinctions between the various entities included in this section tend to wax and wane in their ability to distinguish the specific disorders sufficiently that a practical therapeutic strategy can be made for a given case.[132] Systemic lupus erythematosus (SLE) has many evidences of an autoimmune disturbance affecting almost every tissue and organ structure at various times in various individuals. Several drugs, including hydralazine, procainamide, isoniazid, chlorpromazine, and anticonvulsants, have been associated with a lupus-like syndrome, but in the majority of cases the inciting antigen remains unknown.[132] In both the NZB-NZW mouse and in humans, evidence for a viral etiologic agent of a lupus-like disorder is compelling, but a viral cause has not been established.[132, 133] A characteristic double-stranded DNA and IgG anti-DNA complex is a hallmark of SLE and is expressed in the LE cell test. The interaction of these complexes with complement probably accounts for the severe renal disease and many of the other manifestations of this disorder. Almost all patients with SLE have significant titers of antinuclear antibodies, and particularly anti-DNA and anti-Sm antibodies.[50, 51, 132] A depression of serum complement is commonly found in SLE, particularly in those patients with active nephritis. An hereditary complement deficiency (C2) has been associated with the HLA 10 and HLA 18 tissue types in a typical lupus syndrome in two families.[132] Elevation of gamma globulin is frequently seen and may be associated with a biologically false-positive (BFP) serological test for syphilis. Anticardiolipin antibodies are associated with BFP and an increased incidence of fetal loss, thrombosis, and thrombocytopenia.[50, 134]

Medical management of systemic lupus will depend on the nature and severity of the problems. Steroid therapy is a mainstay in those patients with severe systemic manifestations and may be used in conjunction with immunosuppressive therapy. Patients with mild manifestations and particularly dermatological manifestations may respond to antimalarial therapy, salicylates, or nonsteroidal antiinflammatory drugs.[132, 135]

From a physiatric standpoint there are several problems that may require attention. The arthritis may be extremely painful without objective findings other than joint margin tenderness. It may, on the other hand, be associated with a severe and destructive arthritis—a "rheumatoid cross-over." Polymyositis or myopathy secondary to steroid therapy is frequently seen in association with lupus and is treated as discussed under *Polymyositis*. The severe central nervous system manifestations including coma and hemiparesis or paraparesis are treated initially with high-dose steroids, and ultimately their rehabilitative management will be that required by the persisting neurological deficit. The arthritis *per se* is managed symptomatically along the lines outlined for rheumatoid arthritis.

Progressive Systemic Sclerosis (PSS) or Scleroderma

All of the disorders in this section on systemic vasculitis are associated with Raynaud's phenomenon, and this is particularly true of PSS. Progressive tightening of the skin of the hands, often later progressing onto the forearms, face, trunk, and legs, is characteristic. The onset may be associated with a generalized edematous phase that may subside, leaving minimal skin-fascia adherence or severe progressive sclerodermatous changes. Hyper- and hypopigmentation in the affected areas of the skin are commonly seen; scarring of the fingertips associated with ischemic changes and Raynaud's phenomenon may be painful.[136] Subcutaneous calcification may on occasion be diffuse, and extrusions of calcification through the skin may occur associated with pain and disability, particularly when these occur in the palmar and digital areas. Systemic complications include pulmonary fibrosis, dysphagia secondary to esophageal hypomotility, and malabsorption syndrome.[136] A rare fulminant renal failure with hypertension is often lethal. The so-called CREST syndrome is an acronym for calcinosis, Raynaud's phenomenon, esophageal hypomotility, sclerodactyly, and telangiectasia, all of which may be seen in any given case of PSS.[136] Patients with CREST often demonstrate anticentromere antibodies.[50]

A useful clinical sign for the diagnosis of scleroderma is an inability to pinch a fold of skin overlying the dorsum of the middle phalanges. The sign, when found bilaterally in the absence of previous trauma or generalized edema, is very suggestive of skin-periosteal tethering secondary to scleroderma. The biopsy of the skin tends to be helpful only in those cases in which the clinical diagnosis is obvious and tends to be equivocal when the clinician has the greatest need for pathological confirmation. The laboratory is often not helpful, although antinuclear antibodies with a speckled or nucleolar fluorescence are commonly seen.[50] Rheumatoid factor may be present in about 25 per cent of cases.[136] Recently anticentromere antibodies and more recently a precipitating antibody Scl 70 have been shown to be of diagnostic value in PSS.[50, 68]

The treatment medically is supportive with the use of steroids in those patients with associated myositis. The physiatric treatment consists of exercise and night splinting to prevent contractures and maintain mobility and strength. There is no evidence that the severe deforming contractures

ROBERT L. SWEZEY

can be overcome by any physiatric measure, and in this author's experience, except in those patients in whom the edematous phase of scleroderma has subsided leaving relatively little residua, the results of aggressive exercise and splinting have been disappointing. Raynaud's phenomenon is treated by encouraging the use of gloves, avoidance of cold exposure, and meticulous skin hygiene. Some patients have been reported to respond to control of skin temperature by biofeedback techniques.[137]

Polymyositis (Dermatomyositis)

Polymyositis may accompany SLE, PSS, polyarteritis, or mixed connective tissue disease, and it may occur in association with malignancy or as an idiopathic process in its own right.[138] When the characteristic lavendar (heliotrope) discoloration appears about the eyes and scaling erythematous lesions appear over the extensor surfaces of the knuckles and on the chest in association with proximal muscle weakness, a diagnosis of dermatomyositis can usually be established. Muscle tenderness and a mild symmetrical polyarthritis may be seen in association with this disorder. In children a vasculitis is commonly found, and secondary calcinosis and contractures are frequently seen.[138] The prognosis is generally better in children than in adults.[139] Evidence points to an autoimmune T cell stimulation by muscle tissue as a significant mechanism in the pathogenesis of polymyositis.[140] Clinically in addition to proximal muscle weakness, the elevation of serum muscle enzymes, particularly creatine phosphokinase (CPK), is most helpful in establishing the diagnosis.[140] Other enzymes that are frequently elevated include lactate dehydrogenase (LDH), aspartate aminotransferase (AST), and alanine aminotransferase (ALT). Monitoring of one or two of these elevated enzymes during therapy is extremely useful because they will often revert toward normal or away from normal prior to the clinical remission or exacerbation of muscle weakness. Supporting electromyographical evidence suggesting muscle disease can be helpful, and a muscle biopsy is usually confirmatory.

Medical treatment consists of steroids in an initial dosage of at least 1 mg/kg daily until symptoms are controlled and then gradual tapering to a maintenance dose—usually 20 mg of prednisone daily or greater.[140] If after several months the disease is poorly controlled, immunosuppressive drugs may be required.[140]

The rehabilitative treatment consists of maintenance or restoration of joint mobility and posture, avoidance of contractures, and facilitation of functional activities with the use of assistive devices as required by the degree of muscle weakness. Strengthening exercises in the face of active myositis should be undertaken with caution because the effects of resistive exercises on the existing muscle inflammatory disease have not been adequately assessed.[83] Patients are usually encouraged to increase their activity commensurate with their increasing strength until enzymes are either stabilized or return to normal, at which time resistive exercises can be employed in an effort to obtain maximal muscle strength. It should be remembered that steroid therapy *per se* may be responsible for a proximal myopathy and that full restoration of strength in patients with polymyositis is rarely achieved.[140]

Mixed Connective Tissue Disease (MCTD)

This disorder, which closely resembles SLE and PSS and myositis, has been clinically characterized by the presence of tightly swollen fingers with sclerodermatous changes, Raynaud's phenomenon, hypergammaglobulinemia, and the presence of high titers of ENA (an RNAse-sensitive extractable nuclear antigen).[132, 141] These patients in general less frequently manifest severe chronic renal or CNS disease, but in the aggregate may manifest essentially any and all of the serological or clinical features of SLE, PSS, or polymyositis.[132, 141] The myositis and arthralgias can be controlled by steroids, and the management is essentially that of lupus, scleroderma, or myositis, depending on which symptoms are manifested.[141]

Polyarteritis

There are a number of distinctive disorders associated with autoimmune disturbances that in addition to the previously described entities may be associated with necrotizing lesions in blood vessels ranging from venules to large arteries. The disorders can manifest variously transient skin rashes and include catastrophic multisystem diseases affecting literally every tissue in the body.[142] Joint manifestations are a common accompaniment of many of these disorders, and the arthritis is typically painful but not progressive or destructive.[142] The association of hepatitis B and an immune complex vasculitis that may be transient or chronic has recently been described.[142] Diagnosis is established by muscle or testicular biopsy, and in patients with large vessel vasculitis a celiac angiography may demonstrate arterial aneurysmal lesions in the mesenteric and renal vessels.[142]

Medical treatment consists of steroids or immunosuppressive therapy or both. The physiatrist will be called on to treat patients with residual neurological deficit, myositis, and post-gangrene complications.

Polymyalgia Rheumatica (PRM)

This disorder affects patients usually after the age of 50 years and is more commonly seen in women than in men. Fatigue, severe stiffness, and aching, particularly over the shoulder girdles and pelvic girdle, in association with weight loss, depression, low-grade fever, and a markedly elevated sedimentation rate, are the hallmarks of this disorder. Mild joint manifestations may be distinguished from the generalized stiffness, and the associated giant cell arteritis affecting the temporal and other medium-sized arteries, supplied particularly by the carotid arterial tree, may lead to blindness and stroke.[143, 144] In this age group, the presence of low-titer rheumatoid factor or antinuclear antibodies is not uncommonly found and has no diagnostic significance. The muscle enzymes are normal. Bone scans may show low-grade generalized joint involvement. Diagnosis is usually made on the basis of the clinical features and a very high sedimentation rate.

A therapeutic trial of low-dose steroids, 7.5 to 10 mg of prednisone daily, may produce a marked remission within a few days. Temporal artery biopsy can be performed when the diagnosis remains in doubt, but since the arteritis tends to skip areas, a negative biopsy does not exclude the diagnosis.[143] When temporal or CNS arteritis is suspected, prednisone in a dose of 40 mg daily is administered for six weeks and then reduced to 10 mg or less for maintenance therapy.[143]

Physiatric management consists of range of motion and general reconditioning exercises.

Metabolic Arthropathies

Gout. This is typically an acute monarticular arthritis that will commonly involve the great toe. Rarely it can be chronic and polyarticular and involve small joints in the upper extremities in a manner that closely mimics rheumatoid arthritis.[145] Tophaceous deposits usually occur late and typically occur in the olecranon bursae. Attacks tend to be abrupt in onset, often occurring during the early morning hours and reaching peak intensity within a period of 24 hours. The acute attacks are self-limiting and usually pass off within a matter of one to four weeks. Between attacks the patients are generally symptom free. An elevated serum uric acid is the hallmark of this disorder, and the diagnosis is confirmed by demonstration in the synovial fluid of negatively birefringent crystals of monosodium urate.[146] Crystals may be aspirated from bursae, particularly the olecranon bursae, or scraped from accessible tophaceous deposits, most notably at the first metacarpophalangeal joint and the subcutaneous tophi overlying the ear cartilage. In advanced cases, severe destructive arthritis associated with tophaceous deposits can be seen.

Medical management consists of the use of uricosuric agents, typically probenecid in a dose of 0.5 gm twice to three times daily. This drug should not be used in the presence of renal disease, and is usually not effective when the serum uric acid is consistently above 10 mg per 100 ml.[146] In these cases allopurinol is administered in a once-daily dose of 300 mg. Occasionally uric acid levels below 6 mg per 100 ml can be achieved with allopurinol dosages of 100 mg per day.[147] This agent may be required prophylactically when intensive immunosuppressive therapy is used in the treatment of malignancy.[146] Many patients with mild hyperuricemia (less than 10 mg per 100 ml) may never develop gout and do not require treatment.[146] Conversely, an occasional patient with a "normal" serum uric acid may develop a severe gouty diathesis.[145] Colchicine in a dose of 1 mg stat and 0.5 mg every hour either until symptoms begin to abate, nausea, vomiting, and diarrhea occur, or approximately 10 tablets have been administered can be used as a therapeutic test when the diagnosis cannot be otherwise confirmed. Pseudogout, discussed in the following, may occasionally respond to this regimen as well. Maintenance doses of colchicine of two to four tablets daily may help prevent attacks during the first few months of administration of either uricosuric or allopurinol therapy.

The physiatric management of gout is essentially no treatment in the acute attacks because in general the modalities tend to do nothing to relieve the discomfort, and the attacks respond promptly to nonsteroidal anti-inflammatory drug therapy. The use of canes or crutches as a joint protective measure, however, may facilitate ambulatory activities. Patients with chronic generalized gout may require additional functional retraining and the use of assistive devices and a reconditioning regimen.

Pseudogout (Chondrocalcinosis). Pseudogout consists of a goutlike attack occurring in patients who have either radiographically evident, or sometimes undetectable, chondrocalcinosis.[148, 149] This is a disorder characterized by the deposition of calcium pyrophosphate dihydrate crystals in the articular cartilages.[149] These crystals are weakly positively birefringent and tend to be rhomboid or needle-shaped when observed in the synovial fluid under polarized light.[149] Extrusion of these crystals from the adjacent cartilage precipitates the inflammatory response. Radiographs of the wrists, knees, and symphyses may reveal calcifications on the triangular cartilage, menisci, and symphysis, respectively.[148, 149] Chondrocalcinosis and pseudogout may be associated with hyperparathyroidism, hemochromatosis, and Wilson's disease and may be seen as a familial disorder as well.[149] Most often it is idiopathic in origin, and in contrast to gout it may occur in conjunction with diverse rheumatological conditions, including rheumatoid arthritis, gout, osteoarthritis, and Charcot joints.[149] The acute attacks may respond to local steroid injections or nonsteroidal anti-inflammatory drugs. Chondrocalcinosis may be manifested as a chronic smoldering arthritis often accompanying a severe osteoarthritis. Maintenance therapy may require ongoing nonsteroidal anti-inflammatory drugs, and the use of colchicine may be of value in suppressing the recurrent attacks in some cases.[149] Rehabilitative treatment is symptomatic and supportive.

Miscellaneous Arthritic Disorders

Neuropathic Joint Disease (Charcot Joint). Patients with a loss of sensory innervation or pain sensation, typically in association with tabes dorsalis, diabetes mellitus, or syringomyelia, may develop a disorder of joints that is characteristically marked by a relative lack of pain as compared with the amount of swelling and inflammation manifested. A Charcot joint may rarely present as an inflamed, rapidly destructive process or more typically as an indolent, relatively painless, markedly swollen, unstable crepitant joint.[150] Radiographically, loose bodies, cartilage destruction, and irregular repair with large osteophytes and indeed fractured osteophytes are seen.[150] The association of chondrocalcinosis and pseudogout has been recently noted and may be an aggravating factor.[149] Treatment is symptomatic. The use of stabilizing braces or splints and canes or crutches is frequently helpful in improving function and relieving discomfort. Surgical stabilization and wound healing in general in patients with Charcot joints are fraught with failure, and the status of joint replacement in such cases remains to be determined.[150]

Reflex Sympathetic Dystrophies (Shoulder-Hand Syndrome and Sudeck's Atrophy). A diffuse, usually severe tenderness, swelling, and pain affecting a hand, foot, or entire extremity, causing marked restriction of motion, characterizes these disorders. Typically in the early phases there is edema and there may be some erythema that over a period of weeks evolves into a condition characterized by a cool, clammy, atrophic, and contractured hand, foot, or extremity. This disorder is attributed to a sympathetic or autonomic instability and has been associated with angina pectoris, myocardial infarction, stroke, thoracic surgery, cervical disk disease, fracture, or minor and sometimes inapparent trauma.[151, 152] In the case of the *shoulder-hand syndrome*, typically the hand is involved early and the shoulder later; however, only the shoulder or only the hand may be affected. The elbow is characteristically spared. Dupuytren's contractures are commonly seen in the later stages. Technetium scans have demonstrated diffuse articular involvement and often symmetrical involvement where clinically the disorder is unilateral.[152] Radiographs typically show a severe demineralization with a characteristic patchy, blotchy appearance, and marginal bony erosions may be noted. Synovial biopsy has demonstrated proliferation and increased vascularity of the synovium but minimal inflammation.[152] A peculiar *regional migratory transient osteoporosis* has been shown in one case to be associated with evidence of lower motor neuron denervation by electromyographical studies.[151, 153]

Medical treatment of these disorders includes the use of sympathetic ganglion and epidural blocks in the early phases, which may be repeated serially once or twice a week if symptoms are well controlled, and alternatively or subsequently the use of prednisone.[154] Prednisone administered in a dose of approximately 1 mg/kg for a period of one week, tapered rapidly over the subsequent two or three weeks, appears to suppress the pain and discomfort in both the localized and migrating varieties of this disorder.[151, 153] Analgesics are used as needed, with all due caution to avoid addiction.

Rehabilitative therapy to prevent contractures and deformities in the acute phases consists of appropriate splinting and positioning followed by active assisted to active range-of-motion exercises as soon as they can be tolerated. Functional activities for upper extremity involvement include the use of built-up handles and adapted equipment and activities to encourage joint mobilization and function. Graded activities to encourage "desensitization" of hypersensitive tissues include working with materials of graded textures or wearing stockings or gloves of graded softness. In lower extremity cases, partial relief of weight-bearing by crutches or canes and the use of wading tanks or pools to permit weight-bearing stresses as early as possible is helpful in restoring ambulation. A pool provides a particularly comfortable medium for exercise therapies generally in these cases. With foot involvement, the use of below-knee weight-bearing braces may facilitate ambulation. Transcutaneous nerve stimulation may also relieve pain sufficiently to permit earlier participation in functional and exercise activities. Local steroid injections into the shoulder and manual manipulation of the glenohumeral joint as well as in the distal joints (at a time when the disease is controlled and relatively quiescent and such maneuvers can be tolerated) may help facilitate restoration of mobility and function.

Hypertrophic Pulmonary Osteoarthropathy. This disorder is characterized by painful joint swelling and typically by clubbing of the fingers and toes. Periosteal elevation is usually seen, particularly in the distal radius, ulna, tibia, and fibula, and may be detected by Tc-labeled diphosphate.[155] Painful swelling of the knees, ankles, wrists, and occasionally the finger joints can easily confuse this disorder with rheumatoid arthritis. The synovial fluid findings are noninflammatory. Although this condition may occur as a familial male sex-linked dominant trait, it typically is associated with an underlying systemic disease, most notably primary pulmonary carcinomas.[155, 156] Other disorders that have been associated with pulmonary osteoarthritis include chronic suppurative pulmonary disease, subacute bacterial endocarditis, biliary cirrhosis, ulcerative colitis, regional enteritis, and congenital heart disease. Eradication of the underlying disease can result in remission of the associated pulmonary osteoarthropathy.[156]

In addition to treatment of the underlying disease, the use of analgesics, nonsteroidal anti-inflammatory drugs, and in some cases moderate doses of steroids are given for symptomatic relief. The physiatric treatment *per se* is also symptomatic.

Infectious Arthritis. Septic arthritis may result in a variety of bacterial infections and is typically an acute monarticular process. Synovial fluid analysis, including Gram stain and culture, is the key to the establishment of the diagnosis.[157] Some of the common organisms in acute septic arthritis include streptococci, staphylococci, gonococci, *Hemophilus influenzae*, and Pseudomonas organisms.[157] The last organism is particularly seen in patients who are either drug users or have immunosuppression from any cause, and may produce an acute or indolent arthritis. The chronic infections include tuberculosis, brucellosis, coccidioidomycosis, and other fungal infections and most recently Lyme disease caused by a spirochete, *Borrelia burgdorferi*.[161] Identification of the organism and prompt systemic antibiotic therapy are essential to control the infection.[158] Antibiotics should be accompanied by daily or twice-daily aspirations if necessary to relieve distention and to remove as much debris and infectious material as possible in acute infections.[158] When this cannot be accomplished or when the infection is poorly controlled, surgical drainage may be indicated, and this is particularly true when the hip joint is affected in children.[159] The joints are splinted during the acute phase, and mobilization is commenced as soon as tolerated by pain. The use of ice or cold compresses for control of pain in the early phase is helpful, and subsequently warm compresses or submersion of the affected extremity in a tank or tub can be helpful in restoring mobility. Splinting should be performed in a manner to preserve function, and the splint should be removed once or twice daily for gentle assisted range of motion exercises during the acute phases and more frequently as symptoms abate. More vigorous active or resistive exercises and weight-bearing are best deferred until the signs of infection have been largely brought under control and are stabilized and cultures are no longer positive.

A number of viruses can produce a transient nondestructive arthritis.[160] The only exception to this is smallpox, and at this time it would appear that this disease has been eradicated.[160]

Summation

The rheumatological disorders mentioned here (and numerous others that are either rare or insignificant in their effects on joints) are clearly a highly diverse group of conditions that may be associated at one extreme with lethal complications or severe joint destruction and disability and at the other with an insignificant, almost subliminal, arthralgia. Further, any specific arthritic disease in any given individual, or any given joint in an individual with multiple joints involved, may be highly capricious in its effects. One may see, therefore, severe joint destruction in erosive osteoarthritis, or a minimal, transient PIP joint effusion in one finger in a patient with psoriatic arthritis. An appreciation of the nature of the specific diseases and their spectra of presentations and variable courses is essential to appropriate management. The resources available to the clinician include judicious use of pharmacological therapy, selected use of therapeutic modalities, meticulous attention to joint protective measures, rationally prescribed selective exercise therapy, timely referral for surgical treatment, and a concern with the patient's total psychological, physiological, and socioeconomical functioning. There is clearly a great need to develop in health professionals the skills to meet these enormous challenges.

References

1. Clarke, J. T.: The antibiotic therapy of septic arthritis. *In* Schmid, F. R. (Ed.): Clin. Rheum. Dis., 4:63, 1978.
2. Hines, T. F.: Manual muscle examination. *In* Licht, S. (Ed.): Therapeutic Exercise, 2nd Ed. New Haven, E. Licht, 1965, p. 163.
3. Kendall, H. O., Kendall, F. P., and Wadsworth, G. E.: Muscle Testing and Function, 2nd Ed. Baltimore, Williams & Wilkins, 1971, p. 3.
4. Howell, D. S., Sapolsky, A. I., Pita, J. C., and Woessner, J. F.: The pathogenesis of osteoarthritis. Semin. Arthritis Rheum., 5:365–383, 1976.
5. Sokoloff, L.: The Biology of Degenerative Joint Disease. Chicago, University of Chicago Press, 1969, p. 81.
6. Bennett, J. C. (Ed.): Twenty-third rheumatism review. Arthritis Rheum., 21:R105, 1978.
7. Lee, P., Rooney, P. J., Sturrock, R. D., Kennedy, A. C., and Dick, W. C.: The etiology and pathogenesis of osteoarthritis: A review seminar. Arthritis Rheum., 3:189–218, 1974.
8. Peter, J. B., Pearson, C. M., and Marmor, L.: Erosive osteoarthritis of the hands. Arthritis Rheum., 9:365, 1966.
9. Swezey, R. L.: Arthritis: Rational Therapy and Rehabilitation. Philadelphia, W. B. Saunders Company, 1978, p. 182.
10. Bodyns, J. H. (Ed.): Symposium on total joint replacement: Achievements and expectations, Part I. Geriatrics, 31:45–93, 1976.
11. Dobyns, J. H. (Ed.): Symposium on total joint replacement: Achievements and expectations, Part II. Geriatrics, 31:47–85, 1976.
12. Smillie, I. S.: Diseases of the Knee Joint. London, Churchill Livingstone, 1974, p. 75.
13. Swezey, R. L.: Arthritis: Rational Therapy and Rehabilitation. Philadelphia, W. B. Saunders Company, 1978, p. 184.
14. Peterson, L. F. A., Bryan, R. S., and Combs, J. J.: Surgery for arthritis of the knee. Bull. Rheum. Dis., 25:794–797, 1974–75.
15. Lotke, P. A., Ecker, M. L., McCoskey, J., and Steinberg, M. E.: Early experience with total knee arthroplasty. J.A.M.A., 32:2403–2406, 1976.
16. Hunt, G. C., Fromherz, W. A., Gerber, L., and Hurwitz, S. R.: Leg/hindfoot orthosis: Treatment approach for hindfoot instability and pain. Phys. Ther., 67:1385–1388 (Sep), 1987.
17. Swezey, R. L.: Arthritis: Rational Therapy and Rehabilitation. Philadelphia, W. B. Saunders Company, 1978, pp. 113–118.
18. Bennett, J. C. (Ed.): Twenty-third rheumatism review. Arthritis Rheum., 21:R121–R123, 1978.
19. Swezey, R. L.: Arthritis: Rational Therapy and Rehabilitation. Philadelphia, W. B. Saunders Company, 1978, pp. 133–147.
20. Goldenberg, D. L.: Fibromyalgia syndrome: An emerging but controversial condition. J.A.M.A., 257:2782–2787, 1987.
21. Smythe, H. A., and Moldofsky, H.: Two contributions to understanding the fibrositis syndrome. Bull. Rheum. Dis., 28:928–931, 1977–78.
22. Simons, D. G.: Muscle pain syndromes—Part I. Am. J. Phys. Med., 54:289–311, 1975.
23. Simons, D. G.: Muscle pain syndromes—Part II. Am. J. Phys. Med., 55:15–42, 1976.
24. Awad, E. A.: Interstitial myofibrositis: Hypothesis of the mechanism. Arch. Phys. Med. Rehabil., 54:449–453, 1973.
25. Kraft, G. H., Johnson, E. W., and LaBan, M. M.: The fibrositis syndrome. Arch. Phys. Med. Rehabil., 49:155, 1968.
26. Swezey, R. L., and Spiegel, R. M.: Evaluation and treatment of local musculoskeletal disorders in elderly patients. Geriatrics, 34:56–75, 1979.
27. Travell, J.: Symposium on mechanism and management of pain syndromes. Proc. Rudolf Virchow Med. Soc., 16:1, 1957.
28. Bonica, J. J.: Management of myofascial pain syndromes in general practice. J.A.M.A., 164:732–738, 1957.
29. Copeman, W. S. C.: Fibro-fatty tissue and its relationship to certain "rheumatic" syndromes. Br. Med. J., 2:191–192, 1949.
30. Bland, J. H., Merrit, J. A., and Boushey, D. R.: The painful shoulder. Semin. Arthritis Rheum., 7:21–47, 1977.

31. Carroll, R. E., Sinton, W., and Garcia, A.: Acute calcium deposits in the hand. J.A.M.A., 157:422–426, 1955.
32. Bluestone, R.: Calcific periarthritis and hemodialysis. J.A.M.A., 223:548, 1973.
33. Swezey, R. L.: Pseudo-radiculopathy in subacute trochanteric bursitis of the subgluteus maximus bursa. Arch. Phys. Med. Rehabil., 57:387–390, 1976.
34. Brookler, M. I., and Mongan, E. S.: Anserine bursitis. Calif. Med., 119:8–10, 1973.
35. Smillie, I. S.: Diseases of the Knee Joint. London, Churchill Livingstone, 1974, p. 140.
36. Swezey, R. L.: Arthritis: Rational Therapy and Rehabilitation. Philadelphia, W. B. Saunders Company, 1978, p. 186.
37. Cyriax, J.: Textbook of Orthopaedic Medicine, Vol. 2: Treatment by Manipulation Massage and Injection, 10th Ed. London, Bailliere Tindall, 1980, pp. 11–25.
38. Antich, T. J.: Phonophoresis: The principles of the ultrasonic driving force and efficacy in treatment of common orthopaedic diagnoses. J. Orthop. Sports Phys. Ther., 4:99–102, 1982.
39. Nirschl, R. P.: Tennis elbow. Primary Care, 4:367–382, 1976.
40. Goldie, I.: Epicondylitis lateralis humeri (epicondylalgia or tennis elbow): A pathogenetical study. Acta Chir. Scand. [Suppl.], 339:1–189, 1964.
41. Clark, A. K., and Woodland, J.: Comparison of two steroid preparations used to treat tennis elbow using the hypo spray. Rheumatol. Rehabil., 14:47–49, 1975.
42. Swezey, R. L.: Arthritis: Rational Therapy and Rehabilitation. Philadelphia, W. B. Saunders Company, 1978, p. 86.
43. Turek, S. L.: Orthopaedic Principles and Their Application, 3rd Ed. Philadelphia, J. B. Lippincott, 1977, p. 906.
44. Boyes, J. H.: Bunnell's Surgery of the Hand, 5th Ed. Philadelphia, J. B. Lippincott, 1970, p. 445.
45. Kelikian, H.: Hallux Valgus, Allied Deformities of the Forefoot and Metatarsalgia. Philadelphia, W. B. Saunders Company, 1965, p. 359.
46. Boyes, J. H.: Bunnell's Surgery of the Hand, 5th Ed. Philadelphia, J. B. Lippincott, 1970, pp. 666–670.
47. Boyes, J. H.: Bunnell's Surgery of the Hand, 5th Ed. Philadelphia, J. B. Lippincott, 1970, pp. 225–239.
48. Bennett, J. C. (Ed.): Twenty-third rheumatism review: Juvenile rheumatoid arthritis. Arthritis Rheum., 21:R34–R36, 1978.
49. Brewerton, D. A. (Ed.): Symposium on histocompatibility and rheumatic disease. Ann. Rheum. Dis. 34[Suppl. 1]:1–65, 1975.
50. Fritzler, M. J.: Antinuclear antibodies in the investigation of rheumatic diseases. Bull. Rheum. Dis., 35:1–10, 1985.
51. Smolen, J. S., Klippel, J. H., Penner, E., et al.: HLA-DR antigens in systemic lupus erythematosus: Association with specificity of autoantibody responses to nuclear antigens. Ann. Rheum. Dis., 46:457–462, 1987.
52. Koffler, D.: Immunology of systemic lupus erythematosus and related rheumatic diseases. Clin. Symp., 39:2–36, 1987.
53. Brewerton, D. A.: HLA-B27 and the inheritance of susceptibility to rheumatic disease (Joseph J. Bunim Memorial Lecture). Arthritis Rheum., 19:656–668, 1976.
54. Bennett, J. C.: Future research directions: The infectious etiology of rheumatoid arthritis: New considerations. Arthritis Rheum., 21:531–538, 1978.
55. Bennett, J. C. (Ed.): Twenty-third rheumatism review: Rheumatoid arthritis. Arthritis Rheum., 21:R17–R33, 1978.
56. Ziminski, C. M.: How to use autoantibody testing to diagnose rheumatic disease: Don't depend too heavily on any one test result. J. Musculoskel. Med., 4:13–27, 1987.
57. Linn, J. E., Hardin, J. G., and Halla, J. T.: A controlled study of ANA+ RF− arthritis. Arthritis Rheum., 21:645–651, 1978.
58. Bennett, J. C. (Ed.): Twenty-third rheumatism review: Sjögren's syndrome. Arthritis Rheum., 21:R72, 1978.
59. Mant, M. J., Akabutu, J. J., and Herbert, F. A.: Lithium carbonate therapy in severe Felty's syndrome: Benefits, toxicity, and granulocyte function. Arch. Intern. Med., 146:277–280, 1986.
60. Huskisson, E. C.: Antiinflammatory drugs. Semin. Arthritis Rheum., 7:1–20, 1977.
61. Willkens, R. F.: The use of nonsteroidal antiinflammatory agents. J.A.M.A., 240:1632–1635, 1978.
62. Buckingham, R. B.: Interactions involving antirheumatic agents. Part I. Bull. Rheum. Dis., 28:960–965, 1977–78.
63. Buckingham, R. B.: Interactions involving antirheumatic agents. Part II. Bull. Rheum. Dis., 28:966–971, 1977–78.
64. Bluhm, G. B.: The treatment of rheumatoid arthritis with gold. Semin. Arthritis Rheum., 5:147–165, 1975.
65. Mowat, A. G., and Huskisson, E. C.: D-penicillamine in rheumatoid arthritis. Clin. Rheum. Dis., 1:319–333, 1975.
66. Popert, A. J.: Chloroquine: A review. Rheumatol. Rehabil., 15:235–238, 1976.
67. Situnayake, R. D., Grindulis, K. A., and McConkey, B.: Long term treatment of rheumatoid arthritis with sulphasalazine, gold, or penicillamine: A comparison using life-table methods. Ann. Rheum. Dis., 46:177–183, 1987.
68. Kremer, J. M., and Lee, J. K.: The safety and efficacy of the use of methotrexate in long-term therapy for rheumatoid arthritis. Arthritis Rheum., 29:822–831, 1986.

69. Sherrer, Y., Bloch, D., Strober, S., and Fries, J.: Comparative toxicity of total lymphoid irradiation and immunosuppressive drug treated patients with intractable rheumatoid arthritis. J. Rheumatol., 14:46–51, 1987.

70. Jasani, M. K.: The importance of ACTH and glucocorticoids in rheumatoid arthritis. Clin. Rheum. Dis., 1:335–365, 1975.

71. Fitzgerald, R. H.: Intrasynovial injection of steroids, uses and abuses. Mayo Clin. Proc., 51:655–659, 1976.

72. Balch, H. W., Gibson, J. M. C., El-Ghobarey, A. F., Bain, L. S., and Lynch, M. P.: Repeated corticosteroid injections into knee joints. Rheumatol. Rehabil., 16:137–140, 1977.

73. Halpern, A. A., Horowitz, B. G., and Nagel, D. A.: Tendon ruptures associated with corticosteroid therapy. West. J. Med., 127:378–382, 1977.

74. Gibson, T., Burry, H. C., Poswillo, D., and Glass, J.: Effect of intra-articular corticosteroid injections on primate cartilage. Ann. Rheum. Dis., 36:74–79, 1976.

75. Steinbrocker, O., and Argyros, T. G.: Frozen shoulder: Treatment by local injections of depot corticosteroids. Arch. Phys. Med. Rehabil., 55:209–213, 1974.

76. Swezey, R. L.: Arthritis: Rational Therapy and Rehabilitation. Philadelphia, W. B. Saunders Company, 1978, pp. 103–124.

77. Swezey, R. L.: Arthritis: Rational Therapy and Rehabilitation. Philadelphia, W. B. Saunders Company, 1978, pp. 97–102.

78. Swezey, R. L.: Arthritis: Rational Therapy and Rehabilitation. Philadelphia, W. B. Saunders Company, 1978, pp. 133–148.

79. Kowal, M. A.: Review of physiological effects of cryotherapy. J. Orthop. Sports Phys. Ther., Sept./Oct.:66–73, 1983.

80. Swezey, R. L.: Arthritis: Rational Therapy and Rehabilitation. Philadelphia, W. B. Saunders Company, 1978, pp. 149–154.

81. Halstead, L. S.: Team care in chronic illness. A critical review of the literature of the past twenty-five years. Arch. Phys. Med. Rehabil., 57:507–511, 1976.

82. National attack on arthritis. Congressional Record, Vol. 120, No. 155 (Part II, S–19129), October 11, 1974, pp. 1–10.

83. Swezey, R. L.: Arthritis: Rational Therapy and Rehabilitation. Philadelphia, W. B. Saunders Company, 1978, pp. 21–45.

84. Edington, D. W., and Edgerton, V. R.: The Biology of Physical Activity. Boston, Houghton Mifflin Company, 1976, p. 57.

85. Muller, E. A.: Influence of training and of inactivity on muscle strength. Arch. Phys. Med. Rehabil., 51:449, 1970.

86. Machover, S., and Sapecky, A. J.: Effect of isometric exercises on the quadriceps muscle in patients with rheumatoid arthritis. Arch. Phys. Med. Rehabil., 47:737, 1966.

87. Ekblom, B., Lovgren, O., Alderin, M., Fridstrom, M., and Satterstrom, G.: Effect of short-term physical training on patients with rheumatoid arthritis, II. Scand. J. Rheumatol., 4:87, 1975.

88. Ekblom, B., Lovgren, O., Alderin, M., Fridstrom, M., and Satterstrom, G.: Effect of short-term physical training on patients with rheumatoid arthritis, I. Scand. J. Rheumatol., 5:70–76, 1976.

89. Marbach, J. J.: Arthritis of the teporomandibular joints and facial pain. Bull. Rheum. Dis., 27:918–921, 1976.

90. Bland, J. H.: Rheumatoid arthritis of the cervical spine. J. Rheum., 1:319–342, 1974.

91. Ornilla, E., Ansell, B. M., and Swannell, A. J.: Cervical spine involvement in patients with chronic arthritis undergoing orthopaedic surgery. Ann. Rheum. Dis., 31:364–368, 1972.

92. Linscheid, R. L., and Beckenbaugh, R. D.: Total shoulder arthroplasty: Experimental but promising. Geriatrics, 31:64–69, 1976.

93. Neer, C. S.: Reconstructive surgery and rehabilitation of the shoulder. In Kelley, W. N., Harris, E. D., Ruddy, S., and Sledge, C. B. (Eds.): Textbook of Rheumatology, Vol. 1, 2nd Ed. Philadelphia, W. B. Saunders Company, 1985, pp. 1855–1861.

94. Swezey, R. L.: Arthritis: Rational Therapy and Rehabilitation. Philadelphia, W. B. Saunders Company, 1978, p. 37.

95. Dickson, R. A., Stein, H., and Bentley, G.: Excision arthroplasty of the elbows in rheumatoid disease. J. Bone Joint Surg., 58B:227–229, 1976.

96. Brattstrom, H., and Khudairy, H. A.: Synovectomy of the elbow in rheumatoid arthritis. Acta Orthop. Scand., 46:744–750, 1975.

97. Dobyns, J. H., Bryan, R. S., Linscheid, R. L., et al.: The special problems of total elbow arthroplasty. Geriatrics, 31:57–61, 1976.

98. Ewald, F. C.: Reconstructive surgery and rehabilitation of the elbow. In Kelley, W. N., Harris, E. D., Ruddy, S., and Sledge, C. B. (Eds.): Textbook of Rheumatology, Vol. 1, 2nd Ed. Philadelphia, W. B. Saunders Company, 1985, pp. 1838–1853.

99. Jackson, I. T.: Surgery of the hand in rheumatoid arthritis. Clin. Rheum. Dis., 1:401–428, 1975.

100. Nalebuff, E. A., and Millender, L. H.: Reconstructive surgery and rehabilitation of the hand. In Kelley, W. N., Harris, E. D., Ruddy, S., and Sledge, C. B. (Eds.): Textbook of Rheumatology, Vol. 1, 2nd Ed. Philadelphia, W. B. Saunders Company, 1985, pp. 1818–1833.

101. Cimino, P. M., Brunet, M. E., Riordan, D., Haddad, R. J., Edmunds, J. O., and Davis, M. J.: Wrist arthroplasty: A retrospective study. Orthopedics, 10:337–341, 1987.

102. Swezey, R. L.: Dynamic factors in deformity of the rheumatoid hand. Bull. Rheum. Dis., 22:649–656, 1971.

103. Goldie, I. F.: Synovectomy in rheumatoid arthritis: A general review and an eight year follow-up of synovectomy in fifty rheumatoid patients. Semin. Arthritis Rheum., 3:219–251, 1974.

104. Arthritis and Rheumatism Council and British Orthopaedic Association: Controlled trial of synovectomy of the knee and metacarpophalangeal joint in rheumatoid arthritis. Ann. Rheum. Dis., 35:437–442, 1976.

105. Arthritis Foundation Committee on Evaluation of Synovectomy: Multicenter evaluation of synovectomy in the treatment of rheumatoid arthritis. Arthritis Rheum., 20:765–771, 1977.

106. Robinson, H. S., Kokan, P. J., MacBain, K. P., and Patterson, F. P.: Functional results of excisional arthroplasty for the rheumatoid hand. Can. Med. J., 108:1495–1499, 1978.

107. Brown, P. W.: Hand surgery in rheumatoid arthritis. Semin. Arthritis Rheum., 4:327–363, 1976.

108. Swezey, R. L.: Arthritis: Rational Therapy and Rehabilitation. Philadelphia, W. B. Saunders Company, 1978, p. 182.

109. Haberman, E. T., and Feinstein, P. A.: Total hip replacement arthroplasty in arthritic conditions of the hip joint. Semin. Arthritis Rheum., 7:189–231, 1978.

110. Zarins, B.: Arthroscopy and arthroscopic surgery. Bull. Rheum. Dis., 34:1–4, 1984.

111. Cohen, S., and Jones, R.: An evaluation of the efficacy of arthroscopic synovectomy of the knee in rheumatoid arthritis: 12–24 month results. J. Rheumatol., 48:452–455, 1987.

112. Gschwend, N.: Synovectomy. In Kelley, W. N., Harris, E. D., Ruddy, S., and Sledge, C. B. (Eds.): Textbook of Rheumatology, Vol. 1, 2nd Ed. Philadelphia, W. B. Saunders Company, 1985, pp. 1793–1814.

113. Cracchiolo, A.: Surgery of the knee and foot in rheumatoid arthritis. Clin. Rheum. Dis., 1:383–400, 1975.

114. Williams, R. C.: Rheumatoid Arthritis as a Systemic Disease. Philadelphia, W. B. Saunders Company, 1974, p. 210.

115. Carpenter, J. R., Hattery, R. R., Hunder, G. G., Bryan, R. S., and McLeod, R. A.: Ultrasound evaluation of the popliteal space: Comparison with arthrography and physical examination. Mayo Clin. Proc., 51:498–503, 1976.

116. Steinbach, L., Hellmann, D., Petri, M., Gillespy, T., and Genant, H.: Magnetic resonance imaging: A review of rheumatologic applications. Semin. Arthritis Rheum., 16:79–91, 1986.

117. Thomas, W. H.: Reconstructive surgery and rehabilitation of the ankle and foot. In Kelley, W. N., Harris, E. D., Ruddy, S., and Sledge, C. B. (Eds.): Textbook of Rheumatology, Vol. 1, 2nd Ed. Philadelphia, W. B. Saunders Company, 1985, pp. 1896–1909.

118. Bluestone, R.: HL-A antigens in clinical medicine. Disease-a-Month, 23:1–27, 1976.

119. Romanus, R., and Yden, S.: Pelvo-Spondylitis Ossificans. Chicago, Year Book Publishers, 1955, p. 63.

120. Calin, A., and Fries, J. F.: Striking prevalence of ankylosing spondylitis in "healthy" W27 positive males and females. N. Engl. J. Med., 293:835–839, 1975.

121. Ball, J.: Enthesopathy of rheumatoid and ankylosing spondylitis. Ann. Rheum. Dis., 30:213–223, 1971.

122. Dwosh, I. L.: Reankylosis high in hip patients. Orthop. Rev., 5:77–78, 1976.

123. Swezey, R. L. (Ed.): Straight Talk on Ankylosing Spondylitis. Ankylosing Spondylitis Association, 1985, pp. 9–36.

124. Vatopoulos, P. K., Diacomopoulos, G. J., Demiris, C. S., et al.: Girdlestones operation—Follow-up study. Acta Orthop. Scand., 47:324–328, 1976.

125. Good, A. E.: Reiter's disease: A review with special attention to cardiovascular and neurological sequelae. Semin. Arthritis Rheum., 3:253–286, 1974.

126. Roberts, M. E. T., Wright, V., Hill, A. G. S., and Mehra, A. C.: Psoriatic arthritis. Ann. Rheum. Dis., 35:206–212, 1976.

127. Roux, H., Mercier, P., Maestracci, G., et al.: Psoriatic arthritis and HLA antigens. J. Rheumatol. [Suppl.]3:64–65, 1977.

128. Swezey, R. L., Bjarnason, D. M., Alexander, S. J., and Forrester, D. B.: Resorptive arthropathy and the opera-glass hand syndrome. Semin. Arthritis Rheum., 2:191–244, 1972.

129. Dorwart, B. B., Gall, P., Schumacher, H. R., and Krauser, R. E.: Chrysotherapy in psoriatic arthritis. Arthritis Rheum., 21:513–515, 1978.

130. Harber, L. C.: Photochemotherapy of psoriasis. N. Engl. J. Med., 291:1251–1252, 1974.

131. Haslock, I., and Wright, V.: The arthritis associated with intestinal disease. Bull. Rheum. Dis., 24:750–755, 1973.

132. Bennett, J. C. (Ed.): Twenty-third rheumatism review. Systemic lupus erythematosus. Arthritis Rheum., 21:R51–R70, 1978.

133. Wigley, R. D.: Models of rheumatic disease occurring spontaneously in mice. Semin. Arthritis Rheum., 7:81–95, 1977.

134. Gharavi, A. E., Harris, E. N., Asherson, R. A., and Hughes, G. R. V.: Anticardiolipin antibodies: Isotype distribution and phospholipid specificity. Ann. Rheum. Dis., 46:1–6, 1987.

135. Dubois, E. L.: Antimalarials in the management of discoid and systemic lupus erythematosus. Semin. Arthritis Rheum., 8:33–51, 1978.

136. Campbell, P., and LeRoy, E. C.: Pathogenesis of systemic sclerosis: A vascular hypothesis. Semin. Arthritis Rheum., 4:351–368, 1975.

137. Emery, H., Schaller, J. G., and Fowler, R. S. Jr.: Biofeedback in the management of primary and secondary Raynaud's. American Rheumatism As-

sociation, 40th Annual Meeting, Chicago, June 1976, p. 77.

138. Talbott, J. H.: Acute dermatomyositis-polymyositis and malignancy. Semin. Arthritis Rheum., 6:305–360, 1977.

139. Carpenter, S., Karpat, G., Rothman, S., et al.: The childhood type of dermatomyositis. Neurology, 26:952–962, 1976.

140. Bennett, J. C. (Ed.): Twenty-third rheumatism review. Polymyositis and dermatomyositis. Arthritis Rheum., 21:R83–R89, 1978.

141. Sharp, G. C., Irvin, W. S., May, C. M., et al.: Association of antibodies to ribonucleoprotein and Sm antigens with mixed connective-tissue disease, systemic lupus erythematosus and other rheumatic diseases. N. Engl. J. Med., 295:1149–1154, 1976.

142. Fauci, A. S., Haynes, B. F., and Katz, P.: The spectrum of vasculitis. Ann. Intern. Med., 89:660–676, 1978.

143. Fernandez-Herlihy, L.: Polymyalgia rheumatica. Semin. Arthritis Rheum., 1:236–245, 1971.

144. Huston, K. A., Aunder, G. G., Lie, J. T., et al.: Temporal arteritis. Ann. Intern. Med., 88:162–167, 1978.

145. Talbott, J. A., Altman, R. D., and Yu, T. S.: Gouty arthritis masquerading as rheumatoid arthritis or vice versa. Semin. Arthritis Rheum., 8:77–114, 1978.

146. Klinenberg, J. R. (Ed.): Proceedings of second conference on gout and purine metabolism. Arthritis Rheum., 18:659–894, 1975.

147. Simkin, P. A.: Management of gout. Ann. Intern. Med., 90:812–816, 1979.

148. Rubinstein, H. M., and Shab, D. M.: Pseudogout. Semin. Arthritis Rheum., 2:259–280, 1972.

149. McCarty, D. J.: Diagnostic mimicry in arthritis—patterns of joint involvement associated with calcium pyrophosphate dihydrate crystal deposits. Bull. Rheum. Dis., 25:804–808, 1974.

150. Bruckner, F. E., and Howell, A.: Neuropathic joints. Semin. Arthritis Rheum., 2:47–69, 1972.

151. Swezey, R. L.: Transient osteoporosis of the hip, foot and knee. Arthritis Rheum., 13:858–868, 1970.

152. Kozin, F., McCarty, D. J., Sims, J., and Genant, H.: The reflex sympathetic dystrophy syndrome. Am. J. Med., 60:321–331, 1976.

153. McCord, W. C., Nies, K. M., Campion, D. S., and Louie, J. S.: Regional migratory osteoporosis: A denervation disease. Arthritis Rheum., 21:834–838, 1978.

154. Kozin, F.: Reflex sympathetic dystrophy syndrome. Bull. Rheum. Dis., 36:1–8, 1986.

155. Lokich, J. J.: Pulmonary osteoarthropathy. J.A.M.A., 238:37–39, 1977.

156. Fischer, D. S., Singer, D. H., and Feldman, S. M.: Clubbing, a review with emphasis on hereditary acropachy. Medicine, 43:459–479, 1964.

157. Sommers, H. M.: The microbiology laboratory in the diagnosis of infectious arthritis. Clin. Rheum. Dis., 4:63–82, 1978.

158. Parker, R. H., and Schmid, F. R.: Antibacterial activity of synovial fluid during therapy of septic arthritis. Arthritis Rheum., 14:96–104, 1971.

159. Sledge, C. B.: Surgery in infectious arthritis. Clin. Rheum. Dis., 4:159–168, 1978.

160. Sauter, S. V. H., and Utsinger, P. D.: Viral arthritis. Clin. Rheum. Dis., 4:225–240, 1978.

161. Barbour, A. G.: The diagnosis of Lyme disease: Rewards and perils. Ann. Int. Med., 110:501–502, 1989.

32

Traumatic and Congenital Lesions of the Spinal Cord

MURRAY M. FREED

During the past five decades our understanding of the care of individuals with spinal cord injury has developed and improved more than during the previous 50 centuries. Yet it remains, because of its multisystem involvement, one of the most catastrophic injuries—socially, economically, and physically—that can occur to the young adult.

The earliest available documentary on spinal cord injury is found in the Edwin Smith surgical papyrus, estimated to have been written between 3000 and 2500 B.C., with certain commentaries added 1000 years later.[1] Legend has it that the author was Imhotep, physician to the Pharaoh. He described a man with a broken neck who was paralyzed in all his extremities, whose excretory function was characterized by constant dribbling, and whose muscles were wasting away. Under medical treatment was noted "an ailment not to be treated." This dictum, because the injury's complications were poorly understood, was followed for millennia.

The century prior to World War I saw such advances in surgical procedures for spinal cord injury as laminectomy, nerve section, cordotomy, rhizotomy, and sympathectomy. During the Balkan wars of 1912–1913 there was a mortality rate of 95 per cent within a few weeks.[2] Thompson Walker, commenting in 1917, noted that of approximately 450 British soldiers with spinal cord injuries who had survived evacuation from World War I battlefields and been brought to the Star and Garter and King George hospitals, 179 died of urinary tract infection during a period of two years.[3] Among American troops during World War I, 80 per cent of the 2324 men who had received injury to the spinal cord died before they could be returned from overseas.[4] Of the remainder, who were successfully evacuated to this country, 10 per cent survived the first year; in 1946 it was estimated that less than 1 per cent of those who survived the first year were still alive. Two decades after the end of World War I, Hinman wrote that most fatalities among patients with spinal cord injuries were still due to urinary tract infections and bedsores, and the failure to prevent or control these complications accounted for over 80 per cent of deaths.[5]

Improved understanding of the management of the bladder dysfunction secondary to transverse myelopathy and improved nursing care for the prevention of bedsores accounted for significant changes in survival rates just prior to and during World War II. It was the work of Dr. Donald Munro in the United States and of Sir Ludwig Guttmann in Great Britain that made them prophets in the management of the spinal cord injury and the decrease in its complications.

In 1943, Munro reported a mortality rate of 0.575 in 40 patients during the previous 9 1/2-year period.[6] Sepsis of the genitourinary tract and bedsores accounted for 30.4 per cent of the deaths. In 1946, Kirk stated that there were at that time 1400 paraplegic patients in service hospitals and that the results constituted a tribute to the professional competence of the Army doctors in the war.[7] In 1958, a Veterans Administration study of 5743 patients with spinal cord injuries who survived the immediate handling and the potential early complications in service hospitals and who were subsequently treated, between 1946 and 1955, for their traumatic paraplegia or quadriplegia disclosed an overall mortality rate of 0.139.[8]

717

MURRAY M. FREED

Geisler and co-workers, in studying 1510 spinal cord–injured persons in Canada between 1973 and 1980, recorded 194 deaths. The main causes of death were cardiovascular, renal, respiratory, suicide, and neoplastic. Compared with their 1973 study, mortality had decreased and life expectation had been prolonged. There was a marked decrease in deaths due to renal disease and a marked increase due to suicide and liver disease and the abuse of alcohol.[9]

As the incidence of urinary tract complications declines with progressively better methods of bladder management and with prompt adequate care,[16] the potential longevity of the spinal cord–injured individual will approach normal.

Scope of the Problem

Spinal cord injury occurs most frequently in younger age groups: 80 per cent are under the age of 45 years. The median age is 25, the mean 29.7, and the most common age 19 years. Fifty per cent of the injuries occur in the 15- to 25-year-old group (Fig. 32–1). Fifty-four per cent of the spinal cord–injured have an impairment of quadriplegia, and 82 per cent are male.[10]

In a study during the years 1960 to 1967 in Switzerland, Gehrig and Michaelis concluded that the annual incidence was 15 per million population, with an annual increase of 1.7 per cent.[11] A 1967 Canadian estimate was 12 to 15 per million.[12] In 1969, Young reported estimates that the number of persons experiencing spinal injury in the United States ranged between 3500 and 10,000 annually,

an incidence of between 20 and 50 per million population.[13] Owens and Sharman found an incidence of 12.3 per million in New England in 1970 and predicted an annual increase to 15.6 by 1980 and 17.1 by 1990.[14] Brown gave an incidence of 20 to 30 per million population annually in the 14- to 50-year age group.[15] The National Spinal Cord Injury (SCI) Statistical Center, in a 1986 report, describes an annual incidence of 32 cases per million, excluding those who die within 24 hours of injury.[10]

Young noted that of the roughly 200 million population in the United States in 1969, it was estimated that the spinal cord injury population constituted approximately 500 per million or a total of 100,000 at that time.[13] Sharman and Owens estimated a prevalence of 46,700 in 1970 and predicted 75,200 by 1980 and 108,300 by 1990.[14] In the 14- to 50-year age group, the prevalence was 161 per million for Hawaii in 1971, 121 per million for Nevada in 1970, 119 per million for Maine, and 121 per million for Massachusetts in 1972.[17, 18]

The Gehrig and Michaelis Swiss study disclosed that 36 per cent of spinal cord injuries occurred on the road and in traffic; 35 per cent occurred at work, and 29 per cent occurred at home and in sports.[11] The Nevada study showed 52 per cent resulting from automobile accidents; in Maine the percentage was 51.6,[15] while in Hawaii it was 21.[17, 18] A Canadian study of 1737 cases in 1967–1968 revealed that 37 per cent were due to motor vehicle accidents, 37 per cent to industrial accidents, and 7 per cent to diving.[19] The National SCI Statistical Center reported in 1986 that 47.7 per cent were due to vehicular accidents, 20.8 per cent

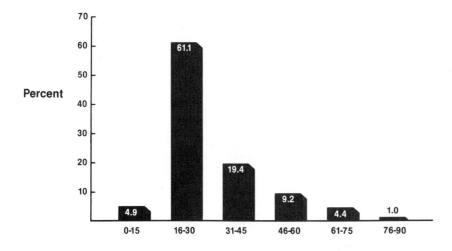

FIGURE 32–1. Age at injury, all levels of spinal cord injury. (From Stover, S. L., and Fine, P. R.: Spinal Cord Injury: The Facts and Figures. Birmingham, AL, University of Alabama-Birmingham, 1986, p. 14.)

to falls, and 9.5 per cent to diving accidents. In the National Pool, acts of violence (gunshot and stabbing) accounted for 14.6 per cent.[10]

Mechanisms of Injury

By definition, paraplegia is paralysis of the lower extremities and all or a portion of the trunk. When the arms are also involved, the term *quadriplegia* is used to describe the impairment.

Fracture-dislocation of the cervical spine is a consequence of sudden and violent flexion or, less frequently, of extension and rotational or horizontal forces. The vertebral fracture-dislocation may result from a direct blow or from acceleration injuries. Motor vehicle accidents are the leading cause of cervical cord trauma, with diving accidents the leading cause in sports injuries. Thoracic spine fractures may result from a direct blow such as occurs in a cave-in, from violent flexion in the seated position, or from a penetrating missile. Thoracolumbar fracture-dislocations are most common at the T 12–L 1 site and follow violent flexion such as occurs in a fall from a height. In such an occurrence, the initial force may strike the calcanei, with the likelihood of fracturing these bony segments, following which the remaining force causes a sufficient degree of flexion at the thoracolumbar junction to produce a fracture-dislocation. The most common sites of fracture-dislocation injuries are the C 5–6, C 6–7, and T 12–L 1 junctions. Certain parts of the spine are relatively protected from injury, namely, the upper thoracic and lower lumbar regions.[21]

Those instances in which radiologic examination shows no fracture or dislocation but in which there is substantial cord damage prove to be hyperextension injuries to the cervical spine in persons with spondylosis.[22] The spinal cord, already compromised by a narrow canal, is compressed by the further narrowing caused by hyperextension of the cervical spine. In addition, Hughes points out, vertebral artery obstruction may occur in the absence of radiologic evidence of fracture and produce a central region of ischemia or infarction in the cervical cord.[22]

In the case of a fracture-dislocation with damage to the entire thickness of the cord, all function at and distal to the site of injury is lost. Thus, there is total sensorimotor loss in the area of the body supplied from the site of injury and below.

Following injury to the cord, vascular and biochemical changes lead to complete infarction and necrosis of the injured segment. The actual mechanism for reduction of spinal cord blood flow after trauma is poorly understood. According to Tator it may be a direct mechanical effect on the blood vessels or there may be a biochemical explanation.[23] There is not only a direct injury to the axons and blood vessels at the time of injury but also a secondary chain of events resulting in hypoxia, edema, and ultimate infarction. Osterholm and his co-workers were of the opinion that norepinephrine release at the site of injury causes severe vasoconstriction that leads to ischemia and hemorrhagic necrosis of the cord.[24]

Early Care

The acute care of the spinal cord–injured individual is directed to stabilization of the medical condition, treatment of associated injuries when present, and appropriate immobilization.

Although steroid therapy is almost universally used for resolution of edema of the injured spinal cord, proof of its beneficial effects is lacking.

In the cervical fracture patient, in lieu of skeletal traction, prolonged bed immobilization may be avoided by posterior fusion, anterior interbody fusion, or halo immobilization in appropriate instances. In the case of thoracic spine fractures, immobilization in recumbency is indicated until the acute period is over, for a period of rest in bed is all that may be required before application of bracing. In those instances of thoracolumbar fracture for which fusion is indicated, Harrington rod application may be the treatment of choice.

Laminectomy is no longer a routine procedure. Any decision for surgical intervention is made after careful consideration of what may be accomplished; when complete paralysis has lasted more than one to two days, there is usually no useful recovery.[25, 26]

Surgery is considered when the paralysis shows a spread of neurological involvement without obvious cause or in the instance of anterior cord syndrome with incomplete paralysis and the finding of anterior compression by radiographic study.

Persistence of instability with or without prior surgery remains an indication for surgical intervention. Neurological improvement as a sole indicator for surgical intervention remains highly controversial; in the same category may be placed decrease of hospitalization time as an indication. The newly developing magnetic resonance imaging techniques may further clarify indications for surgery.

MURRAY M. FREED

For a clearer understanding of the signs and symptoms resulting from spinal cord damage, it is germane to describe the scheme of segmental distribution. The surface regions of the body supplied by the sensory (dorsal) roots of a spinal cord segment through the spinal nerves are called dermatomes. These have been determined by clinical studies and documented (Fig. 32–2). The segmental innervation of voluntary muscles has also been recorded; most muscle groups are innervated from two or more spinal cord segments as shown in Table 32–1.

For better understanding of the complications of spinal cord injury and the prognosis, the description of the impairment is based on the functional level of motor and sensory loss rather than on the anatomical location of the spinal column injury. Thus, "a complete level below C 5" or "a C 5 sensorimotor quadriplegia" denotes that C 5 is the last functioning segment of the spinal cord. This is the terminology in use in the leading spinal cord

TABLE 32–1. Segmental Innervation of Muscles

Neck	Flexion	
	Extension	C 1, 2, 3, 4
	Rotation	
Shoulder	Flexion	C 5, 6
	Abduction	C 5, 6
	Adduction	C 5, 6, 7, 8
	Extension	C 5, 6, 7, 8
Elbow	Flexion	C 5, 6
	Extension	C 7, 8
Forearm	Pronation	C 6, 7
	Supination	C 5, 6, 7
Wrist	Extension	C 6, 7
	Flexion	C 6, 7, T 1
Hand	Gross extension of fingers	C 6, 7, 8
	Gross flexion of fingers	C 7, 8, T 1
	Fine digital motion	C 8, T 1
Back	Extension	C 4 to L 1
Chest muscles, for breathing		T 2 to T 12
Diaphragm		C 2, 3, 4
Abdominal muscles		T 6 to L 1
Hip	Flexion	L 2, 3, 4
	Abduction	L 4, 5, S 1
	Adduction	L 2, 3, 4
	Extension	L 4, 5, S 1
	Rotation	L 4, 5, S 1, 2
Knee	Extension	L 2, 3, 4
	Flexion	L 4, 5, S 1
Ankle		L 4, 5, S 1, 2
Foot		L 5, S 1, 2
Bladder		S 2, 3, 4
Bowel	Rectum and anal sphincter	S 2, 3, 4
Generative system		
Erection	Sacral cord	S 2, 3, 4
Ejaculation	Lumbar cord	L 1, 2, 3

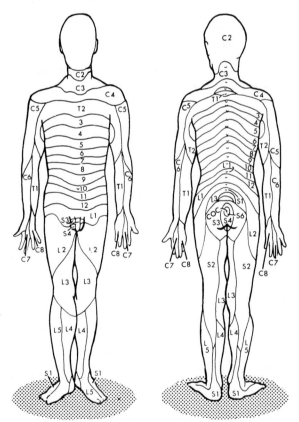

FIGURE 32–2. Spinal nerve dermatomes. (From Tedeschi, C. G., Eckert, W. G., and Tedeschi, L. G.: A Study in Trauma and Environmental Hazards. Philadelphia, W. B. Saunders Company, 1977, p. 78.)

injury centers and is the one propounded by Michaelis.[11] The American Spinal Injury Association (ASIA) proposed that the functional level be the most caudal level with a grade of 3 or F or better.[27] For the pathologist, additional information including the site of bony injury is described so that the pathologist may correlate the neurological or orthopedic findings with the histological findings, since the level of spinal cord involvement may be at variance with the bony injury.

The classification of neurological function promulgated by Frankel and his colleagues in Britain's National Spinal Injuries Centre is becoming widely adopted.[28] The categories are designated A to E:

A. Complete: The lesion is complete, both motor and sensory, below a segmental level.

B. Incomplete: Preserved sensation only; implies that there is some sensation present below the level of the lesion with complete motor paralysis.

C. Incomplete: Preserved motor function but of no practical use to the patient, thus motor useless.

D. Incomplete: Preserved motor function below the level of lesion. Individuals in this group could use lower limbs functionally, and many could walk with or without aids.

E. Recovery: These individuals were free of "neurological symptoms": no weakness, no sensory loss, no sphincter disturbance. Abnormal reflexes may be present.

This classification was proposed since it provided "a system" whereby most cases fall clearly into a specific category, giving results that could be analyzed.

Motor Loss

It is a rare individual who survives complete injury to the third or fourth cervical cord segments, since respiratory difficulties secondary to loss of function ensue. Damage below the fourth cervical segment spares the diaphragm for breathing; the only other significant musculoskeletal functions remaining are neck muscle function and the ability to shrug the shoulders.

Statistically there exist critical levels of spinal cord function (Table 32–2). The described levels of remaining musculoskeletal function are consistent with intact function at the specific spinal cord segment and all those proximal to it, with loss of function to a greater or lesser degree in all distal segments.

The sensory sparing may be determined from the dermatome diagram (see Fig. 32–2).

Functional Significance of Spinal Cord Lesion Level

Although general principles can be mentioned for the management of patients with spinal cord injuries, the specific program for an individual patient must be modified according to the level of

TABLE 32–2. Critical Levels of Spinal Cord Function

C 4	Diaphragm, midcervical extensors and flexors
C 5	Partial strength of all shoulder motions and elbow flexion
C 6	Normal power of all shoulder motions and elbow flexion; wrist extension, which indirectly permits gross grasping by the fingers
C 7	Elbow extension, flexion and extension of fingers
T 1	Completely normal arms and hands
T 6	Upper back extensors, upper intercostal muscles
T 12	All muscles of thorax, abdomen, and back
L 4	Hip flexion, knee extension
L 5	Partial strength of all hip motions with normal flexion, partial strength of knee flexion, partial strength of ankle and foot motion

the lesion. The lower the level of the injury, the greater the amounts of muscle power available to the patient for rehabilitation. Because certain functional groups of muscles are activated at particular levels of the spinal cord, it is possible to categorize the performance to be expected of patients injured at and between these levels (Table 32–2; Figs. 32–3 to 32–11). The understanding of critical levels makes possible the prediction of ultimate function in the absence of complications in the well-trained, well-motivated spinal cord–injured person (Table 32–3).

Fourth Cervical Level

Quadriplegic patients in whom the fourth cervical segment is spared have good use of the sternomastoids and the trapezius and upper cervical paraspinal muscles. They are incapable of voluntary function in the arms, trunk, or lower extremities. The completely paralyzed arms may be supported on balanced forearm orthoses (mobile arm supports; feeders). The patient then uses "body English" and changes in head position to raise and lower the hand. A mouthstick may be useful in typing, writing, dialing, and turning pages.

The most practical method of replacing lost function is by use of "sip-and-puff" pneumatic control for operation of the wheelchair, including the reclining back. It is also appropriate for operation of an environmental control unit (ECU) to manage telephone, radio, television, and cassette tape recorder operation, page turning, and door locking. For those with insufficient ventilatory

Text continued on page 731

C4

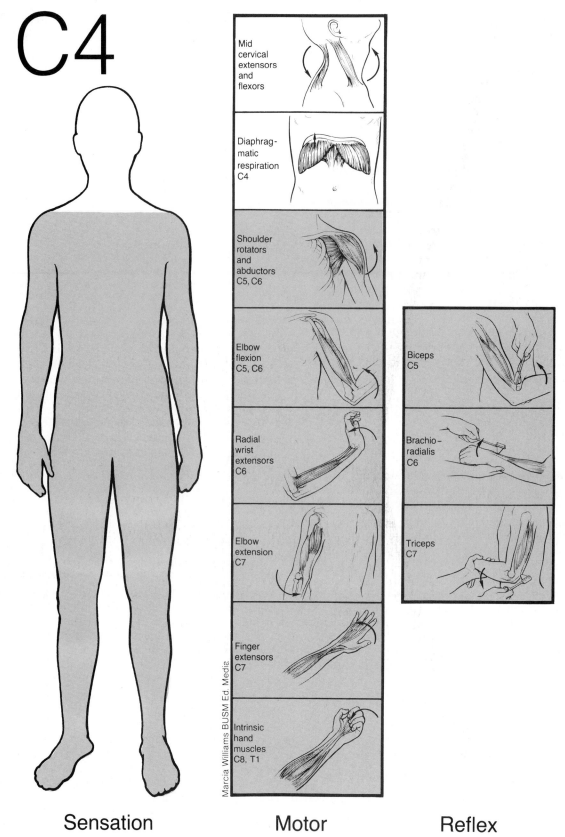

Mid cervical extensors and flexors

Diaphragmatic respiration C4

Shoulder rotators and abductors C5, C6

Elbow flexion C5, C6

Radial wrist extensors C6

Elbow extension C7

Finger extensors C7

Intrinsic hand muscles C8, T1

Biceps C5

Brachio-radialis C6

Triceps C7

Marcia Williams BUSM Ed. Media

Sensation   Motor   Reflex

FIGURE 32–3. Effects of injury with sparing at the fourth cervical level.

722

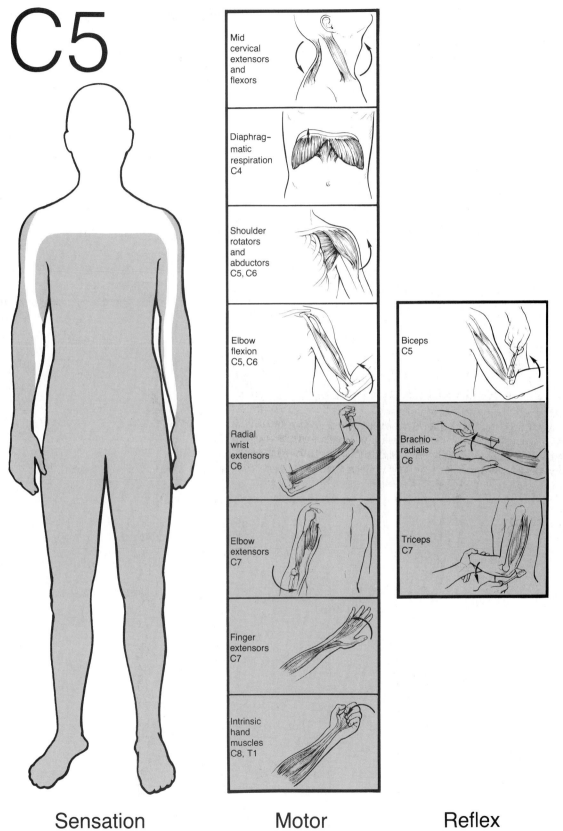

C5

Sensation   **Motor**   **Reflex**

FIGURE 32–4. Effects of injury with sparing at the fifth cervical level.

723

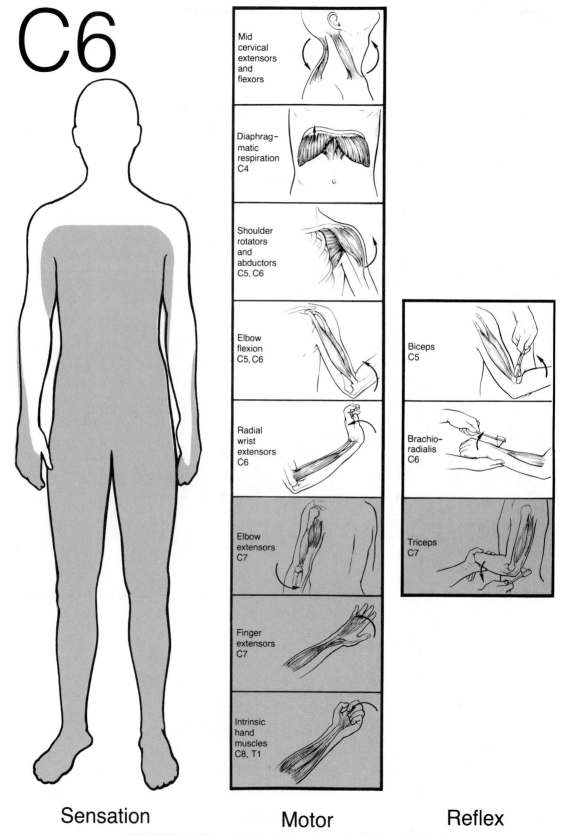

C6

Mid cervical extensors and flexors

Diaphragmatic respiration C4

Shoulder rotators and abductors C5, C6

Elbow flexion C5, C6

Radial wrist extensors C6

Elbow extensors C7

Finger extensors C7

Intrinsic hand muscles C8, T1

Biceps C5

Brachioradialis C6

Triceps C7

Sensation   Motor   Reflex

FIGURE 32–5. Effects of injury with sparing at the sixth cervical level.

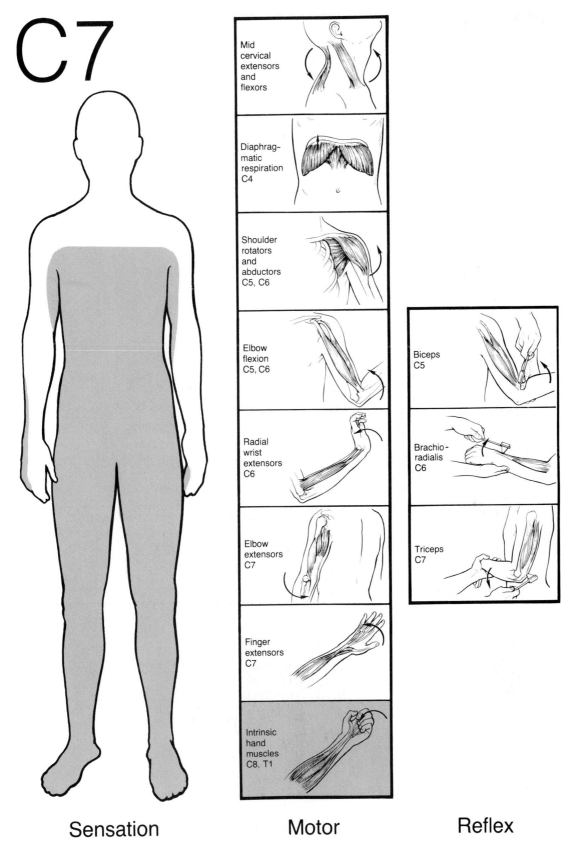

C7

Sensation

Motor

- Mid cervical extensors and flexors
- Diaphragmatic respiration C4
- Shoulder rotators and abductors C5, C6
- Elbow flexion C5, C6
- Radial wrist extensors C6
- Elbow extensors C7
- Finger extensors C7
- Intrinsic hand muscles C8, T1

Reflex

- Biceps C5
- Brachio-radialis C6
- Triceps C7

FIGURE 32–6. Effects of injury with sparing at the seventh cervical level.

725

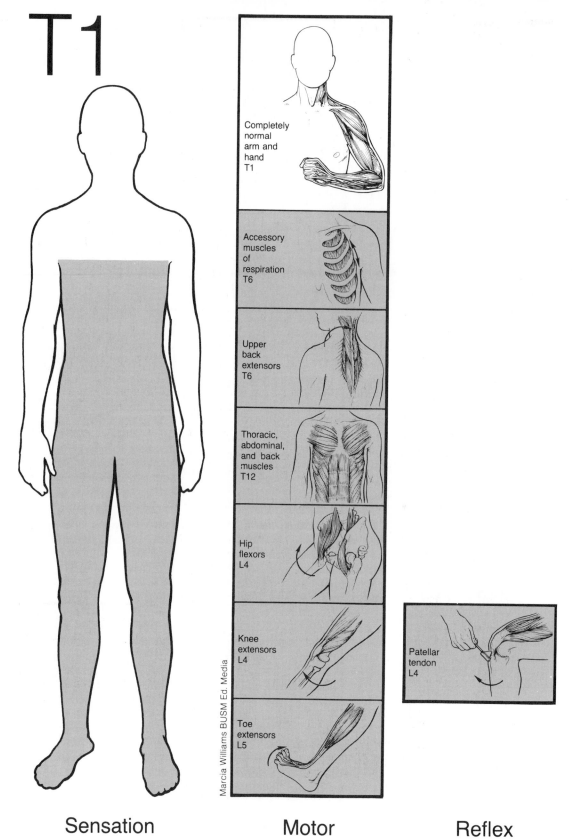

T1

Sensation

Motor

- Completely normal arm and hand T1
- Accessory muscles of respiration T6
- Upper back extensors T6
- Thoracic, abdominal, and back muscles T12
- Hip flexors L4
- Knee extensors L4
- Toe extensors L5

Reflex

- Patellar tendon L4

Marcia Williams BUSM Ed. Media

FIGURE 32–7. Effects of injury with sparing at the first thoracic level.

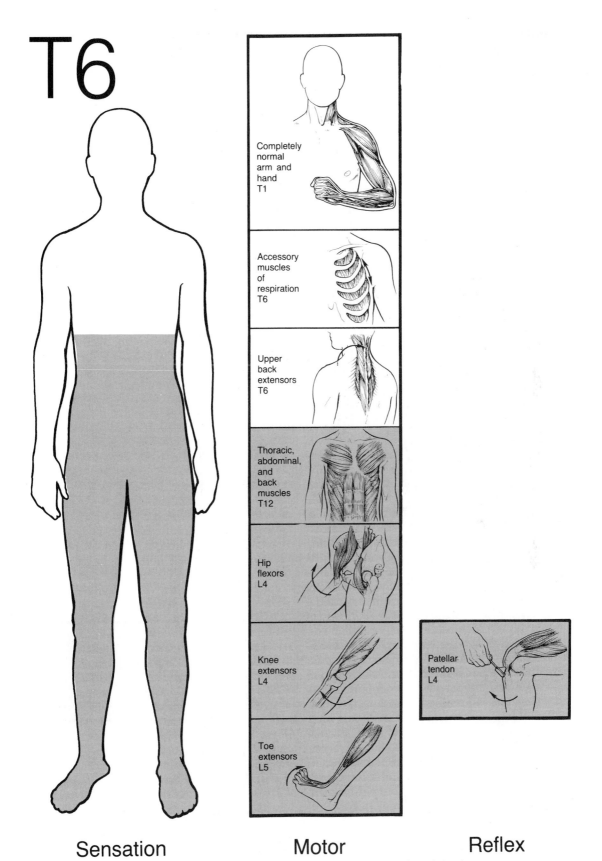

T6

Sensation

Motor

Reflex

Completely
normal
arm and
hand
T1

Accessory
muscles
of
respiration
T6

Upper
back
extensors
T6

Thoracic,
abdominal,
and
back
muscles
T12

Hip
flexors
L4

Knee
extensors
L4

Toe
extensors
L5

Patellar
tendon
L4

FIGURE 32–8. Effects of injury with sparing at the sixth thoracic level.

T12

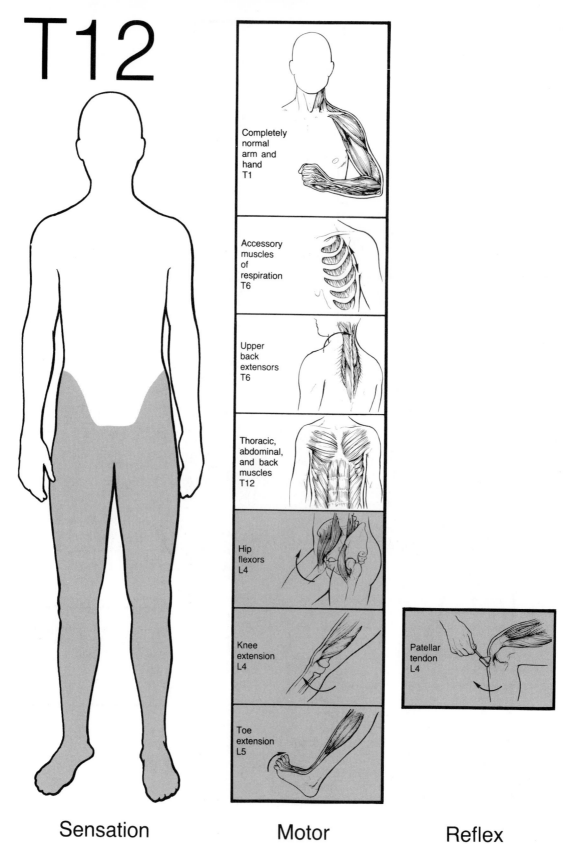

Sensation   Motor   Reflex

FIGURE 32–9. Effects of injury with sparing at the twelfth thoracic level.

728

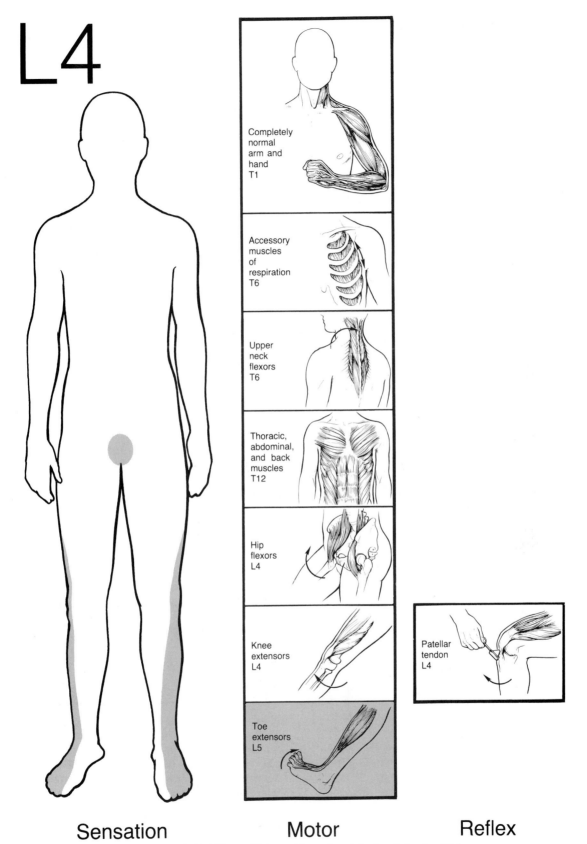

L4

Completely
normal
arm and
hand
T1

Accessory
muscles
of
respiration
T6

Upper
neck
flexors
T6

Thoracic,
abdominal,
and back
muscles
T12

Hip
flexors
L4

Knee
extensors
L4

Toe
extensors
L5

Patellar
tendon
L4

Sensation   Motor   Reflex

FIGURE 32–10. Effects of injury with sparing at the fourth lumbar level.

L5

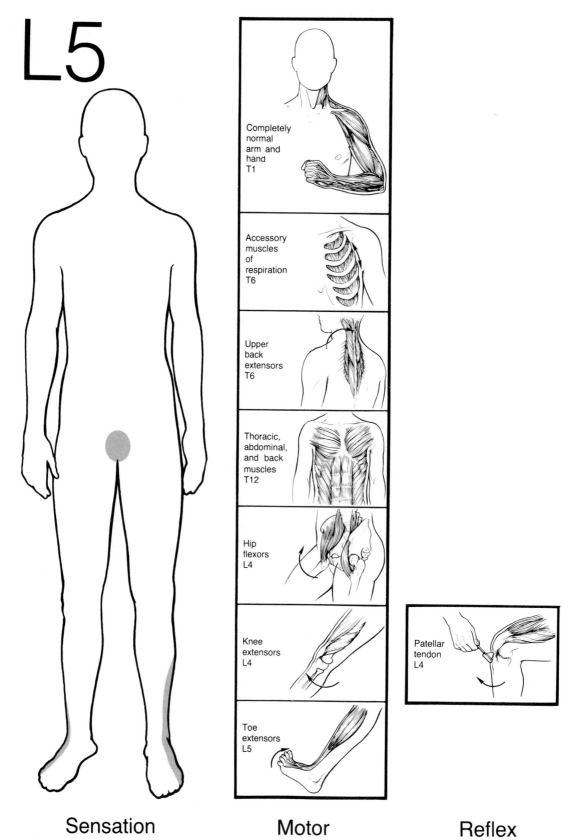

Sensation

Motor

Reflex

- Completely normal arm and hand T1
- Accessory muscles of respiration T6
- Upper back extensors T6
- Thoracic, abdominal, and back muscles T12
- Hip flexors L4
- Knee extensors L4
- Toe extensors L5
- Patellar tendon L4

FIGURE 32–11. Effects of injury with sparing at the fifth lumbar level.

730

TABLE 32–3. Functional Significance of Spinal Cord Lesion Level

ACTIVITIES	C 4	C 5	C 6	C 7	T 1	T 6	T 12	L 4
Self-care								
Eating	−	+	+	+	+	+	+	+
Dressing	−	−	±	+	+	+	+	+
Toileting	−	±	±	+	+	+	+	+
Bed independence								
Rolling, sitting up supine	−	−	±	+	+	+	+	+
Moving about, sitting	−	−	±	+	+	+	+	+
Wheelchair independence								
Transfer to and from	−	−	±	+	+	+	+	+
Mobility	*+	+	+	+	+	+	+	+
Ambulation								
Functional	−	−	−	−	−	±	±	+
Attendant								
Lifting	+	+	±	−	−	−	−	−
Assisting	+	+	±	−	−	−	−	−
Homebound work	+	+	+	+	+	+	+	+
Outside job	+	+	+	+	+	+	+	+
Private car	−	+	+	+	+	+	+	+
Public transportation	±	±	±	±	±	±	±	+
Orthoses or devices	+	+	+	−	+	+	+	+
	EC	Hand	Hand		KAFO	KAFO	KAFO	AFO
Communication skills								
Writing	*+	+	+	+	+	+	+	+
Typing	*+	+	+	+	+	+	+	+
Dictating machine	*+	+	+	+	+	+	+	+
Telephone	*+	+	+	+	+	+	+	+

*Requires pneumatically operated equipment or adaptive devices controlled by mouth.

EC, environmental control; Hand, hand devices; KAFO, knee-ankle-foot orthoses; ADO, ankle-foot orthoses.

strength to manage the pneumatic control, tongue pressure and humidity switches are being developed. Voice-activating mechanisms bode well for the future.[29]

Fifth Cervical Level

The patient with a functioning fifth cervical segment can use the deltoid and biceps muscles to accomplish activities of daily living. Partial continued weakness of the deltoid and biceps may make it necessary to use a balanced forearm orthosis for support of the elbow and shoulder, especially in the early stages of the rehabilitation program. Overhead sling suspension may be used as an interim measure if it appears that permanent orthoses will not be necessary; the patient needs a substitute for nonfunctioning hand and wrist musculature. Fixed support of the wrist and fingers is used, and adapted devices are then applied to the patient's hand by another individual and kept in place until a new activity is started. Skillful use of these devices requires much training and practice.

Quadriplegic patients whose lesion is below the fifth cervical segment can be expected to feed themselves, perform some grooming activities, help with upper extremity dressing, help apply bracing, push their wheelchairs for short distances (with special projections on the wheelchair rims), turn pages, and use the electric typewriter. For these patients, electrically driven wheelchairs are indicated.

Patients with lesions at the fourth and fifth cervical levels require help for lifting and assisting. A hydraulic lift may be necessary to help the family move the patient from bed to wheelchair. Beds for all patients with spinal cord injuries should be adjusted to wheelchair height. Removable armrests are essential components of all wheelchairs for the spinal cord–injured.

Sixth Cervical Level

At the sixth cervical level of involvement, the individual has virtually fully innervated shoulder musculature, elbow flexion, and radial wrist extension; the last permits graded control of the wrist, with gravity performing the flexion movements. Wrist extension can be harnessed through special "tenodesis" splints to drive the fingers into flexion; sometimes a surgical finger flexor tenodesis can be performed for the same purpose. Many patients prefer simply to use leather cuffs strapped to their hands, into which such implements as toothbrushes, forks, and spoons can be inserted.

Patients injured below the sixth cervical segment can perform all the activities of patients with higher-level lesions and in addition can be more helpful in dressing themselves—often doing it completely, can propel their wheelchairs long distances, and usually can transfer themselves from bed to chair using the overhead trapeze or a modified pushup with elbow stabilization by shoulder adduction. Beginning at this level, individuals should be able to drive an automobile with manual controls and additional adaptive equipment.[30] A van with hydraulic lift makes the entire procedure easier in that transfers are eliminated.

Seventh Cervical Level

The major functional additions at the seventh cervical segment are the use of the triceps and the extrinsic finger flexors and extensors. These patients are able to do pushups in the sitting position and therefore can transfer themselves from bed to chair. They can grasp and release and are usually able to operate their hands without splints.

This patient is independent at the wheelchair level.

First Thoracic Level

This individual has normal upper extremities with a strong chain of stabilization to the thorax but lacks trunk musculature for full sitting balance and intercostal and abdominal musculature to supplement diaphragmatic breathing.

However, these individuals should be completely independent of a wheelchair in that they can dress and feed, manage toileting needs, accomplish transfers, drive a car with manual controls, and hold a job away from home requiring self-transportation as can the low-level quadriplegic.

Sixth Thoracic Level

The paraplegic at this level has upper intercostal function and upper back control and thus has an added increment of respiratory reserve. There should be wheelchair independence for activities of daily living.

This individual may be provided with orthoses for standing but should not be expected to walk because of the unusually increased energy demands of such ambulation.

Twelfth Thoracic Level

At this level the individual has full abdominal and virtually full back control as well as intact respiratory reserve. The individual with a T 12 level has normal upper extremities with a chain of strong fixators in the normal trunk to give virtually unlimited function of the upper extremities in the seated position. There should be complete independence in activities of daily living. Functional ambulation continues to be a problem, since the energy demands make it highly impractical for the vast majority. Nevertheless, orthoses should be considered for physiological standing and walking.

Fourth Lumbar Level

This person has the use of the hip flexors and knee extensors and can stand without orthoses and walk without external support. However, because of severe weakness of the glutei coupled with loss of ankle power, there is a laborious waddling and steppage gait. Ambulation is assisted by use of ankle-foot orthoses and by crutches. Failure to use such support will result in genu recurvatum and abnormal lumbar spine strain.

This is a virtually completely independent individual. There is difficulty in stair-climbing and in those activities requiring repetitive changing from seated to standing positions.

As the patient grows older, less functional independence should be expected; reductions in capability vary with the individual, physiological age, and physical abilities.

Congenital Spinal Cord Lesions

The most common group of spinal cord lesions are those resulting from incomplete closure of the vertebral canal. This is commonly seen as posterior spina bifida, in which there is a defect of the laminae; although it may occur at any level, it is most common in the lumbosacral region.[31] When only the laminar defect is present, it is designated spina bifida occulta. Spina bifida denotes an external sac of meninges. When there are adhesions between the cord and connective tissue, cord gliosis, and cavitation, these result in neurological impairments. Meningocele exists when there is a bulging subcutaneous sac containing mainly meninges and fluid; it also may contain nerve roots. In myelomeningocele, the sac contains central nervous tissue, which represents damaged spinal cord with nerve roots; frequently there is a mass of fibrous gliosis with no evidence of intact neurons. In meningomyelocystocele, the meningeal sac contains badly malformed spinal cord. Usually only the anterior half has a semblance of normal anatomy. The central nervous tissue is mainly glial.

Ames and Schut note that 80 per cent of those with meningomyelocele have hydrocephalus and bowel and bladder incontinence.[32] Stark comments that upper motor neuron involvement occurs and that this is the fundamental neurological problem;[33] unexplained by myelodysplasia, it is "probably acquired before, during or shortly after birth."

To develop the potential of those who survive, a well-organized program is required. The contribution of the neurosurgeon is the management of local surgery and the hydrocephalus, and that of the orthopedist the lower extremity deformities. The urologist deals with studies of the urinary tract and corrective reconstructive measures when indicated, and the pediatrician and physiatrist with the child's physical and emotional growth and development.[34] These are joined by a host of co-professional persons to take advantage of the improved life span. This life span has resulted from the slowing of renal damage, by *judicious* use of antibiotics, uterovesicle junction surgical alteration, bladder neck resection, and urinary diversion.

The functional significance of the level of neurological sparing is similar to that of the traumatically spinal cord–injured. The child with spina bifida can usually become ambulatory. Orthoses are prescribed consistent with neurological impairment. Hip and knee deformities may respond to conservative measures, including flexibility exercises and plaster cast wedging; in the former, family members become major participants. Orthopedic surgical correction may be necessary with incomplete results from conservative measures.

Psychological Reaction

On the premise that the spinal cord–injured individual has suffered one of the most physically and socially catastrophic injuries, and appreciating that this person has been physically driven back to infancy in terms of requiring assistance for bathing, dressing, feeding, body elimination, and mobility—there are staggering adjustments to make over the coming weeks, months, and years (see also Chapters 21 to 24 and 38).

Much is accomplished through psychological support therapy and social casework. However, as the length of hospitalization decreases to an average length of stay of 84 to 116 days,[10] the emotional adjustment no doubt will occur after discharge. Treischmann notes that psychological adjustment usually requires 18 to 24 months.[35] Ducharme and Ducharme aver that adjustment to spinal cord injury is multifaceted and an ongoing process that proceeds throughout the patient's life.[36]

Since the physical rehabilitation aspect is carried out over a shorter inpatient stay, depression and denial may make it difficult for the patient to adequately participate in the program. One of the essential tasks of the physician is to facilitate the process by carefully explaining the realities of the injury to the patient and the family. The physician as well as other co-professional personnel needs to be sensitive to how the patient and the family respond to the prognosis. They may not be able to "hear" the prognosis until they can handle the anxiety. Involvement of family and friends is important lest they undermine the treatment and reinforce the denial.

It has been suggested that the "stage theory of adjustment" may no longer be valid.[37] Each new crisis, such as getting out of bed for the first time, the first visit outside the hospital, and the first weekend therapeutic home leave, requires adjustment and coping. The patient may go through all of the stages several times a week or even in a day.

Because depression may manifest itself as self-neglect, attention will need to be directed to ensuring that the spinal cord–injured person is assuming responsibility for scrupulous self-care and for required medical attention.

Bladder Dysfunction

The bladder does not exist as an independent structure but is part of a highly complex reflex mechanism. In normal micturition, there is a balance between the expulsive and retentive forces so that after timely bladder emptying there is no postvoiding residual bladder urine. An understand-

MURRAY M. FREED

ing of this function clarifies the role of the reflex mechanisms in the neurogenic bladder.[38] Bors classified neurogenic bladders into two types on the basis of the neuronal involvement: upper motor neuron and lower motor neuron.[39] The presence of reflex activity in a neurogenic bladder is consistent with an upper motor neuron lesion, and the absence of reflex activity denotes lower motor neuron involvement. He suggested that the bulbocavernosus reflex be used to test the integrity of the spinal sacral reflex arc, thus ruling out trauma to the conus medullaris or cauda equina. Stimulation of the glans penis, of the vesical and urethral mucosa, or of the detrusor produces contraction of the pelvic floor musculature and the anal sphincter. Traction on an indwelling catheter also serves as a stimulus to this reflex. Bors and Comarr note that micturition starts as a purely spinal reflex in infancy and childhood, with the sacral segments of the cord as the only link for transmission of impulses to and from the target structures.[40] Thereafter this develops into a willed process, the spinal activity of smooth and striated muscle becoming integrated with brain function so that the sacral segments, later in life, are the sites for "transmission and modulation" of afferent and efferent impulses between the higher parts of the central nervous system and the so-called target organs.

The upper motor neuron reflex bladder functions without a catheter when there is reciprocation between action of the detrusor and the sphincter. Inability to empty occurs when there is lack of reciprocal action between these two or when voiding reflexes are aborted prior to completion of bladder emptying.

In the lower motor neuron bladder there is lack of reflex detrusor function, and the individual voids by vigorous abdominal straining (see also Chapter 38).

Because of failure of development of an external collecting device for women with neurogenic bladder, prevention of incontinence in women requires special attention. Merritt, Lie, and Opitz[41] have demonstrated a program wherein two thirds were successful in reducing residual volume to less than 150 ml and achieving social continence. The program included intermittent catheterization, fluid intake restriction to 1000 to 1200 ml per day plus sips with medication, addition of neuroactive drugs as deemed appropriate based on urodynamic evaluation, and stimulation techniques (Credé, Valsalva, tapping).[42]

Bowel Dysfunction

The innervation for release of the anal sphincter tone is the same as that for bladder evacuation; the sensory innervation for appreciation of terminal bowel distention is the same as for bladder distention. The stimulus to bowel emptying is distention. Thus, the individual with spinal cord injury, prior to regulation training, experiences alternating phases of constipation and uncontrolled defecation, since the voluntary muscle component inhibits bowel emptying.

Respiratory Dysfunction

The three major motors for breathing are the diaphragm innervated from C 2 through C 4, the intercostal muscles innervated from T 2 through T 12, and the abdominal muscles from T 6 through L 1. The individual with quadriplegia has been spared only the diaphragm. According to Bergofsky, this type of breathing is adequate at rest but requires abnormally large energy expenditure when large tidal volumes are needed to satisfy increased metabolic demands.[43] Thus, the acute and chronic respiratory failure observed in quadriplegic patients arises from two sources: the inefficiency resulting from instability of the costal insertions of the diaphragm and the increased work of breathing due to increased intra-abdominal pressure caused by unusually large excursions of the diaphragm.

Additionally, the lack of abdominal muscle also results in a cough that is feeble at best, with consequent difficulty in clearing secretions in respiratory infections. This same problem with cough is encountered in lower-level injuries down to the point at which there is significant intact function in the lower thoracic cord. Impaired respiratory function, including the inability to cough effectively, is especially hazardous in the patient with high-level spinal cord injury who develops respiratory tract infection; with pooling of secretions, airway obstruction leads to atelectasis.

In those patients whose level of injury is at the C 4 segment or above, there is the likelihood of denervation of the phrenic nerve, resulting in some degree of diaphragmatic paralysis. In addition, there may well be associated thoracic cage injuries. For the newly injured patient, measures are instituted to prevent pulmonary atelectasis, infection, and edema. Ventilator assistance and tracheostomy may be required.

When diagnosis of diaphragmatic paralysis is confirmed, further study is undertaken to assess the state of phrenic nerve transmission so that consideration may be given to phrenic nerve "pacing" after an appropriate trial interval, which may be up to a year, to establish use of accessory muscles and glossopharyngeal breathing.[44-46]

Sexual Dysfunction

Talbot points out that much of the misinformation that has "pervaded society and eventually the medical profession about spinal cord injury patients and their impotence is derived not from medical sources but from a literary source."[47] This source, *Lady Chatterley's Lover*, tells of a World War I paraplegic whom D. H. Lawrence deemed impotent. As Talbot notes, D. H. Lawrence, who was a considerable poet and novelist, was not a physiologist.

Trieschmann states that we must recognize that the onset of a physical disability does not eliminate sexual feelings any more than it eliminates hunger or thirst; that there are many different kinds of sex acts available for satisfaction and a disability may interfere with only a certain number of these; and that the sexuality of the disabled individual must be evaluated in terms of his or her particular pattern of relating to others.[48] Therapeutic efforts must include the disabled individual's partner, since both must learn new patterns of behavior.[49] Hohmann adds that the patient wants to develop attitudes so that he or she is free to engage in whatever sexual behavior is organically possible and psychologically acceptable to him or her and the partner.[50] Cole asks about the paraplegic or quadriplegic man with complete transection, then continues: "His penis may become erect; his nipples may erect. His muscles may develop spasms; his blood pressure, pulse and respiration may increase. The skin of his scrotum may tense. He may develop a skin flush. Emission or ejaculation is unusual." Thus, "the spinal cord patient is capable of most of the sexual responses of the able-bodied."[51] Corresponding responses in the spinal cord–injured female have also been suggested.[49]

The sexual act in the male consists of erection, ejaculation, and orgasm. Erection may be induced by either of two stimuli, central or somesthetic and local tactile, and depends on the integrity of the second, third, and fourth spinal sacral segments for parasympathetic innervation and to a much lesser extent on the segments from T 11 to L 1 for sympathetic innervation.[52] Hyperemia results, through vasodilation and patency of the arteriovenous shunts, from activity of the sacral innervation transmitted through the cauda equina and pelvic nerves (nervi erigentes).

In the spinally injured man, local tactile stimulation provides the mechanism for erection. The success in achieving erection by this method is dependent on the level of the spinal cord injury. In one collected series, the overall success rate has been stated to be 77 per cent.[52] In the Bors and Comarr study of 529 cases, the success rate for erection in complete upper motor neuron lesions was 93 per cent, whereas that in incomplete lesions was 99 per cent.[53] Miller claims that erections occur in 80 per cent of patients with cervical cord lesions.[54] Much remains to be learned about this function in the man with spinal cord injury—certainly with understanding and communicating partners the success rate will be higher.

Ejaculation includes seminal emission and the ejaculation proper.[52] The first, dependent on the peristaltic action of the vasa deferentia, seminal vesicles, and prostate, is mediated through the sympathetic nervous system. The second results from contractions of the pelvic floor muscles and the bulbospongiosus and ischiocavernosus muscles.

Tarabulcy, in his collected series, stated that although 35 per cent had coitus, only 10 per cent achieved ejaculation.[52] The Bors and Comarr study described ejaculation in 5 per cent of those with complete lesions and 32 per cent of those with incomplete lesions.[53]

Orgasm has been described as a sensation resulting from contraction of the smooth muscles of the genitalia and the striated muscles of the pelvic floor coinciding with the ejaculation.[52] Because of the absence of peripheral sensory appreciation, the experience of orgasm is perforce altered in the man with spinal cord injury. Significant numbers of individuals, however, report pleasurable sensations in the genital region and also in an area of intact body surface innervation above the level of injury, particularly the nipple area (T 5) when this is spared.

The estimates of the number of men with spinal cord injuries who have sired children has been on the order of 1 to 5 per cent.[52, 53] To date this has been ascribed to the lesser frequency of successful coitus (35 per cent), to loss of ejaculation and impaired spermatogenesis due to nutritional or hormonal or neurogenic causes or chronic urinary tract infection, and finally to occlusion of seminal passages due to infection.[52]

Recent studies have demonstrated that electric massage of the genitalia has tripled the overall incidence of ejaculation.[55] Use of intrathecal injections of Prostigmin has produced specimens for study as well as for artificial insemination in individuals incapable of ejaculation.[55] These techniques are not without danger, since ejaculations may be accompanied by symptoms of severe autonomic dysreflexia, including hypertension and cardiac arrhythmia.[56]

The male with a cauda equina injury with consequent striated muscle paralysis has a dribbling ejaculation rather than the projectile type. Erection is achieved by some 25 per cent of such men, ejaculation by a lesser number, and progeny by 5 per cent.[53]

In certain instances, with the benefit of careful assessment of the psychological needs and with counseling, there may be indication for a penile endoprosthesis.[57–60]

Less information is available concerning sexual function in the female because fewer women suffer spinal cord trauma. In our clinic the percentage has been under 20. The sequence of events in the sexual act corresponds to that in the male.[52] The tumescence of the clitoris and labia minora is the equivalent of erection. The seminal emission equivalent is contraction of the smooth muscle of the uterus, and the equivalent of ejaculation is the rhythmic contraction of the vaginal sphincter, the ischiocavernosus, and the pelvic floor musculature. Orgasm may be experienced as a pleasurable sensation at the level of demarcation between intact and lost sensation rather than vaginally; in some instances this sensation is vaginal in location.

Following injury, the woman with spinal cord injury may have an interval with loss of menstrual periods or irregularity with eventual return to regularity. The likelihood of pregnancy after spinal cord injury is unchanged, since fertility is unimpaired, and pregnancy and labor may proceed without complications. During labor in women with a lesion at or above the T 4–T 5 level, the manifestations of autonomic dysreflexia may develop and should be distinguished from eclampsia.[61] It may be difficult to know when labor is beginning in patients with injuries above T 10 because of lack of appreciation of uterine contractions.[62]

If the fetus has not been harmed in the accident in which the pregnant woman received the spinal cord injury and if the woman remains free of renal infection, there is all likelihood that a normal child will result.

Pregnancy complicated by paraplegia is threatened more than in normal circumstances by the trauma itself, the immediate post-traumatic situation of the patient and by chronic infections and anemia in pregnancies, following cord injury.[63]

Orthostatic Hypotension

A frequent and dismaying problem encountered by patients with spinal cord injury, particularly those with quadriplegia, is the inability to tolerate the upright position because of orthostatic hypotension. This is characterized by nausea, lightheadedness, and even syncope. For most, this is of a temporary nature and passes with increasing periods in the upright position. For a small number, it persists and requires mechanical or pharmaceutical control. With deprivation of the sympathetic response that prevents pooling of blood in dependent parts and with poor tissue turgor, which allows extravasation of fluid, orthostatic hypotension occurs.

Vallbona and his colleagues have suggested that in cases of complete transection of the cervical spinal cord and loss of orthostatic regulation of sympathetic innervation below the lesion, there is insufficient release of catecholamines in response to sudden positional changes.[64] Slow release of antidiuretic hormone, cortisol, and aldosterone may also play a role.

Temperature Adjustment

Maintenance of body temperature results from a balance of heat production and heat dissipation. Temperature-sensitive structures in the superficial and deep regions of the body act as a warning system to the central temperature-sensitive receptors in the anterior preoptic region of the hypothalamus.[65] A rise in central temperature results in vasodilation and sweating in the periphery, whereas central cooling results in vasoconstriction and shivering. Downey states that the central receptors probably play a dominant role in the thermoregulation, with skin responses functioning mainly in short-term regulation.[66]

According to Guttmann and his colleagues, T 8 is the highest level at which a patient can maintain rectal temperature at 37° C in an environmental temperature from 18° to 40° C.[65] Patients with higher levels are poikilothermic in response to heating or cooling. In patients with spinal injury, shivering occurs only in muscles innervated above the level of the lesion.[67] Miller comments on the presence of rudimentary thermoregulation at the cord level.[54]

Although the mechanism is not fully understood, the person with spinal cord injury does have difficulty adjusting to extremes of ambient temperature, and the higher the level, the greater the difficulty.[68]

Metabolic Alterations

BONE

Prolonged bed rest is known to produce not only muscle atrophy but demineralization of bone as well. In the paralyzed individual this tendency is compounded, particularly in the bony structures below the level of the spinal cord lesion. The development of osteoporosis in the proximal femur makes the individual vulnerable to minimal trauma to the extent that even the ordinary activity of turning in bed may result in a hip fracture. Standing for weight-bearing is of little if any use in prevention or reversal of osteoporosis.

SERUM PROTEIN

In quadriplegics, the median value of the total protein in both the immediate and late postinjury states is at the lower limits of normal.[69] In the later stages there is a gradual increase in the gamma globulin fraction. Once the serum protein changes have occurred, there is rarely return to normal.[70] Attempts to alter this situation in preparation for decubitus ulcer reconstructive surgery have proved fruitless both by nutritional supplement and intravenous albumin infusion. An adequate hemoglobin level has been the most promising preoperative achievement.

HYPERCALCEMIA

Maynard and Imai report immobilization hypercalcemia in growing adolescent quadriplegics.[71] The mechanism is described as an imbalance of osteoblastic and osteoclastic activity in growing adolescents wherein osteoclastic activity with bone resorption is increased and the high increased calcium load is inadequately excreted by the kidneys, with resultant hypercalcemia. This phenomenon must be distinguished from primary hyperparathyroidism. The clinical manifestations of anorexia, nausea, malaise, headache, polydipsia, polyuria, and lethargy are noted most commonly four to eight weeks after injury when the condition occurs in the adolescent spinal cord–injured person. Recommendations for long-term control have been courses of corticosteroids or oral phosphates.[71]

LIVER DYSFUNCTION

Breast enlargement, either unilateral or bilateral, is not uncommon in the patient with spinal cord injury. In our own experience the incidence has been up to 5 per cent. The enlargement has been ascribed to an increase of circulatory estrogens resulting from hepatic dysfunction. Cooper and his colleagues commented that the liver impairment resolves within 8 to 10 weeks.[72] An understanding of this phenomenon will avoid the decision to perform breast biopsy.

Bloom reports that there is elevated ALT in spinal cord–injured persons with mean onset 22 days after injury and mean resolution 67 days after injury. This phenomenon was not correlated with quad-cough or hyperalimentation. The elevation was found in 76 per cent of individuals with quadriplegia and 47 per cent of those with paraplegia.[73]

Cooper and Hoen described temporary elevation of urinary 17-ketosteroid levels during the first 48 hours after spinal injury.[75] Thereafter 50 per cent of paraplegic males showed a decrease for a period of 10 weeks to 7 years. Kaplan and his co-workers noted that in their study of 60 patients, 63.3 per cent showed little or no 17-ketosteroid response to ACTH, and 58.3 per cent showed little or no 17-hydroxysteroid response.[74] Further, testicular atrophy and impaired spermatogenesis have been ascribed to disturbance of pituitary gonadal feedback.[76]

AUTONOMIC DYSREFLEXIA

Autonomic dysreflexia is characterized by elevation of blood pressure on the order of 100 to 200 mm Hg systolic and 50 to 100 mm Hg diastolic, headache, slowing of the pulse, flushing and sweating of the face, and nasal congestion. The possibility of convulsions and cerebral hemorrhage with death exists.[77]

Based on reflex activity, either viscero-vascular or somatovascular, the syndrome occurs because of impaired vascular segmental activity resulting from spinal cord damage above the splanchnic outflow, that is, above levels between T 4 and T 6. Young comments that the autonomic systems (sympathetic and sacral parasympathetic) remain without control from higher regulatory centers. Thus, the reflex mechanisms function in "unrestricted reflex revelry with disastrous consequences to the patient."[78]

Afferent impulses from the offending site enter the posterior gray matter, where they may initiate segmental reflexes and, as well, ascend in the cord to synapse with neurons in the intermediolateral columns of the thoracic cord, initiating autonomic vasoconstrictor reflexes.[79–81] In the able-bodied, inhibitory impulses from higher brain centers regulate the vasoconstriction reflexes. In the high-level spinal cord–injured, the descending inhibitory impulses are blocked at the level of the cord injury, allowing the autonomic reflexes to go uncontrolled. The sole response to the uncontrolled blood pressure elevation is the bradycardia initiated by the baroreceptors in the aorta and carotid sinus and mediated through the medullary vasomotor centers.

Elicited by noxious stimuli to the body parts below the level of injury, the reflex most frequently occurs in response to distention of bladder and bowel. Rossier and his co-workers note that during labor in patients with high thoracic or cervical levels of injury, the manifestations of autonomic dysreflexia should not be confused with preeclampsia.[82]

Bladder calculi, urinary tract infection, and decubitus ulcers have also been implicated.[81] When none of the aforementioned conditions is the cause, presence of an ingrown infected toenail should be sought as the stimulus. Autonomic dysreflexia has already been well documented in patients with high-level spinal cord injuries during cystoscopy.[83] Bors and Comarr note that autonomic dysreflexia may reach a peak after a lapse of time following the spinal cord injury and then subside, but may recur after many years of quiescence.[40]

While seeking a not easily detectable source of the difficulty, chlorpromazine hydrochloride (Thorazine) may be of great assistance. When removal of the noxious stimulus does not result in resolution of the dysreflexia, treatment with amyl nitrite or nitroglycerin should be used initially. Although treatment with guanethidine (Ismelin) has been found useful, concomitant orthostatic hypotension may be a problem. In the instance that blood pressure levels rise above 160 mm systolic and/or 120 diastolic, intravenous therapy with hydralazine hydrochloride (Apresoline) or trimethaphan camsylate (Arfonad) may be indicated. In desperate situations, spinal anesthesia or peripheral (pudendal or sacral) nerve blocks may be considered.

Ramos, Freed, and Marek demonstrated the basis for the transient mild sweating, cutis anserina, coldness, chills, and at times headache that occur at the time of bladder emptying in high-level spinal cord–injured persons with acceptable reflex bladder emptying.[84] Although physical examination, including blood pressure measurement, revealed no abnormal findings, urodynamic studies with concurrent blood pressure and electrocardiographic measurements revealed a drop in heart rate, a rise in blood pressure from $115 \pm 12/70 \pm 11$ to $173 \pm 20/101 \pm 15$ at peak filling ($p < 0.001$). In a small number there was lengthening of the PR interval. In the paraplegic patient the heart rate increased from 72 to 82; the blood pressure rose from $131 \pm 14/77 \pm 10$ to $131 \pm 24/84 \pm 4$ ($p = 0.05$). They have termed this phenomenon *subclinical autonomic dysreflexia*.

Potential Complications

Infection and Calculus Formation

The normal urinary tract is bacteria-free except adjacent to the distal portion of the urethra, and ordinarily the urine is sterile. The neurogenic bladder with large postvoiding residual urine volumes due to obstructive uropathy or impaired expulsive force provides the milieu for bacterial growth. Further, the indwelling catheter, when this is required, provides an entrance mechanism for bacteria from the external environment into the bladder.

The normal bladder mucosa is ordinarily resistant to bacterial entrance; the neurogenic bladder mucosa does not have this protective mechanism.

The person with spinal cord injury is also prone to kidney bacterial infection, since obstruction to urine flow makes the kidney more liable to infection; the neurogenic bladder dysfunction results in bladder infection, which in turn results in kidney infection. The spread of infection is, in a significant number of instances, fostered by the presence of vesicoureteral reflux due to involvement of the intramural portion of the ureters and of the ureteral orifice that is sufficient to interfere with normal function. In the absence of reflux, however, bacteria can reach the kidney by the ascending route.

Urinary stasis favors precipitation of salts resulting in calculus formation. Stones in spinal cord–injured patients consist mainly of phosphates and carbonates of calcium, magnesium, and ammonium. Also, the presence of infection as well as a foreign body in the bladder sets the stage for formation of stones in the bladder and kidney and less commonly in the prostate and seminal vesicles. The presence of calculus also concurrently fosters the infection.

The incidence of urinary tract calculi had been acknowledged to be from 22.5 to 68.7 per cent until after World War II.[85] The most important measure in decreasing calculosis, prevention of infection, has best been achieved by the wide acceptance of intermittent catheterization. Guttmann and Frankel demonstrated an overall incidence of 0.43 per cent in 476 patients treated with intermittent catheterization who were admitted to a spinal cord injury center within 14 days of injury.[86]

Ischemic Ulceration

Decubitus ulcers or ischemic ulcerations are one of the major problems confronting any patient who remains in one position, either sitting or recumbent, for prolonged periods of time.[87] The most frequently involved areas are the sacrum, the trochanters of the hip, the ischial rami, and the malleoli and heels. These are sites with relatively little tissue interposed between the skin and bony prominences. Thus, persons with spinal cord injury, who may be unable to move or turn themselves frequently and who have no sensation of pressure, are especially prone to ulceration because they lack perception of pressure and because circulation to denervated areas is inadequate.

Munro wrote that the propensity for development of ulcers was based on interruption of the autonomic reflex arcs that controlled circulation to the skin; therefore, there was no response to pressure in the normal protective manner.[87] Later Kosiak demonstrated that decubitus ulcers were ischemic in nature and resulted from prolonged tissue ischemia when pressure applied exceeded capillary pressure at sites overlying bony prominences.[88, 89]

Because hydrostatic pressures in capillaries are low and because cessation of flow occurs even in the presence of positive arterial pressure it seems logical that complete tissue ischemia may be present when pressures on the order of capillary pressure are applied.[90]

Thus, an ischemic destructive process occurs with application of high pressure of short duration or prolonged low pressure. According to Kosiak these are localized areas of cellular necrosis; the microscopical changes are characterized by edema, loss of cross-striations and myofibrils, hyalinization of fibers, neutrophilic infiltration, and phagocytosis by neutrophils and macrophages.[89, 90] In animal studies these changes were produced by pressure of 50 mm Hg for one hour in animals with a ligated femoral artery, but did not occur with pressure of 100 mm Hg for two hours in the normal animal.

Deep Vein Thrombosis

Among the complications to which the spinal cord–injured person is subject is deep vein thrombosis. Steinberg[91] points out that more than 100 years after Virchow postulated that "three factors had to cause venous thrombosis: a change in rate of blood flow, vessel wall changes, and a change in blood coagulability, the precise role of each of these factors is poorly understood." Further, "there is no clear-cut evidence at this point in time that prolonged rest by itself, without other contributing factors, predisposes to the development of venous thrombosis."

Although Guttmann and others opined that the most important factor is stagnation of blood flow,[92–94] Wessler's demonstration that it took eight hours before blood trapped between two ligatures of dog's vein fully coagulated indicated that other factors certainly play a role.[95] Clagett and Salzman note that there are elevations in plasma procoagulants and fibrinogen and an increase in platelet number and reactivity following surgery and injuries.[96]

Deep vein thrombosis and its consequence, pulmonary embolism, represent a serious complication in traumatic spinal cord injury, most commonly within the first month after injury.[97, 98] Deep vein thrombosis develops more frequently in complete than in incomplete lesions and with greater frequency in thoracic and cervical injuries.[92, 96] The incidence of deep vein thrombosis has been estimated to be from 12.5 to 58 per cent in the spinal cord–injured[94, 96, 98, 99] and pulmonary embolism on the order of 5 to 10 per cent.[94, 97, 100] Subclinical episodes of pulmonary embolization may occur more frequently than is commonly recognized.[101]

With the generally accepted emphasis on prevention, at least once-daily thigh and calf girth measurements at indelibly marked levels are indicated to detect swelling. Proper application of full leg elastic bandages has proved more valuable than stockings, since the rapid onset of thigh atrophy negates the effectiveness of commercially available full-length elastic stockings. The prophylactic administration of low-dose heparin in the amount of 5000 units twice daily is low in risk and is becoming acceptable although not fully substantiated as a preventive measure. This regimen has been recommended for the first month, followed by Coumadin for the next two months.[102, 103] Aspirin and full anticoagulation carry the risk of increased bleeding at the spinal cord injury site, particularly early after the injury or after spinal surgery, and, in the quadriplegic, increase the likelihood of gastric bleeding where the incidence is already appreciable.

When the presence of deep vein thrombosis is documented, a course of intravenous heparin is indicated for 10 days followed by a 3- to 6-month, or longer, course of Coumadin. When there is the contraindication to anticoagulation, placement of a Greenfield filter or inferior vena cava plication is an alternative method. In considering the use of the Greenfield filter, it should be noted that vigorous chest physical therapy may not be possible because of liability of resultant movement of the filter.[104] Although infrequent, it should be considered in individuals who require a "quad-cough." This maneuver, used to help clear secretions in the quadriplegic or high-level paraplegic patient, results in sudden increase in intrathoracic pressure as a Valsalva maneuver. Such a rise in pressure in the inferior vena cava produces distention of the vena cava, and thus may release the filter and propel it distally.

Heterotopic Bone Formation

Heterotopic bone formation is a not uncommon complication of spinal cord injury but one not possible to predict in a given patient. It has an incidence of 16 to 53 per cent.[105, 106] Heterotopic bone formation is in most instances noted as an incidental finding during the course of x-ray examination. It forms periarticularly below the level of lesion and is associated with hips, knees, shoulders, elbows, and the lumbar paravertebral areas. The most common time for development is in the period from one to four months after injury, with rare occurrence after one year.

The findings may be of the "acute" type, presenting as an inflammatory reaction including local heat, swelling, and redness, or only swelling or induration. To be considered in the differential diagnosis are deep vein thrombosis, cellulitis, joint sepsis, hematoma formation, and fracture. The important consideration is to rule out deep vein thrombosis, for the onset of both thrombosis and heterotopic bone formation is most common in the first months after injury. Heterotopic bone may produce venous obstruction by external compression.

The finding of elevated serum alkaline phosphatase is only suggestive early in the course of heterotopic bone formation. X-ray examination may not reveal positive findings during the first two weeks; a bone scan is the most reliable diagnostic measure and more importantly in late stages as the determinant in deciding on maturity of the process.

It has been accepted that heterotopic bone formation following spinal cord injury requires aggressive passive range of motion[106, 107] for prevention of the ankylosis that severely limits activities of daily living; rest may well increase the joint motion limitations. Disodium etidronate (diphosphonate) has been proposed for the treatment and prevention of heterotopic bone formation. In the therapeutic dosage of 5 mg/kg per day for 12 to 24 weeks, it does not retard healing of any fractures but should prevent further ossification of the process of heterotopic bone formation. In those instances, when there is insufficient response to physical therapeutic measures, surgical intervention is indicated, but only after the bone formation has been demonstrated to be mature.

Spasticity

Every individual who suffers a spinal cord injury develops spasticity to a greater or lesser degree following an interval that may be as short as hours or as long as months. More commonly it occurs within the first two to three weeks following the injury. The development of this phenomenon is an indication that the muscle stretch reflex has become isolated from its supraspinal inhibitory-modulation system so that the alpha and dynamic fusimotor neurons are abnormally excitable.[108] The extensor mechanisms recover first, usually in the lower extremities, with a posture of extension that is difficult to overcome.[108, 109]

Spasticity may have a salubrious effect on activities of daily living in that it provides knee stability in the upright position on a reflex basis, by its effect in expulsion of urinary bladder contents, and by its torque force on bone to maintain bone density. It may, on the other hand, interfere by preventing comfortable wheelchair sitting, by hampering transfer activities and other activities of daily living, and by preventing the bladder from becoming a useful reservoir of urine. Finally, there is the probability of heel cord shortening, pronation deformity at the ankles, and adductor tightness at the hips.

When the spasticity interferes with activities to a sufficient degree and is not overcome by daily routine flexibility exercises, medication should be considered. The most commonly used pharmacological agents are diazepam (Valium), dantrolene sodium (Dantrium), and baclofen (Lioresal). Although diazepam is probably the most widely used and is a polysynaptic inhibitor, it has a short duration.[109] It has been noted that in many instances, a part of its effect may be due to its less specific psychotherapeutic properties.[109] Its addictive properties must be considered in selecting medication for spasticity. Dantrolene sodium requires careful follow-up of liver function because of its side effects, which are dose-related and more common in younger patients. Dantrolene sodium acts on skeletal muscle with a primary effect on extrafusal fibers affecting excitation contraction, coupled with possible effect on intrafusal fibers as well.[110–112]

According to Pedersen, "classification of drugs according to their site of action is often difficult because of incomplete knowledge of the pathophysiology of spasticity and because the agents may have more than one site of action."[109] Further, the site may vary with dosage.

In animal studies, baclofen has shown an inhibitory effect on both monosynaptic and polysynaptic activities.[109] Studies have shown that baclofen's site of action is the Ia fibers, including the alpha motor neurons in the area of presynaptic inhibition.[113] In the past, barbiturates had been used for spasticity. However, the effective intake for relief of the spasticity produced concomitant drowsiness.

Baclofen in four divided doses to the recommended maximum of 80 mg daily is indicated initially for troubling spasticity. When required, small doses of dantrolene sodium may be given for obtaining an adjuvant effect, thus avoiding the side effects of larger doses. Thus, effective preparations are available for spasticity that have proved to be beneficial in improving activities of daily living.

Invasive procedures such as intrathecal alcohol instillation or phenol instillation may resolve the problem of spasticity, but they also damage ventral and dorsal roots and thus preclude development of a reflex bladder and reflexogenic penile erection.[114] Peripheral nerve blocks with phenol, although effective, have demonstrated a side effect of painful paresthesias.[115–117] Awad has proposed the use of an electrical stimulator to localize a motor nerve. The use of an injection needle as the stimulating probe enables the localization of the nerve fibers and simultaneous blockage of these fibers.[117] He feels that phenol has withstood the test of time and is accepted as a local blocking agent, since it is free of local irritation and systemic toxic effects in the 5 per cent solution. Moreover, its immediate onset of action makes it possible to determine the results of the blocks instantaneously. Further, he adds that phenol has the advantages of a reasonably long duration of action, of being easily sterilized without loss of activity, and of ready availability at low cost. When phenol is injected in or around the motor nerve to a spastic muscle, it abolishes the spasticity by interruption of the pathway of the increased activity of the stretch reflex. It does this by blocking the afferent proprioceptive and efferent fibers.[118]

Surgical measures have included obturator neurectomy for adductor spasticity that interferes with nursing care and ambulation, sciatic neurectomy for spastic knee flexors and plantar flexors, and tendon lengthening, particularly for the Achilles tendon and knee flexor.

Malignant Disease

Melzak noted that since infection of the urinary tract is still very common in the patient with spinal cord injury, it would be appropriate to study the incidence of bladder cancer in these individuals.[119] In Great Britain's National Spinal Injuries Centre, his 20-year study beginning in 1944 of 3800 persons with spinal cord injury resulted in the finding of 11 cases of bladder cancer, an incidence of 0.28 per cent. The earliest was diagnosed after 13 years, the latest after 42 years. The youngest patient was 37 years old. Because the vast majority of his patients smoked, he hesitated to accuse smoking as the cause; it is, however, recognized that smokers have a greater incidence of bladder carcinoma. The only common factors proved to be longstanding chronic urinary infection and cystitis, and long-standing catheter drainage. Bors and Comarr found malignant genitourinary tract disease in 0.64 per cent of 2322 patients.[40] The diagnosis was made 10 to 22 years following injury.

Hypertension

In his postmortem study of 122 paraplegics between 1945 and 1962, Tribe found a surprisingly large incidence of hypertension. "Critical assessment of both clinical and pathologic evidence revealed 41 cases of definite hypertension amongst the 122 paraplegics."[120] He concluded that the hypertension was associated with chronic pyelonephritis. Hypertension was an infrequent finding in other studies.[121–125]

Pain

Many patients with injuries to the spinal cord or cauda equina experience pain at some time in early or late course of their illness.[126]

Persistent intractable pain is a problem in a limited number of individuals with spinal cord injury. Gooddy suggests that the pain experienced below the level of the spinal cord lesion may be transmitted through the sympathetic nervous system.[127]

Krueger believed that in most instances the pain originates from lesions of the intraspinal contents, either from intact or partially intact nerve roots or from neuroma formation in severed roots or at the proximal stump of the severed spinal cord, or in the transitional zone immediately above the lesion in cases of nontransecting spinal cord injuries.[126] Pain is more common and more severe in injuries to the lower cord and cauda equina.

Another type of pain has been labeled visceral pain and follows distention by enemas or distention of the urinary bladder.[26] This discomfort is abdominal in nature. Visceral abnormality such as peptic ulcer or cholecystitis may also produce vague nonlocalizing abdominal discomfort.

Bedbrook notes that neurosurgical interruptions have a role in certain intractable pain states in spinal-injured patients but have disadvantages, including unpredictability of immediate beneficial effect, undesirable side effects, and return of pain often within months and usually of a worse type.[128]

Gastrointestinal Function

The transport of products of digestion through the intestine results from peristaltic action that arises from the autonomic plexuses within the bowel wall. Quadriplegic individuals are known to have a high rate of incidence of peptic ulcer that may well be of the stress type. Miller points out that this ulcer phenomenon may be due to unopposed vagal action, as are the ileus and hypermotility.[129]

Superior mesenteric artery syndrome is a complication occurring in the high-level spinal cord–injured, which, although infrequent, is of great importance.[130, 131] The occlusion of the third portion of the duodenum by the superior mesenteric artery in its downward course is produced by traction on this artery on its mesentery or by any downward displacement of the small intestine. This duodenal obstruction results in sudden onset of persistent vomiting of large amounts of fluid. The upper abdomen is distended and tympanitic. Recommended is conservative care, including avoidance of the supine posture after meals, upward manual displacement of the abdominal viscera, and adequate support of the abdominal wall; when these preventive conservative measures are of no avail, then surgical correction becomes necessary.[130]

Degree of Neurological Recovery

Table 32–4 shows the Frankel grade distribution of the 9647 patients reported from the National Spinal Cord Injury Statistical Centre within neurological level groupings at the time of discharge from the initial medical/rehabilitation phases of care.[10] Of those admitted with Frankel grade A, 93.3 per cent were unchanged at discharge; of the remaining 6.7 per cent, two fifths became grade B, one third C, and approximately one quarter D; none recovered. Of those with grade B, 62.7 per cent were unchanged. Of the remaining 37.3 per cent, 10 per cent regressed to grade A, just over one third became C, and just over one half became grade D; 0.7 per cent recovered. Among those with grade C, 46.4 per cent were unchanged at discharge. Of the remaining 53.6 per cent, 2 per cent regressed to A and 0.8 per cent to B whereas 95.6 per cent improved to D, and 1.6 per cent recovered. Of those with Frankel D grades on admission, 93.8 per cent did not change; of the remaining 6.2 per cent, 8.3, 6.7, and 19.2 per cent regressed to A, B, and C respectively whereas 65.8 per cent recovered.

Ditunno and his co-workers concluded that initial biceps strength is a reliable indicator of wrist extensor recovery and most if not all C 5 neurological level patients will gain one full motor level.

TABLE 32–4. Distribution of Patients Within Neurological Groupings at Discharge from Initial Medical/Rehabilitation Phases of Care*

FRANKEL GRADE†	HIGH QUAD C 1–C 4 (%)	LOW QUAD C 5–C 8 (%)	HIGH THORACIC T 1–T 6 (%)	LOW THORACIC T 7–T 12 (%)	LUMBAR L 1–L 5 (%)	SACRAL S 1–S 5 (%)	ALL LEVELS (%)
Complete (A)	45.3	44.7	80.2	66.0	17.5	0.0	51.1
Sensory only (B)	8.0	14.3	6.3	7.2	7.3	0.0	9.7
Motor nonfunctional (C)	12.8	9.0	4.1	6.4	11.4	4.2	8.5
Motor functional (D)	33.7	31.9	9.4	20.4	63.7	95.8	29.6
Recovered (E)	0.2	0.1	0.0	0.0	0.1	0.0	1.1
All grades	100.0	100.0	100.0	100.0	100.0	100.0	100.0

*From Stover, S. L., and Fine, P. R.: Spinal Cord Injury: The Facts and Figures. Birmingham, AL, University of Alabama-Birmingham, 1986, p. 30.

†Neurological level of lesion by degree of preserved function.

Further, this is probably due to overwork hypertrophy and peripheral sprouting of nerve within muscle rather than root level recovery.[132, 132a]

In incomplete upper motor neuron injuries, return of function may go on for 1 to 1½ years, whereas in lower motor neuron injuries the duration may be of several years. However, recovery is progressive during these intervals with degree inversely proportional to time. There is no sudden recovery at the end of these intervals, and this must be made clear to the patient.

Specialized Hospital Units for Care of the Patient with Spinal Cord Injury

The great advantage of using a categorically oriented system of care for the patient with spinal cord injury was first proved by Dr. Donald Munro in the 1930s in his unit in the Boston City Hospital. That a significant number of such patients could not only survive but could also return to a productive and functional life status was later confirmed by Guttmann in England, Weiss in Poland, Cheshire in Australia, Michaelis and Rossier in Switzerland, Bors and Talbot in the United States Veterans Administration, Gregg in Ireland, Meinecke in Germany, and Young and Freed in the United States.[133–143]

The complex nature of the manifestations of spinal cord injury and the potential for life-threatening complications, as well as for complications whose avoidance could decrease the hospital stay and minimize the psychological trauma, makes mandatory the provision of care in a facility especially organized for providing holistic care for this injury.

A lifetime of care begins after discharge from the hospital. The ongoing goals include refinement of physical gains already achieved, maintenance of achieved functional ability and adjustment, and identification of potential or already developed problems. This care includes regular outpatient re-evaluation as well as periodic inpatient study at intervals of 6 to 18 months.

Upon departure from the hospital, the person with spinal cord injury will, when possible, be discharged home, which will have been physically altered. The family will have become familiar with the individual's total needs, and ideally schooling, retraining, and vocational placement will have been arranged.

Special Considerations

Provided with adapted devices to exploit the full potential of their physical functioning and with removal of architectural barriers in the home and community, individuals with spinal cord injury, no matter what the level, can leave their home, make their way by wheelchair (the most essential equipment for mobility) and hand-control–operated motor vehicle, and participate in educational, vocational, recreational, and even social welfare pursuits in behalf of others.

These accomplishments require doors sufficiently wide to permit wheelchair entrance and egress; replacement of entrance stairs by ramps with grades of no greater than 8 per cent; widening of corridors to allow maneuverability of wheelchairs; construction of bathrooms both in public buildings and at home to allow maneuverability in the chair and transfer from the chair onto the toilet and return; and adjustment of public telephones, electric light switches, plugs, elevator operating buttons, and door latches to the height of the person seated in the wheelchair. Internal environmental temperature adjustment is also important in view of the intolerance of the person with spinal cord injury to extremes of heat and cold. Elevator accessibility in multistoried school buildings will permit these individuals to attend regular classroom instruction with their peers.

Prejudice by potential employers and real estate managers remains a problem, as does that of transportation companies. The potential of the person with spinal cord injury, in the absence of medical and psychological complications but even in the presence of multiple physical impairment, is unmeasurable.

Rusk avers:

You don't get fine china by putting clay in the sun. You have to put the clay through the white heat of the kiln if you want to make porcelain. Heat breaks some pieces. Disability breaks some people. But once the clay goes through the white-hot fire and comes out whole, it can never be clay again; once a person overcomes a disability through his own courage, determination and hard work, he has a depth of spirit you and I know little about.[144]

ACKNOWLEDGMENT

Parts of this chapter are taken from Freed, M. M.: Long-term disability from spinal cord injury. *In* Tedeschi, C. G., Eckert, W. G., and Tedeschi, L. G.: Forensic Medicine: A Study in Trauma and Environmental Hazards. Philadelphia, W. B. Saunders Company, 1977, pp. 76–87.

References

1. Elsberg, C. A.: The Edwin Smith surgical papyrus and the diagnosis and treatment of injuries to the skull and spine 5000 years ago. Ann. Med. Hist., 3:271, 1931.
2. Poer, D. H.: Newer concepts in the treatment of the paralyzed patient due to war-time injuries of the spinal cord. Ann. Surg., 123:510, 1946.
3. Thompson Walker, J. W.: Hunterian Lecture on the bladder in gunshot and other injuries of the spinal cord. Lancet, 1:173, 1917.
4. Kuhn, W. G.: The care and rehabilitation of patients with injuries of the spinal cord. J. Neurosurg., 4:40, 1947.
5. Hinman, F.: The treatment of paralytic bladder in cases of spinal cord injury. Surgery, 4:649, 1938.
6. Munro, D.: Thoracic and lumbosacral cord injuries. J.A.M.A., 122:1055, 1943.
7. Kirk, N. T.: Wartime activities of the Army Medical Department. N. Engl. J. Med., 235:182, 1946.
8. Controller, Department of Medicine and Surgery: Mortality Report on Spinal Cord Injury. Reports and Statistics Service, Veterans Administration, Nov. 13, 1958.
9. Geisler, W. O., Jousse, A. T., Wynn-Jones, M., and Breithaupt, M. D.: Survival in traumatic spinal cord injury. Paraplegia, 21:364–373, 1983.
10. Stover, S. L., and Fine, P. R.: Spinal Cord Injury: The Facts and Figures. Birmingham, AL, The University of Alabama-Birmingham, 1986.
11. Gehrig, R., and Michaelis, L. S.: Statistics of acute paraplegia and tetraplegia on a national scale. Paraplegia, 6:93, 1968.
12. Canadian Neurosurgical Society: Report of a Sub-Committee. Paraplegic Care in Canada, 1969.
13. Young, J. S.: The Southwest Regional System for Treatment of Spinal Injury. Proposal to U.S. Department of Health, Education, and Welfare, April 25, 1969.
14. Sharman, G. J., and Owens, K. A. Jr.: Spinal Cord Injury. Report to the National Paraplegia Foundation, Boston, September 1970.
15. Brown, L. M.: Maine's Spinal Cord Injured. Study Report to Bureau of Rehabilitation, Department of Health and Welfare, Augusta, Maine, August 1972.
16. Unpublished data of the National Spinal Cord Injury Model Systems Project, sponsored in part by the National Institute on Disability and Rehabilitation Research and received from the following projects: University of Alabama Spinal Cord Injury System, University of Alabama in Birmingham, Birmingham, AL; Southwest Regional System for Treatment of Spinal Injury, Good Samaritan Hospital–St. Joseph's Hospital, Phoenix, AZ; Northern California Regional Spinal Injury System, Santa Clara Valley Medical Center, San Jose, CA; Southern California Regional Spinal Injury System, Rancho Los Amigos Hospital, Downey, CA; Rocky Mountain Regional Spinal Cord Injury System, Craig Hospital, Englewood, CO; South Florida Regional Spinal Cord Injury System, University of Miami School of Medicine, Miami, FL; Midwest Regional Spinal Cord Injury Care System, Northwestern Memorial Hospital, Rehabilitation Institute of Chicago, Northwestern University, McGaw Medical Center, Chicago, IL; New England Regional Spinal Cord Injury System of University Hospital, Boston University Medical Center, Boston, MA; Missouri Regional Spinal Cord Injury System, University of Missouri School of Medicine, Columbia, MO; New York Regional Spinal Cord Injury System, Institute of Rehabilitation Medicine, New York University, New York, NY; Regional Spinal Cord Injury System of the Delaware Valley, Thomas Jefferson University, Philadelphia, PA; Texas Regional Spinal Cord Injury System, The Institute for Rehabilitation and Research,

ment of traumatic paraplegia and tetraplegia. Paraplegia, 4:63, 1966.

87. Munro, D.: Care of the back following spinal cord injuries. N. Engl. J. Med., 233:391, 1940.

88. Kosiak, M.: Etiology of decubitus ulcers. Arch. Phys. Med. Rehabil., 42:19, 1961.

89. Kosiak, M.: An effective method of preventing decubitus ulcers. Arch. Phys. Med. Rehabil., 47:724, 1966.

90. Kosiak, M.: Etiology and pathology of ischemic ulcerations. Arch. Phys. Med. Rehabil., 40:62, 1959.

91. Steinberg, F. U.: The effects of immobilization on circulation and respiration. In Steinberg, F. U.: The Immobilized Patient: Functional Pathology and Management. New York City, Plenum Medical Book Company, 1980.

92. Guttmann, L.: Venous thrombosis and pulmonary embolism. In Guttmann, L.: Spinal Cord Injuries: Comprehensive Management and Research, 2nd Ed. Oxford, Blackwell Scientific Publications, 1976.

93. Naso, F.: Pulmonary embolism in acute spinal cord injury. Arch. Phys. Med. Rehabil., 55:275, 1974.

94. Shull, J. R., and Rose, D. L.: Pulmonary embolism in patients with spinal cord injuries. Arch. Phys. Med. Rehabil., 47:444, 1976.

95. Wessler, S.: Studies in intravascular coagulation. I. Coagulation in isolated venous segments. J. Clin. Invest., 31:1011, 1952.

96. Clagett, G. P., and Salzman, E. W.: Prevention of venous thromboembolism in surgical patients. N. Engl. J. Med., 290:93, 1974.

97. Watson, N.: Venous thrombosis and pulmonary embolism in spinal cord injury. Paraplegia, 6:113, 1969.

98. Perkash, A., Prakash, V., and Perkash, I.: Experience with management of thromboembolism in patients with spinal cord injury: Part I. Incidence, diagnosis and role of some risk factors. Paraplegia, 16:322, 1978–79.

99. Bors, E., Conrad, C. A., and Massell, T. B.: Venous occlusion of lower extremities in paraplegia patients. Surg. Gynecol. Obstet., 99:451, 1954.

100. Walsh, J. J., and Tribe, C.: Phlebothrombosis and pulmonary embolism in paraplegia. Paraplegia, 3:209, 1965.

101. Wessler, S., Cohen, S., and Fleischman, F. G.: The temporary thrombotic state. N. Engl. J. Med., 254:413, 1956.

102. Watson, N.: Anti-coagulant therapy in the prevention of venous thrombosis and pulmonary embolism in the spinal cord injury. Paraplegia, 16:265, 1978–79.

103. Hachen, H. J.: Anti-coagulant therapy in patients with spinal cord injury. Paraplegia, 12:176, 1974.

104. Sidawy, A. N., and Menzoian, J. O.: Distal migration and deformation of the Greenfield vena cava filter. Surgery, 99:369–372, 1986.

105. Venier, L. H., and Ditunno, J. F., Jr.: Heterotopic ossification in the paraplegic patient. Arch. Phys. Med. Rehabil., 52:475, 1971.

106. Stover, S. L., Hataway, C. J., and Zeiger, H. E.: Heterotopic ossification in spinal cord injured patients. Arch. Phys. Med. Rehabil., 56:199, 1975.

107. Wharton, G. W., and Morgan, T. H.: Ankylosis in the paralyzed patient. J. Bone Joint Surg., 52A:105, 1970.

108. Lance, J. S., and Buchi, D.: Mechanisms of spasticity. Arch. Phys. Med. Rehabil., 55:332, 1974.

109. Pedersen, E.: Clinical assessment and pharmacologic therapy of spasticity. Arch. Phys. Med. Rehabil., 55:344, 1974.

110. Joynt, R. L.: Dantrolene sodium: Long term effects in patients with muscle spasticity. Arch. Phys. Med. Rehabil., 57:212, 1976.

111. Zorychta, E., Esplin, D. W., Capek, R., et al.: Actions of dantrolene in extrafusal and intrafusal striated muscle. Fed. Proc., 30:669, 1971.

112. Monstea, A. W., Herman, R., Meeks, S., et al.: Cooperative study for assessing effects of pharmacologic agents on spasticity. Am. J. Phys. Med., 52:163, 1973.

113. Curtis, D. R., and Felix, D.: GABA and prolonged spinal inhibition. Nature New Biol., 231:187, 1971.

114. Sheldon, C. H., and Bors, E.: Subarachnoid alcohol block in paraplegia. J. Neurosurg., 5:389, 1948.

115. Khalili, A. A., Hammel, M. H., Forster, S., and Benton, J. G.: Management of spasticity by selective nerve block with dilute phenol solutions in clinical rehabilitation. Arch. Phys. Med. Rehabil., 45:513, 1964.

116. Moritz, M. H.: Phenol block of peripheral nerves. Scand. J. Rehabil. Med., 5:160, 1973.

117. Awad, E. A.: Phenol block for control of hip flexor and adductor spasticity. Arch. Phys. Med. Rehabil., 53:554, 1972.

118. Meelhuysen, F. E., Halpern, D., and Quast, J.: Treatment of flexor spasticity of hip by paravertebral lumbar spinal nerve block. Arch. Phys. Med. Rehabil., 49:717, 1968.

119. Melzak, J.: The incidence of bladder cancer in paraplegia. Paraplegia, 4:85, 1966.

120. Tribe, C. R.: Causes of death in early and late stages of paraplegia. Paraplegia, 1:19, 1963.

121. Freed, M. M., Bakst, H. J., and Barrie, D. L.: Life expectancy, survival rates and causes of death in civilian patients with spinal cord trauma. Arch. Phys. Med. Rehabil., 47:457, 1966.

122. Ebel, A.: Discussion of the pathology in selected cases of spinal cord injury. Proceedings: 9th Annual Clinical Spinal Cord Injury Conference, October 1960. Washington, U.S. Government Printing Office, 1961.

123. Finkle, J. R.: Discussion of the pathology in selected cases of spinal cord injury. Proceedings: 9th Annual Clinical Spinal Cord Injury Conference, October 1960. Washington, U.S. Government Printing Office, 1961.

124. Halladay, L. W.: Discussion of the pathology in

selected cases of spinal cord injury. Proceedings: 9th Annual Clinical Spinal Cord Injury Conference, October 1960. Washington, U.S. Government Printing Office, 1961.

125. Lowry, R.: Discussion of the pathology in selected cases of spinal cord injury. Proceedings: 9th Annual Clinical Spinal Cord Injury Conference, October 1960. Washington, U.S. Government Printing Office, 1961.

126. Krueger, E. G.: Management of painful states in injuries of the spinal cord and cauda equina. Am. J. Phys. Med., 39:103, 1960.

127. Gooddy, Y.: On the nature of pain. Brain, 80:118, 1957.

128. Bedbrook, G.: The Care and Management of Spinal Cord Injuries. New York, Springer-Verlag, 1981.

129. Miller, J. M. III: Autonomic function in the isolated spinal cord. In Downey, J. A., and Darling, R. C. (Eds.): Physiological Basis of Rehabilitation Medicine. Philadelphia, W. B. Saunders Company, 1971.

130. Ramos, M. U.: Recurrent superior mesenteric artery syndrome in a quadriplegic patient. Arch. Phys. Med. Rehabil., 56:86, 1975.

131. Raptou, A. D., LaBan, M. M., and Johnson, E. W.: Intermittent arteriomesenteric occlusion of duodenum in quadriplegic patient. Arch. Phys. Med. Rehabil., 45:418, 1964.

132. Ditunno, J. F., Sipski, M. L., Posuniak, E. A., Chen, Y. T., Staas, W. E., and Herbison, G. J.: Wrist extensor recovery in traumatic quadriplegia. Arch. Phys. Med. Rehabil., 68:287–290, 1987.

132a. Ditunno, J. F., Stover, S. L., Freed, M. M., and Ahn, J. H.: A comparison of motor recovery of the upper extremities of C4 and C5 SCI patients. Proceedings of the 15th SCI Meeting. American Spinal Injury Assoc., April, 1989, p. 15.

133. Guttmann, L.: History of the National Spinal Injuries Centre, Stoke Mandeville Hospital, Aylesbury, Paraplegia, 5:115, 1967.

134. Weiss, M.: Fifteen years' experience on rehabilitation of paraplegics at the Rehabilitation Institute of Warsaw University. Paraplegia, 5:158, 1967.

135. Cheshire, D. J. E.: The complete and centralised treatment of paraplegia. Paraplegia, 6:59, 1969.

136. Michaelis, L.: Opening of the Swiss Paraplegic Centre in Basle. Paraplegia, 5:158, 1967.

137. Rossier, A. B.: Organization and function of the French Swiss Paraplegic Centre. Paraplegia, 5:166, 1968.

138. Bors, E.: The Spinal Cord Injury Center of the Veterans Administration Hospital, Long Beach, CA. Paraplegia, 5:126, 1967.

139. Talbot, H. S.: Rehabilitation in a changing world. Paraplegia, 7:146, 1969.

140. Gregg, T. M.: Organization of a Spinal Injury Unit within a Rehabilitation Centre. Paraplegia, 5:163, 1967.

141. Meinecke, F. W.: Opening of the Centre For Spinal Injuries and other severely disabled persons at the Orthopaedic Clinic of Heidelberg University. Paraplegia, 5:104, 1967.

142. Young, J. S.: Development of systems of spinal injury management with a correlation to the development of other esoteric health care systems. Ariz. Med., 27:1, 1970.

143. Freed, M. M.: The Spinal Cord Injury Center, Scope. B.U.M.C., 1:16, 1968.

144. Rusk, H. A.: A World to Care For. New York, Random House, 1972.

33

Aftercare of Fractures

MILAND E. KNAPP

Problems in the aftercare of fractures may arise from causes originating in bone, soft tissue injuries, and edema. Causes originating in bone, such as malunion, delayed union, or nonunion, will not be discussed in this chapter, since they do not properly come under the heading of physical medicine. Soft tissue injuries, including lacerations of nerves, tears of ligaments and joint capsules, and injuries to tendons and muscles, also will not be discussed in this chapter, since they require definitive treatment, often surgical in nature, and although physical measures are commonly useful in their treatment, most of these measures will be discussed under other headings. Persistent edema, in my opinion, is the most common cause of disability following fractures. This problem will be discussed in detail.

Traumatic edema fluid is produced either by the original injury or by mechanical factors following the injury. Extravasation of blood into the soft tissues is a constant accompaniment of fractures. In addition to this, extravasation of edema fluid into the soft tissues may result in so much swelling and interference with normal blood supply that extensive blisters may form, sometimes covering the entire extremity. The extravasated blood and edema fluid must be removed by one of two methods. If return flow circulation is restored adequately and early, both the blood and edema fluid may be removed by absorption into the general body circulation with no undesirable residual effects.

If, on the other hand, the swelling persists longer than a week or two, the swelling may be removed by organization instead of absorption, with the eventual production of fibrous scar tissue. This process is similar to and proceeds at the same time as the organization, which results in the production of fibrous callus in the process of normal bone healing. It is desirable that fibrous tissue develop between the bone ends, since this is the first stage of fixation of the fracture. However, it is not desirable for fibrosis to occur in muscles or between such solid structures as tendon, joint capsule, bone, and strong fascial layers, since these parts are normally movable and the fibrosis limits movement.

"Oedema is glue," says Watson-Jones.[5] Since the fibrous tissue produced between the bone ends and within the soft tissues is developed at exactly the same time, it is obvious that one cannot wait for the bone to heal before treating the soft tissue damage. There are two apparently antagonistic objectives to be obtained simultaneously. First, the bone ends must be held immobile and in constant apposition until healing occurs. Second, the soft tissues must be kept moving to prevent fibrosis and subsequent limited painful motion. However, the objectives are really not as antagonistic as it might appear, since pressure tends to promote bone healing and activity increases circulation to the part and this, too, aids in bone healing. It is necessary at the time of reduction to ascertain that the apparatus that maintains immobility of the bone ends is so arranged that maximal activity of soft tissues can be obtained starting immediately after the reduction of the fracture.

The aftercare of fractures may be divided into early and late stages.

Treatment in the Early Stage

Active Motion. The most effective as well as the most available and the least expensive method of removing edema fluid is active motion. However,

749

MILAND E. KNAPP

in order that this may be accomplished, the surgeon must trim the cast to allow function or apply the retaining apparatus in such a manner that maximal function is possible. For instance, if function of the metacarpophalangeal joints of the hand is to be retained, it is necessary that the immobilizing apparatus not extend distal to the flexion crease of the palm.

Active motion is effective in removing edema fluid because it assists return flow circulation. Normal return flow circulation is carried on to a large degree by muscle activity. The veins are provided with valves that will not allow the blood to flow distally so that when the muscle squeezes down on the vein, blood is forced proximally. The blood cannot return through the valve, so the area fills up from below and blood is again ready to be forced back toward the heart. This same mechanism is present in the lymphatic system.

Elevation. If it is not feasible to remove the edema fluid by active motion, the next best method is elevation. However, it must be remembered that for elevation to be effective, the distal part of the extremity must be above the proximal part and the proximal part above the heart. This is a practical method to use in fractures of the lower extremity when the patient is in bed. Under these circumstances, elevation can be accomplished fairly easily. In the upper extremity, however, elevation is not usually practical because the hand would have to be up in a position above the elbow and the elbow above the shoulder. In fractures of the upper extremity, the patient is not ordinarily restricted to bed, so this method is not available. The use of a sling is not considered to be elevation because the hand and forearm in a sling are below the shoulder by the length of the arm.

Physical Therapy. If neither of these methods is feasible or effective, treatment must be given by what is ordinarily designated as physical therapy. The usual procedures are heat, massage, and motion.

HEAT. The physiological effects of heat may be summarized briefly as relief of pain, increase in the arterial blood supply, increased edema because of the increased capillary pressure that is produced, and softening of fibrous tissue.

The type of heat used is not usually important. Hot packs or hot soaks are quite convenient, as is infrared radiation. In a department of physical medicine, whirlpool baths or similar methods of heat application are usually used. Diathermy is not advisable in the early stages following fractures because, as a result of its greater effectiveness, it often causes increased pain by increasing edema. Heat should always be followed by massage or exercise.

MASSAGE. The physiological effects of massage are relief of pain if the massage is given efficiently and expertly, increase of venous circulation because the stroke of the massage is toward the heart, reduction of swelling as a result of the enhanced return flow circulation, and stretching of fibrous tissue (see Chapter 17).

The massage should be mild so that pain is relieved instead of increased, but it should be firm enough to reduce edema. Violent manipulation or painful types of massage should be avoided because of the possibility of displacing bone fragments before healing has occurred.

EXERCISE. If possible, massage should be followed by active exercise. If it is necessary to remove the supporting apparatus for exercise, the therapist should assist the patient in carrying out the exercise motion, either by overcoming gravity for the patient or by supporting a part of the body while the exercise is being performed. Passive motion should never be used in the early stage after fracture because fear of pain may cause the patient to resist any passive motion, and the so-called passive motion is transformed into resistive motion with the patient doing the resisting. Assisted active exercise is the exercise of choice in early fractures.

To summarize, during the period of immobilization of the fracture, physical treatment is used to reduce swelling as soon as possible and to maintain range of joint motion, muscular strength, and dexterity.

Treatment in the Late Stage

Physical Therapy. If the removal of edema fluid is delayed until the bone is healed, soft tissue adhesions will have become firmly established and may be solid enough to limit motion as well as cause pain. Unfortunately, it is common practice to refer patients for physical therapy two months or more after the original injury, when fibrosis and contractures, painful motion, muscle atrophy and weakness, and persistent brawny edema make the danger of permanent impairment of function obvious. Treatment at this time is entirely different from treatment in the early stage. Now the objectives of treatment are to remove whatever edema is still present, to soften and stretch fibrous tissue, to increase the range of joint motion, to restore circulatory efficiency, to increase muscular strength, and to retrain muscular dexterity.

HEAT. Heat may be used for sedation, to increase circulation, and to soften fibrous adhesions. The type of heat used is not extremely important and depends more upon the availability of the modality and the pathological conditions present in the patient than on any specific properties of the various methods of heat application. In my experience, relaxation is best obtained by the use of moist heat. The whirlpool bath is valuable because heat, massage, and active motion are possible simultaneously in it. Hot packs are often useful, particularly for areas that cannot be treated easily in the whirlpool. Diathermy and short wave diathermy may be used. Infrared radiation is not as effective in the late stage as it is during the early stages.

MASSAGE. Again, heat is followed by massage with emphasis upon deep stroking and compression movements in order to stretch the fibrous adhesions as well as to eliminate any edema that may still be present. This treatment may be considerably more vigorous than that used during the early stage. Tender areas are made less tender by massage. The intramuscular movement produced by the kneading and friction motions helps to stretch adhesions so that a greater range of motion is possible.

EXERCISE. Heat and massage should always be followed by exercise. The most effective regimen begins with assisted active exercise followed by free motion and then resistive exercise as the patient improves. Forced stretching of fibrous bands may be necessary in order to obtain maximal range of motion. It may be done manually or by prolonged stretch, using a weight over a period of a half hour or more (Chapter 18).

Manipulation under anesthesia should be used only if no other method is effective and then should be considered very carefully because of the danger of increasing the disability. If this method is used, it must be followed immediately by physical measures designed to overcome the pain and maintain the range of motion obtained by the manipulation. As the patient gains in range of motion and strength and as pain is decreased, occupational therapy becomes particularly useful because the patient's interest in the productivity of the activity encourages prolonged effort (see Chapter 29). Projects may be chosen to increase range of motion, strength or coordination, and manual dexterity. When the exercise is to be continued for months, the projects should be suitable for home use after discharge from the hospital.

Special Problems

A few special problems seem worth discussing in some detail because physical treatment may prevent serious complications if the condition is recognized before irreversible changes have occurred.

Myositis Ossificans

During the healing process, calcification may occur in the soft tissues as well as around the bone. Frequently, it follows hemorrhage into the muscle or a hematoma in the tissue spaces. The patient usually complains of pain and limited motion. Examination shows palpable localized induration, which may be deep in the tissues. X-ray examination reveals calcification diffusely in the muscle or localized to fascial planes. Continuous hyperemia will assist absorption into the circulation, and the calcification will often disappear without surgical removal.

I have used the following technique: The involved part is wrapped in a bath blanket or other insulating material to prevent heat loss. A gauze bandage holds it in place. Short wave diathermy is then applied to the part as frequently as is convenient. The insulating padding remains in place between treatments to maintain the hyperemia. The diathermy may be applied for a half hour every two hours, all day, if the patient is hospitalized. If the person is an outpatient, it should be repeated at least twice daily for an hour at a time. This treatment must be continued consistently for at least a month. A follow-up x-ray study may show the beginning of absorption at that time, but two or more months of treatment are usually needed. During the treatment period, unusual exercise and stretching of the contracted muscle are prohibited because trauma may further injure the muscle and increase the calcification. When the calcium has nearly disappeared from the muscle itself and the range of motion approaches normal, treatment may be discontinued. Calcification remaining in the fascial planes is of no clinical significance.

Atrophy

Atrophy of Disuse. This form of atrophy follows any prolonged immobilization and involves not only the bone but the muscle as well. X-ray examination may show marked loss of bone density.

Heat is often useful in relieving pain and in softening tissues to overcome contractures, but active exercise is the essential treatment. Roentgenograms should not be used to gauge improvement, because recalcification is extremely slow and the patient will become clinically normal long before the x-ray study shows a normal configuration.

Reflex Sympathetic Dystrophy. This may follow minor fractures. Sudeck's acute post-traumatic bone atrophy, the shoulder-hand syndrome, and causalgia are common examples of reflex sympathetic dystrophy. X-ray studies often show marked bone atrophy with a patchy distribution. It is important to recognize these causes of pain and disability because relief may be greatly accelerated by blocking, with local anesthetics, the sympathetic ganglia supplying the area. Such blocking should be done in addition to the usual physical treatment, as early as the diagnosis can be made, because results improve with early treatment. In these dystrophies, hyperemia is present, as evidenced by swelling, redness of the skin, and bone atrophy. Therefore, heat is not usually beneficial. If heat is desired to relieve pain, it should be used cautiously, and if the pain is not relieved or is increased, as is common, the heat should be discontinued. The essential part of the physical treatment is active exercise. An increase in strength and a decrease in atrophy result, even though active motion may be painful at first.

Volkmann's Contracture

Volkmann's ischemic contracture requires immediate recognition and treatment to prevent severe disability. It usually follows a supracondylar fracture of the humerus but may also follow fracture of both bones of the forearm. Arteriospasm or rupture of blood vessels causes swelling, which compresses the muscles and nerves within the fascial sheath. Necrosis of muscles, of nerves, or even of bone and cartilage may result. The fibrosis produced during healing shortens the muscles on the flexor surface of the forearm, so the fingers contract down into the palm and become nonfunctional. Immediate emergency treatment to relieve pressure or repair arterial injury is imperative. This is a real emergency because even a few hours of delay may result in irreparable damage. When a patient with a forearm or elbow injury complains of pain, sedatives should not be given until the physician has examined the extremity to be sure that this condition is not developing.

If adequate treatment is delayed too long, developing contractures may be prevented or reduced by physical treatment started as early as possible and continued intensively until maximal improvement is obtained. The use of the whirlpool bath followed by massage plus interrupted direct current stimulation to the paralyzed muscles should be started at once. A pancake splint with a malleable wrist section may be adjusted to maintain the length of the flexor muscles as it increases with intensive treatment. The treatment should continue for at least six months to a year. In some cases in which severe damage has occurred, reparative or cosmetic surgery may be needed.

Shoulder Dislocation

Following shoulder dislocation, even though the dislocation is satisfactorily reduced, disability may result.

1. Scapulohumeral contracture may limit motion. Treatment consists of heat, massage, and scapulohumeral motion.

2. The axillary nerve may be injured by pressure of the humeral head as it slips into the axilla. Its motor fibers supply the deltoid and teres minor muscles only, whereas its sensory distribution is to a variable but small area near and slightly posterior to the deltoid insertion. Nerve damage is often unrecognized because the symptoms are masked by a Velpeau bandage or similar retaining apparatus. Removal of the bandage a month or so later reveals that the patient cannot abduct the arm. Then physical therapy is prescribed. The true nature of the injury can be identified by merely stimulating the deltoid muscle with a tetanizing current. If the tetanizing current produces muscle contraction, the nerve is intact. If the muscle does not respond to the tetanizing current, even though some voluntary motion may be present, nerve damage has occurred and the muscle should be treated to prevent fibrosis and limitation of motion.

Treatment consists of interrupted negative direct current stimulation in addition to heat, massage, and scapulohumeral motion. When good voluntary function has returned, the electric stimulation can be discontinued and active exercise prescribed to develop maximal strength.

3. Loss of function at the shoulder joint may also result from rupture of the short rotator tendons. In this case, the head of the humerus, which is normally held in place by the short rotator cuff during abduction, rides upward and strikes the

acromion, which limits abduction. In complete rupture, the only effective treatment is surgical suture. In partial rupture, immobilization in an abducted position and cautious maintenance of range of motion may be adequate to maintain function while the tendon heals.

Hip Fracture

Hip fractures present special problems requiring careful treatment. Intertrochanteric fractures usually heal satisfactorily in about four months because the blood supply is adequate. Open operation with internal fixation secures accurate reduction and maintains contact. However, one must realize that the internal fixation is not intended to support weight-bearing. Many older persons will not walk between parallel bars or on crutches without putting the injured foot to the ground. The plate may break or screws may loosen with weight-bearing. Therefore, if the patient cannot be taught to walk without bearing weight on the fractured extremity, independent ambulation should not be tried until the bone has healed sufficiently to support the patient's weight.

In intracapsular fractures, nonunion is frequent because the major portion of the blood supply comes through the neck of the femur. Since this is broken, the femoral neck and head may not receive an adequate blood supply. Nonunion is common, and aseptic necrosis may supervene even when union is solid. Again, weight-bearing should not be allowed until healing has occurred, and this may take six months. Therefore, the patient must be taught to walk with crutches or a walkerette with a three-point type of gait. It is important to maintain range of motion and strength in both types of fracture. Treatment by whirlpool bath or Hubbard tank, followed by range-of-motion exercise, is helpful and active exercise should be started as early as possible. Gait training in the parallel bars and graduating to underarm crutches should start as soon as the patient can be trusted to keep weight off the injured extremity.

References

1. Knapp, M. E.: Treatment of fracture sequelae. Lancet, 79:106–112, 1959.
2. Knapp, M. E.: Physical medicine in the treatment of fractures. (Panel Discussion, American Medical Association, Atlantic City, N.J., June 12, 1947). J.A.M.A., 137:136–139, 1948.
3. Knapp, M. E.: Physical therapy in fractures about elbow joint. (Read at Annual Session at Cleveland, Ohio, Sept. 3, 1940.) Arch. Phys. Ther., 21:709–715, 1940.
4. Knapp, M. E.: Role of physical therapy in fractures. (Read at American Congress of Physical Therapy. New York, Sept. 8, 1939.) Arch. Phys. Ther., 21:401–407, 1940.
5. Watson-Jones, R.: Fractures and Other Bone and Joint Injuries, 2nd ed. Baltimore, Williams & Wilkins Co., 1941, p. 48.

34

Rehabilitation Management of Diseases of the Motor Unit

WILLIAM S. PEASE
ERNEST W. JOHNSON

Introduction

Persons with diseases and injuries resulting in dysfunction of the motor unit, i.e., motor neurons, peripheral nerves, neuromuscular junction, and muscle fibers, often require rehabilitative care. The management of these patients follows many of the same principles that apply to persons with upper motor neuron dysfunction or other disabilities. However, the particular differences in care are due to the unique pathokinesiology imposed by these diseases.

Diagnosis of the disease process or type of injury must be the first step in proper care. This allows the person's condition to be understood in the context of the prognosis. Diseases of the motor unit may be divided into four categories with respect to prognosis—progressive, transient, static, and recurrent conditions.

Progressive Conditions. Worsening of the pathology occurs at varying rates in these conditions. Amyotrophic lateral sclerosis and infantile spinal muscular atrophy represent rapidly progressive disease. Duchenne muscular dystrophy demonstrates a more intermediate rate of worsening, whereas some processes progress very slowly, such as the hereditary neuropathies and some other myopathies. Anticipation of and planning for the progression of impairment are important features of management in these cases.

Transient Conditions. Disease and injuries in which complete or nearly complete resolution occurs after sudden onset may be termed transient.

Patients with these conditions may recover spontaneously or may require skilled treatment in order to minimize the permanent weakness. Acute inflammatory polyneuropathy, thyrotoxic myopathy, and less severe peripheral nerve injuries are examples of transient conditions.

Management of these conditions requires skill in reversing the pathophysiological process and preventing secondary complications (e.g., contractures) that may lead to impairment after the underlying disease is successfully treated.

Static Conditions. Permanent functional difficulties may occur in some cases while progression of the injury is arrested. Paralytic poliomyelitis, some myopathies, and trauma affecting the conus medullaris, cauda equina, and peripheral nerves typify static conditions. Persons with these long-term impairments need to be monitored for prevention and early treatment of secondary complications, which may take years to develop.

Recurrent Conditions. Many chronic diseases such as polymyositis, myasthenia gravis, and chronic inflammatory polyneuropathy demonstrate recurrent exacerbation and require careful long-term medical and rehabilitative care. Treatment of the underlying pathophysiology, including prevention of exacerbations, takes place concurrently with the physical rehabilitation of the functional deficits imposed by prior episodes.

A distinction must be made between truly progressive diseases and those that apparently progress by the onset or worsening of secondary deformities as growth occurs. Individuals may lose

754

functional abilities by becoming overweight, or children may lose functional abilities as they grow larger or reach a plateau in motor development. Motor unit disease in growing children is more likely to produce deformities whether the condition is progressive or static.

General Principles of Management

Specific treatment of the pathophysiological process is lacking in most motor unit diseases. The ideal approach is prevention—vaccination for viral diseases, education to prevent toxic polyneuropathies, genetic counseling for hereditary diseases, and such measures as desensitization for allergic diseases. If preventive measures have failed or have not been provided, the management is directed largely toward symptoms that appear during the course of the disease.[34] This management should be divided into (1) prospective care and (2) expectant care. Prospective care includes all those measures that should be used irrespective of the chronic disease, such as vaccinations and screening tests, that are given to healthy children and adults. Expectant care includes anticipation of complications that may be expected during the course of a progressive or chronic condition and use of aggressive measures to prevent or minimize these complications. These expected complications may include pain, muscle tightness, deformities of bones and joints, weakness, impaired ventilation, and impaired functional abilities.

Pain. In acute poliomyelitis, acute inflammatory polyneuropathy, and polymyositis, pain may be a significant symptom.[26] Control of pain may require both pharmacological and physical treatment. Salicylates and codeine are often adequate, and narcotics should be used sparingly, as they can produce respiratory depression. Amitryptyline (25 to 50 mg, three times a day [TID], as necessary [prn]) and carbamazepine (100 to 200 mg, twice a day [BID]) may also be useful for neuritic pain. Heat treatment and stretching are often useful as physical modalities.[9, 17, 26] Physical treatment used with or without mild analgesics adequately controls pain in most cases.

Muscle Tightness. Soft tissue shortening may occur at all stages in motor unit disease. Two-joint muscle tightness often appears in the first week and may affect any joint, usually resulting in a flexed position (contracture) (Table 34–1). Physi-

TABLE 34–1. Frequent Areas of Soft Tissue Tightness

Neck flexion	Hip flexion
Shoulder adduction	Hip internal rotation
Elbow flexion	Knee flexion
Forearm pronation	Ankle plantar flexion
Finger adduction	Foot inversion
Finger extension	

cal treatment includes passive, active, and active assisted stretching, usually after the application of heat. A heated pool allows heat and exercise to be combined. Positioning can facilitate prolonged stretch and prevent deformity.[27] Bracing for the prevention of contractures requires careful attention to kinesiology when used to correct deformity so that two-joint muscles are stretched at both joints that they cross (Fig. 34–1).

Deformity. Malalignment of body segments represents a negative aspect of general management. Care must be taken that prescribed equipment is not, in fact, causing progressive deformity. Children are frequently placed in large wheelchairs to allow for growth, often sitting on a sling with one hip higher than the other, with the legs internally rotated and adducted, and leaning on one elbow (Fig. 34–2A). Progression from postural asymmetry to structural deformity is inevitable. A minimal chair prescription should include a firm seat, lumbar support, lateral supports, and adequate arm support (Fig. 34–2B). Malalignments can usually be prevented by positioning, selective stretching, and bracing. If malalignments are fixed or advancing rapidly, they may be corrected or decelerated by surgical procedures or occasionally by mechanical stretching with serial casts and dynamic bracing. At the knee, wedging casts are contraindicated, as they may produce tibial subluxations or supracondylar femoral fractures. Careful continuing observation, particularly during growth spurts, is essential to identify early deformities.

Weakness. Weakness, although present in all motor unit diseases, varies in its presentation and effect on rehabilitation. Proximal weakness interferes with gait, transfers, and gross movement, whereas distal weakness interferes with fine motor skills. Physical treatment can begin with kinesiological and biofeedback techniques and may progress to strengthening exercises in some instances. Progressive resistive exercises may be harmful if they cause fatigue;[17, 21] however, low-intensity exercise may be beneficial for maintenance of

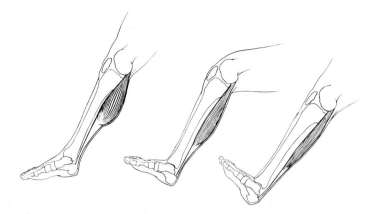

FIGURE 34–1. Stretching of the gastrocnemius muscle: ankle dorsiflexion with knee extension and a midline calcaneus. An example of proper stretch for a two-joint muscle.

strength,[12, 13] for strength gains in some patients with grade four or better strength,[29] and for cardiopulmonary fitness.[16]

Ventilation. With decreasing ventilatory sufficiency, there is a need for mechanical assistance.[1]

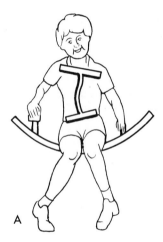

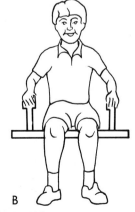

FIGURE 34–2. *A*, Wide hammock seat promotes deformity. *B*, Proper positioning includes a firm seat and correct arm height.

Appropriately prescribed extrathoracic ventilative aids may eliminate the need for tracheostomy and intratracheal volume respiratory support (Fig. 34–3). Early signs and symptoms of hypoxia include sleeplessness, shortness of breath at night, daytime somnolence, and nightmares.[32] As these signs appear, the cuirass or plastic wrap (Fig. 34–4) will enhance gas exchange in the recumbent position.[32] In late stages of motor unit disease, oral positive pressure, pneumobelt, or cuirass ventilators can be used throughout the day, energized from the wheelchair battery. Tracheostomy is rarely needed but may be useful if scoliosis is severe or to aid in controlling aspiration.[2, 3, 32]

Functional Ability. Translation of specific motor and sensory residuals into complicated and practi-

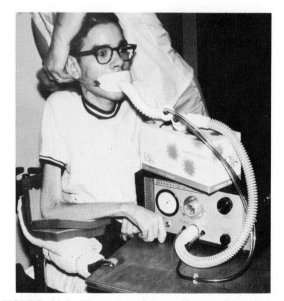

FIGURE 34–3. Home use of intermittent positive-pressure device in a far-advanced case of Duchenne dystrophy. (Note shield to compensate for facial muscle weakness.)

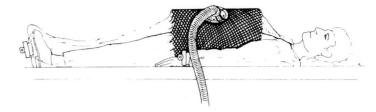

FIGURE 34–4. Plastic wrap (raincoat) respirator uses negative extrathoracic pressure.

cal function is the essence of physical treatment. This ability is often more limited by intelligence and motivation than by actual physical impairments. Participation in regular educational activities should be encouraged. Functional training for locomotion, dressing, eating, and other activities of daily living is practiced as developmentally appropriate. Assistive devices (Fig. 34–5), substitutive training, and selective surgical procedures, e.g., tendon transfer, releases and arthrodeses, all represent management techniques that may be judiciously applied to enhance function. Anticipation of disease progression must be considered when planning future functional needs and adaptations.

Progressive Disease: Duchenne Muscular Dystrophy

This disease is characterized by an insidious onset of weakness and tightness (Fig. 34–6).[3, 22, 23]

Physical Treatment. Vigorous flexibility exercises should be begun early and done intensively under the supervision of a therapist. These exercises must be taught to the parents for the effective use of stretching at home (Fig. 34–7). Suspension and adjustment of the therapeutic exercise program should be determined by periodic rechecks—at least once every three months.[9, 17] Each patient should be examined for muscle tightness, and an individual home program should be prescribed.

Contractures occur early and often are severe, probably because the muscle itself is the site of the pathological lesion. Muscle tightness occurs early in two-joint muscle groups, e.g., gastrocnemius-soleus group, tensor fasciae latae (Fig. 34–8), rectus femoris, and hamstrings in the lower extremities. In the upper extremity, the forearm pronators and wrist and finger flexors often are tight areas. Weakness occurs first in the gluteus maximus; then in the abdominal muscles, foot dorsiflexors, neck flexors, and lower pectorals; and finally in the quadriceps and deltoids.

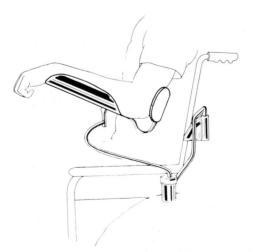

FIGURE 34–5. Balanced forearm orthosis. (From Chyatte, S. B., Long, C., II, and Vignos, P. J.: The balanced forearm orthosis in muscular dystrophy. Arch. Phys. Med. Rehabil., 46:633–636, 1965.)

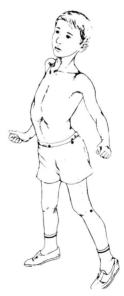

FIGURE 34–6. Characteristic stance of Duchenne dystrophy: increased lordosis, widened stance, and equinus of the feet.

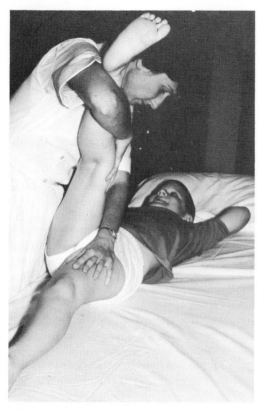

FIGURE 34–7. Stretching the hamstring muscles in a patient with Duchenne muscular dystrophy.

and external torsion of the tibia; and supination deformity of the foot.

The collapsing spine needs careful attention to positioning and support.[19] Extension support of the lumbar spine (Fig. 34–9) helps immobilize the facet joints (Fig. 34–10), providing stability when coupled with a level seat. Exercises to stretch tight spine extensors are counterproductive, since optimally these children's spines should be tight in slight hyperextension.

Strengthening exercises are of unproven value, and clinical impressions suggest that acceleration of the weakness may result.[7, 17] Functional training is helpful as the patient moves from independent ambulation to assisted ambulation and then to wheelchair ambulation.

Bracing and ambulation aids should be minimal, since this is a generalized disease with the individual performing at the maximal energy expenditure. Gowers[20] pointed out that deformities are the principal reason for early loss of ambulation in muscular dystrophy. Hip and knee flexion contractures must especially be guarded against in order to maintain ambulation. If the patient is falling several times each day, long leg braces may prolong limited ambulation for several years.

As ventilatory ability is lost, aids should be introduced. Mouth intermittent positive-pressure breathing may be begun early as a chest expansion exercise and later used additionally to improve nocturnal ventilation.[4, 5] Negative-pressure ventilation is also well tolerated at night.[33] Glossopharyngeal breathing is a useful technique for daytime and in emergencies.[4, 8, 25] Aggressive management of ventilatory failure may add 10 years or more to the patient's life expectancy.[5, 25]

Surgical Management. Selective surgical release

Deformities resulting from asymmetric muscle tightness of an iliotibial band (tensor fasciae latae) are scoliosis (type I, according Bennett's classification); pelvic tilt; subluxation of the opposite hip; flexion contracture, internal rotation deformity, and abduction contracture of the hip; abduction

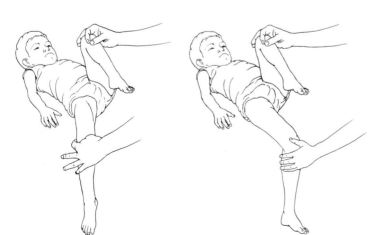

FIGURE 34–8. Iliotibial band—examination for tightness in adduction with hip fully extended.

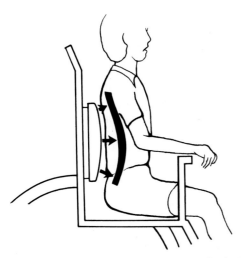

FIGURE 34–9. Lumbar support is provided to maintain extension of the lumbar spine.

of muscle tightness that resists conservative management may prolong and facilitate functional abilities.[15] Rapid convalescence is imperative, i.e., practicing immediate postoperative ambulation in long leg casts after lower extremity surgery and using plastic jackets after spinal fusion to facilitate immediate sitting.[29] One should have the patient measured preoperatively so that the patient can be transferred directly from plaster to an orthosis.

For early inversion instability of the foot, transplantation of the posterior tibial tendon to the lateral dorsum of the foot may be indicated.[28] Another solution is the use of an ankle-foot orthosis. If the deformity is unilateral, lengthening of one side and not the other may result in pelvic obliquity. Achilles tendon lengthening can be disastrous if one does not anticipate the loss of knee stability, which has been maintained by the fixed equinus of the foot.

Surgical release of the iliotibial tract is often quite helpful in prolonging ambulation. The tight tensor fosters knee instability as the patient increases lumbar lordosis to stabilize the weight line behind flexed hips, increasing torque to flex the knee.

The surgical correction of equinovarus foot deformity in a nonambulatory patient is done largely for cosmetic reasons and ease of footwear applications.

In the past, surgical correction of spinal deformity with its surgical risk and prolonged immobilization resulted in excessive morbidity and mortality. Improvement in surgical techniques and the advent of Harrington and Dwyer instrumentation, permitting internal fixation, have improved the risk as well as the surgical outcome. Internal fixation and polypropylene bracing still allow these children to continue to be mobile. The physician can balance the progression of disease and the acceleration of the deformity and in many cases allow the child to continue to sit and to preserve respiratory function that could have been lost through chest wall distortion. The degree of chest restriction due to scoliosis can be gauged by comparing the degree of restrictive lung disease (vital capacity) to the weakness seen elsewhere. A vital capacity of 20 ml per kg or more is considered an acceptable risk. The child's cardiomyopathy should also be considered; however, very little is known about the value of cardiac ejection fraction measurements in Duchenne muscular dystrophy.

General Management. In Duchenne muscular dystrophy, which has an X-linked recessive inheritance pattern, counseling the parents is a neces-

FIGURE 34–10. Extension of spine *(left)* stabilizes facets.

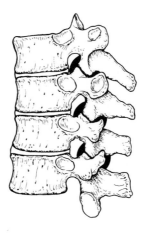
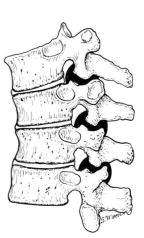

sity.[9] About one third of cases represent new mutations of the gene.[9] The location of the gene is known, and genetic screening for carrier females and male fetuses should be forthcoming. There is a definite association between decreased mental function and muscular dystrophy in specific pedigrees,[11] and one should have realistic expectations of the intellectual skills of patients affected with this condition. Parents of patients are urged to have their names put on the mailing list of the Muscular Dystrophy Association so that the newsletter will provide a means for keeping up with the latest facts. This contact with a reliable source of information is often a deterrent to "doctor shopping" and frustrating trips for "miracle cures" at the urging of well-meaning friends and relatives.

Empathetic attitudes and forthright advice may lessen the fears and frustrations that are inevitable. Periodic checks by a physician conversant with physical management should be done as needed, usually once every three to four months. Attendance at regular school is recommended.

Spinal Muscular Atrophy

This disease offers such a broad spectrum of presentations and rates of survival that great care should be taken to avoid considering this a short-term survival disease. Age of onset, family presentation, and progression of symptoms can be compatible with long-term survival.[30]

Physical Treatment. The hallmark of management is maintenance of mobility and flexibility. Vigorous attention must be given to the potential for muscle tightness in two-joint muscles. Bracing plays some role, but this often takes place later in the course of the disease. A high probability exists for development of scoliosis, and meticulous care must be taken to identify curves and asymmetric tightness and precursors to scoliosis at the earliest possible moment. Patients with these paralytic curves do poorly in Milwaukee braces and do much better in bivalved polypropylene body jackets. Close attention to seating and positioning is indicated, as with the child with Duchenne dystrophy.

Medical Treatment. The same close attention to preventive medicine is warranted as in previous entities. Patients with these syndromes are also subject to the problems of adolescence, as these children often retain mobility and encounter the same crises as their peers. They should all have instruction in human sexuality and, in addition, genetic counseling. This will avoid misunderstanding and obviate some stress.

Surgical Treatment. These children usually benefit from having spinal surgery. Preoperative evaluation of respiratory function allows anticipation of pulmonary problems. Those patients with a vital capacity of 40 per cent or greater rarely require tracheostomy. Internal fixation and fusion to the sacrum are usually required. Rapid postoperative mobilization is accomplished with a bivalved polypropylene body jacket.

General Management. Common sense and cautious optimism are warranted in the older child, and the key phrase is anticipation for prevention.

Amyotrophic Lateral Sclerosis

Physical Treatment. Treatment measures should anticipate progression. Lightweight molded plastic ankle-foot orthoses or canes, or both, are helpful for prolonged and safe ambulation. The patient also should be taught how to fall safely. Positioning and therapeutic exercise are prescribed to prevent deformities and maintain functional ability as well as to facilitate nursing care.

Medical Treatment. When there are bulbar symptoms and a prognosis of continuation for more than several months, a gastrostomy and tracheostomy may be helpful. A suctioning device for home use is often necessary. If there is a short-term prognosis, intramuscular injection of neostigmine (Prostigmin) (1 ml of a 1:1000 dilution) 30 minutes before eating may temporarily facilitate swallowing. Fasciculations will be intensified, however.

Mechanical ventilatory aid may be needed in later stages. The decision to use mechanical ventilatory support should be made by the patient. The subject of assisted ventilation should be discussed as soon as testing shows significant impairment of the vital capacity. In this way, an emergency decision contrary to the patient's wishes can be avoided. Home management is very possible even in the terminal stages with an understanding family. It is important to keep an optimistic attitude in dealing with the patient and the family.

Transient Disease: Guillain-Barré Syndrome (Acute Inflammatory Demyelinating Polyneuropathy)

Weakness is usually reversible over a period of two months to as long as two years. If the onset is acute, ordinarily the recovery is more rapid. An insidious onset may foretell delayed recovery, perhaps over a period of a year or more, and some patients may never regain full strength. The observation of conduction block (neurapraxia) on nerve conduction tests suggests that weakness is not related to axonal degeneration and should be taken as a favorable prognostic sign. The recovery of the amplitude of the muscle-evoked response correlates well with recovery of muscle function.[1] Strengthening exercises and exhaustive activities may aggravate the weakness or result in a relapse. Tightness is prevented and corrected by positioning and early stretching. Pain, often severe, is managed as described previously.

Temporary ambulation aids include dorsiflexion support, temporary splints at the knee, and a light plastic ankle-foot orthosis. Ambulation is begun in the therapeutic pool or in the parallel bars, proceeding to underarm crutches, forearm crutches, canes, and then to only occasional aid as strength returns. Temporary upper extremity aids include the mobile arm support, hand splints, and other adaptive devices.

Pressure ulcerations are frequent preventable complications in this condition, especially if the patient is on a respirator. Ventilatory insufficiency should receive early mechanical support. In acute motor unit illness that affects ventilation, mechanical assistance should usually be started when the vital capacity begins to fall and should be employed in all instances when it reaches 50 per cent.

Static Diseases

Paralytic Poliomyelitis

The literature is replete with excellent descriptions of the proper management of this entity.[6, 8, 26, 35] Prevention is by the Salk vaccine (formalin-killed virus) and the Sabin vaccine (attenuated live virus), the latter used most often in infants and children today. Rare cases of live vaccine–related poliomyelitis are seen in relatives who lack full immunity.

PHYSICAL MANAGEMENT

Most patients have stabilized six months after the onset of paralytic polio. A clear estimation of the probable functional ability and potential sources of deformity is then usually possible. The spine of the growing child should be checked radiographically at least once yearly and more often during periods of rapid growth. Adults need periodic observation for orthotic adjustment and for detection of possible loss of function due to overwork.

There are several general rules of physical treatment. Active exercise should be deferred until the pain is relieved, and selective strengthening exercises should be deferred if there is a significant tightness of the muscle group. Progressive resistive exercises and functional training unavoidably encourage substitutive patterns. Development of substitutive patterns usually inhibits activation of the prime movers; for example, the anterior tibial muscle may drop out of the pattern of dorsiflexion (peroneal flip) if walking is initiated before this muscle is able to carry out its action. Asymmetric strengthening should be avoided because it may aggravate or initiate scoliosis. Overwork can cause further weakness in specific muscle groups. Muscle tightness should be retained if it is symmetric and if weakness is present; for example, back extension tightness in the presence of severe weakness of back extensors.

Orthotic devices are used to prevent deformity (e.g., Hoke's corset), to provide support (e.g., long leg brace), to protect a weakened muscle group (e.g., opponens splint), or to increase function (e.g., mobile arm support).

Attendance at regular school is recommended whenever possible for children. A conference with the teacher to discuss positioning and modification of activities is usually necessary. A forthright but encouraging attitude on the part of the attending physician is essential for both the parents' and the child's well-being. Adult patients' questions regarding prognosis should be answered honestly with encouragement. Early vocational planning is imperative, and the patient's emotional needs should be identified and met at appropriate stages of rehabilitation.

Congenital Myopathies

These myopathies, in the past grouped under benign congenital hypotonia, are usually nonprogressive.[9] Like muscular dystrophy, they require rapid postoperative mobilization and attention to avoiding muscle tightness. With their good prognosis, vigorous efforts should be made to maintain good alignment of the spine (Fig. 34–11). One may lose ambulation after fusion owing to loss of spine mobility, but the potential hazards of the collapsing spine usually outweigh this risk.

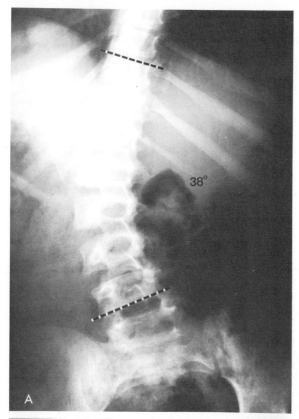

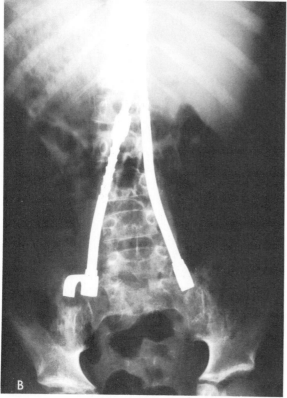

FIGURE 34–11. *A*, Rapidly progressing curve in a patient with fiber-type disproportion. *B*, To retain ambulation, early fusion with Harrington rods and plastic jacket prevented loss of function from immobilization.

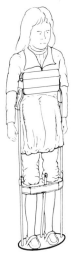

FIGURE 34–12. A static parapodium supports the extended joints against gravity to aid standing.

Arthrogryposis

The syndrome of arthrogryposis multiplex congenita is believed to arise from an absence of fetal movement.[9, 31] Experimental immobilization of the fetus by several techniques has led to this syndrome of soft tissue "ankylosis" and "clubbing" of multiple joints with the articular surfaces remaining intact. Both autosomal dominant and recessive patterns of inheritance have been reported. Counseling of the family and the child at the appropriate age is indicated.

Physical Management. Children with this condition often require early surgical intervention to facilitate standing. The parapodium (Fig. 34–12) is suitable as an initial standing device. Several observers should be evaluating upper extremity function to anticipate problems in activities of daily living. An upper extremity orthosis may be needed to correct deformity as well as to enhance motor function.[14, 18]

Surgical Management. As these children usually have normal intelligence and sensory function, they do well with tendon transfers, such as substitution of the pectoral for the biceps function. These tendon transfers must be done with great care if function is to be improved.

Recurrent Disease

Included in this category are motor unit diseases that may progress, become arrested, or improve.

Polymyositis (dermatomyositis) is a classic example. It appears to be a primary inflammatory disease of the muscle and the muscle vasculature.[9]

Physical treatment is based on the following three principles: maintaining flexibility, minimizing pain through the application of heat (hot tub baths or home baker), and use of minimal bracing or ambulation aids, if needed. Bracing must be done cautiously in cases of proximal weakness, since a rigidly designed ankle brace may aggravate balance problems on uneven surfaces.

In medical management, many authorities feel that high doses of corticosteroids are helpful during an exacerbation or an acute onset of polymyositis.

Summary

The aim in management of progressive motor unit diseases is to prolong functional abilities; in static diseases, to protect the patient from deformity and to increase functional ability; and in transient diseases, to maintain flexibility and to facilitate return of function. The maintenance of the patient's flexibility (especially of the multijoint muscles) and careful follow-up visits are keys to the management of motor unit diseases.

References

1. Albers, J. W., Donofrio, P. D., and McGonagle, T. K.: Sequential electrodiagnostic abnormalities in acute inflammatory demyelinating polyradiculoneuropathy. Muscle Nerve, 8:528–539, 1985.
2. Alexander, M. A., Johnson, E. W., Petty, J., and Stauch, D.: Mechanical ventilation of patients with late stage Duchenne muscular dystrophy: Management in the home. Arch. Phys. Med. Rehabil., 60:289, 1979.
3. Archibald, K. C., and Vignos, P. J.: A study of contractures in muscular dystrophy. Arch. Phys. Med. Rehabil., 40:150–157, 1959.
4. Bach, J., Alba, A., Pilkington, L. A., and Lee, M.: Long-term rehabilitation in advanced stage of childhood onset, rapidly progressive muscular dystrophy. Arch. Phys. Med. Rehabil., 62:328–331, 1981.
5. Bach, J. R., O'Brien, J., Krotenberg, R., and Alba, A. S.: Management of end stage respiratory failure in Duchenne muscular dystrophy. Muscle Nerve, 10:177–182, 1987.
6. Bennett, R. L.: Evaluation and treatment of lower motor unit lesions involving the shoulder, arm, forearm and hand. Arch. Phys. Med. Rehabil., 41:54–61, 1960.
7. Bonsett, C. A.: Pseudohypertrophic muscular dys-

trophy: An anatomical study. Neurology, 13:728–738, 1963.

8. Bosma, J. F.: Significance of the pharynx in rehabilitation of poliomyelitis disabilities in cervical area. Arch. Phys. Med. Rehabil., 38:363–368, 1957.

9. Brooke, M. H.: A Clinician's View of Neuromuscular Diseases, 2nd Ed. Baltimore, MD, Williams & Wilkins, 1986.

10. Chyatte, S. B., Long, C., II, and Vignos, P. J.: The balanced forearm orthosis in muscular dystrophy. Arch. Phys. Med. Rehabil., 46:633–636, 1965.

11. Cohen, H. J., Molnar, G. E., and Taft, L. T.: The genetic relationship of progressive muscular dystrophy (Duchenne type) and mental retardation. Develop. Med. Child. Neurol., 10:754–765, 1968.

12. De Lateur, B. J., and Giaconi, R. M.: Effect on maximal strength of submaximal exercise in Duchenne muscular dystrophy. Am. J. Phys. Med., 58:26–36, 1979.

13. DiMarco, A. F., Kelling, J. S., DiMarco, M. S., Jacobs, I., Shields, R., and Altose, M. D.: The effects of inspiratory resistive training on respiratory muscle function in patients with muscular dystrophy. Muscle Nerve, 8:284–290, 1985.

14. Drumond, D. S., Siller, T. S., and Cruess, R. L.: Management of arthrogryposis multiplex congenita. Chapter 5, Instructional Course Lectures, Am. Acad. Orthopaed. Surg., 23:79–95, 1974.

15. Eyring, E. J., Johnson, E. W., and Burnett, C.: Surgery in muscular dystrophy. J.A.M.A., 58:4–7, 1977.

16. Florence, J. M., and Hagberg, J. M.: Effect of training on the exercise response of neuromuscular disease patients. Med. Sci. Sports Exerc., 16:460–465, 1984.

17. Fowler, W. M., and Taylor, M.: Rehabilitation management of muscular dystrophy and related disorders: I. The role of exercise. Arch. Phys. Med. Rehabil., 63:319–321, 1982.

18. Friedlander, H. L., Westin, G. W., and Wood, W. L.: Arthrogryposis multiplex congenita—A review of forty-five cases. J. Bone Joint Surg., 50A:89–112, 1968.

19. Gibson, D. A., and Wilkins, K. E.: The management of spinal deformities in Duchenne muscular dystrophy. Clin. Orthop. Related Res., 108:41–51, 1975.

20. Gowers, W. R.: Myopathy and a distal form. Br. Med. J., 2:89–92, 1902.

21. Herbison, G. J., Jaweed, M. M., and Ditunno, J. F., Jr.: Exercise therapies in peripheral neuropathies. Arch. Phys. Med. Rehabil. 64:201–205, 1983.

22. Johnson, E. W.: Examination for muscle weakness in infants and small children. J.A.M.A., 168:1306–1313, 1958.

23. Johnson, E. W.: Pathokinesiology of Duchenne muscular dystrophy: Implications for management. Arch. Phys. Med., Rehabil., 58:4–7, 1977.

24. Johnson, E., and Braddom, R.: Overwork weakness in fascioscapulohumeral muscular dystrophy. Arch. Phys. Med. Rehabil., 52:333–336, 1971.

25. Johnson, E. W., Reynolds, H. T., and Stauch, D.: Duchenne muscular dystrophy: A case with prolonged survival. Arch. Phys. Med. Rehabil., 66:260–261, 1985.

26. Knapp, M. E.: The contribution of Sister Elizabeth Kenny to treatment of poliomyelitis. Arch. Phys. Med. Rehabil., 36:510–517, 1955.

27. Lowenthal, M., and Tobis, J. S.: Contractures in chronic neurologic disease. Arch. Phys. Med. Rehabil., 38:640–645, 1957.

28. Milner-Brown, H. S., and Miller, R. G.: Muscle strengthening through high-resistance weight training in patients with neuromuscular disorders. Arch. Phys. Med. Rehabil., 69:14–19, 1988.

29. Moe, J. H., Winter, R. B., Bradford, D. S., and Lonstein, J. E.: Neuromuscular deformities. In Scoliosis and Other Spinal Deformities. Philadelphia, W. B. Saunders Co., 1978, pp. 203–238.

30. Pearn, J. H., Gardner-Medwen, D., and Wilson, J.: A clinical study of chronic childhood spinal muscular atrophy. J. Neurol. Sci., 38:23–37, 1978.

31. Rosenmann, A., and Arad, I.: Arthrogryposis multiplex congenita: Neurogenic type with autosomal recessive inheritance. J. Med. Genet., 2:91–94, 1974.

32. Splaingard, M. L., Frates, R. C., Jefferson, L. S., Rosen, C. L., and Harrison, G. M.: Home negative pressure ventilation: Report of 20 years of experience in patients with neuromuscular disease. Arch. Phys. Med. Rehabil., 66:239–242, 1985.

33. Sutherland, D. H., Olshen, R., Cooper, L., Wyatt, M., Leach, J., Mubarak, S., and Schultz, P.: The pathomechanics of gait in Duchenne muscular dystrophy. Dev. Med. Child. Neurol., 23:3–22, 1981.

34. Swinyard, C. A., et al.: Gradients of functional ability of importance in rehabilitation of patients with progressive muscular and neuromuscular diseases. Arch. Phys. Med. Rehabil., 38:574–579, 1957.

35. Vallbona, C., and Spencer, W. A.: Systematic classification of the chronic sequelae of poliomyelitis. Arch. Phys. Med. Rehabil., 42:114–121, 1961.

35
Rehabilitation for Swallowing Impairment

ARTHUR A. SIEBENS

Introduction

Swallowing is accomplished by forces and motions within the mouth, pharynx, larynx, and esophagus that are synchronized with interruptions in respiration. The forces result from increases in the tension of muscles and the motions from shortening and lengthening of muscles. The synchronization is the result of afferent, efferent, and central nervous system activity, some of which is under volitional control and some of which is not. Because many of the structures of the mouth and pharynx are used in speaking, knowledge of swallowing is related closely to knowledge of oral communication.

Concepts that are generic to rehabilitation apply to swallowing rehabilitation specifically. One of these concepts is the distinction among *impairment, disability,* and *handicap.*[1] Swallowing impairment may be the consequence of alterations in structure (e.g., surgical excisions), in force (e.g., muscle weakness), in motion (e.g., loss of tissue compliance), in afferent activity (e.g., pharyngeal anesthesia), in efferent activity (e.g., motor neuron disease), in central integration of involuntary activity (e.g., brain stem stroke), or in volitional control (e.g., apraxia). The identification of such deficits is crucial to understanding the basis of the patient's complaint. In many instances, however, the impairment, though understood, cannot be altered significantly. The objective of rehabilitation then is a reduction in the effect of impairment on the person, i.e., a reduction of the *disability.* This consists of restoring safe alimentation and hydration by mouth, perhaps by such compensations as

modifications in diet or swallowing pattern. The individual may refuse to eat in public, however, finding these compensations unacceptable except in private settings. A *handicap,* or social implication, is thereby added, for given the importance of eating with friends and colleagues, the individual is unable to meet normal social and professional obligations. By and large, swallowing rehabilitation addresses disability and handicap more effectively than impairment.

General Considerations

It is customary to subdivide the passage of food and drink from mouth to stomach into oral, pharyngeal, and esophageal stages (Table 35–1).[2] Inasmuch as the structures that correspond to these three stages are continuous and particularly inasmuch as the tensions, motions, and nervous system events are not necessarily isolated by stage,[3] these subdivisions are somewhat arbitrary. Generally speaking, however, the oral stage is adapted specifically to creating and transporting a swallowable entity (the bolus), the pharyngeal stage to propelling the bolus from the mouth into the esophagus without contamination of the airways (nasopharynx or larynx), and the esophageal stage to conducting the bolus from the pharynx into the cervical esophagus, through the thorax, and into the stomach. Flow of the bolus throughout its passage is aboral only; retrograde flow is abnormal. Clearance of the passageway is complete and prompt; prolonged residual collections in the mouth, the pharynx, or the esophagus are abnormal.

ARTHUR A. SIEBENS

TABLE 35–1. Swallowing Actions: Relevant Muscles and Their Innervations

SWALLOWING ACTION	MUSCLES*	INNERVATION
Oral Stage		
Lip seal	Orbicularis oris	VII
Cheek control	Buccinator	VII
Vertical chewing	Temporalis	V
	Masseter	V
	Interior pterygoids	V
Horizontal chewing	Exterior pterygoids	V
Lingual mixing	Intrinsics (lingualis)	XII
	Genioglossus	XII
	Styloglossus	XII
Pharyngeal Stage		
Lingual-palatal seal	Styloglossus	XII
	Hyoglossus	XII
Velar seal	Tensor veli palatini	V
	Levator veli palatini	IX,X
Pharyngeal compression	Styloglossus	XII
	Hyoglossus	XII
	Stylopharyngeus	IX,X
	Superior constrictor	IX,X
	Middle constrictor	IX,X
	Inferior constrictor	IX,X
Epiglottic tilt	Aryepiglotticus	IX,X
Laryngeal displacement		
Upward	Thyrohyoid	
	Hyoglossus	XII
	Stylohyoid	VII
	Post digastricus	VII
Forward	Geniohyoid	C 1, 2, 3
	Genioglossus	XII
	Anterior digastricus	V
Glottic seal	Lateral cricoarytenoid	IX,X
	Thyroarytenoid	IX,X
Air flow cessation	Intercostal inhibition	T 1 to T 12
	Diaphragm inhibition	C 3, C 4 (phrenic nerve)
Pharyngoesophageal relaxation	Cricopharyngeal inhibition	IX,X
Esophageal Stage		
Esophageal contractions	Striated muscle fibers	X
	Smooth muscle fibers	X

*Not an exhaustive listing.

It is informative to compare each stage to a mechanical analogue. In the instance of solids, the oral cavity is a mixing chamber in which particles added through the lips are reduced in size and variation by the grinding and chopping actions of teeth, all the while being churned within a salivary fluid by the tongue. Blenders or cement mixers are reasonable comparisons. Because the lingual, masticatory, and emptying functions are all under voluntary control, this stage is uniquely sensitive to cognitive or behavioral abnormalities.

The pharyngeal stage is readily likened to a pump that is valved for unidirectional flow (Fig. 35–1). Compression is a function primarily of the force and motion of the tongue and of the pharyngeal constrictors (Figs. 35–2 to 35–5). Valving requires lip seal (orbicularis oris), lingual seal against the palate to prevent retrograde flow, nasopharyngeal seal by the velum, tracheal seal by complex laryngeal changes, and escape valving through a transiently open pharyngoesophageal union (Fig. 35–6). This stage is relatively involuntary and is completed rapidly (0.5 sec). It is a critical stage in which life can be threatened by

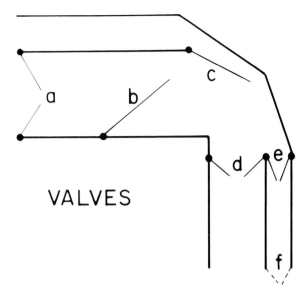

FIGURE 35–1. Valves relevant to unidirectional flow during swallowing: (a) lips, (b) tongue, (c) velum, (d) vocal cords, (e) cricopharyngeus, (f) cardiac sphincter.

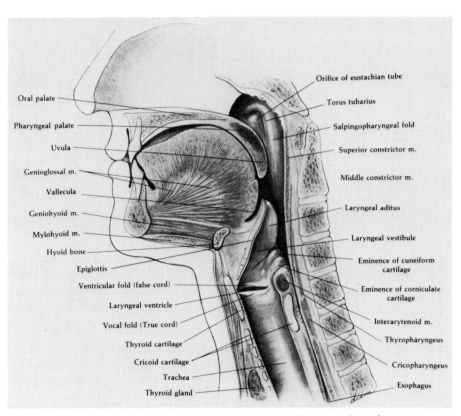

FIGURE 35–2. Sagittal schematic of the pharynx, larynx, and mouth.

ARTHUR A. SIEBENS

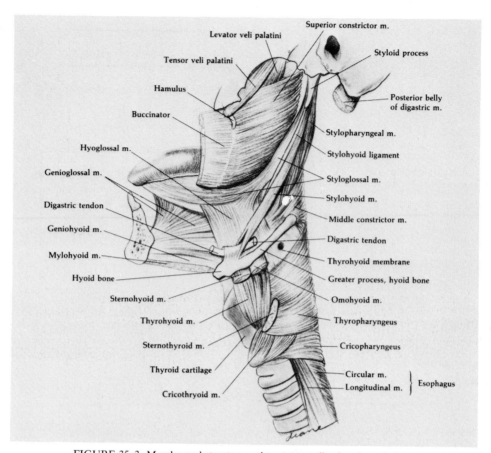

FIGURE 35–3. Muscles and structures relevant to swallowing, lateral view.

abnormal laryngeal valving. The pharyngeal stage is commonly referred to as a reflex because its progression is involuntary.

The esophageal stage[4, 5] begins with the opening of the esophagus and terminates with the passage of the bolus through the esophagogastric junction. Sequential contraction of esophageal muscle fibers contributes to propulsion of the bolus, especially in the recumbent or inverted position. A single peristaltic action or primary wave normally empties the esophagus completely.

Airway Protection

The pharynx is a pathway for both food and air. Preventing the contamination of the larynx, trachea, and bronchi by food products under these conditions is accomplished by remarkably orchestrated forces, movements, and nervous system events. The following are some of the considerations relevant to these essential actions.

Air flow through the pharynx must be interrupted at the instant of bolus flow. Were this not so, the pressure gradients that result in the flow of air through the pharynx and into the larynx and tracheobronchial tree during inspiration[6] would cause the flow of food as well. Aspiration, or laryngeal penetration by food products during inspiration, would be the consequence.

Three events normally protect the airway from such contamination: respiratory interruption, laryngeal seal, and displacement of the larynx. The interruption of air flow occurs whether or not the laryngeal seal is complete. Also, it is independent of the moment in the respiratory cycle at which swallowing happens to fall. The intercostal muscles and diaphragm are not only inhibited but are kept in a "hold" position by a central nervous system event. Air flow ceases at that point, irrespective of whether the larynx is sealed or open and irrespective of the level of inspiration or expiration. Because the pharyngeal and laryngeal musculatures are striated and muscle twitch times are short, the

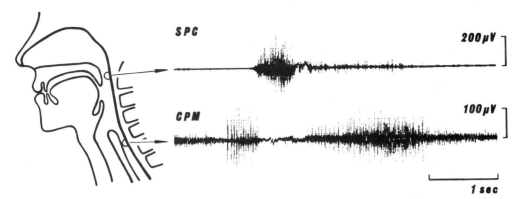

FIGURE 35–7. Myoelectric potentials that have been recorded during one swallow of water. Bipolar surface electrodes are held in place against the pharyngeal wall by suction. SPC, superior constrictor; CPM, cricopharyngeus. Note: Tonic activity of CPM is inhibited synchronously with activation of SPC. The CPM tracing also demonstrates pre-inhibition and post-inhibition activation. (From Tanaka, E., Palmer, J., and Siebens, A.: Bipolar suction electrodes for pharyngeal electromyography. Dysphagia, 1:39, 1986.)

laryngeal sealing motions are quick and the interruption of respiration is correspondingly brief (less than 0.5 sec). At rapid ventilatory rates, however, as in the instance of dyspnea, the interruption of air flow in the interest of swallowing may add a significant limitation for meeting ventilatory requirements.

Tilting of the epiglottis is one of the most dramatic movements associated with swallowing. The angle inscribed by the epiglottis in moving from its resting to its tilted position approximates 135 degrees (see Fig. 35–6). Upward and forward motion of the larynx occurs synchronously with epiglottic tilt, furthering the covering of the laryngeal vestibule achieved by the base of the tongue and the tilted epiglottis. Surprisingly, the presence of the epiglottis itself is not essential for aspiration-free swallowing; its surgical removal is compatible with respiratory health.

The vestibule of the larynx (see Fig. 35–2) is the space in the larynx above the glottis (the opening between the vocal cords). It is bounded superiorly by the epiglottis, laterally by the aryepiglottic folds, and inferiorly and posteriorly by the true and false vocal cords and the arytenoid cartilages. The obliteration of this vestibular or supraglottic space (see Fig. 35–6) is a component of normal laryngeal seal. Its timely accomplishment requires not only the tilting of the epiglottis but a decrease in the transverse and anteroposterior dimensions of the vestibule that is brought about by contraction of the intrinsic muscles of the larynx. Apposition of the vocal cords is synchronous with this folding of the laryngeal vestibule. Penetration of the supraglottic space by food products is considered abnormal but probably occurs normally to

some degree with saliva or other liquids. The folding of the vestibule squeezes contaminants back into the foodway independent of expiratory air flow or cough in many instances of supraglottic penetration, effectively protecting the subglottic airway even if supraglottic mechanisms are impaired.

In summary, airway protection during swallowing exemplifies physiological redundancy in the interest of preserving a vital function. The combination of air flow interruption, laryngeal displacement, and laryngeal seal enhances the likelihood of fail-safe swallowing. Correspondingly, substantial impairment must be assumed to be present when one visualizes penetration of the glottis during swallowing.

How much laryngeal penetration occurs normally is not known. Neither is it known how much airway contamination by food contents is compatible with bronchopulmonary health. It is known, however, that the pH of the contaminant[7] is the critical variable; acidity exceeding pH 2.4 is extremely destructive of lung tissue. Although ciliary action and cough are noteworthy backup systems for failures in airway protection, cough is unreliable in many patients with dysphagia whose neurological condition precludes sensitivity to cough afferents (silent laryngeal penetration) or the capacity for volitional cough, e.g., coma, paralysis of laryngeal or respiratory muscles, and apraxia.

Opening of the Pharyngoesophageal Segment

The ejection of pharyngeal contents into the esophagus (Fig. 35–7) during pharyngeal contraction requires that an opening into the esophagus offer less resistance than the openings to the larynx, nasopharynx, and mouth. The formation of the opening into the esophagus must be a transient event, however, for were the lumen continuously patent, two important functions would be sacrificed: first, the prevention of reflux from the esophagus to the pharynx and second, the prevention of the esophagus being filled with air. Both of these functions derive from the large pressure gradients between the cervical esophagus, at atmospheric pressure, and the thoracic esophagus, which is exposed to pleural pressures.[6] During Valsalva's maneuvers against a closed glottis, at which times intrathoracic pressures may exceed systolic blood pressure, gradients favor regurgitation. During normal breathing, because pleural pressures are subatmospheric, the gradients favor aerophagia. These untoward events are prevented by tonic activity (see Fig. 35–7) of the cricopharyngeus,[8] a small semicircular muscle that clamps the proximal esophagus against the posterior surface of the cricoid cartilage (see Figs. 35–3 and 35–4). Recordings of this muscle's activity (see Fig. 35–7)[9, 10] are unique among those of the muscles of the pharynx. The recordings show continuous activity except during swallowing, at which time potentials transiently cease, only to resume after passage of the bolus. The activity of this muscle serves an important foodway gate-keeping function.

The relaxation of the cricopharyngeus cannot in itself cause the esophageal lumen to expand. A number of mechanisms have been offered to explain this expansion: (1) Pharyngeal constriction may be sufficient to spread the relaxed pharyngoesophageal walls by forcing the bolus through the lumen, an explanation that finds analogues in the opening of the uterine cervix by the fetal head or the opening of the aortic valve by blood during ventricular ejection. The velocity imparted to the bolus by pharyngeal contraction may be sufficient to project the bolus well into the esophagus, especially in the instance of fluids.[11] (2) The pharynx is somewhat funnel shaped, the muscle fibers that form its posterior and lateral walls being oriented obliquely upward and lateral on either side of a median raphe (see Fig. 35–4). Conceivably, contractions of these muscles, together with shortening of the other elevators of the larynx (see Fig. 35–3), result in pulling the lower pharynx and upper esophagus over the bolus, thereby engulfing it.[12] (3) Upper and forward motion of the larynx is a conspicuous swallowing motion (see Fig. 35–6). This motion may widen the distance between the posterior and anterior foodway walls. This explanation requires that the posterior wall be relatively fixed to the prevertebral tissues of the cervical spine and the anterior wall to the cricoid cartilage (see Fig. 35–2). If one accepts this explanation, motion of the larynx upward and forward simultaneously protects the airway, as described above, and assists pharyngeal emptying by widening the relaxed foodway.[13] These three proposed explanations for expanding the foodway lumen at the pharyngoesophageal junction are not mutually exclusive. It is reasonable to believe that each contributes to the entry of food from the pharynx.

Once admitted to the esophagus, the bolus passes through the thorax into the stomach. The roles of gravity, esophageal persталsis, and propulsion (squirting) by the force of pharyngeal contraction vary depending on body position, bolus consistency, bolus volume, and other factors. As discussed above, preventing retrograde flow of acid gastric contents into the pharynx is an important esophageal function.

Rehabilitation of Oral Stage Impairment

Oral stage impairment is detected readily because the structures are all accessible to direct visualization. Moreover, the participation of these structures in speech and their examination by established protocols for the analysis of nonspeech movements and articulation allow an understanding of impairment in terms of strength, motion, coordination, praxis, and cognition.[14] Oral motor exercises include active and passive exercise for the tongue and the lips, which are designed to increase strength, range, velocity, and precision.[15] Although the primary objective of these exercises is improved bolus management, it is likely that they provide improvements in articulation as well. However, because the neural control and synergisms of chewing and oral transport differ from those of articulation, the implications of using oral stage swallowing rehabilitation to correct problems in speech mechanics are not certain.

Drooling of saliva may be decreased by parasympathetic blocking agents such as propantheline. The daily output of saliva is approximately 1.5 liters. The logistics of its disposition by drooling or swallowing is placed in perspective by appreciating that this volume is comparable with the daily output of urine. Insufficient saliva and oral desiccation, sometimes associated with Sjögren's syndrome, can be compensated for by artificial saliva.

If the pharyngeal stage is adequate, loss of food bolus from lip seal failure, pathological cervical flexion, or thoracic kyphosis may be compensated for by positioning the patient so that the floor of the mouth drains toward the pharynx. Retention of food ("squirreling") resulting from oral anesthesia or facial paralysis is correctable by teaching the patient methods of oral clearance or by the avoidance of foods that require extensive oral-stage processing. Retention of food caused by bradykinesia or cognitive impairment may be lessened by the use of liquids and gels. Placing the bolus over the dorsum of the tongue by spoon or straw obviates the patient's need for anterior oral transport. Assuming that the involuntary pharyngeal response is adequate, it is conceivable that the oral stage can be bypassed selectively. The model of infant feeding, i.e., suckling,[16] has been proposed for patients whose cognitive or mechanical oral stage impairment lends itself to presentation of the food bolus to the pharynx directly.

Rehabilitation of Pharyngeal Stage Impairment

Oral feeding without excessive airway contamination by food is the primary goal of swallowing rehabilitation. This goal requires that one identify whether or not airway contamination occurs. Although coughing, choking, and laryngeal stridor associated with swallowing are unequivocal objective evidence of impairment, their absence, regrettably, does not indicate that swallowing is safe. Indeed, recurrent bronchopulmonary infections, rather than coughing or choking, are common presenting symptoms of the patient with a swallowing impairment. In the absence of laryngeal sensation (superior laryngeal nerves, branches of cranial nerve X), penetration of the larynx occurs during inspiration (aspiration) or at any time in the respiratory cycle, the least likely time being during expiration, since air flow sweeps contaminant food from the airway. The sensations of tearing, suffocation, and panic normally associated with penetration of the glottis are not found in many patients with dysphagia. Furthermore, neither the most careful questioning nor the most exacting physical or neurological examination reliably determines that airway contamination is not occurring regularly. One study[17] compared the association between laryngeal penetration that was visualized fluoroscopically in dysphagic patients and (1) the absence of the gag reflex, (2) a wet-hoarse quality of the voice, and (3) the absence of cough. A wet-hoarse quality of the voice after swallowing was found more commonly than the other physical findings. Even wet-hoarseness, however, was not detected in each patient. Nine of eleven patients did not cough when food entered their larynx (silent penetration of the larynx).

Fluoroscopy for Swallowing Rehabilitation. These startling observations have led to the use of fluoroscopy (see Fig. 35–7), recorded either on film (cinefluoroscopy) or videotape (videofluoroscopy), for the routine analysis of swallowing.[18] More important for the field of rehabilitation, this examination allows one to plan effective swallowing rehabilitation[19] by visualizing the consequences of selected interventions. Two important distinctions between rehabilitation studies and the traditional barium swallows are (1) the simulation of normal eating in the fluoroscopy suite and (2) prioritizing the identification of circumstances compatible with safe swallowing in addition to the documentation of swallowing pathology. Accordingly, the patient is seated comfortably and is examined by staff with whom a confident familiarity has been established. The most important variables to work with in designing a rehabilitation program are (1) the patient's position, (2) variations in cervical flexion and extension, (3) food (bolus) characteristics, (4) respiratory modifications, and (5) clearance of residuals of food. The following are brief comments on each of these variables.

POSITIONING. The patient should be comfortable and as much at ease emotionally as possible. The seated position has the following advantages: it allows freedom to modify head and neck relationships for swallowing; it is the position most commonly associated with eating; it is usually optimal for unrestricted breathing and coughing; it permits ready access to the mouth by cups, spoons, and straws for swallowing trials; it allows the effect of gravity to play its customary role on oral, pharyngeal, and esophageal stages; it enables the patient to use either upper extremity; and it presents easy access to tracheostomy tubes for suctioning and other manipulations. If a wheelchair is available that fits the dimensions of the fluoroscopy equipment, the seated position in this chair also obviates the problem of transfer in the Radiology Department. Since many patients with neurogenic dysphagia have mobility impairments, their arrival already positioned for study saves time, effort, and the possibility of accidents in transfer.

ARTHUR A. SIEBENS

The semireclining position is advantageous for at least two circumstances: (1) when fixation of the cervical or thoracic spine in flexion or weak extensors of the neck impose problems in swallowing that are equivalent to those in the prone position at the oral stage and unusual angulation for the pharyngeal stage, and (2) when testing whether or not a hypodynamic pharyngeal stage (e.g., lower motor neuron pathology or myopathy) is compatible with the passage of small liquid boluses around the epiglottis and lateral to the aryepiglottic folds (see Figs. 35–2 and 35–5) into the esophagus without brimming over into the laryngeal vestibule. The supine, prone, or side-lying positions are unusual for swallowing and are unlikely to reduce swallowing disability.

CERVICAL FLEXION AND EXTENSION. The larynx is suspended from the chin, the base of the skull, and the sternoclavicular area (see Fig. 35–3). The tensions of the muscles that compose this suspension system are modified not only by the force of muscle contraction but by the relative positions of the skull, the chin, and the chest. This feature is readily demonstrable to the reader by swallowing when the cervical spine is extended, a position that adds passive tension to the chin-hyoid-chest segment of the suspension. Laryngeal elevation, which contributes to both airway protection and foodway opening, is accomplished against the least resistance when there is slack in the suspension between hyoid-larynx and chest (sternothyroid and sternohyoid muscles). If laryngeal elevators (geniohyoid, digastricus, thyrohyoid) are weak or dystonic, laryngeal elevation and safe swallowing may be assisted by flexing the neck. Whether or not this maneuver is necessary for safe swallowing of all boluses or only of liquid boluses is readily decided by the fluoroscopic study used in swallowing rehabilitation. The visualization that neck flexion is effective must be followed by therapeutic feeding sessions designed to teach the incorporation of this maneuver into swallowing behavior. Cognitive sufficiency compatible with learning is essential to this rehabilitation approach.

BOLUS CHARACTERISTICS. The versatility of the pharynx is reflected in the variability of what is presented at the dining table. Although the oral stage modifies what is placed in the mouth toward a uniform consistency, the spectrum of bolus consistencies presented to the pharynx and esophagus is broad nevertheless. It is reasonable to assume that pharyngeal impairment might only narrow this spectrum rather than place all of the capacity for swallowing in jeopardy. Accordingly, the rehabilitation approach should include identifying bolus options for safe swallowing and capitalizing on these options. A typical study designed for this objective might include presentations of radiopacified thin liquids, thick liquids, puddings, gels, purées, mashed potatoes, and chew-dependent foods such as scrambled eggs and hamburger. These can all be prepared by mixing with barium sulfate.

Bolus-specific dysphagia refers to the fact that swallowing impairment can be defined by the consistency of what is swallowed safely. The study of food consistency is relevant, therefore, to dysphagia. This is the province of engineering science, the terminology of rheology (*rheos* = Greek for flow), and the characterization of foods in terms of viscosity and elasticity. Were it possible to classify foods and swallowing impairments by these objective criteria, the nourishment of the swallowing-impaired patient would be simplified, because the visualization of a few test boluses would suffice to identify swallowing reactions to a large group of foods. One less quantifiable but helpful classification is described in Table 35–2.

A thin liquid usually presents the impaired pharynx with its most trying challenge, this bolus being the most likely one to penetrate the airway. The conversion of liquids to high-water content, low calorie, nonliquid forms may be a successful compensation. Converting liquids to safe swallowing alternatives can be approached through the use of thickening agents, such as arrowroot, gelatin, tapioca, or modified food starch (THICK-IT). When these liquid substitutes are incorporated in the

TABLE 35–2. Liquid and Solid Categories for Patients with Dysphagia

LIQUID CATEGORIES

A. Thin
   e.g., broth, coffee, fruit juices, tea, milk, gelatin
B. Thick
   e.g., cream soup, eggnog, Ensure, hot cereal, nectars
C. Ultra-thick
   e.g., custard, pudding, sour cream, slushies

SOLID CATEGORIES

A. Formable
   e.g., banana, bread, egg salad, mashed potato, puréed meat
B. Particulate
   e.g., cottage cheese, baked fish, chicken salad, cookies, hamburger
C. Multi-textured
   e.g., baked potato, carrots, fruit cup, peas, rice, noodles

patient's diet, the adequacy of hydration should be monitored clinically and by measuring the specific gravity of urine.

RESPIRATORY MODIFICATIONS. The to-and-fro flow of air through the pharynx and larynx tends to sweep food into the larynx during inspiration (aspiration) and out during expiration. Consequently, air flow modifications offer practical approaches to clearing the larynx when swallowing impairment results in its recurrent penetration. The larynx may be cleared between swallows if the individual learns to take a breath before swallowing and to exhale after each swallow. A frequent gentle throat-clearing exhalation may be sufficient to maintain a clear airway. Whether or not these modifications are effective can be visualized as a part of the swallowing study.

Aspiration may be so flagrant that bypassing the mouth, pharynx, and larynx by tracheostomy becomes essential. For some patients who experience laryngeal penetration during inspiration (aspiration), valving the tracheostomy tube to allow inspiration below the larynx and expiration through the larynx allows the continuation of feeding by mouth. This valve also preserves phonation and oral communication despite tracheostomy.

Sealing the airway completely from food is accomplished by tracheostomy with a tube that includes an inflatable cuff. Although such tubes eliminate air flow through the larynx, they do not prevent food from dropping into the larynx from the pharynx. Surgically sealing the larynx through a laryngectomy may become necessary, representing the ultimate failure of compensation for swallowing impairment.

SWALLOWING MODIFICATIONS. Abnormal pooling of liquids or retention of solids is commonly visualized directly in the mouth and, by fluoroscopy, in the pharynx or esophagus of the patient with dysphagia. The vallecula (see Fig. 35–2) and piriform sinuses (see Fig. 35–5) are particularly frequent sites of such bolus residuals. In sufficient volume, liquids in the piriform sinuses may brim over the aryepiglottic folds (Fig. 35–5), giving the voice a wet-hoarse or gurgly quality and predisposing the patient to glottic penetration during inspiration. Clearing these residuals may be accomplished by swallowing more than once per bolus. Residuals of solids may be dislodged by interspersing swallows of liquids. Rotation or bending of the cervical spine may alter pharyngeal relationships sufficiently to prevent or reduce pooling. The effectiveness of these measures can be determined quickly by fluoroscopy.

Pharyngeal Bypass

Airway bypass by tracheostomy is discussed briefly above. Foodway bypass is accomplished most commonly by positioning a nasogastric, orogastric, or gastrostomy tube.

The position of the tube's termination should be decided upon thoughtfully and verified precisely. Most patients with a swallowing impairment are also candidates for rehabilitation for mobility, communication, and self-care. Continuous feeding interferes with these objectives by curtailing freedom of movement. In contrast, bolus feeding, in which a bolus of 250 to 500 ml is instilled into the stomach, requires only a few minutes, provided the tube is of sufficient internal diameter. The bolus must be delivered into the stomach itself. Delivery into the esophagus predisposes the patient to reflux into the pharynx. Delivery beyond the pylorus is incompatible with bolus feeding because the precipitous distention of the small bowel may cause vomiting, diarrhea, perspiration, hypotension, pain, and other disagreeable events associated with the dumping syndrome. Continuous feeding throughout the hours of sleep occasionally may be necessary in order to meet the patient's caloric and fluid requirements. The disadvantage of this approach is that sleep usually requires recumbency, a circumstance predisposing the patient to gastroesophageal reflux and to esophagopharyngeal reflux at a time when the pharynx is particularly vulnerable because of the patient's lack of wakefulness. Continuous feeding is less hazardous if the tube extends beyond the pylorus because reflux into the esophagus is less likely.

Checking gastric residual volume with a syringe is an advisable precaution prior to bolus instillation. This simple procedure can establish how long it takes for the stomach to empty. This information is valuable for deciding how long a patient should be tilted upright after feeding or whether emptying is so delayed and the risk of reflux so great that passage of the tube beyond the pylorus into the small intestine is essential.

Swallowing impairment may facilitate passage of tubes into the airway rather than into the foodway, particularly when tubes are passed over a guide wire. Reduced pharyngeal sensation, absent gag, silent laryngeal penetration, and suppression of cognition all foster the calamities of instilling tube feeding into the lung. Reliable verification of tube placement by x-ray film may be life-saving.

Whether or not a nasogastric tube interferes with swallowing is not clear. On the one hand, it is reasonable to assume that sensory acuity important for swallowing is reduced by accommodation because the initial unpleasantness of the tube disappears within hours of its placement. It is reasonable also to conceive that the tube prevents normal passage of a bolus because of its size or tendency to cling to boluses. On the other hand, clear interference with swallowing is difficult to document by radiofluoroscopic visualization. In any case, the tube should not be a permanent pharyngeal bypass because it is unsightly, obstructs nasal passages, and introduces the possibility of esophageal erosions.

If no progress toward swallowing rehabilitation is likely, a gastrostomy should be performed within days or weeks rather than months after diagnosis. Although endoscopic gastrostomy with a fine tube is practiced commonly,[20] gastrostomy through an incision in the abdominal wall under local anesthesia using a Foley or "mushroom" tube[21] offers the advantage of a larger lumen at no additional cost and no morbidity. The latter also presents the family or nurse with greater ease in tube changing. In both endoscopic and incision alternatives, the gastrostomy should seal itself without surgical closure when the tube is removed. Recovering the ability to be alimented and hydrated by mouth may be arrived at gradually over a period of months. Terminating this period by simply removing the tube and applying dressings until closure occurs is a high point representing success for patient and rehabilitation staff.

Avoidances

The cognitively impaired individual with dysphagia may eat or drink hazardously. Frequently, liquids are assumed falsely to be safely swallowed when other boluses are not. Another form of abuse is filling the mouth more rapidly than it clears. Pharyngeal overload may result in choking. Removal of oral contents and cough assistance by chest and abdominal compression (Heimlich's maneuver) may be necessary.

The individual undergoing swallowing re-education or therapeutic feeding must concentrate. A distracting environment interferes with learning. Moreover, speaking or the expression of emotion can easily invoke foodway and airway mechanisms that override volitional control and enhance the likelihood of aspiration.

The use of faucial stimulation for restoring pharyngeal function has been advocated and practiced widely.[22] A cooled laryngeal mirror is used to touch the base of the anterior arch. Whether or not this time-consuming practice favors the restoration of swallowing capability is conjectural.

The Swallowing Rehabilitation Team

Swallowing rehabilitation requires a knowledge of foods, fluids, fluoroscopy, physiology, pharmacology, phonation, rheology, anatomy, respiration, ingestion, and conceivably other basic disciplines. This knowledge is incorporated in the clinical skills of numerous specialists in both medical and other health-related professions. The swallowing rehabilitation team could have many members, so many that timely and cost-effective patient care would suffer were each involved for all adults and children for whom swallowing rehabilitation is indicated. There is much to say, therefore, for concentrating responsibility among a few individuals whose interest and capability are high, relying on appropriate selective consultation in situations in which additional knowledge is needed and surgical skills are necessary.

The rehabilitation physician qualifies for an important role with respect to both children and adults. Dysphagia frequently occurs in conjunction with other impairments for which rehabilitation is mandatory, e.g., brain injury, cerebral palsy, and stroke. Therefore, a philosophy regarding long-term care; limitation of objectives; and the recognition of family, social, and vocational implications is a necessary part of swallowing rehabilitation. The medical knowledge required for an accurate diagnosis and prognosis and for the appropriate use of medications is essential. Kinesiology,[23] electrodiagnosis,[10] neurophysiology, and the team approach are hallmarks of physiatric expertise and interest that are applicable directly to the rehabilitation of swallowing disorders.

The profession of speech and language pathology has taken a particular interest in patients with swallowing disorders.[22, 24] The initiatives of this profession are in keeping with its special knowledge of the structures, mechanisms, deficits, and treatments applicable to patients with communication disorders.[14, 25] Much of this knowledge is germane to understanding and treating swallowing disability. The rehabilitation nurse is pivotal to the success of a swallowing rehabilitation program, because the feeding of patients and the recognition of swallowing difficulty both fall in the province of this essential profession. The occupational therapist contributes expertise in the rehabilitation of upper extremity function, feeding techniques, and perceptual motor performance. Openness of communication and the willingness to innovate studiously are especially important characteristics for members of all swallowing rehabilitation teams.

ACKNOWLEDGMENTS

A number of colleagues and associates have contributed to the concepts presented in this chapter. Prominent among these are James Bosma, Martin Donner, and Haskins Kashima. Of the members of our swallowing rehabilitation group, I am especially grateful to Patricia Linden, Ann Duchane, Donna Tippett, Jeffrey Palmer, and William Schwarz. Diane Robertson's remarkable drawings add an artistic dimension to this chapter and substitute for thousands of words. Innumerable patients have been silent mentors. The Good Samaritan Hospital administration, the Food Department, and the Department of Radiology under Perry Arnold and Carol Rossi have been most cooperative in making radiopacified foods and allowing open access to the radiology suite. Finally, I am appreciative of the patience of Rose Dalton, Susan Graber, and Alexandra Brzozowski in working and reworking the manuscript during busy office schedules.

References

1. International Classification of Impairments, Disabilities, and Handicaps. Geneva, World Health Organization, 1980.
2. Bosma, J. F.: Physiology of the mouth, pharynx and esophagus. In Paparella, M. A., and Shumrick, D. A. (Eds.): Otolaryngology, Vol. 2. Philadelphia, W. B. Saunders, 1980, pp. 319–329.
3. Donner, M. W., Bosma, J. F., and Robertson, D. L.: Anatomy and physiology of the pharynx. Gastrointest. Radiol., 10:196, 1985.
4. Code, C. F., Creamer, B., and Schlegel, J. F.: An Atlas of Esophageal Motility in Health and Disease. Springfield, Ill., Charles C Thomas, 1958.
5. Vantrappen, G., and Hellemans, J.: Diseases of the Esophagus. New York, Springer-Verlag, 1974.
6. Comroe, J. H.: Physiology of Respiration. Chicago, Year Book Medical Publishers, Inc., 1965.
7. Bartlett, J. G.: Aspiration pneumonia. In Baum, G. L., and Wolinsky, E.: Textbook of Pulmonary Disease. Boston, Little, Brown and Co., 1983, pp. 583–593.
8. Goyal, R. K.: Disorders of the cricopharyngeus muscle. Otolaryngol. Clin. North Am., 17:115, 1984.
9. Doty, R. W., and Bosma, J. F.: Electromyographic analysis of reflex deglutition. J. Neurophysiol., 19:44, 1956.
10. Tanaka, E., Palmer, J., and Siebens, A.: Bipolar suction electrodes for pharyngeal electromyography. Dysphagia, 1:39, 1986.
11. Buthpitiya, A. G., Stroud, D., and Russell, C. O. H.: Pharyngeal pump and esophageal transit. Dig. Dis. Sci., 32:1244, 1987.
12. Negus, V. E.: The mechanism of swallowing. Proc. Royal. Soc. Med., 36:85, 1942.
13. Mendelsohn, M. S., and McConnell, F. M. S.: Laryngoscope, 97:483, 1987.
14. Darley, F. L., Aronson, A. E., and Brown, J. R.: Motor Speech Disorders. Philadelphia, W. B. Saunders, 1975.
15. Netsell, R., and Daniel, B.: Dysarthria in adults: Physiologic approach to rehabilitation. Arch. Phys. Med. Rehabil., 60:502, 1979.
16. Bosma, J. F.: Development of feeding. Clin. Nutr., 5:210, 1986.
17. Linden, P., and Siebens, A.: Dysphagia: Predicting laryngeal penetration. Arch. Phys. Med. Rehabil., 64:281, 1983.
18. Donner, M. W., and Selbiger, M. L.: Cinefluorographic analysis of pharyngeal swallowing in neuromuscular disorders. Am. J. Med. Sci., 251:600, 1966.
19. Siebens, A., and Linden, P.: Dynamic imaging for swallowing re-education. Gastrointest. Radiol., 10:251, 1985.
20. Gauderer, M. W., and Ponsky, J. L.: A simplified technique for constructing a tube feeding gastrostomy. Surg. Gynecol. Obstet., 152:83, 1981.
21. Stamm, M.: Gastrostomy by a new method. Med. News, 65:324, 1984.
22. Logemann, J.: Evaluation and Treatment of Swallowing Disorders. San Diego, College-Hill Press, 1983.
23. Palmer, J., Tanaka, E., and Siebens, A.: Motions of the posterior pharyngeal wall in swallowing. Laryngoscope, 98:414, 1988.
24. Groher, M.: Dysphagia: Diagnosis and Management. Boston, Butterworths, 1984.
25. Netsell, R.: A neurobiologic view of the dysarthrias. In McNeil, M., Rosenbeck, J., and Aronson, A. (Eds.): The Dysarthrias: Physiology, Acoustics, Perception, Management. San Diego, College-Hill Press, 1984.

36

Degenerative Diseases of the Central Nervous System

JEROME W. GERSTEN

With more successful management of acute diseases, there has been a progressive shift in attention toward chronic diseases, especially those classified as degenerative. Degenerative diseases have been characterized by a progressive course and a high incidence in older age groups. Defining degeneration as deterioration adds little to our understanding. The term abiotrophy, the inability of tissue to survive, has often been used to define the degenerative process, but it, too, says little concerning etiology. Some diseases initially categorized as degenerative are now known to be viral in etiology.[6, 35] Creutzfeldt-Jakob disease is an example of this change in categorization. Creutzfeldt-Jakob disease is a spongiform encephalopathy (cerebral and cerebellar), with cortical atrophy and marked neuronal loss in the cerebral cortex, the basal ganglia, the thalamus, the brain stem, the cerebellar cortex, and the spinal cord. Rapidly progressive dementia with motor abnormalities is present. However, the disease is transmissible and is now classified among the slow virus diseases. The physiatrist often is responsible for the management of patients with degenerative diseases and attempts to improve or maintain the functional capacity of these patients. The more common of these diseases are examined in the following discussion.

Dementia

Dementia is an impairment of global cognitive function that results in a decrease in the patient's ability to function in the environment.[10, 28, 30] With the proportionate increase in the population over 65, the dementias have become a serious public health problem with a profound economic impact.[27] It has been estimated that 1.5 per cent to 6 per cent of the population over 65 is severely demented, and 2.5 to 15 per cent mildly to moderately demented. Fifty to seventy-five per cent of dementia is due to Alzheimer's disease (AD), a primary dementia, which is examined later in greater detail. The incidence of AD is 1 per cent per year at age 60, 2 to 3 per cent per year at age 80, and 4 per cent per year above age 80. AD is now the fourth leading cause of death. Secondary dementias, which are often reversible, may result from multiple cerebral infarcts, depression (pseudodementia), metabolic disease (e.g., decreased thyroid function), infection, brain tumor, brain trauma, nutritional deficiencies (e.g., vitamin B_{12}, folate deficiency), severe sensory deficit, heavy metal poisoning, substance abuse (ethanol), and excessive medication. These possibilities should be ruled out during the initial evaluation.[13, 17, 18, 29, 32]

A bimodal distribution in age of onset in AD has been noted, with one peak below age 65 and a second above 65. The former peak was previously referred to as presenile dementia, a distinction that no longer seems helpful. It has been suggested, however, that there is a subgroup with autosomal dominant form of inheritance,[24] especially with onset below age 50. In addition, patients with early onset AD may have more language problems, whereas those with late onset AD may have more visual-constructive problems. Sixty to sixty-five per cent of patients are women.

The brain weight in patients with AD is decreased, and gross atrophy of gyri is present. Sulci are wider and there is ventricular dilatation.[3] Degeneration and neuronal loss are general, although especially marked in the pyramidal cells of the hippocampus[25] and the large pyramidal cells in the association cortex. Degeneration appears early in the nucleus basalis of Meynert and later in the locus ceruleus. The pathology includes the presence of neurofibrillary tangles, neuritic plaques, and granulovacuolar degeneration.[4, 33] Neurofibrillary tangles are intraneuronal masses of cytoplasmic filaments. Two 10-nm filaments are helically wound, with a half period of 80 nm. They consist of an abnormal fibrous protein. Ubiquitin, a protein required for adenosine triphosphate (ATP)-dependent proteolytic system, is a component of the paired helical filament.[39] Neurofibrillary tangles are present in cerebral cortex, pyramidal cells of the hippocampus, and nucleus basalis of Meynert. Neuritic plaques (senile plaques)[31, 46] are extracellular and are found in the frontal and parietal association cortex and the hippocampus. They are focal accumulations of degenerating nerve terminals (axons, dendrites), macrophages, microglia, and astrocytes, surrounding a core of amyloid protein that stains with Congo red. Amyloid is also present in some cerebral and meningeal vessels. Granulovacuolar degeneration consists of cytoplasmic vacuoles containing a central granule. These are present in pyramidal neurons of Ammon's horn of the hippocampus. The degree of dementia has been correlated positively with the number of plaques and tangles that are present.[21]

Cerebral blood flow,[22, 41] oxygen consumption, respiratory rate, and phosphokinase content are reduced in the dementias, with a decrease in cerebral metabolism occurring early with neuronal atrophy[23, 26] and diminished blood flow appearing early in arteriosclerotic dementia. A positive correlation is noted between mean hemisphere flow and the degree of dementia in multi-infarct patients, but no such relationship is recognized in primary dementia.

The cholinergic projection system, originating in cells in the base of the forebrain and terminating in the cerebral cortex and the hippocampus, is affected early.[15, 29] Cholinergic markers, such as choline acetyltransferase and acetylcholinesterase, show early, consistent, and marked decreases.[42] Choline acetyltransferase, an enzyme involved in the synthesis of acetylcholine, may decrease 80 to 90 per cent in the cerebral cortex and the hippocampus. There is a significant correlation between the decrease in choline acetyltransferase and the number of plaques and the decrease in memory.[14, 36]

Other biochemical changes include a decrease in the brain of somatostatin[5, 20] (in the frontal and temporal cortex, correlating with decreased choline acetyltransferase), corticotropin-releasing factor, homovanillic acid, L-dopa, dopamine, and noradrenaline; and a decrease in the cerebrospinal fluid of serotonin, homovanillic acid, gamma-aminobutyric acid, and 5-hydroxyindole acetic acid.

Symptoms of AD are progressive, with a greater decrease in recent memory than in immediate or remote memory.[38] The individual's ability to abstract and calculate decreases.[44] Judgment and orientation are impaired. Somewhat later, dysphasia, dyspraxia, and dysgnosia may appear. Tactile discrimination learning may be impaired.[16] Behavioral symptoms appear early and include apathy, changes in work habits, changes in social relationships, and a tendency to wander. Paranoid delusions may appear in up to one third of patients, depression in up to 20 per cent (or more in some studies), and hallucinations in up to 20 per cent. Late in the course of the disease, there is movement disorder with slow gait, difficulty in the performance of activities of daily living, dyspraxia, and incontinence. The patient is eventually confined to bed, with death occurring 5 to 10 years after onset.

Specific pharmacotherapy for AD has not proved to be of major value. Vasodilators and hyperbaric oxygen produce no significant improvement in symptoms. Dihydroergotamine (Hydergine), a phosphodiesterase inhibitor, in doses of 6 to 12 mg daily, resulted in some beneficial effect on mental alertness, sociability, and memory.[34] In one recent study, Hydergine at a dose of 6 mg per day improved short-term memory but not other cognitive abilities.[43] Acetylcholine precursors, such as choline and lecithin, have not improved cognitive function. Cholinesterase inhibitors, like physostigmine, have been reported to enhance learning in normal young adults and to relieve cognitive dysfunction produced by scopolamine[12] but have not been significantly helpful in AD. Muscarinic agonists thus far have not been effective.[8] Symptomatic treatment is, however, indicated. This includes the use of antidepressants (25 to 75 mg per day of doxepin or desipramine), antipsychotic medication for severe behavioral problems (1 to 2 mg haloperidol per day), and low doses of benzodiazepine for anxiety and restlessness (oxazepam or temazepam, which are metabolized through conjugation).[39, 45]

The major aspects of care are preventive, designed to keep an individual as active and independent as possible in either the home or an institution. To the greatest degree possible, physical activity must be encouraged to maintain strength, range of motion, and alertness; visual, auditory, and social stimuli must be maintained; diet must be kept at an optimal level; and safety must be enhanced.[7, 9] Thirty to forty per cent of the elderly fall each year. In AD the fracture rate from falls is 69 per 1000 falls per year. Falls may be due to associated illnesses (e.g., acute change in cardiac status); confusion and wandering; excessive medication or high dosages, or both; impaired gait and balance; muscle weakness; visual deficit; visual-perceptual deficit; and environmental hazards. The last-mentioned factor includes poor lighting, slippery floors, and scatter rugs. Such environmental hazards must be avoided. In addition, rooms should maintain a familiar layout (do not change the furniture arrangement unnecessarily), and grab bars and hand rails should be installed where needed.

Management of the patient with AD requires consideration not only of purely medical aspects of the disease but also of psychosocial factors.[19] Health must be maintained with appropriate treatment of associated illnesses. The patient, family, and support personnel (nurse, social worker) must be involved early in treatment planning. At an early stage, day care centers can be extremely helpful by providing respite for the family as well as physical activity and socialization for the patient.[40] Recreation therapy can be an important part of the day care program. Counseling should be available at times of crisis, which often involve issues related to nursing home placement.[11]

Parkinson's Disease

Parkinson's disease (PD) is the most common degenerative disease involving the basal ganglia. Although idiopathic disease (paralysis agitans) is currently the most common type observed, postencephalitic, arteriosclerotic, postanoxic, traumatic, or drug (reserpine, phenothiazine, α methyldopa, 1-methyl-4-phenyl-1,2,3,6-tetrahydropyridine [MPTP]) etiologies also may occur.[72] Infectious, genetic, immunological, and environmental etiologies also have been considered.[81] The recent discovery that MPTP, a by-product in the synthesis of a synthetic heroin, could produce a parkinsonian-like syndrome has stimulated the search for environmental factors (e.g., slow toxins) that might produce PD.[52, 63, 90]

Prior to 1918, most known cases of PD were of the idiopathic type. Following the epidemic of encephalitis lethargica (von Economo's disease) from 1918 to 1926, the pattern was altered for a period. From 1920 to 1943, there were two peaks of onset of PD. The first was a small secondary peak in the third decade, representing postencephalitic cases, followed by a larger peak in the sixth or seventh decades, representing the idiopathic type. The incidence of the postencephalitic type of PD has decreased, and the curve representing age of onset is again unimodal, with the peak in the older age group. In the United States, approximately 60,000 new cases are documented per year. The incidence of PD under the age of 50 is approximately 5 to 8 per 100,000 population, rising to 35 per 100,000 population between the ages of 50 and 59, and 100 per 100,000 population between the ages of 60 and 69. Over 1 per cent of the population over 50 may have PD, with a prevalence of over 400,000 persons (approximately 180 persons per 100,000).[65, 68]

The most consistent neuropathological findings are those noted in the melanin-containing cells of the brain stem—the substantia nigra and the locus ceruleus. There is loss of nerve cells with reactive gliosis, especially in the substantia nigra. Degeneration of dopaminergic neurons in the pars compacta of the substantia nigra, with degeneration of an unmyelinated nigrostriatal pathway, results in decreased dopaminergic activity at striatal dopamine receptors. Both D1 and D2 receptors seem to be involved in PD. These changes are related to the motor abnormalities in parkinsonism. In idiopathic PD, eosinophilic inclusions (Lewy's bodies) are present.[61] These bodies are composed of filamentous structures, with a dense core and radially emerging filaments peripherally.

Dopamine (DA), an inhibitory neurotransmitter (membrane stabilizer),[58] is present in highest concentration in the caudate and the putamen. Eighty per cent of the content of DA in the brain is localized at these two sites. In parkinsonism, there is a decrease in the melanin content of substantia nigra cells, a selective decrease of DA in caudate and putamen, and a decrease in homovanillic acid (a monoamine catabolite).[66] A decreased urinary excretion of free DA occurs in PD. The lower the level of free urinary DA, the greater the functional deficit and the more severe the akinesia and the rigidity. Most patients with PD have a decrease in DA release, which is a presynaptic DA deficiency, with a decrease in cerebrospinal fluid homovanillic acid levels. Parkinsonian symptoms may represent an imbalance between inhibitory dopaminergic stimuli and excitatory cholinergic stimuli in the striatum. Symptoms in PD may not appear until at least 60 per cent of the striatal DA has been lost. This factor may be due to increased tyrosine hydroxylase activity and DA release from the remaining dopaminergic terminals.[97] In addition to the decrease in DA, there is a decrease of over 60 per cent in norepinephrine levels in the locus ceruleus and cerebellar cortex.[70]

Dopaminergic inhibition can be demonstrated by the effect of iontophoretically applied DA, via micropipette, on spontaneous electrical activity of caudate nucleus cells. In 50 to 60 per cent of these cells, the firing rate is decreased. In addition, electrical stimulation of the substantia nigra markedly depresses the firing rate of a large number of caudate neurons.[54] In PD, the decrease in inhibition may be related to an imbalance in the activity of the alpha and gamma motor systems, with an increase in alpha activity and a decrease in gamma activity. An increase in excitability of the alpha motor neuron pool has been demonstrated through the examination of the H-reflex—by examination of maximal H/M ratio and the recovery curve of the H response.[54, 59, 64, 79] Excitability of the alpha motor neuron pool is decreased following the administration of L-dopa.[53] With microelectrodes in Ia afferents in humans, increased static fusimotor activity has been demonstrated in patients with parkinsonism. Although overactivity of the fusimotor system is an important part of parkinsonian rigidity, there is no primary defect in this system.

Onset of idiopathic parkinsonism usually occurs after the age of 50 (with a mean of 57.1 years in one study). Motor phenomena are most apparent and for many years have attracted the most attention.[49] These motor phenomena include tremor, rigidity, bradykinesia, disturbances in posture and gait, and decreased facial expression.[91] Tremor may be the earliest symptom, although rigidity and bradykinesia also appear early. The tremor rate is three to six per sec and becomes manifest in distal parts of the extremity. It is present at rest, increased by emotional stress, often inhibited by the initiation of voluntary movement, and perhaps disappears during sleep. Tremor may be initiated when the patient attempts to maintain the upper extremity abducted in an unsupported position. It is probably the result of increased activation of the alpha motor neuron system, with rhythmic discharge through the ventrolateral nucleus of the thalamus. This may be the result of disinhibition in a long loop reflex involving the cortex, the striatum, and the ventrolateral thalamic nucleus.[92]

Rigidity, an early parkinsonian symptom, does not follow the pattern of reciprocal innervation, and increased electrical activity and tone may be present in flexor and extensor muscles simultaneously. This disorder of reciprocal inhibition may also be demonstrated by low intensity stimulation of the tibial nerve. In the normal subject, the tibialis anticus and soleus muscles respond simultaneously in only a small number of instances. In PD, simultaneous responses in these two muscles occur in 77 per cent of patients. Electrical activity may be present in muscles at rest in PD and is not affected by the velocity of motion. There may be, however, excessive reflex response to muscle stretch.[73] Alternating tightening and releasing may produce cogwheel rigidity, i.e., rigidity that gives way in a series of little jerks that occur when passive stretching exceeds the threshold of the static stretch reflex.

Bradykinesia, the slow and difficult initiation of voluntary movements,[86] is independent of rigidity, although the two are often associated. It is noted especially on initiation of voluntary, repetitive acts and may be related to increased central inhibition of the gamma neuron via the ventrolateral nucleus of the thalamus. Slow movement is mainly the result of a motor defect, although the role of arousal or alerting is not clear.

Control of posture is an important function of the basal ganglia, and postural disturbance is frequent in parkinsonism. The classic posture in PD is one of head flexion, thoracic kyphosis, shoulder protraction and abduction, and arm flexion. Postural reflexes are poor, and balance may be lost easily. The patient's gait is slow and shuffling, with difficulty in starting to walk and loss of associated movements. Additional symptoms related to the motor system include weakness and easy fatigue; muscle pain, which may on occasion be severe; and the secondary phenomena of flexion contracture and decreased range of motion.

Autonomic disturbance may exist. This can include excessive salivation (sialorrhea) and sweating, oily skin, chronic constipation, and postural hypotension. Speech disturbance is frequent.[55] A decrease in vital capacity and the loss of vocal intensity are apparent.[94] There is laryngeal impairment, with a decrease in the speed of movement of the lip and the tongue muscles and a decrease in the clarity of articulation occuring later. The precise effect of PD on higher language function has not yet been clarified. Aphasia resulting from vascular lesions of the basal ganglia and internal capsule has been reported.[56, 87]

Visual neglect and impairment in visual-spatial perception are frequent in PD.[50, 93] The latter is noted both in visual-motor tasks that require a complex motor response and in visual-perceptual tasks that require a minimal motor response. Depression is common in PD, occurring in 20 to 60 per cent of patients,[91] as is the deterioration in intellectual function.[78] On the Wechsler's Adult Intelligence Scale, scores are reported to be much lower in performance than in verbal areas, especially in perceptual organization, digit symbol, block design, and object assembly. Dementia, referred to as a subcortical dementia, may be present in 30 to 40 per cent of patients with PD. In recent years, considerable attention has been directed to differences between the dementia of AD and PD.

Treatment of parkinsonism may be pharmacological, physical, or surgical.[51] The basis for major pharmacological therapy is the DA depletion in the striatum in PD and the need to restore DA toward normal levels.[47, 48] DA does not cross the blood-brain barrier. However, the precursor of DA, L-dihydroxyphenylalanine (L-dopa), does cross the blood-brain barrier, can be administered orally, and is then converted to DA in the striatum.[84] Unfortunately, L-dopa is also converted to DA peripherally through the action of dopa decarboxylase. This peripheral decarboxylation may be accelerated by pyridoxine. Dopadecarboxylase inhibitors (carbidopa) block extracerebral conversion of L-dopa to DA and, thus, lower doses of L-dopa are therapeutically effective. Unfortunately, 30 per cent of patients with PD fail to respond to L-dopa. In addition, there may be disturbing side effects (e.g., hypotension; uncontrolled movements of the tongue, the oral or buccal muscles, and the jaw;[95] and depression),[96] on-off effects,[62, 88] and later, a decrease in effectiveness.[82, 83, 85] Thus, there may be a role for ergot alkaloids that selectively inhibit prolactin secretion,[75] such as bromocriptine.[67, 89] Ergot alkaloids penetrate the blood-brain barrier more readily than L-dopa and act directly on DA receptors in the striatum, probably with both presynaptic and postsynaptic effects.[76, 77] Other drugs that may be of value are the anticholinergics (trihexyphenidyl),[71] the antihistamines, beta-adrenergic blockers for tremor, and amantadine, which may increase DA release. It was noted earlier that MPTP could produce a disease closely resembling PD but not identical to it. For cell destruction, MPTP must be converted to MPP+ through the action of monoamine oxidase B. Because of this sequence of events, studies are currently in progress to determine whether or not a monoamine oxidase inhibitor[74] (e.g., Deprenyl) can have a favorable effect on PD.

Drug therapy alone is not sufficient and must be combined with a program of physical therapy.[57] This program is designed to correct faulty posture (or to maintain good posture), to maintain or to increase range of motion, to maintain ambulation and hand function, and to decrease speech dysfunction.[60] With regard to posture, attention must be focused on the tendency toward neck flexion, thoracic kyphosis, and hip and knee flexion. Prevention of contracture is an important element in maintenance of good posture. When necessary, stretching of hip flexors, knee flexors, and ankle plantar flexors must be part of the program. Gait training will be enhanced by successful attempts to improve posture. Ambulation is more functional when there is a slightly broader base, when steps are longer, when there is conscious dorsiflexion of toes on beginning the swing phase, and when associated movements of the upper extremities are gently encouraged. Frequently, gait is improved by painting white lines across the path or placing small obstacles across the path and asking the patient to step over the line or obstacle. Speech training should emphasize deep breathing and strengthening of respiratory muscles to increase audibility. Attention must be given to rhythm and articulation. Singing may be of considerable benefit in improving rhythmic aspects of speech.

Surgery involving pallidocapsular or thalamocapsular lesions is not often used at the present time. However, when tremor and rigidity are severe and not well controlled with oral medication, stereotactic ventralis lateralis thalamotomy is an acceptable option. Results of this procedure are reported to be better in patients with unilateral symptoms and in patients without speech and gait disturbances.[69] Promising results have recently been obtained in PD by grafting tissue of the adrenal medulla into the lateral ventricle in direct contact with the head of the caudate nucleus.[80] This procedure is now being evaluated.

Huntington's Disease

Huntington's disease (HD) is a neurodegenerative disorder, with autosomal dominant transmission. The site of the genetic defect is chromosome 4, and a polymorphic DNA marker has been localized. Prevalence is approximately 5 to 10 persons per 100,000, and there may be about 15,000 to 25,000 persons with HD. Gene carrier prevalence is 1 in 4000 to 1 in 10,000. The average age of onset is 41 years, with the duration of the disease lasting 10 to 20 years. Although HD is characterized by degeneration, atrophy, and cell loss in the cerebral cortex and with gliosis, these changes are especially marked in the caudate nucleus and layers 3, 5, and 6 of the cerebral cortex.[106] The diencephalic-limbic structures, the putamen, and the globus pallidus are involved to a lesser degree, and the pars reticularis of the substantia nigra is relatively spared. There is intense gliosis in regions of neuron loss, with accumulation of lipofuscin in neurons and glia. Morphological abnormalities are noted mainly in dendrites of medium-sized spiny neurons.[103]

The caudate nucleus may show marked loss of choline acetyltransferase activity. There is a decrease in neurochemical markers in spiny neurons, which includes substance P, enkephalins, gamma-aminobutyric acid (GABA), and glutamic acid decarboxylase. The spiny neurons are GABA-ergic or peptidergic (substance P, enkephalin), or both. Nicotinamide adenine dinucleotide phosphate diaphorase neurons are spared. Functionally, there is dopaminergic hyperactivity,[102] which is associated with decreased GABA inhibition. As determined by positron emission tomography, glucose consumption in caudate and putamen are decreased in HD.[107] This decrease does not seem to be related to cognitive deficits. The decrease in neuronal metabolism precedes the anatomical loss of neurons, and the decrease in cerebral blood flow is noted before cortical atrophy appears. In subjects who might be at risk for HD, caudate blood flow is normal.

In the normal subject, the H-reflex is elicited readily in quadriceps, hamstrings, and gastrosoleus muscles. The reflex is infrequently elicited elsewhere. In one study of patients with HD, the H-reflex was elicited in the anterior tibial muscle in eight of nine patients and in five of eight subjects at risk. In the same study, the reflex could be elicited in only 1 of 30 normal subjects in the same muscle.[104] On stimulation of the median nerve at the wrist, somatosensory evoked potentials show a normal cortical latency but a decrease in the amplitude of the N20-P25 component.[101] In a study of auditory event– and visual event–related potentials, 12 of 13 patients with HD had an abnormally increased P3 latency (modal latency at 300 msec).[106] This increase may be related to a delay in stimulus processing. Lymphocytes from patients with HD respond to the presence of brain tissue from these patients by producing migration-inhib-

iting factor. The significance of this observation is not known.

HD is characterized by intellectual deterioration, involuntary choreiform movements, and impairment of voluntary movement.[100] The last-mentioned deficit includes impairment of rhythm and speed of fine motor activity, a wide-based gait, and slow voluntary activity. Symptoms usually begin after the age of 30 (average age of onset, 41 years), initially with abrupt, clumsy, and jerky movements. On occasion, dementia or disturbance of mood or personality may be the first symptom.[106] The abnormal movements are increased by emotional or physical stress and disappear during sleep. Later, choreiform movements (jerking of fingers and wrists) and proximal dystonic movements develop. Ultimately, slurred speech, dementia, and severe functional motor impairment develop, with death occurring 10 to 20 years after onset. During the early phase, the major neuropsychological deficit is severe impairment of memory with relative preservation of IQ scores. The patient has difficulty learning new material. In later stages, a nonfocal deficit is exhibited, with poor performance on all tests except picture-naming,[99] a feature that may differentiate HD from AD, in which naming disorders and aphasia are common. In addition to memory deficit, neuropsychological studies show disorders in visual memory, visual-spatial judgment, and perceptual-motor integration.[105]

Drugs that deplete DA, block DA receptors, or increase acetylcholine also decrease choreiform movement.[102] Symptoms may thus be decreased by reserpine, which depletes the striatum of DA (destroying storage sites), and by haloperidol, which blocks DA receptors (and blocks action of DA). Phenothiazine derivatives, too, may be used to decrease adventitious movements. L-Dopa, on the other hand, increases adventitious movements and has been used in predictive testing for HD. Predictive testing[98] will undoubtedly play an increasingly important role in the management of genetically transmissible diseases. In HD, caudate glucose metabolism and DNA studies have been carried out to determine whether or not asymptomatic individuals who might be at risk of developing symptoms can be identified. Profound ethical and legal issues are associated with the process.

Cerebellar System Degeneration

Classification of cerebellar system degenerations has been difficult and confusing.[110] Two of these disorders are addressed—olivopontocerebellar atrophy (Déjérine-Thomas syndrome)[111] and Friedreich's ataxia (FA) (hereditary spinocerebellar ataxia of Friedreich).

Olivopontocerebellar Degeneration

Olivopontocerebellar atrophy may occur with autosomal dominant or autosomal recessive inheritance, or may even appear in a sporadic fashion. Onset is usually during the fifth decade of life. The abiotrophic process is associated with premature degeneration of neurons, possibly due to enzymatic deficits. Atrophy is noted in the cerebellum, the ventral half of the pons, and the inferior olives. In the cerebellum, there is loss of Purkinje's cells and cells in molecular and granular layers. Demyelination of the middle cerebellar peduncle and the cerebellar hemispheres and involvement of the pontine nuclei and the olives is noted. Occasionally, there is degeneration in the striatum, the posterior columns, and the spinocerebellar pathways, especially in instances with autosomal dominant inheritance (more infrequently in the corticospinal tracts). Cell loss may also be noted in Clarke's column and the cuneate, gracile, hypoglossal, facial, and trigeminal nuclei.

In olivopontocerebellar atrophy, ataxia appears first in the lower extremities, then in the upper extremities, and finally in the bulbar muscles and the trunk. Impairment in equilibrium and gait progresses steadily and results in incapacity within 5 to 10 years. Dementia, cranial nerve involvement (with speech disorder, ptosis, facial muscle atrophy, and dysphagia), and extrapyramidal signs (with muscle rigidity, tremor, and immobile facies) may also be present. The excitatory amino acid transmitters aspartate and glutamate, which are normally high in the cerebellum, are decreased.[108] Some disorder in pyruvate metabolism may be noted. The tonic vibration reflex is weak in olivopontocerebellar atrophy, and evoked potentials (somatosensory, visual, and auditory) may be abnormal.[109]

Friedreich's Ataxia

Friedreich's ataxia, the most common of the spinocerebellar degenerations, occurs at an earlier age than OPCA, with onset usually occurring between 5 and 15 years of age. In one report, onset in patients with autosomal recessive inheritance was set at age 11.75 years, whereas in those with autosomal dominant inheritance, it was set at 20.4 years. The disease is slightly more frequent in males than in females. There is major involvement of the dorsal half of the spinal cord, with atrophy predominating in the dorsal columns but also occurring in the lateral corticospinal tract and the dorsal and ventral spinocerebellar tracts.[113] Degeneration is noted in large myelinated sensory fibers of peripheral nerves. The cerebellum is involved to some degree (Purkinje's cells and dentate nuclei). There is a lesser degree of pathology in the pons, the medulla, Clarke's column, the dorsal roots, and the dorsal root ganglia.

Ataxic gait is usually an early symptom, with incoordination progressing from the lower extremities to the upper extremities and then to the trunk, and is due to cerebellar and proprioceptive deficits. Vibratory sense is lost early in the disease process, and position sense is lost later, with occasional deficits in two-point discrimination and in the perception of pain, temperature, and touch. The small fiber population is relatively unaffected, and thermal thresholds are normal.[108, 115] Awkward movements, intention tremor, slurred speech, and pes cavus usually appear later. Cavus is especially common in patients with corticospinal tract involvement since childhood and is the result of mild hypertonus of long extensors and flexors of the foot and amyotrophy of intrinsic foot musculature. Kyphoscoliosis is present in over 80 per cent of patients and diabetes mellitus in over 10 per cent. Deep tendon reflexes are absent, whereas extensor plantar responses are present. Heart murmurs or cardiac enlargement are not infrequent and may be implicated as the cause of death in these patients. Amplitude of sensory potentials (measured at the wrist or the ankle) is markedly decreased. Sensory conduction velocity in the extremities is reduced, more distally than proximally. Somatosensory and brain stem auditory evoked potentials are rarely normal.[112] Visual evoked responses are abnormal in 67 per cent of patients.[116] Quantitative eye movement recordings show impaired visual-vestibular interaction.[114]

In the presence of distal atrophy in the lower extremities, ankle-foot orthoses may be helpful in prolonging the ability to ambulate. Small weights on the wrists and the ankles may aid in diminishing ataxic movements. The median age of death is approximately 27 years in patients with autosomal recessive inheritance and 40 years in those with autosomal dominant inheritance.

Amyotrophic Lateral Sclerosis

The motor neuron diseases include amyotrophic lateral sclerosis (ALS), progressive muscular atrophy, primary lateral sclerosis, and progressive bulbar palsy—each with a different locus of primary anatomical involvement. In 20 to 25 per cent of patients, the disease does not fit any of the specific patterns suggested by the diagnoses mentioned above. ALS, the most common of the group, involves selective neuronal degenerative loss in the frontal cortex (Betz's cells of the motor cortex), the motor cranial nerve nuclei (except for the oculomotor nuclei), and anterior horn cells in the ventral gray matter of the spinal cord. In addition, there is degeneration of the corticospinal tracts. Affected nerve cells disappear and are replaced by scar tissue (gliosis). No vascular or inflammatory abnormalities and no lipofuscin accumulation are present. There is ongoing end plate modification in ALS, with collateral reinnervation typical of progressive neuropathies and multiple innervations on the same muscle fiber demonstrating a myopathic pattern.[118, 119] Neurofibrillary changes (tangles)[127] have been found in the cerebrum and the brain stem, especially in patients with ALS in Guam. Such tangles are rare in the classic sporadic type of ALS.

The etiology is not known, but suggested factors have included slow virus infection of motor neurons; toxicity (heavy metals, such as lead [Pb] or mercury [Hg]); an autoimmune mechanism,[117] with antibody destruction of the motor neurons; a biochemical abnormality; a genetic defect; an endocrine disturbance; and abiotrophy (premature aging).[120] Serum from patients with ALS has been demonstrated to be toxic to anterior horn cells of the mouse[134] and to suppress terminal sprouting in the botulin-treated mouse. Botulinum toxin induces axonal sprouting in the mouse that is hypothesized to be due to the release of a growth factor. Serum of patients with ALS is hypothesized to contain an antibody that inhibits release of this growth factor. Additional evidence of autoimmune pathogenesis is provided by the high percentage of ALS patients who have an increase in serum IgA and IgE levels and who have Ia antigen on T lymphocytes. Studies of the Chamorro population of Guam, where death rates were 50 to 100 times that of the continental United States, have strongly implicated the toxic seed of the false sago palm *(Cycas circinalis)* in the etiology of ALS. A nonprotein amino acid, β-N-methylamino-L-alanine (L-BMAA) has been isolated from this seed. When L-BMAA is administered orally to macaques, a disease resembling ALS and PD is produced.[132]

The majority of the cases of ALS are sporadic. In 5 to 10 per cent of patients, the disease may be familial, with autosomal recessive inheritance. Worldwide incidence is variable, approximating 0.75 cases per 100,000 persons per year. In Rochester, Minnesota, the incidence ranged between 1 and 1.76 cases per 100,000 persons per year.[124] Temporal variation has also been noted, with a 41 per cent increase in incidence in Israel from 1959 to 1974.[125] Prevalence is about 4 to 6 cases per 100,000 persons. The average age of onset is 57 years, with a 50 per cent mortality rate within three years of onset. Eighty per cent of patients die within five years, and 90 per cent within 10 years.[128] The duration of the illness is less in patients with bulbar involvement. The death rate is approximately 1 in 100,000 persons per year, with an age peak at about 70 years. The age of onset seems to be earlier in hereditary than in sporadic ALS. The male to female ratio varies from 1.5:1 to 2:1 in different studies, whereas the white to nonwhite ratio is approximately 1.7:1.

Atrophy, weakness, fasciculations, and paralysis are characteristic symptoms of lower motor neuron involvement. Atrophy is most often apparent in the hand, either unilaterally or bilaterally. When upper motor neuron involvement is dominant, cramps, muscle pain, increased tone, clonus, and spasticity are present. Weakness in the lower extremities usually involves the dorsiflexors before the plantar flexors and results in footdrop. When intercostal muscles weaken, respiration is impaired and secretions may accumulate in the lungs, with fatal outcome. Speech involvement (dysarthria) usually appears earlier than swallowing difficulty. Bulbar muscle involvement leads to difficulties in swallowing (pharyngeal weakness), chewing, and coughing. Dementia may occur in ALS.[133] Cortical cell loss associated with dementia is mild to moderate in degree. Emotional lability—a pseudobulbar symptom—is frequent, involving 43 per cent of 272 ALS patients in one study. Defects in ocular movement are often detected on electro-oculography and are probably supranuclear in origin. Although clinical sensory deficits are absent, multimodality evoked potential studies have demonstrated dysfunction in sensory systems, with somatosensory evoked potentials abnormal in 59 per cent of patients, brain stem auditory evoked potentials abnormal in 12 per cent, and minor abnormalities in visual evoked potentials in 12 per cent.[126]

JEROME W. GERSTEN

The diagnosis of ALS is essentially a clinical one, but electromyographic studies may be of assistance.[121] These studies show fibrillations, positive waves, and fasciculations, with normal nerve conduction velocity. Recruitment is impaired, with large, polyphasic motor unit action potentials of longer duration. Reinnervation by collateral sprouting may result in larger than normal motor units. Abnormalities of muscle innervation have been reported. There may be decremental response to repetitive nerve stimulation at a rate of 2 to 3 per sec, indicating that there is some defect in neuromuscular transmission. Abnormalities of evoked potentials may be present.

Treatment of the primary problem is not yet possible. Guanidine,[131] neostigmine, and pyridostigmine have been used to increase strength, with some benefit. Amitriptyline or imipramine (50 to 75 mg at bedtime [hs]) may be very helpful in the control of emotional lability. Amitriptyline and trihexyphenidyl may assist in controlling excessive salivation. When spasticity is severe enough to impair function, baclofen should be prescribed. Injection of thyrotropin-releasing hormone has been reported to increase motor function. This process requires further study.

From the earliest phase of the disease, and for as long as possible, attempts must be made to keep range of motion normal and to avoid contracture.[129, 131] Initially, this is achieved by active exercises, assisted when necessary. Later, as the disease progresses, passive exercises must be used. Exercises to maintain or increase strength should be directed toward all muscles needed to maintain the patient's greatest level of function. Involved muscles should be approached cautiously, fatigue should be avoided,[129] and exercise periods should be short. Swimming and bicycling are appropriate at this point. It is possible that excessive exercise of involved muscles may increase weakness. There are some who deny this point and have patients exercise more vigorously.

As weakness progresses and functional impairment ensues, appropriate assistive devices may enable the patient to perform adequately in the home or community for a longer period. These include the short or long opponens hand splint, the foot-ankle orthosis for footdrop, and the soft cervical collar[131] to prevent undue neck flexion. Surgery may be indicated to increase function.[130] The patient must be taught techniques to simplify work and thus conserve energy.[123] Exercise periods may have to be shortened and repeated several times each day. Range-of-motion exercises may require a more aggressive approach, including heat (ultrasound) and prolonged gentle stretching. As weakness progresses and ambulation becomes more difficult, a cane (stick or quad) may prolong the period of erect posture. Devices may assist in rising from a chair, and a wheelchair eventually will be needed. Neck stability may be maintained by a more rigid collar or brace.

Excessive salivation may be a problem. Transtympanic neurectomy has been suggested as a solution. Medication to decrease secretions has been referred to earlier. Suction devices may be necessary to prevent aspiration and pneumonia. Involvement of bulbar musculature may result in swallowing difficulty. This can be managed by medication (neostigmine), by preparing foods that can be swallowed more easily (food processed in a blender), by cricopharyngeal myotomy, or by esophagostomy (more rarely by gastrostomy). When respiratory function becomes severely impaired, with maximal breathing capacity less than 30 l per min, the use of assistive respiratory devices (intermittent positive-pressure breathing, chest respirator) or tracheostomy must be considered.

The importance of the roles of the nurse, the occupational therapist, the physical therapist, the physician, and the speech pathologist in managing the problems noted above is apparent. Psychosocial support is equally important, considering the slow, inexorable progress of symptoms that often last over a very long period of time. The usual sparing of intellectual capacities provides a unique challenge.

References

General

1. Adams, R. D., and Victor, M.: Principles of Neurology, 2nd Ed. New York, McGraw-Hill Book Co., 1981, pp. 815–826.
2. Merritt, H. H.: A Textbook of Neurology, 6th Ed. Philadelphia, Lea and Febiger, 1979.

Dementias

3. Albert, M., Naeser, M. A., Levine, H. L., and Garvey, A. J.: Ventricular size in patients with presenile dementia of the Alzheimer's type. Arch. Neurol., 41:1258–1263, 1984.
4. Bahmanyar, S., Higgins, G. A., Goldgaber, D., Lewis, D. A., Morrison, J. H., Wilson, M. C., Shankar, S. K., and Gajdusek, D. C.: Localization

of amyloid β protein messenger RNA in brains from patients with Alzheimer's disease. Science, 237:77–80, 1987.

5. Beal, M. F., Mazurek, M. F., Tran, V. T., Chattha, G., Bird, E. D., and Martin, J. B.: Reduced numbers of somatostatin receptors in the cerebral cortex in Alzheimer's disease. Science, 229:289–291, 1985.

6. Bockman, J. M., Kingsbury, D. T., McKinley, M. P., Bendheim, P. E., and Prusiner, S. B.: Creutzfeldt-Jakob disease prion proteins in human brains. N. Engl. J. Med., 312:73–78, 1985.

7. Brody, E. M., Kleban, M. H., Moss, M. S., and Kleban, F.: Predictors of falls among institutionalized women with Alzheimer's disease. J. Am. Geriatr. Soc., 32:877–882, 1984.

8. Bruno, G., Mohr, E., Gillespie, M., Fedio, P., and Chase, T. N.: Muscarinic agonist therapy of Alzheimer's disease. A clinical trial of RS-86. Arch. Neurol., 43:659–661, 1986.

9. Buchner, D. M., and Larson, E. B.: Falls and fractures in patients with Alzheimer-type dementia. J.A.M.A., 257:1492–1495, 1987.

10. Council of Scientific Affairs: Dementia. J.A.M.A., 256:2234–2238, 1986.

11. Colerick, E. J., and George, L. K.: Predictors of institutionalization among caregivers of patients with Alzheimer's disease. J. Am. Geriatr. Soc., 34:493–498, 1986.

12. Coyle, J. T., Price, D. L., and Delong, M. R.: Alzheimer's disease: A disorder of cortical cholinergic innervation. Science, 219:1184–1190, 1983.

13. Cummings, J. L., and Benson, D. F.: Dementia of the Alzheimer type. An inventory of diagnostic clinical features. J. Am. Geriatr. Soc., 34:12–19, 1986.

14. Davis, B. M., Mohs, R. C., Greenwald, B. S., Mathe, A. A., Johns, C. A., Horvath, T. B., and Davis, K. L.: Clinical studies of the cholinergic deficit in Alzheimer's disease. I. Neurochemical and neuroendocrine studies. J. Am. Geriatr. Soc., 33:741–748, 1985.

15. Francis, P. T., Palmer, A. M., Sims, N. R., Bowen, D. M., Davison, A. N., Esiri, M. M., Neary, D., Snowden, J. S., and Wilcox, G. K.: Neurochemical studies of early onset Alzheimer's disease. Possible influence on treatment. N. Engl. J. Med., 313:7–11, 1985.

16. Freedman, M., and Oscar-Berman, M.: Tactile discrimination learning deficits in Alzheimer's and Parkinson's diseases. Arch. Neurol., 44:394–398, 1987.

17. Freemon, F. R.: Evaluation of patients with progressive intellectual deterioration. Arch. Neurol., 33:658–659, 1976.

18. Gershon, S., and Herman, S. P.: The differential diagnosis of dementia. J. Am. Geriatr. Soc., 30:558–566, 1982.

19. Glosser, G., Wexler, D., and Balmelli, M.: Physicians' and families' perspectives on the medical management of dementia. J. Am. Geriatr. Soc., 6:383–391, 1985.

20. Greenamyre, J. T., Penney, J. B., Young, A. B., D'Amato, C. J., Hicks, S. P., and Shoulson, I.: Alterations in L-glutamate binding in Alzheimer's and Huntington's diseases. Science, 227:1496–1499, 1987.

21. Greenwald, B., Mohs, R. C., and Davis, K. L.: Neurotransmitter deficits in Alzheimer's disease. Criteria for significance. J. Am. Geriatr. Soc., 31:310–316, 1983.

22. Hachinski, V. C., Iliff, L. D., Zilhka, E., Du Boulay, G. H., McAllister, V. L., Marshall, J., Russell, R. W., and Symon, L.: Cerebral blood flow in dementia. Arch. Neurol., 32:632–637, 1975.

23. Haxby, J. V., Grady, C. L., Duara, R., Schlageter, N., Berg, G., and Rapoport, S. I.: Neocortical metabolic abnormalities precede nonmemory cognitive defects in early Alzheimer's-type dementia. Arch. Neurol., 43:882–885, 1986.

24. Heston, L. L.: Alzheimer's disease, trisomy 21, and myeloproliferative disorders: Associations suggesting a genetic diathesis. Science, 196:322–323, 1977.

25. Hyman, B. T., Van Hyman, G. W., Damasio, A. R., and Barnes, C. L.: Alzheimer's disease. Cell-specific pathology isolates the hippocampal formation. Science, 225:1168–1170, 1984.

26. Johnson, K. A., Mueller, S. T., Walshe, T. M., English, R. J., and Holman, L.: Cerebral perfusion imaging in Alzheimer's disease. Arch. Neurol., 44:165–168, 1987.

27. Katzman, R.: The prevalence and malignancy of Alzheimer disease—a major killer. Arch. Neurol., 33:217–218, 1976.

28. Katzman, R.: Alzheimer's disease. N. Engl. J. Med., 314:964–973, 1986.

29. Katzman, R.: Alzheimer's disease: Advances and opportunities. J. Am. Geriatr. Soc., 35:69–73, 1987.

30. Khachaturian, Z. S.: Diagnosis of Alzheimer's disease. Arch. Neurol., 42:1097–1105, 1985.

31. Kitt, C. A., Price, D. L., Struble, R. G., Cork, L. C., Wainer, B. H., Becher, M. W., and Mobley, W. C.: Evidence for Cholinergic neurites in senile plaques. Science, 226:1443–1445, 1984.

32. Klein, L. E., Roca, R. P., McArthur, J., Vogelsang, G., Klein, G. B., Kirby, S. M., and Folstein, M.: Diagnosing dementia. Univariate and multivariate analyses of the mental status examination. J. Am. Geriatr. Soc., 33:483–488, 1985.

33. Kokmen, E.: Dementia—Alzheimer type. Mayo Clin. Proc., 59:35–42, 1984.

34. van Loveren-Huyben, C. M. S., Engelaar, H. F., Hermans, M. B., van der Bom, J. A., Leering, C., and Munnichs, J. M.: Double-blind clinical and psychological study of ergoloid mesylates (Hydergine) in subjects with senile mental deterioration. J. Am. Geriatr. Soc., 32:584–588, 1984.

35. Manuelidis, E. E., Gorgacz, E. J., and Manuelidis,

L.: Viremia in experimental Creutzfeldt-Jakob disease. Science, 200:1069–1071, 1978.

36. Mohs, R. C.: Clinical studies of the cholinergic deficit in Alzheimer's disease. II. Psychopharmacologic studies. J. Am. Geriatr. Soc., 33:749–757, 1985.

37. Mori, H., Kondo, J., and Ihara, Y.: Ubiquitin is a component of paired helical filaments in Alzheimer's disease. Science, 235:1641–1644, 1987.

38. Ober, B. A., Koss, E., Friedland, R. P., and Delis, D. C.: Processes of verbal memory failure in Alzheimer-type dementia. Brain Cogn., 4:90–103, 1985.

39. Risse, S. C., and Barnes, R.: Pharmacologic treatment of agitation associated with dementia. J. Am. Geriatr. Soc., 34:368–376, 1986.

40. Scott, J. P., Roberto, K. A., and Hutton, J. T.: Families of Alzheimer victims. Family support to the caregivers. J. Am. Geriatr. Soc., 34:348–354, 1986.

41. Tachibana, H., Meyer, J. S., Kitagawa, Y., Rogers, R. I., Okayasu, H., and Mortel, K. F.: Effects of aging on cerebral blood flow in dementia. J. Am. Geriatr. Soc., 32:114–120, 1984.

42. Thienhaus, O. J., Hartford, J. T., Skelly, M. F., and Bosmann, H. B.: Biological markers in Alzheimer's disease. J. Am. Geriatr. Soc., 33:715–726, 1985.

43. Thienhaus, O. J., Wheeler, B. G., Simon, S., Zemlan, F. P., and Hartford, J. T.: A controlled double-blind study of high-dose dihydroergotoxine mesylate (Hydergine) in mild dementia. J. Am. Geriatr. Soc., 35:219–223, 1987.

44. Tierney, M. C., Snow, W. G., Reid, D. W., Zorzitto, M. L., and Fisher, R. H.: Psychometric differentiation of dementia. Arch. Neurol., 44:720–722, 1987.

45. Winograd, C. H., and Jarvik, L. F.: Physician management of the demented patient. J. Am. Geriatr. Soc., 34:295–308, 1986.

46. Wolozin, B. L., Pruchnicki, A., Dickson, D. W., and Davies, P.: A neuronal antigen in the brains of Alzheimer patients. Science, 232:648–650, 1986.

Parkinson's Disease

47. Bauer, R. B., Stevens, C., Reveno, W. S., and Rosenbaum, H.: L-Dopa treatment of Parkinson's disease: A ten-year follow-up study. J. Am. Geriatr. Soc., 30:322–325, 1982.

48. Bianchine, J. R., Shaw, G. M., Greenwald, J. E., and Dandalides, S. M.: Clinical aspects of dopamine agonists and antagonists. Fed. Proc., 37:2434–2439, 1978.

49. Bloxham, C. A., Mindel, T. A., and Firth, C. D.: Initiation and execution of predictable and unpredictable movements in Parkinson's disease. Brain, 107:371–384, 1984.

50. Boller, F., Passafiume, D., Keefe, N., Rogers, K., Morrow, L., and Kim, Y.: Visual impairment in Parkinson's disease. Role of perceptual and motor factors. Arch. Neurol., 41:485–490, 1984.

51. Boshes, L. D., and Doshay, L. J.: Practical management of Parkinson's disease. Geriatrics, 19:644–653, 1964.

52. Burns, R. S., LeWitt, P. A., Ebert, M. H., Pakkenberg, H., and Kopin, I. J.: The clinical syndrome of striatal dopamine deficiency. Parkinsonism induced by 1-methyl-4-phenyl-1,2,3,6-tetrahydropyridine (MPTP). N. Engl. J. Med., 312:1418–1421, 1985.

53. Cherington, M.: Parkinson's disease, L-dopa, and the H-reflex. In Walton, J. N., Canal, N., and Scarlato, G. (Eds.): Muscle Diseases. Proceedings of an International Congress. Milan, May 19–21, 1969. Amsterdam, Excerpta Medica, 1970, pp. 197–200.

54. Connor, J. D.: Caudate unit responses to nigral stimuli: Evidence for a possible nigro-neostriatal pathway. Science, 160:899–900, 1968.

55. Critchley, E. M. R.: Speech disorders in parkinsonism. A review. J. Neurol. Neurosurg. Psychiatry, 44:751–758, 1981.

56. Damasio, A. R., Damasio, H., Rizzo, M., Varney, N., and Gersh, F.: Aphasia with nonhemorrhagic lesions in the basal ganglia and internal capsule. Arch. Neurol., 39:15–20, 1982.

57. Dunne, J. W., Hankey, G. J., and Edis, R. E.: Parkinsonism: Upturned walking stick as an aid to locomotion. Arch. Phys. Med. Rehabil., 68:380–381, 1987.

58. Freed, C. R., and Yamamoto, B. K.: Regional brain dopamine metabolism: A marker for the speed, direction, and posture of moving animals. Science, 229:62–65, 1985.

59. Fujita, S., and Cooper, I. S.: Effects of L-dopa on the H-reflex in parkinsonism. J. Am. Geriatr. Soc., 19:289–295, 1971.

60. Gersten, J. W., Marshall, C., Dillon, T., Schneck, S., Orr, W., and Nelson, C.: External work of walking and functional capacity in parkinsonian patients treated with L-dopa. Arch. Phys. Med. Rehabil., 53:547–554, 1972.

61. Goldman, J. E., Yen, S. H., Chiu, F. C., and Peress, N. S.: Lewy bodies of Parkinson's disease contain neurofilament antigens. Science, 221:1082–1084, 1983.

62. Hardie, R. J., Lees, A. J., and Stern, G. M.: On-off fluctuations in Parkinson's disease. A clinical and neuropharmacological study. Brain, 107:487–506, 1984.

63. Heikkila, R. E., Hess, A., and Duvoisin, R. C.: Dopaminergic neurotoxicity of 1-methyl-4-phenyl-1,2,5,6-tetrahydropyridine in mice. Science, 224:1451–1453, 1984.

64. Herbison, G. J.: H-reflex in patients with parkinsonism: Effect of levodopa. Arch. Phys. Med. Rehabil., 54:291–295, 1973.

65. Hoehn, M. M.: Age distribution of patients with parkinsonism. J. Am. Geriatr. Soc., 24(2):79–85, 1976.

66. Hoehn, M. M., Crowley, T. J., and Rutledge, C. O.: Dopamine correlates of neurological and psychological status in untreated parkinsonism. J. Neurol. Neurosurg. Psychiatry, 39:941–951, 1976.

67. Hoehn, M. M.: Bromocriptine and its use in parkinsonism. J. Am. Geriatr. Soc., 29:251–258, 1981.

68. Hull, J. T.: The prevalence and incidence of Parkinson's disease. Geriatrics, 25:128–133, 1970.

69. Kelly, P. J., Ahlskog, J. E., Goerss, S. J., Daube, J. R., Duffy, J. R., and Kall, B. A.: Computer-assisted stereotactic ventralis lateralis thalamotomy with microelectrode recording control in patients with Parkinson's disease. Mayo Clin. Proc., 62:655–664, 1987.

70. Kish, S. J., Shannak, K. S., Rajput, A. H., Gilbert, J. J., and Hornykiewicz, O.: Cerebellar norepinephrine in patients with Parkinson's disease and control subjects. Arch. Neurol., 41:612–614, 1984.

71. Koller, W. C.: Pharmacologic treatment of parkinsonian tremor. Arch. Neurol., 43:126–127, 1986.

72. Kondo, K., Kurland, L. T., and Schull, W. J.: Parkinson's disease. Genetic analysis and evidence of a multifactorial etiology. Mayo Clin. Proc., 48:465–475, 1973.

73. Landau, W. M., Struppler, A., and Mehls, O.: A comparative electromyographic study of the reactions to passive movement in parkinsonism and in normal subjects. Neurology, 16:34–48, 1966.

74. Langston, J. W., Irwin, I., Langston, E. B., and Forno, L. S.: Pargyline prevents MPTP-induced parkinsonism in primates. Science, 225:1480–1482, 1984.

75. Lawton, N. F., and MacDermot, J.: Abnormal regulation of prolactin release in idiopathic Parkinson's disease. J. Neurol. Neurosurg. Psychiatry, 43:1012–1015, 1980.

76. Lees, A. J., Haddad, S., Shaw, K. M., Kohout, L. J., and Stern, G. M.: Bromocriptine in parkinsonism. Arch. Neurol., 35:503–505, 1978.

77. Lees, A. J., and Stern, G. M.: Sustained bromocriptine therapy in previously untreated patients with Parkinson's disease. J. Neurol. Neurosurg. Psychiatry, 44:1020–1023, 1981.

78. Loranger, A. W., Goodell, H., McDowell, F. H., Lee, J. E., and Sweet, R. D.: Intellectual impairment in Parkinson's syndrome. Brain, 95:405–412, 1972.

79. McLeod, J. G., and Walsh, J. C.: H-reflex studies in patients with Parkinson's disease. J. Neurol. Neurosurg. Psychiatry, 35:77–80, 1972.

80. Madrazo, I., et al.: Open microsurgical autograft of adrenal medulla to the right caudate nucleus in two patients with intractable Parkinson's disease. N. Engl. J. Med., 316:831–834, 1987.

81. Mann, D. M. A., and Yates, P. O.: Pathogenesis of Parkinson's disease. Arch. Neurol., 39:545–549, 1982.

82. Markham, C. H., and Diamond, S. G.: Modification of Parkinson's disease by long-term levodopa treatment. Arch. Neurol., 43:405–407, 1986.

83. Mayeux, R., Stern, Y., Mulvey, K., and Cote, L.: Reappraisal of temporary levodopa withdrawal ("drug holiday") in Parkinson's disease. N. Engl. J. Med., 313:724–728, 1985.

84. Melamed, E., et al.: Aromatic L-amino acid decarboxylase in rat corpus striatum: Implications for action of L-dopa in parkinsonism. Neurology, 31:651–655, 1981.

85. Melamed, E.: Initiation of levodopa therapy in parkinsonian patients should be delayed until the advanced stages of the disease. Arch. Neurol., 43:402–405, 1986.

86. Meyer, C. H. A.: Akinesia in parkinsonism. Relation between spontaneous movement (other than tremor) and voluntary movements made on command. J. Neurol. Neurosurg. Psychiatry, 45:582–585, 1982.

87. Naeser, M. A., Alexander, M. P., Helm-Estabrooks, N., Levine, H. L., Laughlin, S. A., and Geschwind, N.: Aphasia with predominantly subcortical lesion sites. Description of three capsular/putaminal aphasia syndromes. Arch. Neurol., 39:2–14, 1982.

88. Nutt, J. G., Woodward, W. R., Hammerstad, J. P., Carter, J. H., and Anderson, J. L.: The "on-off" phenomenon in Parkinson's disease. Relation to levodopa absorption and transport. N. Engl. J. Med., 310:483–488, 1984.

89. Pfeiffer, R. F., Wilken, K., Glaeske, C., and Lorenzo, A. S.: Low-dose bromocriptine therapy in Parkinson's disease. Arch. Neurol., 42:586–588, 1985.

90. Poirier, J.: Pathophysiology and biochemical mechanisms involved in MPTP-induced parkinsonism. J. Am. Geriatr. Soc., 35:660–668, 1987.

91. Routh, L. C., Black, J. L., and Ahlskog, J. E.: Parkinson's disease complicated by anxiety. Mayo Clin. Proc., 62:733–735, 1987.

92. Teräväinen, H., and Calne, D. B.: Action tremor in Parkinson's disease. J. Neurol. Neurosurg. Psychiatry, 43:257–263, 1980.

93. Villardita, C., Smirni, P., and Zappala, G.: Visual neglect in Parkinson's disease. Arch. Neurol., 40:737–743, 1983.

94. Vincken, W. G., Gauthier, S. G., Dollfuss, R. E., Hanson, R. E., Darauay, C. M., and Cosio, M. G.: Involvement of upper airway muscles in extrapyramidal disorders. A cause of airflow limitation. N. Engl. J. Med., 311:438–442, 1984.

95. Weiner, W. J., and Klawans, H. L., Jr.: Lingual-facial-buccal movements in the elderly. I. Pathophysiology and treatment. J. Amer. Geriatr. Soc., 21:314–320, 1973.

96. Weiner, W. J., Koller, W. C., Perlik, S., Nausieda, P. A., and Klawans, H. L.: Drug holiday and management of Parkinson's disease. Neurology, 30:1257–1261, 1980.

97. Zigmond, M. J., Acheson, A. L., Stachowiak, M. K., and Strickerm, E. M.: Neurochemical compensation after nigrostriatal bundle injury in an animal model of preclinical parkinsonism. Arch. Neurol., 41:856–861, 1984.

Huntington's Disease

98. Bird, S. J.: Presymptomatic testing for Huntington's disease. J.A.M.A., 253:3286–3291, 1985.
99. Butters, N. D. S., Montgomery, K., and Tarlow, S.: Comparison of the neuropsychological deficits associated with early and advanced Huntington's disease. Arch. Neurol., 35:585–589, 1978.
100. Chase, T. N., Watanabe, A. M., Brodie, K. H., and Donnelly, E. F.: Huntington's chorea. Arch. Neurol., 26:282–284, 1972.
101. Ehle, A. L., Stewart, R. M., Lellelid, N. A., and Leventhal, N. A.: Evoked potentials in Huntington's disease. A comparative and longitudinal study. Arch. Neurol., 41:379–382, 1984.
102. Goetz, C., and Weiner, W. J.: Huntington's disease: Current concepts of therapy. J. Am. Geriatr. Soc., 27:23–26, 1979.
103. Graveland, G. A., Williams, R. S., and DiFiglia, M.: Evidence for degenerative and regenerative changes in neostriatal spiny neurons in Huntington's disease. Science, 227:770–773, 1985.
104. Johnson, E. W., Radecki, P. L., and Paulson, G. W.: Huntington disease: Early identification by H-reflex testing. Arch. Phys. Med. Rehabil., 58:162–166, 1977.
105. Josiassen, R. C., Curry, L. M., and Mancall, E. L.: Development of neuropsychological deficits in Huntington's disease. Arch. Neurol., 40:791–796, 1983.
106. Rosenberg, C., Nudleman, K., and Starr, A.: Cognitive evoked potentials (P 300) in early Huntington's disease. Arch. Neurol., 42:984–987, 1985.
107. Tanahashi, N., Meyer, J. S., Ishikawa, Y., Kandula, P., Mortel, K. F., Rogers, R. L., Gandhi, S., and Walker, M.: Cerebral blood flow and cognitive testing correlate in Huntington's disease. Arch. Neurol., 42:1169–1175, 1985.

Olivopontocerebellar Degeneration

108. Bennett, R. H., Ludvigson, P., DeLeon, G., and Berry, G.: Large-fiber sensory neuronopathy in autosomal dominant spinocerebellar degeneration. Arch. Neurol., 41:175–178, 1984.
109. Hammond, E. J., and Wilder, B. J.: Evoked potentials in olivopontocerebellar atrophy. Arch. Neurol., 40:366–369, 1983.
110. Harding, A. E.: The clinical features and classification of the late onset autosomal dominant cerebellar ataxias. A study of 11 families, including descendants of the 'Drew Family of Walworth.' Brain, 105:1–28, 1982.
111. Landis, D. M. D., Rosenberg, R. N., Landis, S. C., Schut, L., and Nyhan, W. L.: Olivopontocerebellar degeneration. Arch. Neurol., 31:295–307, 1974.

Friedreich's Ataxia

112. Caruso, G., Santoro, L., Perretti, A., Massini, R., Pelosi, L., Crisci, C., Ragno, M., Capanella, G., and Filla, A.: Friedreich's ataxia: Electrophysiologic and histologic findings in patients and relatives. Muscle Nerve, 10:503–515, 1987.
113. Fehrenbach, R. A., Wallesch, C. W., and Claus, D.: Neuropsychologic findings in Friedreich's ataxia. Arch. Neurol., 41:306–308, 1984.
114. Furman, J. M., Perlman, S., and Baloh, R. W.: Eye movements in Friedreich's ataxia. Arch. Neurol., 40:343–346, 1983.
115. Jamal, G. A., Hansen, S., Weir, A. I., and Ballantyne, J. P.: The neurophysiologic investigation of small fiber neuropathies. Muscle Nerve, 10:537–545, 1987.
116. Livingstone, I. R., Mastaglia, F. L., Edis, R., and Howe, J. W.: Visual involvement in Friedreich's ataxia and hereditary spastic ataxia. A clinical and visual evoked response study. Arch. Neurol., 38:75–79, 1981.

Amyotrophic Lateral Sclerosis

117. Appel, S. H., Stockton-Appel, V., Stewart, S., and Kerman, R. H.: Amyotrophic lateral sclerosis. Associated clinical disorders and immunological evaluations. Arch. Neurol., 43:234–238, 1986.
118. Bjornskov, E. K., Dekker, N. P., Norris, F. H., and Stuart, M. E.: End-plate morphology in amyotrophic lateral sclerosis. Arch. Neurol., 32:711–712, 1975.
119. Bjornskov, E. K., Norris, F. H., Jr., and Mower-Kuby, J.: Quantitative axon terminal and end-plate morphology in amyotrophic lateral sclerosis. Arch. Neurol., 41:527–530, 1984.
120. Bradley, W. G.: Recent views on amyotrophic lateral sclerosis with emphasis on electrophysiological studies. Muscle Nerve, 10:490–502, 1987.
121. Brown, W. F., and Jaatoul, N.: Amyotrophic lateral sclerosis: Electrophysiologic study (number of motor units and rate of decay of motor units). Arch. Neurol., 30:242–248, 1974.
122. Gurney, M. E., Belton, A. C., Cashman, N., and Antel, J. P.: Inhibition of terminal axonal sprouting by serum from patients with amyotrophic lateral sclerosis. N. Engl. J. Med., 311:933–939, 1984.
123. Janiszewski, D. W., Caroscio, J. T., and Wisham, L. H.: Amyotrophic lateral sclerosis: A compre-

hensive rehabilitation approach. Arch. Phys. Med. Rehabil., 64:304–307, 1983.

124. Juergens, S. M., Kurland, L. T., Okazaki, H., and Mulder, D. W.: ALS in Rochester, Minnesota, 1925–1977. Neurology, 30:463–470, 1980.

125. Kahana, E., and Zilber, N.: Changes in the incidence of amyotrophic lateral sclerosis in Israel. Arch. Neurol., 41:157–160, 1984.

126. Matheson, J. K., Harrington, H. J., and Hallett, M.: Abnormalities of multimodality evoked potentials in amyotrophic lateral sclerosis. Arch. Neurol., 43:338–340, 1986.

127. Meyers, K. R., Dorencamp, D. G., and Suzuki, K.: Amyotrophic lateral sclerosis with diffuse neurofibrillary changes. Arch. Neurol., 30:84–89, 1974.

128. Mulder, D. W., and Howard, F. M., Jr.: Patient resistance and prognosis in amyotrophic lateral sclerosis. Mayo Clin. Proc., 51:537–541, 1976.

129. Sinaki, M., and Mulder, D. W.: Rehabilitation techniques for patients with amyotrophic lateral sclerosis. Mayo Clin. Proc., 53:173–178, 1978.

130. Sinaki, M., Wood, M. B., and Mulder, D. W.: Rehabilitative operation for motor neuron disease: Tendon transfer for segmental muscular atrophy of the upper extremities. Mayo Clin. Proc., 59:338–342, 1984.

131. Smith, R. A., and Norris, F. H., Jr.: Symptomatic care of patients with amyotrophic lateral sclerosis. J.A.M.A., 234:715–717, 1975.

132. Spencer, P. S., Nunn, P. B., Hugon, J., Ludolph, A. C., Ross, S. M., Roy, D. N., and Robertson, R. C.: Guam amyotrophic lateral sclerosis-parkinsonian-dementia linked to a plant excitant neurotoxin. Science, 237:517–522, 1987.

133. Wikstrom, J., Paetau, A., Palo, J., Sulkava, R., and Haltia, M.: Classic amyotrophic lateral sclerosis with dementia. Arch. Neurol., 39:681–683, 1982.

134. Wolfgram, F., and Myers, L.: Amyotrophic lateral sclerosis: Effect of serum on anterior horn cells in tissue culture. Science, 179:579–580, 1973.

Spine: Disorders and Deformities

RENE CAILLIET

Spine disorders and deformities causing pain and disability have many varying etiologies, but most have a common denominator of pain and impairment. The diagnosis, as in all musculoskeletal problems, demands knowledge of normal functional anatomy, knowledge of tissue sites capable of causing pain or dysfunction, and skill in a meaningful examination to ascertain the deviation from normal. Confirmatory tests and their interpretation must specifically relate to the clinical findings. Only then can a specific diagnosis result and meaningful treatment ensue.

The spine is a flexible rod composed of superincumbent functional units supported in equilibrium upon the sacral base. The upright position, held in a balanced equilibrium with minimal muscular effort, is possibly only because the line of the center of gravity falls through the major weight-bearing joints. These are through the first thoracic, twelfth thoracic, and fifth lumbar vertebrae, in front of the knees, and through the hip joints. In a locked knee stance, the center of gravity falls farther in front of all of these joints (Fig. 37–1).

The individual functional unit consists of two vertebral bodies separated by the intervertebral disk designed to bear weight; neural arches that surround and protect the neural tissues; posterior articulations that guide specific movements and prevent other movements; and bone processes that provide mechanical sites for attachment of the musculature (Figs. 37–2 and 37–3).

The functional unit is the basis of structure and function of the total spine. Pain and disability result from injury, inflammation, disease, and infection of elements of the functional unit.

The intervertebral disks have a collagen outer layer (annulus) enclosing a central gelatinous nucleus pulposus. The fibers attach and insert around the circumference of the vertebral end plates and intertwine to permit movement, maintain intradiskal pressure, and keep the vertebral bodies together against distracting forces. They also limit the extent of rotation of one vertebra upon its immediate subjacent vertebra.

The intervertebral disks are formed by an outer series of annular sheets that attach circumferentially from adjacent vertebral end plates in intersecting directions. The nucleus pulposus is located in the inner aspect.

The intrinsic pressure of the nucleus separates the vertebrae and maintains tension in the annular sheets. This forms the anterior weight-bearing portion of the functional unit.

The posterior joints (zygoapophyseal facets) are only slightly weight-bearing. Through their alignment, they permit flexion and extension but restrict lateral flexion and rotation within the unit (Fig. 37–4).

The vertebral column is the erect composite of superimposed functional units that are balanced on the center of gravity.

Erect stance is maintained by ligamentous support, with only occasional righting reflex contractions. The angle of the sacrum maintains the balance of the superincumbent cervical and lumbar lordotic curve and the thoracic kyphotic curve (Fig 37–5). The equality of leg length and horizontal

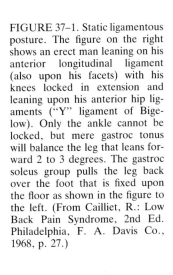

FIGURE 37–1. Static ligamentous posture. The figure on the right shows an erect man leaning on his anterior longitudinal ligament (also upon his facets) with his knees locked in extension and leaning upon his anterior hip ligaments ("Y" ligament of Bigelow). Only the ankle cannot be locked, but mere gastroc tonus will balance the leg that leans forward 2 to 3 degrees. The gastroc soleus group pulls the leg back over the foot that is fixed upon the floor as shown in the figure to the left. (From Cailliet, R.: Low Back Pain Syndrome, 2nd Ed. Philadelphia, F. A. Davis Co., 1968, p. 27.)

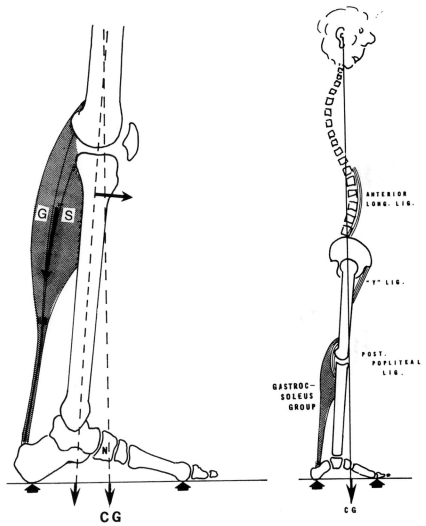

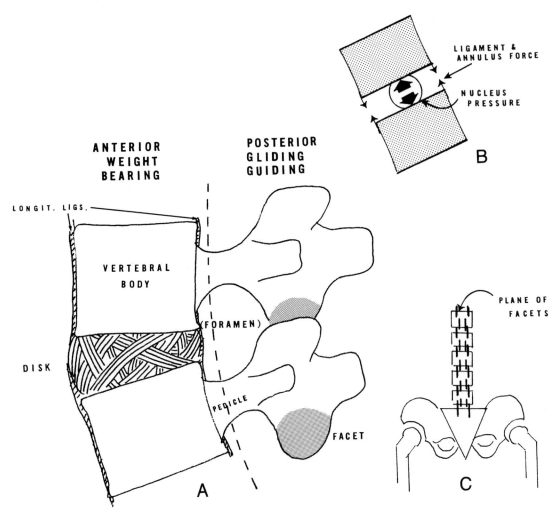

FIGURE 37–2. Functional unit. The anterior weight-bearing portion consists of two adjacent vertebrae separated by the disk. This portion is reinforced by longitudinal ligaments. The posterior portion contains the facets (articulations) that oppose each other in the sagittal plane. The foramina through which emerge the spinal nerves are depicted. The intradiskal pressure within the nucleus separates the vertebrae. This pressure is opposed by the annulus and the longitudinal ligaments. (From Cailliet, R.: Low Back Pain Syndrome, 3rd Ed. Philadelphia, F. A. Davis Co., 1981, p. 3.)

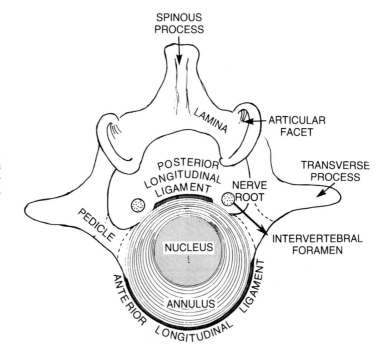

FIGURE 37–3. Functional unit: dorsal view. Lumbar vertebral functional unit viewed from above. (From Cailliet, R.: Low Back Pain Syndrome, 2nd Ed. Philadelphia, F. A. Davis Co., 1968, p. 6.)

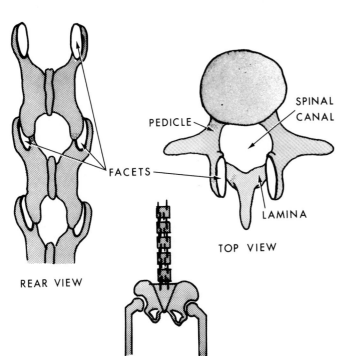

FIGURE 37–4. Plane of posterior articulations. The facets of the lumbar spine are in a sagittal plane, permitting forward flexion and extension but restricting lateral and rotatory motion. The facets glide upon each other but do not bear weight.

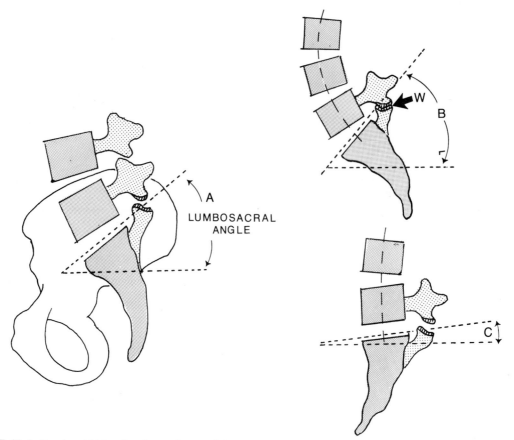

FIGURE 37–5. Facet weight-bearing due to increased lordosis. *A* reveals the normal lumbosacral angle in which the facet surfaces are not abnormally compressed. *B*, Because of the increased sacral angle, the facets become weight-bearing and pain may result. *C* shows the separation of the facets as the sacral angle decreases.

orientation of the pelvis determine the erectness of the vertebral column.

Low Back Pain

The type of low back pain most commonly confronting the physiatrist is of benign mechanical origin. Knowledge of normal functional anatomy and taking a careful history and performing an appropriate examination reveal the deviation that is causing the pain and impairment.

The possibility of organic diseases causing low back symptoms must always be considered. These include entities such as pagetoid changes, metastatic invasion, infection, or referred pain. Appropriate laboratory tests reveal these conditions.

The mechanical benign causes are divided into static (postural) and kinetic (faulty biomechanical) types. Of the static causes, the most prevalent is excessive lordosis (Fig. 37–6), in which there is

exorbitant facet weight-bearing and foraminal closure. Alternatively, prolonged daily flexed postures may cause posterior migration of the nucleus, resulting in low back pain and probably sciatic radiculopathy.

The definitive diagnosis depends on the history and a physical examination in which the pain is reproduced. X-ray studies may reveal disk degeneration and facet arthritis, but the diagnosis is clinical.

Treatment is directed toward the cause of pain. Either flexion or extension is prescribed on this basis. Body mechanics continue to be mandatory to improve posture and modify standing and working positions.

Spondylolisthesis and Spondylolysis

These are structural abnormalities of the spine that can give rise to low back pain.

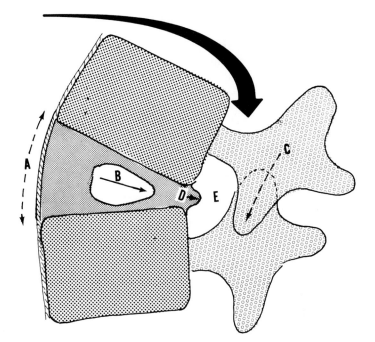

FIGURE 37–6. Static low back pain. Increased lumbar lordosis fully extends the anterior longitudinal ligament (A), compresses the nucleus (B), which then bulges posteriorly (D) and presses upon the sensitized posterior longitudinal ligament. The neural arch approximates (E), compressing facets (C) and narrowing intervertebral foramina (E). (From Cailliet, R.: Low Back Pain Syndrome, 3rd Ed. Philadelphia, F. A. Davis Co., 1981, p. 59.)

SPONDYLOLISTHESIS

Spondylolisthesis, which is a forward slippage of the superior on the immediately inferior vertebra (e.g., L4 upon L5 or L5 upon S1), has numerous etiologies. Normally, L5 is prevented from slipping forward on S1 by the annular fibers of the intervertebral disk, the mechanical block of the posterior facets, and an intact neural arch and pedicles. Defects of any of these structures can permit listhesis.

SPONDYLOLYSIS

A defect in the pars interarticularis, termed spondylolysis, may be evidenced in listhesis (Fig. 37–7). There is some controversy as to whether this is a congenital defect, a neonatal fracture, or a condition acquired in adult life. There is incomplete agreement as to whether the listhesis follows or causes the defect. The pars interarticularis may merely be elongated without a break in continuity.

When there is a deficiency of normal bone mechanics that prevent excessive shear, only the annular fibers of the disk prevent listhesis. In elderly and excessively lordotic patients, disk degeneration may permit listhesis, with secondary facet and isthmus changes.

The finding of excessive segmental lordosis and often a palpable bone prominence of the lumbosacral segment are suggestive of this diagnosis. Specific diagnosis is by anteroposterior, lateral,

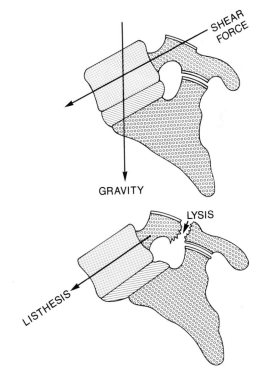

FIGURE 37–7. Mechanism of spondylolisthesis. Gravity compression combined with shear stress of the oblique vertebral angle does not cause forward sliding (listhesis) due to mechanical action of neural arch. With defect in the arch, facet, or pars interarticularis, the shear stress is unopposed, allowing listhesis. (From Cailliet, R.: Low Back Pain Syndrome, 3rd Ed. Philadelphia, F. A. Davis Co., 1981, p. 188.)

and bilateral oblique x-ray studies of the lumbosacral articulation.

Attenuation of the pars interarticularis with or without a break in continuity occurs early in life, at 14 years in girls and at 16 years in boys, and becomes symptomatic. There may be gradual slipping, but onset of pain may be sudden and violent. Neurological involvement, including hamstring spasm, occurs as a result of compression of the cauda equina.

The usual conservative management is reduction of excessive lordosis to decrease the sacral angle. This requires an exercise program, weight reduction, and, occasionally, bracing or corseting. The following exercises are recommended:

1. Instructions in pelvic tilting, in both the prone and the erect position, to decrease lordosis.

2. Low back stretching exercises.

3. Abdominal isometric strengthening exercises.

4. Posture and functional daily activities performed with decreased lordosis.

Severe progression of pain and neurological impairment are indications to consider for surgical intervention. Merely finding a pars interarticularis defect is not an indication for surgery, as many patients with defects found on x-ray study have no symptoms because their defect is held securely by fibrous binding. Other sources of low back pain in the presence of this condition must be considered.

Kinetic Low Back Pain

The spine moves in a specific integrated manner as dictated by the facet alignments, ligamentous limitations, and neuromuscular mechanisms. To permit pain-free movements, daily activities must not exceed these limitations. The normal spine articulates in the following coordinated manner:

1. The lumbar spine flexes and extends in a sagittal plane as directed by the plane of the facets. In forward flexion, the sacrospinal muscles actively elongate until full flexion has been reached, at which point the muscles cease to contract eccentrically, probably by inhibitory impulses arising from the vertebral ligaments. This has been termed the critical point (Fig. 37–8).

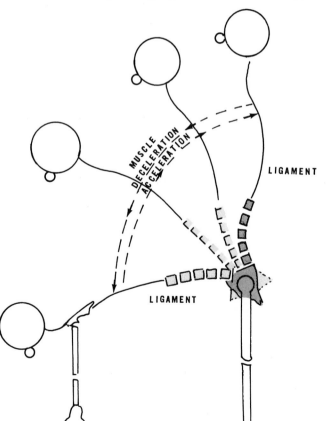

FIGURE 37–8. Muscular deceleration and acceleration of the forward flexing spine from the erect ligamentous support to the fully flexed ligamentous restriction. Muscle eccentric and concentric contraction permits forward flexion and re-extension. (From Cailliet, R.: Low Back Pain Syndrome, 4th Ed. Philadelphia, F. A. Davis Co., 1988, p. 46.)

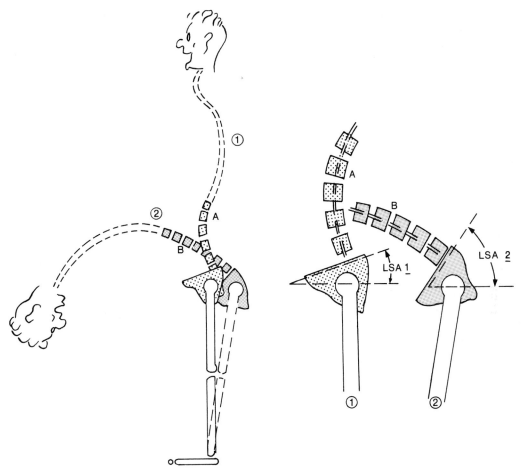

FIGURE 37–9. Lumbar pelvic rhythm. As the lumbar lordosis reverses, there is a simultaneous synchronous pelvic rotation as depicted in LSA1 to LSA2.

2. Forward flexion occurs to the point of reversing the lumbar lordosis; it is limited by the supraspinous ligaments posteriorly and the posterior fibers of the annulus fibrosus.

3. Pelvic rotation occurs about the hip joints to change the sacral angle.

4. The erector spinae muscles elongate eccentrically to gradually decelerate the forward flexion and smoothly contract concentrically to regain the erect lordotic posture.

5. Forward flexion and re-extension physiologically conform to lumbar-pelvic rhythm and must adhere to the direction dictated by the facet joints (Fig. 37–9).

Violation of the pattern of movement discussed earlier can result in low back pain, with or without nerve root entrapment, causing local and, ultimately, radicular pain.

As a result of their alignment, the lumbar spine facets prevent lateral and rotatory movement of the functional unit in the erect or hyperextended position, but in flexion the facets separate and thus place all the rotatory torque stress upon the annular fibers. The rotatory movement in the flexed posture is a major factor in disk herniation and degeneration.

SITES AND CAUSATION OF PAIN

Most anatomical structures of the functional units are capable of eliciting pain. Some tissues are more sensitive as nociceptive sites and can be postulated as the major sites of local or referred pain (Fig. 37–10).

In the functional unit, the following conclusions have been substantiated:

1. The posterior longitudinal ligament is innervated by the posterior recurrent meningeal nerve and has clinically been confirmed as a nociceptive site.[1]

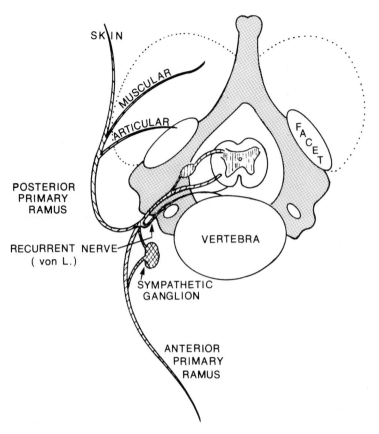

FIGURE 37–10. Innervation of the cervical and lumbar roots: The posterior primary ramus divides into skin, muscular, and articular branches; the anterior primary ramus, with a sympathetic innervation, proceeds to the dermatome and myotome areas. The recurrent nerve supplies the posterior longitudinal ligament and the dura.

2. The nucleus pulposus of the intervertebral disk normally is avascular and aneural except for possible pain ending in the extreme outer layer of the annulus.[2–4] Intradiskal injections of irritating substances have been found to cause low back pain[5] when there has been some herniation of the nucleus into the surrounding annulus.

MECHANISMS OF PAIN

Poor conditioning and faulty biomechanical action probably cause most kinetic low back pain. Weak abdominal muscles impose a great stress upon the disks and allow increased lordosis.[6, 7] Improving the strength of back muscles has not proved to be beneficial except in patients who perform excessively strenuous work and have become debilitated from their usual occupation by an intercurrent illness or injury.

Faulty bending, stooping, and lifting cause the vast majority of low back injuries. In the flexed position, the facets separate and place all the rotatory torque on the annular fibers when flexion is accompanied by rotation. These fibers have limited extensibility and will rupture, pull away

from the end plate, and ultimately permit the normally enclosed nucleus pulposus to escape[8] into the surrounding annulus. In re-extending from the flexed position, if re-extension of the lumbar lordosis occurs before the pelvis is derotated, the facets can lock or the annular fibers of the disk can become torn. Back pain with or without radiculitis can result (Fig. 37–11).

CLINICAL MANIFESTATIONS

A careful history elicits the exact manner in which pain was produced. Distraction of the patient by anxiety, depression, anger, and haste may cause faulty biomechanical function.

CLINICAL FINDINGS

When injury to the low back is caused by mechanical stresses, the findings generally are

1. Erector spinae spasm: this spasm causes the antalgic posture and limited flexion. The exact muscles that are involved are not clearly delineated.

2. Functional scoliosis: usually occurs away from

FIGURE 37–11. Proper and improper flexion re-extension. Upper figure depicts proper re-extension with simultaneous derotation of the pelvis and return of the lumbar lordosis. Bottom figure shows premature return of the lordosis before adequate derotation of the pelvis. Pain occurs from this forward cantilevered excessive lordosis. Faulty re-extension to the erect posture is further aggravated by rotating the lumbar spine, thus causing the facets to become asymmetrically aligned and the disk to be subjected to rotating torque forces. (From Cailliet, R.: Low Back Pain Syndrome, 3rd Ed. Philadelphia, F. A. Davis Co., 1981, p. 77.)

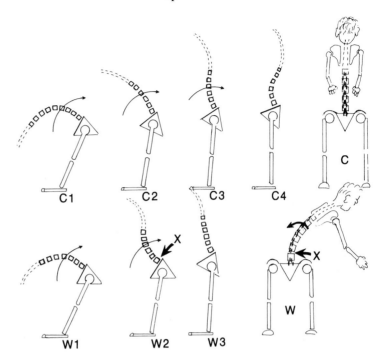

the side of the radicular pain but not necessarily always present in that direction.

3. Positive straight-leg raising: straight-leg raising may be limited due to its effect on rotating the pelvis, protective hamstring spasm, or stretch pain of the irritated sciatic nerve. Pain from simultaneous nuchal flexion, or ankle dorsiflexion, while performing the test, corroborates the positive straight-leg raising to be a nerve pain, as these positions stretch the inflamed meninges.

4. Neurological deficit: objective findings such as sensory or motor impairment of a root(s), or subjective paresthesias or hypesthesia in dermatome areas.

TREATMENT OF ACUTE LOW BACK PAIN

The treatment of acute low back pain includes the following items:

1. Rest in the semiflexed position unless the McKenzie concept, injury to the posterior ligaments by overstretching and tearing, resulting in pain on flexion, has been deduced as the cause; then the prone extension is indicated.[9]

2. Medication for pain.

3. Explanation of the treatment and reassurances to the patient.

4. Frequent local applications of ice to decrease painful muscle spasm.[10]

After the acute condition subsides, gradual ambulation with a carefully outlined manner of bending, stooping, and lifting is taught and initiated. If an acute episode has been one of a number of frequent episodes or if pain remains to a significant degree after a period of bed rest, a back brace or corset may be of value. The brace (1) must be fitted for a specified *limited* time in conjunction with a gradual exercise program and instruction in proper posture and functional habits; (2) must assist by its contour in producing an antalgic lumbar posture;[11] (3) must have an uplifting abdominal support; and (4) must be long enough posteriorly to contact the sacrum and limit thoracolumbar function (Fig. 37–12).

Chronic Low Back Pain

The persistence of disabling pain with equivocal physical findings may require (1) psychological evaluation; (2) consideration of intra-articular facet steroid anesthetic injection; (3) posterior primary division chemical rhizotomy; (4) transcutaneous electrical stimulation; (5) biofeedback for relaxation training; and (6) epidural steroid injection.[12, 13]

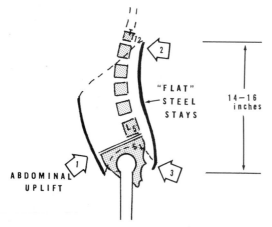

FIGURE 37–12. Corset principle for "flat lumbar spine." The three-point principle of the corset shows the long stays with contact at T12 and low point at sacrum. The stays are flattened. The forward position of the corset presses up against the abdomen and also presses the back against the stays. (From Cailliet, R.: Low Back Pain Syndrome, 3rd Ed. Philadelphia, F. A. Davis Co., 1981, p. 127.)

INDICATIONS FOR SURGICAL REFERRAL

The primary indication for surgery is progressive neurological deficit(s) in spite of a period of adequate conservative treatment. Persistence of incapacitating pain after a prolonged conservative treatment program that causes economic duress to the patient is an indication for surgical consideration. This must follow a psychological as well as a physiological evaluation of the patient.

The presence of urinary retention, indicating a neurogenic bladder, is not a surgical emergency. Urinary retention may be treated conservatively and usually responds well without surgical intervention.

For radiological confirmation of the causative pathology, computed tomography (CT) and magnetic resonance imaging (MRI) have partially replaced myelography, but some surgeons still prefer the older method. There is concern about causing arachnoiditis through the mixture of blood and the injected dye. Careful clinical evaluation and electromyographic localization are useful to localize the precise level of the disk.

Degenerative Disk Disease: "Osteoarthritis"

Dehydration and fragmentation of the intervertebral disk with consequent effects upon the func-

tional unit constitute the entity of degenerative disk disease. Over the years, trauma and possibly inherited vulnerability gradually dehydrate the disk, decreasing its hydromatic effectiveness. The vertebral bodies approximate, causing laxity of the longitudinal ligaments. The intradiskal pressure forces disk matrix between the bodies and ligaments, which gradually forms the nidus for osteophytes (Fig. 37–13).

Anterior compression of the functional unit causes posterior approximation, narrowing the intervertebral foramina and approximating the zygapophyseal joints. Owing to compression, the facet joints undergo degenerative hypertrophic changes. All the tissues capable of pain are made more vulnerable, and the stability and flexibility of the functional unit are impaired. These changes may remain asymptomatic until the back is used in a

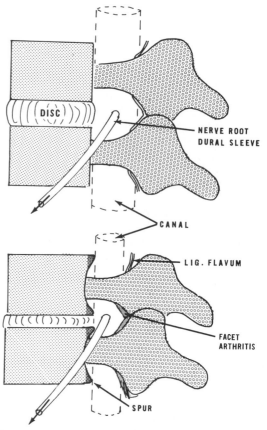

FIGURE 37–13. Spondylosis. Upper figure depicts normal functional unit, lower figure depicts spondylosis. With disk narrowing, spurs form on the vertebrae, narrowing the foramen and compressing the facets. Facet degenerative arthritis results, bulging the ligamentum flavum into the spinal canal. Spinal stenosis results. (From Cailliet, R.: Low Back Pain Syndrome, 3rd Ed. Philadelphia, F. A. Davis Co., 1981, p. 181.)

faulty manner[14] or exposed to severe external forces.

Spinal Stenosis

Narrowing of the spinal canal (see Fig. 37–13) can cause a specific clinical entity termed pseudoclaudication. The patient afflicted with spinal stenosis complains of pain in the distribution of a nerve root (so-called sciatica) after a period of walking or prolonged standing. The onset of pain after a period of walking, if it were true claudication (on a vascular basis), would subside or disappear when the walking stopped. In spinal stenosis, the patient must sit or assume a flexed posture to decrease the lumbar lordosis. The pain subsides and the patient can resume walking.

Pseudoclaudication after prolonged standing also can be relieved by a flexion posture to decrease the lumbar lordosis. This may be accomplished by squatting or sitting.

Conservative management is possible by flat back exercises to decrease the lordosis, by wearing a lumbar brace, or both. The specific diagnosis is made clinically and verified by an x-ray study, a CT scan, or myelography. Surgical decompression may be required when disability persists in spite of conservative management or when the disability increases to an unacceptable level.

Cervical Pain

Pain in the neck, or from the neck, constitutes the second most prevalent musculoskeletal disability confronting the physiatrist. The functional unit in most ways is identical to the lumbar spine segment, except that it glides in an anteroposterior direction. Flexion separates the neural arches, and extension approximates them. Flexion opens the intervertebral foramina, and extension closes them.[15] Rotation opens the intervertebral foramina, and extension closes them.[15] Rotation opens the foramina on the side from which the head is turned and closes those toward which the head is turned.[16] This fact is important in evaluating the clinical history and the physical findings and explains mechanisms of pain in the neck and pain referred in the distribution of the cervical nerve roots.[17]

Pain and disability from the cervical spine can be generally attributed to either trauma or arthritis. Trauma includes (1) hyperflexion-hyperextension injury with soft tissue trauma; (2) posture in which hyperlordosis causes foraminal closure, nerve entrapment, and facet impingement; and (3) chronic tension, postural or emotional, in which the unit and all its tissues, especially the muscular elements, are compressed, resulting in pain. Arthritis is usually of the degenerative type, in which all of the changes described in the lumbar spine are in evidence.

CERVICAL PAIN OR CERVICAL REFERRED PAIN

The history reveals whether the pain is acute or chronic and describes the mechanism considered to cause the pain, and the physical examination reveals which tissues are involved and the degree of injury. Reproduction of symptoms by positions and movements of the head and neck clarify the mechanism and give indication for meaningful treatment. Muscle testing of the upper extremity plays a valuable part in the neurological examination to determine the site and extent of nerve root entrapment.[17]

TREATMENT

The acute condition requires rest, relaxation of tissues, and decrease of inflammation. Rest by reclining is the best method. A collar that is comfortable and custom fitted is of value but does not significantly immobilize the cervical spine. Modalities such as ice, massage, heat, ultrasound, and manipulation have their indications and are beneficial when properly applied. Modifications of posture and daily activities are usually mandatory. Cervical traction essentially decreases lordosis, opens the foramina, and elongates the erector spine. This is of clinical value if it is applied to cause slight flexion of the cervical spine. Isometric exercises to strengthen the short neck flexors and the long neck extensors are valuable. All other modalities listed for the low back, as well as indications for surgical interventions, apply to the cervical spine.

In rheumatoid arthritis, there is definite atlantoaxial instability due to the decrease and the resultant laxity of the supporting ligamentous tissues that encircle the odontoid process. Subluxation of the atlas upon the axis can occur from trauma, and treatment of a moderate severity can similarly cause disruption of the joint. Since the contents of the spinal canal are the cord and its roots, subluxation can result in a high level quadriplegia. The rheumatoid arthritic patient must be protected from such stress by avoidance of specific activities and excessive treatment and should be guarded by a collar or brace.

Scoliosis

Scoliosis is the most deforming orthopedic problem confronting children. It is a potentially progressive condition that affects children during their active growth phase. Ultimate structural changes can only be corrected surgically; thus, early recognition and aggressive treatment are necessary.[18-21]

Scoliosis is unphysiological lateral curving from the midline. Owing to vertebral alignment, the mechanical alignment of the posterior articulations and the ligamentous muscular constraints of the vertebral column, lateral curving is gradually accompanied by simultaneous rotation of the vertebral bodies toward the convex side of the curve. At first, the curvature is functional in that it is reversible and disappears in the recumbent posture, but it gradually undergoes structural changes. A structural scoliosis is a fixed curve that does not correct itself on lateral bending or in the supine position. The lumbar rotation is mild in its cosmetic appearance; however, by virtue of the ribs being firmly attached to the thoracic vertebrae, the ribs undergo rotatory structural deformities in thoracic rotation. Lumbar scoliosis is more apt to cause low back pain.

The symptoms of scoliosis are primarily those of undesirable appearance. The cosmetic sequelae are significant in that scoliosis is more frequent in girls by a ratio of 9:1. Another sequela that justifies treatment is the prevalence of cardiopulmonary complications secondary to rib cage deformity, such as impairment of vital capacity, pulmonary hypertension, and cor pulmonale. Pain is considered to be the third sequela, but there is controversy regarding the incidence of pain in this entity as compared with that in a comparable population of nonscoliotic patients.

Scoliosis is specified as to its site in the vertebral column of its apex: a cervical curve has its apex from C1 to C6; thoracic curve, between T2 and T12; lumbar curve, between L1 and L4, and the thoracolumbar curve, from T12 to L1 (Fig. 37–14). Curves are also designated as primary or compensatory (secondary). They are also termed major or minor, depending on their prominence and significance. By standardization of the Scoliosis Research Society, all curves are now measured by the Cobb method (Fig. 37–15). Recordable measurement of rotation remains unstandardized.

Early examination is best done with the examiner sighting horizontally along the spine of the

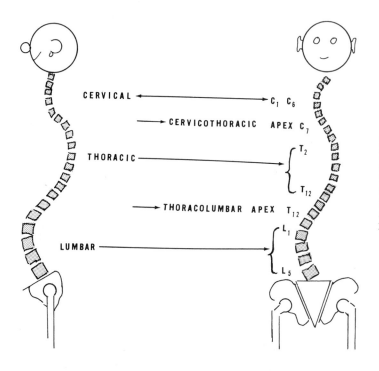

FIGURE 37–14. Spinal level of scoliosis curvatures. The scoliosis is specified to exist at the spinal level related to either the cervical, cervicothoracic, thoracic, thoracolumbar, or lumbar vertebrae. More than one level may be involved. (From Cailliet, R.: Scoliosis: Diagnosis and Management. Philadelphia, F. A. Davis Co., 1975, p. 22.)

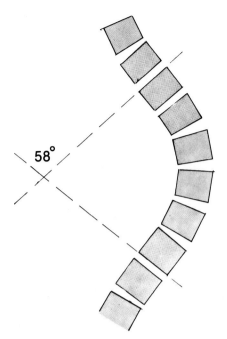

FIGURE 37–15. Cobb method of measuring curvature. A line is drawn along the upper margin of the vertebra that inclines most toward the concavity. A line is also drawn on the inferior border of the lower vertebra with greatest angulation toward the concavity. The angle of these transecting lines is noted and recorded. The apical vertebra is noted but does not enter into the measurement. (From Cailliet, R.: Scoliosis: Diagnosis and Management. Philadelphia, F. A. Davis Co., 1975, p. 29.)

patient, who stands with hips flexed at 90 degrees and legs fully extended. Early minimal curves are frequently seen only in this type of examination (Fig. 37–16).

Curving may progress until epiphyseal closure is completed and the end of growth has been reached. This end point is estimated by viewing the iliac crest apophysis (Fig. 37–17). When the iliac apophysis has completely crested the ilium and has fused, all vertebral growth is considered terminated.[22] Curves of 50 degrees or more are capable of progression even after apophyseal closure by virtue of disk compression on the concave side of the curve.

TREATMENT

In a young child with definite potential for growth, a curve of 10 to 15 degrees can be evaluated at three-month intervals with a standardized x-ray study performed with the patient in a standing position. If the beginning of rotation is found, even with merely 10 to 15 degrees of lateral deviation, a Milwaukee brace is indicated. An unbalanced curve that deviates laterally to the center of gravity is a poor prognostic sign (Fig. 37–18). These curves tend to progress rapidly. The principal aim of treatment is to realign the spine directly above the sacrum (Fig. 37–19).

A 20-degree curve is an indication for bracing. A 50-degree curve is difficult to brace and should be considered for surgical correction and internal fixation with a Harrington rod and fusion. Curves of 50 degrees or more have been shown to progress *after* apophyseal closure and to predispose the patient to cardiopulmonary complications.

Exercises per se *will not deter a curvature that is progressing in a growing child* but will maintain flexibility and improve posture. Children placed in a Milwaukee brace or its equivalent must be given exercises to perform while within the brace and while out of the brace.[23] The Milwaukee brace, or

FIGURE 37–16. Clinical examination method for scoliosis. With the patient bent forward at a right angle (90 degrees) at the hips, the examiner sights horizontally down the entire spine from behind. The patient's legs must be fully extended at the knees, the arms dangling with palms facing, and the feet preferably bare. This method of examination will disclose early minimal scoliosis not easily seen when the patient is erect. (From Cailliet, R.: Scoliosis: Diagnosis and Management. Philadelphia, F. A. Davis Co., 1975, p. 33.)

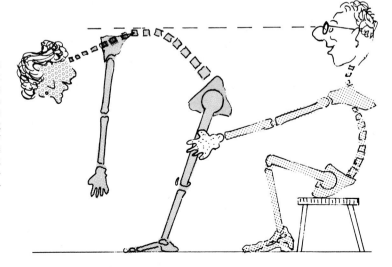

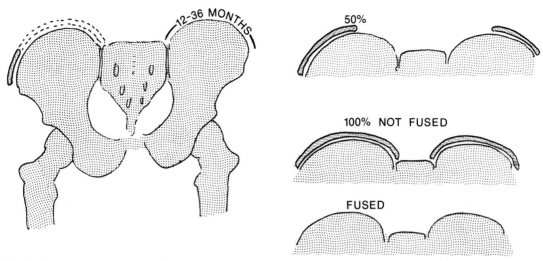

FIGURE 37–17. Closure of iliac apophyseal center. By termination of vertebral growth, the iliac apophyses are also considered to be fused and spinal growth ended. (From Cailliet, R.: Scoliosis: Diagnosis and Management. Philadelphia, F. A. Davis Co., 1975, p. 37.)

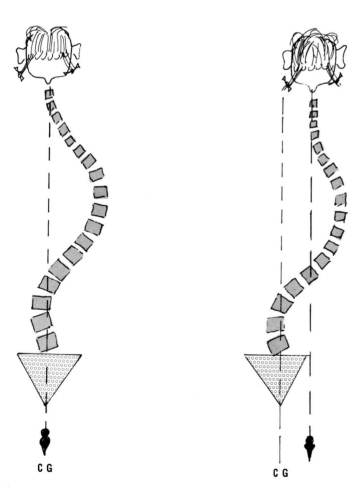

FIGURE 37–18. Balanced and unbalanced curves. With the head directly above the sacrum, a scoliotic curve is considered to be "balanced." Curve shown in figure to right is unbalanced and places stresses upon curves. (From Cailliet, R.: Scoliosis: Diagnosis and Management. Philadelphia, F. A. Davis Co., 1975, p. 91.)

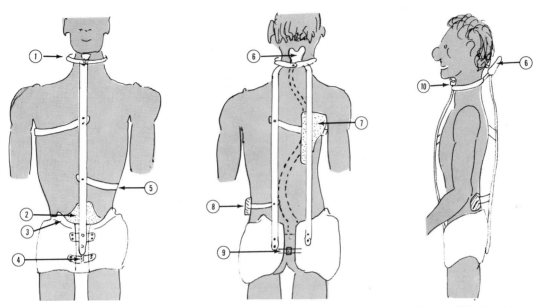

FIGURE 37–19. Milwaukee Brace. 1, Cervical ring. 2, Abdominal pad. 3, Iliac crest band. 4, Closure of iliac band for removal of brace. 5, Lateral band. 6, Occipital pad. 7, Lateral and posterior thoracic pad. 8, Lateral lumbar pad. 9, Posterior fringe. 10, Mandibular pad. (From Cailliet, R.: Scoliosis: Diagnosis and Management. Philadelphia, F. A. Davis Co., 1975, p. 68.)

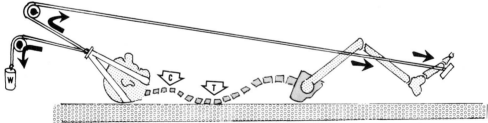

FIGURE 37–20. Cotrel traction. With the patient in the supine position, the cervical head sling passes over a pulley that permits traction by extending the legs against the crossbar attached to the rope. The duration and strength of the traction are graded to the tolerance of the patient under the physician's supervision. When the leg traction force is released, the weight (W) exerts the traction. Cotrel traction (personal observation) distracts the cervical spine (C) with diminution of traction in the thoracic spine (T) and no traction in the lumbar spine. This caudal decrease in traction is undoubtedly due to friction forces of the body on the surface of the bed or plinth. (From Cailliet, R.: Scoliosis: Diagnosis and Management. Philadelphia, F. A. Davis Co., 1975, p. 83.)

its equivalent, is a kinetic, not a static, brace. The lateral pads hold the lateral curves from progressing further but *do not* passively correct the curves. The exercises that entail pulling away from the pads are considered to be the corrective forces.

The pelvic band fits the pelvis and decreases the lordosis. The collar-headband applies distracting forces that elongate the spine, thus decreasing the cervical, thoracic, and lumbar curves. The lateral or posterolateral pads prevent further lateral rotatory deformity and indicate to the patient the direction from which to distract while performing the exercises. In children with round back, an increased dorsal kyphosis, either idiopathic or from Scheuermann's disease, a Milwaukee brace with specific exercises is effective. Traction, specified by Cotrel, has strong European advocacy. This is applied for inpatient, clinical, or home use and is supplemented with exercises (Fig. 37–20). Paraspinal functional electrical stimulation is also being studied at this time with reports of beneficial effects in reducing scoliosis.

CONCLUSION

Early detection of scoliosis or round back and energetic treatment with proper conservative methods prevent the inevitable cosmetic and disabling conditions that usually occur in later life with this condition. These are some of the challenges presented to the physiatrist. After careful clinical evaluation of painful disabling and deforming spinal disorders, treatment must be based on the precise knowledge of functional anatomy.

References

1. Smyth, M. J., and Wright, W.: Sciatica and the intervertebral disc, an experimental study. J. Bone Joint Surg., 40A:1401–1418, 1958.
2. Holt, E. P.: The question of lumbar discography. J. Bone Joint Surg., 50A:720–726, 1968.
3. Hirsch, C.: Etiology and pathogenesis of low back pain. Isr. J. Med. Sci., 2:362–370, 1966.
4. Hirsch, C., Ingelmark, B. E., and Miller, M.: The anatomical basis for low back pain. Acta Orthop. Scand., 33:1–17, 1963.
5. Cloward, R. B.: Cervical diskography: A contribution to the etiology of mechanism of neck, shoulder and arm pain. Ann. Surg., 150:1052–1064, 1959.
6. Bartelink, D. L.: The role of abdominal pressure in relieving the pressure on the lumbar intervertebral discs. J. Bone Joint Surg., 39B:718–725, 1957.
7. Davis, P. R., and Traup, J. D. G.: Effects on the trunk of erecting pit props at different working heights. Ergonomics, 9:475–484, 1966.
8. Cailliet, R.: Soft Tissue Pain and Disability, 2nd Ed. Philadelphia, F. A. Davis Co., 1988.
9. McKenzie, R. A.: The Lumbar Spine. Mechanical Diagnosis and Treatment. New Zealand, Spinal Publications, 1981.
10. Mennell, J. M.: The therapeutic use of cold. J. Am. Osteopath. Assoc., 74:1146–1158, 1975.
11. Morris, J. M., and Lucas, D. B.: Physiological considerations in bracing of the spine. Orthop. Prosthet. Appl. J., 17:37–44, 1963.
12. Delke, T. F. W., Burry, H. C., and Grahame, R.: Extradural corticosteroid injection in the management of lumbar nerve root compression. Br. Med., 2:635–637, 1973.
13. Burn, J. M. B., and Langdon, L.: Lumbar epidural injection for treatment of chronic sciatica. Rheumatol. Phys. Med., 10:368–374, 1970.
14. Epstein, J. A., Epstein, B. S., Rosenthal, A. D., Carras, R., and Lavine, L. S.: Sciatica caused by nerve root entrapment in the lateral recess—the superior facet syndrome. J. Neurosurg., 36:5:584–589, 1972.
15. Cailliet, R.: Neck and Arm Pain. Philadelphia, F. A. Davis Co., 1964.
16. Fielding, J. W.: Cineroentgenography (dentgenography) of the normal cervical spine. J. Bone Joint Surg., 39A:1280–1281, 1957.
17. Jackson, R.: The Cervical Syndrome, 2nd Ed. Springfield, Ill., Charles C Thomas, Publisher.
18. Cailliet, R.: Scoliosis: Diagnosis and Management. Philadelphia, F. A. Davis Co., 1975.
19. Rabin, G. C. (Ed.): Scoliosis. New York, Academic Press, 1973.
20. Hoppenfeld, S.: Scoliosis: A Manual of Concept and Treatment. Philadelphia, J. B. Lippincott, 1967.
21. Roaf, R.: Vertebral growth and its mechanical control. J. Bone Joint Surg., 42B:40–59, 1960.
22. Blount, W. P., and Bolinski, J.: Physical therapy in the nonoperative treatment of scoliosis. Phys. Ther., 47:919–925, 1967.
23. Cailliet, R.: Exercises for scoliosis. *In* Basmajian, J. (Ed.): Therapeutic Exercise, 3rd Ed. Baltimore, The Williams & Wilkins Co., 1978, pp. 430–449.

Supplemental Bibliography

American Academy of Orthopedic Surgeons: Symposium on the Spine. November, 1967, pp. 188–240.
Badgley, C. E., and Arbor, A.: The articular facets in relation to low back pain and sciatic radiation. J. Bone Joint Surg., 23:481–496.
Bennett, R. L.: Recognition and care of elderly scoliosis. Arch. Phys. Med. Rehabil., 42:211–225, 1961.
Bergquist-Ullman, M., and Larsson, U.: Acute low back pain in industry: A controlled study with specific

reference to therapy and confounding factors. Acta Orthop. Scand., Suppl. 170, 1977.

Blount, W. P.: The Principles of Treatment, According to Curve Patterns of Scoliosis and Round Back with the Milwaukee Brace. Postgraduate Course in the Management and Care of the Scoliosis Patient. New York Orthopedic Hospital, 1969.

Bourdillon, J. F.: Spinal Manipulation. New York, Appleton-Century Crofts, 1970.

Cailliet, R.: Low Back Pain Syndrome, 4th Ed. Philadelphia, F. A. Davis, 1988.

Chrisman, O. D., et al.: A study of the results following rotatory manipulation of the lumbar intervertebral disc syndrome. J. Bone Joint Surg., 46A:517–526, 1964.

Cobb, J. R.: Outline for study of scoliosis. Instruct. Lect. Am. Acad. Orthop. Surg., 5:261–275, 1948.

De Palma, A. F., and Rothman, R. H.: The Intervertebral Disc. Philadelphia, W. B. Saunders Co., 1970.

Falconer, M. A., McGeorge, M., and Begg, A. C.: Observations on the course and mechanism of symptom-production in sciatica and low back pain. J. Neurol. Neurosurg. Psychiatry, 2:13, 1948.

Farfan, H. F.: Mechanical Disorders of the Low Back. Philadelphia, Lea and Febiger, 1973.

Harrington, P. R.: Treatment of scoliosis—correction and internal fixation by spine instrumentation. J. Bone Joint Surg., 44A:591–610, 1962.

Hirsch, C.: Studies on the mechanism of low back pain. Acta Orthop. Scand., 24:261, 1951.

Holt, L.: Cervical, dorsal and lumbar spinal syndromes. Acta Orthop. Scand., Suppl. 17, 1954.

Kraus, H.: Clinical Treatment of Back and Neck Pain. New York, McGraw-Hill Book Co., 1970.

Lewin, T.: Osteoarthritis in lumbar synovial joints. Acta Orthop. Scand., Suppl. 73, 1964.

Magora, A.: Investigation of the relationship between low back pain and occupation, age, sex, community, education and other factors. Industr. Med. Surg., 39:465–471, 1971.

Moe, J. H.: Management of idiopathic scoliosis. Clin. Orthop., 20:169–184, 1957.

Morris, J. M., Lucas, D. B., and Bresler, B.: The role of the trunk in the stability of the spine. J. Bone Joint Surg., 43A:327, 1961.

Nachemson, A. L.: Lumbar intradiscal pressure. Acta Orthop. Scand., Suppl. 43, 1960.

Nachemson, A. L.: The lumbar spine: An orthopedic challenge. Spine, 1:59–71, 1976.

Nachemson, A.: Physiotherapy for low back pain patients. Scand. J. Rehab. Med., 1:85–90, 1969.

Norton, P. L., and Brown, T.: The immobilizing efficacy of back braces: Their effect on the posture and motion of the lumbosacral joint. J. Bone Joint Surg., 39A:111, 1957.

Sarno, J. E.: Therapeutic exercise for back pain. In Basmajian, J. (Ed.): Therapeutic Exercises, 3rd Ed. Baltimore, The Williams & Wilkins Co., 1978.

Schmorl, G. H., and Junghanns, H.: The Human Spine in Health and Disease. New York, Grune & Stratton, 1959.

Stern, R. A., Wolf, J. R., Murphy, R. W., and Akeson, W. H.: Aspects of chronic low back pain. Psychosomatics, 14:52–56, 1973.

Turek, S. L.: Orthopaedics. Philadelphia, J. B. Lippincott, 1959.

Williams, P. C.: Conservation management of lesions of the lumbosacral spine. Instruct. Lect., Am. Acad. Orthop. Surg., 10:90–121, 1953.

38

Management of Neurogenic Dysfunction of the Bladder and Bowel

INDER PERKASH

The Bladder

The management of neurogenic bladder dysfunction is too important to be left as a matter for occasional consultation. The urologist should be an active member of the team that follows the patient day by day. By the same token, any physician charged with the overall care of patients with this disorder, whatever his or her own specialty, must have an understanding of the urinary tract dysfunction and the methods available for its treatment according to the needs of the individual patient. Improvement of patient care in the clinical problems of voiding dysfunction lies in a better understanding of neurophysiology and pharmacology of micturition and the ability to apply these principles in the study of micturition (urodynamic evaluation) in such patients.

Neuroanatomy and Neuropharmacology

The essential peripheral components of voiding and continence are the bladder musculature (detrusor), bladder neck mechanism, posterior urethral smooth muscle, and striated pelvic and periurethral muscles. The smooth muscle fibers of the bladder body are described as being composed of three layers—the external and internal longitudinal layers and the middle layer, which is the thickest and is composed of circularly running muscle fibers. All layers intermingle, and the muscular wall of the bladder is to be considered as a continuum of smooth musculature, the vesical detrusor.[1] However, as the detrusor muscles converge on the internal orifice of the bladder, they tend to become oriented into three layers.[2] The most caudal of the middle circular fibers are thickened and prominent, and they form the true bladder neck. This concentric ring of middle circular layer fibers is complete anteriorly, whereas posteriorly it fuses with the trigone. This structure was first described by Heiss in 1915,[3] but later Hutch[4] demonstrated that anatomically and functionally the "fundus ring" or "Heiss ring" fuses with the deep trigone to form a structure that he called the base plate. A considerable amount of smooth muscle from the bladder extends into the posterior urethra. The striated muscle component of the urethra consists of pelvic floor musculature and periurethral extension. In male subjects, the periurethral striated muscle extends between the urogenital diaphragm and the apex of the prostate. This is illustrated in Figures 38–1 and 38–2 (after Hutch).

The female urethra and the posterior urethra in the male essentially resemble each other except for the presence of the prostate in the male urethra, which partly displaces the homogeneous anatomical configuration seen in the female urethra. Recent histochemical and electron microscopic studies[5] show a well-developed circular smooth muscle extension from the bladder into the urethra to the entrance of the ejaculatory ducts in males and a rather less developed extension in females.

810

Management of Neurogenic Dysfunction of the Bladder and Bowel

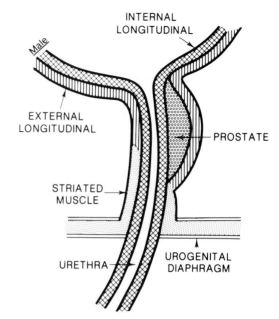

FIGURE 38–1. Sagittal section showing relationship and extent of striated and plain muscles in the male posterior urethra. (After Hutch.)

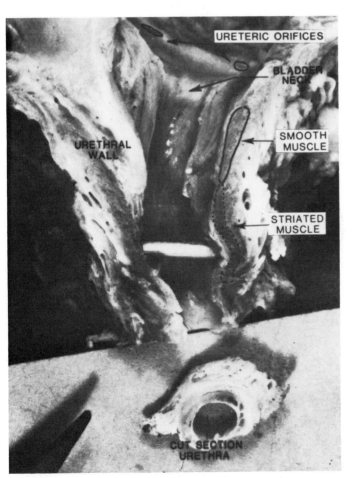

FIGURE 38–2. Musculature and interior bladder neck and cross section of male urethra.

INDER PERKASH

Furthermore, the distribution of sympathetic nerve fibers in the smooth muscle coat is sparse in females in comparison with the male bladder neck region. This finding provides evidence for the necessity for prevention of retrograde ejaculation in the male.

Parasympathetic Nerve Supply. The detrusor muscle is richly supplied by parasympathetic fibers originating from the anterior gray columns of the second, third, and fourth sacral segments of the spinal cord. The third sacral segment seems to contribute most to the bladder wall. Figure 38–3 illustrates the innervation of the bladder. It passes through pelvic splanchnic nerves to synapse in the intramural and extramural bladder ganglia. From these ganglia, postganglionic fibers travel to the detrusor muscle. In view of the peripheral location (mostly in the bladder wall) of the parasympathetic postganglionic cell bodies, damage to the pelvic nerves results largely in decentralization rather than denervation of the bladder (autonomous bladder). The parasympathetic nerves secrete acetyl-

choline at the motor nerve endings and are, therefore, called cholinergic nerves. This innervation to the bladder is so profuse that nearly every smooth muscle cell is individually supplied by one or more cholinergic nerves. Thus, it indicates the importance of the parasympathetic supply initiating and sustaining bladder contraction at micturition.

Sympathetic Nerves. The sympathetic nerve supply originates in cells in the lateral gray column of the spinal cord from the level of T11 to L2. When the sympathetic nerves are stimulated, the nerve endings produce noradrenalin-norepinephrine; the muscles that possess alpha-adrenergic receptors contract when noradrenalin-norepinephrine is present. Those muscles that possess beta-adrenergic receptors relax, however, in the presence of noradrenalin-norepinephrine. In humans, the bladder[5, 6] has a predominance of alpha-adrenergic receptors in the muscles of the bladder neck and the proximal urethra and beta-adrenergic receptors in the detrusor muscle of the bladder. Figure 38–4 diagrammatically illustrates the distribution of

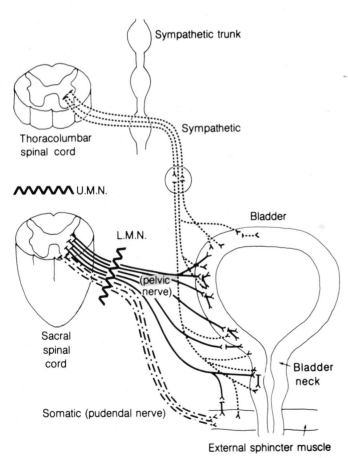

FIGURE 38–3. Innervation of the bladder. (U.M.N. = Upper motor neuron, L.M.N. = lower motor neuron.) (From Perkash, I.: Neuromuscular disorders of the bladder. *In* Friedland, G. W., Filly, R., Govis, M. L., Gross, D., Kempson, R. L., Korobkin, M., Thurber, B. D., and Walter, J.: Uroradiology—An Integrated Approach. London, Churchill Livingstone, 1983, pp. 1291–1316.)

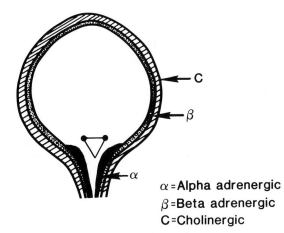

α = Alpha adrenergic
β = Beta adrenergic
C = Cholinergic

Diagramatic illustration of autonomic receptors of the bladder and urethra

FIGURE 38–4. Distribution of autonomic receptors of the bladder and urethra.

autonomic receptors of bladder and urethra. Thus, the effect of sympathetic stimulation is to contract the bladder neck and relax the detrusor muscle. The noradrenalin-norepinephrine that is produced by the sympathetic nerve endings also acts as an inhibitor of the acetylcholine produced by the parasympathetic nerve endings. When the sympathetic nerves are stimulated, the smooth muscle of the prostate, the seminal vesicles, and the ejaculatory ducts contract, resulting in ejaculation. The muscles of the bladder neck simultaneously contract, thereby preventing semen from entering the bladder. A disturbance of this function may result in sterility.

Striated External Urethral Sphincter. There are two components of striated sphincter muscle around the posterior urethra. The circularly arranged fibers surrounding the membranous urethra are usually referred to as external sphincter fibers, and the striated fibers around the prostatic urethra are designated periurethral muscles (see Fig. 38–1). The periurethral striated sphincter is innervated mostly through the pudendal nerve, with fibers originating from the anterior gray columns of the second and perhaps from the third and fourth sacral segments of the cord. The striated sphincter (external sphincter) fibers around the membranous urethra are considered to be slow twitch muscle fibers and are vital for the maintenance of continence. It has also been demonstrated histochemically[7] that the external urethral sphincter (also called a rhabdosphincter by Gil-Vernet[8]

and Winkler[1]) receives triple sympathetic-parasympathetic-somatic innervation. This important study gives a morphological basis to the observation that the action of the external sphincter is normally coordinated with the bladder smooth muscle.[9–11]

Recent neuropharmacological studies indicate antagonistic roles of prostaglandins (PGE_2 and PGF_2) in a variety of organ systems, including the bladder.[12–14] PGE_2 decreases norepinephrine output as well as end-organ responsiveness to norepinephrine and thus is a potent vasodilator and antisympathetic agent. On the other hand, PGF_2 increases norepinephrine output at the synaptic terminals and usually causes vasoconstriction. In relation to the coordinated activity of the bladder, bladder neck, and posterior urethra, prostaglandins may play an important role in modulating activity of sympathetic and parasympathetic fibers.

The Central Innervation. Sensory receptors that primarily detect changes in length and tension have also been found in laboratory animals. They connect directly to the brain stem in the pons where the central micturition center is located.[15–17] A variety of positive and negative feedback loops have been uncovered that are believed to be important in sustaining and then terminating micturition.[18] Although a local reflex arc originating in the bladder, with a sacral micturition center in the conus, produces bladder contractions, the coordination of micturition is known to be influenced by several suprasegmental centers.[19] The cortical centers provide for adequate volitional control of micturition, inhibit uninhibited contractions, and maintain adequate bladder capacity and minimal residual urine. Thus, the normal bladder and the bladder outlet function is maintained by suprasegmental centers through both autonomic and voluntary nervous control. In this system, the urine continues to collect in the bladder that induces gradually increasing feedback through autonomic nerves, which maintain control through cortical awareness and initiate micturition through voluntary effort and the somatic system. Normal micturition is, therefore, entirely a voluntary act secondary to voluntary active contraction of the bladder. Simultaneously, contraction of abdominal musculature and diaphragm takes place to raise intra-abdominal pressure, which is not essential for normal micturition. On the other hand, a patient with a cauda equina lesion and an areflexic (noncontractile) bladder may be able to void only after raising intra-abdominal pressure by suprapubic compression or by bearing down (Credé/Valsalva maneuver).

INDER PERKASH

Normal Voiding

Normal persons can feel when the bladder contains approximately 100 ml of urine. The normal person will also feel a desire to pass urine when the bladder contains 300 to 400 ml of urine. As the bladder fills, the striated muscle sphincter remains contracted; the contraction is mediated through a primitive reflex known as the holding reflex. Normal people do not, however, contract their bladders until they voluntarily trigger the voiding mechanism. The urethral sphincter first relaxes, and then the bladder contracts. A few seconds are required to initiate the voiding process, during which the person must voluntarily get the system working. Thus, if the person feels inhibited or embarrassed (as for example when the patient must void in front of the doctor), the entire process may be slow in starting or may not take place at all.

The first action to take place is the overcoming of the holding reflex. The periurethral striated sphincter is relaxed. At the same time, the bladder neck will relax; immediately thereafter, the detrusor muscle of the dome of the bladder contracts, and voiding takes place through a completely open bladder neck and urethra. Voiding will normally continue until the bladder is empty, but voiding can voluntarily be stopped at any point in the process. This extraordinarily well-coordinated process requires perfect synergy between the sympathetic, parasympathetic, and somatic nerve supplies. Any lesion involving these three nerves will lead to dysfunction.

Study of Micturition (Urodynamic Evaluation)

Urodynamic studies in the broad sense[40] of the term include the urine flow rate, the cystometrogram (CMG), the urethral pressure profile, and the voiding cystourethrogram. Neuropharmacological testing with drugs before and after these tests is also being used increasingly to determine the efficacy of a therapeutic drug. Measurement of urine flow rate is done by asking the patient to void into an instrument that can simultaneously record the peak urine flow and also graphically record the pattern of voiding. The total volume divided by the time gives the flow rate per second. Reduced peak flow and increased voiding time could be due to the obstructing effects of the

prostatic urethra, to neurogenic bladder dysfunction, or to an overdistended areflexic bladder. To resolve whether decrease in flow is due to bladder or urethral factors, a CMG, along with simultaneous electromyography of the periurethral sphincter and the urethral pressure profile, is helpful.[40, 41]

The CMG helps assess bladder function and provides information on the volume-pressure relationship when the bladder is gradually filled with water or carbon dioxide. This test evaluates the contractability of the detrusor muscle, its adjustability to volume, and its capacity to stretch and the patient's sensation of fullness, desire to void, and pain. The pressure in the bladder can be measured by inserting a catheter and using a water manometer or by using a pressure sensor and a multiple channel recorder. A rectal balloon inserted at the same time can discriminate between intravesical and intra-abdominal pressure. The methodology is illustrated in Figure 38–5.

We perform such studies only on patients whose urine is sterile or whose urinary infection is covered adequately with a suitable antibiotic. It is helpful to have the rectum empty. Spinal cord–injured patients should have their bowels emptied on the evening before the studies. The patient is asked to void immediately prior to the study to estimate the amount of the residual urine. The CMG is performed by introducing the catheter into the bladder and emptying it completely. Carbon dioxide or sterile water (at 37° C [98.6° F]) is introduced as the bladder pressure is simultaneously recorded. Patients must inform the physician or nurse as soon as they notice any sensation of fullness in the bladder and must also announce when they feel the desire to void. Patients are then instructed to void, and during voiding, they are asked to cease voiding to observe the voluntary control of the bladder.

The urethral pressure profile is intended to provide an index of urethral resistance to bladder output, to enable an assessment of urinary continence, to allow distinction between a distensible and fibrotic sphincter urethral segment, and to contribute information to enable characterization of detrusor sphincter dyssynergia. However, the intraurethral pressure is a function of the catheter size, the hole size through which fluid is perfused, the fluid perfusion rate, and the distensibility of the urethral sphincter segment; for want of standardization, it is difficult to interpret functionally the value of the peak urethral pressure taken with a certain catheter at a given perfusion rate. A mechanical puller is attached to the catheter to

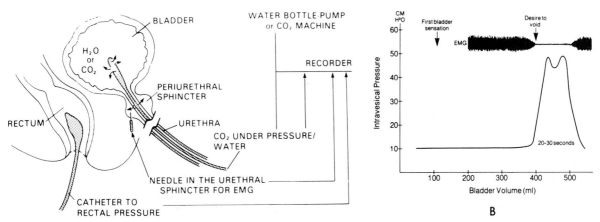

FIGURE 38–5. *A*, Schematic diagram showing method of urodynamic recording of urethral pressure profile, intra-abdominal pressure, and EMG of external urethral sphincter. *B*, Recording of simultaneous normal cystometrogram and EMG of external urethral sphincter. (*A* modified from Ghista, Perkash et al.: Advances in Bioengineering, 1978, 19–23 and Constantinou, C. E.: Urology Digest, 13–21, March 1977.)

pull it through the urethra at a known rate while carbon dioxide or water is introduced. The urethral pressure is simultaneously recorded. The methodology is illustrated in Figure 38–6.

When the normal bladder is filled with increasing volumes of fluid, the intravesical pressure usually rises 10 to 15 cm of water. Figure 38–5*B* illustrates normal CMG and simultaneous electromyography (EMG) of the external urethral sphincter. Any sudden rise in bladder pressure during filling beyond 15 to 20 cm of water is indicative of an unstable bladder. Most incontinent females show this instability with no other associated neurogenic bladder dysfunction. Any long tract disease in the spinal cord leads to increased instability, which becomes manifest as uninhibited bladder contractions over which the patient has no control. Normal

people do not show uninhibited contractions. Complete lesions above the bladder center in the conus lead to a reflex bladder (Fig. 38–7). Lesions in the conus or lesions involving the cauda equina usually lead to a lower motor neuron (areflexic) bladder.

Simultaneous sphincter EMG and CMG are helpful to diagnose complex neurogenic bladder dysfunctions such as detrusor sphincter dyssynergia. This is illustrated in Figure 38–8. Notice that the urethral EMG activity increases with each detrusor contraction (lower tracing). The bladder neck and urethra usually open after repeated suprapubic tapping.

Interpretation of Urodynamic Findings. When normal people are asked to hold their urine, the EMG activity of their periurethral striated sphincter increases significantly, and when asked to pass

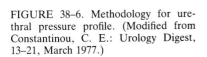

FIGURE 38–6. Methodology for urethral pressure profile. (Modified from Constantinou, C. E.: Urology Digest, 13–21, March 1977.)

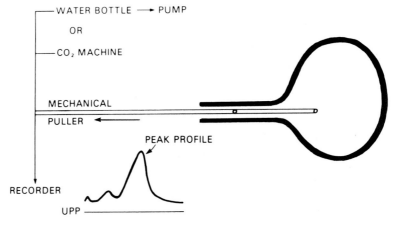

INDER PERKASH

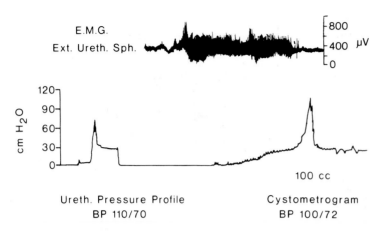

FIGURE 38–7. Reflex bladder contraction when the bladder was filled with 200 ml. (From Perkash, I.: Neuromuscular disorders of the bladder. *In* Friedland, G. W., Filly, R., Govis, M.L., Gross, D., Kempson, R. L., Korobkin, M., Thurber, B. D., and Walter, J.: Uroradiology—An Integrated Approach. London, Churchill Livingstone, 1983, pp. 1291–1316.)

urine, activity decreases markedly. Thus, normal people can usually abolish the external urethral sphincter EMG activity. A sustained voiding pressure on the CMG in excess of 50 cm of water can eventually produce vesicoureteral reflux; this indicates the need for medication with alpha-adrenergic blocking agents or anticholinergic drugs or for sphincterotomy. The beneficial effects of these drugs are easily proved by demonstrating that the voiding pressure falls significantly after the administration of alpha-adrenergic drugs (Fig. 38–9).

During a CMG, normal people will feel full after 100 ml of gas or water has been introduced into the bladder. Normal people will want to void when the bladder contains 400 to 500 ml (see Fig. 38–

5*B*). At no time during bladder filling should the bladder pressure rise above 15 to 20 cm of water in normal people. Patients with hyperreflexia, however, will void spontaneously when the bladder contains about 100 to 200 ml of gas or fluid. Hyperreflexia with no dyssynergia is common in patients with suprapontine lesions during or shortly after an episode of acute cystitis in otherwise normal persons.

When normal people are instructed to void, electrical activity ceases first in the periurethral striated sphincter. Then the bladder pressure increases, and the person voids. At this point, bladder and urethral pressures approximate each other. In patients with detrusor sphincter dyssynergia, the

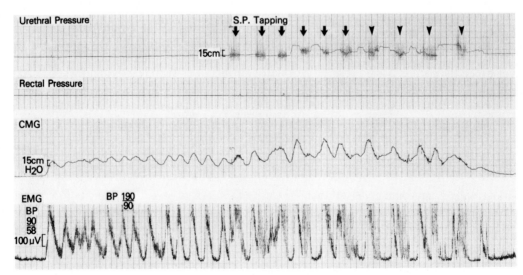

FIGURE 38–8. Simultaneous cystometrogram (CMG) and external urethral sphincter EMG show detrusor sphincter dyssynergia. Urethral pressures done at the same time also show increased pressures with sphincter dyssynergia. Suprapubic tapping (S.P. Tapping) was followed by reduced pressure on CMG and reduction in sphincter activity on EMG (near end of tracing). Patient's rise in BP from 90/58 to 190/90 indicates autonomic dysreflexia.

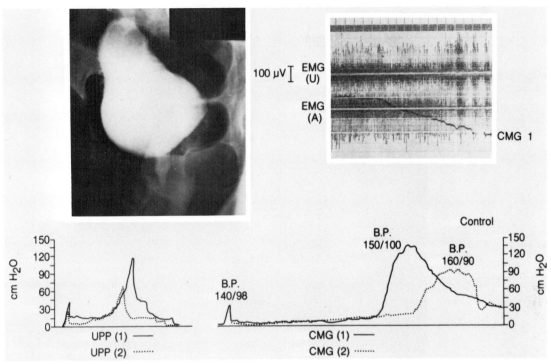

FIGURE 38–9. Urethral pressure peak profile—UPP(2)—after phentolamine shows a drop of 45 per cent and CMG (2) after phentolamine shows a drop of about 35 per cent in maximum voiding pressure. Voiding cystourethrogram shows opened bladder neck but inadequately opened external urethral sphincter. Simultaneous CMG and EMG of external sphincter (U) and anal sphincter (A), and CMG (1) show detrusor sphincter dyssynergia.

striated periurethral sphincter contracts during voiding instead of relaxing, as noted on the EMG.[20] This, in turn, generates high pressures in the bladder, bladder neck, and urethra. Urodynamic studies performed before and after administration of alpha blockers, when demonstrating significant drops both in urethral pressure profile and voiding pressures, can help determine the therapeutic usefulness of these drugs in individual patients.[21]

Types of Neuromuscular Dysfunction of the Bladder

A patient with a neuromuscular dysfunction of the bladder may have either a contractile bladder or a noncontractile bladder. Two main types of contractile bladder are known to exist. The first is called the uninhibited bladder. In this condition, after the bladder has attained a certain volume, which is usually less than normal, the voiding reflex is triggered so that the patient voids and is essentially incontinent. The patient can, however, also void voluntarily. Such patients may be able to avoid incontinence by voiding before the bladder is full enough to trigger the voiding response.

The second type of contractile bladder is called the reflex bladder (see Fig. 38–7). In this condition, there is no voluntary control; voiding occurs through the spinal cord reflex and is completely involuntary. Bladder volumes required to initiate voiding are also less than normal. This type of bladder has also been called the automatic bladder, because it contracts automatically when it has reached a given volume.

The noncontractile bladder may be of three varieties. The first occurs when there is a lower motor neuron lesion, which involves both the sensory and the motor limbs of the reflex arch (Fig. 38–10). Such bladders are cut off entirely from outside control and are, therefore, autonomous or self-governing. Hence the name for this condition: the autonomous bladder. The second variety of noncontractile bladder is that which occurs in a patient who has an upper motor neuron lesion but who has developed overdistention of the bladder (Fig. 38–11). The third variety is due to a loss of the sensory pathway, either the posterior nerve roots or the sensory pathway in the spinal cord.

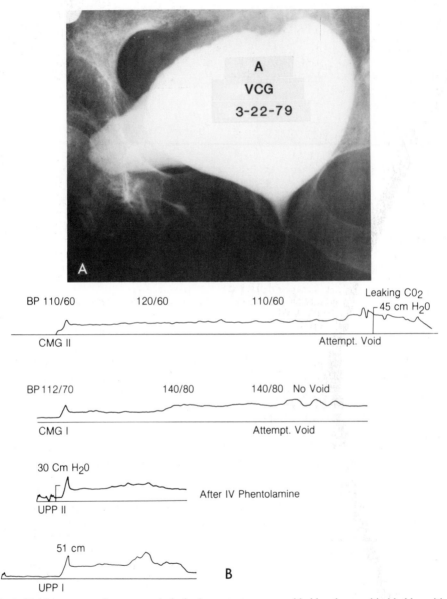

FIGURE 38–10. *A*, Voiding cystourethrogram typical of a lower motor neuron bladder shows a big bladder with a smooth wall that seems to be sinking into the pelvis due to a lax pelvic floor (compare with Fig. 38–8—reflex upper motor neuron bladder). *B*, CMG I and CMG II before and after phentolamine show noncontractile bladder. UPP II after phentolamine shows drop of peak profile pressure from 51 cm to 30 cm of water.

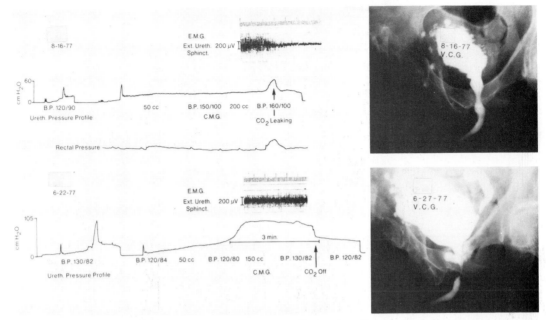

FIGURE 38–11. Simultaneous CMG and EMG external urethral sphincter show (lower tracing) detrusor sphincter dyssynergia, and voiding study shows non-opened external urethral sphincter and reflux. After transurethral sphincterotomy (upper tracing) bladder is noncontractile. Arrow points at the rise in CMG pressure that is simultaneous with an increase in rectal pressure, indicating that this was due to the rise in intra-abdominal pressure. (Reproduced by permission from Perkash, I.: Treatment of voiding dysfunction in spinal cord injured patients: Surgical. *In* Barrett, D. M., and Wein, A. J.: Controversies in neurourology. New York, Churchill Livingstone, 1984.)

Noncontractile bladders are also called areflexic bladders. If a small amount of contractility is still present, they are called hyporeflexic bladders.

Common Causes of Neuromuscular Disorders of the Bladder

Neuromuscular disorders of the bladder are either congenital or acquired. Myelodysplasia is the common congenital cause.

Acquired lesions can affect any part of the central or peripheral nervous system. Common neurological disorders leading to bladder dysfunction are shown in Table 38–1.

Intracranial Lesions. Intracranial lesions affect either the cortical centers or the suprasegmental pathway. Milder lesions usually cause an uninhibited bladder; more advanced lesions usually cause a hyperreflexic bladder with no dyssynergia. Common causes for such disorders are vascular lesions, such as cerebrovascular accidents, ischemia due to arteriosclerosis, intracranial neoplasms, and Parkinson's disease.

Spinal Lesions Affecting the Suprasegmental Pathway. Supraconal lesions in the cord will result in an uninhibited bladder when the suprasegmental pathways are only slightly involved or a reflex neurogenic bladder when the lesion has destroyed all spinal cord pathways to the spinal cord detrusor center. The most common lesions involving the spinal cord are spinal cord injury, spinal cord neoplasm, intervertebral disk disease, and multiple sclerosis.

Cauda Equina Lesions. When the cauda equina is involved, the resultant bladder dysfunction is usually a noncontractile bladder. Common causes are trauma and neoplasms.

Lesions of the Posterior Nerve Roots and Sensory Pathways in the Spinal Cord. These lesions usually cause either a hyporeflexic or an areflexic bladder. The bladder is generally very large in such cases. The most common cause now is diabetes mellitus. All patients with diabetes mellitus who have this lesion also have peripheral neuropathy. Posterior root ganglions may be destroyed due to tabes dorsalis, which is currently rare.

Lesions of the Anterior Horn Cells. These lesions also lead to the development of noncontrac-

TABLE 38–1. Common Neurological Disorders Leading to Bladder Dysfunction*

NEUROLOGICAL DISORDER	USUAL TYPE OF DYSFUNCTION
Suprapontine Lesions	Detrusor hyperreflexia with absent detrusor sphincter dyssynergy
Delayed CNS maturation (childhood)	
	Persistence of uninhibited bladder beyond age 2–3 years. Enuresis later on.
Cerebral atherosclerosis (old age)	Uninhibited bladder
Early multiple sclerosis	Uninhibited bladder
Brain neoplasm	Uninhibited bladder
Pernicious anemia	Uninhibited bladder
Lesions Below the Pons	Usually associated with detrusor sphincter dyssynergy
Spinal cord injuries	Reflex bladder
Spinal cord neoplasms—primary or secondary	Reflex bladder
Syringomyelia	Reflex bladder
Advanced multiple sclerosis	Reflex bladder
Extensive brain neoplasms	Reflex bladder
Extensive brain trauma	Reflex bladder
Conus Lesions	Absent detrusor sphincter dyssynergy
Cauda equina injuries or neoplasms	Areflexic bladder (autonomous bladder)
Acute transverse myelitis	Areflexic bladder (autonomous bladder)
Extensive rectal carcinoma	Areflexic bladder (autonomous bladder)
Following abdominoperineal resection of rectal carcinoma	Areflexic bladder (autonomous bladder)
Perivesical fibrosis following extensive pelvic surgery or trauma	Areflexic bladder (autonomous bladder)
Herniated intervertebral disk	Areflexic bladder (autonomous bladder)
Myelodysplasia and spina bifida	Areflexic bladder (autonomous bladder)
Poliomyelitis	Areflexic bladder (motor-paralytic, sensory intact)
Injury, neoplasms, and herniated disk involving motor nerves to the bladder	Areflexic bladder (motor-paralytic, sensory intact)
Diabetes mellitus	Areflexic bladder (sensory-paralytic bladder, areflexic due to overdistention)
Tabes dorsalis	Areflexic bladder (sensory-paralytic bladder, areflexic due to overdistention)
Guillain-Barré syndrome	Areflexic bladder

*After Perkash, reference 46.

tile bladders. An isolated lesion of the anterior horn cells is usually due to poliomyelitis, which is now rare.

Adverse Drug Effects. Many different drugs that variously affect the autonomic nervous system may cause or prevent bladder dysfunction (Table 38–2). Tricyclic antidepressants, antihistaminics, and phenytoin can all cause incomplete bladder emptying. Clinically significant adverse and unwanted pharmacological effects on voiding function usually appear in patients whose voiding status already borders on being pathological.

TABLE 38–2. Drugs Having a Pharmacological Action on the Bladder, Primarily Through the Peripheral Autonomic Innervation*

DRUGS	MODE OF ACTION	ALTERATION IN BLADDER FUNCTION
Cholinergic Drugs		
Acetylcholine	Physiological neurotransmitter for bladder contractions	Increases intravesical pressure and facilitates voiding
Muscarinic Bethanechol Methacholine	Physiological neurotransmitter for bladder contractions	Increases intravesical pressure and facilitates voiding
Nicotinic Nicotine	Nicotine-like response resembles sympathetic stimulation mediated through release of norepinephrine	
Anticholinergics	Blockage of endogenous transmitter at postsynaptic receptor	Reduces bladder contractility and may lead to urinary retention
Atropine Propantheline D-Tubocurarine	Atropine blocks muscarinic action and d-tubocurarine blocks nicotinic action of acetylcholine. Propantheline blocks muscarinic action and also has a ganglion-blocking action.	
Reserpine Guanethidine	Essentially an adrenergic neuron blocker	
Phenothiazines Antihistaminics	Mild anticholinergic action	
Adrenergic		
Alpha-adrenergic response Phenylephrine	Sympathomimetic response (response mostly on alpha-adrenergic receptors)	Increases bladder outlet and urethral pressure
Ephedrine Imipramine	Action similar to alpha-adrenergic stimulation	
Antiadrenergic		
Alpha blockers Phenoxybenzamine Phentolamine Prazosin HCl	Sympatholytic response	Lower bladder outlet and urethral pressures
Beta stimulants Isoproterenol Progesterone	Sympathomimetic	Lower urethral pressure
Beta blockers Propranolol	Sympatholytic	Increase urethral pressure

*From Perkash, I.: Neuromuscular disorders of the bladder. *In* Friedland, G. W., Filly R., Govis, M. L., Gross, D., Kempson, R. L., Korobkin, M., Thurber, B. D., and Walter, J.: Uroradiology—An Integrated Approach. London, Churchill Livingstone, 1983, pp. 1291–1316.

Evaluation and Management of the Bladder in the Spinal Cord–Injured Patient

Inadequate voiding in patients with spinal injury could be caused by several factors, including an areflexic bladder, detrusor–external urethral sphincter dyssynergia, fixed scarred bladder neck, and enlargement of the prostate. There may also be excess alpha-adrenergic activity demonstrable at the bladder neck leading to bladder–bladder neck dyssynergia and autonomic dysreflexia.

Neurourological Evaluation. A systematic approach to define bladder dysfunction problems during rehabilitation of the spinal cord–injured patient is of utmost importance, since early recognition and management will prevent urological complications and permanent renal damage. Neurological examination should include testing perianal sensations to discover any sacral sparing. The presence of anal tone, anal reflex, and bulbocavernous reflex only indicate intact conus and local reflex arc. However, detection of voluntary contraction of the anal sphincter (determined with a finger in the anal canal) indicates intact voluntary control, and in the presence of quadriplegia, it indicates central cord–type of incomplete lesion. Combined studies such as CMG with EMG of the external urethral sphincter should help determine the neurogenic dysfunction and also discover the presence of significant detrusor sphincter dyssynergia. A drop in urethral pressure profile (about 20 per cent or more) after intravenous phentolamine (5 to 7.5 mg) defines the role of alpha blockers such as phenoxybenzamine for therapeutic use to improve voiding (see Figs. 38–9 and 38–10B). Radiological examination should include initial intravenous urography and voiding cystourethrograms to assess upper tracts and to rule out vesicoureteral reflux. Voiding radiological studies with ciné control are also useful for the diagnosis of bladder neck problems and detrusor sphincter dyssynergy. Linear array transrectal sonography has also been found to be a useful noninvasive modality for the diagnosis of bladder outlet obstruction.[22] When combined with urodynamics, it provides a precise diagnosis of the pathogenesis of voiding dysfunction.[23] It is only with transrectal sonography that a diagnosis of bladder neck ledge can be made with some certainty.

Immediately following injury for a period of one day to usually three to four weeks, all deep reflexes below the level of injury are absent; this is usually referred to as the shock phase. The bladder is areflexic during this period and needs a careful periodic or continuous drainage, and provocative testing such as introduction of 4 oz of sterile cold water at 4° C (39.2° F) does not evoke bladder reflex activity (Fig. 38–12). The ice water test is positive when introduction of cold water is almost immediately followed by rapid rejection of water and catheter out of the bladder. Adequate bladder drainage during the shock phase can prevent the areflexic bladder from developing overdistention and atony:

Intermittent catheterization, rather than leaving a continuous indwelling catheter for drainage of the bladder, when used from the onset reduces incidence of infection and stone disease.[24] If done with regularity, it allows decompression of the bladder and helps monitor the residual urine. It also allows detection of the return of spontaneous voiding on the part of the patient and heralds recovery from the shock phase. Both aseptic and "clean" techniques have been advocated; however, the author prefers an aseptic technique in patients with acute spinal injury, particularly when it is desired to avoid bacteremia in patients prior to or immediately following spinal surgery and also in patients whose condition is complicated by thromboembolism due to deep vein thrombosis. In patients with acute spinal injury with deep vein thrombosis, unsterile intermittent catheterization technique may lead to disseminated intravascular clotting.[25]

Intermittent Catheterization Technique. Intermittent catheterization using a size 12 or 14 cath-

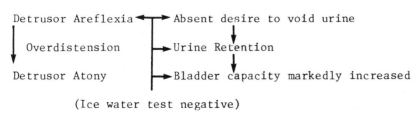

FIGURE 38–12. Bladder overdistention during spinal shock phase. (Reproduced by permission from Perkash, I.: Treatment of voiding dysfunction in spinal cord injured patients: Surgical, 425–435. In Barrett, D. M., and Wein, A. J.: Controversies in Neurourology. New York, Churchill Livingstone, 1984.)

TABLE 38–3. Intermittent Catheterization Record*

| DATE | TIME | INTAKE | REFLEX VOIDING | | RESIDUAL URINE (ml) | TOTAL URINE (ml) | URINE pH |
			Spontaneous	Stimulation (ml)			
10-7-75	11:00 AM	. . .	. . .	80	20	100	7.5
10-15-75	10:30 AM	. . .	. . .	500	180	680	6.5
10-17-75	1:30 PM	. . .	. . .	500	250	750	5.0
10-21-75				300	500	800	5.5

*From Perkash, I.: Intermittent catheterization failure and an approach to bladder rehabilitation in spinal cord injury patients. Arch. Phys. Med. Rehabil., 59:9, 1978.

eter is started every four hours. The patient's fluid intake is restricted to about 2 l in 24 hours. Monitoring is done on a special sheet (Table 38–3). Intake and output are recorded synchronously with the catheterization every day. Table 38–3 shows only pertinent data; therefore, information from several days has been omitted.

Catheterization intervals are extended to six and eight hours with increasing spontaneous voiding between the periods of catheterization. It is preferred not to allow more than 300 to 400 ml of residual fluid, since this may lead to overdistention. Intermittent catheterization is stopped when a balanced bladder is achieved. The bladder is considered to be balanced when (1) the patient can pass adequate urine on reflex or easily with suprapubic tapping and Valsalva's maneuver; (2) residual urine is approximately 100 ml or less; and (3) there are no pathological changes in the genitourinary tract. Long-term intermittent catheterization requires abolishing of the detrusor reflex with anticholinergics to accomplish low pressure in the bladder and continence to obviate the use of external condom-catheter drainage and a leg bag.

An areflexic bladder may retain a fair amount of urine. Therefore, during catheterization when urine flow ceases, the bladder is gently aspirated through the catheter, preferably with a bulb syringe or with suprapubic pressure applied while the catheter is still in the bladder, to empty the bladder completely. After each catheterization, the bladder is irrigated with about 50 ml of normal saline containing 120 μg/ml neosporin and 60 μg/ml polymyxin B. Irrigation is continued while the catheter is being pulled through the urethra. This may be particularly useful when patients are started on intermittent catheterization following removal of an indwelling catheter. Significant reduction in urinary tract infection has been reported in patients whose bladder and urethra were irri-

gated following each catheterization, particularly in a hospital setting.[38, 39] The patient is instructed in bladder retraining using the Credé/Valsalva maneuver following stimulation of the suprapubic region (e.g., by tapping or pulling hairs) between the catheterizations and also prior to intermittent catheterization to trigger voiding. Urine pH is recorded after each catheterization; pH values over 7.0 may invariably be associated with infection due to urea-splitting organisms.

Credé (suprapubic pressure) alone can lead to very high pressures in the bladder and may even lead to vesicoureteral reflux. It is, therefore, recommended only to tap the suprapubic region for about two min, wait, and tap again to accomplish adequate voiding (see Figure 38–8). This leads to contraction of the bladder along with relaxation of the urethral sphincter.

Transient high or low residuals may be noticed with infection.[26] Residuals of less than 50 ml are invariably associated with some degree of bladder infection. True volumes of residuals are seen after eradication of infection. An anecdotal example (see Table 38–3) is a T3 paraplegic patient admitted 21 years after injury with repeated urinary tract infections.[26] Previous transurethral resection of the prostate was carried out in 1969. On admission, residual urine was 20 ml and urinary pH was 7.5; urine culture was positive ($> 10^5$) for *Proteus rettgeri*. After control of infection, residual urine was 180 ml one week later. Two weeks after admission, urine culture showed no growth and residual urine was 500 ml. Transurethral sphincterotomy was performed three weeks after admission. At discharge one month after admission, residual urine was less than 100 ml and no infection was noted.

Patients with spinal cord lesions above the conus on intermittent catheterization for 8 to 10 weeks following injury usually show adequate spontaneous voiding if overdistention of the bladder is prevented and they do not have an enlarged prostate, stricture of the urethra, or dyssynergia of the detrusor-bladder neck smooth muscles or the detrusor sphincter muscles.

Prolonged intermittent catheterization with limitation on fluid intake is frustrating for spinal cord-injured patients with complete lesions and is even a hindrance to their complete rehabilitation. Therefore, the early recognition of patients in whom intermittent catheterization may not be successful is important, and such patients need careful urological intervention to establish an early catheter-free status. Studies of micturition, including simultaneous cystomanometry and periurethral striated EMG and voiding cystourethrography, are

therefore needed to define the dysfunctional neurogenic bladder problems. A trial with alpha-adrenergic blockers and/or striated muscle relaxants may help improve voiding in some patients with minimal sphincter dyssynergia. Therapeutic efficacy of these drugs can be evaluated by repeating the urodynamic study.

An illustration is shown in Figure 38–13. Cystomanometry before phentolamine testing (control), after phentolamine testing, and then 16 days after oral phenoxybenzamine shows marked improvement in voiding. The control study shows sustained detrusor contractions for over 4 min to empty the bladder, as against 3 min after intravenous (IV) phentolamine; also, after oral therapy with phenoxybenzamine, detrusor contractions

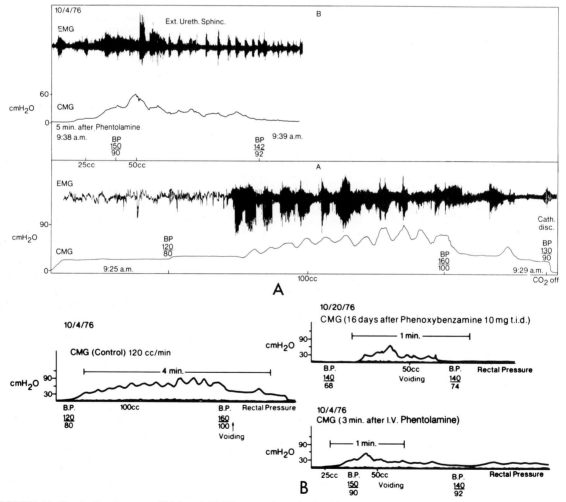

FIGURE 38–13. *A*, Simultaneous CMG and EMG external urethral sphincter recordings show reduced number of bladder contractions and less dyssynergia after phentolamine. A similar result was obtained 16 days later *(B)* with oral phenoxybenzamine when the patient voided more adequately in less time.

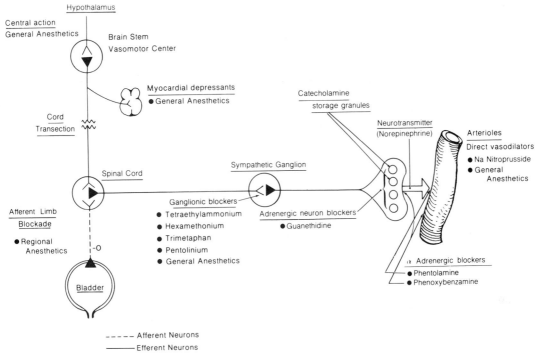

FIGURE 38–14. Principal site of action of hypotensive drugs useful in autonomic dysreflexia. (Reproduced by permission from Schonwald, G., Fish, A., and Perkash, I.: Anesthesiology, 55:550–558, 1981.)

were less sustained and the voiding phase lasted just over a minute. The study shows the usefulness of phentolamine testing in such patients.

Autonomic Dysreflexia and Detrusor Sphincter Dyssynergia. Autonomic hyperreflexia or dysreflexia is an important visceral alarm symptom usually due to a distended bladder or impacted rectum.

An acute episode is associated with throbbing headache, sweating, and bradycardia. There is a generalized sustained increase in sympathetic tone below the level of the lesion, which leads to altered hemodynamics and a rise in arterial pressure by (1) elevating arteriolar resistance, (2) reducing the distensibility of postarteriolar capacity vessels, and (3) directly increasing myocardial contractility. Marked peripheral vasoconstriction below the level of lesion seems to be mediated by norepinephrine. Following an attack of autonomic dysreflexia, there is marked increase of serum dopamine-β-hydroxylase plasma catecholamine, and norepinephrine metabolites (such as normetanephrine) in the urine.[27] Prompt drainage of the bladder usually relieves the acute episode. Local instillation of 0.25 per cent tetracaine hydrochloride 25 to 50 ml in patients with a suprapubic tube or through an indwelling catheter may provide topical anesthesia of the vesical mucosa and reduce triggering impulses to the spinal cord. Gentle evacuation of fecal masses from the rectum and instillation of 1 per cent dibucaine N.F. (Nupercainal) ointment may reduce impulses originating from the rectum.

The control of widespread sympathetic activity below the spinal lesion is the key factor in the management of autonomic dysreflexia. Therefore, spinal anesthesia, ganglion blockers, adrenergic neuron blockers, adrenergic blockers, and drugs acting directly on the blood vessels are useful in controlling hypertension accompanying autonomic dysreflexia.[28] Figure 38–14 diagrammatically illustrates the principal site of action of hypotensive drugs useful in autonomic dysreflexia. Phenoxybenzamine, 10 mg or prazosin hydrochloride 1 mg, three or four times a day, is usually sufficient to control acute dysreflexia. For the immediate control of hypertension with dysreflexia, 5 mg intravenous hydralazine hydrochloride repeated after five min has been found useful in our patients.

Recurrent episodes of autonomic hyperreflexia are usually associated with detrusor sphincter dyssynergia.[27, 28] Therefore, surgical management of detrusor sphincter dyssynergia with adequate transurethral sphincterotomy will provide definitive management of the major primary problem provoking the stimulus for autonomic hyperreflexia. Long-term medical management with guanethidine (Ismelin), 10 to 20 mg/day, does provide relief of hypertension but not adequate control of sweating. It also leads to side effects, such as postural hypotension, nasal stuffiness, and diarrhea, in some patients.

Those patients who show detrusor hyperreflexia as well as detrusor sphincter dyssynergia could run the risk of developing vesicoureteral reflux and silent hydronephrosis.[29] Careful use of the adequate dosage of anticholinergics, alpha blockers, and early transurethral resection of the sphincter may be very rewarding for an adequate and quick rehabilitation of the patient with complete lesions. Also, an alpha blocker such as phenoxybenzamine has been found very useful for long-term treatment of autonomic dysreflexia.[30] Simultaneous cystomanometry and periurethral striated EMG are shown in Figure 38–15A, which illustrates detrusor sphincter dyssynergia and detrusor hyperreflexia in a tetraplegic patient. Strong detrusor contractions are seen after filling the bladder with 50 ml of fluid; the blood pressure rose to 160/100 mm Hg at which time the patient also complained of sweating and headache (autonomic dysreflexia). Following transurethral resection of the sphincter and the use of alpha blockers, marked relief from autonomic dysreflexia was noticed (Fig. 38–15B). During the follow-up for over 10 years, this patient has been voiding easily and has not had any symptomatic infection. Voiding cystourethrogram two and one-half years after surgery showed a well-opened bladder neck and posterior urethra (Fig. 38–15C).

Cauda Equina Lesions. Management of patients with cauda equina lesions needs special consideration. They usually have an areflexic (noncontractile) bladder and void with Credé/Valsalva manipulation. Their lesions are invariably incomplete or mixed and have a potential for recovery. Urodynamic evaluation may indicate an intact external urethral sphincter, and, therefore, such patients with supraconal lesions may not be able to void unless they generate very high intravesical pressures. This could even lead to vesicoureteral reflux. Also, in these patients with damage to the parasympathetic innervation and with reinnervated or intact sympathetic innervation (which emerges above the cauda equina [see Fig. 38–3]), the bladder neck may not open well on voiding. The excess sympathetic activity could be demonstrated on intravenous phentolamine testing. In such patients, voiding can be improved with the use of alpha blockers such as oral prazosin hydrochloride, 1 to 3 mg daily, or by limited bladder neck incision.

Central Cord Syndrome. Neurogenic bladder due to incomplete lesions such as the central cord syndrome[37] may be corrected in over 50 per cent of patients. It is important to separate patients with central cord syndrome from other patients with incomplete tetraplegia. Despite severe neurological dysfunction during the first few weeks, considerable recovery of bladder function can occur, particularly since the bladder fibers are the peripheral ones in the spinal cord. These patients are usually managed with intermittent catheterization and drug therapy. It is possible to cause incontinence by an early transurethral resection of sphincter and thus necessitate an external collecting device. Persisting detrusor sphincter dyssynergia, severe spasticity, and hydronephrotic change may be indications for transurethral sphincterotomy after trial with alpha blockers, anticholinergics, and skeletal muscle relaxants such as baclofen.

Management of the neurogenic bladder in female patients with spinal cord lesions (upper motor neuron) is difficult; however, conal and cauda equina lesions (lower motor neuron) can be easily managed with the Credé/Valsalva maneuver. Intermittent catheterization is started every four to six hours, and with fluid restriction to about 1.5 l a day, these patients may be managed with three catheterizations a day. In supraconal lesions with a hyperreflexic bladder, to reduce stress incontinence between catheterizations, use of an anticholinergic such as oxybutynin 5 mg once or twice a day is helpful. Bladder irritability is increased with infection; therefore, treatment of infection is rather important to prevent leakage of urine. Long-term prophylaxis for urinary tract infection is strongly recommended. The patient is encouraged and trained to empty the bladder by using suprapubic tapping and the Valsalva maneuver periodically. Failure to manage with intermittent catheterization usually results in long-term placement of an indwelling catheter. Neurosurgical procedures such as selective sacral nerve root blocks and rhizotomies may be indicated to convert a reflex (contractile) bladder into an areflexic bladder that, as mentioned above, can be managed easily by the Credé/Valsalva maneuver. Sacral nerve root implants for stimulated voiding are currently being tried in paraplegic patients with contractile bladders.

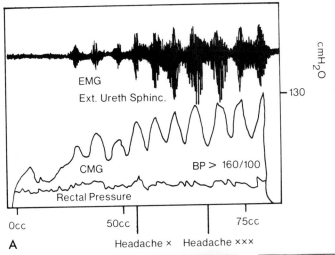

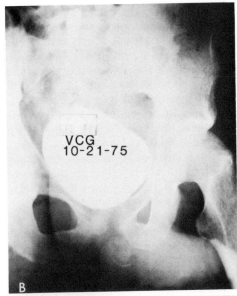

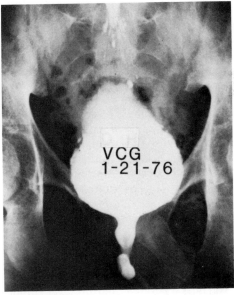

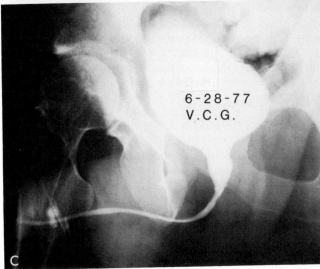

FIGURE 38–15. *A*, Simultaneous CMG and EMG recordings of external urethral sphincter show detrusor sphincter dyssynergia in a C6 tetraplegic about four months after injury. *B*, Voiding cystourethrogram before (10–21–75) and after (1–21–76) transurethral sphincterotomy. *C*, Follow-up voiding cystourethrogram about 18 months later showed well-opened bladder neck and posterior urethra. (Reproduced by permission from Perkash, I.: J. Urol., 131:778, 1979.)

INDER PERKASH

Management of Infection in Patients with Spinal Cord Injury. The use of antibacterial drugs in patients with a neurogenic bladder has been the subject of much debate. There is no disagreement as to the need for antibiotics when there are constitutional manifestions of an acute infection of the urinary tract.

At the start of intermittent catheterization, when the indwelling catheter is being removed, we start patients on a suitable antibiotic for the first three days to prevent dissemination of urethral infection. Both Pearman's[39] study and our own[32, 33] indicate usefulness of bladder and urethal irrigation with antibiotics following each intermittent catheterization. There was significantly lower incidence of bacteriuria, and it also obviated the necessity for prophylaxis during intermittent catheterization. After each catheterization, about 50 ml of polymyxin-neomycin irrigant solution was instilled and removed and then 15 ml of this irrigant was left in the bladder and about 15 ml was used to irrigate the urethra while the catheter was being removed. However, at present we do not recommend the routine use of bladder irrigation with solutions containing neomycin because of the possibility of a toxic reaction. All infections during intermittent catheterization were treated with an appropriate antibiotic.

The most important measure in the prevention of symptomatic urinary tract infection is to ensure adequate bladder drainage. Still, the incidence of bacteriuria with external condom drainage or an indwelling urethral catheter is very high. These patients have heavy perineal and urethral colonization. Fecal incontinence and soiled seating cushions increase the incidence of perineal colonization. Daily thorough perineal washing with plain soap and water and condom change is stressed. Proper laundering of clothes, bedding, and the soiled cushion is also recommended. Our studies indicated a high correlation between bacteriuria and contaminated leg bags.[32] We therefore recommend the use of 0.06 per cent bleach solution for drainage appliance cleaning. Our studies indicate that dilute bleach solution, 2 oz in one quart of water, is a most effective and cost-efficient agent.[34] About 2 oz of this solution is left in the leg bag for about five minutes, and then the leg bag is irrigated with running tap water to remove the bleach solution completely in order to prevent irritation of the skin.

Accurate diagnosis of urinary tract infection in a patient with a neurogenic bladder cannot be achieved by studying symptoms alone. Lack of symptoms, i.e., fever, chills, dysuria, and flank pain in spite of significant bacteriuria ($> 10^5$ colonies per ml), continues to be prevalent in the majority of external condom–wearing spinal cord–injured patients with unobstructed voiding. We documented symptoms in only 3 per cent of 110 patients undergoing a Fairley localization test despite significant bacteriuria ($> 10^5$ colonies per ml).[33] Thus, symptoms *per se* are poorly correlated with significant bacteriuria in spinal cord–injured patients. In addition, use of the Fairley technique, which is reported to accurately localize the site of infection in patients without spinal cord injury, was shown to give less than optimal results in our population.

To assist in the clinical definition of urinary tract infection, quantitation of urine pyuria has proved helpful. It has also been demonstrated that pyuria ($\geq 10^4$ white blood cells per ml of urine) seems to be a useful predictor of urinary tract infection in a group of spinal cord–injured patients on condom catheter drainage.[35] It is suggested that pyuria reflects an inflammatory response and may assist in distinguishing true bladder infection from simple contamination or colonization.

In summary, we recommend treating symptomatic urinary tract infection in patients with fever, chills, and increased signs of dysreflexia. Treatment is also necessary in patients with evidence of vesicoureteral reflux, acute pyelonephritis, or epididymo-orchitis. The patients with symptomatic urinary tract infection are usually not voiding adequately on external condom drainage and are, therefore, placed on intermittent catheterization. Repeated urinary tract infection may necessitate sphincterotomy. All gram-negative infections with urea splitters are treated to prevent calculus disease. Asymptomatic bacteriuria with evidence of tissue infection as exhibited by large numbers of white blood cells in the urine (> 10 white blood cells per high power field) is also treated with an appropriate antibiotic or chemotherapeutic agent. Overzealous use of broad-spectrum antibotics for treatment or for suppressive purposes leads to the emergence of drug-resistant organisms. Availability of quinolones such as norfloxacin and ciprofloxacin may be a boon to the care of urinary tract infection in spinal cord–injured patients.

Our patients who are on external condom drainage with a balanced bladder and who are off intermittent catheterization are prophylactically treated with methenamine or nitrofurantoin (Macrodantin). Patients growing urea-splitting bacteria, such as *Proteus mirabilis*, are given trimethoprim-sulfamethoxazole.

Follow-up. All patients with spinal cord injury

need periodic urological follow-up for the rest of their lives. During the first year after discharge, blood urea nitrogen levels, urine culture (and sensitivities), and the patient's general well-being are reviewed. Unnecessary catheterizations for checking residual urine in a person who shows no clinical evidence of urine retention, infection, or lithiasis may not be warranted. In otherwise asymptomatic patients whose urodynamics had been previously studied, instead of routine annual intravenous pyelography, radioisotope renography for renal function, sonography, and plain x-ray film of the abdomen may be enough for follow-up. Transrectal linear array sonography has been found very useful as a noninvasive modality for follow-up to determine residual urine and any bladder outlet obstruction.[22, 23]

THE BOWEL

Defecation, like the voiding of urine, is under volitional control. The reflex activity starts with the filling and distention of the sigmoid colon and rectum, when afferent impulses thus generated pass to the sacral spinal cord in the conus. Efferent impulses emanate from the spinal cord, leading to the evacuation process when the sigmoid and rectum contract along with a synergistic relaxation of the anal sphincter. Following emptying of the anal canal, the anal sphincter and levator ani contract and there is relaxation of the rectum and lower colon. This process repeats until the entire lower bowel is empty. Under resting conditions, the external anal sphincter shows continuous electrical activity and tonic contraction.[40] However, this activity is absent during the spinal shock phase and following intrathecal injection of alcohol.[41]

Management During the Shock Phase

Complete spinal cord and cauda equina lesions or even severe incomplete transections result in the loss of reflex gastrointestinal function during the shock phase. This may last for two to three days. In some patients, paralytic ileus (which usually involves the stomach and colon also) may be present for several days and bowel sounds will be absent. There is abdominal distention (this is usually absent with lesions below T10), which may lead to regurgitation of food and could interfere with the diaphragmatic movements and, thus, pro-

duce respiratory distress in tetraplegic patients. Such patients need careful monitoring along with gastric tube suction, parenteral alimentation, and fluid replacement. There is widespread venous paralysis during the shock phase, and unless careful fluid balance is maintained, these patients could develop overhydration and pulmonary edema. Intramuscular injections of neostigmine (Prostigmin), 0.3 to 0.5 mg every four hours,[42] or subcutaneous injections of bethanechol, 2.5 mg every six hours, may help restart intestinal activity. A further complication of gastric involvement is mucosal hemorrhages and stress ulceration in the stomach or duodenum. These usually develop within the first two weeks of injury. Patients with a previous history of gastric or duodenal ulceration are particularly susceptible and are, therefore, often given antacids to avoid this complication.

Bowel Retraining

Habit retraining for reflex bowel evacuation may be begun as soon as the patient is out of shock, capable of receiving instructions, and able to take food by mouth. The diet should include foods that produce a stool of normal consistency.

A specific time of day should be established for defecation, such as following breakfast or following the evening meal, to take advantage of the gastrocolic reflex. Until the time when the patient can tolerate sitting in a commode chair, the patient has bowel care performed in bed. The lower rectum is examined and, if it is full, the feces are removed. A suppository may then be inserted (glycerin or bisacodyl USP [Dulcolax]) to stimulate peristalsis reflexly and the movement of feces into the lower bowel or rectal vault. Some patients may need additional digital stimulation, which is accomplished by insertion of the lubricated gloved finger into the rectum and massage of the walls of the rectum in a wavelike motion. Digital stimulation may need to be repeated every 10 minutes for three or four times. Digital stimulation works like the gastrocolic reflex and results in mass peristalsis with evacuation of the colon. Many patients can be managed with digital stimulation only and should be encouraged to experiment. Others may need a combination of a high fiber diet, suppository, and digital stimulation and must use softeners such as dioctyl sodium sulfosuccinate (Colace [Mead Johnson]) to keep their feces from becoming too hard.

INDER PERKASH

Patients who have injuries to the cord at the conus or involving the cauda equina often manage their bowel with manual removal on a daily or every-other-day schedule. These are the patients who may begin having accidental bowel movements as they begin to use a standing frame or to walk in parallel bars. Increasing the frequency of their bowel care from every other day to daily, accompanied by instructions on maintaining firm stool through diet management, may eliminate accidents.

When sitting tolerance permits, the patient should receive bowel care on a commode chair to allow gravity to assist in bowel evacuation. Massage of the abdomen from right to left may also facilitate movement of feces to the lower tract. On those occasions when no feces are evacuated with the standard methods, the patient may need to try a mild laxative and repeat the bowel program 8 to 10 hours later.

Muscular activity is enormously important. The patient who can stand and exercises every day is seldom constipated. In this, as in many other respects, the quadriplegic patient is at some disadvantage because his or her activity is relatively limited. A good bowel habit can still be established, but there is a tendency toward chronic moderate distention, more noticeable, perhaps, on the x-ray film than on physical examination. In the investigation of a patient suspected of having an intra-abdominal lesion, it is important not to interpret this as actual ileus. Once a good bowel habit program has been established, involuntary defecation is unusual as long as the feces remain of normal consistency.

Diarrhea in a spinal cord–injured patient is a sorry experience for the patient and the attendants. It could be associated with impaction. Any such tendency must be promptly and vigorously investigated by a rectal examination. Scybala are prone to produce impactions that require manual extraction. High fecal impaction in the colon could be exhibited as an acute abdomen and may be associated with autonomic dysreflexia, which becomes manifest as a rise in blood pressure and bradycardia and is accompanied by sweating and headache.

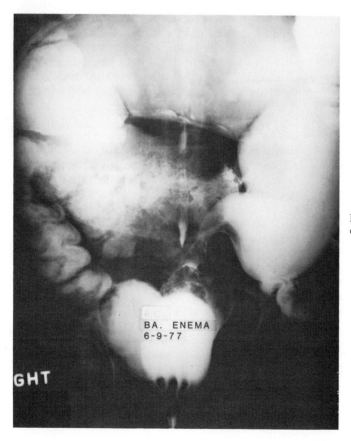

FIGURE 38–16. Barium enema shows megacolon in a quadriplegic patient.

Intra-abdominal Gastrointestinal Problems

In patients with spinal injury, it is sometimes difficult to differentiate acute abdominal lesions from fecal impaction. Rectal examination and palpation of the colon may reveal impaction. Patients using anticholinergics over a long period of time can develop megacolon. Barium enema examination shows a megacolon in a quadriplegic patient (Fig. 38–16) in whom transverse colostomy had to be done to provide adequate bowel evacuation. Transverse colostomy may, therefore, be indicated in patients with a difficult and prolonged bowel program, inadequate bowel emptying, repeated abdominal distention, and vague abdominal symptoms associated with large distended colon. Accidental perforations of the rectum have also been reported following rectal manipulations with enema tips.[43] Also reported are silent perforations of the stomach and appendicitis. Diagnostic criteria for intra-abdominal catastrophe are (1) a history of sudden illness that is out of proportion to the physical signs, (2) associated autonomic dysreflexia, (3) increased abdominal tone or increased generalized spasticity, (4) absent bowel sounds, and (5) shoulder pain due to diaphragmatic irritation with perforated viscus.[44, 45] Urgent intravenous pyelography and blood and urine examination provide additional help to rule out urinary tract pathology. Sometimes root pains may also be confusing. Chest x-ray study, ultrasound B scan, abdominal tap, CT scanning, and even exploratory laparotomy may be necessary to diagnose or rule out intra-abdominal pathology.

References

1. Winkler, G.: Contribucional estudeo de la innervation de la visceras pelvianas. Arch. Esp. Urol., 20:259, 1967.
2. Hutch, J. A.: Anatomy and Physiology of the Trigone, Bladder and Urethra. New York, Appleton-Century-Crofts, 1972.
3. Heiss, R.: Ueber der Sphincter vesicalis internus. Virchows Arch. Pathol. Anat., 220:367, 1915.
4. Hutch, J. A.: The internal urinary sphincters: A double-loop system. J. Urol., 105:375, 1971.
5. Gosling, J. A., and Dixon, J. S.: The structure and innervation of smooth muscle in the wall of the bladder neck and proximal urethra. Br. J. Urol., 47:549, 1975.
6. Nergardh, A., and Boreus, L. O.: Autonomic receptor function in the lower urinary tract of man and cat. Scand. J. Urol. Nephrol., 6:32, 1972.
7. El-Badawi, A., and Schenk, E. A.: A new theory of the innervation of bladder musculature. J. Urol., 111:613, 1974.
8. Gil-Vernet, S.: L'innervation somatique et vegetative des organes genitourinaries. Acta Urol. Belg., 32:265, 1964.
9. Denny-Brown, D., and Robertson, E. G.: On the physiology of micturition. Brain, 56:149, 1933.
10. Ghoneim, M. A., Fretin, J. A., Gagnon, D. J., and Susset, J. G.: The influence of vesical distension on urethral resistance to flow: The collecting phase. Br. J. Urol., 47:657, 1975.
11. Tanagho, E. A., and Smith, D. R.: The anatomy and function of the bladder neck. Br. J. Urol., 38:54, 1966.
12. Weeks, J. R.: Prostaglandins. Ann. Rev. Pharmacol., 12:317, 1972.
13. Hedquist, P.: Autonomic transmission. In Ramwell, P. W. (Ed.): The Prostaglandins, Vol. 1. New York, Plenum Press, 1973, p. 101.
14. Ghoneim, M. A., Fretin, J. A., Gagnon, D. J., et al.: The influence of vesical distension on the urethra resistance to flow: A possible role for prostaglandins. J. Urol., 116:739, 1976.
15. Bradley, W. E., Rockswold, G. L., Timm, G. W., et al.: Neurology of micturition. J. Urol., 115:481, 1976.
16. Urmura, E., Fletcher, T. F., Dirks, V. A., et al.: Distribution of sacral afferent axons in cat urinary bladder. Am. J. Anat., 136:305, 1973.
17. Winter, D. L.: Receptor characteristics and conduction velocities in bladder afferents. J. Psychiat. Res., 8:225, 1971.
18. Bradley, W. E., and Teague, C. T.: Spinal cord organization of micturition reflex afferents. Exp. Neurol., 22:504, 1968.
19. Nyberg-Hansen, R.: Innervation and nervous control of the urinary bladder. Anatomical aspects. Acta Neurol. Scand., 42(Suppl. 20):7, 1966.
20. Quesada, E. M., Scott, F. B., and Cardus, D.: Functional classification of neurogenic bladder dysfunction. Arch. Phys. Med. Rehabil., 49:17, 1968.
21. Awad, S. C., Downie, J. W., Lywood, D. W., Young, R. A., and Jarzylo, S. V.: Sympathetic activity in the proximal urethra in patients with urinary obstruction. J. Urol., 115:545, 1976.
22. Perkash, I., and Friedland, G. W.: Principles of modern urodynamic studies. Invest. Radiol., 22:279–289, 1987.
23. Perkash, I., and Friedland, G. W.: Posterior ledge at the bladder neck: Crucial diagnostic role of ultrasonography. Urol. Radiol., 8:175–183, 1986.
24. Guttman, L., and Frankel, H.: Value of intermittent catheterization in early management of traumatic paraplegia and tetraplegia. Paraplegia, 4:63, 1966.
25. Perkash, A., Prakash, V., and Perkash, I.: Experi-

ence with the management of thromboembolism in patients with spinal cord injury: Part I. Incidence, diagnosis and role of some risk factors. Paraplegia, 16:322, 1978.

26. Perkash, I.: Intermittent catheterization failure and an approach to bladder rehabilitation in spinal cord injury patients. Arch. Phys. Med. Rehabil., 59:9, 1978.

27. Naftchi, N. E., Demeny, M., Lowman, E. W., and Tuckman, J.: Hypertensive crises in quadriplegic patients: Changes in cardiac output, blood volume, serum dopamine-B-hydroxylase activity, and arterial prostaglandin PGE_2. Circulation, 57:336, 1978.

28. Perkash, I.: Pharmacologic Management of Autonomic Dysreflexia. Pharmacology of the Urinary Tract and the Male Reproductive System. New York, Appleton-Century-Crofts, 1982, pp. 285–293.

29. Perkash, I.: Pressor response during cystomanometry in spinal injury patients complicated with detrusor-sphincter dyssynergia. J. Urol., 121:778–82, 1979.

30. Perkash, I.: Detrusor-sphincter dyssynergia and dyssynergia responses: Recognition and rationale for early modified transurethral sphincterotomy in complete spinal cord injury lesions. J. Urol., 120:469, 1978.

31. Perkash, I.: Detrusor-sphincter dyssynergia and detrusor hyperreflexia leading to hydronephrosis during intermittent catheterization. J. Urol., 120:620, 1978.

32. Deresinski, S. C., and Perkash, I.: Urinary tract infections in male spinal cord–injured patients. J. Am. Paraplegia Soc., 8(1):4–6, 1985.

33. Giroux, J., and Perkash, I.: Limited value of the Fairley test in urologic infections in patients with neuropathic bladders. J. Am. Paraplegia Soc., 8(1):10–12, 1985.

34. Giroux, J., and Perkash, I.: In vitro evaluation of current disinfectants for leg bags. J. Am. Paraplegia Soc., 8(1):13–14, 1985.

35. Deresinski, S. C., and Perkash, I.: Urinary tract infections in male spinal cord injured patients. Part Two: Diagnostic value of symptoms and of quantitative urinalysis. J. Am. Paraplegia Soc., 8(1):7–10, 1985.

36. McGuire, E. J., Wagner, F. M., and Weiss, R. M.: Treatment of autonomic dysreflexia with phenoxybenzamine. J. Urol., 115:53, 1976.

37. Perkash, I.: Management of neurogenic bladder dysfunctions following acute traumatic cervical central cord syndrome (incomplete tetraplegia). Paraplegia, 15:21, 1977.

38. Rhame, F. S., and Perkash, I.: Urinary tract infections occurring in recent spinal cord injury patients on intermittent catheterization. J. Urol., 122:669–673, 1979.

39. Pearman, J. W.: Prevention of urinary tract infections following spinal cord injury. Paraplegia, 9:95, 1971.

40. Floyd, W. F., and Walls, E. W.: Electromyography of the sphincter ani externus in man. J. Physiol., 122:599, 1953.

41. Melzak, J., and Porter, N. B.: Studies on the reflex activity of the external sphincter ani in man. Paraplegia, 3:77, 1964.

42. Guttman, L.: Spinal Cord Injuries. London, Blackwell Scientific Publications, 1973, p. 442.

43. Frankel, H. L.: Accidental perforation of the rectum. Paraplegia, 11:314, 1974.

44. Walsh, J. J., Nuseibeh, M. B., and El-Masri, W.: Perforated peptic ulcer in paraplegia. Paraplegia, 11:310, 1974.

45. Dollfus, P., Holderbach, G. L., Husser, J. M., and Jacob-Chia, D.: Must appendicitis be still considered as a rare complication in paraplegia? Paraplegia, 11:306, 1974.

46. Perkash, I.: Neuromuscular disorders of the bladder. In Friedland, G. W., Filly, R., Govis, M. L., Gross, D., Kempson, R. L., Korobkin, M., Thurber, B. D., and Walter, J.:Uroradiology—An Integrated Approach. London, Churchill Livingstone, 1983, pp. 1291–1316.

39

Rehabilitation of Children with Brain Damage

DANIEL HALPERN

The results of brain injury in children are classified as prenatal, perinatal, or postnatal, depending on the age at injury.[1–3] Table 39–1 illustrates the most common etiological factors in each of the important life periods of children.

In the prenatal period, athetosis, which 30 years ago was seen most commonly in the child of an Rh-negative mother, now occurs mainly as a result of prolonged moderate perinatal hypoxia in the mature neonate. As the anoxic process increases in severity, spasticity becomes more prominent. The election of cesarean section to avoid difficult vaginal extractions has reduced the incidence of perinatal anoxic spasticity and traumatic hemiplegia. Biologically active chemicals in the maternal environment are becoming recognized with increasing frequency as a cause of fetal brain injury. Drugs such as alcohol and tobacco, as well as narcotics, have been shown to contribute to fetal incompetence, underdevelopment, and respiratory distress as well as to structural abnormalities. To what extent other mood-altering compounds impair fetal metabolism remains to be defined. Prenatal factors causing prematurity are associated with intracranial hemorrhage and play a significant role in the causation of spastic diplegia.[4] Low birth weight and prematurity continue to represent significant risk factors for brain damage. Maternal malnutrition has been associated with mental subnormality, but no clear relationship has been established between this and brain damage giving rise to motor defects.

In the perinatal period,[5] accidents of the birth process—prolapsing cord, placenta previa, abruptio placentae—remain prominent as causes of acute brain damage. Changes in obstetrical practices have diminished the incidence of traumatic hemiplegia. Changes in the use of maternal sedation have reduced the anoxic damage resulting from respiratory obtundation. The development of sophisticated intensive care systems in newborn nurseries has increased the number of infants surviving prematurity, neonatal respiratory distress syndrome, and other congenital and perinatal abnormalities.[1–3]

Postnatally, bacterial or viral infections, trauma, asphyxia, drownings,[6] and gunshot wounds are causes of childhood brain damage. About one million children each year are injured in automobile accidents. A significant number of these suffer head injury with permanent residual deficits.[7, 8] Many injuries would be totally preventable by use of appropriate seating restraints in motor vehicles and preventive measures against poisoning, falls, and other dangerous impulsive behaviors in children. A recently emphasized hazard is brain damage due to trauma at the hands of parents or other adults in whose care the children are placed. In the rehabilitation of these children, the battered child needs to be identified in order to make appropriate decisions with regard to placement, parental support services, and education that will prevent further injury of the child and siblings.

The purpose of rehabilitation of children with central nervous system impairment is (1) to identify, develop, and train to the optimal level those abilities of which the child is capable and (2) to define the conditions of management under which the child is able to function optimally. This requires an assessment, in the child, of abilities and disabilities of motor function, behavior, receptive and expressive communication, and cognition; and, in

833

TABLE 39–1. Etiology of Brain Damage in Children

PRENATAL	PERINATAL	POSTNATAL
Hereditary	Anoxia	Trauma
Genetically transmitted and present at birth or soon after, e.g., hereditary athetosis, familial tremors, neurological disorders, dermatological syndromes	Mechanical respiratory obstruction	Falls, motor vehicles, gunshot, abuse
	Respiratory distress syndrome	Infections
	Placenta previa	Acute; meningitis, encephalitis (viral or bacterial), thrombophlebitis
	Prolapsed cord	Chronic: brain abscess, bacterial, granuloma, tuberculosis, mycotic-fungal, lues
Acquired *in utero*	Maternal anoxia or hypotension	
Gonadal irradiation	Breech delivery with delayed aftercoming head	
Chromosomal defects	Cerebral hemorrhage	Vascular
Prenatal infections: toxoplasmosis, rubella, lues, or other maternal infections	Trauma: dystocia, obstetrical	Anomalies (with or without hemorrhage): arterial aneurysms, venous aneurysms, malformations, wall dysplasia
	Following anoxia	
Developmental anomalies: meningomyelocele, hydrocephalus, CNS malformation	Constitutional factors	
	Prematurity	Embolus
	Hyperinsulinism	Thrombosis
Prenatal anoxia: maternal anoxia or trauma, anemia, hypertension, placental abnormalities (abruptio, infarcts)	Anemia of newborn	Allergies: vascular occlusion
	Hypoprothrombinemia	Anoxia
		Carbon monoxide poisoning
Chemical toxicity: alcohol, tobacco, prescribed psychoactive drugs and nonprescribed medications, dysmaturity in diabetic mothers		Drowning, food aspiration, croup, and other respiratory obstructions
		Unexplained respiratory arrest (Ondine's "curse")
Prenatal cerebral hemorrhage		Inflammatory-immunological
Toxemia of pregnancy		Lupus erythematosus
Vascular anomalies		Periarteritis nodosa
Maternal bleeding diathesis		Reye's syndrome
Trauma		Toxic
Rh factor		Environmental pollutants
Metabolic disturbances		Lead, other heavy metals
		Organic pollutants
		Maternal drugs or medication
		Metabolic
		Hyperinsulinism
		Electrolyte imbalance
		Post-neoplastic

the community, of family and home resources and needs, schooling facilities, and residential or respite resources.

The Handicapped Child as a Special Person

Intervention for the purpose of habilitation or rehabilitation implies the concept that it is possible to modify the responsiveness of a child with brain damage in a manner that is analogous to that in the normal child. There is much evidence that the developing central nervous system of the child with brain damage has potential for acquiring new responses to stimulation. Van Hof[9] has reviewed the hypothesis that recovery from brain damage in young individuals is better than that in adults. Although there has been wide acceptance as well as experimental support of this concept, he points out that it is still debatable. At the same time, Greenough and co-workers[10] and Yu[11] report that individuals with brain damage show recovery of some functions through environmental modification and experience.

Children have incomplete neuroanatomical structures and neurophysiological processes. The growth of structures is still proceeding. The child is experiencing a broad variety of learning episodes. The child still has not developed learned responses to a large number of experiences and therefore is open to new or different approaches to situations and problems, provided that enough appropriate neural tissue is available. In addition, environmental management to augment learning is easier to provide for the child than it is for the adult.

Neurophysiological Organization of Motor Function

Motor activities are hierarchically organized in the central nervous system. This does not mean, however, that higher levels simply dominate lower levels. The spinal cord, mid-brain, cerebellum, basal ganglia, and cerebral cortex each contribute characteristic motor functions. Each level provides a specific quality of motor organization and responsiveness to the total motor activity. Dysfunction of each level contributes its own special qualities to the abnormality of function that is seen clinically. The clinical manifestations of dysfunction are the result of distortions, deficiencies, and excesses of motor and sensory-motor activities, and the effects of altered experience to modify functional performance. Damage to motor centers or pathways may cause impairment or loss of motor function on the one hand or loss of inhibition or modulation of activities of the residual central nervous system on the other. Sensory performance may be impaired by damage to pathways necessary for reception, perception, processing, or conceptualization. Deficiencies in these functions interfere with motor learning and guidance of coordination. The actual level of functional performance achieved depends on the opportunities for repetition of each motor activity under conscious perception. Each multimuscular activity in the repertory of coordination must be developed by this repetitive practicing. Finally, the attitude and expectations resulting from past experiences determine the willingness of the patient to participate in the learning process, whereas the attitudes and behaviors of family members, peers, and professionals establish the rewarding or nonrewarding social environment in which the patient must work.

Spinal Cord Activity

Independent activity of the spinal cord is characterized by reflex responses to somesthetic stimuli. These responses are based primarily on the muscle spindle stretch-sensitive reflexes, modified by the gamma motor system.[12] A discussion of the spinal and supraspinal reflexes is presented in Chapter 11, page 234.

Clinically, these reflexes are manifested by increased muscle tone or hypertonia. The primary Ia annulospiral fibers respond to rapid stretch with a quick and brief contraction—the myotatic reflex. Animal models indicate that the secondary sensory endings show a prolonged discharge in response to elongation resulting in a persistent contraction, which increases in intensity with stretch. As a result, the muscle shortens progressively, giving rise to persistent contractures with functional shortening of the limb. The flexor musculature is involved preferentially. These two responses taken together constitute the typical patterns of behavior of dynamic and static *spasticity*.

The cutaneous stimuli of touch and pain may directly influence the activity of the anterior horn cells to increase the hypertonia independently of muscle spindles and also, by increasing the activity of the gamma motor system, both to introduce an element of dystonia and to increase muscle spindle spasticity. The Golgi tendon organs inhibit alpha and gamma motor neuron activity and decrease muscular tension. The spinal reflex patterns produced by the long spinal, the crossed extensor-flexor, the extensor thrust, and the Marie-Foix reflexes possess the essential connections to enable the child to carry out effective reciprocation required for quadruped walking. However, the spinal cord does not possess the capacity to integrate these reflexes into an effective walking pattern because it lacks purposeful regulation to achieve balance, equilibrium, and progression. A center with the capacity to initiate reciprocation and support has been reported in the mid-brain by Grillner.[13] Balance, adaptability, and purpose require control from a higher level.

The medulla and mid-brain are sites of centers coordinating reflex activities at a higher level of organization. The symmetrical and asymmetrical neck, tongue, and mouth reflexes and the axio-derotational and labyrinthine reflexes are mediated in the mid-brain, whereas those related to sucking and swallowing have centers at medullary levels. Therefore, these reflex activities may be elicited in response to somesthetic stimulation when there is no response to efforts at volitional movement. Thus, patients with cerebral pyramidal and extrapyramidal impairment may show reflex tongue protrusion and retraction, biting, or a hyperactive gag reflex but not have the ability to chew, manipulate food, or swallow in a coordinated way. Speech may be dysarthric as well. They also may show tonic neck reflexes but be unable to carry out an appropriate reaching effort if the head is

DANIEL HALPERN

restrained. The child with brain damage who manifests hyperactive deep tendon reflexes and generalized persistent flexor posture of all four extremities with inability to extend the neck is demonstrating reflex motor activity originating predominantly from the level of the spinal cord. Some residual volitional supraspinal control may be evident in the form of bowel and bladder continence or restricted stereotyped voluntary motions that utilize the spinal reflex patterns for limited functional purposes.

Mid-Brain Activity—Decerebrate Motor Activity

The vestibular system contributes to extensor dystonia or rigidity owing to uninhibited responsiveness of anterior horn cells to medial vestibular nuclear activity and exaggeration of spasticity by facilitation of muscle spindles through the lateral vestibular nucleus.[14] The patient showing extensor thrust, an opisthotonic posture, and all four limbs held in extension, internal rotation, and adduction shows exaggeration of spindle reflexes by vestibular reflex activity because cerebral and cerebellar brain stem inhibition is deficient. In most patients, therefore, head position and acceleration are not significant contributing elements to the dystonia and spasticity. It is proposed that in these patients, there is failure of inhibition of the response of anterior horn cells to usual vestibular nuclear activity. In those patients who show changes of tone with changes in head orientation, there is loss of inhibition of the vestibular nuclei to postural changes. This response is mediated by activity of the cerebellar vermis. It is conceivable that electrical stimulation of the cerebellum, when it is effective, activates this inhibition.

In patients with lesions in which the functional control of motor activity is essentially at the level of the mid-brain, the extensor dystonia is the characteristic decerebrate posture. Failure of cerebral inhibition of reflexes mediated through the brain stem gives rise to excessive responsiveness to tactile, auditory, visual, or vestibular stimuli. As a result of an uninhibited reticular activating system, startle responses are frequently exaggerated, with a generalized over-response to stimulation. On the other hand, patients with lesions in the reticular activating system show lethargy and impaired responsiveness.

CEREBELLAR REGULATION

The cerebellum[15] contributes elements of control and coordination in terms of force, direction, and distance. The number of motor units contracting in a unit period of time determines the force or speed. The muscles acting synergistically determine the direction; and the length of time they each contract determines the distance. Present concepts regard this control system to be effected by preprogrammed activity.[16] The program has been determined through prior experience and is engaged primarily in the execution of rapid, skilled, volitional, and automatic activities in which feedback is not useful because of the speed of the motion.

Impairment of cerebellar function or interruption of cerebellar pathways to and from the rest of the central nervous system results in dysmetria, dyssynergia, and decomposition of movement. Intention tremor results during attempts to carry out purposeful motions. Taken together, these abnormalities constitute the symptom complex of ataxia. The patient is unable to carry out effective, rapid, accurate, smoothly coordinated or automatic movements or to maintain a stabilized posture.

BASAL GANGLIA

The function of the basal ganglia is to participate in the elaboration of volitional motor activities by organizing current and anticipated support for ongoing activity. Jung and Hassler[17] refer to the activities as ereismatic, referring to postural support for current activity and telekinesis for anticipated activity. Kornhuber[16] and DeLong and Apostolos[18] have shown that the basal ganglia participate in the generation of accurate ramplike motions in which feedback is utilized for positional control. These activities are produced by integration, modulation, and inhibition of selected subordinate reflex motor patterns.

Impairment of function in the basal ganglia, therefore, results in failure of inhibition of reflex patterns of motor activity, and especially impaired performance of automatic postural activity. The patient presents with varying degrees of increased motor tone and uncontrolled inaccurate movements. The increased motor tone is called dystonia. The excessive motion is described as chorea. Together the increased tone and motion may be regarded as dyskinesia. A progression in the clinical spectrum of dyskinesia may be viewed as either nonvoluntary or volition-related activity. *Ballism* is a grossly flailing movement in which the whole limb or side of the body is flung into violent activity. There is no persistent motor tone, and the movements appear to be spontaneous and nonvolitional. This type of movement is not seen in children with brain damage but is seen in adults with damage to the corpus Luysi. *Chorea* consists of flailing or jerky motions of segments of the extremities. There is considerable motion but very little persistent tone. The movements typically are nonvoluntary and are usually seen in Sydenham's or Huntington's chorea. *Choreiform movements* consist of flailing or jerky motions of the limbs, abnormal postures of the head, and facial grimaces that occur during attempts at voluntary movement, on generalized activity, or in response to emotional stimulation because of impaired capacity for inhibition. They are characterized by rapid movements of relatively small range but frequent occurrence and the absence of more than minimal levels of increased persistent tone. *Athetosis* consists of distortions of volition, producing motions that have often been described as writhing, twisting, or wormlike. There is moderate tension and the motions are limited in range. These motions are initiated by voluntary effort or by reflex stimulation. On examination, movement patterns can be recognized as partial or complete expressions of lower level reflexes that have occurred because of inadequate inhibition. *Dystonia* consists of spontaneous motion through a very limited range with a high degree of persistent tone during attempted voluntary activity. Dystonia is characterized by severe co-contraction of antagonistic muscles. The patients often go through severe contortions and gyrations exerting strong motor activity and frequently involving many muscles of the face, head, neck, trunk, and all four extremities. *Rigidity* is the result of constant co-contraction of antagonist muscles. Motion is absent or minimal. The tone is so great that the body part is fixed in position.

MOTOR AND PRE-MOTOR CORTEX

The motor and pre-motor cortex play an important part in the initiation and organization of complex skilled motor activities.[19] They contribute to the adaptability, deftness, complexity, and rapidity that is observed in well-learned motor behaviors in a normal individual. These characteristics of coordination may be encompassed in the general concept of praxis. An individual with a deficiency in the integrated functions of motor activity is regarded as dyspraxic or apraxic.

Dyspraxia is the impairment of ability to perform *learned*, complex voluntary movements. Dyspraxia may be expressed at different levels of complexity. Kinetic or motor dyspraxia represents impaired ability to execute appropriate motor patterns and sequences of muscular activity. Constructional dyspraxia refers to impaired ability to execute manipulative tasks guided by visual or spatial information. Ideomotor dyspraxia describes difficulty in applying motor activity in appropriate functional context. Ideational dyspraxia is an impaired ability to carry out purposeful motor activity in appropriate symbolic context.

Damage to the motor and pre-motor cortex is characterized, therefore, by loss of specific components of the repertory, related to the specific localization of the lesion and proportional to the amount of brain tissue involved. The quality described by Hughlings Jackson as "poverty of movement," or stereotypy, is a major characteristic of cerebral cortical damage.

The stereotyped motor patterns represent an inability to select appropriate muscle groups to carry out motor activity and also to modulate or inhibit synergic patterns generated by lower levels of the central nervous system hierarchy. A familiar example is the flexion of the elbow that occurs during the attempt of a patient with hemiplegia to abduct the shoulder. Another example is the stiffly maintained angle of knee flexion during ambulation, representing inability to coordinate hip extension on the stance leg with knee extension on the swinging leg.

Classification of Motor Symptoms

Understanding of the role of the hierarchical organization of the central nervous system and the integration of motor activity provides for the classification of individuals with brain damage on the basis of clinical features. The motor disability associated with continuing dysfunction occurring in the developmental phase of brain growth is called cerebral palsy. The current classification of motor disorders in cerebral palsy is generally accepted based on the clinical features of the motor impairment of children with brain damage (Table 39–2).

Evaluation of the Child with Brain Dysfunction

The physiatric evaluation of the child with brain dysfunction should include an assessment of the

TABLE 39–2. Clinical Features of Motor Impairment in Brain-Damaged Children

Spasticity	Athetosis
Monoplegia	Nontension
Hemiplegia	Tension
Paraplegia	Choreoathetosis
Diplegia	Dystonic
Quadriplegia	Tremor
Rigidity	Mixed
Ataxia	

capabilities of the child to respond either to stimuli or to instruction. One also needs to differentiate between the ability to respond and the willingness to do so. It is also necessary to distinguish between the failure to respond because motor ability is impaired and the failure to respond because more general systemic or behavioral defects are present. Table 39–3 illustrates the elements to be considered in any evaluation of a child's abilities.

The evaluation of the motor activity of a child with brain injury should correspond to the basic concepts of motor organization that have been outlined in the preceding. *The movements and postures that the individual can achieve constitute the motor repertory, which provides a basis for the prescription of a training program.* The essential characteristic of the motor repertory is that it describes the motor activities of the child and of each of the component limbs in functional terms. The therapeutic program is based on this analysis as it correlates with developmental expectations.

The normal sequence of motor development provides a general guide for the acquisition of new patterns of movement and posture for children with normal systems of motor control. A thorough knowledge of normal motor development is essential in order to make an accurate evaluation. Excellent reviews of this subject are provided by Gesell and Amatruda,[20] Illingworth,[21] and Lowrey.[22] Assessment of motor function in a child should include the history of the age at which key

TABLE 39–3. States Influencing Responsiveness

State of Consciousness
Obtunded consciousness
  Coma, stupor, confusion
  Seizure activity
Hypoactive states
  Somnolence
  Lethargy
  Fatigue
  Febrile or metabolic illness
Hyperactive states
  Mania
  Hyperkinesis
  Hyperirritability
Seizure activity

Sensory and Perceptual Ability
Blindness or impaired visual acuity
Deafness or impaired auditory acuity
Impaired pain perception
Visual-perceptual defects
Language-receptive deficit or auditory imperception
Impaired kinesthesis—touch, proprioception

Cognitive Ability
Situation comprehension
Deficient symbolization
  Passive manipulation
  Gestures
  Verbal impairment

Attentiveness
Ability to orient to significant stimuli
Maintain focus on significant elements
Distractibility
Impulsivity
Stimulus-bound behavior

Affective States
Separation apathy or anxiety
Dejection
Hostility
Rapport
Psychiatric states
  Thought disturbance
  Autism
  Depression
Rigidity to change—novelty rejection
Paucity of rewards or reinforcers

Behavioral Background
Inconsistent discipline
  Nonreinforcement of responding—habituation
  Reinforcement of nonresponding
Promotion of dependency, passivity
Promotion of inattention
Suppression of initiative

Motivation
Inner direction—rejection of external influence
Cooperation
Energy level
Interest level in activities presented
  Previous background
  Rapport
  Value system
  Behavioral drives
  Available reinforcers
Novelty effect
  Positive
  Negative
Rapport—acceptance of nonfamiliar staff personnel

Motor Activity

milestones of function were achieved. The motor developmental history also provides a screening technique to alert the examiner to the existence of a problem. However, it should not be considered to be a rigid track through which each child must pass regardless of the nature and location of the disturbance in the central nervous system. Evaluation of the motor repertory will identify the motor abilities and deficiencies in terms consistent with the neurophysiological diagnosis.

Considerable confusion has been engendered by the manner in which the evaluation of development of function has been used in the assessment and planning of motor training. The motor capacity of a normal child is the result of the biological changes that occur together with the experiential exposure. It is important to distinguish, therefore, between deficits in achievement of motor activities that are the consequence of the injury or dysfunction of specific structures within the central nervous system that control specific types of motor activity; and the failure to develop these activities because of lack of the experiences necessary to establish the appropriate neuronal connections through a learning-developmental process. As an extreme example, it would be inappropriate to consider an adult hemiplegic patient developmentally delayed because the upper extremity is flexed at the elbow, wrist, and fingers, and the thumb is adducted, even though this posture resembles that of a newborn infant. A child who has had an acquired brain injury and shows the same pattern should also be recognized as an individual whose central motor control system is creating these postures. Somewhat more confusing is the child who, as the result of an injury to the cerebellar pathway, has ataxia and does not stand. Lack of standing balance results from the ataxia rather than inability to develop the motor coordination for balance and walking because of "developmental delay."

The developmental sequence in a child with central nervous system damage and dysfunction may differ from that of the child with an intact central nervous system. As an example, it should not be expected that children with hemiparesis will learn to crawl on hands and knees before they learn to stand and walk. The creeping position is much too difficult to assume because of the paralyzed upper extremity, which cannot be extended to provide appropriate support and security. In fact, children with hemiplegia may find that ambulation on their feet is easier after they achieve the coordination necessary for balancing, since the extensor spasticity of the lower extremity assists in providing support. It would be a mistake to restrain these children from walking or to attempt to train them first to creep on hands and knees because they have not followed the "normal" pattern of creeping before walking.

The motor repertory of a child is evaluated by observing the child's posture and movements as they occur spontaneously, in response to verbal or nonverbal instructions, in response to placement in various positions, and in response to the applications of somesthetic stimulation.

VOLUNTARY ACTIVITY

Study of the most recent neurophysiology, as well as clinical observation, indicates that there are three aspects of organization of voluntary motion that require evaluation for the purpose of designing a relevant motor training program. As indicated, contributions to motor organization along these lines are made by the motor cortex, the supplementary motor cortex in the pre-motor frontal area, and, to some extent, the prefrontal cortex, when the elements of purposiveness and functional meaning of a movement are concerned. The basal ganglia, too, have an important role, but it is less well defined.

Specific versus Stereotyped Movement. In observing voluntary activity, the degree to which individuals demonstrate the freedom from or rigidity of association with undesired movements, i.e., stereotyping, must be evaluated. A child with a hemiplegia, for instance, may have difficulty in flexing the elbow without abducting the shoulder or vice versa. The child may have difficulty in extending the hip without excessive adduction and internal rotation. The ability to carry out a specific and precise individual motion at will is an important indicator of the specificity of control and of the range of motor potential for that individual. The greater the stereotyping of function, the fewer are the possibilities for the acquisition of complex gross or fine motor coordination and speed. The normal child, of course, follows a developmental sequence in this regard, progressing from a reach with palmar grasp and the ulnar aspect of the hand down toward the working surface at six months to pronation of the hand with palmar grasp at eight months and eventual radial grasp with pinch and finger prehension at nine to ten months of age. The hemiplegic or quadriplegic child with pronator dystonia is exhibiting stereotypy with limited specific control, and not precocious maturation. Separate individual finger motions for the purpose of complex manipulations may not be acquired until three to four years of age. This specificity develops through practice by learning to inhibit the undesired components of the stereotyped patterns.

Conscious versus Automatic Coordination. The degree to which each motion is carried out by conscious volitional planning or by automatic engrams should also be observed. Automatic engrams are the result of well-established learning and reflect the ability to execute motor activity at a skilled level that does not require the direct attention of the individual once the motion is set into progress. If the central nervous system has never developed the capacity to carry out skilled motor activity at an automatic level, as in many athetoid patients, then it can be carried out only under direct attention. This mode of control is, necessarily, slower; and the number of activities that can be monitored at any time is limited. Prolonged correct practice is essential to develop automatic mechanisms. With continued training, the acquisition of automaticity can be achieved *if the structural substrate for those motions is available.* An assessment of the degree to which such automaticity has been achieved with similar motions or postures can, therefore, give the examiner an idea of the degree to which automaticity training is possible in a proposed skill sequence. As an example, the maintenance of head posture is normally achieved at an early age, and the lack of automaticity is generally a sign of serious impairment of this function. At the same time, it is possible, although unusual, to find individuals who have the ability to either stand or sit in the erect posture without being able to maintain head position, which indicates that lack of head control is not a generalized impairment of balance but that there are specific elements relating to control of individual segments of the body.

Postural Adjustment versus Prime Movers. The third aspect of voluntary motor control to be evaluated is whether the impairment is in the components of postural support or in the control of the prime movers. Whereas individual motions occur utilizing specific or regional muscle groups, the effort may be ineffective because postural activity may be deficient. Similarly, postural coordination may be adequate but voluntary precise activity of those muscles may be impaired when the patient attempts to use them as prime movers. An example of this is the presence of a good extensor support reaction when a patient is placed upright in the standing position, but there is difficulty in getting good reciprocation for stair-climbing because voluntary extension of the hip and knee is inadequate. This difference occurs because reflex mechanisms that are initiated in the support reaction cannot be appropriately inhibited to allow reciprocation or because specific volitional hip extensor activity, which is required for walking or climbing stairs, is not yet available to the child. The decisions for the training program offer the alternatives of exercises to improve the deficient aspects of function, substitution for deficiencies, or recognition that the disability is so great that improvement cannot occur.

Posture and maintenance of position require endurance. Active translational motions should be trained by repetitive motions involving action of the prime and synergic movers. Sensory reinforcement improves motor control. As the characteristic abilities of the voluntary motor activity are identified in each limb, the priorities for the therapeutic program are established.

INVOLUNTARY ACTIVITY

Involuntary activity is the result of uninhibited reflex activity of a simple or complex nature. The degree to which this reflex activity can be modulated is an essential element in the determination of the therapeutic program. The specific reflexes to be observed are discussed in Chapter 11. As a normal individual matures, the reflex activities of the spinal cord, medulla, and mid-brain are integrated into the normal activity and appear as discrete reflex patterns as a rule only during severe exertion when the reflex acts as a facilitating mechanism. Under normal conditions, these reflexes are not apparent, although it is obvious that they are still present within the central nervous system as organized circuits, since they appear clinically when higher-level central nervous system structures are damaged in later life.

Facultative versus Obligatory. Reflexes are considered obligatory if they occur consistently when the appropriate stimulation is applied. They are considered facultative if they occur weakly, intermittently, or inconsistently in response to stimulation or if they can be inhibited by voluntary or automatic activity of the individual. In the rehabilitative program, patients are trained to inhibit excessive tone or excessive reflex activity. Medications like diazepam, baclofen, or dantrolene may be helpful. When uninhibited motor activity is obligatory, intramuscular neurolysis may be useful as a temporary measure to assess the possibilities for learning of inhibition. Tendon lengthening and tendon transfers are effective procedures to decrease sensitivity of the muscle spindle stretch-sensitive endings to reduce obligatory spasticity.

MOTOR CONTROL

The control of accuracy of use of each prime mover muscle needs to be evaluated. Defects in this function are referred to as dysmetria.

Force. Inaccuracy of force giving rise either to dystonia or to abnormal undesired velocity of movement is referred to as dyssynergia. Excessive motor unit activity gives rise to excessive velocity and force of movement.

Synergia. If the prime movers are opposed by co-contraction of antagonistic muscles, this produces dystonic movements. The force is controlled by the temporal organization of the contractions of individual motor units within a muscle. Impairment of the ability to synchronize or desynchronize motor unit contractions, therefore, gives rise to hypotonia, dyssynergia, or dystonia. Impairment of coordination of synergic muscle groups and inhibition of antagonistic muscle groups with the desired motion constitute another aspect of dyssynergia.

Direction. Another component of motor coordination is that of direction, which requires the coordinated contraction of a number of muscles at a specified velocity for a specific period of time to ultimately achieve the desired position. The ability to reach a desired position by the most efficient route requires the coordination of several muscles in an organized correlation of strength and time. A defect in this function produces the clinical picture of ataxia.

Evaluation of Motor Activity

The evaluation of a child's motor activity is carried out topographically. The response of head control in the supine, prone, and sitting positions is observed both in stable positions and during changes of posture. The responses to tilting and to traction on the upper extremities and the closeness of correlation between head raising and lower extremity and upper extremity positions are observed. The characteristics of head responses at the critical developmental ages are well defined, and correlation between age and level of function will give an idea of the severity of involvement. It is helpful to quantify observations by specifying the angle of tilt of the body in each direction that can be applied while the head is held upright. If the head falls, it should be assisted to the erect position, and the length of time the head is held upright when assistance is removed should be observed. In the supine position when the arms are pulled, does the head come with the body, precede, or lag? If the head maintains a linear relationship with the trunk, is this a response to tilt or a function of overall rigidity?

In the recumbent position, the positions of the head, the upper and lower extremities, the spine, and the pelvis are noted. The presence of the ability to roll over either from supine to prone or prone to supine spontaneously or with the facilitation of the body-on-body or head-on-body reflexes is observed. While the child is in the recumbent position, it is useful to look for tonic neck reflexes, either symmetrical or asymmetrical, in response to movement of the head. The symmetrical tonic neck reflexes are observed best in the lateral recumbent position, since the head can be flexed or extended without stimulating vestibular responses, which can overshadow the tonic neck reflexes. Changes in tone of the biceps and triceps may be the most sensitive indicators of persistent tonic reflexes.

Sitting posture is observed in the stable, supported short sitting position, tailor sitting position, and long sitting position. The degree to which sitting posture can be maintained independently by appropriately controlled trunk movements in the anterior, posterior, and lateral directions and the degree to which the upper and lower extremities carry out protective extension and compensatory equilibrium reactions are observed.

In the upright position, the posture of the lower extremities, back, and head is noted both in response to the suspended upright position and during standing. In the suspended upright position, the presence of excessive hip and knee extension and scissoring is indicative of abnormality, as is persistent hip or knee flexion after four months of age. In the weight-bearing position, the presence or absence of a support reaction adequate to maintain body weight is observed. Equinus of the feet or any deficiency in plantigrade foot posture is noted. Weakness of dorsiflexion also is significant. It is important to note whether the support reaction in the lower extremities is reflex or voluntary. When an adequate support reaction is present, are appropriate equilibrium responses available in the head, upper extremities, trunk, hips, and lower extremities? If equilibrium responses are not evident, can they be elicited either through facilitation or through verbal or nonverbal instruction? If adequate support and equilibrium responses are present, the performance of ambulation either with or without assistance is evaluated. While examining for reciprocation, assistance for balance may be given manually at the pelvis to aid a weak gluteus medius. Additional assistance may be given, if needed, for support of the trunk or chest. The requirements for ambulation are (1) support, (2) reciprocation, (3) dynamic equilibrium, (4) segmental coordination, and (5) gait sequence. Each of these components should be evaluated kinesiologically and the training program directed at improving deficiencies.

The function of the upper extremities can be subdivided into reach, grasp, manipulation, placement, and release. Palmar grasp may be ulnar or radial with or without shoulder rotation and forearm pronation or supination. Prehension requires finger and thumb coordination as three-finger pinch, two-finger opposed pinch, and two-finger lateral pinch.

A distinction must be made in the nature and degree of skill of reach and grasp, in impairments due to cerebral disconnection or injury, and in those of developmental delay. The developmentally delayed grasp is considered to be an ulnar type grasp, typical of the normal five- to six-month-old child. Between six and eight months of age, the radial grasp develops. However, the grasp of the child who has damage to the motor cortex is an excessively pronated grasp with weakness of supination.

The persistence of uninhibited reflexes is generally considered a prognostic sign indicating limited potential for motor learning.[23] Nevertheless, when voluntary movements are available or elicitable, they may be used as the basis for the establishment of a training program. Due regard without rigid adherence needs to be given to the level of motor achievement appropriate for age in order to establish appropriate goals.

Bracing and assistive devices may be used to provide support in the functional position if inadequate motor ability in a specific area interferes with functional performance. Thus, children with equinus as a result of a weak anterior tibialis muscle will do well with a dorsiflexion brace if they have the ability to balance the trunk, support weight at hips and knees, and reciprocate. Assistive devices like walkers, axillary or forearm crutches, or canes may also be used to assist balance as well as to provide support. Further assistance for support may be given by blocking the ankle joint of a short-leg brace at 80 degrees to prevent excessive dorsiflexion at the ankle and flexion of the knee. Occasionally a child may be helped by long-leg braces to learn to lock the knees in extension for support while practicing reciprocation and trunk balance. The knees can be unlocked for short periods of time to allow knee control to be practiced while providing the necessary assistance for balance. The basic principle here, as in any learning situation, is to *present a specific task to each child in an isolated form at the level of simplicity and intensity at which the child can succeed and then to increase the complexity, speed, and force as the child's ability to respond increases.*

Some children with poor support reactions have general hypoactivity and show a flexed posture at hips, knees, shoulders, and elbows. They are sluggish in their responsiveness, slow in movement, and have high arousal thresholds. They can be aided by providing a strongly stimulating milieu. Commands should be clear, loud, and rhythmic. Fairly loud, rhythmic music is often useful to provide general reticular system activation. Extensor activity is improved in this way. At the same time, noise and motion that interfere with the child's perception of training activities must be kept to a minimum. The fact that these children are hypoactive does not protect them against distractibility.

Motor Training

Therapeutic management is based on the determination of the level of functional ability represented in the motor repertory, in each of the topographical areas, together with an establishment of priorities for training the functional activities required to meet the patient's needs. As the more basic needs are met by learning improved skills, new goals may be added to the program. The modes of intervention are (1) training of improved motor function, (2) assistance of function by human or specialized devices, (3) substitution for function by specialized devices, (4) limitation of requirements by a modified environment, (5) training of substitute functions to compensate for a deficit, and (6) modification of anatomical or physiological abnormalities by surgical procedures or medication.[24]

Motor training procedures[25] should be carried out in an attitude simulating relaxed play and emphasized by voice, manner, behavior, and ap-

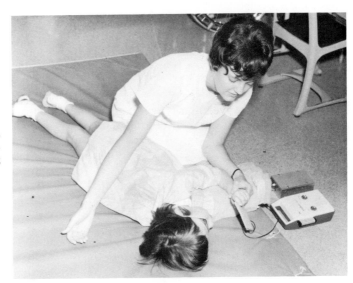

FIGURE 39–1. When the patient is positioned to remove all gravitational demands, she need not attend to body support or balance while concentrating on learning controlled pinch and grasp.

proach that encourage participation in and enjoyment of the activity. At the same time, sufficient structure should be present to ensure that the activity to be performed is clearly discriminated from the background by the child. The milieu should not be overwhelmingly distracting by auditory or visual noise. The activity should be inherently pleasant, attractive, and rewarding to the child. Precise observation of the performance needs to be made by the therapist for recording progress and by the child to recognize the degree of success with which each motion to be trained is being performed. The experience of numerous studies of learning of motor skill in normal adults as well as in handicapped individuals has shown that perception of motor response is important in the learning process.[26, 27] Proper structuring of the training situation will direct the child's attention to the details of each activity. When excessive motor tone is a significant element impairing motor control, volitional inhibition of dystonia—relaxation—should be taught. Techniques for inducing relaxation as advocated by Jacobson,[28] Rood,[29] or Bobath[30] may be used to make the relaxation available for the learning process.

The movements to be trained are selected by evaluation of the motor repertory. Those activities that are inadequate for function are identified, and priorities are set to develop to a more functional level the available but inadequate responses that can be elicited. The kinesiological components of the motion to be trained are then identified. Desynthesis consists of simplifying motions to the level of components that the child can control during each training session (Fig. 39–1). These motions are practiced repeatedly until control is precise and dependable. As precise control of performance of each component is developed, the individual components are combined or resynthesized into progressively more complex activities that gradually approximate the complete motion.

It is important for the child to see that these components are, in fact, useful subordinate units in the final motion. It may be necessary, with some children, to demonstrate this by introducing during a portion of the training session the synthesized motion with sufficient assistance to perform it correctly. One method of isolating a functional component in an activity is to provide assistance by bracing or supporting other components so that the child is able to concentrate on the desired motor component (Fig. 39–2).

The motion to be trained should be isolated under conditions that guarantee optimal attention. Accessory motor activity is allowed only when the motion to be trained is easily performed, automatic, or well learned. The isolation of an activity may be achieved by eliminating the need during training for any accessory motion by positioning the patient, providing assistance, manual manipulation, bracing, or requiring performance only of the single motions to be learned (Fig. 39–3). Progress is achieved by successively chaining components into a re-synthesis of the primary pattern and gradually re-introducing the necessary accessory motor activity, so that the complex functional usefulness is approached[31] (see Chapter 19).

Training of head control may be initiated by

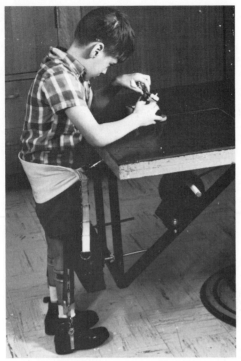

FIGURE 39–2. Minimizing extraneous demands aids in concentration on the assigned task. A short-leg brace, buttock sling, and blocking knee pad decrease demands for attention to support of the lower extremities while attending to a task that requires manual dexterity.

Adequate attention may then be focused on the activity of the hand (see Fig. 39–1). Such isolated activity will of course have limited value in the child's understanding unless it is also clearly related to the training goal of a useful functional activity.

Identify the role of each motor component in the synthesized movement as postural or translational. For postural movements, the training goal will usually be to increase the duration and stability of the motor activity. For the translational or prime mover activity, the criterion would involve accuracy and timing and, to a lesser degree, strength or speed.

Elicit the activity repetitively by

1. Instruction.

2. Carrying out the motion repeatedly in the course of a purposeful act. For instance, in order to extend the neck, the command to look up or to turn the head, "Look at Mommy," may be used.

3. Providing assistance to the motion with instructions to "Move this way," or "I'll help you," or "You help me." For instance, during ambulation training when emphasizing reciprocation and support, assistance may be given for balancing by

providing a wheelchair with adequate trunk support and stabilizing assistance for the head in the erect position (Figs. 39–4 to 39–6). The purpose of passive assistance is to accustom the child to the correct head posture during most of the time while sitting (Figs. 39–7 and 39–8). Short periods of active head control in response to a hinged head halter may then be introduced and carefully timed for endurance (Fig. 39–9).[32] Manual assistance is often necessary for cuing and guidance. As improvement occurs, rewarding auditory or visual feedback systems may be introduced[33] (Fig. 39–10). Stresses in the form of tilting and rocking may be utilized as head control develops to stimulate dynamic as well as static responses.

Upper extremity training may require stabilized posture in a wheelchair, splinting or manual assistance to isolate finger grasp from wrist control, and assistance in carrying or reaching while grasping is being practiced (Fig. 39–11). Another useful technique for practice of hand control is to have the patient recumbent on a mat or table. All postural requirements for the trunk, head, and shoulder are eliminated by appropriate support.

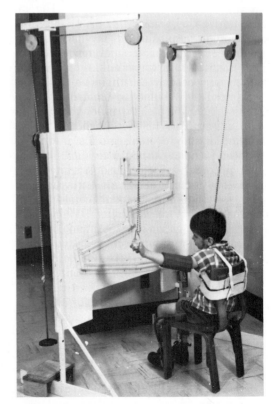

FIGURE 39–3. Assistance to maintain posture allows the patient to concentrate on exerting maximal effort for shoulder depressor activity.

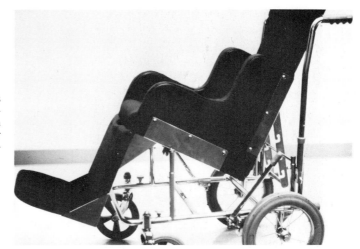

FIGURE 39–4. An adjustable tilting seat orthosis mounted on a Toronto wheel base provides corrected and comfortable support for a child with strong reflex flexion of the trunk and neck, or severe flaccidity with flexor or extensor preponderance.

supporting the child at the trochanters to prevent lateral loss of equilibrium, or by placing one hand on the stance hip and the other under the axilla on the swing side to support against the drop of the pelvis and loss of balance. The child thus learns to carry out an effective compensated Trendelenburg gait.

4. Inducing the activity by facilitation. Ankle dorsiflexion may be induced by exerting resistance against hip flexion (Bechterev's reflex). Head extension may be elicited by tipping the patient forward or by elevating the head and asking the patient to hold it that way. Vestibular stimulation to elicit upper extremity protective extension may be introduced by rolling the child lying prone over a ball or rolling log. Functional electrical stimulation is a useful modality for such motions as wrist extension or elbow extension, or in the lower extremity for hip abduction, hip extension, or knee extension.[34] Elastic bands around the thighs have been used to stimulate abduction. Brushing, icing, or other cutaneous stimulation has been used to facilitate the responses of the underlying muscles.[29] It is important that facilitation techniques elicit a

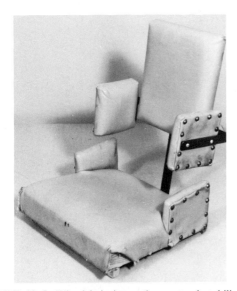

FIGURE 39–5. Wheelchair insert for postural stabilization. The anterior portion of the seat cushion is elevated 15° to 20° to flex the hips. In this way, extensor thrust is reflexly inhibited, and with gravity assisting, the patient remains seated well back in the chair. The upper side pads are adjustable to fit against the lateral thorax at heights corresponding to lateral spinal curves. The lower side pads are thick enough, and set-in to contact the trochanters, giving a three-point pressure system for support.

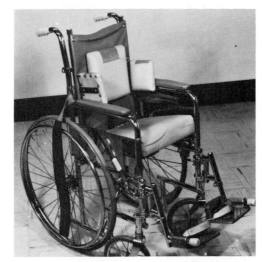

FIGURE 39–6. The wheelchair insert is relatively inexpensive and may be placed in the chair or removed as required for transportation.

DANIEL HALPERN

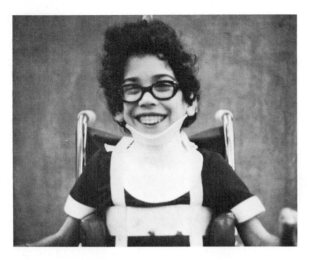

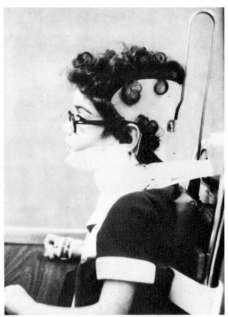

FIGURE 39–7. When a child is unable to sit erect and maintain posture, a molded fitted neck collar may be attached to the chair. Its use should be coordinated with training of volitional head control and should be removed as head balance develops.

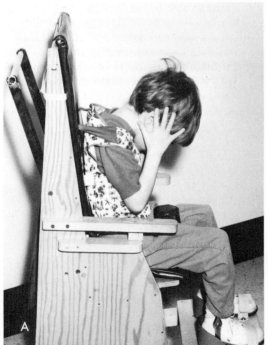

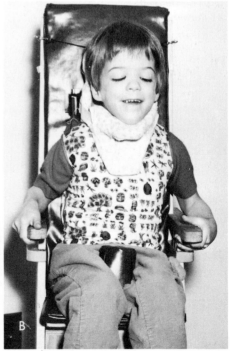

FIGURE 39–8. Phases of training of head control. *A*, Without assistance, the patient allows her head to fall and makes no effort to keep it vertical. *B*, With passive assistance she becomes accustomed to the vertical position as an acceptable one, and with appropriate reinforcement it becomes a desirable one.

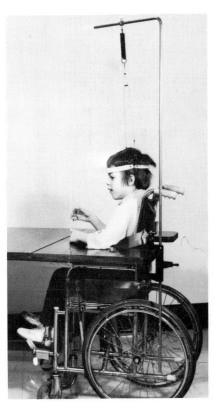

FIGURE 39–9. The hinged head halter provides some active assistance but primarily provides tactile cues regarding correctness of head position.

clear and identifiable activity. When this occurs, the child can participate actively and simultaneously, in attempting to repeat the muscular activity voluntarily, and eventually can perform without the facilitation. If the desired response is not elicited, other more effective techniques should be sought.

Participation should be reinforced by a reward that is *observed* to be effective (Fig. 39–12). In the beginning, this should be done regularly and immediately as the performance meets the minimal criteria. Reinforcement for *cooperation* is a separate issue and should be carried out independently. In some children in whom cooperation is a major issue, especially in the beginning of the training program, reinforcement should be used for any attempt at cooperation, beginning with simply allowing the trainer to manipulate the child. Reinforcement for cooperation may be necessary to achieve and maintain cooperation. However, cooperation in itself does not enhance learning of motor activity. The fact that cooperation fosters repetition is helpful, but the quality of the repetition is governed by careful application of reinforce-

ment or reward to elicit the correct performance of the specific motor activity. It is important, therefore, to set criteria within the ability of the child to succeed and gradually to increase the strictness of standards to be met as they become achievable.

Reinforcement serves also to direct attention to the specific motion and to the criteria for performance. By serving as a sensory feedback mechanism, it aids in developing the ability for self-monitoring. When carried out skillfully, the awareness of the quality of movement that develops becomes associated with the reward or reinforcement. A successful performance, therefore, begins to become rewarding in itself as the awareness of result of the motion becomes its own reinforcement.

With repetition and incorporation of the components of motion into functional, pleasurable, and inherently interesting activities, automaticity can develop as the praxic program becomes established as an engram.[31]

The achievement of criteria in a motor performance is the result of a learning process. Attention is an important element in learning of skilled movements. As learning occurs, automaticity develops through repetition. Automaticity is the result of a well-learned motor program.[27] With the development of automaticity, as the demands for conscious attention diminish, the ability to respond to multiple complex stimuli increases (see Fig. 39–11). Automaticity requires the development of its own neural circuits. If this potential is not present, automaticity will not develop. Not all individuals with brain damage are able to achieve normal levels of automatic motor activity. The achievement of a voluntarily directed motion under conscious attention is not always associated with the later development of automaticity, indicating that the neurocircuitry required for voluntary and for automatic motor activity is different.

Facilitative techniques such as effleurage, tapôtement, muscle percussion, vibration of a specific limb, body or head positioning, passive rocking, tilting, and elastic or nonflexible resistance may be used to assist training.

Functional electrical stimulation is an extremely effective modality for facilitation.[34] Its application requires careful reinforcement. It is best used by applying trains of direct or alternating current impulses simultaneously with voluntary efforts to contract. An instruction like "Help the machine" is useful with children who can understand. The amplitude of the stimulation is determined for *each* contraction by the level needed to achieve a con-

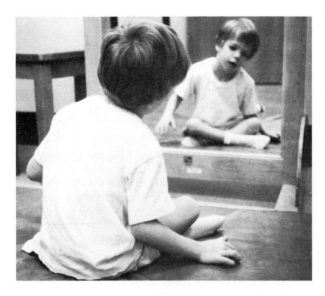

FIGURE 39–10. Visual information as a supplement to proprioception in a teaching format enables the child to progress to independent head posture.

traction. For this purpose, the therapist must have the control rheostat in hand *during* each contraction. Used in this way, there is automatic reinforcement. It is not unusual that in a single session, the amplitude required will decrease with repetition.

By the end of the session, minimal or no stimulation will be required, since the motion will be achieved almost entirely by voluntary effort alone. Nevertheless, by the next day, the procedure will have to be repeated, since long-term motor memory is often deficient in motor dyspraxia (see Chapter 16).

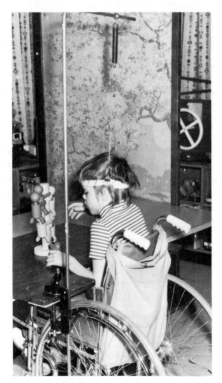

FIGURE 39–11. As ability to maintain an upright head is acquired, other tasks are introduced so that, by practice, automatic engrams of head control develop.

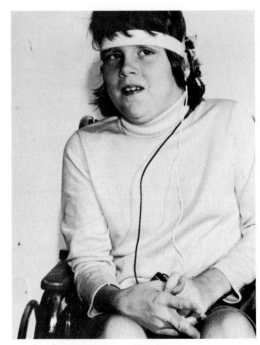

FIGURE 39–12. Mercury switches may be used to provide auditory cues, or music or television can be used as a reward to reinforce the maintenance of upright posture of the head.

These techniques of facilitation generate cutaneous, muscle spindle, kinesiological, or vestibular stimuli. They evoke reflex impulses that converge on anterior horn cells together with volitionally initiated impulses to exceed the excitatory threshold and produce a motor response. In addition, this type of sensory stimulation may also serve to direct attention to the limb being trained, thereby improving the ability of the child to monitor the activity and direct it.

Klein[26] and Keele[35] have shown that during the performance of a highly skilled task, learning and improvement of performance were better in those circumstances in which repetition and attention were higher. According to Klein, knowledge of the criteria of performance was also shown to enhance attention and, with it, to improve learning. See Chapter 19 for a more complete discussion of the training of coordination.

It has been a common observation that during the early teaching of a difficult task, a greatly increased motor tone occurs in patients with motor disorders (Fig. 39–13). In fact, the same thing occurs in normal individuals learning a difficult task, especially when under stress. For the child with brain damage, this uncontrolled motor activity becomes a problem that interferes with learning the desired motor performance. It has been interpreted to be the result of "cortical" participation. Neurophysiological studies, however, have shown that the motor cortex participates in the initiation of a learned motion, but once motion is initiated, activity in related neurons of the motor cortex disappears.[36] It does not follow, however, that learning is carried out best by nonparticipation of the cortex. To the contrary, the cortical neurons are essential to interact with the subcortical structures to produce the coordination pattern. The cortex is required for learning, and the work of Evarts indicates that cortical participation occurs during the initiation of well-learned activities. Pyramidal neurons tend to be continuously active during a motion only when the motion is still being learned. The increased tone occurring during training of motor activities in brain-damaged children is due to increased excitation or insufficient inhibition (Fig. 39–14). Excessive excitation may result from persistence of pre-existing response patterns, inappropriate training techniques, or a distracting milieu. It may also result from the child's efforts to please or the therapist's or parent's exhortation to "try harder." Ability to inhibit irradiation in the nervous system develops with practice, and increased tone represents irradiation that exceeds the capacity for inhibition.

When structure is provided in the therapeutic session to specifically reinforce inhibition of excessive tone and encourage active motion from a state of relaxation, maximal learning of motor skills occurs. Because automatic activities can be carried out without paying attention to them, some programs of training advocate repetition of activity without conscious attention. Studies of motor learning[26] indicate that this is counterproductive. From a practical point of view, it has not been shown to be possible to "eliminate the cortex" from participation in motor learning to develop automatic coordination. More to the point, however, is the concept that learning of a motor skill is more rapid and effective when (1) there is knowledge of criteria for performance; (2) there is knowledge of results; (3) there is active participation of the learner in the motor process; (4) the greater the attention to the criterion-result relationship, the more effective is the learning process; (5) there is massive repetition; and (6) the activity is sufficiently isolated from extraneous requirements to allow successful performance (see Fig. 39–1).

Instruction does not have to be communicated verbally if the child has poor language ability or is immature. By positive reinforcement and passive

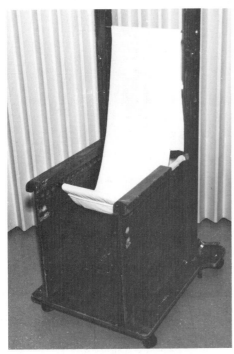

FIGURE 39–13. Special problems require adapted seating. A simple sling chair will prevent severe extensor thrust.

DANIEL HALPERN

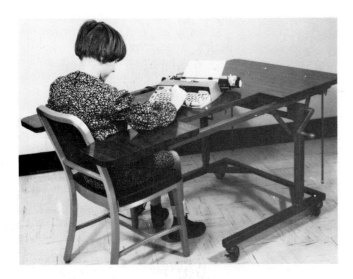

FIGURE 39–14. Even children with mild problems of balance during sitting need stability in order to learn upper extremity motor skills.

structural modeling of the child's activity, communication can be established and the learning process fostered.

Maintenance of musculoskeletal posture and mobility of children with cerebral palsy is essential to the training of control and the development of coordination (Fig. 39–15). The prevention of deformity by regular, careful range-of-motion exercises, stretching, timely orthopedic surgery,[37] and regular observation and accurate measurement is important in management. Intramuscular neurolysis[24] is a useful procedure to achieve muscular relaxation for six months to a year or more while awaiting surgery, or to evaluate the functional benefits that might occur following a surgical procedure to relieve tone. Serial casting is useful to correct recent contractures. Scoliosis may be treated or its advance delayed by the use of an appropriate spinal supportive orthosis. Prompt surgical fusion is extremely useful in preventing serious structural and postural deformity. Special attention should be paid to the hip joints in the presence of simultaneous spasticity of the hip adductor and flexor muscles or adductor and hamstring muscles. This spasticity contributes to early dislocation that may be aggravated by vigorous stretching procedures. Early adductor releases with prolonged night splinting in abduction is often effective in preventing dislocation of the hip. Weight-bearing in the quadruped position also is helpful if feasible.

Cognitive Function

Intellectual function requires synthesis into perception of the stimuli transmitted through the different sensory systems. This is then processed, analyzed, related to other information, and ultimately assigned a meaning to which some response is organized. In assessing cognitive function in children with brain damage, it is important, there-

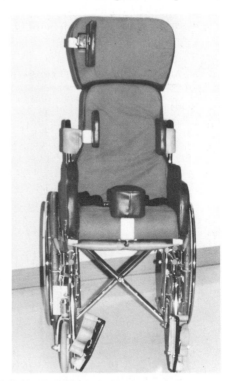

FIGURE 39–15. Difficult positioning problems occasioned by back deformities may be aided by a well-constructed fitted seating orthosis adapted to the needs of the individual child. The seat belt should always be attached at the level at which the seat meets the back of the chair.

fore, to attempt to define these cognitive processes in order to learn which intellectual systems are intact and which are disrupted. Certain tests of intellectual function place relatively strong requirements for performance on noncognitive functions such as behavior, attentiveness, inner drive or energy, and motor coordination. It is, therefore, desirable to identify those behavioral, attitudinal, attentional, and motor functions that are required for the comprehension of the task and for the execution of the response that is supposed to measure the cognitive function that is presumed to be tested.

The preferential processing of linguistic information in the left hemisphere and visual spatial information in the right hemisphere is well known, as is the important role of the corpus callosum for transmitting information between both hemispheres. Proprioceptive information is processed to a large extent in the posterolateral portion of the parietal lobes. As we learn more about the brain, subordinate functions are being localized to certain specific areas of the cortex.[38] It is helpful, when possible, to identify specific deficiencies, since a remedial program may be organized to take into account their influence on the functional capacity of the child. It is of less value to be able simply to identify a child by an averaged IQ level. The intelligence quotient may be useful, for administrative purposes, to place a child with brain damage in a school program. To organize an individualized educational program for a brain-damaged child, knowledge of the individual functional characteristics that affect learning ability in a specific educational area is necessary.

The major sensory areas in which cognitive functioning is mediated are auditory, visual, and somesthetic. Each has an expressive motor aspect as well as receptive aspects—verbal, visual-motor, and kinesthetic. Each may be considered to operate on three levels of abstractness versus concreteness. The most concrete level is that of sensory reception, e.g., hearing, seeing, and touch. A higher level of data processing is that of perception, in which characteristic patterns are identified or recognized: phonemes, sounds, or their combinations; forms, shapes, or designs; or specific body or limb movements. A still higher level of abstraction is reached when these perceptions take on meaning. They begin to be associated with patterns, perceptions, or concepts in other senses. A word becomes associated with a picture or an object; a movement signifies an emotional state or an instruction and becomes a gesture; or a series of standardized shapes on a piece of paper signifies a spoken word, an object or action, a quality, or an idea. Still higher levels of abstraction exist in the form of classification or symbolization.

Among the subordinate processes that have been recognized are those of visual perception—recognition and distinction of shapes and forms; identifying similarities and differences in orientation, shape, size, sequence, order, and spatial relationships; and discriminating a figure on a background. Each process individually contributes important modifications to meanings of visually presented material. A need for multiple tests arises from the fact that in practice, achievement on any of the test batteries and their subtests is influenced by a number of factors in addition to the one nominally being tested. In many cases these factors are not of primary interest in the actual cognitive assessment test, but they interfere with evaluation of significant functions. The problem lies in the fact that most neuropsychological tests are based on normative data, assuming that all children tested are basically similar, and differ only in their position on a bell-curve distribution. Individuals with brain damage, by definition, do not fit into this model, since the assumptions of global similarity are not valid. By a judicious selection of multiple test procedures, it is possible to deduce much information concerning the functional ability of the child in the school situation. It is then necessary to formulate these characteristics in terms that will be useful to the teachers in developing a remedial educational program, and to the therapy staff in selecting the most appropriate teaching methods for motor and perceptual-motor skills. The clinical neuropsychologist can make essential contributions to understanding cognitive processing by the brain-damaged child. The recognition of deficits in identifying or responding to these variables is important for establishing a remedial program.

Personality and Behavior

The child who has suffered brain damage may have distortions of perception of incidents and interpersonal events that carry profound implications for future development of personality and behavior. Damage to specific structures of the brain has been associated with abnormalities of behavior. The frontal lobe, anterior to areas 6 and 8, receives contributions from the dorsal medial nucleus of the thalamus, which conveys impulses from the hypothalamus. These areas are connected by the cingulum and uncinate fasciculus to the anterior portion of the temporal lobe and to parietal and adjacent occipital and temporal association areas. These connections make possible the association of emotional values with sensory or affective input. From experimental evidence it is proposed that this mechanism allows the recognition of events that have an emotional meaning.[39, 40] Rewards or punishments are conceived to be monitored by the hypothalamus and recorded for memory in the frontal cortex. Attention and responses are organized and triggered in the limbic system. Thus, the mechanisms are available for focusing attention on relevant and significant material for the improvement of function and memory with training.

In his review of animal experiments, Isaacson[41] demonstrated that destruction of specific areas in the limbic system gives rise to disorders of concentration affecting the ability to respond appropriately to problem-solving situations. The limbic system is composed of the cingulum, cingulate gyrus, hippocampus, septal nucleus, amygdala, nucleus accumbens, and hypothalamus. The locus ceruleus, mid-brain reticular system, and mid-brain tegmental nuclei are closely related structures. The forebrain structures, septal nucleus, hippocampus, and mid-brain structures are connected by the median forebrain bundle. Deficits in function differ depending on the specific localization of the lesion within the component structures of the limbic system. Laboratory studies[41] in animals have demonstrated that limbic system lesions result in the following abnormalities in behavior: (1) impairment of ability to withhold response to a stimulus, (2) increased activity level, (3) decreased attentive ability, (4) impaired ability to analyze problems systematically, (5) impulsivity, (6) perseveration, and (7) rigidity or resistance to change. Whereas evidence is still insufficient to correlate specific localization of lesions in humans with behavioral changes, these behavioral abnormalities are seen frequently in children with diffuse brain damage. Considerations of the behavioral alterations following limbic system lesions demonstrate that impairments of subordinate functions such as impulsivity or diminished attentive ability may manifest themselves by deficiency in higher cognitive functions.[42] Inability to withhold a response to a stimulus may manifest itself as a premature response to a question. Failure to observe that the response is incorrect because of impulsive behavior may

lead to the conclusion that the child lacks the cognitive information required.

Similarly, inability to attend sufficiently will interfere with the solution to a problem if the problem is presented in a manner that exceeds the duration of attention of the child. The substance of the problem may be satisfactorily managed if the material is presented more succinctly. Attentive ability is limited not only in relation to its duration but in relation to background stimulation. Tests sensitive to figure-background discrimination, either visual or auditory, are useful, therefore, as indices of attentive ability.

Perseveration is another form of responding to previous experience. The child responds to certain criteria given previously without noticing that the conditions may have changed or even refusing to recognize that the conditions have changed. If there is difficulty in recognizing changing conditions, this may provide a reason for responding incorrectly to a problem and may lead to incorrect conclusions concerning the child's ability to comprehend and solve problems. In a group of children with problems in school, the following behaviors were noted to relate closely to disorders of behavior seen in animals with limbic system lesions: tangential responses; distractibility; easy frustration; organizational deficits; visual, spatial, or temporal deficits; limitation of hypothesis formation; and impaired responses to internal cues.

There are conflicting views in the literature on whether deficits of attention represent organic brain damage, an affective disorder, or inadequate prior training. However, as in any other diagnostic exercise, the association of multiple behavioral manifestations of impaired ability to inhibit responses appropriately, a consistent demonstration of the impairment in different situations, and, in addition, signs of organic brain damage may be used as evidence to support an organic basis for the behavior. At the same time, it is necessary to eliminate the possibility of emotional or experiential bases. In practice, it is not unusual to find elements of all three etiological factors operating in the child with brain damage. Management then becomes the problem of dealing with each of the contributory elements in proportion to its significance in the individual child.

PRINCIPLES OF MANAGEMENT IN ATTENTION-DEFICIT DISORDERS

A structured training situation that is consistent in all areas is probably the one essential management technique that applies to attentional deficits of any cause. This structure requires careful establishment of criteria for tasks that provide challenge but are well within the capacity of the child. Distracting competitive stimuli—auditory, visual, social, and motivational—should be reduced to a level manageable by the child. The significant stimulus should be clearly discriminable from the background. There should be a guarantee of success in assigned tasks. This is made possible by a clear definition of the required response at a level at which the child will succeed. This may be done by passively moving the child through the required response, providing a problem-solving protocol to follow with reinforcers of sensory-motor cues as necessary to assure success, e.g., using a series of verbal cues to solve a picture puzzle when verbal skills are better than visual. Assistance is provided at junctures at which blocking occurs during a physical or problem-solving task, and the assistance is diminished as progress is made. A consistent, meaningful reinforcement schedule is provided for correct or successful activity. Monitoring of the effectiveness of the reward is necessary, since not all children respond to the same rewards equally, and satiation may occur. There must be consistent structure, reinforcement techniques and schedules, behavioral management, and disciplinary techniques by all disciplines cooperating in the management of the child. This should include the school teacher, occupational therapist, physical therapist, speech pathologist, nurse, parent, physician, social worker, psychologist, and any other person working with the child. This requires that the therapeutic procedures in physical therapy, occupational therapy, speech therapy, and the schoolroom be homogeneous and provide an appropriate milieu for learning.

Medications are useful for the child with deficits of attention of organic origin. Connors[43] has described a rating scale that is useful for some children with overt brain damage with hyperactivity. The criteria for observation of effects should be defined as precisely as possible. One or more target behaviors may be chosen and incidents counted in a unit period of time. *Ad hoc* rating scales constructed for individual children are preferable. Specific characteristic behaviors are identified and numerical as well as verbal values defined. Observations can be focused on one or two key items that are meaningful in the management plan for that child.

Useful medications have been dextroamphetamine, methylphenidate, amitriptyline, nortripty-line, and trifluperazine. To a lesser extent, the phenothiazines (chlorpromazine, promazine, thioridazine) and minor tranquilizers like hydroxyzine are useful for limited periods of time. Since it is difficult to predict which medications will be effective in any one child, it is useful to proceed with the idea of carrying out a consistent and sequential series of therapeutic trials. A range of dosage levels should be tried to be certain that the best effect with minimal side effects has been achieved. A small percentage of children respond well to one medication for a few months and then proceed to adapt. If the child is followed closely, this may be detected early and a change to another medication may be helpful. Parents need to be educated regarding the rationale for the use of medications. The precise criteria for effectiveness should be defined behaviorally in measureable terms, e.g., number of minutes without reminders on a specific task, number of distractions of gaze per five-minute period, number of impulsive or tangential responses per class hour. Clear distinctions should be made between these measures and "social tolerance," or "tolerable" level of hyperactivity—which are highly subjective measures. The aim of therapy is not to make the child less active, but to permit the child to focus his or her activity for better learning of cognitive as well as motor skills.

All behaviors exhibited by a child need to be recognized as a natural consequence of the interaction of the child with the adults who care for him or her and, later, the peers who are part of his or her environment. The actions of parents, like those of the professionals, depend on their own emotional, cognitive, and attitudinal backgrounds that they bring to the child. Most parents have had little training in child-rearing in general and no training in rearing a handicapped, brain-injured child. Their attempted support or protection often is inconvenient for professionals but does not deserve the epithets of "over-mothering" or "smothering." A realistic assessment of the origins of parental management styles should be included in the development of the program of management for the child.

MANAGEMENT OF EMOTIONAL AND MOTIVATIONAL FACTORS

The most common emotional stress that the brain-injured child experiences during treatment is that of being surrounded by unfamiliar personnel. The immediate involvement of the parents or other familiar adults during the treatment of the child is frequently useful in assisting the transition to the professional. It may be sufficient for the parent to stand by and approve. Some children may do better if the parent handles the child under the direction of the professional in the beginning. Gradual transition to the professional may then be allowed.

However, successful rehabilitation of children cannot be considered to be achieved until the care and handling of the child has been returned to the parents or surrogates. The parents need to be skilled in techniques of management, and the child should behave as well with them as with the therapist, nurse, or teacher. The emotional lability often seen in children with diffuse brain damage of the pseudobulbar type may be managed by maintaining a nonstressful pleasant atmosphere in the educational or therapeutic program. Adequate opportunity for recreation is essential in a management program to provide diversional as well as functional activity in a highly motivating milieu so that there is opportunity to utilize newly learned skills. Emotional problems deriving from interpersonal relationships, familial interactions, disturbances of attitudes, and perspectives secondary to past experience need to be identified and programs of management for retraining of the undesired behavior included in the overall rehabilitation program. Alteration of disturbing behaviors of family members is essential and, although difficult, should be undertaken. Verbal counseling is usually less effective than behavioral management for children. Adolescents and older children may be amenable to verbal mediation, in which case it is a useful adjunct but rarely a mainstay of the program of management.

Programs of Therapeutic Intervention

Since the early 1950s, a number of different schools of thought have developed differing approaches to the therapeutic management of children with brain damage. Each has claimed to be based on neurophysiological concepts selected from the literature to support that particular point of view. Reference has been made to some of these authors in the preceding pages where the ideas developed coincide with the basic approach presented here. Primarily, this approach is based on current concepts of learning theory. The child can change behavior only by a process of learning. The quantity and quality of learning is determined by

the structural and physiological integrity of the entire central nervous system (see Chapter 18). Therefore, an evaluation is required of the specific central nervous system functions that are available in the child for sensation, active participation, and repetitions of performance.[44, 45] If facilitation techniques make an activity available to a child by eliciting a motor response, then a learning process may take place, provided adequate cerebral volitional connections exist.

The reader is referred to discussions by Gillette,[46] Pearson and Williams,[47] and Harris[48] and to the proceedings of the NUSTEP Conference[49] for descriptions of these methods of therapy relating to training of motor activity. A more detailed presentation of the management of motor training based on principles of learning is presented elsewhere.[25, 31] Work by Ayres[50] was originally directed at children with learning disabilities but has been applied to children with mental and motor retardation and developmental disabilities as well. A number of attempts have been made to evaluate treatment techniques advocated by Doman and Delacato.[51] Brunnstrom has described the application of reflex activity for adult hemiplegic patients, which has equal applicability to children with cerebral palsy.[52]

Evaluation of the efficacy of any of the methods proposed has been notoriously inadequate. Only a few studies have been published, and valid controls have been difficult to demonstrate.[53] Evidence for effect has been largely anecdotal. The ideas presented have been subjected to several studies but suffer from similar deficiency in that these studies have not yet been published. Nevertheless, children need to be treated.

Summary

In the present state of knowledge, the most prudent course, and one that is still rooted in a basic respect for each individual as possessing intrinsic human value, is to utilize established principles of learning and behavioral management together with careful neurophysiological diagnosis as a basis for teaching brain-damaged children new motor and behavioral skills. A judgment can be made of the effectiveness of a procedure if one defines the expected goal precisely in measurable terms and maintains accurate records of functional achievement. The strength of a motion, its voluntary range, the number of contractions or repetitions, the duration of activity, the resistance overcome, and the difficulty tolerated may all be used as criteria for measurement of progress. These should show evidence of positive change within a reasonable time. Significant improvement even though small should be demonstrable within two months of consistent application of treatment once appropriate rapport has been established. If this is not seen, it is incumbent upon the professional in charge to identify a reason for failure, change the conditions, change the treatment, or discontinue it as indicated. Even though improvement may be seen in this short time, training of coordination to the optimal level requires months or years. This long period of time essential for the formation of coordination engrams is the basis for the failure of short-term or intermittent therapies. Coordination must be trained until automatic engrams have developed and then been maintained by frequent practice.

When organizing a training program for a child with brain damage, it is important to observe the child's ability to learn. Treatment methods, even if they are proven to be scientifically valid, need to be consistent in their effect upon the child's attentive ability, motivation, and retention, as well as have a demonstrable effect on motor activity. Choices will have to be made that depend on the motor, perceptual, and behavioral characteristics of the child as determined by the lesion in the central nervous system. This development of a plan of management is the responsibility of the physician concerned with the child's habilitation. The specific choices will also be influenced by the previous experience and attitude of the child in a learning situation. Where structure and discipline are required for scholastic work, the imposition of such structure in motor training is equally essential. When training of attentive ability is required for cognitive learning, training and monitoring of attention also should be included in the program of motor training.

For children who do not have problems in attention, motivational energy, or initiative to undertake independent tasks, the "change of pace" provided by recreational periods is beneficial. However, this should not be confused with the therapeutic method selected for its intrinsic ability to develop identified cognitive or motor skills.

Since the children cannot be assigned responsibility for their own activities, the inclusion of parents or other responsible adults is necessary. Family attitudes, goals, and values must be considered. The physical, emotional, intellectual, and financial resources of the family all influence the degree and extent of participation of which the parents are capable. Their instruction in principles and techniques of management should be an on-going process in which the parents work with the child, both under the observation of the professional staff and separately. Simple didactic instruction without hands-on application is insufficient to transfer the performance of the child while under the guidance of the therapist to a home program directed by the parents. It is not until the child is at an optimal level performing at home and at school that it can be said that rehabilitation has been successful.

ACKNOWLEDGMENT

Supported in part by Grant #16–P–56810/5–17 from the Social and Rehabilitation Service, Department of Health and Human Services, Washington, DC, for the University of Minnesota Medical Rehabilitation Research and Training Center.

References

1. Nelson, K. B., and Ellenberg, J.: Epidemiology of cerebral palsy. *In* Schoenberg, B. S. (Ed.): Neurological Epidemiology: Principles and Clinical Applications. Vol. 19, Advances in Neurology. New York, Raven Press, 1978, pp. 421–435.
2. Kiely, J. L., Paneth, N., and Susser, M.: Low birthweight, neonatal care, and cerebral palsy. An epidemiological review. *In* Mittler, P. (Ed.): Frontiers of Knowledge in Mental Retardation. Baltimore, University Park Press, 1981.
3. Hagberg, B., Hagberg, G., and Olow, I.: The changing panorama of cerebral palsy in Sweden 1954–1977. Acta Paediatr. Scand., 64:187–192, 1975.
4. Bennett, F. C., Chandler, L. S., Robinson, N. M., and Sells, C. J.: Spastic diplegia in premature injuries. Etiologic and diagnostic considerations. Am. J. Dis. Child., 135:732–737, 1981.
5. Nelson, K., and Broman, S. H.: Perinatal risk factors in children with serious motor and mental handicaps. Ann. Neurol., 2:371–377, 1977.
6. Moyes, C. D.: Epidemiology of head injuries in children. Child Care Health Dev., 6:1–10, 1980.
7. Brink, J., Ganett, A. L., Hale, W. R., Woo-Sam, J., and Nickel, V. L.: Recovery of motor and intellectual functioning in children sustaining head injuries. Dev. Med. Child Neurol., 12:565–571, 1970.
8. Walker, A. E.: Head injury. *In* Caveness, W. F., and Walker, A. E. (Eds.): Conference Proceedings, Philadelphia, J. B. Lippincott, 1966, p. 15.
9. Van Hof, M. W.: Development and recovery from brain damage. *In* Connolly, K. J., and Prechtl, H.

F. R. (Eds.): Maturation and Development. London, Spastics International Medical Publishers, 1981.

10. Greenough, W. T., Foss, B., and Devoogd, T. L.: The influence of experience on recovery following brain damage in rodents—hypothesis based on developmental research. *In* Walsh, R. N., and Greenough, W. T. (Eds.): Environment as Therapy for Brain Dysfunction. New York, Plenum Press, 1976.

11. Yu, J.: Neuromuscular recovery with training after central nervous system lesions: An experimental approach. *In* Ince, L. P. (Ed.): Behavioral Psychology in Rehabilitation Medicine: Clinical Applications. Baltimore, Williams & Wilkins, 1980.

12. Kottke, F. J.: Reflex patterns initiated by secondary sensory fiber endings of muscle spindles, a proposal. Arch. Phys. Med. Rehabil., 56:1–7, 1975.

13. Grillner, S.: Descending control of spinal circuits. *In* Herman, R. M., Grillner, S., Stein, P. S. G., and Stuart, B. G. (Eds.): Neural Control of Locomotion. New York, Plenum Press, 1975, pp. 351–375.

14. Pompeiano, O.: Vestibulo-spinal relationships. *In* Naunton, R. F. (Ed.): The Vestibular System. New York, Academic Press, 1975.

15. Brooks, V. B., and Thach, W. T.: Cerebellar control of posture and movement. *In* Handbook of Physiology, Section I, The Nervous System—Vol. II, Motor Control, part 2. American Physiological Society. Baltimore, Williams & Wilkins, 1981, pp. 877–947.

16. Kornhuber, H. H.: Cerebral cortex, cerebellum, and basal ganglia: An introduction to their motor functions. *In* Schmitt, F. O., and Worden, F. G. (Eds.): The Neurosciences, Third Study Program. Cambridge, MA, MIT Press, 1974.

17. Jung, R., and Hassler, R.: The extrapyramidal motor system. *In* Field, W., and Magoun, J. (Eds.): Handbook of Physiology, Neurophysiology—Section 1, Vol. II. Washington, DC, American Physiological Society, 1960, pp. 863–927.

18. DeLong, M. R., and Apostolos, P. G.: Motor functions of the basal ganglia. *In* Handbook of Physiology, Section I, The Nervous System—Vol. II, Motor Control, part 2. American Physiological Society. Baltimore, Williams & Wilkins, 1981, pp. 1027, 1039.

19. Evarts, E. V.: Role of motor cortex in voluntary movements in primates. *In* Handbook of Physiology, Section I, The Nervous System—Vol. II, Motor Control, part 2. American Physiological Society. Baltimore, Williams & Wilkins, 1981, pp. 1083–1120.

20. Gesell, A., Amatruda, C. S., Knoblock, H., and Pasamanick, B.: Developmental Diagnosis, 3rd Ed. Hagerstown, MD, Harper & Row, 1974.

21. Illingworth, R. S.: The Development of the Infant and Young Child. Edinburgh, E. & S. Livingstone, 1967.

22. Lowrey, G. H.: Growth and Development in Children. Chicago, Year Book Publishing Company, 1975.

23. Molnar, G., and Taft, E.: Pediatric Rehabilitation I. Curr. Probl. Pediatr., 7:3–155, 1977.

24. Easton, J. K. M., Ozel, A. T., and Halpern, D.: Intramuscular neurolysis for spasticity in children. Arch. Phys. Med. Rehabil., 60:155–158, 1979.

25. Halpern, D.: Therapeutic exercise for cerebral palsy. *In* Basmajian, J. V. (Ed.): Therapeutic Exercises, 3rd Ed. Baltimore, Williams & Wilkins, 1978, pp. 281–306.

26. Klein, R. M.: Attention and movement. *In* Stelmach, G. E. (Ed.): Motor Control, Issues and Trends. New York, Academic Press, 1976.

27. Keele, S. W., and Summers, J. J.: The structure of motor programs. *In* Stelmach, G. E. (Ed.): Motor Control, Issues and Trends. New York, Academic Press, 1976.

28. Jacobson, E.: Progressive Relaxation. Chicago, University of Chicago Press, 1938.

29. Stockmeyer, S. A.: An interpretation of the approach of Rood to the treatment of neuromuscular dysfunction. Am. J. Phys. Med., 46:900–956, 1967.

30. Bobath, K.: A Neurophysiological Basis for the Treatment of Cerebral Palsy. Clinics in Developmental Medicine, No. 75. Philadelphia, J. B. Lippincott, 1980, pp. 1–98.

31. Kottke, F. J., Halpern, D., Easton, J. K. M., Ozel, A. T., and Burrill, C.: The training of coordination. Arch. Phys. Med. Rehabil., 59:567–572, 1978.

32. Halpern, D., Kottke, F. J., Burrill, C., Fiterman, C., Popp, J., and Palmer, S.: Training of control of head posture in children with cerebral palsy. Dev. Med. Child Neurol., 12:290–305, 1970.

33. Harris, F. A.: Treatment with position feed-back controlled head stabilizer. Am. J. Phys. Med., 58:169–184, 1979.

34. Gracanin, F.: Use of Functional Stimulation in Rehabilitation of Hemiplegic Patients. Final Report Research Project No. 19-p. 58395-F-012-66. Dept. of Health, Education and Welfare. Ljubljana, The Institute of the S R Slovenia of Rehabilitation of the Disabled, 1972.

35. Keele, S. W.: Movement control in skilled motor performance. Psychol. Bull., 70:387–403, 1968.

36. Evarts, E. V.: Contrasts between activity of precentral and post-central neurons during movement in the monkey. Brain Res., 40:25–31, 1972.

37. Samilson, R. (Ed.): Orthopedic Aspects of Cerebral Palsy. Clinics in Developmental Medicine, Nos. 52/53. Philadelphia, J. B. Lippincott, 1975, pp. 1–301.

38. Lutey, C.: Individual Intelligence Testing. Greeley, CO, Lutey Publishing Company, 1977.

39. Papez, J. W.: A proposed mechanism of emotion. Arch. Neurol. Psychiatry, 38:725–743, 1937.

40. MacLean, P. D.: The triune brain, emotion, and scientific bias. *In* Schmitt, F. O. (Ed.): The Neurosciences, Second Study Program. New York, The Rockefeller University Press, 1970, pp. 336–349.

41. Isaacson, R.: The Limbic System. New York, Plenum Press, 1974.
42. Kimble, D. P.: The effects of hippocampal lesion on extinction and "hypothesis behavior" in rats. Physiol. Behav., 5:735–738, 1970.
43. Connors, C. K.: Food Additives and Hyperactive Children. New York, Plenum Press, 1979, pp. 113–119.
44. Held, R., and Hein, A.: Movement produced stimulation in the development of visually guided behavior. J. Comp. Physiol. Psychol., 56:872–876, 1963.
45. White, B. L.: Experience and the development of motor mechanisms. *In* Connolly, K. (Ed.): Mechanisms of Motor Skill Development. New York, Academic Press, 1970.
46. Gillette, H.: Systems of Therapy in Cerebral Palsy. Am. Lecture Series No. 762. Springfield, IL, Charles C Thomas, Publisher, 1969.
47. Pearson, P., and Williams, C. E.: Physical Therapy Services in the Developmental Disabilities. Springfield, IL, Charles C Thomas, Publisher, 1972.
48. Harris, F. A.: Facilitation techniques. *In* Basmajian, J. V. (Ed.): Therapeutic Exercise, 3rd Ed. Baltimore, Williams & Wilkins, 1978, pp. 93–137.
49. Bouman, H. D.: Exploratory and analytical survey of therapeutic exercise. Northwestern University Special Therapeutic Exercise Project. Am. J. Phys. Med., 46:1–1108, 1967.
50. Ayres, A. J.: Sensory Integration and Learning Disorders. Los Angeles, Western Psychological Services, 1978.
51. Freeman, R. D.: Controversy over "patterning" as a treatment for brain damage in children. J.A.M.A., 202:385–388, 1967.
52. Brunnstrom, S.: Movement Therapy for Stroke Patients, A Neurophysiological Approach. New York, Harper & Row, Publishers, 1970.
53. Wright, T., and Nicholson, J.: Physiotherapy for the spastic child: An evaluation. Dev. Med. Child Neurol., 15:146–163, 1973.

40

Rehabilitation for Respiratory Dysfunction

H. FREDERIC HELMHOLZ, JR.
HENRY H. STONNINGTON

Disorders of Respiration

Respiration is transport. It is the process of moving oxygen from the air to the alveoli of the lungs by a mass movement of air, called ventilation, and, in turn, removing carbon dioxide from the alveoli by the same mass movement. Ventilation maintains a pressure (concentration) gradient between alveolar gas and venous blood so that gases exchange between blood and alveolar gas by diffusion. The circulatory system provides the transport of oxygen between the lungs and the tissues.

The effort, or cost, of ventilation depends on the elastic properties of the lungs, thorax, diaphragm, abdominal complex, and accessory muscles and the resistance to flow through the multiple air passages between the outside and the alveoli.

Physiological Basis of Disorders of Respiration

Respiratory disorders, then, are conditions that prevent adequate transport of oxygen in and carbon dioxide out of the lungs (exchange), thereby leading to retention of carbon dioxide and to a lack of oxygen. These disorders may be caused by (1) muscle weakness or inefficiency or increasing stiffness of elastic components or (2) increased resistance to air flow through the tracheobronchial tree; hence they are classified as (1) *restrictive* or (2) *obstructive*. A third category, that of conditions

due to an increase in thickness of or a decrease in area of the alveolar diffusing membrane, is usually associated with a restrictive disorder; it leads primarily to low oxygen tension in arterial blood without carbon dioxide retention because of the much greater diffusivity of carbon dioxide in body tissues.

In Figure 40–1 the lung volume relationships and definitions are shown, and the effect of position on the end-expiratory position relative to vital capacity is suggested. The end-expiratory position is that at which elastic recoil of the lung is exactly balanced by the tendency of the chest to expand (point O, for example, in Figure 40–2). This point of equilibrium differs with position: in the supine position, the weight of abdominal contents favors expiration; in the upright position, it favors inspiration. In the weak individual, this change can be used to produce adequate resting ventilation (for example, with the rocking bed).

Restrictive Disorders

Figure 40–2 illustrates the elastic properties of the lung and chest (by which is meant the entire complex of thoracic cage, diaphragm, abdomen, and relaxed abdominal muscles). Normally about 20 cm of water pressure would fill the isolated lung to vital capacity size (curve L, Fig. 40–2). Thus, full inspiration requires a transpulmonary pressure of this magnitude, normally achieved by maintenance of the same pressure below atmospheric in the pleural space, i.e., the space around the lungs

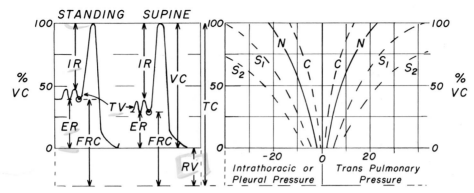

FIGURE 40–1. Subdivisions of total lung capacity (TC) are shown related to pressure (N) in normal respiratory maneuvers. Dotted lines indicate pressures required with different lung compliances. IR = inspiratory reserve volume; TV = tidal volume; ER = expiratory reserve volume; RV = residual volume; VC = vital capacity; FRC = functional residual capacity; C = more compliant than the normal; S_1 and S_2 = less compliant (stiffer) than the normal.

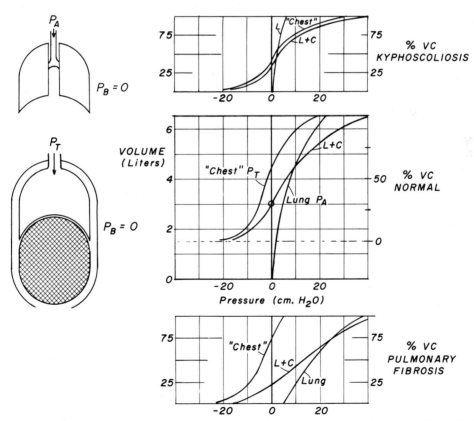

FIGURE 40–2. Pressure-volume diagrams of the lung alone (L; Lung; P_A), of the thoracic cavity alone ("Chest"; P_T), and of the combination (L + C) are constructed to indicate normal relationships and those found in two types of restrictive disorder. P_B = O indicates that the atmospheric (barometric) pressure is the pressure to which the other pressures are referred.

(curves N, Fig. 40–1). The dotted curves indicate the effect of varying the lung compliance (see Fig. 40–1). Curves labeled C are for increased compliance and curves S_1 and S_2, for lungs stiffer than normal.

If the lungs were removed and pressures above and below atmospheric were applied inside the remaining cavity, the characteristic curve marked "Chest" would be obtained (Fig. 40–2).

If, in the paralyzed individual, the combination of lungs and chest were similarly treated, one would obtain the combined curve relating volume to pressure indicated by "L + C" (Fig. 40–2). Such a curve describes the elastic properties of the system and the recoil that must be overcome in breathing. For any given tidal volume, the area between the line of zero pressure and the curve to this tidal volume represents work. If the time required is specified as well, one has an expression of power, or the rate at which work is done.

In Figure 40–2, the chart above the normal indicates the effect of chest deformity in changing the elastic properties of the chest and reducing the vital capacity. Note that the chest curve is the restricting element; thus, intrathoracic (pleural) pressure is never much below atmospheric pressure, because the elastic lung is never stretched sufficiently to produce a large negative pressure.

The chart below the normal chart indicates the effect of increased stiffness of the lung (loss of compliance) in changing the elastic properties of the system and reducing the vital capacity. Note that this disorder leads to pressure well below atmospheric pressure at all lung volumes because of increased elastic recoil of the lung at all volumes.

Restrictive disorders are characterized by an increased energy requirement to overcome elastic recoil of lung or chest structures at any given ventilation. Any disease that stiffens costovertebral or sternocostal connections or causes fibrosis of respiratory, abdominal, or shoulder girdle muscles or of the lungs themselves can lead to restrictive impairment of pulmonary function.

The same effect is produced by the loss of muscle or the loss of nerves that activate the muscles of respiration. The chart marked "normal" in Figure 40–2 shows the relationships that would occur if the vital capacity were reduced by a decrease in both the inspiratory and the expiratory reserve volumes. The restriction in such cases would be the inability to bring force to bear and do work against the recoil of the elastic system.

Obstructive Disorders

In any lung, the air distribution system expands as the lung expands, and, therefore, there is a relationship between lung size and the resistance to gas flow (Fig. 40–3). One of the characteristics of asthma and emphysema is an increase in resistance to air flow as indicated in the curve marked "Emphysema." The dotted curve indicates the behavior in many cases of emphysema when expiration is forced. This is the phenomenon of air trapping, in which the airway develops such high resistance when transpulmonary pressure is high that air flow stops before emptying is complete. It has been shown that the obstructive phenomena in the emphysematous lung are characteristically nonuniform and are primarily brought out on expiration. Asthma tends to produce more uniform obstruction, which is evident to some extent during inspiration.

A simple obstructing lesion of the trachea, when it is intrathoracic, can simulate emphysema if the involved trachea becomes collapsible. This kind of lesion serves here as a model in understanding air trapping (Fig. 40–4). When the lung empties because of its own elastic recoil, the pressure (intrathoracic) around the nonrigid trachea remains below atmospheric levels and the airway remains patent. If forced expiration is attempted and intrathoracic pressure rises above atmospheric pressure, the trachea collapses and prevents egress of the remaining air. It is theorized that multiple small air passages act the same way in emphysema. By obstruction of the airway *outside* the chest during exhalation, the pressure inside these passages is increased and the collapse is prevented. Hence, breathing out through pursed lips or grunting is often beneficial.

Obstructive disease can cause a decrease in arterial oxygen tension and retention of carbon dioxide when obstruction is relatively uniform, as in obstructing lesions of the trachea, for example.

Emphysema, however, and most cases of asthma characteristically cause a reduction in arterial oxygen tension without carbon dioxide retention because of the difference of the carbon dioxide and oxygen dissociation curves. Figure 40–5 illustrates how the retention of carbon dioxide in underventilated areas is compensated for in overventilated areas, whereas so little extra oxygen is taken up in the overventilated areas that the oxygen content and tension of arterial blood are below normal.

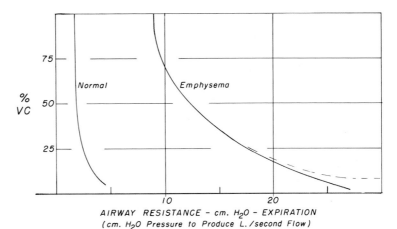

FIGURE 40–3. Resistance to air flow in a normal and emphysematous lung during expiration. Dotted line indicates effect of increased effort during a "forced expiration."

Diffusing Capacity Disorders

The amount of oxygen passing through the alveolar membrane of the lung depends directly on the difference between the alveolar oxygen pressure and the mean oxygen pressure of capillary blood. It depends also on the area of the membrane that separates air and blood; it is reduced by an increased distance between alveolar air and the hemoglobin of the blood (membrane thickness factor). Pulmonary fibrosis in its various forms causes thickening of the membrane and a decrease in alveolar surface, typically without obstructive disease.

Normally, increased oxygen uptake by the lung is caused by a decrease in the oxygen content of venous blood and an increase in pulmonary blood flow, along with an increase in ventilation. A diffusion barrier can be compensated for to some extent by increasing ventilation, which reduces the

carbon dioxide concentration in alveolar gas and thus raises the oxygen concentration (that is, pressure). In these cases the cost of maintaining a low alveolar carbon dioxide pressure is least when a rapid rate of breathing is used. Deep breathing would require excessive work because of decreased compliance.

Diagnostic Characteristics of Disorders

If the vital capacity, the forced vital capacity (maximal expiratory effort following maximal inspiration), and the pattern and volume of ventilation with maximal breathing effort (so-called maximal breathing capacity) are measured with a suitable recording spirometer, the presence of obstructive disease can be detected. If no obstructive phenomena are found but dyspnea is present, the

FIGURE 40–4. Diagram to illustrate one possible mechanism of air trapping and the effect of resistance imposed by pursed-lip or grunting expiration. (This model requires rapid onset of positive intrapleural pressure to show the phenomenon. A resistance interposed between the "alveolus" and the compliant segment of airway converts this to a better demonstration model.)

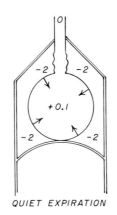

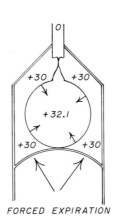

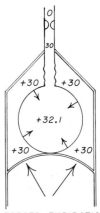

QUIET EXPIRATION   FORCED EXPIRATION   FORCED EXPIRATION
                                                 with EXTERNAL RESISTANCE

H. FREDERIC HELMHOLZ, JR. AND HENRY H. STONNINGTON

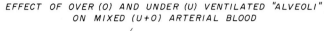

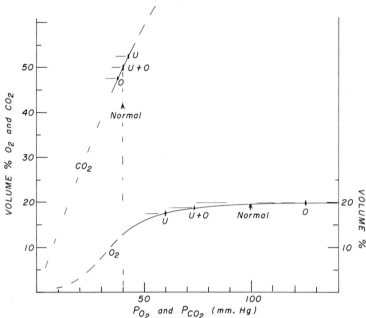

FIGURE 40–5. Plotting of oxygen and carbon dioxide dissociation curves together shows the effect of relative linearity of carbon dioxide solubility contrasted with alinearity of oxygen solubility on content of mixed (U + O) arterial blood content when it is made up of blood perfusing underventilated (U) and overventilated (O) areas of lung.

magnitude of the vital capacity may be used as an index of possible reduction in lung volume. Measurements of diffusing capacity of the lung can be made to detect abnormalities in patients with such conditions. The reader is referred to Comroe and associates[2] for details of testing procedures and, when dealing with children, to Polgar and Promadhat.[3]

Restrictive disorders are inferred when vital capacity and total capacity are reduced and no obstructive disorder is evident. Documentation of such disorders requires special tests that are beyond the scope of this presentation.

The table below gives findings in obstructive and restrictive disorders that can be obtained by a recording spirometer.

Estimates of lung size determined from physical examination and chest roentgenograms will indicate that total capacity is normal or increased in obstructive disorders and reduced in restrictive disorders.

Respiratory Muscles and Their Control

Normal ventilation at rest is accomplished by contraction of the diaphragm with enough activity of the external intercostal muscle to fix the chest cage. Initial shortening of the diaphragm muscle is associated with an outward flare of the lower rib borders and the rise of abdominal pressure, and there is concomitant relaxation of the abdominal muscles. Expiration is caused by gradual relaxation of the diaphragm, with force being provided primarily by the elastic recoil of the lung.

	VITAL CAPACITY	FORCED VITAL CAPACITY* (% in 1 Sec)	MAXIMAL BREATHING CAPACITY
Obstructive	Reduced	Less than 85%	Reduced
Restrictive	Reduced	85% or more	Normal or slightly reduced

*Many modifications of the method of estimating obstruction from a forced vital capacity are used. Any can be used when a recording is obtained.

Increased oxygen demand and carbon dioxide production during muscular activity are accompanied by an immediate increase in ventilation, owing to nervous impulses from active muscles and joints directly. (That due to fever is accompanied by increased ventilation as the result of increased activity of the respiratory center as the temperature rises.) Secondary mechanisms that also can increase ventilation are the effect of increased carbon dioxide tension (or fall of pH) in arterial blood on the respiratory center directly and the effect of a fall in arterial oxygen tension mediated through chemoreceptors (carotid and aortic bodies as well as specialized nerve endings on the surface of the medulla that are sensitive to pH changes in the spinal fluid).

Increased activity of the respiratory center increases both the depth and the rate of breathing, and active expiration (lowering of the ribs by the internal intercostals and contraction of the abdominal muscles) begins. The stimulation of the respiratory center, if sufficiently intense, causes recruitment of accessory muscles of the neck, the shoulder girdle, and the abdomen to aid in inspiration and expiration.

Stimulation of the respiratory center also involves the circulatory centers nearby so that increases in ventilation are accompanied by increases in cardiac output. In addition, with deeper respiration, the decrease in pressure inside the thorax increases the gradient of pressure between the systemic veins and the right atrium, thereby tending to increase venous return, which increases the output of first the right side and then the left side of the heart.

In response to stimulation of the nose, the pharynx, and the tracheobronchial tree, coordinated reflexes are produced, i.e., the sneeze, the gag, and the cough, respectively. These reflexes involve all muscles of ventilation as well as the laryngeal mechanism for blocking the airway as the false vocal cords close the glottis. An effective cough or sneeze requires adequate abdominal muscle activity to raise pressure against the closed glottis so that the sudden release will cause velocity in the tracheobronchial tree adequate to provide turbulent flow. Laminar flow cannot move materials on the wall of the airway. Ciliary action is needed for this function.

When abdominal muscle power is lost or inadequate, an effective cough can be produced by what is called exsufflation, originally introduced by Barach.[4] The proper use of the cough reflex is understood by few, and the procedure is neglected in therapy today. Proper timing of inspiratory and expiratory periods is essential and can be provided by the COF-FLATOR produced to Dr. Barach's specifications.[4, 5]

Basis for Breathing Exercises and Chest Physical Therapy

RESTRICTIVE DISORDERS

When the nerves are intact or remnants of the neuromuscular system are underdeveloped, muscle weakness can be helped by suitable exercise. It should be emphasized that muscles of respiration cannot be put at rest, and, therefore, they should be exercised voluntarily so that the increase in ventilation will make possible lessened activity of the muscles following therapeutic exercise. The margin between activity that will cause damage and activity that will cause hypertrophy can be narrow in patients with restrictive disorders, and due caution should be observed when increased demands are put on respiratory muscles.

Chest deformities disturb the relations between the insertions and origins of respiratory muscles and may tend to flatten the diaphragm by increasing the anteroposterior dimension of the chest. Inefficient use of the diaphragm is demonstrated when the patient pulls in the lower part of the rib cage with inspiration. Often no increase in doming can be achieved in such patients, but the phenomenon should be noted and abdominal muscle exercises should be instituted when benefit is possible. Each case of deformity must be studied carefully before an exercise program is outlined. In many cases, the only possible therapy is mechanical assistance of ventilation.

In treating any fibrosing or sclerosing disease of the chest cage and musculature, the effect of loss of compliance should be kept in mind. Loosening of contractures and stiffened joints, when it is possible, decreases remarkably the work of breathing.

Loss of compliance of the lungs (fibrosis) is difficult to treat by physical means, but further development of respiratory muscles can be tried.

OBSTRUCTIVE DISORDERS

Obstructive disease is accompanied by fixation of the chest in a position larger than the normal end-expiratory level, with an increase in the functional residual capacity and residual volume. This condition tends to produce a flattening of the diaphragm and thus to lessen the usefulness of this muscle in inspiration. In some cases, the abdominal muscles are contracted during inspiration and work against the inspiratory effort of the intercostal, neck, and shoulder muscles. In such cases, help can be afforded by retraining to ensure relaxation of the abdominal muscles during inspiration. The best method is the use of exercises that contract the abdominal muscles during *expiration*.

Because the work of breathing increases rapidly when air velocity increases in obstructive disease, the following formulation is emphasized:

$$\dot{V}_A = (V_T - V_D)\, f$$

in which $\dot{V}_A$ = alveolar ventilation (liters per minute), V_T = tidal volume (liters), V_D = dead space volume (liters), and f = frequency (breaths per minute). Since with each breath the dead space remains constant, the amount of dead space ventilation increases as frequency increases. With each breath, the volume in excess of the dead space inhaled is the effective, or alveolar, ventilation; the greater the tidal volume, the smaller the fraction that is dead space ventilation.

Thus, the minimal total ventilation required for a given alveolar ventilation is attained by slow, deep breathing. Air velocities are also least when a given alveolar ventilation is attained by a *maximal tidal volume* and a *minimal frequency*. Since obstruction is primarily expiratory, fast inhalation ensures the lowest frequency. In addition, the phenomenon of air trapping should be kept in mind and rapid forced expiration should be avoided except through pursed lips or the partially closed glottis or the vocal cords. With these principles in mind, a rational program of breathing exercises can be worked out that will help any patient who normally uses rapid, shallow breathing through an open mouth. The patient who already breathes slowly and deeply and who exhales through pursed lips or grunts during expiration will be helped less but responds positively to reassurance that his breathing pattern is correct. Training can ensure deeper expiration when exercise produces stimulation of the expiratory muscles, if emphasis is put on deeper, faster inhalation and slower exhalation through pursed lips.

Underventilation

When restrictive disorders (including loss of muscle power) and obstructive disorders are of such severity that resting ventilation is insufficient to remove metabolic carbon dioxide, alveolar concentration of this gas rises as carbon dioxide is retained until increased alveolar concentration provides for removal of metabolic production again, according to the following formula:

$$\dot{V}_{CO_2} = \dot{V}_A \times F_{ACO_2}$$

in which $\dot{V}_{CO_2}$ = liters of CO_2 exhaled per minute body temperature, ambient pressure, $\dot{V}_A$ = alveolar ventilation (liters per minute) body temperature, ambient pressure, saturated, and F_{ACO_2} = fraction of CO_2 in alveolar gas.

Underventilation produces respiratory acidosis and, as carbon dioxide rises, oxygen falls to seriously low levels when air is breathed. However, cyanosis cannot be used as an index of adequacy of ventilation because of the variability in the amount of reduced hemoglobin in the superficial (visible) capillary beds. Severe oxygen deficiency in arterial blood is possible with cyanosis (for example, in peripheral vasoconstriction or anemia), and cyanosis occurs frequently in congestive heart failure when arterial blood is sufficiently saturated with oxygen.

Assistance of ventilation is the treatment of choice when the patient is capable of some respiratory effort. It can be accomplished by application of positive pressure to the airway during inspiration by an intermittent positive-pressure breathing inspiration (IPPB[I]) machine. This device is so designed that a slight negative pressure starts a flow of gas, which continues until a preset positive pressure is reached; then the flow stops and the airway is vented to the outside. The pressure setting determines the tidal volume. The patient can slow the rate or speed it up, depending on the ventilation needed. The patient's own respiratory control mechanism thus becomes effective once more in regulating alveolar ventilation to metabolic needs.

When all respiratory activity has ceased, total control of ventilation must be undertaken by applying positive pressure to the airway or negative pressure to the body at regular intervals. It is impossible with the equipment currently available to adjust ventilation as precisely as does the respiratory control system of the body, but estimates made periodically of arterial blood levels of pH and carbon dioxide allow one to check adequacy by the following relationship (Henderson-Hasselbalch equation for the bicarbonate-carbon dioxide system):

$$pH = 6.1 + \log \frac{[HCO_3^-]}{0.03 \, P_{CO_2}}$$

or

$$pH = 6.1 + \log \frac{[Total \, CO_2] - 0.03 \, P_{CO_2}}{0.03 \, P_{CO_2}}$$

The solution indicates that normal values approximate the following:

$$7.4 = 6.1 + \log \frac{20}{1} =$$

$$6.1 + \log \frac{24 \, mEq/l}{0.03 \, (40) \, mM/} =$$
$$l$$

$$6.1 + \log \frac{25.2 - 1.2 \, mM/l}{1.2 \, mM/l}$$

$25.2 = mM/l$ total CO_2 content of blood.
$25.2 \, mM/l = 56.87 \, ml/dl$ or vol %.
$0.03 \, mM/l/mm = $ solubility coefficient for CO_2 at body temperature.

In respiratory acidosis, P_{CO_2} increases and pH decreases. Renal compensation will allow an increase in bicarbonate so that its ratio to P_{CO_2} increases again and pH returns toward normal.

Carbon dioxide retention can be tolerated for relatively long periods of time (although it causes narcosis when excessive), but lack of oxygen cannot; therefore, filling the lungs with high concentrations of oxygen will protect the individual from oxygen lack in emergency situations until definitive treatment can be instituted. Oxygen should always be administered first. When the lung contains only oxygen, carbon dioxide, and water vapor, cyanosis will never intervene if circulation is intact; thus, once oxygen has been administered, cyanosis cannot be an indication of ventilatory insufficiency in any sense at all.

When positive pressure is applied through the airway or when negative pressure is applied around the body to expand the lungs, the intrathoracic pressure relative to systemic venous pressure is inevitably raised and venous return is decreased. The normal circulatory system can compensate for this, but when it is hampered by blood loss or other abnormalities, serious decreases in cardiac output are produced. In those forms of restrictive disorder that are due to decreased compliance of the lungs, positive pressure applied to the airway causes much less circulatory disturbance than does negative pressure around the body. In other restrictive conditions, the two methods affect the circulatory system almost equally. In obstructive disease, the application of positive pressure through the airway may be expected to affect the circulatory system more than would negative pressure around the body.

In those forms of restrictive disorder in which the primary abnormality is a barrier to diffusion of oxygen from alveolar gas to blood, a simple increase in the oxygen concentration of the inhaled gas will provide adequate compensation.

By studying the charts in Figure 40–1, with the additional information that lung compliance is usually within the normal range but the chest curve may be moved to the left in obstructive disease, one can work out the mechanical relationships that may be expected in various forms of pulmonary disorders. The circulatory disorders that affect lung function are those that cause pulmonary venous hypertension (such as mitral stenosis or left-sided heart failure). They produce a decrease in lung compliance and, when pulmonary edema is present, a diffusion barrier.

Proper synchronization of muscular effort in producing ventilation is often lost in patients with obstructive lung disease so that accessory muscles, principally of the neck, are contracted to raise the chest while either the abdominal muscles are simultaneously contracted or there is little or no diaphragmatic contraction taking place. Sometimes the lack of diaphragmatic contraction is due to excessive flattening of the diaphragm, i.e., loss of mechanical advantage. When flattening is severe, one can note drawing in of the lower border of the chest on inspiration (see also discussion of chest deformity above).

Chest Injuries

The special case of chest injuries merits some consideration. Loss of integrity of the lung, which causes pneumothrorax, is an emergency to be handled by a thoracic surgeon, but loss of integrity of the chest cage leads to a mechanical defect that tends to prevent inspiration. For example, negative pleural pressure developed by diaphragmatic contraction causes a nonrigid rib cage to collapse, thus preventing expansion of the lungs. Fixation of the ribs has been the treatment of choice. Positive pressure applied to the airway during inspiration has many advantages in that it ensures ventilation and splints the chest without operative measures. When the ribs are intact but muscle contraction causes pain, inspiration is limited. Therefore, IPPB is the treatment of choice in chest injuries that cause underventilation. It decreases pain as it increases ventilation. An apparatus that delivers a set volume with each breath (volume is pre-set) is usually preferred over pressure pre-set instruments in these cases. A decrease in venous return is the only complication; it should be considered whenever there has been loss of blood. A fall in blood pressure or an increase in pulse rate, or both, indicate the need for blood replacement.

In the use of equipment for the support of or assistance to ventilation, certain principles are often forgotten. Any pneumatic system used is effective only if forces are applied to the elastic system, including the lungs. Any leaks in the system prevent this application. A leak is the most frequent cause of failure and must not be permitted. Devices designed to compensate for leaks are unrealistic and lead to slipshod therapy.

Whenever the nasal passages are bypassed (by the use of tracheal tubes, pharyngeal catheters, mouth breathing, or tracheostomy), sufficient water must be added to the inhaled gas to ensure a relative humidity of 100 per cent at the body temperature of the patient. Gases below this temperature must contain particulate water. In practice, it is necessary to add heat to humidifiers in order to maintain this relative humidity.

The physical therapist is sometimes called upon to assist in the retraining of individuals being weaned from ventilatory support after recovering from paralysis due to disease or weakened by a disease such as tetanus. Since the introduction of techniques of intermittent mandatory ventilation, the incidence of respiratory muscle incoordination following prolonged ventilatory support has decreased. Intermittent mandatory ventilation allows the patient to take breaths on his or her own while still supplying the patient with a determined number of mechanically produced breaths. Retraining involves emphasis on diaphragmatic contraction on inspiration with abdominal extra effort on expiration to increase the doming of the diaphragm.

Note: If ventilatory support has been prolonged or if the diaphragm is weakened by disease, one must remember that the diaphragm cannot be put at complete rest unless ventilatory support is resumed or provided. Any muscle will gain strength (hypertrophy) only if it is given rest periods or periods of minimal activity after being stressed. If a period of relative rest is not provided, the muscle may be damaged. This can, of course, happen to the diaphragm as well as other muscles.

Chest Physical Therapy

It has been known since the days of Hippocrates that if a patient is left in one position for a prolonged period, particularly if depressed by disease (and in modern times by drugs), pneumonia will develop. The actual steps leading to the development of pneumonia are atelectasis in dependent parts of the lung, retention of secretions, and growth of bacteria that ordinarily would be removed with the retained secretions.

Modern blood gas studies identify the first sign of atelectasis as a decrease in arterial oxygen partial pressure without a change in arterial carbon dioxide partial pressure.

All types of chest physical therapy and respiratory therapy techniques providing increased inspiratory effort by direction or incentive spirometry, or increased tidal volume by properly administered IPPB when combined with position changes and activity where possible as well as coughing, will prevent atelectasis and, hence, the pneumonia that so often is a complication in patients after surgery or a severe illness.

Chest physical therapy is the application of physical methods to the respiratory care of patients with pulmonary disease. The range of treatment includes instruction in relaxation and breathing exercises; performance of postural drainage, percussion or clapping, and vibration; and splinting the chest or incision site to facilitate coughing. All these techniques assist in clearing pulmonary secretions. They are particularly indicated in patients with chronic obstructive lung disease that becomes manifested as asthma, bronchitis, emphysema, bronchiectasis, and cystic fibrosis; after major surgery of the upper abdomen, thorax, and cardiovascular system; and in all patients who are dependent on mechanical ventilation. A supportive program of chest physical therapy is necessary to assist patients with neuromuscular disease and a diminished cough reflex or effort who are unable to mobilize their pulmonary secretions. All patients immobilized in bed can benefit from instructions in coughing and breathing exercises. Surgical patients are helped if they have developed confidence in the therapist before the operation. After the operation, it is difficult to gain the cooperation of a patient who is in pain and receiving analgesics.

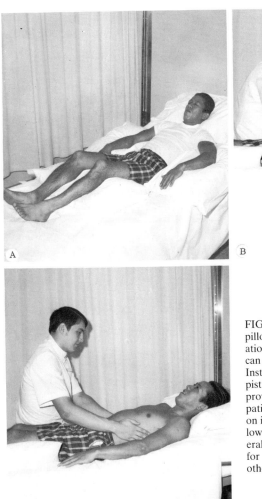

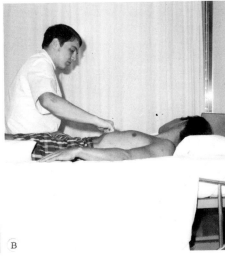

FIGURE 40–6. *A*, Use of bed position and pillows for support helps to effect general relaxation. Once this has been achieved, the therapist can begin instructions in breath control. *B*, Instruction in diaphragmatic breathing. Therapist's knuckles are placed below the xiphoid to provide a resistive pressure, producing in the patient an awareness of diaphragmatic descent on inspiration. *C*, Hands are placed firmly along lower ribs to apply pressure, encouraging bilateral basal expansion of lungs. Similar techniques for localized breathing exercises are applied to other areas of the chest wall.

In the acutely ill patient, chest physical therapy is closely allied with inhalation therapy and intensive-care nursing. A working knowledge of oxygen and humidification equipment, mechanical ventilators, IPPB devices, and endotracheal and tracheostomy tubes is essential.

Breathing Exercises. The therapist should instruct the patient in the techniques of breathing exercises (Fig. 40–6).

Postural Drainage. Optimal use of postural drainage requires a knowledge of the segmental anatomy of the lung.[6–8] References to more detailed manuals are listed at the end of this section. For the patient with a poor cough and widespread pulmonary secretions who is confined to bed, hourly turning from side to side may be inadequate to manage secretions. A modified program of postural drainage, practical even in many critically ill patients, can be developed (Fig. 40–7).

Other Maneuvers. In addition to the basic postural drainage maneuvers that the patient can be taught to do, chest percussion or clapping (Fig. 40–8*A*) and vibration, either manually or mechanically (Fig. 40–8*B*), are necessary and useful adjuncts in clearing secretions.

Other techniques frequently used to help post-operative patients are manual splinting of the chest or abdominal incision by the therapist (Fig. 40–9*A*), patient coughing while hugging a pillow (Fig. 40–9*B*), and use of a blow bottle (Fig. 40–9*C*) for the patient to exhale against resistance in order to encourage increased tidal volume. Adaptations of the techniques can be useful in small children (Fig. 40–10).

H. FREDERIC HELMHOLZ, JR. AND HENRY H. STONNINGTON

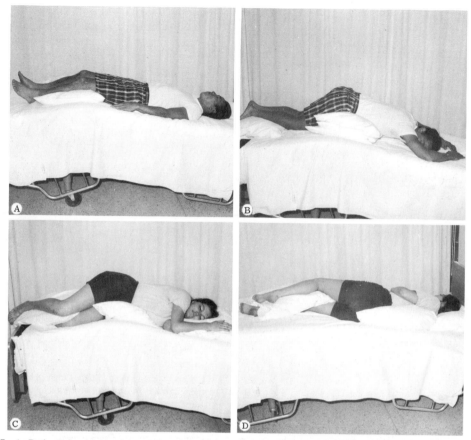

FIGURE 40–7. *A*, Patient should spend some time in the dependent position. Most patients will tolerate 10 to 15 degrees of head-down tilt for a brief period, several times a day. This position facilitates drainage by gravity of the anterior basal segments. *B*, Position used for draining the posterior basal segments. *C*, Position for drainage of right lower lobe and lateral basal bronchus. *D*, Position for drainage of the left upper lobe and for lower division of the superior and inferior bronchi.

Routine Chest Physical Therapy

In the acutely ill patient, chest physical therapy may be given as frequently as every two hours and should be closely coordinated within the overall respiratory program. For routine treatment given two to four times daily, the following sequence and procedures are ordered.

1. Mist Inhalation (20 Min). This will moisten the upper airways and help liquefy secretions. The mist may be cold for febrile patients but preferably is heated to deliver more water. Usually the carrier gas is oxygen-enriched air. Administration via a mask or into a tent may be by humidifier or nebulizer. Instruction for breathing exercises and cough control can be given at this time, if it is convenient for the physical therapist.

2. IPPB (15 Min). These treatments are given by personnel from the inhalation-therapy or the nursing department and result in a period of mild hyperventilation and an increase in lung expansion. IPPB also provides an effective means of delivering bronchodilator, decongestant, and mucolytic agents to the airways and, in addition, continues to add moisture.

3. Chest Physical Therapy (20 Min). After the mist and IPPB are given, postural drainage, combined with vibration and percussion, usually produces good results in clearing secretions. Supplemental maneuvers performed at this time for patients on ventilators are stimulation of cough by direct tracheal suctioning, hyperinflation with oxygen by bag and mask, and instillation of saline through endotracheal and tracheostomy tubes prior to suctioning.

Within the range of respiratory care, chest physical therapy and inhalation therapy have complementary roles. Most patients who receive chest

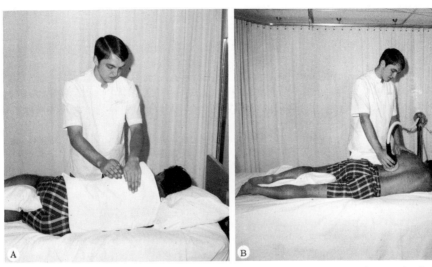

FIGURE 40–8. *A*, Position for chest percussion or clapping. *B*, Position for manual or mechanical vibration.

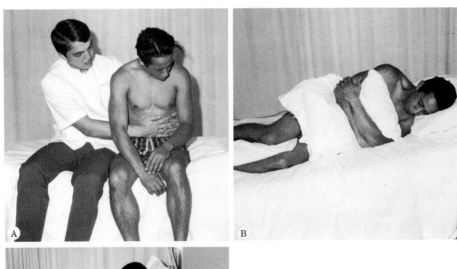

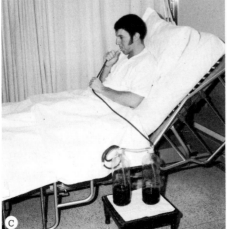

FIGURE 40–9. *A*, Manual splinting of chest or abdominal incision. *B*, While coughing, patient hugs pillow. *C*, Blow bottle helps lung expansion.

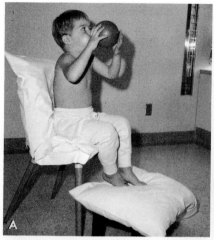
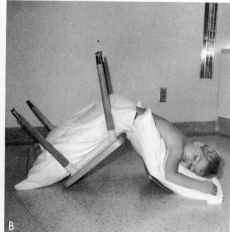
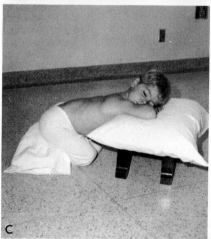

FIGURE 40–10. Techniques useful for small children.

physical therapy also will use one or more pieces of oxygen equipment and likely will receive IPPB therapy as well. The physical therapist must be familiar with the operation of this equipment, just as the inhalation therapist must have experience in the technique of chest physical therapy.

Management of Respiratory Complications in Musculoskeletal Disorders

Patients with disorders seen by the physiatrist frequently have respiratory complications. Conditions such as arthritis, ankylosing spondylitis, muscular dystrophy, and debility, as well as stroke and spinal cord injuries, may lead to poor ventilation, secretion retention, and atelectasis. These compli-

cations are among the main causes of morbidity as well as death in patients with musculoskeletal disorders. It is, therefore, important to provide respiratory care for all of these conditions, but it is particularly important for the quadriplegic patient, and information on this type of care is given in more detail later.

Inspiratory Incentive Spirometry

In recent years, the incentive spirometer has become an inexpensive and effective measure available to the physician and to the patient. Bartlett and co-workers[9] showed how important inspiratory exercises were in treating and preventing atelectasis. They showed that inspiratory incentive spirometers were even more effective than IPPB in conscious and alert patients and that older methods such as blow bottles that employed expiratory methods could actually aggravate atelectasis. The incentive spirometer can help all types of patients, from those who are debilitated and bed bound to those with stroke and spinal cord injuries or muscular dystrophy. In all of these patients, collapse of individual alveoli can be a problem. As more alveoli collapse, significantly larger amounts of right-to-left shunting occur. Also, there is a decrease of the functional residual capacity with a consequent decrease of lung compliance and an increase in the work of breathing. This may not be obvious on clinical observation because the tidal volume may remain constant despite restriction of functional residual volume. The normal individual prevents alveolar collapse with occasional deep breaths and yawns. This mechanism may not be present in some of the disabilities mentioned above. Thus, the regular use of these spirometers maintains the means of maximal lung inflation.

There are many such spirometers on the market. One example is the Voldyne spirometer (Chesebrough-Pond's Incorporated, Greenwich, Connecticut) (Fig. 40–11), which is a hand-held compact spirometer that measures the volume of air inspired up to a maximum of about 4000 ml. Sustained maximal inspiration exercise can thus be combined with volume measurement, and it is the visualization of daily improvement in volume that

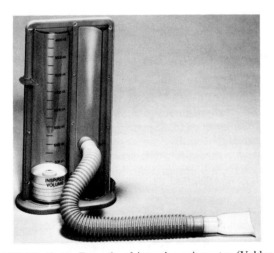

FIGURE 40–11. Example of incentive spirometer (Voldyne, made by Chesebrough-Pond's, Inc.) that allows up to 4000 ml of inspired air to be measured. This is a hand-held device that allows for visualization of daily improvement in volume, as well as giving a means of doing sustained maximal inspiration exercises.

provides incentive to the patient. Other varieties are the Spirocare spirometer (Marion Laboratories Incorporated Pharmaceutical Division, Kansas City, Missouri) and Bartlett-Edwards Incentive Spirometer (McGaw Respiratory Therapy, Division of American Hospital Supply Corporation, Irvine, California).

The Quadriplegic Patient

Bellamy and associates[10] reported a fatality rate of 40 per cent within the first year after injury of the traumatic quadriplegic patient. They were able to show at autopsy that in the vast majority of cases, death was related to pulmonary causes. There are various factors that play a part in this complication. Spontaneous ventilation is impossible if the lesion is above the fourth cervical segment. If the lesion is below the fourth cervical segment, spontaneous respiration is possible and diaphragmatic function is unimpaired but, because of the lack of movement of intercostals and the initial flaccidity of the abdominal musculature, respiratory function is abnormal and respiratory complications occur frequently. As soon as the flaccidity is replaced by spasticity in both the abdominal and intercostal muscles, the patient's respiratory function improves and fewer complications occur. This is particularly so when the patient is in the sitting position. The flaccid abdominal muscles protrude and the diaphragm lowers, with the result that inspiration produces less movement of the diaphragm, and with expiration, no abdominal rebound occurs. In the supine position, the patient has fewer problems. The main complications as a result of these problems are the retention of secretions and atelectasis. McMichan and co-workers[11] describe a careful protocol that effectively prevents these complications from occurring. They stress the importance of turning the patient frequently, having the patient take four deep breathing exercises every four hours, the use of incentive spirometry, and chest percussion. With sputum retention, IPPB is used every four hours, combined with aerosolization of the bronchodilator, isoetharine hydrochloride. Furthermore, once there is radiographic evidence of lobar atelectasis, fiberoptic bronchoscopy and bronchial lavage should be instituted immediately.

Electrophrenic Stimulation

Patients who sustain injuries high in the spinal cord fall into two categories: those who do not

H. FREDERIC HELMHOLZ, JR. AND HENRY H. STONNINGTON

injure the anterior motor neurons of the phrenic nerve and those who do. Thus, if the patient has a cord lesion at C2, C3 and C4 are left intact, and denervation atrophy of the diaphragm does not occur. However, with an injury at C3 and C4, there is likely to be irreparable damage to the phrenic nerve. All of these patients initially need a respirator to stay alive. After a period of time, consideration can be given to the implanting of a phrenic nerve stimulator. Obviously, one cannot stimulate a damaged nerve and the only patients who are likely candidates are those with very high lesions or with incomplete lesions. Therefore, to determine whether or not a patient is a candidate, an electromyogram of the diaphragm is a necessary preliminary study. The presence of a denervated diaphragm is a definite contraindication. Furthermore, one must wait at least six months before considering this alternative. Before that, the flaccidity of the chest wall causes a flail chest syndrome with the movement of the diaphragm and the procedure fails. The chest wall needs to become noncompliant in order to give the diaphragm a chance to provide adequate respiration when stimulated.

The incomplete lesion is an interesting one, and it is important to recognize it. For the importance of this lesion to be understood, one needs to remember that voluntary respiration is controlled by the cerebral cortex and that automatic respiration arises from various areas of the brain stem. These various areas send tracts down to the spinal motor neurons. Thus, it is possible to damage only the automatic tract and leave the voluntary tract intact. If respiration entirely depends upon the voluntary system, sleep apnea occurs. A similar situation can occur in brain stem infarcts as well as in children with the syndrome known as Ondine's curse. This syndrome responds well to electrophrenic pacing.

The modern era of electrophrenic pacing was introduced by Glenn and associates.[12] They used an external battery-powered transmitter. This device transmits trains of pulse-modulated radio frequency energy to a loop antenna. There are two receivers implanted subcutaneously in the right and left sides of the upper anterior chest wall. The receivers are connected to bipolar platinum electrodes that surround each phrenic nerve. The antenna is placed over one of the receivers and only one phrenic nerve is used at one time. For two weeks after installation, no pacing is done, and after that it is started for only short periods of time. Gradually, the system as well as the muscles

are trained and can be used for the full 24 hours, alternating right and left phrenic nerves. The pulse train for the transmitter is fixed to give 34 square impulses in 1.35 sec. This is the inspiratory part of the cycle. There follows a period of 2.65 sec without stimulation during which expiration is allowed to occur. The respiratory cycle lasts four sec, making a rate of 15 breaths per min. It is regulated in such a way that it starts the diaphragmatic contraction with a minimal current that gradually builds up over the inspiratory part of the cycle, giving the muscle a smooth contraction and not a sudden hiccup.

The advantage of this system over the constant use of a ventilator is that it allows the patient to move with much less difficulty; however, the patient still must have a tracheostomy for suction and proper suction equipment must be available at all times. In addition, the patient needs to have some other form of ventilation available in case the system breaks down. There now have been patients who have used this system for many years with few complications. The phrenic nerve does not appear to be damaged by the electrode.

Conclusion

This chapter has dealt with some basic concepts of respiration as well as with what happens during various respiratory disorders. It has touched on the management of some of these disorders. It is clear that this management is complicated particularly in the acute stages of the disorders, and really needs a physician who has specialized in this field. This specialist may well be an anesthesiologist or chest physician. There are, however, prophylactic measures that any physician needs to know about when dealing with these patients.

References

Disorders of Respiration

1. Campbell, E. J. M.: The Respiratory Muscles: And the Mechanics of Breathing. Chicago, Year Book Medical Publishers, Inc., 1958.
2. Comroe, J. H., Jr., Forster, R. E., II, Dubois, A. B., Briscoe, W. A., and Carlsen, E.: The Lung; Clinical Physiology and Pulmonary Function Tests, 2nd Ed. Chicago, Year Book Medical Publishers, Inc., 1962.
3. Polgar, G., and Promadhat V.: Pulmonary Function

Testing in Children. Philadelphia, W. B. Saunders Company, 1971.

4. Barach, A. L., Beck, G. J., Bickerman, H. A., and Seanor, H. E.: Physical methods simulating cough mechanisms. Use in poliomyelitis, bronchial asthma, pulmonary emphysema and bronchiectasis. J.A.M.A., 150:1380, 1952.

5. Barach, A. L., and Beck, G. J.: Exsufflation with negative pressure, physiologic and clinical studies in poliomyelitis, bronchial asthma, pulmonary emphysema and bronchiectasis. Arch. Int. Med., 93:825, 1954.

Chest Physical Therapy

6. Physiotherapy Department, Brompton Hospital, London: Physiotherapy for Medical and Surgical Thoracic Conditions, 1967.

7. Egan, D. F.: Fundamentals of Inhalation Therapy. St. Louis, The C. V. Mosby Co., 1969.

8. Halpern, D.: Techniques of Bronchial Drainage. Department of Physical Medicine and Rehabilitation, University of Minnesota Medical School, Minneapolis, 1967.

9. Bartlett, R. H., Brennon, M. L., Gazzaniga, A. B., and Hansen, E. L.: Studies on the pathogenesis and prevention of postoperative pulmonary complications. Surg. Gynecol. Obstet., 137:925, 1975.

10. Bellamy, R., Pitts, F. W., and Stauffer, E. S.: Respiratory complications of traumatic quadriplegia: Analysis of 20 years experience. J. Neurosurg., 39:596–600, 1973.

11. McMichan, J. C., Michel, L., and Westbrook, P. R.: Pulmonary dysfunction following traumatic quadriplegia. J.A.M.A., 243:528–531, 1980.

12. Glenn, W. W. L., Holcomb, W. G., Shaw, R. K., Hogan, J. F., and Holschuh, K. R.: Long-term ventilatory support by diaphragm pacing in quadriplegia. Ann. Surg., 183:566, 1976.

41

Rehabilitation of the Patient with Heart Disease

THOMAS E. KOTTKE
THERESE H. HANEY
MARGARET M. DOUCETTE

This chapter is written for the physiatrist who is managing the patient with cardiac disease, whether cardiovascular disease is the sole condition or a condition complicating another disease process like diabetes with amputation or stroke. The chapter goals are threefold. The first goal is to provide the reader with a historical perspective on the development of cardiac rehabilitation. The historical perspective helps the reader understand the problems that have been faced and overcome in the management of these patients. It also gives perspective to the further work that needs to be done despite the radical improvements that have occurred over the past quarter century.

The second goal is to provide the reader with the basic management principles for the patient with cardiac disease. The recognition that cardiac rehabilitation is just one, but an essential, facet of the program of comprehensive management will optimize patient outcomes. Cardiac rehabilitation is not designed to replace other interventions, and other interventions cannot replace cardiac rehabilitation. It is expected that the physiatrist working with patients who have cardiac disease will have access to a supportive and interested cardiologist. This teamwork will allow maximum remobilization of the patient with minimum risk of untoward outcomes.

The third goal is to provide the reader with a basic understanding of the principles of comprehensive cardiac rehabilitation—risk factor management, remobilization, and psychosocial reintegration. It is when cardiac rehabilitation is viewed in this perspective that the patient receives the most benefit.

Several comprehensive manuals of cardiac rehabilitation are available. The text by Wenger and Hellerstein[1] is a comprehensive handbook that is recommended as the basic volume. The text by Pollock and Schmidt[2] focuses on the physical activity components of cardiac rehabilitation, and the text by Wilson and colleagues[3] provides advice about day-to-day program management. These three texts are recommended for the professional who is actively involved with the rehabilitation of patients with cardiovascular disease.

The Evolution of Cardiac Rehabilitation

In the last 60 years there has been a revolutionary change in the concepts of care for the patient with acute myocardial infarction. In 1929, it was advised that

The nurse should be carefully instructed to do everything in her power to aid the patient in any physical activity so that all possible movements such as feeding himself or lifting himself in bed are spared. . . . Finally, the patient should be urged to spend at least six weeks, and preferably eight weeks or more, absolutely in bed.[4]

Ten years later, Mallory, White, and Salcedo-Salger[5] wrote,

Thus, our findings support the more or less empirical custom of those who advise for patients with small- to moderate-sized myocardial infarcts, without complications, one month of rest in bed (the first two weeks absolutely complete), and one month of very carefully graded convalescence, with a third month to consolidate recovery and to re-establish good health both of body and mind. To advise less than three weeks in bed is unwise, even for patients with the smallest myocardial infarcts, provided we are sure of the diagnosis; and it is almost equally unwise to advise prolonged bed rest in the absence of complications or when the infarct is not very large, because of the needlessness of so doing and the harm to the patient's health in general and to the morale and happiness of himself and his family.

Levine devoted several paragraphs to warn the reader that much of the treatment of myocardial infarction was based on supposition.[4] The caveat was altogether absent in the paper by Mallory, White, and Salcedo-Salger, however, even though the treatment recommendations were not based on trial but rather on an autopsy series.[5] The ensuing 40 years have been spent trying to wrestle free from the constraints signified by the paragraphs quoted. Only recently has the central question for cardiac rehabilitation changed from "Is activity safe?" to "Does activity help?"

The pioneering papers of the 1950s, 1960s, and 1970s shared a common theme: A group of patients had been subjected to rates of mobilization or levels of exercise intensity previously accepted as unsafe; even so, the patients did not suffer untoward consequences. In 1952, Samuel Levine and Bernard Lown reported that acute myocardial infarction patients could sit up in a chair without problems.[6] In 1968, Tobis and Zohman reported that an in-hospital program of physical training was safe,[7] and in 1974, Bloch and colleagues demonstrated the safety of early mobilization with a controlled trial.[8]

Markiewicz[9] and DeBusk and Haskell[10] demonstrated that patients could be evaluated for physical work capacity as soon as 21 days after acute myocardial infarction, and DeBusk and colleagues[11] and Davidson and associates[12] reported that exercise testing could be used to stratify patients prognostically into low-risk and high-risk groups. In 1986, DeBusk and co-workers[13] reported guidelines for the identification of low-risk patients and patients who might benefit from revascularization (Fig. 41–1).

The safety of outpatient cardiac rehabilitation has been established. In 1986, Van Camp and Peterson reported on the experience of 167 outpatient cardiac rehabilitation programs.[14] Over 50,000 patients exercised for more than 2.3 million hours with only three deaths, 18 cardiac arrests from which the patient was resuscitated, and eight nonfatal myocardial infarctions. The incidence rates per million patient hours of exercise were 8.9 for cardiac arrest, 3.4 for myocardial infarctions, and 1.3 for fatalities.

Although the safety of physical training programs was fairly easy to demonstrate, demonstrating the ability of these programs to reduce the incidence of premature death has been more difficult. Wilhelmsen and associates reported a randomized trial of physical training in 1975.[15] In four years of follow-up, 28 of 158 patients in the training group died, whereas 35 of 157 patients in the control group died. Both Kentala's trial[16] and the National Heart Disease Exercise Program[17] were plagued by low adherence and failed to demonstrate significant program effect. Although all of these trials suffered from sample sizes inadequate to generate statistical significance for the observed differences, meta-analysis (a statistical technique of combining study results) of the studies suggests that exercise after myocardial infarction probably reduces death rates by 20 per cent.[18]

As early as 1968, Naughton and co-workers,[19] Nagle and associates,[20] and others[21] reported that exercise training improved emotional status, and in 1979, Kallio and co-workers[22] reported that their randomized trial of comprehensive cardiac rehabilitation had produced a 60 per cent difference in sudden death and a 40 per cent difference in deaths from coronary heart disease. The major differences between the groups were not in exercise rates and physical work capacity but in blood pressure, serum cholesterol, and weight control.

Cardiac rehabilitation can increase both the length and the quality of life. As described in detail later, life can be prolonged when the patient is treated with beta-adrenergic blocking agents and angiotensin-converting inhibitors and when risk factors are well controlled. Quality of life is optimized when the physician is alert for signs of anxiety and depression while guiding the patient back to the fullest and most active life desired and tolerated by the patient.

Cardiac rehabilitation will be facing another challenge in the future. As the population of the United States grows older, more and more patients will have dysfunction of multiple organ systems.

THOMAS E. KOTTKE, THERESE H. HANEY, AND MARGARET M. DOUCETTE

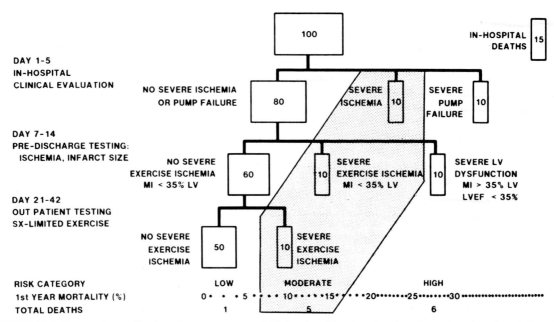

FIGURE 41–1. Prognostic stratification after acute myocardial infarction. The size of each patient subset (numbers in boxes) in the algorithm is approximate and will vary according to the patient population. Stratification of patients into the three main risk categories (low, moderate, and high) is based on the extent of myocardial ischemia (MI) and left ventricular (LV) dysfunction. A variety of clinical observations and tests may be used to detect these abnormalities at various times after acute myocardial infarction. Patients in the shaded area are those most likely to experience a reduction in mortality from coronary revascularization. LVEF denotes left ventricular ejection fraction, and SX symptom-limited. (By permission from DeBusk, R. F., Blomqvist, C. G., Kouchoukos, N. T., Luepker, R. V., Miller, H. S., Moss, A. J., Pollock, M. L., Reeves, T. J., Selvester, R. H., and Stason, W. B.: Identification and treatment of low-risk patients after acute myocardial infarction and coronary-artery bypass graft surgery. N. Engl. J. Med., 314:161–166, 1986.)

These patients will require management by multiple specialists, physiatrists included. The presence of stable cardiovascular disease should not be a barrier to full functioning, but a basic understanding of cardiac pathophysiology and patient care is essential if the physiatrist is to treat the cardiac patient with confidence.

The time course of cardiac rehabilitation has traditionally been divided into phases: phase I has been inpatient cardiac rehabilitation, phase II the first 12 weeks after discharge from the hospital, and phase III the period from 12 weeks to one year after discharge. Each of the four major areas of cardiac rehabilitation—management of cardiovascular pathophysiology, risk factor control, remobilization, and psychosocial adjustment—must be addressed during each phase of the rehabilitation process. The four areas are addressed in this order in the chapter.

Cardiac Pathophysiology

Whereas the majority of patients in a cardiac rehabilitation program will be followed by a cardiologist, both the amount of time that the patient spends in the program and the physical activity of the program will tend to expose the patient's underlying problems. The patient should be referred back to the referring cardiologist when problems arise, but recognition that a problem exists requires that the physiatrist have a basic understanding of cardiac pathophysiology. The next four sections, myocardial energetics, coronary atherosclerosis, congestive heart failure, and dysrhythmia, are written to provide that understanding.

Myocardial Energetics

Physical work requires that oxygen diffuse into the blood in the lungs and be transported to the target tissues by the blood. The heart is the source of energy for oxygen transportation. The work required of the heart closely parallels the systolic blood pressure multiplied by the heart rate (Fig. 41–2).[23] This product is variously referred to as the "double product," the "rate-pressure product (RPP)," or the "pressure-rate product (PRP)."

When patients are performing their activities of daily living, the heart rate alone is a suitable predictor of myocardial oxygen uptake (see Fig. 41–2).

Systolic hypertension increases the myocardial work requirements for any given task. Internal derangements of cardiac anatomy and physiology also increase myocardial oxygen consumption without increasing external work. Stenotic valves between the ventricles and the great vessels require the myocardium to generate higher pressures to force the blood across the valves. In these cases, the double product measured peripherally underestimates myocardial work.

Insufficient ventricular–great vessel valves allow blood to regurgitate from the great vessels into the ventricles during diastole and from the ventricles into the atria during systole. This regurgitation decreases cardiac efficiency because less than 100 per cent of the ventricular output reaches the target tissues.

Cardiac chambers dilate as a compensatory response in congestive heart failure. Because wall tension is proportional to the radius of the ventricle, and oxygen consumption is proportional to wall tension, ventricular dilation results in increased energy consumption at a given level of cardiac output.

Coronary Atherosclerosis

Coronary atherosclerosis is the result of endothelial cell injury, smooth muscle proliferation, and the accumulation of cholesterol by monocytes and macrophages in the subintimal layer of the arteries.[24] Whereas serum cholesterol is a major predictor of atherosclerosis, platelets and platelet-derived growth factor (PDGF) also appear to have a significant role in the development of atherosclerosis.[25]

It is thought that rupture and ulceration of the plaque is one of the mechanisms that leads to the coronary thrombosis that precipitates acute myocardial infarction. Whereas coronary spasm in the absence of atherosclerosis is known to occur, it is seen more frequently at the site of atheromas.

Inadequate coronary blood flow, cardiac ischemia, results in two conditions that are pathological for myocardial cells: oxygen deprivation and the inadequate removal of metabolites.[26] Normal coronary arteries have a flow capacity far in excess of maximum demand, so cardiac ischemia does not develop even under maximum loads when the coronary arteries are normal, but myocardial dysfunction develops rapidly in the presence of ischemia. Humans have been shown to develop collateral circulation in the presence of obstruction, but

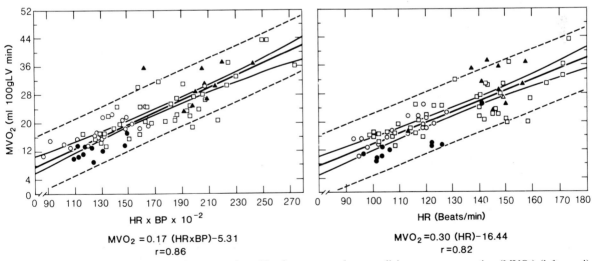

$$MVO_2 = 0.17 \ (HR \times BP) - 5.31$$
$$r = 0.86$$

$$MVO_2 = 0.30 \ (HR) - 16.44$$
$$r = 0.82$$

FIGURE 41–2. Relationship between heart rate times blood pressure and myocardial oxygen consumption (MVO_2) (left panel) and heart rate and myocardial oxygen consumption (MVO_2) (right panel) in 29 subjects. The filled triangles represent combined static and dynamic exercise, the open boxes represent dynamic exercise, the filled circles represent static exercise, and the open circles represent dynamic exercise with propranolol. Heart rate times systolic blood pressure was the best predictor of MVO_2. Heart rate alone also predicted MVO_2. (By permission from Nelson, R. R., Gobel, F. L., Jorgensen, C. R., Wang, K., Wang, Y., and Taylor, H. L.: Hemodynamic predictors of myocardial oxygen consumption during static and dynamic exercise. Circulation, 50:1179–1189, 1974.)

THOMAS E. KOTTKE, THERESE H. HANEY, AND MARGARET M. DOUCETTE

it is not clear that exercise programs can regularly accomplish this task.

Angina pectoris, the squeezing pain of cardiac ischemia that may be present in the chest, neck, jaw, or arms, occurs when myocardial oxygen demand exceeds oxygen supply. Angina during exercise is the result of increasing demand, and angina that occurs at rest may be the result of decreased flow associated with coronary artery contraction or transient obstruction. Angina at rest can also result from increases in cardiac work caused by increases in catecholamine levels during excitement and anxiety.

Congestive Heart Failure

Congestive heart failure develops when the myocardium can no longer supply the energy demanded of it by the body.[27] The etiological factors include hypertension, ischemia, valvular disease, viral infections, infiltrative processes, and idiopathic processes. The therapist should be familiar with the symptoms and signs of worsening congestive heart failure (Table 41–1).

Before the advent of effective diuretics and agents that reduce afterload, bed rest was the mainstay of treatment for congestive heart failure. Diuretics, angiotensin-converting inhibitors, nitrates, and hydralazine eliminate the need for exercise restriction beyond those activities that cause physical distress or symptoms of exhaustion for the patient.

Treatment focuses on lowering output impedance (systolic blood pressure) and thereby cardiac work. The pressures of the accepted definition of systolic hypertension ("borderline," 140 to 160 mm Hg; "definite" >160 mm Hg) are far higher than

TABLE 41–1. Symptoms and Signs of Worsening Congestive Heart Failure

Symptoms
  Waking at night with shortness of breath
  Inability to lie flat without becoming short of breath
  Increasing dyspnea on exertion
Signs
  Increasing weight
  Swelling of the ankles or abdomen
  Decreasing physical work capacity
  Rales in chest
  Third heart sound
  Distended neck veins

optimal for patients with congestive heart failure. It appears that the optimal blood pressure should be at the lowest level that provides for cerebral, visceral, and peripheral circulatory needs. For many patients with congestive heart failure, optimal systolic blood pressure levels are in the 90 to 100 mm Hg range, and few need levels greater than 110 to 120 mm Hg. Whereas most patients will require the administration of diuretics,[28] patients without contraindications should also be on either a combination of nitrates and hydralazine or on an angiotensin-converting enzyme (ACE) inhibitor, as these have been shown to prolong life.[29, 30] Beta blockade has been reported to control congestive heart failure in some trials, but the intervention has not experienced widespread popularity.[31]

Dysrhythmia

It is the rare patient who does not have any dysrhythmia. Few patients have to be physically limited if the dysrhythmia has been treated adequately. Whether fast or slow, ventricular or supraventricular, however, any dysrhythmia that causes syncope, or near-syncope, should be evaluated immediately by a cardiologist.

If dysrhythmia is suggested because of symptoms of palpitations, lightheadedness, near-syncope, or syncope, ambulatory monitoring is more likely than exercise testing to detect rhythm disturbance.[32–34] Because of the day-to-day variability in dysrhythmia during exercise, an exercise test that is negative for dysrhythmia in a patient with syncope does not exclude dysrhythmia as a source of the problem.[35] Patients who have infrequent attacks of palpitations, dizziness, or other symptoms suggestive of dysrhythmia may be given a monitor to carry with them for several weeks so that the rhythm can be recorded or transmitted when the patient is experiencing symptoms.

The therapist should be able to identify the components of the normal rhythm tracing (Fig. 41–3), to identify premature ventricular depolarizations (Fig. 41–4), and to recognize supraventricular dysrhythmias (Fig. 41–5).

Failure to control the ventricular rate in patients with atrial fibrillation can result in impaired exercise performance and frank congestive heart failure. Adequate control of the ventricular rate at rest does not mean that the patient has adequate control of the ventricular rate during exercise.

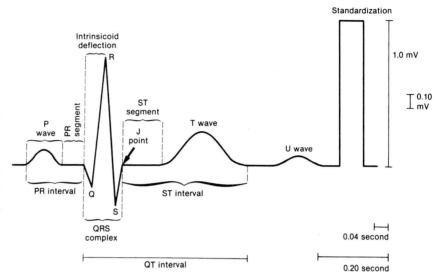

FIGURE 41-3. A normal electrocardiogram showing the morphological character of the P wave, QRS complex, T wave, and U wave as well as the standardization. The P wave results from atrial depolarization, the QRS complex from ventricular depolarization, and the T wave from ventricular repolarization. (By permission from Johnson, R., and Swartz, M. H.: A Simplified Approach to Electrocardiography. Philadelphia, W. B. Saunders Company, 1986.)

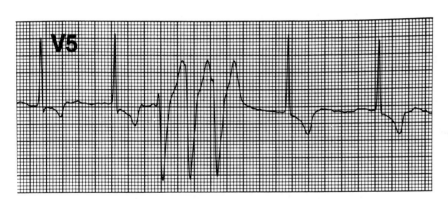

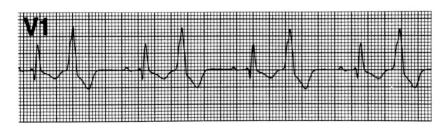

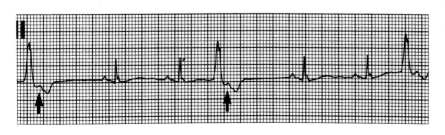

FIGURE 41-4. Ventricular tachycardia is defined as three or more ventricular premature depolarizations in succession (top panel). Ventricular bigeminy is the alternating of supraventricular depolarizations with premature ventricular depolarizations (middle panel). Unifocal premature ventricular depolarizations are demonstrated in the bottom panel. The arrows point to P waves distorting the T waves of the premature ventricular depolarizations. Most cardiac rehabilitation protocols require the cessation of exercise and the notification of a physician if ventricular tachycardia, bigeminy, or more than five unifocal premature depolarizations per minute are observed. (By permission from Johnson, R., and Swartz, M. H.: A Simplified Approach to Electrocardiography. Philadelphia, W. B. Saunders Company, 1986.)

THOMAS E. KOTTKE, THERESE H. HANEY, AND MARGARET M. DOUCETTE

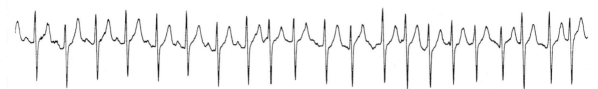

CH 01   11:30AM TUE 8/25/87   MANUAL   25MM/S   DLY   HR=164   GAIN=1   BW=MON

FIGURE 41–5. Supraventricular tachycardia developing in a heart transplant patient. The ninth QRS complex appears earlier than expected and takes off in the middle of the P wave rather than after the P wave as expected. P waves cannot be consistently identified after this depolarization. Exercise should be terminated and a physician should be contacted immediately if supraventricular tachycardia is observed.

Therefore, all patients with atrial fibrillation should have their pulse rates measured during exercise. In the presence of atrial fibrillation, heart rates greater than 120 to 150 beats per minute cause the ventricle to begin contraction before filling adequately, and the cardiac output falls paradoxically. If digitalis fails to control the ventricular rate during exercise, a trial of verapamil or a beta-adrenergic blocking agent is warranted.

Treatment of dysrhythmia is not without side effect. All of the antidysrhythmic agents currently on the market are potentially dysrhythmogenic. It is also important to remember that only beta-adrenergic blocking agents have been shown to prolong life. Therefore, whereas dysrhythmia that causes syncope or near-syncope should trigger an aggressive work-up and therapy, unifocal premature ventricular depolarizations that are asymptomatic or only cause palpitations can be treated with observation alone unless the patient finds them debilitating. Unifocal premature ventricular depolarizations have been shown not to be associated with subsequent coronary events.[32]

Risk Factor Control

Education about risk factor modification should begin during the inpatient phase of cardiac rehabilitation. However, patients are often required to make multiple changes of life style, and participation in an outpatient program can help provide them with further supportive therapy and skill-building for physical activity, diet, cessation of smoking, and management of stress. As described in the following, the entire family unit should be involved in making and supporting these changes.

Blood Pressure

Spontaneous normalization of previously elevated blood pressure after myocardial infarction is a sign of incipient heart failure and indicates poor prognosis.[36] Therefore, systolic blood pressure should be kept in the 100 to 120 mm Hg range. The use of beta-adrenergic blockade agents has been shown to prolong life after myocardial infarction,[18] and ACE inhibitors have been shown to benefit patients with early heart failure.[30] These are the agents of choice in patients without and with heart failure, respectively (Table 41–2).

Diet and Serum Cholesterol

Serum cholesterol is the best predictor of closure of a vein graft of a coronary artery,[37] and control of serum cholesterol reduces the progression[38, 39] or may produce regression of coronary artery stenosis.[40, 41] Whereas total serum cholesterol levels predict coronary heart disease, low-density lipo-

TABLE 41–2. Fundamentals of Blood Pressure Control After Myocardial Infarction

Treat both systolic and diastolic hypertension

Be aware that the disappearance of hypertension after a myocardial infarction is a sign of myocardial dysfunction

The goal for systolic blood pressure should be 100–120 mm Hg

Avoid large doses of diuretics in patients who exhibit repolarization abnormalities on their resting ECG

Use beta-adrenergic blocking agents for patients without heart failure or asthma

Use angiotensin-converting inhibitors for patients with congestive heart failure

protein (LDL) is the fraction directly associated with coronary heart disease. LDL can be calculated by subtracting the high-density lipoprotein level (HDL) and one fifth of the serum triglycerides from the total serum cholesterol level.

Diet is the first-line therapy of hyperlipidemia treatment and control of atherosclerosis. Patients who have clinical sequelae of atherosclerosis should be on a low-fat diet regardless of their serum cholesterol level, for it has been shown that they are susceptible to the effects of dietary fat.

To lower serum cholesterol, patients should be urged to feature fresh fruits and vegetables and whole grain cereal products in their diets (Table 41–3).[42] Skim milk products should be substituted for whole milk products. Patients should avoid sausages, lunch meats, bacon, snack foods, and frozen prepared foods. Meats should be baked or broiled, not fried. Chicken, fish, fresh pork, and lean beef are the meats of choice and should be limited to three to six ounces per day.

If the total serum cholesterol level remains over 200 mg/dl after six months of dietary therapy, the level of the low-density lipoprotein fraction should be calculated. Ideally, the low-density lipoprotein fraction should be less than 130 mg/dl.[43] If it is greater than 160 mg/dl, and the patient is on the lowest fat diet that he or she will tolerate, pharmacological treatment of hyperlipidemia should be initiated (Fig. 41–6).

Unless contraindicated, patients should take one aspirin a day to decrease the progression of coronary artery disease and decrease the risk of coronary thrombosis.[25] Transplant patients deserve special attention to diet and serum cholesterol because of the appetite-inducing and atherogenic properties of corticosteroids.[44]

Smoking

Smoking triples the risk of coronary heart disease for men under 55 years of age.[45] Smoking predicts the appearance of congestive cardiomy-

TABLE 41–3. Dietary Guidelines for Achieving Optimal Lipid Levels

Emphasize	Rationale
Appropriately combined foods of plant origin: beans, cereal grains, vegetables (cooked and raw), fruits	Good-quality protein; low in fat, saturated fat, and cholesterol; low in sodium; low in refined sugar; complex carbohydrates; high in minerals, vitamins, and fiber; lower calorie intake
Fish, poultry, and lean meats, used in small portions and eaten less often as main dish	Good-quality protein; low in fat, saturated fat, and cholesterol; lower calorie intake
Low-fat dairy products for adults	Good-quality protein; high in minerals; low in fat, saturated fat, and cholesterol; lower calorie intake
Less oils and fats used in food preparation and as spreads, with preference for liquid vegetable oils	
De-emphasize	**Rationale**
High-fat meats from domestic breeds as principal protein source	High in saturated fat and cholesterol; high calorie intake
High-fat dairy products (whole milk, cream, cheese)	High in saturated fat and cholesterol; high calorie intake
Whole eggs, unless used as a major source of protein	Egg yolks high in cholesterol
Commercially baked products	High in saturated fat; high calorie intake
Alcoholic beverages	High calorie intake; low in nutrients

From World Health Organization Expert Committee on Prevention of Coronary Heart Disease: Prevention of coronary heart disease. WHO Tech. Rep. Ser. 678, 1982.

THOMAS E. KOTTKE, THERESE H. HANEY, AND MARGARET M. DOUCETTE

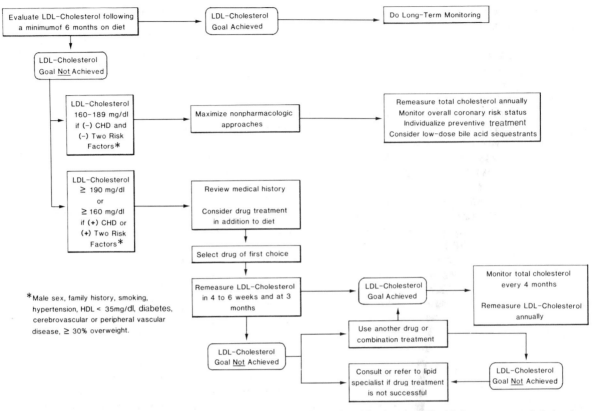

FIGURE 41–6. The National Cholesterol Education Program of the National Institutes of Health has recommended that low density lipoprotein (LDL) be used as the indicator to evaluate whether an individual needs to be placed on lipid-lowering medications. An LDL value of 130 mg/dl or less is the goal. Drug treatment should be initiated at 160 mg/dl if there is a history of coronary heart disease or if other risk factors are present. If the patient has no history of coronary heart disease and has no other risk factors, drug therapy should be initiated at 190 mg/dl.

opathy independently of coronary artery disease.[46] Young women with myocardial infarction are six times as likely to be smokers as are controls.[47]

Continued smoking after myocardial infarction is associated with a doubling of death rates,[48–50] and continued smoking predicts recurrence of sudden cardiac arrest.[51] Smoking causes silent ischemia[52] and reduces the antianginal effects of propranolol, atenolol, and nifedipine.[53] Continued smoking results in higher failure rates for femoral-popliteal artery grafts.[54] Smoking even shortens the survival of patients after bypass grafting of the coronary arteries.[55]

Analysis of the controlled trials of smoking cessation indicates that no one intervention is clearly more powerful than others.[56] The programs that are most likely to succeed use both physicians and nonphysicians to provide the intervention, use multiple modalities of intervention, and provide the intervention over the longest possible time.

As soon as patients enter the hospital, they should be advised to stop smoking. Smoking areas

in hospitals and clinics lead patients to believe that smoking is not a problem.[57] Smoking should not be allowed in any care facility. The entire treatment and rehabilitation team should provide a clear and consistent message that the patient should stop smoking. A therapist should be assigned to work with the patient to develop problem-solving skills to replace the smoking behavior with a more appropriate activity (Table 41–4). The patient can then face urges to smoke with confi-

TABLE 41–4. Guidelines for Smoking Interventions

At each visit, advise the patient that you would like him or her to quit smoking
Ask the patients what they are willing to do about their smoking
Reinforce positive attempts to quit smoking
Reinforce the patient who has quit smoking
Expect that the patient may relapse
Do not give up; most ex-smokers have tried to quit several times before finally succeeding

dence. Although the patient should be reminded that most ex-smokers cannot have a cigarette "now and then" without returning to previous levels of consumption, a "slip" should be viewed after the fact as a learning situation for future abstinence, not as a cause for disabling remorse.

Physical Activity

Evaluation of Physical Work Capacity (Exercise Testing)

Evaluation of physical work capacity requires the combination of three components: type of exercise, intensity of exercise, and duration of exercise. Whereas the ultimate measure of the ability of the heart to do work is the peak double product, the ability of the patient to generate external work will vary with the type of work being done.

The supervising physician must be willing to modify the rate and type of exercise to fit the individual patient's special needs and level of conditioning. Physical work capacity is most frequently evaluated with a multistage treadmill test or a multistage bicycle ergometer test, but arm ergometry, wall weights, free weights, or any other mode of exercise that results in repetitive use of large muscle groups can be used to evaluate cardiopulmonary fitness for the patient who cannot pedal a bicycle or walk on a treadmill.

All patients must be screened for contraindications before exercise testing (Table 41–5).[58] For

TABLE 41–5. Contraindications to Exercise Testing

Acute myocardial infarction
Unstable angina pectoris
Uncontrolled congestive heart failure
Active pericarditis or myocarditis
Recent embolism
Thrombophlebitis or known intracardiac thrombi
Moderate to severe aortic stenosis
Uncontrolled ventricular dysrhythmia
Uncontrolled supraventricular dysrhythmia
Enlarging ventricular aneurysm
Uncontrolled diabetes
Acute systemic illness or fever
Significant emotional distress
Resting blood pressure >120 mm Hg diastolic or >200 mm Hg systolic

Adapted from American College of Sports Medicine: Guidelines for Exercise Testing and Prescription, 3rd Ed. Philadelphia, Lea & Febiger, 1986, pp. 13–14.

patients who can be safely evaluated, several different standardized protocols are available (Fig. 41–7).[59–63] The Bruce treadmill protocol starts at five METS (one MET is considered to be 3.5 ml O_2/kg/minute or the rate of oxygen consumption at rest) and is designed to rule out significant heart disease in otherwise normal patients.[60] Because patients who have heart disease or are deconditioned frequently cannot walk fast enough for even stage one of the Bruce protocol, we prefer the treadmill protocol used by the National Heart Disease Exercise Project.[61] Also referred to as "the Naughton protocol," this protocol starts one at zero grade at two miles per hour. The grade is increased 3.5 per cent every three minutes. The first stage requires two METS of activity, and the requirement is increased by one MET with each succeeding stage. A three-minute stage duration for graded exercise tests allows stabilization of heart rate, blood pressure, and oxygen consumption by the end of the stage and gives a more accurate estimation of physical work capacity than does a stage of shorter duration.

When the reconditioning of the outpatient cardiac rehabilitation patient begins with a bicycle ergometer, a bicycle ergometer should be used to formulate the baseline exercise prescription. The test starts at zero load and increases 12.5 watts every three minutes. For heart and heart-lung transplantation patients, we start at zero load and increase by 12.5 watts every minute. The short stage time allows determination of the patient's strength before the peripheral muscles are overcome by the effects of deconditioning. This protocol also reduces the incidence of severe fatigue following exercise testing.

If ischemia is suspected, the use of multiple indicators including percentage of maximal heart rate achieved, ST-T change, age, and total treadmill time to evaluate the response to exercise is more accurate than the use of ST-T wave depression alone.[64] Resting ST-T wave changes or left bundle branch block precludes the use of the ECG to diagnose exercise-induced ischemia. Exercise thallium studies or multiple gated acquisition (MUGA) studies can be used in these patients. These radionuclide tests are also useful in patients who have equivocal electrocardiographic changes with low double products and low levels of peak physical work capacity.

Arm ergometry can be used to test for ischemia in patients who cannot use their legs (Fig. 41–8).[65] Arms are less efficient than legs at power tasks, so the double product at any given level of external work is higher for arm work than for leg work.[66]

FUNCTIONAL CLASS	CLINICAL STATUS	O₂ REQUIREMENTS ml O₂/kg/min	STEP TEST: NAGLE, BALKE, NAUGHTON* (2 min stages, 30 steps/min)	BRUCE† (3-min stages) mph	BRUCE† %gr	KATTUS‡ (3-min stages) mph	KATTUS‡	BALKE** % grade at 3.4 mph	BALKE** % grade at 3 mph	BICYCLE ERGOMETER** (For 70 kg body weight) kgm/min
NORMAL AND I	PHYSICALLY ACTIVE SUBJECTS	56.0	(Step height increased 4 cm q 2 min)					26		
		52.5						24		
		49.0		mph %gr		4	22	22		1500
		45.5	Height (cm)	4.2	16			20		
		42.0	40			4	18	18	22.5	1350
	SEDENTARY HEALTHY	38.5	36					16	20.0	1200
		35.0	32	3.4	14	4	14	14	17.5	1050
		31.5	28					12	15.0	900
		28.0	24			4	10	10	12.5	750
	DISEASED, RECOVERED SYMPTOMATIC PATIENTS	24.5	20	2.5	12	3	10	8	10.0	
II		21.0	16					6	7.5	600
		17.5	12	1.7	10	2	10	4	5.0	450
		14.0	8					2	2.5	300
III		10.5	4						0.0	150
		7.0								
IV		3.5								

FIGURE 41–7. Several standardized protocols are available to test the physical work capacity of patients known to have or suspected of having coronary artery disease. Oxygen requirements increase from the bottom of the chart to the top. (Reproduced with permission from Exercise Testing and Training of Apparently Healthy Individuals: A Handbook for Physicians (1972). American Heart Association, pp. 32–34.)
*Nagle, F. S., Balke, B., and Naughton, J. P.: J. Appl. Physiol., 20:745–748, 1965.
†Bruce, R. A.: Prescription of exercise in apparently healthy individuals. Dallas, TX, American Heart Association, 1972.
‡Kattus, A. A., Jorgensen, C. R., Worden, R. E., and Alvaro, A. B.: Circulation, 41:585–595, 1971.
**Fox, S. M., Naughton, J. P., and Haskell, W. L.: Ann. Clin. Res., 3:404–432, 1971.

FIGURE 41–8. Weight adjustment is necessary to calculate METS when testing with an arm ergometry protocol. This protocol employs two-minute stages at a crank rate of 60 rpm; 15-second pauses between stages permit accurate ECG and blood pressure recordings. (By permission from Franklin, B. A.: Exercise testing, training and arm ergometry. Sports Med., 2:100–119, 1985.)

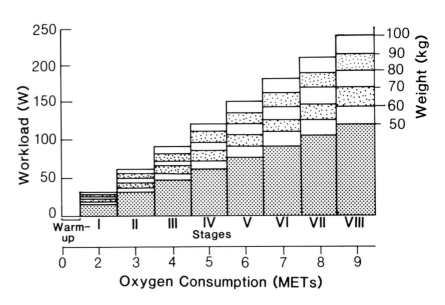

However, maximum rate-pressure product is proportional to the size of the muscle mass doing the external work,[67] and a patient who does not develop myocardial ischemia during leg exercise will rarely, if ever, develop myocardial ischemia with arm exercise.[68] Hung and co-workers tested men under three conditions, treadmill alone, treadmill while carrying a weight, and treadmill after a 1000-calorie meal, and found that patients who did not develop ischemic changes on treadmill alone did not develop ischemia during the other two conditions.[69] Because the prevalence and extent of exercise-induced left ventricular dysfunction, ST-segment depression, angina pectoris, and ventricular ectopic activity did not differ significantly among the test conditions, they concluded that maximal exercise testing on a treadmill or a bicycle ergometer was a sufficient single test to prescribe a program of physical activity.

It is important to remember that not all chest pain during activity is angina pectoris. If the patient is complaining of chest pain during arm activity, arm exercise testing and ambulatory ECG monitoring may be used to satisfy the patient and the physician that the pain is not due to ischemia.[68] If either symptomatic or silent ischemia is observed on ambulatory ECG monitoring, further evaluation is suggested. A correlation between silent ischemia and subsequent coronary events in patients presenting with unstable angina pectoris has been described.[70]

Respiratory Gas Analysis. Measurement of oxygen uptake and carbon dioxide production on a breath-by-breath basis has become commonly available. Metabolic measurement during exercise can help the physician determine anaerobic threshold (i.e., the highest oxygen uptake that can be reached during exercise before an increase in blood lactate occurs) and provide an exercise prescription based on the individual patient's metabolic patterns.[71] The test can also be used to determine the pathological source of low maximum oxygen uptake. For example, low maximum oxygen uptake in the presence of a normal anaerobic threshold indicates poor effort, deconditioning, lung disease, or angina pectoris. The low maximum oxygen uptake and a low anaerobic threshold indicate ventricular dysfunction, pulmonary vascular disease, peripheral vascular disease, or anemia.[71] A decline in the amount of oxygen delivered per ventricular contraction ("oxygen pulse") at peak exercise indicates acute ventricular dysfunction, usually a sign of ischemia.[72]

TABLE 41–6. Guidelines for Inpatient Reconditioning Programs

Frequency:	Two to three times per day
Intensity:	Pulse rise limited to 30 beats per min above resting
Duration:	5 to 20 min per session
Type:	One to five MET upper extremity calisthenics, stair-climbing, bicycling, and walking on a treadmill

Cardiopulmonary Reconditioning

Just as the patient who understands what will happen in the postoperative period needs less pain medication, the patient who has had preoperative instruction regarding postoperative mobilization will respond more quickly and more positively to remobilization efforts. Bed rest itself causes deterioration of function even in normal individuals. In 1949, Taylor and colleagues demonstrated that three weeks of bed rest in six normal individuals raised the pulse while standing from 127 beats per minute to 167 beats per minute.[73] After 16 days of recovery, the pulse while standing had recovered by only 50 per cent. Therefore, there is no role for "rest therapy" in the management of the patient with cardiovascular disease. Early mobilization of the patient hospitalized after myocardial infarction has been demonstrated to be beneficial to the patient's recovery process.[74]

Cardiac rehabilitation should involve the patient in one to two MET exercises as soon as the patient is able to respond appropriately and follow directions.[75] The patient should have two to three exercise sessions per day that last 5 to 20 minutes. The increase of the pulse rate should be limited to 30 beats per minute for patients after myocardial infarction and surgery (Table 41–6).

As soon as patients are able to sit, they should begin spending time in a chair. Pressure monitoring lines, respirator hoses, and intravenous lines can all be manipulated to allow the patient to leave the bed. The patient should be remobilized as rapidly as possible. A five-step program for surgical patients is presented in Table 41–7. Whereas medical patients with congestive heart failure or other complications may take longer to mobilize, the steps are the same.

As soon as patients have left the intensive care unit, they should be encouraged to take their meals sitting in a chair. Every effort should be made to

THOMAS E. KOTTKE, THERESE H. HANEY, AND MARGARET M. DOUCETTE

TABLE 41–7. Five-Step Program of Inpatient Cardiac Rehabilitation for Surgical Patients

STEP	POST-OPERATIVE DAY	NURSING ACTIVITY	OCCUPATIONAL THERAPY ACTIVITIES	PHYSICAL THERAPY ACTIVITIES	WORD OF THE DAY
I	1	Up in chair	Introduce self and program	Introduce self and program	Cardiac rehabilitation
II	2	Self-feeding Bedside commode Walking short distances	Life style assessment Work simplification Energy conservation	Walking short distances, active assisted range of motion, or 1–3 MET calisthenics	Risk factors
III	3	Walk in hall × 3 Bathroom privileges Partial self-bath in bed	Activity precautions Pulse monitoring Smoking cessation	Walk in hall × 3 1–4 MET level calisthenics	MET level
IV	4	Walk *ad lib.* Partial self-bath Out of bed 3–4 hours	ADLs and METS Smoking cessation	Walking *ad lib.* 2–4 MET level calisthenics	Phase II
V	5	Walk *ad lib.* increasing distances	Relaxation training Smoking cessation Work equivalents as appropriate	Walk *ad lib.* 3–5 MET level calisthenics Stair-climbing	Discharge planning

have the patient view the bed as a place to sleep at night and nap for an hour or two in the afternoon, not a place to live. Overly protective family, friends, and health care personnel should be carefully and courteously instructed that all patients will have stiffness and discomfort during the remobilization period, but that the sooner remobilization takes place, the quicker the stiffness will end. We liken the postoperative or postinfarction training period to the training period for athletes; although each has definite guidelines, neither the athlete nor the patient trains for activity by lying in bed.

Specific limits and precautions should replace the vague admonitions "Don't hurt yourself" or "Don't overdo it," since the latter imply to patients that they are at risk but do not give them useful information about how to lower that risk. Figure 41–9 is a decision tree for approaching physical activity. If a patient is asked to or would like to perform a task, he or she must first ask three questions: Is it within my lifting limits? Is it within my MET limits? and Can I do the activity for a limited amount of time? The last question is asked to keep the patient from engaging in an activity from which it is impossible to withdraw (for example, a canoe trip or a long cross-country hike). Tables 41–8 to 41–11 list typical activities.

If the patient can answer "yes" to the first three questions, the patient should perform the activity

for five minutes and take the pulse. If either symptoms of severe dyspnea or chest pain develop, or the pulse limit is exceeded, the patient should either stop or proceed with the task at a lower rate. If the patient does not develop symptoms and the pulse rate is within limits, the patient should continue with an activity for 20 minutes, taking the pulse after 10 minutes and again after 20 minutes. The patient should then stop the activity.

If exhaustion, stiffness, or soreness is experienced in the evening or on the next day, the patient needs to work for shorter time periods, at lower intensity, or with lighter loads. If none of these symptoms is present, the patient should gradually increase the intensity and duration of the activity while periodically monitoring the pulse and keeping alert for new symptoms.

The patient should ideally be exercising large muscle groups at 60 per cent to 70 per cent of maximum heart rate three to five times per week for 10 to 60 minutes per session (Table 41–12). However, if the patient is unable to attain these frequencies or intensities, exercise at lower levels will be helpful. Paffenbarger has written that coronary heart disease death rates could be reduced by 23 per cent if everyone in the population expended more than 2000 kcal per week in vigorous physical activity.[76] These data are frequently but incorrectly interpreted to mean that unless an individual expends at least 2000 kcal per week in

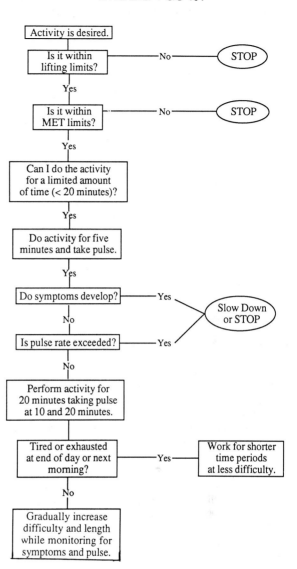

Should I do it?

Activity is desired.

Is it within lifting limits? —No— STOP

Yes

Is it within MET limits? —No— STOP

Yes

Can I do the activity for a limited amount of time (< 20 minutes)?

Yes

Do activity for five minutes and take pulse.

Yes

Do symptoms develop? —Yes—

No

Is pulse rate exceeded? —Yes—

Slow Down or STOP

No

Perform activity for 20 minutes taking pulse at 10 and 20 minutes.

Tired or exhausted at end of day or next morning? —Yes— Work for shorter time periods at less difficulty.

No

Gradually increase difficulty and length while monitoring for symptoms and pulse.

FIGURE 41–9. To determine whether a physical activity can probably be tolerated, the patient checks whether the activity is within lifting and MET limits and whether the activity can be done for less than 20 min. If so, the patient performs the activity for five minutes and stops to evaluate symptoms and pulse. If asymptomatic and below pulse limit, the patient continues the activity for 20 min and evaluates effects of exercise in the evening and the next morning. If asymptomatic, the patient gradually increases the duration and intensity of activity. If symptomatic, the patient should work for a shorter duration and at a lower rate.

TABLE 41–8. Minimal Cardiac Activity

ACTIVITY	POSITION	CARDIAC WORK (CUBS) OR METABOLISM (METS)	CARDIAC OUTPUT (COS)
Leather belt assembly	Sitting at table	1.25	1.10
Leather stamping	Sitting at table	1.35	1.10
Leather tooling	Sitting at table	1.30	1.20
Listening to radio	Sitting in easy chair	1.40	—
Bench assembly, light	Sitting at bench	1.40	1.10
Leather lacing	Sitting at table	1.45	—
Leather lacing	Lateral decubitus	1.55	1.20
Chip carving	Sitting at table	1.60	1.20

CUBS, cardiac work units, ratio to basal; COS, cardiac output, ratio to basal; METS, metabolism, ratio to basal.

887

THOMAS E. KOTTKE, THERESE H. HANEY, AND MARGARET M. DOUCETTE

TABLE 41–9. Light Cardiac Activity

ACTIVITY	POSITION	CARDIAC WORK (CUBS) OR METABOLISM (METS)	CARDIAC OUTPUT (COS)
Eating	Sitting	1.50	—
Sewing	Sitting	1.60	—
Clerical work	Sitting	1.60	—
Setting type	Standing	1.60	1.35
Getting out of and into bed	Bed to chair	1.65	1.45
Leather carving	Sitting on chair	1.70	—
Weaving, table loom	Sitting on stool	1.70	—
Clerical work	Standing	1.80	—
Writing	Sitting	2.00	—
Typing	Sitting on chair	2.00	1.35
Bimanual activity test sanding, 50 strokes/minute	Sitting on chair	2.00	1.40
Weaving, floor loom	Sitting on bench	2.10	1.75
Metal work, hammer	Standing	2.15	1.65
Printing, platen press	Standing	2.30	1.75
Bench assembly, moderate	Sitting	2.35	1.70
Hanging clothes on line	Standing—stooping	2.40	1.80

CUBS, cardiac work units, ratio to basal; COS, cardiac output, ratio to basal; METS, metabolism, ratio to basal.

TABLE 41–10. Moderate Cardiac Activity

ACTIVITY	POSITION	CARDIAC WORK (CUBS) OR METABOLISM (METS)	CARDIAC OUTPUT (COS)
Playing piano		2.50	—
Dressing, undressing		2.50–3.50	—
Sawing, jeweler's saw	Sitting	1.90	2.05
Sawing, hacksaw	Standing	2.55	2.00
Driving car		2.80	—
Bicycling, slowly		2.90	2.45
Preparing meals		3.00	—
Weight lifting, 10 lb lifted 15 inches, 46/minute	Sitting	2.80	2.00
Walking, 2.0 mph		3.20	—
Handsawing, wood	Standing	3.50	2.35
Warm shower		3.50	—

CUBS, cardiac work units, ratio to basal; COS, cardiac output, ratio to basal; METS, metabolism, ratio to basal.

TABLE 41–11. Heavy and Severe Cardiac Activity

ACTIVITY	POSITION	METABOLISM (METS)	CARDIAC OUTPUT (COS)
Bowel movement	Toilet	3.60	—
Bowel movement	Bedpan	4.70	—
Making beds	Standing	3.90	—
Hot shower	Standing	4.20	—
Walking fast (3.5 mph)		5.00	—
Descending stairs		5.20	—
Scrubbing floor	Kneeling	5.30	3.00
Master two-step climbing test		5.70	3.00
Weight lifting, 10–20 lb lifted 36 inches, 15/minute		6.50	3.50
Bicycling, fast		6.90	3.30
Running		7.40	4.0
Mowing lawn		7.70	—
Climbing stairs		9.00	—

METS, metabolism, ratio to basal; COS, cardiac output, ratio to basal.

vigorous physical activity, there is no effect on risk of heart disease. However, the 2000 kcal figure was chosen as a cutpoint. In this data set, the risk of first attack of coronary heart disease begins to decrease at physical activity levels as low as 500 kcal per week (Fig. 41–10).[76] Little benefit accrued from increasing physical activity levels above 4000 kcal per week.

All patients should be encouraged to adopt a walking program. General guidelines are given in Table 41–13. The patient begins walking a quarter mile per day at two miles per hour and works up to two miles a day at four miles per hour (Table 41–14). During inclement weather, the patient can walk in a shopping mall, walk in the halls of a school, or ride a stationary ergometer. Stationary ergometer guidelines are given in Table 41–15. Reading the newspaper or watching television while pedaling can reduce some of the boredom associated with pedaling a stationary ergometer. All patients have a certain number of aches and pains, and a symptom advisory can help the patient distinguish between trivial signs and signs of potential hazards (Table 41–16).

TABLE 41–12. Guidelines for Outpatient Physical Reconditioning Programs

Frequency:	Three to five times per week
Intensity:	Heart rate 60% to 70% of maximum heart rate on treadmill without ischemia
Duration:	10 to 60 minutes per session
Type:	Upper extremity exercises, bicycle ergometer, arm ergometer, stair-climbing, free arm weights, treadmill

In addition to a time devoted to physical activity, all patients should be encouraged to increase physical activity by substituting a low-energy approach to a task with a higher-energy approach. A history should also be taken regarding previous activities involving physical effort (e.g., gardening, bicycling), and the patient should be encouraged to return to these activities as soon as physical conditioning permits. It is far easier to remobilize patients into an activity that they once enjoyed than to attempt to get them to adopt an activity that they have never experienced and may therefore fear. If these activities provide aerobic training, they can replace the walking program.

A manual can opener can be substituted for the electric can opener. The car can be parked at the far end of the parking lot instead of close to the door. Stairs can be taken instead of the elevator. The patient can take a walk during a work break instead of sitting down and eating a snack. Each of these activities contributes toward the physical activity goal.

Strengthening

It has only been in the past 10 years that cardiologists have even considered permitting their patients to perform upper extremity work. Isometric contraction sustained for more than three to four minutes causes marked recruitment of other muscle groups and marked rises in blood pressure.[77] Whereas the blood pressure drops immediately with release of the contraction, it appears

THOMAS E. KOTTKE, THERESE H. HANEY, AND MARGARET M. DOUCETTE

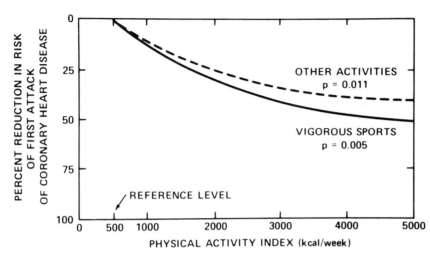

Adjusted for age and follow-up interval

FIGURE 41–10. Reduction in risk of first attack of coronary heart disease by physical activity index. Risk of coronary heart disease begins to decrease as physical activity increases over 500 kcal per week. Risk continues to decrease up to 4000 to 5000 kcal per week. Activity in vigorous (organized) sports has some advantage over stair climbing, walking, and other light activities ("other activities"). About 15 per cent of the population expends fewer than 500 kcal per week during vigorous sports or other activities, the "reference level" in the figure. (By permission from Paffenbarger, R. S. Jr., and Hyde, R. T.: Exercise in the prevention of coronary heart disease. Prev. Med., 13:3–22, 1984.)

TABLE 41–13. Cardiac Rehabilitation Walking Program: General Instructions

1. You may being the walking program on the day after your discharge from the hospital. Day 1 is the day you begin the walking program.
2. When walking outside, use your car to determine distances. If there is a high school near your home, you could use the running track. Once around the outside of a standard track is 1/4 mile. Also, the length of three city blocks is about 1/4 mile.
3. Your walking should be smooth and continuous unless you develop shortness of breath, dizziness, and/or chest pain. You should not stop to window-shop or chat with friends. Do not take your dog with you.
4. For the first few weeks, or until you feel ready, you should walk on level surfaces. Avoid hills and rough ground, and then gradually include low hills and increasing effort as tolerated.
5. Do not walk within one hour after a meal.
6. Use common sense. If the weather is extremely hot or cold, walk indoors. You might walk in a shopping mall or in the local school. When you are outside in the cold, wear a face mask to warm the air before it enters your lungs.
7. If your doctor has prescribed nitroglycerin for you, be sure to have it with you while walking or doing any of the exercises.
8. The walking program is a general guideline. Do the best you can to follow the program, but it is all right to take longer at some of the levels.
9. Take your pulse before, during, and after exercise. Stop and rest if your pulse rate is greater than 120 beats per minute any time during the first six weeks. After six weeks, check with your physician for new pulse rate limits.

TABLE 41–14. Cardiac Rehabilitation Walking Program: Guidelines for Increasing Frequency, Rate, and Distance

LEVEL	DAY	DISTANCE (miles per day)	TIME (min)	DAILY TRIPS	SPEED (mph)
1	1–5	¼	7.5	1	2
2	6–10	¼	7.5	2	2
3	11–15	½	15	1	2
4	16–21	½	15	2	2
5	22–28	¾	22.5	2	2
6	29–35	1	20	1	3
7	36–42	1¼	25	1	3
8	43–49	1½	30	1	3
9	50–63	1¾	35	1	3
		Stay at stage 9 until your doctor tells you to advance			
10	64–77	1½	26	1	3.5
11	78–84	1½	22.5	1	4
12	85–91	1¾	26	1	4
13	92–98	2	30	1	4

TABLE 41–15. Instructions for Stationary Bicycle Exercise Program

1. Use the same precautions that you use for your walking program.
2. Ask your physician to tell you your maximum heart rate, maximum MET level, and target heart rate for 20 min of continuous pedaling.
3. Take your pulse before exercise and every two min thereafter. Stop exercise if you have any cardiac symptoms.
4. Adjust the resistance so that you can pedal at a constant rate of 60 to 80 rpm. Adjust the resistance as required. Set the resistance so that the target heart rate is not exceeded after four min of pedaling. Continue pedaling for 20 min.
5. Re-evaluate your heart rate response weekly. If your pulse is less than 85% of the target pulse, increase the resistance and repeat step 4.
6. At the end of the exercise session, pedal at zero load for three min or until your heart rate drops below 90.

TABLE 41–16. Symptom Advisory for Patients

SYMPTOM	CAUSE	WHAT TO DO
Unusual pulse or heart action may occur while exercising or following an exercise session, e.g., (1) a very irregular or unusually irregular pulse; (2) a fluttering or palpitation in the chest or throat; (3) a sudden burst of rapid heart beats or a very slow pulse; compare these with your normal pulse	An unusual pulse rate may or may not be dangerous; it could indicate extra beats, dropped beats, or problems with the heart rhythm	Check with your doctor before doing more exercising. The doctor can decide if this is harmless or if it needs to be treated.
Pain, discomfort, or heaviness occurs in chest, arm, jaw, or neck during or following an exercise session	This discomfort is possibly angina (heart pain from insufficient blood)	Sit down and rest. If the pain continues and if your doctor has prescribed nitroglycerin, take as your doctor instructed. If the pain continues for 20 minutes, contact your doctor.
Dizziness, lightheadedness, cold sweating, confusion, incoordination, turning white, or fainting occurs during exercise	Not enough blood is reaching the brain	Stop exercising immediately. Lie down with your feet elevated or sit down and put your head between your knees. Stay there until you are feeling better. Check with your doctor before resuming exercises.
The heart rate reaches or exceeds the upper limit set for you; pulse rate stays high after you have stopped exercising	The exercise may be too vigorous	Check your pulse more often during your exercise session. Once your heart rate reaches the upper limit, do not continue to exercise or add new exercises. If this does not control the problem, check with your doctor.
Nausea or vomiting occurs during or right after exercising	Not enough blood and oxygen are reaching the intestine; you could be exercising too hard or stopping the exercise too suddenly	Be sure that you do the exercises correctly and at the right speed. You may have to decrease the speed or length of exercising or drop to a lower level. Include a "cool-down" period.
Uncomfortably short of breath or difficulty catching breath after stopping exercise	The exercises are too hard for your heart and lungs	Follow the procedure for the previous problem. You should be able to hold a conversation while exercising.
Extreme tiredness or fatigue during exercises or up to 24 hours after exercises	The exercises are too strenuous	Follow the procedure for the problem above.
Sleep difficulties develop after starting an exercise program	The exercises are too strenuous	Follow the procedure for the problem above.
Shin splints or pain on the front and sides of foreleg	The tissues of the lower leg are inflamed and irritated	Use shoes with thicker, softer soles. Avoid exercise on concrete.
Pain or cramping in calves only with exercise	Muscle cramps may be due to poor circulation or unconditioned muscles	Use shoes with thicker soles. Cramps should decrease over time. If cramps continue, consult your doctor.
Side stitch or side ache while exercising	Spasm of diaphragm (muscle between the chest and abdomen) or respiratory muscles	Lean forward while sitting and rub your side.
Charley horse or cramping in muscles of arms, legs, or hips	Muscles are out of condition and not accustomed to exercise	Stretch cramped muscles. Take a warm bath and massage cramped muscles. The problem should decrease with conditioning.
Arthritis or gout flares in hips, knees, ankles, toes, or shoulders	Exercises are too hard on these joints	Rest, check with your doctor. Do not restart exercise until the flare is over. Restart at a lower level and increase gradually. Wear good exercise shoes and/or change the type of exercise.

TABLE 41–17. Guidelines for Strengthening
Exercises

Avoid
  Sustained contraction of a single muscle group
  Resistance loads that induce a Valsalva maneuver

Do
  Maintain an exercise heart rate that is ≥ 60% of target
  Set resistance so that 8, 12, or more repetitions of an
    exercise can be performed
  Exercise a muscle group to fatigue and then move on to
    another modality to exercise the next muscle group to
    fatigue; use multiple modalities as a "circuit" that can be
    repeated at least three times per session
  Include a low load cool-down period at the end of exercise

that it is sustained muscular contraction at a resting pulse rate and prolonged muscular contraction with Valsalva's maneuver that increase the risk of ventricular tachycardia and fibrillation during strengthening exercises.[78] Isometric exercise can also cause the ejection fraction of an abnormal heart to fall.

Isometric contraction of either larger or small muscles causes increases in blood pressure, heart rate, and cardiac output.[77] However, the rise in double product is only in proportion to the size of the contracting muscle mass.[67] This is consistent with DeBusk's finding that heart rate, blood pressure, and double product were increased more by forearm lifting than by hand grip.[11]

Whereas cardiac work is determined by the systolic blood pressure, coronary blood flow is determined by the diastolic blood pressure because the majority of coronary blood flow takes place during diastole. Therefore, the patient may be able to exercise to a peak double product value without angina during mixed isometric and dynamic exercise that is higher than the point at which angina develops during purely dynamic exercise.

Myocardial infarction patients can start a strengthening program after four to six weeks, and surgical patients can start as soon as the sternotomy incision has healed. This program should feature exercises that can be performed without the patient's performing a Valsalva maneuver (Table 41–17). The patient should also be exercising at a rate that results in a sinus tachycardia. Lower extremity strengthening can be achieved by having the patient work out on a stationary bicycle with alternating cycles of heavy and light load. Rowing machines, shoulder wheels, and steps have also been used safely to increase strength.[17] Free weights and wall weights are appropriate, as are Nautilus machines. The patient should be given a "circuit" prescription in which a muscle group is exercised until fatigue sets in. The patient then moves on to the next station to exercise another muscle group. Ideally, the patient should be performing at least 8 to 12 repetitions of each exercise before experiencing exhausting fatigue of a muscle group. The difficulty of the circuit should be designed so that the patient is able to complete at least three cycles.

Managing Obligatory Physical Activity

Patients who experience fatigue from their activities of daily living should simplify and plan their work activities (Table 41–18). They should also adopt efficient working postures to decrease fatigue.

There are times when the patient must perform an activity that is above a safe level of sustained rate of physical exertion. Patterson and co-workers have demonstrated that 30-second work-rest cycles accomplish the same amount of work as two- or six-minute work-rest cycles without the concomitant rise in heart rate (Fig. 41–11).[79]

TABLE 41–18. Work Simplification and Energy Conservation Guidelines

1. Set aside time to plan your day's activities. Incorporate rest periods. Organize and prioritize your time to avoid rush.
2. Balance work and rest periods to avoid fatigue.
3. Alternate strenuous tasks with light tasks.
4. Space activities throughout the day, doing some in the morning, some in the afternoon, and some in the evening. Try to perform strenuous activities during the time of day that you feel most energetic.
5. Eliminate steps of a task or a whole task that is not necessary. Have your family help with daily household chores. Ask for help if the job is too difficult for you.
6. Save energy by working with good posture.
7. Use the large, strong muscles of your arms and legs instead of the small muscles of your forearm and back for lifting and pushing.
8. Work at a moderate pace to save energy and feel better at the end of the task.

THOMAS E. KOTTKE, THERESE H. HANEY, AND MARGARET M. DOUCETTE

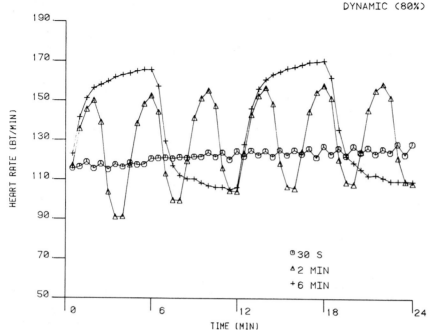

FIGURE 41–11. Whereas work-rest cycle lengths of two and six min result in marked heart rate rises when dynamic work is performed at 80 per cent of voluntary capacity, 30-sec work-rest cycles accomplish the same amount of work and are not associated with a rise in heart rate. The patient should be taught to use short work-rest cycles during heavy physical activity. (By permission from Patterson, R. P., Pearson, J., and Fisher, S. V.: Work-rest periods: Their effects on normal physiologic response to isometric and dynamic work. Arch. Phys. Med. Rehabil., 66:348–352, 1985.)

Practical application means that the patient stuck in the snow should shovel for 30 seconds, rest for 30 seconds, shovel for 30 seconds, and so forth. The same is true for shoveling grain or dirt. The patient who wants to mow the lawn should mow one strip, rest for an equivalent amount of time, mow a second strip, and so forth. This technique can also be applied to sexual activity.

Psychosocial Adjustment

Return to Sexual Activity

It is obvious from a review of the literature on this subject that we know more about the effects of physical activity on humans in space, underwater, and on the athletic field than in the bedroom. This lack of information is even more evident regarding the effects of sexual activity on patients with cardiovascular disease.[80]

Patients and physicians alike tend to equate sexual activity with the risk of sudden death. However, Ueno found that fewer than 1% of sudden deaths in Japan occurred during coitus.[81] Skinner found that among middle-aged, married men, the peak cost of sexual activity does not exceed five METS.[80] Bohlen and co-workers, measuring oxygen uptake, pulse, and blood pressure during four different sexual activities (mastur-

bation, foreplay, intercourse with the man on top, and intercourse with the woman on top), found that intercourse in a familiar position had lower metabolic cost than intercourse in an unfamiliar position.[82] This study also demonstrated that foreplay can be promoted as a metabolically low-cost activity. The previous prohibitions of 8 to 12 weeks between myocardial infarction and sexual intercourse are unnecessary.

A sexual history should be part of the initial work-up of all patients (Table 41–19). Basic therapy includes providing the patient with accurate written material, supporting open discussion of issues, and describing permissible behaviors (Table 41–20).

Because the fear of failure to perform is a frequent cause of failure, couples should be encouraged to postpone sexual intercourse until both partners are comfortable with proceeding. Hugging, cuddling, or noncoital foreplay, since it is relaxing, pleasurable, of low metabolic cost, and without danger to the patient, should be encouraged.

The ideal time for sexual activity is when both partners are well rested. Attempts at sexual activity after heavy eating or drinking predispose the couple to failure. The patient may find that morning or afternoon may be ideal times for sexual activity. If the patient expects to have angina, premedica-

TABLE 41–19. Components of the Brief
Sexual History

A sexual history should include:
  Baseline frequency and type of sexual activity before the
    coronary event
  The patient's expectations about return to sexual activity
  The patient's cardiovascular status
  Health and attitudes of the spouse
  The psychological status of the patient (e.g., fear, anxiety,
    and depression)

tion with nitroglycerin will pre-empt the attack and provide a more satisfactory outcome. If the patient has persistent problems during sexual activity, ambulatory ECG monitoring can be used to detect both dysrhythmia and ischemia.

Complaints of decreased libido or performance may be caused by medications. Drugs specifically known to decrease libido, produce impotence, or interfere with ejaculation include tranquilizers, antihypertensives, beta blockers, antidepressants, thiazide diuretics, phenothiazine, haloperidol, benzodiazepines, alcohol, monoamine oxidase inhibitors, and ganglionic blocking drugs.[1, 80] Hackett and Cassem suggest that sexual dysfunction persisting for more than six or seven months warrants further investigation.[83]

Family Functioning and Social Support

Cardiovascular disease fits the definition of a social disease. The risk factors of coronary heart disease, diet, smoking, weight, and physical activity level are all strongly influenced by the behaviors of the family and peer group. Therefore, the entire family should be included in the rehabilitation effort (Table 41–21).

During the in-hospital phase of cardiac rehabilitation, the spouse should be included in the educational programs for smoking, diet, and physical activity. If the spouse is the food purchaser and food preparer, the intervention to develop skills to prepare low-fat and low-sodium meals should

TABLE 41–20. Guidelines for Basic Sexual Therapy

Give the patient accurate written material about the effects of
  heart disease on sexual functioning
Support the marriage relationship by encouraging open
  communication of feelings and fears about the illness
Describe permissible sexual behaviors

TABLE 41–21. Family and Social Support Activities

Smoking
  All family members should be asked to stop smoking
  The house and family car should be made off limits to
    smoking
  All smoking paraphernalia should be discarded
Nutrition
  All nutrition education should include the family food
    purchaser and preparer
  The family should eat the same meals as the patient
Physical Activity
  The spouse should witness the inpatient exercises
  The spouse should participate in the predischarge exercise
    test
  The spouse should participate in the patient's walking
    program

be directed to the spouse. Because heart disease is known to cluster in families, the entire family should be asked to eat the same meals as prescribed for the patient. Many experts suggest that the entire family should be screened for hypercholesterolemia at the time the patient is enrolled in the rehabilitation program. The entire family should be asked to stop smoking, and both the house and the car should be made off limits to smoking. All smoking paraphernalia should be discarded.

Having the spouse witness and participate in the predischarge exercise demonstration has been shown to reduce anxiety in both the patient and the spouse.[84] The spouse should also be encouraged to participate in the patient's walking program. This both reinforces the patient and allows the spouse and patient time to talk. The spouse must be included in any discussions about sexual activity and should also be included in the discussions of return to work.

Prevention and Treatment of Anxiety and Depression

Although patients with severe myocardial impairment tend to be more depressed than are patients with less severe myocardial impairment, the opposite tends to be true for anxiety.[20] Levels of anxiety and depression correlate poorly with cardiac function (Table 41–22). The therapist must be alert for signs of anxiety and depression in all patients.

Anxiety and depression may focus on finances, sexuality, or physical activity, or they may lack a

THOMAS E. KOTTKE, THERESE H. HANEY, AND MARGARET M. DOUCETTE

TABLE 41–22. Relationship Between Cardiac Dysfunction, Anxiety, and Depression

	SEVERITY OF DYSFUNCTION	MEAN PSYCHIATRIC SCORES	
		Anxiety	Depression
In-hospital	Mild	16.7	6.4
	Severe	14.4	8.2
After discharge	Mild	17.5	8.0
	Severe	14.3	9.1

Anxiety scores ≥21 and depression scores ≥11 are abnormal. From Nagle, R. E., Morgan, D., Bird, J., and Bird, J.: Interaction between physical and psychological abnormalities after myocardial infarction. *In* Stockmeier, B. (Ed.): Psychological Approach to the Rehabilitation of Coronary Patients. Berlin, Springer Verlag, 1976.

focus. A monitored physical activity program for the patient still in the hospital reassures the patient that he or she can still perform the activities of daily living. Before discharge from the hospital, a graded demonstration of exercise capacity will help avoid the development of anxiety and depression. This demonstration also provides the basis for an individualized prescription for exercise and reassures both the patient and the patient's spouse about the safety of physical exertion.[85] In addition to teaching appropriate levels of exercise and producing training effects, outpatient rehabilitation programs provide the patient with a sense of community and generate positive emotional states.[86, 87]

Return to Work

Return to gainful employment is important for both the patient's fiscal status and emotional health. However, only 50 to 80 per cent of patients return to work after a myocardial infarction or heart surgery.[88, 89] Within two years this figure will decline by an additional 10 to 15 per cent.[89]

Angina or other symptoms are not the only determinants of occupational status, because patients treated medically return to work at rates that are as high or higher than surgical patients in spite of poorer symptom control.[90]

Factors that may preclude return to work include previous work status, education, age, continued angina with exertion, length of disability or unemployment, anxiety and depression, congestive heart failure, and retirement benefits. Attitudes of the patient, family, and employer are also powerful predictors of continued employment.[88]

The patients who most need to return to work (laborers and others with relatively little financial reserve and poor disability and illness benefits) are the ones who usually find return most difficult. Employers frequently prefer to hire a younger worker who is at less risk of claiming job-related illness. If there is any question about whether the cardiac patient will be able to return to the previous employment, a vocational rehabilitation consultation should be requested as soon as the problem is identified.

Patients with well-preserved myocardial function and light to moderate physical demands at work are candidates to return to the job as few as four weeks after myocardial infarction.[91] A negative symptom-limited exercise test before return to work should document the safety of occupational activity. If the patient or employer has continued concerns, ambulatory ECG monitoring permits the physician to observe the patient's heart rate and ECG during peak activity and demonstrate the absence of ischemic ECG changes.

Rehabilitation of the Patient with Multiple Problems

Cardiac and Cardiopulmonary Transplantation

Cardiac transplantation is not an option for many patients with ischemic heart disease because of concomitant cerebral vascular disease, peripheral vascular disease, pulmonary disease, or renal disease. For patients with congestive heart failure and without prohibitive disease in other organ systems, however, it represents a life saving intervention. Most patients return to levels of activity that are limited only by their own goals.

After 1977, three-year survival for heart transplant patients living 30 days and receiving cyclosporine was over 70 per cent.[92] Experience with combined heart and lung transplantation is more limited, but of 27 patients receiving transplants at Stanford University, 64 per cent were alive at one year and 39 per cent were alive at four years.[93] Unfortunately, the majority of candidates for heart-lung transplantation die before donor organs become available.

Transplantation patients can use the rehabilitation protocols for coronary bypass patients if two features are kept in mind: the likelihood of severe deconditioning and the denervated heart of the transplantation patient.

Many patients will be so deconditioned and weakened by prolonged bed rest and low cardiac output that they will lack the strength and endurance to walk more than a few steps after their transplant. In cases such as these, the rehabilitation program should be initiated with assisted active range of motion followed by active range of motion plus calisthenics. A stationary bicycle at the bedside can be used for the patient to complete repeated work-rest cycles at zero resistance. When the patient regains adequate strength and endurance, the patient can begin to follow the usual cardiac rehabilitation protocols. The response of the heart rate to exercise is usually slow and limited but can be extremely variable. This slow and limited response of heart rate to exercise and the delayed response of the heart to stopping exercise normally does not cause a problem if adequately long cool-down periods are used.

The Diabetic with Cardiac Disease

Background of the Problem. Diabetes mellitus is a heterogeneous group of disorders characterized by high blood glucose levels, a relative or absolute insulin deficiency, and numerous metabolic and hormonal derangements.[94] Almost six million individuals in the United States carry the diagnosis of diabetes mellitus, and it is estimated that an equal number remain undiagnosed.[95] The two main categories of diabetes mellitus are type I or insulin-dependent diabetes mellitus (IDDM) and type II or non–insulin-dependent diabetes mellitus (NIDDM).

The short-term complications of diabetes mellitus are mainly those of glucose control: hypoglycemia, hyperglycemia, and ketoacidosis. Long-term complications are of three types: macrovascular, microangiopathic, and neuropathic.

The macrovascular complications of diabetes mellitus include hypertension, peripheral vascular disease, cerebrovascular disease, and coronary artery disease. Diabetic patients develop coronary disease at a younger age than do individuals without diabetes and have more extensive vascular involvement, greater mortality, and a relatively greater incidence of asymptomatic ischemia.[96]

Microvascular disease most notably results in retinopathy and nephropathy. Neuropathy may involve virtually any nerve or nerve pathway. Autonomic neuropathy, peripheral motor neuropathy, and sensory neuropathy lead to foot ulcers, amputations, claudication, retinal hemorrhage with blindness, and blunted cardiovascular reflexes.

Diabetes and Exercise. The goal of exercise for the diabetic patient is improved glycemic control, control of obesity and hypertension, and prevention of cardiovascular disease. Increased sensitivity to insulin along with weight loss has been documented in patients with NIDDM.[97, 98] For individuals with IDDM, research has focused on glycemic control and the ability to physically condition these patients.[99]

A thorough history and examination is required before the initiation of any exercise program. The therapist should inquire about previous foot ulcers, and the physical examination should include testing for sensory and structural abnormalities of the lower extremity. The need for an exercise tolerance test is greater for the diabetic patient than for the nondiabetic population owing to the earlier onset of cardiovascular disease and the higher incidence of silent ischemia (Table 41–23).[96] Any diabetic who is at least 30 to 40 years of age, has a history of more than 10 years of diabetes, or has signs or symptoms of cardiovascular disease should have an exercise tolerance test before starting an exercise program.[99, 100] An intravenous dipyridamole-thallium study should be considered if the patient is nonambulatory and ischemia is strongly suspected but cannot be detected with arm ergometry.[101]

One of the most common complications of exercise for patients with IDDM is hypoglycemia.

TABLE 41–23. Evaluation of Physical Work Capacity in Diabetic Patients

Perform exercise test if:
    Duration of diabetes is greater than 10 years
    Patient is more than 30 to 40 years old
    Patient has any signs or symptoms of cardiovascular disease
Select an evaluation mode that parallels planned exercise
    program:
    Treadmill
    Bicycle ergometer
    Arm ergometer
Consider an intravenous dipyridamole-thallium study if the
    patient is nonambulatory and ischemia is strongly suspected
    but cannot be demonstrated with an exercise test
Set the goal-training heart rate at 60% to 70% of maximum
    heart rate achieved on exercise test

THOMAS E. KOTTKE, THERESE H. HANEY, AND MARGARET M. DOUCETTE

Several factors influence this, including the blood sugar at the start of exercise; the site, timing, and type of insulin administered; the duration and intensity of exercise; and the recent caloric intake. Because the body uses blood glucose to replace glycogen stores for up to 24 hours after exercise, hypoglycemia may occur during exercise or up to several hours following exercise.[94]

Diabetic patients should follow specific guidelines during exercise to reduce the risk of hypoglycemia and injury (Table 41–24). Exercise with blood glucose levels over 300 mg/dl or ketosis may actually worsen hyperglycemia owing to a relative hypoinsulinemia that promotes liver glucose output.[94] Exercise should be performed in the morning or at mid-day, because evening exercise sessions may precipitate unrecognized hypoglycemia during sleep. The individual and his or her physician should be prepared to adjust caloric intake, insulin dosing, and time and intensity of physical exercise according to the individual patient's needs and goals.

Special considerations must be given to peripheral neuropathy, both sensory and motor, which increases the risk of foot ulcers and deterioration of Charcot joints. Peripheral vascular disease and claudication may limit the patient from walking at a rate that produces cardiovascular conditioning. Amputations, particularly those with delayed heal-ing, may limit walking and bicycling. Individuals who have had recent laser treatment or retinal hemorrhage secondary to retinopathy may have to have limits placed on tolerable blood pressure rises.

Despite these physical restrictions, a suitable cardiovascular conditioning program can be designed if the basic principles of exercise prescription are followed (Table 41–25). The mode of exercise is the key modification. Swimming laps, other aquatic exercise, bicycling, wall pulley programs, or other low-impact programs can replace high-impact, repetitive activities such as jogging or high-level aerobic exercise classes.

Patient education is critical for the prevention of foot ulcers. Patients should be instructed to make frequent foot checks, particularly as they increase the intensity and duration of the exercise. If feet are anatomically normal, deerskin shoes or commercially available athletic shoes with adequate ventilation, few seams, and good fit are sufficient.

With more severe sensory loss or structural changes such as "clawfoot" or hammer toes, inserts will have to be used. Custom-molded close-cell polyethylene foam inserts molded to the foot distribute weight-bearing forces. These inserts can be used with extra-depth athletic shoes to reduce the probability of foot injury. Composite insoles with a lower layer of microcellular rubber for resilience and reinforced with a cork or Plastazote cradle provide the greatest protection and durability.

TABLE 41–24. Exercise Guidelines for Diabetic Patients

Do Not Exercise:
  If the blood sugar is <80 mg/dl or >300 mg/dl
  If ketosis is present
  Immediately following injection of insulin or at time of
    peak insulin activity
  Late in the evening
When Exercising:
  Check blood sugar prior to exercise
  Carry identification
  During the first two weeks of exercise, or when increasing
    the intensity or duration of exercise, check blood sugar
    four times a day
  Exercise with a friend or notify a partner of plans
  Carry a snack and/or glucagon
  Drink fluids before and after exercise
  Wear protective footwear
  Increase carbohydrate consumption
    15 to 30 gm carbohydrate snack 30 to 60 min before
      exercise
    15 to 30 gm carbohydrate snack per 30 min of moderate
      to heavy exercise
  Decrease insulin dose

Rehabilitation of the Patient with Cardiac Disease: The Future

Comprehensive cardiac rehabilitation means management of ischemia, congestive heart failure, and dysrhythmia; management of nutrition, serum cholesterol, blood pressure, and smoking; and management of physical debility, employment, sexual functioning, and psychosocial adjustment. With comprehensive cardiac rehabilitation, the once-observed deconditioning, pulmonary embolism, shoulder-hand syndrome, and other complications following myocardial infarction need not occur.

An aging population means more patients with multiple organ system dysfunction: renal disease plus heart disease, musculoskeletal disease plus heart disease, pulmonary disease plus heart dis-

TABLE 41–25. Exercise Modifications for Diabetic Patients

CONDITION	RECOMMENDED EXERCISE MODALITY
Peripheral neuropathy Charcot joints	Swimming, aquatic exercise, low-resistance bicycling, upper extremity exercise* Protective footwear
Peripheral vascular disease, claudication (often associated with peripheral neuropathy)	Combined walking and swimming Upper extremity exercises Evaluate for protective footwear
Amputations with delayed healing Foot ulcers	Upper extremity exercise Lower extremity strengthening Avoid weight-bearing

Retinopathy
Recent laser treatment
Retinal hemorrhage
	Walking or bicycling
	Avoid isometric exercise and upper extremity
	  exercise
	Set limits on and monitor maximum systolic blood
	  pressure

*Upper extremity options include arm ergometer, bicycle adapted for arm crank, low-weight wall pulley with quick repetitions, arm and trunk calisthenics while seated.

ease, and diabetes plus heart disease. Exercise has a defined role in the management of many chronic diseases including chronic renal failure.[102, 103]

The rehabilitation of the patient with disease limited to the cardiovascular system has been defined, but it is doubtful that the focus of cardiologists will change to include the rehabilitation of patients with dysfunction in multiple systems. The physiatrist enjoys a professional tradition and interest in managing these patients. Coupled with a basic understanding of cardiac pathophysiology and the back-up of an interested and supportive cardiologist, it is the skills and training of the physiatrist that will provide the answers to these management problems over the next decade.

This chapter has presented protocols that have been tested in randomized clinical trials, protocols tested in trials without control groups, and protocols that are being used with apparent safety but without full evaluation. The reader should view these protocols as a starting point to develop further improvements in patient care rather than as the achievement of an end point, for the observation that Levine and Brown made in 1929 remains true: "It would be presumptuous at the present stage of our knowledge to formulate fixed principles for the treatment of this condition."[4]

References

1. Wenger, N. K., and Hellerstein, H. K. (Eds.): Rehabilitation of the Coronary Patient, 2nd Ed. New York, John Wiley & Sons, 1984.
2. Pollock, M. L., and Schmidt, D. H.: Heart Disease and Rehabilitation, 2nd Ed. New York, John Wiley & Sons, 1986.
3. Wilson, P. K., Fardy, P. S., and Froelicher, V. F.: Cardiac Rehabilitation, Adult Fitness, and Exercise Testing. Philadelphia, Lea & Febiger, 1981.
4. Levine, S. A., and Brown, C. L.: Coronary thrombosis. Medicine, 8:245–418, 1929.
5. Mallory, G. K., White, P. D., and Salcedo-Salger, J.: The speed of healing of myocardial infarction: A study of the pathological anatomy in seventy-two cases. Am. Heart J., 18:647–671, 1939.
6. Levine, S. A., and Lown, B.: "Armchair" treatment of acute coronary thrombosis. J.A.M.A., 148:1365–1369, 1952.
7. Tobis, J. S., and Zohman, L. R.: A rehabilitation program for inpatients with recent myocardial infarction. Arch. Phys. Med. Rehabil., 49:443–448, 1968.
8. Bloch, A., Maeder, J. P., Haissly, J. C., Felix, J., and Blackburn, H.: Early mobilization after myocardial infarction. A controlled study. Am. J. Cardiol., 34:152–157, 1974.
9. Markiewicz, W., Houston, N., and DeBusk, R. F.: Exercise testing soon after myocardial infarction. Circulation, 56:26–31, 1977.
10. DeBusk, R. F., and Haskell, W.: Symptom-limited vs. heart-rate-limited exercise testing soon after myocardial infarction. Circulation, 61:738–743, 1980.
11. DeBusk, R. F., Valdez, R., Houston, N., and Haskell, W.: Cardiovascular responses to dynamic and static effort soon after myocardial infarction. Application to occupational work assessment. Circulation, 58:368–375, 1978.
12. Davidson, D. M., and DeBusk, R. F.: Prognostic value of a single exercise test 3 weeks after uncom-

plicated myocardial infarction. Circulation, 61:236–242, 1980.

13. DeBusk, R. F., Blomqvist, C. G., Kouchoukos, N. T., Leupker, R. V., Miller, H. S., Moss, A. J., Pollock, M. L., Reeves, T. J., Selvester, R. H., Stason, W. B., et al.: Identification and treatment of low-risk patients after acute myocardial infarction and coronary-artery bypass graft surgery. N. Engl. J. Med., 314:161–166, 1986.

14. Van Camp, S. P., and Peterson, R. A.: Cardiovascular complications of outpatient cardiac rehabilitation programs. J.A.M.A., 256:1160–1163, 1986.

15. Wilhelmsen, L., Sanne, H., Elmfeldt, D., Grimby, G., Tibblin, G., and Wedel, H.: A controlled trial of physical training after myocardial infarction. Effects on risk factors, nonfatal reinfarction, and death. Prev. Med., 4:491–508, 1975.

16. Kentala, E.: Physical fitness and feasibility of physical rehabilitation after myocardial infarction in men of working age. Ann. Clin. Res., 4[Suppl. 9]:1–84, 1972.

17. Naughton, J.: The national exercise and heart disease project. Cardiology, 63:352–367, 1978.

18. Furberg, C. D., and May, G. S.: Effect of long-term prophylactic treatment on survival after myocardial infarction. Am. J. Med., 76:76–83, 1984.

19. Naughton, J., Brunn, J. G., and Lategola, M.: Effects of physical training on physiologic and behavioral characteristics of cardiac patients. Arch. Phys. Med. Rehabil., 49:131–137, 1968.

20. Nagle, R. E., Morgan, D., Bird, J., and Bird, J.: Interaction between physical and psychological abnormalities after myocardial infarction. In Stockmeier, B. (Ed.): Psychological Approach to the Rehabilitation of Coronary Patients. Berlin, Springer Verlag, 1976, pp. 84–88.

21. Sanne, H.: Exercise tolerance and physical training of non-selected patients after myocardial infarction. Acta Med. Scand. [Suppl.], 1–124, 1973.

22. Kallio, V., Hamalainen, H., Hakkila, J., and Luurila, O. J.: Reduction in sudden deaths by a multifactorial intervention programme after acute myocardial infarction. Lancet, 2:1091–1094, 1979.

23. Nelson, R. R., Gobel, F. L., Jorgensen, C. R., Wang, K., Wang, Y., and Taylor, H. L.: Hemodynamic predictors of myocardial oxygen consumption during static and dynamic exercise. Circulation, 50:1179–1189, 1974.

24. Ross, R.: The pathogenesis of atherosclerosis—an update. N. Engl. J. Med., 314:488–500, 1986.

25. Eichner, E. R.: Platelets, carotids, and coronaries. Critique on antithrombotic role of antiplatelet agents, exercise, and certain diets. Am. J. Med., 77:513–523, 1984.

26. Braunwald, E., and Sobel, B. E.: Coronary blood flow and myocardial ischemia. In Braunwald, E. (Ed.): Heart Disease. Philadelphia, W. B. Saunders Company, 1980, p. 1279.

27. Mancini, D. M., Le Jemtel, T. H., Factor, S., and Sonnenblick, E. H.: Central and peripheral components of cardiac failure. Am. J. Med., 80:2–13, 1986.

28. Young, J. B., Leon, C. A., and Pratt, C. M.: Potentially deleterious effects of long-term vasodilator therapy in patients with heart failure. Chest, 91:737–744, 1987.

29. Sutton, F. J.: Vasodilator therapy. Am. J. Med., 80:54–58, 1986.

30. The CONSENSUS Trial Study Group: Effects of enalapril on mortality in severe congestive heart failure: Results of the Cooperative North Scandinavian Enalapril Survival Study (CONSENSUS). N. Engl. J. Med., 316:1429–1435, 1987.

31. Fowler, M. B., and Bristow, M. R.: Rationale for beta-adrenergic blocking drugs in cardiomyopathy. Am. J. Cardiol., 55:120D–124D, 1985.

32. DeBusk, R. F., Davidson, D. M., Houston, N., and Fitzgerald, J.: Serial ambulatory electrocardiography and treadmill exercise testing after uncomplicated myocardial infarction. Am. J. Cardiol., 45:547–554, 1980.

33. Faris, J. V., McHenry, P. L., Jordan, J. W., and Morris, S. N.: Prevalence and reproducibility of exercise-induced ventricular arrhythmias during maximal exercise testing in normal men. Am. J. Cardiol., 37:617–622, 1976.

34. Soyza, N. D., Murphy, M. L., Bissett, J. K., and Kane, J. J.: Detecting ventricular arrhythmia after myocardial infarction: Comparison of Holter monitoring and treadmill exercise. South. Med. J., 70:403–404, 1977.

35. Sami, M., Kraemer, H., and DeBusk, R. F.: Reproducibility of exercise-induced ventricular arrhythmia after myocardial infarction. Am. J. Cardiol., 43:724–730, 1979.

36. Kannel, W. B., Sorlie, P., Castelli, W. P., and McGee, D.: Blood pressure and survival after myocardial infarction: The Framingham Study. Am. J. Cardiol., 45:326–330, 1980.

37. Bourassa, M. G., Fisher, L. D., Campeau, L., Gillespie, M. J., McConney, M., and Lesperance, J.: Long-term fate of bypass grafts: The Coronary Artery Surgery Study (CASS) and Montreal Heart Institute experiences. Circulation, 72[Suppl. V]:V71–V78, 1985.

38. Levy, R. I., Brensike, J. F., Epstein, S. E., Kelsey, S. F., Passamani, E. R., Richardson, J. M., Loh, I. K., Stone, N. J., Aldrich, R. F., Battaglini, J. W., et al.: The influence of changes in lipid values induced by cholestyramine and diet on progression of coronary artery disease: Results of NHLBI Type II Coronary Intervention Study. Circulation, 69:325–337, 1984.

39. Brensike, J. F., Levy, R. I., Kelsey, S. F., Passamani, E. R., Richardson, J. M., Loh, I. K., Stone, N. J., Aldrich, R. F., Battaglini, J. W., Moriarty, D. J., Fisher, M. R., Friedman, L., Friedewald,

W., Detre, K. M., and Epstein, S. E.: Effects of therapy with cholestyramine on progression of coronary arteriosclerosis: Results of the NHLBI Type II Coronary Intervention Study. Circulation, 69:313–324, 1984.

40. Malinow, M. R.: Atherosclerosis: Progression, regression, and resolution. Am. Heart J., 108:1523–1537, 1984.

41. Blankenhorn, D. H., Nessim, S. A., Johnson, R. L., Sanmarco, M. E., Azen, S. P., and Cashin-Hemphill, L.: Beneficial effects of combined colestipol-niacin therapy on coronary atherosclerosis and coronary venous bypass grafts. J.A.M.A., 257:3233–3240, 1987.

42. World Health Organization Expert Committee on Prevention of Coronary Heart Disease. Prevention of coronary heart disease. WHO Tech. Rep. Ser. 678, 1982.

43. Gotto, A. M. Jr.: Treatment of hyperlipidemia. Am. J. Cardiol., 57:11G–16G, 1986.

44. Nashel, D. J.: Is atherosclerosis a complication of long-term corticosteroid treatment? Am. J. Med., 80:925–929, 1986.

45. Rosenberg, L., Kaufman, D. W., Helmrich, S. P., and Shapiro, S.: The risk of myocardial infarction after quitting smoking in men under 55 years of age. N. Engl. J. Med., 313:1511–1514, 1985.

46. Hartz, A. J., Anderson, A. J., Brooks, H. L., Manley, J. C., Parent, G. T., and Barboriak, J. J.: The association of smoking with cardiomyopathy. N. Engl. J. Med., 311:1201–1206, 1984.

47. Slone, D., Shapiro, S., Rosenberg, L., Kaufman, D. W., Hartz, S. C., Rossi, A. C., Stolly, P. D., and Miettinen, O. S.: Relation of cigarette smoking to myocardial infarction in young women. N. Engl. J. Med., 298:1273–1276, 1978.

48. Wilhelmsson, C., Elmfelut, D., Vedin, J. A., Tibblin, G., and Wilhelmsen, L.: Smoking and myocardial infarction. Lancet, 1:415–419, 1975.

49. Salonen, J. T.: Stopping smoking and long-term mortality after acute myocardial infarction. Br. Heart J., 43:463–469, 1980.

50. Mulcahy, R.: Influence of cigarette smoking on morbidity and mortality after myocardial infarction. Br. Heart J., 49:410–415, 1983.

51. Hallstrom, A. P., Cobb, L. A., and Ray, R.: Smoking as a risk factor for recurrence of sudden cardiac arrest. N. Engl. J. Med., 314:271–275, 1986.

52. Deanfield, J. E., Shea, M. J., Wilson, R. A., Horlock, P., de Landsheere, C. M., and Selwyn, A. P.: Direct effects of smoking on the heart: Silent ischemic disturbances of coronary flow. Am. J. Cardiol., 57:1005–1009, 1986.

53. Deanfield, J., Wright, C., Krikler, S., Ribeiro, P., and Fox, K.: Cigarette smoking and the treatment of angina with propranolol, atenolol, and nifedipine. N. Engl. J. Med., 310:951–954, 1984.

54. Myers, K. A.: Relationship of smoking to peripheral arterial disease. Aust. Fam. Physician, 8:765–768, 1979.

55. Hermanson, B., Omenn, G. X., Chromal, R. A., and Gersh, B. J.: Beneficial six-year survival outcomes from smoking cessation in older men and women with coronary artery disease: Results from the CASS study. N. Engl. J. Med., 319:1365–1368, 1988.

56. Kottke, T. E., Battista, R. N., DeFriese, G. H., and Brekke, M. L.: Attributes of successful smoking cessation interventions in medical practice: A meta-analysis of 39 controlled trials. J.A.M.A., 259:2883–2889, 1988.

57. Kottke, T. E., Hill, C. S., Heitzig, C., Brekke, M., Blake, S., Arneson, S., and Caspersen, C.: Smoke-free hospitals. Attitudes of patients, employees, and faculty. Minn. Med., 68:53–55, 1985.

58. American College of Sports Medicine: Guidelines for Exercise Testing and Prescription, 3rd Ed. Philadelphia, Lea & Febiger, 1986, pp. 13–14.

59. Committee on Exercise, American Heart Association: Exercise Testing and Training of Apparently Healthy Individuals: A Handbook for Physicians. Dallas, TX, American Heart Association, 1972.

60. Bruce, R. A.: Multi-stage treadmill test of submaximal and maximal exercise. In Exercise Testing and Training of Apparently Healthy Individuals: A Handbook for Physicians. Dallas, TX, American Heart Association, 1972, pp. 32–34.

61. Nagle, F. S., Balke, B., and Naughton, J. P.: Gradational step tests for assessing work capacity. J. Appl. Physiol., 20:745–748, 1965.

62. Fox, S. M., Naughton, J. P., and Haskell, W. L.: Physical activity and the prevention of coronary heart disease. Ann. Clin. Res., 3:404–432, 1971.

63. Kattus, A. A., Jorgensen, C. R., Worden, R. E., and Alvaro, A. B.: S-T-segment depression with near-maximal exercise in detection of preclinical coronary heart disease. Circulation, 41:585–595, 1971.

64. Kansal, S., Roitman, D., Bradley, E. L. Jr., and Sheffield, L. T.: Enhanced evaluation of treadmill tests by means of scoring based on multivariate analysis and its clinical application: A study of 608 patients. Am. J. Cardiol., 52:1155–1160, 1983.

65. Franklin, B. A.: Exercise testing, training and arm ergometry. Sports Med., 2:100–119, 1985.

66. Balady, G. J., Schick, E. C., Weiner, D. A., and Ryan, T. J.: Comparison of determinants of myocardial oxygen consumption during arm and leg exercise in normal persons. Am. J. Cardiol., 57:1385–1387, 1986.

67. Buck, J. A., Amundsen, L. R., and Nielsen, D. H.: Systolic blood pressure responses during isometric contractions of large and small muscle groups. Med. Sci. Sports Exerc., 12:145–147, 1980.

68. Balady, G. J., Weiner, D. A., McCabe, C. H.,

and Ryan, T. J.: Value of arm exercise testing in detecting coronary artery disease. Am. J. Cardiol., 55:37–39, 1985.

69. Hung, J., McKillip, J., Savin, W., Magder, S., Kraus, R., Houston, N., Goris, M., Haskell, W., and DeBusk, R.: Comparison of cardiovascular response to combined static-dynamic effort, post-prandial dynamic effort and dynamic effort alone in patients with chronic ischemic heart disease. Circulation, 65:1411–1419, 1982.

70. Gottlieb, S. O., Weisfeldt, M. L., Ouyang, P., Mellits, E. D., and Gerstenblith, G.: Silent ischemia predicts infarction and death during 2 year follow-up of unstable angina. J.A.C.C., 10:756–760, 1987.

71. Wait, J.: Cardiopulmonary stress testing. A review of noninvasive approaches. Chest, 90:504–510, 1986.

72. Patterson, R. P., and Remole, W. D.: The response of the oxygen pulse during a stress test in patients with coronary artery disease. Cardiology, 67:52–62, 1981.

73. Taylor, H. L., Henschel, A., Brozek, J., and Keys, A.: Effects of bed rest on cardiovascular function and work performance. J. Appl. Physiol., 2:223–239, 1949.

74. Abraham, A. S., Sever, Y., Weinstein, M., Dollberg, M., and Menczel, J.: Value of early ambulation in patients with and without complications after acute myocardial infarction. N. Engl. J. Med., 292:719–722, 1975.

75. Lindquist, R. D.: Providing patient opportunities to increase control. Dimens. Crit. Care Nurs., 5:304–309, 1986.

76. Paffenbarger, R. S. Jr., and Hyde, R. T.: Exercise in the prevention of coronary heart disease. Prev. Med., 13:3–22, 1984.

77. Ramos, M. U., Mundale, M. O., Awad, E. A., Witsoe, D. A., Cole, T. M., Olson, M., and Kottke, F. J.: Cardiovascular effects of spread of excitation during prolonged isometric exercise. Arch. Phys. Med. Rehabil., 54:496–504, 510, 1973.

78. Atkins, J. M., Matthews, O. A., Blomqvist, C. G., and Mullins, C. B.: Incidence of arrhythmias induced by isometric and dynamic exercise. Br. Heart J., 38:465–471, 1976.

79. Patterson, R. P., Pearson, J., and Fisher, S. V.: Work-rest periods: Their effects on normal physiologic response to isometric and dynamic work. Arch. Phys. Med. Rehabil., 66:348–352, 1985.

80. Skinner, J. B.: Sexual relations and the cardiac patient. In Pollock, M. L., and Schmidt, D. H.: Heart Disease and Rehabilitation, 2nd Ed. New York, John Wiley & Sons, 1986, p. 583.

81. Ueno, M.: The so-called coition death. Jpn. J. Leg. Med., 17:333–340, 1963.

82. Bohlen, J. G., Held, J. P., Sanderson, M. O., and Patterson, R. P.: Heart rate, rate-pressure product,

and oxygen uptake during four sexual activities. Arch. Intern. Med., 144:1745–1748, 1984.

83. Hackett, T. P., and Cassem, N. H.: Psychologic aspects of rehabilitation after myocardial infarction and coronary artery bypass surgery. In Wenger, N. K., and Hellerstein, H. K. (Eds.): Rehabilitation of the Coronary Patient, 2nd Ed. New York, John Wiley & Sons, 1984, p. 449.

84. Ewart, C. K., Taylor, C. B., Reese, L. B., and DeBusk, R. F.: Effects of early postmyocardial infarction exercise testing on self-perception and subsequent physical activity. Am. J. Cardiol., 51:1076–1080, 1983.

85. Taylor, C. B., Bandura, A., Ewart, C. K., Miller, N. H., and DeBusk, R. F.: Exercise testing to enhance wives' confidence in their husbands' cardiac capability soon after clinically uncomplicated acute myocardial infarction. Am. J. Cardiol., 55:635–638, 1985.

86. Taylor, C. B., Houston-Miller, N., Ahn, D. K., Haskell, W., and DeBusk, R. F.: The effects of exercise training programs on psychosocial improvement in uncomplicated postmyocardial infarction patients. J. Psychosom. Res., 30:581–587, 1986.

87. McPherson, B. D., Paivio, A., Yuhasz, M. S., Rechnitzer, P. A., Pickard, H. A., and Lefcoe, N. M.: Psychological effects of an exercise program for post-infarct and normal adult men. J. Sports Med. Phys. Fitness, 7:95–102, 1967.

88. Stern, M. J., Pascale, L., and McLoone, J. B.: Psychosocial adaptation following an acute myocardial infarction. J. Chronic Dis., 29:513–526, 1976.

89. Kronmal, R. A., Davis, K., Fisher, L. D., Jones, R. A., and Gillespie, M. J.: Data management for a large collaborative clinical trial (CASS: Coronary Artery Surgery Study). Comput. Biomed. Res., 11:553–566, 1978.

90. Oberman, A., Wayne, J. B., Kouchoukos, N. T., Charles, E. D., Russell, R. O. Jr., and Rogers, W. J.: Employment status after coronary artery bypass surgery. Circulation, 65(7 Pt 2):115–119, 1982.

91. DeBusk, R. F., and Dennis, C. A.: Occupational work evaluation of patients with cardiac disease: A guide for physicians. West. J. Med., 137:515–520, 1982.

92. Modry, D. L., and Kaye, M. P.: Heart and heart-lung transplantation: The Canadian and world experience from December 1967 to September 1985. Can. J. Surg., 29:275–279, 1986.

93. Starnes, V. A., and Jamieson, S. W.: Current status of heart and lung transplantation. World J. Surg., 10:442–449, 1986.

94. Richter, E. A., Ruderman, N. B., and Schneider, S. H.: Diabetes and exercise. Am. J. Med., 70:201–209, 1981.

95. Diabetes in America. National Diabetes Group. NIH Publication No. 85–1468, 1985.

96. Ewing, D. J., Campbell, I. W., and Clarke, B. F.: Assessment of cardiovascular effects in diabetic autonomic neuropathy and prognostic implications. Ann. Intern. Med., 92:308–311, 1980.

97. Rönnemaa, T., Mattila, K., Lehtonen, A., and Kallio, V.: A controlled randomized study on the effect of long-term physical exercise on the metabolic control in type 2 diabetic patients. Acta Med. Scand., 220:219–224, 1986.

98. Boden, G.: Treatment strategies for patients with non-insulin-dependent diabetes mellitus. Am. J. Med., 979[Suppl. 2B]:23–26, 1985.

99. Schneider, S. H., and Ruderman, N. B.: Exercise and physical training in the treatment of diabetes mellitus. Comp. Ther., 12:49–56, 1986.

100. Hanson, P., and Kochan, R.: Exercise and diabetes. Primary Care, 10:653–662, 1983.

101. Leppo, J., Boucher, C. A., Okada, R. D., Newell, J. B., Strauss, W. H., and Pohost, G. N.: Serial thallium 201 myocardial imaging after dipyridamole infusion: Diagnostic utility in detecting coronary stenoses and relationship to regional wall motion. Circulation, 66:649–657, 1982.

102. Kottke, T. E., Caspersen, C. J., and Hill, C.: Exercise in the management and rehabilitation of selected chronic disease. Prev. Med., 13:47–65, 1984.

103. Miller, T. D., Squires, R. W., Gau, G. T., Ilstrup, D. M., Frohnert, P. P., and Sterioff, S.: Graded exercise testing and training after renal transplantation: A preliminary study. Mayo Clin. Proc., 62:773–777, 1987.

Management of Vascular Disease

GARY FELL   D. E. STRANDNESS JR.

The clinical management of patients presenting with peripheral vascular disease is dependent on an understanding of the natural history of the disease process combined with an accurate diagnosis of the degree of severity of the patient's disease. Recently, advances have been made in the noninvasive assessment of the pathophysiological state of the limb circulation that are of assistance in the clinical assessment of the patient with regard to both the diagnosis and the therapy.

Arterial Disease

Acute Arterial Occlusion

Acute arterial occlusion secondary to embolus, acute thrombosis, or trauma may result in severe ischemia and gangrene of the limb. The major factors that affect the outcome in acute arterial occlusion are the location of the obstruction, the available collateral circulation, and the extent to which thrombus propagation occurs. Emboli most commonly lodge at sites of branches or bifurcations of major vessels, which is also the most common area for the development of atherosclerotic plaques. Propagation of thrombus proximal and distal to the obstruction may occur, resulting in further reduction in flow to the distal limb.

The heart is the most common source of emboli to both the upper and the lower limbs. Less common sources of emboli include ulcerated atherosclerotic plaques and aneurysms of proximal major arteries. In the lower limb, emboli most commonly lodge in the superficial femoral and popliteal arteries, although occlusion of the abdominal aorta is seen in about one sixth of all cases.

If the distal perfusion is inadequate to sustain viability, cutaneous sensation is usually lost within one hour, and after six hours the calf muscles become edematous and tender and begin to undergo ischemic contracture. Shortly thereafter, fixed staining of the skin occurs, which is a certain sign of inevitable tissue loss.

The symptoms and signs that develop in response to acute occlusion are in large part related to the site and extent of the occlusion. The five major features of acute arterial occlusion are pain, paresthesia, paralysis, pallor, and pulselessness. If the collateral circulation is adequate, numbness is the most prominent early symptom and may rapidly disappear. Pain in the foot or hand clearly indicates that the collateral circulation is inadequate and should prompt immediate action. Physical examination with this degree of ischemia reveals a cool, pale distal limb with absent palpable pulses distal to the site of occlusion.

The proximal extent of the obstruction can usually be localized by tracing out the major vessels with a Doppler ultrasonic velocity detector. In addition, the measured ankle pressure can help in deciding the most appropriate course of action. It is rare for a patient with an acute arterial occlusion and an ankle pressure of 40 mm Hg or greater to proceed to loss of tissue with nonoperative therapy.

The diagnosis of acute arterial occlusion with evidence of an inadequate collateral circulation demands urgent operation to restore an adequate circulation. Failure to operate will lead to the onset of tissue death in as little as six hours after the onset of symptoms.[1] If viability of the limb is not in question, then the indications for operative intervention will depend on the location of the occlusion. If the occlusion is proximal to or in the popliteal artery, claudication will result. Thus, for obstructions in these locations, operation is generally indicated because removal of emboli is most easily accomplished in the first 48 to 72 hours after the event.

Embolectomy is usually easily accomplished with an inflatable balloon-tipped catheter under local anesthesia. The operative mortality is in the 15 to 30 per cent range, with cardiac disease being the most common cause of death. In survivors, limb salvage occurs in 80 to 90 per cent in most reported series.[2, 3]

Full systemic anticoagulation with heparin initially and oral anticoagulants later may reduce the extent of propagation of secondary thrombosis and is not a problem should the patient require operation. Pain relief usually is required along with the correction by intravenous fluids of metabolic acidosis and hypovolemia. Protection of the extremity is very important, since the ischemic limb is very susceptible to even minor trauma, both mechanical and thermal. The application of direct heat is inappropriate and may produce significant thermal damage to the skin. In addition, the raised temperature increases the metabolic requirement of a limb unable to maintain even the basic metabolic requirements. The head of the bed should be raised 6 to 8 inches, thereby increasing tissue perfusion with the aid of gravity. Vasodilator drugs have not been found to be useful.

Acute thrombosis may occur in patients with marked arteriosclerosis obliterans, as a complication of peripheral aneurysms (popliteal, femoral), or as a result of compression associated with thoracic outlet or popliteal artery entrapment syndromes. The degree of ischemia is variable, and therapy is more difficult than with acute embolism. In addition to noninvasive studies to measure the perfusion pressure to the limb, arteriography should be performed, since direct arterial surgery is often required.

Arteriosclerosis Obliterans (ASO)

Atherosclerosis involves primarily the large and medium-sized arteries, in which progressive stenosis may lead to occlusion of the most severely involved vessels. Limb survival is possible because of the extensive network of pre-existing collateral vessels that increase in size in response to disease. These collateral pathways are high-resistance conduits that produce an abnormal pressure drop across the diseased segment. Multisegmental stenoses and occlusions are common and in ASO result in an even greater decrease in the perfusion pressure to the distal limb. The most common site of disease is the superficial femoral artery at the level of the adductor canal, followed by involvement of the aortoiliac segment.

Patients with arteriosclerosis obliterans typically present with a slow progression of symptoms unless the disease process is complicated by acute thrombosis on a pre-existing plaque. Intermittent claudication, the ischemic pain related to exercise, is the most common symptom of arteriosclerosis obliterans. The amount of exercise required to induce the pain remains relatively constant on a day-to-day basis, and pain usually subsides rapidly upon cessation of walking. As the disease progresses to involve more than one segment, exercise tolerance is progressively reduced. The terminal stage of the disease is manifested by the appearance of ischemic rest pain of the foot and digits, which may be partially or completely relieved by dependency. Ulceration and gangrene are common when the perfusion pressure falls below 40 mm Hg at the level of the ankle or digit.[4]

It should be noted that claudication always involves a more distal limb segment than the actual level of occlusion. Therefore, superficial femoral artery occlusion is associated with calf claudication, whereas aortoiliac disease may produce thigh and buttock pain in addition to that which occurs in the muscles of the calf.

In recent years, it has been recognized that there are nonvascular conditions that can mimic intermittent claudication. These usually involve the back and hip and include neurospinal stenosis, degenerative joint disease, herniated nucleus pulposus, and, rarely, a spinal cord tumor. From a clinical standpoint, the history is often important in making this differentiation. With intermittent claudication due to arterial disease, the walk-pain-rest cycle from day to day is very constant. In contrast with nonvascular causes, this cycle may vary considerably from day to day. In addition the patient may develop the pain while sitting or standing, something that never occurs with claudication secondary to arterial disease. Another important clue is found on physical examination. If there are sensory or reflex changes in the limb,

GARY FELL AND D. E. STRANDNESS JR.

one must be very suspicious that arterial disease is not the problem.

The physical examination usually supports the clinical diagnosis made from the patient's history. The appearance of the limb in single-segment disease is normal, but absent or diminished pulses may be noted. In more advanced stages of disease, dependent rubor and delayed capillary filling may be noted together with evidence of poor skin nutrition with the absence of hair, skin ulceration, and perhaps gangrene of the digits or foot. Careful auscultation for the detection of bruits in the abdomen and over the common femoral and popliteal arteries may confirm suspected arteriosclerotic vascular disease.

NONINVASIVE ASSESSMENT

Noninvasive evaluation and confirmation of the presence, severity, and rate of progression of ASO and of the results of reconstructive vascular surgery are now possible with simple, relatively inexpensive bedside equipment. A number of techniques have been developed, including strain gauge plethysmography, pulse volume recording, and Doppler ultrasonic velocity detection. The sensor is usually placed over the digits, the foot (plethysmography), or the dorsalis pedis or posterior tibial artery (ultrasonic velocity detector). The systolic blood pressure can be estimated at the level of the ankle and then compared with the brachial systolic pressure.[5] The ankle systolic pressure is normally equal to or above the brachial systolic pressure. Arterial occlusions at one or more sites result in a pressure drop that can be expressed as a ratio of arm/ankle pressure that is less than 1.0. This arm/ankle index is used to adjust for changes in systemic blood pressure. The absolute level of the ankle or digit pressure is of importance in alerting the physician to the development of rest pain. Pressures at or below 40 mm Hg are marginal in terms of tissue perfusion.

The measurement of ankle systolic pressures after exercise on a treadmill can be very useful in making the diagnosis of true claudication. Normally, with the amount of stress associated with walking on a treadmill at two miles per hour on a 12 per cent grade there should be no drop in the ankle systolic pressure. However, in the presence of arterial disease, the ankle blood pressure falls often to very low levels and may require up to 20 minutes to return to the pre-exercise level. This simple test is very useful in defining the basis for a patient's complaint with exercise.

The recordings and measurements can be used to confirm the clinical suspicion of occlusive vascular disease, to assist in differentiating vascular from neurogenic pain, to follow patients on medical regimens, and to evaluate the patency and effectiveness of reconstructive vascular surgery.

THERAPY

The patient and the patient's family must be fully acquainted with the natural history of the disease, in particular the expected chance of loss of a limb or the indications for and outcome of reconstructive vascular surgery. The expected rate of a major amputation after the onset of intermittent claudication is 1.4 per cent per year; the prospect of dying inside five years is about 15 per cent.[6] Diabetics, however, have a much increased risk of amputation, 34 per cent in 10 years in one study.[7]

Medical management, which is always required whether surgery is performed or not, is palliative, supportive, and preventive, but not curative. Surgical intervention is not indicated for those patients with intermittent claudication that does not limit employment or the ability to maintain usual daily activities. Of course, after surgery, the basic atherosclerotic disease process is still present, and continuing care is necessary to prevent progression and the potential threat of limb loss.

Clearly, for the patient with symptoms, the elimination or reduction of risk factors is mandatory. The cessation of smoking and recognition and control of diabetes, hypertension, and hyperlipidemias may, if properly managed, contribute to the reduced progression of the disease. Vasodilating drugs and long-term anticoagulation have not been found to be efficacious in the treatment of chronic arteriosclerosis obliterans.

Exercise on a daily basis to the limit imposed by claudication may result in an increased walking distance. If there are no contraindications, it is advisable to ask patients with intermittent claudication to walk up to their limit twice to three times daily. Fungal infections, minor wounds, contusion, scratches, blisters, rubbing from shoes, and minor surgical operations around the toes frequently precipitate episodes of local skin necrosis, ulceration, and sepsis and must be avoided or recognized and treated promptly.

Patients with severe lower limb ischemia, as evidenced by rest pain, cyanosis, rubor, ulceration, or gangrene, in whom surgical reconstruction is not feasible require bed rest in a warm environment with the head of the bed elevated 6 to 8 inches. Analgesia is often required, although the necessity for using narcotics may be an indication for amputation. Protection of the feet from trauma—mechanical, thermal, or chemical—is mandatory or healing of damaged tissue will have even less of a chance of occurring.

Daily physical therapy is used to prevent disuse atrophy and joint contractures, particularly of the hip and knee joints. Patients who remain in bed because of severe ischemia are at considerable risk of developing ulceration secondary to the effects of pressure on the heels.

There are two major treatment modalities available to improve blood flow to the limbs. These include transluminal angioplasty or direct arterial surgery. To evaluate patients for these procedures has in the past required arteriography. With the development of duplex scanning it is now possible to evaluate the important arterial segments noninvasively to determine which approach is applicable and most likely to succeed.

Reconstructive vascular surgery is indicated for rest pain, nonhealing ulcers, and severe progressive disabling intermittent claudication. Moderate or mild intermittent claudication that is incompatible with the patient's work is only a relative indication for operation. All patients must be fully acquainted with the risks of surgery, particularly the 1 to 5 per cent mortality rate associated with aortoiliac reconstruction and the prospect of graft occlusion of 15 per cent at 5 years.[8, 9] For femoropopliteal revascularization, the mortality rate is considerably less, although the rate of graft failure is higher, approximately 40 to 50 per cent at five years.[10, 11]

Operation is contraindicated in the absence of threatened tissue loss if the patient is sedentary or unable to walk for other reasons such as paralysis or general debility. Significant extracranial cerebrovascular and ischemic coronary artery disease should be fully evaluated and treated prior to revascularization of the lower extremities.

Amputation is considered when there is no alternative procedure available and it is certain that the patient will benefit from the proposed operation. Indications include gangrene of the limb with sepsis, nonhealing ulceration, and intractable rest pain. Dry gangrene of individual digits or ulceration on non–weight-bearing areas can be managed expectantly and amputation withheld.

Further consideration prior to amputation should be given to the expected quality and length of life. One third of vascular amputees will be dead within two years and two thirds within five years; loss of a limb poses a further threat to the enjoyment of remaining life. The early mortality associated with below-knee amputation is approximately 5 per cent, although with advancing age and increasing numbers of associated illnesses, the figure may be higher.

Thromboangiitis Obliterans (Buerger's Disease)

In contrast to arteriosclerosis obliterans, which is multisegmental and involves the large and medium-sized arteries, Buerger's disease has a different distribution. Thromboangiitis obliterans commences in the smaller arteries of the feet and hands and progresses proximally to involve the medium-sized vessels. It is primarily an inflammatory process involving the entire neurovascular bundle.

The typical patient with thromboangiitis obliterans is a male cigarette smoker in the 20- to 40-year age range. The first symptom is usually intermittent claudication, often of the instep initially and of the calf with further progression of the disease. Recurrent episodes of superficial thrombophlebitis in short nonvaricose segments of veins are seen in about 40 per cent of patients. Upper extremity involvement and cold sensitivity are seen frequently. Ischemic rest pain in the digits is often associated with ulceration and then frank gangrene.

The clinical course of the disease is greatly influenced by whether or not the patient stops smoking. Unfortunately, many patients with Buerger's disease continue to smoke in the face of progressive disease, and first minor and then major amputations are required to remove the gangrenous tissue.

Venous Disorders

Acute venous thrombosis remains the most common vascular disease that develops in the hospital. The disease is most feared for its two major complications, which are pulmonary embolism and the post-thrombotic syndrome.[12] Pulmonary embolism remains a major problem in terms of both morbidity and mortality. It is a fact that 80 per cent of patients who die of pulmonary emboli will do so in less than two hours, making it impossible to do much in the way of salvage given these time constraints. The major problem with deep venous

GARY FELL AND D. E. STRANDNESS JR.

thrombosis is our inability to make an accurate diagnosis at the bedside. It is now well established that for all patients who present with symptoms or signs suggestive of acute venous thrombosis, the bedside diagnosis is accurate only half the time. The only exception to this is in cases of iliofemoral thrombosis. When this occurs, there is massive swelling of the limb, severe pain, cyanosis, and coldness, which is difficult to confuse with any other condition.

When the diagnosis of venous thrombosis is suspected, it must be confirmed by some independent means. There are now a variety of testing procedures available in the vascular laboratory that can be used to confirm the status of the deep venous system.[13, 14] These include Doppler, impedance plethysmography, and, more recently, ultrasonic duplex scanning. Each of these methods is sufficiently accurate to permit the diagnosis to be ruled in or out, and the appropriate therapy to be applied. In those cases in which the noninvasive tests are indeterminant, it will be necessary to resort to the use of phlebography. The major problem with this invasive test is that it is painful and carries with it a small but ever present risk of producing a chemical phlebitis because of the irritating nature of the contrast material. When this occurs, it is necessary to institute heparin therapy to limit the amount of thrombosis that results.

Superficial thrombophlebitis is an entity distinct from and unrelated to involvement of the deep veins. It presents with exquisite local tenderness, cutaneous erythema, and a palpable thrombosed vein. Propagation into the deep venous system rarely occurs, and it does not lead to the development of pulmonary emboli. Its recognition is primarily on physical examination. If it is confused with cellulitis, examination with the Doppler will confirm thrombosis of the involved vein.

Therapy

The treatment of acute superficial thrombophlebitis includes rest, elevation of the limb, and local heat in the early inflammatory period. Ambulation may be begun as soon as the pain subsides.

Established deep venous thrombosis is treated by full systemic heparinization. The heparin is administered by continuous intravenous infusion after an initial loading dose is administered.[15] The partial thromboplastin time is checked prior to the commencement of therapy and then on a daily basis to maintain a value of at least two times that of the control. Intravenous heparin is continued for 10 days, at which point oral anticoagulants commenced prior to the cessation of heparin should be in the therapeutic range.

The duration of oral anticoagulant therapy is unsettled, although recent evidence suggests a six-week course for uncomplicated isolated calf vein thrombosis.[16] Following major iliofemoral vein thrombosis or pulmonary embolism, a three- to six-month course of anticoagulants is required.

In the acute phase of the deep venous thrombosis, the patient should remain in bed with the foot of the bed elevated. No other local measures are required. Ambulation should be encouraged early, and no patient should be allowed to remain sitting or standing still; the patient should either be actively walking or resting with the legs elevated. During ambulation, support stockings should be used if edema develops.

Post-Thrombotic Syndrome

Following single or multiple episodes of deep venous thrombosis, the deep and perforating veins are often subject to both obstruction and destruction of the venous valves. Blood in the deep veins is thereby forced by the calf muscle pump via abnormal pathways into the superficial venous system during exercise, when in the normal situation the reverse occurs. Over a prolonged period, chronic interstitial edema and rupture of small subcutaneous vessels occurs; hemosiderin (stasis pigmentation) deposition occurs along with fibrosis, cutaneous atrophy, and lymphatic obstruction. These chronic changes in the skin of the leg may lead to the development of stasis ulceration.

The first clinical manifestation of chronic venous insufficiency is the development of dependent edema of the limb, which is worse at the end of the day and tends to clear after a period of recumbency and elevation. Secondly, stasis pigmentation is noted followed by induration and less resolution of the edema with elevation of the limbs. Ulceration is common and usually develops following minor episodes of trauma. The ulcers commonly occur in the region of the medial malleolus but may extend all the way around the ankle. Multiple organisms can often be cultured from the base of the ulcer and secondary infection may occur, leading to episodes of cellulitis, further fibrosis, induration, and the prevention of healing of the ulcer.

Therapy

The major goal in all patients with the post-thrombotic syndrome is to reduce the ambulatory venous pressure. This may usually be accomplished by the wearing of tailored, graduated pressure support stockings, bandages, or both, combined with elevation of the legs whenever possible.

In cases with ulceration, healing can always be achieved by persistent, prolonged bed rest and elevation. For most patients this is not feasible, and the ulcer must be healed while the patient remains active and ambulatory. Healing can usually be achieved by the use of the Unna boot applied from the base of the toes to below the knee. The dressing is applied directly to the ulcer and changed weekly or sooner if drainage is excessive. The patients remain ambulatory, and when complete healing has occurred, a tailored pressure gradient stocking is used. For large ulcers that do not respond to this form of therapy, skin grafting may become necessary.

Lymphatic Disorders

Lymphedema occurs secondary to congenital or acquired lymphatic obstruction. It always involves the dorsum of the digits, foot, or hand, which is rare with edema secondary to venous obstruction. It is often brawny in nature and does not respond as rapidly to elevation. Ulceration is rare, but cellulitis secondary to streptococcal infection is not uncommon. For this reason, prophylactic penicillin is commonly used, since repeated episodes of cellulitis lead to edema that is worse after each episode.

Since the edema is difficult to manage once it gets out of control, it is essential that daily care include the following: (1) limb measurements recorded in a diary; (2) graded, heavy elastic support; (3) prophylactic penicillin; and (4) the use of intermittent pneumatic compression devices at night to assist in the control of the edema.

Lymphangiography has been recommended to confirm the diagnosis, but this is rarely required. Further, if lymphangitis occurs secondary to the procedure, the edema is always worse. The lifetime nature of the problem must be emphasized to the patient, and frequent medical follow-up is mandatory to ensure compliance with recommended therapy. Surgical removal of the involved tissue is only rarely required if proper conservative therapy has been used and followed.

References

1. Tibbs, P. J.: Acute ischemia of the limbs. Proc. R. Soc. Med., 55:593, 1962.
2. Levy, J. F., and Butcher, H. R.: Arterial emboli: An analysis of 125 patients. Surgery, 68:968, 1970.
3. Blaisdell, F. W., Steele, M., and Allen, R. E.: Management of acute lower extremity arterial ischemia due to embolism and thrombosis. Surgery, 84:822, 1978.
4. Strandness, D. E. Jr.: Diagnostic considerations in occlusive arterial disease. Vasc. Surg., 11:271, 1977.
5. Carter, S. A.: Role of pressure measurements in vascular disease. *In* Bernstein, E. F. (Ed.): Noninvasive Diagnostic Techniques in Vascular Disease. St. Louis, C. V. Mosby, 1978.
6. Boyd, A. M.: The natural course of arteriosclerosis of the lower extremities. Proc. R. Soc. Med., 53:591, 1962.
7. Silbert, S., and Zazeela, H.: Prognosis in arteriosclerotic peripheral vascular disease. J.A.M.A., 166:1816, 1958.
8. Mozersky, D. J., Sumner, D. S., and Strandness, D. E. Jr.: Long term results of reconstructive aortoiliac surgery. Am. J. Surg., 123:503, 1972.
9. Hill, D. A., McGrath, M. A., Lord, R. S. A., and Tracy, G. D.: The effect of superficial femoral artery occlusion on the outcome of aortofemoral bypass for intermittent claudication. Surgery, 87:133, 1980.
10. Reichle, F. A., Rankin, K. P., Tyson, R. R., Finestone, A. S., and Shuman, C.: Long term results of 474 arterial reconstructions for severely ischemic limbs: A fourteen year followup. Surgery, 85:93, 1979.
11. Szilagyi, D. E., Hageman, J. H., Smith, F. R., Elliott, J. P., Brown, F., and Dietz, P.: Autogenous vein grafting in femoro-popliteal atherosclerosis: The limits of its effectiveness. Surgery, 86:836, 1979.
12. Strandness, D. E. Jr., Ward, K., and Krugmire, R. Jr.: The present status of acute deep venous thrombosis. Surg. Obstet. Gynecol., 145:433, 1977.
13. Sumner, D. S., and Lambeth, A.: Reliability of Doppler ultrasound in the diagnosis of acute deep venous thrombosis both above and below the knee. Am. J. Surg., 138:205, 1979.
14. Strandness, D. E. Jr.: Invasive and noninvasive techniques in the detection and evaluation of acute venous thrombosis. Vasc. Surg., 11:205, 1977.
15. Salzman, E. W., Deykin, D., Shapiro, R. M., and Rosenberg, R.: Management of heparin therapy: Controlled prospective trial. N. Engl. J. Med., 292:1046, 1975.
16. Hull, R., Delmore, T., Genton, E., Hirsh, J., Gent, M., Sackett, D., McLoughlin, D., and Armstrong, P.: Sodium versus low-dose heparin in the long-term treatment of venous thrombosis. N. Engl. J. Med., 301:855, 1979.

GARY FELL AND D. E. STRANDNESS JR.

Suggested Reading

Haimovici, H. (Ed.): Vascular Surgery, Principles and Techniques, 2nd Ed. New York, McGraw-Hill Book Company, 1984.

Rutherford, R. W. (Ed.): Vascular Surgery, 2nd Ed. Philadelphia, W. B. Saunders Company, 1985.

Knox, R. A., and Strandness, D. E. Jr.: Ultrasound techniques for the evaluation of lower extremity arterial occlusion. Semin. Ultrasound, 2:264, 1981.

Hershey, F. B., Barnes, R. B., and Sumner, D. S.: Noninvasive Diagnosis of Vascular Disease. Pasadena, Appleton Davies Inc., 1984.

Strandness, D. E., and Thiele, B. L.: Selected Topics in Venous Disease. Mt. Kisco, NY, Futura Publishing Company, 1984.

Jager, K. A., Ricketts, H. A., and Strandness, D. E. Jr.: Duplex scanning for the evaluation of lower limb arterial disease. *In* Bernstein, E. F. (Ed.): Noninvasive Diagnostic Techniques in Vascular Disease, 3rd Ed. St. Louis, C. V. Mosby, 1985.

Kinmonth, J. B.: The Lymphatics. London, Edward Arnold, 1982.

43
Reconstructive Surgery of the Extremities

JOACHIM L. OPITZ

With the advent of total joint replacement during the last 20 years, reconstructive surgery of the extremities has entered a new and promising era. Substantial advances also are being made in tendon transfers and in post-traumatic reconstruction of extremities. The following chapter outlines the principles related to common reconstructive procedures in the extremities and to their subsequent postoperative management.

Total Joint Replacement

General Considerations

Purposes. The purposes of total joint replacement are to relieve pain, to correct deformities, to reestablish function, and to prevent or ameliorate painful secondary effects on adjacent joints. The combination of high-density polyethylene and highly polished resilient metal alloys (nickel, chrome, molybdenum, titanium), as first described by Charnley[5] in his total hip prosthesis, has led progressively to replacement of all major joints in both lower and upper extremities. Many different prostheses of various degrees of constraint are being used, most of which have the combination of high-density polyethylene and metal in their components or are joint spacers made of special Silastic rubber elastomers. Clinical experience of more than 15 years has indicated very little wear of the polyethylene-on-metal prostheses, approximately 0.15 mm per year in total hip arthroplasty, maintenance of the low-friction features, and no foreign body reactions. The optically polished metal components have usually satisfactory resilience, excellent tissue acceptance, and no appreciable wear. Long-term follow-up of 5 to 12 years in patients who have the Charnley-type low-friction total hip arthroplasty has revealed excellent or good results in 80 to 88 per cent.[8, 22, 36] In patients with total semiconstrained or resurfacing knee arthroplasties, long-term follow-up of between 5 and 10 years has indicated excellent or good results in 88 to 90 per cent.[17, 40, 44, 45]

Limitations. The greatest, initially unanticipated, source of late failures relates to loosening of cemented prosthetic devices at the bone-cement interface.[18] Methyl methacrylate, a cementing compound, provides major advantages over the press fitting of components. The methacrylate is well tolerated by tissues, although it is less than ideal as a grouting agent. The higher the degree of constraint built into a total joint replacement and the rougher its use in the absence of pain in the young and in the overweight person, the higher the incidence of late loosening tends to be.

Infection in total joint replacements, even though of low incidence, is also a worrisome cause of failure. Hematogenous spread of organisms is the usual cause of late infection and often necessitates the temporary removal of the prosthetic components. Therefore, the prophylactic use of antibiotics is justified in total joint replacements when transient bacteremia is to be expected, such as with tooth extractions, thorough professional dental cleansing, urinary tract infection, and systemic infections.

Because of the worrisome, slowly increasing incidence of subclinical and clinical loosening of total joint prostheses with increasing years of heavy

JOACHIM L. OPITZ

use, including revision total arthroplasties,[19] the biological method of fixation by ingrowth of bone into a porous surface of the prosthesis has been developed. Harris[16] recently described the factors controlling optimal bone ingrowth of total hip components. Among such factors are an optimal pore size (100 to 150 μ), press fitting of the prosthesis into cancellous bone, and avoidance of weight-bearing during the first months after placement to ensure rigid initial fixation and undisturbed ingrowth of bone. Early results (five years of follow-up) of maintained fixation by bone ingrowth in total hip arthroplasties are encouraging.[14]

Long-term results in total replacements of shoulders,[6] elbows,[33] and wrists[9] are not as good as of those of hips and knees, but overall they are successful.

Long-term results in total replacements of digital joints and of the ankle have been less successful.[2, 46]

Indications. The main indications for total joint arthroplasties exist in patients afflicted with degenerative joint disease, destructive rheumatoid arthritis, and, to some extent, post-traumatic arthritis. Total joint replacement for post-traumatic arthritis is currently limited to the hip, knee, thumb, shoulder, and elbow.

In destructive polyarthritis, the indications for total joint replacements of the lower extremities have precedence over those of the upper extremities, except on the occasion when a patient otherwise would be totally dependent in feeding and self-care. Often, joints of the upper extremity improve remarkably once they are relieved of the severe stress of assisting the lower extremities in weight-bearing after total hip or knee replacement.

Contraindications. Absolute contraindications for total joint arthroplasties exist in patients with recent septic arthritis, paralysis about the joint to be replaced, and neuropathic joint disease. Relative contraindications exist in patients with severe osteoporosis, severe and incorrectable ligamentous defects about the joint, and other physiological or psychological deficiencies of proportion.

Goals. The goals of postoperative physiatric management need to be in line with the purposes of total joint replacement. They are relief of pain, redevelopment of comfortable musculoskeletal functions, and development of living habits that avoid excessive stress on the joint replacement.

RELIEF OF PAIN. For practical purposes, pain can be defined for the patient and therapist as the degree of discomfort that causes motor incoordination, such as unreasonable cocontraction of the antagonistic muscle groups (splinting). This defi-

nition allows for a gradual increase in strain of therapeutic exercises as the patient maintains smooth neuromuscular function about the replaced joint. The patient who undergoes total joint replacement usually has had years of progressive pain about the joint in question. Long-term expectation and experience of joint pain, progressive limitation of range of motion, and the decrease of strength due to diminished use of the extremity, often have led to deep-seated changes in coordination and motor behavior. Muscle misuse, that is, unreasonable cocontraction of antagonistic muscles, usually has become firmly established before total joint replacement. The effects of muscle misuse tend to perpetuate vicious circles of pain. As a result of muscle misuse, a number of undesirable effects evolve. Range of motion becomes unnecessarily limited by heavy cocontraction of antagonistic muscle groups. Joints are exposed to high compression forces because such cocontractions occur during attempted motion, causing increased wear and synovial irritation. Last, the involved muscles themselves become overused. With chronic joint pain, muscle contractions often last much longer than needed. Continued lowgrade to moderate muscle contraction, therefore, may result in chronic muscle overuse with associated tension myalgia, muscle attachment pain, and tenosynovitis. Such pernicious interrelationships contribute substantially to the increase in pain and the limitation of functions. Because pain is also a very effective inhibitor of muscle contraction, it causes progressive decrease of strength as a result of muscle misuse.

When the patient is seen postoperatively in the department of physical medicine and rehabilitation, the motor behavior of muscle misuse usually has been further reinforced by the substantial bone and soft-tissue trauma during the joint replacement procedure and by the apprehension of the patient, who often expects the postoperative program to be a painful experience. The examination tends to be less threatening to the patient if the evaluator first takes inventory of the uninvolved extremities and then inspects the involved extremity. Slow, passive motion of the involved limb follows in order to explore the pain-free range of motion. Testing for clinically apparent deep venous thrombosis, peripheral nerve injury, deep infection, and substantial hematoma usually can be done without considerable and potentially threatening movements of the involved extremity. The assessment of the total passive range of motion is of questionable value at this point, because it is usually limited by muscle guarding, which should be avoided. Thus, during the evaluation process, the patient can be relieved of some anxiety and can become better prepared to work for improvement of normal function. The negative effects of muscle misuse on the joint, periarticular structures, range of motion, strength, and normal joint function make it logical that the first and perhaps the most important therapeutic goal after an operation is to eliminate abnormal motor behavior resulting from expected or actual pain.

Pain usually can be eliminated because the total joint replacement has rendered the joint itself free of pain. The patient should know and experience that the therapeutic exercises and subsequent therapeutic functional activities can be practiced smoothly and without pain.

Priorities of successive exercises in activities should be carefully considered (Table 43–1). These priorities need to be adhered to in order to eliminate pain, to avoid muscle misuse and substitution patterns, and to ensure the efficient attainment of the overall goals of total joint replacement. Generally, it is advisable first to reestablish a functional territory of pain-free motion, then to redevelop normal motor behavior and a satisfactory pain-free range of motion, and then to maintain normal motor behavior before gentle, prolonged stretching, which may be done six weeks after total arthroplasty, and before advancing to formal strengthening (if indicated).

REESTABLISHMENT OF NORMAL FUNCTION. Neuromuscular re-education is the initial therapeutic exercise system that is designed to assist the patient in the reestablishment of pain-free, well-coordinated motor activities. In neuromuscular reeducation, the patient's undesirable old pattern of muscle misuse is consciously dismissed by allowing the therapist to move the extremity passively through the pain-free range of motion. The patient should permit passive movement without interference through many repetitions. As the patterns of

TABLE 43–1. Priorities of Successive Exercises and Activities After Total Joint Replacement*

Passive relaxed motion and neuromuscular reeducation
Active (assisted) range-of-motion exercises
Light functional activities of daily living, hobby, and self-care
Redevelopment of maximal desirable range of motion (with gentle, prolonged stretching)
Formal strengthening (if indicated)

*Modified from Opitz, J. L.: Total joint arthroplasty: Principles and guidelines for postoperative physiatric management. Mayo Clin. Proc., 54:602–612, 1979. By permission.

muscle misuse are eliminated in this fashion, the therapist then, through various techniques, coaches the patient to contract the prime mover of a specific motion, free of associated, undesirable cocontraction of antagonistic muscles. Motion through the pain-free arc is then accomplished by gentle contraction of the prime mover while assistance is given by the therapist. In this way, normal motor behavior is reestablished and incorporated in range-of-motion exercises and light functional activities of daily living. Dysfunctional motor behaviors, if they reappear, are recognized at their inception by experienced therapists. These behaviors are promptly and gently discouraged. Usually, motor tasks that cause motor incoordination should temporarily be made simpler for the patient. If this measure is unsuccessful, techniques of neuromuscular re-education need to be reapplied. Often, simply a temporary reduction in speed, force, and perhaps arc of motion permits the return of an acceptable motor pattern. In this way, the patient progresses most efficiently to more difficult tasks while the comfortable motor capacity of the joint is not violated and is allowed to increase.

Because the potentially available range of motion can be developed at mild to moderate, usually pain-free muscle contractions, and because strengthening exercises usually require potentially painful, strong muscle contraction, strengthening exercises are best postponed until the full range of motion has been redeveloped. For strengthening exercises, muscle contractions about the joint should be free of pain and should have become nonthreatening to periarticular structures.

Some uncertainty exists concerning when stretching exercises can be applied safely to increase the range of motion more efficiently than by the active-assisted or active range-of-motion exercises alone. The reasons for such uncertainty relate to the difficulty in estimating the tensile strength of periarticular structures and that of the ingrowing bone as ingrowth progresses and to the degree of stretching force applied by the individual therapist during stretching exercises.

When exposed to pain-free, mild to moderate stretching forces for 15 to 30 min several times a day, maturing scar tissue should elongate without injury. Such stretching forces can be applied four to six weeks after operation without threatening essential periarticular structures. In fact, such gentle, prolonged stretching forces are probably important for the proper alignment of collagen bundles and, thus, lead to better connective tissue

JOACHIM L. OPITZ

structures about the joint as healing progresses. Forceful stretching should be avoided because it is likely to result in pain, splinting of the muscles being stretched, and irritation of the joint. Such stretching also threatens the integrity of periarticular structures and causes protective motor behavior (muscle misuse) with its negative consequences.

When rapid increases in range of motion are not forthcoming, the daily measurement of active range of motion (goniometry) at the end of the last exercise period of the day with the patient in a gravity-eliminated position of the joint is helpful in assessing progress (Fig. 43–1). Results of goniometry are likely to be reproducible only if the motion is done actively by the patient without assistance. The results of daily goniometry are particularly helpful in motivating the patient for range-of-motion exercises, because the patient is then challenging himself or herself. If the daily results are recorded on a graph, the patient, the therapist, and the physician can easily follow and appreciate advances in range of motion. Slowing of progress, lack of progress, or actual regression of performance is recognized early.

After increases in range of motion have stopped, further increases often may be achieved by heating the connective tissue to be stretched with ultrasound at the time of gentle, prolonged stretching. This technique was described by Lehmann and associates.[25] For practical purposes, ultrasound may be applied safely in the presence of metallic or plastic implants.

Restrengthening of the involved extremity, as mentioned earlier, is last on the list of priorities because of the associated strong muscle contractions, which are potentially painful and possibly injurious to periarticular structures and interfaces of ingrowing bone. Often, formal strengthening exercises are not necessary because the extremities with total joint replacements, when kept free of pain, strengthen spontaneously to substantial levels as they are made to perform the daily functional activities during the first three to six months after operation. Because of the relatively high incidence of loosening of components in total joint replacement when the extremities are exposed to heavy mechanical stresses, formal restrengthening to a maximal degree may be unnecessary or even contraindicated. If strengthening is needed, it should be postponed until it can be done comfortably. Pain is a very potent inhibitor of muscle contraction and prohibits strengthening.

ADEQUATE RELIEF OF WEIGHT-BEARING. Reliable reduction of weight-bearing after hip, knee, and ankle replacements continues to be of concern. Examinations of reproducibility of reduction in weight-bearing in biomechanical laboratories have shown that the only consistently reproducible method for relief of weight-bearing identified is to "touch only" with the involved lower extremity during gait. This reduces weight-bearing to 20 lb (9 kg) or less. "Touch-only" weight-bearing can be checked simply by the physician and therapist during gait training of the patient. In order to

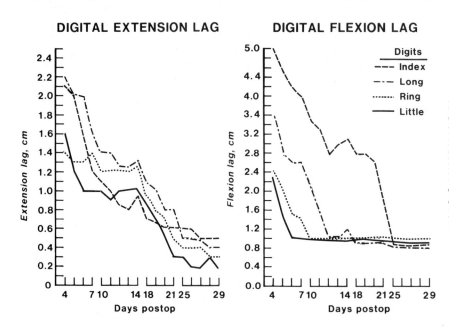

FIGURE 43–1. Graphs showing decreasing active extensor and flexor lags of digits after total metacarpophalangeal joint replacement in a patient with rheumatoid arthritis. (From Opitz, J. L.: Total joint arthroplasty: Principles and guidelines for postoperative physiatric management. Mayo Clin. Proc., 54:602–612, 1979. By permission.)

check touch-only weight-bearing, one assesses the friction between the shoe and the floor resulting from the superimposed body weight of the patient by means of a few gentle, rapid knocks against the heel of the patient's shoe by the examiner's foot during the stance phase. Weight-bearing is minimal (touch only) if the patient's foot is easily (and minimally) displaced by gentle knocking during stance. The foot cannot be displaced by this method if weight bearing is substantial. Touch-only weight-bearing is indicated generally for three months in total joint replacement of the lower extremity with biological fixation.

Often, however, weight-bearing can be reduced enough postoperatively for the patient with cemented components to be free from discomfort. Such an order might read: "Weight-bearing on the left (or right) lower extremity as tolerated comfortably." It permits progressive increase in weight-bearing without overly stressing recently operated soft tissues, provided that, in the patient with cemented total hip replacement, the greater trochanter has not been osteotomized and reattached. If substantial muscle or bone had to be divided and reapproximated, the formal method of touch only is the only reliable method of preventing overexposure to the mechanical stresses of weight-bearing.

Evaluation before starting physical therapy and occupational therapy (when indicated) requires review of the written referral, of the operative report, and of the appropriate preoperative and postoperative roentgenograms in order to determine whether unusual circumstances exist that necessitate modification of the postoperative program. Any personal input from the surgeon by word or (preferably) in writing helps serve the same purpose. Nevertheless, the operative report and roentgenograms still should be reviewed carefully. If any question remains, clarification by the surgeons is imperative before a treatment program is started.

Lower Extremities

Total Hip Arthroplasty. Total hip replacements are done routinely in patients with painfully decompensating primary or secondary degenerative joint disease, rheumatoid arthritis, or congenital hip disease. Total hip replacement also may be done to salvage other arthroplasties of the hip if the hip has become painful or to salvage arthrodeses of the hip, provided that the hip mus-

culature is adequate. Since 1961, when Charnley[5] reported on total hip arthroplasty, low-friction arthroplasty with a high-density acetabular polyethylene component and the corresponding optically polished Vitallium femoral head prosthesis, progress in total joint replacement has been phenomenal. The advantages of metalloplastic prostheses have been confirmed for several of the major joints in terms of no pain, no wear, good mobility, adequate stability, and durability if not overly stressed. Several total hip prostheses are available for fixation of both components by cementing with methyl methacrylate or by ingrowth of bone (Fig. 43–2). A prosthesis for replacement of the proximal femur after intracapsular femoral neck fractures is the bipolar Bateman prosthesis, which is often inserted by press fitting without cement.[3, 24]

Special long-stemmed femoral components as part of a total hip arthroplasty may replace en bloc resection of tumors involving the proximal femur where amputation of the lower extremity by hip disarticulation was previously necessary.

The patient is referred to physical medicine and rehabilitation during the third or fourth day after total hip arthroplasty. The exercise program consists of individual brief periods of neuromuscular re-education for active-assisted range of motion of ankle, knee, and hip. Gait training should be started with parallel bars as soon as the patient is free of orthostatic hypotension when sitting up. Initially, the therapist should check the patient's pulse during sitting and during standing to identify orthostasis by noticing the development of tachycardia. After standing balance has been achieved with the help of parallel bars, neuromuscular re-education reestablishes proper motion of the involved extremity during the swing phase in the parallel bars. Also, the stance phase of the involved lower extremity is practiced (noted as "touch only" or "weight-bearing as tolerated comfortably") with parallel bars. If several repetitions of the isolated swing phase and stance phase are performed satisfactorily, the patient is asked to take a single step. If the single step is performed well, the patient should attempt to take two consecutive steps. The number of consecutive steps is increased progressively as acceptable performance permits. A decrease in speed and accuracy of performance indicates fatigue and signals the need for a short pause or a longer rest period. Once an uninterrupted gait with the help of parallel bars has become smooth and acceptable (three-point gait for unilateral and four-point gait for bilateral

JOACHIM L. OPITZ

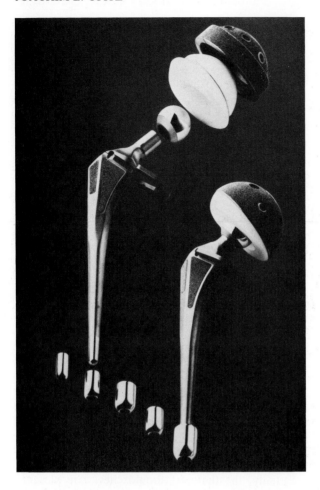

FIGURE 43–2. Modular total hip prosthesis designed for bony ingrowth.

hip involvement), the patient is advanced to the use of crutches. Again, one should start and advance with the same sequence as was done with the use of parallel bars before beginning gait training on curbs and stairs. Touch-only weight-bearing is usually required for three months with total hip replacements with biological fixation.

Isometric contraction of the quadriceps muscle of the involved extremity against gravity through 10 repetitions is usually tolerated well. Formal isometric strengthening of the quadriceps muscle of the uninvolved side, however, also may be very beneficial for rapid development of a safe gait, especially in relation to curbs and stairs.

If postoperative dislocation of the hip is to be prevented, restriction of hip flexion to 90 degrees and of adduction requires the patient to use assistive devices for dressing below the waist, an elevated toilet seat, and a pillow between the knees when lying on the side and to avoid sleeping on the operated side. Such antidislocation measures are indicated for about three months until new

capsular tissues have formed and the periarticular muscle tone has substantially increased (Fig. 43–3).

Written home instructions should provide direction on the restrictions of weight-bearing and a maximum of 90 degrees of hip flexion (usually during the first three months), as related to the usual activities of daily living and of self-care. A program of range-of-motion exercises is generally not necessary, since pre-existing hip flexion contractures are usually released surgically and hip flexion increases with sitting. Written home instructions and isometric strengthening of quadriceps may be indicated or may be contraindicated (in the presence of biological fixation). The patient is usually ready for dismissal within two weeks after surgery.

Preventive care to avoid loosening of cemented prosthetic parts should include avoidance of obesity, running, jumping, and heavy lifting. Swimming, walking, bowling, or cycling may be done.

Preventive care to avoid hematogenous late infection of the replaced joint requires the prophy-

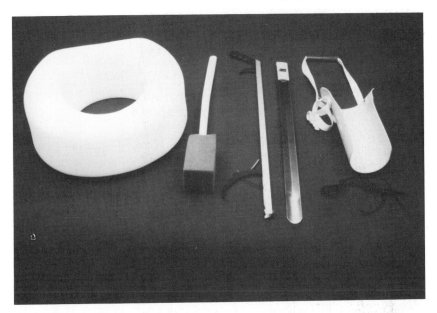

FIGURE 43–3. Assistive devices initially used by patients after total hip replacement.

lactic temporary use of antibiotics whenever periods of bacteremia are expected, such as during dental work, systemic illnesses, and tonsillitis.

During recheck visits, deficits of function are identified and are treated on an individual basis with physical therapy. Transition from crutches to canes occurs usually at 4 to 12 weeks after operation. For the patient to have adequate support during the stance phase on the involved side with the use of a cane, the quadriceps muscle of the involved side should have an isometric 10 repetition maximum of at least 8 kg (approximately 18 lb).

Total Knee Arthroplasty. Severe progressive gonalgia with increasing instability and increasing deformity in primary or secondary degenerative joint disease and destructive rheumatoid arthritis are the usual indications for total knee arthroplasty. En bloc resections of low-grade neoplasms of the distal femur or proximal tibia may be replaced with fully constrained prostheses, whereas previously above the knee amputations had to be done. Total knee prostheses are available with minimal constraint (polycentric, anatomical, and similar designs), partial constraint (anametric, total condylar, UCI, and several others), and full constraint (the kinematic rotating hinge and others) (Figs. 43–4 to 43–6).

Usually, the patient can be referred to the physical medicine and rehabilitation department between the second and fourth postoperative day. Initial therapeutic exercises consist of neuromuscular re-education to gentle, active-assisted range-of-motion exercises. There is a substantial advantage if range-of-motion exercises can be begun from a fully extended knee position if the knee has been immobilized postoperatively in full extension. Difficulties in achieving full active extension of the knee are common in patients in whom the knee was immobilized postoperatively in flexion. Adhesions, which form rapidly between the quadriceps mechanism and the surrounding tissues, are likely to be the cause of the difficulties. These adhesions can be stretched, reduced, and eliminated much more easily by the weight of the leg during assisted flexion from full extension than by the proximal pull of the quadriceps muscle alone in a proximal direction if the knee had been kept

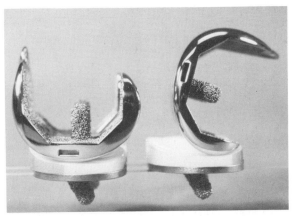

FIGURE 43–4. Porous-coated total knee prosthesis. Note resurfacing features of components and beaded surfaces for biologic fixation.

JOACHIM L. OPITZ

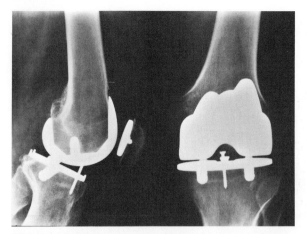

FIGURE 43–5. Porous-coated total knee arthroplasty with biological fixation. *Left,* Lateral view, showing three components. *Right,* Anteroposterior view.

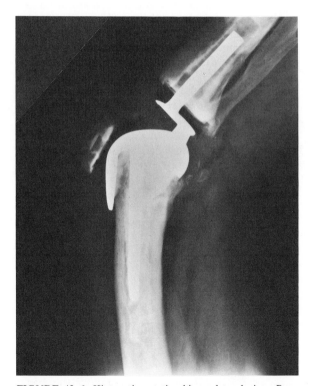

FIGURE 43–6. Kinematic rotating hinge, lateral view. Prosthesis allows rotation of metallic axis in the polyethylene component, cemented in proximal tibia. Also, it allows for flexion and extension of metalloplastic hinge joining the tibial and femoral components. Resurfacing of the patella is also accomplished. The prosthesis is used when periarticular support has become insufficient so that full internal constraint has to be provided.

previously in flexion. Under such circumstances, adhesions of the quadriceps mechanism, which formed with the knee in flexion, often effectively block the transmission of quadriceps power for full knee extension to the patellar tendon and tibia. For this reason, if the knee is immobilized postoperatively, immobilization in full knee extension is strongly advised.

The use of a constant passive motion apparatus during the early postoperative period greatly enhances remobilization of the knee after total knee arthroplasty (Fig. 43–7). Constant passive motion generally is well accepted by patients during the early postoperative period.

Gentle, pain-free, prolonged stretching (10 to 20 min four times per day) to increase knee flexion or extension usually may be started after the second postoperative week if progress is inadequate with range-of-motion exercises. The force of stretching must, of necessity, be very mild. For increase of knee flexion, part of the weight of the leg is borne in an antigravity position by the therapist. For increase of knee extension, part of the weight of the lower extremity is supported by the plinth, bed, or chair, with the patient in a semisitting position.

The principles for gait training are the same as those outlined for total hip arthroplasty. Usually, they involve the touch-only process. Redevelopment of adequate knee flexion and ankle dorsiflexion during the swing phase, along with adequate knee extension during the stance phase, is emphasized.

At times, mild isometric quadriceps strengthening can be started toward the end of the second postoperative week, when satisfactory range of motion has been developed and gait training on the level is essentially complete. Isometric strengthening should not be painful and should not increase joint stiffness or swelling or cause joint effusion. Also, the opposite quadriceps muscle is strengthened, if desirable.

Patients are usually ready for dismissal within two to three weeks after operation. The written home program consists of active assisted range-of-motion exercises and mild isometric quadriceps strengthening (10 repetitions per day), with weekly increases in resistance that are comfortably tolerated without producing evidence of joint irritation.

During recheck visits, the transition from crutches to a cane is done when adequate healing of bone and soft tissues has progressed and antigravity quadriceps strength has progressed to at least 8 kg (approximately 18 lb).

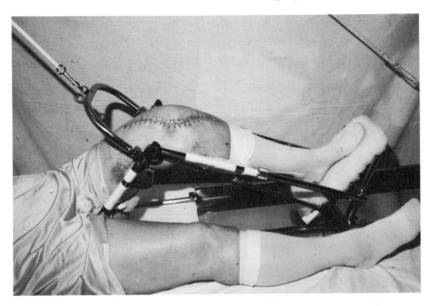

FIGURE 43–7. Constant passive motion apparatus. The knee is being moved slowly through its pain-free arc of motion. Resistance to motion by muscle guarding interrupts the cycle. Range of passive motion, speed, and the degree of resistance that interrupts the motion are adjustable. When used correctly, the apparatus has met with excellent patient acceptance.

Upper Extremities

Total Shoulder Arthroplasty. Total shoulder arthroplasty is indicated when previously one would have considered fusion of the glenohumeral joint for pain and lack of function in primary or secondary degenerative joint disease, rheumatoid arthritis, avascular necrosis, and similar conditions of the shoulder. Special long-stem prostheses are available to replace large humeral bone defects after en bloc tumor resection.[43] Generally, pain relief, shoulder function, and cosmesis are better with total shoulder arthroplasty than with shoulder arthrodesis. The incidences of loosening of the glenoid component have improved with the use of semiconstrained or nonconstrained total shoulder prostheses that provide larger surfaces for anchorage in the scapula with methyl methacrylate (Neer) or with ingrowth of bone and initial screw fixation (English-McNab).[6, 29, 35] Because the stability of the shoulder joint with decreasing degrees of internal constraint relies on the stability of the repaired rotator cuff, particular care should be taken during the postoperative management. Heavy use of the upper extremity should be permanently avoided. With the resurfacing total shoulder arthroplasty (Fig. 43–8), satisfactory relief of pain can be anticipated in approximately 90 per cent of patients. Also, in 90 per cent of patients, active range of motion can be anticipated to degrees that permit the usual activities of daily living and light work.[43] Contraindications to total shoulder arthroplasty are related to paralysis, recent septic arthritis, poor bone or soft-tissue structures, and other substantial physiological or psychological inadequacies.

Referrals for gentle mobilization occur at about the fourth postoperative day. During the initial two weeks after the arthroplasty, the upper extremity is held in a neutral position in a shoulder immobilizer along the thorax, with the elbow in flexion, except during the therapeutic exercises, which are done twice daily. The therapeutic exercise program consists of gentle, passive, relaxed range-of-motion exercises in the supine position with the avoidance of pain as well as of neuromuscular re-education of the shoulder groups for active, gentle, assisted range-of-motion exercises. Combinations of external rotation, abduction, and extension are carefully avoided with the usual anterior surgical approach to the joint.

During the first two weeks, all shoulder exercises are done in the supine position for better relaxation of the shoulder girdle musculature during exercises. Active range-of-motion exercises are also done for the elbow, wrist, and hand.

During the second week, sitting posture is practiced in order to achieve a balanced position of the head in relation to the upper part of the back. Once the head no longer represents overhanging weight, the nuchal muscles and the trapezius muscles are likely to relax spontaneously. As the trapezius muscles relax, the pectoral muscles also tend to relax spontaneously. Postural relaxation of the shoulder girdle musculature is desirable during

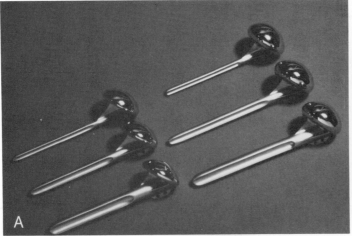

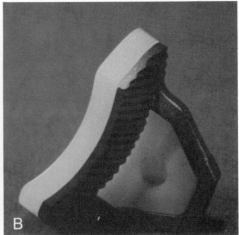

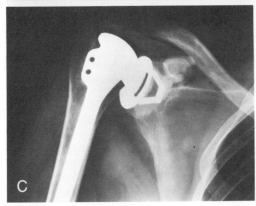

FIGURE 43–8. *A*, Neer total shoulder prosthesis. Note different available sizes of humeral head. *B*, Polyethylene glenoid component viewed from its side. Note metal backing. *C*, Total shoulder arthroplasty with a Neer prosthesis. (Courtesy of Dr. R. H. Cofield.)

the postoperative phase, especially when, during the third postoperative week, the supine shoulder exercises are also done in the sitting position (with assistance given by the therapist). During the third postoperative week, light functional hand activities (such as light assembly work, knitting, mosaic work, puzzles, and the like) are started in occupational therapy, with the upper extremity supported in a deltoid aid (Fig. 43–9). Throughout the postoperative period, passive, relaxed range-of-motion exercises, however, are continued; range-of-motion exercises are done twice daily with the elbow flexed and the patient in the supine position.

The patient is usually dismissed toward the end of the third week. The home exercise program consists of the aforementioned passive, relaxed (supine), active-assisted (supine and sitting) range-of-motion exercises. The patient continues to use a balanced sitting posture and light functional activities of the upper extremity. Frequent rest periods are advisable (semisitting or supine). Fur-

ther, the use of a headrest and a backrest when riding in a car or watching television is helpful for ongoing relaxation of neck and shoulder girdle musculature.

During recheck visits, the exercise program is updated in terms of emphasizing advancement of certain ranges that are particularly needed and shoulder girdle relaxation. Gentle, comfortable, prolonged stretching in gravity-eliminated positions (supine and side-lying) is added to range-of-motion exercises, if necessary. If tolerated without discomfort, pain-free isometric contractions (10 repetitions) of the shoulder abductors, adductors, external rotators, and internal rotators, with the shoulder in neutral position, may be started at 12 weeks. In occupational therapy, the patient advances to light self-care, dressing, and household activities when these activities can be performed free of substitution patterns (free of discomfort) without the use of much force.

During additional recheck visits, the exercises may be further modified for needed increases of

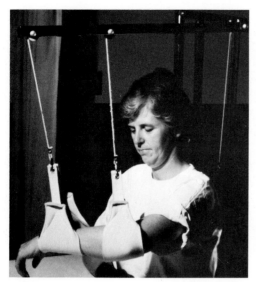

FIGURE 43–9. Deltoid aid as used after total shoulder replacement. (From Opitz, J. L.: Total joint arthroplasty: Principles and guidelines for postoperative physiatric management. Mayo Clin. Proc., 54:602–612, 1979. By permission.)

range of motion and for some further increase in strength. Careful emphasis is placed on relaxation, freedom from substitution patterns, freedom from pain, and an increase in range of motion. Strengthening can be done isometrically against absolute resistance with the shoulder in an adducted and otherwise neutral position.

Patients with substantial repairs of the rotator cuffs, especially when fascial grafts are needed, may require that the upper extremity be kept in an airplane splint for four to six weeks. During this period, only passive, relaxed (supine) range-of-motion exercises are done above the splint level. The mobility of the distal joints is also maintained while the extremity is resting on the splint. Sitting posture for enhancement of nuchal and shoulder girdle release is especially important in these patients. Gradual mobilization of the shoulder after removal of the splint follows the guidelines previously described.

Total Elbow Arthroplasty. The usual indications for total elbow arthroplasty are severe pain and permanent limitation of essential function that are not amenable to synovectomy and resection of the radial head in rheumatoid arthritis or to nonresection arthroplasty in degenerative arthritis. Semiconstrained or resurfacing prostheses, usually interfacing polyethylene with metal, are available. The minimal or nonconstrained prosthesis is preferred when periarticular structures can be

adequately repaired. When a nonconstrained prosthesis fails, usually there is the option of changeover to a resectional arthroplasty, which allows the elbow to remain fairly stable and with fairly satisfactory, pain-free flexion-extension ranges.

Postoperatively, once the swelling has definitely begun to subside, static and dynamic elbow splints are made in occupational therapy, usually between the fourth and the sixth postoperative days (Fig. 43–10). The dynamic splint has plastic hinge joints, which allow flexion and extension to occur in a fixed neutral plane. Usually during the next day, neuromuscular re-education for active, gentle, assisted elbow flexion and extension (pronation and supination if the prosthesis allows) is started. Range-of-motion exercises are done with gravity eliminated by means of a raised powder-board. Active, gentle, assisted range-of-motion exercises are done to maintain shoulder mobility in the supine position. Active ranging is done also for wrist and hand at the same time.

Initially, active-assisted range-of-motion exercises of the elbow allow flexion only to about 60 degrees. The range of flexion thereafter is only slowly allowed to advance to 100 degrees in order to preserve the reattachment of the triceps muscle. No forcing, no stretching, no painful movements, and no resistance to the triceps muscles are permitted during the first two weeks (or longer).

During the third postoperative week, light activities of daily living and light diversional activities are practiced in occupational therapy, and the patient should be free of substitution patterns.

If indicated, gentle, prolonged stretching utilizing only the weight of the upper extremity distal to the elbow and free of any pain may be started after the third week and may be included in the home exercise program, if tolerated without evidence of joint irritation.

The home exercise program consists of active, gentle, assisted range-of-motion exercises and gentle, prolonged stretching (15 to 20 min two to four times daily), if indicated. Formal strengthening usually is not emphasized at this point, but it may become part of the home program during later recheck visits.

Total Wrist Arthroplasty. Arthritic and post-traumatic conditions of both wrists may be amenable to total joint replacement to relieve pain, to salvage function, and to improve cosmesis. Total wrist arthroplasty can be done when other surgical procedures, such as synovectomy, soft-tissue repair, and other arthroplasties, are inadequate.

JOACHIM L. OPITZ

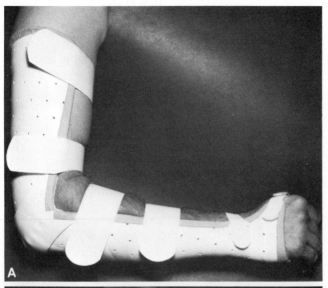

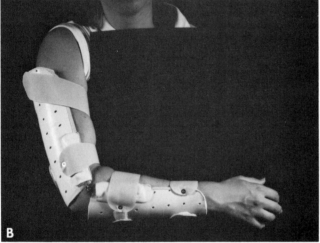

FIGURE 43–10. Static (*A*) and dynamic (*B*) splints used after total elbow replacement. (From Opitz, J. L.: Total joint arthroplasty: Principles and guidelines for postoperative physiatric management. Mayo Clin. Proc., 54:602–612, 1979. By permission.)

Periarticular structures should be sufficiently strong or adequately repairable to assure stability and a balanced transmission of power across the replaced joint. Total wrist arthroplasty has come of age, mostly in its semiconstrained version (Volz) and in its nonconstrained version (Meuli), both of which interface polyethylene with metal components (Fig. 43–11). Relief of pain and improvement of range of motion usually are satisfactory.[1] Potential loosening of the components requires permanent restriction of forceful engagement of the upper extremity.

Postoperatively, the wrist is kept immobilized in slight extension and in neutral abduction for approximately 10 days. During this period, the extremity distal to the elbow is usually elevated.

Because reestablishment of tensile strength of periarticular connective tissue in a proper position is of utmost importance for proper functioning of the semiconstrained (Meuli) and the nonconstrained (Volz) total wrist prostheses, particular care and proper balancing of tendon pull during surgery continue postoperatively during mobilization and functional training.

At approximately the 10th postoperative day, an isoprene (Orthoplast) resting splint with 20 to 40 degrees of wrist extension and with the thumb positioned in abduction is made. In addition, a dynamic Orthoplast wrist splint (Fig. 43–12) is made with a plastic hinge on each side. This splint permits only wrist flexion and extension to occur in a neutral abduction-adduction stance, so that

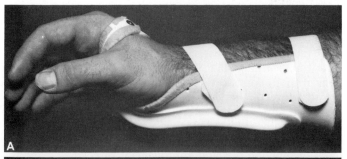

FIGURE 43–11. Total wrist prostheses. *A,* Volz (semi-constrained). *B,* Meuli (nonconstrained).

the second and third metacarpals are aligned in the direction of the long axis of the radius.

On the same day, active control of edema is started, with wrapping and rewrapping of the digits, the hand, and the wrist with soft rubber wrappings. Decongestive massage to the same area may

be added (except for the incisional area) and continued until the postoperative edema has subsided. The hand, wrist, and forearm can be maintained in an elevated position during rest.

Therapeutic exercises are started on the same or the following day. They consist of neuromuscular re-education to redevelop active, gentle, assisted flexion and extension of the wrist with a dynamic splint in place. Active, gentle, assisted digital flexion, extension, intrinsic-minus and intrinsic-plus positions of the digits, and opposition of the thumb are also practiced free of substitution patterns. Active range-of-motion exercises are done for the elbow and the shoulder.

As soon as patterns of isolated hand movements and of isolated wrist flexion and extension are acceptable, the dynamic splint may be left off during some of the exercises. Neuromuscular re-education is then started to redevelop a balanced wrist function, including radial and ulnar abduction.

The next goal of therapeutic exercises is the redevelopment of properly coordinated digital flexion with wrist extension and of digital extension with wrist flexion in a proper wrist abduction-abduction stance. Last, isolated digital and thumb movements are practiced with the wrist in various positions of extension (and flexion) and ulnar (and radial) abduction.

Light functional hand activities are started (at first in the dynamic splint) as soon as synergistic hand-wrist movements, as well as the basic hand

FIGURE 43–12. Static (*A*) and dynamic (*B*) splints used after total wrist replacement. (From Opitz, J. L.: Total joint arthroplasty: Principles and guidelines for postoperative physiatric management. Mayo Clin. Proc., 54:602–612, 1979. By permission.)

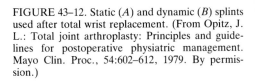

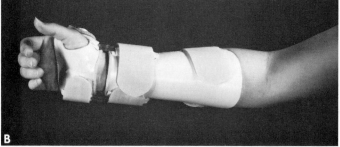

functions, are smooth in various wrist positions. The patient usually accomplishes this within the third postoperative week. The light functional hand and wrist activities consist of simple placement of objects, to light assembling (leather work, mosaics, puzzles), to simple painting, feeding, and simple knotting. Great care is taken to ensure that the light functional hand activities are free of substitutional patterns, such as undesirable associated elbow and shoulder motions, inappropriate wrist flexion with digital flexion, and inappropriate radial abduction instead of slight ulnar abduction stance of the wrist. When the patient is not in therapy, the dynamic wrist splint continues to be worn most of the time. The patient is dismissed when, under supervision, the exercises can be done securely and smoothly, without evidence of stress and increasing joint irritation. Written instructions are provided for the coordinated wrist-hand exercises, range-of-motion exercises, and light functional hand activities described earlier.

At six weeks (if necessary), gentle, prolonged (15 to 20 min, four times a day) stretching is taught during several sessions to gain missing ranges, especially wrist flexion and ulnar deviation. If necessary, mild isometric strengthening of wrist extensors also can be added. Exercises for further advancement of proper combined wrist and hand motions, as well as of light-to-moderate activities of daily living (complete dressing, self-care, and kitchen, household, and diversional activities), are added progressively.

Total Metacarpophalangeal Joint Replacement. Total arthroplasty of metacarpophalangeal joints may be useful in patients with destructive rheumatoid arthritis who have metacarpophalangeal subluxation, usually associated with ulnar drift. Total metacarpophalangeal arthroplasties can be done if the tendons can be repaired satisfactorily, the structure of the skin is adequate, the neurovascular status is satisfactory, and the patient is physiologically and psychologically stable. Usually, one can expect to obtain relief of pain, improvement of function,[37, 46] and improvement of cosmesis. At the present time, pinch force and power grip are not improved over preoperative levels.[37] For metacarpophalangeal joint replacement, the most common prostheses are those made of silicone rubber (Swanson) (Fig. 43–13). The Swanson prosthesis acts as a joint spacer. Careful reconstruction of capsular and ligament structures about the metacarpophalangeal joint is very important. Semi-constrained cemented metal-on-plastic prostheses (Steffe, Shultz, Walker) are less fre-

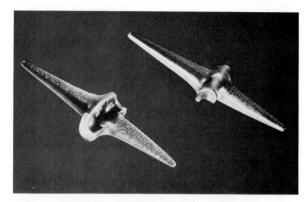

FIGURE 43–13. Total metacarpophalangeal joint prosthesis: Swanson silicone rubber joint spacer. *Left,* Volar aspect. *Right,* Dorsal aspect. Prosthesis is shaped to provide an extension assist to the replaced joint.

quently used today because of problems with loosening.

After the acute postoperative tissue responses have subsided adequately with the hand kept elevated, static and dynamic Orthoplast splints are made (Fig. 43–14). The splints should fit comfortably and should be checked daily for proper fit. Adjustments are made as swelling decreases and range of motion increases. The resting splint needs to support the metacarpophalangeal joints in moderate extension and in proper radioulnar alignment. Swan-neck deformity of the proximal interphalangeal joints is prevented by providing support for the digits in the neutral abduction-adduction stance at the metacarpophalangeal joints and in moderate flexion at the interphalangeal joints. Ulnar deviation is prevented, if necessary, by incorporating dividers at the proximal phalangeal level. The dynamic splint assists metacarpophalangeal extension by supporting function of the extensor digitorum communis with elastic slings across the proximal phalanges, and it allows the digits to track properly in a radioulnar alignment. Care should be taken to provide gentle dynamic metacarpophalangeal extension assistance by adjusting and readjusting the elastic pull to degrees that can be tolerated comfortably over time. The dynamic splint is worn for 6 to 12 weeks. The patient may remove the splint only for exercises and bathing activities and during dressing, when the splint would be in the way.

Antiedema measures are started promptly on referral as needed. These have already been described in the section on total wrist arthroplasty.

The initial therapeutic exercise program consists of neuromuscular re-education for active, gentle,

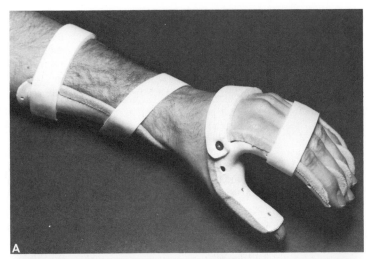

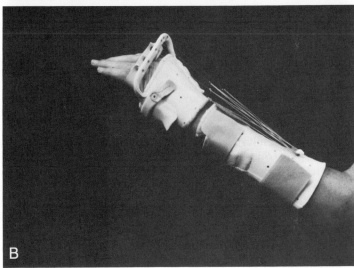

FIGURE 43–14. Static wrist and hand splint (*A*) and dynamic metacarpophalangeal extension-assist splint (*B*) used after total metacarpophalangeal joint replacement. (*A* From Opitz, J. L.: Total joint arthroplasty: Principles and guidelines for postoperative physiatric management. Mayo Clin. Proc., 54:602–612, 1979. By permission.)

assisted exercises, especially digital extension and flexion, of which digital extension has definite priority so that as much opening as possible for grasp can be achieved. The size of grasp in the rheumatoid hand is usually substantially decreased because of the dislodgment of the metacarpophalangeal extensor hood mechanism and the adduction contracture of the thumb. Neuromuscular re-education is also concerned with the redevelopment of smooth execution of the intrinsic-plus and intrinsic-minus digital positions, of digital radial abduction, and of thumb opposition. All of these movements constitute the six classic digital exercises practiced routinely and are included in the home program for the subsequent 6 to 12 months.

A number of common substitution patterns are encountered by patients after metacarpophalangeal replacement (Table 43–2). Substitution patterns indicate motor incoordination and should be avoided carefully in their early beginnings. Retraining uses the basic techniques of neuromuscular re-education. Once the exercises are progressing, basic grasp functions of the hand (tip or power prehension, lateral prehension or key grip, cylindrical grasp, and spherical grasp) are also practiced.

Active, gentle, assisted range-of-motion exercises are also given for the more proximal joints of the upper extremities, as indicated. Light functional hand activities are started as soon as the basic grasp functions of the hand are performed smoothly in slow but correct motion. The light functional hand activities have been described in the section on total wrist arthroplasty. Forceful use of the hand is carefully avoided in order to maintain the repaired periarticular structures in

TABLE 43–2. Common Hand and Forearm Substitution Patterns After Total Joint Replacement of the Wrist and the Hand*

TASK	SUBSTITUTION BY USE OF SPECIFIC MUSCLES AND MOVEMENTS
Digital flexion	Intrinsic muscles at metacarpophalangeal joint with interphalangeal joint in extension
Digital extension	Intrinsic muscles at interphalangeal joint with metacarpophalangeal joint in flexion
Thumb abduction	Ulnar digital intrinsic muscles for associated digital ulnar abduction
Thumb opposition	Thenar muscles for thumb adduction and flexion
Grasp opening	Wrist flexors for associated wrist flexion
Forearm supination	Associated shoulder external rotation and adduction
Forearm pronation	Associated shoulder internal rotation and abduction

*From Opitz, J. L.: Total joint arthroplasty: Principles and guidelines for postoperative physiatric management. Mayo Clin. Proc., 54:602–612, 1979. By permission.

their optimal positions as much as possible. Special instructions are given and practiced to protect the hands from unnecessary strain during common activities of dressing, self-care, kitchen and other housework, and avocational activities, in part by using different techniques and in part by using assistive devices. Written home instructions for work simplification may be helpful.

Very gentle, prolonged stretching (20 min four times per day) may be added after three to six weeks if the redevelopment of range of motion is lacking. Pain should be carefully avoided. The patient can be started on a home program of exercises, usually after the third postoperative week. The home program consists of active, gentle, assisted range-of-motion exercises, light functional hand activities, and work simplification to avoid overuse of the hand. Strengthening in the form of progressive resistive exercise is contraindicated in rheumatoid arthritis because of the loss of tensile strength of tendon attachments and other periarticular soft tissues.

Tendon Transfers

General Considerations

Purposes. Tendon transfers can be most helpful for the reestablishment of power in patients with isolated, nonprogressive deficits of the lower motor neuron (such as peripheral nerve injuries), tetraplegia in spinal cord injury, and post-traumatic reconstruction of the upper extremities. Especially in post-traumatic reconstruction, the use of tendon transfers has increased substantially during the past decade. However, tendon transfers in stable upper motor neuron deficits such as hemiplegia or cerebral palsy are not as common and need to be highly individualized. Their long-term outcome is usually difficult to predict.

Surgical Considerations. Since tendon transfers are usually the final step in reconstructive surgical efforts, other applicable procedures for correction of deformities (capsulotomies, osteotomies, tendon lengthening), for stabilization (arthrodeses, tenodeses, insertion of bone blocks), or for reconstruction of peripheral nerves (neurolysis, nerve reanastomosis, nerve transfer, nerve graft) usually should be done before or at least at the time of tendon transfer. Likewise, prior to tendon transfer, sufficient range of motion and maximal strength of muscles involved in tendon transfers, as well as maximal redevelopment of sensation to touch, pain, and kinesthesis, need to have been developed by appropriate nonsurgical and possibly surgical methods.

Transfer of spastic muscles is often contraindicated. If selected for transfer, they should function fully in phase with that of the lost voluntary motor power because of otherwise insurmountable difficulties later with neuromuscular re-education in the presence of spasticity.

Poor results in tendon transfers also can be expected if the patient is still bedridden, does not really want surgery, is mentally inactive, or has not yet adequately accepted his or her major physical disability for a lifetime.

As Moberg[31] has pointed out, sensory function in the area of the tendon transfer is very important. In the absence of other than ocular afference, only a single, simple transfer can be expected to develop satisfactory function. Further, no tendon transfer should impair any existing function. Moberg believes that a tendon transfer should be fully reversible if the result is unsatisfactory. Having received a tendon transfer, the patient should retain the option of being returned to the preoperative condition.

Optimal team intercommunication before and after tendon transfers is important among the specialties involved, such as the primary service, orthopedics, physical medicine and rehabilitation, neurology, and neurosurgery. Such interrelationships usually take time to develop, but they are of utmost importance for optimal decision-making, patient motivation, postoperative management, follow-up care, and the management of possible complications.

Decisions regarding tendon transfers in traumatic tetraplegia should be delayed at least for one year in order to have full return of function present, all spasticity apparent, and maximal strength developed in all muscles to be used in transfer. Patients should have sufficiently progressed educationally, emotionally, sociovocationally, and physically in their readaptation to spinal cord injury. In peripheral trauma, similar considerations are often true, depending on extent and severity of injury and the resulting impairment.

Orientation of the patient prior to tendon transfers involves a realistic description of the limited goals of the procedure itself, time and cost involved, the necessary preoperative and postoperative efforts of the patient, and the number and duration of needed follow-up visits.

A two-tier decision-making process, involving the reconstructive team, the patient, and a significant other person, with the two evaluations and related decision-making conferences conducted three to nine months apart, is the basis for the development of a sound plan for treatment, follow-up care, and the authorization of cost.

Preoperative Program. Ideally, the preoperative program concentrates on three basic issues: reestablishment of the needed passive range of motion for the expected function of the transfer; maximal strengthening of the presumptive new muscle power; and initial training of conscious perception of kinesthetic sensations relating to neuromuscular re-education of the transfer.

Preoperative mobilization reestablishes the passive motion of the expected function. Shortened connective tissue about the joint capsule, intra-articular connective tissue, and adhesions about tendons and muscle bellies usually can resist even strong stretching forces of short duration. Therefore, stretching needs to be done gently over prolonged periods (20 to 30 min, four times per day). Within limits, connective tissue usually can elongate without trauma during gentle prolonged stretching. If needed, serial, static splinting or casting or prolonged, gentle pull of rubber bands may, in time, assist in providing adequate passive range of motion. If not, combined ultrasound heating with stretching of the area[25] is likely to give further increase in range of motion.

Graphic recording of daily measurements of range of motion is helpful in motivating patients to continue their stretching exercises for weeks as well as for the therapist's quick orientation regarding progress of range of motion.

With early and persistent use of such range-of-motion exercises, surgical release procedures often can be limited substantially, or even avoided, thus lessening trauma and increasing chances of successful tendon transfers.

Before transfer, the muscle to be transferred should be as strong as possible. Once the muscle is transferred, its effective strength usually decreases by one grade owing to the change in routing of its tendon. During the postoperative period of complete immobilization (usually three weeks), the strength of the transferred muscle decreases exponentially to approximately half of its preoperative strength. Adhesions form between the tendon at the site of its anastomosis and wherever vascular injury to tendon or muscle occurred, causing segmental necrosis. Although assistive power can mobilize such adhesions of the tendon in a distal direction, the proximal mobilization of the tendon can be done only by the power of the transferred muscle itself. For such reasons, maximal preoperative strengthening is highly desirable. Maximal restrengthening of muscles to be used in second-stage transfers is also essential. For the same reason, postoperative immobilization should be in the position of the shortest resting lengths of the transferred muscle.

Kinesthetic sensory training can be started preoperatively in preparation for neuromuscular re-education of the transferred muscle. Conscious perception of related joint movement, joint position, related muscle contraction and relaxation (with augmented sensory feedback through the palpating free hand of the patient), force of muscle contraction, and conscious perception of tendon tapping and stroking of the skin overlying the muscle to be transferred can be practiced preoperatively in order to increase the kinesthetic awareness of the patient.

In the selection of a suitable muscle for transfer, if at all possible, a synergistic muscle should be chosen, especially in patients with upper motor neuron deficit and with transfers in the lower extremity. During transfer, the routing of the tendon should be done with the least possible disturbance of its mesotenons, as noted, in order to avoid segmental tendon necrosis with the associated formation of adhesions and possible stretching of the necrotic tendon segment during mobilization.

Routing of the transferred tendon should be as straight and as superficial as possible since adhesions tend to be more extensive and firmer at tendon angulations and in deeper tissues.

Tendon anastomosis should be done with non-constrictive suturing and with the least irritating suture possible in order to lessen adhesions at that site.[20]

Strength and amplitude of the muscle to be transferred should be equal to or, if possible, larger than that of the original muscle.

Immobilization after tendon transfer should be kept at a safe minimum so that the adhesions that form regularly about the transferred tendon are capable of elongation with gentle range-of-motion exercises. Thus, they can, in a nontraumatic fashion, mature to become mesotenons of adequate length and provide adequate blood supply to the transferred tendon.[20]

Early prolonged tension of the transferred tendon should be avoided in order to prevent gap formation at the site of tendon anastomosis, which predisposes the anastomosis to rupture during remobilization. Gap formation also increases the formation of adhesions.[21]

Postoperative Management. Postoperative management usually consists of the following components: antiedema measures; gentle, prolonged passive range-of-motion exercises; neuromuscular re-education of basic movements; gentle, active (assistive) range-of-motion exercises; redevelopment of the proper use of the transferred muscle in light functional activities; and redevelopment of accuracy and speed (coordination).

The postoperative antiedema measures are the same as those used after total wrist or metacarpophalangeal joint replacement. If hydrotherapy is being used for cleansing and relaxation purposes, one should carefully avoid causing increases in edema during immersion by keeping the duration of hydrotherapy relatively short (10 to 15 min) and the water temperature relatively low initially (35° C [95° F] or less).

As mentioned previously, gentle, well-controlled, small, passive movements can be used to cause progressive elongation of adhesions around the tendon without rupturing. In this fashion, new mesotenons of adequate length are being formed at a time when the new fibrovascular tissue is still immature, without embarrassing the tendon anastomosis. This may be started as early as three or four days to one week after the operation.[27] Such gentle passive motions may be done four times a day, without pain, through a very small range that

is increased in very small increments during the subsequent two weeks. As mentioned previously, gentle, early passive motion provides the greatest advantage if the limb is immobilized postoperatively in a position with the transferred muscle at its shortest resting length.

Three weeks after the operation, neuromuscular re-education of the transferred muscle is started. Passive range of motion of approximately 30 degrees (as needed for neuromuscular re-education) has been developed by that time. During neuromuscular re-education of the transferred muscle, one should never ask the patient primarily for the performance of the motion for which the tendon transfer has been done. Rather, the patient should be asked to produce that motion for which the transferred muscle was originally responsible. The original motion then is being blocked manually by the therapist, so that the transferred tendon can now execute the new motion. In this fashion, the patient will be able to perceive the new set of kinesthetic sensations: the feeling of muscle contraction, the tendon tension of the transferred muscle, and the sensation of the new motion affected. This new set of combined kinesthetic input, when consciously perceived, recalled, and reproduced by the patient through many correct repetitions, forms the new engram and the intended new motor skill. The old engram then is being progressively forgotten and left with the function of previously synergistic muscles of the transfer.

As soon as the new, basic movements can be executed deliberately in clear and acceptable patterns actively (usually in physical therapy), functional training with light functional activities is started (usually in occupational therapy). Six weeks after operation, the resistance demanded during functional activities can be increased to moderate levels, if they can be performed without pain or fatigue. Performance should always be kept fully acceptable and at its peak, because negative training with deterioration of the new engrams or motor patterns is likely to occur, with increasing synergistic and antagonistic recruitment of muscles, if functional training is done until the patient is fatigued (with increasing effort and decreasing accuracy and speed).

After successful neuromuscular re-education, increases in range of motion may be accomplished by active, gentle, assistive range-of-motion exercises between three and six weeks after operation. After six weeks, gentle prolonged (10 to 20 min, four times per day) stretching exercises may be added to the daily program. As mentioned before, daily graphing of active ranges is particularly helpful for the maintenance of motivation of the patient and for the quick orientation regarding success (see Fig. 43–1). Ultrasound heating in combination with stretching may be used when increases in range of motion have leveled off.[25] If needed, operative tenolysis rarely is indicated before completion of tendon healing, at approximately six months.

Strengthening of the transferred muscle best occurs with its use in functional activities after two weeks. Single transfers may be strengthened formally with progressive resistive exercises after tendon healing is complete. However, the associated overflow of motor activities, which is likely to occur with maximal or near-maximal efforts, may weaken or destroy the new engrams, especially when done with multiple tendon transfers or single transfers that either are spastic or are transferred out of phase. Usually, formal strengthening exercises are neither needed nor advisable.

Upper Extremities

In patients with deltoid paralysis, numerous attempts at transfer of biceps, triceps, trapezius, and other muscles have been made; yet when such transfers are accomplished, not the desired substitution of deltoid function but rather effects of tenodesis may be noted around the glenohumeral joint.

Arthrodesis of the shoulder in painful, flail shoulders with presence of major portions of the scapular rotators still is likely to be the best reconstructive choice. In medial winging of the scapula due to serratus anterior paralysis, the pectoralis minor muscle, lengthened by a fascial graft, may decrease winging and stabilize the scapula when transferred to its inferior angle. When lateral winging of the scapula is caused by trapezius paralysis, levator scapulae may be transferred to a more lateral position on the scapula in association with fascial fixation of the vertebral border of the scapula to the thorax.

Biceps Paralysis. Missing biceps function often can be replaced in part by proximal advancement (by 3 to 4 cm) of the common origin of flexor carpi radialis, flexor carpi ulnaris, and palmaris longus muscles (Steindler's procedure), if these muscles are strong. Since these muscles normally cross the elbow, proximal transfer of the origin further lengthens the lever arm for elbow flexion. The

muscles, however, should be opposed by strong wrist and digital extensors at the wrist.

Commonly used tendon transfers in peripheral nerve injuries have been well described.[28]

Radial Nerve Paralysis. Radial nerve paralysis results in the absence of extension of the wrist, thumb, and proximal finger joints and the loss of brachioradialis and thumb abductor muscles. Suggested transfers are pronator teres to extensor carpi radialis longus and brevis; flexor carpi ulnaris or flexor digitorum superficialis to extensor digitorum communis; and palmaris longus to translocated extensor pollicis longus.

Ulnar Nerve Paralysis. Ulnar nerve paralysis may result in absent or inadequate lateral stability of the index finger (first dorsal interosseus muscle). Lateral stability of the index finger is essential for tip and lateral prehension between the thumb and the index finger. To substitute for a paralyzed first dorsal interosseus muscle, the tendon of the extensor indicis proprius or the tendon of the extensor pollicis brevis may be transferred to the tendon of the first dorsal interosseus. Paralysis of the fourth and fifth digits may not require any transfer of tendons.

Median Nerve Paralysis. Median nerve paralysis results in loss of sensation of the medial surface of the palm. Every attempt should be made to restore sensation. In low median nerve paralysis, the motor loss of consequence may be opposition of the thumb. The pronator teres or adductor pollicis muscle may be used in transfer for opposition of the thumb. High median nerve paralysis results in loss of finger flexion of the first, second, and third digits (flexor pollicis longus muscle, flexor digitorum superficialis muscle, and the radial half of flexor digitorum profundus muscle) and loss in opposition of the thumb (opponens pollicis, flexor pollicis brevis, abductor pollicis brevis, and flexor pollicis longus muscles). Possible tendon transfers in high median nerve paralysis may be as follows: the ulnar half of the flexor digitorum profundus muscle or the brachioradialis to the flexor tendons of the second and third digits, the extensor carpi radialis longus muscle to the flexor pollicis longus muscle, and to the opponens pollicis muscle. Arthrodesis of the metacarpophalangeal joint of the thumb may be necessary. Other combinations of tendon transfers are possible.

Forearm and Hand Trauma. Repair of cut or crushed tissues, such as arteries, nerves, tendons, ligaments, muscles, or bones in the hand or forearm, is a challenging, often formidable, problem both in surgical repair and in rehabilitation follow-

930

ing surgery. There is a rapidly increasing understanding of the anatomy of vascular supply to tendons, pulley systems, maintenance and replacement of peritendinous structures, tendon grafting, and principles of early mobilization.[27] The postoperative management follows principles similar to those described earlier.[41]

Spinal Cord Injury

Reconstruction of the upper limb in cervical spinal cord injury is actively being pursued by teams in several countries with increasing success.[32]

In spinal cord injury that spares C5 and C6, active elbow extension can be restored to moderate antigravity levels using the mobilized posterior deltoid muscle in transfer to the olecranon, with interposition of a tendon graft from toe extensors.[30] Elbow extension is essential for independence in reaching above the level of the shoulder, driving, and when further power is needed in transfers. During the postoperative mobilization of elbow flexion and re-education of the posterior deltoid for triceps muscle function, one needs to progress extremely slowly to avoid stretching of the tendon graft. If the graft elongates, it compromises the limited contractile amplitude of the deltoid muscle for elbow extension. Various static and dynamic elbow splints are used to allow increments of only 10 degrees of elbow flexion per week from a fully extended position after initial immobilization of six weeks, until tendon healing is complete after six months.

In spinal cord injury that spares C5 in which only a fairly strong brachioradialis muscle is available in the forearm, wrist extension and key grip (lateral prehension) can be restored through transfer of the brachioradialis muscle to the extensor carpi radialis brevis muscle, tenodesis of the flexor pollicis longus muscle at the distal radius with resection of the annular ligament, allowing the involved tendon to bowstring, and through arthrodesis of the interphalangeal joint of the thumb.[30] Sensory function at this level of deficit is often preserved in the thumb. This procedure allows for moderate grip opening of lateral prehension during passive wrist flexion and fairly adequate key grip prehension during active wrist extension in persons who otherwise would have no hand or wrist function. The postoperative re-education of the brachioradialis to wrist extension usually is not difficult, especially if elbow flexion is opposed by newly developed active elbow extension, as described

earlier. Fine tuning of tension of the thumb flexor tenodesis may require a simple reoperation.

In spinal cord injuries that spare C6, strong extensor carpi radialis longus and brevis, pronator teres, and brachioradialis functions may be preserved. It may be possible to restore digital extension, digital flexion, and lateral prehension of the thumb through transfer of the extensor carpi radialis longus muscle to the extensor digitorum communis muscle and the extensor pollicis longus muscle (first stage) and through transfer of the pronator teres muscle to the flexor digitorum profundus muscle and of the brachioradialis muscle to the flexor pollicis longus muscle (second stage).[26] Sufficient time should elapse between the two stages to allow for neuromuscular re-education of extensor carpi radialis longus to extensor digitorum communis and extensor pollicis longus function, restrengthening of pronator teres and brachioradialis, and remobilization of the wrist and hand with careful preservation of flexion contracture at the metacarpophalangeal joints of the digits.

Other tendon transfers in the tetraplegic patient are possible and have been proposed.[7, 23, 47] All tendon transfers into the tetraplegic hand may be doomed to failure unless, by some means, clawing of the hand as a result of intrinsic muscle paralysis is prevented. The prevention of the claw-hand deformity should be started at the onset of tetraplegia through deliberate development of metacarpophalangeal joint flexion contractures. Such flexion contractures may develop with the use of static forearm- and hand-based splints. Later, the hands should be used as fists during mat activities and transfers. It may be necessary to wear a hand-based splint during such activities in order to elevate the rest of the hand 2 to 3 cm from the supporting surface so that the metacarpophalangeal and interphalangeal joints may remain in flexion. In patients with an inadequate metacarpophalangeal flexion stance in the tetraplegic hand, metacarpophalangeal flexor tightness can be regained by long flexor tenodesis or by volar metacarpophalangeal capsulorrhaphy (Zancolli) or by both. However, neither procedure will prevent overstretching of the metacarpophalangeal joints again if the reestablished metacarpophalangeal flexion contractures are not protected from overstretching. This is especially likely to happen during independent transfer activities.

Lower Extremities

Hip Group Paralysis. In hip abductor paralysis, two tendon transfer procedures are available. Tensor fasciae latae may be freed, together with a strip of fascia lata. The strip of fascia lata is then attached to the greater trochanter, is continued posteriorly, and is anastomosed to the lateral two thirds of the mobilized erector spinae muscles. The erector spinae muscles can be placed in such a position as to act more as an extensor or more as an abductor of the hip. Usually, the effect of this transfer is predominantly that of a tenodesis, providing increased stability during stance phase. Only in partial paralysis of gluteus medius can one expect to abolish the typical abductor lurch by transfer of tensor fasciae latae.

In 1952, Mustard[34] described the transfer of the iliopsoas muscle through a large window in the iliac wing to the greater trochanter for the same purpose. Adequate function of the sartorius and rectus femoris muscles, however, is essential to provide adequate hip flexion.

Quadriceps Paralysis. In isolated quadriceps paralysis, the transfer of the biceps femoris and of one of the medial hamstring muscles into the quadriceps tendon gives power for climbing stairs, getting in and out of chairs, and walking up and down hills. Care should be taken to avoid this transfer in patients with weakness of the posterior thigh and leg muscles because further weakening of these groups by the described transfer will result in genu recurvatum and its associated gait disturbance.

Cerebral Palsy

Tendon transfers in cerebral palsy[13] and hemiplegia are often unpredictable in their final outcome because movement patterns rather than individual muscle functions are represented in the brain and remain unchanged by tendon transfers. Often, the immediate results appear to be satisfactory, only to regress back to a similar abnormal postural stance. Severe spasticity, athetosis, mental retardation, and ataxia are usually regarded as contraindications to tendon transfers.

The pronation deformity of the upper extremity in hemiplegia may be improved by transfer of the flexor carpi ulnaris muscle across the dorsal aspect of the forearm to the extensor carpi radialis longus muscle,[42] with release of the pronator teres muscle. Knee flexion deformity may be improved by transferring the hamstring insertions proximally to the femoral condyles.[12] In rotational deformities of the thigh in patients with cerebral palsy, derotational femoral osteotomy again brings the long axis of

the foot parallel to the line of progression. A similar procedure can be done at the tibia, if indicated. Both procedures can be very helpful adjuncts in the corrective treatment of cerebral palsy. Rebalancing of the spastic ankle and foot deformities by transferring tendons needs to be considered individually. Oftentimes, it requires combinations with bone stabilization procedures, tendon lengthening, tenotomy, or neurectomy.[39] Spastic equinovarus deformity due to overactive gastrocnemius-soleus muscles often can be improved by sectioning of the gastrocnemius origin, with subsequent reattachment of the gastrocnemius in a shortened length distally. Often, it is advisable to weaken the gastrocnemius muscle at the same time, with selective sectioning of parts of its motor nerves in the popliteal fossa. If a contracture of the soleus muscle or of both the soleus and gastrocnemius muscles is present, the preferred operation is the Z-plasty of the Achilles tendon. Judicious, regular stretching of the posterior calf muscles remains essential for maintenance of the achieved dorsiflexion range at the ankle.

Other Reconstructive Procedures

Shoulder

Arthrodesis of the shoulder may be done unilaterally in severe degenerative joint disease, provided that scapular rotator muscles of the shoulder are normal and the other shoulder is essentially unimpaired. Arthrodesis of the shoulder is not advisable in women because of its anticosmetic effects and should not be done in persons whose occupation requires humeral rotation of that side. Today, total shoulder arthroplasty has become a viable alternative in many instances.

Recurring dislocation of the shoulder often happens in a downward and anterior direction. The Bankart operation repairs the anteroinferior portion of the capsule, especially when it is often torn away from the glenoid rim. The Putti-Platt operation, in addition, reinforces the tendon of the subscapularis muscle to prevent the forward and downward dislocation of the humeral head. Postoperatively, until tendon healing is complete, shoulder mobilization should avoid stretching of the repaired structures in abduction or external rotation (or both). General principles of mobilization are the same as those in total shoulder arthroplasty.

Wrist and Hand

In unilateral, severe, painful, post-traumatic degenerative arthritis of the wrist, arthrodesis may still be a good choice, since it provides pain-free stability, especially when forceful use of the upper extremity is required.

Boutonnière, swan-neck, and other rheumatoid hand deformities of digits and thumb may be amenable to highly skillful tissue reconstruction procedures (especially when done early), in addition to total joint replacement or arthrodesis (or both) of digital joints or thumb joints.[10]

Painful degenerative joint disease of the trapeziometacarpal joint of the thumb is usually associated with ligamentous laxity of the supporting soft tissues. Ligamentous reconstruction with tendon interposition arthroplasty is yielding excellent or good results in a very high percentage of patients,[4, 11] whereas results after silicone rubber joint replacements have been discouraging.[38] Postoperatively, even moderate to heavy functional hand activities need to be delayed until tendon healing is complete or longer. Protective hand care is advisable indefinitely.

Dupuytren's contracture of the palmar fascia, often involving the flexor tendon sheaths, may be excised. Early postoperative mobilization, including gentle prolonged stretching for digital extension, is essential for optimal outcomes of the procedure. The digital extension ranges, however, need to be maintained indefinitely, if possible, by a reasonable stretching routine.[15]

Hip and Thigh

Spasticity of the hip adductor muscles may result in impairment of gait owing to scissoring of the lower extremities. When scissoring is excessive, it may impair the accessibility of the perineum. Adductor tenotomy or obturator neurectomy (or both) may relieve the hip adductor contractures. Postoperative stretching is essential for the maintenance of gains made in range of motion.

Decreased leg length may occur, with predominantly unilateral impairment of a lower extremity in the growing child. The most commonly used corrective measure is designed to slow down the growth of the uninvolved lower extremity. The procedure should be done some years before the growth centers are closed, usually between the ages of 10 and 12 years. Steel staples are placed in the epiphysis of the lower portion of the femur or upper part of the tibia. They may be removed at any time as required. The operation is usually considered if the leg length discrepancy is in excess of 2.5 cm. If growth is complete, excision of a segment of the femur may be done to accomplish equal leg length.

Knee

Ligaments, menisci, and articular surfaces of the knee are often subject to injury. Repair of these structures is done frequently in common surgical procedures of the knee, such as removal of a torn medial or lateral meniscus, internal fixation of fractured bone segments involving the joint surfaces, or repair of torn cruciate or collateral ligaments. Torn major ligaments of the knee may be successfully repaired if operated on soon after the injury occurred. Later repairs often are not successful in restoring good stability of the knee. Remobilization after adequate healing of repaired tendons should be done initially strictly in planes of motion that do not injure the repaired structures yet provide slowly increasing flexion range of the knee that had been immobilized in an extended position. Mobilization of a knee that had been immobilized in a semiflexed or flexed position may be difficult because of adhesions of the quadriceps mechanism, which a deconditioned, weak quadriceps muscle cannot mobilize proximally. In such a case, passive extension of the knee may be regained relatively easily, yet active extension is not forthcoming adequately. Eventually, tenolysis of the quadriceps mechanism may be required.

Operations to restore reasonable function in knees damaged by degenerative joint disease or rheumatoid arthritis, yet not requiring total joint replacement, include debridement of hypertrophic joint ridges, synovectomy, and osteotomy. The principles of postoperative remobilization and of quadriceps and hamstring strengthening are, in general, the same as those described for total knee arthroplasties.

Ankle and Foot

Several arthrodeses are available to prevent footdrop or to prevent and correct deformities of the foot (or both). Usually, the arthrodeses are delayed until the growth centers are closed. Among the most common procedures is the triple arthrodesis. It is a classic operation in which the three major joints of the posterior part of the foot (the talocalcaneal, the calcaneocuboid, and the talonavicular joints) are fused. The procedure may be used for any condition in which the posterior part of the foot is unstable or in a varus or valgus position. It may be combined with tendon transfers. An arthrodesis of the tibiotalar joint will prevent the dropping of the foot into an equinus position. However, a fused ankle causes a definite limp and requires pain-free mobility of the foot to allow a reasonably good gait.

Resection of part of the proximal phalanx of the first toe (Keller's procedure) may be done for the usual hallux valgus deformity with or without bunionectomy. Resectional arthroplasties of other metatarsophalangeal joints also may be helpful in treating painful, destructive arthritis or metatarsalgia (usually affecting the digital nerves in the third and fourth metatarsal spaces).

The deformity of hammer toe consists of dorsiflexion of the proximal phalanx, plantar flexion of the middle phalanx, and flexion or extension of the distal phalanx. Usually, the deformity affects most severely the second toe and to lesser degrees the third to fifth toes. Treatment is either by partial resection or by arthrodesis of the proximal interphalangeal joints.

References

1. Beckenbaugh, R. D.: Total wrist arthroplasty: The wrist. Mayo Clin. Proc., 54:513–515, 1979.
2. Bolton-Maggs, B. G., Sudlow, R. A., and Freeman, M. A.: Total ankle arthroplasty. A long-term review of the London Hospital experience. J. Bone Joint Surg., 67B:785–790, 1985.
3. Bowman, A. J., Jr., Walker, M. W., Kilfoyle, R. M., O'Brien, P. I., and McConville, J. F.: Experience with the bipolar prosthesis in hip arthroplasty. A clinical study. Orthopedics, 8:460–467, 1985.
4. Burton, R. I., and Pellegrini, V. D., Jr.: Surgical management of basal joint arthritis of the thumb. Part II. Ligament reconstruction with tendon interposition arthroplasty. J. Hand Surg., 11A:324–332, 1986.
5. Charnley, J.: Arthroplasty of the hip: A new operation. Lancet, 1:1129–1132, 1961.
6. Cofield, R. H.: Total shoulder arthroplasty with the Neer prosthesis. J. Bone Joint Surg., 66A:899–906, 1984.
7. Curtis, R. M.: Tendon transfers in the patient with spinal cord injury. Orthop. Clin. North Am., 5:415–423, 1974.
8. Dall, D. M., Grobbelaar, C. J., Learmonth, I. D., and Dall, G.: Charnley low-friction arthroplasty of the hip. Long-term results in South Africa. Clin. Orthop., 211:85–90, 1986.
9. Dennis, D. A., Ferlic, D. C., and Clayton, M. L.: Volz total wrist arthroplasty in rheumatoid arthritis: A long-term review. J. Hand Surg., 11A:483–490, 1986.
10. Dobyns, J. H., and Linscheid, R. L.: Rheumatoid hand repairs. Orthop. Clin. North Am., 2:629–647, 1971.
11. Eaton, R. G., Glickel, S. Z., and Littler, J. W.: Tendon interposition arthroplasty for degenerative arthritis of the trapeziometacarpal joint of the thumb. J. Hand Surg., 10A:645–654, 1985.
12. Eggers, G. W. N.: Transplantation of hamstring tendons to femoral condyles in order to improve hip extension and to decrease knee flexion in cerebral spastic paralysis. J. Bone Joint Surg., 34A:827–830, 1952.
13. Eggers, G. W. N., and Evans, E. B.: Surgery in cerebral palsy. J. Bone Joint Surg., 45A:1275–1305, 1963.
14. Engh, C. A., Bobyn, J. D., and Glassman, A. H.: Porous-coated hip replacement. The factors governing bone ingrowth, stress shielding, and clinical results. J. Bone Joint Surg., 69B:45–55, 1987.
15. Fietti, V. G., Jr., and Mackin, E. J.: Dupuytren's disease. In Hunter, J. M., Schneider, L. H., Mackin, E. J., and Bell, J. A. (Eds.): Rehabilitation of the Hand. St. Louis, The C. V. Mosby Co., 1978, pp. 147–153.
16. Harris, W. H.: Factors controlling optimal bone ingrowth of total hip replacement components. Instr. Course Lect., 35:184–187, 1986.
17. Insall, J. N., and Kelly, M.: The total condylar prosthesis. Clin. Orthop., 205:43–48, 1986.
18. Johanson, N. A., Bullough, P. G., Wilson, P. D., Jr., Salvati, E. A., and Ranawat, C. S.: The microscopic anatomy of the bone-cement interface in failed total hip arthroplasties. Clin. Orthop., 218:123–135, 1987.
19. Kavanagh, B. F., Ilstrup, D. M., and Fitzgerald, R. H., Jr.: Revision total hip arthroplasty. J. Bone Joint Surg., 67A:517–526, 1985.
20. Ketchum, L. D.: Primary tendon healing: A review. J. Hand Surg., 2:428–435, 1977.
21. Ketchum, L. D., Martin, N. L., and Kappel, D. A.: Experimental evaluation of factors affecting the strength of tendon repairs. Plast. Reconstr. Surg., 59:708–719, 1977.
22. Lachiewicz, P. F., and Rosenstein, B. D.: Long-term results of Harris total hip replacement. J. Arthroplasty, 1:229–236, 1986.
23. Lamb, D. W., and Landry, R.: The hand in quadriplegia. Hand 3:31–37, 1971.
24. Lausten, G. S., Vedel, P., and Nielsen, P. M.: Fractures of the femoral neck treated with a bipolar endoprosthesis. Clin. Orthop., 218:63–67, 1987.
25. Lehmann, J. F., Masock, A. J., Warren, C. G., and Koblanski, J. N.: Effect of therapeutic temperatures

JOACHIM L. OPITZ

on tendon extensibility. Arch. Phys. Med. Rehabil., 51:481–487, 1970.

26. Lipscomb, P. R., Elkins, E. C., and Henderson, E. D.: Tendon transfers to restore function of hands in tetraplegia, especially after a fracture-dislocation of the sixth cervical vertebra on the seventh. J. Bone Joint Surg., 40A:1071–1080, 1958.

27. Mackin, E. J., and Maiorano, L.: Postoperative therapy following staged flexor tendon reconstruction. *In* Hunter, J. M.., Schneider, L. H., Mackin, E. J., and Bell, J. A. (Eds.): Rehabilitation of the Hand. St. Louis, The C. V. Mosby Co., 1978, pp. 247–261.

28. Magness, J. L., and Elkins, E. C.: Tendon transfer: A review of patient selection and commonly used procedures. Arch. Phys. Med. Rehabil., 48:1–11, 1967.

29. McElwain, J. P., and English, E.: The early results of porous-coated total shoulder arthroplasty. Clin. Orthop., 218:217–224, 1987.

30. Moberg, E.: Surgical treatment for absent single-hand grip and elbow extension in quadriplegia: Principles and preliminary experience. J. Bone Joint Surg., 57A:196–206, 1975.

31. Moberg, E.: Helpful upper limb surgery in tetraplegia. *In* Hunter, J. M., Schneider, L. H., Mackin E. J., and Bell, J. A. (Eds.): Rehabilitation of the Hand. St. Louis, The C. V. Mosby Co., 1978, pp. 304–311.

32. Moberg, E.: The present state of surgical rehabilitation of the upper limb in tetraplegia. Paraplegia, 25:351–356, 1987.

33. Morrey, B. F., and Bryan, R. S.: Total joint replacement. *In* Morrey, B. F. (Ed.): The Elbow and Its Disorders. Philadelphia, W. B. Saunders Co., 1985, pp. 546–569.

34. Mustard, W. T.: Iliopsoas transfer for weakness of the hip abductors: A preliminary report. J. Bone Joint Surg., 34A:647–649, 1952.

35. Neer, C. S., II, Watson, K. C., and Stanton, F. J.: Recent experience in total shoulder replacement. J. Bone Joint Surg., 64A:319–337, 1982.

36. Older, J.: Low-friction arthroplasty of the hip. A 10–12-year follow-up study. Clin. Orthop., 211:36–42, 1986.

37. Opitz, J. L., and Linscheid, R. L.: Hand function after metacarpophalangeal joint replacement in rheumatoid arthritis. Arch. Phys. Med. Rehabil., 59:160–165, 1978.

38. Pellegrini, V. D., Jr., and Burton, R. I.: Surgical management of basal joint arthritis of the thumb. Part I. Long-term results of silicone implant arthroplasty. J. Hand Surg., 11A:309–324, 1986.

39. Phelps, W. M.: Long-term results of orthopaedic surgery in cerebral palsy. J. Bone Joint Surg., 39A:53–59, 1957.

40. Ranawat, C. S.: The patellofemoral joint in total condylar knee arthroplasty. Pros and cons based on five- to ten-year follow-up observations. Clin. Orthop., 205:93–99, 1986.

41. Schutt, A. H., and Opitz, J. L.: Hand rehabilitation. *In* Goodgold, J. (Ed.): Rehabilitation Medicine. St. Louis, C. V. Mosby Co., 1988, pp. 646–659.

42. Steindler, A.: Postgraduate Lectures on Orthopedic Diagnosis and Indications, Vol. 2. Springfield, Ill., Charles C Thomas, Publisher, 1951, pp. 32–51.

43. Total Joint Arthroplasty Symposium: Part I. Mayo Clin. Proc., 54:489–526, 1979.

44. Total Joint Arthroplasty Symposium: Part II. Mayo Clin. Proc., 54:557–612, 1979.

45. Townley, C. O.: The anatomic total knee resurfacing arthroplasty. Clin. Orthop., 192:82–96, 1985.

46. Vahvanen, V., and Viljakka, T.: Silicone rubber implant arthroplasty of the metacarpophalangeal joint in rheumatoid arthritis: A follow-up study of 32 patients. J. Hand Surg., 11A:333–339, 1986.

47. Zancolli, E.: Surgery for the quadriplegic hand with active strong wrist extension preserved: A study of 97 cases. Clin. Orthop., 112:101–113, 1975.

44

Diagnosis and Rehabilitation of Auditory Disorders

JEROME D. SCHEIN
MAURICE H. MILLER

More than 17 million persons in the United States suffer a significant hearing impairment.[58, 59] Of these, over two million have profound losses preventing the discrimination of speech: they are *deaf*. Despite its substantial prevalence and harsh consequences, hearing impairment does not receive the attention it merits from rehabilitation personnel, government agencies, and the general public.

In the sections that follow, we first consider the numerical and social significance of impaired hearing. Then we discuss the auditory system from a functional-anatomical viewpoint. The various causes of hearing loss are preceded by a review of techniques for diagnosis of hearing impairment. The remaining sections turn from diagnosis and evaluation to remediation of hearing problems, considering, in turn, aural rehabilitation, hearing aids, education, and related matters.

Extent and Nature of Hearing Impairment

Impairment of hearing is the most prevalent chronic physical disability in the United States. There are more common acute conditions (e.g., the common cold), and mental illness reportedly occurs more frequently than any physical disability. But arthritis, heart conditions, blindness, and other chronic physical disabilities do not individually strike as many of our citizens as does hearing impairment.

Table 44–1 summarizes some recent comparative data on impaired hearing. Even over the brief span of six years that is shown, there is a significant increase in the population rates: from 690 per 10,000 in 1971 to 702 per 10,000 in 1977. This upward trend in the rates for impaired hearing has prevailed in studies by the National Center for Health Statistics conducted since at least 1962, and it is expected to continue until 2050, when more than 10 per cent of the United States population will be hearing-impaired.[58, 59]

Table 44–1 also illustrates other important points. Note the age-relatedness of the data—rates of hearing impairment increase with age, dramatically after 44 years. For the youngest age group, 3 to 16 years of age, the rate for the sexes combined is 1.63 per cent in 1977, increasing over six times for the 45-64 age group to 10.73 per cent and increasing more than 15 times for the 65 and over age group to 26.19 per cent.

Sex differences are also evident in Table 44–1. Hearing impairment predominates in males at all ages. The extent of differences is curvilinear, with smaller differences between rates for men and women in the youngest and oldest age groups. Both genetic and environmental explanations for the male predominance have been proposed,[21] but regardless of the reasons for it, state rehabilitation planners should recognize the sex difference in making provisions for services.

Hearing impairment ranks high in its severity of consequences. When it occurs early in life, a hearing impairment, even a relatively mild one, tends to interfere with education, especially speech and language development.[7, 15, 56] A conductive impair-

935

JEROME D. SCHEIN AND MAURICE H. MILLER

TABLE 44–1. Rates per 10,000 Persons Three Years of Age and Over Reporting Impaired Hearing, by Age and Sex: United States, 1971 and 1977*

SEX AND AGE (IN YEARS)	RATES PER 10,000 POPULATION	
	1971	1977
Both sexes, all ages 3 years+	690	702
3–16	162	163
17–24	265	205
25–44	447	414
45–64	1000	1073
65 and over	2741	2619
Males, all ages 3 years+	809	832
3–16	178	183
17–24	349	229
25–44	557	564
45–64	1286	1414
65 and over	3262	3134
Females, all ages 3 years+	581	580
3–16	145	141
17–24	189	181
25–44	345	274
45–64	741	764
65 and over	2359	2257

*Modified from Ries, P. W.: Hearing ability of persons by sociodemographic and health characteristics: United States. Vital and Health Statistics, Series 10, No. 140, 1982.

ment that raises the threshold in the better ear by as little as 20 decibels (dB) above the normal threshold can markedly interfere with the acquisition of both verbal and nonverbal learning, particularly if sustained during the first two years of life when the child is biologically programmed for rapid language development.

Profound hearing losses that occur during or before speech development are associated with failure to acquire intelligible speech—a frequent, although not a necessary, correlate.[10, 34] Delay in language acquisition, too, is a usual concomitant of early hearing losses. Later onsets of hearing impairment, although less likely to affect speech and language, may result in social isolation, loss of principal occupation, and major emotional upheavals—all consequences that are dependent, to some degree, upon the extent of impairment and the remedial steps taken to counteract it.[1, 55, 80]

Hearing loss poses barriers to human communication. The result of impaired hearing, then, is frequently a social handicap. Because it attacks the base of interpersonal relations, disruption of communications is no trivial matter. Without vigorous, effective rehabilitation, the hearing-impaired person suffers as much as does one afflicted by any other physical disability—typically more. This chapter focuses on what are now considered sound rehabilitation practices. To understand them, however, the reader must address the prior considerations that are presented in the following discussion.

Functional Anatomy of the Ear

The auditory system is composed of the peripheral mechanism (the outer, middle, and inner ear) that activates a series of intricate connections within the central nervous system through the eighth nerve and terminates in the auditory receptive areas of the temporal cortex. The anatomy and physiology of this complex system are reviewed briefly here as a basis for understanding the different types of hearing loss. The reader desiring more detailed information should consult the relevant references.*

Figure 44–1 schematizes the human ear. The *outer ear* consists of the *pinna* or *auricle* and the *external auditory canal*. The pinna adds slightly to sensitivity for high frequencies and helps to direct sound waves into the external auditory canal.

The *tympanic membrane* or *eardrum* divides the outer ear from the middle ear. The *middle-ear cavity* contains a chain of three tiny bones, the *ossicles,* whose names are *malleus, incus,* and *stapes.* Suspended in the cavity by a system of ligaments, the ossicles increase the effective pressure of sounds conveyed to the inner ear, because of the large difference between the area of the tympanic membrane and the footplate of the stapes, which is attached to the oval window (*condensation effect*). The ossicles function as a lever, because the length of the manubrium and neck of the malleus is greater than that of the long process of the incus, so that the force at the tympanic membrane is increased by a factor of 1.3 at the stapes. Thus, the pressure increase by a factor of 17, resulting from the area difference of the tympanic membrane and stapes footplate, is further amplified by 1.3, resulting in a theoretical maximum total pressure increase of 17 × 1.3, or 22, which corresponds to 27 dB.[90]

Dividing the middle ear from the inner ear are two membranes: the *oval window*, to which the stapes is attached, and the *round window*. The latter compensates for the changes in pressure caused by impression and expression of the oval

---

*See references 2, 3, 14, 22, 83–87, 91.

Diagnosis and Rehabilitation of Auditory Disorders

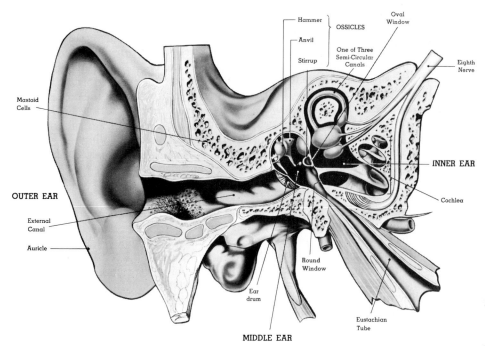

FIGURE 44–1. Sectional diagram of the human ear. (Reproduced with permission of the Sonotone Corp.)

window. Encased in the temporal bone is the *inner-ear cavity*, which houses a series of canals in the bone foundation called the *osseous labyrinth*. It is filled with *perilymph*, a liquid similar in chemical composition to cerebrospinal fluid. The perilymph circulates through the three principal subdivisions of the labyrinth: the *semicircular canals*, the *vestibule*, and the *cochlea*. The semicircular canals are arranged so as to provide the stimuli an individual uses to orient himself or herself in space. The conch-shaped cochlea contains the *organ of Corti*. The conversion of mechanical to electrical (neural) energy takes place at this point. The organ of Corti has over 30,000 hair cells on its inner and outer portions. The auditory nerve interacts with the hair cells by synaptic junctions. Vibrations of the inner ear fluids bend the cilia of the hair cells, initiating a change of neural potential. The resulting impulses are transmitted along the auditory pathways to the temporal cortex.

Theories of Hearing

The exact manner in which the cochlea functions as an analyzer of sound is the subject of vast research and continuing discussion. Four theories predominate as explanations of how hearing takes place.

The *place theory* states that pitch perception is related to the point of maximal stimulation along the basilar membrane of the organ of Corti. This theory proposes that the hair cells function as a series of tuned resonators. It is generally accepted for stimuli with a frequency at or above 5000 Hz.

The *frequency theory* relates pitch perception to the frequency of a current of impulses in the auditory nerve. For example, a sound with a frequency of 500 Hz would cause the fibers within the auditory nerve to fire at a rate of 500 times per sec. Since no auditory nerve fiber is capable of firing faster than 1000 times per sec, this theory could account for pitch perception only at frequencies around 1000 Hz or less.

A compromise between the place and frequency theories is the *volley theory*. It holds that pitch perception for frequencies up to 1000 Hz can be explained primarily on the basis of the frequency theory and that the place theory accounts for pitch perception at the higher frequencies.

The *traveling wave theory* postulates, on the basis of meticulously performed experiments with cochlear models, that sound is propagated in the form of a wave traveling from the base to the apex of the cochlea. The maximum amplitude of the wave occurs at a point on the basilar membrane corresponding to the frequency of the stimulus.

These four theories of hearing cover present-day

views. They appear here for two purposes. First, the fact that four different explanations persist indicates the complexity of the process. The rehabilitator can use this perspective in approaching hearing impairment. Second, these theories serve to introduce the next topic, the measurement of hearing and diagnosis of hearing impairment.

Introduction to Audiometry

Two common-sense aspects of sound have sophisticated analogues in the measurement of hearing: pitch and loudness. Objectively, *sound* is a form of wave motion resulting from a change in pressure or particle displacement in an elastic medium, such as air. The wave form is characterized by alternate pressure peaks and valleys called *compressions* and *rarefactions*. One successive compression and rarefaction constitute one cycle of a sound wave. The more rapidly these vibrations occur, the higher the *frequency*, symbolized by the abbreviations Hz (for *hertz*) or cps (for *cycles per second*). A sound wave whose cycles occur 500 times per second would be designated as 500 Hz; one vibrating twice as fast would be written 1000 Hz. The psychological equivalent of frequency is *pitch;* the more rapidly the wave oscillates, the higher the pitch is perceived by the listener, although pitch is affected by other factors. Middle "C" on the piano, for example, has a frequency near 256 Hz, while the next higher octave is 512 Hz. The human ear is theoretically capable of hearing sounds as low as 20 Hz and as high as 20,000 Hz. For purposes of hearing and understanding connected discourse in quiet surroundings by persons whose hearing was normal early in life, however, the critical frequencies range from 500 to 3000 Hz. This point has considerable importance for the testing of hearing and for rehabilitation, as is discussed later.

The *intensity* (loudness) of sound is measured by the amount of its pressure. *Sound-pressure level* is the difference between a given pressure and 0.0002 dynes per cm^2, the standard reference. The amount of the difference is expressed in decibels (dB), a log unit in which 0 dB = 0.0002 dynes per cm^2, the standard value. The reader unfamiliar with logarithms should note that to increase from 1 dB to 100 dB requires 100,000 times more energy, not a mere 100 times. This relative measure can also be confusing, because the same unit, dB, is used in measuring hearing sensitivity. However, in the latter case, the standard reference is not 0.0002 dynes per cm^2 but is a statistically determined amount of energy needed by a "normal" person to hear that particular sound (the *hearing-threshold level*). To avoid confusing the two concepts, decibel values should carry the reference level as part of the notation, e.g., 40 dB sound-pressure level (abbreviated as SPL) or 40 dB hearing-threshold level (abbreviated as HTL). The amount of energy expressed by the former differs significantly from that expressed by the latter.

The weakest amount of sound pressure that the human ear experiences as sound is a very small quantity, but the range of sound pressure that the ear can perceive is extremely large. Subjectively, a listener may describe some sounds as causing a tickling or painful sensation. The sound pressure that corresponds to very loud sounds is 1,000,000,000,000 (10^{12}) times greater than the sound pressure of barely audible sounds. That is why a log scale is used to express this tremendous range of pressures that the human ear can experience as sound. The range on the decibel scale would be expressed as 0 to 120 dB hearing-threshold level, a more manageable set of numbers.

Another term of importance in measuring hearing is *threshold,* the point at which correct responses are elicited 50 per cent of the time. Hearing sensitivity is defined by the amount of energy (in decibels) required by a listener to respond appropriately to the stimulus half the time. It follows, then, that the higher the threshold, the poorer the hearing. A person whose threshold is 0 dB hearing-threshold level has no deviation from normal and, therefore, has more sensitive hearing than someone whose threshold for the same stimulus is, say, 20 dB hearing-threshold level. That a larger number signifies poorer hearing sensitivity must be borne in mind as audiograms are read.

The Audiometer and the Audiogram

Audiometry is the measurement of hearing. Basic testing to determine the degree and type of hearing loss is performed with a *pure-tone audiometer,* an instrument for measuring hearing sensitivity that provides pure tones of selected frequencies at calibrated sound-pressure levels. The results of such testing are recorded on an *audiogram,* which is a graph showing hearing sensitivity as a function of frequency.

In the audiogram shown in Figure 44–2, "Zero

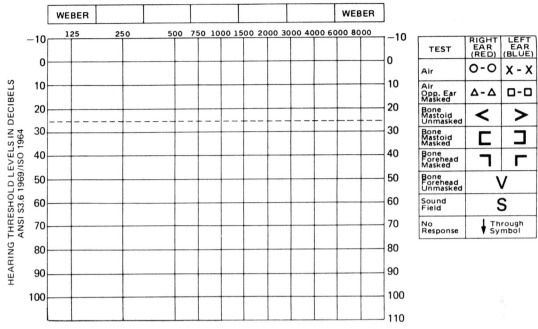

FIGURE 44–2. Pure tone audiogram showing hearing-threshold levels as a function of tonal frequency.

dB hearing-threshold level" represents the zero reference level. The range between −10 dB and 25 dB in the audiogram is considered to be within normal limits. This definition has been appropriately questioned in relation to the hearing of children going through major periods of speech and language development, when a threshold increase even to 20 or 25 dB may significantly impede language acquisition and the development of academic skills.

At thresholds above this normal-hearing range, differing degrees of hearing impairment are indicated by higher numbers. The audiogram in Figure 44–3 shows normal hearing throughout the tested range in the left ear. However, at 4000 Hz in the right ear, the hearing threshold is 35 dB greater than that of the normally hearing person — a deviation indicative of a problem in the auditory system, albeit a small one in this example.

The test results shown in Figure 44–3 represent thresholds for *air conduction*, i.e., for stimuli transmitted to the external ear through earphones. Another way of presenting stimuli to the ear is *bone conduction*, in which a vibrator is placed on portions of the skull, usually on the mastoid process.

The general anatomical area of the ear that is involved in the patient's hearing impairment can be determined by comparing air-conduction to bone-conduction thresholds. Bone-conduction measurements must be performed with the judicious use of *masking,* i.e., presenting a complex signal to the contralateral ear to prevent it from picking up the sound presented to the ear under test. Through the bone-conduction test an attempt is made to bypass the middle-ear system and conduct sound directly to the inner ear. Judicious use of masking, particularly for assessing bone conduction, is critical to the validity of this important procedure.

Acoustic Impedance (Immittance) Evaluation

Impedance or immittance measurements are not hearing tests in the usual sense, and the term *audiometry* should not be employed to describe them. These procedures have become an essential component of the evaluation of persons with auditory problems and constitute one of the most powerful diagnostic tools available. Some clinicians use impedance measurements at the beginning of the evaluation to determine which audiological procedures are indicated, whereas others use them to obtain site-of-lesion data and to provide additional diagnostic information.[29, 43]

Impedance measurements are an objective

JEROME D. SCHEIN AND MAURICE H. MILLER

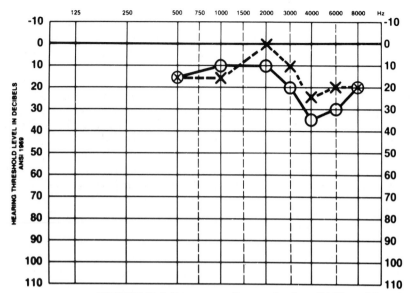

TEST	RIGHT EAR	LEFT EAR
AIR	O-O	X-X
AIR OPP EAR MASKED	△-△	☐-☐
BONE MASTOID MASKED	<	>
BONE MASTOID UNMASKED	⊏	⊐

FIGURE 44–3. Pure tone audiogram showing mild bilateral loss above 3000 Hz.

method for assessing the integrity and performance of the peripheral auditory system. The electro-acoustical impedance meter contains a probe tip that is sealed in the external auditory meatus. The probe tip has three holes: (1) one for a probe tone of about 220 Hz, (2) one for a cavity air-pressure control, and (3) one for a pick-up microphone to compare the sound-pressure level in the ear canal with reference to the sound-pressure level in the impedance meter. A test tone is introduced, and the sound that is reflected by the tympanic membrane is measured. The amount reflected depends upon the mass and stiffness of the system and the acoustical resistance of the air.

The basic immittance battery includes *tympanometry, static compliance,* and measurement of the *acoustical reflex.* Each of these tests provides valuable information, although static compliance is the least useful of the three measurements. The index of diagnostic accuracy is significantly improved when the entire immittance battery is used, especially in relation to other audiological and nonaudiological site-of-lesion studies. Tympanometry is probably the most sensitive indicator of middle-ear function available today. Acoustical-reflex and stapedial-reflex decay tests are useful in the differential diagnosis of cochlear and retrocochlear lesions and in evaluating patients with suspected functional hearing problems. Reflex levels can be used in selection and adjustment of hearing aids for difficult to test children. Some abnormality in the acoustical reflex (i.e., elevated

or absent reflex or the presence of significant reflex decay) is related to an acoustical tumor in as many as 85 per cent of cases.

Speech Audiometry

Speech audiometry is a measure of overall hearing performance for functional speech stimuli. It is also used to estimate the degree of actual handicap imposed by the auditory deficit. Calibrated speech materials are used to assess two aspects of auditory performance: speech-reception thresholds (or spondee thresholds) and speech discrimination.

Speech-reception thresholds or spondee thresholds are obtained by asking the patient to repeat a series of spondee words (those that have roughly equal stress on the two syllables, e.g., "cowboy," "mushroom," "airplane"). The materials are presented at successively louder levels by monitored live voice or a recording into earphones worn by the patient. Threshold is the level at which the patient is able to repeat just 50 per cent of the words correctly.

Speech discrimination or, more correctly, *word discrimination* is a test of the patient's ability to understand speech when the level of presentation is not a factor in determining the number of words repeated correctly. Lists consisting of 50 words are presented that theoretically reflect the frequency of occurrence of the various phonetic elements in everyday conversational speech (i.e., they are phonetically balanced). The level of presentation is usually 30 to 40 dB above the patient's speech-reception threshold, although in some cases it is important to obtain a complete articulation function test reflecting the patient's ability to understand speech as the intensity of the signal is gradually increased. Word discrimination is widely used in differential diagnosis and hearing-aid evaluation. Jerger and his associates developed lists of synthetic sentence material consisting of seven-word sentences that are grammatically correct but meaningless ("Small boat with a picture has become").[82] They can be presented with a competing speech message introduced into the contralateral or ipsilateral ear. The procedure has been suggested for diagnosis of brain stem and cortical lesions as well as for hearing-aid evaluation.

Pure-tone air-conduction and bone-conduction audiometry, speech audiometry, and the impedance (immittance) battery compose the basic audiological evaluation that should be performed on all persons with known or suspected auditory problems. On the basis of the results of these tests and the case history, some or all of the procedures described next may be indicated.

The Audiological Site of Lesion Battery

An impressive array of audiological procedures is now available to elucidate the nature of the auditory problem and to determine, in conjunction with nonaudiological procedures, the site of a lesion within the auditory system. Although each test has a different index of accuracy in predicting the locus of pathology, the accuracy increases significantly when each test is viewed as part of a comprehensive battery and carefully evaluated with a recognition of the advantages and weaknesses of each procedure for different groups of hypacusic patients. A number of audiological procedures have been sensitized to provide additional diagnostic information, particularly in difficult to diagnose early and mild lesions. These modifications will not be discussed in the following brief review of some of the audiological site of lesion studies now in use.

Loudness Balance Tests. A tone of a given frequency is presented alternately to the two ears of the patient, who is asked to match its relative loudness. This procedure, called the *Alternate Binaural Loudness Balance* test, allows the demonstration of recruitment in certain ear pathologies. *Recruitment* is an abnormal growth in the loudness of sound when its intensity is increased above the impaired threshold. It is characteristically present in persons with cochlear lesions (e.g., Ménière's disease, ototoxic deafness, noise-induced hearing loss) and frequently, but not invariably, absent in persons with eighth-nerve tumors and other lesions affecting the auditory nerve. The test is optimally suited for cases of unilateral sensorineural losses but can be used in persons with asymmetrical losses in whom the difference in hearing sensitivity between ears exceeds 30 to 40 dB at some frequencies and when the better, reference ear is known to be nonrecruiting.[9]

A loudness balance test that can be used when there is no difference in sensitivity between the ears and both have a symmetrical loss of approximately equal degree is called the *Monaural Loudness Balance* test or the *Alternate Monaural Loudness Balance* test. It involves a comparison of the relative loudness of two frequencies, one at an impaired and one at an unimpaired frequency, presented alternately to the same ear of the patient. The test is more difficult for the patient than the Alternate Binaural Loudness Balance test because a comparison of two sounds of disparate frequencies is involved, and results can be affected by the musical sophistication of the subject and, to a greater extent than with some other audiological tests, by a practice effect. Persons with eighth-nerve lesions, a major concern of the diagnostician, are more likely to show a unilateral or asymmetrical loss, in which the Alternate Binaural Loudness Balance test is the procedure of choice, rather than bilateral, symmetrical losses, in which the Alternate Monaural Loudness Balance test would be employed.

Short Increment Sensitivity Index. The short increment sensitivity index measures the patient's ability to detect small changes in intensity. A pure tone is presented to the patient at 20 dB above the threshold. Twenty-one–dB increments are superimposed upon the constant tone at periodic intervals. Persons with pathological cochleas are able to detect these small increments, whereas those with lesions elsewhere usually cannot.[30]

Békésy's Audiometry. Békésy's audiometry uses a self-recording technique to determine pure-tone thresholds. The patient is told to push a button and keep it depressed as long as the signal is heard and to release it when the tone is no longer audible. The audiometer is connected to an X-Y recorder that traces the patient's audiogram as a series of vertical excursions of the marking pen. In a version widely used today, thresholds are established first for periodically interrupted and then for continuous pure tones. The relationship of thresholds for the two types of stimuli is compared to differentiate various pathologies, including pseudohypacusis.[9] The Alternate Binaural Loudness Balance test, the short increment sensitivity index, and Békésy's test have fallen into some disrepute of late because of their failure to detect many cases of acoustical neurinomas and to an increasing degree are being replaced by newer techniques, e.g., stapedial reflex measurements and brain stem evoked-response audiometry.

Abnormal tone decay or auditory adaptation is a loss of sensitivity that occurs during exposure to an auditory stimulus. It is a symptom that in its most bizarre forms is characteristic of eighth-nerve lesions, although various degrees and patterns of abnormal tone decay can occur in cochlear and brain stem lesions. Tone decay of 30 dB or more is generally considered to reflect retrocochlear pathology. However, the likelihood of a retrocochlear lesion increases when tone decay of only 30 dB is found in association with normal or near-normal thresholds at the frequency at which the test is performed. Any conventional audiometer can be used to perform this test, which is a powerful screening and diagnostic tool in differential diagnosis.[24]

Electrophysiological (Neuroelectric) Tests of Auditory Function

For many patients, tests that do not involve active cooperation in the form of voluntary, conditioned responses are essential. Among the patients in whom objective procedures are most useful are children who are too young or too involved to respond to standard pediatric audiological measures (e.g., children under 18 months of age and those who are retarded, neurologically impaired, or severely disturbed psychologically) and persons with suspected functional auditory problems. For the latter, such tests may play an important but still controversial role in medicolegal proceedings. Finally, some forms of electrophysiological measures are extremely sensitive detectors of eighth-nerve, brain stem, and cortical lesions and, thus, compose an important part of the site of lesion battery.

Electroencephalic audiometry quantifies changes in the electroencephalogram that result from auditory stimulation. *Evoked-response audiometry* is a general term used for the different forms of audiometry that tap a number of electric responses that can be evoked from different parts of the auditory system by auditory stimulation. All of these responses are very small and require repetitive stimulation and the summation of many responses with the use of a response-averaging computer. The responses, which are time-locked to the acoustical stimuli, add in the memory of the computer, and the random background activity of the brain and muscles is canceled out. The most widely used of the electric auditory responses today is *brain stem evoked-response audiometry*.[26, 37]

With brain stem evoked-response audiometry, a measurement is made of auditory-evoked potentials believed to originate between the eighth nerve and the inferior colliculus. The responses appear quite reliable and not difficult to identify. Brain stem evoked-response audiometry has become the most accurate noninvasive procedure in the diagnosis of acoustical neurinomas and has the lowest false-positive rate.[6] For purposes of determining hearing thresholds, brain stem evoked-response audiometry can measure within 10 dB of the individual's psychophysical threshold for the stimulus used, when appropriate signal characteristics and recording techniques are used.

Electrocochleography measures the electrophysiological activity that originates within the cochlea or the auditory nerve. The compound action potential of the auditory nerve is the basis for most electrocochleography studies. Recording sites are the transtympanic membrane, where needle electrodes make contact with the promontory of the cochlea, the intrameatal surface, and the surface of the external auditory canal. For the uncooperative patient, an anesthesiologist is necessary to monitor and control levels of anesthesia, and life-support equipment must be available should complications of general anesthesia occur. An otolaryngologist inserts the electrodes and is responsible for pre- and postrecording medical care of the patient. The test procedure is carried out by an audiologist. The action potential response appears to be a sensitive indicator of cochlear and auditory nerve activity. *Cochleograms* can be obtained that reflect recruitment, sensorineural losses of various degrees and configurations, and total hearing impairment. Recordings obtained from sites other than the promontory of the cochlea appear to be of limited value.[11] This invasive technique has been largely replaced by brain stem evoked-response audiometry in most laboratories, although electrocochleography provides data on certain aspects of cochlear function not yielded by brain stem evoked-response audiometry.

Classification of Types of Hearing Impairment

Peripheral, organic hearing impairments can be usefully divided into three categories for rehabilitation purposes. These three categories are based on the locus of the lesion responsible for the impairment. *Conductive impairments* prevent or interfere with transmission of sound to the cochlea. Such lesions occur in the outer or middle ear. Hearing loss resulting from damage to the cochlea, or the auditory nerve or both is called *sensorineural impairment.* When these structures are defective, interpretation of the auditory stimulus may be difficult or impossible. When both conductive and sensorineural impairments are present, the loss is referred to as *mixed* or *combined.*

The value of this three-part classification of peripheral hearing impairment is that some rehabilitative strategies are directly associated with them. These strategies will be discussed later. Here we concentrate on the procedures for determining the site of the lesion.

Pure-tone air-conduction audiometry provides quantitative information about hearing sensitivity only. To determine the type of hearing impairment present, other tests are required. Table 44–2 relates the degree of hearing loss on the pure-tone audiogram to the degree of difficulty in understanding conversational speech. This relationship is far from an exact one, because the ability to understand speech cannot be directly predicted from responses to pure-tone stimuli. Difficulty in understanding speech is also related, in part, to the configuration of the audiogram and to the amount and type of distortion present. Persons with significantly greater losses in the high frequencies (above 1000 Hz) usually have noticeable problems in speech discrimination, although low-frequency sensorineural losses can also be related to poor speech discrimination, e.g., Ménière's disease. The degree of difficulty in understanding speech with or without amplification is also dependent upon the type of hearing loss present, the age at onset, and other factors. Nonetheless, the table relates the approximate degree of difficulty that most persons in each category will experience.

Figure 44–4 shows the air-conduction thresholds of an individual with an average pure-tone loss of 60 dB. Bone-conduction measurements fall entirely within normal limits. This individual has a *conductive* hearing impairment. A conductive hearing impairment reflects damage or disease to the outer or middle ear. Conductive hearing impairments are potentially correctable by a variety of medical and surgical means.

Hearing-conservation programs in schools often do not detect many auditory problems, especially those associated with secretory otitis media (see later). The schools set screening levels for air conduction at 20 or 25 db hearing-threshold levels, levels too high for early detection. The hearing tests are given too infrequently to uncover many fluctuating losses. Most critically, a better test than air conduction for such problems would be tym-

TABLE 44–2. Relation of Degree of Hearing Loss to Ability to Understand Speech

CLASS	CLASSIFICATION CATEGORY OF HEARING LOSS	AVERAGE HEARING THRESHOLD LEVEL FOR 500, 1000, AND 2000 Hz IN THE BETTER EAR*		ABILITY TO UNDERSTAND SPEECH
		More Than	Not More Than	
A	Within normal limits		25 dB	No significant difficulty with faint speech
B	Slight or mild	26	40 dB	Difficulty only with faint speech
C	Moderate	41	55 dB	Frequent difficulty with normal speech
D	Moderately severe	56	70 dB	Frequent difficulty with loud speech
E	Severe	71	90 dB	Can understand only shouted or amplified speech
F	Profound	91		Usually cannot understand even amplified speech

*Re: 1969 ANSI reference threshold. Adapted from Davis, H.: Guide for the classification and evaluation of hearing handicapped. Trans. Am. Acad. Ophthalmol. Otolaryngol., 69:740–751, 1965.

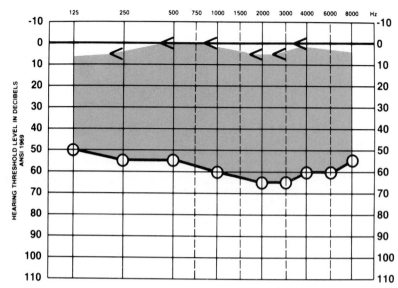

FIGURE 44–4. Conductive hearing impairment in right ear with large air-bone gap (shown in shaded area) associated with otosclerosis.

panometry, a measure of the change in eardrum compliance that has been described above.

Figure 44–5 shows a bilateral *sensorineural* hearing impairment in a noise-susceptible individual who has worked in a very noisy environment without using personal hearing-protective devices. Note that there is no air-bone gap; i.e., bone-conduction values closely parallel the air-conduction thresholds.

Figure 44–6 shows a *mixed* hearing impairment. In this case, the loss of hearing below 1000 Hz is primarily conductive and secondary to otitis media, whereas the loss above 1000 Hz is primarily sensorineural and secondary to presbycusis. Specifying

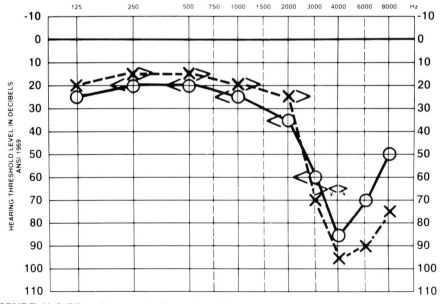

FIGURE 44–5. Bilateral symmetrical sensorineural hearing impairment secondary to noise exposure.

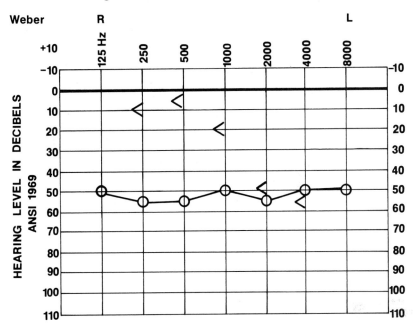

FIGURE 44–6. Vertical mixed or combined hearing impairment.

the cause of the impairment, of course, requires more than an audiogram. An inferential diagnosis involves acquiring a careful history and additional nonaudiological tests, as well as thorough physical examination.

Major Causes of Hearing Impairment by Locus of Lesion

In the following discussion, the principal causes of hearing impairment are arranged in the order of the anatomical structures involved. The first group describes impairments associated with the outer ear. Note, however, that a given patient may simultaneously suffer more than one disorder, although this presentation treats each disorder separately.

Outer Ear

Disorders of the outer ear may affect sound conduction. They generally are amenable to treatment restoring normal functioning of the auditory system. They may be associated with middle- and inner-ear problems whose management is considered in subsequent sections.

Congenital Atresia of the External Auditory Canal. Failure to develop an opening in the external meatus affecting sound conduction to the tympanum is often associated with microtia and multiple rudimentary or auricular tags of accessory auricles. These obvious malformations may be accompanied by deformities of the middle ear or inner ear as well as of other organs, e.g., the kidneys. These conditions may be unilateral or bilateral and may present both auditory and cosmetic problems.

Foreign Bodies. Tumors involving skin, cartilage, and bone are found in the external auditory canal and may require surgical removal. By far the most common problem is impacted cerumen (ear wax), which can cause up to a 40-dB conductive loss. As long as a pinhead opening of the tympanic membrane remains visible, cerumen is unlikely to affect hearing significantly. However, when the eardrum is completely obstructed by cerumen, removal by an otologist is indicated. Osteomas, hyperostoses, and exostoses require surgical management only when they completely obstruct the external meatus or present other problems to the patient.

Collapsed Canal. Some persons have an anatomical variant of the outermost portion of the cartilaginous portion of the external canal and tragus. The pressure of the earphone used to test air-conduction thresholds can produce a collapse of the meatus. Although this is not a lesion *per se*, it may cause a pseudoconductive loss to appear on the audiometric test, unaccompanied by any complaint of auditory difficulty. Such problems do not

JEROME D. SCHEIN AND MAURICE H. MILLER

occur in tuning-fork measurements. These patients will require "propping" of the ear canal with an earmold or other plug to prevent this false conductive hearing loss from contaminating the results of audiological measurements performed with earphones. The problem occurs quite frequently in elderly persons.

External Otitis. External otitis is usually the result of a bacterial infection in the skin of the external auditory canal. Redness, swelling, and discharge may accompany the infection. The hearing loss, when present, is conductive.

Treacher Collins Syndrome. Treacher Collins syndrome combines abnormalities of the mandible with hearing loss resulting from the first-branchial-arch origin of the mandible, malleus, and incus. The loss is conductive.

Middle Ear

A variety of congenital lesions of the middle ear may occur, including absent or fused ossicles, congenital fixation of the stapedial footplate, and occasionally a complete immobilization of the ossicular chain. Again, hearing losses resulting from these disorders are conductive, unless other auditory structures are involved. These conditions often respond well to surgical management.

Otitis Media. Acute infections of the middle ear are accompanied by pain, fever, and malaise. Widespread use of antibiotics has dramatically reduced the incidence of acute mastoiditis arising from otitis media, but their use may mask the classic symptoms of infection and lead to a latent form (*silent* or *occult otitis media*) accompanied by varying degrees of conductive hearing loss.

Serous or *secretory otitis media* is by far the most prevalent cause of conductive hearing loss in preschool-age and school-age children. The child suffering from this condition is typically not constitutionally ill and attends school but experiences a fluctuating conductive hearing loss that is often not detected by hearing-conservation programs in the school (see earlier discussion of tympanometry).

Among the complications of inadequately treated serous otitis media is *cholesteatoma,* a squamous cyst that begins in the middle ear and extends into the mastoid antrum, often to the mastoid tip. Cholesteatomas can destroy the ossicular chain and are potentially fatal. Irreversible sensorineural hearing losses may also occur in children with silent, inadequately treated serous otitis.[17, 21, 45] In long-standing cases of serous otitis

media, conservative management is usually ineffective, and surgery, consisting of adenoidectomy, myringotomy, and insertion of ventilation tubes into the eardrum to replace a malfunctioning eustachian tube, is the treatment of choice. Treatment of an underlying allergy, often to food rather than inhalants, may be required for some intractable cases.

Otosclerosis. Otosclerosis is a common cause of hearing loss in adults. The disease affects the otic capsule and in its early stage often involves a softening of the oval window anterior to the stapes footplate. It is twice as common in women as in men and is relatively rare among blacks. The condition can also involve cochlear structures and may even have its primary effect on the inner ear, a form of the condition known as *labyrinthine* or *cochlear otosclerosis.*

Persons with otosclerosis whose lesions involve primarily the oval window and who audiometrically show large air-bone gaps and good speech discrimination are typically excellent candidates for stapedectomy, a surgical procedure in which the involved portion of the stapes is removed and the ossicular chain is reconstructed in a variety of ways. Stapedectomy can restore hearing to within 10 dB of the preoperative bone-conduction curve in 80 to 90 per cent of carefully selected patients. Some patients with far advanced otosclerosis who may have unmeasurable air-bone gaps may be helped through stapes surgery to regain sufficient hearing to allow them to use amplification or to allow the use of ear-level rather than body-mounted instruments. The specific objectives of surgery in such cases must be carefully explained to these patients, so that they are not led to believe that the surgery can eliminate the need for hearing aids. Moderate doses of fluorides with a calcium supplement and vitamin D, although still constituting a controversial treatment, should be considered for patients with rapidly progressive forms of cochlear otosclerosis.[74, 76]

Discontinuities of the Ossicular Chain. Mechanical damage to the ear from blows to the head (as in vehicular or bicycle accidents) can cause a dislocation of the ossicular chain and varying degrees of conductive hearing loss. Surgical procedures are available to reconstruct the ossicular chain and restore hearing, often to normal or near-normal levels. Impedance evaluation is extremely helpful in distinguishing ossicular-chain discontinuities from otosclerosis, an important consideration in cases involving medicolegal litigation.

Inner Ear

By far the largest number of hearing-impaired persons in the general population have disease or damage to the cochlea. A smaller number have lesions affecting the eighth nerve, whereas some have combinations of cochlear and eighth-nerve involvement. Conditions such as acoustical tumors have serious life-threatening implications, and early diagnosis and management are essential. Lesions affecting the cochlea, in general, are not correctable by medical or surgical techniques, and patients with such lesions represent the largest population of candidates for hearing aids and various forms of audiological rehabilitation. They are suffering from sensorineural hearing impairments.

Noise-induced Hearing Loss. Noise, both in and out of the work place, is believed to account for more cases of hearing impairment than all other causes combined. It is certainly the major cause of new cases of hearing loss. Over five million individual work areas have been identified as having potentially hazardous noise levels. More than 40 million workers are exposed each work day to a noise level of over 90 dBA (the "A" network; see definition in the next paragraph), and 16.5 million persons have already sustained some permanent sensorineural hearing loss from noise exposure. The federal government, through the Occupational Safety and Health Administration of the Department of Labor, passed a final regulation on occupational noise exposure which became effective on August 22, 1981. It requires a hearing-conservation program for all workers exposed to noise level equal to or greater than 85 dBA for a time-weighted equivalent of eight hours.[38] Exposures greater than 90 dBA are permitted for various periods of time (e.g., 100 dBA for two hours and 105 dBA for one hour), but the cumulative noise exposure in any eight-hour period must not exceed an average of 90 dBA. The hearing-conservation program must include noise monitoring, audiometric testing, worker education, and use of personal hearing-protective devices.[36A, 40]

Noise-level measurements are made on a *sound-level meter,* an instrument that measures noise at the source. It consists of a microphone, an amplifier, a calibrated attenuator, an indicating meter, and a series of circuits (networks) which adjust the overall frequency characteristics of the input. The "A" network (signified in the symbol dBA) simulates the response of the normal ear to low-frequency sounds; it is the most commonly used setting for studies of work place and environmental noise.

Noise exposure first damages the outer hair cells of the organ of Corti and later involves its inner hair cells, the sensory and vascular epithelium of the cochlea, and the capillary vessels. Eventually the organ of Corti disappears and is replaced by a layer of simple epithelial cells. Audiometrically, a threshold elevation is first noted at 4000 Hz and less often at 3000 and 6000 Hz. As exposure increases in susceptible individuals, particularly those not using any personal hearing-protective devices, the noise-induced loss increases and spreads to lower and higher frequencies. In addition to the hearing loss, *tinnitus* (noises heard without external stimulation) becomes a major symptom and often precedes hearing loss or is present when changes in hearing occur (vide infra).

While occupational noise exposure accounts for the greatest incidence of noise-induced hearing loss, excessive noise exposure affects people in virtually every area where they live or play. Rock-music concerts and discotheques, trap and skeet shooting, power lawn mowers, chain saws, snowmobiles, motor-driven bicycles, garbage disposals, blenders and ice-jets, personal earphones attached to stereo cassettes and radio devices, and home stereo units are a few of the avocational sources of significant noise exposure. An example of auditory damage from gunfire exposure is shown in Figure 44–7. The illustration on the bottom shows damage to the sensory elements of the cochlea responsible for reception of high-frequency stimuli. The figure on the top shows an intact sensory mechanism on the contralateral nonexposed side.

Presbycusis is the term applied to the various ways in which the auditory system degenerates with age. All portions of the system are subject to such changes from atrophic alterations in the skin of the external auditory canal and a flaccidity of the tympanic membrane to a nonspecific osteitis and sclerosis of the auditory ossicles. However, auditory changes with age involve primarily the sensorineural and central mechanisms and not the conductive system.

Audiologically, age changes associated with presbycusis are usually characterized by a gradual loss of pure-tone sensitivity in the high frequencies. Figure 44–8 displays data based on eight different studies from four countries, with hearing level for 25-year-old adults used as a reference. Note that males lose hearing for high frequencies more rapidly than females, but the general trend applies to both sexes.

JEROME D. SCHEIN AND MAURICE H. MILLER

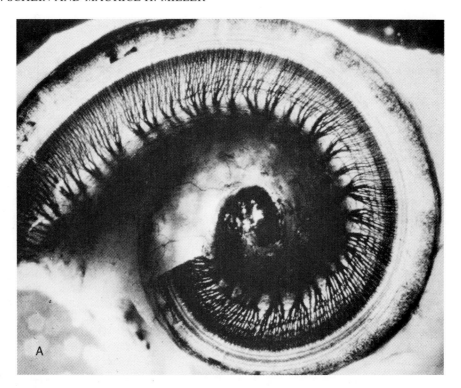

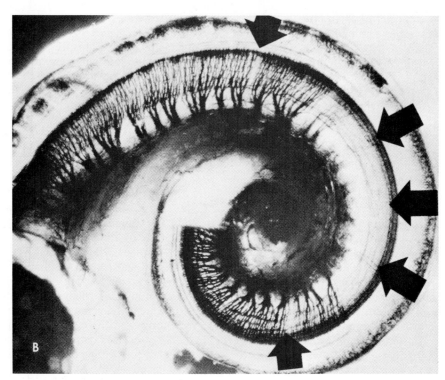

FIGURE 44–7. *A,* The cochlea of a normal, healthy ear seen under an electron microscope. *B,* Noise-damaged cochlea. Further deterioration from noise exposure may be prevented by use of hearing protection.

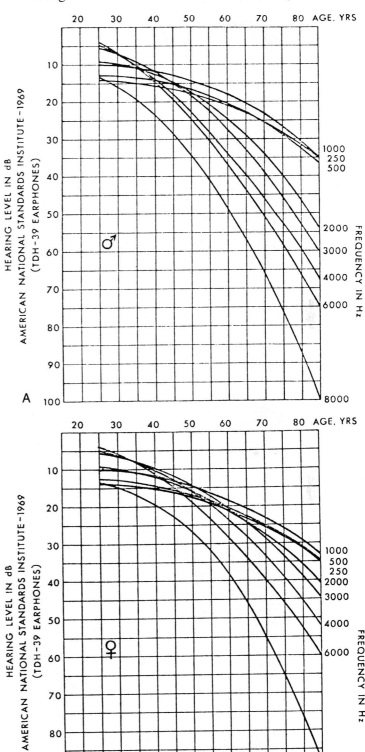

FIGURE 44–8. *A,* Composite presbycusic curves for males, according to Spoor, modified to conform to ANSI-1969 standard. *B,* Composite presbycusic curves from females, according to Spoor, modified to conform to ANSI-1969 standard. (From Lebo, C. P., and Reddell, R. C.: The presbycusis component in occupational noise-induced hearing loss. Laryngoscope, 82:1399–1409, 1972.)

JEROME D. SCHEIN AND MAURICE H. MILLER

More significant than the decrease in high-frequency sensitivity among the elderly is the disproportionate drop in speech discrimination that is frequently encountered in this population, particularly in the presence of noise. Such an abnormal breakdown in the understanding of speech has been termed *phonemic regression* and has important rehabilitative implications. Persons having this condition benefit less from hearing aids and require more intense audiological rehabilitation than those with good discrimination.

A neural form of presbycusis involves a loss of neurons in the central nervous system and is often seen in persons with severe arteriosclerosis. This variety of the condition does not lend itself to simple correction by existing forms of electroacoustical amplification. Specifically designed geriatric audiological rehabilitation programs using a team approach and involving both individual and group sessions are required to achieve success with such cases. However, the neural form of presbycusis is only one of at least four forms of the condition that have been identified, and each group shows a different potential for audiological rehabilitation. A *sensory form* involves degeneration of the sensory and supportive cells of the basal turns of the cochlea. Atrophy of the stria vascularis, which is believed to be the site of endolymph production, produces a *metabolic type* of presbycusis. *Mechanical presbycusis* results from a disorder of the motion mechanics of the cochlear duct caused by stiffening of the basilar membrane.[72, 73] Each of these forms of presbycusis is accompanied by a different constellation of audiological findings and by varied histories. The patient with metabolic presbycusis has an excellent prognosis for successful use of amplification, often with relatively short periods of audiological rehabilitation. In contrast to this group, the neural form requires massive rehabilitation, and amplification alone will play a less decisive role in achieving any success. Combinations of these forms of presbycusis often coexist.

The presbycusic population, which represents the largest number of new patients seen by audiologists, has not been adequately served by many hearing professionals, who have tended to view presbycusis as a single entity, usually unresponsive to hearing aids and audiological rehabilitation. Since over 20 million hearing-impaired persons over the age of 65 are expected by the year 2030,[59] it is critical that the most creative and resourceful professional talent available be mobilized to provide services to this challenging population. For-

tunately, signs of such efforts are beginning to emerge.

Ototoxic Drugs. Inner-ear structures are susceptible to damage by a wide variety of pharmaceutical agents. Some drugs, such as aspirin and quinine, exert transient effects on the auditory system, whereas others, such as the aminoglycoside antibiotics (neomycin, kanamycin) can cause irreversible changes. Isoplatinum and other drugs used in cancer chemotherapy may be ototoxic. Even those drugs whose ototoxic effects are reversible may produce permanent hearing loss through interactions with other factors, e.g., noise exposure. A factor that complicates the relationship between drugs and hearing damage is the delayed effect that some medications have on the auditory system. Dihydrostreptomycin, for example, may produce damage to the auditory system up to six months after cessation of therapy.

Virtually all ototoxic effects are signaled by tinnitus, which characteristically precedes audiometric changes. High-frequency audiometry (at and above 10 kHZ) may uncover auditory changes before tinnitus occurs. Patients taking any known or suspected ototoxic drug should be told to inform their physician at once if tinnitus occurs so that adjustments in medication can be made when feasible. Serial audiometric monitoring and vestibular studies using electronystagmography are essential in such instances. Since ototoxic drugs affect primarily the cochlear hair cells, the potential for severe irreversible sensorineural hearing loss from these agents should be considered whenever they are prescribed, particularly to patients with any of the noted risk factors.

Ménière's Disease. Ménière's disease, although not nearly as frequent as any of the causes of sensorineural hearing loss previously described, probably causes more suffering and anguish than all other auditory disorders combined. The typical patient complains of a true *rotary vertigo* (illusion of movement); a fluctuating, low-frequency sensorineural hearing loss; tinnitus; nausea and vomiting; and a sensation of fullness in the ear. Attacks come in clusters, with periods when the patient is free from symptoms. The hearing loss is unilateral in about 80 per cent of cases, but some patients with this disorder show bilateral involvement if studied over a period of many years. Audiologically, patients show evidence of a cochlear lesion, and speech discrimination is markedly affected during the Ménière's attack. Ménière's disease is believed to involve a dilatation of the endolymphatic spaces (endolymphatic hydrops) resulting from an inability to absorb endolymph or a hypersecretion of endolymph, and a specific etiological agent can be established in 55 per cent of affected patients.[53] Patients should be evaluated for food allergy with one of the newer diagnostic procedures (radioallergosorbent test [RAST], cytotoxic test) as well as for possible endocrine disturbances, including impaired glucose metabolism.[33, 52, 75]

Ménière's disease has been called the number one unsolved problem in clinical otology. It has been treated with an extraordinary array of medical and surgical approaches, few subject to controlled investigation of any kind. Some patients with intractable forms of the disease require surgical intervention. The long-term benefits of surgery, particularly those procedures designed to preserve hearing, are controversial. There is a persistent danger that a patient who has had a total ablation of cochlear and vestibular function may at some time in the future develop symptoms in the opposite ear. In addition to ongoing care by the otolaryngologist, patients with Ménière's disease should be evaluated and managed by audiologists who can select and adjust specially designed hearing aids for use during periods when hearing sensitivity and speech discrimination are sufficiently depressed to warrant assistance. Special modifications of existing hearing-aid circuits may be required by these patients to compensate for various forms of nonlinear distortion and for severely reduced tolerance. Auditory training and speechreading are strongly indicated for many of these patients.

Viral and Bacterial Disease. The most common viral cause of unilateral sensorineural hearing loss is *mumps*, which typically produces a total unilateral loss without involvement of the vestibular system. *Measles* and *chicken pox* can cause bilateral hearing impairment. *Bacterial meningitis* may damage both the cochlear and vestibular systems. Other bacterial diseases implicated in sensorineural hearing loss are *typhoid fever, diphtheria,* and *scarlet fever*. Scarlet fever can cause a purulent otitis media in addition to inner-ear damage, resulting in a mixed hearing loss. The importance of immunization against diseases such as measles and mumps cannot be overemphasized. Prenatal rubella is discussed later.

Sudden Deafness. Although most sensorineural hearing loss is typically characterized by insidious onset, some persons lose their hearing suddenly, often reporting the condition upon awakening. The etiology is obscure but is believed to result from either a viral labyrinthitis causing inner-ear changes, similar to those occurring in mumps deafness, or a vascular occlusion (spasm, embolism) affecting the blood supply to the inner ear. Some persons report sudden loss of hearing after exposure to cold. Since approximately 50 per cent of affected persons show spontaneous hearing recovery, often to within normal limits, it is difficult to evaluate the efficacy of any therapeutic regimen. Audiologists, by the performance and interpretation of sophisticated site of lesion studies, can usually determine whether the cochlea, the eighth nerve, or both are involved, and treatment can be based in part upon such diagnostic data. Since sudden deafness is a dramatic, frightening condition, most otologists advocate vigorous treatment including vasodilation, anticoagulation, and corticosteroids, the latter particularly when audiological tests localize the lesion in the auditory nerve.

Familial and Congenital Hearing Loss. There are over 60 types of hereditary hearing loss that can be separated from one another by type of impairment, age at onset, severity, mode of genetic transmission (dominant, recessive, and sex-linked), and associated abnormalities in other systems caused by the same genetic agent. Forty per cent of profound childhood deafness is autosomal recessive in origin, 10 per cent is by autosomal dominant transmission, and 3 per cent is by sex-linked gene. A large proportion of affected persons have profound, bilateral sensorineural hearing loss and require special educational facilities. In many cases, the auditory problem is progressive. Genetic counseling represents the major approach to prevention of these conditions.[20]

Congenital hearing losses arise from conditions affecting the birth process, such as birth trauma, or those appearing in the first few days of life, such as icterus neonatorum and kernicterus. Congenital hearing loss also applies to impairments secondary to viruses and other agents that affect the mother during pregnancy. *Maternal or prenatal rubella* is the best example. In the 1963–1964 rubella epidemic, at least 45 per cent of the children born of mothers with confirmed prenatal rubella showed significant hearing loss, either as the primary deficit or in association with heart and eye defects. Almost any infection, particularly if contracted during the first trimester of pregnancy, can damage the fetus' auditory system.

The Joint Committee on Infant Hearing Screening recommended that the hearing of infants who exhibit any item on the following list of risk factors should be screened under the supervision of an audiologist prior to three months of age but no later than six months after birth:

1. Family history of childhood hearing impairment.

2. Congenital perinatal infection (e.g., cytomegalovirus, herpes, rubella, toxoplasmosis, syphilis).

3. Anatomical malformations involving the head or neck (e.g., dysmorphic appearance, including syndromal and nonsyndromal abnormalities of the pinna).

4. Birth weight less than 1500 gm.

5. Hyperbilirubinemia at a level exceeding indications for exchange transfusion.

6. Bacterial meningitis, especially with *Haemophilus influenzae*.

7. Severe asphyxia that may include infants with Apgar scores of 0 to 3, infants who fail to institute spontaneous respiration by 10 min, and infants with hypotonia persisting up to two hours post partum.[31]

Lesions of the Eighth Nerve. Acoustical neurinomas account for over half of all tumors involving the cerebellopontine angle.[18] The tumor is believed to produce signs and symptoms typically between 30 and 40 years of age and older. However, with modern diagnostic techniques, the identification of these tumors can be made at an early age, and it is not unusual for these conditions to be diagnosed in the second decade of life.

The usual site of origin of an acoustical tumor is the vestibular portion of the eighth cranial nerve in the region of Scarpa's ganglion. These tumors are believed to originate frequently in the internal auditory canal. They enlarge slowly within the canal and can produce bone erosion extending toward the cerebellopontine angle. The initial symptoms of these tumors are hearing impairment, unsteadiness of gait, and tinnitus. Tinnitus typically develops in association with hearing impairment but can be the only presenting symptom. Patients may report only a distortion or alteration of the quality of sound in the affected side (especially noticeable when using a telephone), with no significant impairment in hearing sensitivity. Abnormal tone decay and abnormalities of the stapedial reflex are often present. Dizziness in the form of an unsteadiness occurs as an early symptom in about 80 per cent of patients. True vertigo is less common, occurring in about a third of patients, but may become a significant symptom as the tumor enlarges. Other early complaints are a prickling sensation, an itching sensation, pain in the affected ear, and difficulty understanding speech.

Diagnostic evaluation of these conditions includes an audiological battery with tests for abnormal auditory adaptation and brain stem evoked-response audiometry, vestibular evaluation using electronystagmography, neuroradiological studies using CT screening with contrast media and magnetic resonance imaging (MRI) and posterior fossa myelography with contrast media when the suspicion of a tumor is high. Abnormalities in the stapedial reflex are found in 83 to 85 per cent of acoustical tumors. However, brain stem evoked-response audiometry is believed to be the most accurate audiological method of identifying tumors, with a reported success rate of 95 to 98 per cent. It is important to note that audiological site of lesion studies cannot determine the *nature* of the lesion at this stage, although the *site* of the lesion is correctly identified in an impressive percentage of patients. Degenerative, inflammatory, and vascular lesions of the eighth nerve often show a constellation of audiological responses identical to those found in space-occupying lesions of the eighth nerve.

Persons with Exaggerated Hearing Levels. Emotionally based hearing problems are of two types: psychogenic and malingering. *Psychogenic deafness* is a form of conversion hysteria in which a serious emotional problem is converted into an apparent inability to hear. *Volitional hearing impairment* or *malingering* is a conscious simulation of hearing loss on the part of an individual who wishes to convince the examiner that the hearing problem is greater than is actually the case. The wide variety of tests used for the detection of these conditions (also referred to as *nonorganic* or *functional* hearing impairments or *pseudohypacusis*) include various forms of electrophysiological audiometry, such as brain stem evoked-response audiometry, that do not involve any voluntary response on the part of the patient under evaluation.

Central Auditory Impairments. Central auditory impairments result from lesions affecting the brain stem pathway in the lateral lemniscus and the primary auditory project area on the superior temporal gyri of the temporal cortex (Heschl's gyrus). In general, tests of auditory function that are used in the evaluation of peripheral auditory disorders are useless in the demonstration of a central auditory lesion. Patients with unilateral temporal lobe disease typically show a deficit in understanding distorted speech on the ear contralateral to the affected temporal lobe. Tests for central auditory lesions involve a variety of frequency-distorted word tests, speech in the presence of a competing message presented either ipsilaterally or contralaterally, periodically interrupted speech stimuli, and other methods of reducing the external redundancy of the speech message.[5, 33, 50]

Tinnitus

Tinnitus is a subjective sensation of sound in the head that may be localized in one or both ears or perceived in the cranial area. It may be described as a throbbing, hissing, whistling, booming, clicking, buzzing, roaring, or high-pitched tone or as noise. Tinnitus may result from an auditory impairment in any location within the auditory pathway. It may have a vascular, muscular, or hormonal origin. Any disease or injury capable of affecting the auditory system may be accompanied by tinnitus.

Tinnitus is believed to affect over 37 million Americans. For some 6 to 7 million of these individuals, tinnitus may be as disabling as a hearing loss or more so. Desperate sufferers have submitted to a variety of surgical procedures that sometimes involve sacrificing the hearing of the affected ear, and some patients have not obtained relief of tinnitus even after such destructive procedures have been performed, suggesting a central rather than a peripheral basis for the symptom. Suicides and suicide attempts have been reported in some tinnitus sufferers unable to obtain relief from the condition.

Occasionally, tinnitus is objective and can be heard by the examiner. Among the reported causes of objective tinnitus are palatal myoclonus, tensor-tympani or stapedial myoclonus, and an abnormally patent eustachian tube. Vascular abnormalities can also cause objective tinnitus and include arteriovenous fistulas and hemangiomas of the external ear. A plaque in the internal carotid artery may also cause this condition. It is *subjective tinnitus,* also called static, nonvibratory, or intrinsic tinnitus, that accounts by far for the largest number of patients suffering from the condition.

Tinnitus is a symptom that may reflect a wide array of otic and auditory problems, many of which are treatable or controllable by medical, surgical, and rehabilitative measures. All patients complaining of this condition should receive a complete diagnostic evaluation, including a careful case history, physical examination, audiological site of lesion studies, and, when indicated, neuroradiography and vestibular studies.

A large number of patients have disabling tinnitus related to noise exposure, head injury, or ototoxic medication. Some patients obtain relief by medical management. Vasodilators, histamine, large doses of vitamin A, xylocaine, and carbamazepine (Tegretol) are among the substances that have been tried, with generally discouraging results. Patients who are borderline hearing-aid candidates may obtain relief from a hearing aid that masks the tinnitus when the instrument is in use. The hearing aid should be used in the ear in which the tinnitus is more severe, and binaural aids should be considered for patients with bilateral tinnitus.

Biofeedback and tinnitus maskers are now employed for some patients with intractable tinnitus unresponsive to other therapies. Biofeedback seeks to achieve muscle relaxation and increased circulation.[28] An electromyographic device allows the patient to experience the electrical output of the frontalis muscle by viewing a voltmeter and listening to clicks relayed to him or her by earphones. The peripheral vasculature is dilated by raising the temperature of the finger. Some patients can learn muscle relaxation in 12 one-hour visits. Biofeedback appears to be most useful in patients who are extremely anxious about the condition. Tension appears to exacerbate the patient's perception of the tinnitus, causing it to become subjectively louder. When the patient learns to relax physically, it is hoped, the patient is able to reduce the apprehension and tension and achieve greater control of his or her response to the problem.

Tinnitus maskers are usually built into either a postauricular or an all in the ear housing. The object is to mask the patient's tinnitus with a band of white noise.[51] A volume control allows the patient to adjust the gain of the instrument to a level that just masks the tinnitus. The majority of tinnitus sufferers match their tinnitus with a frequency of 2000 Hz or higher. The tinnitus masker is a relatively innocuous, noninvasive method of providing relief from this condition and should be considered for patients whose auditory problems have been comprehensively evaluated by competent specialists who have ruled out significant organic and psychological pathology. Double-blind studies are necessary to determine whether or not the masker provides significant improvement rather than a distraction or a placebo effect. Long-term follow-up of patients using the maskers is essential to determine persistence of the benefits and any as-yet-unknown side effects. As yet, no significant adverse effects on residual hearing have been reported; nonetheless, hearing should be

JEROME D. SCHEIN AND MAURICE H. MILLER

closely monitored audiologically in patients using tinnitus maskers.

Another approach designed to provide relief for persons with severe, disabling tinnitus is *external electrical stimulation*. One such device uses two generators, one producing a low radiofrequency carrier signal that easily penetrates the skin and the other a sweep-frequency sine wave whose output modulates the carrier signal. The combined electrical signal is delivered by two electrodes placed on the skin over the mastoid bone. The patient applies the external electrical stimulation at home on a cumulative, progressive time schedule. Success rates reported by different investigators vary widely, and no double-blind studies have been made. At present, these devices are not available in the United States.[78, 79]

Additional Disabilities

The patient's presenting complaint, hearing impairment, or deformity of the ears may so occupy the rehabilitator's attention that secondary disabilities are overlooked. Yet these additional problems are often critical factors in the patient's rehabilitation. Another disability tends to multiply, rather than add to, the problems of hearing loss. As a rule, the presence of a hearing impairment raises the probability of another disability. Among deaf school children, for example, about one in three has an additional educationally handicapping condition.[62] Similar findings emerge in studies of hearing-impaired adults. Of critical importance is whether or not the patient's visual functioning is intact. The more impaired the individual's hearing, the more dependent he or she becomes on vision.[66] Planning for auditory rehabilitation must take into account all of a patient's limitations and assets, and hearing ability should not be viewed as an isolated factor.

Treatment of Hearing Impairment

Treatment of hearing impairment depends generally on three factors: type of loss (conductive, sensorineural, or mixed), degree, and age at onset. Available treatments, in turn, fall into three large categories: surgical-medical intervention, corrective amplification, and education. These treatments often overlap, of course, with patients receiving two or more procedures from among these broad categories. The management of hearing impairment should also include counseling at every stage. Because of the ubiquitous need for it, counseling is alluded to in each section.

Surgical-Medical Intervention

Conductive losses are generally amenable to medical and/or surgical management of impairment. The degree of conductive impairment and the status of the patient's bone conduction and speech discrimination influence the decision to operate. However, the age at onset does not, except for some elderly persons with serious medical problems. Regardless of how long or short the duration of the loss, its reversal is considered worthwhile. Procedures range from repair and reconstruction of the tympanic membrane (*myringoplasty*) to replacement of the ossicles. In some instances, plastic surgery on the outer ear may be indicated to construct an absent pinna or otological surgery may be required to open the external canal. The vastly increased ability to surgically correct conductive hearing problems reinforces the value of prompt, accurate diagnosis. Mixed losses do not result in the same degree of hearing recovery that conductive losses do. Nonetheless, consideration should be given to removing the conductive component of the loss, thus restoring a portion of the hearing ability.

Many eighth-nerve tumors are surgically removed and, depending on the surgical route employed, hearing may be preserved. However, hearing preservation may not be the primary objective of such procedures. Various surgical procedures are employed by some otologists for patients with Ménière's disease, but the primary objective in these cases is relief from intractable vertigo. The extent to which surgery improves hearing is controversial. Prevention is critical in the case of noise-induced hearing loss, ototoxicity, and prenatal rubella, but medical-surgical treatment is of little avail for conditions such as presbycusis. (Inner-ear surgery to improve hearing is not provided by most otologists; however, see the section discussed later on cochlear implants, a procedure now being used.)

In addition to surgery, medication, and related tactics, complete management should include counseling directed at the patient's adjustment to the emotional impact accompanying sensory impairment and preparing the patient to accept limitations and overcome handicaps that remain after treatment (see earlier). In particular, patients should be given an opportunity to realistically appraise their condition and any therapeutic limitations.

The Cochlear Implant

The object of the cochlear implant is to provide hearing in a deaf ear by electrical stimulation of the auditory nerve. Efforts have been directed at implanting one or more electrodes permanently in the cochlea of patients with no residual hearing. The indwelling prosthesis connected to an external transducer is designed to deliver electrical stimuli to remaining nerve fibers and to provide selective stimulation, related to acoustical frequency, for different nerve fibers through multiple electrodes—a goal that has not yet been successfully achieved. Implants in use in the United States employ either single or multiple intracochlear electrodes. One or more fine-wired electrodes are introduced through the round window or through holes drilled into the scala tympani. Intensity discrimination in implanted individuals is usually good, but frequency discrimination is often poor. Controversy surrounds the evaluation of patients with implants, with questions largely about how effectively they learn to understand connected discourse without visual cues. Less debate is attached to claims that patients with implants tend to improve their lipreading when the implant signals *supplement* visual cues. Most patients learn to recognize familiar environmental sound, and most appreciate the auditory contact they regain with the implant.

At this time, the use of cochlear implants is a therapeutic option for selected patients with profound sensorineural hearing losses. Some implant subjects are initially pleased by their ability to detect certain sounds but later become frustrated by their inability to discriminate speech. Others report satisfaction extending over years. Candidates for implants should be adults with adventitious hearing loss, no measurable residual hearing, and the inability to benefit from available hearing aids. Only patients with sensory rather than neural deficits should be considered. Candidates should be told to expect some improvements in auditory awareness and gross discrimination but not in speech discrimination. The human cochlea contains 25,000 to 30,000 nerve fibers working together to allow the auditory discriminations necessary for normal function. We are not yet near

the point at which this system can be reproduced with a cochlear prosthesis. Special, intensive audiological rehabilitation is indicated for patients with implants.

To implant or not to implant stirs the greatest controversy when the subjects of the question are children. Introducing an electrode into the cochlea possibly causes damage to residual hearing that is irreversible.[27] Extracochlear implants that are placed on the medial wall of the middle-ear cavity might yield results equal to or better than those achieved with an intracochlear implant, and they would have the likely advantage of not damaging viable intracochlear neurons and not promoting bone growth in the otic capsule. Comparative studies of children with implants and those fitted with high-quality conventional amplification or sophisticated multichannel, portable tactile aids have not been conducted as yet. It may be that the quality and intensity of the audiological rehabilitation children receive contribute more to their progress rather than the particular devices used.

Such information is difficult to impart to parents whose children are threatened by deafness and who are encouraged by popular accounts of "bionic hearing aids." In assisting them to reach a decision, the auditory rehabilitationist must undertake an intensive investigation of the child's hearing, searching for residual auditory capacity. Testing should be repeated until no doubts remain as to the nature of the child's hearing status. Then appropriate trials with other treatment options should be made before electing the irreversible consequences of the implant.

In our judgment, the present state of the art requires that no child undergo implant surgery unless she or he can be given extensive postimplant rehabilitation. The evidence so far suggests that the success of implantation, in children as in adults, depends more heavily upon the rehabilitation program than upon the type of implant.

Hearing Aids

The hearing aid is the major tool of audiological rehabilitation and should be considered for all persons with medically irreversible forms of hearing impairment. A hearing aid is any device that brings sound more effectively to the ear of the listener and, by this broad definition, includes the ear trumpet, the hand cupped behind the ear, and the acoustical fan.

With rapid development of various forms of

JEROME D. SCHEIN AND MAURICE H. MILLER

electroacoustical amplification, few persons with hearing impairments seriously consider the non-electronic forms. Microminiaturized transistor circuits allow us to present speech at a comfortable and tolerable level to virtually all hearing-impaired persons, except to those with profoundly impaired speech discrimination and no measurable hearing responses. Persons whose hearing impairment is too severe to enable them to comprehend speech may still benefit from amplification sufficient for detection of low-frequency components of some of the vowels as well as nonspeech sounds, thus improving contact with their auditory environment and providing clues that can aid speechreading.

Many persons with borderline auditory problems who would not have accepted a body-mounted hearing aid (Fig. 44–9) now derive significant benefit from small, easily carried hearing aids mounted entirely in or near the ear and used for selected listening situations. Because of improvements in hearing-aid design during the last 20 years, virtually all individuals with any degree of significant difficulty in social or professional listening situations can derive substantial benefit from ear-level amplification. Increasingly, audiologists reject the classic indications for hearing-aid candidacy (a pure-tone average of 40 dB or more in the better ear) and evaluate suitable forms of wearable amplification for *all* persons reporting difficulty in listening situations important to their daily lives.[39]

All hearing aids have the following basic components: a microphone that converts sound into electrical energy, an amplifier that increases the strength of the electrical signal, and a receiver or an earphone that converts the amplified signal back into acoustical energy. The system is energized by a battery. The output may be fed into either an air-conduction receiver or a bone-conduction vibrator.

The basic types of electroacoustical hearing aids are described in the following sections.

Behind the Ear or Postauricular Hearing Aid. This type of instrument accounts for about 20 per cent of hearing aids purchased today and is shown in Figure 44–10. Postauricular hearing aids do not interfere with the wearing of eyeglasses, so the hearing aid can be used with or without spectacles, an advantage for persons whose use of hearing aids and eyeglasses does not coincide. Figure 44–11 pictures an *eyeglass* hearing aid in which the amplifier, microphone, and receiver are built into the temple of the spectacles.

All in the Ear Hearing Aids. These hearing aids have grown in popularity enormously in recent years and now account for over 70 per cent of new hearing aids purchased (Fig. 44–12). A form of in the ear hearing aid is the canal type. This is the smallest of the existing forms of wearable amplification and fits entirely in the external auditory meatus (Fig. 44–13). Improvements in design significantly reduce the problems of acoustical feedback, expand the frequency response, reduce distortion, and allow the incorporation of features formerly available only with larger instruments, e.g., compression circuits to limit the saturation sound-pressure level of the instrument.

Body-worn Hearing Aids. These were the predominant method of mounting hearing aids in the pretransistorized era, but they have shown a sharp

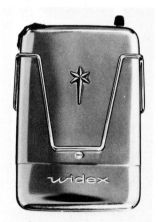

FIGURE 44–9. A body-mounted hearing aid.

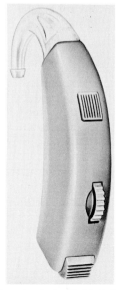

FIGURE 44–10. A postauricular (behind-the-ear) hearing aid.

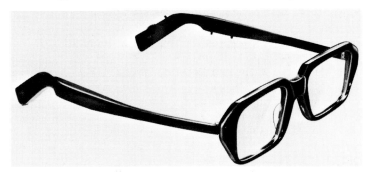

FIGURE 44–11. An eyeglass hearing aid.

decrease in popularity and now account for only 2 to 3 per cent of hearing aids purchased (see Fig. 44–9). The decline in the use of these instruments has paralleled the improved performance of ear-level aids. True binaural hearing is not possible with body-mounted hearing aids, one of a number of advantages of mounting the entire instrument in or near the ear. Other disadvantages of the body-type aid are the noise that results from layers of clothing rubbing against the microphone and the awkward position required for use of the telephone with this type of instrument.

In terms of its functions, the hearing aid must also have the following characteristics:

Gain. A hearing aid must provide sufficient amplification to compensate for the degree of hearing loss present. The gain of an amplifying system refers to the difference between the input (microphone) and output (receiver) of the system.

Output. Output is the level of the input signal plus the gain of the hearing aid. *Maximal output* or *saturation sound-pressure level* refers to the maximal power-handling capacity of the aid. Every amplifying system must impose a restriction on the strength of the signal delivered by the hearing aid so that the user's tolerance level for loud sounds

is not exceeded. Maximal output must be achieved without excessively distorting the speech signal. *Peak clipping* (eliminating the crests of sound waves) has traditionally been used to achieve output control, but this is often accomplished at the sacrifice of speech intelligibility, particularly when only the positive portion of the sound waves is clipped. Various forms of compression amplification are now available in which the gain of the hearing aid is automatically reduced when the intensity of the input signal reaches a predetermined level. Time constants must be carefully specified to prevent degradation of the speech signal and a "flutter" or "thump" sound in the system. Careful selection of the appropriate maximal-output levels represents a critical factor in determining successful adjustment to a hearing aid, especially in hearing-impaired persons with *recruitment* (an abnormal increase of the loudness of the sound as its intensity is raised above the impaired threshold) and a restricted range of comfortable loudness. Patients who are "overfit" will find the hearing aid an unpleasant and uncomfortable experience. The recognition of the significance of this factor in affecting hearing-aid performance and the conduction of tests of tolerance as part of

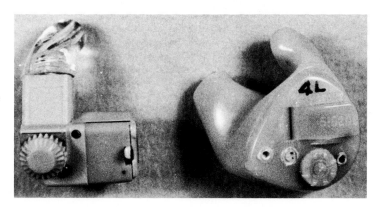

FIGURE 44–12. Two types of in-the-ear hearing aids.

JEROME D. SCHEIN AND MAURICE H. MILLER

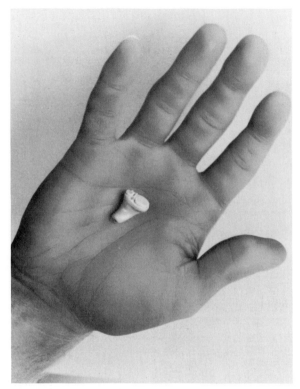

FIGURE 44–13. An in-the-canal hearing aid. (Courtesy of Argosy Electronics, Inc.)

the hearing-aid evaluation has led to successful use of hearing aids by many previously "unfittable" patients.

Frequency Response. Frequency response refers to the range of frequencies that a particular hearing aid amplifies. The microphone generally limits the low-frequency response of the system, whereas the receiver limits the high-frequency response. There is a strong relationship between the high-frequency response of the hearing aid and the user's ability to discriminate speech in quiet and in noise. Since frequencies over 1000 Hz contribute 60 per cent of the intelligibility of speech (but account for only 5 per cent of total power), excessive amplification in the low frequencies can mask the weak consonant sounds and adversely affect the understanding of speech. Furthermore, many hearing-aid users have relatively good unaided hearing for low frequencies and require less amplification in this portion of the range. Appropriate modification of the frequency response so that greater amplification is provided in the high-frequency range (through 6000 to 7000 Hz, when indicated) is, second only to proper control of maximal output, the most important determinant of successful hearing-aid use.

Distortion. Distortion occurs when the output of an amplifying system is not a faithful reproduction of the input signal. All amplifying systems distort to some extent and the relatively low fidelity of portable hearing aids tends to produce significant distortion. To add to the problem, current hearing-aid users are invariably persons with some form of sensorineural hearing loss for whom even low levels of distortion may be unacceptable.

In the field of audiology, most attention has been directed to *harmonic distortion.* This occurs when signals other than the input are produced at the output. When a tone of 1000 Hz is introduced into a hearing-aid microphone, other frequencies, such as 2000 and 3000 Hz, which are integral multiples of the basic frequency, may occur at the output. *Intermodulation distortion* occurs when the output contains a greater number of components than the input. These frequencies are arithmetic sums and differences of two or more frequencies. *Transient distortion* is present whenever the hearing aid is unable to duplicate accurately the initial onset or sudden decay of a sound. The result is a "lingering" of the wave form, causing a ringing sound. Many speech sounds such as /p/ and /k/ are transient in nature, and the ringing referred to can seriously hamper speech discrimination. Transient distortion, which appears related to the presence of sharp resonant peaks in the frequency response, is probably a critical factor in the ability of persons with sensorineural hearing loss to discriminate speech in noise. Unfortunately, current hearing-aid standards do not specify the conditions for measurement of this form of distortion, and manufacturers generally do not include transient distortion data in their specifications.

New Developments in Hearing Aids. A detailed discussion of the various developments in hearing aids is beyond the scope of this chapter, and the reader is urged to consult one or more of the excellent references on the subject.[4, 8, 51] Among these advances are directional microphones, the electret condensor microphone, various sophisticated output-limiting circuits, and open earmolds. Hearing aids that pick up a signal from the side of a poorly or nonfunctioning ear and reroute it to the side of the ear with better hearing (Contralateral Routing of Signals, or CROS, aids) have been developed in an almost endless number of variations, providing great assistance for persons with audiograms characterized by precipitous high-frequency dropoffs as well as those with other hard-to-fit configurations. Wearable, ear-level, binaural hearing aids are available and are in widespread use by many hearing-impaired persons, including pre-lingually hearing-impaired children and blind-deaf persons. Their use should be evaluated by audiologists who can make appropriate selections in relation to specific audiological manifestations and in carefully controlled sound-field evaluations with different systems. Hearing aids should always be evaluated both in a quiet and in noisy environments; the signal-to-noise ratios should simulate those the patient will be likely to encounter in everyday listening.

An impending revolutionary advance in wearable amplification will be made by the introduction of *digital hearing aids.* Controlled by a microprocessor, these new devices automatically adapt to the auditory environment, discriminating speech and noise on an ongoing basis. By identifying the frequency range that the noise occupies, it can tune itself to reduce that noise and enhance the speech signal. This feature of digital hearing aids answers the most frequently voiced complaint of hearing-aid users: difficulty understanding speech in noisy surroundings. Unlike conventional hearing aids, the digital instruments do not amplify all signals, wanted and unwanted, simply because of sound-pressure level and proximity to the microphone. These "smart" hearing aids promise a new era in auditory rehabilitation.[23]

Management of the Sensorineural Hearing-Impaired Patient. After a complete diagnostic evaluation has been done and the patient's sensorineural hearing impairment is established as medically irreversible, the audiologist is a key professional in meeting the patient's audiological rehabilitative needs. Under controlled conditions, the audiologist determines first whether or not the use of a hearing aid is justified. If such indication is established, the audiologist will, through tests of aided performance in properly sound-isolated environments, seek the answers to a series of important clinical questions. On which ear should the hearing aid be used, or should the aid be alternated from one ear to the other? Is a binaural hearing aid indicated? Air conduction or bone conduction? Earmold type? Special circuit modifications? In one widely used system of hearing-aid evaluation, the specialist will then select from representative samples of current hearing aids several that are appropriate for the type and degree of hearing loss present. On the basis of the patient's performance with these instruments in a *hearing-aid evaluation,* the audiologist will recommend an amplifying system that meets the needs of the patient. He or she will either sell the hearing aid to the patient or

refer the patient to a reliable hearing-aid dealer in the patient's community. The subtle interactions between the many varieties of impaired hearing and the multiple forms and characteristics of currently available hearing aids strongly indicates that audiologists who sell their own hearing aids, rather than hearing-aid merchants, will best serve these patients. Follow-up services after the hearing aid is obtained are critical to the overall success of the rehabilitation process and should be arranged when the aid is acquired.[24, 52]

Emotional Impact

The rehabilitator who ignores the emotional impact of hearing loss cannot hope to be optimally effective. Wright[89] has illuminated the natural history of any acquired physical disability: from initial shock to mourning to revised values and eventual positive adjustment. At each phase, the rehabilitator has an important role to play. Most important, the rehabilitator must be aware of any tendencies to pass over or move too quickly through any phase. Wright's thesis, supported by subsequent research, is that the phases are *natural*; newly disabled persons need to go through them and resolve the powerful emotions aroused at each step. An important task of rehabilitators, in addition to implementing the technical knowledge at their command, is to assist the patient to gain emotional acceptance of the new status imposed by the impairment. Without that acceptance, rehabilitation will be impeded.[55, 77]

Dealing with the emotional concomitants of acquired physical disability may require skills beyond those the rehabilitator has acquired. In such instances, competent psychiatric and psychological assistance should be sought. Counseling or psychotherapy may be conducted in one-to-one, group, or a combination of individual and group sessions.[66] It may precede other therapeutic intervention, follow it, or be coincident with it. Even if the rehabilitator manages the counseling personally, consultation with mental health experts may prove to be a valuable therapeutic adjunct.

What about congenital hearing impairments? The gradual awareness that typically occurs tends to cushion the emotional shock for the born-deaf and pre-lingually deafened child. That is not true, however, for parents who are told that their young child is deaf.[42] For them, it is a shock. Parental counseling should be routinely offered to parents who receive such information. They will tend to

JEROME D. SCHEIN AND MAURICE H. MILLER

pass through the same phases mentioned earlier, even though their child, not they, has suffered the loss. Attempting to undertake education and rehabilitation of young children without first attending to the parents' emotional adjustment will prove partially, if not wholly, ineffective.[71] Parents frequently report that they heard nothing the professional said after giving them the child's diagnosis, despite vigorous efforts on the practitioner's part to inform them about critical next steps in treatment.

Most unfortunate are parents who have been told of their child's deafness by a diagnostician whose entire demeanor suggests a death sentence rather than a diagnosis. Equally incongruous is being cheerful when confronting parents with what they regard as very bad news. The appropriate attitude might best be characterized as *understanding* and *hopeful*—understanding of the parent's bitter feelings and hopeful about the child's future.[42] Above all, the practitioner must recognize the function of time. Parental adjustment will not be instantaneous even in the most competent practitioner's hands. Some time is essential for recovery from depression, working through of anger, and resolving the value hierarchy they have acquired over years. How much is needed will vary from person to person. The practitioner must monitor the reactions, set aside or provide time for counseling, and in these ways assist the clients and parents to acquire facilitating attitudes toward their own or their child's rehabilitation. If an emotional disorder co-exists with a hearing impairment, it will require the special skills of psychologists and psychiatrists in its management. Hearing impairment and psychosis may be present in such disorders as prenatal rubella.

Auditory Training

After the aid has been selected, the audiologist will schedule a series of visits to work with the patient on initial adjustment to the hearing aid. Trial or rental periods are often arranged so that the hearing aid can be returned with a minimum of expense to the patient if a satisfactory level of performance cannot be achieved. An extended period of audiological rehabilitation will be necessary for some individuals. Patients with very poor discrimination, excessive recruitment, and a narrow dynamic range should not be issued a hearing aid unless first enrolled in an extensive audiological rehabilitative program in which adjustment to various amplifying systems is carefully monitored (see earlier discussion of phonemic regression). Systematic training in speech discrimination in various listening situations will be necessary for many persons with sensorineural hearing impairments. For others, acceptance of and adjustment to hearing aids are realized early.

The hearing-aid user should be counseled about the limitations of amplification in relation to his or her particular auditory problems and needs. The patient's concerns and fears about the hearing loss and its interaction with the hearing aid must be managed with consummate professional skill. The initial fear that many persons feel about using an electronic apparatus must be confronted. The loss of manual dexterity, particularly among elderly persons, affects their ability to manipulate the small controls of the hearing aid, to change the battery, and to insert the earmold into the ear. These seemingly simple mechanical operations must be demonstrated to them over and over again, with support and assistance offered until success is finally achieved. The audiologist's role in the patient's acceptance of and adjustment to amplification and his or her ability to improve receptive listening skills through special training are potent determinants of the successful use of hearing aids. In a very real sense, the audiologist's responsibility to the hearing-impaired patient *begins* on the day when the patient obtains the recommended hearing aid.

Other Assistive Devices

Hearing impairments diminish or eliminate the ability to use telecommunications. Also, hearing losses affect many everyday activities that involve devices that emit auditory signals. Recently, means have been developed to surmount auditory barriers to using the telephone and to enjoying television,[69] as well as to compensate for hearing loss in other mundane activities.

Telephone Adaptation Devices. Telephone adaptation devices for deaf people send audible signals over the telephone lines to machines at the receiving end, which convert the signals to visible form. At present, there are a half dozen versions. Each has a keyboard, a coupler that attaches to the telephone mouthpiece, and a message display. The machines differ in size, portability, type of keyboard, and display. They are important to deaf people, because they provide easy access to facilities not otherwise possible. Deaf people, of course, can make telephone calls through interpreters, friends, and relatives. Telephone adaptation devices give deaf people added independence and increased employability. As more and more telephone adaptation devices come into being, the social and economic disadvantages the telephone imposes on deaf people will be lifted.[60]

Captioned Television. Since early 1980, many television programs have carried *captions*—printed versions of the spoken transmission. The captions are "hidden;" i.e., they are broadcast over the vertical blanking interval (line 21 on American television sets), so they are seen only on sets equipped with a special decoder. Organizations interested in hearing-impaired people, particularly the National Association of the Deaf, have fought vigorously to win this concession from the television industry. Captioned television helps alleviate the social isolation caused by severe hearing impairment.[64]

Home Appliances. Appliances can usually be fitted with light-signaling adaptations to replace the auditory signal. The doorbell can be wired so that when it is rung it flashes the lights in any or all rooms in the house. Alarm clocks can turn on lights or activate a vibrator placed under the deaf person's pillow. The National Association of the Deaf (814 Thayer Avenue, Silver Spring, MD, 20910) issues a catalogue describing a variety of these and other pieces of equipment for the deaf householder. Merely knowing such devices are available can give the newly hearing-impaired person a psychological boost, for their abundance and ready availability indicate that many people share the same problem.

Education and Training

Loss of hearing confers no compensatory gains on the afflicted individual. What must be done to overcome the disability must be learned. The task of the rehabilitator is to teach the adaptive means for coping with the problems hearing loss engenders and for using devices, especially hearing aids and assistive listening devices, designed to compensate for the loss. Hearing aids and other adaptive devices have been discussed above, along with auditory training. What follows are educational strategies for living with a hearing loss.

Since hearing loss principally interferes with interpersonal communication, these strategies are directed toward the communication barriers and their emotional accompaniments. The age of the

individual at the time hearing is impaired heavily affects educational and rehabilitation planning. This fact is indicated with respect to each of the ensuing discussions of educational intervention.

Speech. Speech, once established, is usually not lost because of a hearing impairment, but articulation and voice quality may deteriorate in cases of progressive or sudden hearing loss.[47, 80] Early, severe hearing loss does, however, affect speech development. Pre-lingually deaf children can learn to speak well, but few currently do.[10, 34] These frequent failures, in view of the occasional successes, are more likely due to lack of adequate education than to inherent inability to acquire speech (see the section on language that follows). Readers may wrongly infer that the preceding statement unfairly condemns the valiant teachers who struggle so hard to develop deaf children's speaking abilities. Readers might alternatively assume the statement merely urges that more of the educational day be devoted specifically to developing speech. Neither position reflects our view. We recognize the awesome task of teaching speech through the use of proprioceptive, tactual, and visual clues in the absence of auditory feedback. To us, the solution to pre-lingually deaf children's present lack of success in developing more intelligible speech lies not in the amount of time expended but in the methods selected to teach speech. When success is not attained, the procedures, not the child, should be suspected, and new approaches should be sought to attain the educational objectives.[10, 34, 41] Admittedly, excellent speech development for every born-deaf child may be an overly idealistic goal for educators. However, even a little facility in speech can be useful in our highly oral culture. Socioeconomic success has been, and probably can continue to be, attained without it.[68] The development of language, however, is another matter, for we distinguish between speech (a motor ability) and language (a symbol system).[12]

For the person who becomes deaf after speech has been established, the problem becomes one of maintaining its good quality. Post-lingually deafened children must not only be encouraged to continue using their speech but they must also be given feedback to assist them with melody, rhythm, articulation, and loudness. Although less critical as age at onset increases, speech conservation retains an important place in rehabilitation of children and adults.[80] Patients need instruction on how to adjust the volume of their speech in response to extra-auditory cues, to avoid misarticu-

JEROME D. SCHEIN AND MAURICE H. MILLER

lations, and to retain normal voice quality. Retention of good speech after hearing impairment is far less difficult than developing speech without auditory feedback; however, the value of retaining this ability makes the provisions for speech conservation critical in the rehabilitation process for hearing-impaired adults.

Speechreading refers to determining what a speaker is saying by observation rather than hearing *per se.* An older term, *lipreading,* suggests that the observations are of the lips alone. However, other cues, especially situational and contextual ones, are usually critical in deciphering a particular message. For that reason, we prefer the term *speechreading,* because it implies that a broader range of stimuli are involved. That information other than lip movements is essential to speechreading is established by the disparity between the 40 or more phonemes in spoken language and the 16 discriminable shapes of the lips.[3] By observing one's own lips in a mirror while successively saying "time" and "dime" or "bare," "pair," and "mare," one quickly can grasp the speechreader's major difficulty—*homophenes*, words that look exactly or almost alike on the lips.

To what extent can speechreading be taught? Some people seem to acquire the skill readily, others not.[3, 44, 49] Since less than half the visual differentiation of speech can be determined from the principal source, the lips, the good speechreader must make use of other information. Knowledge of the language appears critical, as does familiarity with the culture. If a well-dressed stranger stops you on the street and asks, "Do you have (a dime)/(the time)?" the latter choice is the likely one. At a party, you would have little difficulty choosing the correct choice from among "Do you want a (bear)/(mare)/(pair)/(beer)?" Of the four homophenes, the last has the highest probability in the circumstances. Making use of cultural-linguistic cues is easier for the person who loses hearing later in life than for the born-deaf person. The former has more exposure to language and generally more acquaintance with the culture. That is why, contrary to popular belief, normally hearing adults, as a group, are better speechreaders than the average pre-lingually deaf person.

Prospective speechreaders can be taught to make use of their residual hearing. They need to be alerted to variations in speech rhythms and to ways of combining visual information with whatever auditory information they can perceive. In addition, they can learn to imitate what they see in order to make use of proprioception. Such instruc-

tion can bolster the speechreader's confidence, another major factor. Good speechreaders appear to be good linguistic gamblers; they bet on the most likely outcome. When subsequent reactions indicate it, they must also be willing to drop an apparently poor guess and make another.

Sharpening visual perception and sensitizing the speechreader to language nuances can be achieved in the instructional setting. The personality qualities contributing to speechreading may not be developed in the classroom. Some rehabilitation programs use group strategies to help speechreaders overcome their reluctance to approach a conversational situation flexibly and with minimal embarrassment. Sharing frustrations and emotional upset with similarly affected persons seems to increase many speechreaders' confidence in their eventual ability to succeed.

There are a number of methods of teaching speechreading. Each offers its own emphases, sequence of lessons, and drills.[3, 44, 49] No one method will be optimal for all persons. The speechreading instructor should have a variety of methods and materials to meet the varying needs of hearing-impaired students. Counseling must help avoid the disastrous consequences of overly high expectations. Speechreading cannot fully compensate for a hearing loss. The hearing-impaired person who continually finds that the precise information is not being received may feel depressed by his or her own inadequacy. The person must understand that the process itself is not wholly adequate; it is a good supplement but a limited one. Understanding the limitations of speechreading will add to, not subtract from, its usefulness.

Language. Language deficits are common among pre-lingually deaf persons. On standardized tests of English, the average deaf 18-year-old student scores at about a fourth-grade level—a score indicating virtual illiteracy.[56] The extent of the language deficit correlates with age at onset, as well as degree, of hearing impairment. As noted above, even relatively mild losses of hearing may give rise to academic retardation.

Linguists now recognize that American Sign Language (Ameslan), used by most early deafened adults, meets all the criteria for a language.[61] As will be discussed next, the language deficit found among early deafened persons is an English-language deficit. The same individuals may be fluent in Ameslan. Thus, their language deficiency, as with their speech defects, may be due more to inadequate educational strategies than to any inherent weakness in learning potential. Indeed, considerable ancillary evidence supports this conclusion.[41] Most instruction in public schools is auditory; instruction by visual means has not received the same attention from educators.

The language deficits associated with early hearing impairments call for special education. Where to provide this education—in residential schools, day schools, special classes, or regular classes and resource rooms—depends upon many factors: the child, the family, and available community resources.[7] Regardless of where it is given, special attention to language is critical to the academic development of deaf children.

Manual Communication. A great deal of emotion has clouded the consideration of manual communication in rehabilitation. "Talking with one's hands" has negative connotations in our culture. Manual communication, however, has undeniable advantages for some profoundly hearing-impaired persons. It requires no special equipment. It is entirely visual. Anything that can be expressed through speech can be expressed manually.

Manual communication basically takes two forms in the United States: Manual English and Ameslan. Manual English has a number of variations, but they all present English on the hands. *Fingerspelling* is a special type of Manual English: it represents each letter of the alphabet with a distinct hand configuration To communicate by fingerspelling, one spells each word letter by letter. Almost all manual communicators make some use of fingerspelling, whether or not they also use signs; it is useful at least to indicate proper names.

Signs are hand-motion configurations that represent concepts. In Manual English signs generally stand for words. Signs in Manual English follow English syntax. In the most elaborate forms of Manual English, the appropriate linguistic forms are differentiated by adding signs for the suffixes.[61]

Ameslan does not follow English syntax. A single sign may represent a fairly complex thought, i.e., be appropriately translated by an English phrase or sentence.[61] The nature of Ameslan probably grows from its visual, as opposed to English's auditory, mode of presentation. It is likely that Ameslan suits the visual information-processing system as English does the auditory system.

To learn Ameslan requires as much involvement as learning any other language. Acquiring proficiency in Manual English is less demanding. For adults with late-onset deafness, Manual English is probably preferable to Ameslan, because it closely resembles their native language. As with any language, Ameslan has its dialects. These occur as frequently and are as distinct as American English dialects in this country. Furthermore, Ameslan is not taught in schools and classes for deaf children. It is passed from person to person with all the possibilities for variation that attend an unwritten language that is not formally taught. This situation, however, is about to change as educators and linguists take more interest in it. Notational systems are coming into use, grammars are being written, and curricula are being prepared for Ameslan.[61]

The rehabilitator should properly conclude from the preceding discussion that deaf clients will not necessarily know sign and that, if they do know sign, they will not necessarily understand all varieties of sign. Because the Rehabilitation Act Amendments of 1978 (P.L. 95–602) require that all rehabilitation personnel communicate with the client "in his own language or preferred mode of communication," interpreters will be called upon more frequently to assist in the rehabilitation process. *Manual interpreters* who are properly qualified know several forms of Manual English and Ameslan and are adept at determining the client's communication preferences. Rehabilitation personnel who are not proficient in manual communication and who have deaf clients will need to learn how to use interpreters effectively. A good beginning will be made with the realization that employing an interpreter introduces a new element in rehabilitation and that teamwork will be enhanced by consultation with the interpreter before the client is seen. In that way, many problems can be avoided, and the client-interpreter-rehabilitator interaction can be smoothed.[58]

The Self-Help Movement

Beginning in 1980, a new element entered the rehabilitation of hearing-impaired people: the development of self-help groups. Foremost among these new organizations is Self Help for Hard of Hearing People, Inc., whose chosen acronym is SHHH. Begun by a severely hearing-impaired, ex-CIA agent, Harold E. Stone, Self Help for the Hard of Hearing, Inc., has grown rapidly in less than a decade into a national organization with over 25,000 members, a bimonthly magazine, and a national headquarters: 7800 Wisconsin Avenue, Bethesda, MD 20814. It also has affiliate chapters in several foreign countries. As a self-help organization, Self Help for the Hard of Hearing, Inc., bases its actions on the principle that hearing-impaired persons should first seek, through individual and group actions, to help themselves before they turn to government and voluntary agencies for assistance. The organization is important to auditory rehabilitation. First, it is important because its meteoric growth reflects the increased prevalence of hearing impairment in the population and the greater burden imposed by hearing loss in this information age. Second, it offers auditory rehabilitators a resource for providing that scarce, but essential, ingredient in successful auditory management—counseling. Through its membership, Self Help for the Hard of Hearing, Inc., provides peer counseling as well as extensive information about assistive listening devices and other matters of particular interest to hearing-impaired people. In addition, the organization serves as a rallying point for advocates seeking improved conditions for hearing-impaired people.

References

1. Alpiner, J. G. (Ed.): Handbook of Adult Rehabilitative Audiology. Baltimore, Williams & Wilkins, 1978.
2. Bast, T. H., and Anson, B. J.: The Temporal Bone and the Ear, Springfield, Ill., Charles C Thomas, Publisher, 1949.
3. Berger, K. W.: Speechreading Principles and Methods. Baltimore, National Educational Press, 1972.
4. Berger, K. W., and Millin, J. R.: Hearing aids. In Rose, D. E. (Ed.): Audiological Assessment, 2nd Ed. Englewood Cliffs, N.J., Prentice-Hall, Inc., 1978.
5. Bolla, E., and Calearo, C.: Central hearing processes. In Jerger, J. (Ed.): Modern Developments in Audiology. New York, Academic Press, Inc., 1963.
6. Brackman, D. E., Selters, W. A., and Don, M.: Electric response audiometry. In Paparella, M., and Shumrich, D. A. (Eds.): Otolaryngology. Philadelphia, W. B. Saunders Company, 1980.
7. Brill, R. G.: The Education of the Deaf. Washington, D.C., Gallaudet College Press, 1974.
8. Briskey, R. J.: Binaural hearing aids and new innovations. In Katz, J. (Ed.): Handbook of Clinical Audiology, 2nd Ed. Baltimore, Williams & Wilkins, 1978.
9. Brunt, M. A.: Békésy audiometry and loudness balance testing. In Katz, J. (Ed.): Handbook of Clinical Audiology, 3rd Ed. Baltimore, Williams & Wilkins, 1985.
10. Calvert, D. R., and Silverman, S. R.: Speech and Deafness. Washington, D.C., A. G. Bell Association for the Deaf, 1975.
11. Crowley, D. E., Davis, H., and Beagley, H.: Clinical use of electrocochleology: A preliminary report. In Ruben, R. J., Elberling, C., and Salomon, G. (Eds.): Electrocochleology. Baltimore, University Park Press, 1976.
12. Cutting, J. E., and Kavanagh, J. F.: On the relationship of speech to language. Asha, 17:500–506, 1975.
13. Dallos, P.: The Auditory Periphery: Biophysics and Physiology. New York, Academic Press, Inc., 1973.
14. Davis, H.: Anatomy and physiology of the auditory system. In Davis, H., and Silverman, S. R. (Eds.): Hearing and Deafness, 4th Ed. New York, Holt, Rinehart and Winston, 1978.
15. Downs, M. P.: The handicap of deafness. In Northern, J. L. (Ed.): Hearing Disorders. Boston, Little, Brown and Company, 1976.
16. Durrant, J. D.: Anatomic and physiologic correlates of the effects of noise on hearing. In Lipscomb, D. M. (Ed.): Noise and Audiology. Baltimore, University Park Press, 1978.
17. English, G. M., Northern, J. L., and Fria, T. J.: Chronic otitis media as a cause of sensorineural hearing loss. Arch. Otolaryngol., 98:17–22, 1973.
18. Evans, V., and Courville, C. B.: The nervus acusticus. Pathologic conditions involving the eighth nerve and cerebello-pontine angle. Laryngoscope, 42:432–455, 1932.
19. Feldman, A. S.: Acoustic impedance admittance battery. In Katz, J. (Ed.): Handbook of Clinical Audiology, 2nd Ed. Baltimore, Williams & Wilkins, 1978.
20. Fraser, G. R.: The Causes of Profound Deafness in Childhood. Baltimore, Johns Hopkins University Press, 1976.
21. Ganzer, A. W., and Kleinmann, H.: Sensory neural hearing loss in mucous otitis. Arch. Otolaryngol., 215:91–93, 1977.
22. Gelfand, S. A.: Hearing. An Introduction to Psychological and Physiological Acoustics. New York, Marcel Dekker, 1981.
23. Graupe, D., Grosspietsch, J. K., and Taylor, R. T.: A self-adaptive noise filtering system. Hearing Instruments, 37:29–32, 1986.
24. Green, D. S.: Tone decay. In Katz, J. (Ed.): Handbook of Clinical Audiology, 3rd Ed. Baltimore, Williams & Wilkins, 1985.
25. Hodgson, W. R.: Hearing aid counseling and orientation. In Katz, J. (Ed.): Handbook of Clinical Audiology. Baltimore, Williams & Wilkins, 1978.
26. Hood, L. J., and Berlin, C. I.: Auditory evoked potentials. In Halpern, H. (Ed.): The Pro-Ed Studies in Communicative Disorders. Austin, TX, Pro-Ed, 1986.
27. House, J. W.: Effects of electrical stimulation of tinnitus. Paper given at Second International Tinnitus Seminar, New York, 1983.
28. House, J. W., Miller, L., and House, P. R.: Severe tinnitus: Treatment with biofeedback training. (Results in 41 cases.) Trans. Am. Acad. Ophthalmol. Otolaryngol., 84:697–703, 1977.
29. Jerger, J. F., and Northern, J. L. (Eds.): Clinical

Impedance Audiometry, 2nd Ed. Hudson, New Hampshire, American Electromedics Corp., 1980.

30. Jerger, J., Shedd, J., and Harford, E.: On the detection of extremely small changes in sound intensity. Arch. Otolaryngol., 69:200–211, 1959.

31. Joint Committee on Infant Hearing. 1982 statement. ASHA, 24:1017–1018, 1982.

32. Keith, R.: Central Auditory Dysfunction. New York, Grune and Stratton, 1977.

33. Kinney, S. E.: The metabolic evaluation in Ménière's disease. Otolaryngol. Head Neck Surg., 88:594–598, 1980.

34. Ling, D.: Speech and the Hearing-impaired Child: Theory and Practice. Washington, D.C., A. G. Bell Association for the Deaf, 1976.

35. Lybarger, S. F.: Earmolds. In Katz, J. (Ed.): Handbook of Clinical Audiology, 3rd Ed. Baltimore, Williams & Wilkins, 1985.

36. Margolis, R. H., and Shanks, J. E.: Tympanometry. In Harvey Halpern (Ed.): The Pro-Ed Studies in Communicative Disorders. Austin, TX, Pro-Ed, 1986.

36A. Miller, M. H.: Occupational hearing conservation. In Halpern, H. (Ed.): The Pro-Ed Studies in Communicative Disorders. Austin, TX, Pro-Ed, 1986.

37. McCandless, G. A.: Neuroelectric measures of auditory function. In Rose, D. E. (Ed.): Audiological Assessment, 2nd Ed. Englewood Cliffs, N.J., Prentice-Hall, Inc., 1978.

38. Miller, M. H.: OSHA Hearing Conservation Amendment: 1910. 95, Occupational noise exposure. In Miller, M. H. (Ed.): Occupational Hearing Conservation: State of the Art. Upper Darby, Pa., Instrumentation Associates, Inc., 1981.

39. Miller, M. H.: Hearing Aids. Indianapolis, Bobbs Merrill, 1972.

40. Miller, M. H., and Harris, J. D.: Hearing testing in industry and hearing conservation in industry. In Harris, C. M. (Ed.): Handbook of Noise Control, 2nd Ed. New York, McGraw-Hill Book Company, 1979.

41. Moores, D. F.: Educating the Deaf. Boston, Houghton Mifflin, 1978.

42. Naiman, D., and Schein, J. D.: For Parents of Deaf Children. Silver Spring, Md., National Association of the Deaf, 1978.

43. Northern, J. L., and Grimes, A. M.: Introduction to acoustic impedance. In Katz, J. (Ed.): Handbook of Clinical Audiology, 2nd Ed. Baltimore, Williams & Wilkins, 1978.

44. O'Neill, J. J., and Oyer, H. J.: Visual Communication for the Hard of Hearing. Englewood Cliffs, N.J., Prentice-Hall, Inc., 1961.

45. Paparella, M. M., and Brady, D. R.: Sensorineural hearing loss in chronic otitis media and mastoiditis. Arch. Otolaryngol. 74:108–115, 1970.

46. Paparella, M. M., and Davis, H.: Medical and surgical treatment of hearing loss. In Davis, H., and Silverman, S. R. (Ed.): Hearing and deafness, 4th Ed. New York, Holt, Rinehart and Winston, 1978.

47. Penn, J.: Voice and speech patterns with the hard of hearing. Acta Otolaryngol., Suppl. 124, 1955.

48. Penrod, J. P.: Speech discrimination testing. In Katz, J. (Ed.): Handbook of Clinical Audiology, 3rd Ed. Baltimore, Williams & Wilkins, 1985.

49. Perry, A. L., and Silverman, S. R.: Speechreading. In Davis, H., and Silverman, S. R. (Eds.): Hearing and Deafness. New York, Holt, Rinehart and Winston, 1978.

50. Pinheiro, M. L., and Musiek, F. E.: Assessment of Central Auditory Dysfunction. Foundations and Clinical Correlates. Baltimore, Williams & Wilkins, 1985.

51. Pollack, M. C.: Special applications of amplification. In Pollack, M. C. (Ed.): Amplification for the Hearing Impaired, 3rd Ed. New York, Grune and Stratton, 1987.

52. Proctor, C. A.: Abnormal insulin levels and vertigo. Laryngoscope, 91:1657–1662, 1981.

53. Pulec, J. L.: Ménière's disease. In Northern, J. L. (Ed.): Hearing Disorders. Boston, Little, Brown and Co., 1976.

54. Pulec, J. L., House, W. F., and Hughes, R. L.: Vestibular involvement and testing in acoustic neuromas. Arch. Otolaryngol., 80:677–681, 1964.

55. Ramsdell, D. A.: The psychology of the hard-of-hearing and deafened adult. In Davis, H., and Silverman, S. R. (Eds.): Hearing and Deafness, 4th Ed. New York, Holt, Rinehart and Winston, 1978.

56. Ries, P.: Further studies in achievement testing, hearing impaired students. United States; Spring 1971 Series D, No. 13, Washington, D.C., Office of Demographic Studies, Gallaudet College, 1973.

57. Sanders, D. A.: Hearing aid orientation and counseling. In Pollack, M. C. (Ed.): Amplification for the Hearing Impaired, 2nd Ed. New York, Grune and Stratton, 1980.

58. Schein, J. D.: The demography of deafness. In Higgins, P., and Nash, J. (Eds.): Understanding Deafness. Springfield, IL, Charles C Thomas, 1987.

59. Schein, J. D.: Effects of hearing loss in adults. In Alberti, P. W., and Ruben, R. J. (Eds.): Otologic Medicine and Surgery. New York, Churchill Livingstone, 1987.

60. Schein, J. D.: Telecommunications for the deaf, Inc. (TDI). In Van Cleve, J. (Ed.): Gallaudet Encyclopedia of Deaf People and Deafness. New York, McGraw-Hill, 1986.

61. Schein, J. D.: Speaking the Language of Sign. Revised. Silver Spring, MD, TJ Publishers, Inc., 1987.

62. Schein, J. D.: Multiply handicapped hearing-impaired children. In Bradford, L. J., and Hardy, W. G. (Eds.): Hearing and Hearing Impairment. New York, Grune and Stratton, 1979.

63. Schein, J. D.: Hearing disorders. In Kurland, L. T., Kurtke, J. F., and Goldberg, I. D. (Eds.): Epidemiology of Neurologic and Sense Organ Disorders. Cambridge, Mass., Harvard University Press, 1973.

64. Schein, J. D.: From zero to line 21: Closing the TV

gap for deaf viewers. J. Educ. Technol. Systems, 9(3):241–245, 1980.

65. Schein, J. D.: How well can you see me? Teaching Exceptional Children, 12:55–58, 1980.

66. Schein, J. D.: Group techniques applied to deaf and hearing-impaired persons. *In* Seligman, M. (Ed.): Group Psychotherapy and Counseling with Special Populations. Baltimore, University Park Press, 1982.

67. Schein, J. D.: Model State Plan for Rehabilitation of Deaf Clients. Silver Spring, MD., National Association of the Deaf, 1980.

68. Schein, J. D., and Delk, M. T.: The Deaf Population of the United States. Silver Spring, MD., National Association of the Deaf, 1974.

69. Schein, J. D., and Hamilton, R.: Impact 1980. Telecommunications and Deafness. Silver Spring, MD., National Association of the Deaf, 1980.

70. Schill, H. A.: Thresholds for speech. In Katz, J. (Ed.): Handbook of Clinical Audiology, 3rd Ed. Baltimore, Williams & Wilkins, 1985.

71. Schlesinger, H. S., and Meadow, F. P.: Sound and Sign. Berkeley, CA., University of California Press, 1972.

72. Schuknecht, H.: Presbycusis. Laryngology. 65:402–419, 1955.

73. Schuknecht, H.: Further observations on presbycusis. Arch. Otolaryngol., 80:369–382, 1964.

74. Schuknecht, H.: Stapedectomy. Boston, Little, Brown, 1971.

75. Shambaugh, G. E., and Wiet, R. V.: The diagnosis and evaluation of allergic disorders with food intolerance in Ménière's disease. Otolaryngol. Clin. North Am., 13(4):671–679, 1980.

76. Shambaugh, G. E., Jr., and Causse, J., Jr.: Ten years' experience with fluoride in otosclerotic (otospongiotic) patients. Ann. Otol. Rhinol. Laryngol., 83:635, 1974.

77. Shontz, F. C.: Physical disability and personality. *In* Neff, W. S. (Ed.): Rehabilitation Psychology. Washington, D.C., American Psychological Association, 1971.

78. Shulman, A.: External electrical stimulation in tinnitus control. Am. J. Otolaryngol., 6:110–115, 1985.

79. Shulman, A., Tonndorf, J., and Goldstein, B.: Electrical tinnitus control. Acta Otolaryngol., 9:318–325, 1985.

80. Silverman, S. R.: Conservation and development of speech. *In* Davis, H., and Silverman, S. R. (Eds.): Hearing and Deafness, 4th Ed. New York, Holt, Rinehart and Winston, 1978.

81. Sims, D. G.: Visual and auditory training for adults. *In* Katz, J. (Ed.): Handbook of Clinical Audiology. Baltimore, MD., Williams & Wilkins, 1978.

82. Speaks, C., and Jerger, J.: Method for measurement of speech identification. J. Speech Hear. Res., 8:185–194, 1965.

83. Stevens, S. S. (Eds.): Handbook of Experimental Psychology. New York, John Wiley and Sons, 1951.

84. Tobias, J. V. (Eds.): Foundations of Modern Auditory Theory, Vol. 1. New York, Academic Press, Inc., 1970 and 1972.

85. Von Békésy, G.: Experiments in Hearing. New York, McGraw-Hill, 1960.

86. Wever, E. G.: Theory of Hearing. New York, John Wiley and Sons, 1949.

87. Wever, E. G., and Lawrence, M.: Physiological Acoustics. Princeton University Press, 1954.

88. Wiley, T. L., and Block, M. C.: Overview and basic principles of acoustic immitance. *In* Halpern, H. (Ed.): The Pro-Ed Studies in Communicative Disorders. Austin, TX, Pro-Ed, 1986.

89. Wright, B. A.: Physical Disability—A Psychological Approach. New York, Harper and Row, 1960.

90. Yost, W. A., and Nielsen, D. W.: Fundamentals of Hearing. An Introduction. New York, Holt, Rinehart and Winston, 1977.

91. Zemlin, W. R.: Speech and Hearing Science. 2nd Ed. Englewood Cliffs, N.J., Prentice-Hall, 1981.

45

Footwear and Footwear Modifications

RITA BISTEVINS

General Considerations

Shoes consist of the upper, the sole, and, in most cases, an added heel. The material and style of each of these components contribute to the overall appearance and utility of the shoe. The commonly worn footwear styles include the oxford, pump, sandal, moccasin, tennis shoe, clog, and various types of boots (Fig. 45–1). The heel height varies from a negative heel that is lower than the forefoot position (Fig. 45–1b) to 2 or 3 inches high (Fig. 45–1c). The shoe upper is made of a flexible material—leather, woven fabrics, or synthetic materials such as urethane or vinyl. Leather is the most suitable of all available materials, as it has the ability to "breathe," is moisture absorbent, and tends to mold to the shape of the foot with wear.[19] This is not the case with most synthetic materials. Because of their poor ability to handle moisture, the manmade materials may be more useful for open style shoes such as sandals. In the oxford style shoe, the upper consists of at least three pieces that are cut from a pattern. The anterior part, covering the instep and toes, is known as the vamp. The pieces that make up the posterior part of the shoe are known as the quarters. Prior to lasting, these pieces are sewn together and fitted with a lining made of leather or canvas. The cut of the upper determines the fastening style of the shoe, which may be open to the toe, balmoral, blucher, or convalescent type (Fig. 45–2). The sole consists of three layers—the insole, the outsole, and the filler between them. The insole may be made of thin leather or manmade material. The filler usually consists of cork dust and latex.

The outsole may be made of leather, rubber, crepe, plastic, wood, or other materials. The same variety of materials is available for the heels. The structural stability of the shoe is enhanced by the heel counter, the shank, and the toe box (Fig. 45–3). The heel counter, which is made of firm leather or other stiff material, supports the posterior part of the shoe. The shank, usually made of steel, is used to provide additional support for the shoe in the region corresponding to the arch of the foot. The toe box may be hard, made of synthetic materials, or soft, made of cloth coated with latex. Some work boots, in addition, have a protective steel cap reinforcement over the toes.

Shoes are constructed over a last, which is a footlike form made of plastic or wood. The last determines the desired dimensions and style features of the shoe.[19] The usual last has a slight forefoot inflare. However, the suitability of the inflared last form has been questioned. Bleck[2] found that 85 per cent of normal feet in children were straight. According to observations by Holscher and Hu,[15] a last with a straight medial border may be more suitable for the general population. Shoes made according to a straight last are available from some manufacturers. In addition, combination lasts are used to produce footwear of combined dimensions such as a medium width forefoot and a narrow fitting heel. During the lasting process, the insole is temporarily tacked to the bottom of the last. After positioning of the heel counter and the toe box, the upper is applied snugly over the last so that the shoe upper adapts to the form of the last in every detail. It is then secured to the insole. Some steps of the lasting process include handling of the materials in a high-

967

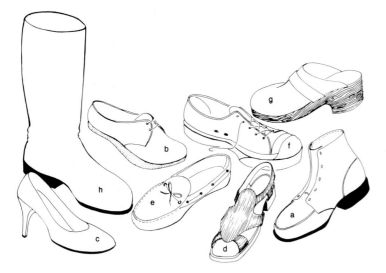

FIGURE 45–1. Commonly worn footwear styles. *a,* Laced work shoe; *b,* oxford — shown here with a negative heel; *c,* pump; *d,* sandal; *e,* moccasin; *f,* tennis shoe; *g,* clog; *h,* boot.

humidity environment. This softens the leather for shaping. The lasting process is followed by attachment of the outsole and the heel. In most footwear manufactured today, the upper is secured to the sole by rubber-based adhesives. The heel is attached by either gluing or nailing. For some outdoor footwear, heavy duty workshoes, and tennis shoes, a rubber or plastic sole is applied with vulcanizing or injection molding utilizing plastic materials.[19] In the so-called welt construction shoe, first a strip of leather known as the welt is sewn to the upper, the lining, and the insole. After the shank is attached, the outsole is stitched to the welt, followed by heel attachment and trimming of the heel and edges of the sole to the required contour. The welt construction shoes are quality shoes. They provide comfort because of a seam-free insole. They hold their shape well and have good structural stability, but they may be somewhat heavier and less flexible.

Shoes are worn for protection of the feet from rough terrain, cold, moisture, and dirt. Shoes are also important fashion items and are usually selected according to the current fashion trends.

Our footwear requirements change from infancy to old age. The infant needs shoes for protection from cold only. At other times, the shoes may be left off. When the child is just beginning to stand, his or her shoes should have a firm heel counter,

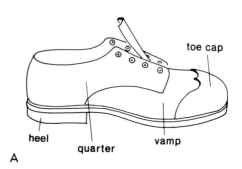

A

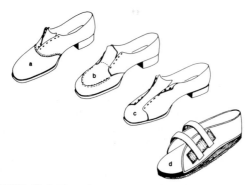

FIGURE 45–2. Fastening styles of oxford shoes. *a,* balmoral; *b,* blucher; *c,* open to the toe; *d,* convalescent.

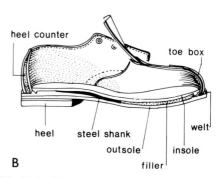

B

FIGURE 45–3. Component parts of oxford style shoe. *A,* External view; *B,* longitudinal section.

a soft leather top, and soft flexible sole approximately ⅛ inch thick.[9] The soft flexible sole is also of advantage for the crawling child, as shoes with stiff soles tend to roll into a toe-in or toe-out orientation, thus aggravating any toe-in or toe-out tendencies.[20]

As the child begins to walk, he or she should have a shoe with a firm heel counter and a firm sole approximately ¼ inch thick.[9] The heel height may be ¼ inch or ⅜ inch. During the first two years of life, a high top shoe will fit more securely. After this age, the foot and the heel have developed sufficiently to stay in a low shoe, although the heel width in many children's shoes is too great. For ages 3 years to 9 years, a round toe shoe is recommended to accommodate the growing foot. The heel height may be ¼ to ⅜ inch. The shoe should have a steel shank, but flexibility should be allowed for the forefoot. The shoe of the active adolescent also should have a steel shank and a firm heel counter to prevent rapid shoe breakdown. Shoes for the growing foot should be fitted to allow ½ to ¾ inch distance between the longest toe and the end of the toe box during weight-bearing. In all cases, the counter should fit the heel snugly. Frequent evaluation of footwear fit is needed, as children may outgrow their footwear in three to four months. The shoes should be replaced when the foot size has increased so that the toes approach the end of the toe box or when there is other evidence of tightness or loss of shape of the shoes.

A shoe with a firm heel counter and a snug fit at the heel is recommended for adults of all ages. In weight-bearing, there should be ½ inch distance between the toes and the end of the toe box to ensure adequate length. In a shoe of proper width, there should be no bulging at the welt. Tested over the widest portion of the foot, the upper should be loose enough to permit grasping a small fold of the material between the forefinger and thumb.

With increasing age, the foot tends to become wider and less flexible. A wider shoe with a soft flexible sole and a soft upper is recommended for the elderly person. A cushioned insole and a low heel may provide a more comfortable fit. However, shoes with soft soles are not suitable for elderly persons who tend to shuffle their feet when walking. The soft soles, especially those made of crepe, may cause tripping. To ensure maximal stability and safety in walking, special care must be taken to have the elderly person's footwear always securely fastened.

Shoe sizes are indicated by numbers referring to the length and by letters referring to the width. In the United States, children's shoe sizes range from 1 (infant size) to 13, starting again at size 1 on the adult scale. Although this is variable, men's shoes up to size 14 or 15 and women's shoes up to size 12 or possibly size 13 are available in shoe stores. Larger sizes may need to be ordered from the manufacturer or specialty houses. The width ranges from A (narrow) to E (wide). Some manufacturers record the width as N (narrow), M (medium), or W (wide). With each increase in the length or the width of the shoe there will be an increase in both the length and the width. The shoe retailer may not stock all sizes in all widths, so extra narrow or extra wide shoes may need to be ordered specially. Lasts and sizes change with the manufacturer and with changing fashions, so correct fit can be determined only by trying the shoe on the foot. Functionally, the shoe should be comfortable for several hours of uninterrupted wear. The shoe should bend easily where the foot normally bends and remain rigid where the foot is normally rigid.[20] The shoe should not interfere with the normal lateral stability of the foot and should not cause loss of balance due to insecure fit.

These important functional considerations have been disregarded in the design of some fashion footwear. The thick inflexible platform sole limits the normal motion of the foot during walking. The normal lateral stability of the foot is reduced if the shoe is constructed with a convexity in the sole, permitting the foot to rock from side to side. The narrow base of a high heel also contributes to instability. Backless shoes tend to slide off the feet and cause loss of balance. In addition, the shank curve and a forward slanting heel seat permit the foot to slide forward in the shoe, crowding the toes in the toe box and causing skin irritation and foot deformities. The negative heel may cause discomfort due to tension on the triceps surae.

These undesirable consequences of fashion footwear are by no means limited to women's shoes. Some problems related to footwear result from the materials used for modern shoe construction or the processing of these materials. Common allergens in footwear are rubber-based adhesives, coloring agents, and, in leather shoes, chrome and formaldehyde present in most leathers as tanning agents.[10] Moisture from perspiration may leach chemicals out of one area and transfer them to distant sites, thus causing apparent spread of the dermatitis. White buck or other undyed leather or tennis shoes may need to be substituted. When the tanning agents are at fault, vegetable-tanned or glutaraldehyde-tanned leather shoes may be needed. Excessive moisture is a particular problem with synthetic materials and some specialy treated leathers. Ventilation holes similar to those in some tennis shoes may need to be made in the upper by using a leather punch. Wearing two pairs of cotton socks is also helpful. Prospective allergy testing of shoe components may be appropriate in some cases.[10]

In general, the adult has a wide choice of footwear materials and styles. Time spent in selection of a well-fitting shoe is time well invested, as the result will be comfort and walking ease during many months.

Footwear Modifications

Welt process shoes are best suited for modifications because the sole and the upper can be separated and reattached without disturbing the structural stability of the shoe. This type of shoe can support orthotic devices, including metal braces. The so-called orthopedic shoe is a welt shoe. In addition, it has an extended heel on the medial side known as the Thomas heel, an extended medial heel counter, and a rigid steel shank. Shoes that have soles attached by adhesives do not lend themselves to modifications that require separation of the sole and the upper because of the difficulty of reattaching the soles. However, some shoes of this type may be suitable for simple external modifications such as heel elevations or metatarsal bars. Various internal shoe modifications can be fabricated from a heat-moldable polyethylene foam (Plastazote).[14] A full-molded insole requires an extra-depth shoe. In the manufacture of these shoes, extra depth has been provided to accommodate a removable insole of ¼- to ⅝-inch thickness in the different shoes. The insole can be removed to provide extra space in the shoe to accommodate deformities, or it can be replaced by an insole individually molded for each patient. Sandals can be made of a heat-moldable soft insole material, microcellular rubber soling, and the appropriate materials for the upper. The inventive physician or orthotist will adapt them to a variety of conditions.

Footwear modifications should be detailed in a written prescription that defines the type of footwear to be modified and the desired modifications. A simple diagram attached to the prescription may convey added information and clarify the request.

If the shoes are to be supplied by the orthotist, the prescription should indicate the freedom the patient may be permitted in shoe selection, for example, in the selection of color, lacing, or style. When the situation warrants it, and often it is a regular practice in some clinics, the physiatrist and the orthotist may examine the patient together. It is the physician's responsibility to evaluate the modified shoe to confirm that the desired effect has been achieved.

The style and appearance of the shoe are of great importance to the patient and should never be disregarded in the prescription of shoes and shoe modifications. It is common sense to use the simplest and most cosmetically acceptable modification that will achieve its purpose. The patient should clearly understand the purpose of the modification and have an opportunity to communicate his or her preferences to the physiatrist and the orthotist. The following paragraphs contain some practical guidelines for footwear selection and modification in the conditions commonly seen in the physiatrist's practice.

Elevations. Heel and sole elevations, also known as heel and sole lifts, are prescribed when there is a need for length adjustment of the lower limb. A lift of ⅜ inch or less can be worn under the heel inside a suitable shoe. This type of lift may be made of felt, firm rubber, or other materials and lightly glued into its position. Higher elevations will require external modification. For adjustments of up to 1 in, heel elevation alone will be sufficient. When the length adjustment exceeds 1 in, both heel and sole elevations are used. Care should be taken to maintain the heel height greater than the sole height in order to avoid a negative heel effect. Tapering of the distal portion of the sole upward will aid in walking by allowing easier weight transfer over the forefoot, as the elevated sole is usually not flexible (Fig. 45–4). Although the usual soling materials can be used for heel and sole elevations, lightweight materials such as cork are recommended if the lift is relatively high. When covered with leather matching the shoe upper, the elevated portion is less conspicuous.

Forefoot Deformities. Deformities of the forefoot such as a bunion require a wide shoe with a soft upper. Extra room for the deformity may be provided by slitting the upper close to the sole or along seams or excising a portion of the upper. A patch of material similar to the upper material is then sewn into place over the excised portion, ensuring that the needed width adjustment has been achieved. This simple modification can be

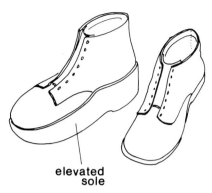

FIGURE 45–4. Sole and heel elevations. Note the upward tapered distal portion of the elevated sole.

done in most shoe repair shops. It will provide comfortable walking in a shoe of acceptable appearance.

Painful Heel Spurs and Plantar Fasciitis. In most cases, heel pain will subside with a decrease in the amount of weight-bearing and the addition of an insert of soft rubber or soft-grade polyethylene foam (Plastazote) cut to fit under the heel inside the shoe. This provides a cushion under the heel and slightly relieves tension on the plantar fascia. Various inserts and heel cups are also available without a prescription in foot care and athletic shops. Campbell and Inman[7] report good success in resistant cases using the University of California Biomechanics Laboratory shoe insert that provides an alternate method to elevate the arch. The theory of the University of California Biomechanics Laboratory shoe insert is to hold the foot in a position that relieves tension on the plantar fascia. By holding the heel in inversion with forces against the navicular bone and the outer border of the forefoot, this position is maintained without direct pressure on the soft tissues under the longitudinal arch. The insert is a plastic shell made by laminating layers of nylon and fiberglass, constructed according to a plaster cast. The cast is made from a negative that is taken with the leg externally rotated while the forefoot is held in pronation and slight adduction.

Flat Feet. Adults with mildly pronated feet that are asymptomatic require no special shoes or shoe modifications. If there is evidence of longitudinal arch strain, a Thomas heel shoe that also has a long medial heel counter will provide some support despite the fact that the Thomas heel extends only part way under the arch. Supports of the longitudinal arch can be added. Although some commercially available supports may fit, individually molded arch supports made of polyethylene foam may be better tolerated. Only the flexible flat foot will adjust to these modifications. The rigid flat foot needs to be fitted for comfort only. In the usual case, this means selection of a wide shoe with a comfortable fit. A molded polyethylene foam insole backed by microcellular rubber may increase the patient's comfort. If the molded insole is used, an extra-depth shoe is also needed. The insole should be molded to the foot as is without incorporating an arch support, as the arch support may produce undesirable pressure and cause pain under the inflexible arch.

Footwear modifications using a Thomas heel and a medial heel wedge are recommended for children with flexible flat feet who have leg pain in the evening following a long day of activity. Pain may be expected to subside as early as within two to three days. Cowell[9] believes that the Thomas heel and medial heel wedge are most appropriately used for the flexible flat foot. This type of correction should not be used for flexible flat feet that do not form an arch in either a sitting or a standing position, as pressure in the arch region will aggravate the discomfort.[9] The need for footwear corrections for children with asymptomatic flat feet is questionable.

For the medial heel wedge and the Thomas heel to be effective, the shoe fit should be satisfactory and the heel counter should fit snugly and resist distortion.[1] If the heel of the shoe is too wide, a fitted heel counter will be needed. The medial heel counter should be extended but not as far forward as the navicular bone if spot pressure on this bone is to be avoided. The medial heel wedge should be placed between the outsole and the insole (Fig. 45–5). The wedge should be highest on the medial side, tapering to 0 laterally. For children up to age 2 years, the wedge should measure 1/16 inch; from age 2 to 5 years, 1/8 inch; after age 5 years, 3/16

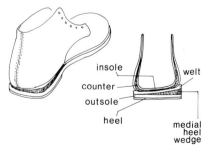

insole
welt
counter
outsole
heel
medial
heel
wedge

FIGURE 45–5. Medial heel wedge. The medial heel wedge is positioned between the insole and the outsole. The wedge tapers to 0 laterally.

inch.[9] In some cases, a small pad just anterior to the os calcis weight-bearing area may be needed to maintain the heel in its proper position.

The Insensitive Foot. Impaired lower extremity sensation may result from peripheral nerve or spinal cord injury, myelodysplasia, stroke, neuropathies, and other conditions seen in the physiatrist's practice. The foot with impaired sensation requires a careful evaluation prior to footwear selection. The evaluation should include assessment of skin condition and the distribution of plantar pressure during standing and walking. Attention must be paid to the thickness of fat pads, calluses, and scarring on the plantar surface of the foot. With the use of the Harris mat, the plantar pressure evaluation can be carried out in the physiatrist's office. The footprint made by the patient bearing weight on the inked mat indicates areas of high pressure that may need to be protected by special shoe modifications. A thin form of the Harris mat can be used inside the shoe for additional evaluation.[4, 21] The Microcapsule Sock Test developed at the United States Public Health Service Hospital at Carville, Louisiana, also may be used for the evaluation of pressures inside the shoe.[4, 12]

If the evaluation reveals that the sensory-impaired foot has no soft tissue or skeletal deformity, carefully fitted regular shoes are acceptable.[12] In cases in which an area of concentrated pressure has been demonstrated by plantar pressure evaluation, a microcellular rubber insole will distribute the stress over a larger area. An extra-depth shoe may or may not be needed. If the foot is scarred on the plantar surface from previous trauma, the risk of further injury is increased. In this case, a combination insole of molded polyethylene foam backed by microcellular rubber is recommended for the active patient. Molded polyethylene foam with latex cork backing is another useful combination of materials. Soft-grade and medium-grade Plastazote may be used for the same insole (Fig. 45–6). The insoles are fitted inside extra-depth shoes. If a bone deformity on the plantar aspect of the foot is also present, a soft molded insole of polyethylene foam is recommended, with areas of relief under the prominences to prevent plantar ulceration.[12] A variety of other insole materials are available and may be useful alone or in combination. In a clinical study, Leber and Evanski evaluated the ability of seven commonly used shoe insole materials to relieve areas of high plantar pressure.[16] Of the materials tested, polyurethane foam, Plastazote, and Spenco decreased the pres-

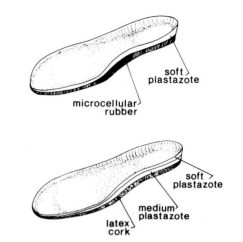

FIGURE 45–6. Insoles for use inside extra-depth shoes. Note combinations of materials.

sure most effectively. A metatarsal bar attached to the flexible sole in its correct position with the high point of the bar located just proximal to the metatarsal heads will relieve stress on the metatarsal heads. When the sole is rigid, a rocker bar can be fitted by the orthotist.[4] This allows the substitution of a rocking motion for direct pressure on the metatarsal region (Fig. 45–7). A sandal with a soft molded insole can be made from a kit or from assembled materials in a relatively short time and may be of value for patients who need temporary footwear during healing of foot lesions (Fig. 45–8). Individually made rigid-soled rocker shoes are used in special cases for patients with Hansen's disease.[4] Unfortunately, the expert craftsmanship and experience required to make these shoes, as well as the appropriate facilities, may not be available in all locations.

Regardless of whether the sensory impairment is considered permanent or transient, the patient must be taught techniques of preventive foot care. Because of decreased or absent sensory feedback, the patient may not be aware that his or her footwear is too tight or that skin breakdown is

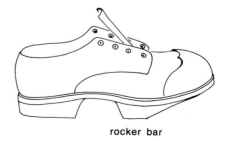

FIGURE 45–7. Oxford shoe with a rocker bar.

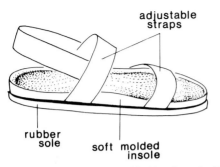

FIGURE 45–8. Sandal with soft molded insole and adjustable straps. It is similar to sandals made from a kit.

imminent from trauma due to other causes. For the same reason, he or she is not able to adjust the gait to lessen the repetitive pressure of walking on the skin areas that may be already inflamed.[3] The preventive program includes daily foot examination to detect areas of tissue trauma and the examination of shoes and socks.[21] In the hospital setting, diagnostic aids such as thermography and volumetric studies may be available to detect signs of inflammation. At home, however, the patient will need to monitor for these signs visually and by touch. Particular attention must be paid to the areas that receive the greatest pressure, especially the region of the metatarsal heads. This region is particularly vulnerable, as the forefoot carries the greatest load in walking by sustaining the weight for a longer period of time than the heel.[11] The multiply handicapped patient may not be able to carry out the examination independently and may require assistance from a member of the family. In some cases, gait training may be needed to minimize the effects of repetitive stress. Usually, this involves teaching the patient to walk slowly and to take shorter steps. Shoes should be changed at midday and again in the evening.[3] At first, new shoes should not be worn longer than two hours without examining the feet. If spasticity complicates the clinical picture, additional trauma to the foot may result as the spastic muscles force the foot against the shoe. When the patient exerts effort in ambulation, the level of spasticity may increase; therefore, the fit of the shoe may be different in ambulation than during non–weight-bearing or while standing. Repeated evaluation of the footwear and of orthotic and assistive devices, combined with judicious use of medication or intramuscular neurolysis for control of spasticity, may be necessary in the management of the difficult case. Inquiry into the patient's daily activities often reveals the need for work simplification tech-

niques in order to reduce the total distance walked each day. The skin of the insensitive foot may lack the normal perspiration moisture, leading to scaling and fissuring. Daily foot soaks followed by application of an emollient to retain skin moisture may be needed.[21] We have found Albolene, with its main ingredients of mineral oil, petrolatum, and paraffin, useful for this purpose. It also seems to be well accepted by patients.

The Arthritic Foot. The foot is involved in 90 per cent of all patients who have had rheumatoid arthritis for any period of time.[18] The metatarsophalangeal joints are affected early in the disease, and tenosynovitis, rheumatoid nodules, and inflamed bursae are common. Atrophy of fat pads also occurs. A wide shoe with a soft upper is recommended to avoid painful mediolateral compression of the metatarsophalangeal joints. It should have a flexible sole. A soft heel counter is useful for those patients who have heel pain due to rheumatoid nodules and inflamed bursae. The common abnormalities of the foot in advanced arthritis include hallux valgus, clawing of the toes, spread of the forefoot, and a rigid flat foot. When there is clawing of the toes, an extra-depth shoe should be prescribed to avoid pressure on the dorsum of the toes. The shoe should be wide and have a soft toecap that can adjust to the deformities. Spot stretching may be needed to further enlarge the upper. A commonly prescribed modification for relief of pressure on the painful metatarsal heads is a metatarsal pad attached inside the shoe. This localized modification has disadvantages. As the shoe loosens with wear, the pad may no longer be in its correct location and can cause undesirable pressure in other areas of the weight-bearing surface of the foot. For this reason, a full-molded insole is preferable to distribute weight over the entire weight-bearing surface. As for the insole used for the insensitive foot, heat-moldable or a combination of moldable and nonmoldable materials may be used. External modification in the form of a metatarsal bar applied to a flexible sole may serve to reduce pressure over the painful metatarsophalangeal region.

The severely deformed foot requires a custom-made shoe. The shoe is made according to a plaster cast of the foot. Whenever possible, leather should be used for the upper. Also of value for indoor use and in warm climate outdoors are sandals with soft soles, with the straps adjusted or altered so that they avoid pressure on sensitive areas. High heel shoes are not suitable for the arthritic foot, since in the high heel shoe extra weight is placed on the already painful metatarsal heads.[13] Also, in general, the arthritic foot is not flexible enough to fit well into a high heel shoe. The use of physical therapy measures to maintain foot flexibility is of advantage to the patient, as the patient with a flexible foot will have a greater choice of footwear styles and in some instances may even tolerate a moderate heel. The choice of suitable footwear and footwear styles for the patient with severe deformities such as hallux valgus and fixed deformities of the toes may be increased by corrective surgical procedures that restore the foot to near-normal shape.[22] The patient with severe rheumatoid arthritis and decreased function of the hands often requires assistive devices for dressing his or her feet and adaptations for closure of the shoes.

Athletic Shoes

With increasing numbers of men and women participating in distance walking and running for aerobic conditioning, the physiatrist may be consulted for advice regarding proper footwear for these activities, as well as for prevention and treatment of running injuries. Therefore, he or she must become familiar with the characteristics of a good running shoe and its role in injury prevention. Wearing poorly constructed running shoes or sneakers may contribute to injury, since they lack the protective features of a good running shoe.[5]

A well-designed training shoe must be comfortable, fit well, and provide sufficient cushioning and stability to protect the limbs from the trauma of repetitive heel strikes of running. At the same time, the shoe should be fairly lightweight and flexible. The upper, which is usually made of nylon and leather, should have a laced vamp and a well-padded tongue to prevent irritation of the dorsum of the foot. A well-molded Achilles pad prevents irritation of the Achilles tendon. The toe box should be at least 1½ inches high to allow toe motion without pressure on the toenails. The shoe should have a firm heel counter for hindfoot stability. The midsole should be flexible, and there should be a soft, raised heel wedge to absorb impact on heel strike. The heel should be slightly flared for additional stability and beveled to help rapid roll-off. A studded outer sole increases shock absorption and traction in wet conditions.[5] The shoes must be kept in good condition, and any lateral or medial wear on the heel or sole should be repaired to maintain stability. In general, the foot with a tendency toward hyperpronation re-

quires a firmer shoe for support than does a cavus foot.[17] These general guidelines may help the patient to select the proper training shoe from the wide variety of styles and materials available. However, the final choice must be individualized, recognizing that each individual has a distinct walking and running gait, specific training goals, and a unique anatomy of the feet.

The shock-absorbing characteristics of running shoes decrease significantly with use.[8] This was demonstrated in various shoe models exposed to simulated running by mechanical heel strikes and in two types of running shoes worn by volunteer runners during normal training. In the shoes worn by the volunteer runners, the shock absorption capacity decreased approximately 20 per cent after the first 150 miles and about 30 per cent at 500 miles. It was also noted that the shock absorption capability of the shoes was severely lowered when the shoes were wet with rain or perspiration; therefore, running in adverse weather conditions may permit greater forces to be transmitted to the body. After drying, the shock absorption level recovered to that consistent with the shoe mileage.[8]

When shoe modification or orthotic prescription appears necessary because of pain or injury related to running, the clinician must remember that the majority of injuries occur because of training errors.[5] Some examples of training errors include excessive mileage, inadequate warm-up, and hard, irregular, or sloping running surfaces. Correction of the training errors may avert the need for shoe modifications or expensive orthotic devices.

Whenever possible, the simplest and most lightweight modification should be used. For a leg-length discrepancy, a heel lift may be worn inside the shoe. Alternately, a full sole lift may be added just under the outer sole. In cases of recurrent Achilles tendinitis, an additional heel wedge of sponge rubber in the midsole area can be used to elevate the heel. This modification lessens the impact on the heel on heel strike and protects the Achilles tendon. In metatarsalgia, a sponge rubber rocker bottom insert in the midsole area of the shoe is recommended. Such adjustments should be done bilaterally to maintain balance.[5, 6]

Orthotic devices in the form of shoe inserts are worn to compensate for biomechanical problems, most often to correct hyperpronation. For the cavus foot the orthosis may provide greater cushioning. Simple, commercially available supports, suitable for temporary use, can be purchased without a prescription according to shoe size. The insole of the shoe is usually removed to accommodate the insert. The orthosis prescribed for permanent use is made according to a plaster cast of the foot to ensure an accurate fit. The appropriate corrections to achieve a neutral foot position are added at the orthotic laboratory. Usually, either a flexible orthosis made of leather and rubber or a semi-rigid type made of materials such as polyethylene is prescribed. However, a rigid polypropylene orthosis occasionally may be used for a very flexible foot or for high mileage runners who need increased foot control.[5, 6] Follow-up evaluation of the orthosis along with the appropriate shoes is necessary to ensure that the desired effect has been achieved.

Conclusion

The changing styles and materials of fashion footwear make the selection of suitable shoes an ongoing challenge for everyone, including persons whose feet are considered normal. This challenge is considerably greater for persons whose feet require special consideration because of deformity, disease, or nonconformity to the usual last. The amount of experimental data relating to the usefulness and long-term effects of various types of footwear and footwear modifications is limited. For the most part, the clinician will need to rely on his or her own evaluation and clinical judgment regarding footwear selection and modification. In addition, the clinician must recognize the importance of the patient's preference and acceptance of the modified footwear. Patient education regarding the individual footwear needs is of paramount importance. It should always be available to the patient, as it may help to avoid future disability.

ACKNOWLEDGMENT

The author wishes to express thanks to Winkley Orthopedic Laboratories of Golden Valley, Minnesota, for information regarding currently available adaptations for shoes and to Jean Magney for preparing the illustrations for this chapter.

References

1. Allison, J. D.: Change in heel width following support of pronated foot. Arch. Phys. Med. Rehabil., 48:195–200, 1967.

2. Bleck, E. E.: The shoeing of children: Sham or science? Dev. Med. Child. Neurol., 13:188–195, 1971.

3. Brand, P. W.: Management of the insensitive limb. Phys. Ther., 59:8–12, 1979.

4. Brand, P. W.: Repetitive Stress on Insensitive Feet: The Pathology and Management of Plantar Ulceration in Neuropathic Feet. U.S. Public Health Service Hospital, Carville, Louisiana, 1975.

5. Brody, D. M.: Running injuries. Clin. Symp. 32 (4):1–36, Ciba Pharmaceutical Company, USA, 1980.

6. Brody, D. M.: Rehabilitation of the injured runner. Am. Acad. Orthop. Surg. Instruct. Course., 33:268–278, 1984.

7. Campbell, J. W., and Inman, V. T.: Treatment of plantar fasciitis and calcaneal spurs with the UC-BL shoe insert. Clin. Orthop., 103:57–62, 1974.

8. Cook, S. D., Kester, M. A., and Brunet, M. E.: Shock absorption characteristics of running shoes. Am. J. Sports Med., 13:248–253, 1985.

9. Cowell, H. R.: Shoes and shoe corrections. Pediatr. Clin. North Am., 24:791–797, 1977.

10. Dahl, M. V.: Allergic contact dermatitis from footwear. Minn. Med., 58:871–874, 1975.

11. Grundy, M., Tosh, P. A., McLeish, R. D., and Smidt, L.: An investigation of the centres of pressure under the foot while walking. J. Bone Joint Surg., 57B:98–103, 1975.

12. Hampton, G. H.: Therapeutic footwear for the insensitive foot. Phys. Ther., 59:23–29, 1979.

13. Haslock, D. I., and Wright, V.: Footwear for arthritic patients. Ann. Phys. Med., 10:236–240, 1970.

14. Hertzman, C. A.: Use of Plastazote in foot disabilities. Am. J. Phys. Med., 52:289–303, 1973.

15. Holscher, E. C., and Hu, K. K.: Detrimental results with the common inflared shoe. Orthop. Clin. North Am., 7:1011–1018, 1976.

16. Leber, C., and Evanski, P. M.: A comparison of shoe insole materials in plantar pressure relief. Prosthet. Orthot. Int., 10:135–138, 1986.

17. McKenzie, D. C., Clement, D. B., and Taunton, J. E.: Running shoes, orthotics and injuries. Sports Med., 2:334–347, 1985.

18. Potter, T. A.: Correction of arthritic deformities. In Hollander, J. E., and McCarty, D. J.: Arthritis and Allied Conditions. Philadelphia, Lea & Febiger, 1972, pp. 629–672.

19. Rossi, W. A.: Shoes and the shoe industry—reality versus illusion. J. Am. Podiatry Assoc., 68:215–229, 1978.

20. Schuster, R. O.: The effects of modern footgear. J. Am. Podiatry Assoc., 68:235–241, 1978.

21. Shipley, D. E.: Clinical evaluation and care of the insensitive foot. Phys. Ther., 59:13–18, 1979.

22. Thomas, W. H.: Surgery of the foot in rheumatoid arthritis. Orthop. Clin. North Am., 6:831–835, 1975.

46

Prevention and Rehabilitation of Ischemic Ulcers

MICHAEL KOSIAK
FREDERIC J. KOTTKE

Ischemic ulcers are localized areas of cellular necrosis and vascular destruction that have suffered prolonged exposure to pressures high enough to cut off the local circulation. Weight-bearing bone prominences that are subcutaneous or padded only by a thin layer of subcutaneous tissue or muscle are especially susceptible. Prolonged anemia due to pressure that collapses the microcirculation cuts off the oxygen and nutrition essential for the maintenance of metabolism and causes the death of the cells in the areas of supravascular pressure. Any other factors that impair the metabolic activity of these cells increase their susceptibility to pressure necrosis. Diabetes mellitus, circulatory impairment from any cause, protein malnutrition, anemia, old age, and other conditions that reduce cellular metabolism all increase the susceptibility to cellular necrosis in the presence of supracapillary pressure. The location of the ischemic ulcers depends upon inactivity that exposes certain pressure points to supracapillary pressure without relief for prolonged periods of time. Bedfast patients most frequently develop ischemic ulcers over the sacrum and trochanters, but they may also develop ulcers on the posterior part of the heels, the back of the head, the malleoli, the crests of the pelvis, the borders of the scapulae, the lumbar spine, and the areas of prolonged contact when one leg lies on top of the other. The ischial areas and sacrum are most frequently at risk for patients confined to a wheelchair or for other patients who sit for prolonged periods of time without moving. When the episodes of ischemia are repeated, the damage to

cellular metabolism is cumulative. Patients who are debilitated, semicomatose or unconscious, have areas of analgesia, or have paralysis so that they cannot move freely and frequently are most likely to develop ischemic ulcers.

Incidence

The exact incidence of ischemic ulcers is unknown. Studies in the past would indicate that up to 28 per cent of the hospital population might be afflicted.[35] In patients with spinal cord injuries, an incidence of 24 to 85 per cent has been reported, with 7 to 8 per cent of the deaths in these patients being attributed to complications arising from the presence of ischemic ulcers.[2, 16, 29] Most readmissions to spinal cord injury centers are for treatment of ischemic ulcers.[9]

Etiology

Primary Factors

PRESSURE

Ischemic ulcers arise from prolonged tissue ischemia caused by pressure exceeding the tissue capillary pressure. Studies of the changes in capillary blood flow using several experimental methods have established important facts regarding vascular hemodynamics. Remarkable instability in capillaries at low perfusion pressures with cessation or

976

temporary reversal of flow at a low positive pressure has been demonstrated.[4, 37]

Because the hydrostatic pressures in capillaries are relatively low (from 13 to 32 mm Hg) and because cessation of flow occurs even in the presence of positive arterial pressure, it would seem that complete tissue ischemia should occur when pressures of the order of capillary blood pressure are applied to the body.[30] However, the data from multiple experiments indicates that the perfusion of the area of compression continues at pressures considerably higher than that.[13, 25, 26] Kosiak's early experiments on dogs produced ischemic ulcers only when pressure of 140 mm Hg or higher was maintained for hours.[26] Dinsdale, working with pigs, could not produce pressure ulcers at pressures below 290 mm Hg, although pressure plus intermittent abrasive trauma caused lesions until the pressure dropped below 45 mm Hg.[13] Holloway and co-workers found that blood flow through the skin continued at pressure above 60 mm Hg.[20] Newson and Rolfe reported that oxygen tension at the skin surface decreased less than 20 per cent when pressure up to 200 mm Hg was applied to the surface of the skin.[36] However, there is a methodological error in their method of measurement of pressure that varies with the surface measured. Patterson and Fisher found that, during their usual period of sitting, paraplegics were exposed to pressures of approximately 100 mm Hg for up to 12 hours without pressure relief of more than 1 second's duration more frequently than every 10 minutes or pressure relief of 5 sec or longer more frequently than every 30 min without developing decubiti.[39] The pressures reported in these studies are in the range of capillary pressure during reactive hyperemia, which may have a significant protective effect.[31] The end result is that while pressure occluding circulation is a *sine qua non* for the production of ischemic ulcers, we lack a full and precise understanding of the amount and duration of that pressure. It is known that the pressure that will produce necrosis due to ischemia is far below the extreme pressures necessary to cause mechanical crushing damage to the cells.[22] Most of the studies of the effects of pressure have been of single incidents. It is to be expected that the cumulative effects of repeated incidents of pressure will make the site increasingly susceptible to necrosis.[13, 18, 20, 21] In view of the uncertainties regarding the level of pressure at which cellular damage begins and because of the high incidence of ischemic ulcers occurring in patients at risk, the best advise still remains to establish a regimen in which

there is complete relief of pressure for approximately 5 sec every 15 min.

Pathological changes following ischemia have been shown to be due to disturbances in capillary circulation. The presence of edema and cellular infiltration 24 hours after the application of moderate pressure would indicate changes in capillary permeability due to capillary membrane ischemia. By electron microscopy, Dinsdale demonstrated edema in endothelial cells obstructing the capillaries as the result of pressure ischemia[13] (Fig. 46–1). Increasing the degree or duration of ischemia not only increases the changes in capillary membrane permeability but also interferes with cellular metabolism to a degree sufficient to produce cellular necrosis and an inflammatory reaction in muscle tissue.[18]

The application of 60 mm Hg pressure for one hour has been shown to produce edema, cellular infiltration, and extravasation in the tissue of dogs. An inverse relationship, resembling a parabolic curve, was found to exist between the amount and the duration of pressure that normal tissue could tolerate before pathological changes would occur (Fig. 46–2).[25]

Microscopic examination of rat muscle 24 hours after being subjected to 70 mm Hg pressure for one hour demonstrated a decrease or loss of cross striations and myofibrils, hyalinization of fibers, and neutrophilic infiltrations (Figs. 46–3 and 46–4).

When complete relief of pressure was provided at regular five-min intervals, such as in an alternating pressure support system, the tissue showed consistently less evidence of ischemic change or no change at all when compared with tissue subjected to an equivalent amount of constant pressure. This was true even at pressures as high as 240 mm Hg for three hours (Table 46–1).[26]

In the sitting position, resting pressures can assume alarming magnitudes, although the pressures encountered by the patient in the prone and supine positions may also exceed capillary pressure.*

FRICTION AND SHEARING

The importance of shearing force as a factor in the production of ischemic ulcers was first reported by Reichel.[40] Although his work was primarily a clinical study, it clearly showed that shearing and stretching of blood vessels tended to compound

---

*See references 5, 32, 33, 21, and 44.

MICHAEL KOSIAK AND FREDERIC J. KOTTKE

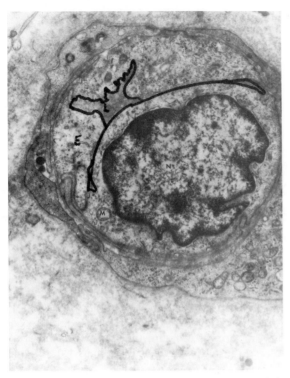

FIGURE 46–1. Edema of the capillary endothelium of the dermis resulting from exposure to intermittent friction and constant pressure of 227 mm Hg over three 1.5 hour periods. The endothelial nucleus (N) and the endothelial cytoplasm (E) are so swollen that the lumen of the capillary (L, outlined in black) is almost completely obliterated (× 30,000). (Courtesy of Sidney M. Dinsdale: Mechanical Factors in Pathogenesis of Ischemic Ulcers in Swine. Ph.D. Thesis, University of Minnesota, 1970.)

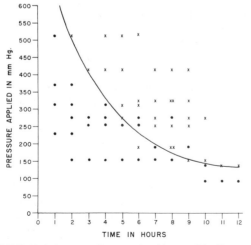

FIGURE 46–2. Pressure-time relationship noted in 62 separate experiments in 16 dogs: X = ulceration; • = no ulceration.

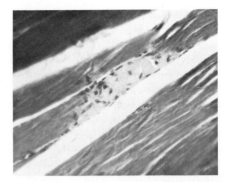

FIGURE 46–3. Muscle of normal rat's leg after application of 115 mm Hg constant pressure for two hours. The section shows early involvement of an isolated fiber consisting of hyaline degeneration and phagocytosis. Stained with hematoxylin and eosin. Magnified 380 ×.

the ischemic changes produced by external pressure, thereby increasing the rate of tissue breakdown.

Dinsdale,[13] working with swine, demonstrated significant skin breakdown when the tissue was subjected to both pressure and friction, at a pressure significantly less than that when necrosis was caused by pressure alone (45 mm Hg versus 290 mm Hg). The data from these studies conducted on normally innervated and paraplegic pigs deserve special consideration, because the skin and the subcutaneous soft tissues of the pig are more like those of the human histologically than are those tissues of other experimental animals. There is one major difference, however. A necrotic ulcer of the skin and subcutaneous tissues of the pig is highly resistant to infection and heals spontaneously regardless of how it is treated. Therefore, it does not present a suitable model to use when comparing differences of the various treatment modalities

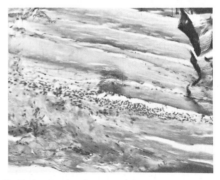

FIGURE 46–4. Muscle of paraplegic rat's leg subjected to 70 mm Hg constant pressure for four hours. The section shows an isolated fiber undergoing necrosis associated with extensive phagocytosis by neutrophils and macrophages. Stained with hematoxylin and eosin. Magnified 170 ×.

TABLE 46–1. Microscopic Changes Noted in Muscle of Animals 24 Hours After Application of Pressure*

PRESSURE TRANSMITTED TO MUSCLE	TIME IN HOURS	NORMAL		PARAPLEGIC	
		Constant Pressure	Alternating Pressure (5 min intervals)	Constant Pressure	Alternating Pressure (5 min intervals)
35 mm Hg	1	None	None	None	None
	2	None	None	None	None
	3	None	None	None	None
	4	None	None	None	None
70 mm Hg	1	None	None	None	None
	2	Moderate	None	Moderate	Minimal
	3	Moderate	Minimal	Moderate	Minimal
	4	Moderate	Minimal	Marked	Minimal
115 mm Hg	1	None		None	
	2	Minimal		Moderate	
	3	Marked		Marked	
	4	Moderate		Moderate	
155 mm Hg	1	None	None	None	None
	2	Moderate	None	Minimal	None
	3	Marked	Minimal	Minimal	None
	4	Moderate	Moderate	Moderate	Minimal
190 mm Hg	1	None		Minimal	
	2	Minimal		Moderate	
	3	Marked		Marked	
	4	Marked		Marked	
240 mm Hg	1	Minimal	None	Moderate	None
	2	Moderate	Minimal	Moderate	None
	3	Moderate	None	Moderate	Minimal
	4	Moderate	Moderate	Marked	Minimal

*None = No microscopic change.

Minimal = Involvement of isolated fibers.

Moderate = Involvement of up to 10 per cent of muscle examined.

Marked = Involvement of more than 10 per cent of muscle examined.

to produce healing of ischemic ulcers. Bennett and associates compared the pulsatile blood flow through the skin with the compressive pressure and the shear force of normal adults, geriatric subjects, and paraplegic subjects while they sat on a special wheelchair with a hard plastic seat. All subjects showed the same range of sitting pressures, but median paraplegic and geriatric shear forces were approximately three times those of the normal controls, and rates of pulsatile blood flow through the skin were less than one third of those of controls.[3]

Using another paradigm to compare tangential frictional force on the skin to impairment of cutaneous blood flow, Bader and co-workers calculate that the shear forces on the skin of the buttock of the patient in a semi-reclining position in bed at an angle of 30 degrees with the knees extended would exert an effect adequate to decrease blood flow 50 per cent.[2]

TEMPERATURE

The effect of increased temperature that increases cellular metabolism and, therefore, increases the risk of ischemic necrosis has attracted attention recently. Since the metabolic rate increases 10 per cent with every 1° C (1.8° F) rise in tissue temperature, any increase in temperature in conjunction with tissue ischemia may further compromise the metabolism and survival of the ischemic cells. This relates particularly to the composition and conformity of seat cushions and mattress surfaces, which may retain heat and moisture.[15]

Studies of temperature differences of the skin of paraplegic patients when sitting on five different

MICHAEL KOSIAK AND FREDERIC J. KOTTKE

kinds of cushions showed a great variation of thermal insulation of these cushions of up to 10° C (18° F) under the ischial tuberosities and the thigh.[44]

AGING

The incidence of ischemic ulcers appears to increase with age. After the third decade, a progressive decrease in skin pliability and elasticity has been reported, whereas after the fifth decade, a rapid decrease in blood flow through the skin occurs.[1, 24]

Other reasons for the increased incidence of ischemic ulcers in the elderly could be attributed to a greater lack of mobility, poorer state of nutrition, higher incidence of complicating medical problems impairing cellular metabolism, and longer periods of confinement than in younger patients.[14]

Contributing Factors

NUTRITION

Recently, increased emphasis has been placed on the role of nutrition during the acute and convalescent phases of illness, especially on the negative nitrogen and calcium balances that inevitably appear after an acute insult. After almost any illness or injury, such as a fracture, tooth extraction, or even a mild infection, negative nitrogen, phosphorus, sulfur, and calcium balances with evidence of osteoporosis, wasting of tissue, and loss of weight generally result. The reaction is much more pronounced, of course, in a severe insult than in a mild one. This negative balance reaches its peak in about two days to two weeks and does not return to normal for several months. No dietary product can completely reverse the negative balance, although the degree of negativity of the nitrogen balance can be reduced.[11]

Because of the severe alteration of body metabolism produced by almost any illness and the additional changes produced by the bed rest associated with injury or illness, the dietary intake should be increased to counterbalance the metabolic losses.

Poor dietary habits must be considered. Among adolescents and accident-prone individuals it is common to find bad dietary habits. Many of these individuals have become accustomed to living on junk foods or eating in fast food establishments. They may eat an insufficient amount of protein and decline to eat meat or other protein in the hospital diet. Protein insufficiency inhibits or prevents healing of ulcers. Sterling[44a] noted that if paraplegic patients had a serum protein of less than 3.0 gm/dl, their decubital ulcers would remain indolent with no sign of healing. For a good metabolic response, the patient with an ischemic ulcer should be eating 80–100 gm of protein each day. This usually requires high protein supplements in addition to the three daily meals.

EDEMA

Edema of varying degrees is undoubtedly a contributing factor in the production of ischemic ulcers. An increased amount of interstitial fluid increases the distance from the capillary to the cell. Since the rate of diffusion of oxygen and food from the capillary to the cell decreases geometrically in proportion to this distance, it is clear that edema has a profound influence on the supply of nutrients to the cell. Even before there is frank necrosis or persistent hyperemia, grossly visible edema is present that impairs the transportation of oxygen and nutrition to the cell. The presence of edema during recurrent ischemia compounds the impairment of metabolism.

ANEMIA

Anemia is also a contributing factor of great significance in determining whether or not cellular hypoxia and necrosis will occur. It is obvious that the possibility for ischemic tissue to survive is greatly enhanced when the hemoglobin content and the supply of oxygen within the blood are normal, even though blood flow is reduced. If in ischemia there is also a decreased oxygen content in the blood, cellular metabolism is further restricted.

ENDOCRINE DISORDERS

Hormonal imbalances upset metabolism and delay healing. Diabetes mellitus is the most frequent hormonal problem. Careful management of the insulin requirement is essential for prevention of ischemic ulcers as well as healing. Adrenal cortical insufficiency or excess interferes with protein metabolism by the cell. Today, adrenal corticoid excess that is the result of therapy is encountered more frequently than adrenal insufficiency, which is rare. Administration of adrenal corticoids to patients who have ischemic ulcers should be avoided if possible. Euthyroidism should be maintained; either hypothyroidism or hyperthyroidism interferes with the cellular metabolism needed for healing.

Prevention

Ischemic ulcers are entirely preventable. They need not and should not occur. Some aspect of avoidable negligence is found when they do occur. However, prevention requires knowledge of the correct techniques of management of patients at risk and then the conscientious and continuous application of those techniques, which may require significant expense. Since ischemia lasting only 30 to 60 min causes metabolic impairment that may lead to necrosis of cells, the program of preventive maintenance must be continuous. Patients who have multiple etiological factors that impair cellular metabolism are at greater risk than those with a healthy metabolism, but all are threatened by cellular necrosis if the tissues are exposed to complete ischemia for a period of somewhat less than one hour. Moreover, the effects of exposure to repeated ischemia are cumulative. The results of allowing ischemic ulcers to develop are devastating. Ulcers are always disabling; if their healing is prolonged, they are debilitating and occasionally lead to the patient's death.[12] Treatment of ischemic ulcers after they have developed is difficult, time-consuming, and very expensive.

General Preventive Measures

EDUCATION

Education is the basis of any comprehensive preventive program. Intensive, informative educational efforts that are repeated frequently for hospital personnel as well as for the patient and the family are absolutely essential. All persons involved must be kept continuously aware and informed regarding the primary cause of pressure sores, the serious consequences that can develop if the sores are not cared for, and the patient morbidity that invariably results.

New equipment and adaptations must be thoroughly evaluated by the medical and nursing personnel, and information regarding new materials and improved methods must be provided to all the hospital staff. Above all, the patient and the medical staff must be made to realize that ischemic ulcers can be prevented but that no device or treatment measure, regardless of its cost or design,

can effectively substitute for informed, conscientious skin care.

IDENTIFICATION OF THE HIGH-RISK PATIENT

Because of the critical time-pressure relationship, it is essential at the time of admission to the hospital or nursing facility that efforts be made to identify every patient whose mobility is limited or restricted. Those persons with impaired mobility, especially in combination with decreased sensation or alteration in the level of mental awareness, are obvious candidates for skin breakdown if they are neglected. A single episode of neglect of a comatose or anesthetized patient for even an hour may result in ischemic necrosis. Identification of these persons at the time of admission to the hospital and institution of appropriate, preventive skin-care programs will effectively preclude development of ichemic ulcers.

Special consideration must be given to patients who require sedation or mood-altering drugs. In the process of providing relief of pain and limiting mental anguish and anxiety, the patient's mobility and response to the discomfort of pressure are depressed, with the result that the patient may not move frequently enough to relieve the pressure on the areas at risk.

The comatose, decerebrate, anesthetized or spinal cord–injured patient is a prime candidate for skin breakdown because of the above-mentioned factors. These people must be identified at the time they are admitted to the medical-care facility, and intensive measures for preventive skin care must be instituted immediately.

The postsurgical or multiply traumatized patient also falls into this category because extensive surgical procedures, casting, and postoperative sedation all tend to interfere with the patient's capacity for mobility, thereby promoting skin breakdown.

RECOGNITION OF IMPENDING SKIN BREAKDOWN

All personnel working with these patients must be taught how to recognize early those skin changes that are an indication of an impending breakdown of the skin. The earliest clinical evidence of damage to the skin is indicated by inflammation of the skin, which blanches on the application of digital pressure. This process originally presents as a hyperemic response except that the inflammation, unlike the hyperemic response, persists for a longer period of time. Whereas hyper-

MICHAEL KOSIAK AND FREDERIC J. KOTTKE

emia lasts up to one half to three fourths as long as the occlusion, this pre-ulcer inflammatory reaction may persist for several hours after the pressure has been relieved. At this stage, the condition is usually a completely and readily reversible process. Prevention of progression to more serious damage can be effected by the immediate complete elimination of pressure to the involved area. The time needed for complete resolution of the inflammation depends on the length of time the tissue has been subjected to pressure that has occluded the circulation. Without prompt attention, this condition progresses to increasing inflammation and erythema that persists for more than 24 hours and does not blanch on digital pressure. The skin and underlying tissue become indurated by edema, and there may actually be some vesicle formation. However, even at this stage, prompt preventive measures are generally effective.

Failure to recognize the skin changes noted above and to immediately relieve the involved area of all pressure will result in rapid progression to frank ulceration. The ability to recognize clinically the development of skin changes involving only the dermis, with its associated inflammatory response, is infinitely more important than any classification of the deep, undermined, and infected ulceration. Early recognition of the impending skin changes and the institution of immediate preventive measures can lead to prevention of frank breakdown.

Specific Preventive Measures— Elimination or Reduction of Pressure

If we accept the proposition that pressure in excess of capillary pressure is the chief cause of ischemic ulcers, then our primary preventive efforts must be directed toward reducing or eliminating pressure over susceptible areas.

Intermittent relief of pressure must be provided for all patients, but especially for those who have been identified as highly susceptible to skin breakdown because of other metabolic impairments. Position changes must be made not less frequently than every two hours around the clock. Patients with multiple risk factors must be turned or shifted more frequently. The skin must be carefully assessed each time the position is changed, and areas showing evidence of inflammation must then be completely relieved of compression.

Because of the relationship of body weight to the supporting surface area of the body, there are areas of pressure in excess of capillary pressure when the patient is lying motionless on a standard mattress with the weight distributed as uniformly as possible. The areas of greatest pressure and at greatest risk are usually over the sacrum when supine and over the greater trochanter of the side on which the patient is lying. Complete relief of pressure for each resting surface must be provided at regular intervals. An intermittent pressure support system appears to offer the greatest advantage because relief from pressure is provided to each resting surface at regular predictable intervals.[24]

Extremes of pressure on alternating pressure relief surfaces exceed those resting pressures on static surfaces but do not have the destructive effect of pressures exceeding capillary pressure that are applied for prolonged periods of time.[22] Alternatively, when the patient floats on a loose-surface water bed[46] or an air-flow bed, on which the patient is supported by microbeads continually suspended in a column of flowing air,[41] the body is allowed to float in such a system at a surface pressure below capillary pressure. Even on these beds, patients at extreme risk because of multiple factors interfering with normal metabolism may need frequent turning.

Management

General Measures

Since any major infectious or traumatic process requiring enforced bed rest results in dramatic changes in body metabolism, appropriate dietary measures must be initiated if only to counteract the effects of infection and bed rest. Wound repair is influenced by the nutritional disorders stemming from the altered metabolic processes associated with severe injury as well as by the patient's previous nutritional status.

Superimposed on these disturbances are other problems posed by contaminating microorganisms and compromised blood supply to the injured tissues. Obviously, maintenance of the patient in a good state of nutrition and hygiene should be of high priority both to sustain healing and to avoid infection.

Specific Measures

CONSERVATIVE MEASURES

Conservative treatment methods share three common objectives: pressure relief, wound debridement, and infection control.

Pressure Relief. Since pressure is the primary cause of ischemic ulcers, complete relief of pressure from the involved area is essential if healing is to take place. The ulcerated area should never be subjected to any pressure unless absolutely necessary for resting support.

When multiple ulcers involve several areas that are required for support of the body, these areas must be provided complete relief of pressure at regular intervals. This can be accomplished physically by frequent turning of the patient or mechanically by means of an alternating pressure support system. The alternating-pressure air mattress is a good and economical mechanical method of providing pressure relief for the supine patient. However, over areas of maximal support, the pressures often may exceed capillary pressure so that even the patient cared for in this manner must be turned.

As mentioned earlier, the air-flow type of bed allows the patient to float on a mass of microbeads suspended in a column of rapidly flowing air with pressure less than capillary pressure on all supporting surfaces.[41] Therefore, ischemic ulcers begin to heal even though they are a part of the supporting surface of the body. Flotation water beds provide a similar type of low-pressure flotation support and are much less expensive than the air-flow beds.[14, 19, 42, 46] They require a heater with a thermostat to keep the water at body temperature so that the patient does not become hypothermic. When first introduced, water beds were widely used on rehabilitation wards and other units of acute care hospitals for patients with ischemic ulcers or for patients who were at risk for developing the lesions. Water beds have gradually lost ground in favor to the air-flow bed in hospitals because they are heavy and difficult to move, but they still commonly are used by spinal cord–injured patients in their homes.

Debridement. Because all eschemic ulcers exhibit some degree of tissue necrosis, cleansing of the ulcer and the surrounding area is important.

MECHANICAL DEBRIDEMENT. Various forms of mechanical debridement are accepted in the treatment of ischemic ulcers. Cleansing of the ulcer and the surrounding tissue is best accomplished through the use of a bland antiseptic soap and warm water. The area can then be rinsed well with warm water and normal saline.

Hydrotherapy in the form of whirlpool or Hubbard tank baths is beneficial in assisting in the cleansing of large necrotic ischial or sacral ulcers. Minor surgical debridement is frequently necessary in small necrotic lesions, whereas major surgical debridement, requiring the facilities of the operating room, may be needed in the treatment of the larger lesions.

CHEMICAL DEBRIDEMENT. Enzymes in the form of ointments, solutions, powders, and sprays have been used in the treatment of pressure sores with varying degrees of reported success. Enzymes physiologically debride eschar and necrotic tissue, thus tending to reduce infection.

Enzymatic substances are either fibrinolytic (capable of dissolving fibrin), proteolytic (capable of splitting protein by hydrolysis), or collagenolytic (capable of dissolving collagen). Although these enzymes assist in wound debridement, they have no healing effect *per se*.

Enzymatic measures are indicated especially when simple mechanical debridement is ineffective and surgical debridement is not indicated. Repeated, prolonged use of enzymatic compounds causes progressive lysis of normal protein as well as necrotic material and actually may enlarge wounds as well as delay healing. Enzymatic solutions are usually equally as effective as pastes or ointments with fewer undesirable side effects.

OTHER DEBRIDING AGENTS. Numerous other agents, usually in the form of packs, poultices, and baths, have been used in the treatment of ischemic ulcers. The physiological actions of some of these substances have been debated and the end results have, at times, been of questionable value. Almost without exception, the primary action of these methods of treatment is simple mechanical debridement combined with relief of pressure.

Control of Infections. Persisting superficial infection prevents or retards adequate healing of an ulcer even though pressure is removed and adequate circulation and nutrition are restored. For an ulcer to heal to become functional skin again, it must regain a covering of epithelium of normal thickness and durability and develop a subcutaneous layer of loose connective tissue with adequate capillary circulation to meet all of the metabolic demands placed on that area of skin. Unless durable epithelium, adequate loose connective tissue in the subcutaneous layer, and adequate capillary circulation are restored, the healed defect will be structurally inadequate to tolerate the mechanical and physiological stresses to which it will be exposed.

Infection in the superficial layer of the ulcer prevents all three aspects of healing from occurring normally. A culture of the ulcer will demonstrate that it harbors a number of types of bacteria that

MICHAEL KOSIAK AND FREDERIC J. KOTTKE

grow in the superficial layer, stimulating both serous and purulent secretions proportional to the degree of infection. Granulation tissue composed of capillary buds and loops surrounded by loose connective tissue is stimulated to proliferate by the infecting organisms and continues to proliferate until the infection is suppressed. The infection also promotes development of a dense meshwork of collagen fibers, called a scar, over the base of the ulcer that will cut off the capillary circulation necessary to support the metabolism of the skin as it contracts. If infection is prevented, healing begins to occur promptly and rapidly. The borders of a large uninfected wound will close in, both by formation of new epidermal cells and by contraction or shortening of connective tissue at a rate of 0.5–1.0 mm per day if the wound is not exposed to abrasion, which wipes away the newly formed epidermal cells.[7, 38] As the diameter of the wound decreases, for reasons which are not understood, the rate of closure slows progressively. The newly formed epithelial cells float on the fluid secretion at the edge of the ulcer and become adherent slowly as collagen fibers become attached to the undersurfaces of the wound.[8] Any mechanical wiping or scrubbing of a wound reduces or stops healing by wiping away these newly forming epidermal cells. Likewise, gauze bandages that adhere to the wound as well as debridement of the edges of the ulcer remove the newly formed epidermis and retard healing. A clean ulcer with minimal infection shows a healthy red base, no accumulation of angry red granulation tissue, and minimal serous secretion.

Systemic antibiotics are of benefit to combat invasive pathogenic organisms and to prevent bacteremia but are essentially ineffective when applied to the surface of the ulcer where the less invasive organisms continue to multiply as well as being continually reintroduced from the surrounding environment. Over many years a diverse variety of compounds have been advocated for direct application to decubital ulcers to control infection. In general, the problem with all of these substances is that they usually are only bacteriostatic (although occasionally they are bactericidal), but at the same time they are irritating to the bodily tissues and promote a dense fibrosis in the bed of the ulcer, inhibit capillary budding, and suppress growth of the epidermal cells, all of which interfere with the growth necessary to close the ulcer.

Any severely infected ulcer will show extensive production of serous or purulent exudate. Excessive build-up of granulation tissue may occur, e.g.,

capillary buds and loops with surrounding collagen and fibrocytes and inflammatory exudate called exuberant granulation, which always indicates extensive superficial infection and subsides when the infection is controlled. Until the infection is controlled, the ulcer will not heal. On the other hand, any agent or treatment that inhibits both bacterial and tissue metabolism leaves a wet or nearly dry indolent ulcer that shows no sign of healing. These indolent ulcers tend to increase in size over time owing to the mechanical trauma of washing and cleansing and may become extensively undermined as they persist for months or even years. Such persistent purulent foci promote amyloidosis, which may destroy the kidneys or other vital organs and be the proximate cause of death.[12]

Substances that have been advocated because of their suppression of purulent drainage, although they also inhibit healing, are Dakin's solution, mercurochrome solution, weak iodine solutions, soap and water, plain water (which is destructive because of its hypotonicity), and pHisoHex. Also, other procedures have been suggested, such as packing the wound with sucrose, dried red cells, or chlorophyll or using saturated rock salt baths to produce a hyperosmotic environment. Various metallic ions, such as copper, silver, zinc, tin, gold, which show the typical effects of bacteriostasis, impairment of metabolism, and promotion of fibrosis have been advocated.

On a cycle of about every 20–30 years, abandoned methods are rediscovered and advocated again. Occasionally, one of these methods will be useful, although most of them go through a cycle of producing enthusiastic support because they suppress purulence, followed by the emergence of skepticism when the ulcer remains indolent; they are finally abandoned because of the failure of healing. One such method has been the use of a very weak silver ion solution, either as the nitrate or as a proteinate. This method of treating ischemic ulcers and burns was very popular in the second decade of the 20th century and then fell into disuse until it was reintroduced in the 1960s.[34] Another method very recently reintroduced as useful to accelerate wound healing is low-intensity direct electrical current applied to the wound.[6] This technique also is a resurrection of an old method advocated by manufacturers of electrotherapy equipment at the turn of the century that was rejected by the conventional wisdom of general medicine. After many nonscientific investigations for many purposes, it was concluded that electrotherapy was nonscientific quackery because it lacked convincing scientific evaluation. At that time, the electrical direct current was promoted as a method of iontophoresis to deliver copper, zinc, silver or other metallic ions from the cathode.[17, 27, 28] It was stated that the cathode would cause hardening of the underlying tissues because the metallic ions released into the tissues would result in a decrease of exudation, and the anode would cause softening of the tissues that would result in an increase in the rate of healing. In 1985, Carley and Wainapel report essentially the same results, this time in a controlled study.[6] If prolonged follow-up shows good healing with a well-vascularized and flexible scar and a durable epidermis, this method has much to offer. If the cicatrization of the connective tissue under the healing skin cuts off capillary circulation so that the skin remains friable, this method will be added to the long list of unsatisfactory treatments.

A third method that appears highly effective clinically because it is bactericidal without delaying the metabolism for healing of either epidermal cells or fibroblasts is the use of ultraviolet radiation for the treatment of ischemic ulcers. The technique was developed empirically and passed on by preceptorship. However, it has not been validated by control studies and does not fall within the sphere of conventional wisdom. This method of treating and healing of ischemic ulcers with all degrees of infection was taught to the author by repeated clinical demonstration 40 years ago by Miss Helen Dexter, the Physical Therapy Supervisor at the Minneapolis Veterans Administration Hospital who had learned of the method by clinical demonstration 20 years earlier. Studies of the effects of ultraviolet radiation show a bactericidal band peaking at 2540Å.[27, 28] Twice the minimal effective dose of cold quartz ultraviolet radiation is effective to destroy all motile forms of bacteria on the surface of the ulcer.[23] Since the bacteria reside superficially on a wound rather than within the tissues, the destruction of those superficial bacteria quickly cleans the wound. Although the spores of spore-forming bacteria are more resistant to ultraviolet radiation, they have no effect until they develop into the motile form. Therefore, the daily application of ultraviolet radiation is effective as a bactericidal agent for superficial wounds. Twice the minimal effective dose daily of cold quartz ultraviolet radiation by a grid source over the surface of the wound or by an orificial applicator in fistulas or under undermined edges of the ulcer is effective for bactericidal benefit without the inhibition of tissue metabolism needed for healing

(Fig. 46–5). Cold quartz ultraviolet radiation above five times the minimal effective dose definitely begins to inhibit tissue healing and to delay epithelial growth. Greater than ten times the minimal effective dose of ultraviolet radiation causes destruction of tissue.

It has been reported that treatment of ischemic ulcers by a hydrocolloid occlusive dressing, which is kept in place for a number of days, promotes faster healing than the usual wet or dry gauze dressings.[47] This dressing provides a moist milieu in which epithelial cells can grow and spread more easily. The occlusive barrier protects these new epithelial cells, which float on the edges of the ulcer, from being wiped away by friction and abrasion or from being pulled away by adhering to a dry dressing. If the hydrocolloid does not cause irritation to the ulcer bed or the epithelial border, as is indicated by an increase of serous or purulent exudate, it would appear to be an excellent method of management. A number of these dressings are now produced commercially, but some do cause undesirable irritation of cells in the wound.

Surgical Measures

Although conservative measures are obviously the treatment of choice whenever indicated, surgical intervention plays a very important part in the treatment of ischemic ulcers.

No attempt will be made to review or discuss the technical nature of surgical intervention. Since this subject has been thoroughly discussed and reviewed in the surgical literature, the reader is referred to the surgical journals for a more complete and comprehensive assessment of the problem.

Summary

Ischemic ulcers continue to constitute a major medical problem that interferes with the care of elderly and debilitated patients and patients with paralysis and anesthesia, such as spinal cord–injured patients. In spite of the great advances made in modern medical care, too little attention has been paid to the prevention of pressure ulcers. As a result, even though pressure ulcers are completely preventable, a great number still develop in patients in hospitals and nursing homes as well as in those at home.

Preventive measures must be based on education

MICHAEL KOSIAK AND FREDERIC J. KOTTKE

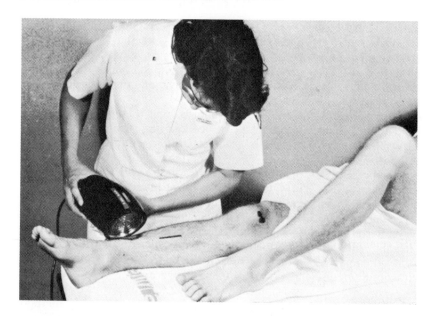

FIGURE 46–5. "Cold quartz" ultraviolet source being used in treatment of chronic ulcer.

of the patient, the family, and all involved professional personnel. Patients and personnel must be constantly reminded of the etiology, pathology, and cost of ischemic ulcers. They must also be convinced that ischemic ulcers can be prevented through diligent and enlightened nursing attention and self-care. The importance of providing pressure relief to the areas supporting the weight of the body must continue to be stressed, and materials and methods must never be substituted for sound nursing care.

References

1. Alexander, H., and Cook, T.: Variations with age in the mechanical properties of human skin in vivo. *In* Kenedi, R. M., Cowden, J. M., and Scales, J. T. (Eds.): Bedsore Biomechanics. Baltimore, University Park Press, 1975, pp. 109–117.
2. Bader, D. L., Barnhill, R. L., and Ryan, T. J.: Effects of externally applied skin surface forces on tissue vasculature. Arch. Phys. Med. Rehabil., 67:807–811, 1986.
3. Bennett, L., Kavner, D., Eng, D., Lee, B. Y., Trainor, F. S., and Lewis, J. M.: Skin stress and blood flow in sitting paraplegic patients. Arch. Phys. Med. Rehabil., 65:186–190, 1984.
4. Burton, A. C., and Yamada, S.: Relation between blood pressure and flow in human forearm. J. Appl. Physiol., 4:329–339, 1951.
5. Bush, C. A.: Study of pressure in skin under ischial tuberosity and thighs during sitting. Arch. Phys. Med. Rehabil., 50:207–212, 1967.
6. Carley, P. J., and Wainapel, S. F.: Electrotherapy for acceleration of wound healing: Low intensity direct current. Arch. Phys. Med. Rehabil., 66:443–446, 1985.
7. Carrel, A., and Hartmann, A.: Cicatrization of wounds. I. The relation between the size of a wound and the rate of cicatrization. J. Exper. Med., 24:429–450, 1916.
8. Christopher, E.: Kinetic aspects of epidermal healing. *In* Maibach, H. I., and Rove, D. T. (Eds.): Epidermal Wound Healing. Chicago, Year Book Medical Publishers, Inc., 1972, pp. 53–69.
9. Conference on care of patients with spinal cord injury. Palo Alto, CA., Veterans Administration Hospital, 1975.
10. Dewis, L. S., Caplan, H. I., and Pache, H. L.: Treatment of decubitus ulcers by use of a water mattress. Arch. Phys. Med. Rehabil., 49:290–293, 1968.
11. Dietrick, J. E.: Effects of immobilization on metabolic and physiological functions of normal men. Bull. N.Y. Acad. Med., 24:364–375, 1948.
12. Dietrick, R. B., and Russi, S.: Tabulation and review of autopsy findings in fifty-five paraplegics. J.A.M.A., 166:41–44, 1958.
13. Dinsdale, S. M.: Decubitus ulcers in swine. Light and microscopy study of pathogenesis. Arch. Phys. Med. Rehabil., 54:51–56, 1973.
14. Exton-Smith, A. N.: Prevention of pressure sores: Monitoring mobility and assessment of clinical condition. *In* Kenedi, R. M., Cowden, J. M., and Scales, J. T. (Eds.): Bedsore Biomechanics. Baltimore, University Park Press, 1975, pp. 133–139.
15. Fisher, S. V., Szymke, T. E., Apte, S. Y., and Kosiak, M.: Wheelchair cushion effect on skin temperature. Arch. Phys. Med. Rehabil., 59:68–72, 1978.
16. Freed, M. M., Bakst, H. J., and Barrie, D. L.: Life

expectancy, survival rates and causes of death in civilian patients with spinal cord trauma. Arch. Phys. Med. Rehabil., 47:457–463, 1966.

17. Friel, A. R.: Electric Ionization. A Practical Introduction To Its Use In Medicine and Surgery. New York, William Wood & Co., 1922.

18. Harman, J. W.: A histological study of skeletal muscle in acute ischemia. Am. J. Pathol., 23:551–565, 1947.

19. Harris, C.: Flotation as an aid to treatment of decubitus ulcers. J. Am. Geriatric Soc., 15:605–610, 1967.

20. Holloway, G. A., Jr., Daly, C. H., Kennedy, D., and Chimoskey, J. E.: Effects of external pressure loading on human skin blood flow measured by ^{133}Xe clearance. J. Appl. Physiol., 40:597–600, 1976.

21. Houle, R. J.: Evaluation of seat devices designed to prevent ischemic ulcers in paraplegic patients. Arch. Phys. Med. Rehabil., 50:587–594, 1969.

22. Hussain, T.: Experimental study of some pressure effects on tissues with reference to the bed sore problem. J. Pathol. Bacteriol., 66:347–358, 1953.

23. Koller, L. R.: Ultraviolet Radiation. New York, John Wiley & Sons, 1952.

24. Kosiak, M.: A mechanical resting surface: Its effect on pressure distribution. Arch. Phys. Med. Rehabil., 57:481–484, 1976.

25. Kosiak, M.: Etiology and pathology of ischemic ulcers. Arch. Phys. Med. Rehabil., 40:61–69, 1959.

26. Kosiak, M.: Etiology of decubitus ulcers. Arch. Phys. Med. Rehabil., 42:19–29, 1961.

27. Kovacs, R.: Electrotherapy and Light Therapy. Philadelphia, Lea & Febiger, 1932.

28. Krusen, F. H.: Physical Medicine. Philadelphia, W. B. Saunders Co., 1941.

29. Kuhn, W. G., Jr.: Care and rehabilitation of patients with injuries of spinal cord and cauda equina. J. Neurosurg., 4:40–68, 1947.

30. Landis, E. M.: Micro-injection studies of capillary blood pressure in human skin. Heart, 15:209–228, 1930.

31. Lewis, T., and Haynol, I.: Observations relating to the tone of the minute vessels of the human skin. Heart, 14:177, 1928.

32. Lindan, O., Greenway, R. M., and Piazza, J. N.: Pressure distribution on the surface of the human body: 1. Evaluation in lying and sitting positions using a "bed of springs and nails." Arch. Phys. Med. Rehabil., 46:378–385, 1965.

33. Mooney, V., Eisbund, M. J., Rogers, J. E., and Stauffer, E. S.: Comparison of pressure distribution qualities in seat cushions. Bull. Prosthet. Res., (Spring) 129–143, 1971.

34. Moyer, C. A., Bretano, L., Gravens, D. L., Margraf, H. W., and Monafo, W. W.: Treatment of large human burns with 0.5% silver nitrate solution. Arch. Surg., 90:812–867, 1965.

35. Munro, D.: Care of the back following spinal-cord injuries. N. Engl. J. Med., 223:391–398, 1940.

36. Newson, T. P., and Rolfe, P.: Skin surface PO$_2$ and blood flow measurements over ischial tuberosity. Arch. Phys. Med. Rehabil., 63:553–556, 1982.

37. Nichol, J., Girling, F., Jerrard, W., Claxton, E. B., and Burton, A. C.: Fundamental instability of small blood vessels and critical closing pressures in vascular beds. Am. J. Physiol., 164:330–344, 1951.

38. Orentreich, N., and Selmanowitz, V. J.: Levels of biological functions with aging. Trans. N.Y. Acad. Sci., Series II, 31:992–1012, 1969.

39. Patterson, R. P., and Fisher, S. V.: Pressure and temperature patterns under the ischial tuberosities. Bull. Prosthet. Res., 17:5–11, 1980.

40. Reichel, S. M.: Shearing force as a factor in decubitus ulcers in paraplegics. J.A.M.A., 166:762–763, 1958.

41. Scales, J. T., Lunn, H. F., Jeneid, P. A., Gillingham, M. E., and Redfern, S. J.: The prevention and treatment of pressure sores using air support systems. Paraplegia, 12:118, 1974.

42. Siegel, F. J., Vistnes, L. M., and Labu, D. R.: Use of the water bed for prevention of pressure sores. Plast. Reconstr. Surg., 51:31–37, 1973.

43. Souther, S. G., Carr, S. D., and Vistnes, L. M.: Pressure, tissue ischemia and operating table pads. Arch. Surg., 107:544–547, 1973.

44. Souther, S. G., Carr, S. D., and Vistnes, L. M.: Wheelchair cushions to reduce pressure under bony prominences. Arch. Phys. Med. Rehabil., 55:460–464, 1974.

44a. Sterling, H. M.: Personal communication.

45. Tsuchida, Y., and Tsuya, A.: Measurement of skin blood flow in delayed deltopectoral flaps using local clearance of ^{133}Xenon. Plast. Reconstr. Surg., 62:763–770, 1978.

46. Weinstein, J. D., and Davidson, B. A.: A fluid-support in the prevention of treatment of decubitus ulcers. Am. J. Phys. Med., 45:283–290, 1966.

47. Yarkony, G. M., Lakone, C., and Carle, T. V.: Pressure sore management: Efficacy of a moisture-reactive occlusive dressing. Arch. Phys. Med. Rehabil., 65:597–600, 1984.

47

Rehabilitation of Problems of Sexuality in Physical Disability

THEODORE M. COLE   SANDRA S. COLE

If one reflects on the images that may come to mind when the word "sex" is spoken, many people would think pleasant thoughts such as lovemaking, fun, warmth, and pleasure—both giving and taking. On the other hand, if one considers the imagery evoked by the word "disability," it would not be surprising for many people to think of such concepts as alone, ugly, incapable, and painful. A significant realization may occur when these two sets of concepts are put into juxtaposition. The emotional reaction to the concepts of sex and disability together might include such thoughts as impossibility, frustration, withdrawal, disinterest, or vulnerability. It is clear that a conscious effort will be needed by health professionals and disabled people alike to alter the attitudes that lead to such thoughts.

Although physicians are generally informed about the pathophysiology of genitourinary and reproductive function, they may not be informed about contemporary sexual behavior. The information they do possess may be colored by personal preferences, aversions, and taboos that may further foster ignorance. The uneasiness and anxiety that result from misinformation may make it difficult for the physician to hear or treat the patient's complaints. Patients and their families can also be ill-informed or uncomfortable with sexuality, thereby impeding the physician's ability to obtain a cogent sexual history or initiate a referral for sexual intervention. The presence of a physical disability does not erase the years of socialization that may make it difficult for patients and families to discuss sexuality with the physician. That same discomfort or anxiety may lead to sexual dysfunction and marital strife, and the foundation for

sexual dysfunction may be passed on to children. However, a patient's unwillingness to talk about sexuality does not necessarily mean disinterest. Unwillingness may mean that the patient is anxious or fearful about the sexual implications of the physical disability. The physician may be able to reduce the anxiety by taking positive actions to facilitate comfort and set the expectation with the patient that sexuality, like any other important aspect of living, is an appropriate area of concern for physicians and the patients who seek their services.

While studying human sexuality curricula in American medical schools, Ebert and Lief[1] pointed out that although reproductive physiology and pathology were commonly taught, sexuality training programs for medical students were almost non-existent before 1954. In the early 1960s there were only three programs. However, by 1968 there were 30 medical schools offering sexuality curriculum and by 1975 nearly all medical schools reported substantial sex education programs for their students. Interest in sexuality and physical disability has followed a similar course of recent expansion.

A physical disability is the result of an impairment that can usually be described by a physician. A handicap is a collective result of all the hindrances that a disability places between an individual and optimum functional potential. It is more accurate to refer to an individual with a disability rather than a disabled person because the term "disabled" subordinates all areas of function to the disabling aspect. These are not irrelevant attitudinal distinctions. The degree to which a physical disability is handicapping is relative to each situation and social role. Not all people perceive the same disability as particularly handicapping, especially with respect to sexuality. A physical condition that is not necessarily disabling or handicapping may become so owing to social stigmatization. Roberts and Roberts[2] conclude that a physical attribute becomes a handicap only when it is seen as a significant obstacle to the accomplishment of a particular goal, and that a physical attribute may become handicapping not because it imposes actual limitations but because it interferes with social relations or is in conflict with the individual's value systems.

Sexuality: Its Meaning for Rehabilitation

Some physical disabilities affect sexuality directly by disablement of genital function. However, most do not. Blindness does not affect genital function, but it certainly affects communication. Myocardial infarction is frequently followed by impotence in a high percentage of males and may also affect the libido and activities of the patient's partner because of fear of sudden death precipitated by sexual activity. The individual with a disfiguring burn may want acceptance and contact but instead withdraws and covers up. In these examples sexuality is defined by and expressed in how people present themselves—their bodies, activities, relationship preferences, and aversions. Understood in broad terms, it becomes clear that sexuality may influence and be influenced by physical disability. Sexuality is an avenue toward intimacy.[3] The imposition of a life devoid of intimacy may have a devastating effect upon the person with a physical disability and may compound the health care problems with which the physician must deal.

Medical rehabilitation has been defined in many ways. For the purposes of this chapter, it is defined as a process that promotes a stabilization of the disabling condition, maximizes restoration of lost functions, and institutes adaptive mechanisms that allow resumption of responsibility for part or all of one's own life. If a physical disability is complex and moderately severe, pursuit of these goals will require the efforts of an integrated team of practitioners who can provide an array of health care services in medical, psychosocial, vocational, and educational areas. Such a team will discover that fruitful work with a person with a physical disability mandates a rapport of trust and openness that must be maintained over the duration of the handicap and its treatment. Trust is not easily achieved and may be hampered by aloofness, impaired communication, or distance between the physician and the patient. Sensitive attention given to sexuality, however, can play a facilitating role in building rapport by emphasizing caring, comprehensiveness, and openness, while minimizing aloofness and barriers to communication.

Foundations of Sexual Health

When one accepts a broad definition of human sexuality, one can better see and understand the sexuality of people with handicapping conditions. One may then understand when and in what ways the handicapped person may have concerns about expressing sexuality.

As for any other aspect of health care, the practitioner should be trained in how to initiate questions and interventions relative to sexuality. Consideration of the physician's own sexuality may help him or her become more effective in dealing with the sexuality of others. Lief[4] points out that a physician learns about sexuality differently than he or she learns about other scientific topics. One can effectively employ a body of knowledge about chemistry without emotionally understanding one's own chemistry. However, one cannot effectively employ a body of knowledge about sexuality and apply it to a patient without thinking about one's own sexuality. The absence of self-understanding about sexuality may lead the physician to do harm to the patient and disservice to the medical profession.

Sexuality is a health issue. Rehabilitation, perhaps more than most other medical specialties, concerns itself with the whole patient. Sexuality is part of the whole and is a natural function. However, naturalness may be impeded by many things, including previous experiences or physical conditions. The physician can be helpful as diagnostician, educator, or therapist by employing the medical model. The medical model should not be abandoned when dealing with the area of sexuality. It is not sufficient for a physician to ask, How is your sex life? A similar abandonment of the medical model would cause the physician to ask a patient with ulcerative colitis, How is your defecation life? Specific questions and answers can lead to diagnoses and therapy.

Sexual health is different for different people.

THEODORE M. COLE AND SANDRA S. COLE

However, there are several components of sexuality that are common to a state of sexual health. These include a positive self-esteem, freedom from prohibiting attitudes and ignorance, and a willingness to risk intimacy with another person. For some people sexual health also involves a measure of physical competence. Like other physical activities, sex requires a certain amount of practice and skill. Unfortunately, our culture does not provide physically disabled people with a sufficient array of sex education materials to allow them to become educated about themselves and the world in which they live. Thus, many people with physical disabilities either learn little about themselves or possess spotty if not erroneous information about their physical capabilities. Remediation of this misinformation is clearly within the province of the physician.

Psychosexual Development of Children

During infancy and the first decade, boys experience penile erections at regular intervals. These may be reflexogenic during infancy but later on result from deliberate self-stimulation. Females also engage in self-stimulation. Their early sexual character is described as being more diffuse than that of the male. The early sexual experiences of girls may result from a wider assortment of stimuli than direct genital stimulation. During these years, both boys and girls are having their attention drawn to sex with such tasks as toilet training, learning sex differences between parents, siblings, and friends, and learning or adopting sexual modesty codes. During these same years, the child is developing a language base that will include "acceptable" and "dirty" words for conveying sexual information. Facility with sexual language becomes exceedingly important if the youth is to understand the world, communicate with peers, and avoid problems that arise from ignorance.

Learning differences between right and wrong is a major task during these growing years. It is hoped that the child will build wholesome attitudes toward self while at the same time learning how to get along with peers. The development of a conscience becomes evident at a time when the child is learning appropriate sex roles, acquiring moral and ethical standards, and beginning to project attitudes toward social groups and institutions that have direct sexual associations.

The child grows within the framework of a society that adopts, projects, and enforces a set of attitudes that impact back on the child's sexuality. Both the able-bodied and the physically disabled child must contend with society's attitudes toward menstruation, wet dreams, masturbation, and sexual fantasies. Society's admiration of the "perfect body" may convey the message that physical disability desexualizes the child. The family's efforts to protect the child from rejection or exploitation may lead to avoidance of the topic of sex and normal family interactions. The child may thus be insulated from exposure to sexual situations and may be thought of by peers as "less than" other children. The gaps in the sex education of a child may lead to problems that can become insurmountable in later years. Parents, in turn, may be isolated by the child's fear of admitting ignorance or of revealing fantasies and concerns. Like able-bodied children, the disabled child worries about being normal, over- or undersexed, attractive or unattractive. It is clear that the physician can help to provide the child with an adult role model that recognizes sexuality in the formative years and helps the child and the family develop a growing sense of sexual health.

Sexual Physiology and Responsivity

It is not the purpose of this chapter to provide a comprehensive discussion of the physiological and behavioral aspects of sexuality. For such information the reader is referred to appropriate texts.[5-10] However, a brief review is appropriate to establish a common basis of understanding between the authors and readers.

The sexual response cycle has been described by many workers. The work of Masters and Johnson may be the best known and identifies four phases of the cycle.

The excitement phase can be psychological or physical. It begins when the person is first aware of being sexually stimulated. Both men and women show increases in muscle tension, heart rate, blood pressure, and breathing rate. If stimulation continues in the male, erection of the penis occurs. In the female, vaginal lubrication begins with continued stimulation. If stimuli cease to be effective, the next phase will not occur and the body will return to the unaroused state. If sexual stimulation continues, however, the second phase begins.

The plateau phase is the second phase and extends from the end of excitement until the beginning of orgasm. Owing to neurovascular influences, congestion of the primary sexual organs occurs. If stimulation is ineffective or ceases, the body will show a gradual reduction of the physiological phenomena that are part of this phase. With continued effective stimulation, the third phase will commence.

Orgasm is the third phase. If no psychological or physical discomfort occurs, the person will progress through one or more orgasms. Orgasms customarily last from 30 to 60 seconds but have been described as lasting from as little as a few seconds to as long as several minutes. Most often, the male ejaculates during orgasm and is aware of a rhythmic contraction of his perineal muscles. Women also experience rhythmic contractions of the pubococcygeal muscles, and in both sexes anal sphincter contraction occurs synchronously with contractions of the pelvic floor. Immediately after orgasm, a refractory period commences during which time more stimulation will not produce further sexual arousal. The refractory phase may last from minutes to days, depending on such factors as age and intensity of sexual arousal. Women have brief refractory periods and may be multiorgasmic.

The fourth phase is called resolution. During this phase the body returns to its prearoused and relaxed state.

Inability to achieve orgasm is often equated with sexual dysfunction. However, as can be seen from the description of the sexual response cycle, dysfunction can occur at any phase in the cycle. Educating patients about their natural responsiveness and physiological functioning while encouraging them to become comfortable with themselves and their sexuality, can be very therapeutic for people with or without physical disabilities.

Although sexuality, intimacy, and genital function can be separated, they are usually interconnected. It is helpful, therefore, to define the more common genital dysfunctions so that one can understand how they can cause or be caused by personal or interpersonal problems. It should be kept in mind that genital aspects of sexual function have an impact on the entire personality. Changes in genital function will almost always create reverberations throughout the personality structure of the individual.

Female Sexual Dysfunctions

Preorgasmia. Women who have never experienced an orgasm by any means are considered preorgasmic. In the absence of physical disability, the roots of preorgasmia are usually found in the religious upbringing, the family environment or childhood sexual trauma.

Secondary Nonorgasmia. Secondary nonorgasmia is often situational. Women who experience orgasm with masturbation or with a partner's stimulation but not with sexual intercourse are included in this group. Also included are women who experience physical orgasm but do not experience a psychological component and women who experienced orgasm during an earlier part of their life but not currently.

Dyspareunia. Women who experience disabling pain during intercourse are considered to have dyspareunia. Prior to counseling, a woman should receive a thorough medical examination to exclude organic causes of vaginal pain.

Sexual Aversion. Women who are repulsed or terrified by sex are described as being sexually aversive. Etiologic factors may include one or more of the following: doubts about her own sexual adequacy; overreaction to body odors, penis size, or semen; early traumatic sexual experience; or extremely prohibiting religious views leading to feelings of guilt and shame regarding sex.

Vaginismus. Vaginismus occurs during attempted penetration of the vulva by the erect penis and is characterized by involuntary spasms of the muscles of the pelvic floor that surround the outer third of the vagina. This dysfunction is also frequently associated with sexual fears and anxieties about intercourse. Its roots can frequently be found in the woman's lack of self-acceptance, an underdeveloped ability to form sexual relationships, inability to trust a partner, religious prohibitions, or previous sexual trauma.

Male Sexual Dysfunctions

Premature Ejaculation. A man is said to prematurely ejaculate if he ejaculates before he wishes. This is one of the most common sexual dysfunctions of men, and, fortunately, one of the easiest to treat.

Primary Erectile Dysfunction. A condition of primary erectile dysfunction exists when a man states that he has never been able to maintain an erect penis for the purpose of sexual penetration. He may, however, be capable of having erections during masturbation and may report erections during sleep. Physical examinations should be carried out to eliminate organic causes, which will be

THEODORE M. COLE AND SANDRA S. COLE

described later. Anxieties, which may be rooted in sexual trauma in early life, male sex role stress, feelings of inadequacy, or prohibiting religious or moral views may also be etiologically significant.

Secondary Erectile Dysfunction. Men who have been able to achieve erections on some occasions but not on others are said to have secondary erectile dysfunction. Erection may be possible during foreplay but may disappear as coitus is attempted. Some men report achievement of erections with some partners but not with others. Common causative factors include excessive use of alcohol, relationship stresses, and secondary effects of some therapeutic medicines to be described later.

Retarded Ejaculation. Men whose ejaculatory reflexes are inhibited while erection remains are experiencing retarded ejaculation. Such men sometimes experience ejaculation through manual or oral stimulation but are unable to ejaculate while the penis is contained in the vagina. Etiologic factors often include guilt feeings surrounding sex in general or guilt feelings with specific sexual partners. Sexual identity conflicts, fear of pregnancy in a partner, and moral and ethical considerations also may play a part.

As this brief description of the more common sexual dysfunctions shows, the causation is often related to dysfunctional sexual attitudes, behavioral problems, relationship problems, or early traumatic sexual experiences. However, none of them presupposes the presence of a physical disability as a causative factor or an initiating event leading to sexual dysfunction. Any of these sexual dysfunctions can be seen in a physically disabled adult. In addition, a sexual dysfunction may have its onset after the occurrence of a physical disability. The physician should therefore be acquainted with the ways in which sexual function may be altered by a physical disability.

Sexual Evaluation of the Disabled Patient

Why Ask?

The physician asks questions of the patient in order to make diagnoses, develop a plan of management, assess effectiveness of therapy, and make modifications in relation to progress. The goal is restoration to optimal function as an individual in the community. Specific diagnoses of sexual dys-

functions that are amenable to correction can be made by an alert clinician who asks the right questions in a sensitive way.

Masters and Johnson have asserted that sexual dysfunction occurs at one time or another in at least 50 per cent of the general population. There is a probability that problems of sexuality are even more frequent in persons with disabilities. Many sexual dysfunctions are treatable if identified. The problems associated with sexual dysfunction often are substantive and concrete. Although many sexual dysfunctions become intertwined with the personality structure, there are often functional problems that can be remedied by brief therapy.

How to Ask

The rehabilitation model serves us well in the area of sexuality. Just as with rehabilitation issues such as mobility, self-care, and weakness, which are treated within the context of the disabilities, questions about intimacy may be integrated into the medical history. Information may be gained with inquiries and questions dealing with pain, alterations in bodily sensations, disfigurements, and so on. Segregating questions about sexuality from the medical and rehabilitation history conveys the message that sex is not really a health issue or is less acceptable to the physician than other aspects of the patient's health.

Since in our culture discussion of sex usually carries an emotional loading that is stressful to the patient, questions should be discreetly and privately asked, and an understanding of confidentiality should be established early in the interview. Difficult questions can often be made easier if the physician will frankly ask the patient for permission to delve into personal and even sensitive areas. When the patient understands that informing the physician is helpful and allows treatment of the problems that stem from the physical disability, then willingness is usually freely expressed. Identifying personal areas as sensitive is a useful technique for eliciting the patient's permission. The patient may be more prepared to answer questions if there is a clear relationship between the question and the disability under consideration. Thus, questions to an arthritic patient about pain on movement, especially freedom of movement of the hips, can easily be seen to be a sex-related topic. Similarly, the medical ramifications of diabetic peripheral neuropathy should properly include questions relative to erections in the male, vaginal lubrication in the female, and orgasmic function in both.

The physician can make the socially stressful situation of the medical interview more comfortable by indicating to the patient that it may seem awkward when a person is asked to reveal personal areas of self to a relative stranger. Simply saying so may do much to allay anxiety and allow a sensitive exploration of sexual issues.

Some physicians are reluctant to commence a sexual interview because they fear that, once begun, a comprehensive review of material with which they are not familiar must be carried out. However, most physicians do not need to conduct a comprehensive sexual interview in order to go over information useful for the rehabilitation team. Specific questions may be all that are needed to identify the sexual problems and concerns of some patients. Lief[4] points out that perhaps 25 per cent of patients with sexual dysfunctions can be benefited solely by providing information within an atmosphere of friendliness and permission to talk. The sexual partner of the patient is an important person to be interviewed, either separately or with the patient. Not only may the physician gain new and important insights about the patient's sexuality, but bringing the partner along at the same rate as the patient may avoid future pitfalls created by unevenness of information and expectations between the patient and the sexual partner.

Reactions from the patient or partner may indicate areas of need. Thus, the patient who displays apparent indifference after questions about sexuality may really be displaying anxiety or fear of discovery. Very few people are genuinely disinterested in their own sexuality. A skilled clinician can return in the future with further questions if the indifference persists throughout the initial interview. Denial of sexual concerns may genuinely reflect a lack of concern on the part of the patient. However, the lack of concern may stem from lack of information rather than an informed reason to be unconcerned. For example, a patient in the early stages of severe stroke may believe that he or she will return to the pre-morbid vocation, and may not recognize until weeks later that a vocational disability has resulted. So, too, a return to questions of sexuality and intimacy at a later date may reveal that the denial has been replaced by a genuine interest, or even by fear of dysfunction. The use of comfort-producing techniques such as brief anecdotes about similar situations can do much to forge a basis for subsequent productive discussions on intimate issues.

Some patients may react with frank hostility. Often hostility is strong evidence of a serious problem that deserves further exploration if not consultation by professionals skilled in human sexuality and physical disability. All the while, the physician must remember to avoid becoming defensive or to feel a need for lengthy explanations of sexually related questions.

The language of sex may be as personal as the activities themselves. The physician should make an effort to understand the patient and provide a language that is comfortable and communicative. Resorting to strictly medical terms is often as undesirable in the area of sexuality as it is in any medical area where accurate communication is essential. However, the physician may learn that the patient's sex-related words and language are different from his or her own. The physician should be prepared to use the patient's preferred language in order to communicate. Thus, for some people "come" may be a more effective word than orgasm and "hard-on" may be more communicative than erection.

What to Ask

The patient should be encouraged to express his or her needs, concerns, and fears about the disability and expressions of intimacy. The type and duration of the disability are important, since a disability having its onset during childhood usually has a different effect upon sexuality than a disability that has its onset after psychosexual development has been completed. Information having to do with sexual techniques, frequency, sexual fantasy, and personal values and ethics is important to gather in order to be helpful. The physician should remember not to put persons into conflict with their God, their morals, or their ethics in the area of sexuality. Specific questions should be asked in order to gain an understanding of a couple's sexual patterns. Information about sexual practices, either solitary or with the sexual partner, should be gathered. Masturbation, anal sex, oral genital stimulation, manual genital manipulation, and use of sexual devices are frequently practiced among adults in Western culture. The patterns of sexual expression are important for a physician to know, just as it is important to know about a patient's daily living activities or vocational interests in setting goals for a rehabilitation plan. The physician must not overlook the fact that some

THEODORE M. COLE AND SANDRA S. COLE

people engage in homosexual activities either exclusively or in addition to heterosexual activities. Thus, the sexual orientation of the patient should be determined. Questions about sexual partners other than the primary partner should also be asked, especially in cases of erectile dysfunction or loss of libido.

In interviewing a physically disabled person, as with a person without an apparent disability, sex should be considered in a broad sense, not only as genital function. Sex is a major avenue of communication between people and involves not only coitus and self-pleasuring but any other physical activity that is mutually acceptable and pleasurable. The physician's inquiries about sexual history should be made in a way that is acceptable and satisfying to both the patient and the physician. An interview can be not only diagnostic but sometimes therapeutic as well.

The physician's examination should also assess the patient's general knowledge about sexuality. The physician can help patients by having available, for educational purposes, printed material and examples of equipment or devices used by disabled persons. This may include not only items that a disabled person may use to accomplish activities of daily living, such as catheters, fecal drainage bags, and the like, but also equipment related to sexual function, such as an electrical vibrator.

Physical Examination

As with any other aspect of the physical examination, the physician's examination of the patient with respect to sexual function should be organized and systematic.

Sensory testing should include testing of the genitals and the perineal area. In addition, other erogenous zones, whether identified by the patient or believed to be important by the physician, should also be examined for sexual function. In many cases of spinal cord injury, erogenous zones change dramatically after sensory paralysis. Frequently, the dermatomal levels just above the anesthetic area of the body become erogenous, whereas they may not have been so prior to the disability. Sensory examination should also include the urinary and rectal sphincters, and special attention should be paid to the S 1, S 2, and S 3 dermatomes on the buttocks and legs.

Motor testing should include the S 1 to S 3 motor segments of the lower extremities as well as sphincter tone strength of the pelvic floor and the rectum. The bulbocavernosus reflex should be tested in both the male and the female. Its absence may indicate a lesion of the reflex arc between the pelvic floor and the spinal cord. The force of the urinary stream, either audibly or visibly monitored, may help to provide information about detrusor S 1 to S 3 function, which can be influenced in a parallel way with organic sexual function. Motor testing must also address impairments of mobility—ability to voluntarily move body parts in order to accomplish sexually related positions and movements. In addition to joint motion and strength, it will also be important to consider the presence of pain on movement or posture, coordination, and endurance.

Vascular lesions in the large vessels of the legs and pelvis may explain the lack of pelvic congestion following sexual stimulation. They may also be responsible for erectile dysfunctions in both men and women. The shaft of the penis should be examined for the plaques of Peyronie's disease, and the vagina should be examined for mechanical obstructions and inflammation.

Examination of the urinary tract should include not only a thorough examination of the external genitals but also electrical studies of the bladder and the pelvic floor. A cystometrogram can provide the physician with important information about the function of the bladder, which is served by many of the same nerve roots that serve sexual function. EMG studies of the external urinary or rectal sphincter may also help to diagnose upper or lower motor neuron disease, which in turn may affect not only erectile function but ejaculation in the male and lubrication in the female as well. Investigation of nocturnal penile tumescence is a technique that has become popular in recent years and may be useful to the physician in diagnosing erectile dysfunction in the male. Erections varying in length from 15 to 30 minutes occur several times a night during periods of rapid eye movement (REM) sleep in the neurologically intact male. The absence of such a phenomenon may indicate an organic basis for the erectile dysfunction.

The physician should also examine the patient for target organ disease elsewhere, as in patients with diabetes mellitus. A history of changes in bowel function, loss of esophageal motility, or gastric atony may help confirm the autonomic neuropathy of diabetes. Ten to 25 per cent of diabetics have disturbances of pupillary function. Decreased sudomotor function is also seen in the peripheral neuropathy of diabetes mellitus. Orthostatic hypertension, changes in peripheral pulse rate with positional changes of the body, alterations in the R-R interval on the ECG during and after the Valsalva maneuver, and cardiovascular responses to forceful gripping are all measures of autonomic nervous system function.

Classification of Physical Disabilities

For purposes of a construct of disability and sexuality, physical disabilities can be grouped into four categories, depending on age of onset and the progressive or stable nature of the disability.

Type I Disabilities— Preadolescent Nonprogressive

Type I disabilities are those that begin before puberty and are not progressive. Congenital brain injury, limb amputation in early life, and congenital loss of organs of special sensation are examples. People with these disabilities experience a lifetime of being different from their peers. Protective or guilt-laden attitudes by society or parents may have an inhibiting effect on their sexual maturation. They may be deliberately or inadvertently deprived of important adolescent experiences. Such individuals may emerge from adolescence with maturational deficits and lack of social skills. They may find themselves in an adult world, wanting to be sexually sophisticated but lacking the requisite education.

DEVELOPMENTAL DISABILITIES

Public Law 94–103 states that a developmental disability is a physical or mental impairment resulting in limitations of major life activities. It is manifested before the age of 22 years and is likely to continue. It often produces a lifelong need for special or extended care. Public Law 94–142 specifically provides for public education for all school-age children who are physically disabled. The education is mandated to occur in the least restrictive manner.

Easton[11] points out that addressing the sexuality of such a person may require considerable and continuing effort. The individual who has been disabled from birth or early childhood has been different for a lifetime. Together with the usual self-consciousness of adolescence, the developmental disability may prevent the child from mixing with other children. The child may focus much energy into academic achievement. Many children are delayed in reaching independence owing to physical, mental, or emotional barriers occurring within themselves. Added to this is the fact that growing up takes place in a society that is uneasy about sex, where sexual activity begins at earlier and earlier ages, and where there is not enough communication between the child and the adult world. Robinault[12] states that the physician can take the role of healer, educator, and counselor. However, the role of healer may be conflicted by the chronicity of the disease, the role of educator by the diversity in which the child lives, and the role of counselor by the many options for sexual education and expression that are available and practical in our society.

Easton[11] states that the handicapped child may not learn because of limited physical and social experience, low demands or expectations from the family and school, and limited teaching in the skills of adolescence and adulthood. Learning may also suffer from a lack of honest feedback about inappropriate behavior, problems attendant to separation from the family, and informational deficits in street language and innuendo. The child may lack an orientation to peer values and may manifest egocentricity and preoccupation with physical or academic activities that are encouraged by the family and society. Added to these may be learning or perceptual problems, deficits in special sensation, and expressive or receptive communication problems. The mosaic may be complicated by a limited supply of energy that is drained by demands placed on the child for independence and mobility. The result is often a child who does not know how to take responsibility for his or her own social and sexual success.

Example: A 15-year-old girl with cerebral palsy was brought by her mother to the physician ostensibly to receive a prescription for new orthopedic shoes. On questioning by the physician, the mother was found eager to be provided with birth control information because she recognized that her daughter knew little, asked less, and had no sexual experience with boys. She reasoned that one day opportunity would either develop or be pressed upon the young woman. Referral to a clinic for developmentally disabled teenagers was made. Not only did both mother and daughter receive helpful information about fertility, but also age-appropriate sex education material was provided. The family found a mechanism for ongoing consultation relative to becoming an adult woman in an increasingly explicit society.

Example. A 22-year-old male college student with spina bifida was referred to a psychiatrist for episodes of rage that were directed at anyone in his vicinity. Evaluation found an extremely frustrated young man, feeling the need for information but lacking any experience with an adult or peer who would view his sexuality in a positive manner. Thus, he had never been told accurate or appropriate information relative to his desires and fears, and eventually he became a behavior problem as a method of striking back at an alien and unresponsive society. Therapeutic sex education was provided as part of a rehabilitation program, and his family and he were aided in how to more constructively avoid heightening his frustration by answering questions and providing information.

The physician must understand the very real limitations imposed by the child's disability and at the same time make use of the child's environment and strengths. The child whose family provides healthy, warm, and loving support will generally do better in psychosexual development. Most important is the need to consider the child as a sexual person from the very beginning. School personnel may also play a role as the child progresses to a larger world. The goals of education may need to be different for the child with a physical handicap, and more emphasis may have to be placed on social abilities than on pure academics. In providing services to such a child and family, the physician should respect the family's value system. Sensitive issues or different standards of ethics, religion, and sex will require sensitivity from the physician.

DEAFNESS

Deafness is the most common chronic disability in the United States today (see Chapter 44). In approaching the deaf child and the family, the physician should recognize that 90 per cent of deaf children have parents with normal hearing abilities. Usually children with congenital deafness receive their education and much of life's experiences in residential schools where they may stay until 21 years of age.

Since the average deaf child achieves a reading level between the fourth and fifth grade, deaf children are handicapped by a dearth of sex education material available at that level. The deaf child or young adult may have had difficulties in

learning about sexuality because of limited auditory observational opportunities. Added to this is the fact that sex-related sign language is very regional in the United States and very private and personal. It is often not readily available to the developing child. In those few schools for the deaf in which sex education is provided, it is necessary that the signing interpreter be comfortable with sexuality. Graphics have been found to be helpful, especially when prepared specifically for deaf children.

The physician's approach to a deaf child and family must be directed toward helping the child achieve social skills and a positive self-image while encouraging the caretakers in the family and schools to facilitate the sexualization of the child as a normal and healthy development.

ADVICE TO CLINICIANS

1. When the clinician includes sexuality in the assessment, it will provide an opportunity to gather information regarding beliefs, attitudes, behavior, and experiences in sex education and sexual behavior. In addition, it provides the opportunity to educate and discuss topics of sexuality. This type of communication is more effective if it is done over a period of time and not all at once, since discussion about sexuality may be awkward, embarrassing, or difficult.

2. Be aware and respectful of the fact that older children and teenagers may have only a superficial knowledge about sexuality and sexual behavior, even though they may have already been sexually active. Generally, one must consider that children may present themselves as knowledgeable and "savvy" but may have a thin veneer of knowledge.

3. During discussion, explore the level of social maturity, assessing how much the person knows, has been exposed to, or has experienced in situations such as intercourse, sexual exploitation, molestation, pregnancy, parental divorce, and so on.

4. Expect to find deeply embedded personal and family beliefs and attitudes about disability, sexuality, sex behavior, and religion. Values must be considered and respected by the clinician, particularly if the nature of the discussions evokes some of these values.

5. A certain amount of rebelliousness may be anticipated as normal adolescent behavior that may also be reflected in reactions to sexuality and discussion.

6. Encourage the development of communication skills that will be helpful to the individual in

the adult world of sexuality. Be prepared to provide information on anatomy, physiology, socialization, privacy, appropriate and inappropriate touch, refusing unwanted sexual activity, and the basic language of sex. When you are working with a minor, it is recommended that you discuss with the family the importance and necessity of the topic of sexuality as a part of daily living in order to enhance the skills, knowledge, and comfort of the individual as he or she matures. Your interest is to gain the acknowledgment and support of the family so they can continue this education.

7. Involve the parents and encourage them to address the sexual development of their child. Promote education and socialization opportunities, which are crucial pieces of healthy sexual development. Many parents are hesitant and tend to be protective when it comes to sexuality.

8. Be sensitive to the possibility of previous or existing sexual abuse. If you discover the possibility or existence of sexual abuse, contact an authority and the local child protection team in your facility. Be aware that you are legally required to report all suspected cases to the state child protection agency, which will assume responsibility to investigate the case.

Where administratively at all feasible, *do not* assign personal hygiene duties to a male nurse or attendant when the patient is a female minor. It is well established that 99 per cent of sexual exploitation is committed by someone known to the disabled individual. Institutions, programs, and facilities should act preventively to support sexual health.

9. Family counseling might be considered when, in your estimation, the presence in the family of a child or adolescent with a disability is affecting the dynamics of family behavior and perhaps creating difficulties within the family structure. Emotional strain may cause a rift in the relationship between the parents or may be negatively directed toward the child or adolescent.

10. Attempt to learn the value system of the family and work within it.

11. Be "sex positive" in words, attitudes, and actions.

12. Be prepared to recommend peer counseling where appropriate and useful.

13. Normal sexual development for disabled individuals, just as for able-bodied people, may include active fantasies, language skills, masturbatory behavior with or without orgasm, and expectations of having sexual partners.

14. Try to reflect the perspective that all people

are sexual and that sexual feelings are natural. Avoid sublimating the topic of sex and encourage the patient to develop naturally. Some disabled individuals divert normal sexual energy to "alternative" thoughts or activities (e.g., concentrating on therapy or mobility issues at the expense of interpersonal skills, becoming everyone's "best" friend, and avoiding intimate personal relationships).

Type II Disabilities— Preadolescent Progressive

Type II disabilities also begin before puberty and may produce effects similar to those of type I. However, these disabilities are progressive, and the child becomes more dysfunctional with time. Examples include juvenile rheumatoid arthritis, childhood-onset diabetes mellitus, muscular dystrophy, and cystic fibrosis. Because of the nature of the disability, these patients are involved in regular treatment programs that require much of their energy. This produces an inadequate body image, a feeling of being sick, and an unwillingness to regard their bodies as able to provide sensual pleasure.

Neuromuscular diseases are typical examples of type II physical disabilities. A child who is growing up with muscular dystrophy may experience many of the physical difficulties described in type I and, in addition, is handicapped by progressive deterioration of physical abilities.[13, 14] The child may face loss of mobility, reduced endurance, and difficulties with muscular coordination. Contractures may necessitate special and conspicuous external equipment such as a wheelchair and orthotic devices. The physician should recognize that the child's orientation may be toward a continually declining base of health and physical and emotional expectations.

Example. A 28-year-old female with cystic fibrosis was in the pre-terminal stage of her illness, experiencing severe limitations of her function and requiring frequent medical interventions for progressive pulmonary insufficiency. Shortly before her death, she revealed to her parents her painful years as an adolescent, unaware of sexual information, unable to understand sexual innuendo in the media, fearful of reaching out to a peer, and harboring deep resentments at having been excluded from the development she wished she had been allowed to have.

THEODORE M. COLE AND SANDRA S. COLE

ADVICE TO CLINICIANS

1. Talk honestly and frankly with parents while being informative, helpful, and respectful.

2. Help the family and patient set realistic, sequential, and attainable short-term goals, the achievement of which will reinforce positive self-esteem and body image.

3. Offer sex information that is educational. Not to do so implies that the person has no sexual expectations or potential.

4. Information may be designed not to change sexual behavior so much as to help the individual understand the world around him or her.

5. Family counseling may be offered to help set realistic expectations for family members.

6. Be "sex positive" in words and attitudes.

7. Attempt to learn the value system of the family and work within it.

8. Consider recommending peer counseling to patient or family.

9. Refer to recommendations previously stated in type I for further suggestions.

Type III Disabilities— Postadolescent or Adult Nonprogressive

Type III disabilities are those that occur in adolescent or adult life and are nonprogressive. Examples include traumatic spinal cord injury, amputation, and disfiguring burns. Individuals with these disabilities have already experienced a "normal" adolescence and have probably been sexually socialized. This reference point may be helpful in their efforts to reestablish their psychosexual identity. Further, they may already have learned the interpersonal skills necessary for the development of healthy adult sexual relationships. These skills may serve them after they become disabled.

SPINAL CORD INJURY

Injury to the spinal cord usually has its onset after puberty and is nonprogressive. The concept of self is severely stressed by spinal cord injury.[15] Soon after the injury, depression frequently becomes a dominant personality pattern as the patient begins a relative acceptance of an unpleasant reality.[16] Teal and Athelstan[16] state that depression is primarily due to the perception of a diminished self-worth. They point out that the paralyzed person's sexuality can have a powerful effect on a

sense of self-worth. Similarly, self-worth can have a significant effect on sexuality. They followed 256 patients for 2 to 20 years after spinal cord injury and learned that sexual satisfaction is often lacking. In comparison to other aspects of post-disability adjustment, their subjects showed less satisfaction with their sexual lives than they did with their employment situations, living arrangements, social lives, and general health.

Bregman and Hadley[17] report that only 50 per cent of spinal cord–injured women whom they studied had received even the basic information about sexuality during their initial hospitalization and rehabilitation. Cole and his co-workers[18] compared able-bodied single and married medical students to a group of single and married men and women with spinal cord injury living in the community. They found that spinal cord–injured people were more ready than the medical students to talk about sex and displayed less defensiveness and more openness. They also found that the role of fantasy was stronger in the spinal cord–injured population than in the medical students.

Cole[19] and his co-workers studied sexual attitudes and experiences of spinal cord–injured people at the time of discharge from their initial hospitalization, one year later, and again two years after injury. Approximately one fourth to one third of their patients reported that the importance of sex declined within the first year after injury, but at the end of the second year interest had returned to the pre-injury level or had become heightened. Approximately one third of the patients reported that the spinal cord injury did not produce a change in the sexual activity they enjoyed the most, but many expressed a wish for more sexual counseling while in the hospital. Fifty per cent considered their sexual adjustment to be good two years after their injury, but more than half of the patients reported that they were not as sexually active as they would have liked. The most common reason offered one year after injury was lack of partners. Two years after injury, lack of activity was attributed not only to lack of partners but also to fear of rejection, health concerns, and problems with erections. Three years after injury, males listed problems with erections as being the major reason for lack of activity.

Berkman[20] worked with veterans in the United States military and tested the hypothesis that improved sexual adjustment would be accompanied by proportionate increases in psychological, social, physiological, and vocational adjustment. She applied an Index of Sexual Adjustment to 104 sexually active spinal-injured adults living in the community and found that sexual adjustment was more favorable among the young and among those whose financial resources were greater. She also found that the Index of Sexual Adjustment varied directly with companion indices measuring physical function and community participation. Lastly, the ability of the person to function in the worker role also varied directly with scores obtained on her Index of Sexual Adjustment.

EXAMPLE

A 23-year-old male paraplegic college senior returned for an office visit to the physician who had directed his rehabilitation five years earlier. The young man advised the physician to provide more comprehensive and useful sexual information to future patients, saying that information that he had received proved of limited utility. On his own initiative, he had contacted the Center for Independent Living in his college community where he learned important information about his sexuality and his sexual options. Like his able-bodied college classmates, his expanded knowledge base fostered a greater willingness to explore his self-concept and his ability to compete with fellow students on campus.

McClure[21] studied contraceptive practices of spinal cord–injured women through questionnaires to the women and to rehabilitation physicians. Although most physicians she sampled had not seen complications from contraceptives, those who had seen them described phlebitis or complications secondary to the use of intrauterine contraceptive devices. She also questioned 227 spinal cord–injured women, 25 per cent of whom were sexually active paraplegic women and 57 per cent of whom were sexually active quadriplegic women, and found that 21 per cent of the paraplegic women had become pregnant, as had 7 per cent of the quadriplegic women. The most frequent methods of contraception were oral contraceptives and intrauterine devices.

Advice to Clinicians

1. Initiate discussion early. Be supportive as a rehabilitation team and uniform with the information provided. Be sure information gathered is exchanged with the team, since a patient may select only one member of the team in whom to confide such personal issues. Discuss with the team the most appropriate and capable member to provide counseling and education.

2. Regard the patient as a sexual person and show respect and sensitivity to issues such as loss of femininity or masculinity, fear of abandonment, feelings of shame because of body changes or loss, and decreased body image or self-esteem.

3. It has become a medically responsible obligation to provide to patients current, accurate, and factual information about sex education and activities including safe sex in a sensitive manner. Provide resource material to reinforce discussions initiated by appropriate team members. (See reference 24 and *Patient Resources* list at end of chapter.)

Specific information about birth control, pregnancy, fertility, and *safe sex techniques* should be explicitly provided, and, where possible, written information should reinforce verbal discussion.[40] All State Departments of Public Health have information and brochures available on sexually transmitted diseases, including AIDS.

4. Provide peer counseling where appropriate.

5. Be "sex positive." Discuss sexual options and diversity. Try to avoid negative discussions about loss and limitation. Although loss is real, sexual enrichment and sexual enhancement need not be eliminated or regarded as "substitution."

6. Educate that it is natural to have erotic feelings and to be sexually aroused. Identify for the patient the possibility that the previously erogenous areas of sensitivity of the genitals may be re-experienced in different areas of the body in which injury has not impaired sensation. It is frequently reported that heightened sensitivity to innervated areas of the back of the neck, ears, nipples, and forearms can create erotic sensations similar to those previously experienced in the genitals.

7. Provide couple counseling where appropriate.

8. Speak directly and educate about the myths regarding sexual performance. Many people focus exclusively on genital activity in sexual expression and limit their sexual activities to intercourse. Understandably, in these instances, sexual dysfunction caused by the disability will be perceived as a severe problem. Re-education would be appropriate to expand the definition of sexual enhancement and enrichment to include foreplay, pleasuring, massage, kissing, hugging, holding, and any other form of intimacy that would increase the pleasure factor of sexual satisfaction in addition to sexual intercourse. In most cases, vaginal containment of a flaccid penis is possible with instruction, practice, and counseling.

THEODORE M. COLE AND SANDRA S. COLE

BRAIN INJURY

Injury to the brain by trauma or vascular disease falls in the category of type III disabilities. The sexual correlates of damage to the frontal lobe are related to learning and behavioral problems. Loss of fantasy and loss of moral and ethical restraints are often seen. However, increases in libido have not been described. Temporal lobe dysfunction is associated with a change in the sexual activation system. Usually this is associated with a decreased libido and decreased genital and sexual arousal. Rarely, excessive libido may be seen.

Other correlates of brain dysfunction are associated with hemianesthesia, which may accompany left or right hemispheric damage. Patients may be unaware of touch, or touch may be perceived as painful or uncomfortable. If the language centers are damaged, the ability of the patient to participate in the verbal communication of sex may be impaired. Urinary and bowel continence may not be reliable. Autonomic nervous system abnormalities may lead to alterations in tumescence of the sex organs or lubrication of the vagina. Added to these are the kinesiosexual dysfunctions that can result from weakness, spasticity, incoordination, limitation of motion, or pain associated with the physical activities and postures associated with sexual expression.

Patients may manifest several sexual concomitants during the stages of recovery from brain damage. During the coma phase, no recognizable sex focus is seen. However, during progression from the vegetative to the community reintegration stages, a progression of sexual foci can be seen. Early in the awakening stage, patients may manifest sexual interest through autostimulation of the genitals. Coital interest and masturbatory activity begin to appear as the patient becomes more alert. Efforts by the staff to appropriately channel these interests can be useful.

Family education is extremely important at this point. As the patient is reintegrated into the community, the main sexual focus is to increase the psychosexual skills of the patient. A fuller understanding of pleasuring and an appreciation of the consequences of actions can also be taught to many patients. As with all other aspects of sexuality, it is important to establish awareness of the self as worthwhile and deserving of physical and intimate experiences. Most patients can be taught to express their desires and to focus them on appropriate people.

Advice to Clinicians

1. Early in the treatment program, initiate discussion about sexuality and sexual changes. Work directly with the family and the staff to reduce stress created by the impact of brain injury on the family and the rehabilitation team.

2. Discuss sexual matters openly with the family and with the team to provide information and to set expectations, particularly where inappropriate behavior may be apparent.

3. Shape and control appropriate behavior related to sexuality. This may help avoid embarrassment as a result of inappropriate or outrageous sexual behavior from the patient to family members or staff.

4. Be prepared to provide family peer counseling (family to family). Local head injury associations can be very helpful as resources.

5. *Later* in the treatment program, discussion is indicated regarding issues of birth control, fertility, and safe sex with the patient and/or partner.

6. Be "sex positive" even when discussing limiting inappropriate behavior.

7. Provide information and education regarding increased options and diversity in sexual expression.

8. Work on communication skills with the family and with the team on discussion of difficult sexual topics, particularly those of inappropriate behavior. Discuss, when appropriate, the possibility or presence of decreased sexual desire of the brain-injured patient or the partner.

9. If possible, provide for sex education instruction and perhaps opportunities for private experiences for the head-injured patient and partner so that difficult or stressful sexual situations related to the injury can be addressed directly by the rehabilitation team. Many institutions and facilities have found that a weekend pass or an overnight in a private suite has been helpful to begin to address the transitional issues of intimacy when the patient returns home or transfers to a facility, regardless of the type of disability experienced by the patient.

10. Provide spouse counseling if indicated.

Type IV Disabilities— Postadolescent Progressive

Type IV disabilities include the degenerative diseases that affect most adults who live to be old. They may also affect younger adults who are coping with advancing disease processes. Examples include degenerative heart disease, stroke, cancer, and chronic renal disease. Their onsets are often gradual and their courses progressive, thus allowing slow adjustment to the disabling process. However, like type II disabilities, the type IV disabilities produce an unstable base from which one can plan a lifetime. People with these disabilities may find it necessary to invest considerable energy in maintaining their health and thus have great difficulty in looking upon themselves as "well," even though physically disabled.

HEART DISEASE

Hellerstein and Freidman[22] have found that the postcoronary sexual activity will depend on such factors as precoronary sexual drive and performance, the customary effects of aging, pre-illness personality, emotional reaction to heart disease, current socioeconomic status, and the health attitudes and decisions of the sexual partner. The physician should investigate these factors in addition to focusing on the contractile functions of the heart. Furthermore, pharmacological management of heart disease, edema, and hypertension may require use of medications that also can affect sexual function. Hellerstein and Freidman have proposed a social class hypothesis that describes individuals who may be at lower risk for coronary heart disease. These people are not only more sexually active but are better educated, more affluent and verbally fluent, less obese, and less hypertensive.

With proper sexual counseling and taking into account age and other medical conditions, the development of fears in both the patient and the mate can be averted. Depression, reduced self-esteem, and preoccupation with life or death are obvious deterrents to sexual health. Patient and family education should point out that postcoronary sexual activity is feasible in 80 per cent of patients. The nature of the physical activity can be altered if resumption of precoronary patterns of sexual activity produces angina or respiratory symptoms. Episodes of sexual contact can be shorter and less physically strenuous so as not to place excessive demands on the heart. The cardiac demand of sexual activity can be held down to that experienced by other customary activities of everyday living and work.

ARTHRITIS

Arthritis may be associated with chronic pain, depression, and disfigurement, and these characteristics may produce sexual dysfunctions as part of the clinical picture. Chronic pain may produce or be produced by depression, and the libido may be affected. Some patients may experience enough pain on joint motion that physical activities of sexual expression may sometimes be precluded. It should be noted, however, that some patients describe a dramatic reduction in pain following genital stimulation and orgasm. The possible role of endorphins has been implicated, as has been the psychological role of caring and being cared for by another person.

Ehrlich[23] reports that specific locations of arthritis may be more commonly associated with sexual dysfunctions. A prime example is arthritis of the hips in a woman, causing inability to abduct and externally rotate them for intercourse in the traditional male-on-top position. Arthritis of the spine may cause pain on motion and arthritis of the knees may limit leg flexion or kneeling for men and women during sexual intercourse. Deforming arthritis of the hands not only may be unattractive but may also limit manual dexterity for purposes of stroking, caressing, and genital manipulation. Interferences in hygiene may result from arthritic involvement of hips and hands, preventing adequate toileting of the perineum and genitals.

Some arthritides are associated with rashes or ulcers of the skin or mucocutaneous areas, for example, psoriatic arthritis, Sjögren's syndrome, or Behçet's disease. Dryness of the vagina may also occur in Sjögren's syndrome.

LUNG DISEASE

Chronic progressive lung disease generally includes chronic bronchitis, emphysema, chronic obstructive pulmonary disease (COPD), and chronic obstructive lung disease (COLD). The distinguishing factor of all four is the progressive destruction of the lungs' ability to adequately exchange gases and clear excess mucus. The result is increasing shortness of breath in association with anxiety and chronic cough.

Chronic progressive lung disease is a dramatic example of a physical condition that may produce sexual disabilities. With the progression of lung disease, the patient's ability to perform even the simple daily activities of bathing, dressing, and household chores may be affected. Patients can often benefit from a medical regimen that also includes instruction in relaxation, diaphragmatic breath control with pursed lip breathing, and postural drainage techniques. Specific kinesiological instruction in sexual expression is also helpful. Positions that have been found effective for postural drainage of the lungs can be adapted for methods of sexual expression. Patients and partners can be counseled in options to traditional positions so that sexual intercourse can be accomplished in the sitting, standing, side-lying, and kneeling positions. Simultaneous use of oxygen in association with deliberate relaxation is also helpful. Sometimes a period of preparation with nebulization of bronchodilators and bronchial drainage may be helpful immediately preceding sexual activity.

DIABETES MELLITUS

Diabetes mellitus usually has its onset in adult life and is progressive. It has been reported that half of all male diabetics have erectile dysfunction and about one third of diabetic women experience orgasmic dysfunction. Although diabetic neuropathy appears to be the primary etiologic factor in a majority of cases, some sexual problems in diabetics are due to correctable causes such as vascular occlusions.

In the diabetic male, erectile dysfunction may have an abrupt onset, but more commonly the onset is gradual. In 85 per cent of cases, the erectile dysfunction is due to organic causes and is the most common sexual disturbance.[24] Usually libido is unaffected, as is ejaculation in the diabetic male.

The physician may be able to separate the psychological from the physiological causes for erectile dysfunction by the use of nocturnal penile tumescence testing, although this method is not entirely accurate. The diabetic patient is no less susceptible to psychogenic reasons for erectile dysfunction than is the nondiabetic male, and, thus, it is important to consider nervous, vascular, and psychic functions simultaneously. In many men the organic dysfunction is accompanied by a psychological one, and the clinician should think of both causes rather than simply one or the other. In the male, retrograde ejaculation may also occur owing to diabetic neuropathy and is, of course, associated with the impaired fertility. Sensation of orgasm is usually retained, however, as is the sense of light touch and pinprick on the genitals.

It has been reported[24] that 35 per cent of diabetic women have orgasmic dysfunction, whereas only 6 per cent of nondiabetic women report this problem. Usually the onset in women is five to seven years later than sexual dysfunction in the man, and its occurrence is often associated with the decrease in vaginal lubrication, chronic vaginitis, and dyspareunia. Libido is usually unimpaired.

The treatment of sexual dysfunction in diabetes includes metabolic regulation of the diabetes, correction of localized vascular disturbances, sexual counseling, and, in the male, consideration of implantation of a penile prosthesis.

END-STAGE RENAL DISEASE

Sexual rehabilitation of the hemodialysis patient has been described by Levy.[30] There are over 30,000 new cases of end-stage renal disease occurring each year in the United States, most of which are a result of chronic pyelonephritis and glomerulonephritis. Although 15 years ago most of these patients would have died, most are now able to live on the artificial kidney and, thus, are coming to the attention of clinicians who are concerned about sexual function. A number of metabolic disturbances accompany this syndrome, including bone pain, chronic anemia, peripheral neuropathies, anorexia, and fatigue. Most patients receive treatment six hours a day, three times a week, and many have to go to a medical care facility to receive it. Only 30 per cent of men on chronic hemodialysis return to full vocational productivity.

The sexual dysfunction that was first recognized in this patient population was erectile dysfunction among men. However, lubrication problems and anorgasmia have recently been described in women on chronic hemodialysis. The prevalence of impotence in men on hemodialysis is probably 70 per cent, and the lack of improvement on hemodialysis is all the more remarkable because the same patients usually sustain improvements in all other physical functions during the same period of time. Although endocrinological abnormalities have been described, there is no evidence that they correlate directly with sexual dysfunctions. Another factor that may play a role is the frequent necessary use of antihypertensive medications, which, by themselves, may adversely influence sexual function by decreasing tumescence in males and libido in both sexes.

As for the other disabilities, psychological factors also play an important role. A man's sense of his masculinity and a woman's sense of her femininity may be severely stressed by inability to function in traditional or previous roles, inability to assume previous employment, or dependency on outside support mechanisms. For men, role reversal is often experienced as the wives go back to work to help support their families. Role reversal may affect the man's sense of his masculinity. As with other progressive disabilities, depression, anxiety, and chronic fatigue may play important roles in sexual activity and satisfaction.

Treatment must take into consideration the medical and the psychological components. Recent research has shown that depletion of trace amounts of zinc may be linked to reduced testosterone production in patients on hemodialysis.[31] Probably the most important treatment is prevention of future difficulties and counseling with the patient and the sexual partner.

GENERAL ADVICE TO CLINICIANS

1. Obtain printed pamphlets and literature for patient education. These are becoming increasingly available. Recommended references appear in the *Patient Resources* list at the end of this chapter.

2. Give medically sound, informative, and endorsing advice on what people can do sexually and safely so that they are not fearful or compromised unnecessarily.

3. Be creative in your thinking and discussion. If what is "traditional" for the patient or couple is no longer available because of the disability, encourage exploration and experimentation within the value system of the patient and partner. Be validating and respectful.

4. Provide couple counseling where appropriate. Include the partner or spouse of the patient in your discussions whenever possible. Always consider the partner of the patient when planning case management. Educate and counsel *early* in the assessment process and rehabilitation program.

5. Be prepared to make a referral to community resources that can be supportive to the patient or couple if your facility is unable to provide these services on an ongoing basis.

6. People are not fragile. Although the topic of sexuality may be difficult to initiate and discuss, it is almost always regarded with great respect and appreciation by the patient and family. These personal sexual issues can be worrisome and frightening to everyone involved (patient, partner, and family) at a time of crisis. Omitting discussion could negatively reinforce the fears and anxieties that may currently exist in the patient's thinking. Initiation of discussions about sexuality can reflect dignity when done with genuine concern and respect.

Effects of Medications on Sexuality

Increasingly, physicians are becoming aware of the host of effects that some drugs may have on the body. Some drugs have a potentiating effect on one another, whereas others have an inhibiting effect.

If one regards sexuality in a broad sense, not limited to genital function, one can see that many medications are capable of affecting sexual function. Any drug that produces or reduces pruritus or a skin rash will have a sexual effect through affecting appearance and distractability. Drugs that treat bone pain caused by neoplasms or osteoporosis or that reduce inflammation of joints and permit greater range of motion will have a sexual effect. Medications that control spasticity, increase strength, or reduce muscle pain will have a salutary effect upon kinesiosexual function. Medications that control seizures, diminish the rigidity of Parkinson's disease, or alter a mood may affect sexual function in obvious ways. Heart and lung disease treated by pharmacological agents that reduce circulatory symptoms, heart pain, and shortness of breath may affect sexuality. Medications used to treat peptic ulcer may produce dryness of the mouth and thus affect oral activities associated with sex. Medications that are used to treat diarrhea or that influence rectal sphincter function may play a role in sexual activities. Contraceptives or antibiotics that weaken resistance to the development of vaginitis may produce dyspareunia and thus affect sexual function. Drugs thought to be sexually innocuous may in fact have significant side effects. When a patient believes that he or she is experiencing an iatrogenic, drug-induced sexual difficulty, the drug may simply be stopped without informing the physician and the patient will become a silent noncomplier.

Antihypertensive diuretic drugs may produce an effect on sexual function by depleting potassium stores and producing fatigue. Thiazide diuretics may also produce diabetes. If taken for a long period of time they may contribute to the diabetic syndrome described earlier. Spironolactone, on the other hand, has a potassium-conserving effect but produces other sexual side effects such as breast tenderness, galactorrhea, and gynecomastia, which is not always reversible in the male. In large doses, spironolactone may reduce circulating testosterone and increase circulating progesterone.[32] In 25 to 40 per cent of men, spironolactone is known to produce erectile dysfunction and decrease sperm production. Spironolactone also may influence the hormonal events of the menstrual cycle.

Reserpine produces depression in 5 to 15 per cent of patients and in this group may adversely affect the libido. Guanethidine is a ganglionic

THEODORE M. COLE AND SANDRA S. COLE

blocker that in two thirds of male patients may lead to a reduction of ejaculatory ability. Propranolol, a beta blocker, has been known to produce erectile dysfunction in some men.

Hydralazine is considered to be innocuous as measured by its effect on sexual function. Although it produces an increase in heart rate when used with propranolol, heart rate changes alone may not be deleterious. Sexual side effects often associated with other antihypertensive medications may be reduced in up to 85 per cent of patients thus treated. Alpha-methyldopa is one of the most widely used antihypertensives. In doses of less than 1 gm per day, erectile function, libido, and ejaculatory ability are seldom affected. However, as daily dosages approach 1.5 to 2 gm per day, up to half of men questioned report erectile dysfunction and decrease in libido. The physician must be sensitive to the direct as well as to the peripheral side effects of medications on sexual function. Therapy can include adjustments in medication schedules and dosages as well as counseling to minimize or prevent the effects of anxiety or depression that may follow alterations of sexual function.

Almost all men with traumatic spinal cord injury are interested in regaining their potency and fertility. Ninety per cent of spinal-injured men are unable to ejaculate using physical stimulation of the penis. Early work by Guttman and Walsh[33] described the intrathecal injection of neostigmine (Prostigmin), which produced ejaculation in some spinal-injured males. However, side effects, including autonomic hyperreflexia and hypertension, have been severe in some cases, making physicians and patients reluctant to employ this method. More recently, Chapelle and co-workers[34] have reported a larger series in which autonomic hyperreflexia occurred but was medically managed without reported complications. The European literature has reported successful electroejaculation in the human male.[35-37] Even more recently, Bennett and her associates[38] presented a report on successful pregnancies after electroejaculation in spinal cord–injured males. Their series of 37 spinal cord–injured men yielded a 59 per cent rate of successful ejaculations in patients with the mean age of 30 years and duration of time since injury of 11 years. Four pregnancies were achieved in 10 women who were artificially inseminated. Bennett concluded that it is no longer appropriate to assume that all spinal cord–injured males should be considered infertile.

Although the methods used have not yet found widespread application, there is now the possibility that electrostimulation may be effective in paraplegic and quadriplegic men, even those injured many years ago.

Effects of Surgical Procedures on Sexuality

Penile Prostheses

The urological surgeon can implant a penile stiffener or penile prosthesis when there is organic erectile dysfunction, and some urological surgeons are willing to install the device in selected cases of psychogenic erectile dysfunction. Confirmation of the presence of erectile dysfunction requires an adequate history and physical examination, a search for localized vascular insufficiency, and examination of the abdomen, penis, and scrotum. Manual dexterity also is important if the surgeon is installing a hydraulic stiffener as described by Scott, Bradley and Timm.[25] If the surgeon is considering a semirigid prosthesis, such as developed by Small and Carrion,[26] Finney,[27] or Jonas,[28] then the absence of prostatic obstruction must be assured. Bladder instrumentation may be difficult or impossible after the semirigid prosthesis is installed. In the hands of some surgeons the surgical success rate is greater than 90 per cent, and mechanical complications are negligible with a semirigid device. Although the surgical success rate may also be greater than 90 per cent with the inflatable prosthesis, mechanical complications may be as high as 15 per cent.

However, the penile prosthesis should not be adopted without adequate assessment and evaluation of each individual case. Maddock[29] has emphasized the importance of preoperative evaluation even though the patient himself may adamantly request implantation of the device. Maddock points out that there is no such thing as a totally organic erectile dysfunction. A psychological component is always present in the form of a discrepancy between male performance standards and the reality of any physical limitation. He also points out that in some men in whom sexual dysfunction coexists with diabetes, the dysfunction may be a psychological defense mechanism against anxiety or threat rather than linked only to the complications of diabetes.

Maddock found that problems of self-esteem and overall psychological disturbances of patients treated surgically were generally greater than for patients treated with psychotherapy. There was also a greater incidence of excess alcohol consumption among the VA population who were treated surgically. Although surgery did not appreciably increase the frequency of sexual intercourse after adequate time for healing, most patients were satisfied with the result. Surgery did not significantly affect self-esteem levels or personal adjustments of patients with their wives, even though motivation for surgery appeared to be largely interpersonal, i.e., probably related to feelings of self-worth or "manliness" and/or relational rather than "sexual" *per se*. Maddock concluded that the outcome of surgery and possibly even the motivation to have the surgery were strongly linked to the attitudes and behavior of the female partner. Whether the surgery was deemed to be successful by the patients, particularly the married patients, was a function of how the female partner responded sexually after procedure.

Gynecological Problems

Surgical procedures frequently performed by the gynecologist include vulvectomy, hysterectomy, tubal ligation, abortion, vaginal repair, cystocele repair, hymenectomies, and clitoral hood resections. In each of these cases a mechanical alteration of the women's genitals may bring about changes in libido as well as in sexual activity. When the ovaries are removed, circulating testosterone is reduced and the woman may experience a decrease in libido. A loss of the uterus may result in a change of pelvic sensation for women who have been accustomed to feeling the penis touch the uterine cervix during sexual intercourse. Vaginal repair must be carried out by a surgeon who is sensitive to reconstruction of the vagina without making it either too tight or too short for sexual intercourse. Vulvectomy can have a severe psychological effect on the inadequately prepared woman and her sexual partner. Grief, depression, fear, and mood swings have been described by vulvectomized women, many of whom have expressed fear of establishing new sexual relationships. Those who are married state that they are glad that they are married so that they do not have to risk rejection in the establishment of a new sexual relationship. Some women have described a dramatic decrease in libido, self-image, and sexual activity following vulvectomy. Most women have asked for better preoperative counseling and education, especially of their husbands.

Physician Involvement in Problems of Sexuality

A number of new texts have recently been published that may be useful to clinicians.

Depending on skills, interest, and job responsibilities, each physician can find a level of involvement appropriate to himself or herself. Annon[44] has suggested a four-tiered scheme of involvement (the PLISSIT model). The first tier—level 1, P represents permission—is that level at which the physician generates an attitude wherein the disabled person senses permission to express and discuss sexual concerns. This can be done by asking leading questions, by initiating talk about sensitive subjects, or simply by listening to the spoken or body language of the patient. All physicians should be able to function at level 1. Not to do so may deny patients permission to discuss the very real problems and concerns that they may be facing.

The second tier—LI represents limited information—is a level at which the physician provides limited information for general problem-solving. Typically, the limited information is educational and nonpersonal and deals with the disability and its implications on sexual health in a general sense.

The third tier—SS represents specific suggestions—is the level at which the physician provides specific suggestions about sexual concerns and dysfunctions. This implies that the physician has taken a sexual history and is knowledgeable about sexuality and the particular physical disability under consideration.

The fourth tier—IT—is the level of intensive therapy. This is provided by professionals who have been thoroughly trained in sex counseling and who also understand physical disabilities. Intensive therapy often involves intrapersonal and psychological issues and frequently requires relationship counseling. It goes well beyond providing permission, limited information, or even specific suggestions. It implies a thorough understanding and training in psychodynamics, especially as they relate to sexuality. It also implies a thorough understanding of physical disabilities, medical rehabilitation, and personal and family reactions to disability in the rehabilitation environment.

THEODORE M. COLE AND SANDRA S. COLE

Guidelines for Working with People with Physical Disabilities

The following are a few guidelines that may help the physician and the patient in the area of sexuality and physical disability.

1. Genital function alone does not make a functional relationship.

2. Urinary incontinence does not mean genital incontinence.

3. Absence of sensation does not mean absence of feelings.

4. Inability to move does not mean inability to please or be pleased.

5. The presence of deformities does not mean the absence of desire.

6. Inability to perform does not mean inability to enjoy.

7. Loss of genitals does not mean loss of sexuality.

8. Sexual dysfunction is not synonymous with personal inadequacy.

References

1. Ebert, R. K., and Lief, H. I.: Why sex education for medical students? In Green, R. (Ed.): Human Sexuality, A Health Practitioner's Text. Baltimore, Williams & Wilkins, 1975, pp. 1–6.
2. Roberts, M., and Roberts, A.: Psychosocial Rehabilitation of the Handicapped. Proc. 1st International Conference on Lifestyle and Health. A. S. Leon and G. T. Amundson (Eds.). Minneapolis Dept. of Conferences, University of Minnesota, 1979.
3. Cole, T. M., and Glass, D. D.: Sexuality and physical disabilities. Arch. Phys. Med. Rehabil., 58:585–586, 1977.
4. Lief, H. I.: New developments in the sex education of the physician. J.A.M.A., 212:1864–1867, 1970.
5. Kolodny, R. C., Masters, W. H., and Johnson, V. E.: Textbook of Sexual Medicine. Boston, Little, Brown & Company, 1979.
6. Sandler, J., Myerson, M., and Kinder, B. N.: Human Sexuality: Current Perspectives. Tampa, Mariner Publishing Company, 1980.
7. McCary, J. L.: McCary's Human Sexuality, 3rd Ed. New York, D. Van Nostrand & Company, 1978.
8. Katchadourian, H. A., and Lunde, D. T.: Fundamentals of Human Sexuality, 2nd Ed. New York, Holt, Rinehart & Winston, 1972.
9. Kaplan, H. S.: The New Sex Therapy. New York, Brunner Mazel Publication, 1974.
10. Kelly, G. F.: Sexuality: The Human Perspective. Woodbury, Barron's, 1980.
11. Easton, J.: Children, parents, and schools. Paper presented at Sexuality and Physical Disabilities: Medical Aspects and Clinical Care Seminar, University of Michigan Medical Center, November 1980.
12. Robinault, I.: Sex, Society and the Disabled—A Developmental Inquiry into Roles, Relationships, and Responsibility. Hagerstown, Harper & Row, 1978.
13. Anderson, F., Bardach, J., and Goodgold, J.: Sexuality in Neuromuscular Diseases. Monograph 56, New York Institute of Rehabilitation Medicine, 1979.
14. Goodgold, J., Bardach, J., and Anderson, F.: A Study of Sexuality in Muscular Dystrophy and Related Diseases. Muscular Dystrophy Association. 1979.
15. Nagler, B.: Psychiatric aspects of cord injury. Am. J. Psychiatry, 107:49–56, 1950.
16. Teal, J. C., and Athelstan, G. T.: Sexuality and spinal cord injury: Some psychosocial considerations. Arch. Phys. Med. Rehabil., 56:264–268, 1975.
17. Bregman, S., and Hadley, R. G.: Sexual adjustment and feminine attractiveness among spinal cord injured women. Arch. Phys. Med. Rehabil., 57:448–450, 1976.
18. Cole, T. M., Chilgren, R. A., and Rosenberg, P.: A new programme of sex education and counseling for spinal cord injured adults and health care professionals. Int. J. Para., 11:111–124, 1973.
19. Cole, T. M.: Unpublished data for Regional Spinal Cord Injury Center of Minnesota, Theodore M. Cole, M.D., Director, 1977.
20. Berkman, A. H., Weissman, R., and Freilich, M. H.: Sexual adjustment of spinal cord injured veterans living in the community. Arch. Phys. Med. Rehabil., 59:29–33, 1978.
21. McClure, S.: Contraception and the spinal injured woman. Paper presented at Sexuality and Physical Disabilities: Medical Aspects and Clinical Care Seminar, University of Michigan Medical Center, November 1980.
22. Hellerstein, H. K., and Freidman, E. H.: Sexual activity and the post coronary patient. Arch. Intern. Med., 125:987–999, 1970.
23. Ehrlich, G. E.: Sexual problems of the arthritic patient. In Ehrlich, G. E. (Ed.): Total Management of the Arthritic Patient. Philadelphia, J. B. Lippincott, 1973, pp. 193–208.
24. Kolodny, R. C., Masters, W. H., and Johnson, V. E.: Textbook of Sexual Medicine. Boston, Little, Brown & Company, 1979.
25. Scott, F. B., Bradley, W. E., and Timm, G. W.: Management of erectile impotence. Use of implantable, inflatable prosthesis. Urology, 2:80, 1973.
26. Small, M. P., Carrion, H. M., and Gordon, J. A.: Small-Carrion penile prosthesis. Urology, 5:479, 1975.

27. Finney, R. P.: New hinged silicone penile implant. J. Urol., 118:585, 1977.
28. Jonas, U., and Jacobi, G. H.: Silicone-silver penile prosthesis: Description, operative approach, and results. J. Urol., 123:865, 1980.
29. Maddock, J. W.: Assessment and evaluation protocol for surgical treatment of impotence. Sexual. Disabil., 3:39–49, 1980.
30. Levy, N. B.: The sexual rehabilitation of the hemodialysis patient. Sexual. Disabil., 2:76–81, 1979.
31. Antoniou, L. D., Sudhakar, T., Shalhoub, R. J., et al.: Reversal of uremic impotence by zinc. Lancet, 2:895–898, 1977.
32. Caminos-Torres, R., Ma, L., and Snyder, P. J.: Gynecomastia and semen abnormalities induced by spironolactone in normal men. J. Clin. Endocrinol. Metab., 45:255–260, 1977.
33. Guttman, L., and Walsh, J. J.: Prostigmin assessment test of fertility in spinal-injured man. Paraplegia, 9:38–51, 1971.
34. Chapelle, P. A., Roby-Brami, A., Yakovleff, A., and Bussel, B.: Neurological correlations of ejaculation and testicular size in men with complete spinal cord section. J. Neurol. Neurosurg. Psychiatry, 51:197–202, 1988.
35. Francois, N., Maury, M., Jouannet, D., David, G., and Vacant, J.: Electroejaculation of a complete paraplegic followed by pregnancy. Paraplegia, 16:248–251, 1978.
36. Brindley, G. S.: Electroejaculation and the fertility of paraplegic men. Sexual. Disabil., 3:223–229, 1980.
37. Hachen, H. J.: Bilan endocrinien et spermatogenese chex le traumatise medullaire. Ann. Med. Phys., 21:403–417, 1978.
38. Bennett, C. J., Seager, S. W., Vasher, E. A., and McGuire, E. J.: Sexual dysfunction and electroejaculation in spinal cord injured male: A review. J. Urol., 139:453–457, 1987.
39. Deegan, M. J., and Brooks, N. A.: Women and Disability: The Double Handicap. New Brunswick, NJ, Transaction Books, Inc., 1985.
40. Neinstein, L. S., and Katz, B.: Contraception and Chronic Illnesses: A Clinician's Sourcebook. Atlanta, GA, American Health Consultants Books, 1986.
41. Trieschmann, R. B.: Aging with a Disability. New York, Demos Publications, 1987.
42. Neistadt, M. E., and Freda, M.: Choices: A Guide to Sex Counseling with Physically Disabled Adults. Malabar, FL, Robert E. Krieger Publishing Company, 1987.
43. Dechesne, B., Pons, C., and Schellen, A. (Eds.): Sexuality and Handicap: Problems of Motor Handicapped People. Springfield, IL, Charles C Thomas, 1986.
44. Annon, J.: The Behavioral Treatment of Sexual Problems: Brief Therapy. New York, Harper & Row, 1976.

Patient Resources

Duffy, Y.: All Things Are Possible. A. J. Garvin and Associates, P.O. Box 7525, Ann Arbor, MI 48107, 1981.
Mooney, T., Cole, T., and Chilgren, R. A.: Sexual Options for Paraplegics and Quadriplegics. Boston, MA, Little, Brown & Company, 1975.
Rabin, B.: The Sensuous Wheeler: Sexual Adjustment for the Spinal Cord Injured. Barry Rabin, Ph.D., 5595 East 7th Street, Suite 353, Long Beach, CA 90804, 1980.
Toward Intimacy: Family Planning and Sexuality Concerns of Physically Disabled Women. By the Task Force on Concerns of Physically Disabled Women. New York, NY, Human Sciences Press, 1980.
Zimmerman, D.: Sex Can Help Arthritis. Atlanta, GA, Arthritis Foundation, 1975.
Anderson, F., Bardach, J., and Goodgold, J.: Sexuality and Neuromuscular Disease. The Institute of Rehabilitation Medicine and The Muscular Dystrophy Association (Rehabilitation Monograph No. 56), 1979.
Levy, N.: Sex and Intimacy for Dialysis and Transplant Patients. Virgil Smirnow Associates, Health and Public Affairs, 8501 Burdette Road, Washington, DC, 1978.
Corbet, B. (Ed.): National Resource Directory: An Information Guide for Persons with Spinal Cord Injury and Other Physical Disabilities. Newton, MA, National Spinal Cord Injury Association, 1985.
Treadwell, M. C., and Patrias, R. L.: Growing Up With Spina Bifida. A Book About Puberty, Independence and Caring. Department of Physical Medicine and Rehabilitation, University of Michigan Hospitals, Ann Arbor, MI 48109, 1981.
Hossler, C. J., and Cole, S. S.: Intimacy and Chronic Lung Disease. Department of Physical Medicine and Rehabilitation, University of Michigan Hospitals, Ann Arbor, MI 48109, 1983.
Intimacy and Disability. Emerging Issues in Rehabilitation, Institute for Information Studies, Suite 104, 200 Little Falls Street, Falls Church, VA 22046, 1982.
Ostomates: Sex and the Male Ostomate; Sex, Courtship and the Single Ostomate; Sex, Pregnancy and the Female Ostomate. United Ostomy Association, Inc., 1111 Wilshire Blvd., Los Angeles, CA 90017. Telephone: (213) 481–2811.
Strodtman, L., and Knopf, R.: Sexual Health and Diabetes. Michigan Diabetes Research and Training Center, University of Michigan, Ann Arbor, MI 48109, 1983.
About Sexuality and People with Disabilities. A Scriptographic Booklet, Channing L. Bete Co., Inc., South Deerfield, MA, 1985.
McKee, L., Kempton, W., and Stiggall, L.: An Easy Guide to Loving Carefully. Planned Parenthood of

THEODORE M. COLE AND SANDRA S. COLE

Contra Costa, 1291 Oakland Blvd., Walnut Creek, CA 94596, 1980.

Ferreyra, S., and Hughes, K.: Table Manners. A Guide to the Pelvic Examination for Disabled Women and Health Care Providers. Sex Education for Disabled People, 477 Fifteenth St., Oakland, CA 94612, June 1982.

White, S. C.: The Sensuous Heart: Guidelines for Sex After a Heart Attack. Atlanta, GA, Pritchett & Hull Associates, Inc., 1984.

What Everyone Should Know About People With Disabilities. A Scriptographic Booklet, Channing L. Bete Co., Inc., South Deerfield, MA, 1982.

48

Upper Extremity Prosthetics

LEONARD F. BENDER

The absence of all or part of the limb comes about either from congenital skeletal deficiency or from amputation by trauma or surgery. The word *amputation* should be reserved for surgical, traumatic, and disease-created limb losses. Avoidance of the confusing term *congenital amputation* would help to clarify the distinction between congenital skeletal deficiencies and amputations.

Congenital Skeletal Deficiency

Of cases of skeletal deficiency involving the upper extremity, in all age groups, the deficiency is congenital in 22 per cent.[1] Analysis of the age group from birth to 10 years shows that 75 per cent of limb losses are congenital and only 25 per cent traumatic or surgical. Then, as children grow to adulthood, traumatic amputation and tumors account for an increased percentage of upper limb deficiencies, and when all age groups are considered together, trauma is the etiologic agent in 70 per cent.

The reasons for congenital malformations are largely unknown. Hereditary abnormalities identified as leading to limb deficiency are extremely rare.[2] Teratogenic agents have received considerable attention as a result of the thalidomide catastrophe in Europe between 1960 and 1963. Excessive radiation is often implicated;[3] cortisone and tolbutamide are highly suspect. Positive proof of the teratogenic effect of many chemical agents and environmental pollutants remains to be demonstrated.

The most common congenital skeletal deficiency in the upper limb is absence of the distal two thirds of the forearm, the wrist, and the hand. According to the Dundee classification promulgated in 1974, this would be a transverse deficiency, forearm, upper one third. Previous classifications used the term *hemimelia,* and later *meromelia*, combined with the type and level of deficiency. The latest classification was developed at an international conference held in Dundee, Scotland.[4] It simplifies the terminology and divides all congenital skeletal deficiencies into transverse or longitudinal. Transverse is defined as absence of all skeletal elements distal to the deficiency along a designated transverse axis; the axis is described by a two-letter abbreviation of the area of the limb (SH, shoulder; AR, arm; FO, forearm; CA, carpals; MC, metacarpals; PH, phalanges) plus the level in that area (total, upper one third, middle one third, distal one third). Longitudinal deficiency is an absence extending parallel to the long axis of the limb; all bones missing are named in two-letter abbreviations plus the term *partial* or *total*. Arranged in order of decreasing frequency, congenital upper limb skeletal deficiencies in the United States are forearm, upper one third; wrist, total; arm, lower one third; forearm, total; arm, total; and metacarpal, middle one third.[1]

Causes of Acquired Limb Loss

Amputation of upper limb segments in children below 10 years of age is rare; motor vehicle accidents, tumors, and trauma from natural disasters such as earthquakes and high winds are among the etiologic agents. Children 10 to 20 years old subject themselves to more hazardous situations than

1009

LEONARD F. BENDER

younger children do, and malignancy is also more likely to develop in this age group.

Trauma is the cause of upper limb amputation in 70 per cent of patients over age 18. In Michigan, the preponderance of amputations in adults is caused by stamping presses, conveyor mechanisms, and farm machinery such as corn pickers, threshers, and balers. Diseases account for only 6 per cent of all arm amputations, which is in sharp contrast to lower limb amputations, 40 per cent of which are necessitated by peripheral vascular syndromes. Malignancies constitute one half of the disease-related causes of arm amputation and appear predominantly in the 10- to 20-year age group.

Amputation

Levels of Amputation

Upper extremity amputation stumps are classified by level of amputation, using terminology different from that used for congenital skeletal deficiency. First, the length of the stump must be measured. Above-elbow stumps are measured from the tip of the acromion to the bone end; this measurement is compared with the sound side distance from acromion to the lateral epicondyle and is expressed as a percentage of normal side length. Below-elbow measurement is made from the medial epicondyle to the end of the ulna or radius, whichever is longer in the stump, and to the ulnar styloid tip on the sound side. Levels of amputation are as follows (see also Fig. 48–1):

PERCENTAGE OF NORMAL	CLASSIFICATION
Above-Elbow	
0	Shoulder disarticulation
0–30	Humeral neck
30–50	Short above-elbow
50–90	Long above-elbow
90–100	Elbow disarticulation
Below-Elbow	
0–35	Very short below-elbow
35–55	Short below-elbow
55–90	Long below-elbow
90–100	Wrist disarticulation

In bilateral amputations, where no normal segment remains for comparative measurement, the normal upper arm length is estimated by multiplying the patient's height by 0.19, and normal forearm length is estimated by multiplying by 0.21.[5, 6]

Elective Amputation

Elective amputations may be performed when the hand or the entire limb is sensationless and functionless. The hand may also be swollen, painful, and limited in range of motion. The most frequent cause is brachial plexus injuries or multiple cervical root avulsions.

Preoperative Rehabilitative Care

Only on rare occasions do the physiatrist and therapists knowledgeable in prosthetics have an opportunity to examine and to advise a patient prior to amputation. When such an occasion does arise—in elective amputation, for instance—the patient can be instructed in postoperative range-of-motion exercises and shown some of the prosthetic components available to amputees. One-handed techniques for some basic activities of daily living can be demonstrated, and a degree of psychological support can be developed through this early contact.

Postoperative Rehabilitative Care

The immediate postoperative period offers a few days during which the physician, physical and occupational therapists, and nurses may provide specialized care and give instructions to the patient, which will shorten the period of stump conditioning and help to reduce psychological depression. Range-of-motion exercises for the remaining joints of the arm, one-handed ways of performing activities of daily living, and proper skin care techniques can be taught early.

A variety of methods are utilized by surgeons to care for the stump. Some begin application of elastic stump shrinkers or elastic bandages the day after amputation; others wait until the stitches are out. Rigid plaster dressings may be used instead of elastic bandages. When applied properly, elastic bandages are effective in shaping the stump and reducing edema. Six to eight weeks of wrapping usually will bring the stump to satisfactory condition for fitting with a definitive prosthesis, but wrapping must be continued until the prosthesis is received. However, we prefer to fit all suitable stumps with immediate or early postoperative prostheses.

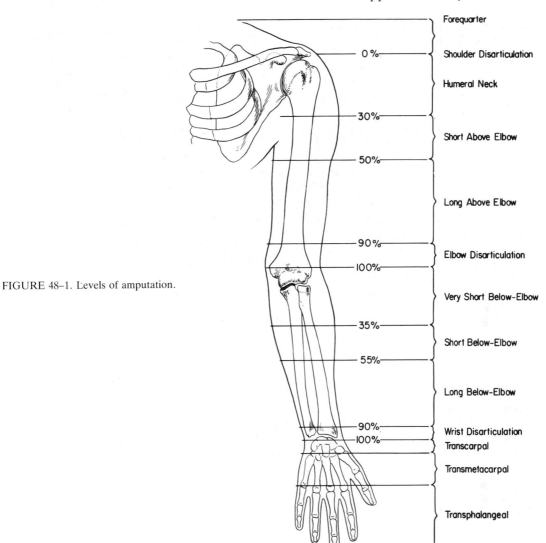

Forequarter

0% — Shoulder Disarticulation

Humeral Neck

30%

Short Above Elbow

50%

Long Above Elbow

90% — Elbow Disarticulation
100%

Very Short Below-Elbow

35% — Short Below-Elbow

55%

Long Below-Elbow

90% — Wrist Disarticulation
100% — Transcarpal

Transmetacarpal

Transphalangeal

FIGURE 48–1. Levels of amputation.

Immediate Postoperative Fitting

The advantages of immediate postoperative fitting were first described for lower extremity amputations.[7] A similar procedure has been tried during elective amputation in the forearm or arm when it was possible for the physician and prosthetist to make arrangements in advance.[8] When prior arrangements cannot be made, it is possible to make an early postoperative prosthesis a day or two after surgery. The application of a prosthesis immediately after amputation minimizes pain and edema in the stump, facilitates healing, and re-duces waiting time for the preparatory or training prosthesis. It also precludes the development of one-handedness.

Persons with simultaneous bilateral upper extremity amputations are ideal candidates for immediate or early postoperative fitting with a plaster prosthesis. The frustration of being totally dependent on others can largely be avoided by use of a temporary prosthesis on one or both sides.

The construction of an immediate postoperative plaster prosthesis is usually done in the operating room or an adjoining cast room (Fig. 48–2). Sterile technique is maintained until the inner wall of the plaster socket is completed. The surgical incision

LEONARD F. BENDER

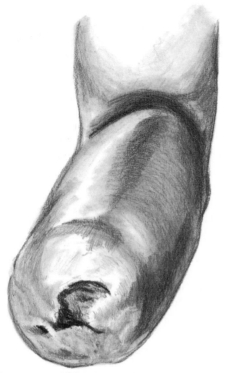

FIGURE 48–2. Early postoperative below-elbow stump.

is first covered with one layer of nonadhering gauze and one or two 4 × 4 inch gauze pads. The stump is covered with stockinette and plaster or resin-impregnated bandage (e.g., Scotch cast or fiberglass bandage), creating a thin-walled, rigid plaster socket (Fig. 48–3). Cotton webbing straps for suspension of the prosthesis and splayed polyvinyl chloride tube attached to either a wrist unit or an elbow unit are placed in the proper positions relative to the socket and are secured to the thin-walled socket with adhesive tape and are reinforced with Elastoplast (a type of elasticized adhesive tape). The prosthetist can then incorporate a baseplate laterally on the plaster socket and proceed to construct and fit a harness and control cable (Fig. 48–4). In a week to 10 days, the socket

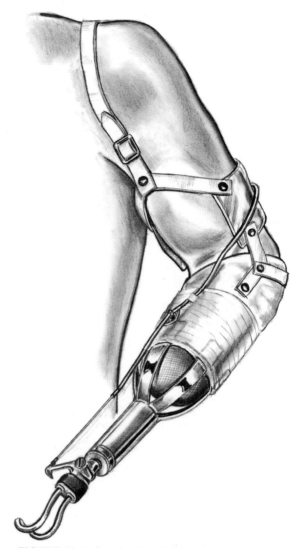

FIGURE 48–4. Completed early below-elbow prosthesis.

should be removed by slipping it off. The wound can be examined and either the first socket replaced on the stump if it is still a good fit or a new plaster socket constructed in a process similar to that just described. When the stump is well healed and appropriately contoured, the preparatory prosthesis can be constructed.

Prosthetic Sockets

The most important component of the prosthesis is the inner wall of the socket. If it does not fit satisfactorily, the prosthesis may not function effectively and may be uncomfortable. Almost all

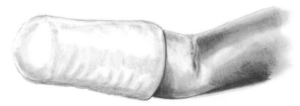

FIGURE 48–3. Stump dressing prior to attachment of prosthetic components.

sockets are made with two walls: an inner wall that fits the amputation stump comfortably and an outer wall that has the general contour of the normal arm or forearm. In special cases, such as elbow disarticulation, there may be no space between the inner and outer walls, and the socket is considered to have a single wall.

With infants, it is customary in our clinic to use a three-walled socket. The inner wall fits the stump. A middle wall is constructed over a thin wax build-up and is designed to fit the stump a year or two after the prosthesis is first fitted to the patient. The outer wall again corresponds to the normal contour of that segment of the arm. The inner wall of such a socket can be removed by the prosthetist as the child grows and needs more room inside the socket. This extends the useful life of the prosthesis considerably and reduces cost.

The upper rim of the usual below-elbow socket should be located 1.5 cm below the epicondyles of the humerus when the elbow is held at a right angle. The trimline should come straight volarly from the ulnar side and then curve distally on the volar surface to allow adequate room for the tendon of the biceps brachii muscle. Long stumps may have a longer volar relief area.

Very short below-elbow stumps will often be fitted with a modified Munster type of socket. In this socket, the trimline comes proximal to the epicondyles and the socket is fitted while the elbow is held slightly flexed. The posterior portion of the socket presses above the olecranon on the triceps tendon as the elbow is extended. The anterior portion of the socket is contoured snugly around the biceps tendon. When this design of socket is fitted properly, a suspension harness may not be necessary; this makes it well suited for electronic hands and hooks with myoelectronic control systems.

Very short below-elbow stumps with limited range of motion at the elbow may benefit from a split socket with a step-up hinge; the forearm outer shell moves 2 degrees for each degree the stump moves at the elbow. The gain in motion in this type of prosthesis is accompanied by reduction in power, whereas the Munster socket retains power through a limited range of motion. Very short below-elbow stumps with marked reduction in strength may also be fitted with a split socket, but the motion of the stump is utilized to operate an elbow-locking mechanism instead of utilizing it for elbow flexion and extension.

For short and long above-elbow stumps, the standard socket is trimmed approximately 1 cm lateral to the acromion on a line that runs around to the axilla anteriorly and posteriorly. If the above-elbow stump is less than 35 per cent of humeral length (humeral neck), the socket will have to be constructed so that it extends 2.5 cm medial to the acromion.

Sockets for shoulder disarticulation level of amputation require extensions over a portion of the scapula posteriorly and over a small portion of the rib cage anteriorly. Sockets for forequarter amputations require a large area of contact over the rib cage anteriorly and posteriorly.

Terminal Devices

Terminal devices are made in the shape of a hand or a variety of hooks. Some are functional, and others are not. Special terminal devices are also available in the form of adapted standard or special tools.

Voluntary opening terminal devices are opened by tension placed on the control cable and are closed by rubber bands or springs. They have a two-cycle action: pulling the control cable opens the device, and releasing the control cable permits the device to be closed by its rubber bands or springs. Voluntary opening devices operate quickly with a minimum of control motions and are preferred by most persons with amputations. All Dorrance hooks and hands are voluntary opening devices (Fig. 48–5).

Voluntary closing terminal devices provide a degree of graded prehension that is generally not

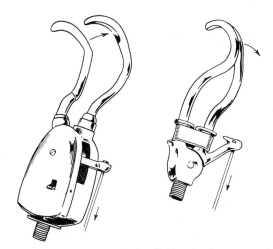

FIGURE 48–5. Voluntary closing (left) and voluntary opening (right) terminal devices. Tension applied to the control cable closes VC devices and opens VO devices.

LEONARD F. BENDER

possible with voluntary opening devices. They usually have a four-cycle action: pulling the control cable closes the hook partially or fully; releasing the control cable tension causes the hook to lock in the attained position; a slightly stronger pull unlocks the hook; and release of the pulling force allows the hook to spring open.

Motor-driven terminal devices are manufactured primarily in Europe, England, and Canada and are operated by a small electric motor. Both opening and closing of the hands and hooks are provided by the reversible electric motors.

Cosmetic hands are nonfunctional hands constructed of rigid or semirigid material and covered by a cosmetic glove. They may also be molded out of a semirigid material in the size and shape of a normal hand. They may have the standard stud that screws into a friction wrist unit or they may be secured to the stump by a zipper on the volar surface of the glove. They are available in many color shades to match the appearance of the skin.

Which Terminal Device to Use

In the United States it is convenient to select a Dorrance voluntary opening hook and hand. The Dorrance hand is frequently used because the thumb moves away from the palm simultaneously with finger extension as tension is exerted through the control cable. No passive prepositioning of the thumb by the other hand is necessary, as is done with the APRL hand. Dorrance hands are available in four sizes from glove size 6 through 8.

The selection of appropriate terminal devices for a patient is part of writing the prescription for a prosthesis. The team needs detailed information about the patient in order to perform this function; this information includes the patient's size, level of amputation, previous occupation and future vocation, avocational interests, and the willingness to accept a functional terminal device.

An infant needs a small hook, such as a Dorrance 12P, which is the smallest available. There are functional hands small enough for an infant; they are available in mechanical and myoelectronic systems. As the child grows, a slightly larger hook will be needed, the Dorrance 10X or 10P. P indicates plastisol coating and X indicates neoprene lining of the hook. Depending on the child's size, a larger hook may be needed at about six years of age. A Dorrance Model 99X is 1.3 cm longer than a 10X; a Dorrance 88X is 2.5 cm longer than a 10X. Either the 99X or 88X may be

used up to age 12 or 13 years. The two most popular hooks for adults are the Dorrance Models 5XA and 7. Model 5XA is used for light activities (Fig. 48–6), since it is made of aluminum, and Model 7, made of steel, is used for heavy work (Fig. 48–7). If it is important to have the terminal device lock firmly around a handle or other cylindrical objects, the Dorrance Model 6 superlock hook may be preferred. For wrist disarticulation and long below-elbow length stumps, it may be necessary to use a shorter hook, such as Dorrance Models 88X or 8, to avoid having the hook-fingers lower than the tip of the thumb on the normal side.

Electric hands are available in a wide spectrum of sizes accommodating toddlers two years of age or even younger and all other ages up to adult. The electric hand is customarily controlled myoelectronically and is applied to short or long below-elbow or above-elbow stumps.

All hooks and hands made in the United States have the same ½-inch, 20-thread stud for attachment to wrist units, and all are interchangeable. Most foreign-manufactured terminal devices also use the same stud and, therefore, are also interchangeable. A patient who wishes a cosmetic or functional hand need only select the proper size of hand and color of cosmetic glove. It can then easily

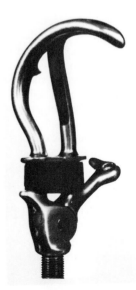

FIGURE 48–6. The Dorrance 5XA hook is light in weight, neoprene lined, and popular with adults for desk work. (From Bender, Leonard F.: Prostheses and Rehabilitation after Arm Amputation, 1974. Courtesy of Charles C Thomas, Publisher, Springfield, Illinois.)

cially adapted standard and special tools are also available for direct insertion into terminal devices or into the wrist unit. Detailed descriptions of these terminal devices are available in catalogues provided by various prosthetic component manufacturers and in textbooks.[9]

Wrist Components

Terminal devices must be attached to a below-elbow socket or to a forearm shell in the case of above-elbow amputations. Wrist units provide a mechanism for the attachment of terminal devices in either case. A wrist unit is laminated into and becomes an integral part of a below-elbow socket or a forearm shell. There are two basic designs of mechanical wrist units. Most are threaded sockets that limit rotation of the terminal device through a friction ring but do not lock in any position. Other units provide both a locking feature and a mechanism for quickly changing from one terminal device to another. These quick-change wrist units require a metal adapter that is screwed onto the stud of each mechanical terminal device and fits snugly into the wrist unit. Quick-change wrist units are preferred by persons who need to lock the terminal device to prevent rotation of it as they lift and manipulate heavy objects and by those who frequently change from one terminal device to another. Quick-change wrist units for electronic terminal devices have made use of electric-pow-

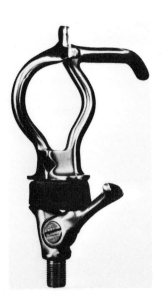

FIGURE 48–7. The Dorrance 7 hook is used by many male adults because it is durable and can hold a number of tools or a knife or a nail. (From Bender, Leonard F.: Prostheses and Rehabilitation after Arm Amputation, 1974. Courtesy of Charles C Thomas, Publisher, Springfield, Illinois.)

and quickly be interchanged with a functional hook-type terminal device.

In addition to commercially available hands and hooks, devices to meet special requirements are sometimes needed. A locking tool chuck screws into standard wrist units or can be adapted to quick-disconnect wrist units. Many different tools can be held in this chuck (Fig. 48–8). Many spe-

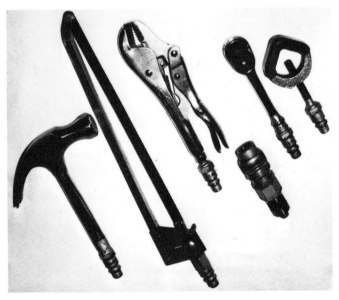

FIGURE 48–8. A tool chuck with a rotating locking ring accepts a hexagonal shaft that can be attached to many different tools. (From Bender, Leonard F.: Prostheses and Rehabilitation after Arm Amputation, 1974. Courtesy of Charles C Thomas, Publisher, Springfield, Illinois.)

LEONARD F. BENDER

ered hooks and hands far simpler for amputees with both these devices. They are available only for adults.

Friction wrist units are available in various sizes, from infant through adult, and in two shapes, circular and oval. Quick-change wrist units are all circular. A thin friction wrist unit is available for use with wrist disarticulation stumps; it reduces the length of the socket by nearly 1 cm.

A unit that provides flexion at the wrist may be added to a standard wrist unit or may be an integral part of a special wrist unit. This unit permits the terminal device to be positioned close to the body and is appropriate for persons with bilateral short above-elbow amputations because some dressing, grooming, and toileting activities require it. Most other amputees find that they do not need it.

A few wrist units have been developed that enhance pronation and supination of the terminal device through either mechanical linkage or electric power. Whereas the mechanical ones have found limited acceptance, the electric-powered units are highly desired. They provide 360 degrees of rotation, giving the amputee considerably increased function.

Elbow Components

Most persons with below-elbow amputations require a harness for suspension of the prosthesis and for control of the terminal device. The straps that fasten the below-elbow socket to the harness are generally termed *hinges*. A Munster type of below-elbow socket with a myoelectronically controlled terminal device does not require a control cable and should not need the suspension portion of a harness. All other below-elbow sockets require either flexible or rigid hinges. Rigid hinges are made of metal and are preferred by some for short stumps to provide stability of the socket on the stump in all positions of the elbow. Flexible hinges are customarily made of synthetic fabrics rather than leather so they do not stretch or absorb perspiration. Rigid hinges are available with a single pivot, a polycentric pivot, a multiple-action or step-up mechanism, and a locking device. Selection of the appropriate hinge depends largely on the characteristics of the below-elbow stump and the type of harness used.

Above-elbow prostheses for all levels of above-elbow amputation except elbow disarticulation utilize either an elbow unit that locks in different positions between 5 and 135 degrees of elbow flexion or an electric elbow. The mechanical elbow has a friction plate turntable above the elbow that permits the forearm shell to be positioned through a limited range of rotation that simulates internal and external rotation of the arm. An adjustable spring mechanism mounted on the medial aspect of the unit assists elbow flexion by partially counterbalancing the weight of the prosthesis distal to the elbow (Fig. 48–9).

Elbow disarticulation stumps require rigid hinges on the outside of the socket, since the customary elbow unit, when installed distal to the socket, would place the axis of elbow motion at least 5 cm lower than that on the sound side. A number of electronic elbows are available for toddlers up to adults. They use clutches for locking in position, offer a wide variety of control systems, including myoelectronic and mechanical, provide significantly increased control and versatility over mechanical elbows, and are sought by most above-elbow amputees. No longer considered experimental, they should be utilized whenever the appropriate criteria are met[10] (Fig. 48–10).

Shoulder Components

Shoulder units are needed for forequarter levels of amputation as well as for shoulder disarticulations and some amputations at the level of the

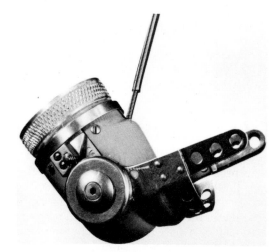

FIGURE 48–9. Hosmer positive locking elbow with forearm lift assist. (From Bender, Leonard F.: Prostheses and Rehabilitation after Arm Amputation, 1974. Courtesy of Charles C Thomas, Publisher, Springfield, Illinois.)

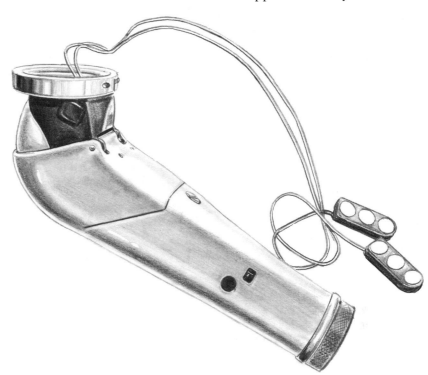

FIGURE 48–10. Utah myoelectronic elbow.

humeral neck. Shoulder units may be either a ball joint or two friction hinges or plates that create a universal joint. In the completed prosthesis, their position is not changed by control cables or electric motors; they must be prepositioned with the sound arm or by pressing the prosthesis against a solid object.

A cosmetic shoulder pad may be all some patients desire rather than a functional upper extremity prosthesis. Such a pad can be constructed from a block of polyfoam and held on with a chest strap. It will provide a normal shoulder contour.

Prosthetic Suspension and Control

The prosthesis must ordinarily be held on the stump through some arrangement of straps called a harness. In addition to suspension of the prosthesis, the harness provides an attachment for the control cable, which operates the terminal device and, in above-elbow amputations, the elbow unit. The harness most commonly used is shaped like the figure eight (Fig. 48–11). The straps should cross in back just to the sound side of the lowest cervical vertebra, and they are sewn to each other

at that point. If a ring is inserted at the point at which the straps cross, the length of each strap can be adjusted through a buckle and the harness is called an O-ring harness. The anterior strap, which lies in the deltopectoral groove on the amputated side, attaches directly to the socket of an above-elbow prosthesis or to the Y-strap and triceps pad of a below-elbow prosthesis. The posterior strap on the amputated side provides the attachment for the proximal end of the control cable. In some persons, the loop that runs through the sound axilla creates compression of the neurovascular components on that side when the prosthesis is used for heavy lifting; this occurs because the harness transfers the pull on the suspension strap of the prosthesis across to the axillary loop.

Persons who do heavy work may prefer a modified shoulder saddle harness (Figs. 48–12 and 48–13). It suspends the prosthesis through a Bowden cable (a braided steel cable inside a tubular housing), which runs over the top of the shoulder on the amputated side, attaching anteriorly and posteriorly to the socket of an above-elbow prosthesis with the cable housing anchored through baseplates and retainers on the anterior and posterior aspects of the saddle. In a below-elbow prosthesis, the suspension cable attaches to the Y-strap ante-

LEONARD F. BENDER

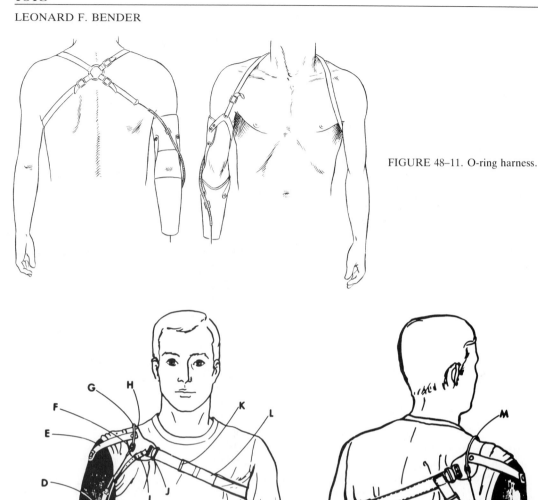

FIGURE 48–11. O-ring harness.

FIGURE 48–12. Modified shoulder saddle harness for above-elbow prosthesis. *A,* Button placed midline to dorsum of socket. *B,* Turntable aligned perpendicular to parasagittal line, and as close to the body as possible. *C,* Strap and buckle for adjustment. *D,* Retainer for elbow lock cable. *E,* Elastic "V" strap to eliminate excessive internal rotation and to hold top of socket snugly against shoulder. *F,* Point in cable where sharp angle must be avoided. *G,* Suspension cable. *H,* Polyethylene saddle 1½ inches wide. *I,* Strap and buckle for adjustment. *J,* Snap buckle. *K,* Three-prong safety buckle. *L,* Nylon webbing 1⅜ inches wide and ¹⁄₁₆ inch thick. *M,* Suspension cable housing should not touch saddle. *N,* Slit, do not cut out piece of cross-bar hanger strap. *O,* Use two rivets on cross-bar hanger strap. *P,* Attach base plate here. *Q,* Dual control cable. (From Bender, Leonard F.: Prostheses and Rehabilitation after Arm Amputation, 1974. Courtesy of Charles C Thomas, Publisher, Springfield, Illinois.)

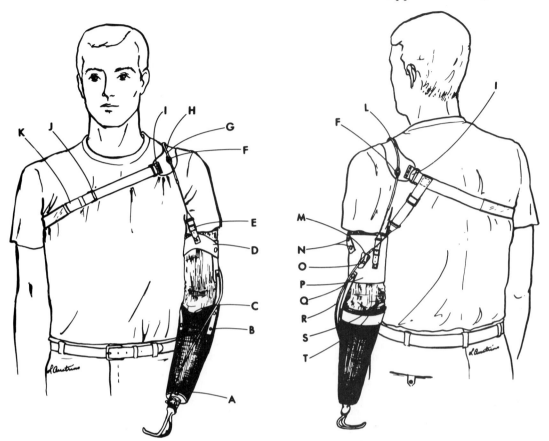

FIGURE 48–13. Modified shoulder saddle harness for below-elbow prosthesis. *A*, FM wrist with release button placed in midline. *B*, Rivets fastening the flexible elbow hinges. *C*, Cut-out for biceps tendon. *D*, Polyethylene Y-strap, 1/8 inch thick. *E*, Strap and buckle for adjustment of suspension cable. *F*, Point in cable where sharp angle must be avoided. *G*, Bowden suspension cable and housing. *H*, Polyethylene saddle 1½ inches wide. *I*, Snap buckle for chest strap fastener. *J*, Three-prong safety buckle for chest strap adjustment. *K*, Nylon chest strap. *L*, Suspension cable housing should not touch saddle. *M*, Slit, do not cut out a piece of cross-bar hanger strap. *N*, Use two rivets. *O*, Use two rivets on cross-bar hanger strap. *P*, Polyethylene triceps pad. *Q*, Use one rivet to attach flexible elbow hinge to triceps pad. *R*, Single control cable. *S*, Flare socket to avoid pressure on olecranon. *T*, Place hinge cross-strap (proximally) within ¼ inch of edge of socket. (From Bender, Leonard F.: Prostheses and Rehabilitation after Arm Amputation, 1974. Courtesy of Charles C Thomas, Publisher, Springfield, Illinois.)

riorly and to the triceps pad posteriorly. The shoulder saddle, Y-strap, and triceps pad all may be constructed of clear polyethylene, and a chest strap must be used to hold it in the correct position over the top of the shoulder. The shoulder saddle provides a large weight-bearing area and permits the lifting of heavy axial loads with comfort and without pull being transferred to the sound axilla.

In forequarter amputations, shoulder disarticulations, and humeral neck amputations, a chest strap alone will usually provide adequate suspension and a proper attachment for the control cable. This chest strap attaches both anteriorly and posteriorly to the socket of the prosthesis.

Mechanical control of functional terminal devices and elbow units is achieved by metal cables

running through a housing that guides the cable from its point of origin to the point of attachment on the device (Fig. 48–14). The cable is composed of braided stainless steel wire with a smooth surface; the housing is stainless steel wire tightly wound to form a small tube. The housing is attached to the socket and to the forearm shell of an above-elbow prosthesis through retainers and baseplates. In a below-elbow prosthesis, the control cable housing is attached to the triceps pad through a crossbar hanger assembly and to the socket through a baseplate and retainer. A Bowden control system utilizes a single control cable inside a single piece of housing attached at two or more points to the prosthesis or the harness.

The fair-lead control system is similar to a Bow-

LEONARD F. BENDER

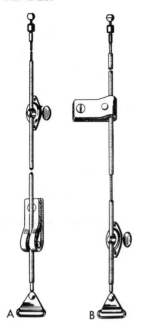

FIGURE 48–14. *A*, Bowden control. *B*, Fair-lead control. (From Bender, Leonard F.: Prostheses and Rehabilitation after Arm Amputation, 1974. Courtesy of Charles C Thomas, Publisher, Springfield, Illinois.)

den control except that the single control cable slides through two separate pieces of cable housing. This system provides two actions: (1) a force transmitted to the terminal device to operate it, and (2) a force applied to move the two pieces of housing toward each other. The second force can be used to flex the elbow, as long as it requires less force to flex the elbow than it does to operate the terminal device. A single control cable thereby becomes a dual control system for above-elbow prostheses.

Myoelectronic control has been utilized to operate electric motor-driven hands, hooks, wrists, and elbows. Surface electrodes are placed inside the inner wall of the socket and press against the skin over analogous or appropriate muscles. The electromyographical signal that is detected by these electrodes when the muscle beneath them contracts can be amplified and utilized to control the flow of current from a battery to an electric motor (Fig. 48–15). This type of control is most frequently used in below-elbow prostheses to operate an electric hand or hook. Newer electronic control systems permit sequential operation of electric-powered elbow motion, wrist rotation, and hand or hook operation through use of multilevel EMG signals and electronic switches that are responsive

to speed of muscle contraction or to muscle co-contraction and a mixture of these functions.

Prosthetic Prescription

Both the amputee and the prosthetist are served best by having an amputee clinic or team compose the elements of a prescription. The team may consist of a social worker, a prosthetist, an occupational therapist, a rehabilitation nurse, a physical therapist, an orthotist, a vocational counselor, and a physician. Their roles are consistent with their background and training. To write an appropriate prosthetic prescription, the team must have adequate information about the patient; this should include educational achievements, previous jobs, age, distance from home to the clinic or prosthetist's office, motivation and aptitude for further educational or vocational training, level of interest in wearing a prosthesis, psychological adjustment to amputation, secondary diagnoses, and the status of the stump. Based on this information, the team should decide when the stump is ready to be fitted with a prosthesis. The written prescription should specify each structural component. Additionally, it is helpful to order one extra harness, one extra control cable assembly, a pair of band appliers, and as many driving rings as indicated. A driving ring is a metal loop that attaches to a steering wheel and accepts the hook fingers of a terminal device in its center; these are needed particularly by the left arm amputee for each motor vehicle driven. The extra harness makes it possible to wash one harness while wearing the other. The extra control cable provides a spare in case one

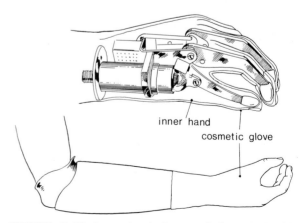

FIGURE 48–15. A myoelectrically controlled prosthesis with electric hand.

inner hand

cosmetic glove

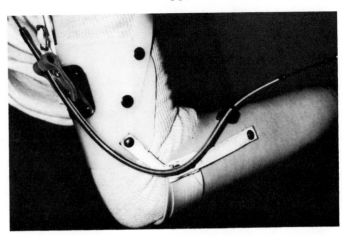

FIGURE 48–16. A standard prosthesis for a short below-elbow stump using a polyethylene triceps pad with attachments of flexible Dacron below-elbow hinges, polyethylene Y-strap, and leather cross-bar hanger strap. (From Bender, Leonard F.: Prostheses and Rehabilitation after Arm Amputation, 1974. Courtesy of Charles C Thomas, Publisher, Springfield, Illinois.)

breaks. Band appliers allow the amputee to put additional rubber bands on the terminal device.

The following is a typical prescription for a short below-elbow stump in a person who has good to normal range of motion and strength at the elbow and shoulder, who wishes to use the prosthesis in farming, and who also desires a cosmetic hand for social events:

Socket: Double-wall, below-elbow with trimline just below epicondyles.

Terminal device: Dorrance Model 7 hook and Dorrance Model 4 hand plus cosmetic glove.

Wrist: Hosmer FM (quick-disconnect).

Elbow: Flexible Dacron elbow hinges.

Harness: Polyethylene shoulder saddle, triceps pad, and Y-strap; Bowden control system (Fig. 48–16).

It could be equally appropriate to write the following prescription:

Socket: Double-wall, below-elbow, self-suspending type.

Terminal device: Otto Bock Greiffer plus Otto Bock electric hand.

Wrist: Otto Bock electric quick-disconnect and Otto Bock wrist rotator with myoelectric control.

Similar specific prescriptions can be written for each level of amputation and for each set of constraints.[9]

Prosthetic Check-out and Training

If one has been able to see the amputee within 30 days or possibly a few weeks after amputation, the first prosthetic socket should be a preparatory socket with an inner wall of clear plastic, the prescribed terminal devices, and other components but without the outer wall. This allows observation of the skin and adjustment of the socket.

After the prosthesis has been fabricated, it should be delivered to the amputee team for initial check-out on the amputee. The initial check-out takes only a few minutes and involves primarily an inspection of the components and their function. Conformance with the prescription should be checked along with the efficiency and workmanship of the prosthesis. After the patient dons the prosthesis, the fit of the socket and the position of the harness on the amputee should be observed.

Training proceeds during the completion of the check-out process. The amputee is taught to don the prosthesis by slipping it on like a jacket or a pull-over sweater. Control of each of the mechanisms of the prosthesis is then taught. When isolated movements have been mastered, the amputee moves on to performing specific integrated activities of daily living. Finally, skills useful in vocations and avocations are taught. During check-out and training, the team members will agree on final contour and specifications. Then the definitive prosthesis should be fabricated and checked out.

When a satisfactory level of control and use dexterity has been achieved, the training process is terminated and the amputee is asked to come back for periodic rechecks at lengthening intervals. These rechecks help provide preventive maintenance when the wearer does not recognize declining efficiency of the prosthesis and also provide continuing contact with the amputee during readjustment.

Partial Hand Amputations

Amputation of part of a hand creates significant functional limitations and special prosthetic or orthotic problems. A variety of patterns of partial hand amputation can be observed, and the needs

LEONARD F. BENDER

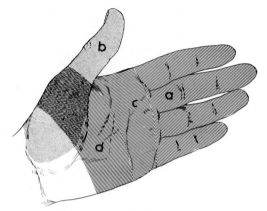

FIGURE 48–17. Levels of partial hand loss: *a,* transphalangeal; *b,* thenar; *c,* transmetacarpal, distal; *d,* transmetacarpal, proximal.

ers, threshers, power saws, shredders, and corn pickers. They may also be caused by bullet wounds, explosions, freezing, and burning. Congenital skeletal deficiencies of the hand occur in many forms and add to the confusing variety of partial hand losses.

Analysis of these losses permits development of a classification of losses that will help guide the amputee clinic team toward the most appropriate prosthetic or orthotic solution. Levels of loss can conveniently be classified as follows (Fig. 48–17):

a. Transphalangeal with involvement or sparing of the thumb.
b. Thenar.
c. Transmetacarpal distal with involvement or sparing of the thumb.
d. Transmetacarpal proximal with involvement or sparing of the thumb.

Transphalangeal levels of amputation usually require no device. The amputee may desire cosmetic fingers or even a portion of a cosmetic glove. These are available in a variety of skin tones, but they will provide little or no increased function. If the need can be defined, an orthosis may be specially designed to permit a needed function.

for devices vary considerably. Some persons are interested primarily in appearance, whereas others desire function.

The causes of partial hand amputation are primarily traumatic and may involve such devices as punch presses, metal shears, conveyor belts, grind-

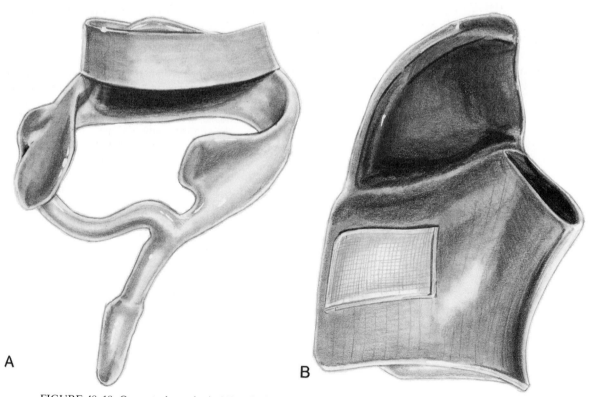

FIGURE 48–18. Open steel prosthesis *(A)* and mitt-shaped prosthesis *(B)* used in transmetacarpal amputations.

Thenar amputations are infrequent. Loss of only the distal phalanx usually necessitates nothing other than possibly a cosmetic thumb tip. Loss of part of or the entire proximal phalanx usually is best handled by constructing a prosthetic thumb of epoxy resins with a neoprene volar surface and a strap around the wrist to hold it in place.

Transmetacarpal distal and proximal levels of amputation can be fitted with three different devices: a cosmetic glove, a mitt-shaped prosthesis, or an open steel prosthesis shaped like an opposition semicircle. The mitt-shaped prosthesis is constructed like other double-walled sockets, but the exterior contour is that of slightly flexed fingers with no separation between the digits. It may be constructed with no strap to hold it on so that the amputee can merely slide the partial hand stump into the prosthesis and easily remove it when there is no need for it. The open steel prosthesis has a foundation shaped like a hand orthosis but has a steel rod attached to the foundation that extends out approximately in the contour of the previous fingertip positions; the intact thumb can then use it as an opposition device (Fig. 48–18). The more proximal the level of amputation, the more difficult it is to construct the device.

In proximal transmetacarpal amputations, it may be possible and desirable to utilize functional fingers that can be attached to a short double-wall socket and controlled by a Bowden cable coming from a standard O-ring harness.

References

1. Davies, E. J., Friz, B. R., and Clippinger, F. W.: Amputees and their prostheses. Artif. Limbs, 14:19, 1970.
2. Lamy, M., and Marteaux, P.: The genetic study of limb malformations. *In* Swinyard, C. A. (Ed.): Limb Development and Deformity: Problems of Evaluation and Rehabilitation. Springfield, IL, Charles C Thomas, Publisher, 1969, pp. 170–175.
3. Cohlan, S. Q.: A review of teratogenic agents and human congenital malformations. *In* Swinyard, C. A. (Ed.): Limb Development and Deformity: Problems of Evaluation and Rehabilitation. Springfield, IL, Charles C Thomas, Publisher, 1969, pp. 161–170.
4. Kay, H. W.: Clinical applications of the new international terminology for the classification of congenital limb deficiencies. Inter-Clinic Information Bull., Vol. XIV, No. 3, 1975.
5. Carlyle, L.: Using body measurements to determine proper lengths of artificial arms. Artificial Limbs Research Project, UCLA, Pamphlet Series No. 2, 1951.
6. Carlyle, L.: Fitting the artificial arm. *In* Klopsteg, P. E., and Wilson, P. D. (Eds.): Human Limbs and Their Substitutes. New York, McGraw-Hill, 1954, pp. 637–652.
7. Weiss, M.: Neurological implications of fitting artificial limbs immediately after amputation surgery. Report of Fifth Workshop Panel on Lower-Extremity Prosthetics Fitting, Committee on Prosthetics Research and Development, National Academy of Sciences, February 1966.
8. Malone, J. M., Fleming, L. L., Robertson, J., Whitesides, T. E. Jr., Leal, J. M., Poole, J. U., and Grodin, R. S.: Immediate, early, and late postsurgical management of upper-limb amputation. J. Rehabil. Res. Dev., 21:33–41, 1984.
9. Bender, L. F.: Prostheses and Rehabilitation after Arm Amputation. Springfield, IL, Charles C Thomas, Publisher, 1974.
10. Sears, H. H., Andrew, J. T., and Jacobsen, S. C.: Clinical Experience with The Utah Artificial Arm. Canadian Association of Prosthetists and Orthotists Yearbook, 1984.

49

Rehabilitation of the Lower Extremity Amputee

LAWRENCE W. FRIEDMANN

The exact incidence and prevalence of amputation is unknown. In the United States, about 43,000 new major amputations a year occur. Most of these are due to vascular disease, with 90 per cent involving the legs. In the author's experience, approximately 5 per cent are partial foot and ankle amputations, 50 per cent are below the knee amputations, 35 per cent are above the knee, and 7 to 10 per cent are at the hip.

Limb absence or loss may occur from many causes. Among them are congenital absence, limb reduction deformity, reduplication of parts, thermal or electrical burns, crush, vascular occlusions or injuries, infections, tumors, traumatic loss, and neurogenic resorption. The most frequent indication for amputation of the lower limb is gangrene resulting from occlusive arterial disease. In the upper limbs of adults, the most common cause of amputation is trauma. The injury is most commonly due to misuse of power tools at work and at play. In children, congenital absence or deformity of limbs is the most common cause, with malignant tumors, infections, and trophic changes being relatively rare causes of amputation.

Principles of Physiatric Management

Preparation for Amputation

Preoperative evaluation and consultation by a physiatrist who has special skills and knowledge of amputations and their sequelae is highly desirable. In cases in which amputation is not an emergency, physical and psychological preparation of the patient and family is important. The potential amputee should be counseled on the following:

1. The physicians are doing their best to save the limb. The natural course of the disease may cause loss of the body part. If it cannot be saved, every effort will be made to leave a stump of the optimal length consistent with good healing to obtain the best possible function with a prosthesis.

2. The range of motion and strength of the stump and of the sound limbs need to be maintained. Strengthening of the upper limbs is important for the use of crutches or a walker. Breathing and trunk exercises are required before and after surgery.

3. The care of the general health and the other limbs is vital. Walking may often be achieved with one leg amputated but is extremely difficult with both legs amputated above the knees. Continuing medical supervision will be required for care of the residual limb, protection of the other limbs, management of any other complications of systemic arterial disease and any concurrent diseases, and modifications of the artificial limb.

Amputation Levels

The selection of surgical level for the amputation is probably one of the most important decisions that must be made for the amputee. The pathological process dictates most of the decisions. In malignancies, if chemotherapy with local resection is inadvisable, amputation above the proximal joint is advised. In other conditions, the viability of the remaining tissues determines the most distal possible level. Functional considerations then determine whether to amputate more proximally. All of these considerations go into the surgical judgment.

The level of amputation for vascular disease is best chosen in the operating room by the vascular surgeon, who observes whether and how well the skin bleeds. Skin closure should be done by an experienced member of the amputation team, since the skin is the crucial interface between the musculoskeletal structures and the prosthetic socket. Because skin adherent to bone will tend to tear at its edge, prevention of adhesions is important at the time of amputation. After healing, gentle stroking and friction massage help to mobilize any minor degree of adherence. The level of amputation for the lower limb may be classified on an anatomical or functional (prosthetic) basis. Some important technical information may thus be summarized. The patient utilizes a leg prosthesis like a stilt, balancing the full superincumbent body weight over the prosthesis with each step. Body weight is applied to a relatively small surface area, predisposing to skin irritation and breakdown if the stump is not fashioned as a functional weight-bearing end-organ for use in a person-machine interface.

For forefoot surgery, it may be possible to remove only the necrotic tissue, with successful healing. When distal metatarsal and toe amputations are contemplated, one should save only bone for which healthy full-thickness skin coverage can be provided. Split-thickness and insensate grafts on the foot are unsatisfactory because persistent pressure from foot wear usually causes skin breakdown. Toe amputation and transmetatarsal amputation need mobile plantar sensate skin. The major foot ablations are Lisfranc's tarsometatarsal amputation and Chopart's tarsotarsal amputation. Both lead to almost inevitable foot deformity causing further disability and should usually be avoided. Only in selected circumstances is Chopart's amputation useful in children and certain adults.[14]

True ankle disarticulation is done mainly as an open amputation and drainage procedure in adults. In infants it may replace Syme's amputation. The supra-articular cut in Syme's amputation should not be perpendicular to the long axis of the tibia

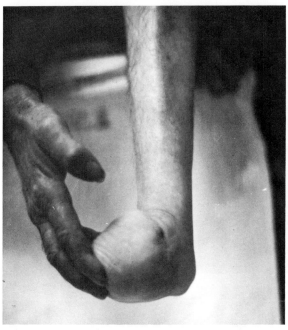

FIGURE 49–1. Syme's amputation stump with dislocation of the heel pad.

but parallel to the ground when that patient stands so as to provide a flat surface for weight-bearing. Rounding the bones, except for rasping slightly the sharp edges of the bone, reduces the area for bearing the weight of the body and is a surgical error. The traditional Syme's amputation remains the best. The heel pad must adhere to the tibia. If it does not, weight-bearing capacity is reduced (Fig. 49–1). Using a calcaneal fragment delays healing. If the fragment slips, weight-bearing is impossible (Fig. 49–2).

Amputation between the ankle joint and the junction of the lower and middle thirds of the tibia is called a long below-knee amputation (the healing rate at this level in vascular disease is reduced). Between that point and the junction of the upper and middle thirds of the tibia, transection produces a standard below-knee amputation. Amputation above that results in a short below-knee amputation. An ultrashort below-knee amputation has a stump only from the tibial plateau to just below the tibial tubercle. The healing rate improves inversely with stump length.

The choice between an above-knee and a below-knee amputation is often a difficult decision, since healing of the amputation stump is nearly ensured for above-knee amputations, but use of the below-knee prosthesis is much more likely to meet with

LAWRENCE W. FRIEDMANN

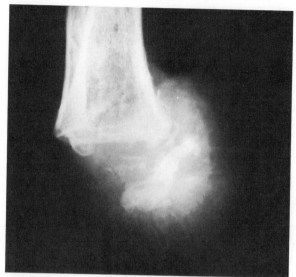

FIGURE 49–2. Syme's amputation with dislocation of the calcaneal fragment and heel pad.

success in the older patient. With modern amputation methods, between 75 and 90 per cent of vascular cases amputated below the knee may be successful.[14] The value of retaining the knee is so great that it is wise to amputate just below the knee even in questionable cases. Skin vascularity is the crucial factor in limb survival, and methods of evaluation of circulation are being upgraded. There are times when the 10 per cent risk of possibly having to revise a failed ultrashort below-knee amputation must be accepted in order to try to optimize the patient's future functional capacity.

When a below-knee amputation is necessary, it is best done at the junction of the middle and upper thirds of the tibia, usually between 8 and 18 cm below the tibial plateau. A stump as short as 3 cm below the tibial plateau can be fitted with a below-knee prosthesis.

A knee disarticulation is an anatomical transection. There are various surgical modifications. The true knee disarticulation is a much better amputation level than above the knee, since it is much less traumatic for frail patients, it is fully weight-bearing distally, the prosthesis needs no ischial seat, and the gait is better. The knee disarticulation formerly was rightfully denigrated because the artificial limbs were so cumbersome. With newer knee designs, an excellent prosthesis can now be made.[32] The patient has full weight-bearing through the knee and excellent prosthesis control. Using a long anterior flap under the femoral con-

dyles requires that the anterior skin be very long. If the long flap has an adequate blood supply, a very short below-knee amputation can usually be performed. If the blood supply is mediocre, it is advisable to perform the disarticulation using shorter equal medial and lateral flaps with a suture line between the femoral condyles. That scar does not interfere with weight-bearing.

An above-knee amputation should be performed in such a way that an available prosthetic device can be utilized. Distal weight-bearing is not tolerated. An amputation 10 cm above the knee joint is desirable. A longer amputation, such as the Gritti-Stokes or supracondylar, will require that the prosthetic thigh be longer than the unamputated side because almost 7 cm is needed for the internal knee joint mechanism. However, the higher the amputation, the greater the loss of socket control.

The long above-knee amputation is at 55 to 75 per cent of the length of the normal femur. That is an excellent functional length. Amputation at 35 to 55 per cent of the femoral length is called a medium above-knee amputation. From the groin to 35 per cent of the length of the femur is a short above-knee amputation. Above this point is functionally a hip disarticulation amputation even when part of the femur remains. The hip disarticulation amputation preserves the ischial tuberosity and pelvis. The patient can bear weight through the ischial tuberosity; there is no effective bony lever to move a prosthesis. Amputation through the pelvis is defined as hemipelvectomy, or hindquarter ablation. The hindquarter amputee must bear weight on the soft tissues and chest cage.

The surgical levels of greatest utility are the transmetatarsal, the Syme's, and the standard below-knee amputations. The vascular supply is relatively good, provided the surgical level is well chosen. The next best level is the ultrashort below-knee amputation. These patients, with a bone stump 3 to 7 cm long, measured from the tibial plateau, require removal of the fibula and all of the muscles originating below the knee (Fig. 49–3). Hamstring section is frequently required for accurate prosthetic fitting. The patients bear weight on the patellar tendon and both tibial flares. Specially constructed artificial limbs are required, but function is far superior to that of the above-knee amputation.

The higher the amputation level, the more energy must be expended for ambulation. The below-knee amputee walking on level ground uses between 10 and 40 per cent more energy than does

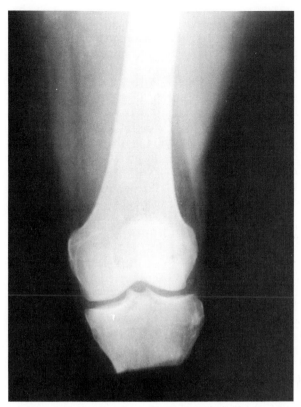

FIGURE 49–3. Ultrashort, below-knee amputation with removal of the fibula.

a nonamputee walking the same distance.[19, 21] The above-knee amputee under the same conditions uses between 60 and 100 per cent more energy.[39] Thus, a bilateral below-knee amputee uses less energy for walking than does a unilateral above-knee amputee.

The sensory implications of lower limb amputation level are frequently ignored. An amputee loses the sensory input from the skin, joints, tendons, and muscles. If the muscles are not reattached over the bone end at the normal length/tension relationship, the information given to the central nervous system is erroneous as well as diminished. This interferes with the central excitatory state and thus motor control.

The removal of a joint markedly decreases the sensory information provided to the patient. When one amputates above the knee, the patient does not know where the prosthetic foot is when walking in the dark. The patient with an ultrashort below-knee stump always knows that the prosthetic foot is directly below the stump in a straight line from the tibial segment to the floor.[14]

Postoperative Care

The main objective is to ensure rapid wound healing with minimal scarring and adhesion of the skin to the underlying bone. The usual method is to place a soft dressing on the wound over the drain, and allow the incision to heal. An elastic bandage may be used over the dressing.

The principle of the rigid dressing used alone is excellent. The socket prevents edema, protects the stump, and helps the stump to heal.[14] A method that is now diminishing in popularity is the rigid total-contact dressing with a prosthesis attached immediately. It is still the method of choice for children and some clean traumatic ablations.[5] For vascular cases in the elderly, pressure produced by the rigid dressing and immediate ambulation can cause serious ischemic damage except under the most meticulous circumstances, and an amputee team must be available 24 hours a day, seven days a week.[14] A better technique for vascular cases is the Unna semirigid dressing (Fig. 49–4). It is easily changed, and there are few instances of wound breakdown.[18]

Other methods of postoperative care include (1) the "controlled environment treatment,"[34] which utilizes a machine that supplies bacteria-free air to the wound with controlled humidity and temperature. This provides a perfect environment for primary wound healing. The technique is still experimental (Fig. 49–5).

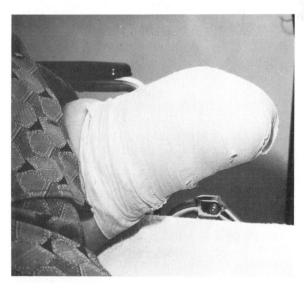

FIGURE 49–4. Unna semirigid dressing made with gauze impregnated with Unna paste. It provides a firm conforming inelastic support that helps prevent and reduce edema while keeping the skin moist *without maceration.*

LAWRENCE W. FRIEDMANN

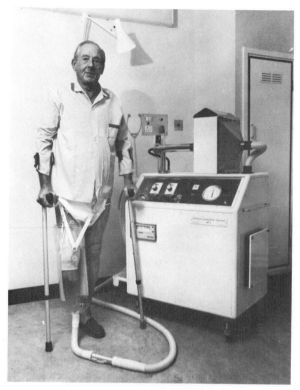

FIGURE 49–5. Controlled environment treatment on standing patient. (Photograph courtesy of Professor Ernest Burgess.)

Less desirable is (2) an inflated transparent plastic bag placed on the stump so the skin can be observed while edema is kept low. In the author's experience, it causes skin maceration, and in the above-knee amputee keeps the thighs abducted and flexed, fostering a hip flexion and abduction contracture. A variation is to use a temporary prosthesis with an airbag inside it.

The therapist will perform a prosthetic evaluation and report any problems to the clinic team. The therapist will train the amputee in the donning and doffing of the prosthesis and in use of the limb in self-care, ambulation, recreation, and the patient's job.

The therapist will serve as a prime source of information to the team regarding the type of permanent prosthesis the patient should have. Aside from the length and condition of the residual limb, there are many other situations that modify what component is optimal for which individual. The therapist will report the patient's responses to various component and alignment changes so the optimum final prescription can be given.

There may be conditions apart from the stump that affect the use of a prosthesis. It may be inadvisable to provide a patient having serious cardiorespiratory disease with any prosthesis inasmuch as the effort required may jeopardize survival. Provision of a wheelchair, walker, or crutches may be safer. Stress testing is needed, and a trial with an ultralight provisional limb may be done carefully. Hemiplegia on either side may prevent a patient from using an artificial leg unless additional stability is built into the leg. Amputation of the leg on the side opposite an arm amputation may dictate a special harness or control or contraindicate use of a prosthesis.

Postoperative Conditioning

Deconditioning of the patient and the residual limb must be avoided or reversed. This deconditioning has physical, mental, emotional, social, economical, and vocational components, all of which should be worked with as soon as the amputee is ready to work with the various members of the team.

To prevent contractures, the stump must be moved through its full range of motion at least four times daily. The prone position helps to discourage knee and hip flexion contractures. Active assistive and active exercises against resistance are important for strengthening muscles. Endurance is best enhanced by use of a temporary limb. Facilitation exercises are excellent, especially for correction of contractures, but expensive in therapists' time. If contractures exist, splinting should be used. The dial lock orthosis maintains during the night and on weekends the range of motion that the therapist obtained during the treatment sessions.

In high amputations, personal hygiene may be impaired. After hemipelvectomy, a patient may have difficulty sitting on the toilet seat. Bilateral amputees need to learn transfer techniques into and out of a wheelchair and bed and onto the toilet.

Unilateral amputees can balance on one leg and walk with crutches or use a prosthesis. The more proximal the amputation, the more difficult ambulation will be, especially on rough, uneven terrain. The use of a cane or crutches is very important. Irregular pavement is just as difficult to walk on as is rocky ground. Unilateral hip disarticulation and hemipelvectomy patients often abandon their prostheses because crutch ambulation is faster and easier. Approximately 85 per cent of young men with this level of amputation will abandon their prostheses. Fifty per cent of women retain the prostheses, primarily for cosmesis.

Bilateral amputees walk much more poorly than do unilateral amputees because most of the functional adjustments to prosthetic use are made by the remaining limb. If there is a second prosthesis, these adjustments cannot be made. Bilateral above-knee amputees frequently do not ambulate. The energy costs are great, and they find wheelchair use preferable.

Vascular disease is systemic. The vessels of the other leg, coronary arteries, cerebral arteries, and ophthalmic arteries all are involved. Each complicates rehabilitation.

Treatment should be conceived of as part of a continuum in the natural history of the disease, vascular or otherwise, from prevention to cure or compensation for loss. Amputation is not a failure of medical or surgical knowledge and skill. It is an inevitable phase in the natural history of the illness.

Following amputation, there is often a muscular imbalance; some muscles are weakened by surgical removal of the insertion, whereas their antagonists remain intact. Muscular imbalance leads to development of contracture, which impairs the use of the prosthesis.

We exercise the patient thrice daily to counteract the tendency toward contractures, but the best way to avoid contractures and to build up the stump is the early use of a temporary articulated prosthesis.

Exercise all the remaining limbs to maintain range of motion and muscle power. I believe proprioceptive neuromuscular facilitation to be most valuable in combating joint contractures. Exercise equipment is helpful as a supplement to manual resistive exercises. For lower limb amputees, balancing exercises are needed to learn to stabilize the superimposed trunk on the prosthetic socket. Strong abdominal, paraspinal, and hip muscles are needed for this action. Since the amputee will need crutches, exercises of the shoulder girdle and arms should be prescribed. Massage of the stump of any type helps lessen the almost universal fear of handling it. Centripetal massage helps reduce edema, improve circulation, and prevent adhesions.

Components of Lower Extremity Prostheses

THE PARTS OF A PROSTHESIS

The socket partially encloses the stump to form a union between it and the artificial limb. Its function is to provide stability and to transmit forces as accurately as possible between the device and the patient's body.

The prosthesis must be held on by some form of suspension, e.g., suction (atmospheric pressure), a strap, condylar clamping, muscular grasp, or friction. Various straps may be used over bone prominences, over the shoulders, or around the waist. Garter belt and corset suspension may be advisable in special circumstances.

The terminal device is that part of the artificial limb that contacts the environment. In the leg it is the foot.

The activating force for the prosthesis is usually muscular power, but external power is being used experimentally for artificial legs. Control over the leg prosthesis is transmitted from body power.

The length of the prosthesis is obtained by structural elements, either internal, analogous to bone, or external. They are referred to as endoskeletal or exoskeletal.

One important aspect of prosthesis fabrication is alignment, the relationship of parts of the prosthesis to each other. The alignment of the different components determines much of the comfort and the ability of the patient to use the prosthesis. Flexion contractures of the hip and knee may thwart the achievement of successful alignment. Alignment varies with the heel heights of shoes. Patients must purchase all shoes with the same heel heights. For a woman who wishes to change from low heels to high heels for social occasions, the prosthetist must be informed prior to fabrication of the prosthesis so the artificial feet can be made interchangeable.

FOOT AND ANKLE MECHANISMS

An artificial foot may have ankles that are rigid or allow motion in one or more planes. The SACH (solid ankle cushion heel) foot can be obtained for heels of various heights, with or without toes, and for the level of Syme's amputation (Fig. 49–6). Single-axis ankles move in the flexion-extension plane with the axis of rotation parallel to the floor and at 105 degrees to the line of progression. Plantar flexion is controlled by resistance of a rubber posterior bumper, and dorsiflexion is controlled by resistance of an anterior bumper (Fig. 49–7). The dual-axis ankle has two degrees of freedom, i.e., flexion-extension and inversion-eversion. A "universal ankle" allows rotation in addition to the other two axes. Separate rotators are available.

With increasing ability to move the ankle, there is decreasing stability. The precise "trade-off" that

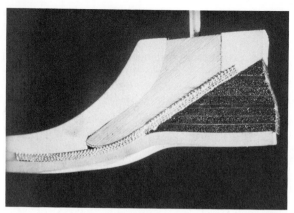

FIGURE 49–6. Cross-section of SACH foot. (Photograph courtesy of the late Mr. William Tosberg.)

one makes depends on the patient's individual needs. Patients who walk on uneven terrain may want a dual- or triple-axis ankle, despite their noisiness, heavier weight, costliness, and need for frequent repairs. The dual-axis is prescribed most frequently for golfers who need the wide stance. Other athletes often wish these more sophisticated ankles also.

Newer feet are now coming on the market. The Seattle (Fig. 49–8), Flex (Fig. 49–9), Carbon Copy II, STEN-foot (Fig. 49–10), and SAFE feet allow

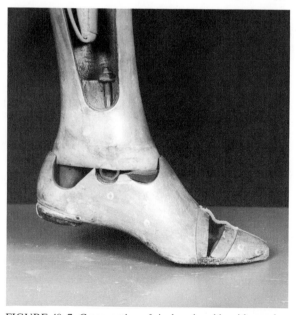

FIGURE 49–7. Cross-section of single-axis ankle with wooden foot with toe break.

some push off by storing energy and releasing it later in the stance phase of gait. The Carbon Copy II foot is lighter and said to be more functional than the SACH foot. The rest, except for the Greissinger five-way foot, are heavier than the SACH, but lighter than the single-axis foot. The precise indications and contraindications have yet to be clarified, but the feet are good for running on a flat surface, but not irregular terrain. The Flex-Foot is the best for jumping, but very poor on irregular surfaces. Active young patients benefit from energy-storing feet, which are an expensive waste in the elderly. The Carbon Copy II foot is inexpensive. Women prefer feet with toes for open shoes. The SACH foot is most commonly used. Feet with mechanical axes are used only for special situations after a trial on a provisional limb.

SHANK AND THIGH MATERIALS

There are two basic designs for thighs and shanks. The traditional is the exoskeletal, in which there is a hard external form of the shank that supports the body's weight. The newest is the endoskeletal, in which there is a supporting central member going from the socket to the ankle. This may or may not have joints or be surrounded by a soft cosmetic cover. Exoskeletal legs are stronger and more durable. Endoskeletal limbs look nicer, have a more pleasant feel, and are less noisy when accidentally struck.

SOCKETS

The socket is used to transmit the weight of the body and may be used to suspend the device. It transmits muscular forces to the limb and inertia, floor reaction, and gravity to the stump. The socket is the most important determinant of comfort. The fit determines the pressure distribution between the patient's body and the device, and the control of the device. The most commonly used socket materials are plastic laminate and wood.

Stumps have areas that are pressure sensitive and others that are pressure resistant. Weight must be borne proportionally on those areas that are most tolerant of pressure.

Partial Foot Amputation

For patients who have had toe excision, either no prosthesis or a filler for the shoe to prevent the foot from sliding forward in the shoe is all that is needed. If the first toe or transmetatarsals have

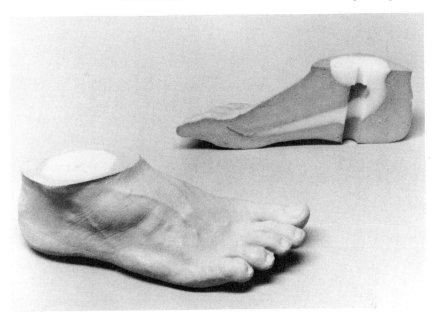

FIGURE 49–8. Seattle Foot with cross-section. (Photograph courtesy of the Seattle Foot Co.)

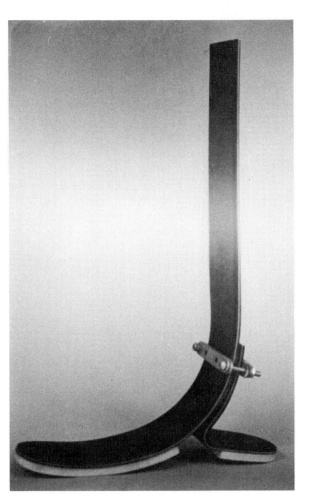

FIGURE 49–9. Flex-Foot. (Photograph courtesy of the Flex-Foot Corp.)

LAWRENCE W. FRIEDMANN

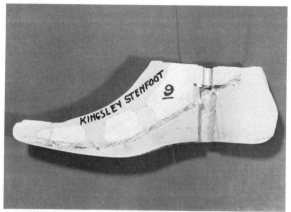

FIGURE 49–10. Section of Kingsley STEN-foot. (Photograph courtesy of the Kingsley Manufacturing Co.)

been amputated, a long steel shank, a rigid leather sole, or a foot orthosis may be used to improve toe off and to prevent unsightly curling of the front of the shoe.

The Syme's Amputee

The Canadian Syme's socket has a weight-bearing end pad and a patellar tendon–bearing bar, since prolonged total end-bearing is not tolerated. There is a medial trap door over the distal shank that allows the bulbous distal end of the stump to enter the prosthesis and acts as a condylar suspension clamp over the malleoli (Fig. 49–11). An elastic inner wall may replace the trap door. If the bulbous terminal end of the stump is removed, the opening may be omitted. This limb needs a special low-profile SACH foot.

The Below-Knee Amputee

The Conventional Socket. The shape of the socket determines the name and weight-bearing characteristics of the below-knee prosthesis. The "conventional" socket must be fitted so that it does not exert pressure over the distal anterior end of the tibial stump, the fibular head, or the tibial crest. Although a superior prosthetist can make a wooden leg in the patellar tendon–bearing (PTB) shape, most are less than adequate. The anterior brim of the socket supports the body weight on the patellar tendon. It may be fabricated as a molded socket for patients who must kneel a lot, and then is more comfortable than a PTB limb. The conventional wood socket requires the use of external knee joints and a thigh lacer that transfers part of the body weight from the socket to the skin

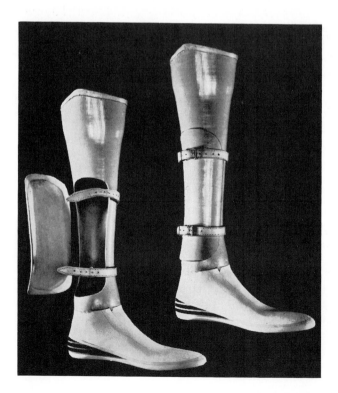

FIGURE 49–11. Canadian Syme's prostheses.

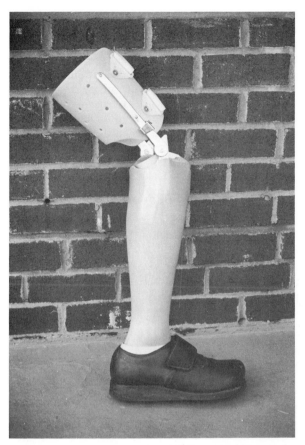

FIGURE 49–12. Specially designed PTB prosthesis for a sculptor in Mexico. Note the plastic perforated thigh corset with lockable knees and single-axis foot. The perforations and plastic thigh corset were for perspiration in the hot, humid environment. The lockable knees and single-axis ankle were so that he could lean into his sculpture as he used his hammer and chisel.

to 1.22 kg/cm^2 on descending a 3-degree incline. At the kickpoint, the distal end of the cut tibia, on level walking the pressure maximum is 0.86 kg/cm^2, but it goes to 1.40 kg/cm^2 on 3-degree descending, and to 0.65 kg/cm^2 on 3-degree ramp ascending.[8] Relief from pressure must be provided for the fibular head, the hamstrings, and the tibial crest. The socket brim comes to the middle of the patella anteriorly with the sides at the same level or higher.

The patellar tendon–bearing socket may be used with a plastic liner for resiliency. The liner may be soft or semisoft, fabricated, poured, or foamed. Shrinkage is rapid and local pads should be added to the liner, both to take up the extra space and to redistribute the pressure so that sensitive areas of the stump are protected. Some long-term amputees prefer the hard socket used with wool stump socks.

A total-contact pad of sponge rubber, felt, or silicone helps prevent stasis of blood and lymph in the distal stump. By doing so, it helps prevent chronic dermatitis, ulceration, and pain due to edema and congestion.[4] It is useful in patients with skin problems, impaired proprioception, edema, cerebellar or vestibular imbalance, or phantom limb sensation.

An unusual total-contact socket may be used to provide even pressure distribution in very difficult-to-manage cases with varying edema. A water bag supported by an adjustable height-lifting platform may be used. The platform is usually elevated and depressed by a screw adjustment.

The Slip Socket. Skin lesions due to friction when skin is adherent to bone, tendon, or a plastic

of the thigh (Fig. 49–12). The socket is customarily left open at the bottom, and for those with perspiration problems this makes evaporation easier. Skin irritation from friction and stump "choking" (edema and its sequelae) from constriction by the superior portion of the socket while the bottom is left open is fairly common (Fig. 49–13).

The Patellar Tendon–Bearing (PTB) Socket. This design is made of plastic over a mold of the stump held with the knee in flexion of 5 to 10 degrees. It bears weight primarily on the area of the patellar tendon and on the medial tibial flare. A popliteal prominence holds the stump forward on the patellar bar to ensure that weight is borne on the patellar tendon (Fig. 49–14). The pressure on the patellar tendon during level walking is a maximum of 1.67 kg/cm^2. The pressure decreases

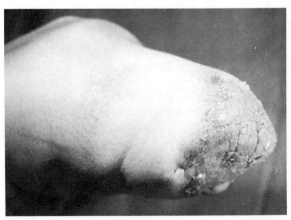

FIGURE 49–13. Below-knee stump with severe chronic and acute "choking" with blisters and cracked, fungoid, discolored skin.

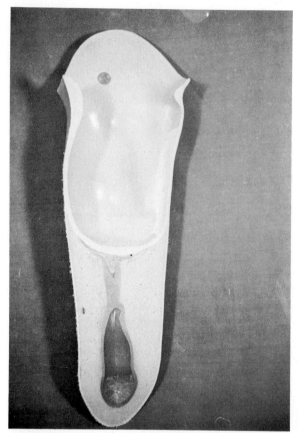

FIGURE 49–14. Cross-section of double-wall, total contact patellar tendon–bearing socket with endoskeletal tube surrounded by lightweight filler and outer laminated shank.

vascular graft are lessened by a slip socket (Fig. 49–15). It has the two layers of the socket separated. The inner layer is kept near the stump by elastic bands, a ball, or a spring, while allowing the outer layer to piston during swing, when gravity pulls the foot and shank away from the stump.

The Bent or Kneeling Prosthesis. For severely contracted knees, the socket may be flexed on the prosthetic shank, but with a long stump it is unsightly. For men with extremely short stumps with flexion contractures, the bent-knee prosthesis may be necessary, although it has a number of serious disadvantages. The knee provides an excellent weight-bearing surface when the knee is flexed 90 degrees. The external knee hinges damage clothing. The thigh is longer than normal when sitting, the gait is mediocre, and the protrusion is uncosmetic for women wearing skirts (Fig. 49–16).

Other Socket Modifications. The total-contact socket helps reduce the concentration of stress on a delicate stump by distributing weight-bearing

evenly over the entire skin of the stump. It may use air compression to reduce edema, as well as giving support for the tissues of the stump, as in the air chamber socket, in which a sealed chamber of air is compressed by the stump through an elastic membrane during stance phase.

Friction may be reduced by a gel socket. The gel socket has a double-layered flexible leather liner with a gel-like substance encased between the layers. Interlayer movement is in the gel.[36] This is most valuable when the skin is adherent, especially after burns (Fig. 49–17).

A diagonal posterior wall relieves medial hamstring pressure.

SUSPENSIONS FOR BELOW-KNEE PROSTHESES

Many below-knee socket designs have suspension built in. They do not modify the weight-bearing characteristics of the socket.

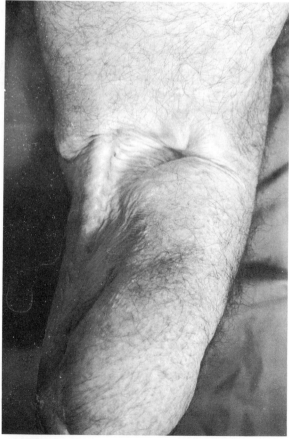

FIGURE 49–15. Patient with below-knee amputation with residual Dacron graft covered by adherent insensate scar tissue.

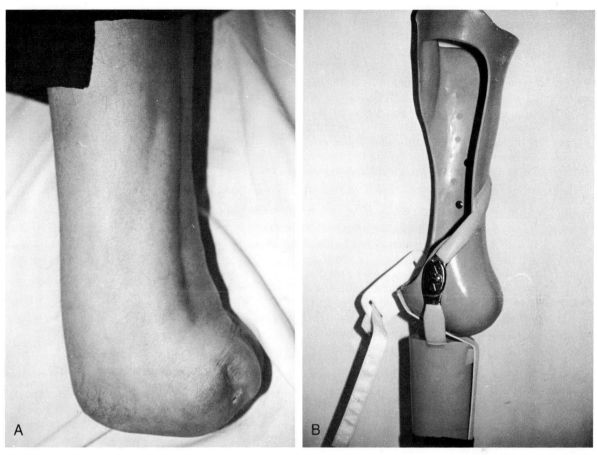

FIGURE 49–16. *A*, Patient with short below-knee stump with irreversible flexion contractures. *B*, Prosthesis for the patient with polycentric joint and elastic knee extension aid.

FIGURE 49–17. Patient with insensate scar adherent to the underlying bone with pull-in gel insert.

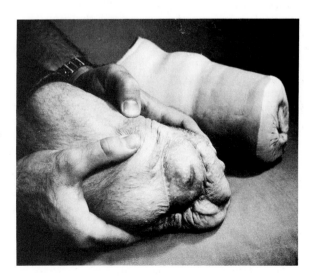

LAWRENCE W. FRIEDMANN

The suprapatellar cuff is the most common suspension. It is a strap that goes from the prosthesis to above the patella and around the lower thigh. It is used for patients with normal knees.

The thigh corset with side joints (Fig. 49–12) is an old suspension. It is a partial weight bypass device that has some suspension features, if the side bars are curved in over the femoral condyles. It gives mediolateral stability. The weight-bearing capacity is important for patients who are obese, for patients who have arthropathy of the knees, for those who are athletes, for those who climb, and for those who lift and carry weights. It may be a valuable addition despite its clumsiness, the thigh atrophy it causes, the excessive wear on clothing, and the discomfort in hot weather.

The KBM or wedge socket uses a wedge condylar clamp to provide suspension. Removable wedges are most common, but a removable medial wall is excellent. Flexible walls may also give condylar clamping.

The suprapatellar-supracondylar (SP/SC or PTS) suspension uses supracondylar clamping and has a high anterior wall that cups over the superior pole of the patella for additional suspension during swing phase (Fig. 49–18).

A rubber sleeve suspension of latex or neoprene, developed at the University of Michigan, is useful for suspension, especially if used concurrently with a gel insert liner. It suspends by friction and suction.[9] Some patients get contact dermatitis, and it must only be used with those in whom good hygiene can be ensured. It may be used alone, or in addition to other suspensions.

A socket with "pockets" for the bellies of contracted muscles is an experimental method to try to use muscular grasp to suspend the limb (Fig. 49–19).

Shoulder or waist belts and corset suspension are occasionally used for patients with ostomies, abdominal scarring or masses, or gross obesity. Suction suspension has not proved successful below the knee, but new efforts are under way. The "suction suspension socket" functions mainly through friction. It is useful for stumps with distal adhesions.

Bypass Prostheses. For amputees who have lesions in the shank, knee, or femur, a complete bypass of weight-bearing may be needed. An ischial weight-bearing socket prosthesis with an open end is required. The knee is locked during the stance phase, but may be bent when the patient sits. A rocker foot or patten bottom is essential

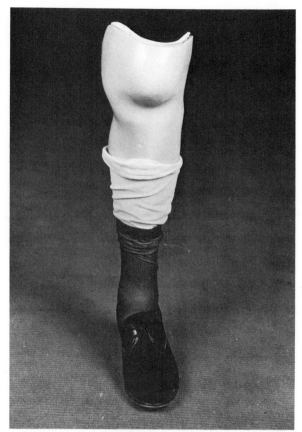

FIGURE 49–18. Supracondylar-suprapatellar suspension socket.

(Fig. 49–20). In the case of a distal lesion, an open PTB socket with brace bars and a patten may be sufficient (Fig. 49–21). It has a back that can be removable or hinged at the top or side.

Knee Disarticulation

Knee disarticulation stumps are tough, give excellent muscular control of the artificial limb, and last a lifetime. Although the stumps are bulbous and long, functional gains exceed the cosmetic problem now that polycentric knees with hydraulic friction and extension aid shorten the prosthesis when sitting and improve the swing phase characteristics. Narrowing the condyles has proved unwise.[32]

For the disarticulated knee, the prosthesis is composed of a socket with a thin flexible brim that ends below the ischium if all of the weight can be

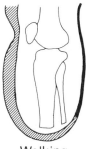

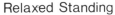

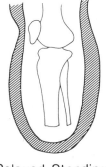
Relaxed Standing

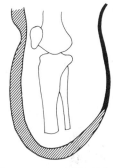
Walking

FIGURE 49–19. *Upper,* Conventional PTB socket does not allow contracting muscles to expand. *Lower,* PTB socket using muscular grasp suspension has "pocket" in the back so that contracting muscles fill the space. The circumference at the midcalf is greater than the circumference at the patellar tendon, thus suspending the prosthesis.

Relaxed Standing   **Contracted Walking**

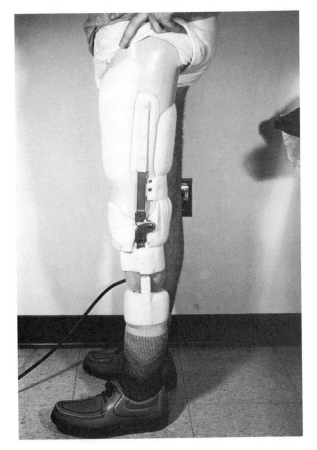

FIGURE 49–20. Below-knee bypass prosthesis of the ischial weight-bearing type. Note openings to relieve perspiration and suprapatellar bar for suprapatellar suspension. Also note offset knee joint and fixed ankle.

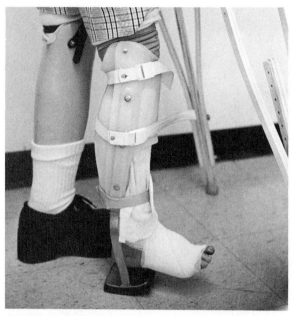

FIGURE 49–21. Below-knee bypass of patellar tendon–bearing type with superior hinge and posterior flap closure.

adherent to the bone, pulling on the suture line causes the skin to break down frequently. The tissues displaced proximally form an uncomfortable roll of flesh over the medial brim of the socket, called an "adductor roll," under which hidradenitis suppurativa frequently occurs.

The most common socket is an ischial weight-bearing quadrilateral shape, which is modified to relieve pressure over the sensitive muscles and tendons. The patient bears weight on the ischium, which is held on the ischial seat by a counterforce through the femoral triangle bulge on the antero-medial wall (Fig. 49–23).

Patients who have irregular, tender, adherent, postoperative scars or masses in the femoral triangle may not be able to withstand the pressure from the bulge over the femoral triangle of a quadrilateral socket. If this is the case, a plug-fit or narrow mediolateral dimension socket may be desirable.

The socket has a rounded anteromedial corner for the conjoint tendon of the adductor longus and gracilis muscles, and a posteromedial one for the

taken by the femoral condyles, or an ischial weight-bearing socket if not. Ancillary suspension is not required because an anterior trap door is utilized to provide condylar clamping, as well as allowing entry. Alternatively, an expandable inner sleeve may be used so that the condyles can expand the liner while it is pushed down into the socket. Then the liner contracts, gripping the condyles and preventing displacement in swing.

The older knee unit consisted of external hinge joints. They wear clothing severely, they are wide and unsightly, and there is no friction. This leads to excessive heel rise and terminal swing impact during walking.

Above-Knee Sockets

The above-knee stump is circular when relaxed, so sockets were originally conical. That shape is a "plug-fit" socket. The thigh has a different shape when the muscles contract. Newer sockets take the form of the active thigh.

In the "plug-fit socket," the pressure is distributed evenly by friction to the surface, pushing the skin proximally (Fig. 49–22). Since the bottom of the socket is not supported, edema and stump skin irritation at the terminal end due to "choking" may cause considerable difficulty. If the scar is

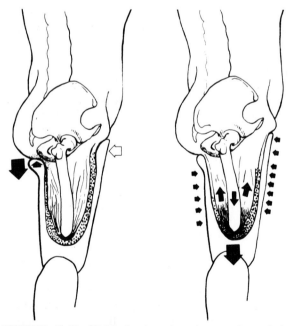

FIGURE 49–22. Weight-bearing above-knee sockets. *Left,* Quadrilateral socket. The skeletal support is on the ischium, which is held on the ischial seat by pressure from the bulge over the femoral triangle anteriorly. *Right,* The plug-fit socket compresses the soft tissues of the stump, stopping them from descending farther into the socket. The residual femur is held by this sling mechanism's supporting weight through the femoral head in contrast to the quadrilateral socket. Atrophy is great in the plug-fit socket and minimal in the quadrilateral socket.

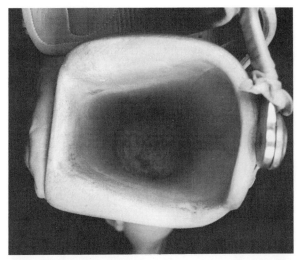

FIGURE 49–23. Quadrilateral socket seen from the top. The ischial seat is to the left bottom. The femoral triangle bulge is to the left top. The medial wall is thin. The lateral anterior wall is high. There is relief anteromedially for the conjoint tendon and posteromedially for the hamstrings. There is a pocket laterally for the greater trochanter.

hamstring tendons. Relief for the gluteus maximus and the rectus femoris is provided by large, hollowed out areas on the posterior and anterior walls, respectively.

Since the abductors of the femur are intact while the adductor muscles have been sectioned, the abductors are relatively stronger. This produces an abducted gait. The socket must be aligned in adduction to place the abductors on stretch to prevent a Trendelenburg lurch. Inadequate socket adduction is a very common fabrication fault.

Planned initial flexion is provided to allow sufficient extension range for a normal stride. Since muscles contract best at a slightly elongated length, the initial flexion provides adequate strength and range for the hip extensors to extend the thigh. This is an important consideration with mechanical knee joints, since the prime force causing knee extension is extension of the thigh on the pelvis. It also compensates for hip flexion contracture.

If the socket is too snug at the brim, the stump will swell distally. If the socket is tight anteromedially, the patient will walk with the leg externally rotated. If the anteroposterior dimension is too great, the ischial tuberosity will fall inside the socket. If the patient is too far into the socket for any reason, there will be pain over the ramus of the ischium and the adductors.

In Germany, the older triangular socket is making a comeback owing to perceived deficiencies in the quadrilateral socket design.[27] The corners are the conjoint tendon anteromedially, the hamstrings posteromedially, and the greater trochanter laterally.

The contoured adducted trochanteric–controlled alignment method (CAT–CAM)[35] (Fig. 49–24) and the normal shape–normal alignment (NSNA)[29] sockets are said to be more comfortable and functional than the quadrilateral socket. They are part of a series of experimental socket designs with a narrow mediolateral dimension, and a longer anteroposterior dimension. There is no ischial seat, but the ischium sits inside an indentation in an attempt to prevent lateral socket movement. There is no Scarpa's femoral bulge. The designers stress socket adduction, which was part of the quadrila-

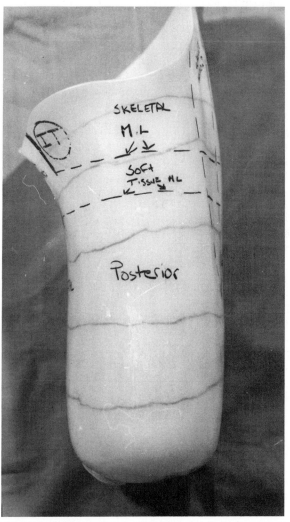

FIGURE 49–24. The C.A.T.–C.A.M. socket. Note the attempt to enclose the ischium.

teral design also, but often ignored. Patients did not like the resultant genu valgum, and do not like it with the new designs either. The designs are still evolving. They seem to be useful for those with scars or internal prostheses in Scarpa's triangle.

Newer materials such as carbon filament or fiberglass act as reinforcement in the polyester or acrylic for structural strength of a supporting frame that may be closed or with openings (ISNY socket).[25] They are often combined with flexible inserts of polyethylenes, Surlyn, or silicone elastomer.[24] Flexibility makes the socket more comfortable. Our limited experience to date has been that since these sockets are usually used without stump socks, sweating is increased in warm weather. The flexible brim is much more comfortable when the patient sits, especially for those with large abdomens. The thin inserts have had a breakage problem. When the inserts are made thicker to decrease breakage, the flexibility is markedly decreased, thus reversing the comfort advantage. We have used a one-piece socket made of flexible laminate on top. It is very comfortable when sitting, it is functionally the same as a rigid socket, and the durability is excellent.

The "ship's funnel" socket is used for patients born with proximal focal femoral deficiency (see Fig. 49–38).

The total-contact principle is used in above-knee sockets and has the same benefits as in the below-knee limb.

KNEE UNITS FOR THE ABOVE-KNEE PROSTHESIS

One may have no joint at all at the knee, or a single-axis joint that is locked while standing, but which may be unlocked for sitting. Locked joints are used for patients who are infirm and unstable, especially those just learning to use an above-knee prosthesis (Fig. 49–25).

Knee locking during stance may be obtained by a weight-activated knee lock, often called a "safety knee." It inhibits buckling at heel strike (Fig. 49–26).

Joint stability is determined by the location of the single axis at the knee relative to the weight line. The farther the joint is located behind the weight line, the more stable the knee is (and the harder it is to flex for heel and toe off). Polycentric knee units are used to raise the instantaneous axis of rotation to be nearer to the hip joint and thus markedly improve the stability during stance phase

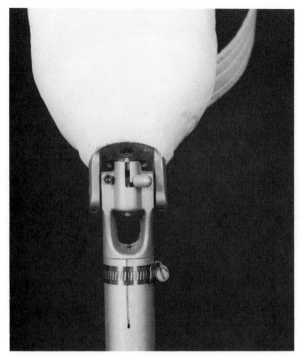

FIGURE 49–25. Knee lock for endoskeletal provisional limb. Note the handle in the reverse "J" slot. Keeping the handle where it is shown keeps the knee joint open. Pushing it to the left into the long slot causes automatic locking.

while walking. Polycentric units are more expensive, noisier, and heavier than single-axis knee units (Fig. 49–27). They are used in the knee disarticulation limb to improve the cosmesis during sitting.

Extension aids are added to a prosthesis to reduce heel rise at the beginning of swing phase. They accelerate the shank after toe off. They may be elastic, flexible wooden hickory sticks, coiled and wrapped springs, compressed air, or a hydraulic fluid (Fig. 49–26).

A friction mechanism reduces excessive heel rise in early swing, and reduces terminal swing impact at the end of swing. Variable friction improves the cosmesis of swing phase more than constant friction. The friction may be provided mechanically, by compressing air, by restricting the flow of a hydraulic fluid, or even, experimentally, by electromagnetic forces.

Hydraulic and pneumatic variable friction knee units are cadence responsive to improve swing phase for young, active, muscular individuals who want to walk at different speeds (Fig. 49–28). The

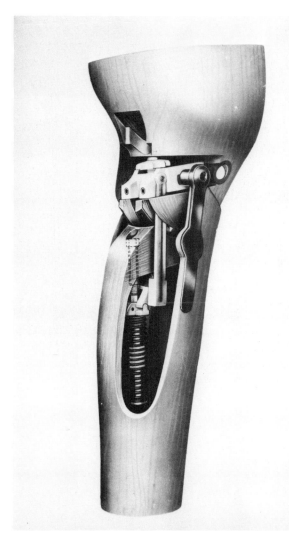

FIGURE 49–26. Drawing of Otto Bock "safety knee." Note spring extension aid on bottom, knurled knob for friction adjustment, and brake mechanism. (Drawing courtesy of the Otto Bock Co.)

Henschke-Mauch S-N-S unit also has stance phase stability and locking when desired.

SUSPENSION MECHANISMS

One suspension for the above-knee amputee is a plastic or metal pelvic band. There is a joint over the ipsilateral greater trochanter, which is near the axis of rotation of the hip in the sagittal plane. The lower bar is attached to the socket. From the joint, a molded T-shaped bar extends upward and surrounds the pelvis between the greater trochanter and the iliac crest. This is used for elderly and

very unstable individuals. The disadvantage is that it pinches the abdominal fat during sitting. It should be avoided as unnecessarily restrictive unless the Silesian bandage is inadequate (Fig. 49–29).

A more comfortable but less stable suspension is a Silesian bandage. It is a flexible webbing that is attached to the lateral side of the thigh socket. It is brought by the patient across the back, over the contralateral pelvis between the iliac crest and the greater trochanter, and is attached anteriorly. A variant is a waist belt, which goes over the iliac crest. A Neoprene belt is more secure and quite comfortable.

Still less stable but more functional for young, agile individuals is the suction suspension. A spring valve is placed in the lower part of the socket, which allows air to be expelled when the patient puts weight on the stump but does not allow air re-entry during swing (Fig. 49–30). When worn without a stump sock, the suction socket is held on by atmospheric pressure during swing. There is a slight positive pressure during stance, which minimizes distal edema. Whereas it is not necessary in each case, total contact eliminates most problems associated with terminal edema. Good balance, back flexibility, hamstring elasticity, and hand strength are required for donning of the suction socket, since the patient must bend at the waist to 90 degrees and pull the stump into the

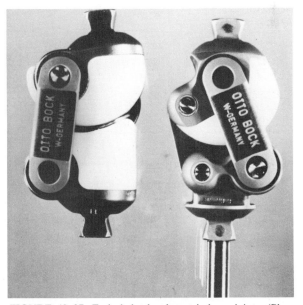

FIGURE 49–27. Endoskeletal polycentric knee joints. (Photograph courtesy of the Otto Bock Co.)

LAWRENCE W. FRIEDMANN

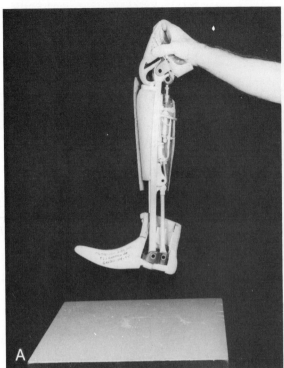

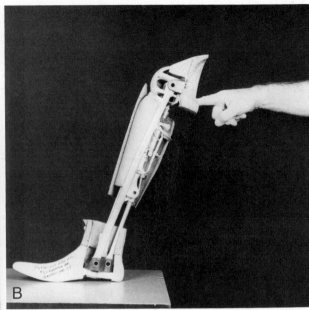

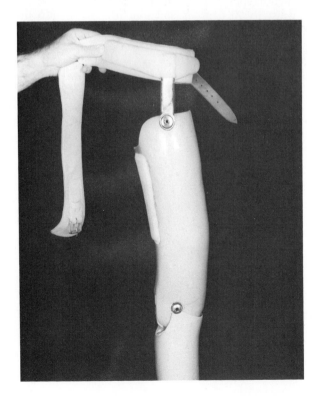

FIGURE 49–28. Hydracadence knee. *A,* Note ankle dorsiflexion accompanying knee flexion. This assists with foot clearance during swing phase. *B,* Note ability to plantar flex foot when patient is sitting. This improves cosmesis. (Prosthetic section courtesy of Orthopedic Aids, Inc.)

FIGURE 49–29. Pelvic band suspension.

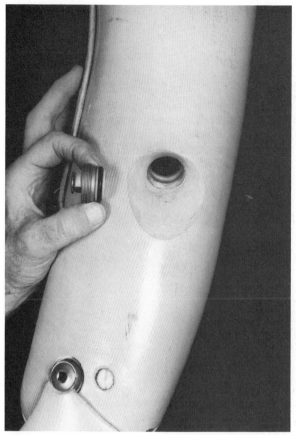

FIGURE 49–30. Suction valve and insert. Note pull-valve on left of valve to allow air to enter socket.

socket with stockinette while inserting and withdrawing the stump alternately. It should not be attempted by the elderly, the infirm, or patients with poor balance. It cannot be used for many patients with severely scarred stumps, or if the stump varies in volume owing to gain or loss of weight, treatment for malignancy, cardiac or renal edema, and so on. The concomitant use of partial suction using a thin stump sock and a Silesian bandage for suspension is an excellent way to treat young individuals soon after their amputation. Corset or shoulder harness suspensions are rarely needed except for patients with a colostomy, ileostomy, late pregnancy, or abdominal mass.

Hip Disarticulation Prostheses

The hip disarticulation socket is cast to bear weight on the ischial tuberosity, and encloses the ilii for control. The hemipelvectomy socket bears weight on the remaining soft tissues and the lower rib cage. The socket is attached to a thigh piece by means of a Canadian hip joint, which is parallel to the ground, transverse to the line of progression, and anterior to the socket. When the patient stands, the body weight is entirely behind the hip joint. There is a posterior stop so that there is stability of the pelvic socket on the prosthetic femoral segment. The center of gravity is aligned anterior to the knee joint to provide stability for the knee. A lightweight SACH foot is usual. The prosthesis is activated by active pelvic tilt or by trunk rotation (Fig. 49–31).

Hemicorporectomy

Hemicorporectomy patients are rare, the procedure mostly being reserved for pelvic malignancy. A sitting bucket bearing weight on the rib cage allows the patient to sit in a wheelchair. Cosmetic legs, not suitable for ambulation, are best for the elderly. In young, very active, muscular individuals, some may try to use lockable articulated prostheses for ambulation with a two-point gait similar to the paraplegic patient. This gait requires a tremendous amount of energy. Therefore, most patients will abandon walking after a short time and use a wheelchair.

Principles of Prescription Writing

A prosthesis can be fitted as soon as the wound is healed. If wound healing is delayed or is expected to last more than four weeks, I prescribe a bypass prosthesis so that training may progress, and the person may go home walking while the wound is healing.

The preliminary examination will determine the nature of the patient's stump, the general physical condition, and any special problems there may be physically, emotionally, or vocationally. The patient must decide whether the prosthesis will be used for heavy or light work and for what types of recreation. If the patient lives far from a prosthetic center, then only those components should be used that are durable and do not require much maintenance.

The hobbies of the patient may also determine which devices are to be provided. A golfer with an amputated leg may benefit from a dual- or universal-axis ankle.

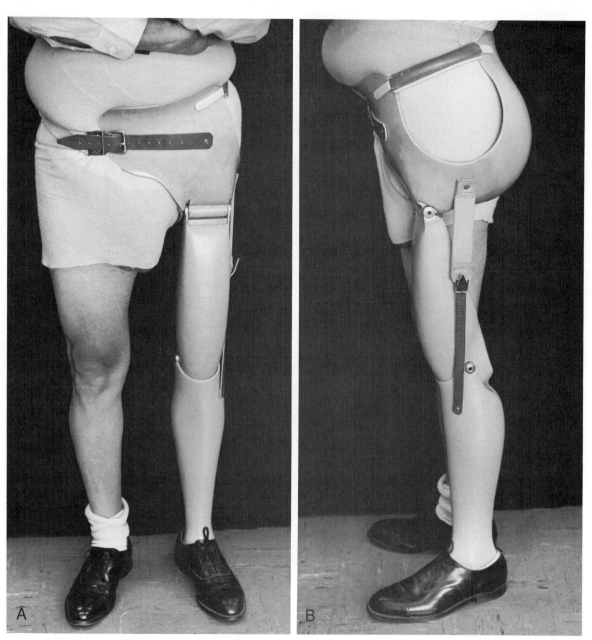

FIGURE 49–31. Canadian hip disarticulation prosthesis. Note anterior joint and elastic stride length control in *B*.

The prescription for the leg amputee depends on many factors in addition to stump length, e.g., stump shrinkage, range of motion and the strength of the stump, scarring or "dog ears," and so on. The climate and the culture of the person modify the prescription. The precise nature of the work and hobbies should be factors in the choice of components.

The prime purpose of an artificial leg is to diminish functional disability during standing, walking, climbing stairs and hills, pulling, carrying, working, running, and jumping. The specific disability a patient feels most inhibiting may not be one that the prosthetic team envisions. Since our efforts are to restore the individual to a specific subculture in optimal condition, we must know and modify the patient, the environment, and the person-machine interface between them.

The basic principle in devising a machine to enable amputees to walk is that their center of gravity must be over the base of support to prevent falling. The essence of walking is that patients fall off one leg and catch themselves on the other. This alternating process of propulsion (acceleration) and reception (deceleration) is basic. Both mobility and stability of the limb depend on muscular activity, gravity, and inertia. The joints are stable when they are inhibited from further motion in one direction and the center of gravity is so located that it moves the joints in that direction, usually with little or no muscular activity.

Body build is important. An obese individual uses an artificial appliance less well than does a wiry person. The socket is further from the bone that must control it. A patient's coordination must be good. The patient's opposite leg may well determine whether the patient can and should walk with an artificial leg.

There are a number of patients who want an artificial leg despite their inability to use it for walking. Cosmesis is a form of function. In rare cases, leg cosmesis is an important vocational need. When cost is a factor, the legs used to model stockings in store windows may be purchased for attachment to the wheelchair seatboard (Fig. 49–32).

Fitting

The forces acting on the stump and the device are determined by the available muscle power, gravitational forces, and inertia. There is always

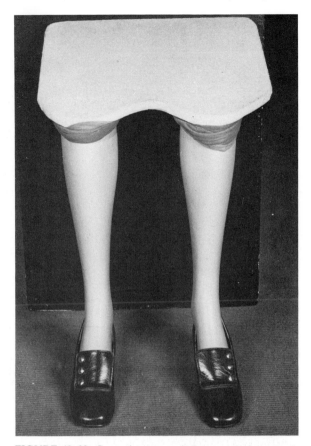

FIGURE 49–32. Cosmetic mannequin legs attached to wheelchair seat board.

some motion between any socket and the underlying skin, muscle, and bone. Work is force exerted over a distance. The work output of a prosthesis is equal to the work the patient puts into it (work input), minus frictional and other mechanical losses. Thus, for a prosthesis to be effective, both the muscular force that the stump can impart to it and the distance through which the part can move (range of motion) are important.

The effective use of an artificial limb depends to a considerable extent on the degree of neuromuscular coordination of the patient. The amputee who is agile, who learned to dance and play sports easily, has little difficulty in learning to use a new artificial limb. The patient who was always clumsy may have difficulty in learning. I would prefer to err on the side of overprescribing provisional artificial limbs rather than neglect to provide for the patient who needs one. I give the patient a chance to prove whether the limb is feasible for him or

LAWRENCE W. FRIEDMANN

her. My concern for safety has led me to prescribe devices that improve stability, such as thigh corsets, and knee friction locks. For the amputee over 55 years of age, I also prescribe a wheelchair for convenience and for conservation of energy.

If a patient with medical complications needs to be stood, a prefabricated pylon prosthesis may be used to aid standing, but because a pylon has no joints, it results in a poor gait pattern.

Prescription by Level of Amputation

For toe amputation, no replacement is needed.

For the partial or complete transmetatarsal, a shoe filler and perhaps a stiff sole for the shoe are all that is required.

Transtarsal amputation of Chopart's type is rarely indicated, but in those few cases for which it is beneficial, the prosthetic need is for a high collar shoe and a toe filler.[14]

For Syme's amputation, the Canadian Syme's prosthesis should be prescribed, usually with a medial trap door for ventilation. A closed prosthesis can be obtained with an elastic inner wall for suspension. The disadvantages are that it has a wide stovepipe shape and inhibits evaporation of perspiration.

For the below-knee amputee, there are many choices. The socket is usually of the total-contact PTB type with an insert of polyethylene. An air chamber is used if the end of the stump is tender. If friction causes lesions, a gel insert or slip socket is provided. If there is discomfort during sitting or walking, increased flexibility of the brim and possibly the walls might improve comfort. In that situation, the ISNY socket might be prescribed.

Suspension is usually the suprapatellar cuff, but a supracondylar wedge is effective if the patient does not have fat knees. The supracondylar/suprapatellar suspension is especially good for women. Elastic sleeve suspension (neoprene or latex) is very helpful, but only for those without skin allergies and who practice good hygiene. For heavy work and active sports, a thigh corset with side joints markedly improves endurance. The thigh corset is required for all patients with unstable knee joints.

The person with a true knee disarticulation has only a few choices. The socket has a flexible brim ending in the upper thigh. It can have either a trap door or an elastic inner sleeve. External joints should not be used because then the knee protrudes excessively when the patient sits and is thus unsightly. The only choices are which polycentric joint to use, and whether to use a hydraulic unit with it. The foot components are the same as for the below-knee individual.

The above-knee amputee now has many types of sockets from which to select his or her preference. While the quadrilateral socket is still the standard, the person with a scar in the femoral triangle may use the plug-fit, the NSNA, or a CAT–CAM socket. For flexibility and comfort, the ISNY is a good choice. The three last-mentioned sockets are expensive, and when cost is a significant factor, they should be eliminated from consideration. Suspension is relatively simple. Most new amputees can use a Silesian bandage. Young people can switch to suction sockets. Unstable elderly patients need pelvic bands if Silesian bands prove insufficient. The choice of knee unit is difficult. Recent amputees, unstable people, and the elderly need lockable joints, which can be unlocked for sitting. Young people need open joints with variable friction, preferably hydraulic. Adults past 50 years of age need constant friction knees, sometimes with a weight-activated friction lock. The same foot components are available as discussed previously.

For the bilateral above-knee amputee, stubby prostheses are used for evaluation and training before full-length limbs are prescribed. They will be used at home later as well, to reduce energy costs despite their poor appearance (Fig. 49–33).

The Canadian is the only prosthesic design at the present time used for the hip disarticulation or for the hemipelvectomy.

Prosthesis Final Evaluation

When the prosthesis is completed, it must be inspected for fulfillment of the prescription, workmanship, fit, and alignment by the prosthetist. It is then functionally re-evaluated by the physical therapist and then by the physiatrist. A complete evaluation cannot be done when the patient first receives the prosthesis, since the preliminary alignment is an approximation. If there is a question whether the socket is truly total-contact in nature, or whether the fit is appropriate, xeroradiography of the patient's stump inside the socket with and without weight-bearing settles the issue. This technique is invaluable, since it accentuates margins

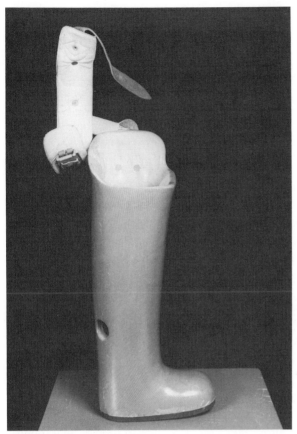

FIGURE 49–33. Stubby prostheses for bilateral above-knee amputee. Note that the projection on the lower right is posterior and not a toe. The lower part is curved like a rocker bottom.

bandages are used, they must be reapplied carefully at least four times a day. Elastic socks, or shrinkers, are preferable to shrink stumps in order to avoid window edema and proximal constriction greater than distal compression, which increases stump edema by its tourniquet action. The stump shrinkers should be worn whenever the patient does not wear the artificial limb. A garter belt prevents the elastic sock from rolling down and producing proximal constriction. If more compression is desired, a smaller size can be used, a five-ply wool stump sock can be worn under the shrinker, or elastic bandages can be applied over the shrinker. One may use two different stump shrinkers, one over the other, a Bessco stump shrinker next to the skin, and a Truform stump shrinker over it. The Bessco sock is smooth and has more distal pressure than proximal. The Truform sock gives much more compression, but it has a pad at the distal end that usually slips down, allowing some distal induration. By using them together, more compression is attained, and distal induration is avoided. A Daw sheath next to the skin avoids tension on the wound margin and makes the shrinkers easier to don.

Shrinkage should continue until the prosthesis is worn regularly, which is the best method of shrinking and shaping a stump. The use of a temporary articulated prosthesis after the wound is healed should be routine. The weight of the patient's body in the socket is far more pressure than can be applied by any elastic material. It is pressure that causes the subcutaneous fat to atrophy as well as edema fluid to be resorbed. The temporary artificial limb also assists in general conditioning and permits training for walking. The early construction of the permanent leg is not advisable since rapid shrinkage is common, and early replacement of the socket would be necessary. It is better both medically and economically to use a temporary provisional prosthesis until the stump has shrunk to its functional size. The temporary socket is attached to leased components, which the patient eventually returns to the prosthetist when the permanent prosthesis is finished.

The patient is discharged to ambulate with the temporary limb for three to six months until the stump is almost at its final size, depending on the patient's weight and activity level. The effective use of an artificial limb depends on the patient's neuromuscular coordination. The best test of feasibility to use a prosthesis is a trial. It is better to prescribe a temporary artificial limb and to use the

and interfaces and shows the edges of the bone structures, muscles, skin, stump socks, and both the soft and the hard parts of the prosthetic socket.

Amputee Training

The size of the stump depends on the muscle mass, its fluid content, and the amount of subcutaneous fat. Any edema can be squeezed out by short-term pressure. The fat disappears rapidly with socket pressure, proportional to the amount of pressure and the frequency with which the pressure is applied. Shrinkage is necessary to reduce the stump volume for the most efficient use of the permanent prosthesis.

Stumps may be shrunk with elastic bandages. When a space occurs between turns of an elastic bandage, "window edema" is frequent. This is common as the patient turns in bed. When elastic

limb for its predictive value of successful walking than to try to go without one. Patients and families are reluctant to trust a physician's judgment that a prosthesis will not be useful in the absence of such a trial. Failure to be able to walk using a provisional limb makes nonprescription of a permanent limb more acceptable. The provisional limb also allows accurate evaluation of the patient's potential as a prosthesis user and permits use of various prosthetic components to determine which would be best for each individual. The permanent prosthesis can be worn between one and one-half and two years before replacement.

Stump and skin care are vital, since the patient's comfort is dependent more on the integrity of the skin than it is on anything else. The patient cannot use the prosthesis if skin lesions are tender. Prostheses invariably interfere with the normal functions of the skin. Careful maintenance of the skin must be taught.

The skin requires toughening where it comes into contact with the device. This toughening is best done by progressive use of the device.

Stump hygiene is taught, since this is the single most important factor in the prevention of skin problems (see p. 1051). The patient is taught to wash the skin and prosthetic components with a bland soap and water at night so that all have time to dry before the socket is donned in the morning. The stump must be rinsed thoroughly and dried by patting rather than by vigorous rubbing. The stump socks should be washed daily with a mild soap in lukewarm water. They must be rinsed thoroughly, allowed to dry flat (not hung up), and allowed to rest for three or four days before being used again. The inner surface of the socket must be cleansed each evening with a warm, soapy cloth and rinsed thoroughly with a clean, damp cloth. The socket is dried with a towel and left open to dry overnight. If there is a soft insert, it should be ascertained from the prosthetist whether it can be cleansed in this manner without absorbing water.

Donning and doffing are taught. Crutch-walking is continued with the prosthesis, stressing balance and rhythm. A forearm crutch is desirable to avoid axillary pressure; the forearm band should open on the lateral side. The patient must learn to appreciate the difference in sensation between a proper and an improper gait. Trunk movement to compensate for poor balance should be minimized. The patient is also taught to hop in the home.

Unless the patient is going to need a walker permanently for safety, gait-training should not include the use of a walker. It is impossible to walk with equal step lengths using a walker unless it has two wheels.

For the above-knee amputee, teaching balancing and weight-shifting is more difficult because the patient does not have proprioception in the artificial knee. Active prosthetic adduction and abduction as well as flexion and extension must be taught to demonstrate how the leg is manipulated and so that the patient can become familiar with the amount of muscular movement and range of motion required to raise the foot off the ground and to swing the artificial leg. The length of the step and the weight borne with each leg should be equal.

After walking on the level is safe, the patient should be taught to ascend and descend curbs, steps, ramps, and irregular terrain. The above-knee amputee ascends ramps and steps with the normal leg first followed by the prosthesis. When descending, the amputee leads with the prosthesis.

Gait

The reader should review the chapter on gait (Chapter 4) by Lehmann. Any changes in the determinants of gait that exaggerate the motion of the center of gravity by an increase in amplitude and by more rapid acceleration or deceleration of limb segments will increase energy consumption. For any deviation from normal, it is important to determine not only what the deviation is and what parts of the body it involves, but also at what point it occurs during the gait cycle. An abnormal gait may be symmetrical or asymmetrical, a limp.

Appraisal of gait observes the following: (1) symmetry of movements of body parts throughout the gait cycle (length of stride, armswing, movement of trunk); (2) smoothness of movements (staggering, loss of balance, incoordination); (3) width of gait; and (4) presence or absence of pain.[12]

Each part should be observed systematically as follows: (1) the head and shoulders, noting whether they dip or are elevated, depressed, protracted, retracted, or rotated; (2) the arms, paying particular attention to armswing, noting any asymmetry in abduction or motion; (3) the trunk, checking any forward or backward lurch, list to either side, or absence of normal lumbar motion; (4) the pelvis, noting anterior or posterior tilt, hiking of the hip, and whether the sides stay level or drop; (5) the hips, checking motion in extension, flexion, rotation, dropping, circumduction, abduction, and adduction; (6) the knees, evaluating stability, flexion, and extension; and (7) the ankles and feet, noting dorsiflexion, plantar flexion, eversion, and inversion, during both swing and stance.

Observations by videocamera with slow motion and stop frame capability from the front, back, and side provide the viewing time necessary to evaluate each of these components of gait.

Gait Deviations of Below-Knee Amputees

HEEL STRIKE DEVIATIONS

Excessive knee flexion at heel strike may occur from multiple causes; usually it is due to a heel cushion that is too stiff. The socket may be too far anterior relative to the foot. The patient may not adequately resist flexion of the knee because there is discomfort over the distal tibia. The patient may have weak quadriceps muscles, or poor gait-training. The opposite faults will cause inordinately delayed knee flexion at heel strike. If the patient puts the center of gravity forward at heel strike by bending at the waist, this is commonly due to pain over the distal end of the tibia, or weakness of the quadriceps.

MID-STANCE DEVIATIONS

The basic deviations are a medial or lateral thrust of the knee. This is usually due to misplacement of the prosthetic foot relative to the socket. Excessive knee flexion at mid-stance may be due to foot dorsiflexion, anterior tilt of the socket, or anterior displacement of the socket over the prosthetic foot.

PUSH OFF DEVIATIONS

Abrupt knee flexion is usually due to excessive anterior tilt of the socket, the socket being too far forward over the foot, or the foot set in too much dorsiflexion. Abrupt knee extension at toe off is caused by the opposite faults.

Gait Deviations of Above-Knee Amputees

Above-knee amputees may have deviations similar to those of below-knee amputees. In addition, they may have the following problems.

HEEL STRIKE DEVIATIONS

Toe rotation of the prosthetic foot when the heel strikes the ground is generally due to a flabby stump, excessive amount of soft tissues, or inadequate fit of the socket. It may occur when the prosthetic heel is too stiff. Occasionally, a patient attempts to increase knee stability by digging the heel into the ground or intentionally rotating the prosthetic foot, since the knee of the prosthesis cannot flex unless its axis is perpendicular to the line of progression. Knee instability occurs when the knee joint is forward relative to the weight line. The progressive increase of a hip flexion contracture may accentuate this problem.

MID-STANCE DEVIATIONS

Lateral trunk bending occurs when there is discomfort in the crotch or at the distal lateral aspect of the femoral stump. Less commonly, it occurs when there is an abduction contracture. Functional length is the combined length of the prosthesis, stump socks, and stump. If the prosthesis is functionally too short because the patient sinks too far into the socket, the patient will bend the trunk laterally. A patient who is insecure or has poor balance will also do the same. Excessive lordosis at mid-stance is generally due to a hip flexion contracture. Other causes may be weak hip extensors or weak abdominal muscles. The ischial tuberosity may not be well seated on the ischial seat because of insufficient support from the bulge of the socket over the femoral triangle. All bilateral above-knee amputees have excessive lumbar lordosis because of impaired hip extension.

PUSH OFF DEVIATIONS

The major deviation at heel off is the whip, i.e., rotation of the heel in either direction. It is most commonly due to flabby musculature. The patient may have put on the prosthesis in an incorrect position, especially if using a Silesian bandage suspension. More rarely, the whip may be due to poor alignment or poor contouring of the socket. The major deviation at toe off is inability to flex the prosthetic knee. This is due to a foot that has been excessively plantar flexed or the presence of excess knee friction.

SWING DEVIATIONS

The major deviation occurring during swing is an uneven step length with an uneven armswing. These occur because the patient has a fear of committing weight to the prosthesis for fear of falling, or because of pain. The patient takes a long step and brief stance with the prosthesis (which may be compounded because of a hip flexion contracture) and a short step with prolonged stance on the sound leg. This may also occur because of an incorrect amount of knee friction to provide smooth cadence. Excessive heel rise early in swing is generally due to inadequate extension aid or inadequate knee friction. Another deviation is called vaulting, elevation of the entire body on the sound extremity by excessive plantar flexion of the foot so the patient does not stub the toe of the prosthesis. It happens when the patient attempts to walk very fast. The cause is a functionally long limb because of inadequate tightness of the suspension. The limb may be functionally too long because of gain of weight, edema, or too many stump socks. Other causes may be that the extension aid is too tight or the knee friction is too great.

The more obvious faults in mid-swing are the variations of abducted gait (the patient keeps the prosthesis farther lateral but parallel to the line of progression than the sound leg). This occurs when the prosthesis is functionally too long. Rarely it may be due to errors in fabrication. Another cause may be pain in the groin from the medial brim of the socket, especially if the patient has an adductor roll, or if the patient sinks too far into the prosthetic socket. Inadequate adduction of the lateral wall also causes this abnormality. Alignment of the prosthetic foot too far from the midline, a pelvic joint that is abducted, a contracture of the hip in abduction, insecurity, and inadequate gait-training also are other causes. A circumducted gait is related to an abducted gait. In this gait, stance is relatively normal, but the patient swings the leg through in a semicircular fashion. This may be caused by a prosthesis that is too long or may be a residual training fault.

The major deviation during deceleration is an excessive impact at the end of the swing phase. This causes jarring accompanied by a loud noise as the knee bangs into full extension just before heel strike as the shank strikes the bumper forcefully. This may be due to insufficient friction at the knee or to an excessively strong extension aid. Occasionally, the knee bumper has fallen out. Most frequently, it is a habit that patients establish when they are insecure, attempting to dig the heel into the ground to ensure knee extension before committing weight to the prosthesis.

Prognosis

Every patient must accept that all amputee gaits are abnormal. Only pre-amputation nonambulators can be restored to their former physical activity level. The disadvantages of a prosthesis include discomfort, heaviness, difficulty in donning and doffing, a somewhat ungainly appearance, noise during operation, and disagreeable texture to touch. The discomfort can be diminished by proper fit and stump conditioning. The weight of the prosthesis usually is about half the weight of the body segment it replaces, from 3 to 7 lb (1.18 to 3.18 kg) for a below-knee prosthesis, and from 7 to 12 lb (3.18 to 5.45 kg) for an above-knee prosthesis. Lightweight prostheses are available for those who need them. There is usually a trade-off in strength, durability, and cost. The patient often complains of prosthetic "dead weight," which is not due to a defect in fabrication.

The lower limb prosthesis gives a somewhat unnatural gait pattern, which is not cadence responsive, except for the hydraulic and pneumatic swing phase units. All units present difficulties when the amputee tries to go up or down inclines or steps. The higher the amputation, the greater the energy cost on level ground. At subject-specific chosen rates of walking, the unilateral below-knee amputee used 9 per cent more energy, the unilateral above-knee patient used 50 per cent more calories, and the bilateral above-knee amputee used 280 per cent more energy on level ground.[21] For above-knee single amputation, a prosthesis is less costly of energy than are crutches, provided the patient is well trained. The pulse rate of crutch-walkers is higher than that of prosthetic ambulators.[11] Walking up and down inclines and steps and on irregular surfaces costs more energy proportionately for the limbless than for the normal. More precise studies under these conditions to determine the energy required are needed.

Prosthetic use depends on many factors. For example, body build determines size and weight of the limb. A fat person has to carry a much heavier prosthesis, since it has a larger circumference, and therefore contains more plastic. A weak person needs a lighter limb. Agility is a factor, as motor skill allows a patient to manipulate a more complex device, and to use it more adroitly. The cardiovascular reserve determines how much work the person can do when walking. The more efficient the prosthetic machine, the more walking the person can do. The attitude of the amputee and the family helps to determine whether the person is satisfied with what we can give him or her. No artificial limb can replace what has been lost, and while it may be acceptable to many people, there are some who demand a perfect replacement, which we are unable to provide. Although a leg of reasonable appearance can be provided and a trained gait may show little limp, some persons' desire for cosmesis and function, especially early after amputation, is such that they cannot be satisfied.

Economics plays a part in both provision of a limb and repairs. The cost of limbs, training, and repairs is high, both in money and in expenditure of time. Special legs may need to be designed for irregular terrain, hot damp climate, or other conditions.

Figures on the survival of patients after amputation caused by vascular disease of the legs vary. Hansson found that the survival of patients after amputation caused by vascular disease of the legs was only 1.5 years; from 30 to 50 per cent of patients die within a year after amputation.[20] One of four patients will lose the other lower extremity prior to death. If the first limb is ablated above the knee, and if the patient has not learned to walk with a prosthesis by the time of the second amputation, it is unlikely that the patient will succeed in ambulation with two prostheses, even if the second limb is below the knee. Patients with bilateral below-knee amputations usually walk. Even cardiac patients can often walk for short distances after appropriate training and conditioning.[1] Training should include demonstrating to family members and caretakers how well the patient can walk and what the daily activity level at home should include.[37]

Maintenance and Repair

The prosthesis is a tool that may be damaged if it is used incorrectly. Artificial limbs are expensive, and their maintenance is important. The joints should be cleaned of dirt and lint and lubricated every two or three weeks with a silicone spray. A good-quality saddle soap should be used to clean the leather parts at least weekly. Adjustment or repair of deteriorating or breaking parts should be made by the prosthetist as often as needed. Prostheses do wear out and need to be replaced.

The average durability has been reported by World War II veterans to be 3.50 ± 1.1 years for below-knee prostheses and 3.15 ± 1.2 years for above-knee prostheses.[29]

Problems of Amputees and Their Treatment

Skin Problems

The human skin has complex functions and extraordinary abilities to adapt to changes in demands placed on it. The skin is an important regulator of body temperature. A significant amount of heat is lost through the digits. The amputation of digits puts an extra strain on all of the remaining sweat glands. In an amputee, the remaining extremities are primarily responsible for heat dissipation to control body temperature. Perspiration will therefore be increased over the rest of the body, and although this is annoying, it is not detrimental. Use of an artificial limb requires increased energy expenditure and thus also increases sweating to dissipate this increased heat. Sweating of the stump is also increased, and since it is covered by an impervious socket, the sweating causes maceration. The maceration predisposes to infection by bacteria and fungi and injury by outside forces.

To prevent maceration, the skin requires exposure to the air. This can be achieved by using porous rather than nonporous materials, perforated construction, and stump socks made of absorbent natural fibers to wick away the sweat. Sweating can be diminished also by antiperspirants or by iontophoresis with copper sulfate or formalin. Cornstarch and unscented talc are excellent absorbers of perspiration and good lubricants, leaving the skin supple, smooth, firm, and dry. The powders are used in the socket and after the evening bath. Astringents and rubbing alcohol dry the skin excessively, causing it to flake. They should not be used.

Some patients prefer soft skin. For them, lanolin or cocoa butter can be used. These should be washed off in the morning. Liquid skin emollients and petroleum jelly predispose to maceration and should not be used.

The socket and other prosthetic materials dissolve in the sweat and as solutes may act as irritants or antigens and cause allergic problems in the stump. Skin is fairly resistant to abrasive action, but this resistance decreases when the skin is moist. The function of the skin as an exchanger of gases

LAWRENCE W. FRIEDMANN

and as a sensory organ is impaired by the perspiration and the socket. The sense organs accommodate rapidly and sensation diminishes.

Weight-bearing in the socket causes many mechanical stresses on the skin, e.g., intermittent stretching and friction. Friction on the skin causes both abrasion and heat, both of which are destructive. Mechanical stresses are highest at the junction of a rigid and a flexible part of an object; thus, tearing of gland orifices and capillary damage are most severe where the edge of the socket holds the skin in a rigid manner, whereas the skin immediately adjacent to and not enclosed in the socket has a great amount of flexibility. The same problem occurs inside the socket where it is not in total contact with the skin.

Skin ulceration may occur through maceration, excessive pressure, friction, shear, and concentrated stresses. A pressure sore will heal if the cause is removed. Modification of the device is necessary, and only rarely is surgery necessary—for example, removal of a sharp bone ridge or spicule. When there is ulceration, the limb should not be worn until healing is complete. In rare instances, a "bypass" device will be necessary so the patient can walk prior to healing of an ulcer.

When the skin is adherent to underlying bone, concentration of stresses occurs with stretching and weakening of the skin, and with deposition of hemosiderin at the juncture between flexible and adherent skin. Pulling the stump into the socket rather than pushing it in helps by pre-stressing the skin (Fig. 49–34). Friction massage helps loosen the skin attachment. If ulceration recurs, friction-reducing measures are indicated, as described previously.

Tight proximal brims, especially in suction sockets, may cause "mushrooming" with the socket holding the soft tissue up away from the socket bottom, resulting in engorgement of the small blood vessels of the skin with resultant rupture and extravasation of blood (Fig. 49–35). The dark pigmentation frequently seen at the end of the stump is the result of such bleeding. Pulling the tissues into the socket prevents the problem.

Blocking of the eccrine temperature-controlling sweat glands by the socket or by keratin, especially when the patient perspires profusely, may cause rupture of the sweat ducts, which, if superficial, develops small blisters. If they are deeper, it causes "prickly heat." Where the rupture is still deeper, papules form. Sweating is under autonomic control; efforts to control the sweating with anticho-

linergic agents are sometimes successful. When general perspiration diminishes too much, the temperature control of the body may be compromised. Local excessive perspiration may be diminished after copper sulfate or formalin ion transfer.

Apocrine glands are important only in the groin and axilla; the groin may be irritated by the socket of the above-knee amputee, and the axilla during crutch-walking. These adrenergic glands respond to painful stimuli. Their involvement may cause a stubborn disease of the skin called "hidradenitis suppurativa" with a foul discharge from painful cysts. The emotional state of the amputee is therefore also of physical importance.

Sebaceous glands seldom cause skin problems, since the back pressure of the sebum usually stops further production. Epidermoid cysts may occur when small keratin plugs develop in the skin of the adductor region of the thigh at the upper edge of the prosthesis. They may become infected and prevent the wearing of the prosthesis. Infections, primarily those caused by staphylococci, are most frequent during the summer. Good stump hygiene will diminish the incidence of infections, which are treated in the usual manner when they do occur.

Allergic manifestations of the skin are common in the amputee and may be due to the plastics and resins used in finishing the prosthesis. Sometimes a new cleansing agent—cream or lubricant—or the use of a foam rubber cushion or plastic-covered pad in the bottom of the socket may produce contact dermatitis. Incompletely cured epoxy resins may produce an irritation dermatitis. The pink pelite often causes irritation, whereas the white never does.

A fungus infection secondary to excessive perspiration is manifested by a reddish-brown incrustation with weeping. The socket should be washed with 5 per cent formalin and rinsed off with alcohol. Fungicidal solutions, powders, or ointments should be used on the stump. Tinactin, Desenex, and Asterol are examples. The application of liquid medication at night and powder in the morning is the best regimen. Perspiration should be decreased.

Ingrown or infected hair follicles can be treated by plucking. Sometimes the infection may be so severe as to require antibiotics along with incision and drainage of the abscess. If this is a recurring problem, the prosthesis should be checked for excessive piston action. If it persists, epilation, either chemical or electrolytic, should be performed. If sebaceous cysts interfere with socket

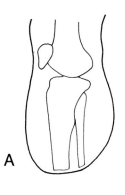

A

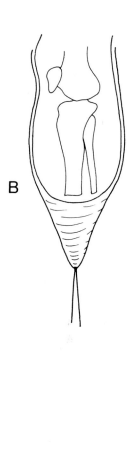

B

FIGURE 49–34. Pulling on the strings shown in *B* and *C* pulls the soft tissues to stretch them distal to the bone end. This narrows the soft tissues while making them longer. This technique is used often in prosthetics: after open amputation, it aids closure; it is used to don the suction socket; it prevents the adductor roll in above-knee socket use; it is used to pre-stress the tissues for suspension; and it is used as a treatment for bony overgrowth in children.

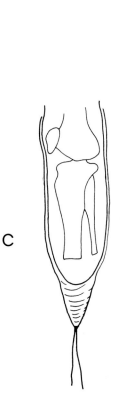

C

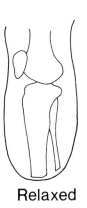

Relaxed

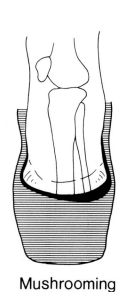

Mushrooming

FIGURE 49–35. If a stump mushrooms in a socket, carving out the socket will be insufficient. Pre-stressing of the soft tissues by pulling them into the socket is required.

fit, they should be removed. If they become infected, they should be treated with incision and drainage. If they recur, excision is the treatment of choice. Chafed areas point to piston action or poor socket fit.

If the stump has had split-thickness skin grafts, either because of extensive burns or for surgical considerations, hypersensitivity of the skin may be a problem. Pressure should be avoided over such areas, but surgical reconstruction may become necessary. Removal of the grafts and replacement by full-thickness sensate skin can sometimes be done by skin expansion methods. Occasionally the use of an elastic garment or pressure from an Unna dressing whenever the limb is not worn may help. Friction reduction with polyamide sheaths, gel inserts, cornstarch, "second skin," and the like may be of value.

Infections

Stump infections, if open, require antibiotic treatment; if closed, they must be opened along with associated antibiotic treatment.

Bone Problems

Bypassing weight-bearing through the remaining skeletal system, such as ischial weight-bearing in an above-knee prosthesis, causes osteoporosis. The remaining periosteum may develop bone spurs, which cause pressure on the skin.

The most common type of bone overgrowth is bone spurs due to remnants of periosteum left in the stump at the time of surgery. Generally, socket modifications can compensate for it. On occasion, a pull-in socket is needed. Surgical removal of the spur and periosteum is sometimes required. Xeroradiography with weight- and non–weight-bearing with the prosthesis will show both the relationship of the spur to the socket and skin and exactly how "total-contact" the socket really is.[23]

In the child, an amputation through a long bone before bone maturity increases the bone length due to endosteal and periosteal growth, while the skin does not grow as much. The bone end becomes pointed and pushes through the skin. Skin traction is the preferred treatment to prevent stump shortening (Fig. 49–34). If surgery is required, the techniques of Marquardt, in which the spur is removed and replaced by a fragment of cartilage or epiphysis or a special metal and plastic, are best. This prevents repeated surgery, which shortens the bone.

Scoliosis

Patients who have unequal leg lengths may develop scoliosis. Usually this is a functional scoliosis that can be corrected by the length of the prosthesis. In the absence of daily stretching exercises, the scoliosis may become fixed. Therefore, exercises for range of motion are advised for the growing child.

Neuromas

The cut end of every nerve becomes a neuroma, which is usually painless if adequately protected. Neuromas exposed to pressure may give great pain and may require revision. Capping of the nerve ends is of occasional benefit. Burial in bone and injection of the nerve with destructive chemicals are of no use.

Psychological Problems

Management of the behavioral aspects of the patient is important. Because of the massive assault on the patient's body, self-image, and way of life, the entire psychic defense mechanism is stressed. The patient is highly vulnerable at this time, but also amenable to psychic change. The concept of amputation as punishment for sin persists. A feeling of guilt and shame often accompanies an amputation, either congenital or acquired. The timing, depth, and sequence of the emotional reactions vary from individual to individual.[15] The artificial limb hides the amputation and the "sin" that "caused" the amputation and also the functional loss. Understanding the psychosocial factors is important in prosthesis prescription, since a prosthesis serves psychological and social as well as functional needs. Even a lower limb prosthesis serves cosmetic functions.

Patients are looked upon more adversely if they have an obvious physical deformity than if they do not. Limb provision is vocationally important, since it is easier for a patient with an artificial leg to get a job than it is for a person using crutches.

Anger and frustration are extremely common. The anger is self-directed at first, and later it is directed toward the people who contributed to the limb loss, or toward the medical staff. The staff's reactions may inhibit the rehabilitation process if they personalize the anger.

Traumatic amputees have a sudden emotional shock without preparation. Those with premonitory mourning with chronic occlusive arterial disease or malignancy adjust in a different way and take amputation better. All amputees live in dread of disease or injury to the contralateral limb.

Worry about the limitation of function, although expressed very commonly, is possibly the least important psychological reaction. Reality testing is the best treatment.

Except in extreme cases, the psychological reactions to amputation are best handled by the physiatrist and the surgeon and, when properly trained, the therapists who work with the patient. Among the psychological defense mechanisms commonly utilized by amputees are withdrawal, obliteration, compensation, and substitution, depending to some extent on their preamputation personalities.

Psychological adjustment to a prosthesis depends on the realization that the prosthesis is a tool for performing certain activities. The efficacy of a tool depends on its appropriateness for the job to be done and the skill with which it is used.

In rehabilitation, the patient does the work; the "team" gives advice and guidance. The acceptance of advice depends on interpersonal relations, and that is why the advice of the aide or therapist may be taken over that of the physiatrist. The patient usually has far more contact with the former, and likes and trusts them more.

At least as important as encouragement, we must give the amputee the truth. We must tell the patient that all prostheses have deficiencies in their present state of development. They have an unstable attachment that makes them feel heavier than the limb they are replacing, even though they are considerably lighter. The instability may cause skin irritation aggravated by perspiration. The friction of the harness is also irritating. Gait with a prosthesis is always abnormal at best, and cosmesis is never as good as we would like it to be.

Phantom Sensation

"Phantom sensation" is a normal occurrence after amputation of a limb. This is the sensation of the presence of the amputated part. The patient experiences the sensations as though from an intact limb, which is now missing. It may be accompanied by not unpleasant tingling. At first the phantom sensation can be so deceptive that the patient may attempt to scratch the chin with an absent hand or to walk on a missing leg. With the passage of time, phantom sensation tends to diminish in a manner that has been described as "telescoping into the stump," but occasionally it may persist for decades. The last sensations to disappear are those that originate from the missing thumb or index finger, or from the great toe, which may be perceived as directly attached to the stump.

Almost all amputees except young children and those with brain damage have phantom sensation. Patients with congenital limb deficiencies, or those who have had a surgical or traumatic amputation before the age of four years, do not usually experience phantom sensation. For some patients, the phantom sensation assists them in learning to use the prosthesis.

A number of theories have been proposed for the phenomenon. A limb is an integral part of the body, continuously bombarding the sensory cortex with tactile, proprioceptive, and occasionally painful stimuli, which are remembered largely subconsciously as part of the body image. After amputation, these remembered perceptions produce phantom sensation, which may even include the feeling of a ring, wristwatch, or bracelet worn on the phantom hand or wrist.[15] Deformity of a limb present before amputation usually continues to be perceived in the phantom. Anesthetic limbs leave no phantom after amputation, and gradual loss of an extremity, as in leprosy, usually is not associated with phantom sensation. Surgical amputation of a body part in leprosy gives rise to phantom sensation of the whole part even after partial resorption has not resulted in a phantom.

Pain

Pain may occur in a number of forms. Pain may originate in the stump itself and is referred to as local pain. It may occur as pain referred to the stump. There also may be phantom pain, or pain apparently referred into the absent part. Additionally, there may be pain in other areas that interferes with prosthetic use.

Local pain may be due to an unprotected neuroma that is being pressed upon. Generally, desensitization by tapping and socket relief will alleviate the pain. Occasionally, injections of local anesthetic with or without corticosteroids or ultrasound may be required to help desensitize the neuroma. Rubbing, tapping, and massaging should be continued. If these measures are not successful, acupressure, transcutaneous electrical nerve stimulation, or phenol nerve blocks may be used. Excision of the neuroma or placing the residual nerve in a more protected location may be required. Adherent scars and bone spurs may be tender and require socket modifications or surgical revision. Skin and bone pain, as well as ischemic pain, may occur.

Sometimes referred pain is felt either within the stump or beyond the end of the stump, which originates from a distal site. A patient who has a herniated intervertebral disk may feel referred pain in the lateral side of the calf, and toes, even though those parts have been removed. Deep pain may be referred in a segmental distribution to an amputated limb just as it is to an intact limb. Pelvic congestion may be referred to the leg, stump, or phantom leg. Pain in the hip joint may be referred down the leg. This may be due to arthritis in the hip or merely biomechanical problems. The cause of referred pain must be determined by investigation in which the patient is treated as though he or she were not an amputee.

Biomechanical pain in joints, muscles, tendons, and ligaments other than the amputated limb must also be given consideration. These pains are due to the biomechanical abnormalities that develop secondary to the mechanics of walking with a prosthesis. The abnormal gait should be evaluated to see whether it is due to the prosthesis, improper training, or some other problem of the patient. Improving prosthetic alignment, and compensatory exercises, may help to resolve the problem or indicate further treatment. Careful examination by a physician skilled in both prosthetic use and biomechanical problem-solving is necessary.

Phantom Pain

Phantom pain must be distinguished from phantom sensation, stump pain, and referred pain. If the sensation of the absent limb is painful and disagreeable, with strong paresthesias, it is referred to as phantom pain. Phantom sensation usually occurs and is to be expected; phantom pain is not. Parts that have been crushed and those in which ablation has been delayed are more frequently painful than those removed promptly for nonpain-

ful conditions. Phantom pain may be constant or intermittent and may be of any degree of severity.

One of every two or three patients complains of phantom pain at some time. It is severe early after amputation in 5 to 10 per cent of patients. At that stage, it is hard to determine whether the pain is stump pain or more proximal pain referred distally, or phantom pain. Phantom pain is variously described as cramping, crushing, burning, or shooting and may be intermittent or continuous, frequently waxing and waning in cycles of several minutes' duration. It is localized in the phantom, not the stump. It is often perceived as a painful twisting or distortion of the part, as, for example, a clenching of the fist with the fingernails digging into the palm. It remains severe in fewer than 1 per cent of amputees, but in those it may disrupt the entire personality.

Phantom pain may be precipitated or intensified by any contact, not necessarily painful, with the stump or with a "trigger area" on the trunk, contralateral limb, or head. A neuroma in the stump may be tender, but 80 per cent of patients with phantom pain have no detectable abnormal tenderness of the stump. Phantom pain may also be triggered by urination, defecation, sexual intercourse, angina pectoris, or cigarette smoking.

Phantom pain has often been associated with emotional disturbance, but it has been difficult to determine whether the emotional disturbance preceded or resulted from the phantom pain. Some studies indicate that after amputation there is no greater incidence of neuroses among patients with phantom pain than there is among those without such pain. Amputations necessitated by war wounds or other trauma are less likely to be followed by phantom pain than are amputations for other reasons, even though the emotional trauma understandably might be greater in the former group.

Nevertheless, psychogenic factors may be suspected in patients who experience phantom pain "immediately" after amputation, who complain bitterly about their physical disfigurement, who have excessive difficulty in learning to use their prosthesis, or who refuse to use their prostheses. Those who are chronically maladjusted at home and in society, or who complain of increased pain after discussion of disturbing events, after contact with other patients having had amputations, or after an interview with a staff member concerning some significant conflict or interpersonal relationship, are also suspect. In these patients, the phantom pain may represent an emotional response to the loss of the limb, which may be helped by skillful psychiatric management.

Despite considerable research, the cause of phantom pain remains elusive. The most likely explanation, consistent with recent understanding and theories of pain and of the structure and function of the central nervous system, relates phantom pain to the loss of inhibitory influences normally initiated through the afferent impulses from the limb and their associated central connections. The spinothalamic tract was thought to be the principal pathway to the sensory cortex for the afferent impulses from the limbs. However, recent information suggests that the multisynaptic afferent system (MAS) carries much more afferent information through the spinal cord to the brain than does the oligosynaptic spinothalamic tract. The bilateral MAS crosses and recrosses the midline, eventually ending in the reticular formation of the brain stem.

Melzack has proposed a model to explain phantom limb pain consistent with these considerations and the gate control theory of pain.[33] He believes that a portion of the brain stem reticular formation acts as a "central biasing mechanism" by exerting a tonic inhibitory influence, or bias, on transmission at all synaptic levels of the somatic projection system. When a large proportion of sensory fibers is destroyed by amputation of a limb, thereby decreasing the amount of input into the reticular formation, the inhibitory influence decreases. This results in self-sustaining activity at all neural levels that can be triggered repeatedly by the remaining fibers. Pain occurs when the output of the self-sustaining neuron pools reaches or exceeds a critical level. This model helps to explain not only the failure of surgical interruption to produce lasting relief of phantom pain, but also the frequent temporary success of various therapeutic procedures that influence the central excitatory state of the nervous system at different levels.

For ease of understanding and treatment, it is helpful to classify phantom pain into different categories of sensation. In the author's experience, four common types, with variants, exist.

Of the four types, the most common is a cramping sensation—pain similar to that of muscle spasm. Patients say that their fist or foot remains in an uncomfortable position and that they would be comfortable if they could just move it. This pain seems to be relieved by simultaneous bilateral exercise of the contralateral normal limb together with the phantom. Occasionally, surging sinusoidal electrical stimulation of the stump assists voluntary exercise and relieves the pain. In addition, massage of the stump may help relieve the pain. Muscle relaxants or heat is occasionally of help. The proponents of the osteomyoplastic amputation insist that cramping phantom pain is much less common with that surgical method than with other procedures. Percussion of the stump by the fingers (tapôtement) in a progressively more vigorous manner by the therapist or the patient, and "therapeutic abuse" by pounding with a rubber mallet or stimulating with a mechanical vibrator, may be used to desensitize the part and the pathways for pain. The nervous system accommodates to stimuli fairly rapidly. Superficial and then deep kneading massage also reduces tenderness. When the stump can tolerate it, a temporary socket should be applied, and gentle partial weight-bearing should be started with graduated increased weight-bearing as tolerated by the patient.

The second type of phantom pain is an electric shock–like discomfort in the phantom limb that lasts for a few seconds. It is lancinating and episodic, superimposed upon either painless sensations or some other type of phantom pain. It appears to be a neuritic pain. If the pain is due to the pressure of a poorly fitting prosthesis and can be corrected by refitting or alignment, that is not phantom pain. If injection of the neuroma with a steroid is effective, again that is stump pain and not phantom pain. Desensitization by both "therapeutic abuse" and prosthesis use is helpful in true phantom pain. The application of cold decreases the central excitatory state of the pathways in the spinal cord. Cold may be applied with ice packs or by ethyl chloride spray. Ultrasound over the nerve trunk may offer some relief from this type of phantom pain. Since the pain lasts a short period of time, narcotics should not be used. Systemic analgesics are pointless for a pain that lasts only a few seconds and comes intermittently. Most patients can ignore it.

The third and most severe type of phantom pain is a burning, agonizing discomfort throughout the stump and the phantom limb. The stump generally feels hot, but it may feel cold. It may look normal, red, or cyanotic. It is exquisitely tender. Clothing or a gust of air touching the stump can trigger the pain. The patient often wraps the stump in protective clothes or towels to avoid irritation. It often occurs after crushing or stretching trauma to the nerves. This is the pain of causalgia or reflex sympathetic dystrophy. Conservative treatments the same as for causalgia are indicated. Early temporary blockade of the autonomic nervous system by injection of a local anesthetic is desirable.

LAWRENCE W. FRIEDMANN

Other treatments include sympathetic blocking agents such as dibenzyline and guanethidine, nonnarcotic analgesics, TENS, acupuncture, electrical stimulation, and the physical measures for desensitization. Pain is ameliorated by the use of measures that decrease the central excitatory state in the central nervous system. These measures are rubbing, tapping, heating, or cooling the stump, or spraying with ethyl chloride spray. Gradual and increasing prosthetic use may be helpful. Sympathectomy may be helpful. Because the condition may become increasingly severe, it has been treated with drastic surgical procedures, such as rhizotomy and even prefrontal lobotomy, the value of which is doubtful at best. Since most surgical methods of treatment are not successful, they should not be used except in cases in which suicide may be anticipated.

The fourth type of phantom pain is a squeezing, wrenching, "hot poker" type pain, not as easily classified as the other three. All of the measures that have been found useful for the other three types of phantom pain should be tried for relief.

MANAGEMENT OF THE PATIENT WITH PHANTOM PAIN

Treatment for phantom pain should proceed from simple noninvasive to more complex or invasive measures and be based on general principles of good management. One should not consider destructive surgical procedures until all simpler alternative methods have failed to provide lasting relief. The following 10 points summarize a practical program of management for pain.

1. Preoperatively, prepare patients by informing them that following amputation they can expect phantom sensation, which is normal and not harmful.

2. Postoperatively, examine the stump regularly, checking its appearance, sensation, and function. Use the words "stump" and "residual limb" in conversations with patients to get them used to both terms.

3. Postoperative care is as important as surgical technique in healing of the incision; any evidence of infection should be treated vigorously.

4. When the wound is sufficiently healed, the therapist should instruct the patient in massaging the stump with an emollient lotion and afterward applying tincture of benzoin to toughen the skin. The patient may also be instructed in gentle pounding or slapping of the stump and in use of a mechanical vibrator, taking care not to traumatize the scar.

5. The patient should exercise the stump muscles through imaginary movement of the phantom limb (for example, peddling an imaginary bicycle using the stump and good leg in reciprocal fashion, or rowing an imaginary boat using the stump and good arm simultaneously).

6. Provide a functional as well as a cosmetic prosthesis as soon as possible, since this can often prevent or relieve phantom pain. Immediate postoperative fitting of a temporary prosthesis is used to reduce the incidence of phantom pain.

7. A number of measures may be tried to block neural conduction and relieve phantom pain: ethyl chloride spray; local procaine injection of sensitive areas in the stump; injection of peripheral nerve or dorsal nerve roots with procaine, which, although providing only temporary anesthesia, may be followed by long-lasting relief; ultrasound; and hypertonic saline injection to interspinous ligaments (which acts as a counterirritant).

8. Many neurosurgical procedures have been advocated; none is permanent. Probably the best results reported have been with anterolateral cordotomy. Electrostimulation of the dorsal column in the spinal cord by implanted subdural electrodes and activated by a subcutaneous radiofrequency stimulator control has been used. The long-term value is still debated, and adverse effects of erosion of the dorsal columns have been reported. Frustratingly, pain recurs after section of peripheral nerves or of dorsal nerve roots and even after amputation of the limb at a higher level. Neurosurgical procedures on the spinal cord may provide initial relief but often are followed by late recurrence of phantom pain, even after bilateral high thoracic or cervical cordotomies. Surgical ablation of the cerebral somatosensory cortex and injury to this area of the brain have been observed to abolish both phantom pain and phantom sensation.

9. Psychiatric treatment may be necessary in some cases. Hypnosis, distraction conditioning, imagery, and psychotherapy have been utilized. The value of early hands-on treatment is that the patient is distracted early, and body image is consciously manipulated in a positive direction while the patient is most malleable soon after the surgery. It is mainly in those patients in whom early intervention was not done that more intensive psychological manipulation becomes necessary.

10. When any procedure results in relief of phantom pain, the patient should resume handling and normal movement of the stump, prescribed exercises, massage, and use of the prosthesis in order to decrease the likelihood of recurrence of phantom pain.

Edema

Edema of the stump after amputation is usual. Total-contact sockets prevent edema, especially if they are inelastic.[13] Edema may be controlled by elastic bandaging, a plaster cast, air bags, or an Unna dressing. An Unna dressing is made like a cast by using a commercially available impregnated gauze. It is placed directly on the skin. In contrast to a plaster cast, the gauze is not folded on itself when reversing direction, but is cut. When the prosthesis is being worn, edema usually indicates that there is constriction of the proximal stump. This may be due to the stump's sinking too far into the prosthesis, too many stump socks, cardiac or renal failure, chemotherapeutic agents for malignancy, weight gain, or excessive suction by the socket. The edema causes an indurated, red mass acutely, progressing to chronic eczema and fungoid lesions, and possibly ulceration. It also increases sensitivity and pain in the end of the stump.

Contractures

Contractures of joints usually occur prior to or immediately after an amputation. Fibroblasts do not sleep. For this reason, every limb requires a full joint range of motion at least four times a day. Even in the presence of pain and severe injury, most limbs can be moved passively with care. Prevention of contractures is easier than corrective treatment. Hip contractures are generally in flexion, abduction, and external rotation; contracture at the knee is usually in flexion. It is extremely difficult to walk with either of these contractures.

For correction, serial casting, progressive passive or dynamic splinting, proprioceptive neuromuscular facilitation, stretching of the antagonist to produce reciprocal inhibition, and traction are useful. Surgery may be necessary as a last resort.

Acceptance or Rejection of Prostheses

The acceptance and use of a prosthesis reflects the patient's evaluation of its relative advantages and disadvantages. The advantages of the leg are that it improves appearance and the patient's body image, that it frees the hands from crutches, and that it permits easier transfer, standing, and ambulation. The prosthetic gait is slower than most crutch gaits and may be even more costly in energy expenditure. Ambulation with the above-knee prosthesis is considerably slower and more laborious than propelling a wheelchair.

The extent to which the rehabilitation team can minimize the disadvantages and maximize the advantages of a prosthesis will determine acceptance by the patient. The patient evaluates the limb on a cost:benefit continuum. Cost includes economics, comfort, time lost from work and play, appearance, and so on. The team should utilize successfully rehabilitated patients as volunteer patient counselors to help in this endeavor.

In our enthusiasm for prosthetic fitting, we should not delude patients into believing that they will be "almost normal" after fitting and training with an artificial limb.

Vocational Aspects

A prospective employee has only two things to sell: the work of his or her mind and the work of his or her body. Mental work can be expressed by the mouth or hands. Neither is impaired after leg ablation.[16] For the leg amputee, any vocation requiring prolonged standing or walking, carrying of heavy loads, and running will present difficulty. There is no contraindication to any type of physical work that the amputee can perform, with the exception of that requiring fine balance. Thus, construction work at high altitudes will be contraindicated, even if just part of the foot is missing. With higher levels of amputation, such as the Syme's and the below-knee, heavy work can frequently be performed provided that the prosthesis is adequate for the patient's need. With above-knee amputations, walking for long distances and the ability to carry heavy weights become progressively diminished. Sedentary jobs are possible for such patients. Following bilateral lower extremity amputations, the problems increase by geometric progression. Most amputees who were doing manual work prior to the limb loss change jobs to sedentary or managerial type work. Others retire. Only a few continue to do manual work, and most of those need many job modifications.

The Juvenile Amputee

Treatment Goals

The goal of all treatment for limb anomalies is getting the patient to function optimally in the

LAWRENCE W. FRIEDMANN

family and in society. There is no doubt that if it were possible, we would like all congenital amputees to live with loving parents. Where this is not possible, optimal function in sheltered communal living is desirable. Society has not begun to provide adequate sheltered communal living for the disabled, except in parts of Europe. Although having the disabled live in communities and buildings with the nondisabled is desirable, provision should be made for the severely disabled to live together in apartments with no architectural barriers. Patients with different disabilities can help each other in a mini-community in which each individual may have a disability but the community itself is independent.

The Differences Between Adult and Child Amputees

Amputations in children are usually congenital or traumatic but may be due to malignant disease. Vascular disease, the most common cause in adults, is very rare in children. For the congenital limb reduction or reduplication defects that we cavalierly refer to as amputations, we need to consider that many of these lesions occur in children with anomalies in other limbs and organs. They often have not only the obvious physical defects with their associated functional losses, but sometimes intellectual, cognitive, educational, social, and later sexual and vocational difficulties. These children live a normal life span unless associated problems intervene. For that reason, treatment must be seen as a continuum, with what we do now as an integral part of what we wish to accomplish for the 40-year-old or 60-year-old person the child will inevitably become.

The major difference in treatment between the child amputees and the adult amputees is the maturation factor. Growth occurs not only in size but also in intellectual capacity and neuromusculoskeletal maturation. Emotional problems are found in congenital amputees if feelings of guilt and inadequacy of the parents are transmitted to the youngster. At first the child with congenital amputation does not miss the absent limb and is usually unconcerned with appearance until starting school, or the onset of puberty. Parents are frequently very concerned with appearance very early. They feel that they were not capable of producing a normal child, and so they are inferior. To hide their own "inferiority," they hide the child or the anomaly.

In most aspects of growth and development, the limb-deficient child is similar to normal children except that the limb grows more slowly and thus is shorter. The limb is abnormal in its bone structures, its articulations, its musculature, and often its nerves. Disuse atrophy makes it smaller in circumference. Crawling may or may not be possible. If not, since the nervous system maturation is dependent on sensory feedback and practice, neuromuscular development is slowed markedly. Between the ages of 9 and 15 months, the child usually begins to stand. A child with a congenital lower limb deficiency will use the arms and the normal lower limb, if there is one, for pulling up and standing. If, before the age of 9 months, an artificial limb that supplies adequate length and stability is provided, the child will start to walk with it independently. At no subsequent age will an amputee learn to utilize a device as well.

Treatment Implications

The personality of the child develops to its greatest degree before the age of one year; for this reason, informed help should be given to the parents so that they will accept the limb-deficient child as an integral part of the family and develop a relationship between the child, the family, and the clinic team. Part of the problem is that often the parents and the professionals have different goals, or at least emphases, which often are unexpressed. Whereas the professionals are usually more concerned with the functional losses the child has, the parents are usually more concerned with the appearance of the child. This conflict, if hidden, may result in sabotage of the team's efforts. Cosmesis must be recognized as an important function in life. Satisfactory understanding can be worked out only if the issue is raised and aired.

Prostheses will need frequent adjustments in the first two years. The second major growth spurt occurs between the ages of 11 and 13 years in girls and 13 and 15 years in boys. During periods of rapid growth, frequent visits to the clinic will be necessary to adjust the length and form of the prosthesis.

Evaluation of the juvenile amputee is more difficult than that of adults. Since the child has difficulty in communication, rapport may take a longer time to establish. Whereas an adult can frequently be evaluated in one session, the young amputee commonly requires many sessions in order to gain the relaxation and cooperation needed to determine ranges of motion, muscle tone, and strength. Whereas congenital amputees frequently have coexisting anomalies, other abnormalities may be attributed to the absence of the limb itself. Congenital scoliosis is far more frequent in patients with unilateral limb deficiencies than in otherwise normal children. In the absence of a lower limb, if the growth of the normal limb is not compensated for by frequent prosthetic adjustments, the child may develop a compensatory scoliosis.

Active exercises prevent contractures. Positioning to prevent contractures is of less benefit for an active child than for an adult. Flexion contractures following traumatic amputation are almost unknown in young amputees, but the congenitally limb-deficient child frequently has limitations of movement of the adjacent joints due to contractures or abnormally formed structures. These may need correction by casting, stretching, dynamic splinting, or surgery. Slow, steady orthotic stretching should be aided by manual stretching on an intermittent basis, rather than the reverse.

Certain lower limb anomalies need no treatment. Shoe modifications such as lifts, molds, and extensions or more complex orthotic devices may be required to modify weight-bearing. Still others need prostheses to equalize leg length and to modify weight-bearing through the skeletal system. Others require therapeutic surgical correction in lesser or more major degrees. Surgical correction will not be discussed in this chapter except briefly and as a possibility of the treatment of each specific defect.

Surgical ablation should be deferred if possible, since the amputated extremity tends to grow at a slower rate than the congenitally deformed limb would otherwise have done. Thus, a long above-knee amputation in the young child, performed for deformity at the knee, becomes a short above-knee stump by the time of skeletal maturity. Usually, the longer the amputation can be deferred, the better the physical end result. In order to avoid early amputation of the lower limb, special weight-bearing prostheses may be constructed for patients with an abnormal femur, tibia, or foot.

Overgrowth of the bone of the stump with lack of compensatory lengthening of the skin and subcutaneous tissues is frequent after transection of long bones of juvenile amputees, especially the humerus and the tibia. Conservative treatment by traction at night and in the prosthesis is the initial approach.[17] Marquardt uses epiphysis, cartilage, or artificial materials implanted at the bone end to correct the problem, with much success.[31]

The removal of terminal skin tabs is advisable if they interfere with the fit of the prosthesis. The removal of abnormal digits in the lower limb is usually of little significance except to help with fitting of the shoe. Correction of foot deformities to ensure a plantigrade foot for weight-bearing must be started very early at the time when the plasticity of the connective tissues shows a good response to prolonged stretch.

Prostheses and Components

Most prosthetic devices have been designed for adult war casualties. When children's prostheses are made, many designers make small models of adult prostheses, which are usually far from optimal. They do not take into account the immature neuromusculoskeletal system of the child with its limited sources of power for transfer, the limited ability to learn techniques for control, or the frequent prosthetic changes and replacements required because of growth. In contrast to the adult, for whom shrinkage of the stump requires frequent changes in the socket, the stump of the child undergoes rapid growth and increased muscular bulk that exceeds the atrophy of subcutaneous fat from the pressure of the socket. The proportionally greater amount of soft tissue around the bone of the stump causes instability, and harnessing becomes more difficult. Changes in growth may require rechecks every one to three months to make sure that the socket and harnessing still fit. Children's prostheses must be individually designed with the components appropriate for optimal function at each stage of neuromuscular development.

Older amputees may be fitted with conventional prostheses of the adult type. The below-knee amputee may be fitted with a standard or modified patellar tendon–bearing prosthesis with suprapatellar cuff suspension and SACH foot. The SACH foot and now the energy-storing feet have been a boon to children's prosthetics. The use of a thigh corset is advised for the young below-knee amputee to prevent genu recurvatum, which occurs frequently after prolonged use of a cuff suspension.

For the above-knee amputee, conventional prostheses can be used. Suspension is usually by Silesian bandage. Although true suction suspension is rarely possible before the age of seven years, because of rapid change in size, ancillary suction may make use of the prosthesis more effective. Children learn to use lower limb prostheses quickly. For patients with deformed lower limbs, the foot may be able to take some weight-bearing even with a false joint proximally. Gluteal weight-bearing is often a great assist. True ischial weight-bearing is very difficult to attain in the young child because of baby fat and the fact that the ischial tuberosity is anterior to its usual location in patients with proximal focal femoral deficiency. Patients with very short lower limbs or complete absence of both lower limbs can be taught to walk in bucket sockets with stubby legs, without knee joints. These can be lengthened as the child grows, changing to the Canadian type hemipelvectomy design with modifications. Amputees with unilateral hip disarticulation are managed the same as are adults and fitted with prostheses as early as possible.

In order to plan proper treatment, one must understand the natural course of a congenital anomaly throughout the patient's life. A number of problems and the necessary management are presented in the following.

Congenital deformities of the feet are best treated with external or internal shoe corrections.

Proximal Focal Femoral Deficiency

The most common major lower limb reduction deformity is proximal focal femoral deficiency (PFFD). The problems caused by PFFD are (1) leg length discrepancy, (2) unstable hip, (3) muscles with abnormal origins and insertions, resulting in weakness, loss of endurance, and abnormal motion, (4) malrotation of the limb, and (5) associated defects, including fibular hemimelia in 69 per cent and other limb deficiencies in 51.7 per cent. Conservative treatment is advised for most patients with unilateral PFFD and should consist of shoe lifts or foot platforms to equalize the length of the extremities. As length discrepancy increases, a brace-type prosthesis with gluteal and ischial weight-bearing should be used. Later, a prosthesis of plastic with a "ship's funnel" socket is used if ischial weight-bearing is needed. These sockets are markedly different from quadrilateral sockets for adult amputees. The lateral wall is very much higher and goes almost to the iliac crest for lateral support. The medial wall is narrow. This is especially important for boys so as not to damage the genitalia between the medial socket walls. Boys should be told to wear hard athletic supporters early. Marquardt[31] has found that the ischial tu-

berosities of children with proximal focal femoral deficiency are farther anterior than normal. The ischial seat must thus be placed farther forward. Gluteal weight-bearing is more important, so the posterior wall of the socket is at least as high as the anterior wall. The socket does not provide for flexion of the patient's knee, and a prosthetic knee joint at or below the patient's heel with the foot in maximum plantar flexion is best (Fig. 49–36). Corrective alignment and SACH feet should be used. When the toes of the plantar flexed foot extend to the level of the contralateral mid-calf, no cosmetic prosthetic knee unit is feasible. A prosthetic limb that bears weight on the patellar tendon is advisable (Fig. 49–37).

The treatment for bilateral PFFD should be conservative for all those able to walk without prostheses. These are patients with almost equal length legs. Amputation should not be considered for these children, since it destroys their ability to walk without prostheses at home with minimal expenditure of energy and in emergencies. Prostheses are provided for use in school and for social occasions to raise the child to a more normal height (Fig. 49–38). Those with markedly unequal leg lengths must be treated as unilateral or as bilateral amputees with the appropriate prosthesis for extremity.

Surgical Possibilities

Amputation may be considered for a cosmetically grotesque deformity. Chopart's amputation is preferable in order to preserve maximal possible length prior to bone maturity. Delaying amputation until maturity is advised unless serious psychic abnormalities arise. After bone maturity, a Syme's amputation is preferred. In the author's experience, weight-bearing on the foot should be performed as long as possible to delay the skin problems so frequently associated with lifelong prosthetic irritation. In most cases, nonsurgical management can be prolonged or even permanent, albeit not without some functional and cosmetic defects during sitting.

Van Nes[39] proposed tibial rotation osteotomy of 180 degrees, converting the ankle into a knee joint with the reversed foot acting as the below-knee stump (Fig. 49–39). A thigh corset is mandatory. Ankle plantar flexion gives prosthetic knee extension, and ankle dorsiflexion causes prosthetic knee flexion. This procedure has been successful in

Text continued on page 1067

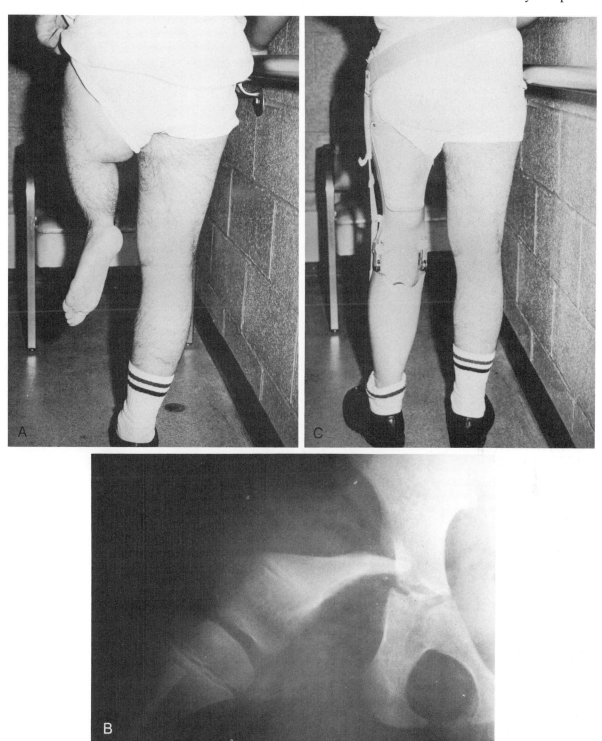

FIGURE 49–36. *A*, This 23-year-old male with proximal femoral focal deficiency (PFFD) has his heel just above the axis of rotation of his normal knee. *B*, The patient has no acetabulum and no femoral head, a class "D" PFFD. *C*, A ship's funnel socket encloses the lower extremity with ischial and gluteal support. Notice the heel above the knee joint and the foot plantar flexion. A knee lock is used.

LAWRENCE W. FRIEDMANN

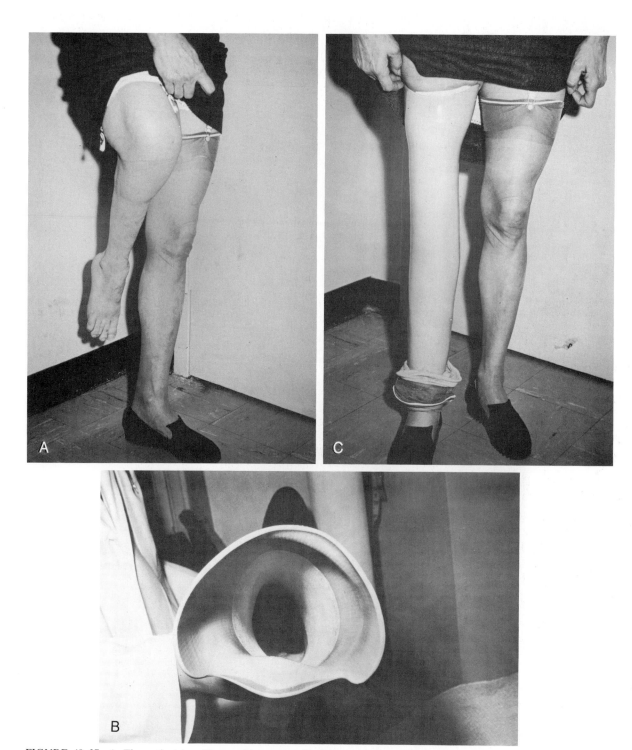

FIGURE 49–37. *A,* The patient is a 71-year-old woman with PFFD with leg and foot of normal length. *B,* The PTB-type prosthesis has an elastic inner sleeve to avoid an unsightly suspension. *C,* Sitting is uncosmetic without a knee joint.

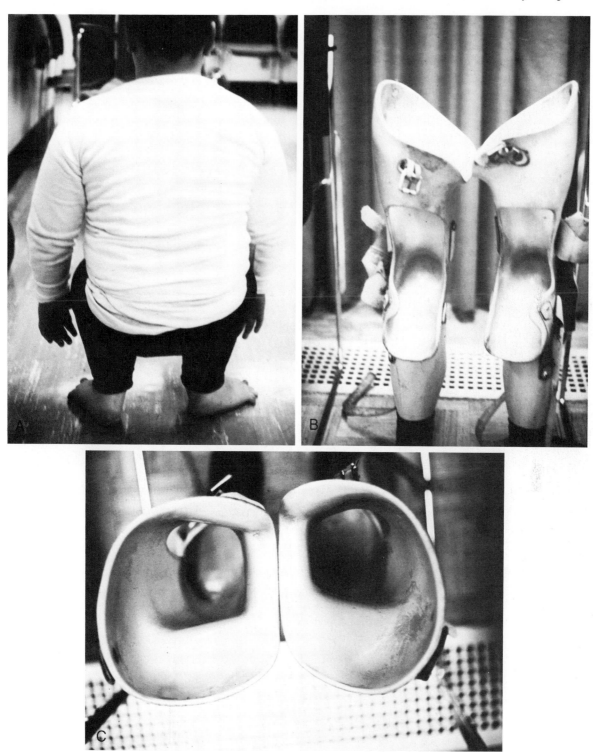

FIGURE 49–38. *A*, Patient with bilateral PFFD. *B*, Uses bilateral ship's funnel prostheses with additional weight-bearing on his feet. *C*, Note that the weight-bearing is both ischial on the anteriorly placed ischial seats and on the gluteus.

LAWRENCE W. FRIEDMANN

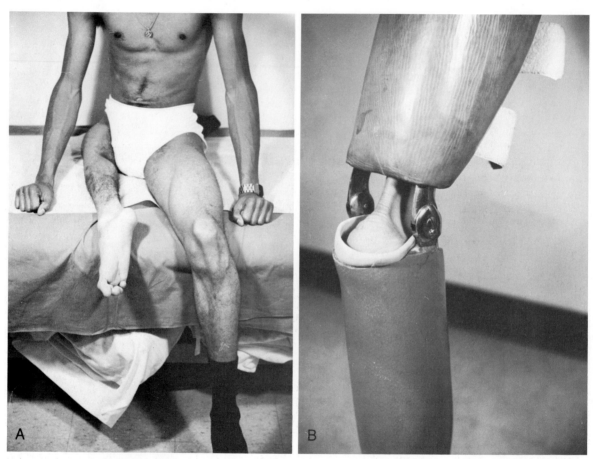

FIGURE 49–39. *A*, Adult after a Van Nes rotation osteotomy, converting the ankle to a joint at the level of the knee. *B*, The heel is anterior in the socket.

many cases. The normal range of motion at the ankle permits only 60 to 75 degrees of total motion, providing motion of the reconstructed "knee" between 170 and 105 degrees. Even if 10 degrees of flexion at the knee is provided, the knee cannot be flexed to more than 100 degrees. The strength of the reconstructed "knee" is poor, and ankle instability is frequent. There is a relatively high derotation rate in this complex procedure in inexperienced hands. Fabrication of the prosthesis is difficult. The appearance of the undressed person is bizarre.

On occasion, arthrodesis of the knee is advisable to provide a rigid end-bearing stump. Arthrodesis of the knee is rarely required, since the exoskeletal socket usually provides adequate support for the enclosed natural knee. Reconstruction of the hip should be attempted only if the acetabulum and femoral head are present. It is performed only to correct the deformities of abduction, flexion, and

external rotation. Bone grafting is usually required. Arthrodesis of the hip is functionally poor. Correction of contractures is only moderately successful.

The term "hemimelia" means congenital absence of half of the limb. The part that is partially or totally absent is named, so that tibial hemimelia means absence of the tibia. A transverse defect means part of the limb is gone as if it had been cut off by a guillotine. A paraxial hemimelia means that a longitudinal ray is gone. If an intermediate part is gone, but a terminal part remains, that is called intercalary.

Fibular hemimelia often allows weight-bearing on the foot. Usually there is anterior tibial bowing with a dimple in the skin over the bow. Shortening of the limb requires adaptations mentioned previously. Partial or total amputation of the foot is common, since the foot often is markedly deformed. As an example, a 72-year-old man with

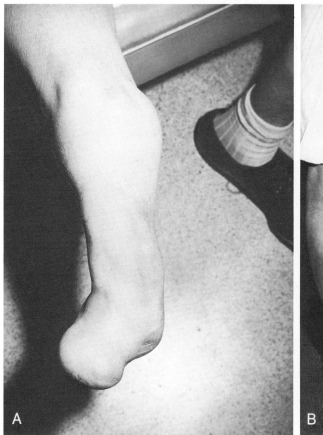 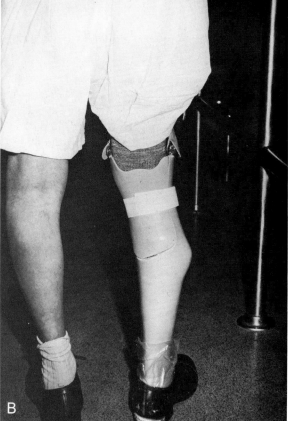

FIGURE 49–40. *A*, Adult male with fibular hemimelia and amputation of the forefoot. Note the irritation of the skin over the medial side of the ankle and minimal callus on the patellar tendon. *B*, The prosthesis has a posterior trap door with an inferior hinge and is molded for the residual foot.

LAWRENCE W. FRIEDMANN

partial terminal paraxial fibular hemimelia and a partial amputation of the foot performed 40 years earlier now has scoliosis that is most likely due to unequal leg length. There is degenerative arthritis in the right hip, probably secondary to proximal focal femoral deficiency rather than osteoarthritis, since an amputee almost invariably puts greater weight on the normal leg. Partial foot ablation has given rise to irritation over the metatarsal heads and Achilles tendon, but the partial weight-bearing for many years helped protect the skin over the patellar tendon better than either a below-knee or Syme's amputation would have (Fig. 49–40).

In patients with intercalary complete longitudinal tibial hemimelia, the soles of the feet are pointed to the groin. Ambulation without reconstruction is possible only with massive prostheses. Aitken[2] says that complete tibial hemimelia should be treated by knee disarticulation. In selected cases, the proximal end of the fibula is transplanted under the femur.[7] Incomplete tibial hemimelia may be treated by tibiofibular synostosis with subsequent disarticulation of the ankle, or by disarticulation of the knee.

In amelia, the complete absence of the limb, and for those who have dislocated hips so that no weight-bearing is feasible through the deformed limbs, no prosthesis may be required for sitting, but one is necessary if the child wants to walk. If the child cannot sit, a bucket prosthesis can be fabricated, letting the feet protrude. If the patient has inadequate upper limbs for crutch-walking, a reciprocating-type walker is required. At the beginning, footboards to elongate the shoes are used to provide balance. Later these are eliminated. Many designs of walkers have been used.

Rehabilitation Involves Total Function

The treatment of children and adults who have amputations requires consideration of all of their problems: physical, emotional, educational, social, vocational, and sexual. It demands ingenuity and a willingness to modify standard methods for fitting and training. Active involvement in childhood activities should be encouraged. All patients should be urged to participate in recreational activities, sports, and games, including swimming, which is too frequently neglected.

Because of the multiplicity of problems, large and small, encountered in the rehabilitation of amputees, the demands on the physiatrist are great, but the rewards are immeasurably greater.

References

1. Adler, J. C., Mazzarella, N., Puzsier, L., and Alba, A.: Treadmill training program for a bilateral below-knee amputee patient with cardiopulmonary disease. Arch. Phys. Med. Rehabil., 68:858–861, 1987.
2. Aitken, T.: Tibial hemimelia. *In* Selected Lower Limb Anomalies: Surgical and Prosthetic Management. Proceedings of the National Academy of Sciences Symposium, 1971, pp. 1–19.
3. Atlas of Limb Prosthetics. St. Louis, C. V. Mosby, 1981, pp. 277–314.
4. Bakalim, G.: Sponge rubber pad in the prosthesis in cases of chronic dermatitis and ulceration in the stump. Acta Orthop. Scand., 34:117–122, 1964.
5. Bender, L.: Personal communication, 1985.
6. Bowker, J. H., and Thompson, R. G.: Management of musculoskeletal complications. *In* Atlas of Limb Prosthetics. St. Louis, C. V. Mosby, 1981, pp. 448–458.
7. Brown, W.: The Brown operation for total hemimelia tibia. *In* Selected Lower Limb Anomalies: Surgical and Prosthetic Management. Proceedings of the National Academy of Sciences Symposium, 1971, pp. 20–28.
8. Chino, N.: Interface pressures in below-knee (B-K) prosthesis upon ramp walking. Jpn. J. Rehabil. Med., 12:57–64, 1975.
9. Chino, N., Pearson, J. R., Cockrell, J. L., Mikishko, H. A., and Koepke, G. H.: Effect of Rubber Sleeve Suspension on Negative Pressure in Below the Knee Prostheses. Kenny-Michigan Rehabilitation Foundation & Social and Rehabilitation Service Grant RD–2604–M, 1972.
10. Ducroquet, R., Ducroquet, J., and Ducroquet, P.: Walking and Limping—A Study of Normal and Pathological Walking. Philadelphia, J. B. Lippincott, 1968.
11. Erdman, W. J. II, Hettinger, Th., and Saez, F.: Comparative work stress for above-knee amputees using artificial legs or crutches. Am. J. Phys. Med., 39:225–232, 1960.
12. Friedmann, L. W.: Rehabilitation of amputees. *In* Licht, S. (Ed.): Rehabilitation and Medicine. New Haven, Elizabeth Licht, Publisher, 1968, pp. 349–376.
13. Friedmann, L. W.: Lower Limb Prosthetics. New York University Post-Graduate Medical School, 1975 revision, pp. 221–232.
14. Friedmann, L. W.: The Surgical Rehabilitation of the Amputee. Springfield IL, Charles C Thomas, Publisher, 1978, pp. 205–209.
15. Friedmann, L. W.: The Psychological Rehabilitation of the Amputee. Springfield, IL, Charles C Thomas, Publisher, 1978, pp. 127–140.

16. Friedmann, L. W.: Amputation. *In* Stolov, W. C., and Clowers, M. R. (Ed.): Handbook of Severe Disability. U.S. Department of Education, Rehabilitation Services Administration, 1981, pp. 169–188.

17. Friedmann, L. W., and Friedmann, L.: The conservative treatment of the bony overgrowth problem in the juvenile amputee. Inter-Clinic Information Bull., 20:17–23, 1985.

18. Ghiulamila, R. I.: Semi-rigid dressing for postoperative fitting of below-knee prostheses. Arch. Phys. Med. Rehabil., 53:186–190, 1972.

19. Gonzalez, E. G., Corcoran, P. J., and Reyes, R. L.: Energy expenditure in below knee amputees: Correlation with stump length. Arch. Phys. Med. Rehabil., 55:111–119, 1974.

20. Hansson, J.: The leg amputee—a clinical followup study. Acta Orthop. Scand. [Supp.], 69:1–104, 1964.

21. Huang, C. T., Moore, N. B., Jackson, J. R., Fine, P. R., Kuhlemeier, K. V., Traugh, G. H., and Saunders, P. T.: Energy cost of ambulation for amputees, a study using the mobile automatic metabolic analyzer. Arch. Phys. Med. Rehabil., 58:521, 1977.

22. Inman, V. T., Ralston, H. J., and Rodd, F.: Human Walking. Baltimore, Williams & Wilkins, 1981, pp. 1–117.

23. Irwin, G. A. L., Friedmann, L. W., and Shapiro, D.: Prosthetic fit in below-knee amputation: Evaluation with xeroradiography. Am. J. Roentgenol., 148:99–101, 1987.

24. Jendrzejczyk, D.: Flexible socket systems. Clin. Prosthetics Orthotics, 9:27–31, 1985.

25. Kawamura, I., and Kawamura, J.: Some biomechanical evaluations of the ISNY flexible above-knee system with quadrilateral socket. Orthotics Prosthetics, 40:17–23, 1986.

26. Klopsteg, P. E., and Wilson, P. D.: Human Limbs and Their Substitutes. New York, Hafner Publishing Company, 1968, pp. 481–619, pp. 653–738.

27. Lehneis, H. R.: Beyond the quadrilateral. Clin. Prosthetics Orthotics, 9:6–8, 1985.

28. Levy, S. W.: Skin problems of the leg amputee. Arch. Dermatol., 85:65–81, 1962.

29. Long, I. A.: Normal shape–normal alignment (NSNA) above-knee prosthesis. Clin. Prosthetics Orthotics, 9:9–14, 1985.

30. Lowry, R.: Durability of lower extremity prostheses. Arch. Phys. Med. Rehabil., 47:742–743, 1966.

31. Marquardt, D.: Personal communication, 1976.

32. Mazet, R. Jr., and Hennessy, C. A.: Knee disarticulation: A new technique and a new knee-joint mechanism. Orthop. Prosthet. Appl. J., 20:39–53, 1966.

33. Melzack, R.: The Puzzle of Pain. New York, Basic Books, 1973.

34. Redhead, R. G., and Snowdon, C.: Report on controlled stump environment. British Research and Development Unit Bulletin, St. Mary's Hospital, Roehampton, England, 1971.

35. Sabolich, J.: Contoured adducted trochanteric–controlled alignment method (CAT–CAM): Introduction and basic principles. Clin. Prosthetics Orthotics, 9:15–26, 1985.

36. Sonck, W. A., Cockrell, J. L., and Koepke, G. H.: Effect of liner materials on interface pressures in below-knee prostheses. Arch. Phys. Med. Rehabil., 51:666–669, 1970.

37. Stephen, P. J., Hunter, J., and Aitken, R. C. B.: Morbidity survey of lower limb amputees. Clin. Rehabil., 1:181–186, 1987.

38. Traugh, G. H., Corcoran, P. J., and Reyes, R. L.: Energy expenditure of ambulation in patients with above knee amputations. Arch. Phys. Med. Rehabil., 56:67–71, 1975.

39. Van Nes, C. P.: Rotation-plasty for congenital defects of femur: Making use of ankle of shortened limb to control knee joint of prosthesis. J. Bone Joint Surg., 32B:16, 1950.

50
Rehabilitation for Burn Patients

ELIZABETH A. RIVERS
STEVEN V. FISHER

In this chapter, the classification, the pathology, and the surgical treatment of burns are discussed, since this background is needed to understand burn rehabilitation. The overlapping stages of healing and varied treatment modalities create a unique opportunity for the members of the rehabilitation and surgical teams to cooperate through their specific contributions to obtain the best possible function and cosmesis for the patient.

Incidence

Each year, about 1 per cent of the population sustains a burn despite excellent burn prevention programs conducted by many fire departments in the United States.[1] One in every 70 burned adults is hospitalized annually.[2] Except for children from one to five years of age who receive scalds, the majority of burn accidents occur in males 17 to 30 years of age.[3] Home-related accidents account for 66 per cent of all burn injuries.[4] The ramifications in the costs of hospital treatment, in pain, long frightening hospital stays, loss of loved ones, job displacement, the stigma of disfigurement or permanent disability, and in impoverishment (hospital treatment costs $2000 a day) affect every community member.[5] An organized, positive approach to rehabilitation that is initiated immediately can reduce the final degree of disability.

Classification by Physical Characteristics

Burn severity is classified according to the patient's age, the agent causing cell damage, the per cent of the cutaneous surface injured, the depth of tissue destruction, the body areas injured, and types of associated injuries or illnesses. For this reason, burn patients undergo triage for treatment at a burn center, a local hospital, or an outpatient center, depending on the severity of the injury (Fig. 50–1).[6]

Injuring Agent

The depth and per cent of tissue destruction caused by an injuring agent vary widely, depending on the duration and the intensity of exposure to the agent. Therefore, the mechanism of the burn should be immediately documented. Burns are of mixed depths and may be affected positively by early treatment, so that seconds count in initiating first aid.

Caustic chemical agents may cause liquefaction necrosis (alkalines) or coagulation necrosis (acids).[7] Massive, prolonged flushing with water dilutes and removes these chemicals. Hazardous substances hotlines and poison control hotlines are excellent community resources for information on the proper treatment of exposure to other chemicals.

Thermal injury can result from the extremes of heat or cold. The procedure that directs the patient to "drop, roll, and cool" (without causing frostbite) interrupts the process of a flame burn. Immediate cooling limits tissue destruction in heat injuries.[8] In a cold injury, crystallized frozen cells may survive if handled gently until rapid rewarming in water at 38.2°C (100.8°F) is completed.

Electrical burns are deceptive because the cur-

TRIAGE OF THE BURNED PATIENT

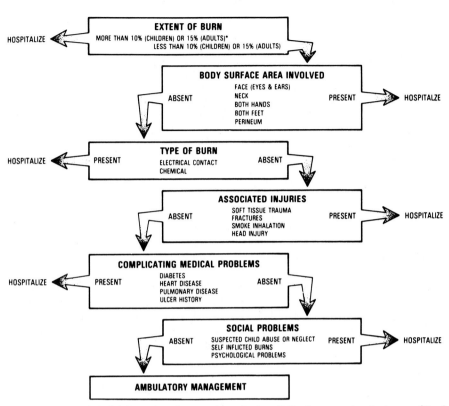

FIGURE 50–1. A decision tree is helpful to triage burn patients for hospitalization or out-patient care. (Used with permission from Wachtel, T. L.: Epidemiology, classification, initial care and administrative considerations for critically burned patients. Crit. Care Clin., 1:11, 1985.)

rent density concentrates heat damage at comparatively small entrance and exit sites. However, the current flows invisibly throughout the body along tissues with minimal electrical resistance, including neurovascular bundles and blood vessels. Sances and co-workers[9] calculate that the rise in tissue temperature is proportional to the square of the current flowing in each of the tissue compartments, multiplied by its resistivity, times the cross-sectional area, multiplied by the duration of current application. Lee and Kolodney[10] calculate joule heating seen in electrical contact burns, including the differing effects of series or parallel tissue arrangement, and heat transfer from warmer areas to cooler areas by conduction and at the skin surface by convection. The rate of cooling after an electrical injury is remarkably affected by blood flow to the tissue. They also postulate[11] that current flow causes cell death independent of heating effects through perforations in the plasma membrane. Injured cells produce inflammatory media-

tors such as thromboxane that cause microvascular coagulation, ischemia, and cell death. Robson[12] postulates that upsetting intercellular mediators such as prostaglandins leads to excess production of thromboxane and, in turn, marked microvascular vasoconstriction.

Compartment pressure syndromes may result from edema from the injury, necessitating early fasciotomies. Immediate microvascular thrombosis may necessitate amputation of involved limbs. After cardiac or respiratory arrest, with successful resuscitation, a person with an electrical injury may experience additional severe disabilities after the burn because of the associated episode of anoxia. In electrical injuries, cataracts are common if the entrance or exit of the electrical current is near the head, but these may not be noted until as late as three years following the injury.

Radiation overdose accidents by the Therac 25 linear accelerator have stimulated renewed interest in treatment of burns from radiation. Additional information is available from the Atomic Energy Agency.[13]

Body Surface Area

In burn centers, the extent of the burn is documented by a detailed chart such as the Lund-Browder chart.[14] As a rough estimate, the patient's palm print, excluding the fingers, is approximately one per cent of the body surface area. Another estimate for the adult is the rule of nines, in which the head, each arm, the front of the chest, the back of the chest, the abdomen, the lumbar back and buttocks, the front of the lower extremity, and the back of the lower extremity are each considered to be nine per cent of the body.

Associated Trauma

Other injuries associated with burns include transection of arteries, tendons or nerves; brain injury; fractures; intrathoracic or abdominal injuries; and inhalation injury. Respiratory involvement is suspected when the patient exhibits restlessness, lethargy, wheezing, rhonchi, rales, carbonaceous sputum, hoarseness, dyspnea, stridor, and mouth and nose burns. If needed, endotracheal intubation and assisted ventilation are a priority, because airway edema worsens as fluid resuscitation progresses. An additional benefit of early intubation is the freedom to administer narcotics without undue concern about respiratory depression.

Wound Depth

Most wounds treated in a hospital are of mixed depths, and even experienced surgeons have difficulty accurately determining the depth of injury by its appearance at the time of examination.[15] Burn depth (Fig. 50–2) may be reliably determined by the 21st day after the injury. Areas healed by this time are partial-thickness burns (second degree). Full-thickness areas remain unhealed and need a skin graft. Deep dermal burns may regenerate from epithelial remnants at the base of sweat and oil glands and hair follicles. However, this type of injury, which does not heal in 10 to 14 days, usually scars heavily unless excised and grafted early (Fig. 50–3).

Pathophysiology

Systemic Response

The systemic response to a large burn is observed in every organ system.[3] Skin damage impairs the body's barrier to water, bacteria, and foreign bodies and results in loss of temperature control. The cardiovascular system exhibits hypovolemic shock followed by hyperdynamic activity. Capillaries become nonselectively permeable for the first 24 hours after the injury. The hematocrit increases, and circulating platelets become more adhesive. Hyperventilation and increased oxygen consumption are noted in the pulmonary system, and later, the complications of pneumonia, pulmonary edema, or emboli may develop. Increased catabolism followed by increased anabolic activity is mediated by the endocrine system. In burns greater than 40 per cent of the body surface area, maximal rates of catecholamine synthesis are noted. Core and mean skin temperatures are well above normal because exogenous pyrogen from bacteria cell walls and endogenous pyrogen liberated from phagocytic cells circulates to the thermoregulatory area in the cerebral sympathetic center.[16] Hypermetabolism is greater following a burn than in any other injury and does not regress until the wound is closed, subsurface remodeling subsides, and hyperemic tissue begins to mature.[17] Urine urea may be as high as 40 gm per day in fed patients. Replacement by a combination of glucose and nitrogen-containing nutrients as well as lipids and insulin must be provided to avoid muscle wasting and to provide energy for healing.[17] Initially, the gastrointestinal system becomes adynamic. Ileus is not unusual, often making parenteral nutritional support necessary. Immunosuppression alters the host defense system. Kidney function may be impaired by shock, infections, antibiotic toxicity, or circulating myoglobin.

Fluid resuscitation has decreased mortality by restoring tissue perfusion. There are many formulas, for example, Parkland, Baxter, Brooke, for successful fluid replacement, based on the amount of body surface area burned and patient weight. Normal vital signs, a urine output of 50 ml per hour in adults, a normal central venous pressure, acceptable blood gas values, and normal pulmonary artery wedge pressure indicate adequate fluid administration. However, generalized edema usually necessitates escharotomies in full-thickness or circumferential burns[6] (see Fig. 50–4). Fascioto-

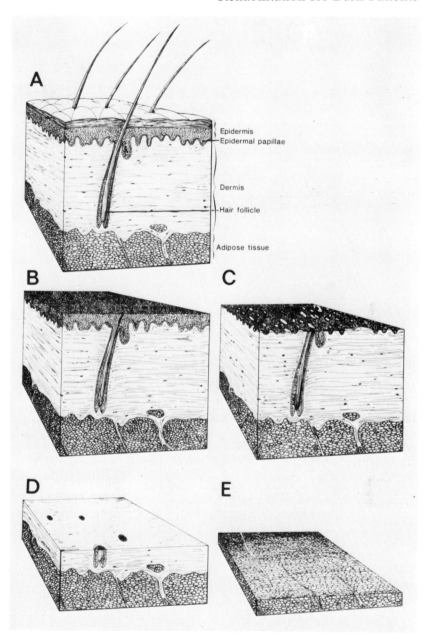

FIGURE 50–2. Depth of burns. *A,* Normal skin. *B,* Superficial partial-thickness (first degree). *C,* Superficial partial thickness (second degree). *D,* Deep partial-thickness (second degree). *E,* Full-thickness (third degree). (Used with permission from Fisher, S. V.: Rehabilitation management of burns. In Basmajian, F. V., and Kirby, R. L. [Eds.]: Medical Rehabilitation. Baltimore, Williams & Wilkins, 1984, p. 306.)

mies may be necessary to avoid compartment syndromes in electrical or very deep burns.[18]

Local Response

The local response to cell injury includes the liberation of vasoactive agents (histamine, serotonin, bradykinin, prostaglandins, leukotrienes, platelet-activating factors) and an immediate increase in interstitial osmolality.[19] Local edema and thrombosis increase ischemia and may convert partial-thickness burns to full-thickness injuries. Plasma loss through the wound accounts for 25 per cent of the total daily nitrogen loss. Heat loss through vaporization in a burn greater than 40 per cent of the total body surface area is influenced by ambient environmental temperature and by the

ELIZABETH A. RIVERS AND STEVEN V. FISHER

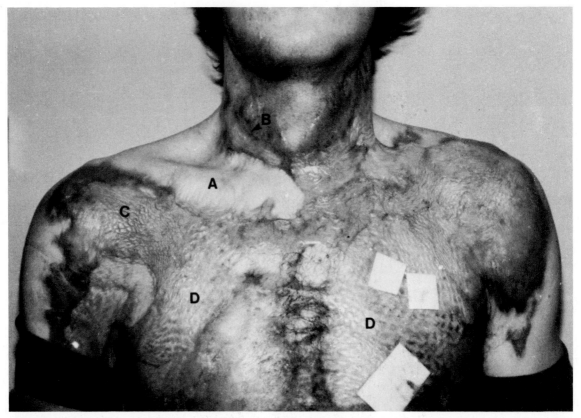

FIGURE 50–3. The appearance of grafts nine months after injury demonstrates the value of early excision. *A,* Right subclavian area excised and grafted with 1.5:1 mesh on the third day at the same time hand grafts were placed. All other grafts were placed six weeks later when the patient stabilized medically. *B,* Sheet grafts are very wrinkled. *C,* Graft made of 1.5:1 mesh is wrinkled and scarred. *D,* Graft made of 3:1 mesh took 12 months to heal durably and appears very wrinkled and scarred.

patient's inability to vasoconstrict, insulate the body, or limit heat transfer from the body's core to the surface. Therefore, the patient's treatment environment must be kept warm.[16]

Wound Healing

The goal of therapeutic wound management is to restore an intact integument. Patients with burns of up to 75 per cent of the body surface area and who are treated in a burn center may anticipate healing with skin durable enough to allow return to a meaningful role in their community. Important contributions to this improved outcome include new, safer, and more effective methods of early surgical debridement and skin grafting by experienced skilled surgeons and anesthesiologists; decreased loss of body mass and positive nitrogen balances from individualized parenteral or enteral nutritional support; improved antibiotics; individ-

ualized pharmacokinetic dosing; and early individualized rehabilitation consonant with the patient's goals.

Mechanical Cleansing

Debridement, a term coined by Napoleon's surgeon general for aggressive removal of devitalized tissue and foreign bodies, is now done in the operating room. Epluchage is the removal of devitalized burned tissue by sharp dissection performed serially with premedication for pain.[21] Gentle, bloodless eschar removal with scissors and forceps is accomplished after daily hydrotherapy. Hartford[22] compared mortality, incidence of positive blood cultures, and length of hospital stay for patients treated with immersion versus rinsing and found no statistically significant differences. The time-honored procedure of submersion[23] in the Hubbard tank provides reasonably comfortable

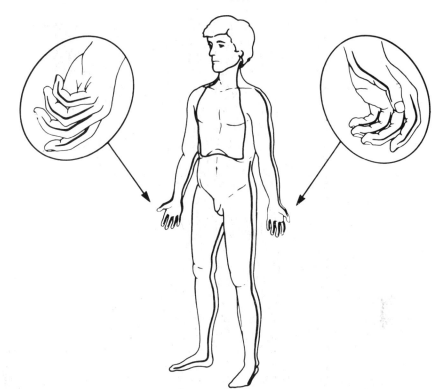

FIGURE 50–4. Preferred sites for escharotomy are shown. Incisions through the eschar on the neck are made over and parallel to the sternocleidomastoid muscle, avoiding the external jugular vein. The escharotomies may be extended onto the chest if the burn restricts respiratory excursions. (Used with permission from Wachtel, T. L.: Epidemiology, classification, initial care, and administrative considerations for critically burned patients. Crit. Care Clin., 1:16, 1985.)

soaking to remove dressings and a warm, antigravity environment for exercise. Disadvantages include contact with intestinal bacteria, which multiply in the bath water (avoided by water rinse over a tub or in bed); edema, if a body part is held in a dependent position in warm water; chilling, if the patient's entire body is exposed while leaving the tub; exposure of disfigurement, which is especially frightening to children; increased itching from edema and drying; and rebound stiffness one hour after the immersion.

Control of Systemic Infection

Infection is the most common cause of death for burned patients. The patient's immunosuppressed condition, protein-rich eschar, and loss of the protective skin barrier invite bacterial, viral, or fungal invasion. Increased attention to nutrition through the use of high-protein diets perfused enterally has improved immune function and has increased survival.[24] Circulation to the wound is compromised and, therefore, systemic antibiotics are prescribed for specific cultured infections, for positive blood cultures, or for gram-negative sepsis. Rapid excretion and hypermetabolism necessitate use of individualized, pharmacokinetic dosing to maintain adequate blood levels with minimal toxicity.

Topical Antimicrobials

Topical antimicrobials decrease wound flora. No one topical chemotherapy has been found superior to any other in terms of patient survival. Broadspectrum silver sulfadiazine is the most commonly used topical antimicrobial. It is easy to apply as a thin film over the wound or on longitudinal strips of fine mesh gauze and is the least painful agent, but sensitivity and leukopenia resulting from the use of this agent are not uncommon. Mafenide acetate (Sulfamylon) penetrates eschar well, but causes metabolic acidosis and is painful. One half per cent silver nitrate solution, nitrofurazone (Furacin), povidone-iodine, and bacitracin are also available for topical use.

Surgical Debridement and Coverage

In the 1970s, Janzekovic demonstrated that burn wounds accept skin grafts if they are tangentially excised to produce uniform punctate bleeding before infection develops. This technique has become widely accepted because it preserves dermal collagen and patent capillaries in the partially injured zone between necrosis and hyperemia.[25] In addition, the presence of inflammatory tissue or eschar on the burn surface produces hypermetabolism and immune deficiency that can lead to death. The possibility of the developement of this complication further supports the practice of early wound closure.[3] Early (1st to 10th day) excision and grafting of deep dermal burns results in a better cosmetic and functional outcome than is seen in patient's with similar wounds that are permitted to heal spontaneously. In the thin-skinned elderly patient or infant, extreme caution must be used regarding donor depth, and care must be taken to avoid a full-thickness defect. Heimbach[15] reported a decrease in the duration of hospitalization, patient mortality, sepsis, and improved pain management as additional benefits of early excision.

The experienced surgeon completely excises all necrotic tissue with sequential dermatome passes (set at $\simeq 0.010$ in) over the eschar in an attempt to minimize blood loss and operating time. Uniform punctate bleeding is seen if viable dermis remains. Excision into fat, which is less vascular, is common. Tendons and patent veins are preserved, if possible. Hemostasis is achieved with epinephrine solution, topical thrombin, pressure wraps, and the judicious use of cautery. This procedure is followed by placement of a split-thickness sheet or a meshed autograft for definitive wound closure, or an artificial skin or a temporary skin substitute. Autograft (transfer of the patient's own skin from one site to another) provides permanent coverage. The graft is secured by staples, Steristrips, or sutures and is protected with an absorptive, immobilizing, compressive bandage. Prompt wound coverage prevents desiccation. If bleeding is not well controlled or if residual devitalized epithelium is suspected, autografting may be delayed for 24 hours. The wound must be covered with a biocompatible dressing to prevent formation of a new eschar. No more than a maximum of 20 per cent of the body surface area may be excised at a time because of bleeding.

Another method of burn wound closure is the excision to the fascia followed by grafting. This method is associated with decreased blood loss and a higher percentage of graft survival.[26] However, the contouring fat does not regenerate, which leaves cosmetic disfigurement, and distal lymphedema is often seen in extremity burns that are circumferentially grafted. Grafts that permanently adhere to fascia may also limit range of motion. In addition, wrinkling makes the defect more obvious when the patient moves the underlying muscle or tendon (Fig. 50–5).

Initially, fibrin serves to adhere free grafts to the recipient bed, and cellular nourishment occurs by osmosis until inosculation (union of two vessels) and capillary penetration from the granulation bed take place. Thick grafts need more nourishment and therefore graft acceptance is less certain. Full-thickness sheet grafts are reserved for reconstructive procedures, since a full-thickness donor area must be primarily closed or closed by a split-thickness graft. For an improved cosmetic outcome, the face, neck, hands and other exposed areas may be grafted onto fat, which is vascular enough in these areas to nourish a graft and which preserves contours. When adequate donor skin for sheet grafts is available, split-thickness sheets may be aligned in units along the lines of relaxed skin tension for optimal cosmesis. Difficulty in draining seromas or hematomas is a disadvantage of sheet grafts, and, therefore, the recipient bed must be meticulously dry.

Skin-meshing devices allow even expansion of the donor skin to cover large body recipient areas. The cutaneous mesh sizes range from 1.5:1 to 9:1; the smaller expansion produces more attractive results and more rapid healing because interstices heal by epithelial migration from the margin of cutaneous decussations (intersection in the form of an X). The mesh pattern remains permanently visible. In addition, the wound heals by contraction. The raised collagen scars leave a permanent irregular surface with varied pigmentation (see Fig. 50–5). The donor skin shrinks about 20 per cent because of its elasticity, thereby concentrating the melanin, which causes it to appear darker than the original epidermis. Even grafts from areas with similar pigmentation, such as the scalp to the face, differ slightly in appearance. Final repigmentation in a deep dermal injury is often dark and unnecessarily protective.

Biological dressings substitute for skin until autografting is undertaken or until partial-thickness burns heal. Cadaver skin homografts and pigskin xenografts have been widely used to decrease pain and to improve autograft survival. These grafts permit immediate excision of massive burns, even when autografts are unavailable. Biological dressings inhibit bacterial invasion, promote granulation tissue growth, and protect exposed tendons or nerves. Cadaver homograft,[27, 28] known as allograft,

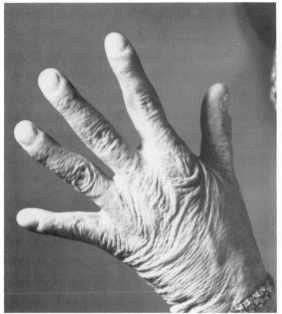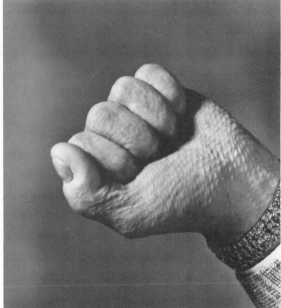

FIGURE 50–5. Appearance of 1.5:1 meshed grafts nine years after healing. Wrinkles from grafts tethered on underlying tendon, fascia, or bone call attention to disfigurement. Mesh interstices produce permanently raised scars with undesirable texture. Irregular pigmentation also makes the defect more obvious.

is temporarily vascularized, and short-term wound closure is obtained because of this vascularization. It must be removed after 7 to 21 days to prevent difficult removal or a rejection reaction. When available, fresh skin has more viable cells present, but frozen skin is also effective. The homograft functions as skin, and theoretically, at least, early excision[29] covered with homograft decreases burn hypermetabolism and its associated complications. Pigskin is a nonvascularized cover that serves as an outer epidermal barrier and an inner collagen scaffold for the granulation bed.[30] It must be changed every three to seven days to prevent a rejection reaction, difficult removal, or an infection. Sticking and drying of the graft may make exercise painful. BioBrane is a useful synthetic temporary skin substitute.[31] It is a nonallergenic and permeable membrane, which is stapled over the excised full-thickness or partial-thickness wound with slight tension to achieve contact. The outer layer is Silastic and is bonded to the tissue contact layer of collagen covered nylon. Opsite and N-Terface are other types of synthetic films. The use of artificial skin is still experimental.[32] The artificial skin graft has two layers. The dermal layer is made from cowhide collagen and shark cartilage chondroitin-6-sulfate. The patient's fibroblasts migrate into this scaffolding to form a neo-

dermis. The outer layer is composed of medical grade Silastic. When autografts become available, an equivalent portion of the Silastic is peeled away and a very thin (0.003 in) autograft is placed. Eventually, the dermal layer is absorbed. There is no permanent mesh pattern visible in the grafted tissue. This system offers great promise, especially for massive injuries for which minimal donor skin is available.

Role of Physical Medicine and Rehabilitation

The Goals of Rehabilitation

Research and practical experience have broadened knowledge of wound healing, resulting in improved care and shorter hospital stays for patients. However, the phase of wound maturation is variable, determined in large part by the person's genetic make-up. Long-time observers[34] of wound healing note that each person's course of healing is unique. Scar maturation is a long process that ends when the healed wound has no further abnormal collagen deposition, the blood vessels decrease to near-normal size, and the surface is ideally soft, flat, supple, mobile, and of proper color and durability. The skin that is severely burned will be permanently changed. It has a new texture and has obvious color changes—either hypopigmentation or hyperpigmentation. It is dry if sweat and oil glands are absent. Durability and elasticity are lessened if the dermis has been destroyed. Sensation is diminished in grafted areas and is changed in bulky or flat scars. Amputations, nerve injuries, or brain damage permanently change physical function. The rehabilitation team undertakes to minimize the effects of these changes.

Members of the physical medicine team are uniquely trained to recommend, devise, and implement cost-effective rehabilitation modalities. The physiatrist, occupational therapist, physical therapist, psychologist, social worker, and vocational counselor contribute a specific frame of reference for successful independence. The colloquial saying, "Life is what happens to you while you are planning your future" characterizes the recovery process of burn victims. Patients and families caught up in their reaction to the severe trauma find future independence difficult to imagine. Patient participation in both the healing process and independent living programs has long been encouraged by physiatrists. However, some patients who participate in rehabilitation during early wound healing view discharge as a welcome termination of burn care and pain. Often, patients eagerly anticipate what they believe is a well-deserved rest. The recalcitrant patient who endures scar control and exercise in the hospital may abandon custom-made elastic stockings, traction, total contact splints, and recommended physical activity once he or she feels safe at home. The patient's dream is that home will magically bring back the previous physical and emotional status. However, it quickly becomes obvious that achieving adequate epithelial healing for safe home care is only the beginning.[33] Returning to a productive, satisfying life in the home, the family, the work place or the school, and the community is the intensely challenging goal of rehabilitation therapy.

For the sake of discussion, rehabilitation management is divided into three overlapping phases. The first phase of recovery begins with the burn incident. It continues through the process of epithelial healing in partial-thickness injury or through debridement in full-thickness tissue destruction. Superficial burns that heal in two weeks mature during this phase. The second phase of burn recovery is the period requiring immobilization for grafting. This period begins with the application of a skin graft and continues until that graft has vascularized. The third or final recovery phase begins with the establishment of a stable epithelium covering either the healed partial-thickness or the grafted wound. This wound maturation period continues for up to two years. The recovery process continues over several years. Throughout this period, the frequent changes of a patient's condition require a process of ongoing evaluation and appropriate adjustments in the therapy program.[35]

Initially, the rehabilitation team conducts a history and physical examination to document previous injuries, the evaluation of neuromuscular and musculoskeletal function, medical conditions, left- or right-handedness, occupation, architectural barriers in the home, and who will be helping with home care.

Rehabilitation Management During Acute Care

During the early or pre-grafting burn recovery period, the goals of rehabilitation management are the following: (1) to promote wound closure and prevent infection; (2) to control edema; (3) to maintain joint and skin mobility; (4) to maintain strength and endurance; (5) to facilitate patient and family participation in therapeutic procedures that bring about wound healing and rehabilitation; and (6) to improve self-feeding and independent personal hygiene.

EXERCISE

Ambulation and active range-of-motion exercises are the most important rehabilitation modalities to introduce immediately after the injury. During this early rehabilitation phase, supervised active range-of-motion exercises orient the patient toward recovering mobility. In several burn centers, intubated patients ambulate with the aid of nurses. Transferring to a chair and walking, in addition to slow active movement through the full range of motion for each joint, will speed healing by reducing edema and also will improve the patient's confidence. Use of the Invacare wheeled walker equipped with an overhead bar (Fig. 50–6) provides upper extremity elevation and a hand grasp to reduce edema, stretch tight connective tissue on the flexor side of affected joints, and to lift the body or transferring to a chair. A progressive ambulation program is encouraged and docu-

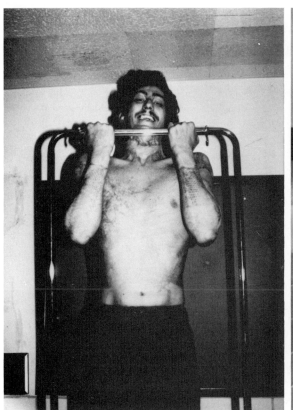
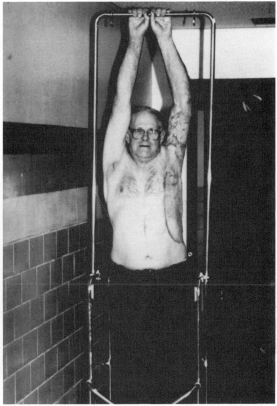

FIGURE 50–6. Invacare overhead bar with wheeled walker. *Left,* supervised pull-up exercise. *Right,* pumping overhead bar assists shoulder, elbow, and hand motion; walking laps distracts patient from discomfort.

mented. Multiple repetitions are painful and unnecessary, as is heavy resistance, at this stage of recovery. However, if the injured tissue is maintained in one position for a prolonged time, the collagen fibers begin to contract, scar tissue grows into the edematous tissues, and contractures develop rapidly.

POSITIONING

Positioning is defined as the proper arrangement of body parts. Burn patients have a high risk of developing contractures, and supervised positioning attempts to limit this complication. The patient often assumes a flexed, adducted position in an attempt to withdraw from pain. An extended position is no more painful, but moving to that position is uncomfortable. The therapist can help the patient become aware that changing positions actually relieves pain. Antideformity positioning may assist in the reduction of edema. Clinitron or KinAir beds distribute pressure on the tissue. However, they promote protraction of the shoul-

ders and thoracic kyphosis, with a subsequent reduction in vital capacity as well as flexion contractures of the hips and knees. Wedge pillows, over-bed suspension bars, deltoid aids, and elevating tables assist in alternating positions.

ORTHOSES

It is beyond the scope of this chapter to discuss all orthotic devices used for burn patients, and the reader is directed to other excellent sources.[36–41] Orthoses are an extension of positioning. They also provide tissue protection and reduction of edema. A few specific examples follow. In the burned hand, a resting wrist, finger, and thumb orthosis is used for positioning when the patient is unconscious or uncooperative. Antigravity elevation is universally used for the reduction of edema (Fig. 50–7) and orthoses are designed as adjuncts to this method. In addition, a continuous passive motion machine may be helpful to decrease swelling in the hand. Protection is given by a finger extension trough, secured with a pressure distrib-

ELIZABETH A. RIVERS AND STEVEN V. FISHER

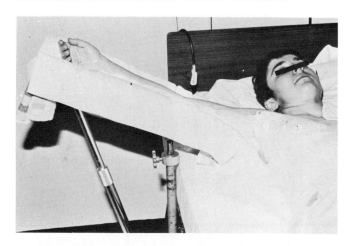

FIGURE 50–7. Abduction trough. Abduction aides attached to narrow beds are necessary to maintain proper antigravity positioning.

uting bandage, if the proximal interphalangeal joints or dorsal hoods are exposed. Other hand structures that may need protection during inactive periods are the tendons in the carpal tunnel, the oblique retinacular ligament, and the deep finger flexors. Similarly, in the lower extremities, the anterior tibialis and Achilles tendons may need protection during rest and orthotic support during activity or exercise.

When the soles of the feet are burned, double-depth, adapted footwear protects the foot by reducing pressure, which decreases pain during walking. The foam ankle-foot orthosis overcomes the weight of bedding and supports the ankle in the neutral position.

In the case of a circumoral burn, the microstomia correction orthosis should be judiciously used for exercise and for positioning.

Rehabilitation During the Period of Immobilization

During the period of immobilization in burn wound care, rehabilitation therapy goals include the following: (1) to provide an exercise program to prevent complications such as phlebitis, pneumonia, and contractures; (2) to design orthoses and to plan positioning, especially if the graft extends over a joint; (3) to decrease the incidence of hallucinations and confusion by helping family and staff provide appropriate sensory stimulation, especially if the person is on a Rotobed, KinAir, or Clinitron bed or is sensorily deprived in other ways; and (4) to reassure and educate the patient and family about the appearance of grafts and scars and the normal processes of wound healing.

EXERCISE

When a severe inflammatory process surrounds a joint, the results of three to seven days of immobility needed to allow skin graft vascularization may be disastrous. If at all possible, supervised, gentle active motion is instituted on the third to fifth day after autografting. Active antigravity exercise can usually begin earlier with other biological dressings. Range-of-motion exercises can continue in all body parts up to one joint proximal and one joint distal to the grafting.

ORTHOSES

Orthoses primarily help to immobilize and position a body part after grafting. In centers using the exposure method of graft healing, elevation, support, and protection of the grafted areas are accomplished with pillows, slings, skeletal traction, or thermoplastic splints designed to expose the graft. Safely securing a thermoplastic splint without impairing circulation may be a challenge if the burn is circumferential and extends beyond the borders of the graft.

When the healed wound is expected to be especially fragile, as it is after grafts with artificial skin, overhead, balanced suspension of the body part by skeletal traction is indicated (Fig. 50–8). The proper use of skeletal immobilization is reviewed elsewhere.[42, 43] Precautions noted include use of the proper counterbalancing weight for each individual and thoroughly investigating patient complaints.

In centers where grafts are covered with a postoperative bandage, a frequently used dressing is the bulky wrap (Fig. 50–9). This gauze pressure bandage decreases swelling and, therefore, pre-

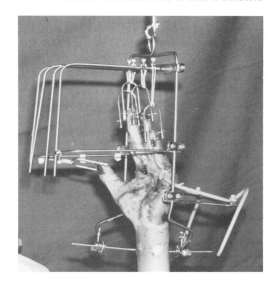

FIGURE 50–8. Hay rake traction. This configuration allows the fingers to be moved throughout the entire arc of range of motion.

vents fibroplastic proliferation into the edema and functions as an orthosis. The authors have decided to describe the bulky wrap of the hand since its management is difficult. The bandaging technique can readily be generalized for use in other body parts, especially in the extremities. Many surgeons use a single layer of nonadherent gauze that is in contact with the graft. Two dozen completely opened gauze 4 × 4 sponges are then placed into the palm, between the interdigital webs, and into the thumb web space. A dozen fluffed gauzes are

placed dorsally, and the entire bandage is held in place with a snug gauze wrap. Stability is increased if the whole bandage is reinforced with a dorsal or a palmar plaster splint, or both. The plaster should not contact the skin. A single layer of Webril cotton wrap simplifies later removal of the plaster. The orthosis may be secured with an elastic bandage wrapped with gradient pressure.

When thermoplastic splints are used, they may be fitted over a single layer of nonadherent gauze, a bulky wrap, a stent-dressing, or a wet fine-mesh

FIGURE 50–9. The bulky hand wrap. *Left,* grafts with nonadherent gauze in interdigital spaces. *Right,* finished gauze wrap ready for Webril and plaster reinforcement, if desired.

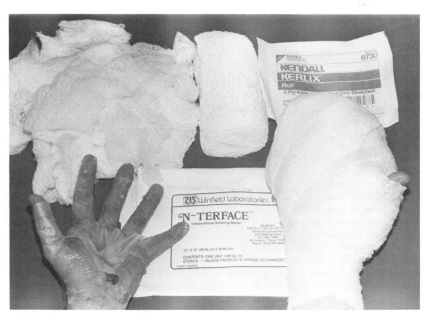

ELIZABETH A. RIVERS AND STEVEN V. FISHER

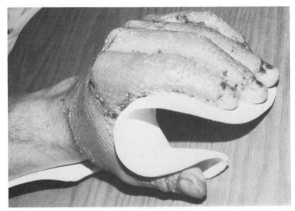

FIGURE 50–10. The postoperative hand orthosis. Wrist, metacarpophalangeal joints, interphalangeal area, and thumb are immobilized in a safe position.

gauze dressing. Any plastic splint can be cut open so wetting fluid or drainage can escape. Very wet dressings cause maceration, which may result in superficial infection. When the patient is fitted with the positioning splint under anesthesia, it is important for the body parts to be correctly aligned. It is often easier for the patient to adjust to wearing a splint after surgery, during the time maximum pain medication is being administered. After that period of adjustment, the splint often feels more comfortable, which increases patient compliance with therapy.

The postoperative hand orthosis is positioned with wrist extension at 20 degrees, metacarpophalangeal flexion at 65 degrees, interphalangeal extension at 0 degrees, and thumb abduction and rotation (Fig. 50–10). It is convenient to elevate the whole arm and splint, secured with a gauze wrap, above heart level on a foam wedge. The splint will rest inflamed tissue in the position of maximum venous return, prevent wristdrop, prevent finger metacarpophalangeal hyperextension with flexion of the proximal interphalangeal joint, and prevent thumb adduction and thumb interphalangeal hyperextension. If the patient has a complete or partial laceration of any flexor tendons in addition to the burn, the wrist must be placed in flexion to prevent the muscle tone from rupturing the healing flexor tendon. An elbow extension splint combined with a foam wedge immobilizes grafts of the antecubital or olecranon areas. Burns of the shoulders are more difficult to manage and require team consultation to achieve maximal ease of wound care with minimal trauma or shearing to the healing graft. Commercially available foam ankle-foot orthoses are convenient for immobili-

zation of the lower extremity graft. The position of this orthosis should be watched to avoid pressure on the peroneal nerve at the head of the fibula.

Rehabilitation During the Period of Maturation

During the wound maturation phase of burn healing, the goals of rehabilitation are as follows: (1) to promote return of normal strength and endurance and improve dexterity and coordination; (2) to assist in regaining full active range of joint motion; (3) to fit total contact, stretching orthoses; (4) to successfully control edema and provide antigravity positioning; (5) to minimize hypertrophic scar formation; (6) to improve independent living skills; (7) to teach compensation techniques for exposure to friction, trauma, ultraviolet light, chemical irritants, and extremes of weather or temperature; (8) to make the patient aware of sensory changes, especially in the case of denervation; (9) to have the patient successfully return to full-time participation in all school or work activities except contact sports; (10) to encourage taking part in recreational activities; (11) to help the patient return to vocational duties; and (12) to assist the patient in initiating a discussion of sexuality.

EXERCISE

Full active range of motion returns most quickly when inflammatory processes are minimal, when grafts are on dermal defects, and when the patient continues hourly elevated active motion during the day. With encouragement, the patient can move through the extremes of motion, which prevents loss of joint function and better nourishes the cartilage and the surrounding soft tissue. The object of exercise is to speed healing by improving circulation, decreasing edema, and decreasing the inflammatory response. Reciprocal pulleys, two-handed calisthenics, slow bicycling, and dowel exercises are the safest methods for providing self-directed, passive motion early after the injury. The therapist, as the coach, provides many choices, and graded programs may be written that break activity down into small enough component parts to document improvement (Fig. 50–11). Active motion and gentle terminal stretching exercises are continued despite the presence of open tendons, except for the dorsal hood mechanism over the proximal interphalangeal joint. That joint is im-

**Do exercises at least
four times a day.**

Remove splint, exercise.
Wash skin and splint; dry well.
Reapply splint after exercise.
Do not leave splint off longer
than 10 minutes.
Repeat exercises for both sides
of face.
Hold each stretch for at least
two minutes.
When skin will tolerate more
stretch, increase case size.

To keep facial tissue loose and mobile,
slowly stretch the cheek by placing a
syringe case between the teeth and into
the pouch of one cheek. The corner of the
lips on the opposite side of the mouth is
also stretched.

Stretch both corners of the lips backward.
Pull them into a large "EEE" by placing
the syringe case between the teeth and
pulling backward at the corners of the
mouth. This is the second exercise to do
with the cone-shaped stretching device
or syringe case.

The third exercise stretches the corner of the mouth.
Slide the cone between the cheek and the teeth. This
stretches one side of the lips and cheek pouch. Hold
the stretch on each side for a count of 60.

The fourth stretch uses two cones, one in
each side of the mouth. Slide one syringe
case between the teeth and the corner of
the lips on the most difficult side. Then
slide the second device in, crossing the
syringe cases at first. Both corners of
the lips and both cheek pouches stretch.
Hold for a count of 100 or longer.

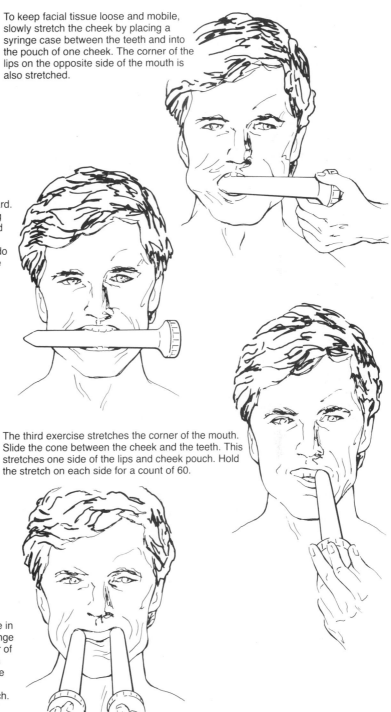

FIGURE 50–11. Written facial exercise program. It is graded by using varied circumference cylinders.

mobilized in extension until skin coverage is complete if the dorsal hood is destroyed. Otherwise, it is kept in extension until it heals or until a reconstructive surgeon recommends an alternate position.

The eyelids, mouth, neck, axilla, elbow, wrist, thumb, ankle, and hip are particularly vulnerable to contracture from the patient's inadvertent assumption of the flexed, adducted posture and from normal wound contraction (Fig. 50–12). Cocontraction of muscles in anticipation of pain slowly exacerbates progressive joint contractures.

The use of gentle terminal stretching exercises administered by the therapist helps the patient understand that the joint will slowly move further after participation in active motion exercises. Also, as the patient holds a gentle prolonged stretch, the soft tissues are lengthened and discomfort decreases. Each patient can learn to do his or her own terminal stretching exercises with the other hand or with environmental surfaces, such as stretching the heel cord by performing wall push-off exercises with the heels flat on the floor (Fig. 50–13). Prolonged, gentle manual or mechanical stretching is needed to reduce severe contractures (Fig. 50–14). The entire length of the scar band must be elongated by combined stretching of the

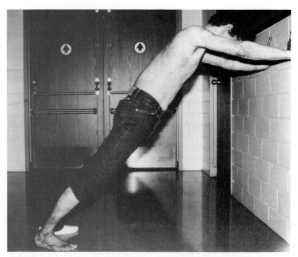

FIGURE 50–13. Wall push off. Patient with healed burn over 70 per cent of the body surface area simultaneously lengthens heel cords and improves arm strength and range of motion.

joints involved. Microscopic tears in the connective tissue will increase the inflammatory process and will slow complete healing. Therefore, the force must be gentle but must progress daily as the patient's tolerance increases and frequently needs to be accompanied by an orthosis, which preserves the increased range of motion.

Patients with greater than 50 per cent of surface area burned or who are immobile for prolonged periods are likely to develop heterotopic ossification.[44] When this complication is suspected, x-ray studies or bone scans should be performed and treatment changed accordingly.

Manual resistive exercises, progressive or regressive resistive exercises, Cybex, BTE, bicycle riding, and other therapeutic modalities done daily help the patient regain strength and endurance. Outpatient treatments have the additional benefit of establishing a pattern of leaving the protective home environment every day. Objectively documented improvement is encouraging. Attending a health club increases social contacts and may improve self-esteem as strength and endurance increase.

POSITIONING

Antigravity positioning of the burned extremities, maintained with slings, traction, and wedge pillows, assists venous return and prevents blisters and decubiti. If changed often, antigravity positioning also prevents contractures. Initially, dependent positioning will be painful. Later, a timer, set

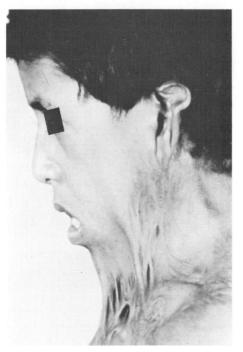

FIGURE 50–12. The end stage of hypertrophic scar and contractures. The natural course of hypertrophic scarring results in major physical and cosmetic disability.

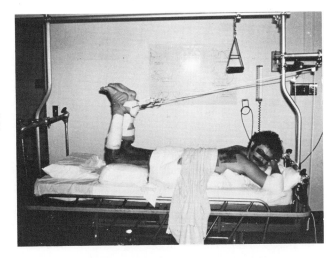

FIGURE 50–14. Active exercise. The patient may engage in active progressive strengthening exercises while still confined to bed, if the resistance is minimal.

to ring every hour reminds the patient to change the positioning of the part.

ORTHOSES

A wide variety of orthotic materials and designs are available to assist the patient in regaining functional mobility of contracted joints. Splints painlessly maintain increased range of motion and are greatly appreciated by the patient. Daily half-hour periods of painful, aggressive stretching administered by a therapist to achieve elongated connective tissue by itself are ineffective. The splint blocks undesirable motion and encourages active motion away from the restrictive orthosis. The patient controls the speed and number of repetitions of stretch. The tissue becomes warm and moist under the total contact orthosis. Skin that is softened in this way is more comfortable to stretch.

Microstomia correction appliances may be dynamic[45] or static.[46] Hartford and co-workers[47] describe an adjustable appliance that is still commercially available from Horst Buckner, Life Like Laboratories in Dallas, Texas. This splint may be used for exercise several times a day or as a night maintenance device. Rivers and colleagues[48] suggest the use of an acrylic splint (Fig. 50–15) made by a dental laboratory to conform to a dentist's positive cast of the patient's teeth. This splint preserves dental alignment when the patient is wearing a transparent orthosis or an elastic hood with a silicone insert for scar control.

Rivers[33] described a transparent orthosis for the face and neck, which has proved very successful for the management of hypertrophic scarring. The four-step process[49] of fabrication, including taking a negative facial impression, forming a positive plaster cast, fabricating a transparent plastic total contact orthosis, and fitting the orthosis, is time consuming. In the properly fitting orthosis, the scar tissue is flattened against the underlying skeletal structure, thereby minimizing hypertrophic scars. The facial contours are well preserved. An elastic hood, worn with a silicone insert, also controls facial scars (Fig. 50–16). The patient must be observed for complications of sleep apnea[50] or mandibular retraction.[33]

The patient needs nasal conformer inserts if scars develop inside the nostril. Corneal domes provide temporary protection and humidity when the patient is unable to close the eyelids either because of coma or because the skin is contracted. A microstomia stretching orthosis is used to correct microstomia and to preserve dental alignment when the scar is over the upper teeth. When any of these methods are prescribed, the patient needs two sets of facial orthoses to accommodate them. The patient benefits from written instructions (Fig. 50–17), especially when many splint combinations are used. The facial orthosis must also fit with the neck splint if both are needed (see Fig. 50–15).

In a 10 year study, Feldman and MacMillan[51] documented a declining need for reconstructive procedures related to the increased use of transparent and molded polyvinyl chloride neck orthoses. Initially, a soft foam neck splint may be an adequate reminder to extend the neck. If numerous bulky, strong scars appear, the foam compresses, allowing neck flexion, and, progressive contraction of the scars. A vinyl tubing splint has slightly greater stability, allows exercise, and

ELIZABETH A. RIVERS AND STEVEN V. FISHER

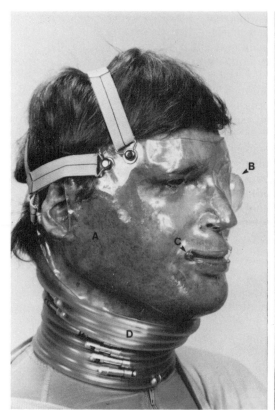 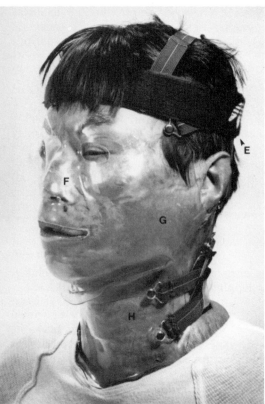

FIGURE 50–15. A variety of transparent face and neck orthoses. *A,* W-Clear night face mask maintains facial contours with added humidity domes for corneal humidification. *B,* ExpoBubble for corneal humidity and protection. *C,* MacFarlane microstomia correction appliance worn with the mask. *D,* Clear plastic tubing, secured in same order in each application, gives flexibility with some contracture control. *E,* Athletic headband may control forehead scars even without plastic. *F,* A nostril conformer controls internal scar growth. *G,* Day face mask controls scars and preserves facial contours. *H,* W-Clear total-contact neck orthosis preserves neck contours by conforming to musculature and underlying bony structure.

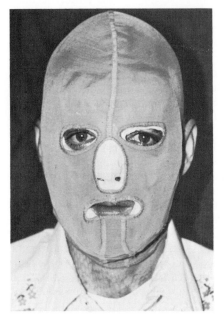

FIGURE 50–16. Elastic cloth face mask maintains pressure when combined with a silicone insert. However, patients often reject wearing it because of the grotesque appearance and because casual observers may fear the sinister appearance.

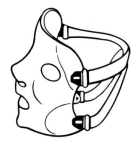

Transparent day splint.

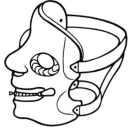

Transparent night splint.

Worn with mouth spreader, nose cones, and eye humidity domes as needed for scars.

PURPOSE: The splint maintains normal face contours, decreases pain and itching, prevents contractures, minimizes scars, and moisturizes tissue.

WEAR: Continuously, except to bathe, eat, and exercise. (20 hrs/day.)
NEVER LEAVE MASK OFF FOR LONGER THAN ONE HOUR!

APPLY: Directly to skin. (Kerlix patch if needed.)
Over or under elastic hood.

SPLINT CARE: Splint is plastic. Wipe with soapy cloth and cool water. Rinse well.
Dry thoroughly before reapplying.
Clean splint hourly, decreasing to daily.

SKIN CARE: Observe face for swelling or poor circulation. Observe skin under splint for reddened areas.
Call therapist if rash or breakdown is observed.
Do exercises thoroughly before applying splint to prevent rubbing.
Wipe splint and dry skin as needed. Reapply splint quickly.
Normal skin will gradually decrease perspiring.
Burned skin will not sweat.
Do not perforate splint in any red areas!

If you will be in sunlight, **wear sunscreen under splint** when removing for exercise.

SPLINTS ARE **FLAMMABLE.** DO NOT EXPOSE TO SOLVENTS, OPEN FLAME, OR CIGARETTES.
Problems with splint, contact: _____

FIGURE 50–17. Written face mask instructions. These clarify the use of orthoses during the frustrating time when the patient takes charge of implementing scar control.

toughens skin (Fig. 50–15). A hard plastic splint is needed 23 hours a day to preserve body contours. The anterior border of the mandible should be left free to allow neck rotation and to prevent mandibular retraction (Fig. 50–15).

The anterior and posterior axillary folds are compressed with a figure-of-eight clavicle strap. When the tissue is durable enough not to blister from friction, the strap may be worn at all times. Total contact axillary splints may be needed when the patient is inactive, preferably during sleep. Soft inserts or overlays of silicone, Hollister odor absorbent dressings, felt, or similar materials improve total contact of the splint.

Scars of the antecubital or olecranon area are challenging due to the difficulty of compressing the tissue without causing blisters or decubiti. A plaster fall-out splint improves supination as well as elbow flexion or extension, depending on the application. Later, a thermoplastic splint, secured wrist to elbow, may be used as a fall-out splint, which blocks motion in the direction of the contracture and allows relaxation away from the splint to stretch the contracture. Splints must be removed daily for active exercise, especially when the inflammatory process is active.

Hand and wrist contractures are often improved with the use of overnight plaster splints that stretch and compress the most severe contractures (Fig. 50–18). Bell[52] provides an excellent overview of

ELIZABETH A. RIVERS AND STEVEN V. FISHER

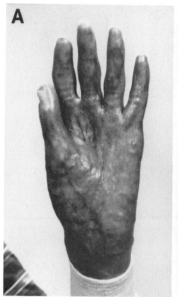
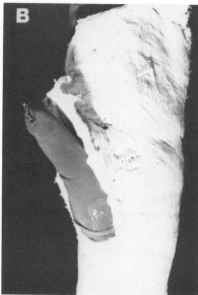
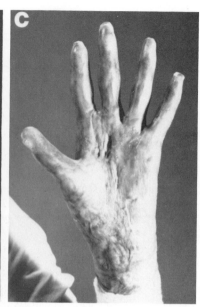

FIGURE 50–18. Contracture reduction. *A,* Decreased motion and fragile, sensitive skin at initiation of treatment. *B,* Hs cast with cut-outs for thumb carpometacarpal and metacarpophalangeal and finger extension exercise. (Prolonged stretch before application.) *C,* One week of night casting increases motion.

plaster casting for patients with hand injuries. A severe dorsal and volar burn usually needs to be stretched in both flexion and extension. Advantages of plaster splinting are its low cost and the prevention of slippage. The cast is removed, followed by prolonged stretching and active exercise and strengthening for several hours. The cast is then reapplied, stretching the tissue away from the tightest residual contractures. Used as an early adjunct to the use of active motion or a continuous passive motion machine, plaster serial casting prevents many contractures and decreases pain. The cast is usually fitted over wrinkle-free elastic gloves or tightly wrapped Webril. This method avoids edema of parts that are not included in the cast. Elastomer silicone has been used for total contact stretching. Disadvantages of this method include the development of blisters, maceration, and difficulty in keeping the elastomer odor free. Practice by the patient and family decreases risks of pinching, misplacement, and slippage when the patient independently removes and reapplies splints.

Hand-based splints control scars within the hand, including cupping, tight web space contractures and thenar eminence and hypothenar eminence contractures. These are often stretched out with a cast and later maintained by a total contact thermoplastic splint (see Fig. 50–18). Otoform K, elastomer, silicone, thermoplastic, felt, Betapile, Webril, lambs wool, Tubiton, or any soft material

may successfully stretch the thumb web and interdigital spaces. These splints are usually applied between two Isotoner gloves if the tissue is fragile. The spacers are attached to a button on the Tubigrip sleeve. This avoids a tight wrist band, which produces distal edema and also irritates the base of the thumb. Single-finger trough splints of silicone or thermoplastic are helpful in stretching flexion contractures or protecting unstable proximal interphalangeal joints (see Fig. 50–18). These splints are often worn with night casts or splints.

If scoliosis or other trunk contractures develop that are resistant to active exercise, a spinal orthosis may be indicated. Hip orthoses are rarely needed, although spica serial casting is effective, when indicated, in increasing hip motion.

Knee contractures are seldom noted when early ambulation is instituted. However, they can be treated in a manner similar to the treatment for elbow contractures. Toe extension contractures develop in growing children if the scar tissue is dense and graft interstices are relatively large. During the day, sheepskin-lined, high-top tennis or orthopedic shoes flex the toes. A steel shank prevents upward metatarsal hyperextension and a curled-toe position. This shoe needs a rocker bottom to move from foot flat to toe off. When the foot resists stretching and is serial casted into ankle dorsiflexion and toe flexion, a temporary lift on the opposite shoe will prevent hip and knee strain

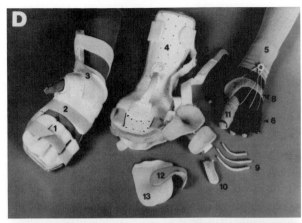

FIGURE 50–18 *Continued D,* Orthosis used seven months later to maintain softening, improved durability, and stretching. 1, Total-contact Aquaplast finger extension spacers. 2, Palmar conformer with thumb "C" bar secured to dorsal splint with elastic Velcro and "D" rings, stretching thenar/hypothenar area as well as thumb radial abduction. 3, Adjustable elastic Velcro straps with "D" ring. 4, Dorsal low temperature isoprene splint for left hand (Made by K. Russo, OTR. St. Barnabas, New Jersey.) 5, Tubigrip shaped support bandage used to secure spacers from wrist "button." 6, Isotoner glove worn over and under spacers. 7, First interosseous spacer PEG elastic wrapped over glove. 8, Elastic interdigital spacers worn over glove. 9, Otoform-K interdigital spacers wrapped in Webril worn under glove. 10, Otoform-K silicone finger trough. 11, Trough secured with elastic wrap. 12, Otoform-K day thumb web spacer worn under glove. 13, Palmar Otoform-K night compression orthosis. *E,* Hand demonstrates increased motion after four months of night casting that was accompanied by active day exercise.

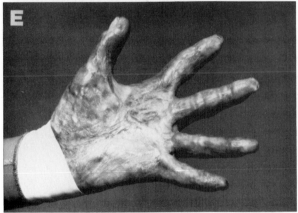

during ambulation. Usually, the cast is applied for one to four weeks at a time and is continued until active motion is maintained. Active children need a fiber glass cast reinforcement for durability. If healed tissue on the sole of the foot remains fragile, a varied density soft orthotic insert, made to conform to a plaster foot model by an orthotist, is the most satisfactory solution. The patient may need several inserts to keep the tissue dry and comfortable. Taking time to change the orthosis, the stocking, and the shoe helps prevent skin breakdown, and subsequent forced rest and immobility may prevent pain and prolonged time off from work for the healing of blistered skin.

Prosthetic fitting is outside the scope of this presentation. The interested reader is directed to an excellent overview by Meier.[53]

TISSUE COMPRESSION AND VASCULAR SUPPORT

Elevated postioning combined with external vascular support usually provides adequate control of swelling. However, for the severe circumferential burn, lymphedema may become progressively worse as the time spent in standing increases. Chronically impaired circulation with a venous stasis ulcer can be protected using Unna's paste boot under an elastic bandage. For severe unresponsive swelling, a Wright linear compression pump, may be needed. Some patients need lifelong vascular support. The least expensive commercially available support is usually successful. Moisturizing the underlying tissue several times daily is required.

CONTROL OF HYPERTROPHIC SCAR

A hypertrophic scar is a hard, red, collagenous bundle of connective tissue raised above the surface of the burn wound. Myofibroblasts remain active 24 hours a day in this hyperemic, dynamically remodeling wound until some currently unknown factor causes their regression approximately 18 months after healing.

The decrease in nourishment and oxygen supply

to the scar has been hypothesized for the hypertrophic scar coming to maturity earlier when compression is used, but this theory is undocumented.[54] An excellent review of the effects of pressure is presented elsewhere.[55] Good outcomes in controlling this type of scar tissue can be expected if the patient, family, and burn team maintain intensity, tenacity, and persistence in the care of the wound. A sense of humor is helpful to reduce patient anger during this rigorous period.

An elastic bandage wrapped in a figure-of-eight configuration is the most supportive and the least shearing technique used for fragile, newly healed epithelium. Unna's paste boot, Xeroform, or fine-mesh gauze can protect open or blistered areas. Severely damaged, edematous fingers may tolerate individual spiral Elset wraps over Unna's paste boot when a figure-of-eight bandage, Coban, PEG, or an Isotoner glove would be too abrasive. As skin becomes more durable, soft elastic cloth such as Tubigrip[56, 57] or Isotoner gloves can be donned without damage. If needed, patients may be fitted with more expensive, custom-fitted elastic garments. Barton-Carey, Bioconcepts, Medi, and Jobst are some companies that supply these garments.

The burn team must remain alert to delayed growth in children wearing elastic pressure garments for a long time period.[58]

INDEPENDENT LIVING SKILLS

Patients regain skills for activities of daily living most quickly when their goals are ascertained early in treatment (Fig. 50–19) and when a written program for practice is provided (Fig. 50–20).

COMPENSATION TECHNIQUES FOR EXPOSURE TO FRICTION OR TRAUMA, ULTRAVIOLET LIGHT, CHEMICAL IRRITANTS, AND EXTREMES OF WEATHER OR TEMPERATURE

Healed epithelium never regains its original durability, elasticity, or pigmentation (Table 50–1). In addition, many seriously burned individuals lose a considerable amount of subcutaneous fat, especially if the injury is on the palm of the hand or the sole of the foot. The subcutaneous tissue acts as a shock absorber in the unburned person and protects the underlying nerves and blood vessels. In its absence, a slight blow may cause severe pain. The radial aspect of the thumb, the elbow, the anterior tibia, and the heel and the ball of the foot

are areas especially vulnerable to injury when overlying tissue has been destroyed. A thin pad such as Lois M. Barber finger pressure wraps or padded Tubigrip under the vascular support garment improves comfort. Spenco dermal pads or biker's gloves can be used as a substitute for lost skin durability during activities. Custom orthoses are needed to cushion feet.

The skin may remain unusually fragile for a prolonged period of time. Friction or trauma of scratching, rubbing of bandages, swelling of a dependent part, chemical irritation, tape contact, or excessive heat can cause blisters. If small blisters are left intact, the protein fluid will speed healing and the external dried epithelial cells will be protective. Large blisters that spread or trap infection should be drained and the dead matter removed to speed healing. Mercurochrome is painful when applied to open areas. When applied to the surrounding healed epithelium, it may increase durability. Common sense is needed in regard to discontinuing vascular support garments. A piece of Xeroform over the open area and a small, temporary opening in the elastic garment may aid healing. Providing instruction for use of sunblock protection is very important for areas that do not regain pigment.

SENSORY CHANGES AND DENERVATION

Neuropathies and sensory abnormalities are common complications in the burn patient. Interested readers are referred to other sources for their multiple etiologies and treatment.[39, 59–61] Elderly patients have a greater risk of neuropathy.[62] Patients who are more severely burned and maintained for long periods on parenteral hyperalimentation also tend to exhibit more severe peripheral neuropathy and pain. If complaints of dysesthesias and pain are misinterpreted by the staff as manipulative behavior at about the same time pain medications are being tapered, cooperation with therapeutic modalities is undermined. Short continuance of narcotics combined with desensitization techniques undoubtedly reduce the problem. Most neuropathies resolve slowly. However, in addition to being taught desensitization and compensation techniques, the patient appreciates assistance with the reintegration of sensory information. Benson's relaxation response (discussed later) practiced daily, helps the person tune out sensations arising from the accident.[63] For some patients dysesthesias from the healed tissue become a cen-

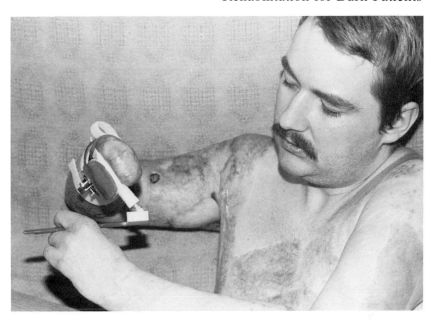

FIGURE 50–19. Inpatient practice of self-care. The patient chooses daily living activities he or she considers important. When needed, orthotics can be revised for optimal function.

tral, compelling part of their awareness. Individual counseling as well as reassurance by the physician and therapist help the patient accept that the return of sensation is a positive sign, even if the sensation is temporarily distorted. Patients slowly come to realize that the emergency has passed, and by using vision as well as tactile sensation from the burned and unburned parts, the sensory information is more quickly reintegrated.

SEXUALITY

Many patients report that regaining their sexual identity is their most important goal for recovery. They have been suddenly and traumatically shocked into realizing their vulnerability in this industrialized society. They want to deepen and strengthen relationships with a domestic partner and are afraid of rejection. They now seek satisfying, relaxing intimacy, even if that was not important before the accident. They find it reassuring when their physician initiates a matter-of-fact discussion of sex and birth control in the same way he or she discusses pain or appetite. It is important for the burned person to discuss his or her new family role as well as physical changes. Feeling secure in the family, despite physical changes, facilitates reintegration of the person's changed body image. With emotional support, the patient can assume responsibility for initiating communication with a domestic partner. Appearance, behavior, and personal hygiene reflect the level of the patient's self-esteem. Camouflage makeup[64] covers some unattractive scars or blemishes, but the person must adjust to the permanently altered texture of scars and mesh grafts. The patient's new self-image influences his or her attitude toward sex. This attitude is quickly communicated to the spouse. The partner appreciates openness. The spouse is often fearful, especially of hurting the burned partner, but is also interested in finding ways to resume mutually satisfying, pleasurable sexual activity. Understanding, communication, imagination, and experimentation can open opportunities to resume an exciting, loving relationship. Patients need reassurance that blisters caused during sexual contact are not dangerous and need not impede continuing sexual activity. Specific activities carried out leisurely, such as allowing plenty of time, holding, gentle stroking, and discussing mutual desires, will enhance intimacy between the partners.[65] For the sexually active female, birth control should be considered before menstruation resumes; the hormones produced during pregnancy increase the size and density of burn scars. Mature scars rarely interfere with pregnancy; however, scarred or lost mammary tissue may interfere with nursing. Direct injury to the penis or female genitalia is rare. When scars are present, remodeling can be assisted by compression with elastic supports and bikini-type garments that do not tent away when the patient sits down. The use of commercially available scrotal supports with wide legbands and waistbands and foam inserts and the

ELIZABETH A. RIVERS AND STEVEN V. FISHER

PATIENT'S DAILY SKILLS CHECK LIST
By discharge, all burn patients will have learned to do the following tasks independently:

	YES	NO	NEEDS MORE PRACTICE	PHN OR RELATIVE	OTHER
I. HYGIENE/GROOMING:					
Wound Care:					
Wash wound					
Apply medication					
Apply gauze					
Tub bath					
Shower					
Appropriately wash					
healed and unburned skin					
Lotion and massage					
self appropriately					
Care of overgrafted tissue					
and sweat and oil gland regrowth					
Buff-n-Puff					
Grit Soap					
Shampoo:					
Wash					
Rinse and dry hair					
Trim around open areas					
Comb and brush					
Shave:					
Remove ingrown hairs					
Toileting:					
Approach and sit on stool					
Raise and lower clothing					
Wipe self					
Clean hands					
Oral Hygiene:					
Brush teeth					
Stretch mouth					
Lotion lips					
II. DRESSING:					
Independent applying aces					
Independent in bra					
Independent donning custom (top)					
elastic garment (bottom)					
Independent					
dressing lower body,					
including tying shoes					

FIGURE 50–20. A daily living skills checklist modified for burn patients. Asking the family to assist in completing the daily skills checklist alerts them to the staff's expectation of independence.

PATIENT'S DAILY SKILLS CHECK LIST *Continued*

By discharge, all burn patients will have learned to do the following tasks independently:

	YES	NO	NEEDS MORE PRACTICE	PHN OR RELATIVE	OTHER
III. EATING:					
Feed self					
Cut meat, open milk carton,					
sugar package, butter, bread					
IV. HOMEMAKING:					
I. Meal Preparation:					
Safe with cold meal					
(milk, sandwich, apple)					
Safe with hot liquids					
(coffee, soup, etc.)					
Safe with stove top and oven					
2. Kitchen Care:					
Wash dishes					
Put away dishes					
Empty dishwasher					
Sweep floor					
Clean counters					
Clean stove and oven					
Defrost refrigerator					
3. Other:					
Make bed					
Change bed linen					
Vacuum					
Dust					
Wash windows					
Change light bulbs					
Carry and put away groceries					
Do laundry					
Mop floors					
4. Miscellaneous:					
Set and wind clock, watch					
Put coins in machines					
Handle wallet					
Sign name					
Write letter					
5. Clean bathroom					
Change toilet paper roll					

FIGURE 50–20 *Continued*

Illustration continued on following page

ELIZABETH A. RIVERS AND STEVEN V. FISHER

PATIENT'S DAILY SKILLS CHECK LIST *Continued*
By discharge, all burn patients will have learned to do the following tasks independently:

	YES	NO	NEEDS MORE PRACTICE	PHN OR RELATIVE	OTHER
V. MOBILITY:					
Walk for 10 minutes					
Run					
Stair climbing					
Ride bike					
Safe motor vehicle operation					
Safe riding bus and public transportion					
VI. RECREATIONAL ACTIVITIES:					
1. Knows precautions regarding:					
A. Fragile healed skin					
B. Sensory changes					
C. Pigmentation changes					
D. Circulatory changes					
E. Exposure to irritants, e.g., petroleum products, concrete, animal waste					
2. Initiates old or new social contacts					
3. Initiates stress-reducing physical recreation three times a week or more					
4. Initiates discussion of desires in social interaction					
5. Initiates doing things for others in family or social contacts					
VII. WORK ACTIVITIES:					
Return to old job (usually in 6 to 12 months)					
Find a new job					
Work with Vocational Rehabilitation Counselor					
VIII. RETURN TO SCHOOL:					
Able to concentrate on learning					
Takes part in non-contact sports					
IX. SEXUALITY:					
Resolving changed body image					
Initiates discussion of desires					

*Note: Patients burned and grafted to all five extremities (both arms, both legs, and head) will routinely be offered intensive therapy in the Ramsey Rehabilitation Center, supervised by Dr. Steven Fisher. They will also be offered public health nurse assistance to achieve independence at home. The parents or caretakers of all children under five years of age will be offered public health nurse assistance. Contact your social worker for help if you are interested in these services.

FIGURE 50–20 *Continued*

TABLE 50–1. Altered Wound Morphology*

ABSENT OR IMPAIRED MORPHOLOGY	CONSEQUENCES OF WOUND
Epidermis	
Stratum basale	Source for proliferating cells
Stratum spinosum	Decreased protection
Stratum granulosum	Water loss
Stratum corneum	Water loss, microorganism growth, entry of noxious agents
Melanocytes	Repeated sunburn
Dermis	
Altered collagen	Decreased tensile strength
Increased collagen	Scarring
Aging collagen	Altered surgical response
Nerves	
Affected?	Pruritus/paresthesias
Absent from affected area	Decreased sensation
Vascular System	
Impaired	Impaired
Absent from affected area	No healing (depends on area)
Fragility	Reinjury
Basement Membrane Zone	
Basal decidua and densa	Blisters
Rete pegs and dermal papillae	Blisters, fragility
Epidermal Appendages	
Sweat ducts	Impaired thermoregulation
Sebaceous glands	Loss of hair root, duct, sweat and oil glands
Hair follicle	
External lubrication?	
Fingernail bed	Malformed or absent nail
	Basal cells for proliferation absent

*From Johnson, C. L.: Wound healing and scar formation. Top. Acute Care Trauma Rehabil., 1(4):1–14, 1987.

frequent induction of erections aid in reducing penile contractures. Vigorous stretching and frequent massage with a nonviscous moisturizer are beneficial.

Interested professionals may find Milton Erickson's sexual counseling approach helpful. Erickson's approach, as described by Haley,[66] was to help couples focus on positive action. He believed that couples who have worked out an amiable way of living together before a stressful event, with positive support and commitment to each other, could resolve sexual difficulties. One of Erickson's basic premises is that the art of marriage includes achieving independence while simultaneously remaining emotionally involved with one's partner. This type of adjustment is crucial for the burned person, whose full recovery is dependent on his or her ability to capitalize on family resources.

Pain and Itch Management

Even small burns are painful and interfere with satisfying life activities while they are healing. The use of adequate analgesia without the side effect of emotional highs, to aid in comfortable exercise and self-care is influential in successful rehabilitation and patient satisfaction. Marvin[67] proposes that as myths about narcotic addiction are dispelled among health care workers and as newer drugs are developed, prevention or controlling pain using non–pain-contingent therapies will increase. Allowing cancer patients to administer their own medication and use slow-release oral morphine or pain cocktails permits a reduction in the total amount of medication needed. As more humane approaches such as this are initiated for burn patients, stress is reduced for the rehabilitation team. Specific pharmacological interventions are suggested by Ahrenholz and Solem.[68] Sometimes, when the patient requests sleeping pills and pain pills, careful physician inquiry will reveal that antidepressants, anti-inflammatory drugs or antihistamines are indicated. It is important for one doctor to be in charge of dispensing medications, since prescriptions as well as street drugs or alcohol may be inappropriately ingested by a patient. Some studies have confirmed that burn victims who are likely to abuse drugs, alcohol, or both did so before the accident.[69] Outpatient treatment in these situations may be indicated.

Behavioral interventions such as hypnosis, visualization, or relaxation procedures enhance the effect of drugs and have the additional benefit of speeding wound maturity, because improved attitudes increase rehabilitation program participation. Feelings of anger, fear, loneliness, or helplessness bring pain acutely to the patient's awareness.[70] Patients benefit from sharing personal experiences of pain relief in a trauma group led by a professional trained in group behavioral interventions.

Interventions for itching are based on the etiology of the wound. Patients are relieved to learn that the pruritus that accompanies healing deceases spontaneously in 12 months. As wound healing progresses, alternating antihistamine medications every two hours may be necessary to prevent scratching. Itchy scales, crusts, and soap residue are avoided by meticulous hygiene using plain water. Hot water is contraindicated because swelling and sweating increase pruritus. Dry tissue is moisturized with an unscented lotion. Rubbing improves venous circulation and prevents fingernails, which are prophylactically kept clean and trimmed short, from opening the skin. Lubrication and moisturization are continued, even if the rubber in compression garments deteriorates. Elastic wraps, Tubigrip, or custom garments decrease stimulation of the nerve endings by exhausting receptors and by decreasing edema. Patting, use of a vibrator or a transcutaneous electrical nerve stimulator, or cool pack application may relieve itching for several hours. Discomfort from sweat in plugged pores is reduced by air conditioning. To relieve itching, especially during stressful situations, patients should practice daily the following behavioral intervention of the relaxation response, which is modeled on the work of Benson[63]:

1. Sit quietly in a comfortable position. Choose a place where you will not be disturbed.

2. Practice while sitting on a comfortable chair with the feet flat on the floor, the hands on the legs, and the head unsupported.

3. Close your eyes.

4. Breathe through your nose. As you breathe out, say the word, "one," silently to yourself. Breathe easily and naturally.

5. Continue for approximately 20 min. You may open your eyes to check the time, but do not use an alarm. When you finish, sit quietly for several minutes, at first with your eyes closed and later with your eyes opened. Do not stand up for a few minutes.

6. Do not worry about whether you are successful in achieving a deep level of relaxation. Maintain a passive attitude and permit relaxation to occur at its own pace. Distracting thoughts are normal. When these thoughts occur, return to repeating "one."

7. Some patients report that it is difficult to judge for themselves whether this technique is working. Often after a week of consistent practice, they report feeling more alert and either losing their discomfort or becoming less aware of discomfort.

8. Patients also report that if they practice this procedure within two hours after a meal, the relaxation does not seem as satisfactory. Deep relaxation can often occur best just after awakening when the body is well rested and before any food is eaten. You may be familiar with increased dreaming when you have eaten a large meal just before going to sleep. That is one example of increased activity of the mind in response to digestion.

9. Also, this procedure may interfere with your sleep if done within three to four hours of bedtime.

Emotional Issues

Extensive burns produce one of the most devastating and dehumanizing injuries a human being can experience.[71] In addition, pre-morbid personality disorders, alcohol problems, and organic brain syndromes are observed more often in burned patients than in other patient populations.[72] Psychiatric morbidity present before the burn is associated with poor psychosocial adjustment after the occurrence of the burn.[73] It is interesting that, in an Australian pilot study, Tucker[73] found that burn severity does not efficiently predict psychosocial outcome.

The person's attributes before the burn, including physical, emotional, intellectual, social, and spiritual histories, provide initial coping skills. Additional skills are needed. Psychologists help the person to focus on the present, to regain as much control as possible, to redefine the meaning of the accident, to desensitize themselves to reminders of the injury, to deal with stress in a positive way,[74] and to gradually accept loss and trauma in a matter-of-fact way and to relegate these problems as part of the past. "Getting their feelings out," is discouraged.[75] Repeated discussion of the injury may increase the severity of post-traumatic stress disorder. Initially patients need to preserve fragile but useful coping mechanisms, including denial.[76] Anvi[77] points out that conflicts between patients and family and staff are expected in the stressful, highly technical, intensive care areas where burn injuries are treated. Mental health professionals address staff expectations as well as patient needs.

Tucker[73] also observed a high incidence of post-traumatic stress disorders among recently burned patients. This syndrome is defined in The Third Edition of the Diagnostic and Statistical Manual of Mental Disorders (abbreviated DSM III) with specific criteria.[78] The burn patient responds to a recognizable stressor that evokes the distress symptoms. In addition, the patient often experiences vivid, intrusive dreams or recollections of the incident. Other frequently noted characteristics are an exaggerated startle response, impaired memory, a reduced capacity for concentration, avoidance of reminders of the accident, and withdrawal from normal social interaction and from work. Treatment is aimed at giving the patient as many choices as reasonably possible, thereby relieving a sense of helplessness. Stress reduction strategies and goal-directed individual counseling are also beneficial. Short-term pharmacological intervention may also be appropriate.

Permanent Partial Disability

Appraising the extent of the burn injury and objectively estimating residuals that affect performance are most accurate when based on an objective evaluation[79] by an experienced physician. Rating permanent impairment is a physician's function. Disability or handicap is related to performance loss, age at occurrence of the injury, amount of education completed, economic and social situations, sexual function, and the burned person's attitude toward recovery. It is the patient's responsibility to contact both the supervisor and the physician regarding return to work. However, the physician has the final responsibility in determining when it is medically safe for the patient to resume work.

The following questions summarize burn residuals to be considered in the appraisal of the extent of disability: Do the employee's open areas contain pathogens? Is the skin intact, blistering, or thinned? Is the skin moist, supple, and resistant to low humidity? How durable is the partial thickness healed skin? How fragile are the sheet and meshed grafts? Can the skin tolerate exposure to extremes of heat and cold?[80] Does unfiltered ultraviolet light cause sunburn? How is protective repigmentation progressing? How sensitive is the healed skin to chemicals and dust? Does the employee have residual pain? Is chronic edema a problem in dependent tissues? Are joint contractures present? Do these contractures interfere with job performance? Does the employee exhibit decreased coordination and poor endurance? Is the employee's sensation changed and has he or she learned to compensate for this? Is visual impairment present? Does it interfere with job performance? Are there any changes in hearing capacity? Are scar control garments still needed? Do these garments interfere with work? Is there loss of respiratory capacity? Is grotesque disfigurement present, especially in the facial and hand areas? Can it be camouflaged? Does it interfere with job performance? Are amputations present? Is cognitive brain function changed? Is there a fear of returning to work or places where cues, such as the place of injury, are

encountered? Is the employee taking medications that interfere with alertness? When would the employee be able to safely drive an automobile?

The answers to each of the questions above, considered individually, will influence the patient's return to a former line of work. Burned or not, about one worker in 10 changes his or her occupation each year, and preparing for a new job requires a considerable investment of time and money.[81] When work site accommodations and job modifications will allow return of the injured worker to the initial position, work and income stability can be regained quickly. Safety requirements of the industry, flexibility of employers, creativity of rehabilitation counselors, and the worker's perseverance all influence the outcome of job modification.[82]

Attorneys often encourage the patient to delay return to work because of pending litigation; however, the patient sacrifices a sense of mastery and fulfilling productivity during the prolonged period of inactivity. Delaying the return to work maintains the person in a role of a patient and robs the burned person of the opportunity to improve self-esteem by contact with co-workers.[83] Chronic incompetence, loss of all expectation of regaining former status, and resignation to being honorably disabled, including accepting the stigma of reduced social and sexual adequacy, need not be inevitable.[84] The risk of this disability syndrome is decreased by early rehabilitation team intervention aimed at returning the person to a job consistent with his or her level of physical recovery. Psychological assistance to alter dreams, standards, and expectations; positive experiences; and early involvement of attorneys help patients find resilience to cope with their physical and emotional changes, overcome depression, and feel pride in themselves again. Burned people represent a tremendous economic resource. Their productivity has been interrupted, at an immense cost to all. Initiating enough rewarding activity to help them regain their satisfying pre-injury life style and prestige is the professional's challenge.

Children's Issues

Burns are one of the most common forms of child abuse seen by a physician. When the burn is a result of negligence or abuse, the child should be treated in the hospital while arrangements are made for proper care at home. The history related by the parents and the pattern of the burn are often incompatible. If this is true, the physician must report this suspicion to the hospital child investigation team. In states in which there is a child protection law, the hospital staff is freed from doing investigational tasks by the law enforcement team. Burn staff is then able to treat the child and be supportive of positive parental interaction, if it is observed.

The care of children is a challenge. Their needs differ in several ways from those of the adult. Historically, they have been undermedicated for pain. Parents may not be able to be available for much of the day. The young child's outcome is best when rehabilitation is done by the parent as much as possible, with the therapist acting as the parent's partner.

When a child is developing a contracture, some type of intervention is indicated. However, the child unrelentingly moves and wiggles in any immobilization device. It is difficult to contour a splint, cast, or dressing around the chubby arm, hand, or fingers of a young child. Catching the edge of a solid appliance against the crib sometimes dislodges even a well-fitted orthosis. Blisters, pain, and decubiti do not deter young children from persistent attempts at bandage removal. Pounding the splint or cast against a table or door is common. Stuffing food or toys into the bandage is another difficult situation. If the child removes the dressings, sucking or biting at the numb areas of injury is common. Therefore, a well-fitted, lightweight long arm or leg cast, secured to the extremity by a closed long sleeve or pajama leg, offers a relatively safe immobilization appliance.

In the hand splint, simple abduction and extension of all digits with a slight palmar arch preserves the healing tissue length as well as possible. A silicone mitt may be formed over the hand by adhering the healed tissue to a plastic sheet or a temporary positioning splint using two-sided carpet adhesive tape while pouring the dorsum of the mitt. When the silicone is set, the splint and adhesive are gently removed and the palmar part of the mitt is formed. Once the hand is immobilized in the splint or mitt, the child may ignore the injured extremity, allowing it to heal.

After the healing tissue is dry, specific contractures, such as finger flexion and thumb adduction, are noted. Serial casting is often the only way to preserve tissue length without causing blisters or distal edema. It takes 8 to 12 months of casting to achieve stable tissue. In pre-school children who need serial hand casting, the cast should extend above the elbow to prevent slippage. The cast must be tight enough to stay in place but with adequate dressing to absorb perspiration and to protect underlying tissue during cast removal.

Children desire to be active and enjoy doing things as independently as possible. They participate more willingly in the rehabilitation program when offered realistic choices, such as "Do you want to exercise your arm or your leg first?" or "Do you want to walk to the bathroom or to the TV room now?" They often prefer describing what is happening in their own words, if this is allowed. During a dressing change, it is considerate to give the child a choice, such as, "I do not know how this will feel to you. I want you to tell me what it is like—if it is cold, if it pinches, if it itches, or how it feels." Unnecessary fears are created by an adult bluntly stating that something is going to hurt and by a child's partial understanding of the treatment. It is helpful to remember that a child's ability for abstract reasoning is not well developed. For example, a child whose pet was "put to sleep" by a veterinarian may not be reassured that skin grafting will not hurt because he or she will be put to sleep. Adult therapists and physicians can reassure children by simple, clear, honest explanations of the expected course of treatment and by demonstrating genuine concern for the child's point of view.

Social Issues

Burns can happen to you, your friends, your children, or your family. Society reacts negatively to the burned person's scars and stiff gait, making it difficult to maintain an attractive, lovable, capable identity. Mass media advertising emphasizes flawlessness, and television shows sometimes portray characters in unrealistic medical situations, such as receiving perfect results from plastic surgery. America's love affair with perfect skin supports the multibillion dollar fashion and cosmetic industries. Patients recovering from burns have to learn to live comfortably in imperfect skin. These people report feeling sad and embarrassed when observers stare and make condescending or cruel remarks. They say the approval and encouragement of friends, family, and acquaintances are most influential in regaining the opportunity to experience a full and satisfying life. Despite a changed external appearance, burned persons think and feel like any other person. Professionals set the example for community members to treat the healed burned person like anyone else.

References

1. Maley, M. P.: Burn education and prevention. *In* Hummel, R. P. (Ed): Clinical Burn Therapy. Boston, John Wright-PPSG, Inc., 1982, pp. 509–540.
2. Accident Facts. Chicago, Ill. National Safety Council, 1983.
3. Demling, R. H.: Burns. N. Engl. J. Med., 313:1389–98, 1985.
4. O'Shaughnessy, E. J.: Burns. *In* Stolov, W. C., and Clowers, M. R. (Eds.): Handbook of Severe Disability. U.S. Dept. of Ed., Rehabil. Serv., 1981, pp. 409–418.
5. Eisenberg, M. G.: Burn rehabilitation introduction. *In* Eisenberg, M. G., and Grzesiak, R. C. (Eds.): Advances in Clinical Rehabilitation. Vol 1. New York, Springer, 1987, p. 176.
6. Wachtel, T. L.: Epidemiology, classification, initial care, and administrative considerations for critically burned patients. Critical Care Clin., 1:3–25, 1985.
7. Achauer, B. M., and Martinez, S. E.: Burn wound pathophysiology and care. Crit. Care Clin. 1:50, 1985.
8. Ofeigsson, R., Mitchell, R., and Patrick, R. S.: Observations on the cold water treatment of cutaneous burns. J. Pathol., 108:145, 1972.
9. Sances, A., Myklebust, J. B., Larson, S. J., Darin, J. C., Swiontek, T., Prieto, T., Chilbert, M., and Cusick, J. F.: Experimental electrical injury studies. J. Trauma, 21:589, 1981.
10. Lee, R. C., and Kolodney, M. S.: Electrical injury mechanisms: Dynamics of the thermal response. Plast. Reconstr. Surg., 5:663, 1987.
11. Lee, R. C., Kolodney, M. S.: Electrical injury mechanisms: Electrical breakdown of cell membranes. Plast. Reconstr. Surg., 5:672, 1987.
12. Robson, M. C.: Discussion. Plast Reconstr. Surg., 5:680, 1987.
13. What the General Practitioner (MD) Should Know about Medical Handling of Overexposed Individuals. IAEA-TECDOC-366 (A technical document issued by the international atomic energy agency), Vienna, 1986.
14. Lund, C. C., and Browder, N. C.: The estimation of areas of burns. Surg. Gynecol. Obstet., 79:352, 1944.
15. Heimbach, D. M., and Engrav, L. H.: Surgical Management of the Burn Wound. New York, Raven Press, 1984, p. 1.
16. Wilmore, D. W.: Metabolic changes in burns. *In* Artz, C. P., Moncrief, J. A., and Pruitt, B. A. (Eds.): Burns—A Team Approach. Philadelphia, W. B. Saunders Company, 1979, pp. 120–125.
17. Goodwin, C. W.: Metabolism and nutrition in the thermally injured patient. Crit. Care Clin., 1:97–117, 1985.
18. Masten, F. A.: Diagnosis and management of compartment syndromes. J. Bone Joint Surg., 62A:286, 1980.
19. Pruitt, B. A.: Pathology of the burn wound. *In* Wound Healing Symposium, 19th Annual Meeting, American Burn Association, Washington, D.C., April 29, 1987.
20. Johnson, C. L.: Wound healing and scar formation. Top. Acute Care Trauma Rehabil., 1:1–14, 1987.
21. Haynes, B. W., Jr: Epluchage. *In* Wound Healing Symposium, 19th Annual Meeting, American Burn Association, Washington, D.C., April 29, 1987.
22. Hartford, C. E., Panoc, C. L., and Swennson, A.: To tub or not to tub. (Abstract.) 12th Annual Meeting, American Burn Association, San Antonio, Tx., 1980.
23. Carter, P. R.: Common Hand Injuries and Infections. Philadelphia, W. B. Saunders Company, 1983.
24. Alexander, J. W., MacMillan, B. G., Stinnett, J. D., Agle, C. K., Bozlan, R. C., Fischer, J. E., Acker, J. B., Morris, M. J., and Krummel, R.: Beneficial effects of aggressive protein feeding in severely burned children. Ann. Surg., 192:505–17, 1980.
25. Warden, G. D., Saffle, J. R., and Kravitz, M.: A two-stage technique for excision and grafting following thermal injury. J. Trauma, 22:98–106, 1982.
26. Deitch, E. A.: Full fascial excision. *In* Wound Healing Symposium, 19th Annual Meeting, American Burn Association, Washington, D.C., April 29, 1987.
27. Graham, W. P., Hamilton, R. W., and Lehr, H. B.: Versatility of skin allografts—desirability of a viable frozen tissue bank. J. Trauma, 11:494–501, 1971.
28. Carney, S. A.: Generation of autograft: The state of the art. Burns Incl. Therm. Inj., 12:231, 1986.
29. Echinard, C. E., Sajdel-Sulkowska, E., Burke, P. A., and Burke, J. F.: The beneficial effects of early excision on clinical response and thymic activity after burn injury. J. Trauma, 22:560–65, 1982.
30. Silverstein, P.: The development of porcine cutaneous xenograft as a biologic dressing. *In* Wound Healing Symposium, 19th Annual Meeting, American Burn Association, Washington, D.C., April 29, 1987.
31. Robson, M.: Synthetic skin dressings: Round table discussion. J. Burn Care Rehabil., 6:66, 1985.
32. Burke, J. F., Yannas, I. V., Quimby, W. C., Bondoc, C. C., and Jung, W. K.: Successful use of a physiologically acceptable artificial skin in the treatment of extensive burn injury. Ann. Surg., 194:413, 1981.
33. Rivers, E. A.: Rehabilitation management of the burn patient. *In* Eisenberg, M. G., and Grzesiak, R. C. (Eds.): Advances in Clinical Rehabilition, Vol 1. New York, Springer, 1987, p. 177–214.
34. Brand, P., Yancy, G.: In His Image. New York, Zondervan, 1984, p. 47.
35. Giuliani, C. A., and Perry, G. A.: Factors to consider in the rehabilitation aspect of burn care. Phys. Ther., 65:619–23, 1985.
36. Wright, P. C.: Fundamentals of acute burn care and

physical therapy management. Phys. Ther., 64: 1217–31, 1984.

37. Mackin, E. J.: Prevention of complications in hand therapy. Hand Clin., 2:429–47, 1986.

38. Covey, M. H., Prestigiacomo, M. J., and Engrav, L. H.: Management of face burns. Top. Acute Care Trauma Rehabil., 1:40–49, 1987.

39. Helm, P. A., Kevorkian, C. G., Lushbaugh, M., Pullium, G., Head, M. D., and Cromes, G. F.: Burn injury: Rehabilitation management in 1982. Arch. Phys. Med. Rehabil., 63:6–16, 1982.

40. Van Straten, O., Ben Meir, P., Greber, B., and Mahler, D.: New ideas in splinting of burns. Burns. Incl. Therm. Inj., 13:66–8, 1987.

41. Pullium, G. F.: Splinting and positioning. In Fisher, S. V., and Helm P. A. (Eds.): Comprehensive Rehabilitation of Burns. Baltimore, Williams & Wilkins, 1984, pp. 64–95.

42. Harnar, T., Engrav, L., Heimbach, D., and Marvin, J. A.: Experience with skeletal immobilization and grafting of severely burned hands. J. Trauma., 25:299–302, 1985.

43. Johnson, C., O'Shaughnessy, E., Ostergren, B.: Burn Management. New York, Raven Press, 1981.

44. Teperman, P. S., Hilbert, L., Peters, W. J., and Pritzker, K. P. H.: Heteroptopic ossification in burns. J. Burn Care Rehabil., 5:283–287, 1984.

45. Conine, T. A., Carlow, D. L., and Stevenson-Moore, P.: Dynamic orthoses for the management of microstomia. J. Rehabil. Res. Dev., 24:43–48, 1987.

46. Carlow, D. L., Conine, T. A., Stevenson-Moore, P.: Static orthoses for the management of microstomia. J. Rehabil. Res. Dev., 24:35–42, 1987.

47. Hartford, C., Kealey, G., Lavelle, W. E., and Buchner, H.: An appliance to prevent and treat microstomia from burns. J. Trauma, 15:356–360, 1975.

48. Rivers, E., Collin, T., Solem, L. D., Ahrenholz, D., Fisher, S., and Macfarlane, J.: Use of a custom maxillary night splint with lateral projections in the treatment of microstomia. Proceedings of American Burn Association's Annual Meeting, Orlando, FL, 1985. (Abstract)

49. Rivers, E. A.: Management of hypertrophic scars. In Fisher, S. V., Helm, P. A. (Eds.): Comprehensive Rehabilitation of Burns. Baltimore, Williams & Wilkins, 1984, pp. 177–217.

50. Robertson, C. F., Zuker, R., Dabrowski, B., and Levinson, H.: Obstructive sleep apnea: A complication of burns to the head and neck in children. J. Burn Care Rehabil., 6:353–357, 1985.

51. Feldman, A. E., and MacMillan, B. G.: Burn injury in children: Declining need for reconstructive surgery as related to use of neck orthoses. Arch. Phys. Med. Rehabil., 61:441–449, 1980.

52. Bell, J.: Plaster of Paris, In Fess, E. (Ed.): Hand Splinting, Principles and Methods, 2nd Ed. St Louis, Mo, C V Mosby, 1985.

53. Meier, R. H., III: Amputation and prosthetic fitting. In Fisher, S. V., and Helm, P. A. (Eds.): Comprehensive Rehabilitation of Burns. Baltimore, Williams & Wilkins, 1984, pp. 267–310.

54. Page, R. E., Robertson, G. A., and Pettigrew, N. M.: Microcirculation in hypertrophic burn scars. Burns Incl. Therm. Inj., 10:64–70, 1983.

55. Jensen, L. L., and Parshley, P. F.: Postburn scar contractures: Histology and effects of pressure treatment. J. Burn Care Rehabil., 5:119–123, 1984.

56. Bruster, J. M., and Pullium, G.: Gradient pressure. Am. J. Occup. Ther., 37:485–488, 1983.

57. Rose, M. P., and Deitch, E. A.: The clinical use of a tubular compression bandage, Tubigrip, for burn-scar therapy: A critical analysis. Burns Incl. Therm. Inj., 12:58–64, 1985.

58. Leung, K. S., Cheng, J. C. Y., Ma G. F. Y., Clark, J. A., and Leung, P. C.: Complications of pressure therapy for post-burn hypertrophic scars: Biochemical analysis based on 5 patients. Burns Inc. Therm. Inj., 10:434–438, 1983.

59. Helm, P. A., Pandian, G., and Heck, E.: Neuromuscular problems in the burn patient: Cause and prevention. Arch Phys. Med. Rehabil., 66:451–453, 1985.

60. Helm, P. A.: Neuromuscular considerations. In Fisher, S. V., and Helm, P. A. (Eds.): Comprehensive Rehabilitation of Burns. Baltimore, Williams & Wilkins, 1984, pp. 235–241.

61. Jackson, L., and Keats, A. S.: Mechanism of brachial plexus palsy following anesthesia. Anesthesiology, 26:190–194, 1965.

62. Helm, P. A., Johnson, E. R., and Carlton, A. M.: Peripheral neurological problems in the acute burn patient. Burns, 3:123–125, 1976.

63. Benson, H.: Beyond the Relaxation Response. New York Times Books, 1984, p. 150.

64. Seidel, L., and Copeland, I.: The Art of Corrective Makeup. Garden City, N. Y., Doubleday & Co, 1984.

65. Mooney, T. O., Cole, T. M., and Chilgren, R. A.: Sexual options for paraplegics and quadriplegics. Boston, Little, Brown & Co, 1975.

66. Haley, J.: Uncommon Therapy. New York, W. W. Norton and Company, 1973.

67. Marvin, J. A.: Pain management. Top. Acute Care Trauma Rehabil., 1:23, 1987.

68. Ahrenholz, D. H., Solem, L. D.: Management of pain after thermal injury. In Eisenberg, M. G., and Grzesiak, R. C. (Eds.): Advances in Clinical Rehabilition, Vol 1. New York, Springer, 1987, pp. 215–229.

69. Krach, L. E., Fisher, S. V., Butzer, S. C., Rivers, E. A., Solem, L. D., Essling, M. M., and Snyder, B. D.: Electrical injury: Long-term outcome. (Abstract.) Arch. Phys. Med. Rehabil., 60:533, 1979.

70. Thompson, T. L., and Steele, B. F.: The psychological aspects of pain. In Simmons, R. C. (Ed.): Understanding Human Behavior in Health and Illness, 3rd Ed. Baltimore, Williams & Wilkins, 1985, pp. 60–67.

71. Tollison, C. D., Still, J. M., and Tollison, J. W.: The seriously burned adult: Psychologic reactions, recovery and management. Georgia Medical Assoc J. 69:121–124, 1980.

72. Kolman, P. A.: The incidence of psychopathology in burned adult patients: A critical review. J. Burns Crit. Care., 4:430–436, 1983.

73. Tucker, P.: Psychosocial problems among adult burn victims. Burns Incl. Therm. Inj., 13:7–14, 1987.

74. Bernstein, D. A., and Borkovec, P. D.: Relaxation training: A manual for the helping professions. Champaign, Il., Research Press, 1973.

75. Patterson, D. R.: Psychologic management of the burn patient. Top. Acute Care Trauma Rehabil., 1:24–39, 1987.

76. Cooper-Fraps, C., and Yerxa, E. J.: Denial: Implications of a pilot study on activity level related to sexual competence in burned adults. Am. J. Occup. Ther., 38:529–534, 1984.

77. Anvi, J.: Severe burns. Adv. Psychosom. Med. 10: 57–77, 1980.

78. American Psychiatric Association: Desk Reference to the Diagnostic Criteria from DSM-III,. Washington, D.C., American Psychiatric Association, 1982, pp. 111–112.

79. American Medical Association's Council on Scientific Affairs: Guide to the Evaluation of Permanent Impairment. Chicago, American Medical Association, 1984.

80. Ben, S. C., Tsur, H., Keren, G., and Epstein, Y.: Heat tolerance in patients with extensive healed burns. Plast. Reconstr. Surg., 67:499–504, 1981.

81. Merchandising Your Job Talents. US Dept of Labor, Employment & Training Adminstration, 1983.

82. Rivers, E.: Vocational considerations with major burn patients. Top. Acute Care Trauma Rehabil., 1:74–80, 1987.

83. Mumford, E.: The social significance of work and studies on the stress of life events. *In* Simmons, R. C. (Ed.): Understanding Human Behavior in Health and Illness, 3rd Ed. Baltimore, Williams & Wilkins, 1985, pp. 402–413.

84. Weinstein, M. W.: The concept of the disability process. Psychosomatics, 19:96, 1978.

51
Rehabilitation of Patients with Cancer

MYRON M. LaBAN

There are many complex problems that arise in the management of the cancer patient as the disease progresses from one stage to another. The specialist in physical medicine and rehabilitation, joining with medical and surgical colleagues, can contribute special skills to both the diagnosis and the management of complications related to neoplastic diseases and their treatment. The multifaceted team approach—blending the skills of the physiatrist and the physical, occupational, and speech therapists, as successfully employed in the rehabilitation of chronic neuromuscular disability—can with equal facility be utilized in the management of the cancer patient. Although the rehabilitative goals of caring for patients with syndromes of hemiplegia, paraplegia, quadriplegia, amputation, neuropathy, and myopathy may remain essentially the same, treatment time is often telescoped by progressive disease requiring frequent alterations in the staging of functional levels of locomotion and self-care. The direct or remote effects of the cancer itself, the residual effect of radical surgery, and the toxic side effects of chemoprophylaxis and radiotherapy, combined with a sympathetic understanding of the dying process, individually or collectively are challenges the physiatrist must master to become a successful member of the oncology treatment team.

Direct Involvement of an Organ

Brain

Cerebral metastasis is the most frequent neurological complication of systemic neoplasia.[1] The number of patients with brain metastasis is increasing as systemic cancers are more effectively controlled and as longevity increases. Lung and breast carcinoma are the most frequent primary tumors metastasizing to the brain, with large bowel, pancreas, and renal carcinoma also important primary tumors. Approximately 20 to 40 per cent of all tumors eventually metastasize to the brain, with 10 per cent of these cases demonstrating multiple sites of metastasis. In more than half the cases, patients with carcinoma of the lung and malignant melanoma also develop brain metastasis.

Primary tumors of the central nervous system together account for 2 to 5 per cent of all tumors, with 80 per cent of those involving the brain. Gliomas account for 50 per cent of all primary brain tumors, the majority of which are glioblastomas. Meningiomata are the most prevalent of the nongliomatous tumors. Pituitary adenomas, primarily chromophobic in origin, represent 12 to 18 per cent of intracranial neoplasms.

Most primary brain tumors of children are located in the posterior cranial fossa. Medulloblastomas and astrocytomas are each present in 30 per cent of cases, with ependymomas found in only 12 per cent.[2]

Approximately 40 per cent of patients presenting with hemiplegia secondary to brain metastasis can be restored to greater independence and to an improved quality of life during their period of survival. An additional 30 per cent gain some degree of palliation with early tumor identification followed by surgical decompression, corticosteroids, and external irradiation.[3] The symptoms of hemiparesis and aphasia may clear dramatically when compared with the often slower resolution

1102

of symptoms following a vascular occlusive episode.

Rehabilitation treatment should be initiated as soon as medically feasible. The prescription must be accommodated to reasonable goals. When an intracranial metastasis is rapidly progressive and associated with symptoms of headache, intractable focal seizures, mentation changes, and debilitating vomiting, palliative treatment programs to prevent the development of contractures, decubiti, thrombophlebitis, and malnutrition as well as bladder or bowel complications are most appropriate. Restorative or supportive rehabilitation goals utilizing proven techniques successfully employed in the noncancer patient are appropriate in those patients whose level of mentation and cardiopulmonary reserve are sufficient to tolerate the physical stress of activity. The patient's dignity and self-esteem can be maintained by encouraging self-care and recognizing often unexpressed fears of an impending loss of mentation as well as of death by acknowledging and responding to the patient's needs and wishes.

Spinal Cord

Four thousand new cases of primary spinal cord tumor are detected annually. Meningiomas and neurofibromas account for 50 per cent of all spinal cord tumors and occur most frequently at thoracic cord levels. Gliomas, primarily of the ependymoma type, represent another 23 per cent, with half arising in the filum terminale or conus medullaris. Less common are those of a miscellaneous group, which include the epidermoid and dermoid cysts as well as hemangioblastomas and chordomas.[4]

Epidural metastases with spinal cord compression are all too frequent complications of systemic cancer. Autopsy studies have demonstrated epidural metastases in over 5 per cent of all cancer patients. The most common primary sources are breast, lung, Hodgkin's disease, and prostatic carcinoma. Ninety per cent of these patients initially present with pain localized to the site of spinous metastasis. Too often, weeks to months pass before a radicular pattern of pain and weakness develops sufficient to warrant intensive diagnostic study. In 50 per cent of patients with metastatic disease, initial negative findings on x-ray studies and nuclear scan examinations can delay appropriate treatment.[5, 6] In these early stages, electromyographic examination can be useful in suggesting the presence of paraspinous muscle metastasis when the neurological, nuclear scan, and x-ray examinations are otherwise normal.[7] Computed axial tomography scanning, with or without myelography, often yields the most significant information on pathology present at the osseous-neurological interface. Magnetic resonance imaging complements both types of studies by providing superior soft tissue definition. Earlier identification and aggressive surgical or radiotherapeutic treatment of spinal metastasis are more likely to maintain independent, ambulant patients than is expectant delay. The neurological deficit can be produced by direct mechanical compression of the spinal cord or cauda equina by the tumor itself through direct hematogenous spread, usually via the venous epidural plexus of Batson or by vertebral collapse and subsequent neural compression.

Paraplegia secondary to the pressure of an epidural metastasis responds poorly to decompressive laminectomy by itself except at the level of the cauda equina, where prolonged pressure is tolerated better. Wright reported on 38 patients who were paraplegic or severely paraparetic prior to treatment. Of the 17 treated with combined radiotherapy and surgery, 50 per cent were ambulant following therapy. Twenty-one were treated by surgery alone, and only three (14 per cent) were ambulant postoperatively.[8]

A pathological fracture-dislocation compromising the spinal cord or associated with painful vertebral instability secondary to an infiltrative carcinoma should be stabilized by metallic fixation devices, sometimes in conjunction with methyl methacrylate cement. Wiring of adjacent cervical vertebral processes combined with bone fusion is used to stabilize the neck, whereas at thoracic and lumbar levels, Harrington or Knodt compression rods are similarly employed (Fig. 51–1).[9] External supports, including corsets, braces, and molded plastic jackets, are often poorly tolerated, particularly when metastases are generalized.

The prognosis for functional recovery is much better for primary spinal canal tumors such as meningiomas and neurofibromas than for metastatic tumors, even after treatment with additional high-voltage irradiation. Similarly, metastatic tumor types demonstrate a marked variability of response to treatment. Prostatic carcinoma and myeloma both are often responsive to combined surgery, chemotherapy, and irradiation, whereas breast and lung carcinomas are less so. Both of these tumors have an additional propensity for early and widespread metastasis. Radio-sensitive

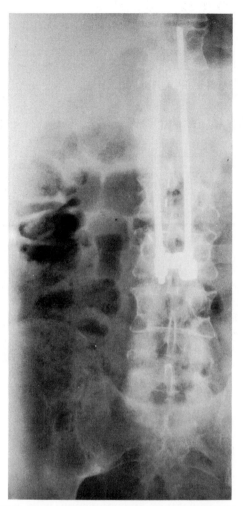

FIGURE 51–1. Surgical decompression and stabilization by Harrington rods of vertebra invaded by metastatic renal cell carcinoma.

tumors within the spinal canal, such as Ewing's sarcoma, lymphomas, neuroblastomas, and leukemias, may be effectively treated with irradiation therapy without laminectomy.[10, 11]

The paraparetic patient with cancer requires the same immediate attention to bladder, bowel, and skin care that all patients with spinal cord dysfunction demand.[12] A rehabilitation program should be initiated immediately, adjusted to the postoperative limitations of a decompressive laminectomy and the associated debilitating effects of irradiation and chemotherapy. In this regard, therapeutic decisions related to mobilization, sitting, and lower extremity weight-bearing must be made with full knowledge of the primary malignancy and evaluation of any metastases that might cause a patho-

logical fracture if therapy is too vigorous (Fig. 51–2).

Although the mechanics of rehabilitation treatment are similar to those utilized for spinal cord–injured patients, the cancer patient often has more pain and less endurance for physical treatment. An initial rapid improvement in functional self-sufficiency may be followed by a steady decline. In this regard, all equipment for activities of daily living should be ordered with the potential of managing a patient who has a disability that is likely to progress further than when initially evaluated.

Pain

To the layman, cancer is synonymous with prolonged intractable pain. Segmental neuromuscular or musculoskeletal pain is a concomitant of bone metastases, and pain may be the harbinger of an occult metastasis. Successful management of this debilitating and demoralizing symptom depends upon the identification of the anatomical site of neoplastic involvement. This task can be expedited by an understanding of the natural history of the type of tumor (Fig. 51–3).

Spinal metastases, with or without involvement of the paraspinal muscles, have associated local pain in 96 per cent of patients. Radicular or regional pain is present in 80 to 90 per cent of patients with cervical and lumbar lesions and in 55 per cent of thoracic tumors. Pain usually precedes and may mask other neurological signs and symptoms by several weeks. There may be rapid progression from minor motor deficits to total paralysis.[13] Bone metastases can cause pain, but development of this and other neurological symptoms and signs should not be attributed to the bone metastases without at least considering an associated epidural metastasis. An expanding epidural metastasis can cause a rapid and often permanent loss of motor function if not identified early and if the cord is decompressed. Well-intended but misguided treatment, including cervical traction therapy, also has the potential for accelerating paresis when an occult extradural metastasis is masked by cervical osteoarthritis (Fig. 51–4).[14]

Spinal metastasis may be vertebral, epidural, or paraspinal. Metastases that cause instability of bone produce excruciating pain by distortion of the rich supply of pain endings in the periosteum or the more meager supply of pain endings in the

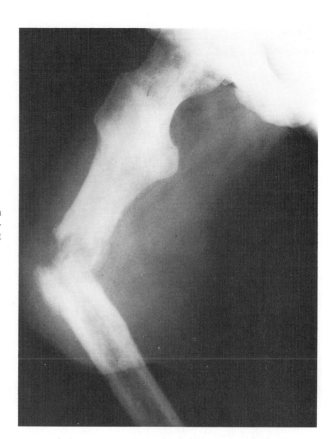

FIGURE 51–2. Flexibility exercises with stretching in a patient with chronic multiple sclerosis produced a pathological fracture in a femur invaded by metastases from occult carcinoma of the breast.

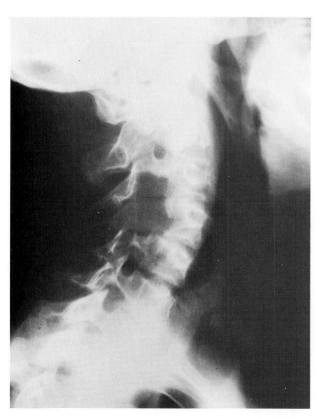

FIGURE 51–3. Invasion of cervical vertebrae by metastases from carcinoma of the esophagus one month after normal x-ray studies.

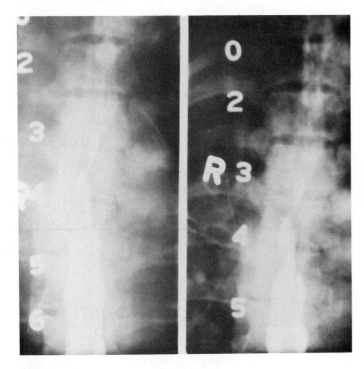

FIGURE 51–4. Epidural metastases from an occult prostatic carcinoma in a patient who developed quadriparesis while being treated with traction therapy for cervical radiculopathy.

endosteum. Metastases to vertebrae or other bones, with or without fractures or dislocations, may be identified radiographically and confirmed both by radioisotope scanning and by bone biopsy (Fig. 51–5). Epidural metastases may cause distortion of pain endings or may be silent until symptoms of myelopathic loss due to compression become evident; once suspected, confirmation can be made by myelography.

Paraspinal muscle metastasis may be identified electromyographically, even when unassociated with neurological dysfunction or x-ray evidence of metastasis.[15] A pattern of segmental paraspinal muscle denervation confined to the distribution of the posterior primary rami with sparing of the anterior rami may be the earliest objective evidence of paraspinal muscle metastasis (Fig. 51–6).

Locally invasive carcinomas of the bladder, cervix, lung, and prostate can produce lumbosacral or brachial plexus dysfunction as well as extremity-compressive mononeuropathies that can also be localized electromyographically (Fig. 51–7). In each instance, the electrodiagnostic abnormalities are confined to the anterior rami distribution, whereas the posterior rami are spared.

Whenever metastases invade a vertebra, producing sufficient instability to allow distortion of the periosteum, excruciating pain is produced. Fracture lines may or may not be evident on x-ray study. Appropriate spinal bracing to prevent this distortion gives prompt relief of pain, allowing relaxation of the associated muscle spasm and resumption of sitting and ambulation by the patient (see Chapter 27, Spinal Orthoses). Heat and massage have been used effectively since the time of Hippocrates for analgesia and the relief of muscle spasm and are followed by mobilizing exercises, leading to ambulation and the resumption of more than sedentary activity. As long as the patient is adequately braced so that there is no periosteal distortion, he or she is relatively free from pain. Transcutaneous electrical stimulation plays a role in the physiological blockade of pain perception in a significant proportion of patients. Beyond this, narcotics given on a timely schedule rather than on demand provide a steady state of analgesia.[16] Various psychotropic tricyclic drugs have also been successfully utilized in achieving a comfortable state of function. As pain is ameliorated, the patient is able to relax, to sleep at night, and to participate in his or her own rehabilitation program while concurrent high-voltage radiation or chemotherapy is used for a direct attack on the tumor.

When pain is no longer responsive to radiation therapy or chemotherapy and increased narcotics are required for comfort, ablative surgical procedures may be useful.[17] They should always be directed initially at the peripheral rather than the

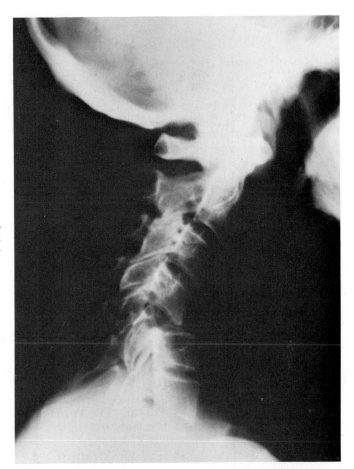

FIGURE 51–5. Vertebral collapse from metastases from primary carcinoma of the lung presenting as neck stiffness without pain in a neurologically normal patient.

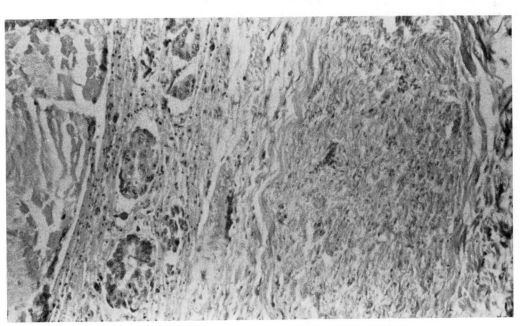

FIGURE 51–6. Metastatic adenocarcinoma in paraspinal muscle adjacent to nerve.

MYRON M. LaBAN

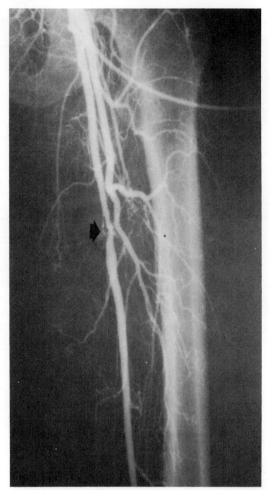

FIGURE 51–7. Adenocarcinoma associated with a partial vascular occlusion of the deep femoral vessels was identified initially by electromyographic compromise of a branch of the femoral nerve to the vastus medialis.

central nervous system. Preferred surgical procedures include chemical rhizotomy, or celiac block with alcohol. Infrequently, surgical thoracic chordotomy may be required.

Percutaneous cervical chordotomy and dorsal column electroanalgesia are both relatively new procedures. Percutaneous cervical chordotomy, unlike the open thoracic procedure, can be performed under local anesthesia. Both procedures have the potential of compromising sphincter and lower extremity control, especially when done bilaterally. Chordotomy, either percutaneous or open, is generally reserved for patients with a life expectancy of less than one year. The resultant anesthetic block fails in 40 per cent of open thoracic chordotomy procedures in less than one year

and in 100 per cent of all percutaneous cervical procedures.

Direct dorsal column electrostimulation of the low threshold touch and proprioceptive fibers of the spinal cord theoretically should inhibit pain transmitted over C fibers. Electrodes are placed on the thoracic spinal cord four to eight segments above the level of entrance of pain impulses into the cord and stimulated with one milliamp pulse at 0.3 msec duration at a frequency of 50 to 200 hertz with a subcutaneously implanted stimulator. Although direct dorsal column stimulation can raise the pain threshold 60 to 100 per cent, there are serious risks associated with subdural implantation, and this technique has been superseded largely by transcutaneous electrical stimulation.[18]

Secondary Effects of Carcinoma

Neuropathy, polymyositis, and myasthenic syndrome are frequently associated with neoplasia and may be present preceding its clinical identification. Each syndrome can be identified by electrodiagnostic studies.[19, 20]

Carcinomatous neuromyopathy, the combined clinical presentation of proximal extremity weakness and atrophy with a distal reduction of deep tendon reflexes, has been found associated with many types of neoplasms. It is, however, more likely to occur with ovarian or lung carcinoma. Evidence of neuromyopathy has been identified in 16 per cent of patients with these two neoplasms. Electrodiagnostic studies demonstrating slowing of nerve conduction velocities with proximal myopathic and distal neuropathic motor units are typical of carcinomatous neuromyopathy.

Twelve per cent of all patients with dermatomyositis have an associated malignancy. However, over the age of 50, half or more will have an associated neoplasm. In the vast majority of cases, the combined symptoms of periorbital rash and proximal extremity weakness precede those of an underlying tumor. An electromyographic pattern of muscle membrane hyperirritability associated with myopathic motor units, histologic evidence of muscle necrosis, and elevated serum enzymes is typical of this syndrome. Although there has not been a specific tumor type associated with dermatomyositis, carcinomas of the breast, lung, stomach, ovary, and uterus have been frequently reported.[21, 22]

The myasthenic syndrome most often associated

with oat cell carcinoma of the lung, although similar in its curare sensitivity and initial symptomatic complaint of weakness, differs from typical myasthenia gravis in several important features. These include sparing of the cranial muscles, decreased or absent deep tendon reflexes, and no diagnostic response to neostigmine. Tetanic nerve stimulation tests at or in excess of 20 stimuli per sec produce an increment of evoked action potentials rather than a decrement typical of myasthenia gravis at slower rates of stimulation.[23] Guanidine hydrochloride has been more effective than anticholinesterases in the management of this syndrome.

Complications of Treatment

Radiotherapy

Progressive radiation myelopathy or plexopathy following radiotherapy of malignant disease near the vertebral column is a well-recognized complication of treatment (Fig. 51–8). An irreversible transverse myelitis usually begins 9 to 12 months after irradiation. Two per cent of patients receiving

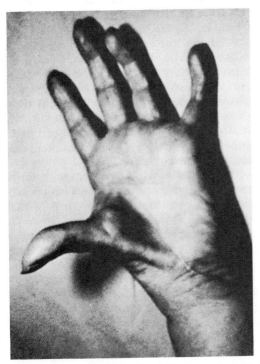

FIGURE 51–8. Postirradiation brachial plexopathy with impairment of hand function.

over 4000 rads to the spinal cord will develop paresis at the level of treatment.[24]

Less disabling but occurring with greater frequency are complaints of pain and stiffness in previous fields of irradiation treatment, especially in and around the pelvis. Arthralgias from the sacroiliac joints and the pubic symphysis are not uncommon following irradiation for endometrial carcinoma. Radiographic evidence of osteoarthritic degeneration of the underlying joints may be accompanied by electromyographic evidence of prolonged insertional potentials, and increased resistance to electrode insertion suggests fibrosis of the irradiated muscles. This particular group of patients often responds well to a combination of interarticular steroids, diathermy, and flexibility exercises.

Radiotherapy to the neck and chest has the potential for producing both progressive neurological and vascular complications. In the former instance, a denervating brachial plexopathy may develop and, in the latter case, a stenosing carotid arteritis may precipitate a late stroke syndrome.[25]

Chemotherapy

Chemotherapy of systemic cancer utilizing a multidrug approach assumes that drug effectiveness will be additive, whereas the toxicity of the individual drugs will be diminished as well as diversified.[26] Among the host of side effects of common chemotherapeutic agents are drug-specific neurological disorders, such as sensorimotor peripheral neuropathy, cranial nerve dysfunction, meningoencephalopathy, cerebellar ataxia, paraplegia, and cerebral dysfunction.[27] The use of some myelosuppressive drugs results in hemorrhages, especially when the platelet count falls below 10,000 per mm³. Disseminated intravascular coagulation and direct tumor invasion also have this potential for hemorrhage. Each can produce a secondary neurological dysfunction, especially when bleeding occurs in a closed area such as the retroperitoneal space.[28] Although usually dose-related, complications of drug therapy are highly unpredictable, with some patients demonstrating severe toxic side effects with only modest treatment dosages. When an early neuropathy is suspected, electromyography and nerve conduction velocity studies are appropriate. These studies can be both diagnostic and prognostic, permitting a more judicious administration of drug and rehabilitation therapy. Patients with a clinically symptomatic neuropathy are managed with flexibility, co-ordination, and strengthening exercises and the use of ambulatory aids and lightweight bracing when indicated.

Surgical Therapy

Surgical resection of a primary or metastatic neoplasm, whether performed as a cure or as a palliative measure, is associated with the inherent risk of complications. Cervical nerve lesions associated with facial and neck surgery and intractable cervical pain as a result of loss of supporting shoulder girdle muscle following a radical neck dissection remains a continuing challenge to reconstructive and rehabilitation treatment. Peripheral nerve and nerve plexus palsies are occasionally products of the risk associated even with meticulous dissection. Although occurring less frequently than in the past, they still occur even with less radical surgical procedures. Lymphedema following radical mastectomy may require management, but its incidence has been greatly reduced by the recent acceptance of the modified mastectomy procedure. Even in this group of patients, however, trauma to the shoulder or postoperative infection can produce lymphedema requiring intermittent pneumatic pumping supplemented by a retention sleeve and hand gauntlet.[29]

Amputation surgery may vary from localized extirpation to radical and massive amputation. Hemicorporectomy with its attendant ostomy management problems and plastic jacket supports is among the most radical of these procedures.[30] The long-established doctrine for extremity amputation for a neoplasm was transection above the joint proximal to the lesion. Today some surgeons are suggesting amputation only 5 to 8 cm proximal to a lesion visualized by x-ray film or bone scan.[31] In other instances, segmental bone resection rather than amputation has been used, with the bone segment replaced by an intramedullary rod or bone grafts in an effort to preserve the length of the extremity. These approaches have been made acceptable by the effective combination drug therapies.

The technique of immediate postoperative prosthetic fitting of the cancer patient has resulted in a faster physical and psychological recovery for both the patient and the family.[32] An additional benefit is the ease with which the temporary and permanent sockets can be modified to accommodate stump shrinkage attendant with early ambulation and ongoing chemotherapy. Although expensive, the prosthetic fitting of the young above-knee cancer amputee is no more costly than providing a prosthesis for the elderly vascular amputee. Prosthetic wearing time in both is roughly equivalent at 2.2 years.[33]

Coping

Complete restoration of function should always be the objective of rehabilitation. When not obtainable, the maintenance of functional capacity to its fullest extent remains the goal. The efforts of the rehabilitation team often can return the cancer patient to an active and productive life. Accommodative rehabilitation goals should be adapted to each patient and, if necessary, altered to the changing needs of the patient. The goals can be identified as preventive, restorative, supportive, and palliative. The goals are preventive when the complications of the malignancy or treatment can be predicted and circumvented by anticipatory treatment, e.g., contractures and decubiti. They are restorative when the disability can be managed by adequate treatment and the patient can accommodate sufficiently to minimize any residual handicap. They are supportive when daily interventional therapy improves function, preserves the patient's ability to meet self-care needs, and permits a sense of self-worth in spite of progressive disease or sustained disability. The goals are palliative when they are used to anticipate the potential for malnutrition, to retard problems of bed rest with its attendant loss of 3 per cent of physical strength per day, to manage respiratory and bowel and bladder problems, and to limit contractures and decubiti.

Accommodative rehabilitation goals can best be staged with reference to levels of care that include diagnosis and pretreatment, definitive therapy, convalescence, and transition. Each phase in the special problem of cancer requires frequent reevaluations that are necessary for the adaptation to increasing disability. The initial efforts may be directed toward ambulation and self-care. Later, it may be necessary to reorient the patient to wheelchair and assisted self-care activity.[34] Finally, supportive care of the nonmobile patient may be the objective. Early in the evaluation, every effort should be made to mobilize family and community resources to provide assistive and supportive care at home if discharge planning is to be expedited.[35] Family involvement, which is necessary at all levels of function, is imperative during final states of supportive care. Equipment such as hospital beds, wheelchairs, lifts, and other nursing items can be obtained on loan through the "cancer closet" of the local unit of the American Cancer Society. Nursing assistance provided by the Visiting Nurse Association is an invaluable adjunct to the management of the patient at home. Although instruction in patient bed care, including nutrition and skin care as well as ostomy and catheter management, should be provided to the family prior to hospital discharge, continuing supervision by the visiting nurse is essential.[35]

An awareness of the status of the cancer patient depends once again upon close and attentive follow-up. Pain during assistive joint range-of-motion exercise may be the first indicator of a new metastasis or pathological fracture. Increased weakness may be a sign of an increasing pressure myelopathy or neuromyopathy.

Through a positive, supportive approach to therapy, the rehabilitation team can help overcome the sense of despair and helplessness that accompanies the diagnosis of disseminated cancer. The patient may be less fearful of death itself than overwhelmed by the process of dying with its attendant anxieties, increasing dependency, and fear of abandonment. Patients who do not receive adequate support may withdraw completely and refuse all therapeutic overtures. However, most patients never lose hope and welcome all emotional and physical support. A continuing major effort must be made by the rehabilitation team to bridge the gulf between those who treat and cannot cure and those who will otherwise die abandoned to grief and loneliness. At the terminal stage of cancer, all medical and rehabilitation team members need to continue the efforts to maintain contact with and support of the patient so that he or she will not feel abandoned and alone.[36, 37]

Waiting is a therapeutic component of this process. Finding the right moment to provide support for the patient's concerns of family welfare—including finances, children and spouse, and finally death—may or may not occur. Once we are able to accept our own inadequacies to cure and adopt proximal waiting as a loving concomitant of the dying process, we as treating specialists can become more secure the next time we wait.[38]

References

1. Markesberg, W. R., Brooks, W. H., Gupta, G. D., and Young, A. B.: Treatment for patients with cerebral metastasis. Arch. Neurol., 35:754–756, 1978.
2. Simionescu, M. D.: Metastatic tumors of the brain. J. Neurosurg., 17:361–373, 1960.
3. Posner, J. B., and Shapiro, W. R.: The management of intracranial metastasis. In Morley, T. P. (Ed.): Current Controversies in Neurosurgery. Philadelphia, W. B. Saunders Co., 1976, pp. 356–366.
4. Epstein, B. S.: Spinal canal mass lesions. Radiol. Clin. North Am., 4:185–202, 1966.
5. Gilbert, H., Apuzzo, M., Marshall, L., Kogan, A. R., Crue, B., Wagner, J., Fuchs, K., Rush, J., Rao, A., Nussbaum, H., and Chan, P.: Neoplastic epidural spinal cord compression—A current prospective. J.A.M.A., 240:2771–2773, 1978.
6. Moersch, F. P., Winchell, McK. C., and Christoferson, L. A.: Spinal cord tumors with minimal neurologic findings. Neurology, 1:39–47, 1951.
7. LaBan, M. M., and Grant, A. E.: Occult spinal metastasis—early electromyographic manifestation. Arch. Phys. Med. Rehabil., 52:223–225, 1971.
8. Wright, R. L.: Malignant tumors of the spinal extradural space—results of surgical treatment. Ann. Surg., 157:227–231, 1963.
9. Raycroft, J. F., Hockman, R. P., and Southwick, W. O.: Metastatic tumors involving the cervical vertebrae: Surgical palliation. J. Bone Joint Surg., 60A:763–768, 1978.
10. Barron, K. D., Hirano, A., Araki, S., and Terry, R. D.: Experiences with metastatic neoplasms involving the spinal cord. Neurology, 9:91–106, 1959.
11. Millburn, L., Hibbs, G. G., and Hendrickson, F. R.: Treatment of spinal cord compression from metastatic carcinoma. Cancer, 21:447–452, 1968.
12. Dietz, J. H.: The physician's viewpoint. In Symposium on Rehabilitation and Cancer Proceedings. New York, American Cancer Society, 1969, pp. 16–22.
13. Harrington, K. D.: Metastatic disease of the spine. J. Bone Joint Surg., 68-A:1110–1115, 1986.
14. LaBan, M. M., and Meerschaert, J. R.: Quadriplegia following cervical traction in patients with occult epidural prostatic metastasis. Arch. Phys. Med. Rehabil., 56:455–458, 1975.
15. LaBan, M. M., Meerschaert, J. R., Perez, L., and Goodman, P. A.: Metastatic disease of the paraspinal muscles: Electromyographic and histopathologic correlation in early detection. Arch. Phys. Med. Rehabil., 59:34–36, 1978.
16. Foley, K. M.: The treatment of pain in the patient with cancer. CA, 36:194–215, 1986.
17. Leavens, M. E.: The neurosurgeon's role in rehabilitation of the cancer patient. In Rehabilitation of the Cancer Patient. Chicago, Year Book Medical Publishers, Inc., 1972, pp. 139–156.
18. Sykes, N. P.: Pain control in terminal cancer. Int. Disabil. Stud., 9:33–37, 1987.
19. Richardson, E. P. Jr.: Neurologic effects of cancer. In Holland, J. F., and Frei, E. III (Eds.): Cancer

Medicine. Philadelphia, Lea & Febiger, 1982, pp. 1240–1251.

20. Stefansson, K., and Arnason, G. W.: Paraneoplastic syndromes of the brain—spinal cord, nerves, and the striated muscle. *In* Moosa, A. R., Robson, M. D., and Schimpff, S. C. (Eds.): Comprehensive Textbook of Oncology. Baltimore, Williams & Wilkins, 1986, pp. 410–416.

21. Bohan, A., and Peter, J. B.: Polymyositis and dermatomyositis. N. Engl. J. Med., 292:344–347, 1975.

22. Bohan, A., and Peter, J. B.: Polymyositis and dermatomyositis. N. Engl. J. Med., 292:403–407, 1975.

23. Lambert, E. H.: Defects of neuromuscular transmission in syndromes other than myasthenia gravis. Ann. N.Y. Acad. Sci., 135:367–384, 1966.

24. Coy, P., Baker, S., and Dolman, C. L.: Progressive myelopathy due to radiation. Can. Med. Assoc. J., 100:1129–1133, 1969.

25. Lipaztein, R., Dalton, J. F., and Bloomer, W. D.: Sequelae of breast irradiation. J.A.M.A., 253:3582–3584, 1985.

26. Krakoff, I. H.: Cancer chemotherapeutic agents. CA, 27:130–143, 1977.

27. Riggs, C. E. Jr.: Clinical pharmacology of individual antineoplastic agents. *In* Moosa, A. R., Robson, M. C., and Schimpff, S. C. (Eds.): Comprehensive Textbook of Oncology. Baltimore, Williams & Wilkins, 1986, pp. 210–215.

28. Belt, R. J., Leite, C., Haas, C. D., and Stephens, R. L.: Incidence of hemorrhagic complications in patients with cancer. JAMA, 239:2571–2574, 1978.

29. Stillwell, G. K., and Redford, J. W. B.: Physical treatment of postmastectomy lymphedema. Proc. Mayo Clin., 33:1–8, 1958.

30. Easton, J. K. M., Aust, J. B., Dawson, W. J., and Kottke, F. J.: Fitting of a prosthesis on a patient after hemicorporectomy. Arch. Phys. Med. Rehabil., 44:335–337, 1963.

31. Sim, F. H., Ivins, J. C., and Pritchard, D. J.: Surgical treatment of osteogenic sarcoma at the Mayo Clinic. Cancer Treat. Rep., 62:205–211, 1978.

32. Sarmiento, A., May, B. J., Sinclair, W. F., McCullough, N. C., and Williams, E. M.: Lower-extremity amputation. The impact of immediate postsurgical prosthetic fitting. Clin. Orthop., 68:22–31, 1970.

33. Aitken, G. T.: Prosthetic fitting following amputation for bone tumor: A preliminary report. Inter-Clinic Information Bull., 3:1–2, 1964.

34. Dietz, J. H. Jr.: Rehabilitation of the patient with cancer. *In* Calabresi, P., Schein, P. S., and Rosenberg, S. A. (Eds.): Medical Oncology: Basic Principles and Clinical Management of Cancer. New York, Macmillan, 1985, pp. 1501–1522.

35. DeLisa, J. A., Miller, R. M., Melnick, R. R., Mikulic, M. A., Gerber, L. H.: Rehabilitation of the cancer patient. *In* DeVita, V. T. Jr., Hellman, S., and Rosenberg, S. A. (Eds.): Cancer; Principles and Practice of Oncology. Philadelphia, J. B. Lippincott, 1985, pp. 2155–2188.

36. Kubler-Ross, E.: On Death and Dying. New York, Macmillan Publishing Co., 1969.

37. Vanderpool, H. Y.: The ethics of terminal care. J.A.M.A., 239:850–852, 1978.

38. Connelly, J. E.: The right moment. J.A.M.A., 258:832, 1987.

52

Rehabilitation's Relationship to Inactivity

EUGEN M. HALAR / KATHLEEN R. BELL

The cardinal goal of rehabilitation medicine is to improve physical and psychosocial function in individuals with chronic disease and disability so they can attain the optimal level of independence. To achieve this aim, one must not only make a diagnosis and treat pathology and functional losses but also monitor for potential complications that could cause additional problems or disability. The prevention and treatment of complications, therefore, are among the basic tenets of the rehabilitation professional.

The complications of prolonged bed rest, immobilization, and inactivity have not always been recognized as a common cause of dysfunction. Only within the last four decades have clinicians become aware of the deleterious effects of prolonged bed rest and inactivity and of the beneficial effects of activity and exercise.

Hippocrates was the first to affirm that exercise strengthens the body, whereas inactivity leads to deterioration. Throughout early medical history, many physicians advocated activity and motion as useful tools in preserving mental and physical well-being. However, Hilton, in 1863, and later Thomas, Johns, and others profoundly influenced clinicians' attitudes in respect to activity by promoting bed rest and immobilization as a basic principle in tissue healing.[15] The "rest until healed" attitude prevailed in Western medicine during the first four decades of this century,[66] despite little evidence to support these views.[15] Until 1960, for example, it was believed that 6 weeks were necessary for complete healing of infarcted myocardium based on postmortem studies by White, and for this reason, at least six weeks of bed rest were prescribed for treatment of myocardial infarc-

tions.[123] Postural hypotension and deep venous thrombosis were quite commonly encountered in these patients. Over time, clinical experience has dictated a move toward earlier mobilization, with a resultant decrease in length of hospitalization and in the incidence of major morbidity associated with the period after myocardial infarction. The present practice of early mobilization began after World War II and was promoted by the studies of Deitrick and Taylor.[28, 113] The onset of space travel in the 1960s has given a new impetus for further investigation of the deleterious effects of prolonged inactivity. It is commonly accepted today that inactivity can cause a wide range of adverse effects on multiple organs and systems (Table 52–1).

Although these complications do not spare any age or gender, the chronically ill, aged, and disabled populations are particularly susceptible.[10] With prolonged immobilization, a normal, healthy person will develop tightness of back and extremity musculature, weakness, and osteoporosis as well as cardiovascular deconditioning. The patient with a pre-existing neurological or other chronic disease will develop the same complications but at a much accelerated rate. In this population that does not have a margin of reserve, such adverse results can cause additional functional losses.

Initially, immobility produces a reduction of functional capacity in a single organ and later affects multiple organs and body systems (Fig. 52–1). When functional capacity falls to dangerously low levels, new symptoms and signs appear.[74] For instance, reduced capacity of the musculoskeletal system will produce weakness and disuse atrophy, which will eventually produce a reduction in en-

1113

TABLE 52–1. Effects of Prolonged Bed Rest and Inactivity

SYSTEM	EFFECTS
Musculoskeletal:	Muscle weakness, atrophy, contractures, immobilization, degenerative joint disease, and osteoporosis
Cardiovascular:	Cardiovascular deconditioning, postural hypotension, and thromboembolic phenomena
Respiratory:	Ventilatory dysfunction, upper respiratory infections, and hypostatic pneumonia
Metabolic:	Androgen, growth hormone, parathyroid, insulin, electrolyte, protein, and carbohydrate metabolism changes
Genitourinary:	Stasis, urinary tract infections, and stones
Gastrointestinal:	Constipation, loss of appetite, and loss of weight
Nervous:	Sensory deprivation, anxiety, depression, confusion, intellectual dysfunction, incoordination, and motor control loss
Skin:	Pressure sore

durance, cardiovascular deconditioning, and osteoporosis.

In general, deconditioning is defined as reduced functional capacity of a body system or systems and should be considered as a separate condition (disuse syndrome) from the original process that led to curtailment of normal activity. The antithesis of deconditioning is body fitness; the maintenance of fitness should be as much a goal of the physician as treating the primary disease. Full physical fitness for daily activities and work should be part of every rehabilitation program. And so, prescribed inactivity must be specific to the affected organ and should be reversed as soon as possible.

The objective of this chapter is to review those deleterious effects of bed rest and inactivity as opposed to the beneficial effects of physical activity.

The Musculoskeletal System

Early and common manifestations of prolonged immobility are encountered in the musculoskeletal system. The deterioration of the musculoskeletal system reflects its basic purposes: standing in an erect position, performing bipedal ambulation, and utilizing the upper limbs for activities of daily living. Static standing results in a 16 to 19 per cent increase in energy expenditure as compared with lying quietly. During locomotion or strenuous physical activity, the metabolic rate of muscle can increase 50 to 100 times that at rest.[14, 20, 56] This increase in the metabolic rate, in turn, causes a 15- to 20-fold increment in muscle blood supply and triggers a strong cardiopulmonary response. The efficiency of the cardiopulmonary response to muscle work depends upon the frequency with which the maximal functional capacity of muscle is approached. Because of this interaction, the maximal cardiovascular response gradually declines with reduced physical activity.[89, 93, 109] This decline of musculoskeletal functional capacity is enhanced in the chronically ill or disabled individuals who are maintained at bed rest because of pain or pathology of other organs.

Prolonged inactivity and bed rest will invariably cause a wide range of adverse musculoskeletal effects, among which disuse weakness, contractures, degenerative joint disease, and immobilization osteoporosis are the most prominent.

VICIOUS CIRCLE OF INACTIVITY

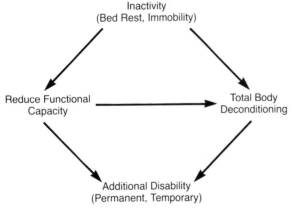

FIGURE 52–1. Prolonged inactivity and bed rest cause a reduction in the functional capacity of organs and systems until new symptoms and signs of body deconditioning appear. If inactivity is not replaced with activity, the reduction of function will lead to disability.

Weakness and Disuse Atrophy

Inactivity directly affects muscular strength, endurance, and stamina. In the recumbent position, muscle activity is minimal and the force exerted by gravity on the bones and supportive connective tissues is reduced. At complete and prolonged bed rest, a muscle will lose 10 to 15 per cent of strength per week and 50 per cent in three to five weeks. In two months, muscle bulk may shrink to half the original size.[89] The histological changes seen in muscle by electron microscopy after six weeks of immobilization are fiber degeneration and an increased proportion of fat and fibrous tissue.[12, 87] The first muscles to become weak and atrophic are the muscles of the lower extremities and trunk that are used to resist gravity. In a classic study, Deitrick described muscular weakness in healthy subjects after four to six weeks of enforced bed rest.[28] The greatest loss of strength was in the gastrocnemius-soleus muscle (20.8 per cent), followed by the anterior tibialis muscle (13.3 per cent), and the shoulder girdle and biceps muscles (8.7 and 6.6 per cent). There was no detectable loss in strength of the intrinsic hand muscles. This reduction in strength was accompanied by muscular atrophy, demonstrated by circumference and cross-sectional measurements (Table 52–2).

Weakness of the quadriceps, glutei, and back extensor muscles particularly affects climbing stairs or prolonged ambulation. Difficulty in performing activities of daily living and poor work tolerance may result from generalized muscle weakness. Other common consequences include muscular pain, backaches, unsteadiness of gait, and falls.*

*See references 29, 30, 38, 41, and 58.

TABLE 52–2. Histochemical and Metabolic Changes in the Muscle Following Prolonged Inactivity*

CHANGES IN MUSCLE FOLLOWING INACTIVITY
Reduced:
    Cross section of biopsied muscle fiber size (42 per cent)
        Predominant type I muscle fiber atrophy
    Oxidative enzymes
        Succinyl dehydrogenase
        Creatine phosphokinase
    Storage of fuel sources
        Creatine
        Glycogen
        VO_2 max consumption
    Intracellular water content
        Increase in extracellular water content

*Morphological changes predominate, although histochemical changes are also found.

A number of alterations in physiological parameters can be seen in muscle with prolonged inactivity. Oxidative enzymatic activity, in particular, is adversely affected, resulting in lowered tolerance to oxygen debt and earlier and longer accumulation of lactic acid.[37, 65]

Early studies[3, 26] demonstrated that bed rest was associated with a catabolic state, resulting in increased urinary elimination of nitrogen. The trigger for this negative nitrogen balance is still unknown; degradation of muscle protein and reduced synthesis of contractile proteins have been implicated. Recently, evidence for calcium-activated proteolytic enzymes located on the sarcolemma has emerged. Still other theories for muscular atrophy and degeneration have included alterations in the influence of growth factors (for instance, fibroblast or epidermal growth factor) or a reduction in sarcolemmal binding sites.[11, 12, 50]

Muscular strength varies widely in each individual and is directly related to the activity of the neuromuscular system. Exercise is the specific physiological stimulus that can increase functional capacity and reverse disuse atrophy and muscular weakness if the appropriate intensity, frequency, and duration are used.[93, 109]

Using submaximal exercise (65 to 75 per cent of maximum), one can reverse disuse weakness at a rate of 6 per cent per week, a significantly slower rate than is seen for the original loss.[89] Isometric exercises produce an increase in muscle strength but their effects on endurance and cardiovascular conditioning are suboptimal. Isotonic exercises, on the other hand, significantly improve the functional capacity of the musculoskeletal and cardiovascular systems.[55, 57] The increase in power can be as high as 20 to 40 per cent per week in healthy subjects.[9, 14, 109]

After a few weeks' delay, an increase in muscular size will follow an increase in power. This increase in muscular mass is mainly due to the enlargement of individual fibers, which can reach a 50 per cent increase in the cross-sectional examination, and an increase in the capillary density of muscle. Histochemical analysis has demonstrated that the mitochondrial volume per muscle fiber and oxidative enzymatic activity are also increased (Table 52–3).*

Several mechanisms are responsible for the increase in muscle functional capacity. Higher capillary density and increased blood flow through the muscle prolong the transit of blood, allowing in-

*See references 8, 11, 12, 37, and 65.

EUGEN M. HALAR AND KATHLEEN R. BELL

TABLE 52–3. Known Effects of Aerobic Exercise on Body Systems

SYSTEM	EFFECTS
Muscle	
Increased:	Muscle strength, endurance, and work and exercise tolerance
	Oxygen utilization
	Capillary density
	Oxidative enzyme activity
Reduced:	Lactic acid production at given VO_2 max
Cardiovascular	
Increased:	Left ventricular end-diastolic volume
	Heart stroke volume
	Peripheral blood flow
	Cardiac muscle efficiency
	Fibrinolysis
Reduced:	Heart rate at given oxygen uptake
	Blood pressure
	Heart rate/blood pressure product
	Peripheral vascular resistance
	Platelet aggregation
Metabolic (hormonal)	
Increased:	High-density lipoprotein
	Utilization of free fatty acid
	Tolerance to heat
	Endorphins
Reduced:	Triglycerides
	Fasting plasma glucose level
General:	Increase in work capacity
	Prevention of osteoporosis

creased absorption of nutrients and oxygen. The muscle itself shows elevated oxidative enzyme activity, with improved utilization of pyruvates, fatty acids, and ketones. The proportional increase in free fatty acid utilization reduces the demand for glucose, thus preserving the storage and reserves of glycogen. This increase in reserves, together with better utilization of high-energy nutrients, significantly contributes to muscular endurance.[95] Muscles should be used regularly if their normal functional capacity is to be maintained.

PREVENTION AND REMOBILIZATION

Disuse weakness and atrophy are most effectively treated by prevention, particularly since the extent of weakness and atrophy in subjects with pre-existing chronic disease is difficult to ascertain. Early mobilization, therapeutic exercises, and functional training are the simplest and most effective methods of prevention. Contraction of a muscle at 20 to 30 per cent of maximal strength for a few seconds a day will maintain its strength. In healthy subjects, contractions at half of maximal strength for one second a day have also been shown to be effective.[89, 108, 109] Electrical stimulation may

be used in the case of an isolated immobilized muscle or muscle group to prevent loss of strength and bulk. For instance, stimulation could be applied to the quadriceps muscle if it is encased in a long leg cast, preserving strength and shortening the rehabilitation period after immobilization.[51]

Contractures

In general terms, a contracture is defined as the lack of full passive range of motion resulting from joint, muscle, or soft tissue limitations. Contractures can be divided into three categories according to the anatomical location of pathological changes: arthrogenic, muscular (myogenic), and connective tissue contractures (Table 52–4). Of these groups, myogenic and soft tissue contractures are most frequently associated with immobility. Although other conditions predispose the patient to contracture, the single most frequent causative factor is the absence of mobilization at a joint. Three basic factors play an important role in the development of contracture: limb position, duration of immobilization, and mobilization of unaffected parts. The addition of contracture at any joint will reduce

TABLE 52–4. Effects of Immobility and Musculoskeletal Conditions on the Development of Contractures*

PRIMARY FACTORS	SECONDARY FACTORS	ADVERSE EFFECTS
1. Muscle Conditions		
A. Intrinsic	Pain, muscle fibrosis, lack of stretch and mobility	1. Myogenic contractures
1. Trauma		
2. Inflammation		Structural
3. Degeneration		
B. Extrinsic Factor		
1. Spasticity	Imbalanced muscles, ill-adapted joint position, and reduced mobility	Extrinsic
2. Flaccid paralysis		
3. Positional, mechanical		
2. Joint Conditions		
A. Cartilage damage	Pain, effusion, splinting, and lack of motion	2. Arthrogenic contracture
1. Trauma		
2. Inflammation		
3. Infection		
4. Immobilization		
B. Capsular fibrosis	Pain, splinting, and lack of stretch	Capsular
C. Joint soft tissue, ligaments	Pain and lack of stretch (mobility)	Joint soft tissue
3. Soft Tissue Conditions		
A. Skin, subcutaneous fibrosis (burns)	Mechanical resistance to motion and pain	3. Soft tissue contracture
B. Tendon, aponeurosis	Pain, fibrosis, and reduced motion	Tendinous, soft tissue
1. Trauma		
2. Inflammation		
C. Calcifications (heterotopic)	Resistance to motion and pain	

*Pathological changes in tissue and body immobility together enhance the onset and progression of joint contracture. For example, if pain is present and splinting occurs, reduced mobility leads to the development of contractures. If the joint is placed in a full-flexed position and range of motion is not allowed, shortening of the muscles and soft tissue around the joint causes contracture.

mobility and the ability to perform activities of daily living, especially in persons with disabling neuromuscular conditions.

Contracture of the hip flexors reduces extension, shortens stride, and requires the patient to walk on the ball of the foot with an increased lumbar lordosis and a subsequent increase in energy consumption. For biomechanical reasons, flexion contractures of the hip cause the hamstring muscle to become relatively shorter, which, in turn, flexes the knee. It is not uncommon to see the patient with a contracture at the hip develop knee and ankle-joint limitations (Fig. 52–2). Hip extension contractures with marked limitation of flexion are not encountered frequently. Both wheelchair mobility and car transfers are impaired in advanced extension contractures of the lower extremity.

The most common causes of contractures of the knee joint are shortening of the hamstrings and soft tissue tightness behind the knee. If a flexion contracture of the knee is 30 degrees or greater, the quadriceps, hamstrings, and gastrocnemius muscles must work harder during the stance phase of the gait cycle (e.g., the work of the quadriceps muscle is increased by 50 per cent). This increases overall energy consumption during ambulation and reduces endurance.

Tightness of the gastrocnemius-soleus muscle is the most frequent cause of plantar flexion contracture (Fig. 52–3). If a contracture causes plantar flexion of the ankle, two adjacent joints, the knee and metatarsal joints, withstand greater stress during weight-bearing. Tightness of the gastrocnemius-soleus muscle pulls the knee joint into extension, leading to genu recurvatum and degenerative changes in the knee joint. Plantar flexor contracture causes an absence of heel strike and reduces the push off phase of gait.

Contracture of the upper extremity may cause impairment of functions such as reaching, dressing,

EUGEN M. HALAR AND KATHLEEN R. BELL

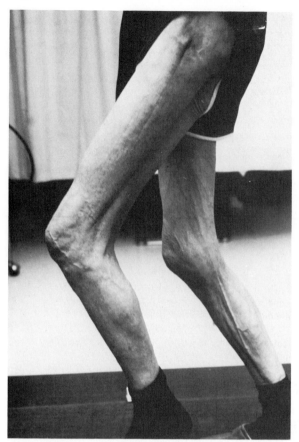

FIGURE 52–2. Patient with hip and knee flexion contracture having difficulties in ambulation. The patient developed hip flexion contracture after an intertrochanteric fracture. Subsequent tightness of the hamstrings, and the development of soft tissue behind the knee followed.

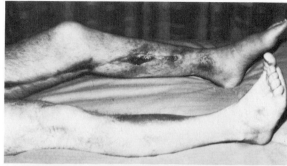

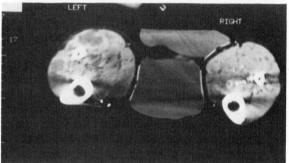

FIGURE 52–3. A patient with knee and plantar flexion contracture due to ischemic infarction of the gastrocnemius muscle. The patient developed a sudden onset of foot drop with no apparent cause. Subsequently, he developed a myocardial infarction and underwent coronary artery bypass graft surgery. His donor site on the left leg showed no healing, and secondary closure was allowed. Several weeks later, the patient developed swelling and a palpable, painful mass in the left gastrocnemius muscle. Computerized tomography (CT) showed infarcted gastrocnemius and anterior tibialis muscles. The patient underwent femoral-to-femoral bypass graft surgery. The patient's open wound healed, but he continued to have fixed contractures of the ankle and left knee. CT scan shows the infarcted area in the anterior tibialis and gastrocnemius muscles.

grooming, eating, and the performance of fine motor tasks.

It is important to determine which structures in the joint, muscle, or soft tissue are contracted and what underlying mechanisms play a part in the development of contracture so that treatment can be appropriately directed.

MUSCULAR CONTRACTURES

Muscular contractures may be secondary to intrinsic or extrinsic factors. An *intrinsic muscular contracture* is structural in nature and can be associated with inflammatory, degenerative, ischemic, or traumatic processes in the muscle itself. Myositis and other inflammatory diseases lead rapidly to the development of muscular fibrosis. Muscular dystrophies are classic examples of a degenerative process. Histological changes in the

dystrophies include muscle fiber loss, segmental necrosis of muscle fibers, abnormal appearance of residual muscle fibers, and increased lipocytosis and fibrosis.[71] The final result is the degeneration of muscle and the proliferation of new connective tissue subsequent to muscle shortening. Fibrosis is also implicated as a sequela of ischemic changes or direct trauma to the muscle (see Fig. 52–3). Immediately after hemorrhage, deposition of fibrin occurs at the site of bleeding. Two to three days later, the fibrin fibers are replaced by reticular fibers, which form a loose meshwork of connective tissue. If the muscle is kept immobilized, dense tissue is formed as early as seven days. In three weeks' time, wide bands of dense fibrous tissue will resist stretching, limiting range of motion of the joint.

Among the causes of intrinsic muscular shortening, heterotopic ossification results from metaplasia of collagen to bone. In injuries to the spinal cord and other structures of the central nervous system or after surgeries of the hip, heterotopic ossification is not uncommon.[73] The cause is unknown; however, a local alteration in metabolism or blood flow (stasis) in conjunction with the systemic alteration in calcium metabolism brought about by immobility are considered contributing factors. Although effective treatment for relief of the heterotopic calcification is not available, aggressive maintenance of range of motion is generally accepted as the cornerstone of preventive therapy.[103]

Extrinsic or positional muscular contracture may be due to spasticity, paralysis, or the mechanical (positional) restriction of motion. Spastic muscles cause a dynamic imbalance of muscle control in the involved extremities. The usual length of spastic muscle is reduced, which encourages a flexed posture in the upper extremity and plantar flexion and inversion in the lower limb. If these positions are allowed to persist and full range of motion is not provided, then shortening results. Early spastic contracture can be overcome by applying lengthening tension to the muscle for several seconds. More severe contractures associated with spasticity are characteristically difficult to treat but may respond to a combination of passive range of motion with prolonged stretch, heat or cold application to the spastic muscle, antispasticity medication, motor point blocks, or specific nerve blocks.

If paralyzed muscle groups cannot provide adequate balance to opposing muscles, a contracture may result. For instance, in chronic peroneal palsy, the antagonist, the triceps surae, is commonly contracted, causing inversion of the ankle and impaired ambulation. Prolonged stretching to maintain motion of the triceps surae and strengthening or support of the weak peroneal muscles to restore normal functional activity is essential.

Mechanical factors commonly cause contracture in bedridden and inactive patients. Some degree of muscular shortening is present, even in the healthy sedentary person, especially in those muscles that cross multiple joints. Intrinsic disorders of the muscle may increase the effect of positional factors in the development of muscular tightness. In muscular dystrophy, for example, plantar flexion contractures are a product of early intrinsic muscular shortening and improper positioning of the limb. Extensors of the hip are often very weak, forcing the patient to develop excessive lumbar lordosis and to walk on the toes in order to position

the center of gravity behind the hips and in front of the knees. However, walking on the toes prevents the stretching of the triceps surae usually achieved during the stance phase of gait, thus encouraging fibrotic tissue to shorten even more. If this sequence is not recognized, one might assume that fibrosis is the only reason for the plantar flexion contracture. The surgical lengthening of the Achilles tendon in such a case shortens the muscle belly, thereby weakening the plantar flexors and diminishing the ability of the patient to walk on the toes. Since walking on the toes in these patients is not only a result of the contracture but also is done to facilitate ambulation, decreased function may result from inadequate intervention.

Two-jointed muscles are usually the first to become shortened when normal range of motion is not maintained. The hamstrings, back muscles, tensor fascia latae, rectus femoris, and gastrocnemius muscles are among the most common types affected. For patients on bed rest, the tendency to develop tightness is promoted by the typical position of comfort, that is, flexed hips and knees and plantar-flexed ankles.

In those patients with inflammatory arthritides, positions of comfort may be particularly dangerous. Intra-articular pressure measurements and pain assessment studies indicate that pressure and pain in the joint are least at 35 to 45 degrees of hip and knee flexion and at 15 degrees of ankle plantar flexion. Therefore, during periods of maximal joint swelling and synovitis, these patients tend to assume positions of biomechanical disadvantage for these two-jointed muscles, resulting in extrinsic muscular shortening as well as intrinsic fibrosis of the joint capsule.

Another group of patients with a tendency to develop mechanically induced contractures are amputees. Flexion contracture of the hip in above-knee amputees is mainly due to prolonged sitting in a flexed position. Surgically weakened hip adductors and hamstrings in these patients also contribute to faulty positioning and to fixed flexion and abduction contractures. The below-knee amputee with a tendency toward prolonged sitting and immobility develops shortening of the hamstrings owing to prolonged knee flexion. Application of a rigid postoperative dressing with the knee held in extension allows a knee extension contracture to develop with restricted knee flexion due to tightness of the quadriceps muscle.

Controversy is still found in the literature regarding the contribution of the components of muscle to the resistance to passive stretch. Four

EUGEN M. HALAR AND KATHLEEN R. BELL

factors are considered important: (1) the inherent passive viscoelastic property of muscle fiber; (2) intramuscular collagen; (3) the level of gamma motor neuron activity; and (4) the state of central nervous system excitation. The influence of prolonged bed rest and inactivity on these factors has not been fully investigated. It appears that muscles undergo contracture during inactivity because there is a change in the nature and content of collagen fibers that surround and intermingle with muscle fibers (collagen of endomysium, perimysium, and epimysium). The results of all investigations indicate that muscle fiber, at least in the beginning of contracture, contributes very little to its formation.

Individual muscle fibers follow Hook's law and elongate linearly. Studies on muscle fiber components, in which only the sarcolemma was left intact, indicate that although the muscle membrane possesses elasticity, it is only a fraction of the total elasticity of a single muscle fiber. Furthermore, during passive tension, the sarcolemma begins to elongate when about 40 per cent of the elongation of muscle fiber has already occurred. The consensus, therefore, is that myofibrils rather than muscle membranes are the principal contributors to the elasticity of the muscle fiber.

An isolated muscle fiber can be maximally elongated up to 300 per cent of the resting length as opposed to the whole muscle, which is able to elongate only up to 30 per cent of its resting length.[102, 107] Intracellular muscular structure, studied in a single muscle fiber preparation during initial elongation, shows elasticity that is ascribed to have a value of 5×10^6 dynes per cm^2 as compared with 5×10^3 dynes per cm^2 for sarcolemma. However, the elasticity for collagen fibrils is significantly higher, 10^{10} dynes per cm^2. Thus, the collagen fiber meshwork is the most important factor in restricting passive elongation of the whole muscle. The progressive contribution of the collagen fiber meshwork to passive tension as the muscle is stretched can be explained by the fact that at higher tension, there is a progressive recruitment of slack collagen fibers contributing to the increased resistance. All of the collagen fibers in a resting muscle are not oriented parallel to the longitudinal axis of muscle fiber and in the direction of the muscle pull. As passive tension is increased, progressively greater numbers of collagen fibers straighten in the direction of pull and become more effective in providing passive resistance.[13, 45] Furthermore, during elongation, most of the collagen fibers are maximally stretched even before muscle fiber elements become involved, indicating that the collagen fibrils play a major role in passive resistance to stretch.[102, 107]

Under normal conditions, collagen fibers are coil shaped and loosely arranged to allow full range of motion. However, if a foreshortened position of the muscle is maintained for longer than five to seven days, the loose connective tissue in the muscle belly becomes shortened and then gradually changes into dense connective tissue. The relative proportions of loose to dense collagen fibers may also be altered in the soft tissue surrounding a joint, further compounding the problem. In cases such as burns, immobility will promote the proliferation of new collagen tissue, causing a rapid development of multiple joint contractures.

PREVENTION OF MUSCULAR CONTRACTURES

Flexibility exercises performed three times a week for 10 to 15 min in healthy but inactive subjects are sufficient to maintain the optimal resting length of the long muscles, which may not be stretched during normal daily activity or locomotion. Active range of motion with terminal stretch must also be directed to the two-jointed muscle if effective maintenance of full joint motion is a goal. For mild muscular contractures, passive range of motion with a sustained terminal stretch is effective if applied for 20 to 30 min twice a day.

In severe contractures, prolonged stretching continuously applied for at least 20 to 30 min is required. The prolonged stretching is usually accompanied by heat application. For muscular contractures, heat is applied to the muscle belly or musculotendinous junction. Ultrasound as a deep heating modality is recommended for structural (intrinsic) contractures. It will raise muscle temperature to 40 to 43° C (104 to 109.4° F) which will influence viscous properties of connective tissue and maximize the effect of stretching.[46] Whenever muscle is stretched, proximal body parts should be well stabilized. For instance, the pelvis should be stabilized before vigorous hip flexion stretching is applied to prevent excessive strain on the low lumbar area.

Dynamic splinting or serial casting is an approach that may be used if prolonged passive stretch does not produce the desired results. By applying a serial cast or dynamic splint, a sustained stretch can be achieved for several days. The cast is applied immediately after passive stretching to obtain the best possible effects. Reapplication of the cast is usually done every third or fourth day, each time following stretching and repositioning. Serial casting is commonly used in severe plantar and knee flexion contracture. For the smaller joints of the hands or elbows, dynamic splinting is indicated. Elastic bands are used to provide the deserved tension in the appropriate direction. Dynamic splints will allow functional use of the limb while stretch is applied.

Contracture of the Connective Tissue of the Joint

Arthrogenic contractures are usually the result of inflammation, infection, degenerative joint disease, or repeated trauma. The pain, which is due to synovial effusion or is associated with inflammation and arthritis, often culminates in joint splinting (voluntary and involuntary) and immobility. Prolonged splinting or immobility allows the collagen of joint capsule and soft tissue to shrink. In degenerative joint diseases, cartilage loss is the initiating factor of joint pain and impaired range of motion (Table 52–4).

Although pain is usually a major aspect of joint disease, patients with a loss of pain sensation and proprioception may develop severe degenerative joint disease (Charcot's joint). However, they may have relatively well-preserved joint mobility because of the lack of pain and splinting.

Capsular tightness is a common outcome of prolonged immobilization. If a joint capsule and the adjacent soft tissue are not repeatedly stretched by joint motion, the collagen fibers will become shortened and restrict full range of motion. If collagen tissue proliferation occurs, even greater capsular tightness may result. Tightness of capsular pattern compromises full range motion in all directions. The shoulder is a common site of joint capsule contracture that usually is induced by bicipital tendonitis, subdeltoid bursitis, and rotator cuff degenerative changes with subsequent joint splinting. Progression of capsular contracture may lead to a frozen shoulder and to the loss of arm function. The posterior knee capsule is another example of capsular shortening, which is also a consequence of prolonged flexion. Infrapatellar contracture syndrome is a proliferation of fibrous tissue below the patella after knee surgery, which is promoted by prolonged immobility restricting flexion.

Soft tissue around a joint can also become shortened by inflammation, trauma, or faulty positioning of an extremity. The shortening and proliferation of collagen fibers in soft tissue usually limit movement in only one direction of joint motion.

PREVENTION OF JOINT CONTRACTURE AND RESTORATION OF JOINT MOTION

Two basic principles are used in the prevention of arthrogenic and soft tissue contractures—optimal positioning of the involved joint and early joint mobilization. If a contracture is present, the immobilized extremity should be positioned in such a way that optimal physiological stretch is maintained. The literature provides no clear-cut guidance on when to initiate active or passive range of motion to the joint with diminishing signs of acute infection or inflammation. Recently, a more aggressive approach of remobilization has been introduced for prevention of contractures in infected or operated joints. The continuous passive motion approach uses specifically designed devices for different joints to provide passive continuous motion to the joint immediately after joint surgery or during infection.[7] The basic principle of the approach is to provide a painless passive motion to the affected joint without the use of the muscles in order to prevent compression of cartilage during strong muscle contractures.

When applying terminal stretch manually to a joint with a contracture, slight distraction of the joint may prevent soft tissue impingement and compression of the joint. This maneuver is particularly applicable in joints with a large range of mobility, for instance, in the case of the shoulder joint. In the shoulder adduction and internal rotation contracture, the normal downward gliding of the humeral head in the glenoid fossa is prevented by tight adductors. Therefore, forced abduction may cause impingement of the rotator cuff tendons against the acromion. Stretch applied in the direction of forward flexion and external rotation should be attempted before forceful abduction.

Effects of Immobilization on the Development of Degenerative Joint Disease

Immobilization degenerative joint disease is a term used to define severe degenerative joint changes produced by prolonged immobilization in

EUGEN M. HALAR AND KATHLEEN R. BELL

experimental animals and has a clinical significance.

Limitation of full range of motion can be the result of pathological processes in the joint itself, that is, due to cartilage or synovial changes coupled with pain and immobility. It should be mentioned here that long-term immobilization of a joint in experimental animals produces clinically well-known degenerative joint changes, as well as capsular tightness with the development of a fixed joint contracture. In one study on animals, both periodic and continuous immobilization for 30 days induced severe degenerative joint changes, i.e., cartilage destruction with thickening and a contracted joint capsule.[39, 42] The current belief is that both the shrunken capsule and joint immobilization in a fixed position cause prolonged compression of the cartilage sites of contacts and their degeneration. This results in a reduction of cartilage water content, a decrease in hyaluronate and chondroitin sulfate content, and a loss of hexamines from periarticular tissue. In chronic arthrogenic contractures, proliferation of intracapsular and periarticular connective tissue occurs along with cartilage thinning, vascular engorgement, and trabecular bone resorption.[39, 42]

Effects of Immobilization on the Development of Osteopenia and Hypercalcemia

Although the phenomenon of bone loss during prolonged periods of immobilization is well known, it is often clinically silent for years. Routine radiographs do not reveal the presence of osteoporosis until a 40 per cent loss of total bone density occurs. The bone scan may be positive, particularly at long bone metaphyses and throughout the axial skeleton, due to increased regional blood flow.[18, 19] In neurological diseases accompanied by paralysis, such as spinal cord injuries, osteopenia may become so advanced that fracture of long bones may occur with relatively little force. This problem should be considered when designing an exercise program for paraplegic, quadriplegic, or other paralyzed persons. A person with alterations in bone metabolism, such as occurs in postmenopausal osteoporosis or Paget's disease, may also be at increased risk for similar fractures if kept at prolonged bed rest.

The syndrome of immobilization hypercalcemia is not uncommon in children and young adults; studies have indicated that up to 50 per cent of healthy children with single fractures of the lower limb (in a cast or held in traction) on bed rest will have hypercalcemia that is confirmed by positive findings on laboratory tests.[91] Symptomatic hypercalcemia occurs approximately four weeks after the onset of bed rest. Early signs include anorexia, abdominal pain, constipation, nausea, and vomiting. Progressive neurological signs are weakness, hypotonia, emotional lability, stupor and, finally, coma. Severe hypertension may also accompany this syndrome.[35, 64, 76, 124] The diagnosis should be considered in the face of prolonged recumbency of a child or young adult with a fracture. Laboratory aids in diagnosis are elevated serum and urine calcium levels, a calcium and creatine ratio greater than 0.40 on a 24-hour urine specimen, normal parathyroid hormone, and increased urine hydroxyproline levels. Serum alkaline phosphatase, phosphate, creatinine, and urea nitrogen levels are generally normal.[91]

Wolff's law states that bone morphology and density are dependent upon the forces that act on the bone.[75, 88, 116] Normal forces are disrupted during immobilization and non–weight-bearing situations. Studies performed on animals indicate that bone resorption is the primary alteration in bone kinetics;[125] this is particularly true of trabecular bone, although cortical bone loss may be significant.[70] Evidence in animals and human studies with long-term immobilization supports the notion that different phases of bone loss exist.[70] The initial stage is a rapid loss of bone with equally rapid reversal. The second stage of bone loss begins about 12 weeks after immobilization in dogs and is slower but longer lasting. The final phase is one in which the volume of bone is maintained at 40 to 70 per cent of the original volume. The rate of loss is higher in younger individuals and in weight-bearing bones.

Increased bone resorption during immobilization appears to be a major factor in bone loss despite the lack of suppression of the parathyroid hormone. Total serum calcium concentration generally remains normal, as does serum phosphorus.[33, 62] However, urinary calcium, phosphorus, and hydroxyproline are significantly increased, resulting in a negative mineral balance.[106] Urinary calcium excretion is maximal by seven weeks of immobilization. During a 30- to 36-week period of bed rest, it is estimated that 4.2 per cent of the total body calcium is lost.[33, 49, 96]

The Cardiovascular System

The impairment of cardiovascular functional capacity is another common complication of prolonged bed rest with inactivity. Four major adverse manifestations are encountered in the cardiovascular system: (1) redistribution of body fluids, (2) postural hypotension, (3) cardiovascular deconditioning, and (4) thromboembolic phenomena.

The pressure of the blood column in the vessels of the trunk and lower extremities during standing is responsible for shifting 700 ml of blood into the legs. In the supine position, this hydrostatic pressure is eliminated, causing 500 to 700 ml of blood to return to the lungs and right side of the heart, thus increasing the central blood volume and distention of high pressure baroreceptors. This results in the suppression of antidiuretic hormone release. In animal experiments, this suppression of antidiuretic hormone is mediated by the vagus nerve. However, in patients who have received a cardiac transplant, suppression of antidiuretic hormone is also present, even though the vagus nerve to the heart is cut. A few days of bed rest produces significant diuresis, resulting in an 8 to 12 per cent loss of plasma volume during the first two weeks of bed rest. During the second to fourth week of bed rest, the plasma loss may reach 15 to 20 per cent. The cardiac response to redistribution of blood volume is different initially and later during prolonged bed rest. The augmentation of central blood volume that occurs on lying down causes an increase in heart rate, stroke volume, and cardiac output.[44, 72, 121] The activation of baroreceptors in the atrium causes the reversal of these initial cardiogenic responses, resulting in a progressive reduction of stroke volume and cardiac output of 6 to 13 per cent.

An elevated hematocrit level and a minimal reduction of red blood cell mass was also found after prolonged bed rest. However, since the reduction of the plasma volume is greater than the reduction of red cell mass, blood viscosity is increased, possibly triggering thromboembolic events. Other studies have also shown a significant reduction of plasma protein after prolonged inactivity. The reduction of plasma volume and plasma protein can be minimized by exercise. Isotonic exercises have been shown to be maximally effective in preventing the reduction of plasma volume during bed rest.*

As noted previously, a large shift of extracellular fluid occurs on assuming the upright position, causing an initial reduction of cardiac output (25 per cent), a reduction of heart stroke volume (40 per cent), and a compensatory increase in heart rate (25 per cent). Ten to fifteen per cent of the blood volume is shifted into the legs (mainly into deep intramuscular and intermuscular venous systems), increasing venous pressure to 120 cm of water. A 10 to 20 per cent increase in plasma volume in the extracellular space of the lower limbs further contributes to the overall effect of the redistribution of body fluid. Despite this process, blood pressure in normal subjects is not changed or becomes slightly elevated on arising. However, the normal compensatory response of vasoconstriction, increased heart rate, and blood pressure on assuming an upright position may be significantly altered after extended bed rest.[113] Severe *postural hypotension* is a common hazard of prolonged inactivity and bed rest. Several possible mechanisms play a role in the development of postural hypotension. An excessive shift of blood from the lungs and heart to the legs may be the initial causative factor. The sympathetic adrenergic system appears to respond inadequately and is unable to maintain normal blood pressure when an individual assumes the upright position. Increased beta-adrenergic sympathetic activity during bed rest may also contribute to postural hypotension upon assuming upright position.[85, 112]

Symptoms and signs of postural hypotension include pallor, sweating, dizziness, lightheadedness, decreased systolic pressure (more than 20 mm Hg), increased heart rate (usually more than 20 beats per minute), and decreased pulse pressure. Fainting may result. In patients with coronary artery disease, anginal pain may be triggered, since inadequate coronary blood supply results from reduced diastolic filling.[40] In healthy subjects, the ability to adjust to the upright position may be completely impaired after three weeks of bed rest. Only a few days of bed rest may also produce orthostasis in patients with major trauma, systemic disease, and advanced age.

It takes more time to restore normal cardiovascular postural responses than to disrupt them. The process of reconditioning depends on the duration of bed rest and can last weeks or months.

The differential diagnosis of orthostatic hypotension includes the autonomic neuropathy associated with diabetes mellitus, Addison's disease, or idiopathic chronic orthostatic hypotension. Quadriplegic patients are particularly susceptible to developing postural hypotension. Their normal increase

---

*See references 52–54, 57, 60, and 72.

EUGEN M. HALAR AND KATHLEEN R. BELL

in plasma norepinephrine on assuming the upright position is delayed in addition to dependent blood pooling. The efficiency of antigravity suits to treat postural hypotension of quadriplegic patients indicates that blood pooling may be the most important factor of their orthostatic intolerance.[118]

During prolonged bed rest and inactivity, a progressive reduction of *cardiovascular efficiency* occurs, which is associated with a progressive reduction of cardiac output and stroke volume. The end-diastolic ventricular volume declines 6 to 11 per cent after two weeks of bed rest. The resting pulse rate increases progressively during prolonged recumbency. During the first two months, the resting pulse rate usually increases a half a beat per day. Taylor found an average increase in the resting pulse rate of 12 to 23 beats per minute after 10 days of strict bed rest.[112, 113] This decrease in cardiac efficiency can be clinically demonstrated by the changes observed in heart rate for a given physical activity. For instance, walking at the rate of 3.6 miles per hour on a 10 per cent incline for 30 min after three weeks of bed rest can result in an increase in a heart rate that is 35 to 45 beats per minute higher than the baseline rate obtained for the same exertion. This is approximately a 25 per cent reduction in cardiovascular performance.[56, 108, 114]

Cardiac insufficiency can also be demonstrated when a person is tilted to an upright position. The increase in pulse rate of 60 beats per minute upon tilting to an upright position is twice the normal response of 15 to 25 beats per minute.

Exercise tolerance and work capacity are both significantly reduced following bed rest and inactivity. Many studies have demonstrated a decrease in the maximal oxygen uptake (17 to 28 per cent). It appears that the increased duration of inactivity is negatively correlated with changes in VO_2max. After ten days of bed rest, a 5.2 per cent reduction of VO_2max occurs, whereas by 26 days, a 19.5 per cent decline is seen.[56, 59] Maximal exercise duration testing, using either a treadmill or a bicycle ergometer, may also demonstrate reduced ability to perform exercises and work. Total transport and utilization of oxygen could be the reason for this insufficiency. The reduction in musculoskeletal functional capacity, decrease in muscle strength and endurance, reduced pumping effect of the lower extremity muscles, poor venous return, and overall lower muscle metabolic activity contribute to this work intolerance. Several studies have shown clearly that a period of bed rest for as little as three to five days leads to cardiovascular deconditioning.[6] The studies on weightless conditions also reveal a reduction of exercise capacity (10 to 50 per cent) and a loss of left ventricular volume (5 to 50 per cent) in astronauts during long flights.

Early mobilization of patients after major surgical procedures, obstetric deliveries, and major trauma have reduced the incidence of *thromboembolic events* when compared with previous medical practices entailing prolonged bed rest. Studies on factors relating to the occurrence of thromboembolic events reveal a direct relationship between the frequency of deep vein thrombosis and the duration of bed rest.[36, 48, 86, 97] Virchow's triad consists of stasis, increased blood coagulability, and damage to the blood vessel wall. Two of these three factors are influenced by prolonged immobility. Stasis of blood flow in the lower extremities is directly related to the reduced pumping effect of the calf muscles. A hypercoaguable state is induced by plasma volume reduction and dehydration. A high degree of clinical suspicion of deep vein thrombosis is in order when clinical evidence of localized edema, erythema, calf pain, palpable cords, or Homans' sign is present in the immobile patient.[115] Laboratory studies such as Doppler ultrasound, radionuclide venography, and contrast venography, which is the accepted standard for diagnosis, should be considered to confirm clinical suspicion. Unfortunately, the last test is time-consuming and painful and may irritate the intima, inducing thrombophlebitis.[16, 84] Pulmonary embolism is a life-threatening disorder that is clinically diagnosed by the sudden onset of dyspnea, tachycardia, tachypnea, and cardiac murmur or pleural rub.[97] The diagnosis is confirmed by tests of arterial blood gases, ventilation-perfusion scan, and pulmonary angiography. Prevention of thromboembolic complications during prolonged immobility may be accomplished with low-dose heparin injections (5000 units twice a day) and intermittent active exercises of the calf, thigh, and abdominal muscles.

PRINCIPLES OF PREVENTION AND RECONDITIONING

Several measures are routinely implemented to prevent orthostatic hypotension. Early mobilization to counteract the effects of bed rest and progressive strengthening exercises to the major muscle groups are most effective. Contraction of the abdominal and leg musculature is used for promoting venous blood return and reducing pooling. If swelling in the lower extremities is present, elevation of the legs in the supine and reclining positions and supportive garments are beneficial (Ace bandage wrapping, full-length elastic stockings, and abdominal binders).[98, 118]

In patients with severe postural hypotension and paraplegia or quadriplegia, it may be necessary to use a tilt table to restore tolerance to the upright position. A gradual increase in the angulation of the tilt allows closer control of blood pressure and pulse before and immediately after each position change.[59, 60] If blood systolic pressure after 15 min is persistently lower than 50 mm Hg, expect that the patient will faint. The desired goal for using the tilt table is obtaining a position of 75 degrees for 20 min without orthostatic changes. Ephedrine and other sympathetic agents may be necessary to maintain blood pressure. Mineralocorticoids (Florinef) with adequate salt and fluid intake are other supportive measures used to reduce or eliminate postural hypotension.

The intensity of exercise at the beginning of cardiac reconditioning should be at 65% or less of the maximal heart rate and should be raised later to 70 to 80 per cent. In general, a 20-beat increase in the heart rate during periods of exercise is a good guideline to use to assess whether or not the exercises will induce an adequate increase in cardiovascular fitness. If a deconditioned individual exercises at that level, the endurance and work capacity may increase 20 to 40 per cent per week. The frequency and duration of exercise training (conditioning) depend upon the goals that are set for each patient and should be based on the patient's general condition; warm-up exercises should always be a part of conditioning training programs. In 60 to 70 per cent of healthy men, sudden vigorous exercises were found to cause a significant S-T depression or hypokinetic ventricular wall motions and a decrease in ejection fraction but, interestingly, could be prevented by warm-up exercises. In the same respect, cool-down exercises enhance venous return, prevent postexercise hypotension, provide better elimination of lactic acid, and induce the postexercise increase of catecholamines and heat.[9, 14, 27]

At a given level of activity after exercise training, the heart rate becomes significantly reduced. With exercise training, the cardiac output and maximal oxygen uptake (VO_2max) gradually increase. However, at a given oxygen uptake level, the cardiac output before and after the exercise training is unchanged because the heart stroke volume is increased but the heart rate is reduced. The blood pressure may initially increase at the beginning of the exercise period. After exercise training, blood pressure decreases, possibly owing to a reduction in peripheral blood vessel resistance.[56, 67, 104]

The Metabolic and Endocrine Systems

The musculoskeletal and cardiovascular complications of inactivity are routinely associated with alterations in the reactions of the metabolic and endocrine systems. Characteristically, metabolic and endocrine changes of inactivity have a slow and insidious onset and a delayed recovery period after the resumption of activity. In fact, many of the metabolic and endocrine complications become clinically apparent during remobilization (Table 52–5 and Fig. 52–4).

Negative Nitrogen Balance

Inactivity produces an increase in the excretion of urinary nitrogen (average loss may reach 2 gm per day), leading to hypoproteinemia, edema, and weight loss. Diuresis, which is due to the suppression of antidiuretic hormone, results in weight loss that is accelerated by a loss of appetite for protein-rich food. It is interesting to notice that exercises performed during bed rest (for two weeks) cause a greater weight loss than bed rest alone (1.77 kg versus 0.4 kg).[53, 54] This loss of body weight during inactivity is mainly due to loss in lean body mass rather than to loss of fat. When inactivity is associated with starvation or major trauma, for instance, long bone fractures, the daily loss of nitrogen can reach significant proportions—as much as 8 or 12 gm daily.[21, 63, 83]

Nitrogen excretion usually begins on the fifth or sixth day of recumbency, peaks during the second week, and lasts during the entire period of immobilization. The restoration of normal nitrogen balance becomes progressively more difficult as the duration of bed rest increases. Only one week is needed to restore nitrogen balance after three weeks of bed rest; however after seven weeks of bedrest, about seven weeks of activity and retraining are required. A single reason for the occurrence of nitrogen loss is not obvious. Both a reduction of protein synthesis and an increase in protein breakdown have been found. Tryptophan and niacin are abnormally low after two weeks of immobility. Butterworth found that half of chronically hospitalized patients suffer from tryptophan

EUGEN M. HALAR AND KATHLEEN R. BELL

TABLE 52–5. Metabolic and Endocrine Changes: Effects of Bed Rest and Inactivity on Healthy Subjects

METABOLITES/ HORMONES	EFFECTS/CHANGE	ONSET/DURATION OF CHANGE	RECONDITIONING
Antidiuretic hormone	Inhibited/diuresis	Second and third day and entire bed rest period	
Sodium	Excretion increased	First and second day, becoming normal later	
Potassium	Excretion increased	End of first week, becoming normal later	
Nitrogen	Excretion increased/2.0 gm daily Hypoproteinemia	Fifth and sixth week or entire bed rest period	One week of retraining needed after three weeks of bed rest
Nitrogen after trauma*	8.0 gm daily loss/ hypoproteinemia	Immediately after trauma	
Sulfur, phosphorus	Increased excretion	Entire period of recumbency	
Calcium	Increased urinary excretion	Second and third day, with peaks at fourth and fifth weeks, months, years or entire duration bed rest period	Months, years
Calcium in spinal cord injury patients*	Hypercalcemia		
Parathyroid hormone	Increased blood levels		
Thyroid hormone	Increased diurnal variation		
Insulin	Increased serum level	Entire bed rest period	
C-peptide (Proinsulin)	Increased levels		
Adrenocorticotropic hormone	Increased (three times normal level) adrenal unresponsiveness		One month of inactivity followed by 20 days of activity
Carbohydrates	Increased intolerance	Entire bed rest period	
Androgen hormones	Decreased		
Spermatogenesis	Decreased		
Cholesterol content	Increased (membrane)		One month of bed rest followed by 14 days of activity
Low-density lipo- proteins	Decreased		
Cortisol	Increased urinary excretion		

*Metabolic changes due to major trauma or diseases associated with inactivity.

and niacin insufficiency.[17] However, it is not clear whether this insufficiency is caused by inadequate diet, inactivity, or both.

Negative Balance of other Minerals

It is well known that both major trauma and inactivity may be associated with excessive losses of sodium, potassium, sulfur, phosphorus and magnesium (Fig. 52–3).[47, 82]

Initially, the inhibition of antidiuretic hormone is triggered by an increase in central venous pressure, producing a significant diuresis with increased loss of sodium. This sodium loss is prominent during the first two days of recumbency. Potassium loss usually occurs toward the end of the first week of immobility. Both serum sodium and potassium levels are normal during the entire period of bed rest, although their excretion is increased. It is not clear whether or not the increase in sodium excretion due to immobilization could result in the hyponatremia in elderly patients, which is known to cause significant medical problems.

Endocrine Changes

The basal metabolic rate is decreased during the entire period of bed rest. Deitrick's study of immobilized healthy subjects in leg casts demonstrated a reduced basal metabolic rate starting on the second day of recumbency and lasting three

COMPOUND EFFECT OF TRAUMA AND INACTIVITY
ON METABOLIC BALANCE

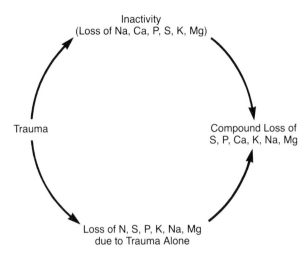

Inactivity
(Loss of Na, Ca, P, S, K, Mg)

Trauma

Compound Loss of
S, P, Ca, K, Na, Mg

Loss of N, S, P, K, Na, Mg
due to Trauma Alone

Negative metabolic balance induced by trauma can be aggravated by
negative metabolic balance produced by prolonged bed rest and immobility.

FIGURE 52–4. Major trauma or disease causes well-known
metabolic imbalances (N, Ca, K, Na, Mg, S, P). Prolonged
inactivity, bed rest, and immobilization also cause negative
metabolic balances. The combined effect may be devastating.

weeks after six to seven weeks of immobilization.[28]
In other studies, the thyroid hormone concentrations were normal during bed rest but have been characterized as being very unstable. Diurnal variations of thyroid hormone activity during bed rest have a greater variability than those in healthy active subjects.[4, 120, 121]

During bed rest, significant carbohydrate intolerance has been found. Glucose tolerance tests in immobilized subjects revealed hyperglycemic and hyperinsulinemic responses. Levels of insulin were twice as high in these subjects as compared with controls with normal activity levels. Proinsulin C-peptide concentrations were also increased, clearly indicating that the release of insulin from the pancreas was normal but its effectiveness was diminished.[120, 123] During the entire first month of recumbency, the levels of insulin gradually become higher, although plasma glucose levels remain normal. This finding should not be confused with the hyperglycemic response upon glucose loading found in the same subjects. The progressive increase in insulin levels peaks at the end of the first month and starts to decline thereafter but does not reach normal values as long as inactivity persists.

The plasma glucose level after prolonged bed rest (one month or more) may even drop below normal levels, leading to hypoglycemic crises. In chronic bedridden subjects, carbohydrate intolerance may mimic brittle diabetic conditions. From this evidence, it appears that inactivity increases tissue resistance to endogenous insulin.*

The level of corticosteroids in the serum during bed rest has varied in different studies.[77, 85] However, urinary cortisol excretion is increased. The adrenal glands become less responsive to the stimulation of adrenocorticotropic hormone following prolonged bed rest. In studies of bed rest of more than one month, adrenocorticotropic hormone levels were three times higher than the baseline and required about 20 days of activity to return to normal. During bed rest and immobility, the cholesterol level is increased. However, the low-density lipoprotein level decreases. Lipoproteins were noted to return to the normal level 14 days after remobilization. Serum parathyroid hormone is increased during immobilization and is a factor in hypercalcemia of immobility.[80] Androgen levels and decreased spermatogenesis have also been reported.[22]

The Respiratory System

The respiratory system is the site of life-threatening complications during prolonged immobility.

The mechanical restriction to ventilation caused by recumbency reduces tidal volume, minute volume, and functional ventilatory reserve capacity. Pulmonary capillary blood volume and total lung diffusing capacity are also decreased. Vital capacity is usually unchanged, although it may be reduced after prolonged recumbency. Several factors account for these ventilatory alterations. Diaphragmatic and intercostal movements during recumbency are diminished (reduced chest expansion). Breathing becomes shallower, and alveolar respiration is reduced with a relative increase of carbon dioxide in the alveoli. Consequently, the rate of respiration increases. Clearance of secretions is more difficult in a recumbent position. Secretions are not evenly spread around all sides of the bronchial walls. The dependent side of the bronchial wall accumulates more secretions than the upper part of the wall, which becomes dry, rendering the cilia ineffective in clearing the secretions. This results in pooling of the secretions in

---

*See references 31, 32, 79, 81, and 111.

the lower parts of the bronchial tree.[15] Coughing is also ineffective in the supine position. Reduced diaphragmatic and intercostal motion, compounded by abdominal muscle weakness and ineffective ciliary function, predisposes the patient to upper respiratory infections and hypostatic pneumonia. The ventilation/perfusion ratio may significantly change in dependent areas of the lungs with poor ventilation and overperfusion, leading to arteriovenous shunting and to a reduced arterial oxygenation.[95, 108, 110]

If a patient must be kept in a recumbent position, frequent changes in position should be made. Meticulous pulmonary toilet should be maintained with deep breathing and coughing and adequate hydration. An incentive spirometer may be necessary to prevent atelectasis. Chest percussion and postural drainage with oropharyngeal suctioning can ameliorate bronchial pooling of secretions. The presence of pre-existing pulmonary disease requires an aggressive program of pulmonary toilet, and the need for bronchodilators should be assessed.

The Genitourinary System

In a recumbent position, both renal blood flow and renal water elimination (diuresis) are increased. This is followed by an increase in sodium and potassium excretion. Calcium and phosphorus loss also occurs, persisting long after remobilization has begun. Hypercalciuria and phosphaturia of immobilized subjects fosters the development of bladder and kidney stones, leading to hematuria, urinary tract infections, and urosepsis. In addition, urinary drainage from the renal pelvis and ureters is diminished without gravitational assistance, resulting in stagnation of urine, which further promotes kidney stone formation.[106]

Bladder emptying is impaired in the supine position, as it is much more difficult to generate intraabdominal pressure. Weakened abdominal muscles, restricted diaphragmatic movement, and incomplete pelvic floor relaxation all occur, culminating in partial urinary retention.

Bladder stones, especially struvate and carbonate-apatite stones, are commonly found (15 to 30 per cent of immobilized patients). Hypercalciuria and urinary retention combine, providing an ideal environment for stone formation. Retained urine permits an overgrowth of urea-splitting bacteria, increasing urinary pH and ammonia and allowing precipitation of calcium and phosphorus. Once formed, bladder stones create a nidus for bacterial growth, completing a cycle of stone-bacterial proliferation. Stones also cause microtrauma to the mucosal lining of the bladder, increasing the likelihood of bacterial infection. The presence of bladder stones decreases the effectiveness of antimicrobial treatment and may result in recurrent urinary tract infections. A dysfunctional urinary bladder with poor contractility of the detrusor muscle and deficient sphincter coordination will exacerbate any of the problems described above.

Adequate fluid intake and acidification of urine will reduce bacterial colonization in the immobilized patient. Complete bladder emptying should be encouraged by using an upright position for voiding. If retention is suspected, residual volumes should be obtained after voiding. Indwelling urinary catheters may be necessary for medical reasons in some patients but should be removed as soon as possible.

The Gastrointestinal System

Common effects of inactivity on the gastrointestinal tract are a loss of appetite (especially for protein-rich food) and reduced peristalsis, causing slower absorption of nutrients. These factors may result in measurable hypoproteinemia. The slower rate of peristalsis is thought to be caused by a high level of adrenergic activity. This factor, along with the loss of plasma volume and dehydration that accompanies bed rest, often results in constipation. Constipation may be worsened by a patient's inability to use a bedpan; its use requires both unphysiological positioning and social embarrassment. The end point of this process is fecal impaction, requiring enemas, manual removal, or finally, surgical attention.[69]

To prevent constipation due to inactivity, a neurogenic bowel condition, or both, it is important to implement a bowel training program. This program may consist of supplying a fiber-rich diet and adequate fluids, scheduled post-meal toileting, and the use of glycerin or suppositories, stool softeners, and a bedside commode or toilet.

The Central Nervous System

Prolonged physical inactivity may produce sensory and psychosocial deprivation. The lack of environmental, physical, mental, and social stimulation may lead to a wide range of central nervous system dysfunctions.* A patient on prolonged bed rest has reduced exposure to such basic social and chronological cues as the time of day, movement through space, and personal orientation.[5] Social isolation alone with preserved physical activity can cause anxiety and emotional lability but will not usually cause intellectual deterioration.[43, 61] In contrast, studies have clearly shown that, when physical inactivity is present in conjunction with social isolation, cognitive processing is impaired.[61] In 1961, Litman demonstrated that patients who are socially inactive are less motivated to participate in rehabilitative efforts than those who are socially active. Hammer and Kenan found that socially inactive patients are less likely to seek help and participate in the rehabilitation process.[59] Prolonged social isolation and inactivity may become manifested as irritability, hostility, reduced cooperation, and a lack of emotional stability, including anxiety, neurotic behavior, and depression. Judgment, problem solving and learning ability, memory, psychomotor skills, and alertness all may be impaired. Perceptual impairment can be found even after seven days of immobilization. If the patient on prolonged bed rest and social deprivation is also disabled, the problems can be further compounded. Lack of concentration and motivation, depression, and reduced psychomotor skills and coordination may drastically affect the patient's ability to achieve the highest possible level of functioning and independence.

An important strategy in the prevention and treatment of these complications is to apply appropriate physical and psychosocial stimulations early in the course of illness. It is often difficult to distinguish the effects of the primary disease from those of prolonged inactivity and psychosocial deprivation. Options for the prevention of these effects include group therapy sessions, attention to socialization and avocational pursuits during evenings and weekends, and encouragement of family interaction.

In some rehabilitation centers, physical restoration is stressed without adequate concern for psychosocial functioning. In such situations, patients are discharged while they are still socially inactive and isolated.

ACKNOWLEDGMENT

We would like to acknowledge David DeGroot, B.S., for his contribution of the figures and tables.

*See references 20, 34, 92, 99, and 100.

References

1. Abramson, A. S., and Delagi, E. F.: Influence of weight-bearing and muscle contraction on disuse osteoporosis. Arch. Phys. Med. Rehab., 42:147–152, 1961.
2. American Heart Association Committee Report: Statement on Exercise. Circulation, 64:1327A–1329A, 1981.
3. Arnold, J. S., and Bartley, M. H.: Skeletal changes in aging and disease. Clin. Orthop., 49:17–38, 1966.
4. Balsam, A., and Leppo, L. E.: Assessment of the degradation of the thyroid hormones in man during bedrest. J. Appl. Physiol., 38:216–219, 1975.
5. Banks, R., Cappon, D.: Effect of reduced sensory input on time perception. Percept. Mot. Skills, 14:74, 1962.
6. Bassey, E. J., and Fentem, P. H.: Extent of deterioration in physical condition during postoperative bed rest and its reversal by rehabilitation. Br. Med. J., 4:194–196, 1974.
7. Bentham, J. S., Brereton, W. D. S., Cochrane, I. W., and Lyttle, D.: Continuous passive motion device for hand rehabilitation. Arch. Phys. Med. Rehab., 68:248–250, 1987.
8. Bergstrom, J.: Muscle electrolytes in man. Scand. J. Clin. Invest., 14(68):1–110, 1962.
9. Blomqvist, C. G., and Stone, H. L.: Cardiovascular adjustments to gravitational stress. In Geiger, S. R. (Ed.): Handbook of Physiology; Section 2: The Cardiovascular System; Shepherd, J. T., and Abboud, F. M. (Eds.): Handbook of Physiology, Volume III, Peripheral Circulation and Organ Blood Flow, Part 2. Bethesda, Md., American Physiological Society, 1983.
10. Bonner, C. D.: Rehabilitation instead of bed rest? Geriatrics, 24(6):109–118, 1969.
11. Booth, F. W.: Effect of limb immobilization on skeletal muscle. J. Appl. Physiol., 52(5):1113–1118, 1982.
12. Booth, F. W., and Gollnick, P. D.: Effects of disuse on the structure and function of skeletal muscle. Med. Sci. Sports Exerc., 15:415–420, 1983.
13. Bornstein, P., and Byers, P. H.: Collagen Metabolism; Current Concepts (Pamphlet). Kalamazoo, Mich., Upjohn, 1980.
14. Brooks, G. A., and Fahey, T. D.: Exercise Physiology. New York, John Wiley & Sons, 1984.
15. Browse, N. L.: The Physiology and Pathology of Bed Rest. Springfield, Il., Charles C Thomas Publishing, 1965, pp. 1–221.
16. Browse, N. L.: Diagnoses of deep vein thrombosis. Br. Med. Bull., 34:163–167, 1978.
17. Butterworth, C. E., Jr.: Editorial: Malnutrition in the hospital. J.A.M.A., 230(6):879, 1974.
18. Cann, C. E., and Adachi, R. R.: Bone resorption and mineral excretion in rats during spaceflight. Am. J. Physiol., 244(3):R327–R331, 1983.

EUGEN M. HALAR AND KATHLEEN R. BELL

19. Cann, C. E., Genant, H. K., and Young, D. R.: Comparison of vertebral and peripheral mineral losses in disuse osteoporosis in the monkey. Radiology, 134:525–559, 1980.

20. Chase, G. A., Grave, D., and Rowell, L. B.: Independence of changes in functional and performance capacities attending prolonged bed rest. Aerospace Med., 37:1232–1238, 1966.

21. Chobanian, A. V., Lillie, R. D., Tercyak, A., and Blevins, P.: The metabolic and hemodynamic effects of prolonged bedrest in normal subjects. Circulation, 49(3):551–559, 1974.

22. Cockett, A. T., Elbadawi, A., and Zemjanis, R.: The effects of immobilization on spermatogenesis in subhuman primates. Fertil. Steril., 21:610–614, 1970.

23. Colquhoun, W. P.: Effects of personality on body temperature and mental efficiency following transmeridian flight. Aviat. Space Environ. Med., 55(6):493–496, 1984.

24. Convertino, V. A., Hung, J., Goldwater, D., and Busk, R. F.: Cardiovascular responses to exercise in middle-aged men after 10 days of bedrest. Circulation, 65:134–140, 1982.

25. Corrodi, H., Fuxe, K., and Kokfelt, T.: The effect of immobilization stress on the activity of the central monoamine neuron. Life Sci., 7:107–112, 1968.

26. Cuthbertson, D. P.: Influence of prolonged muscular rest on metabolism. Biochem. J., 23:1328–1345, 1929.

27. Debusk, R. F., and Hung, J.: Exercise conditions soon after myocardial infarction: Effects on myocardial perfusion and ventricular function. Ann. N. Y. Acad. Sci., 382:343–354, 1982.

28. Deitrick, J. E., Whedon, G. D., and Shorr, E.: Effects of immobilization upon various metabolic and physiologic functions of normal men. Am. J. Med., 4:3–32, 1948.

29. Demida, B. F., and Machinski, I.: Use of rehabilitation measures for restoration of human physical work capacity after the prolonged limitation of motor activity. Kosm. Biol. Aviakosm. Med., 12(1):74–75, 1979.

30. Deyo, R. A., Diehl, A. K., and Rosenthal, M.: How many days of bed rest for acute low back pain? N. Engl. J. Med., 315:1064–1092, 1986.

31. Dolkas, C. B., and Greenleaf, J. E.: Insulin and glucose responses during bedrest with isotonic and isometric exercise. J. Appl. Physiol., 43(6):1033–1038, 1977.

32. Dolkas, C. B., and Sandler, H.: Countermeasure effectiveness of abnormal glucose tolerance during bedrest. Washington, D.C., Aerospace Med. Assoc. Preprints, 1974, pp. 169–70.

33. Donaldson, C. L., Hulley, S. B., Vogel, J. M., et al: Effect of prolonged bed rest on bone mineral. Metabolism, 19:1071–1084, 1970.

34. Downs, F. S.: Bedrest and sensory disturbances. Am. J. Nurs., 74:434–438, 1974.

35. Drivas, G., Ward, M., and Kerr, D.: Immobilization hypercalcemia in patients on regular hemodialysis. Br. Med. J., 3(5981):468, 1975.

36. Eastman, N. J.: The abuse of rest in obstetrics. J.A.M.A., 125:1077–1079, 1944.

37. Eichelberger, L., Roma, M., and Moulder, P. V.: Effects of immobilization on the histochemical characterization of skeletal muscle. J. Appl. Physiol., 12:42–50, 1958.

38. Eldrige, L., Liebhold, M., and Steinback, J. H.: Alterations in cat skeletal neuromuscular junctions following prolonged inactivity. J. Physiol. (London), 313:529–545, 1981.

39. Enneking, W. F., and Horowitz, M.: The Intraarticular effects of immobilization on the human knee. J. Bone Joint Surg., 54:973–985, 1972.

40. Fareeduddin, K., and Abelmann, W. H.: Impaired orthostatic tolerance after bed rest in patients with myocardial infarction. N. Engl. J. Med., 280(7):345–350, 1969.

41. Ferguson, A. B., Vaughn, L., and Ward, L.: A study of disuse atrophy of skeletal muscle in the rabbit. J. Bone Joint Surg., 39-A:583–596, 1957.

42. Finsterbush, A., and Friedman, B.: Early changes in immobilized rabbit's knee joint: A light and electron microscopic study. Clin. Orthop., 92:305–319, 1973.

43. Fraser, T. M.: The Effects of Confinement as a Factor in Manned Space Flight. NASA Report CR-511. Washington, D.C., NASA, 1966.

44. Fuller, J. H., Bernauer, E. M., and Adams, W. C.: Renal function, water and electrolyte exchange during bedrest with daily exercise. Aerospace Med., 41(1):60–72, 1970.

45. Garcia-Bunuel, L., and Garcia-Bunuel, V. M.: Connective tissue metabolism in normal and atrophic skeletal muscle. J. Neurol. Sci., 47:69–77, 1980.

46. Gersten, J. W.: Effect of ultrasound on tendon extensibility. Am. J. Phys. Med., 34:362–369, 1955.

47. Giannetta, C. L., and Castleberry, H. B.: Influence of bedrest and hypercapnia upon urinary mineral excretion in man. Aerospace Med., 45(7):750–754, 1974.

48. Gibbs, N. M.: Venous thrombosis of the lower limbs with particular reference to bedrest. Br. J. Surg., 191:209–235, 1957.

49. Globus, R. K., Bikle, D. D., and Morey-Holton, E.: Effects of simulated weightlessness on bone mineral metabolism. Endocrinology 114:2264–2270, 1984.

50. Goldspink, D. F.: The influence of immobilization and stretch on protein turnover in rat skeletal muscle. J. Physiol. (Lond), 264:267–282, 1977.

51. Gould, N., Donnermeyer, D., Pope, M., and Ashikaga, T.: Transcutaneous muscle stimulation as a method to retard disuse atrophy. Clin. Orthop., 164:215–220, 1982.

52. Greenleaf, J. E., Bernauer, E. M., Morse, J. T.,

et al: +Gz tolerance in man after 14-day bedrest periods with isometric and isotonic exercise conditioning. Aviat. Space Environ. Med., 46(5):671–678, 1975.

53. Greenleaf, J. E., Bernauer, E. M., Young, H. L., et al: Fluid and electrolyte shifts during bedrest with isometric and isotonic exercise. J. Appl. Physiol., 42(1):59–66, 1977.

54. Greenleaf, J. E., Greenleaf, C. J., Van Derveer, D., et al: Adaptation to Prolonged Bedrest in Man: A Compedium of Research NASA TM-X-3307. Washington, D.C., NASA, 1976, pp. 1–183.

55. Greenleaf, J. E., and Kozlowski, S.: Exerc. Sport Sci. Rev. 10:83–119, 1982.

56. Greenleaf, J. E., and Kozlowski, S.: Reduction in peak oxygen uptake after prolonged bedrest. Med. Sci. Sports Exerc., 14(6):477–480, 1983.

57. Greenleaf, J. E., Young, H. L., Bernauer, E. M., et al: Effects of isometric and isotonic exercise on body water compartments during 14 days bed rest. Washington, D.C., Aerospace Med. Assoc. Preprints, 1973, pp. 23–24.

58. Haggmark, T.: A study of morphologic and enzymatic properties of skeletal muscles after injuries and immobilization in man. Stockholm, Sweden, Thesis Karolinska Institute, 1978.

59. Steinberg, F. U. (Ed.): Immobilized Patient: Functional Pathology and Management. New York, Plenum Medical Book Co., 1980.

60. Hargens, A. G., Tipton, C. M., Gollnick, P. D., Mubarak, S. J., Tucker, B. J., and Akeson, W. H.: Fluid shifts and muscle function in humans during acute simulated weightlessness. J. Appl. Physiol., 54(4):1003–1009, 1983.

61. Haythorn, W. W.: The Mini World of Isolation: Laboratory Studies. In Rasmussen, J. F. (Ed.): Man in Isolation and Confinement. Chicago, Il., Aldine Publishing 1973, pp. 218–239.

62. Heath, 3d, H. J., Earll, J. M., Schaaf, M., et al: Serum ionized calcium during bed rest in fracture patients and normal men. Metabolism, 21:633–640, 1972.

63. Heilskov, N. C. S., and Schonheyder, F.: Creatinuria due to immobilization in bed. Acta. Med. Scand. 151:51–56, 1955.

64. Henke, J. A., Thompson, N. W., and Kaufer, H.: Immobilization hypercalcemia crisis. Arch. Surg., 110(3):321–323, 1975.

65. Henriksson, J., and Reitman, J. S.: Time course of changes in human skeletal muscle succinate dehydrogenase and cytochrome oxidase activities and maximal uptake with physical activity and inactivity. Acta Physiol. Scand. 99:91–97, 1977.

66. Walls, E. W., and Philips, E. E. (Eds.): Rest and Pain, London, Bell, 1950.

67. Holmgren, A., Mossfeldt, F., Sjostrand, T., and Strom G.: Effect of training on work capacity, total hemoglobin, blood volume, heart volume and pulse rate in recumbent and upright positions. Acta Physiol. Scand. 50:73–83, 1960.

68. Issekutz, B., Jr., Blizzard, J. J., Birkhead, N. C., et al: Effect of prolonged bed rest on urinary calcium output J. Appl. Physiol. 21:1013–1020, 1966.

69. Ivy, A. C., and Grossman, M. I.: Gastrointestinal function during convalscence. Fed. Proc. 3:236–239, 1944.

70. Jaworski, Z. F. G. (Ed.): Proceedings of the First Workshop on Bone Histomorphometry. Ottawa, University of Ottawa Press, 1976, pp. 254–256.

71. Johnson, E. W.: Pathokinesiology of Duchenne muscular dystrophy: Implications for management. Arch. Phys. Med. Rehabil., 54:4–7, 1977.

72. Johnson, P. C., Briscoll, T. B., and Carpentier, W. R.: Vascular and extravascular fluid changes during 6 days of bedrest. Aerospace Med., 42:875–878, 1971.

73. Klein, L., Player, J. S., Heiple, K. G., Bahniuk, E., and Goldberg, V. M.: Isotopic evidence for resorption of soft tissue and bone in immobilization of dogs. J. Bone Joint Surg., 64(3):225–230, 1982.

74. Kottke, F. J.: The effects of limitation of activity upon the human body. J.A.M.A., 196:117–122, 1966.

75. Krohlner, B., Toft, B., Nielsen, S. P., and Tondevold, E.: Physical exercise as prophylaxis against involutional vertebral bone loss: A controlled trial. Clin. Sci., 64(5):541–546, 1983.

76. Lawrence, G. D., Loeffler, R. G., Martin, I. G., and Conner, T. B.: Immobilization hypercalcemia: Some new aspects of treatment and diagnosis. J. Bone Joint Surg., 55:87–94, 1973.

77. Leach, C. S., Hulley, S. B., Rambaut, P. C., and Dietlein, L. F.: The effect of bedrest on adrenal function. Space Life Sci., 4(3):415–423, 1973.

78. Leadbetter, W. F., Engster, H. E.: Problems of renal lithiasis in convalescent patients. J. Urol., 53:269–281, 1945.

79. Lecocq, F. R.: The Effect of Bedrest on Glucose Regulation in Man. NASA SP-269. Washington, D.C., NASA, 1971, p. 268.

80. Lerman, S., Canterbury, J. M., and Reiss, E.: Parathyroid hormone and the hypercalcemia of immobilization. J. Clin. Endocrinol. Metab., 45(3):425–488, 1977.

81. Lipman, R. L., Schnure, J. J., Bradley, E. M., Lecocq, F. R.: Impairment of peripheral glucose utilization in normal subjects by prolonged bed rest. J. Lab. Clin. Med., 76:221–230, 1970.

82. Long, C. L., Bonilla, L. E.: Metabolic effects of inactivity and injury. In Downey, J. A. (Ed.): Physiological Basis of Rehabilitation Medicine. Philadelphia, W. B. Saunders Company, 1971, pp. 209–227.

83. Mack, P. B., and Montgomery, K. B.: Study of nitrogen balance and creatine and creatinine excretion during recumbency and ambulation of five young adult human males. Aerospace Med., 44(7):739–746, 1973.

84. McDonald, G. B., Hamilton, G. W., Barnes, R.

W., et al: Radionuclide venography. J. Nucl. Med., 14:528–530, 1973.

85. Melada, G. A., Goldman, R. H., Luestscher, J. A., and Zager, P. G.: Hemodynamics, renal function, plasma renin, and aldosterone in man after 5 to 14 days of bedrest. Aviat. Space Environ. Med., 46(9):1049–1055, 1975.

86. Micheli, L. J.: Thromboembolic complications of cast immobilization for injuries of the lower extremities. Clin. Orthop., 108:191–195, 1975.

87. Miller, M. G.: Iatrogenic and neurogenic effects of prolonged immobilization of the ill aged. J. Am. Geriatr. Soc., 23(8):360–369, 1975.

88. Moore Ede, M. C., and Burr, R. G.: Circadian rhythm of urinary calcium excretion during immobilization. Aerospace Med., 44:495–498, 1973.

89. Müller, E. A.: Influence of training and of inactivity on muscle strength. Arch. Phys. Med. Rehabil., 51:449–462, 1970.

90. Piemme, T. E.: Effects of two weeks of bed rest on carbohydrate metabolism. In Murray, R. H., and McCally, M. (Eds.): Hypogravity and Hypodynamic Environments. NASA SP-269. Washington, D.C., NASA, 1971, pp. 281–287.

91. Rosen, F. J., Woolin, D. A., and Finberg, L.: Immobilization hypercalcemia after single limb fracture in children and adolescents. Am. J. Dis. Child., 132:560–564, 1978.

92. Ryback, R. S., Lewis, O. F., and Lessard, C. S.: Psychobiologic effects of prolonged bed rest (weightlessness) in young healthy volunteers (study II). Aerospace Med., 42:529–535, 1971.

93. Saltin, B., and Rowell, L. B.: Functional adaptation to physical activity and inactivity. Fed. Proc., 39(5):1506–1513, 1980.

94. Sandler, H: Effects of bedrest and weightlessness on the heart. In Bourne, G. H. (Ed.): Hearts and Heart-Like Organs, Vol. 2. New York, Academic Press, 1980, pp. 435–534.

95. Sandler, H., Vernikos, J., et al: Effects of inactivity on muscle. In Sandler, H., and Vernikos, J. (Eds.): Inactivity: Physiological Effects. Orlando, Academic Press Inc., 1986, pp. 77–97.

96. Schneider, V. S., and McDonald, J.: Skeletal calcium homeostasis and counter measures to prevent disuse osteoporosis. Calcif. Tissue Int., 36:S151–S154, 1984.

97. Sevitt, S., and Gallagher, N.: Venous thrombosis and pulmonary embolism: A clinico-pathological study in injured and burned patients. Br. J. Surg., 48:475–489, 1961.

98. Sieker, H. O., Burnum, J. F., Hickman, J. B., and Penrod, K. E.: Treatment of postural hypotension with a counterpressure garment. J.A.M.A., 161:132–135, 1956.

99. Smith, M. J.: Changes in judgment of duration with different patterns of auditory information for individuals confined to bed. Nurs. Res., 24(2):93–98, 1975.

100. Smith, S.: Studies of small groups in confinement. In Zubek, J. P. (Ed.): Sensory Deprivation: Fifteen Years of Research. East Norwalk, CT, Appleton-Century-Crofts, 1969, pp. 374–403.

101. Spector, S. A.: Effects of elimination of activity on contractile and histochemical properties of rat soleus muscle. J. Neurosci., 5(8):2177–2188, 1985.

102. Spector, S. A., Simard, C. P., Fournier, S. M., Sternlicht, E., and Edgerton, V. R.: Architectural alterations of rat hind limb skeletal muscle immobilized at different lengths. Exp. Neurol., 76:94–110, 1982.

103. Spielman, G., Gennarelli, T. A., Rogers, C. R.: Disodium etidronate: Its role in preventing heterotopic ossification in severe head injury. Arch. Phys. Med. Rehabil., 64:539–542, 1983.

104. Staniloff, H. M.: Current concepts in cardiac rehabilitation. Am. J. Surg., 147:719–724, 1984.

105. Steinberg, F. U.: The Immobilized Patient: Functional Pathology and Management. New York, Plenum Press, 1980, pp. 1–156.

106. Stewart, A. F., Adler, M., Byers, C. M., Segre, G. V., and Broadus, A. E.: Calcium homeostasis in immobilization: An example of resorptive hypercalciuria. N. Engl. J. Med., 306:1136–1140, 1982.

107. Stolov, W. C., Fry, L. R., Riddel, W. M., and Weilepp, T. G., Jr.: Adhesive forces between muscle fibers and connective tissue in normal and denervated rat skeletal muscle. Arch. Phys. Med. Rehabil., 54:208–213, 1973.

108. Stremel, R. W., Convertino, V. A., Bernauer, E. M., and Greenleaf, J. E.: Cardiorespiratory deconditioning with static and dynamic leg exercise during bedrest. J. Appl. Physiol., 41(6):905–909, 1976.

109. Stremel, R. W., Convertino, V. A., Greenleaf, J. E., Bernauer, E. M.: Response to maximal exercise after bed rest. (Abstract.) Fed. Proc., 33:327, 1974.

110. Svanberg, L.: Influence of posture on lung volume ventilation and circulation in normals: A spirometric and bronchospirometric investigation. Scand. J. Clin. Lab. Invest. 9(525):1–195, 1957.

111. Takayama, H., Tomiyama, M., Minagawa, A., Imasaki, T., and Tanaka, K.: [The effect of physical exercise and prolonged bedrest on carbohydrate, lipid and amino acid metabolism (author's transl)]. Jpn. J. Clin. Pathol., 22(Suppl):126–136, 1974.

112. Taylor, H. L.: The effects of rest in bed and of exercise on cardiovascular function. Circulation, 38(6):1016–1017, 1968.

113. Taylor, H. L., Henschel, A., Porozek, J., and Keys, A.: Effects of bedrest on cardiovascular function and work performance. J. Appl. Psychol., 2:223–29, 1949.

114. Parker, J. F., Lewis, C. S., and Christensen, D. G. (Eds.): Conference Proceedings of Spaceflight Deconditioning and Physical Fitness. NASA Pub-

lication NASW–3469. Washington, D.C., NASA, 1981, pp. 13–81.

115. Todd, J. W., Frisbie, J. H., Rossier, A. B., et al: Deep venous thrombosis in acute spinal cord injury: A comparison of 1251 fibrinogen leg scanning, impedance plethysmyography and venography. Paraplegia, 14(1):50–57, 1976.

116. Uhthoff, H. K., and Jaworski, Z. F. G.: Bone loss in response to long-term immobilization. J. Bone Joint Surg., 60-B:420–429, 1978.

117. Vallbona, C.: Bodily responses to immobilization. *In* Kottke, F. J., Stillwell, G. K., and Lehmann, J. F. (Eds.): Krusens's Handbook of Physical Medicine & Rehabilitation, 3rd Ed. Philadelphia, W. B. Saunders Company, 1982, pp. 963–976.

118. Vallbona, C., Spencer, W. A., Cardus, D., Dale, J. W.: Control of orthostatic hypotension in quadriplegic patients with the use of a pressure suit. Arch. Phys. Med. Rehabil., 44:7–18, 1963.

119. Vernikos, J.: Stress response as a function of age and sex. *In* Cullen, J., Siegrist, J., Wegman, H. M. (Eds.): Breakdown in Human Adaptation to Stress, Vol. I, Part 2. Boston, Kluwer Academic Publishers, 1984, pp. 509–521.

120. Vernikos-Danellis, J., Winget, C. M., Leach, C. S., and Rambaut, P. C.: Circadian endocrine and metabolic effects of prolonged bedrest: two 56-day bedrest studies. NASA Technical Bulletin TMX-3051. Washington, D.C., NASA, 1974, pp. 1–45.

121. Vernikos-Danellis, J., Dallman, M. F., Forsham, P., Goodwin, A. L., and Leach, C. S.: Hormonal indices of tolerance to +Gz acceleration in female subjects. Aviat. Space Environ. Med., 49:886–889, 1978.

122. White, P. D., Mallory, G. K., Salcedo-Salger, J.: The speed of healing of myocardial infarcts. Trans. Am. Clin. Climatol. Assoc., 52:97–104, 1937.

123. Wirth, A., Diehm, C., Mayer, H., Mört, H., Vogel, I., Björntorp, P., and Schlierf, G.: Plasma C-peptide and insulin in trained and untrained subjects. J. Appl. Physiol., 50:71–77, 1981.

124. Wolf, A. W., Chuinard, R. G., Riggins, R. S., et al: Immobilization hypercalcemia. Clin. Orthop., 118:124–29, 1976.

125. Young, D. R., Niklowitz, W. J., Brown, R. J., and Jee, W. S.: Immobilization-associated osteoporosis in primates. Bone, 7:109–117, 1986.

53

Rehabilitation of Patients with Lymphedema

PAUL A. NELSON

Edema is the abnormal accumulation of fluid in the body and is usually caused by cardiac, hepatic, or renal disease. Lymphedema is swelling of soft tissues due to an accumulation of lymph, the fluid carried in the vessels that accompany arteries and veins and that, like the latter, possess smooth muscle and valves to aid in centripetal flow of lymph. The lymphatic system retrieves plasma proteins filtered out through blood capillary walls and transmits them back into the venous circulation via the regional lymph nodes and the thoracic duct. Aided by the normal action of skeletal muscles, the lymph fluid can move from the feet to the thoracic duct in just a few minutes.[1] This flow may be assisted by pulsation of adjacent blood vessels, by the thoracic pump, and by gravity.[2]

Lymphatic vessels compose a closed, endothelium-lined system, originating in capillaries that are more permeable than those of blood to microscopic particles and protein molecules and that are bathed on the outside by tissue fluid. Although it contains fibrinogen and thrombin, lymph does not normally contain thromboplastin substance, a constituent of platelets; for this reason, lymph clots more slowly, in 10 to 20 minutes, than does blood, which clots in 4 to 8 minutes. However, when bacteria or traumatized cell fragments, which contain thromboplastin, are present in lymph, thrombosis in a lymph vessel may readily occur. This thrombus soon contracts, separating itself from the vessel wall, thereby leaving some space for lymph to flow around the clot. Subsequently, however, recurrent thromboses may completely block the vessel.[3]

Primary Lymphedema

In the fetus there may be aplasia of the lymphatic system in some part of the developing body, and as a consequence the infant is born with marked swelling of one or more limbs. This condition, which is quite rare, is called lymphedema congenita. More frequently, swelling of an extremity develops during childhood or adolescence without any history of trauma to the limb or previous evidence of impaired circulation; this is lymphedema praecox. When a similar situation occurs in an adult, it is termed lymphedema tarda. These three forms of primary lymphedema presumably are all caused by deficient development *in utero* of the lymphatic system.

Secondary Lymphedema

Among 300 cases of lymphedema of the lower extremity studied at the Mayo Clinic, approximately one third had been diagnosed as primary lymphedema (lymphedema praecox in 93 and congenital lymphedema in 12). In another third of the 300 patients, the onset of lymphedema was considered unrelated to inflammation, occurring after surgical removal of inguinal lymph nodes in 61, after occlusion of lymphatic trunks by malignant growths in 32, after radiotherapy with secondary scar tissue formation in three, and after prolonged compression in one. In the remaining 98 patients, inflammation apparently was the major cause of swelling of the lower limb; diagnosis of thrombo-

1134

phlebitis, lymphangitis, or cellulitis was made in 41, of some injury to soft tissues in 33, of venous insufficiency in 12, of trichophytosis in five, of unspecified systemic disease in five, and of filariasis in one patient.[4]

Among 247 cases of lymphedema of the upper extremity studied at the Cleveland Clinic, swelling was associated with surgical removal of the breast necessitated by malignant tumor in 231 patients. Four of the remaining 16 patients had been diagnosed with idiopathic lymphedema: two, lymphedema praecox; and one each, axillary vein occlusion, Cushing's disease, Hodgkin's granuloma, lupus erythematosus, melanoma, obesity, scar tissue, trauma, use of depilatory cream, and vascular hematoma.[5] Because of its predominant role, postmastectomy lymphedema of the upper extremity deserves the physician's special attention.

Etiologic Factors in Postmastectomy Lymphedema

At a site of severe inflammation, particles of colloidal size or larger will pass through the capillary endothelium into the tissue spaces but will not be removed because of the formation of fibrin thrombi in the lymphatic vessels, which will obstruct the flow of lymph.[6] When the protein content of lymph increases, collagen is laid down more rapidly. This fibrosis contributes to further stasis of lymph flow. As a result of the accumulation of lymph fluid and protein in the tissues, there is increased susceptibility to infection. Thus, a vicious cycle is set up with progressive thromboses in lymph vessels, more stasis of lymph, more fibrosis, and progressive enlargement of the limb.

Lymphatic vessels have remarkable powers of regeneration. When a large lymphatic vessel is cut, a new channel develops through the scar tissue with physiological restoration of lymph flow as early as the eighth day.[7] Collateral vessels also develop extensively. However, if lymph flow is too great, it causes dilation of the collateral vessels with incompetent lymphatic valves and accumulation of lymphatic fluid and may even cause reversal of lymph flow due to the effect of gravity.

Infection

Halsted[8] ascribed elephantiasis chirurgica to wound infection, cellulitis, and necrosis of skin flaps at the suture line. He believed that decreasing

the postoperative "dead space" reduced the incidence of infection. Resulting from removal of pectoral muscles and axillary tissue, this space soon becomes filled with bloody serum, an excellent medium for growth of bacteria, which eventually is replaced by fibrous tissue. Guthrie and Gagnon[9] advocated reconstruction of a "high" axilla as a preventive measure of infection in postmastectomy lymphedema. Supporting Halsted's concept, Habif[10] emphasized the importance of avoiding skin lesions of the hand and arm, which might introduce infection; he noted even in the absence of obvious cellulitis that a lymphedematous arm decreases in size when the patient receives antibiotic therapy. Britton and Nelson[11] reported that the onset of lymphedema of the upper extremity was precipitated by acute erysipeloid cellulitis in one third of 94 patients.

Surgical Obliteration of Lymphatics

A radical mastectomy involves the extensive removal of pectoral muscles and lymph nodes and lymphatic vessels in the anterior portion of the axilla, which procedure may not leave sufficient channels for adequate lymph drainage from the upper extremity. After lymphangiography in eight patients with postmastectomy lymphedema, Danese and Howard[12] reported marked dilation of the lymphatics of the forearm and arm, extending into subdermal and even intradermal plexuses, with backflow and reflux filling of radial, medial, and ulnar channels, regardless of which channel had been cannulated. They stated that with longstanding lymphostasis, fibroblastic proliferation causes obliteration of additional lymph vessels, increased lymphatic obstruction in the axilla, and consequently progressive lymphedema and induration in the limb.

Mustard and Murillo[13] compared two operative series of patients with breast cancer: (1) 96 patients who had had a radical mastectomy between 1940 and 1945, in which there had been close dissection of tissue around the axillary vein; and (2) 121 patients who had had a radical mastectomy between 1945 and 1949, in which there had been special care taken to preserve the areolar tissue surrounding the axillary vein and the closely associated lymphatic trunk. Of the first series, 53 per cent developed lymphedema; of the second series, only 4 per cent developed postmastectomy lymphedema. The five-year survival rates were almost identical: 54 per cent for the first and 58 per cent for the second group of patients.

From these studies it is clear that in surgical removal of the breast for cancer, the surgeon should make every attempt to preserve lymphatic trunks in order to avoid postoperative lymphedema of the upper extremity.

Scar Tissue Formation After Irradiation

Possible benefit to the patient from prophylactic irradiation after radical mastectomy is still being debated. Patterson and Russell[14] found no difference in the five-year survival rates in a group of 1461 patients between those who had received routine prophylactic radiotherapy following mastectomy and those who had received radiotherapy only when there was evidence of metastatic carcinoma at the time of operation. Analyzing a group of 1007 patients with postmastectomy lymphedema, Treves[15] found the incidence of lymphedema twice as great among patients who had been irradiated as among those who had not. Several investigators have associated acute, weeping radiodermatitis with early subsequent massive lymphedema of the entire upper extremity. Such skin reactions occurred more frequently in individuals exposed to 250 kilowatt x-ray irradiation who were especially sensitive to radiation.

Quite possibly, irradiation may increase the likelihood of postmastectomy lymphedema by causing scar tissue to form in the axillary region, which may result in gradual obstruction of remaining lymphatic trunks. On the other hand, Britton and Nelson[11] reported that in 72 per cent of 114 patients, the onset of postmastectomy lymphedema had no apparent relationship to radiotherapy.

Venous Obstruction

Although Smedal and Evans[16] related postmastectomy lymphedema to thrombophlebitis of the axillary vein with accompanying lymphangitis of the perivascular sheath, venous obstruction does not appear to be an important factor in causing lymphedema. Venograms by Schorr, Hochmann, and Fraenkel[17] failed to show correlation between venous occlusion and swelling of the arm. Caution must be taken in interpreting phlebograms so as not to confuse "kinking" of the axillary vein,

occurring with adduction of the arm, with actual venous occlusion.

Treatment of Lymphedema

Elevation of the arm, application of elastic bandages, massage, hydrotherapy and exercises, mechanical compression, and other nonsurgical measures have usually helped reduce swelling temporarily but have rarely achieved lasting control of severe lymphedema either in the upper or in the lower limb. These methods are impractical for an active person and after a limited trial are usually abandoned.

Recognition of the role of infection and training the patient to avoid trivial infections have been emphasized by Guthrie and Gagnon[9] and by others. Habif[10] achieved a low incidence of lymphedema with a program of meticulous surgery, prompt treatment of infection, and instruction of the patient in proper care of the hand or foot.

Surgical Measures

In 1908 Handley[18] introduced a surgical procedure (lymphangioplasty) for alleviation of lymphedema of the upper extremity, which consisted of subcutaneous insertion of silk threads from the forearm to the shoulder designed to serve as "wicks" to assist lymphatic drainage by capillary action. Using this technique, a number of surgeons, including Treves[19] and Zieman,[20] reported early improvement in several patients, but how much benefit was due to the operation and how much to elevation and bandaging of the arm is not clear. Recurrent acute infections with marked swelling have been reported following the Handley procedure, which have necessitated extensive surgical excision of infected thread and subcutaneous tissue.

In 1912 Kondoleon[21] attempted to improve lymph drainage in the arm by attaching edematous tissue to muscle to effect communication between the superficial and deep lymphatic channels. Unfortunately, this technique proved unsatisfactory from a cosmetic point of view, resulting in increased swelling of the forearm and hand.

Numerous other surgical procedures have been advocated for correction of lymphedema of the upper extremity. Treves[22] employed Gelfoam rolls along the axillary vein; Guthrie and Gagnon[9] utilized celloidin strips inserted subcutaneously from the forearm to the shoulder. Other surgeons employed flaps from the latissimus dorsi, pectoralis minor, or teres minor muscles designed to regenerate lymphatic pathways below the axilla. Gillies and Mallard[23] reported favorable results in relief of lymphedema of the arm by re-routing lymphatic drainage by means of rotated skin flaps or full-thickness skin grafts. Goldsmith, de los Santos, and Beattie[24] advocated transmitting a long strip of omentum through a subcutaneous tunnel from the abdomen up into the arm and laying it out over the muscles. Although each of the various surgical procedures has had its advocates, none has achieved wide acceptance. If surgery is considered, it should be reserved only for patients who are greatly disabled by massive lymphedema.

Physiatric Measures

A program for management of lymphedema consists essentially of five steps:

1. Explanation to the patient of factors causing lymphedema to ensure full cooperation.

2. Vigorous initial treatment of infection with antibiotic therapy and prompt treatment of subsequent infection when it recurs.

3. Emphasis on proper care of the hand and arm or, in the case of lymphedema of the lower extremity, on proper foot care.

4. Provision of a custom-fitted, gradient-pressure elastic sleeve and gauntlet (or long and/or short elastic stockings), which the patient is expected to wear continuously when up and about.

5. Encouragement of normal use of the extremity within the patient's tolerance and of moderate elevation of the arm or leg when the patient sits for an extended time or is recumbent.

At the time of initial interview with the patient, the physician should describe the surgical procedure the patient has undergone, the usual response of tissue both to surgery and to irradiation, when it is given, and the role each procedure plays in the subsequent onset of lymphedema. The physician must emphasize what the patient can do to reduce or minimize the swelling. Some patients may develop lymphedema for the first time many years after their operation following some unusually strenuous activity, such as painting the kitchen, taking brass rubbings in a cathedral, or trimming rose bushes. Such activities, of course, must be avoided.

A swollen limb is an excellent culture medium for bacteria entering through some break in the skin. With compromised blood and lymph circulation, the swollen limb is unable to combat infection as effectively as a normal extremity. An infection may vary in appearance from an acute erysipeloid reaction with massive swelling of the arm and systemic symptoms to a faint blush and detectable induration of the skin over the inner surface of the arm and the extensor surface of the forearm. An acute cellulitis can cause thrombosis of remaining lymphatic vessels, with increased stasis of lymph and progressive fibrotic changes in connective tissue. Because of the prevalence of infection in patients with postmastectomy lymphedema (in one series of 94 patients, 53 per cent had a history of recurrent cellulitis and 77 per cent on initial examination had evidence of chronic subclinical infection[11]), initial treatment with 250 mg erythromycin four times daily for one week is justified for all patients. On rare occasions patients will require a longer period of antibiotic therapy or an alternative broad-spectrum antibiotic.

Emphasis must be placed on proper care of the swollen extremity. This may be made clearer to the patient by a *do's* and *don'ts* reminder sheet (Table 53–1). The patient is instructed to avoid all cuts, scratches, pinpricks, hangnails, insect bites, burns, and strong soaps and detergents. Specific "don'ts" are holding a cigarette in the swollen

TABLE 53–1. Instruction Sheet for Proper Hand Care To Be Given Patient with Postmastectomy Lymphedema

---

The arm may swell after a radical mastectomy because lymph vessels and nodes have necessarily been removed and the body is therefore less able to combat infection in this extremity.

Every effort must be made by you to avoid all cuts, scratches, pinpricks, hangnails, insect bites, burns, and strong detergents, as these may lead to serious infection and increased swelling.

Do not pick at or cut cuticles or hangnails.
Do not dig in the garden or work near thorny plants.
Do not reach into a hot oven.
Do not permit injections to be given in this arm.
Do not permit blood specimens to be drawn from this arm.
Do not permit your blood pressure to be taken on this arm.

Do wear loose-fitting rubber gloves when washing dishes.
Do wear a thimble when sewing.
Do apply a good lanolin-base hand cream several times daily.

Do contact your doctor if your arm appears red, warm, or unusually swollen.

Do return for a two-month check-up and measurement for a new sleeve.

hand, wearing a wristwatch, reaching into a hot oven, carrying a heavy purse, or arranging a bouquet of roses. Physicians are cautioned not to allow injections to be given into or blood to be drawn from this arm or to take blood pressure determinations on this extremity. To prevent chapping of the hand, the patient should apply hand cream liberally several times daily and wear a loose-fitting rubber glove when washing dishes. The patient should use her arm and hand normally but avoid strenuous activities.

After a week's treatment with an antibiotic, the patient returns, at which time the swollen limb is usually perceptibly reduced in size. If there is no evidence of infection at this time, the limb is inserted into an inflatable sheath and intermittent pneumatic compression is applied at 30 mm Hg pressure in three-minute cycles (2.5 minutes on and 0.5 minutes off) for five or six hours. Some centers using the same pumping device prefer 60 mg Hg pressure for a shorter time (from 30 minutes to 2 hours).[25] At the beginning of the treatment period, the patient may be given a mild diuretic (20 mg furosemide) to aid excretion of fluid. Following treatment, the therapist uses a special tape to measure circumferences of the extremity at 1.5-inch intervals from the wrist or ankle to the axilla or groin. These measurements provide the pattern for fabrication of the gradient-pressure elasticized Dacron support.

With proper care, an elastic sleeve, stocking, or tights should provide excellent support for the limb and prevent progressive swelling for two to three months of daily use. The patient should apply it each morning as soon as possible after arising and wear it continuously throughout the day when up and about. After each day's use it should be washed carefully in mild soapsuds (not detergent), rinsed thoroughly, and hung up to dry without being wrung out. If the patient has difficulty pulling on the sleeve or stocking, the limb can be dusted with baby powder. Some patients prefer to draw on their elastic stocking or sleeve over a sheer nylon hose, which then may be removed.

The elastic support should fit snugly over the involved extremity; if the material can be gathered by pinching and lifted from underlying skin, it is too loose and does not provide optimal support to the limb. In such case, the patient should receive another session of intermittent pneumatic compression and measurement for a better-fitting elastic support (Fig. 53–1).

For at least a year after the initial treatment, the patient should return at two- or three-month intervals for a recheck by the physician, intermittent pneumatic compression for three hours, and measurement for a new elastic support, which is then mailed directly to the patient's home.

Patients with lymphedema of the lower extremity are instructed to wash their feet daily with mild soap and warm water. After gentle and thorough drying—blotting, not rubbing, between the toes—they should apply a small amount of lanolin cream to the skin. If there is cracking of the skin

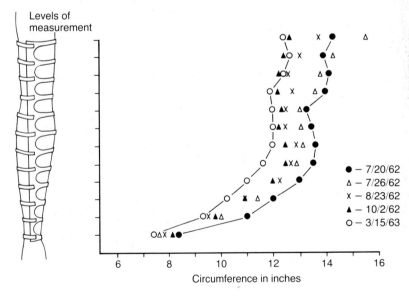

FIGURE 53–1. A series of measurements of circumference of upper extremity at various levels are required in patient with postmastectomy lymphedema. Lines joining measurements taken 7/20/62 and 3/15/63 emphasize decrease in size of arm over period of eight months.

● — 7/20/62
Δ — 7/26/62
x — 8/23/62
▲ — 10/2/62
○ — 3/15/63

between the toes, a fungicidal medicament is prescribed. They are told to cut their toenails straight across, since this decreases the likelihood of infection.

The encouraging success in the physiatric management of lymphedema has been gratifying both to patients afflicted with this distressing condition and to their physicians. Stillwell[26] has summarized the physiatric management of postmastectomy lymphedema as follows: elevation of the arm on an adjustable wooden support, manual massage, pneumatic pumping, active exercises, elastic bandaging, and instructions for home treatment. In a survey of late results of treatment in 385 patients with postmastectomy lymphedema seen over a 13-year period at the Cleveland Clinic, 183 patients were still living. Of this group, 96 patients reported that they wore their elastic sleeve every day and 25 that they wore it occasionally; and 123 patients (67.2 per cent) stated that they had benefited from the treatment program.[27]

References

1. Elkins, E. C., Herrick, J. F., Grindlay, J. H., Mann, F. C., and DeForest, R. E.: Effect of various procedures on the flow of lymph. Arch. Phys. Med. Rehabil., 34:31–39, 1953.
2. Ladd, M. P., Kottke, F. J., and Blanchard, R. S.: Studies of the effect of massage on the flow of lymph from the foreleg of the dog. Arch. Phys. Med. Rehabil., 33:604–612, 1952.
3. Opie, E. L.: Thrombosis and occlusion of lymphatics. J. Med. Res., 29:131–146, 1913.
4. Allen, E. V., Barker, N. W., and Hines, E. A., Jr.: Peripheral Vascular Diseases, 3rd Ed. Philadelphia, W. B. Saunders Company, 1962, p. 695.
5. Nelson, P. A.: Recent advances in treatment of lymphedema of extremities. Geriatrics, 21:162–173, 1966.
6. Menkin, V.: Biochemical Mechanisms in Inflammation, 2nd Ed. Springfield, IL, Charles C Thomas, Publisher, 1956.
7. Middleton, P. S.: Congenital lymphangiectatic fibrous hypertrophy (elephantiasis congenita fibrosa lymphangiectatica). Br. J. Surg., 19:356–361, 1932.
8. Halsted, W. S.: Swelling of arm after operations for cancer of breast—elephantiasis chirurgica—its cause and prevention. Bull. Johns Hopkins Hosp., 32:309–313, 1921.
9. Guthrie, D., and Gagnon, G. P.: Prevention and treatment of postoperative lymphedema of arm. Ann. Surg., 123:925–936, 1946.
10. Habif, D.: Edema of arm. In Haagensen, C. D.: Diseases of Breast. Philadelphia, W. B. Saunders Company, 1956, pp. 645–656.
11. Britton, R. C., and Nelson, P. A.: Causes and treatment of postmastectomy lymphedema of arm: Report of 114 cases. J.A.M.A., 180:95–102, 1962.
12. Danese, C., and Howard, J. M.: Postmastectomy lymphedema. Surg. Gynecol. Obstet., 120:797–802, 1965.
13. Mustard, R. L., and Murillo, C.: Prevention of arm lymphedema following radical mastectomy. Ann. Surg., 154[Suppl.]:282–285, 1961.
14. Patterson, R., and Russell, M. H.: Clinical trials in malignant disease. Part III. Breast cancer: Evaluation of postoperative radiotherapy. J. Fac. Radiologists (London), 10:175–180, 1959.
15. Treves, N.: Evaluation of etiological factors of lymphedema following radical mastectomy: Analysis of 1,007 cases. Cancer, 10:444–459, 1947.
16. Smedal, M. I., and Evans, J. A.: Cause and treatment of edema of arm following radical mastectomy. Surg. Gynecol. Obstet., 111:29–40, 1960.
17. Schorr, S., Hochmann, A., and Fraenkel, M.: Phlebographic study of swollen arm following radical mastectomy. J. Fac. Radiologists, 6:104–108, 1954.
18. Handley, W. S.: Lymphangioplasty; new method for relief of brawny arm of breast cancer and for similar conditions of lymphatic oedema. Lancet, 1:783–785, 1908.
19. Treves, N.: Management of swollen arm in carcinoma of breast. Am. J. Cancer, 15:271–276, 1931.
20. Zieman, S. A.: Re-establishing lymph drainage for lymphedema of extremities. J. Int. Coll. Surg., 15:328–331, 1951.
21. Kondoleon, E.: Die operative Behandlung der elephantiasteschen Oedema. Zentralbl. Chir., 39:1022–1025, 1912.
22. Treves, N.: Prophylaxis of postmammectomy lymphedema by use of Gelfoam laminated rolls. Cancer, 5:73–84, 1952.
23. Gillies, H., and Mallard, D. R., Jr.: The Principles and Art of Plastic Surgery, Vol. I. Boston, Little, Brown & Company, 1957, pp. 175–177.
24. Goldsmith, H. S., de los Santos, R., and Beattie, E. J., Jr.: Omental transposition in control of chronic lymphedema. J.A.M.A., 203:1119–1121, 1968.
25. Tinkham, R. G., and Stillwell, G. K.: The role of pneumatic pumping devices in the treatment of postmastectomy lymphedema. Arch. Phys. Med. Rehabil., 46:193–197, 1965.
26. Stillwell, G. K.: Physiatric management of postoperative lymphedema. Med. Clin. North Am., 46:1051–1063, 1962.
27. Ziessler, R. H., Rose, G. B., and Nelson, P. A.: Postmastectomy lymphedema: Late results of treatment in 385 patients. Arch. Phys. Med. Rehabil., 53:159–166, 1972.

54

Physiatry in Sports Medicine

JAMES C. AGRE

Physical activity and participation in sports activities is an important component of normal daily living in able-bodied and disabled individuals. Historically, at least since the time of the ancient Greeks, physical exercise has been praised as an adjunct to good health. Physical activity is known to bring about many beneficial changes both physiologically and psychologically.

Beneficial physiological adaptations resulting from endurance exercise include the following:[35] (1) increased physical work capacity; (2) increased muscular endurance; (3) reduction in adiposity; and (4) blood lipid and lipoprotein changes. All of these changes will result in a more healthy individual.

The psychological benefits of regular exercise are difficult to measure objectively; however, regular exercise is known to help relieve muscular tension, makes one feel and sleep better, increases one's alertness and level of vigor, and may aid in motivation for improving other health habits including dietary changes and cessation of cigarette smoking.

In contrast, limitation of physical activity and exercise results in a progressive deterioration of cardiovascular and musculoskeletal performance and efficiency, metabolic disturbances, and difficulty in maintaining normal body weight. Unquestionably, the physiological and psychological benefits of regular physical exercise do improve the quality of life. Although participation in sports and physical activity has not been proved to increase the years of one's life, it certainly will add life to the years. Unfortunately, participation in sports and physical activities can lead to injuries. However, in comparing the risk of physical activity (that may lead to injuries) with the risk of inactivity (that leads to adverse effects upon one's health), one may easily conclude that it is much better to be active (with its inherent risks) than to be inactive.

Since participation in sports and activities is a vital component in health maintenance, health care professionals should assist individuals in their exercise programs. The role of the health care professional in caring for the injured athlete is twofold. The health care professional should (1) advise individuals of ways to decrease the risk of injury during activity, and (2) when an injury does occur, assist the individual to achieve as complete recovery as possible.

Rehabilitation of athletic injuries is an old rather than a new concept. The use of therapeutic exercise had been recommended as early as 1000 B.C. by the Hindus and Chinese. The trainers who provided care to early Greek athletes were expected to be well versed in diet, massage, and exercise therapy. The use of hydrotherapy and weightlifting were recommended for postsurgical patients as early as the fifth century A.D.[54]

The importance of proper and adequate rehabilitation of the injured athlete constitutes one of the major focuses of sports medicine. As has been discussed by Smodlaka,[52] the treatment of most athletic injuries is nonsurgical, requiring the usage of common sense, medications where needed, and therapeutic exercise. A small percentage of athletic injuries require surgical intervention followed by appropriate and adequate rehabilitation. According to two noted orthopedic surgeons, "Rehabilitation of the athlete following injury or surgery is perhaps the most important aspect of treatment, for often the degree of rehabilitation determines the ability of the athlete to safely and effectively return to competition,"[5] and ". . . much of sports medicine is, indeed, rehabilitation."[44] For these reasons, it is important that specialists in the field of physical medicine and rehabilitation be involved in the care of injured athletes. It is hoped that the physicians in the future will be able to prescribe specific therapeutic exercise programs for their injured patients in just the same way drug prescriptions are made today. (Included in the prescription should be the specific exercises, indicating their frequency, intensity, and duration.)

In this chapter it will not be possible to cover the entire field of sports medicine, or, for that matter, the area of rehabilitation following musculoskeletal injuries. It will be the purpose of this chapter to briefly review the basic pathophysiological mechanisms of soft tissue injuries, the adverse effects of rest upon fitness, and the general principles of treatment and rehabilitation, and to provide some information on injury prevention.

The Pathophysiology of Soft Tissue Healing

Most sports-related injuries occur to the soft tissues. There are two major mechanisms for sports injuries. The injuries may be acute in nature (such as a result from a blow) or may be caused by repeated microtrauma, eventually leading to an overuse injury. Regardless of the causes of injury, an understanding of the healing process of soft tissue is needed so that the injuries can be treated intelligently and the athlete may return to his or her sport safely and quickly. The process of soft tissue healing has been recently reviewed by Medoff[39] and is summarized later.

Composition of Soft Tissues

The composition of muscles, tendons, ligaments, and other soft tissues varies, but all are composed of cellular and noncellular elements. Approximately 70 per cent of the weight of any soft tissue is water.

MUSCLE

Muscle is composed of cells which provide the contractile force that results in movement. These muscle cells, or fibers, are bonded together with a three-dimensional lattice of collagen, which connects the muscle to the skeleton. The collagen lattice has a treelike structure, starting as small filaments arising from individual muscle fibers, which coalesce and eventually fuse into a single tendon, which attaches the muscle to bone. Although "muscle pull" or muscle strain injuries are frequently diagnosed, the exact pathophysiological mechanism underlying this disorder is unknown but may be due to failure of the collagen lattice network rather than a primary rupture of the muscle fibers themselves.[39]

TENDON

Tendon is a highly structured and organized soft tissue composed of collagen fibers and connects muscle to bone. The collagen fibers in tendon run parallel from muscle to bone, and this results in a tissue with great tensile strength. Tendinitis is a commonly diagnosed inflammatory process within a tendon and is usually due to a failure of collagen fibers secondary to the application of repetitive tensile forces that exceed the biomechanical yield strength of the tendon. The inflammation within the tendon is a response to, rather than a cause of, the injury.

LIGAMENT

Ligaments are soft tissue structures that connect bone to bone. The function of ligaments is to provide resistive tensile forces that allow normal joint motion while preventing abnormal joint motion. Tendons and ligaments are almost identical in chemical and histological composition, although ligaments have a slightly higher elastin content. The collagen fibers of tendons run in a regular linear fashion, whereas those of the ligaments tend to have more of a weave, which in general allows the ligament to be more elongated at the expense of stiffness.

Healing of Soft Tissues

The healing of soft tissues can be divided conceptually into four separate phases: injury, inflammation, repair, and remodeling.[19, 24, 39, 45] Although this division is useful from a conceptual standpoint, there is a great deal of overlap of the phases.

INJURY PHASE

All soft tissue injuries occur primarily as a result of the tensile failure of collagen fibers. Several aspects of fiber composition of a given tissue are important in its biomechanical characteristics and include the following: fiber orientation, the num-

JAMES C. AGRE

ber of fiber crosslinks, the resting length, and the cross-sectional area.[64] Tissues with highly linear deposition of collagen (such as tendons) are much stiffer than is tissue with an intrinsic braid (such as the anterior cruciate ligament) when compared by equal cross-sectional areas.

Research has shown that the strength of tissues is dependent on the history of application of stress to the tissue. As little as two weeks of disuse can cause a significant decline in the strength of a soft tissue and also lead to metabolic changes in the tissue.[6] Six months or more of strenuous training may be required to increase the strength of normal tendons.[43, 59] The intensity and frequency of training has a significant influence on the strength of the collagenous components of the soft tissue. Recovery from even short periods of disuse is difficult and prolonged.[43]

The biomechanics of the collagen fiber to a large degree determines whether a given stress will result in injury. Normal collagen fibers have been stressed to the point of failure experimentally and have demonstrated several reproducible characteristics. Initially, as stress is applied to collagen, deformation of the tissue (strain) exceeds the change in stress as the fibers become oriented to the applied force (stress) (Fig. 54–1). Following this, the fibers show a linear change in deformation with increased stress (representing the functional range of the tissue). As a certain force is exceeded, deformation again exceeds increases in stress. In this stage, microfailure of fibers occurs. This plastic deformation of the tissue will not allow the tissue to return to its previous resting length and represents the initial stage of injury.[17, 38, 42, 63, 64] Noyes and colleagues[42] have shown plastic deformation to occur in a ligament up to twice the usual resting length prior to frank rupture. With further increase in stress, rupture of the tissue occurs.

INFLAMMATORY PHASE

The inflammatory phase follows injury and is an extremely complex and not well understood phenomenon. This phase peaks at about the third day following an injury. Rupture of collagen fibers and blood vessels leads to hemorrhage and an immediate humoral response (including the clotting cascade and release of chemotactic and vasoactive factors). Edema formation results from vasodilation and an increase in vascular permeability. Within hours, macrophages appear in the injured area and remain present for several weeks. The macrophages mediate fibroblast proliferation,[34]

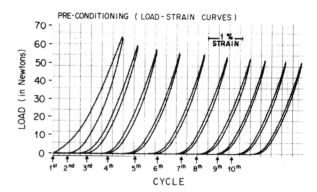

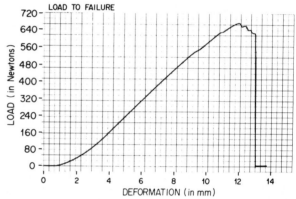

FIGURE 54–1. The stress-strain relationship of normal collagen. (From Woo, S.L.-Y., Gomez, M. A., Seguchi, Y., et al.: Measurement of mechanical properties of ligament substance from a bone-ligament-bone preparation. J. Orthop. Res., 1:22–29, 1983.)

and fibroblasts are important in the repair phase as they produce new collagen. Within a few days of injury, the first signs of revascularization appear, apparently stimulated by reduced oxygen tension and increased acidity in the area of the lesion.[10]

REPAIR PHASE

Increasing numbers of fibroblasts are found in the injured area toward the end of the inflammatory phase. The primary function of the fibroblasts is to produce collagen microfibrils.[60] Collagen is synthesized in much the same manner as are other proteins with the exception of a few unique steps. The presence of ascorbic acid is vital to the formation of collagen. In the absence of ascorbate, underhydroxylated collagen is produced, and little of this peptide escapes from the fibroblast cell; that which does escape fails to form characteristic collagen.[8]

REMODELING PHASE

By the end of the repair stage, which may take several weeks in lower extremity ligament injuries, new collagen fibers bridge the area of the injury. Although this occurs, and clinical symptoms are markedly decreased, the lattice of the collagen is a completely disorganized gel structure with very little tensile strength. The turnover of collagen is maximal at this time. This turnover may proceed for two years and accounts for the increases in strength that occur during this time. The degree of strength is dependent on many factors briefly discussed previously. In surgically created wounds to the medial collateral ligament, wound strength has been reported to be approximately 50 per cent of normal strength after 12 months.[24, 45, 64]

The increase in wound strength that occurs over time has been attributed largely to the re-orientation of collagen fibers to the lines of stress, although the development of crosslinks probably plays an additional role. How this orientation occurs is unknown, but application of small stresses on the healing wound produces significant increases in strength when compared with wounds that are completely immobilized.[11, 43, 59] For instance, in 1953, Buck sectioned the Achilles tendons of rats and allowed them to retract without suturing. In rats in which the muscles were denervated at the time the tendon was cut, the collagen fibers developed into a distorted pattern rather than in parallel bundles, as were found in the rats that had normally innervated triceps surae musculature (Fig. 54–2).

The acquisition of wound strength is a slow process, and a rational treatment of clinical injuries should consider these factors.[39] Complete immobilization appears deleterious, but too rapid an increase in stress across the area of injury will lead to re-injury, if the applied stress exceeds the strength of the healing tissue. To date, quantitative assessment in the clinic of the biomechanical parameters of an injured area is unavailable. Early *pain-free* mobilization with graduated resistive exercise in small increments should be pursued.

Adverse Effects of Rest upon Physical Fitness

Rest is an important part of the first-aid treatment and is a vital component in the care of all injuries. Immediately following injury, immobilization of the injured part will help reduce hemorrhage, edema formation, and the risk of further injury. The use of rest in the treatment of athletic injuries, however, does not come without cost. The adverse effects of rest upon the human body

should be recognized so they may be minimized as much as possible when rehabilitating the injured athlete. Complete rehabilitation of athletic injuries entails not only the rehabilitation of the injured part, but also rehabilitation of the adverse effects of rest upon the body.

The effects of inactivity and rest have been reviewed by many others in the past.[14, 20, 32, 40, 50, 58] Rest leads to impairment of muscular strength and endurance, mobility, metabolism, cardiorespiratory fitness, and neurological function (such as balance and coordination).

Effect on Muscle Strength and Endurance

It has been well established that muscular strength is maintained by frequent contractions of the muscle that produce tension.[23, 49] The stimulus to increase strength appears to be due to the maximum tension or maximal rate of metabolic activity produced during the contraction of the muscle. It has been stated that daily isometric contractions at a tension that is 20 to 30 per cent of maximal are just sufficient to maintain the strength of muscle for normal daily activities.[32] In the absence of activity, Mueller has reported a decline in strength of approximately 3 per cent per day.[40] Muscular strength and endurance are also related. As strength decreases through disuse, muscular endurance also decreases. This results from a reduction in muscular strength, circulation, and concentration of oxidative enzymes in the mitochondria of the muscle.[18, 32]

Effect on Mobility

Mobility may be impaired by shortening or fixation of connective tissues as a result of immobility. Connective tissue is constantly changing in the body, with removal, replacement, and reorganization being continuous processes within the body. Where there is frequent motion, loose areolar connective tissue is laid down as a loose meshwork of randomly oriented fibers that allows considerable range of motion to occur between moving body parts. The collagen meshwork normally shortens to the length to which the connective tissue is frequently stretched. If a part is immobilized, dense connective tissue is formed instead of areolar connective tissue. Significant reorganization of areolar connective tissue causing restriction of mo-

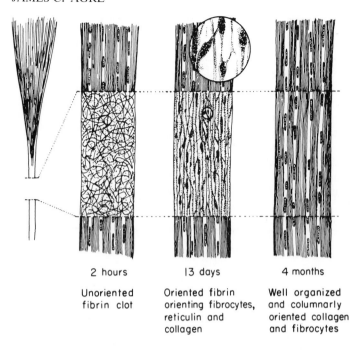

2 hours
Unoriented
fibrin clot

13 days
Oriented fibrin
orienting fibrocytes,
reticulin and
collagen

4 months
Well organized
and columnarly
oriented collagen
and fibrocytes

FIGURE 54–2. Diagram of healing of Achilles tendon of rat when cut and not sutured. (From Kottke, F. J. Therapeutic exercise. *In* Krusen, F. H., Kottke, F. J., and Ellwood, P. M.: Handbook of Medicine and Rehabilitation, 2nd Ed. Philadelphia, W. B. Saunders Company, 1971. Data of Buck.[11])

tion will occur in less than a week of immobilization, and in the presence of trauma or edema, additional collagen fibers will be laid down in as short a time as three days to even further impair motion.[32] Perkins has described the deleterious effect of limitation of motion in the clinical setting on the development of contracture of the shoulder.[46] If the injured shoulder is not immobilized, recovery of full range of motion occurs in 18 days. If the shoulder is immobilized for 7 days, recovery occurs in 52 days. If the shoulder is immobilized for 14 days, recovery occurs in 121 days. If the shoulder is immobilized for 21 days, recovery occurs in 300 days.

Effect on Cardiorespiratory Fitness

Limitation of activity, especially limitation associated with bed rest, produces significant impairment in cardiorespiratory fitness. Taylor and colleagues studied six normal and healthy young men through a control period, three weeks of bed rest, and a recovery period of up to 10 weeks. Following three weeks of bed rest, there was a marked decrease in the adaptability of the cardiovascular system to the upright posture, as well as decrease in the ability to do aerobic work and anaerobic work.[58] Similar findings were reported by Saltin

and co-workers, who studied the response to exercise after three weeks of bed rest and after training in five normal, healthy young males. Following three weeks of bed rest, lean body mass decreased while total body weight remained constant; maximal oxygen uptake fell by 27 per cent on the average (Fig. 54–3); at submaximal exertion, cardiac output declined 14 per cent; stroke volume fell by 24 per cent, while heart rate increased by 20 per cent. Calculated heart rate at an oxygen uptake of 1.5 liters per minute increased from 145 beats per minute to 180 beats per minute (Fig. 54–4). Up to eight weeks of intensive physical training was required to restore these individuals to their pre–bed rest level of cardiorespiratory fitness.[50]

Effect on Metabolism

Metabolic imbalance also occurs as a result of inactivity and bed rest. A negative protein nitrogen balance has been reported during immobilization with a loss of up to 3.5 gm of nitrogen per day.[14, 58] Deitrick and colleagues reported that a recovery period of seven weeks was required to regain the nitrogen that had been lost in normal subjects during a seven-week period of immobilization. They also showed a loss of 13 gm of calcium during the seven-week period of immobilization. In the

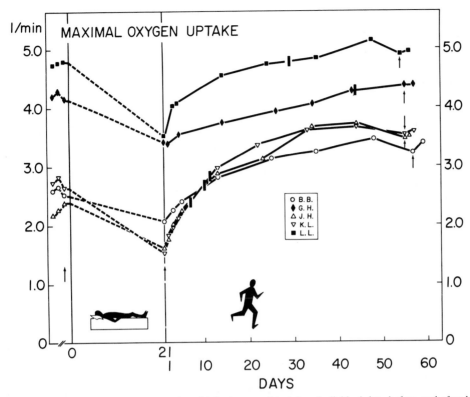

FIGURE 54–3. Changes in maximal oxygen uptake with bed rest and training. Individual data before and after bed rest and at various intervals during training. Arrows indicate circulatory studies. Heavy bars mark the time during the training period at which the maximal oxygen uptake had returned to the control value before bed rest. (From Saltin, B., Blomquist, G., Mitchell, J. H., Johnson, J. L., Wildenthal, K., and Chapman, C. B.: Response to exercise after bed rest and after training: A longitudinal study of adaptive changes in oxygen transport and body composition. Circulation, 37[Suppl. 7]:1–78, 1968. By permission of the American Heart Association, Inc.)

first three weeks of activity after bed rest, an additional 4 gm of calcium were lost. This calcium was apparently lost from the bone that did not receive stress during the bed rest period. Years may be required to restore the structure of osteoporotic bone after a period of immobilization.[14]

Effect on Coordination

The functional integrity of the nervous system is also highly dependent on activity. As discussed by Kottke, sensory-motor coordination is a delicately balanced relationship between sensory inflow, reflex augmentation and modification of muscular contraction, supraspinal modulation of performance, and cerebral regulation of coordinated motor activity.[32] Limitation of activity by rest changes sensory input of all types, especially of proprioceptive stimuli that are responsible for regulating neuromuscular performance. Studies in sensory

deprivation demonstrate reduction in sensory perception, intellectual function, and motor coordination following prolonged sensory deprivation.[9, 36, 61]

Rehabilitation of Athletic Injuries

There are two major mechanisms for sports injuries. Injuries may result from frequent microtrauma (overuse injuries) or from acute trauma.

Rehabilitation of Overuse Injuries

Overuse injuries commonly result from sports activities, especially of the endurance type, and may account for half of all sports injuries.[47, 55] The common etiologic factor of all overuse injuries is

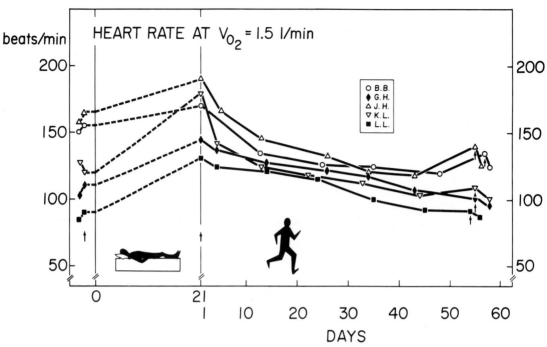

FIGURE 54-4. Heart rate during exercise at a standard submaximal oxygen uptake before and after bed rest and at various intervals during training. Heart rates at $\dot{V}_{O_2}$ 1.5 l/min calculated by linear interpolation from measurements at several submaximal oxygen uptake levels. Arrows indicate circulatory studies. (From Saltin, B., Blomquist, G., Mitchell, J. H., Johnson, J. L., Wildenthal, K., and Chapman, C. B.: Response to exercise after bed rest and after training: A longitudinal study of adaptive changes in oxygen transport and body composition. Circulation, 37[Suppl. 7]:1–78, 1968. By permission of the American Heart Association, Inc.)

repetitive trauma that exceeds the tissue's ability to repair itself. Damage to tissue from overloading is not surprising when biomechanical factors are considered.[39] For instance, the ground reactive force at mid-stance in running is 250 to 300 per cent of body weight. Thus, an average 70-kg runner will absorb well over 200 tons of force per mile run.[37] In competitive swimmers, males perform over 400,000 overhead strokes in a season, whereas females perform over 600,000 strokes.[21] Not surprisingly, over 50 per cent of world class swimmers complain of shoulder pain, most of which is due to overuse.[48]

The great frequency with which overuse injuries occur in sports indicates that anyone dealing with sports injuries should be comfortable with caring for such injuries. Factors leading to overuse injuries have been divided into intrinsic and extrinsic categories by Renstrom and Johnson[47] (Table 54-1). Intrinsic factors include problems with malalignment, which may be due to excessive femoral anteversion, pronation of the foot, or other structural causes. These factors may lead to abnormal stress being placed on bones, joints, or soft tissues,

and lead to tissue breakdown. Muscle imbalance, weakness, and poor flexibility are other intrinsic factors that may lead to athletic injuries by overstressing tissues.[2, 7, 47] Another intrinsic factor leading to overuse injuries is poor technique. This is not an uncommon cause of injury in running or swimming. For instance, in breast strokers, im-

TABLE 54-1. Factors in Overuse Injury

EXTRINSIC	INTRINSIC
Training errors	Malalignment
Time	Excessive pronation
Overdistance	Femoral neck anteversion
Repetitions	Orthopedic disorders
Intensity	Leg length discrepancy
Hills	Muscular imbalance
Technique	Muscular weakness
Fatigue	Flexibility
Surfaces	
Hard	
Soft	
Canted	
Footwear and equipment	
Environmental conditions	

proper technique for the whip-kick has been reported to cause medial knee pain.[57] Extrinsic errors are very common in running injuries.[12] In fact, James and colleagues report that 60 per cent of running injuries result from training errors.[26] These errors include increasing the time spent running, the distance of the run, or the intensity of the run too quickly. In view of the fact that over 200 tons of force will be absorbed per mile run in the average runner, it becomes readily apparent how these errors may lead to overuse running injuries.[37] Changing the surface upon which one runs, or running on a slanted surface, may also lead to overuse injuries by increasing the ground reactive forces or altering the biomechanics. Improper equipment selection (such as running shoes that provide inadequate support) may also lead to overuse running injuries.

The treatment of overuse injuries, as with other injuries, begins with rest of the injured part. Whenever possible, relative rest should be used so that the injured part may be protected and rested while the individual continues with activities to maintain as high a level of fitness as possible, but does not aggravate the injury. The use of nonsteroidal anti-inflammatory medications in addition to rest may be helpful when inflammation is a contributing factor to the overuse injury.[21] Corrections of intrinsic and extrinsic factors contributing to the overuse injury should be made through appropriate therapy and education. As the injury resolves, a gradual increase in activity in a carefully designed program, which is always subalgenic (pain-free), should be instituted.

Rehabilitation of Acute Athletic Injuries

At the time of the acute injury, pain, edema, and the extravasation of blood, lymph, or synovial fluid (depending on the tissues injured) will restrict movement and enforce immobilization. This natural immobilization, or the immobilization provided by the splint or cast, will immediately result in the onset of deconditioning and atrophy.[14, 32, 40, 50, 58] The presence of extravasated blood and lymphedema in and around joints, ligaments, muscles, and tendons will lead to the formation of adhesions and fibrosis.[30, 32] Histological evidence of fibrosis and decreased range of motion of a joint may be seen as soon as four days following injury.[11, 25] The initial phase of the rehabilitation

program is designed to minimize these problems as much as possible.

Rehabilitation means to restore to a normal or an optimal state of health. Rehabilitation of an athletic injury is the process of returning the athlete to a high level of conditioning for competition. Because athletes are immediately restricted in their movements and partially or totally immobilized after an acute injury, rehabilitation should begin with first aid and continue until the athlete is able to return to competition. The rehabilitation program for acute athletic injuries can be divided conceptually into four separate phases as outlined in the following.

PHASE 1: ACUTE TREATMENT

The first phase of rehabilitation is the immediate treatment of the acute sports injuries (such as muscle strains, joint sprains, contusions). The goals of this treatment should be directed at reducing pain, preventing further injury, and minimizing hemorrhage and edema formation (which will lead to a reduction in tissue fibrosis and, thus, expedite the healing process and the athlete's return to training and ultimately to competition). Basic principles should be followed at this time to minimize hemorrhage and edema formation (Table 54–2). Immediately following the injury, the affected part, or the entire body, if necessary, should be immobilized or placed at rest to prevent further injury. Ice or cold compresses should be applied to the injured part for 10 to 30 minutes periodically for at least the first 24 to 72 hours. The use of ice serves two purposes: it reduces pain and it results in vasoconstriction, which reduces hemorrhage and edema formation.[33] The application of a compression wrap using elastic bandage as well as elevating the injured part above the level of the heart also aids in the reduction of hemorrhage and edema formation. The use of a Jobst stocking with 50 to 100 torr of alternating air pressure has also been advocated for treating acute ankle sprain injuries.[52] When large hematomas result from an injury, aspiration has been suggested, if possible, to reduce the amount of adhesion formation and fibro-

TABLE 54–2. First-Aid Treatment for Athletic Injuries

R	est and immobilization
I	ce
C	ompression
E	levation

JAMES C. AGRE

sis.[53] In addition to these measures, the use of analgesics may aid in the reduction of pain.

PHASE 2: SUBACUTE TREATMENT

The second phase of rehabilitation follows acute treatment. The promotion of the reparative processes is the goal of this phase of rehabilitation, while at the same time, great care must be taken to avoid further damaging the injured tissues. In this phase, gradual and careful mobilization is performed. As was discussed by Perkins in his 1952 Robert Jones Lecture in London: "It is difficult to say when the inflammation has ceased and repair (of the injured part) has begun. It is difficult clinically to determine when to switch from one treatment to the other."[46] Thirty-five years later, we still face the same problem. There is no objective test that can be performed that will provide this information. The use of common sense, as was advised by Perkins and by others, continues to hold true today. Clinical experience and judgment are necessary, since there is no reliable clinical research available to answer this problem. Knowledge of the healing process of tissues, as discussed previously, is necessary in making the decision to advance treatment.

The use of early exercise is essential in the athlete's rehabilitation program. The use of exercise will facilitate the healing process,[27–29] whereas the lack of exercise may lead to permanent disability.[13] Great care must be taken, however, since exercise that is too vigorous can result in further injury and possibly permanent disability. The optimal conditions for healing depend on a balance between activity and protection of the injury from stress. Clinical experience has shown that pain is a reliable indicator for a too vigorous therapy program. The therapy program must be kept subalgenic at all times.

As the pain and induration resolve, a slowly progressive and pain-free program of passive and active mobilization of the injured part is begun to stimulate venous and lymphatic return and to prevent adhesion formation and fibrosis. As resorption continues, the use of heat may be added to induce local hyperemia and stimulate circulation in the area of the injury. The rationale for different types of heating is discussed in detail in Chapter 13. Ultrasound is the best heat modality of therapeutic benefit for deep-lying tissues and especially for heating soft tissues at bone junctions (i.e., the joint capsules). When heat treatment is initiated (waiting at least 72 hours after injury is recom-

mended), one must observe the injury site very carefully to be certain that the use of heat does not lead to further hemorrhage or induration, since this will prolong the healing time. In the first several days when heat is used, it should be combined with elevation of the extremity and compression to aid in the prevention of the development of further edema formation. Gentle, pain-free, isometric muscle strengthening exercises for the muscles at the site of the injury may be added to the program of gentle mobilization as soon as they can be performed in an absolutely pain-free fashion. This will reduce, to some extent, the loss of muscle strength associated with the injury and the mandated rest. When the induration resolves and pain-free range of motion returns to normal, dynamic strengthening exercises may be carefully initiated. Initially, manual resistive exercise with a physical therapist is recommended so that the program can be carefully monitored and the patient educated to the importance of maintaining a pain-free program (so that further injury can be prevented). The range of motion through which the resistive exercise is carried out initially should be well within the limits of pain-free motion. The range may be increased gradually as the program progresses. When manual resistive exercise through the entire range of motion can be performed without pain, progressive resistive exercises with free weights or the use of gym equipment or isokinetic equipment may be initiated.

The importance of pain-free mobilization, stretching, and strengthening exercise must be emphasized to the patient. If the therapy program provokes pain, it indicates that tissues are being damaged. This will only prolong the healing process and the therapy time. Additionally, if strengthening exercises provoke pain and the patient does not heed this signal, the patient will learn to recruit muscles improperly. This will lead to uncoordinated muscle contractions, which will definitely impair the patient's progress in the rehabilitation program.

Throughout the first two phases of the rehabilitation program the athlete should be allowed to be as active as possible, as long as the site of injury is protected so that further injury cannot be induced. This will help minimize the deleterious effects of rest and maintain, as much as possible, the athlete's level of fitness.

PHASE 3: SUPERVISED PROGRESSIVE EXERCISE PROGRAM

The third phase of the rehabilitation program is begun when manual resistive exercise of the injured part can be performed throughout the entire range of motion without provoking pain. The goals of this phase are to achieve complete return in flexibility, muscular strength, muscular endurance, muscular speed, muscular power, coordinated movement patterns and agility, and cardiorespiratory fitness so that the athlete can return to competition.

Flexibility. During any period of immobilization, flexibility is reduced and needs to be treated with a stretching program. Static stretching, proprioceptive neuromuscular facilitation (PNF) techniques (static stretching interspersed with isometric contraction of the agonist muscle),[31] and static stretching interspersed with isometric contraction of the antagonist muscle are all effective means of improving flexibility. An example of each technique for stretching the hamstring muscles is described in the following.

Static stretching entails applying tension to the hamstring muscles in a lengthened position within the range of tolerance to discomfort for 30- to 60-second intervals with short breaks between intervals. This is repeated several times, each time with the muscle held at its maximal tolerated length.

PNF stretching usually requires the use of a partner. The partner passively flexes the subject's hip (with the knee straight) until the hamstring muscles are brought to their maximal tolerated length; the hip is then slightly extended (to minimally reduce the length of the hamstrings). The subject then isometrically contracts the hamstrings, building up to maximal force over one to two seconds, and then holds this maximal effort for approximately five seconds. The subject relaxes, and then the partner passively flexes the hip until the hamstrings again reach the tolerated point of lengthened position, and this is held for 15 to 30 seconds. This cycle is repeated several times. This technique makes use of Golgi tendon organ excitation, which inhibits both the alpha motor neurons of the motor units and the gamma motor neurons of the extrafusal muscle fibers.

When stretching the hamstring muscles using isometric contraction of the antagonist muscle, the hip is flexed with the knee extended until the hamstrings reach their maximal tolerated stretched length. The subject then isometrically contracts the ipsilateral quadriceps muscles, following which the hamstrings relax to allow further stretching of the hamstring muscles. This is also repeated several times. This technique makes use of reciprocal inhibition.

The neurophysiology of these stretching techniques has been reviewed by Stanish in greater detail.[56] The stretching program is more effective if a period of warm-up precedes the stretching so that the tissues are warmer, and if stretching is also performed during the cool-down period.[62] All stretching must be performed carefully so that flexibility is improved while the risk of injury from the stretching program is minimized.

Muscular Strength and Endurance. Progressive resistive exercise is performed to improve muscular strength and endurance. Therapeutic exercises to develop strength and endurance are discussed in detail by De Lateur (Chapter 20). During strength training, both sides of the body should be worked independently, since this prevents the injured limb from depending on the noninjured limb. Once strength of the injured side is 90 to 95 per cent of the strength of the noninjured side, emphasis of the program should be changed to the development of endurance.

Muscular Speed. Muscular speed can be developed by participation in sport-related exercises in the athlete's sport. Participation in exercises at approximately half speed, gradually increasing to three-fourths speed, and finally up to full speed, can be begun once muscular strength has returned to at least 90 per cent of normal (or of the noninjured side). Isokinetic equipment can also be used to develop muscular speed, but sport-specific speed training will also enhance coordination and help re-develop the skill patterns required for the athlete's sport.

Coordinated Movement Patterns. Only the repetitive practice of sport-specific skill patterns in training can develop the coordinated movement patterns required. Coordination is developed along with muscular speed by using increasingly complex exercises and slowly increasing speed. The athlete should be very carefully observed to be certain that the activities are being performed correctly. During this training, it is often necessary to isolate specific parts of the skill pattern to work on each one individually until the movements are sufficiently coordinated so that they may be integrated together. These concepts are very similar to those of training individuals with neuromuscular impairment, which is described in detail by Kottke (Chapter 19).

Cardiorespiratory Fitness. As muscular endurance develops, the activities will also develop the athlete's cardiorespiratory fitness. A much greater time may be needed for the athlete to achieve return to complete cardiorespiratory fitness than was the time of immobilization.[50] Therefore, every effort should be given in the earlier phases of rehabilitation to minimize the loss in cardiorespiratory fitness.

PHASE 4: RETURN TO COMPETITION

The fourth phase of the rehabilitation program begins when the athlete returns to competition. This phase should not begin until the athlete has achieved a complete recovery (or as complete a recovery as is possible) in flexibility, muscular strength, muscular endurance, muscular speed, muscular power (a combination of strength and speed), agility and coordinated movement patterns, and cardiorespiratory fitness. Return to competition prior to this will only place the athlete at much greater risk of sustaining another, and possibly more severe, injury. Some of the variables (such as flexibility, muscular strength, and cardiorespiratory fitness) can be objectively measured, and it is advisable to do so whenever possible. Flexibility can be measured goniometrically (Chapter 2). Muscular strength can be estimated from manual testing (Chapter 2), but precise, quantitative measurement with isokinetic or isometric devices is recommended whenever possible, since subtle deficits can be missed with manual muscle testing that might predispose the athlete to recurrent injury.[3, 4] Cardiorespiratory fitness can be measured with treadmill exercise testing.[4, 50] Following return to competition, the athlete needs to maintain a high level of training to maintain the gains made in the rehabilitation program and reduce the risk of future injury.

Injury Prevention

The easiest injuries to treat are the injuries that do not occur. This, however, is much easier said than done. There are data to indicate that the incidence of athlete injuries can be reduced. For instance, many years ago, Abbott and Kress reported that a program of thigh muscle strengthening in military academy cadets reduced both the re-injury rate and the rate of original injuries to the knee.[1] The severity of injuries that did occur was also minimized as a result of the strengthening program. Ekstrand and Gillquist prospectively studied injuries and mechanisms of injuries in soccer players.[16] They reported several interesting findings. Traumatic leg injuries occurred in players with inadequate or no shin guards. Noncontact knee injuries usually occurred in players with a history of knee injury and existing instability. A study of injury sequence revealed that a minor injury was often followed within two months by a major injury. And severe injuries that were incurred during fouls occurred to the individual causing the foul. In another study, Ekstrand and colleagues studied the efficacy of an injury prevention program in a randomized trial.[15] Twelve adult soccer teams were allocated at random to two groups of six teams, one being given a prophylactic program and the other serving as control. The prophylactic program consisted of the following:

1. Correction of training (including proper warm-up and stretching before training and a cooldown program following the training sessions).

2. Provision of optimum equipment (such as shin guards).

3. Prophylactic ankle taping (for all players with previous ankle sprains or clinical instability).

4. Controlled rehabilitation following injuries (with return to practice and games only after full pain-free range of motion and at least 90 per cent of muscle strength were achieved).

5. Players with grave knee instability were excluded.

6. Information was given to the coaches and players at training camp about the importance of disciplined play and the increased risk of injury with undisciplined play.

7. Correction and supervision of these measures were regularly made by the physician or physiotherapist.

With this program, the injuries in the test teams were 75 per cent fewer than in the controls. The most common types of soccer injuries, strains and sprains to the knees and ankles, were all significantly reduced. It was concluded that the proposed prophylactic program, including close supervision and correction by physicians and physiotherapists, significantly reduced the incidence of soccer injuries. Agre and Baxter prospectively studied a collegiate soccer team for two years.[3] The use of a well-designed warm-up and stretching program before training sessions and matches completely eliminated hamstring and hip adductor muscle strain injuries, which were very common prior to the onset of the program. It can be concluded that simple measures, as described, can be used to reduce the incidence of athletic injuries, and such preventive measures should be advocated.

The clinical use of musculoskeletal profiling is also becoming much more common.[3, 4, 22, 51] Profiling may indicate where an athlete may have a musculoskeletal abnormality that could lead to injury, if appropriate rehabilitation is not instituted. Once a particular area is determined to be at risk for injury, intervention may be undertaken to reduce the risk of injury. Preventive rehabilitation measures may include stretching or strengthening exercises, equipment modification, alteration in training technique, or other measures.

Conclusion

Physical activity and participation in sports activities is an important component of normal daily living. Unfortunately, injuries will occur from time to time as a result of sports activities. The treatment of most athletic injuries is nonsurgical, requiring the usage of common sense, medications where needed, and appropriate therapeutic exercises with proper supervision. Rehabilitation of the athlete following injury or surgery is the most important aspect of treatment. It is usually the quality and degree of rehabilitation that determine whether the athlete can safely and effectively return to competition. For this reason, specialists in physical medicine and rehabilitation need to be involved in the treatment of athletic injuries.

References

1. Abbott, H. G., and Kress, J. B.: Preconditioning in the prevention of knee injuries. Arch. Phys. Med. Rehabil., 50:326–333, 1969.
2. Agre, J. C.: Hamstring injuries: Proposed aetiological factors, prevention and treatment. Sports Med., 2:21–33, 1985.
3. Agre, J. C., and Baxter, T. L.: Musculoskeletal profile of male collegiate soccer players. Arch. Phys. Med. Rehabil., 68:142–150, 1987.
4. Agre, J. C., Casal, D. C., Leon, A. S., McNally, M. C., Baxter, T. L., and Serfass, R. C.: Professional ice hockey players: Physiologic, anthropometric, and musculoskeletal characteristics. Arch. Phys. Med. Rehabil., 69:188–192, 1988.
5. Allman, F. L.: Rehabilitation following athletic injuries. In O'Donoghue, D. H. (Ed.): Treatment of Injuries to Athletes, 4th Ed. Philadelphia, W. B. Saunders Company, 1984, p. 677.
6. Amiel, D., Akeson, W. H., Harwood, F. L., et al.: Stress deprivation effect on metabolic turnover of the medial collateral ligament collagen. Clin. Orthop., 172:265–270, 1983.
7. Baker, B. E.: Current concepts in the diagnosis and treatment of musculoskeletal injuries. Med. Sci. Sports Exerc., 16:323–327, 1984.
8. Barnes, M. J.: Function of ascorbic acid in collagen

metabolism. Ann. N. Y. Acad. Sci., 258:264–277, 1975.
9. Bexton, W. H., Heron, W., and Scott, T. H.: Effects of decreased variation in sensory environment. Can. J. Psychol., 8:70–76, 1954.
10. Branemark, P. I.: Experimental biomicroscopy. Bibl. Anat., 5:51–55, 1965.
11. Buck, R. C.: Regeneration of tendon. J. Pathol. Bacteriol., 66:1–18, 1953.
12. D'Ambrosia, R., and Drez, D. (Eds.): Prevention and Treatment of Running Injuries. Thorofare, NJ, Charles B. Slack, 1982.
13. Dehn, E., and Torp, R. P.: Treatment of joint injuries by immediate mobilization. Clin. Orthop., 77:218–231, 1971.
14. Deitrick, J. E., Whedon, D., and Shorr, E.: Effects of immobilization upon various metabolic and physiologic functions of normal men. Am. J. Med., 4:3–36, 1948.
15. Ekstrand, J., Gillquist, J., and Liljedahl, S. O.: Prevention of soccer injuries, supervision by doctor and physiotherapist. Am. J. Sports Med., 11:116–120, 1983.
16. Ekstrand, J., and Gillquist, J.: Soccer injuries and their mechanisms: A prospective study. Med. Sci. Sports Exerc., 15:267–270, 1983.
17. Frank, C., Woo, S. L.-Y., Amiel, D., et al.: Medial collateral ligament healing: A multidisciplinary assessment in rabbits. Am. J. Sports Med., 11:379–389, 1983.
18. Grimby, G., and Einarsson, G.: Muscle morphology with special reference to muscle strength in postpolio subjects. Birth Defects: Original Article Series, 23:265–274, 1987.
19. Gross, L., and Smith, L. W.: Wound healing and tissue regeneration. In Barnothy, M. F. (Ed.): Biologic Effects of Magnetic Field. New York, Plenum Press, 1964, pp. 140–145.
20. Herbison, G. J., and Tabbot, J. M.: Muscle atrophy during space flight: Research needs and opportunities. Physiologist, 28:520–527, 1985.
21. Herring, S. A., and Nilson, K. L.: Introduction to overuse injuries. Clin. Sports Med., 6:225–239, 1987.
22. Hershman, E.: The profile for prevention of musculoskeletal injury. Clin. Sports Med., 3:65–84, 1984.
23. Hettinger, T., and Mueller, E. A.: Muskelleistung und Muskeltraining. Arbeitsphysiologie, 15:111–126, 1953.
24. Hunt, T. K., and Van Winkle, W., Jr.: Wound healing. In Hepenstall, R. B. (Ed.): Fracture Treatment and Healing. Philadelphia, W. B. Saunders Company, 1980, pp. 1–34.
25. Jackson, D. S., Flickinger, D. B., and Dunphy, J. E.: Biomechanical studies of connective tissue repair. Ann. N. Y. Acad. Sci., 86:943–947, 1960.
26. James, S. L., Bates, B. T., and Ostering, L. R.:

Injuries to runners. Am. J. Sports Med., 6:40–50, 1978.

27. Jarvinen, M.: Healing of a crush injury in rat striated muscle. 2. A histological study of the effect of early mobilization and immobilization on the repair process. Acta Pathol. Microbiol. Scand., A83:269–282, 1975.

28. Jarvinen, M.: Healing of a crush injury in rat striated muscle. 3. A microangiographical study of the effect of early mobilization and immobilization on capillary ingrowth. Acta Pathol. Microbiol. Scand., A84:85–94, 1976.

29. Jarvinen, M.: Healing of a crush injury in rat striated muscle. 4. Effect of early mobilization and immobilization on the tensile properties of gastrocnemius muscle. Acta Chir. Scand., 142:47–56, 1976.

30. Knapp, M. E.: Practical physical medicine and rehabilitation: Lecture 5: Late treatment of fractures and complications, part 1. Postgrad. Med., 40:A109–A113, 1966.

31. Knott, M., and Voss, D. E.: Proprioceptive Neuromuscular Facilitation, Patterns and Techniques. New York, Harper & Row, 1965.

32. Kottke, F. J.: The effects of limitation of activity upon the human body. J. A. M. A., 196:825–830, 1966.

33. Lehman, J. F. (Ed.): Therapeutic Heat and Cold, 3rd Ed. Baltimore, Williams & Wilkins, 1982, pp. 563–602.

34. Leibovich, S. J., and Ross, R.: A macrophage dependent factor that stimulates the proliferation of fibroblasts in vitro. Am. J. Pathol., 84:501–514, 1976.

35. Leon, A. S., and Blackburn, H.: The relationship of physical activity to coronary heart disease and life expectancy. Ann. N. Y. Acad. Sci., 301:561–578, 1977.

36. Lilly, J. C.: Mental effects of physical restraint and of reduction of ordinary levels of physical stimuli of intact, healthy persons. Psychiatr. Res. Rep. Am. Psychiatr. Assoc., 5:1–9, 1956.

37. Mann, R. A.: Biomechanics of running. In Mack, R. P. (Ed.): American Academy of Orthopedic Surgeons Symposium on the Foot and Leg in Running Sports. St. Louis, C. V. Mosby, 1982.

38. Marinozzi, G., Pappalardo, S., and Steindler, R.: Human knee ligaments: Mechanical test and ultrastructural observation. Ital. J. Orthop. Traumatol., 9:231–240, 1983.

39. Medoff, R. J.: Soft tissue healing. Ann. Sports Med., 3:67–70, 1987.

40. Mueller, E. A.: Influence of training and of inactivity on muscle strength. Arch. Phys. Med. Rehabil., 51:449–462, 1970.

41. Nigg, B. M.: Biomechanics, load analysis and sports injuries in the lower extremities. Sports Med., 2:367–379, 1985.

42. Noyes, F. R., DeLucas, J. L., and Torvik, P. J.: Biomechanics of anterior cruciate ligament failure: An analysis of strain-rate sensitivity and mechanisms of failure in primates. J. Bone Joint Surg., 56A:236–253, 1974.

43. Noyes, F. R., Torvik, P. J., Hyde, W. B., et al.: Biomechanics of ligament failure. II. An analysis of immobilization, exercise, and reconditioning effects in primates. J. Bone Joint Surg., 56A:1406–1418, 1974.

44. O'Donoghue, D. H.: Treatment of Injuries to Athletes, 4th Ed. Philadelphia, W. B. Saunders Company, 1984.

45. Peacock, E. E., Jr., and Van Winkle, W., Jr.: The biochemistry and the environment of wounds and their relation to wound strength. In Peacock, E. E., and Van Winkle, W. (Eds.): Surgery and Biology of Wound Repair, 2nd ed. Philadelphia, W. B. Saunders Company, 1976, pp. 81–203.

46. Perkins, G.: Rest and movement. J. Bone Joint Surg., 35B:521–539, 1953.

47. Renstrom, P., and Johnson, R. J.: Overuse injuries in sports: A review. Sports Med., 2:316–333, 1985.

48. Richardson, A. B., Jobe, F. W., and Collins, H. R.: The shoulder in competitive swimming. Am. J. Sports Med., 8:159–163, 1980.

49. Rose, D. L., Radzyminski, S. F., and Beatty, R. R.: Effect of brief maximal exercise on strength of the quadriceps femoris. Arch. Phys. Med. Rehabil., 38:157–164, 1957.

50. Saltin, B., Blomquist, G., Mitchell, J. H., Johnson, J. L., Wildenthal, K., and Chapman, C. B.: Response to exercise after bed rest and after training: A longitudinal study of adaptive changes in oxygen transport and body composition. Circulation, 38[Suppl. 7]:1–78, 1968.

51. Sapega, A. A., and Nicholas, J. A.: The clinical use of musculoskeletal profiling in orthopedic sports medicine. Phys. Sportsmed., 9:80–88, 1981.

52. Smodlaka, V. N.: Rehabilitating the injured athlete. Phys. Sportsmed., 5:43–52, 1977.

53. Smodlaka, V. N.: Rehabilitation of injured soccer players. Phys. Sportsmed., 7:59–67, 1979.

54. Snook, G.: The history of sports medicine. Am. J. Sports Med., 12:252–257, 1984.

55. Sperryn, P. N., and Williams, J. G. P.: Why sports injury clinics? Br. Med. J., 5966:364–365, 1975.

56. Stanish, W. D.: Neurophysiology of stretching. In D'Ambrosia, R., and Drez, D. (Eds.): Prevention and Treatment of Running Injuries. Thorofare, NJ, Charles B. Slack, 1982.

57. Stullberg, S. D., Shulman, K., Stuart, S., and Culp, P.: Breaststrokers knee: Pathology, etiology, and treatment. Am. J. Sports Med., 8:164–171, 1980.

58. Taylor, H. L., Henschel, A., Brozek, J., and Keys, A.: Effects of bed rest on cardiovascular function and work performance. J. Appl. Physiol., 2:223–239, 1949.

59. Tipton, C. M., Mathes, R. D., Maynard, J. A., et al.: The influence of physical activity on ligaments and tendons. Med. Sci. Sports, 7:165–175, 1975.

60. Van Winkle, W., Jr.: The fibroblast in wound healing. Surg. Gynecol. Obstet., 124:369–386, 1967.

61. Vernon, J., and Hoffman, J.: Effect of sensory deprivation on learning rate in human beings. Science, 123:1074–1075, 1956.

62. Warren, C. J., Lehmann, J. F., and Koblanski, J. N.: Elongation of rat tail tendon: Effect of load and temperature. Arch. Phys. Med. Rehabil., 52:465–474, 1971.

63. Woo, S. L.-Y.: Mechanical properties of tendons and ligaments. Biorheology, 19:385–396, 1983.

64. Woo, S. L.-Y., Gomez, M. A., Seguchi, Y., et al.: Measurement of mechanical properties of ligament substance from a bone-ligament-bone preparation. J. Orthop. Res., 1:22–29, 1983.

55

Treatment of Spasticity by Neurolysis

ESSAM A. AWAD   DENNIS DYKSTRA

Intramuscular Neurolysis Using Phenol

Spasticity, manifested as involuntary contraction of paretic muscles, is a major problem in the rehabilitation of patients afflicted with diseases or injury of the central nervous system. This is commonly seen in patients with cerebral palsy, multiple sclerosis, spinal cord injury, myelopathy, familial spastic paraplegia, stroke, and lateral sclerosis. These patients show varying degrees of functional impairment and disability. At the University of Minnesota Hospital and Clinic, treatment of spasticity by phenol blocks has been utilized for over 25 years, providing good control of spasticity in a rapid and cost-effective manner. In a selected population of patients with spasticity, phenol blocks allow restoration of useful function in the extremities.

Spasticity as a Problem

Patients with central nervous system disorders usually manifest spasticity in the flexor muscle groups, although the extensors may also be affected. Spasticity in the upper extremity in the hemiplegic patient results in adduction and internal rotation of the shoulder, flexion of the elbow, pronation of the forearm, and flexion of the wrist and fingers. In the lower extremity, spasticity results in hip and knee flexion as well as plantar flexion of the foot. The plantar flexion of the foot results in apparent lengthening of the lower extremity, which forces the patient to circumduction during ambulation. The heel often slips out of the shoe. Shuffling of the forefoot further interferes with walking and predisposes the patient to fall. Spasticity of the arm renders the hand useless, particularly in cases in which there is some voluntary muscular strength in the flexors of the fingers, which is usually exaggerated by the involuntary spasticity. Often, in these patients, there is some return of strength in the extensor muscles of the fingers and the wrist that is difficult to assess because of excessive finger and wrist flexor spasticity and spasms. Thus, these patients not only are unable to use their hands but also have difficulty in dressing, grooming, self-feeding, writing, grasping, or wearing gloves in order to go outside in cold weather.[1] Similar statements could be made regarding multiple sclerosis patients, although spasticity usually affects the lower extremities, particularly the hip adductors and flexors as well as the hamstrings and the plantar flexors of the feet. Bilateral hip adductor spasticity interferes with perineal hygiene, catheterization, and sexual intercourse.[2] In the cerebral palsy patient, the same muscles are usually spastic, resulting in the classic spastic diplegic gait. Thus, the problems resulting from spasticity could be summarized as difficulty in activities of daily living and in ambulation.

Treatment of Spasticity

Several methods for control of spasticity have been used in this patient population. Perhaps the most common is the use of drugs. These are useful in cases of excessive widespread spasticity. However, many patients on antispasticity drugs tend to become drowsy, and spasticity is never completely abolished while the patient is fully conscious. Drawbacks of drugs include toxic reactions, hypersensitivity, and intolerance.

Surgical procedures such as tenotomy or neurectomy have been utilized.[3] These expose the patient who is already disabled to surgical risk as well as postoperative restriction of motion. Selective posterior rhizotomies have been performed in cerebral palsy children with fair results.[4] Peripheral nerve blocks have the disadvantage of loss of sensation in the distribution of the nerve block; in some cases they also result in severe neuritic pain that lasts for several months.[5]

Motor Point Blocks

Motor point blocks, or intramuscular neurolysis, have been used at the University of Minnesota Hospitals since 1963. We have accumulated an extensive experience over many years and modified the procedure continually to achieve the best possible results for our patients. This procedure taxes the patient less heavily than any other method for control of spasticity. It is performed for adult patients in the outpatient clinic without anesthesia. For children, however, an anesthetic is needed in order to enable the physiatrist to properly localize the motor points and the terminal branches of the intramuscular nerves. This requires the patient not to move the limb involved. The most important advantage of this technique is that it can be tailored to the needs of the individual patient so that one can eliminate the undesirable involuntary spasticity and at the same time retain the proper function in the particular muscle. This is impossible to achieve if peripheral nerve blocks, surgical intervention, or antispasticity drugs are used.

Intramuscular neurolysis is most effective in patients when the problem of spasticity is well localized to a limited number of muscles. It is not as effective and is difficult to perform when all the extremities are severely spastic. It should also be stated clearly that this procedure will not reduce a severe contracture. However, it will assist the therapist in stretching and overcoming a mild to moderately severe contracture, a condition that often underlies spasticity of long duration.

How much blocking can one do? To answer this question, the patients may be divided into two groups according to the spastic extremity's being functional or nonfunctional. If the extremity to be blocked is functional, even with minimal function present, extreme care and a very limited approach is pursued. On the other hand, if the part is nonfunctional and the prognosis for return of function is definitely nil, then more liberal blocks are performed.

Apparatus

Two types of stimulators have been used.

TECA Ch3 Chronaximeter and Variable Pulse Generator. This stimulator generates electrical stimuli of adjustable intensity, duration, and intervals between pulses. Prior to the development of sophisticated electromyographical equipment, it was commonly used for quantitative electrodiagnostic procedures such as chronaxie and the strength-duration curves. The instrument utilizes 110 volts, 60-cycle power. Adjust the selector switch to chronaxie. In this position, the instrument generates pulses of adjustable duration and intervals. The output switch could be positioned to run continuously, manually, or through the use of a foot switch.

Portable Block Stimulator. A small, portable constant-current stimulator was built by our engineers especially for this purpose. This instrument is easy to carry to the patient anywhere. The output is a square wave pulse, 0.25 msec in duration, and the output intensity is 0 to 10 mA. The frequency of stimuli is set at 2 Hz. The instrument is powered by a 9-volt battery. This stimulator has proved satisfactory in our experience during the past 16 years.

Patient Preparation

After selection of the patient, the procedure is explained in detail to the family and the patient. They are told that there will be some discomfort with the needle-probing and with the use of electrical stimulation for localization of the intramuscular nerves. The solution to be used is described as phenol or carbolic acid, 5 per cent solution in water, a highly toxic substance not harmful in the small doses used. Since phenol is excreted in the urine, it may make the urine appear smoky. Vigorous stretching or excessive use of the extremity is to be avoided for 48 hours following the procedure. The patient is asked to report any pain or

ESSAM A. AWAD AND DENNIS DYKSTRA

paresthesias during or following the block. As a routine, the patient is asked to report by phone one week following the block any noticeable improvement, difficulties, or problems. The patient is also warned that immediately following blocks on the lower extremity muscles, stiffness may be eliminated and some muscular weakness may follow. Return of spasticity is to be anticipated in three to nine months. A consent form for the procedure is signed. Occasionally, we have asked the patient to discontinue the use of antispasticity medications for two to three days prior to the procedure. This was felt to assist the physiatrist in better localization of the innervation of the spastic muscles. The patient is then undressed and put in a comfortable position so that the muscles to be blocked are easily accessible and the distal part of the extremity is in full view of the operator.

Technique

Intramuscular neurolysis to control spasticity is a relatively simple procedure that could be applied to any spastic skeletal muscle. However, it requires good knowledge of anatomy, particularly the innervation and architecture of muscle. There are basically three steps to follow.

1. Localization of the motor point. This point is defined as the most irritable point of a given muscle, or the point on the skin at which an electrical stimulus of minimal amplitude and duration will result in a visible contraction of that muscle. The motor points of superficial muscles are easily defined. Motor point charts are available and serve as a good guide for the beginner.[6] Some muscles, such as the gastrocnemius, that have two heads also have two motor points; the physiatrist as well as the physical therapist is capable of performing this step. The chronaximeter is used for this purpose. It is more difficult to localize the motor points of deeper muscles. The author relies on identification of the muscular nerves to a specific muscle by reviewing an anatomy atlas and the dissected cadavers in the anatomy laboratory.

2. Insertion of the needle electrode slightly proximal to the motor point, aiming at the intramuscular nerve and its branches. We have essentially discontinued the practice of insertion of the needle electrode at the motor point, since the denervation induced in that manner is not long-lasting. Reinnervation and, hence, recurrence of spasticity depend on the length of the distal segment of the denervated nerve fibers. We have

found that within the length of the intramuscular nerve, the more proximal the site of the block, the longer the duration of the block. Another advantage of this modification of the procedure is that it becomes easier for the physiatrist to block one or more branches of the intramuscular nerve rather than attempting to block at the motor point, which requires many injection sites to achieve the same result. The injection needle is coated with an insulating substance except for its tip and is connected to the output of the chronaximeter. The frequency of the stimuli is usually 2 per second, the current intensity is 1 mA or less, and the duration is 0.1 to 0.2 msec. The stimulus is repeated automatically. When the needle tip is in close contact with the motor nerve or one of its branches to the muscle, fascicles of that muscle will contract and relax rhythmically at the same rate as the electrical stimuli. The current intensity is reduced to obtain a minimal contraction, and attempts at improving localization are repeated by looking for stronger contractions induced by less current.

3. Phenol injection. The injection of a trace (usually 0.1 to 1.0 ml) of 5 per cent phenol solution in water at this time will be followed by cessation of the contractions despite continued stimulation. Then the needle is inserted farther into the muscle or withdrawn to the subcutaneous tissues and reinserted slightly medial or lateral to the first injection site, in search for other branches of the intramuscular nerve. Accurate localization of the branches of the intramuscular nerve is repeated as in step 2. It is important to bear in mind the relationship of the origin and termination points of the intramuscular nerve as well as the architecture of the muscle in a three-dimensional fashion. The immediate effect of the injected phenol on the spastic muscle is assessed, and a decision is made whether to perform further injections. Thus, the results of the procedure are essentially instantaneous. It is important, however, to realize that the injection of one site results in denervation of only one fascicle in the muscle. If spasticity is severe, often the physician has to block several points until the desired effect is achieved, e.g., the abolition of clonus.

Indications

Patients selected for intramuscular neurolysis can be generally divided into two groups. The first is the functional patient who is able to perform certain activities with the spastic extremity, for example, ambulation. In this group, neurolysis has to be tailored extremely carefully in order to eliminate the spasticity and not interfere with the functions that the patient already has been able to perform. The second group are the patients who are unable to use the extremity involved. The procedure is then performed to facilitate nursing care or improve hygiene. In this latter group, extensive neurolysis can be performed.

Neurolysis is indicated in the following conditions:

1. Undesirable localized spasticity such as in the gastrocnemius muscle in stroke, spinal cord injury, muscular sclerosis, or cerebral palsy patients.

2. Severe hip adductor spasticity and spasms that interfere with perineal hygiene, urinary bladder care, and sexual intercourse.

3. Involuntary movements such as sudden spasms of the arm or leg and spontaneous sustained ankle clonus.

4. Genu recurvatum in the hemiplegic patient, in order to prevent progression of knee hyperextension, which results from gastrocnemius spasticity and shortening.

5. In the treatment of decubitus ulcer in order to facilitate correct positioning of the lower extremities, particularly prior to plastic surgical repair. Sudden hip flexor spasms may stretch the gluteal skin and interfere with approximation of skin flaps, and thus delay healing.

6. In the treatment of the spastic hand and wrist in hemiplegia, cerebral palsy, or multiple sclerosis.

Contraindications

Contraindications to neurolysis are as follows:
1. Poor general health.
2. Presence of severe excessive contractures of the spastic muscles, since this procedure will not change the clinical picture significantly.
3. Do not block the quadriceps femoris muscle in a patient who is ambulatory or who is able to use the lower extremity for pivot transfers. Spasticity of the quadriceps is beneficial to these patients, although the leg may be extended when they sit down.

Complications

Phlebothrombosis of the Calf or Thigh Muscles. This usually follows repeated indiscriminate prob-ing and the injection of large quantities of phenol solution by the novice. The patient may complain of pain and develop swelling and tenderness of the part injected. Swelling of the thigh may lead to edema of the lower extremity. Swelling of the calf may lead to edema of the foot. Thrombosis could be avoided by minimizing probing and the quantity of phenol used.

Peripheral Nerve Injury. This may occur if localization is not carefully done, particularly in the forearm, since the flexors of the wrist and fingers are closely related to the median and ulnar nerves. Observation of the hand during electrical stimulation prior to injection is mandatory. If the intrinsic muscles of the hand respond to stimulation in the proximal forearm, the site should be avoided.

Muscular Weakness. A certain degree of muscular weakness is expected following the procedure. If extensive neurolysis is performed, excessive muscular weakness will result that may interfere with the patient's ability to function. Thus, the neurolysis has to be titrated carefully to suit the particular individual's needs.

Lightheadedness. Occasionally, a patient will complain of lightheadedness immediately following the procedure. This is usually transient, and spontaneous recovery occurs within 5 to 15 minutes.

Increased Spasticity in the Antagonist Muscles. In certain patients, spasticity will appear following neurolysis of the agonist muscles; for example, following successful block of the hamstring muscles, the quadriceps may show evidence of spasticity with extension of the leg. This effect occurs because of the reduction of reflex reciprocal inhibition in the antagonist when there is reduction of reflex activity in the agonist.

Advantages of Phenol

Phenol has been widely used as a neurolytic agent.[7] It causes indiscriminate aseptic necrosis of tissues depending on its concentration. We prefer and use a 5 per cent solution in water, after having experimented with other concentrations. The immediate action of phenol renders it possible for the physiatrist to determine the results of the block instantaneously. Thus, the physiatrist can make a judgment as to whether to proceed with further injections. Phenol has passed the test of time and is accepted as a local blocking agent, since, in the quantities used, it is free of local irritation and systemic toxic effects. It is easily sterilized, it is available at low cost, and its action is of reasonably long duration.

Phenol Preparation

The 5 per cent phenol solution is not available commercially. The pharmacist in your hospital should be able to prepare it. The ingredients include crystalline phenol USP 50 gm, sodium bisulfate 1 gm, disodium ethylene diamine tetra-acetate 0.5 gm, and water for injection, 100 ml. The sodium bisulfate and sodium EDTA are dissolved in approximately 900 ml of water for injection. The phenol is dissolved in this solution using a magnetic stirrer. The solution is then filtered through a chemically resistant membrane filter (Solvinert or Fluoropore) of sterilizing porosity into a sterile evacuated 1-liter container using aseptic technique. The solution is packaged by gravity into presterilized 10-ml serum vials that are fitted with presterilized stoppers. These are sealed with a tear-off seal. The vials are labeled 5 per cent phenol in water for injection, sterile, single dose, expire in one year.

Halpern[8] described the histological effects of intramuscular injection of phenol in animals. There was nerve destruction with secondary denervation, muscular atrophy, and muscle necrosis. Both nerve and muscle showed evidence of regeneration. The volume of tissue necrosed was observed to be about one third of the volume of solution injected.

The duration of relaxation after a phenol block varies from 3 to 12 months, with an average of 6 months. This is essentially a process of chemical denervation, the extent of which depends entirely on the practitioner. The physiatrist should aim at maintaining the delicate balance between abolishing excessive spasticity and retaining the desirable function. Recurrence of spasticity is to be anticipated and depends on the following factors: (1) the nature of the primary disease and whether its course is stationary or progressive; (2) the severity and extent of spasticity; (3) the extent of the block performed; and (4) the presence or absence of other factors that aggravate spasticity, such as skin breakdown or urinary tract infections.

Phenol blocks for control of spasticity are an excellent method of treatment. An ankle clonus, hip adductor spasticity, or wrist and finger flexor spasticity could be easily eliminated. In nonprogressive disorders, a permanent effect may be achieved following two or three blocks over a period of two years. Gains in activities of daily living and ambulation are immediate, often surprisingly good, and gratifying and enhance the total rehabilitation of the patient rapidly.

Neuromuscular Blockade by Botulinum Toxin

Botulinum toxin produces paralysis of skeletal muscle by blocking the release of acetylcholine at motor end plates; therefore, appropriate local application can be used to obtain localized reduction of spasticity.[10]

Botulinum toxin was identified as a neuroparalytic, thermolabile exotoxin produced by the anaerobic spore-bearing bacillus *Clostridium botulinum* in 1897 by Van Ermengen.[9] This exotoxin is a protein appearing as seven antigenically distinct types. The most common form, botulinum A toxin, was first used therapeutically in 1981 to correct strabismus[11] and has since been reported in treatment of blepharospasm,[12] torticollis,[13] spastic dysphasia,[14] and detrusor-sphincter dyssynergia of the urinary bladder.[15]

In vertebrates, the toxin produces a flaccid paralysis of skeletal muscles leading to a respiratory death. Botulinum toxin is thought to act by interfering with cholinergic transmission in the peripheral nervous system at ganglionic and postganglionic synapses, and at neuromuscular junctions.[16] The toxin's action at the neuromuscular junction points to uncoupling of the excitation-secretion mechanism at the axon terminal. More precisely, the toxin appears to alter the ability of intracellular calcium to trigger exocytosis.[17, 18]

Botulinum toxin binds very rapidly and quite firmly to muscle.[19, 20] Intramuscular injection produces a prolonged effect. Very small doses injected into a skeletal muscle are rapidly and firmly bound to that muscle, and little toxin is available to pass into the circulatory system to produce a systemic effect.[11] The maximum blockade occurs after three to four days. The effects of repeated toxin administration are cumulative, as the toxin binds with more and more axon terminals. The release of acetylcholine from the end plate is at first diminished and then inhibited.[20, 21] Changes in botulinum-treated skeletal muscles are similar to the effects of denervation.[22]

In physical medicine and rehabilitation, botulinum A toxin has been used experimentally to treat detrusor-sphincter dyssynergia in patients with spinal cord injuries, torticollis, and spasticity of the gastrocnemius and soleus muscles. The most extensive use of the toxin in human patients has been to treat excessive activity of extraocular muscles.[11]

The LD_{50} (Oculinum) for the monkey is approximately 39 units of toxin per kilogram of body weight. Monkeys and humans respond similarly to the same doses per body weight of this preparation injected into the eye muscles,[11] and it is considered that the LD_{50} dose for the monkey applies comparably to man. The maximum one-time dose administered to patients in our experience for blockade of any skeletal muscle has been less than 10 per cent of the LD_{50} for the monkey.

Botulinum A toxin has been injected into the spastic striated sphincter muscle of patients with spinal cord injury who suffered from detrusor-sphincter dyssynergia. In 10 of 11 patients, electromyography indicated sphincter denervation after the injection of toxin; bulbosphincteric reflexes[23] were more difficult to obtain and showed a decreased amplitude and a normal latency. The urethral pressure profile decreased an average of 33 cm of water after toxin injection in seven patients. Postvoiding residual urine volume decreased by an average of 115 ml after toxin injection in 11 patients. In the seven patients in whom it could be determined, the blocking effects of the toxin lasted an average of 59 days. Botulinum toxin also decreased the incidence and severity of autonomic hyperreflexia in five patients.

A double-blind study of effectiveness of botulinum toxin on detrusor-sphincter dyssynergia in five patients with high spinal cord injuries showed that after three weekly injections of the sphincter with botulinum toxin, electromyography of the voluntary sphincter revealed partial denervation; the urethral pressure profile decreased an average of 25 cm of water; and postvoiding residual urine volumes decreased an average of 125 ml. Bladder pressure on voiding decreased an average of 30 cm of water. The bulbosphincteric reflexes were more difficult to obtain and showed a decreased amplitude with normal latency. These parameters were unchanged from baseline values in two patients who received three weekly injections of normal saline. These two patients subsequently were injected with botulinum toxin and showed the expected responses. The toxin's effects were not permanent but persisted for an average of 60 days.

Botulinum A toxin has been used to block spasms of the sternocleidomastoid and trapezius muscles of patients with torticollis, resulting in increased range of motion. In one patient, the toxin was effective in reducing pain and tremor.

The toxin's effects lasted approximately 50 days in these patients. The procedure is described at the end of this section.

Spasticity of the gastrocnemius and soleus muscles that developed after a closed head injury, and resulted in persistent toe-walking on the spastic lower extremity, has been blocked to produce foot flat–walking by four injections of botulinum toxin at weekly intervals. Injections into multiple sites were necessary to reduce spasticity in these large muscles. Again the effects are not permanent but diminish and disappear in about 60 days.

Undesirable side effects of paresis of other muscles have developed in some patients. Three patients with detrusor-sphincter dyssynergia experienced upper extremity weakness that made transfers and some activities of daily living more difficult for two to three weeks. Blurred vision, difficulty in swallowing or breathing, or gastrointestinal upset did not occur. Patients with torticollis have experienced mild generalized weakness, difficulty in holding their heads erect, or difficulty in swallowing on the side injected, lasting two to four weeks. Single-fiber electromyography studies after botulinum toxin blockade revealed increased jitter and fiber density as an effect on distant muscles.[24] Circulating toxin was not detected in the serum, and antitoxin antibodies could not be detected after recovery.

A number of questions remain regarding the use of botulinum A toxin to reduce muscle spasticity. Appropriate injection techniques and doses remain to be established for various conditions. Possible long-term effects of the toxin and possible interactions of toxin with other medications must be investigated. However, limited experience indicates that botulinum A toxin is effective to produce a controllable reduction of muscle spasticity lasting several months.

The procedure used for blocking the external urethral sphincter in sphincter-detrusor dyssynergia has been as follows: The striated muscle sphincter is injected with an initial dose of 140 units of toxin in 5.5 ml of normal saline in at least four different sites through a cystoscope using a 23-gauge, 35-cm, Teflon-coated monopolar electrode needle connected to an electromyography machine.[15] The use of electromyography has allowed us to inject the toxin into the areas of maximum muscle activity. Patients' blood pressures are monitored for autonomic hyperreflexia, and 10 mg of nifedipine is administered by mouth if the systolic blood pressure increases to more than 180 mm Hg, the diastolic blood pressure increases to more than

ESSAM A. AWAD AND DENNIS DYKSTRA

110 mm Hg, or the patient complains of increasing headache, flushing, sweating, or blurred vision. The procedure is continued 15 minutes after nifedipine is given.[17] After cystoscopy, a Foley catheter is left in place for 24 hours, and the patient is treated prophylactically for four days with trimethoprim and sulfamethoxazole or nitrofurantoin. A second injection of 240 units of toxin in 5.5 ml of normal saline is given 7 to 10 days later. One week after the second injection, postvoiding residual urine volume and sphincter denervation are evaluated. After the effects of the toxin have worn off, in approximately 50 to 60 days, the patient is reinjected with 240 units of toxin. Effects of this injection typically last 50 to 60 days.

The procedure for blocking the trapezius, sternocleidomastoid, or splenius muscles for spastic torticollis has been the injection of 140 units of toxin in 5.5 ml of normal saline into the area of maximal activity of the spastic muscles as identified by electromyography using a 3.75-cm, 23-gauge insulated needle. No attempt is made to inject at the motor point of the muscle, but rather the toxin is diffused throughout the muscle. Two weeks later, 140 units of toxin in 5.5 ml of normal saline is injected into the previously injected trapezius, sternocleidomastoid, or splenius muscles. After the second injection, the patient is encouraged to begin range-of-motion and stretching exercises for the neck muscles. The effects last 50 to 60 days. If reinjection is needed again, 140 units in 5.5 ml of normal saline is injected into the spastic muscles. This technique of toxin diffusion may not work well with large muscles. In such cases, locating the motor points with a stimulator, and injecting at those sites, may prove to be a more effective technique.

References

1. Awad, E. A.: Intramuscular neurolysis for stroke. Minn. Med., 55:711–713, 1972.
2. Awad, E. A.: Phenol block for control of hip flexor and adductor spasticity. Arch. Phys. Med. Rehabil., 53:554–557, 1972.
3. Freeman, L. W., and Heimburger, R. F.: Surgical relief of spasticity in paraplegic patients. J. Neurosurg., 5:556–561, 1968.
4. Laitinen, L. V., Nilsson, S., and Fugl-Meyer, A. R.: Selective posterior rhizotomy for treatment of spasticity. J. Neurosurg., 58:895–899, 1983.
5. Khalili, A. A., Harmel, M. H., Forster, S., and Benton, J. G.: Management of spasticity by selective peripheral nerve block with dilute phenol solutions in clinical rehabilitation. Arch. Phys. Med. Rehabil., 45:513–519, 1964.
6. Walthard, K. M., and Tchicaloff, M.: Motor points. In Licht, S. (Ed.): Electrodiagnosis and Electromyography, 3rd Ed. New Haven, CT, E. Licht, Publisher, 1971, pp. 153–170.
7. Wood, K. M.: The use of phenol as a neurolytic agent: A review. Pain, 5:205–229, 1978.
8. Halpern, D.: Histologic studies in animals after intramuscular neurolysis with phenol. Arch. Phys. Med. Rehabil., 58:438–443, 1977.
9. Van Ermengen, E.: Ueber einen neuen anaeroben Bacillus und seine Beziehungen zum Botulismus. Ztschr. Hzg., 26:1–56, 1897.
10. Burgen, A. S. V., Dickens, F., and Zatman, L. J.: The action of botulinum toxin on the neuromuscular junction. J. Physiol. (London), 109:10–24, 1949.
11. Scott, A. B.: Botulinum toxin injection of eye muscle to correct strabismus. Trans. Am. Ophthalmol. Soc., 79:734–770, 1981.
12. Scott, A. B., Kennedy, R. A., and Stubbs, H. A.: Botulinum A toxin injection as a treatment for blepharospasm. Arch. Ophthalmol., 103:347–350, 1985.
13. Tsui, J. E., Eisen, A., Mak, E., Carruthers, T., Scott, A., and Calne, D. B.: A pilot study on the use of botulinum toxin in spasmodic torticollis. Can. J. Neurol. Sci., 12:314–316, 1985.
14. Blitzer, A., Brin, M. F., Fahn, S., Lange, D., and Lovelace, R. E.: Letter to the Editor. Laryngoscope, 11:1300–1301, 1986.
15. Dykstra, D. D., Sidi, A. A., Scott, A. B., Pagel, J. M., and Goldish, G. D.: Effects of botulinum A toxin on detrusor-sphincter dyssynergia in spinal cord injured patients. J. Urol., 139:919–922, 1988.
16. Simpson, L. L.: Studies on the mechanism of action of botulinum toxin. In Ceccarelli, B., and Clementi, F. (Eds.): Advances in Cytopharmacology, Vol. 3., Neurotoxins: Tools in Neurobiology. New York, Raven Press, 1979, pp. 27–34.
17. Simpson, L. L.: The origin, structure and pharmacological activity of botulinum toxin. Pharmacol. Rev., 33:155–188, 1981.
18. Sugiyama, H.: Clostridium botulinum neurotoxin. Microbiol. Rev., 44:419–488, 1980.
19. Simpson, L. L.: The neuroparalytic and hemagglutinating activities of botulinum toxin. In Simpson, L. L. (Ed.): Neuropoisons: Their Pathophysiological Actions, Vol. 1. New York, Plenum Press, 1971, pp. 303–324.
20. Drachman, D. B.: Botulinum toxin as a tool for research on the nervous system. In Simpson, L. L. (Ed.): Neuropoisons: Their Pathophysiological Actions, Vol. 1. New York, Plenum Press, 1971, pp. 325–347.
21. Brooke, V. B.: The action of botulinum toxin on motor nerve filaments. J. Physiol. (London), 123:501–515, 1954.
22. Fex, S., Sonesson, B., Thesleff, S., and Zelena, J.:

Nerve implants in botulinum poisoned mammalian muscle. J. Physiol., 184:872–882, 1966.

23. Dykstra, D., Sidi, A., Cameron, J., Magness, J., Stradal, L., and Portugal, J.: The use of mechanical stimulation to obtain the sacral reflex latency: A new technique. J. Urol., 137:77–79, 1987.

24. Lange, D. J., Brin, M. F., Warner, C. L., Fahn, S., and Lovelace, R. E.: Distant effects of local injection of botulinum toxin. Muscle Nerve, 10:552–555, 1987.

25. Dykstra, D. D., Sidi, A. A., and Anderson, L. C.: The effect of nifedipine on cystoscopy induced autonomic hyperreflexia in patients with high spinal cord injuries. J. Urol., 135:1155–1157, 1987.

56

Management of Chronic Pain

DIANA D. CARDENAS   KELLY J. EGAN

Pain complaints are one of the most common symptoms that bring patients to a treating physician. Pain that occurs at the time of tissue injury and during the healing process is known as acute pain. Pain that persists beyond the predicted time of healing is known as chronic pain. The distinction between acute and chronic pain is one of time rather than intensity. Under certain conditions such as rheumatoid arthritis, there may be episodes of recurrent tissue damage or inflammation associated with recurrent episodes of acute pain. The importance of distinguishing between these types is that the treatment used for one may not be helpful for the other. Indeed, treatment modalities used for acute pain sometimes actually worsen chronic pain.[1] This chapter focuses primarily on chronic pain associated with prior tissue damage or injury but begins with a general description of pain transmission. Discussion of chronic pain associated with spinal cord injury is found elsewhere in this volume.

Pain Transmission and Modulation: Current Concepts

Nociception or the detection of injury by peripheral nerve fibers[2] involves chemical mediators that are released or synthesized in response to tissue damage.[3] These chemical mediators include prostaglandins and leukotrienes, which sensitize nociceptive afferents, and bradykinin and histamine, which directly activate the nociceptors.[3] Nonsteroidal anti-inflammatory drugs (NSAIDs) such as acetylsalicylic acid block the production of prostaglandins and thus reduce pain. Leukotriene synthesis, however, is not blocked by NSAIDs.[3] Once the nociceptor is stimulated, a variety of chemical

neurotransmitters are involved in transmitting the signals toward the cortex. These neurotransmitters include a group of polypeptides, the best studied being substance P (SP). Experimental depletion of SP in rat spinal cord produces thermal analgesia.[4] A synthetic antagonist to SP, (D-Pro^2, D-Trp$^{7, 9}$)-SP, blocked *in vivo* SP-induced excitation of locus ceruleus (LC) neurons in the rat but did not block the response of the LC to noxious stimuli.[5] Other synthetic analogues of SP have been developed. (D-Pro^2, D-Phe^7, D-Trp^9)-SP has been shown to block the vasodilator effect of SP in response to electrical stimulation of the inferior alveolar nerve of the cat.[6]

In addition to the polypeptides, the neurotransmitters involved in pain transmission and modulation include acetylcholine, norepinephrine, serotonin, and the more recently discovered endorphins. Serotonin is of special interest because lowered cerebrospinal fluid levels are implicated in certain cases of depression. Tricyclic antidepressants (TCAs) are found not only to benefit depression at usual therapeutic doses by affecting central serotonin levels[7] but also to reduce pain.[8] Endorphins are endogenous opioid substances found in the brain, anterior pituitary, adrenal gland, gut, and sympathetic nervous system. Endorphins are found diminished after chronic narcotic use[9] and increased by strenuous exercise. The so-called runner's high is chemically related to an increase in central nervous system (CNS) endorphin levels.

Melzack and Wall have eloquently described modulation of pain by the CNS as the gate control theory of pain.[2, 10] Briefly, the activated nociceptor transmits information by way of small myelinated (A-delta) and unmyelinated (C) axons into the dorsal horn of the spinal cord and on to higher brain centers.[11] The large-diameter sensory axons

(A-beta fibers) can activate inhibitory interneurons in the spinal cord to dampen the pain signal. In addition to segmented interactions within the dorsal horn, the brain transmits descending signals that "open" or "close" the gate.[2] Examples of peripheral nonpainful stimulation that tend to close the gate include counterstimulation with transcutaneous electrical stimulation or massage, acupuncture, stretching, and heat and cold application. Whereas these modalities are useful in many instances in which nociception plays a major role, other overriding mechanisms tend to lessen their usefulness in chronic pain. Descending signals from higher centers that can dampen or "close" the "gate" include central inhibition produced by distraction and relaxation, cognitive relabeling, regular aerobic exercise, and treating depression. These techniques may be very beneficial to the patient with chronic pain. The opposites of these (focusing on pain, anxiety, inactivity, depression) are thought to "open" the gate and augment the pain signal.

Development of Chronic Pain

Despite many recent advances, pain is still a poorly understood phenomenon. Physicians are generally taught the "disease/medical" model of pain in which organic causes are to blame. If no organic cause can be found, then the pain is called psychogenic. Such a dichotomy represents the extreme ends of the spectrum and does not consider the effect of pain on the environment or the effect of the environment on expressions of pain.

Certain factors contribute to the development of chronic pain: (1) an unclear diagnosis; (2) inappropriate, delayed, or prolonged treatment of acute pain; and (3) psychosocial influences. Although a clear diagnosis is not always possible, reasonable effort should be made to determine the cause or contributing factors to pain. In cases of low back pain, the etiologic factor is said to be unclear 85 per cent of the time.[12] Whereas mechanical and musculoskeletal factors are often causative factors, establishing their contribution may require treatment first. Each patient may have a possible combination of organic disease, psychopathological disorder, disuse, or learned pain behaviors. The more "chronic" the problem (duration), the more likely it is that nonorganic factors have come into existence and play a contributing role in the maintenance of the pain problem. Without a clear diagnosis, the patient may not receive timely treatment

of the causative factors. Even in face of a clear diagnosis, patients may not be treated appropriately, especially with regard to the underutilization or overutilization of narcotics during acute pain. Prolongation of bed rest or analgesics or sedatives can lead to chronic pain by producing secondary complications from disuse and drug dependence. Psychosocial influences may include positive reinforcement of pain behavior by friends or family, compensation or disability payments, and "time-out" from the stresses and responsibilities of daily life.[13, 14]

Simply categorizing chronic pain as organic versus psychogenic or lumping all chronic pain complaints in a category of "learned pain" is not useful. Chronic pain is usually multidimensional in its cause, and each patient carries a possible combination of nociception, disuse, and learned pain. In addition, the environmental factors are different for each patient. A careful detailed history and physical examination by a physician and psychological assessment by a trained psychologist are important in determining etiologic factors and in planning an effective treatment program.

Chronic Low Back Pain

Evaluation and Management

Low back pain is, of course, the most common chronic pain problem in the United States. It is estimated that 1400 days are lost from work per year per 1000 workers in the United States owing to low back pain.[15] Although the treatment of acute low back pain most commonly involves bed rest, controversy exists as to the optimal duration of such rest. Objective data to support the efficacy of bed rest are lacking. Wiesel and colleagues concluded that bed rest decreases time loss from work after randomly treating a group of army recruits for acute low back pain with either bed rest or limited activity.[16] However, secondary consequences of this form of treatment may have had an effect on the results. The recruits at bed rest were allowed to return to full duty once they became symptom-free. Those who were undergoing limited activity were assigned to restricted duty status that eliminated all physical exercise, but they were required to observe their peers in training. It is possible that the recruits at bed rest found enforced rest more distressing than did recruits who were allowed to be on restricted duty status. In another study, Deyo and co-workers found that two days of bed rest were as good as seven days of bed rest as regards pain resolution in a group of civilians with acute low back pain.[17] No bed rest was found to be as good as four days of bed rest in a group of 252 patients with acute low back pain randomized to four days of bed rest or physiotherapy and education.[18] Bed rest patients took 42 per cent longer to report a "normal level of activities" (p = 0.004). Those randomized to physiotherapy and education reported they stopped taking drugs "46 per cent sooner" (p = 0.048).[18] In all of these studies, patients were without motor deficits.

The significance of the duration of bed rest for acute low back pain is that repeated prescriptions for bed rest or continued bed rest are often recommended for pain that has become chronic. The adverse effects of such immobilization include muscle atrophy and tightness. Muscle atrophy produced by immobilization does not produce a loss of muscle fibers[19] and, hence, is reversible. Hettinger and Mueller demonstrated up to a 20 per cent loss of muscle strength for each week of bed rest.[20] The rate of recovery, however, is much slower, i.e., only 10 per cent increase of initial strength per week occurs despite daily exercise at 100 per cent of maximal muscle strength. Chronic pain patients often present with a history of prolonged inactivity and benefit from education on the effects of immobilization on the muscular system as well as the other systems of the body. Details of the effects of immobilization are found in other chapters in this volume.

History and Physical Examination

The patient with chronic pain may be complaining of any or all of the following: low back pain, neck pain, abdominal pain, pelvic pain, headache, or other musculoskeletal pain. In the case of low back pain, the underlying pathological process is not often identifiable. Any of the anatomical structures of the spine, including ligaments, muscles, skin, facet joints, vertebrae, and nerve roots, may produce low back pain. Postural and structural abnormalities may alter the physiological curves of the spine and result in, or aggravate, back pain. Metabolic conditions may play a part and must be determined. Thorough history-taking should reveal the pattern of daily activity, usage of analgesic medications or sedatives, sleep pattern, and evidence of depression or other affective disorders and give a preliminary idea of the degree of psychosocial and environmental factors that are influencing the pain. Although the physician will obtain this type of information during the history, a comprehensive and in-depth psychological assessment needs to be conducted too. The physical examination and diagnostic tasks that are performed are said to result in a solid cause in only 12 to 15 per cent of the cases of low back pain. These causes include acute disk herniation, compression fractures, spinal stenosis, and spondylolisthesis. However, abnormalities may be unrelated to pain symptoms, and it is known that 25 per cent of asymptomatic patients have positive myelograms.[21] The vast majority (90 per cent) of patients who experience an acute attack of back pain become symptom-free within eight weeks.[22] Nachemson reports that six months after an acute episode, there are only 2 to 3 per cent left suffering.[22]

In examining the patient with chronic low back pain, nonorganic physical signs are useful. Waddell standardized a group of five types of physical signs that correlated with the hypochondriasis, depression, and hysteria scores of the Minnesota Multiphasic Personality Inventory in a group of 84 low back pain patients.[23] None of these nonorganic signs was observed in 50 normal subjects; however, false-positives were found in elderly patients who had difficulty standing because of pain. The five types of physical signs are as follows: (1) tenderness in a superficial or nonanatomical distribution; (2) positive simulation tests in which back pain is produced by axial loading over the patient's skull or by rotating the shoulders and pelvis in the same plane; (3) the distraction test during straight leg raising or during other portions of the examination; (4) regional weakness or sensory disturbances that cannot be explained on a localized neurological basis; (5) overreaction during the examination. Patients may have a high number of Waddell's signs in combination with organic findings. Although over-reaction or exaggeration of signs and symptoms may be found in the chronic pain patient, those with hysterical paralysis of the upper or lower extremities require a special approach with strong emphasis on behavioral shaping.[13, 24] Details of the musculoskeletal examination are found in other sections of this text.

Drug Withdrawal

The majority of patients admitted to chronic pain services are found to be taking narcotics, sedative drugs, or both.[25, 26] Such drugs impair patients intellectually, physically, and socially.[27] They also affect the patient's ability to distinguish between pain and the need for medication. One of the most important aspects of the management of chronic pain is the withdrawal of narcotics and sedative drugs. Tolerance to the effect of these medications may lead to the escalation of drug usage. The most common method for prescribing such medications, particularly narcotics, is on a "prn" or as needed basis. This leads to fluctuating blood levels and peaks and valleys in symptom relief.[1]

Drug withdrawal is safest when done on an inpatient basis. This not only provides greater observation for potential withdrawal symptoms, but also reduces the accessibility to medications. A safe regimen that has been used successfully at the University of Washington includes, in addition to a toxicology screen when indicated, a 48-hour inpatient drug profile, i.e., a period of time when the patient is allowed to take usual medications on a prn basis. At the end of the 48-hour drug profile, the total equivalencies of narcotics and sedatives are tallied up. Methadone is used to substitute for the narcotic analgesics, and phenobarbital for the sedatives (Tables 56–1 and 56–2).

The pain cocktail is a system used for drug withdrawal and for delivering medication on a

TABLE 56–1. Narcotic Conversion Tables

| DRUG | DOSE (mg) EQUAL TO 1 NARCOTIC EQUIVALENT (= 10 mg ORAL METHADONE) | |
	Oral	IM
Butorphanol (Stadol)		2.0
Buprenorphine (Buprenex)		0.3
Codeine	200	130
Diacetylmorphine (heroin)		3.0
Hydromorphone (Dilaudid)	7.5	1.5
Meperidine (Demerol)	400	100
Methadone (Dolophine)	10	8.0
Morphine	60	10
Oxycodone (Percodan)	30	15
Oxymorphone (Numorphan)		1.5
Pentazocine (Talwin)	180	60
*Propoxyphene HCL (Darvon)	260	
*Propoxyphene napsylate (Darvon-N)	400	

*Never need more than 40 mg methadone for 24 hours for Darvon replacement.

Steven H. Butler and Terence M. Murphy, unpublished material, 1987.

TABLE 56–2. Sedative/Hypnotic/Tranquilizer Conversion Tables

DRUG	DOSE (mg) EQUAL TO 1 BARBITURATE EQUIVALENT (= 30 mg ORAL PHENOBARBITAL)
Benzodiazepine*	
Alprazolam (Xanax)	1.0
Chlordiazepoxide (Librium)	25
Clonazepam (Clonopin)	4.0
Clorazepate (Tranxene)	15
Diazepam (Valium)	10
Flurazepam (Dalmane)	15
Lorazepam (Ativan)	2.0
Oxazepam (Serax)	10
Barbiturates	
Amobarbitol (Tuinal)	100
Butabarbitol (Butisol)	100
Butalbital (Fiorinal)	100
Pentobarbital (Nembutal)	100
Phenobarbital (Phenobarbital)	30
Secobarbital (Seconal)	100
Glycerol	
Meprobamate (Miltown)	400
Ethyl alcohol	
Whiskey (100 proof)	90 ml

*Patients taking large doses or on long-term usage of benzodiazepines may require direct tapering and may not tolerate conversion to phenobarbital.

Steven H. Butler and Terence M. Murphy, unpublished material, 1987.

time-contingent basis. The major components of the pain cocktail include, in addition to the long-acting oral narcotic methadone or the long-acting oral sedative phenobarbital, a taste- or flavor-masking vehicle such as cherry syrup or Maalox. Acetaminophen and hydroxyzine are often added to enhance the other ingredients. Although the half-life for methadone is 24 hours, the analgesic effect is only six hours; hence, the pain cocktail containing methadone is given every six hours. The benefits to administering the pain cocktail on a time-contingent basis rather than as needed are (1) "flying" and "crashing" are avoided, and (2) the pain behavior is disassociated from the medication.

Because there may be considerable stress on transferring a patient from short-acting prn medications to a long-acting time-contingent pain cocktail, it is best to start with 120 per cent of the patient's calculated daily dose. The doses there-

DIANA D. CARDENAS AND KELLY J. EGAN

after are tapered at the rate of 10 to 20 per cent per day for methadone and 10 per cent per day for phenobarbital. Patients are aware that they are being tapered but not of when doses are changed. At the same time that the pain cocktail is used to taper the patient from narcotics and sedatives, the patient will be engaged in a process of learning new strategies for dealing with chronic pain. It is important to remember that without alternatives to medication, simply withdrawing the patient from such drugs will result in only short-term success. Tricyclic antidepressants are often prescribed for treatment of depression associated with chronic pain, and evidence supports an analgesic effect of TCAs independent of their psychological effects in chronic pain patients with and without depression.[28, 29]

Reactivation

Since bed rest and the dictum to "take it easy" are all too commonly prescribed to chronic pain sufferers, it is not surprising that a vicious cycle of pain leading to immobilization leading to further pain is set into motion. To counter the situation, reactivation is necessary. Passive treatment such as hot packs and massage, which may be useful in the initial treatment of a muscle pain problem, will only reinforce the immobilization mode and does not counteract the detrimental effects of chronic disuse. Similarly, whereas trigger point injections may be quite helpful to the patient in the context of active remobilization, they should not be regarded as a separate and independent treatment, nor given on a prn basis. At all points in the treatment program for chronic pain, the plan and its rationale should be discussed with the patient to increase cooperation as well as to educate the patient to be his or her own best advocate in future bouts with the chronic pain problem.

Exercises properly prescribed to increase strength and endurance and to increase flexibility need careful structuring. The physiatric examination helps to define the upper limits of performance for the patient.[14] The optimal method is to use a quota system in which, following a baseline, each exercise is increased by a pre-set amount in small bite-size portions. During the baseline period, the patient exercises to his or her own tolerance, letting pain or fatigue be the guide.[30, 31] Patients are thus more likely to succeed in reaching a desired goal and they are less likely to overdo and then fail if given an exact pre-set increment for each exercise each session. Although rewards from staff in the form of verbal encouragement are useful, the very act of recording the day's quota in simple graphs is reinforcing to the patient. Such a system helps to restore any loss of range of motion and strength but, more important, demonstrates to the patient that it is safe to move. The patient learns that "hurt" is not the same as "harm."[32] Failure to reach such quotas must be promptly discussed with the patient, and either the quota must be readjusted or the program should be terminated. The successful outcome is dependent on participation in all aspects of a pain program, and the reactivation program is a very important aspect.

Psychological Issues in the Management of Chronic Low Back Pain

Illness Conviction

As essential as reactivation is in the rehabilitation of the individual with chronic low back pain, convincing the patient to participate fully in a rigorous, demanding, and, almost inevitably, painful physical therapy program is often one of the most difficult tasks facing the treatment team. If the individual's "illness conviction" is not adequately and effectively addressed to the patient's satisfaction, the patient either will refuse to carry out the prescribed program or will do so in a half-hearted, reluctant fashion and will leave the treatment program convinced that he or she was fortunate not to have seriously damaged anything. Any gains made through physical therapy will be lost by the patient when rest is again the order of the day. As with any intervention aimed at remobilizing and redirecting the chronic pain patient, the best approach tends to consist of a series of strategies all designed to chip away at the patient's conviction that reactivation is dangerous.

1. General education regarding low back pain, relationship between back pain and physical findings. The more "credible" the source from the patient's point of view, the more likely it is that the patient will accept the information. When thesame type of information comes from several sources, more headway is gained than with only one source.

2. Specific information using the patient's own x-ray films, EMGs, and the like to reassure the patient about his or her back's stability.

3. General education about chronic pain itself, the difference between acute and chronic pain, and the distinction between "hurt" and "harm."

4. Examples of other patients, farther along in their treatment, who also admit to having had the same fears as the beginning patient.

5. Selective social attention by staff focused on gains rather than on limitations or pain complaints.

6. Use of gradually increasing "quotas" along with patient monitoring in the form of graphs whereby the individual can see gains in activity level, rather than focusing on increased pain.

7. Frank discussion of potential consequences of continuing to search for the "quick fix."

Typically, with these strategies, the individual's illness conviction will gradually decline in strength as physical capacities increase. The actual improvement in stamina, strength, and flexibility contributes most to the individual's confidence in the treatment program, but without intensive attention paid to laying to rest the patient's deepest fears, a significant number of patients' programs will be doomed from the start.

Consequences of Improved Functioning

Once a patient begins to observe improvement in strength, stamina, and flexibility, new concerns may emerge. Behavior tends to be maintained by its consequences; the consequences of being labeled ill or disabled have different meanings for different patients, but giving up the disabled role clearly means changes in the individual's life. The psychological evaluation prior to treatment should have identified the consequences of being "disabled by pain" and the likely obstacles to improving physical status. The balance of each of the consequences can be weighed with respect to strength and direction. The more positive (to the patient) the consequences of remaining disabled and the more negative (to the patient) the consequences of reactivation, the more difficult the rehabilitation process will be unless changes in the consequences can be manipulated to help ensure maintenance of treatment gains.

Vocational Goals

For the individual with chronic low back pain, vocational issues are often paramount in treatment planning. Typically, the pain has resulted in the patient's being unable to perform a former job. Early in treatment, it is advisable to begin planning for and working toward a return to the former functioning level if that seems possible. The vocational counselor can help the physician and the psychologist more thoroughly evaluate the relevant vocational issues and the individual's skills, and give a realistic picture of what work might be available taking all the information and the community needs into consideration. A clear vocational goal arrived at as early as possible gives the treatment team and the patient a direction as well as the expectation that some type of gainful employment is possible. Work is important, not only for economical reasons, but also because it defines one's social status, provides nonfinancial rewards (such as regular contact with others), and often has a major impact on the individual's perception of self. The vocational goals for an older worker who formerly held a very physically demanding job and who has few years of formal education are clearly going to be very different from the vocational goals for a younger, better educated worker, but each individual needs a vocational plan in place as soon as it is feasible. Just as physical therapy for the inactive patient with chronic pain depends for its ultimate success on gradually increasing activity level, so does vocational planning depend on a gradual return to work and "work hardening" activities.

Summary

The patient with a chronic pain problem typically has a complicated medical and psychological history. An adequate comprehensive treatment of the problem requires a careful and multidisciplinary assessment. The goal of the assessment is to identify nociceptive factors that may be correctable, psychological factors that can be addressed (pharmacologically or behaviorally), the contribution of disuse to the pain problem, and the socioenvironmental context in which the pain problem is maintained. The distinction between acute and chronic pain management strategies cannot be overemphasized when attempting to help the individual to achieve a more functional life. The management of chronic pain requires a much broader approach than that of acute pain problems, in which the context of the pain is not necessarily relevant to its maintenance. When chronic pain problems are treated with a unidimensional acute pain approach (such as with narcotics or immobilization), the problem is further complicated and the chronicity is maintained.

References

1. Black, R. G.: The chronic pain syndrome. Surg. Clin. North Am., 55:999–1011, 1975.
2. Wall, P. D.: Introduction. *In* Wall, P. D., and Melzack, R. (Eds.): Textbook of Pain. New York, Churchill Livingstone, 1984, pp. 1–16.
3. Fields, H. L., and Levine, J. D.: Pain-mechanisms and management. West. J. Med., 141:347–357, 1984.
4. Yaksh, T. L., Farb, D. H., Leeman, S. E., and Jessell, T. M.: Intrathecal capsaicin depletes substance P in the rat spinal cord and produces prolonged thermal analgesia. Science, 206:481–483, 1979.
5. Engberg, G., Svensson, T. H., Rosell, S., and Folkers, K.: A synthetic peptide as an antagonist of substance P. Nature, 293:222–223, 1981.
6. Rosell, S. K., Olgart, B., Gazelius, G., Panopoulos, P., Folkers, K., and Horig, J.: Inhibition of antidromic and substance P–induced vasodilatation by a substance P antagonist. Acta Physiol. Scand., 111:381–382, 1981.
7. Sternbach, R. A., Janowsky, D. S., Huey, I. Y., and Segal, D. S.: Effects of altering brain serotonin activity on human chronic pain. *In* Bonica, J. J., and Abbe Fessard, D. (Eds.): Advances in Pain Research and Therapy I. New York, Raven Press, 1976, pp. 601–606.
8. Monks, R. C.: The use of psychotropic drugs in human chronic pain: A review. Sixth World Congress of the International College of Psychosomatic Medicine, Canada, Sept. 15, 1981.
9. Jacquet, Y. F.: B-Endorphin and ACTH-opiate peptides with coordinated role in the regulation of behavior? Trends Neurosci., 2:140–143, 1979.
10. Melzack, R., and Wall, P. D.: Pain mechanisms: A new theory. Science, 150:971–978, 1965.
11. Heinbecker, P., Bishop, G. H., and O'Leary, J.: Pain and touch fibers in peripheral nerves. Arch. Neurol. Psych., 29:771–789, 1933.
12. Nachemson, A., and Bigos, S.: The low back. *In* Cruess, R. L., and Rennie, W. R. J. (Eds.): Adult Orthopaedics. New York, Churchill Livingstone, 1984, pp. 843–844.
13. Trieschmann, R. B., Stolov, W. C., and Montgomery, E. D.: Approach to treatment of abnormal ambulation resulting from conversion reaction. Arch. Phys. Med. Rehabil., 51:198–206, 1970.
14. Fordyce, W. E., Fowler, R. S., Lehmann, J. F., de Lateur, B. J., Sand, P. L., and Trieschmann, R. B.: Operant conditioning in the treatment of chronic pain. Arch. Phys. Med. Rehabil., 54:389–408, 1973.
15. Nachemson, A. L.: The lumbar spine: An orthopaedic challenge. Spine, 1:59–71, 1976.
16. Wiesel, S. W., Cuckler, J. M., Deluca, F., Jones, F., Zeide, M. S., and Rothman, R. H.: Acute low-back pain: An objective analysis of conservative therapy. Spine, 5:324–330, 1980.
17. Deyo, R. A., Diehl, A. K., and Rosenthal, M.: How many days of bed rest for acute low back pain? A randomized clinical trial. N. Engl. J. Med., 315:1064–1070, 1986.
18. Gilbert, J. R.: Clinical trial of common treatments for low back pain in family practice. Br. Med. J., 291:791, 1985.
19. Cardenas, D. D., Stolov, W. C., and Hardy, R.: Muscle fiber number in immobilization atrophy. Arch. Phys. Med. Rehabil., 58:423–426, 1977.
20. Hettinger, T., and Mueller, E. A.: Muskelleistung und muskeltraining. Arbeitsphysiologie, 15:111–126, 1953.
21. Wiesel, S. W., et al.: Industrial Low Back: A Comprehensive Approach. Charlotsville, The Michie Company, 1985, p. 492.
22. Nachemson, A. L.: Natural course of low back pain. *In* White, A. A., and Gordon, S. L. (Eds.): Symposium on Idiopathic Low Back Pain. St. Louis, C. V. Mosby, 1982, pp. 46–51.
23. Waddell, G., McCulloch, J. A., Kummel, E., and Venner, R. M.: Nonorganic physical signs in low-back pain. Spine, 5:117–125, 1980.
24. Cardenas, D. D., Larson, J., and Egan, K. J.: Hysterical paralysis in the upper extremity of chronic pain patients. Arch. Phys. Med. Rehabil., 67:190–193, 1986.
25. Maruta, T., Swanson, D. W., and Findlayson, R. E.: Drug abuse and dependency in patients with chronic pain. Mayo Clin. Proc., 54:241–244, 1979.
26. Turner, J. A., Calsyn, D. A., Fordyce, W. E., and Ready, L. B.: Drug utilization patterns in chronic pain patients. Pain, 12:357–363, 1982.
27. Buckley, F. P., Sizemore, W. A., and Charlton, J. E.: Medication management in patients with chronic non-malignant pain: A review of the use of a drug withdrawal protocol. Pain, 26:153–165, 1986.
28. Couch, J. R., and Hassansin, R. S.: Migraine and depression effect of amitriptyline prophylaxis. Trans. Am. Neurol. Assoc., 101:1–4, 1976.
29. Lascelles, R. G.: Atypical facial pain and depression. Br. J. Psychiatry, 122:651–659, 1966.
30. Fordyce, W. E.: Behavioral concepts in chronic pain and illness. *In* Davidson, P. O. (Ed.): Behavioral Management of Anxiety, Depression, and Pain. New York, Brunner/Mazel Press, 1976, pp. 147–188.
31. Fordyce, W. E.: Behavioral Methods for Chronic Pain and Illness. St. Louis, C. V. Mosby, 1976.
32. Fordyce, W. E.: Learning processes in pain. *In* Sternbach, R. A. (Ed.): Psychology of Pain, 2nd Ed. New York, Raven Press, 1987, pp. 49–66.

Osteoporosis

VELIMIR MATKOVIC
REBECCA D. JACKSON
WALTER J. MYSIW
ROBERT WHITTEN
DARINKA DEKANIC

With increases in life expectancy and in the number of elderly people, bone loss and fractures are becoming more common in the United States, as they are elsewhere. The problems associated with bone loss and aging are not only medical; there are also social, cultural, and economic ramifications that affect the life of a community or a nation. In 1980, the number of people in the world age 60 years and above was estimated at 291 million, or 8 per cent of the world's population. By the year 2000, this number is expected to reach 585 million, increasing this proportion to 9 per cent. By the middle of the next century, there will be up to 100 million people over the age of 55 years in the United States (Fig. 57–1).[1] As a consequence, an epidemic of bone fractures among the elderly should be expected (Fig. 57–2). In many countries, even now most of the orthopedic beds are occupied by hip fracture patients, and total expenses for the community are enormous. The annual cost of osteoporosis in the United States is estimated to be about 7 to 10 billion dollars.[2] Whereas osteoporosis is the major underlying cause of fractures of the long bones, neuromuscular instability in elderly individuals is an important contributor to the fall that usually produces the fractures. In this context, the benefit of exercise and maintenance of physical fitness not only would contribute to the prevention of bone loss but also should improve protective responses in muscle strength all over the body, thereby leading to a reduction in the incidence of fractures. Based on this, specialists in physical medicine and rehabilitation should be more and more involved in the prevention program for and chronic care of the osteoporotic population.

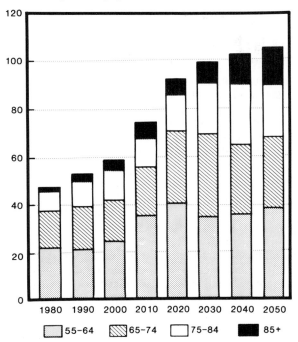

FIGURE 57–1. Number of people (in millions) in the United States over 55 years of age. (Bureau of Census, 1983.)

1169

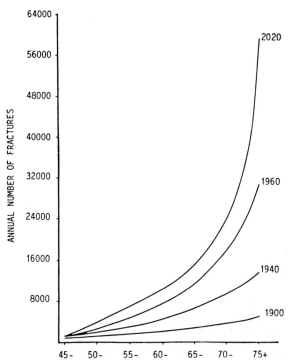

FIGURE 57–2. Annual number of hip fractures in the United States calculated by applying current incidence to the census of the population at a particular time.

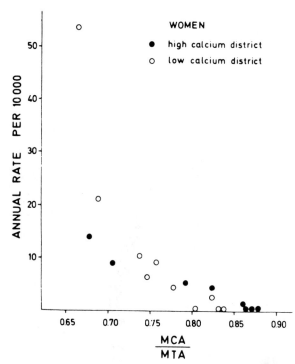

FIGURE 57–3. The relationship between bone density and annual hip fracture rates. (From Matkovic, V., Kostial, K., Simonovic, I., Buzina, R., Brodarec, A., and Nordin, B. E. C.: Bone status and fracture rates in two regions of Yugoslavia. Am. J. Clin. Nutr., 32:540–549, 1979.)

Definition

Osteoporosis is a bone disease characterized by a reduction of bone tissue relative to the volume of anatomical bone that increases susceptibility to fracture. Current understanding of osteoporosis indicates that the disease is present when bone mass lies more than two standard deviations below the mean of young adults of the same sex. This indicates that all women and men become osteoporotic if they live long enough. Whether a bone breaks depends on the relationship between the severity of the trauma and the strength of bone; what osteoporosis does is to increase the fracture risk—not cause the fracture. Fracture risk rises as bone density falls[3] (Fig. 57–3). The chemical composition of osteoporotic bone is considered to be normal. The skeleton is composed of a mineral component, calcium hydroxyapatite (60 per cent); and organic material, mainly collagen (40 per cent). In osteoporosis, the bone is of normal size but contains less bone tissue without change in the ratio of mineral component to organic material. In osteomalacia, for example, the amount of bone may be normal or even increased, but it has reduced mineral content. In some patients, osteo-porosis and osteomalacia could coexist, and in those cases, the ash content of bone and the amount of bone tissue per unit volume are reduced (Fig. 57–4).

Classification

Osteoporosis can be classified according to localization in the skeleton and according to etiology (Table 57–1). Localized osteoporosis affects part of the skeleton; generalized osteoporosis affects, to a greater or lesser extent, different parts of the

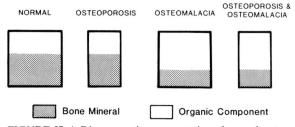

FIGURE 57–4. Diagrammatic representation of normal, osteoporotic, and osteomalacic bone.

TABLE 57–1. Classification of Osteoporosis

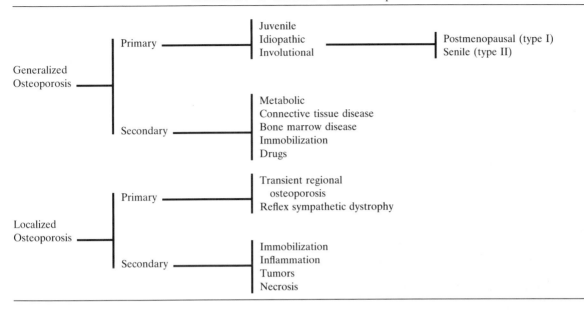

whole skeleton. Both types of osteoporosis can further be classified into primary and secondary osteoporosis. The causative agent in primary osteoporosis usually is not fully known; in secondary osteoporosis the predisposing factor, either local or systemic, is always present. Finally, generalized osteoporosis can further be classified according to the age of the patient when clinical signs are presented into juvenile or idiopathic osteoporosis and involutional osteoporosis. Juvenile osteoporosis affects children and adolescents of both sexes; idiopathic osteoporosis affects premenopausal women and middle-age men. Involutional osteoporosis is, by far, the most common form of osteoporosis and includes postmenopausal osteoporosis (type I) and aging-associated osteoporosis (type II), previously termed *senile osteoporosis*. Type I osteoporosis affects postmenopausal women between the ages of 50 and 65 years, and type II osteoporosis affects individuals over the age of 70 years.[4]

Primary Involutional Osteoporosis

Epidemiology

Primary involutional osteoporosis is the most common form of osteoporosis. It begins in middle life and becomes increasingly more common with advancing age. We now recognize the three main sites of fracture associated with bone loss: wrist, spine, and hip.[5] The epidemiology of spinal osteoporosis is difficult, because vertebral fractures can occur without symptoms,[6] but about 8 per cent of women will be affected by 80 years of age. A vertebral fracture may be classified as either a partial vertebral deformity, which is the partial loss of height of the anterior edge or middle section of the vertebral body, or a complete compression fracture, which is the collapse of the entire vertebral body. Approximately half a million cases of vertebral osteoporosis occur every year.[7] The majority of patients with compression fracture syndrome are postmenopausal women, age range 50 to 70 years, and as such are classified as type I osteoporosis.

The incidence of wrist fractures starts to rise immediately after menopause with a cumulative prevalence of about 15 per cent by the age of 80 (Figs. 57–5 and 57–6). The approximate annual number of patients with wrist fractures is about 172,000 cases. Wrist fractures are the result of moderate trauma and occur during rapid postmenopausal bone loss and, therefore, could be classified as type I osteoporosis. These fractures are very uncommon among men. Female to male ratio is 5:1. Incidence of fractures is similar among different populations (Fig. 57–7). Only about 18 per cent of forearm fractures result in hospitalization, and most patients require no rehabilitation

VELIMIR MATKOVIC ET AL.

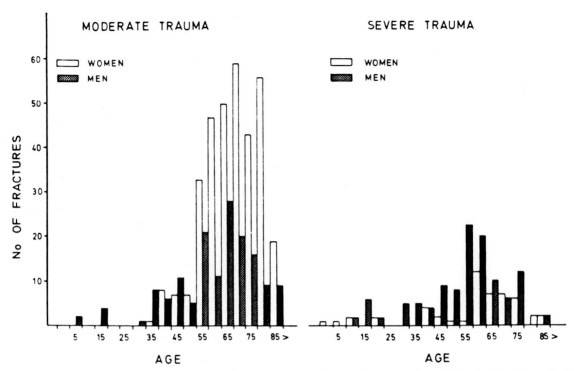

FIGURE 57–5. Number of wrist fractures according to age, sex, and type of trauma. (From Matkovic, V., Ciganovic, M., Tominac, C., and Kostial, K.: Osteoporosis and epidemiology of fractures in Croatia. An international comparison. Henry Ford Hosp. Med. J., 28:116–126, 1980. Copyright 1980 by Henry Ford Hospital.)

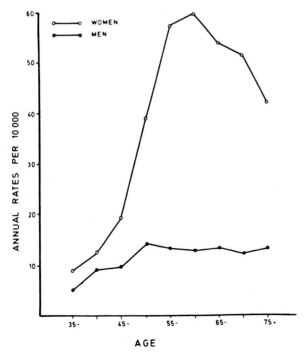

FIGURE 57–6. Annual wrist fracture rates according to age and sex. (From Matkovic, V., Ciganovic, M., Tominac, C., and Kostial, K.: Osteoporosis and epidemiology of fractures in Croatia. An international comparison. Henry Ford Hosp. Med. J., 28:116–126, 1980. Copyright 1980 by Henry Ford Hospital.)

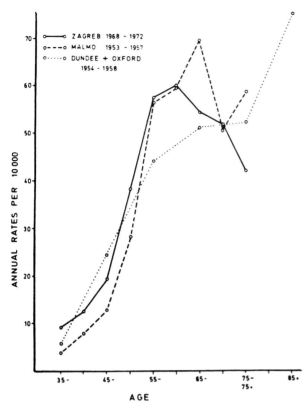

FIGURE 57–7. Annual wrist fracture rates among women from different countries. (From Matkovic, V., Ciganovic, M., Tominac, C., and Kostial, K.: Osteoporosis and epidemiology of fractures in Croatia. An international comparison. Henry Ford Hosp. Med. J., 28:116–126, 1980. Copyright 1980 by Henry Ford Hospital.)

services. These fractures are rarely fatal and cause much less disability than do the other two osteoporotic syndromes.[8]

Hip fractures tend to occur later in life with a cumulative prevalence of about 6 per cent by the age of 80. There is 20 to 25 years' delay in time between the peak incidence of wrist fractures and hip fractures (Fig. 57–8). Hip fractures are twice as common in women as in men, but the female to male ratio is not as high as for wrist and compression fractures. The majority of patients with hip fractures sustain the fractures after moderate trauma (Fig. 57–9), and those patients also tend to have less cortical bone (Fig. 57–10). Approximately 200,000 hip fracture cases occur every year in the United States.[7] Adult white women who live to age 80 have a 15 per cent lifetime risk of suffering a hip fracture. In contrast, a white male who has a 75-year life expectancy has only a 5 per cent lifetime risk of hip fracture. An 80-year-old woman who has an average of nine years of

remaining life expectancy still has about a 50 per cent chance of suffering a hip fracture before she dies.[8] Hip fractures are associated not only with high morbidity but also with high mortality. About 12 to 30 per cent of patients with hip fractures will die within one year after the accident (Fig. 57–11). In the majority of cases, mortality occurs within the first three months after the trauma.[9] Advanced age, presence of chronic illness, and disability are responsible for this. Hip fractures are classified as type II or senile osteoporosis. They are more common among Caucasians and Orientals than in Blacks (Fig. 57–12). The reason for this could be the difference in the peak bone mass level among these groups, as well as the level of physical activity in the population.[10]

The majority of patients with hip fractures are referred from nursing homes; the presence of vitamin D deficiency and secondary hyperparathy-

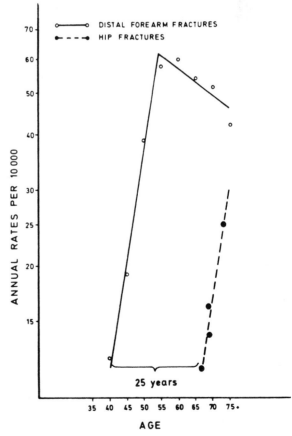

FIGURE 57–8. Annual wrist and hip fracture rates for women in Croatia. (From Matkovic, V., Ciganovic, M., Tominac, C., and Kostial, K.: Osteoporosis and epidemiology of fractures in Croatia. An international comparison. Henry Ford Hosp. Med. J., 28:116–126, 1980. Copyright 1980 by Henry Ford Hospital.)

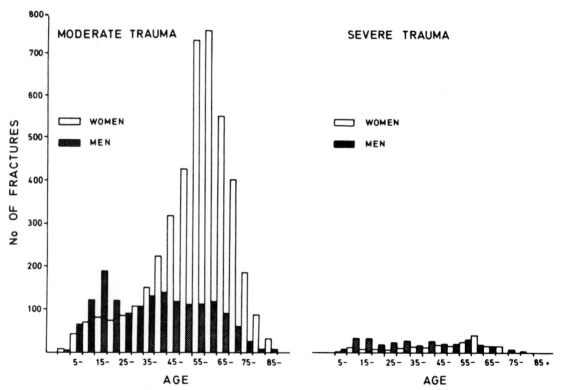

FIGURE 57–9. Number of hip fractures according to age, sex, and type of trauma. (From Matkovic, V., Ciganovic, M., Tominac, C., and Kostial, K.: Osteoporosis and epidemiology of fractures in Croatia. An international comparison. Henry Ford Hosp. Med. J., 28:116–126, 1980. Copyright 1980 by Henry Ford Hospital.)

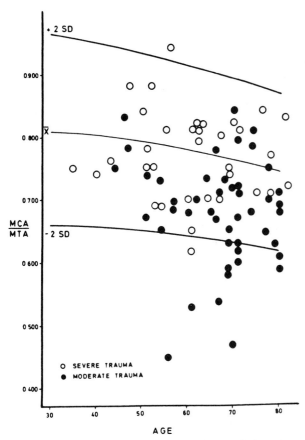

FIGURE 57–10. Metacarpal cortical/total area ratio in patients with hip fractures after moderate and severe trauma. (From Matkovic, V., Ciganovic, M., Tominac, C., and Kostial, K.: Osteoporosis and epidemiology of fractures in Croatia. An international comparison. Henry Ford Hosp. Med. J., 28:116–126, 1980. Copyright 1980 by Henry Ford Hospital.)

roidism could be a contributing factor to the rising incidence of these fractures among elderly people. Recent studies fail to show consistent differences in bone mass, measured at a number of skeletal sites, in patients with hip fractures compared with controls.[11] The most likely explanation is that as bone mass declines, the risk of fractures increases. Another hypothesis is that the primary cause of hip fractures in the elderly is impaired balance, resulting in falls, rather than reduced bone mass. A normal neuromuscular response that protects the skeleton against trauma and subsequent fractures would be *abnormal* in those patients. Based on this, public health measures should be directed not only at prevention of bone loss but also at the prevention of falls. A third explanation could be that a hip fracture is a result of the summation of multiple microfractures secondary to the abnormality in tissue repair and bone turnover.

Pathogenesis

The human skeleton reaches a peak bone mass between late adolescence and the early 20s. Thereafter, bone loss occurs, gradually resulting in increased fracture risk with minimal or moderate trauma (Fig. 57–13). It seems logical, then, to conclude that the main determinants of osteoporosis will be the peak bone mass level reached at skeletal maturity and the subsequent rate of bone loss. Besides the bone mass level, the abnormality in microstructure and bone tissue repair could lead to bone fragility and change in bone quality, which can contribute to the overall incidence of fractures among the elderly. Each determinant of osteoporosis will be considered separately.

PEAK BONE MASS

Since bone mass is the principal determinant of fracture, high bone mass at skeletal maturity is

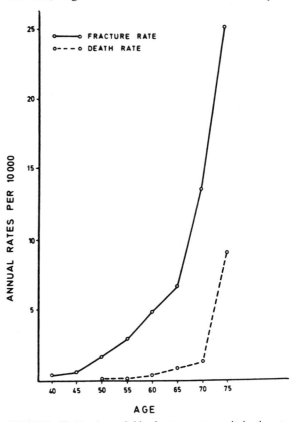

FIGURE 57–11. Annual hip fracture rate and death rate, according to age, in Croatia. (From Matkovic, V., Ciganovic, M., Tominac, C., and Kostial, K.: Osteoporosis and epidemiology of fractures in Croatia. An international comparison. Henry Ford Hosp. Med. J., 28:116–126, 1980. Copyright 1980 by Henry Ford Hospital.)

VELIMIR MATKOVIC ET AL.

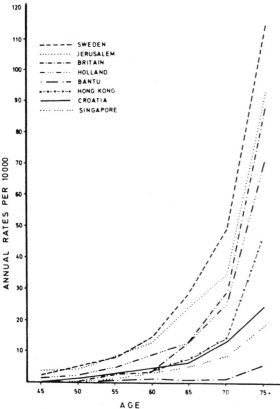

FIGURE 57–12. International comparison of the incidence of hip fractures among women. (From Matkovic, V., Ciganovic, M., Tominac, C., and Kostial, K.: Osteoporosis and epidemiology of fractures in Croatia. An international comparison. Henry Ford Hosp. Med. J., 28:116–126, 1980. Copyright 1980 by Henry Ford Hospital.)

considered the best protection against age-related bone loss.[12, 13] Besides well-known factors influencing body stature, very little is known about mechanisms increasing peak bone mass. Peak bone mass is clearly the result of age, sex, and probably other genetically determined factors.[14, 15] Men have more bone mass than women, and blacks have heavier skeletons than Caucasians.[16] As a direct consequence of this, men and blacks have a lower incidence of fractures than their counterparts. It has been suggested recently that peak bone mass could be related to nutrition as well. It was shown that calcium intake is an important determinant of peak bone mass in young adults[17, 18] (Fig. 57–14).

The period between 9 and 20 years of age seems to be critical for achievement of peak bone mass. From birth until about age 20, bones are in a phase of rapid growth and bone modeling. After this period, the skeleton is in the process of constant

remodeling throughout life. Among the mentioned ages, the most important years are probably during the adolescent growth spurt, when rapid bone modeling occurs. This is the time when bone mineral content increases at the rate of about 8.5 per cent per year.[19, 20] The average male begins his growth spurt at around 12 years of age, and reaches his maximum velocity and height growth at about 14 years of age. At this time, he will be growing

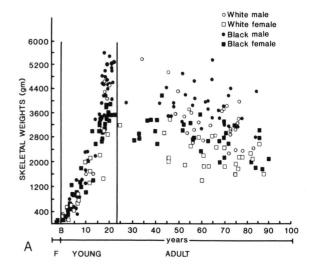

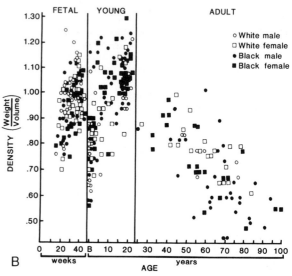

FIGURE 57–13. Skeletal weights (A) and density (B) according to age, sex, and race. (From Trotter, M., and Hixon, B.: Sequential changes in weight, density, and percentage ash weight of human skeletons from an early fetal period through old age. Anat. Rec., 179:1–18, 1974.) (Trotter, M., Hixon, B., 1974, by permission of Anatomical Records, a publication of the Wistar Press[16].)

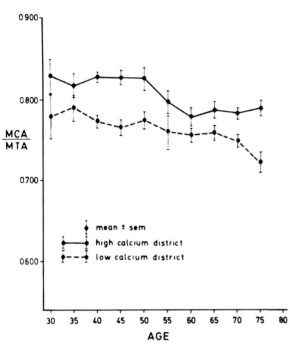

FIGURE 57–14. Two populations of men with different peak bone mass (density). (From Matkovic, V., Kostial, K., Simonovic, I., Buzina, R., Brodarec, A., and Nordin, B. E. C.: Bone status and fracture rates in two regions of Yugoslavia. Am. J. Clin. Nutr., 32:540–549, 1979.)

at nearly twice his childhood or preadolescent rate. His growth will be almost completed by age 18. Females begin puberty approximately two years earlier (8 to 10) and will reach maximum velocity in their height growth around 12 years of age. Cessation of linear growth in girls will be around age 16. Thereafter, in both boys and girls, body length increases by about 2 per cent; this increase continues into the early 20s, or the young adult period. This increase is accounted for primarily by continued vertebral growth.[21]

Maximum skeletal bone mass based on skeletal weight measurements is achieved by the beginning of the third decade.[16] Total body calcium as determined by neutron activation analysis is highest at the age of 20.[22, 23] Total body bone mineral, as well as total body bone density, as determined by a dual-photon absorptiometry technique, peaks at the age of 20 and declines thereafter.[24] Looking at tubular (cortical) bone envelopes, we can conclude that the external diameter of tubular bones, as an indicator of periosteal growth, reaches a plateau by the age of 20 in males and a few years earlier in females. Medullary area is constantly increasing in males after the age of 20. In females, however, during this adolescent growth spurt, there is an

endosteal apposition of cortical bone. Cortical bone mass, as represented by cortical width and cortical area, is at its maximum by the age of 20, at least as reflected in radiogrammetry studies of the second metacarpal bone.[25] By the beginning of young adulthood (the third decade), bone mineral content of the forearm, as assessed by the single-photon absorptiometry technique, is approaching its highest level—a fact that indicates, once again, that adolescence could be a critical period for cortical peak bone mass formation.[26]

There is little data regarding changes in trabecular bone mass in the adolescent period, but present literature suggests that the peak bone mass at the vertebral column has been achieved by the age of 20. Postmortem data, using bone ash measurements and compressive strength measurements, indicate an increase in those figures through the beginning of the third decade with a decline thereafter.[27, 28] The determination of bone mineral density at the lumbar spine with the use of the dual-photon technique also indicates that bone mineral content is declining after its maximum at the age of 20 in both males and females.[29] Iliac crest bone biopsies show that trabecular peak bone mass is reached between late adolescence and 20 years of age.[30]

Over a period of 20 years, in order to accumulate a total body calcium level of about 1000 gm and 1200 gm, respectively, females need an average daily accretion of calcium into the skeleton of 140 mg/day and males need 165 mg/day. During the adolescent growth spurt, the required calcium retention (mg/day) is two to three times higher than the average value. The calcium accretion to the skeleton can go up to 500 mg/day for males and up to 400 mg/day for females.[25, 31, 32] Mineral deficiency during this period could reduce the degree of positive calcium balance, with a resultant reduction in the level of bone mass reached by skeletal maturity.[18, 32, 33] Presumably, such low bone mass at skeletal maturity would contribute to low bone mass at menopause and subsequent increased risk for fracture (Fig. 57–15).[18] Currently, there is a great emphasis on the research in this subject, primarily involving environmental factors that might modulate peak bone mass formation.[34–36]

RATE OF BONE LOSS

After peak bone mass has been reached, bone loss begins and persists until age 85 to 90 years. Lifetime losses range from 20 to 30 per cent for males and up to 45 to 50 per cent for fe-

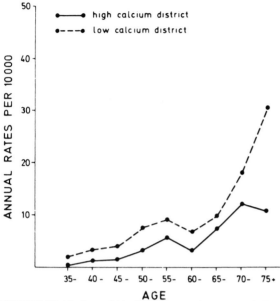

FIGURE 57–15. Annual hip fracture rates in two populations of men with different peak bone mass. (From Matkovic, V., Kostial, K., Simonovic, I., Buzina, R., Brodarec, A., and Nordin, B. E. C.: Bone status and fracture rates in two regions of Yugoslavia. Am. J. Clin. Nutr., 32:540–549, 1979.)

males.[4, 34, 37] Loss of bone with advancing age is a universal phenomenon present in almost every population studied so far, and the rate of bone loss seems to be equal among different populations. Bone loss begins earlier and proceeds more rapidly in females than in males, with an accelerated phase in postmenopausal years. The rate of age-related bone loss is about 0.5 to 1 per cent *per annum* in both sexes. It increases in women in the immediate postmenopausal period to approximately 2 to 3 per cent per year for 3 to 15 years after menopause.[4, 37] After the age of 70, there is a decline in the rate of bone loss to 0.5 to 1 per cent per year. At that time, the rate of bone loss is equal between men and women (Fig. 57–16). This accelerated bone loss in females is attributed to the loss of estrogen function and is responsible for the development of type I osteoporosis (wrist fractures and compression fractures of the spine). The sex ratio of the incidence of involutional osteoporosis between the ages of 50 and 70 is 5:1 and is a direct reflection of the rapid postmenopausal bone loss in females, which is two to four times higher in comparison to males. After the age of 70, the rate of bone loss declines and, as explained before, there is no sexual difference in the rate of bone loss. Sex ratio of the incidence of involutional osteoporosis after the age of 70 is,

therefore, 2:1 (hip fracture incidence).[4, 10] This phase of bone loss is considered to be related to the aging process. Since men do not have menopause, the aging process is considered to be the only reason for the bone loss.

Menopause is associated with clear-cut changes in the metabolism of estrogens and calcium, which subsequently reflect the loss of bone that starts at menopause. Bone loss may be attributed to an increase in sensitivity of the skeleton and, in the absence of estrogen, to the resorbing action of parathyroid hormone (PTH), as originally suggested by Heaney and Nordin in 1965.[38, 39] Menopause is associated with a profound fall in plasma estradiol and to a lesser degree in plasma estrone (Fig. 57–17). Estradiol is the main estrogen secreted by ovaries during the premenopausal period. Depending on the phase of the menstrual cycle, the plasma range in postmenopausal women is between 100 and 1000 pmol/liter. During the postmenopausal period, the level is below 60 pmol/liter. Plasma estrone level in premenopausal women (one half comes from ovaries and one half from adrenals) is about 150 to 600 pmol/liter, and between 50 and 250 pmol/liter in the postmenopausal period.[40] After cessation of ovarian function, the main source of estrogens in the postmenopausal period is the adrenal glands, and estrone then becomes the main circulating estrogen derived from androstenedione by peripheral conversion.

This abrupt fall in the secretion of sex hormones is followed by the rise in plasma gonadotropins, particularly the follicle-stimulating hormone (FSH). There is also a decline in adrenal androstenedione production with age; the decline suggests the existence of adrenopause, which might further contribute to the estrogen deficiency status and influence the rate of bone loss.[40, 41]

As a result of increased bone resorption due to menopause, there is a small rise in plasma calcium concentration, and as a direct reflection of this there is an increase in urine calcium excretion as judged by the calcium creatinine ratio in a two-hour fasting urine test. The indices of bone turnover that indicate increased bone resorption/formation are elevated; the indices are urinary hydroxyproline, serum alkaline phosphatase, and osteocalcin.[42] The rise in plasma calcium concentration suppresses a parathyroid hormone secretion, and this leads to the increase in tubular resorption of phosphate and rise in plasma phosphate after the menopause. As a result of estrogen deficiency, there is also a slight fall in vitamin D

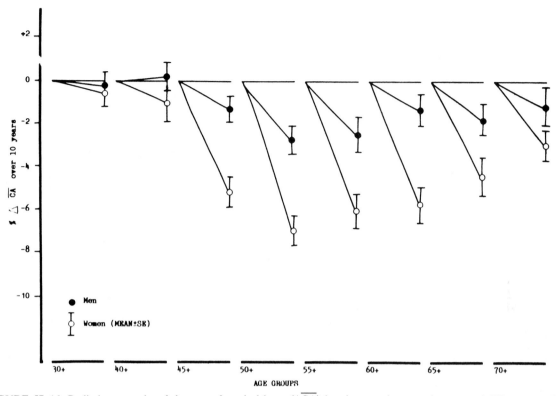

FIGURE 57–16. Preliminary results of the rate of cortical bone ($\Delta\overline{CA}$) loss in normal men and women of different age (473 subjects).

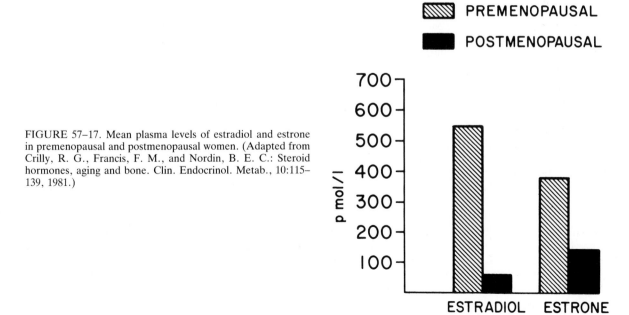

FIGURE 57–17. Mean plasma levels of estradiol and estrone in premenopausal and postmenopausal women. (Adapted from Crilly, R. G., Francis, F. M., and Nordin, B. E. C.: Steroid hormones, aging and bone. Clin. Endocrinol. Metab., 10:115–139, 1981.)

VELIMIR MATKOVIC ET AL.

level $(1,25(OH)_2D_3)$ and a fall in calcium absorption, which contributes to the negative calcium balance at lower calcium intakes. This might aggravate postmenopausal bone loss induced by estrogen deficiency.[43]

It is still not known if patients with crush fracture syndrome (type I osteoporosis) represent a population of patients with osteoporosis secondary to increased rate of bone loss (fast bone-losers) or if they are simply a combination of decreased peak bone mass level with the same or increased rate of bone loss.[44] Because estrogen deficiency is the main cause of the accelerated phase of bone loss, estrogen supplementation in women seems to be the ideal prevention against type I osteoporosis.

BONE CELL FUNCTION, BONE TURNOVER, AND TISSUE REPAIR

Creation of peak bone mass, as well as bone loss, is the ultimate event of bone remodeling mediated by bone cells throughout our lifetime. Exchange of bone tissue, which allows bone growth and skeletal development, is usually called *bone modeling*. The net bone tissue balance during bone modeling is positive (formation exceeds resorption) until cessation of growth and formation of peak bone mass. During late adolescence, after growth is being completed and peak bone mass and density are being reached, the exchange of bone tissue is called bone remodeling. Bone tissue is being remodeled internally without significant change in the shape of the bone as an organ. During the process of aging, bone remodeling creates negative net bone tissue balance where bone resorption exceeds formation. The main factors responsible for bone remodeling are well-differentiated bone cells: osteoclasts, which resorb the microscopic quantum of bone tissue and osteoblasts, which repair the resorption-mediated defect. The osteoclasts and osteoblasts are coupled together in a basic multicellular unit (BMU).[45, 46] Cortical bone undergoes remodeling through a BMU represented in a haversian system. Trabecular bone undergoes remodeling within a BMU called a trabecular osteon.[47] A typical bone remodeling sequence in a trabecular bone is represented in Figure 57–18.[48] The local remodeling cycle begins with activation of quiescent cells at the bone surface. Remodeling stimulus (either hormones, local tissue factors, or physical force) influences lining cells to contract and to expose bone surface, which then attracts osteoclasts. Osteoclasts originate from bone marrow monocytes and migrate to the exposed bone surface to resorb a packet or quantum of bone. A resorption site can be identified histologically by the presence of a cutting cone in cortical bone or a resorption cavity (Howship's lacuna) on endosteal and trabecular bone surfaces. After resorption is completed, osteoblasts that originate from bone marrow mesenchymal cells invade the area and start to synthesize new bone matrix. Biochemically this is reflected in serum bone alkaline phosphatase that originates from osteoblasts. Subsequently bone matrix becomes mineralized. Some osteoblasts are being incorporated into newly formed bone and become osteocytes. When resorptive cavity is being repaired, bone remodeling ceases, and bone surface becomes quiescent again. The entire remodeling cycle from activation to complete repair lasts about three months. There are two million remodeling units active throughout the human skeleton at any one time. The resorption and formation in a remodeling cycle are coupled with bone resorption being followed by bone formation. At skeletal maturity, at which bone loss is negligible (age between peak bone mass formation and menopause), bone formation is equal to or slightly less than bone resorption with a net bone balance of zero or slightly less than zero. During aging, bone formation cannot follow bone resorption (uncoupling between formation and resorption), with the creation of negative bone balance ultimately leading to osteoporosis (Fig. 57–19).[49, 50]

The main functions of the bone remodeling process are the repair of skeletal microfractures and the release of calcium into the circulation as a part of the homeostatic control mechanism. During constant stress, every material is susceptible to fatigue fracture. Since the main role of the skeleton is to support the body and, as such, it is constantly being stressed, the development of microfractures (fatigue fractures) is probably a normal event. In normal situations when the stress is relatively short, these microfractures will heal quickly through the process of bone remodeling. If stress lasts long enough, multiple microfractures can develop, which ultimately could result in a bone fracture (typical march fractures of the metatarsal bones in runners and soldiers). The speculation is that with aging, the ability of bone tissue to repair microdamage (trabecular perforation) is not sufficient; this could contribute to the development of different fracture syndromes by changing the quality of the bone.

Microfractures have been described in the proximal part of the femur as well as in the spine.[51, 52]

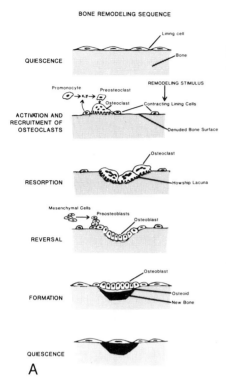

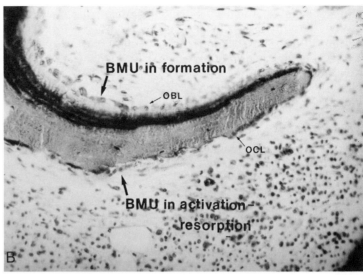

FIGURE 57–18. *A,* Bone remodeling sequence at trabecular bone surface (x, y = tissue factors that stimulate preosteoclasts.) (After Parfitt[48] and Rodan, G. A., and Martin, T. J.: Calcif. Tissue Int., **33**:349, 1981.) *B,* Bone remodeling sequence at trabecular bone surface *in vivo* in parathyroid bone disease. Notice formation on one side of the trabecular surface and bone resorption on the other. Two BMU are in different phases of activity. (OBL, osteoblast; OCL, osteoclast.)

Inability of bone tissue to repair microdamage can explain occurrence of fractures due to moderate trauma in patients who have normal bone mass in comparison to age- and sex-matched controls.[53]

Bone remodeling is under the influence of various systemic hormones and local tissue factors. Activators of bone remodeling or bone resorption are parathyroid hormone (PTH), prostaglandin (PGE), $1,25(OH)_2$ vitamin D_3, thyroid hormone, vasoactive intestinal peptide (VIP), and phosphate through creation of secondary hyperparathyroidism. It was recently discovered that interleukin-1, which comes from macrophages, can also stimulate bone resorption. The inhibitors of bone resorption are calcitonin, estrogens, diphosphonates, and calcium by suppression of PTH. The only currently

FIGURE 57–19. Pathogenesis of trabecular bone loss with age and reversal of bone loss with ADFR therapy, at BMU level. At maturity, resorption (R) equals formation (F). During aging there is disbalance between resorption (R) and formation (F_1). ADFR therapy restores bone mass by activation and suppression of resorption (r) and by new bone formation (f). (Adapted partially from Courpron, P., et al.: *In* Jee, W. S. S., and Parfitt, A. M. (Eds.): Bone Histomorphometry. Armour Montagu, Levallois, 1981, pp. 323–329.

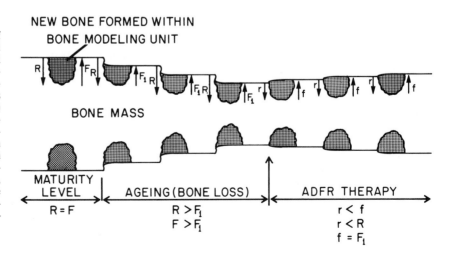

VELIMIR MATKOVIC ET AL.

known agent that can stimulate bone formation outside the BMU is sodium fluoride. There is intensive research going on involving different bone growth factors (matrix proteins) that might have applicability in the treatment of various osteoporotic conditions in the near future by correction of abnormal coupling between resorption and formation.

Risk Factors for Peak Bone Mass Formation and Rate of Bone Loss

There are many factors that influence acquisition and maintenance of peak bone mass as well as the rate of bone loss. They all eventually can determine who is at risk of osteoporosis. Risk factors can be divided into endogenous and exogenous origin (Table 57–2).

GENETIC FACTORS

Bone mass acquired at maturity is an important determinant of bone mass at any given subsequent time. Prevalence of osteoporosis is low in groups with a high peak bone mass; such sex/ethnic groups include men versus women and blacks versus Caucasians as previously explained. According to the international studies of bone mass among different population groups, it seems that the rate of bone loss is the same among different ethnic groups. Therefore, it is likely that the racial differences in the incidence of osteoporosis reflect differences in peak bone mass rather than in rates of bone loss. Several twin studies also suggested that bone mass is under genetic influence.[14, 54] It was suggested recently that heredity influences acquisition of bone mass rather than rate of bone loss.[15, 55] Because the mother and father probably contribute equally to the acquisition of bone mass by the child, screening should include both parents.[15] There is a higher genetic linkage for body size parameters than for body density. This linkage indicates that the petite body habitus should be at greater risk for the development of osteoporosis.[55, 56] It has also been known for quite some time that osteoporosis might run in families; therefore, family history should be a part of a screening process.[57] The interaction between genetic factors and environment is still not known. One of the reasons black people have denser skeletons is due to more favorable calcium economy in the body (less calcium excretion in the urine), but blacks have a greater resistance to the bone-resorptive effects of PTH and $1,25(OH)_2D_3$. This resistance may allow them to accumulate more bone during growth.[58]

AGE

Age seems to be one of the most important determinants of bone loss and fractures. Aging appears to be encoded in our genes and reflected by the wide range of maximal life span potential that humans possess. It appears likely that the genetic basis of aging involves two types of species-specific differences. The first difference is in range of maturation and programmed timings of developmental stages. The second type relates to biochemical systems involving self-maintenance.[59] The first type applies to the skeletal growth, maturation, and differentiation, all of which result in a peak bone mass formation. The second type relates to the skeletal integrity and maintenance throughout a lifetime at the basic multicellular unit level. As Down's syndrome may have the greatest number of features associated with the senescent phenotype, it can be considered a human genetic model for the aging process. It was noticed several years ago that young patients with Down's syndrome have a reduced percentage of cortical area in comparison to the age-matched controls.[25]

TABLE 57–2. Risk Factors for Osteoporosis

Endogenous
  Genetic factors
    Caucasian and Oriental
    Petite body habitus
    Family history
  Age
    Advanced
  Sex
    Female
  Loss of ovarian function
    Premature menopause
    Amenorrhea (not induced)
  Medical diseases
Exogenous
  Nutrition
    Calcium
    Phosphate
    Protein
  Life style
    Smoking
    Caffeine intake
    Inactivity
  Immobilization
  Medications
    Glucocorticoids

LOSS OF OVARIAN FUNCTION

Premature menopause, either idiopathic or surgically induced, can be considered a risk factor for early bone loss. A normal woman who undergoes oophorectomy at the age of 40 (normal expected age of menopause is 50) should have bone mass 10 years later at the same level as a normal woman at age 60. Late menarche is also associated with a lower than average bone mineral content.[60] Prolonged amenorrhea secondary to excessive physical exercise in young female athletes and heavy cigarette smoking with depressed estrogen levels in postmenopausal women can cause osteoporosis; therefore, excessive physical exercise (leading to hormonal abnormalities) and heavy smoking can be considered risk factors for the development of osteoporosis through interference with adequate plasma estrogen levels.[61, 62]

Women who have been taking oral contraceptives have higher forearm densities, but definitive studies involving other skeletal sites are still lacking.[63]

Estrogen deficiency is a major pathogenetic factor in the development of postmenopausal osteoporosis (type I). Retrospective and prospective studies indicate that postmenopausal estrogen use protects against osteoporotic fractures; there is ample evidence that postmenopausal bone loss is reduced by this therapy.[64–68]

Parity and lactation seem to have no adverse effect on bone mass.[25, 69, 70]

NUTRITION

Among nutritional factors, low calcium, low vitamin D, high protein, high phosphate, and caffeine intakes have been considered to be risk factors for the development of osteoporosis. These factors can influence peak bone mass formation and subsequent rate of bone loss. Experiments with laboratory animals have established that calcium deficiency can cause osteoporosis.[71] In the majority of the experiments, animals were fed a low-calcium diet during the growing period, and skeletons were examined when the animal reached adulthood.[17, 72] The results indicated that calcium deficiency can cause osteoporosis by decreasing peak bone mass formation, rather than affecting adult bone mass.[33, 73] Experimental calcium deficiency can cause growth retardation in animals and bone volume and density decrease.[73] There is no clear-cut evidence that growing human skeletons react in the same way, although some older studies suggest they could. At the turn of the century, a

group of British children who received milk supplementation grew taller in comparison to a non-supplemented group.[74] Unfortunately, bone mass measurements were not done in this study. The Ten State Nutrition Survey of children of different socioeconomical backgrounds reveals that children of greater affluence had a 5 per cent higher skeletal mass and bone formation rate than did children from lower socioeconomical classes.[75] From these studies, it is not quite clear if those differences were due to inadequate protein or mineral nutrition. Malnutrition certainly can lead to growth retardation, and with correction of nutritional deficit, children can rapidly regain lost growth.[76] It is not known at the present time if there is adequate "catch-up mineralization" of the skeleton, particularly after the growth spurt period. It was also reported recently that some of the children who suffered an accidental fracture have decreased bone mineral density as determined by single-photon absorptiometry technique, as well as decreased calcium intake.[77] A study of the calcium intake, bone mass, and fracture rates in two populations in Croatia, Yugoslavia, revealed that people with higher calcium intake over their lifetime (1000 to 1200 mg/day) have denser skeletons and fewer hip fractures than do people who have lower calcium intake (400 to 500 mg/day) (Figs. 57–14, 57–15, 57–20, and 57–21).[18] Because differences were present at the age of 30, the study indicated that calcium is probably more important for peak bone mass formation than for decreased bone loss.

The difference between mean calcium intake and net skeletal calcium accretion is lower for adolescent females than for other females or for males of any age (Figs. 57–22 and 57–23) indicating that inadequate mineral nutrition can occur easily in female adolescents.[78] To satisfy high skeletal retention, allowing for obligatory calcium excretion into the urine and variable absorption efficiency, calcium intake during adolescence should exceed 1000 mg/day.

Calcium metabolism during adolescence is presented in Figure 57–24. The average hydroxyproline (OHPr) excretion of females is 1.5 to 2 times higher during adolescence than at maturity (30 mg/24 hours). On a 1200 mg/day calcium intake (RDA), adolescent females should have a fecal calcium of about 800 mg/day, a urine calcium of about 150 mg/day, and, depending on activity level, a total calcium pool of about 550 mg of which 250 mg is incorporated into the skeleton. Digestive juice calcium, which depends on body size and dietary phosphorus, should be about 150

VELIMIR MATKOVIC ET AL.

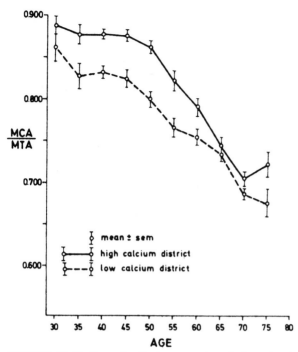

FIGURE 57–20. Bone density (metacarpal cortical area/total area) among two populations of women with lifetime difference in calcium intakes. (From Matkovic, V., Kostial, K., Simonovic, I., Buzina, R., Brodarec, A., and Nordin, B. E. C.: Bone status and fracture rates in two regions of Yugoslavia. Am. J. Clin. Nutr., 32:540–549, 1979.)

mg/day. Exact data for the amount of calcium that comes to the pool by the process of bone resorption are not known, but the values certainly depend on rate of bone modeling. In this case, it was calculated to be 1.5 to 2 times the adult value as judged by OHPr excretion. In normal metabolic circumstances, this amount of calcium should be matched by bone formation.

If, for example, the calcium intake will be lower than 1200 mg/day with subsequent decrease in calcium retention by 100 mg/day for 5 years, this should lower the peak whole-body calcium by 182 gm. The same amount of bone calcium will allow the postmenopausal women to be in a negative calcium balance of 30 mg/day for 16 years and 15 mg/day for 32 years.

The hypothesis is that residents of a low-calcium district in Croatia did not have adequate calcium intake during adolescence and ended the bone modeling period with decreased peak bone mass level.[18] It was also recently reported that postmenopausal women who had decreased dairy product consumption during adolescence had decreased bone mass in the postmenopausal period.[79]

High calcium intake in the postmenopausal period cannot completely prevent bone loss. Calcium intake below 1000 mg/day in postmenopausal women can potentiate negative calcium balance and aggravate postmenopausal bone loss, which could ultimately result in osteoporosis.[43] Longitudinal studies show definite beneficial effects of estrogens but not so pronounced an effect of calcium. In one study, calcium supplementation reduced slightly the rate of cortical bone loss as determined by single-photon absorptiometry of the forearm and whole-body calcium analysis.[80] Given that 80% of the whole body calcium is present on cortical bone, this finding may be particularly significant. There is no question that some percentage of the human population is calcium deficient and responds to calcium supplementation, but isolation of this segment of the population by simple noninvasive screening methods is almost impossible.[81]

Vitamin D deficiency can cause rickets in children and calcium malabsorption and osteomalacia in adults. Vitamin D deficiency can be the result of either inadequate exposure to sunlight or inadequate dietary intake of vitamin D. In elderly

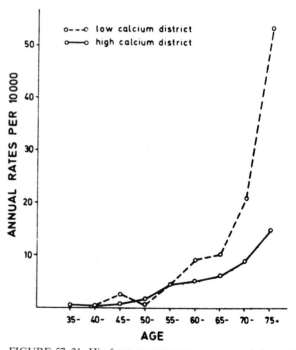

FIGURE 57–21. Hip fracture rates among two populations of women with different calcium intakes and different peak bone mass. (From Matkovic, V., Kostial, K., Simonovic, I., Buzina, R., Brodarec, A., and Nordin, B. E. C.: Bone status and fracture rates in two regions of Yugoslavia. Am. J. Clin. Nutr., 32:540–549, 1979.)

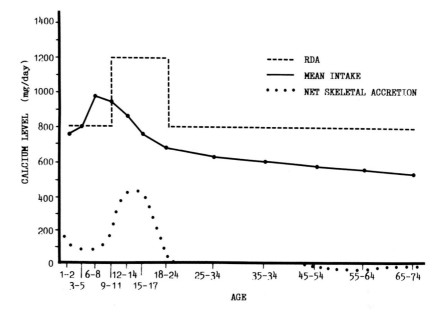

FIGURE 57–22. Recommended dietary allowance for calcium (RDA), mean calcium intake of women in the United States (DHHS Publ. No. [PHS]83–1681), and calcium accretion into the skeleton according to age.

patients, however, low plasma $1,25(OH)_2D_3$ levels could also be due to impaired 1-alpha hydroxylation by the aging kidney. It was reported that a substantial number of patients in England with hip fractures have osteomalacia and that this disease can contribute to the incidence of hip fractures. Vitamin D deficiency can also cause myopathy, which can further contribute to the hip fracture incidence through increased risk of falling second-ary to neuromuscular instability.[82] So far, there is no convincing evidence that vitamin D status is an important determinant of peak bone mass or age-related bone loss in the general population.

High phosphate intake and abnormally low calcium to phosphate ratio (1:6) was implicated in the development of osteoporosis and secondary hyperparathyroidism in laboratory animals. This has not been rigorously studied in humans, but it

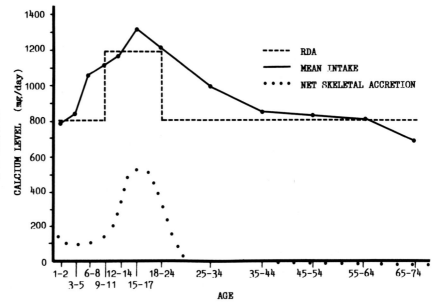

FIGURE 57–23. Recommended dietary allowance for calcium (RDA), mean calcium intake of men in the United States, and calcium accretion into the skeleton according to age. Notice that male teenagers follow RDA line.

VELIMIR MATKOVIC ET AL.

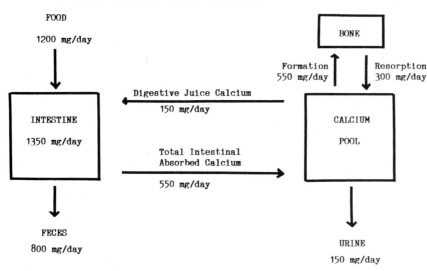

FIGURE 57–24. Scheme of calcium metabolism for normal teenage girl on calcium intake of 1200 mg/day (RDA).

has been suggested that excessive consumption of phosphate through soft drinks could be a risk factor for the development of osteoporosis.[83]

Protein-calorie malnutrition during childhood can cause growth retardation and decreased formation of cortical bone, and therefore can interfere with peak bone mass formation. On the other hand, excessive protein intake (in excess of 120 gm/day) can cause hypercalciuria and can increase the demand for calcium in postmenopausal women.[84]

Excessive caffeine consumption can also contribute to increased calcium excretion in the urine and, therefore, potentiate negative calcium balance and increase calcium requirements.[85]

Alcoholism is probably a risk factor of greater relative importance than has been commonly recognized. Prevalence of significant alcohol abuse in the adult U.S. population ranges between 8 and 16 per cent. It was demonstrated several years ago that bone mass is seriously depleted in both male and female alcoholics.[86] Defective osteoblastic function rather than increased bone resorption has been reported in patients with alcoholism.[87] Compression fractures in elderly men strongly indicates chronic alcohol consumption.

BODY HABITUS

Slenderness or petite body habitus is considered a risk factor for osteoporosis. On the other end of the spectrum, obesity and increased muscle mass are present in patients with degenerative arthritis.[88]

Obesity through its weight-bearing action and favorable estrogen metabolism in fat tissue has always been associated with increased bone density. Owing to estrogen status, obese women are protected from osteoporosis but have a higher incidence of cancer of the uterus.

PHYSICAL ACTIVITY

The incidence of osteoporosis is higher in the Western hemisphere; this could be partially due to the lack of physical activity in the population.[89] The bone loss that occurs with prolonged immobilization suggests also that physical exercise might help to prevent osteoporosis.[90] Bone density, at least in cortical bone, is higher in athletes than in their nonathletic counterparts; increase in total body calcium and vertebral bone mineral content has been reported recently after moderate exercise in patients with postmenopausal osteoporosis.[91–93] All of this indicates that daily weight-bearing activity is essential to skeletal health. Mechanical weight-bearing stress is probably the most important exogenous factor affecting bone development and peak bone mass formation, as well as affecting the maintenance and integrity of bone mass later on through its action on bone remodeling. A hundred years ago, a famous Berlin anatomist, Julius Wolff, was the first to recognize the relationship between mechanical stress and bone remodeling. In his publication *The Law of Bone Transformation,* which was printed in 1892, Wolff stated: "Every change in the function of bone is followed by definite changes in internal architecture and external confirmation according to mathematical law." He indicated that form follows function.[94] Almost 100 years since this discovery, we still do not know the mechanisms that lead to increased bone formation and increased bone density secondary to increased level of stress. Since electrical fields influence bone growth, it has been suggested that endogenous piezoelectricity generated by stress could be involved in osteoblastic stimulation and new bone formation.[95] It was also suggested recently that increased plasma levels of calcitonin found during acute physical exercise could be involved in the process as well.[96] Daily physical exercise contributes to the prevention of osteoporosis, not only by increasing bone mass but also by improving neuromuscular function and coordination, thereby decreasing falls that can cause hip fractures.[97] In one study, persons with hip fractures were significantly less active than normal controls, especially in household and job activities.[98]

Clinical Presentation

The main clinical signs and symptoms of osteoporosis are back pain, loss of height, spinal kyphosis, and multiple fractures, usually of the vertebrae, wrists, and hips. Back pain is the most common symptom in patients with compression fracture syndrome. Fractures of the vertebrae may be spontaneous but often occur after some ordinary activity such as bending or lifting. Pain may be mild or severe and may last for days or weeks before subsiding. After multiple compression fractures have occurred, however, chronic pain may develop in association with spinal deformity and progressive dorsal kyphosis, also known as a "dowager's hump." Multiple wedge-type compressions are responsible for the development of dorsal kyphosis. Loin pain is also common in spinal osteoporosis and is the result of bruising of the ribs over the iliac crests. Compression fractures are most commonly located between the end of the thoracic spine and the beginning of the lumbar spine (T 8– L 3). The majority of patients with spinal osteoporosis later in life (type II osteoporosis) have asymptomatic vertebral compression that may be detected only by radiographic examination. Loss of body height or the development of kyphosis may be the only sign of multiple vertebral fractures. Discomfort, debility, and sometimes depression secondary to the constant fear of hip fracture

may accompany thoracic shortening. ADL functions could be restricted. Loss of skin thickness, constipation, and abdominal bloating are frequent concomitant signs of the disease. In spite of the patient's multiple vertebral compressions, the incidence of radiculopathy and spinal cord trauma is negligible.

Wrist fractures are usually the result of moderate trauma or a fall from a standing position. They tend to occur outside the house and are more frequent during the winter months.[70] Sometimes reflex sympathetic dystrophy or Sudeck's bone atrophy will develop after the wrist fracture and immobilization in a plastic cast.

Hip fractures are another important clinical manifestation of osteoporosis. Patients with hip fractures are more likely to be elderly and female than are patients with vertebral fractures. The majority of hip fractures occur at home after moderate trauma. The majority of patients have a tendency to fall backward or to the side as a result of a balance problem. In the majority of cases, the fall precedes the fracture, but in some cases a sudden increase in movement will cause a fracture, provoking a fall. Fractures occur either in the neck of the femur or at the intertrochanteric region. Patients with hip fractures tend to be debilitated, senile with the presence of multiple chronic diseases, and on multiple medications including psychotropic drugs. Fractures tend to promote fear of loss of independent living, fear of additional falls and fractures, and depression.

Diagnostic Approach and Screening Methods

The diagnostic approach includes a medical history, physical examination, anthropometry, blood and urine chemistry, metabolic studies, bone mass measurements, and bone biopsy (Table 57–3).

MEDICAL HISTORY

The medical history is an essential part of the diagnostic work-up and screening of osteoporosis in the general population. The medical history should include questions pertinent to bone mass maintenance and bone loss including the risk factors previously mentioned. Part of the medical history should also be a nutritional evaluation by dietary interview (recall method) to obtain adequate assessment of protein, calcium, phosphate, and vitamin D consumption, as well as coffee and

VELIMIR MATKOVIC ET AL.

TABLE 57–3. Diagnostic Approach and Screening Methods Available

Medical history	Dietary interview
Physical examination	
Anthropometry	Total height, sitting height, armspan, weight, nutritional anthropometry
CBC/urinalysis	
Blood chemistry	Ca, P, Ca^{++}, creatinine, albumin, electrolytes, 25(OH)D$_3$, 1,25(OH)$_2$D$_3$, PdTH, alkaline phosphatase, osteocalcin
Fasting urine test	Ca/creatinine, TmP/GFR
	Nephrogenous c′AMP
	OHPr/creatinine
24-hour urine	Ca, creatinine, OHPr, free cortisol
Metabolic studies	Calcium balance
	Calcium absorption
	Calcium skeletal kinetics
Bone mass measurements	X-ray, radiogrammetry
	Single-photon absorptiometry
	Dual-photon absorptiometry
	CT, neutron activation analysis
	UTV, bone scan
Bone biopsy and	Static histomorphometry
histomorphometry	Dynamic—tetracycline labeling

alcohol intake. Dietary history should be taken by a skilled nutritionist. Information about life style is essential as well.

PHYSICAL EXAMINATION

Physical examination is, again, very important for diagnosis. Previously described signs and symptoms of the disease should be looked for.

ANTHROPOMETRY

Basic anthropometry should include total height, sitting height, armspan, and body weight. Loss of height is one of the features of osteoporosis primarily due to compression fractures of the spine and kyphosis. The ratio of sitting height to total height is abnormal in the osteoporotic population. Sometimes elderly patients cannot recall their height of 20 to 30 years earlier; measurement of armspan (or of tibial length) could be of help in this regard. There is a good correlation between total height and armspan, as well as total height and tibial length. The discrepancy between the armspan and the current height could provide some estimate of the degree of height loss. This applies primarily when studying a group of people rather than when studying the dynamics of height loss in one individual. As weight has a protective effect on bone tissue, it will be highly unlikely to find obese patients with compression fractures secondary to generalized primary osteoporosis. Weight and height measurements are also important for

calculation of body surface area necessary for metabolic study.

BLOOD AND URINE CHEMISTRY

A complete blood count as well as urine analysis should be a part of the general screening. Low hemoglobin or anemia could be present in diseases that also affect the skeleton and are responsible for the development of secondary osteoporosis (multiple myeloma, sickle cell disease, and others). Examination of urinary sediment can indicate the presence of chronic renal diseases and kidney stones.

Blood chemistry should include measurements of plasma calcium, ionized calcium, serum phosphate, creatinine (renal function), albumin, and total protein as well as electrolytes and calcium-regulating hormones. Plasma calcium is usually normal in patients with primary involutional osteoporosis, and any abnormality in blood calcium could indicate the presence of some other metabolic bone disorder such as hyperparathyroidism (PHP), osteomalacia, metastatic bone disease, and others. If ionized calcium is not available, plasma calcium should be corrected per albumin or total protein.[99] Albumin not only is helpful for the evaluation of blood calcium but also can indicate malnutrition. Low albumin values were found in debilitated patients with hip fractures; such values suggest protein malnutrition. Serum phosphate is borderline high in postmenopausal women secondary to suppression of parathyroid function and increased tubular reabsorption of phosphate. Serum phosphate is low in patients with osteomalacia, primary hyperparathyroidism, and phosphate diabetes (vitamin D resistance). Serum creatinine is essential for baseline renal function but also for expression of various indices of tubular reabsorption of calcium, phosphate, and $c'AMP$. Determination of $25(OH)D_3$ could help in distinguishing patients with osteomalacia secondarily due to nutritional deficiency. Low $25(OH)D_3$ levels could be found in patients with hip fractures as well as in nursing home residents. Determination of $1,25(OH)_2D_3$ is not essential in routine clinical practice except when patients are part of the research protocols, a situation in which determination of this vitamin is essential. Determination of PTH could help in screening for primary hyperparathyroidism or in patients with mild secondary hyperparathyroidism. Another screening test for parathyroid bone disease could be the determination of nephrogenous $c'AMP$ based on blood and two-hour fasting urine measurements. The $c'AMP$ of renal origin is under parathyroid hormone influence and therefore serves as a biological marker of PTH activity on renal tubules as well as of maximum tubular reabsorption of phosphate (TmP/GFR).[100, 101]

Urine tests should include two-hour fasting urine tests (after 10 to 12 hours' overnight fast) as well as the collection of 24-hour urine for determination of calcium, creatinine, phosphate, sodium, and OHPr. Patients with osteoporosis usually have a normal excretion of calcium during 24 hours. Any type of hypocalciuria (less than 70 mg Ca per 24 hours) could indicate the presence of malabsorption and osteomalacia. Any hypercalciuria (greater than 300 mg Ca per 24 hours) could indicate the presence of excessive bone resorption secondary to destructive bone disease or hyperabsorptive state. Increased calcium creatinine ratio in fasting urine is usually high in patients with postmenopausal osteoporosis (type I) as well as in other conditions in which bone resorption is higher than normal. It serves also as a bone turnover index. When the calcium absorption process is completed, fasting urine tests reflect overnight changes in the skeleton and therefore indicate input of calcium from bone to extracellular fluid volume pool.[102]

BONE TURNOVER INDICES

Bone turnover indices are biochemical (noninvasive) markers of the bone remodeling process. Some markers indicate bone resorption (calcium/creatinine ratio in fasting urine; urinary OHPr, and potentially acid phosphatase of bone origin osteoclast-containing enzyme), and some indicate bone formation (bone alkaline phosphatase and osteocalcin, also called bone GLA protein or BGP). As bone resorption is coupled with bone formation, the indices of resorption highly correlate with indices of bone formation; therefore, both reflect bone turnover status.

Calcium/creatinine ratio reflects bone resorption after an overnight fast as previously explained. OHPr is a product of collagen metabolism. Urine collection requires a collagen-free diet. Values tend to be normal in osteoporotic patients (30 to 40 mg per 24 hours) or slightly elevated in fast bone-losers. Values are high during growth in patients with PHP, Paget's disease, and renal osteodystrophy. Alkaline phosphatase originates from osteoblasts and tends to be normal in patients with osteoporosis or slightly elevated when bone turnover increases (postmenopause, very elderly). If alkaline phosphatase is highly abnormal, indications will be acute fracture, Paget's disease, osteomalacia, renal osteodystrophy, or PHP. Bone alkaline phosphatase is heat labile and therefore can be distinguished from liver enzyme. If isoenzyme is not available, screening the liver function with gamma-GGT could help in the differentiation of the origin of total alkaline phosphatase (if elevated only). Alkaline phosphatase is also high during growth and declines after cessation of puberty, the same as excretion of OHPr in urine.

Osteocalcin is a protein that contains gammacarboxyglutamic acid. This is a calcium-binding vitamin K–dependent protein. BGP originates from bone cell synthesis rather than from bone matrix degradation and therefore reflects bone formation. It is elevated in postmenopausal osteoporosis with high bone turnover and generally follows the other markers.[103, 104]

METABOLIC STUDIES

Calcium balance technique, calcium kinetics, and calcium absorption are considered to be a part of the research protocol. They are very difficult to perform and cannot be applied in daily routines. The calcium balance technique requires the presence of a metabolic ward and sophisticated personnel. The technique measures calcium input and output from the body. A continuous fecal marker has to be used to correct calcium excretion into the stool.[105] The calcium balance is positive during

VELIMIR MATKOVIC ET AL.

bone modeling and is negative during the period of bone loss. Negative calcium balance of about 30 mg/day over 20 to 30 years could lead to osteoporosis Calcium kinetics uses radioactive calcium isotopes (^{47}Ca, ^{45}Ca) and can determine skeletal calcium dynamics or bone tissue remodeling.[106] The calcium absorption technique could be useful in studying patients with hypercalciuria and renal stones as well as in patients with all kinds of malabsorption including those with osteoporosis. The study can be done using either radioactive calcium isotopes (single or dual technique) or stable calcium isotopes (^{42}Ca, ^{44}Ca, ^{46}Ca, ^{48}Ca). This technique could also provide some data about bioavailability of calcium from different calcium sources in the gastrointestinal system.[107, 108]

BONE MASS MEASUREMENTS

There are currently several methods available to study skeletal pathological processes and bone mass. These range from classical skeletal radiology to new sophisticated techniques with excellent precision and accuracy suitable for mass screening of osteoporosis in the general population.

Skeletal Radiology and Radiogrammetry

Standard radiographs are available and essential for the establishment of the diagnosis of osteoporotic fractures of spine, wrist, hip, or other bones. However, these radiographs are insufficient for the study of bone loss and for determining the risk of fractures. At least 30 per cent of bone mineral has to be lost before changes are seen on classical bone radiographs.

To evaluate axial osteoporosis, lateral films of the thoracic and lumbar spine are needed. The shape and density of each vertebral body should be evaluated. Density grade is based on the comparison of density within the vertebral body with that of intervertebral space (disk space–soft tissue). If there is a significant difference between the density, this indicates that severe osteoporosis probably is not present. When there is no difference between density of the two compartments, bone loss is more significant. The first signs of trabecular bone loss within the vertebral body are loss of horizontal trabeculae and accentuation of vertical trabeculae, followed by accentuation of the terminal plates resulting from loss of intravertebral-trabecular architecture. Further bone loss leads to the changes in the shape of the vertebral body; such changes include biconcavity, wedging, and subsequent full compression (Fig. 57–25). It is normal for anterior vertebral height to be 10 to

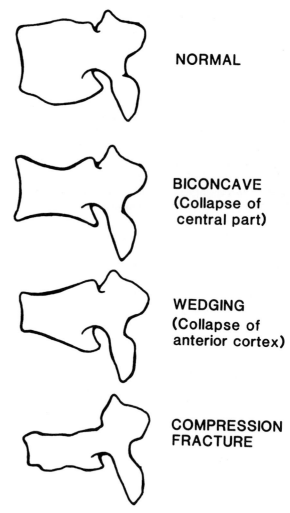

NORMAL

BICONCAVE (Collapse of central part)

WEDGING (Collapse of anterior cortex)

COMPRESSION FRACTURE

FIGURE 57–25. Abnormal shapes of vertebral body in spinal osteoporosis.

16 per cent less than posterior vertebral height. Therefore, if a wedge fracture is defined as a difference of 15 per cent, overdiagnosis of osteoporosis may result.

Examination of the trabecular pattern of the proximal femur, known as Singh's index, could help us in evaluation of the bone mass in that region. According to Wolff's law of tissue response to stress, trabecular bone loss in the femur (as well as in the vertebrae) precedes other changes. In maturity, there is almost no trabecular bone loss and thus no pattern can be distinguished. Ward's triangle is not visible. With aging, loss of trabeculae proceeds in the following manner: loss of horizontal trabeculae (intertrochanteric), loss of trabeculae that originate from the lateral femoral cortex, and subsequent loss of supporting trabeculae that originate from the medial femoral cortex (Fig. 57–26). Score 6 indicates good bone density and score 1 indicates osteoporotic hip bone. Measurement of the calcar femorale was used in the past to establish the degree of cortical bone loss in the hip (thickness of the medial cortex at the intersection with the intertrochanteric line).

Study of the cortical bone mass based on plain radiographs has been used extensively in the past. The technique is also known as radiogrammetry. Prior to the 1970s, radiogrammetry of the metacarpal bones was a dominant method in epidemiological studies of bone loss as well as in clinical trials. The technique involves x-ray study of the nondominant hand in the posteroanterior position. At the mid-point of the metacarpal bones, the width of the medullary (MW) canal as well as the total width (TW) has to be measured. From basic measurements, cortical area (CA), total area

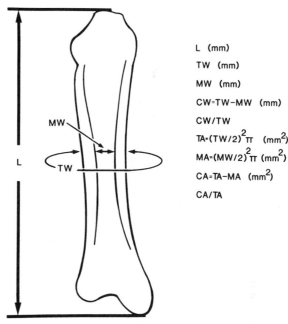

$$L \ (mm)$$
$$TW \ (mm)$$
$$MW \ (mm)$$
$$CW = TW - MW \ (mm)$$
$$CW/TW$$
$$TA = (TW/2)^2 \pi \ (mm^2)$$
$$MA = (MW/2)^2 \pi \ (mm^2)$$
$$CA = TA - MA \ (mm^2)$$
$$CA/TA$$

FIGURE 57–27. Radiogrammetry of the metacarpal bone.

(TA), and CA/TA ratio can be calculated (Fig. 57–27). CA represents bone mass, and CA/TA ratio represents bone density.[110] Density of the cortical bone mass correlates quite well with that of the forearm (based on single-photon absorptiometry) and the spine (based on dual-photon absorptiometry), and even with the whole-body calcium analysis.[111] Although the technique does not take into account intracortical porosity, it is noninvasive and reveals changes in the endosteal and periosteal envelopes with age. In the study of bone mass in children, hand radiographs are useful in determining the ratio of skeletal age to maturation.[112]

Hand radiographs may be helpful in the diagnosis of primary hyperparathyroidism. One of the main features of this disease is subperiosteal cortical bone resorption and intracortical porosity secondary to increased BMU number and size.

To rule out metastatic bone disease and multiple myeloma, x-rays of the spine, pelvis, hips, and skull should be screened for signs of localized bone resorption and increased bone sclerosis secondary to osteoclastic and osteoblastic metastatic changes. In multiple myeloma there may be bone resorption cavities without evidence of surrounding bone tissue formation (salt and pepper skull).

Radiographic examination is not used for mass screening for osteoporosis because it is not sufficiently sensitive and accurate. It is also rather

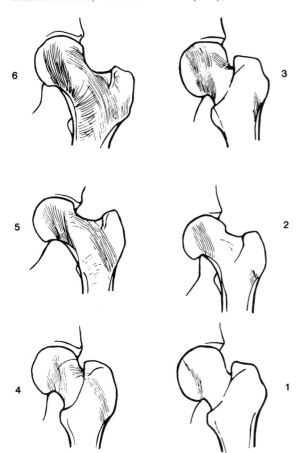

FIGURE 57–26. Trabecular pattern of proximal femur (six osteoporotic grades). (Adapted from Singh, M.: J. Bone Joint Surg., 52A:457–467, 1970.)

expensive and radiation exposure is quite high (10 to 300 mrem per study).

Single-Photon Absorptiometry

Single-photon absorptiometry (SPA) was discovered in 1960 by Cameron and Sorenson and, since then, has been used extensively to study bone loss.[113] The technique is based on the absorption of a collimated beam of photons in the skeleton. For that purpose, either ^{125}I or ^{261}Am has been used. The technique can determine bone mineral content or bone mineral density in grams per centimeter or square centimeter in the bones of the peripheral skeleton (forearm—proximal site with greater than 95 per cent cortical bone; distal site, 50 per cent cortical, 50 per cent trabecular bone; calcaneus—predominant trabecular bone). Mineral content in the forearm is relatively well correlated with the mineral content of the hip and the whole skeleton but is only moderately correlated with the amount of trabecular bone in the spine.

SPA satisfies almost all the criteria for the mass screening for osteoporosis in the population: sensitive enough, accurate, relatively inexpensive, and minimal radiation exposure (3 to 10 mrem). The weakness of this technique is that it measures bone mineral density at the forearm, which sometimes does not correlate quite as well with bone mineral density of the axial skeleton. In a patient with osteoporosis of the spine, it is necessary to measure bone density or bone mass in the spine. The machine that scans the forearm at different levels is probably more precise than are the other machines that have the ability to scan only at one site. Precision is 1 to 2 per cent, which allows relatively easy detection of postmenopausal bone loss.

Dual-Photon Absorptiometry

This method is similar to SPA except that it measures transmission of two separate photon energies through a medium of bone and soft tissue.[114] Gadolinium (^{153}Gd) serves as a source of photon energies. Dual-photon absorptiometry (DPA) allows measurements of bone mineral in the axial skeleton (L 1–L 4 of lumbar spine) and in the hips, and whole-body mineral analysis. Bone mass is usually expressed in terms of bone mineral content (grams) and bone mineral density in grams per centimeter or grams per square centimeter. The negative side of DPA is that it cannot distinguish bone mineral content of the vertebral body only, due to superimposition of the spinal transverse processes, osteophytes, and calcified aorta. Short-term precision of DPA with a spine phantom is about 1 to 2 per cent. Short-term precision of

DPA in humans, which includes variation due to subject positioning, moving during scan, a more difficult analysis, and instrument error, is between 2.6 and 3 per cent. Long-term precision is mostly affected by the source activity (age) and change of the isotope. Scanning the same phantom with different bone densitometers produced by independent manufacturers gives different values for bone mineral density up to 10 to 15 per cent; such measurements indicate difficulty in comparison of the results between centers.[115]

Recently, a new dual absorptiometry technique has been developed for the measurement of bone mineral density in the skeleton, dual-energy x-ray absorptiometry (DEXA). The principle is similar to gadolinium absorptiometry, but the advantage of this technique is that it requires shorter measurement time (5 to 15 minutes), provides better image detail, improves measurement precision (less than 1 per cent), and reduces radiation exposure (1 to 3 mrem) (Figs. 57–28 and 57–29). In addition, the technique eliminates the use of radioactive isotopes and solves licensing and disposal requirements. In the future, DEXA may replace gadolinium DPA as the procedure of choice for bone density measurement in osteoporosis screening. Two types of x-ray based systems are considered: *K-edge filtered system,* which operates at a fixed kilovoltage and uses filter materials having K-edges to create two peaks in their output spectra; and *switched-kV system,* which uses conventional filter material but alternates between two different kilovoltages for sequential dual-energy measurements. In the long run, this technique will be less costly because it will eliminate the cost of the gadolinium.[116, 117]

Indications for Bone Densitometry

The following are clinical justifications for measuring bone mineral density in the skeleton.

1. To screen postmenopausal women who are going to take estrogens.

2. To screen for low bone mass in persons with major risk factors.

3. To establish the diagnosis of osteoporosis in mild cases with minimal bone loss and some vertebral deformities.

4. To determine the severity of bone loss in newly diagnosed osteoporotic patients with vertebral fractures so that the most appropriate therapy can be selected.

5. To monitor efficiency of a new medication in a research trial.

6. To evaluate the degree of bone loss and the effect of treatment in other metabolic bone disor-

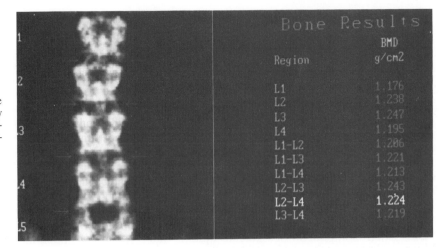

FIGURE 57–28. Scan of the spine obtained by the new dual x-ray absorptiometry machine. (Courtesy of Dr. R. Mazess, Lunar Corporation, Wisconsin.)

ders like osteomalacia, renal osteodystrophy, parathyroid bone disease, and others.[118]

Computed Tomography

Computed tomography of the spine is currently the only technique that allows the radiologist to record the density of the interior trabecular por-

tions of bones separately from their cortex. Computed tomographic scans are widely available but are more expensive and involve larger doses of radiation (over 200 to 1000 mrem); therefore, such scans are not convenient for mass screening in osteoporosis.

Neutron Activation Analysis

Bombardment of the entire body with neutrons transforms a small proportion of stable calcium isotope ^{48}Ca to a radioactive form, ^{49}Ca. The energy released by the decay of ^{49}Ca in the body is counted by whole-body scintillation counters, and this provides an estimate of the quantity of calcium in the body. Since about 99 per cent of calcium is in the bone, it is assumed that total body calcium accurately represents the total quantity of the skeletal mineral. Neutron activation analysis is useful for assessing the skeletal response to experimental therapies but is available only in a few research centers and is associated with substantial radiation exposure (2000 mrem); therefore, it is not practical for mass screening. The results of this technique correlate very well with the results of single-photon absorptiometry of the forearm and radiogrammetry as well.

Ultrasound Transmission Velocity

Depending on elastic modules, ultrasound transmission velocity (UTV) in bone is a function of both bone mass and intrinsic bone quality. In theory UTV provides more information about bone fragility than does the determination of bone mass alone. As a substantial number of osteoporotic patients overlap with nonfractured patients, the evaluation of bone quality could be of tremendous help; the use of ultrasound would be ideal in this regard. At this time UTV can only be meas-

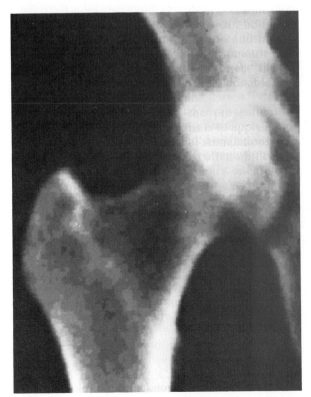

FIGURE 57–29. Scan of the hip obtained by the new dual x-ray absorptiometry machine. (Courtesy of Dr. R. Mazess, Lunar Corporation, Wisconsin.)

ured in bones without overlying soft tissue, such as patella or calcaneus. A recent study in which the patella was measured in patients with mild spinal osteoporosis (less than three fractures, anterior compression greater than 20 per cent) revealed that UTV was significantly more sensitive than were bone mineral content measurements of the spine using dual-photon absorptiometry.[119, 120]

Bone Scan

Technetium (^{99m}Tc) diphosphonate bone scan can be used to evaluate patients with osteoporosis. Bone scan is based on skeletal uptake of bone-seeking agent represented in diphosphonate labeled with ^{99m}Tc. Bone scan is dependent on vascular supply to the bone as well as to the nonvascular component of skeletal uptake and retention. Diphosphonate is absorbed to calcium phosphate crystals and is deposited in the zone of mineralization as well as along the resorption cavities of the bone. Diphosphonate is more likely to be adsorbed to the immature calcium phosphate crystals than to the mature calcium hydroxyapatite crystals.[121] A common indication to use bone scans in a patient with osteoporosis is to establish the age of the fracture. In acute compression fractures of the spine, the bone scan should be positive, but it will be negative in chronic cases. The bone scan can also pick up the small percentage of patients with hip fractures in whom the fracture line is not visible on plain films. Bone scan can also be used for the diagnosis of local osteoporosis such as migratory osteoporosis or reflex sympathetic dystrophy. The uptake in the involved extremity is increased secondary to increased blood flow but also due to retention in the bone tissue.

Bone Biopsy and Histomorphometry

A bone biopsy is an invasive procedure performed usually on the iliac crest for the purpose of analysis of bone tissue, bone cells, and bone turnover dynamics. A bone biopsy can be done as an outpatient procedure and is associated with minimal discomfort and risk to the patient.[122] Intact bone cylinder with cortical and trabecular part may be obtained from the ilium using a special bone biopsy trephine (Fig. 57–30). The specimen must be prestained in Villanueva osteochrome stain and then embedded in hard plastic (methyl methacrylate). The bone has to be cut in the undecalcified state with a heavy-duty microtome to preserve cellular and structural details. Only an experienced histomorphometrist can assess the structural and dynamic changes. It is believed that the iliac crest bone biopsy reveals the same pathophysiological changes found in the axial skeleton. Bone biopsy in osteoporotic patients reveals thin cortices and

reduction in the number of trabecular profiles (Figs. 57–31 and 57–32).

Before the biopsy, two separate courses of tetracycline are administered to the patient. Since tetracycline chelates amorphous calcium phosphate crystals, it is bound at the site of mineralization (active calcification) and can be detected by fluorescence under ultraviolet light. Patients usually take the tetracycline in a dose of 250 mg three times a day for three days, and then 11 days off with a repeated course for another three-day period. The bone biopsy is usually done after the fourth day from the last dose.[123] By measuring the distance between the two tetracycline labels, it is possible to calculate the mineral apposition rate, from which the bone formation rate can be derived (Figs. 57–33 and 57–34). Bone cells, resorption, and formation samples can be measured and create a basis of bone histomorphometry.

Histomorphometric analysis of the iliac crest bone biopsies suggests that postmenopausal osteoporosis is a heterogeneous disorder with a spectrum of bone-remodeling activity that ranges from accelerated to reduced bone turnover.[124] Some physicians consider bone biopsy to be a necessary part of the work-up so that therapy for the underlying disorder can be adjusted to the fundamental pathophysiological process.[125]

In general, bone biopsy should not be used to establish the diagnosis of osteoporosis. The indications for bone biopsy are to determine the presence of osteoporosis in a relatively young patient, to rule out osteomalacia or parathyroid bone disease, or to monitor the effect of treatment in a special research protocol (Figs. 57–35 and 57–36).

Prevention

Factors that can reduce the rate of postmenopausal bone loss or increase peak bone mass formation would be the ideal agents for the prevention of osteoporosis in the general population. Those agents are estrogens, adequate nutrition (calcium), and weight-bearing exercises. Elimination of risk factors that contribute to the incidence of falls among the elderly should also be considered as a part of the global prevention program for the reduction of the number of fractures in the population.

ESTROGENS

Estrogens can effectively treat symptoms associated with menopause, such as vasomotor flushes,

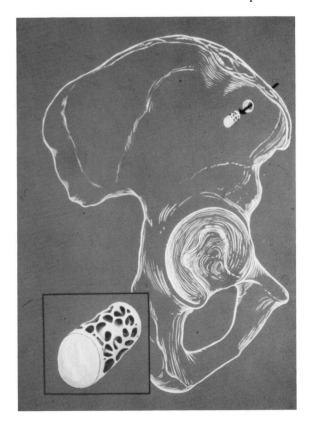

FIGURE 57–30. Transiliac crest bone biopsy. *Inset,* Cylinder and trabecular bone. (Courtesy of Dr. A. M. Parfitt, Bone and Mineral Metabolism Laboratory, Henry Ford Hospital, Detroit, Michigan.)

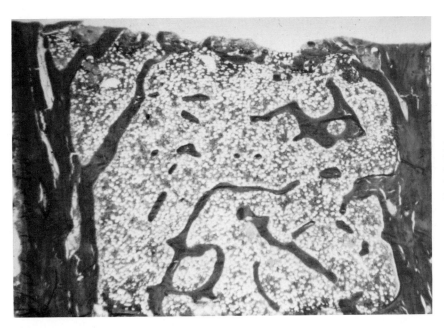

FIGURE 57–31. Section of bone biopsy specimen in a normal woman (Goldner stain). Notice thickness of the cortex and the number of trabeculae.

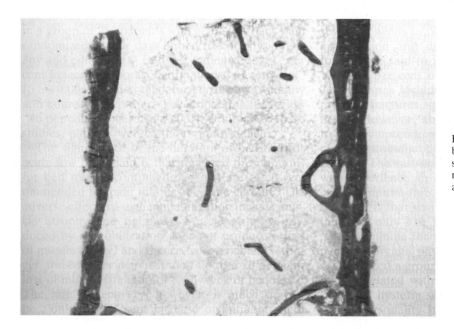

FIGURE 57–32. Section of bone biopsy specimen in a patient with severe spinal osteoporosis (Goldner stain). Notice thin cortices and absence of trabeculae.

FIGURE 57–33. Bone formation with osteoblasts (OBL), osteoid, and zone of mineralization (Villanueva osteochrome stain). Patient previously labeled with tetracycline.

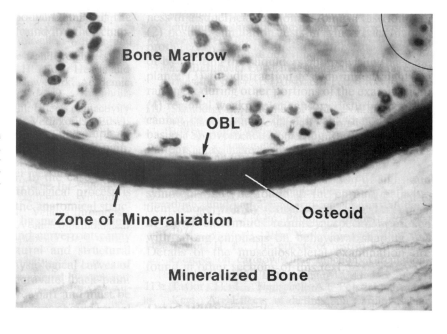

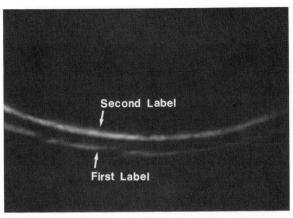

FIGURE 57–34. The same specimen as in Figure 57–33 under UV light. Notice first and second labels and the bone formed in-between labels over the three-week period.

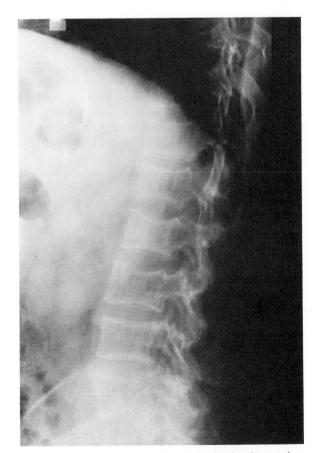

FIGURE 57–35. X-ray film of the lateral spine in a patient with severe osteomalacia secondary to phosphate diabetes. Signs typical of spinal osteoporosis. (From Massumi, M., et al.: Arch. Phys. Med. Rehabil., 68:615A, 1987.)

sweating, and dyspareunia. Estrogens are also effective agents in the prevention of postmenopausal bone loss. If treatment can be initiated early enough, estrogens can practically keep bone mass at the same level and prevent bone loss and the incidence of fractures later on.[66–68]

Guidelines for Estrogen Therapy

1. Estrogen therapy can be considered for the prevention of osteoporosis in women who are at high risk for developing the disease.

2. Low-dose estrogens can be used effectively to prevent bone loss (0.625 mg) during three weeks out of four. The fourth week, progestin (10 mg of medroxyprogesterone) could be added, which would reduce the incidence of cancer of the uterus.

3. Patients on estrogen therapy should undergo regular gynecological examinations annually, including mammography and breast examinations.

4. Estrogen therapy should be continued for at least 5 to 15 years beyond the onset of postmenopausal symptoms. If women have bilateral oophorectomy at an earlier age, they should continue treatment for a relatively longer period of time.[36]

The exact mechanism of estrogen action at the bone level is not completely known. The action does block bone resorption and improve calcium absorption in the gastrointestinal system. Estrogen receptors have been found recently in osteoblasts, but the meaning of this is still unknown.[126] Contraindications to estrogen use should be estrogen-dependent malignancy (breast cancer), thrombophlebitis and other disorders of increased coagulability, and certainly unexplained vaginal bleeding. Cancer of the uterus is the main risk associated with estrogen treatment. Estrogen increases the risk of endometrial cancer three to eight times. This increase in the incidence of cancer is diminished with cyclic or continuous progestin treatment. In addition to cancer prevention, progestins may have a beneficial effect on bone that is independent of estrogens.[127]

CALCIUM

Adequate calcium intake is certainly essential for bone growth and development. The recommended dietary allowances for calcium are 1200 mg/day for adolescents and for pregnant women, 1000 mg/day for children, and 800 mg/day for adults. Not only can adequate calcium intake contribute to peak bone mass formation with subsequent reduction in the incidence of osteoporosis in the population, but also the intake can partially suppress postmenopausal cortical bone loss. Adequate calcium intake in the postmenopausal period

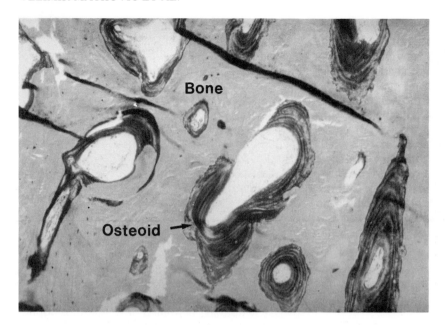

FIGURE 57–36. Bone biopsy from the patient presented in Figure 57–35 (Villanueva osteochrome stain). Notice wide osteoid seams as a result of mineralization defect secondary to osteomalacia. (From Massumi, M., et al.: Arch. Phys. Med. Rehabil., 68:615A, 1987.)

can also reduce the requirement for estrogen supplementation to a minimum of 0.325 mg. Calcium can be obtained either through natural dietary sources or from calcium supplements. The main dietary sources of calcium are milk and dairy products. One glass of milk (200 ml) has about 250 mg of calcium. The most common and least expensive calcium supplement is calcium carbonate, but probably the best bioavailability is from calcium citrate or calcium citrate-malate.[128] The bioavailability of calcium from calcium carbonate among elderly patients with achlorhydria is decreased.[129]

For most adults, cutaneous vitamin D synthesis mediated by sun exposure, as well as a balanced diet, can assure adequate vitamin D nutrition. There is no clear-cut evidence that vitamin D can either contribute to peak bone mass formation or effectively reduce the rate of bone loss; but without any question, adequate vitamin D intake is important for calcium absorption. Housebound or nutritionally deprived elderly people are particularly susceptible to vitamin D deficiency and may develop signs and symptoms of osteomalacia. The RDA for vitamin D is 400 IU per day.

EXERCISE

Weight-bearing exercise may increase bone density and strength during growth and maturation and reduce bone loss with advancing age. Accumulated data so far indicate that exercise over many years as judged by physiological parameters can contribute to greater bone density. Recent studies suggest that even relatively short-term (9 to 12 months) weight-bearing exercise programs may enhance vertebral bone density among elderly individuals. Until further information is available about type, duration, and frequency of weight-bearing exercise, walking (three to four times weekly) is a reasonable recommendation. Swimming does not satisfy weight-bearing requirements and may not have the same effect as walking or running.[130–134]

IMPROVEMENT OF ACTIVITIES OF DAILY LIVING (ADL)

In an attempt to prevent fractures, one must design measures that aim at the prevention of falls, which increase with aging. The main factors leading to the tendency to fall are decline in vision or hearing, generalized decrease in muscle strength and coordination, loss of balance, presence of multiple chronic diseases, common use of sedatives, or consumption of alcohol. There are also numerous environmental hazards that contribute to the tendency to fall. Increasing home safety, therefore, should be a part of the overall prevention program. The aim is to exclude all factors contributing to an unsafe home; and improvements include the following: provide optimal lighting, eliminate slippery floor surfaces, and ensure adequate hand supports in key home areas. Home visits by occupational therapists would be the most efficient way of initiating improvements in home safety among the geriatric population.

Treatment of Spinal Osteoporosis

SYMPTOMATIC MEASURES

Someone needing treatment for osteoporosis indicates that bone has been lost already to the point of developing fractures. Acute compression fracture in the spine creates pain that lasts about one to two weeks and sometimes requires bed rest. Plain analgesics on a regular schedule, as well as on a prn basis, could be initiated. Sometimes the application of local heat could be of help. A TENS unit might also help in the treatment of chronic back pain secondary to spinal osteoporosis of type II. After a two-week period, ambulation should be initiated if possible. In some cases, a thoracic orthosis (perhaps the rigid shell type) should be prescribed. The main reason for the application of a thoracic orthosis is to prevent further fracture by limiting motion in the spine. The period of time a patient should wear a spinal orthosis is still unknown. There is some evidence that spinal fracture can contribute to immobilization and that immobilization can further contribute to bone loss.[135] Therefore, back braces should not be prescribed for a long period of time. Lying on a flat surface for 30 minutes daily with a bath towel inserted below the lumbar spine would help correct kyphosis and the loin pain that is the result of severe kyphosis.

CALCITONIN

Calcitonin is a 32–amino acid protein produced by thyroid C cells. Several studies have demonstrated that calcitonin therapy decreases the rate of bone loss in osteoporotic patients. This was proved by DPA or SPA, as well as whole-body calcium analysis.[136] Calcitonin works through the inhibition of bone resorption. The main disadvantage of calcitonin treatment is that it has to be given parenterally (subcutaneously). The usual dose is 50 to 100 IU daily or every other day. Flushing and local irritation are common side effects.

SODIUM FLUORIDE

Sodium fluoride is the only agent known to increase bone mass. It stimulates bone formation independently of BMU function. In large doses sodium fluoride can cause an increased production of abnormal bone that has less torsional strength than normal bone. Widened osteoid seams and increased bone resorption are noticed. The dose should not exceed 75 mg/day, and calcium supplements should be given (500 mg Ca/day). The main side effects are nausea, gastrointestinal bleeding, and joint pains. The FDA still has not approved sodium fluoride for general use.[137]

ADFR THERAPY

In 1979, Frost proposed coherence, or ADFR, therapy for osteoporosis (A, activate; D, depress; F, free; R, repeat). The basic principle of treatment is the sequential and intermittent administration of drugs that will bring into synchronization the bone areas that are otherwise in random phases of bone turnover. According to the ADFR theory, the remodeling process is first pharmacologically (A) activated by an agent that initiates osteoclastic activity, then (D) depressed with a second agent, and finally followed by a period (F) free from treatment to allow osteoblasts to fill in the resorptive cavity. The cycle can then be (R) repeated according to life cycles of bone cell lines[138, 139] (Fig. 57–19). The agent used to activate BMUs is PTH (1–34 peptide) or oral phosphate as an indirect activator (secondary hyperparathyroidism). Etidronate disodium (diphosphonate) was used to suppress bone resorption. This treatment gave some excellent preliminary results in patients with spinal osteoporosis and seems to be very promising.[140, 141]

ANABOLIC STEROIDS

It was shown that anabolic steroids (stanazolol) can prevent bone loss or actually increase bone mass. Unfortunately they are associated with masculinization, with toxic liver effects if used orally, and with abnormality in lipid metabolism that can promote atherogenesis. The dose used was 2 mg three times daily for three weeks out of four.[142] They are not approved by the FDA for osteoporosis therapy.

Treatment of Hip Fractures

The main goal is to prevent hip fractures rather than to treat the disease. When a fracture develops, the most common methods of treatment are internal fixation or Austin-Moore hemiarthroplasty. Sometimes debilitated patients who are at high risk for surgery need bed rest and traction treatment, but they will be at high risk for developing pneumonia and pressure sores. The mortality in this group will be substantially higher; therefore, early operative management that increases mobility is widely practiced. After surgery, movement should begin relatively soon, when patients are almost recovered from anesthesia and all tubes and drains are removed. Complications of surgical procedures are non-union, avascular necrosis, and infection as well as failure of the device. Usually patients with hip fractures want to be able to enjoy quiet living, to be able to sit (90 per cent of hip flexion), to stand or walk (with some extension of the hips if possible), and to perform all kinds of ADLs including toileting (30 per cent abduction). A much greater range is desirable but not essential. Regarding muscle power, patients have to be encouraged to practice sitting, standing, or walking. The quadriceps, hamstrings, and gluteal muscle groups are therefore the most important to increase and maintain strength. Adequate nutrition support is also essential in the rehabilitation program. If osteomalacia is discovered, vitamin D therapy should be initiated. After implementation of the prospective payment system, the mean length of hospitalization for hip fracture patients fell from 17 to 10 days, and the mean number of physical therapy sessions received decreased substantially (4.9 to 1.7). Concomitantly, the proportion of patients discharged to nursing homes increased from 21 to 48 per cent. This increase in long-term nursing home placement suggests that the quality of care of elderly patients with hip fractures has deteriorated. This certainly interferes with the quality of life of the patients and is associated with substantial immobility.

Secondary Osteoporosis

There are many systemic and metabolic diseases that can cause bone loss in the whole skeleton (Table 57–4). These include Cushing's syndrome, hypogonadism, hyperthyroidism, and primary hyperparathyroidism. Hyperparathyroidism can cause excessive bone resorption and bone fractures, but currently with biochemical and other mass screening procedures (blood calcium), parathyroid bone disease is usually detected at a very early stage; bone fractures are uncommon. Also,

TABLE 57–4. Secondary Causes of Osteoporosis

Hormonal and metabolic disorders
Hypogonadism
Cushing's syndrome
Hyperthyroidism
Hyperparathyroidism
Homocystinuria
Connective tissue disorders
Osteogenesis imperfecta
Ehlers-Danlos syndrome
Diseases of bone marrow
Multiple myeloma
Lymphoproliferative diseases
Mastocytosis
Immobilization
Medications
Glucocorticoids
Thyroid hormone (excessive dose)
Long-term heparin therapy

it is very rare to see patients with hyperparathyroidism and compression fractures in the spine, because those patients primarily suffer from cortical bone loss.

Osteogenesis imperfecta of adult onset can sometimes mimic osteoporosis, but those patients tend to have more fractures and they are relatively younger. Some of them have clinical features of the disease such as blue sclerae. Multiple myeloma is a relatively common condition and has to be ruled out by performing protein electrophoresis.

The most common form of secondary osteoporosis is corticosteroid-induced osteoporosis. It has long been recognized that superphysiological doses of corticosteroids cause severe bone loss, which is more predominant in trabecular bone and metabolically more active than in the cortical bone. As a result, compression deformities of the vertebrae, as well as pelvic bones, are very common.[143] Corticosteroids will decrease bone formation rate by depressing osteoblast function but also will increase bone resorption manifested by an increase in osteoclast number and resorption sites. There is speculation that bone resorption activity is mediated by parathyroid hormone, because parathyroidectomy abolishes osteoclastic response to steroids in laboratory animals. Malabsorption of calcium is another feature of corticosteroid therapy. It can cause secondary hyperparathyroidism and potentiate negative calcium balance. The exact mechanism of this is still unknown, but some data suggest the steroids might directly impair vitamin D metabolism or synthesis of carrier protein responsible for calcium transport in the gut. Discontinued steroid therapy should be encouraged because recent animal studies suggest that alternate-day steroid application may produce less severe bone loss than daily treatments. The treatments also should be aimed to correct calcium malabsorption and partially to correct secondary hyperparathyroidism. The patient should take vitamin D, 50,000 units three times weekly, and 500 mg of calcium per day.[144] Recent clinical trials with a new heterocyclic glucocorticoid, deflazacort, revealed that this steroid contains systemic anti-inflammatory potency that is equivalent to prednisone with relatively less adverse effect on calcium metabolism. In recent clinical studies, deflazacort did not induce to the full extent the metabolic features of secondary hyperparathyroidism. The study suggested that the skeletal effects of prednisone therapy are mediated, at least in part, by increased parathyroid hormone activity and that the deflazacort is less potent in this regard.[145]

Osteoporosis Due to Immobilization

Complete immobilization of the whole body or of an extremity leads to osteoporosis, either generalized or local. Initially, this condition was described in patients who were immobilized for fractures, paraplegics, polio patients, and hemiplegics secondary to a cerebrovascular accident, and even normal individuals who volunteer to stay in bed for long periods of time. Bone loss can be detected by classical radiological methods within three months of the onset of immobilization. The affected bone never recovers completely, even after the full restoration of movement. Studies using newer techniques of bone mass measurements including single-photon absorptiometry, dual-photon absorptiometry of the spine, and histomorphometry of the iliac crest showed that the bone loss proceeds about 4 per cent per month during the initial phase of bed rest.[146] Non–weight-bearing bones such as the radius and bones of the hand demineralize at a much lower rate than do the weight-bearing parts of the skeleton. The same amount of bone loss (4 per cent) could be expected only in normal postmenopausal women and over the 12-month period.

Patients with diffuse osteoporosis secondary to immobilization could lose up to 30 or 40 per cent of their total bone over a relatively short period of time; this is almost the same as the loss in patients with primary involutional osteoporosis over a lifetime. After a substantial amount of bone

has been lost, the rate of bone loss subsides as in the osteoporosis of the aging. Subjects with high initial bone mass lose more bone than those who start with less bone so that all immobilized patients end up with much the same bone mass. PTHs have been implicated in the pathogenesis of bone resorption secondary to immobilization, but PTH activity is being suppressed during the phase of acute immobilization secondary to increased level of blood calcium in extracellular fluid.[147]

Histological examination reveals a predominant number of osteoclastic bone resorption sites. Bone trabeculae become thin, but by about the fifth week of immobilization the bone volume reaches a new steady state.

The main clinical presentation of bone loss due to immobilization is certainly the fracture. Bone that is osteoporotic from immobilization is more liable to fracture than is normal bone, and it is therefore common for a fracture that has been treated by immobilization to be complicated by further fractures of the same limb when immobilization ceases. Usually, an osteoporotic limb does not cause tenderness, pain, or any other symptom.

The abnormality in calcium metabolism is directly proportional to the amount of bone tissue immobilized. Or, speaking in terms of BMUs, the abnormality is directly proportional to a number of those units present at a time in the immobilized bone. Patients in whom one extremity is paralyzed usually do not develop hypercalciuria or hypercalcemia, but quadriplegic patients, in general, develop significant hypercalciuria and mild hypercalcemia. This is more pronounced in young patients who became paralyzed (during the bone modeling period) than among the elderly. Also, it is very well known that patients with Paget's disease of the bone will develop hypercalcemia upon bed rest for any reason. The main explanation for this is the number of activated BMUs present in the immobilized skeleton. Normally, up to two million BMUs are working at a time; this number is substantially higher in growing individuals and in patients with Paget's disease of the bone. After acute immobilization, particularly in young persons, urine calcium can rise for several weeks and may reach 600 to 800 mg/day before it returns to normal.[148] This hypercalciuria is not regularly reversed by mobilization of the patient. Plasma calcium is also rising, but malignant hypercalcemia is relatively rare (blood calcium of greater than 14 mg/100 ml). In the majority of patients, plasma calcium is within normal range or borderline high. Plasma phosphate tends to be high with evidence of increased tubular absorption of phosphate. This probably indicates PTH suppression secondary to elevation in blood calcium in spite of a belief that PTHs might be necessary for bone resorption. Immobilization could increase the sensitivity of bone to PTH action, but other local tissue factors might be involved.

Hypercalciuria could facilitate kidney stone formation; however, even in paraplegics the incidence of renal stones is not very high.[149] Kinetic studies reveal that during acute immobilization, the rate of bone resorption is two to three times higher than in normal individuals. Bone formation in this stage is also slightly elevated but cannot compensate for the rate of bone resorption; thus, there is a disbalance in coupling between bone formation and resorption. During the chronic phase, patients are in calcium equilibrium and resorption; formation rates are close to normal (Table 57–5).[150] This is also a time period when substantial amount of bone tissue has been lost and the rate of bone loss declines.

So far, there is no satisfactory treatment for this type of osteoporosis. High calcium intake certainly is contradictory in patients who develop hypercalcemia because this can aggravate the symptoms of elevated blood calcium and can further increase calcium excretion in the urine leading to kidney stone formation. Phosphate, diphosphonates, and thiazide diuretics have been given in the hope of reducing the bone loss resulting from bed rest.

Several of these have diminished hypercalciuria, but none has been shown to reduce bone loss as judged by photon absorptiometry.[151] Some studies indicated that passive movement on a tilting table could reduce urinary calcium, but other studies have suggested that active muscular action is required to counteract the resorption process.

Early rehabilitation of disabled individuals certainly might help in reversing the trend of bone loss and substantially decrease the incidence of osteoporosis in disabled individuals.

Localized Osteoporosis

Among the localized osteoporotic conditions, the most common are reflex sympathetic dystrophy—Sudeck's bone atrophy—and transient regional osteoporosis.

Reflex Sympathetic Dystrophy

Reflex sympathetic dystrophy is a clinical entity with numerous synonyms that all describe a disorder of either upper or lower extremity characterized by neuromuscular disturbances and dystrophic changes of the skin, subcutaneous tissues, bones, and joints. The disease is also known as the *shoulder-hand syndrome* or *post-traumatic osteoporosis*. The main clinical characteristics of this

TABLE 57–5. Calcium Balance and Kinetic Data in Acute and Chronic Immobilization, Compared with Normal Subjects

CASE	DIET Ca	FECAL Ca	URINE Ca (gm/day)	BALANCE	BONE FORMATION (gm/m²/day)	BONE RESORPTION (gm/m²/day)
ACUTE GROUP						
P.C.	0.260	0.370	0.327	−0.437	0.485	0.772
A.A.	0.518	0.660	0.285	−0.427	0.491	0.759
D.W.	0.233	0.322	0.236	−0.325	0.543	0.772
L.M.	0.913	0.931	0.303	−0.321	0.442	0.663
W.K.	0.602	0.605	0.446	−0.449	0.473	0.745
CHRONIC						
L.N.	0.419	0.329	0.064	+0.026	0.154	0.139
B.S.	0.359	0.212	0.131	+0.016	0.194	0.183
D.D.	0.337	0.247	0.067	+0.023	0.275	0.257
NORMAL SUBJECTS						
R.M.	0.846	0.741	0.100	+0.005	0.250	0.247
R.R.	0.233	0.180	0.117	+0.064	0.303	0.340
S.G.	0.628	0.449	0.105	+0.074	0.338	0.290
C.L.	1.125	0.965	0.196	−0.036	0.347	0.368

From Heaney, R. P.: Radiocalcium metabolism in disuse osteoporosis in man. Am. J. Med., 33:188–200, 1962.

condition are local pain and tenderness, swelling, decreased range of motion, increased redness and vasomotor instability, trophic skin changes, and localized osteoporosis. The disease usually goes through different stages. Stage I (acute form) lasts a few weeks to six months. The patients have pain, decreased range of motion, and redness in the involved extremity. The skin may be hyperesthetic and tender. At this point, we cannot see evidence for osteoporosis based on x-ray examination. Stage II follows and lasts another three to six months. The swelling decreases, but stiffness and decreased range of motion become more pronounced. Also, there is an atrophy of subcutaneous tissue and muscles. Early signs of contractures are seen as well. An x-ray examination usually shows localized patchy osteoporosis. In Stage III, which lasts for months and goes to irreversible alterations, the features are progressive atrophy of skin, muscle, bone, and joints. Pain may be decreased but there is a severe reduction in the range of motion. At this time, blood flow to the extremity is diminished, as is the skin temperature. Radiography shows diffuse osteoporosis with spotted decalcification.[152, 153]

ETIOLOGY

The majority of patients with reflex sympathetic dystrophy have had trauma as the initiating cause, cerebrovascular accident with hemiplegia, or myocardial infarction and cervical disk disease; in some cases, the disease could be without any underlying reason.

HISTOLOGY

During the stage of bone resorption and skeletal demineralization, increased numbers of osteoclasts can be seen lining the resorption holes.[154] This indicates that there might be bone resorption mediated by osteoclasts. The ultimate biochemical stimuli that trigger bone resorption certainly are not known. For almost one century, this condition has been attributed to the abnormality in sympathetic nerve discharge.

DIAGNOSIS

Diagnosis of reflex sympathetic dystrophy is usually made by clinical observation. A bone scan could be of help because it can show increased uptake in the involved extremity. For the hand, this means increased uptake in carpal and metacarpal joints. In the later stage of the disease and after three months, x-ray changes in the form of cortical subperiosteal resorption can be seen.

Bone density analysis using SPA also reveals a substantial amount of bone loss in hemiplegic patients.[155, 156]

TREATMENT

In the acute phase, the majority of patients respond to systemic corticosteroids. Usually, larger doses (up to 100 mg/day) are started and tapered over a 10-day to two-week period. Sometimes nonsteroidal anti-inflammatory agents or local application of heat can be of help. Recently a few European studies showed beneficial effects of intravenous diphosphonates as well as application of calcitonin treatment of more chronic bone atrophy.[157, 158] Intravenous diphosphonates probably block bone resorption by an adsorption to calcium phosphate crystals. Calcitonin blocks bone resorption and treats the pain secondary to endogenous secretion of endorphins in the brain.[159] Stellate ganglion blocks may also be helpful.

Transient Regional Osteoporosis

This is a relatively uncommon condition. The disease is characterized by localized migratory osteoporosis involving one of several joints with a predominance of hip involvement. The disease is usually self-limiting and lasts up to six to nine months. The diagnosis is based on clinical observations, x-ray changes, and increased radioisotope uptake on the bone scan. The diagnosis is also per exclusion. Conditions such as osteomyelitis, collagen disorders (rheumatoid arthritis), and cancer metastasis must be ruled out. The cause of this condition is not known. There is a possibility that this is also a form of reflex sympathetic dystrophy.[160]

Management of transient regional osteoporosis is determined by the severity of pain and disability, with the goal of maintaining some use of the involved part until the disease resolves spontaneously. Some patients respond to nonsteroidal anti-inflammatory agents or other pain medications. Use of oral corticosteroids has been rapidly effective in the majority of patients. Again, relatively large doses are started and tapered over a 7- to 10-day period. Physical therapy measures should be consistent with joint protection with slow initiation of gradual ambulation.[161]

References

1. Old age—a problem for society as a whole. WHO Chron., 28:487–494, 1974.

VELIMIR MATKOVIC ET AL.

2. Cummings, S. R., et al.: Bone mineral densitometry. Ann. Intern. Med., 107:932–936, 1987.

3. Nordin, B. E. C.: The definition and diagnosis of osteoporosis. Calcif. Tissue Int., 40:57–58, 1987.

4. Riggs, B. L., and Melton, L. F.: Involutional osteoporosis. N. Engl. J. Med., 314:1676–1677, 1986.

5. Nordin, B. E. C.: Clinical significance and pathogenesis of osteoporosis. Br. Med. J., 1:571–576, 1971.

6. Gershon-Cohen, J., Rechtman, A. M., Schraer, H., and Blumberg, N.: Asymptomatic fractures in osteoporotic spines of the aged. J.A.M.A., 153:625–627, 1953.

7. Iskrant, A. P., and Smith, R. W.: Osteoporosis in women 45 years and over related to subsequent fractures. Public Health Rep., 84:33–38, 1969.

8. Cummings, S. R., Kelsey, J. L., Nevitt, M. C., and O'Dowd, K. J.: Epidemiology of osteoporosis and osteoporotic fractures. Epidemiol. Rev., 7:178–208, 1985.

9. Alffram, P. A.: An epidemiologic study of cervical and trochanteric fractures of the femur in an urban population. Acta Orthop. Scand. [Suppl.]:65, 1964.

10. Matkovic, V., Ciganovic, M., Tominac, C., and Kostial, K.: Osteoporosis and epidemiology of fractures in Croatia. An international comparison. Henry Ford Hosp. Med. J., 28:116–126, 1980.

11. Cummings, S.: Are patients with hip fractures more osteoporotic? Am. J. Med., 78:487–494, 1985.

12. Nowton-John, H. F., and Morgan, D. B.: The loss of bone with age, osteoporosis and fractures. Clin. Orthop., 71:229–252, 1970.

13. Garn, S. M., Rohman, C. G., and Wagner, B.: Bone loss as a general phenomenon in man. Fed. Proc., 26:1729–1736, 1967.

14. Smith, D., Nancy, W., Won Kang, K., Christian, J., and Johnston, C.: Genetic factors in determining bone mass. J. Clin. Invest., 52:2800–2808, 1973.

15. Matkovic, V., and Chesnut, C.: Genetic factors and acquisition of bone mass. J. Bone Mineral Res., 2[Suppl.]:329A, 1987.

16. Trotter, M., and Hixon, B.: Sequential changes in weight, density, and percentage ash weight of human skeletons from an early fetal period through old age. Anat. Rec., 179:1–18, 1974.

17. Matkovic, V., Kostial, K., Simonovic, I., Brodarec, R., and Buzina, R.: Influence of calcium intake, age and sex on bone. Calcif. Tissue Res. [Suppl.], 22:393–396, 1977.

18. Matkovic, V., Kostial, K., Simonovic, I., Buzina, R., Brodarec, A., and Nordin, B. E. C.: Bone status and fracture rates in two regions of Yugoslavia. Am. J. Clin. Nutr., 32:540–549, 1979.

19. Mazess, R., and Cameron, J.: Skeletal growth in school children: Maturation and bone mass. Am. J. Phys. Anthropol., 35:399–403, 1971.

20. Christiansen, C., Rodbro, P., and Thoger Nielsen, C.: Bone mineral content and estimated total body calcium in normal children and adolescents. Scand. J. Clin. Lab. Invest., 35:507–510, 1975.

21. Tanner, J. M.: Growth at Adolescence. With a general consideration of the effects of hereditary and environmental factors upon growth and maturation from birth to maturity. Oxford, Blackwell Scientific Publications, 1962.

22. Ott, S., Murano, R., Lewellen, T. K., and Chesnut, C.: Total body calcium by neutron activation analysis in normals and osteoporotic populations: A discriminator of significant bone mass loss. J. Lab. Clin. Med., 102:637–645, 1983.

23. Aloia, J., Vaswani, A., Ellis, K., Yuen, K., and Cohn, S.: A model for involutional bone loss. J. Lab. Clin. Med., 106:630–637, 1985.

24. Gotfredsen, A., Hadberg, A., Nilas, L., and Christiansen, C.: Total body bone mineral in healthy adults. J. Lab. Clin. Med., 110:362–368, 1987.

25. Garn, S. M.: The earlier gain and later loss of cortical bone. In Nutritional Perspectives. Springfield, IL, Charles C Thomas, Publisher, 1970.

26. Mazess, R. B.: On aging bone loss. Clin. Orthop., 165:239–252, 1982.

27. Arnold, J. S.: Amount and quality of trabecular bone in osteoporotic vertebral fractures. Clin. Endocrinol. Metab., 2:221–238, 1973.

28. Weaver, J., and Chalmers, J.: Cancellous bone. Its strength and changes with aging and evaluation of some methods of measuring of its mineral content. I: Age changes in cancellous bone. J. Bone Joint Surg., 48A:289–298, 1966.

29. Riggs, B., Wahner, H., Dunn, W., Mazess, R., Offord, K., and Melton, L.: Differential changes in bone mineral density of the appendicular and axial skeleton with aging: Relationship to spinal osteoporosis. J. Clin. Invest., 67:328–335, 1981.

30. Meunier, P., Courpron, P., Edouard, C., Bernard, J., Bringuier, J., and Vignon, G.: Physiological senile involution and pathological rarefaction of bone. Quantitative and comparative histological data. Clin. Endocrinol. Metab., 2:239–256, 1973.

31. Leitch, I., and Aitken, F.: The estimation of calcium requirements: Reexamination. Nutr. Abstr. Rev., 29:393–411, 1959.

32. Matkovic, V., Fontana, D., Tominac, C., Lehmann, J. F., and Chesnut, C.: Influence of calcium on peak bone mass. A pilot study. J. Bone Mineral Res., 1 [Suppl.]:168A, 1986.

33. Matkovic, V., Dekanic, D., and Kostial, K.: Calcium, teenagers and osteoporosis. In Osteoporosis: Current Concepts. Report of the Seventh Ross Conference on Medical Research. Columbus, OH, Ross Laboratories, 1987, pp. 64–66.

34. Consensus Conference: Osteoporosis. J.A.M.A., 252:799–802, 1984.

35. Osteoporosis. Lancet, 2:833–835, 1987.

36. Peck, W. A., Riggs, L. B., Bell, N. H., Wallace, R. B., Johnston, C. C., Gordon, S. L., and Shulman, L. E.: Research directions in osteoporosis. Am. J. Med., 84:275–282, 1988.

37. Riggs, L. B., Wahner, H. W., Melton, L. J., Richelson, L. S., Judd, H. L., and Offord, K. P.: Rates of bone loss in the appendicular and axial skeletons of women. J. Clin. Invest., 77:1487–1491, 1986.

38. Heaney, R. P.: A unified concept of osteoporosis. Am. J. Med., 39:877–880, 1965.

39. Jasani, C., Nordin, B. E. C., Smith, D. A., and Swanson, I.: Spinal osteoporosis and the menopause. Proc. R. Soc. Med., 58:441–444, 1965.

40. Crilly, R. G., Francis, F. M., and Nordin, B. E. C.: Steroid hormones, aging and bone. Clin. Endocrinol. Metab., 10:115–139, 1981.

41. Albright, F.: Osteoporosis. Ann. Intern. Med., 27:861–882, 1947.

42. Delmas, P. D., Wahner, H. W., Mann, K. G., and Riggs, L. B.: Assessment of bone turnover in postmenopausal osteoporosis by measurement of serum bone glu-protein. J. Lab. Clin. Med., 102:470–476, 1983.

43. Heaney, R. P., Recker, R. R., and Saville, P. O.: Menopausal changes in calcium balance performance. J. Lab. Clin. Med., 92:953–963, 1978.

44. Christiansen, C., Riis, B. J., and Rodbro, P.: Prediction of rapid bone loss in postmenopausal women. Lancet, 1:1105–1108, 1987.

45. Frost, H. M.: Tetracycline based histological analysis of bone remodeling. Calcif. Tissue Res., 3:211–237, 1969.

46. Parfitt, A. M.: Quantum concept of bone remodeling and turnover: Implications for the pathogenesis of osteoporosis. Calcif. Tissue Int., 28:1–5, 1979.

47. Parfitt, A. M.: The action of parathyroid hormone on bone. Metabolism, 25:809–844, 1976.

48. Parfitt, A. M.: The cellular basis of bone remodeling: The quantum concept reexamined in light of recent advances in the cell biology of bone. Calcif. Tissue Int., 36:37, 1984.

49. Parfitt, A. M., Mathews, C., Rao, D., Frame, B., Kleerekoper, M., and Villanueva, A. R.: Impaired osteoblast function in metabolic bone disease. In DeLuca, H. F., Frost, H. M., Jee, W. S. S., Johnston, C. C., and Parfitt, A. M. (Eds.): Osteoporosis—Recent Advances in Pathogenesis and Treatment. Baltimore, University Park Press, 1981, pp. 321–330.

50. Arlot, M., Edouard, C., Meunier, P. J., Neer, R. M., and Reeve, J.: Impaired osteoblast function in osteoporosis: Comparison between calcium balance and dynamic histomorphometry. Br. Med. J., 289:517–520, 1984.

51. Parfitt, A. M.: Trabecular bone architecture in pathogenesis and prevention of fracture. Am. J. Med., 82:68–72, 1987.

52. Frost, H. M.: Mechanical microdamage, bone remodeling, and osteoporosis: A review. In DeLuca, H. E., Frost, H. M., Jee, W. S. S., et al. (Eds.): Osteoporosis: Recent Advances in Pathogenesis

and Treatment. Baltimore, University Park Press, 1981, pp. 185–190.

53. Frost, H. M.: Bone remodeling and its relationship to metabolic bone disease. Springfield, IL, Charles C Thomas, Publisher, 1973.

54. Pocock, N. A., Eisman, J. A., Hopper, J. L., Yeates, M. G., Sambrook, P. N., and Eberl, L.: Genetic determinants of bone mass in adults: A twin study. J. Clin. Invest., 80:706–710, 1987.

55. Christian, J. C., Slemenda, C., and Johnston, C. C.: Heritability of adult bone density and the loss of bone mass in aging male twins. J. Bone Mineral Res., 3[Suppl.]:587A, 1988.

56. Saville, P. D.: Observations on 80 women with osteoporotic spine fractures. In Barzel, U. (Ed.): Osteoporosis. New York, Grune & Stratton, 1970.

57. Seeman, E., Bach, L., and Cooper, M.: Bone mass in offspring of patients with osteoporosis. J. Bone Mineral Res., 3[Suppl.]:72A, 1988.

58. Bell, N. H., and Epstein, S.: Effects of body habitus and race on Vitamin D and mineral metabolism. In Osteoporosis: Current Concepts. Columbus, OH, Ross Laboratories, 1987, pp. 11–18.

59. Brown, W. T.: Human genetic models for aging research. In Kent, B., Butler, R., (Eds.): Human Aging Research. New York, Raven Press, 1988, pp. 163–183.

60. Johnell, O., and Nilsson, B. E.: Lifestyle and bone mineral mass in perimenopausal women. Calcif. Tissue Int., 36:354–356, 1984.

61. Drinkwater, B. L., Nilson, K., Chesnut, C. H., Bremner, W., Shainholtz, S., and Southworth, M. B.: Bone mineral content of amenorrheic and eumenorrheic athletes. N. Engl. J. Med., 311:277–281, 1984.

62. Jensen, J., Christiansen, C., and Rodbro, P.: Cigarette smoking, serum estrogens and bone loss during hormone replacement therapy early after menopause. N. Engl. J. Med., 313:973–975, 1985.

63. Goldsmith, W. F., and Johnston, J. O.: Bone mineral effects of oral contraceptives, pregnancy and lactation. J. Bone Joint Surg., 57A:657–668, 1975.

64. Weiss, N. S., Ure, C. L., Ballard, J. H., Williams, A. R., and Daling, J. R.: Decreased risk of fractures of the hip and lower forearm with postmenopausal use of oestrogen. N. Engl. J. Med., 303:1195–1198, 1980.

65. Hutchinson, T. A., Polansky, S. M., and Feinstein, A. R.: Postmenopausal oestrogens protect against fractures of hip and distal radius. Lancet, 2:705–709, 1979.

66. Meema, S., Bunker, J. L., and Meema, H. E.: Preventive effect of oestrogen on postmenopausal bone loss. Arch. Intern. Med., 135:1436–1440, 1975.

67. Lindsay, R., Hart, D. M., Forrest, C., and Baird, C.: Prevention of spinal osteoporosis in oophorectomised women. Lancet, 2:1151–1154, 1980.

68. Ettinger, B., Gennant, H. K., and Cann, C. E.:

Long term oestrogen replacement therapy prevents bone loss and fractures. Ann. Intern. Med., 102:319–324, 1985.

69. Walker, A. R. P., Richardson, B., and Walker, F.: The influence of numerous pregnancies and lactation on bone dimensions in South African Bowtu and Caucasian mothers. Clin. Sci., 42:189–193, 1972.

70. Matkovic, V.: Influence of age, sex and nutrition on bone loss. Ph.D. Thesis, University of Zagreb, 1976.

71. Nordin, B. E. C.: Osteoporosis, osteomalacia, and calcium deficiency. Clin. Orthop., 17:235, 1960.

72. Matkovic, V.: Influence of age, sex and nutrition on the bone of rats. Master of Science Thesis, University of Zagreb, 1974.

73. Sherman, H. C.: Calcium and phosphorus in foods and nutrition. New York, Columbia University Press, 1947.

74. Leighton, G., and Clark, M. L.: Milk consumption and growth of school children. Lancet, 1:40, 1929.

75. Garn, S., and Clark, D.: Nutrition, growth, development and maturation: Findings from the ten-state nutrition survey of 1968–1970. Pediatrics, 56:306–319, 1975.

76. Ashworth, A., and Millward, D.: Catch-up growth in children. Nutr. Rev., 44:157–175, 1986.

77. Chan, G., Hess, M., Hollis, J., and Book, L. S.: Bone mineral status in childhood accidental fractures. Am. J. Dis. Child., 138:569–570, 1984.

78. Matkovic, V., and Dekanic, D.: Developing strong bones—the teenage female. In Kleerekoper, M., Krane, S. (Eds.): Clinical Disorders of Bone and Mineral Metabolism. New York, Mary Ann Liebert Inc., 1989.

79. Sandler, R., Slemenda, C., LaPorte, R., Cauley, J., Schramm, M., Baresi, M., and Kriska, A. M.: Postmenopausal bone density and milk consumption in childhood and adolescence. Am. J. Clin. Nutr., 42:270–274, 1985.

80. Riis, B., Thomsen, K., and Christiansen, C.: Does calcium supplementation prevent postmenopausal bone loss? A double-blind, controlled study. N. Engl. J. Med., 316:173–177, 1987.

81. Burnell, J. M., Baylink, D. J., Chesnut, C., Mathews, M. W., and Teubner, E. J.: Bone matrix and mineral abnormalities in postmenopausal osteoporosis. Metabolism, 31:1113–1119, 1982.

82. Aaron, J. E., Gallagher, J. C., Anderson, J., and Nordin, B. E. C.: Frequency of osteomalacia and osteoporosis in fractures of the proximal femur. Lancet, 1:229–233, 1974.

83. Krook, L., Whalen, J. P., Lesser, G. V., and Lutwak, L.: Human periodontal disease and osteoporosis. Cornell Vet., 62:32–52, 1972.

84. Kim, Y., and Linkswiler, H.: Effect of level of protein intake on calcium metabolism and on parathyroid and reuse function in the adult human male. J. Nutr., 109:399–404, 1979.

85. Heaney, R. P., and Recker, R. R.: Effects of

nitrogen, phosphorus, and caffeine on calcium balance in women. J. Lab. Clin. Med., 99:46–55, 1982.

86. Saville, P. D.: Changes in bone mass with age and alcoholism. J. Bone Joint Surg., 47A:492–499, 1965.

87. DeVernejoul, M. C., Bielakoff, J., Herve, J., Gueris, J., Hott, M., Modorowski, D., Kuntz, D., Kuravet, L., and Ryckewaert, A.: Evidence for defective osteoblastic function. A role for alcohol and tobacco consumption in osteoporosis in middle age men. Clin. Orthop. Rel. Res., 179:107–115, 1983.

88. Dequeker, J., Goris, P., and Uytterhoeven, R.: Osteoporosis and osteoarthritis. J.A.M.A., 249:1448–1451, 1983.

89. Chalmers, J., and Ho, C. K.: Geographical variations in senile osteoporosis. J. Bone Joint Surg., 52B:667–675, 1970.

90. Dietrick, J. E., Whedon, G. D., and Shorr, E.: Effects of immobilization upon various metabolic and physiologic functions of normal men. Am. J. Med., 4:3–36, 1948.

91. Nilsson, B. E., and Westlin, N. E.: Bone density in athletes. Clin. Orthop., 77:179–182, 1971.

92. Dalen, N., and Olsson, K. E.: Bone mineral content and physical activity. Acta Orthop. Scand., 45:170–179, 1974.

93. Aloia, J. F., Cohn, S. H., Bab, T., et al.: Skeletal mass and bony composition in marathon runners. Metabolism, 27:1793–1796, 1978.

94. Kaplan, F. S.: Osteoporosis. Clinical Symposia. West Caldwell, New Jersey, Ciba-Geigy, Vol. 35, No. 5, 1983.

95. Bassett, C. A. L.: Biologic significance of piezoelectricity. Calcif. Tissue Res., 1:252–272, 1968.

96. Aloia, J. F., Ransulo, P., Deftos, L., Vaswani, A., and Yeh, K. J.: Exercise-induced hypercalcemia and the calciotropic hormones. J. Lab. Clin. Med., 106:229–232, 1985.

97. Sandler, R. B.: Muscle strength and skeletal competence: Implications for early prophylaxis. Calcif. Tissue Int., 42:281–283, 1988.

98. Astrom, J., Ahnquist, S., Beertema, J., and Jonsson, B.: Physical activity in women sustaining fracture of the neck of the femur. J. Bone Joint Surg., 69B:381–383, 1987.

99. Payne, R. B., Little, A. J., Williams, R. B., and Milner, J. R.: Interpretation of serum calcium in patients with abnormal serum proteins. Br. Med. J., 4:643–646, 1973.

100. Broadus, A., Mahaffey, J. E., Bartter, F. C., and Neer, R. M.: Nephrogenous cyclic AMP as a parathyroid function test. J. Clin. Invest., 60:771–783, 1977.

101. Bijvoet, O. L. M.: Kidney function in calcium and phosphate metabolism. In Avioli, L. V., and Krane, S. M. (Eds.): Metabolic Bone Disease, Vol. I. New York, Academic Press, 1977.

102. Nordin, B. E. C.: Assessment of calcium excretion

from the urinary calcium/creatinine ratio. Lancet, 2:368, 1959.

103. Price, P. A., Parthemore, J. G., and Deftos, L. J.: New biochemical marker for bone metabolism: Measurement by radioimmunoassay of bone GLA protein in the plasma of normal subjects and patients with bone disease. J. Clin. Invest., 66:878–883, 1980.

104. Brown, J. P., Malaval, L., Chapuy, M. C., et al.: Serum BGP: A specific marker for bone formation in postmenopausal osteoporosis. Lancet, 1:1091–1093, 1984.

105. Albright, F., and Reifenstein, E. C.: The parathyroid glands and metabolic bone disease. Baltimore, Williams & Wilkins, 1948.

106. Bauer, G. C. H., Carlsson, A., and Lindquist, B.: Evaluation of accretion, resorption and exchange reaction in skeleton. Kgl. Fysiograf. Sallskap. Lund. Forh., 25:1, 1955.

107. Heaney, R. P., and Recker, R. R.: Estimation of true calcium absorption. Ann. Intern. Med., 103:516–521, 1985.

108. Neer, R., Tully, G., Schatz, P., and Hnatowich, D. J.: Use of stable ^{48}Ca in the clinical measurement of intestinal calcium absorption. Calcif. Tissue Res., 26:5–11, 1978.

109. Davies, K. M., Recker, R. R., and Heaney, R. P.: A vertebral radiogrammetric standard. J. Bone Mineral Res., 3[Suppl.]:223A, 1988.

110. Barnett, E., and Nordin, B. E. C.: The radiological diagnosis of osteoporosis: A new approach. Clin. Radiol., 11:166–174, 1960.

111. Manzke, E., Chesnut, C. H., Wergedel, J. E., Baylink, D. J., and Nelp, W. B.: Relationship between local and total bone mass in osteoporosis. Metabolism, 24:605–615, 1975.

112. Greulich, W. W., and Pyle, S. I.: Radiographic Atlas of Skeletal Development of Hand and Wrist, 2nd Ed. Stanford, CA, Stanford University Press, 1949.

113. Cameron, J. R., and Sorenson, J. A.: Measurement of bone mineral in vivo. An improved method. Science, 142:230–232, 1963.

114. Mazess, R. B.: The noninvasive measurement of skeletal mass. In Peck, W. A. (Ed.): Bone and Mineral Research Annual 1. Amsterdam, Excerpta Medica, 1983, pp. 223–279.

115. Shipp, C. C., Berger, P. S., Deehr, M. S., and Dawson-Hughes, B.: Precision of dual photon absorptiometry. Calcif. Tissue Int., 42:287–292, 1988.

116. Sorenson, J. A., Hanson, J. A., and Mazess, R. B.: Precision and accuracy of dual energy x-ray absorptiometry. J. Bone Mineral Res., 3[Suppl.]:230A, 1988.

117. Stein, J. A., Waltham, M. A., Lazewatsdy, J. L., and Hochberg, A. M.: Dual energy x-ray bone densitometer incorporating an internal reference system. Radiology, 165P:313, 1987.

118. Riggs, L. B., and Wahner, H. W.: Editorials: Bone densitometry and clinical decision-making in osteoporosis. Ann. Intern. Med., 108:293–295, 1988.

119. Avioli, L. V., Brandenburger, G., Chesnut, C. H., Gallagher, J. C., Heaney, R. P., Lappe, J., and Recker, R. R.: Ultrasound transmission velocity in screening for bone fragility. J. Bone Mineral Res., 3[Suppl.]:588A, 1988.

120. Rubin, C. T., Pratt, G. W., Porter, A. L., Lanyon, L. E., and Poss, R.: Ultrasonic measurement of immobilization-induced osteopenia: An experimental study in sheep. Calcif. Tissue Int., 42:309–312, 1988.

121. Fogelman, I.: Bone Scanning in Clinical Practice. New York, Springer-Verlag, 1987.

122. Rao, S. D., Matkovic, V., and Duncan, H.: Transiliac bone biopsy. Complications and diagnostic value. Henry Ford Hosp. Med. J., 28:112–115, 1980.

123. Parfitt, A. M.: Personal communication, 1987.

124. Meunier, P. J., Sellami, S., Briancon, D., and Edouard, C.: Histological heterogeneity of apparently idiopathic osteoporosis. In DeLuca, H. F., Frost, H. M., and Jee, W. S. S. (Eds.): Osteoporosis: Recent Advances in Pathogenesis and Treatment. Baltimore, University Park Press, 1980, p. 321.

125. Kleerekoper, M., Frame, B., Villanueva, R. A., Oliver, I., Rao, D. S., Matkovic, V., and Parfitt, A. M.: Treatment of osteoporosis with sodium fluoride alternating with calcium and vitamin D. In DeLuca, H. F., Frost, H. M., Jee, W., Johnston, C., and Parfitt, A. M. (Eds.): Osteoporosis: Recent Advances in Pathogenesis and Treatment. Baltimore, University Park Press, 1981, pp. 441–448.

126. Eriksen, E. F., Berg, N. J., Graham, M. L., Mann, K. G., Spelsberg, T. C., and Riggs, B. L.: Evidence of estrogen receptors in human bone cells. J. Bone Mineral Res., 2[Suppl.]:238A, 1987.

127. Weinstein, M. C.: Estrogen use in postmenopausal women—costs, risks and benefits. N. Engl. J. Med., 303:308–316, 1980.

128. Nicar, M. J., and Pak, C. Y. C.: Calcium absorption from calcium carbonate and calcium citrate. J. Clin. Endocrinol. Metab., 61:391–393, 1985.

129. Recker, R. R.: Calcium absorption and achlorhydria. N. Engl. J. Med., 313:70–73, 1985.

130. Dalsky, G. P., Stocke, K. S., Ehsani, A. A., Slatopolsky, E., Lee, W. C., and Birge, S. J.: Weight bearing exercise training and lumbar spine bone mineral content in postmenopausal women. Ann. Intern. Med., 108:824–828, 1988.

131. Krolner, B., Toft, B., Pors Nielson, S., and Tondevold, E.: Physical exercise as prophylaxis against involutional vertebral bone loss: A controlled trial. Clin. Sci., 64:541–546, 1983.

132. Smith, E. L., and Raab, D. M.: Osteoporosis and physical activity. Acta Med. Scand., 711:149–156, 1984.

133. Aloia, J. F., Cohn, S. H., Ostuni, J. A., et al.:

Prevention of involutional bone loss by exercise. Ann. Intern. Med., 89:356–358, 1978.

134. Pocock, N. A., Eisman, J. A., Yeates, M. G., et al.: Physical fitness is a major determinant of femoral neck and lumbar spine bone mineral density. J. Clin. Invest., 78:618–621, 1986.

135. Heaney, R. P., Avioli, L. V., Chesnut, C. H., Recker, R. R., and Gallagher, J. C.: Is bone loss the cause of osteoporotic fracture or its consequence? J. Bone Mineral Res., 3:79A, 1988.

136. Gruber, H. E., Ivey, J. L., Baylink, D. J., Matthews, M., Nelp, E. B., Sisom, K., and Chesnut, C. H.: Long term calcitonin therapy in postmenopausal osteoporosis. Metabolism, 33:295–303, 1984.

137. Dambacher, M. A., Ittner, J., and Ruegsegger, P.: Long term fluoride therapy of postmenopausal osteoporosis. Bone, 7:199–205, 1986.

138. Frost, H. M.: Treatment of osteoporosis by manipulation of coherent bone cell populations. Clin. Orthop. Rel. Res., 143:227–244, 1979.

139. Frost, H. M.: Editorial: The ADFR concept revisited. Calcif. Tissue Int., 36:349–353, 1984.

140. Anderson, C., Cave, R. D. T., Crilly, R. G., et al.: Preliminary observations of a form of coherence therapy for osteoporosis. Calcif. Tissue Int., 36:341–343, 1984.

141. Miller, P. D., Neal, B. J., McIntyre, D. O., Yanover, M. J., and Kowalski, L.: The effect of cyclical ADFR therapy on axial bone density in postmenopausal osteoporotic women. J. Bone Mineral Res., 3[Suppl.]:378A, 1988.

142. Chesnut, C. H., Ivey, J. L., Gruber, H. E., et al.: Stanozolol in postmenopausal osteoporosis: Therapeutic efficacy and possible mechanism of action. Metabolism, 32:571–580, 1983.

143. Kleerekoper, M., Rao, D. S., Matkovic, V., Whythe, L., and Avioli, L.: Endogenous Cushing's disease in two adults presenting with osteoporosis as the major clinical manifestation. In Barzel, U. S. (Ed.): Osteoporosis II. New York, Grune & Stratton, 1979, p. 244.

144. Peck, W., et al.: Corticosteroids and bone. Calcif. Tissue Int., 36:4–7, 1984.

145. Gennari, C., Imbimbo, B., Montagnani, M., Bernim, M., Nardi, P., and Avioli, L. V.: Effects of prednisone and deflazacort on mineral metabolism and parathyroid hormone activity in humans. Calcif. Tissue Int., 36:245–252, 1984.

146. Anonymous: Osteoporosis and activity. Lancet, 2:1365–1366, 1983.

147. Donaldson, C. L., Hulley, S. B., Vogel, J. M., Houttmer, R. S., Bayers, J. H., and McMilan, E.: Effect of prolonged bed rest on bone mineral. Metabolism, 19:1071–1084, 1970.

148. Plum, F., and Dunning, M. F.: The effect of therapeutic mobilization on hypercalciuria following acute poliomyelitis. Arch. Intern. Med., 101:528–536, 1958.

149. Kohli, A., and Lamid, S.: Risk factors for renal stone formation in patients with spinal cord injury. Br. J. Urol., 58:588–591, 1986.

150. Heaney, R. P.: Radiocalcium metabolism in disuse osteoporosis in man. Am. J. Med., 33:188–200, 1962.

151. Lockwood, D. R., Vogel, J. M., Schneider, V. S., and Hulley, S. F.: The effect of the diphosphonate EHDP on bone metabolism during prolonged bed rest. J. Clin. Endocrinol. Metab., 41:533–561, 1975.

152. Escobar, P. L.: Reflex sympathetic dystrophy. Orthop. Rev., 15:41–46, 1986.

153. Plewes, L. W.: Sudeck's atrophy in the hand. J. Bone Joint Surg., 38B:195–203, 1956.

154. Lenggenhager, K.: Sudeck's osteodystrophy. Minn. Med., 54:967–972, 1971.

155. Bekerman, C., Genant, H. K., Hoffer, P. B., Korin, F., and Ginsberg, P.: Radionuclide imaging of the bones and joints of the hand. Radiology, 118:653–659, 1975.

156. Genant, H. K., Kozin, F., Bekerman, C., McCarthy, D. J., and Sims, J.: The reflex sympathetic dystrophy syndrome. Radiology, 117:21–32, 1975.

157. Nordin, B. E. C.: Personal communication, 1988.

158. Devogelaer, J. P., Dall'Armellino, S., Huaux, J. P., and Nagant deDeuxchaisnes, C.: Dramatic improvement of intractable reflex sympathetic dystrophy syndrome by intravenous infusions of the second generation bifosphonate APD. J. Bone Mineral Res., 3[Suppl.]:213A, 1988.

159. Gennari, C., Bocchi, L., Orso, C. A., Francini, G., Civitelli, R., and Maioli, E.: The analgesic effect of calcitonin in active Paget's disease of bone and in metastatic bone disease. Orthopaedics, 7:1449–1452, 1984.

160. Lakhampal, S., Ginsberg, W. W., Luthra, H., and Hunoler, G. G.: Transient regional osteoporosis. Ann. Intern. Med., 106:444–450, 1987.

161. Arnstein, R. A.: Regional osteoporosis. Orthop. Clin. North Am., 3:585–600, 1972.

58

Physiatric Rehabilitation and Maintenance of the Geriatric Patient

CHANG-ZERN HONG   JEROME S. TOBIS

There is a vast variability in the capacity of the elderly. Most of the elderly population (over the age of 65) live independently in the community without functional losses. Many of the presumed decremental changes seen with aging may result from underlying chronic diseases, such as those involving the musculoskeletal and cardiovascular systems, and may not be due to the intrinsic aging process itself. Chronic disease increases in frequency with age, with 80 per cent of the elderly having at least one chronic condition. But it does not follow that every older person suffers from disease processes. Aging itself is a relatively benign process that is compatible with independence in all physical activities when minimal chronic illness is present.

On the other hand, 45 per cent of those persons over the age of 65 have some limitation in the performance of activities of daily living, and of those over 85 years of age, 60 per cent show such limitations. Rehabilitation medicine seeks to reduce these limitations by improving the functional capacity of the elderly disabled person. Based on this principle, rehabilitation in the elderly population should emphasize "prevention through training" to preserve unimpaired functions and to restore those functions that are impaired.

Biology of Aging

As shown in Figure 58–1, many physiological functions gradually decrease after age 30. Much of the decrement in function may be related to de-

conditioning or disuse.[2] However, through appropriate training, the curve may shift upward (i.e., toward better function). The biological changes of each organ system[20] are listed in Table 58–1. Some of these changes are due to pathological processes or diseases rather than to aging itself. To epitomize this principle, it seems appropriate to relate the humorous adage of an elderly patient told by her physician that her right knee pain is due to aging. The patient protests this explanation with, "How about my left knee, which is the same age as my right knee but never hurts?"

Special Considerations in Care of the Elderly

The elderly patient is more likely to have pathological lesions in many organ systems. As a result,

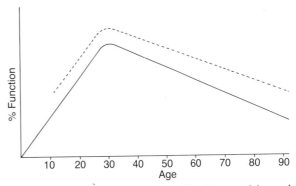

FIGURE 58–1. Deterioration of function in general in aged subjects (solid curve) and the influence of training (dotted curve).

1209

CHANG-ZERN HONG AND JEROME S. TOBIS

TABLE 58–1. Biological Changes Associated with Aging*

ORGAN SYSTEM	MORPHOLOGICAL CHANGES	PHYSIOLOGICAL CHANGES
Nervous System		
Brain	Cortical atrophy	Reaction time prolonged
	Nerve cell loss	Memory ↓ (especially short-term)
	Lipofuscion deposition	Cognition ↓
	Crystalloid is maintained	
	Fluid is ↓ slightly	Vision ↓, taste ↓, smell ↓
Peripheral Nerve	Myelin ↓	Conduction velocity ↓ (disease?)
Muscle	Size of muscle cells ↓	Strength ↓
	Interstitial fat and collagen	Endurance ↓
	Lipofuscion deposition	Speed ↓
Skeletal System		
Bone and Joints	Kyphosis	Postural changes
	Disk degeneration	Body height ↓
	Osteoarthritis (disease)	Range of motion ↓
	Osteoporosis	
Cardiovascular System		
Heart	Myocardial hypertrophy	Cardiac output ↓ (disease)
	Coronary arteriosclerosis (disease)	Coronary blood flow ↓
	Stiffness of heart valve	
Blood Vessels	Stiffness of vessel wall	Peripheral resistance ↑
	Elastocalcinosis	Blood pressure ↑ (disease)
Respiratory System		
Chest Wall	Deformity (kyphosis)	Compliance of chest wall ↓
	Calcification of cartilage	
Lungs	Number of alveoli ↓	Maximal breathing capacity ↓
	Dilatation of bronchioles	Emphysema (disease)
	Elasticity ↓	
	Parenchyma ↓	
Gastrointestinal System		
Teeth	Loosening	Soft diet required
	Alveolar atrophy	
Stomach	Atrophy	Reduced motility and secretion
Intestine	Atrophy	Reduced motility and secretion
Liver	Size reduced	No change in liver function
Pancreas	Fat content ↑	Volume and concentration of
	Functional tissue ↓	enzymes ↓
Excretory System		
Kidney	Atrophy of the glomeruli	Glomerular filtration rate ↓
	Renal tubular cell mass ↓	Tubular function ↓
Endocrine System		
Sex hormones	Estrogen ↓	Infertility in female
	Androgen ↓ (?)	Loss of tumescence in male
Pituitary	Weight ↓	
	Follicle-stimulating hormone ↑	

*It is difficult to differentiate how much of each change is solely the result of aging and what contribution is due to disease.
(↓ = Decreased; ↑ = increased.)

the rehabilitation program for a specific functional disability may be complicated by several concurrent medical problems. Thus, for example, the elderly stroke victim may not only suffer from cerebrovascular disease but also may have osteoarthritis, coronary heart disease, and peripheral vascular disease. The physiatrist concerned with the elderly patient should take all health factors into account in developing a rehabilitation plan for the individual patient. With the multiplicity of organ systems involved, an interdisciplinary approach is highly recommended. The team conference should involve as many professional disciplines as required. However, in many rehabilitation settings, not all disciplines may be available, such as a vocational counselor, a dentist, or a dietitian. The physiatrist then must take the responsibility to coordinate the whole rehabilitation management program by contacting the other professionals as indicated.

It must be anticipated that the elderly patient has functional limitations and a margin of safety narrower than that of younger adults. In many situations, one may not expect recovery of full function in the elderly. Occasionally, maintenance of the remaining function may be more realistic than achieving the functional status the patient enjoyed before the onset of the disability, since the potential physical capacity may be markedly limited. For example, the elderly stroke victim with cardiac failure may become ambulatory but will be restricted in the distance he or she can walk or the cadence achieved.

The quality of life during the period of survival is a primary concern of the physiatrist. Some elderly disabled patients may have limited functional reserve, which limits the goal that may be achieved through the rehabilitation program. For such patients, the realistic goal should include improving the quality of life. A bedridden, chronically ill elderly patient may become socially isolated, leading to depression and withdrawal from social contact. On the other hand, a geriatric patient may become more active socially after a short course of rehabilitation. An effective rehabilitation program helps these patients to live a more independent and socially involved life.

Comprehensive rehabilitation is cost efficient as well as effective in improving the quality of life. The expense entailed in prolonged nursing home or home health care may far exceed the cost of an effective inpatient rehabilitation program. Even in the narrow domain of fiscal considerations, the provision of a rehabilitation program that enables an elderly patient to live independently at home rather than staying in a nursing home may result in significant savings for the patient and the institution.

The geriatric patient may be expected to suffer impairments of cognition, emotional stability, confusion, and loneliness. In the very elderly, impairment in short-term memory and reduced learning capacity and attention span may result in the patient's being labeled as "hard to train." However, after the rehabilitation team evaluates the patient carefully and designs the program appropriately, a rehabilitation program can usually be carried out within these limitations. For example, one should try to avoid introducing any complicated task that is new to the patient. Whenever feasible, activities should be those that previously were familiar to the patient. The instructions must be clear and concise. Repetition may be required for reinforcement to make certain the desired activity becomes an established behavior pattern. There is a high incidence of depression and anxiety in the disabled elderly population, retarding the rehabilitation process. The rehabilitation psychologist may play an important role in helping such patients develop behavior-supporting programs. Antidepressant medication may be warranted for some patients, in which case consultation with a geropsychiatrist may be desirable. Some elderly patients may experience confusion and not be able to adjust readily to the unfamiliar fast-changing hospital environment. The staff must be sensitive to these factors and facilitate the adjustment of the patient. The orientation program for each patient by the staff may require repeated training regarding the hospital environment, reintroduction to staff members, and discussion of local and general events to help each patient re-establish and maintain his or her orientation.[29] Due to limited mobility and lack of close relatives, the elderly patient may suffer from social isolation. The lonely geriatric patient should be encouraged to participate in social activities. A strong social support system is invaluable for successful rehabilitation of the elderly.

Physiological Changes in the Elderly

The decrease in muscle strength, endurance, and speed seen in the aging process has been shown to be due to a corresponding decrease in both the size and the number of muscle fibers, especially the type II fibers (fast fibers),[10, 14, 26] a decrease in muscle enzyme activities,[8, 9, 13, 25, 30] and also disturbances of the neuromuscular junction.[6, 11, 12] Based on these changes alone, one may anticipate that the trainability of older individuals declines in old age. However, this is not supported in some recent studies. Moritani and deVries found that there was a significant increase in the maximal voluntary strength of the older subjects with exercise that was comparable to that of the young, when expressed as a percentage change with respect to the initial strength.[16, 17] Therefore, they concluded that the trainability of muscle function of the older subject does not differ greatly from that of young people. The biological changes seen in skeletal muscles of older individuals, as mentioned above, may be due to inactivity rather than to the aging process, since one can see similar changes in disuse resulting from immobilization.[15, 18]

In studies of the nervous system, it was found that the changes seen in the elderly on the electroencephalogram, such as slowing of the dominant frequency, were similar to those seen as the result of inactivity[2, 33, 35] probably owing to prolonged sensory and perceptual deprivation. An exercise program prevented these abnormalities on the electroencephalogram.[34] Other similar neurological functional changes that occur in both the aging process and inactivity include increased auditory threshold, decreased taste sensitivity, alterations in behavior, and depression.[2] Recently, Dustman and co-workers demonstrated that older individuals who were trained with aerobic exercise for four months had significantly greater improvement in a neuropsychological test battery than did controls.[7] Vogt and Vogt found that an exercise program was also capable of delaying the involutional changes of the spinal cord and the peripheral nerves.[31]

Physical activity is important to stimulate bone metabolism to maintain the skeletal system.[1, 22, 24] The density of bone is positively related to physical activity. Immobilization leads to excessive loss of mineral content of the skeleton. The high incidence of osteoporosis in the geriatric population is probably due, in part, to inadequate activity, since physical exercise effectively increases the bone mineral content in the elderly.[22]

In the cardiopulmonary system, left ventricular function and, therefore, stroke volume decrease with age and inactivity and increase with exercise.[2, 21] Since the heart rate also declines with age, the maximal cardiac output and the cardiac output at each level of work also decrease with age and inactivity. A program of physical activity reduces the decline of aerobic capacity (maximal oxygen consumption) in the aging process due to less decline in maximal cardiac output.[4, 5] The total peripheral resistance increases with age and weightlessness (similar to inactivity) and, thus, blood pressure shows similar changes.[2] It is reported that long-term exercise training may reduce blood pressure in hypertensive subjects but not in normotensive individuals.[27]

From studies of hormonal regulation in the aged, it has been claimed that poor glucose tolerance occurs with aging and inactivity.[2] The degree of this abnormality is proportional to the degree of immobilization. Exercise ameliorates this finding. This reversal is probably related to an increase of insulin-binding sites and, thus, an increase of insulin sensitivity seen after a period of physical training.[23] Decreased activity of the sympathomedullary axis was found in aged and inactive individuals.[2] This may affect the alertness and behavior of elderly individuals. Exercise may increase the activity of the sympathomedullary axis. The effects of aging, inactivity, and exercise on the regulation of sex hormones have not been well studied. Briggs and associates found that ambulatory men had a higher level of mean serum androgen than did immobilized men.[3]

Based on the analyses mentioned above, the functional deterioration in the elderly is presumed to be at least partly due to inactivity. Therefore, physical exercise becomes an important therapeutic approach to improve general function in the elderly disabled person.

Therapeutic Exercise for the Elderly Disabled

Therapeutic exercises may be prescribed in a variety of ways and for various purposes. Submaximal aerobic exercise, without the anaerobic component seen in maximal exercise to tolerance, is the appropriate type of exercise for elderly subjects because of their limited cardiopulmonary fitness. The submaximal exercise loads can be judged more accurately by determining how far the patient is from his or her maximum.[32] In exercise exceeding aerobic capacity, the exercise accumulation of lactate may cause the patient to feel too exhausted to exercise further so that a training effect cannot be achieved. Static (isometric) exercise may cause significant hypertension that overloads the cardiovascular system.[19, 32] Therefore, dynamic exercise (either isotonic or isokinetic) is preferred for the elderly patient.

Interval training, consisting of a physical conditioning program of short exercise periods alternated with regular rest pauses, has been advocated by most cardiologists as part of the training for cardiac patients. We found this to be applicable to geriatric patients in general. Intermittent exercise prevents a high serum lactate level throughout the exercise period and, thus, is more tolerable to the geriatric patient than is continuous physical activity. For general conditioning exercises, it is desirable to have all muscle groups involved in activity in order to improve the general fitness level. Elderly patients should be involved in such activity on a regular basis as their capacity permits.

An elderly disabled person may be encouraged to continue an exercise program on a regular basis after being discharged from hospital care. The therapist plays a role in helping the patient to organize the program for the home setting in a practical manner. For example, ambulation in parallel bars can be achieved by placing two sets of chairs back-to-back with a three-foot space between (Fig. 58–2). For ease in learning, remembering, and performance, complicated activities

should be avoided for the elderly disabled patient. This is particularly important for a home exercise program. For example, most functional activities of daily living are already familiar to the elderly disabled patient and, thus, are easy to understand and are practical to include as a form of exercise to improve motor function. Designation of a measurable quantity of exercise is desirable, with progression to a greater amount as the patient improves. When functional activities are prescribed, the intensity level of the activity is not as critical to the assessment as the duration or frequency of the activity. For example, the number of step-up exercises on a stair or stand-up exercises from a chair may be recorded.

Until recently, most athletes and their coaches have believed that warm-up and cool-down exercises are essential for avoiding athletic injury. The scientific basis for that principle is still obscure. The long-held opinion that muscles are likely to be injured until the temperature of the muscle has increased is clearly not true. It is more likely that after a period of inactivity, light exercise re-establishes neuromuscular coordination and then muscle and connective tissue tears are not caused by errors in performance. At the end of the exercise period,

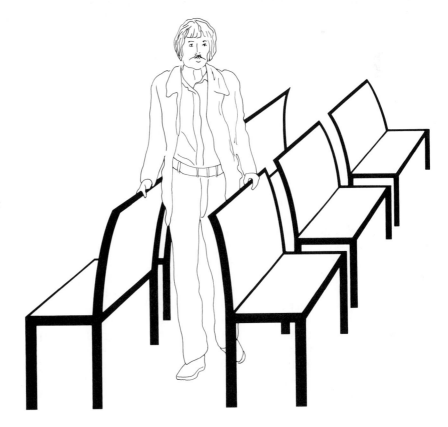

FIGURE 58–2. Home setting for the practice of ambulation.

CHANG-ZERN HONG AND JEROME S. TOBIS

light activity that is continued for a few minutes maintains intramuscular circulation at a level that aids in the removal of metabolites produced by the exercise.

Involving a debilitated elderly person in a rehabilitation program entails risks, such as the possibility either of an accidental fall that results in a fracture or of excessive strain on an impaired cardiovascular system. However, in most cases, the risks are warranted, since the alternative is debilitation; immobilization with the sequelae of depression, osteoporosis, and decubiti; and decline. However, the elderly patient requires close supervision during physical activity training to avoid undue risk.

Prescription of Physical Medicine Modalities for the Elderly Patient

Some physical medicine modalities are very useful for geriatric patients. However, they should be prescribed carefully, with special consideration of particular problems in this age group. Thermotherapy is indicated for soft tissue lesions, such as a sprain, a strain, bursitis, myofascial pain syndrome, fibromyalgia, chronic arthritis, or pain and stiffness occurring after surgery. Some aged patients have reduced thermal sensation, and precautions should be taken to avoid blisters or burns that may occur on the lower extremities in the presence of peripheral neuropathy. Geriatric patients who have cardiovascular disease or renal failure may have an exacerbation of their problems if vigorous heat therapy is used. Patients may have a coagulopathy or other blood dyscrasia and may develop bleeding if the heat is applied over a hemorrhagic site. Patients with malignancy have at least the hypothetical risk of spread of the malignant cells if heat is applied directly over the area containing a malignant growth. The patient with a nonlocalized infection may be at risk of developing bacteremia or septicemia if the heat is applied directly over the site of infection. On the other hand, heat is an excellent way to facilitate the drainage of an abscess or a boil. Heat applied to an ischemic area in the case of peripheral vascular disease may precipitate gangrene if the rise in local metabolism exceeds the concomitant increase in local blood flow and oxygenation of local tissue.

Special precautions must be taken with the patient suffering from dementia or a disturbance of consciousness and who is not able to feel pain from overheating and may suffer a burn.

Hydrotherapy at a moderate temperature of 39.0 to 41.2° C (102 to 106° F) is indicated for joint contracture or stiffness; systemic or local chronic arthritis; soft tissue lesions involving large areas of the limbs or trunk such as sprains, strains, or burns; postoperative stiffness and pain; and chronic ulcers.

Geriatric patients who have an open infected wound or an acute dermatological lesion require appropriate management to prevent nosocomial infections. In using generalized heat therapy (Hubbard tank), precautions must be taken against overheating any patients who have impaired cardiac function or adrenal insufficiency. If the patient has an ostomy, the stoma should be shielded for sanitary reasons before submersion in the whirlpool or Hubbard tank.

Electrotherapy may be indicated to obtund pain by transcutaneous electrical nerve stimulation, to improve motor function, as with biofeedback techniques used in hemiplegia, or to prevent atrophy in peripheral neuropathy. Patients with sensory impairment may not perceive the intensity of the stimulation and may develop burns owing to poor electrode contact on the skin or a current of excessive intensity. If the patient has a pacemaker, application of electrodes near the heart should be avoided.

Massage is indicated to relieve edema, pain, and swelling of soft tissue lesions and to reduce scars and adhesions. If a patient has deep vein thrombosis or acute thrombophlebitis, massage over that area may induce an embolus. Massage should be avoided over localized infections or malignant lesions to prevent the breakdown of local tissue and lymphatic barriers, resulting in the spread of the lesion.

Traction and manipulation may be effective in restoring motion or relieving pain of spondylosis, degenerative joint disease, or soft tissue scars or contractures. Spinal manipulation may be hazardous for patients with spondylosis with osteophytes impinging on nerve roots or directly on the cord. If the vertebrae are osteoporotic, traction or manipulation requires special care. Geriatric patients have a high incidence of carotid arteriosclerosis or atherosclerosis, and sudden forceful manipulation may induce carotid artery insufficiency or the spread of emboli into the cerebral circulation.

The rehabilitation program for each specific problem in the elderly patient is based on the same general principles as the rehabilitation for a specific disorder, such as hemiplegia, paraplegia, fracture, arthritis, or amputation, which have been described in other chapters in this book. Geriatric patients are likely to have multiple problems, which make rehabilitation in these cases more complicated than that for younger patients. In the assessment of the elderly patient, in addition to the traditional testing of self-care activities, emphasis should be placed on instrumental activities of daily living, which include skills that are necessary for the patient to remain independent in community living: the ability to travel, to shop, to use money appropriately, and, of course, to communicate effectively. Comprehensive assessment followed by coordinated management and use of the members of the rehabilitation team as necessary results in the restoration and preservation of a high quality of life for geriatric patients until they reach far advanced old age.

References

1. Aloia, J. F.: Exercise and skeletal health. J. Am. Geriatr. Soc., 29:104–107, 1981.
2. Bortz, W. M.: Disuse and aging. J.A.M.A., 248:1203–1208, 1982.
3. Briggs, M. H., Garcia-Webb, P., and Scheung, T.: Androgen and exercise. Br. Med. J., 3:49–50, 1973.
4. Dehn, M., and Bruce, R.: Longitudinal variations in maximal oxygen intake with age and activity. J. Appl. Physiol., 33:805–807, 1972.
5. DeVries, H.: Physiological effects of an exercise training regimen upon men aged 52–58. J. Gerontol., 25:325–336, 1962.
6. Drahota, Z., and Guttman, E.: The effect of age on compensatory and "post-functional hypertrophy" in cross-striated muscle. Gerontology, 6:81–90, 1962.
7. Dustman, R. E., Ruhling, R. O., Russell, E. M., Shearer, D. E., Bonekat, H. W., Shigeoka, J. W., Wood, J. S., and Bradford, D. C.: Aerobic exercise training and improved neuropsychological function of older individuals. Neurobiol. Aging, 5:35–42, 1967.
8. Ermini, M.: Aging changes in mammalian skeletal muscle. Gerontology, 22:301–316, 1976.
9. Ermini, M., and Verzar, F.: Decreased restitution of certain phosphate in white and red skeletal muscles during aging. Experimentia, 24:902–903, 1967.
10. Guttmann, E., and Hanzlikova, V.: Motor unit in old age. Nature, 209:921–922, 1966.
11. Guttmann, E., Hanzlikova, V., and Jakoubek, B.: Changes in the neuromuscular system during old age. Exp. Geront., 3:141–146, 1968.
12. Guttmann, E., Hanzlikova, V., and Vyskocil, F.: Age changes in cross-striated muscle of the rat. J. Physiol., 219:331–343, 1971.
13. Guttmann, E., and Syrovy, I.: Contraction properties and myosin-ATPase activity of fast and slow senile muscles. Gerontologia, 20:239–244, 1974
14. Larsson, L., Sjodin, B., and Karlsson, J.: Histochemical and biochemical changes in human skeletal muscle with age in sedentary males, age 22-65 years. Acta Physiol. Scand., 103:31–39, 1978.
15. MacDougall, J. D., Ward, G. R., Sale, D. G., and Sutton, J. R.: Biochemical adaptation of human skeletal muscle to heavy resistance training and immobilization. J. Appl. Physiol., 43:700–703, 1977.
16. Moritani, T.: Training adaptations in the muscles of older men. In Smith, E.L. and Serfass, R. C. (eds.): Exercise and Aging: The Scientific Basis. Hillside, NJ, Enslow Publishers, 1981.
17. Moritani, T., and DeVries, H. A.: Potential for gross muscle hypertrophy in older men. J. Gerontol., 35:672–682, 1980.
18. Patel, A. N., Razzak, A., and Dastur, D. K.: Disuse atrophy of human skeletal muscles. Arch. Neurol., 20:413–422, 1969.
19. Petrofsky, J. S. and Phillips, C. A.: The physiology of static exercise. Exerc. Sport Sci. Rev., 14:1–44, 1986.
20. Rossman, I.: The anatomy of aging. In Rossman, I. (Ed.): Clinical Geriatrics, 2nd Ed. Philadelphia, J. B. Lippincott Company, 1979, pp. 3–22.
21. Sidney, K. H.: Cardiovascular benefits of physical activity in the exercising aged. In Smith, E. L. and Serfass, R. C. (Eds.): Exercise and Aging: The Scientific Basis. Hillside, NJ, Enslow Publishers, 1981, pp. 131–147.
22. Smith, E. L.: Bone changes in the exercising older adult. In Smith, E. L. and Serfass, R. C. (eds.): Exercise and Aging: The Scientific Basis. Hillside, NJ, Enslow Publishers, 1981, pp. 179–186.
23. Soman, V. R., Koivisto, V. A., Deibert, D.: Increased insulin sensitivity and insulin binding to monocytes after physical training. N. Engl. J. Med., 301:1200–1204, 1979.
24. Stillman, R. J., Lohman, T. G., Slaughter, M. H., and Massey, B. H.: Physiological activity and bone mineral content in women aged 30 to 85 years. Med. Sci. Sports Exerc., 18:576–580, 1986.
25. Syrovy, I., and Guttmann, E.: Changes in speed of contraction and APTase activity in striated muscle during old age. Exp. Gerontol., 5:31–35, 1970.
26. Tauchi, H., Yoshika, T., and Kobayashi, H.: Age changes in skeletal muscles of rats. Gerontologia, 17:219–227, 1971.
27. Tipton, C. M.: Exercise, training, and hypertension. Exerc. Sport Sci. Rev., 12:245–306, 1984.
28. Tobis, J. S.: Rehabilitation of the geriatric patient. In Rossman, I. (Ed.): Clinical Geriatrics, 2nd Ed. Philadelphia, J. B. Lippincott Company, 1979.
29. Tobis, J. S.: The hospitalized elderly. (Editorial.) J.A.M.A., 248:874, 1982.

CHANG-ZERN HONG AND JEROME S. TOBIS

30. Versar, F., and Ermini, M.: Decrease of creatine phosphate restitution in old age and the influence of glucose. Gerontolgia, 16:223–230, 1970.
31. Vogt, C., and Vogt, O.: Aging of nerve cells. Nature, 158:304–308, 1946.
32. Zohman, L. R., and Tobis, J. S.: Cardiac Rehabilitation. New York, Grune & Stratton, 1970.
33. Zubek, J. P., and Wilgoch, L.: Prolonged immobilization of the body: Changes in performance and in the EEG. Science, 140:306–307, 1963.
34. Zubek, J. P., and Wilgoch, L.: Counteracting effects of physical exercise performed during prolonged perceptual deprivation. Science, 142:504–506, 1963.
35. Zubek, J. P., and Wilgoch, L.: Effect of immobilization behavior and EEG changes. Can. J. Psychol., 20:316–334, 1966.

59

The Rehabilitation of Traumatic Brain Injury

D. NATHAN COPE

The patient with traumatic brain injury (TBI) or closed head injury is an increasingly prominent problem in rehabilitation. Although traumatic brain injury is by no means a new condition, it is only during the past decade that specialized approaches and programs have been developed to address the unique needs of this population. Rehabilitation of the TBI patient is now known to require a combination of medical and psychological approaches provided over an increasingly extensive length of time. This factor, in turn, has led to the development of an array of specialized categorical programs addressing aspects of this need (Table 59–1). The rapid proliferation of these programs has been one of the most pronounced recent events in the evolution of clinical rehabilitation. These categorical programs are oriented in various ways toward some specific aspect of the treatment of

TABLE 59–1. Categories of Rehabilitation Programs for Patients with Head Injuries

Acute rehabilitation
Behavior management
Coma treatment
Day treatment
Extended intensive rehabilitation
Family support
Higher support
Higher education facilities
Independent living
Individual service providers
Life-long residential
Long-term rehabilitation
Nursing homes, skilled nursing care and young adult
Referral centers
Transitional living

the brain-injured patient. Demand for reliable information about the availability and characteristics of these new programs led the National Head Injury Foundation to catalogue and publish a national directory of services,[1] which currently lists programs under 13 distinct categories of service (Fig. 59–1). This list includes programs for medical-physical restoration, cognitive remediation, behavioral management, resocialization, family support, and education. The 1989 edition of this directory contains more than 400 individual program listings.

Incidence, Prevalence and Demographics

Definitive figures regarding the incidence and associated epidemiological features of TBI are difficult to obtain, although without question it is a problem of enormous magnitude. A number of local and national surveys have produced estimates of these figures, which have been recently summarized.[23] The death rate from TBI in the United States is between 20 and 30 per 100,000. The overall total incidence of head injury is more difficult to determine, in part, owing to lack of agreement on an operational definition of what features should operationally define brain injury. At the less severe end of the spectrum, TBI undoubtedly can occur with subtle and only recently recognized sequelae, which health statistics, primarily hospital records, have not adequately captured.[4] Bearing in mind this bias toward underestimation, currently accepted approximations of

1217

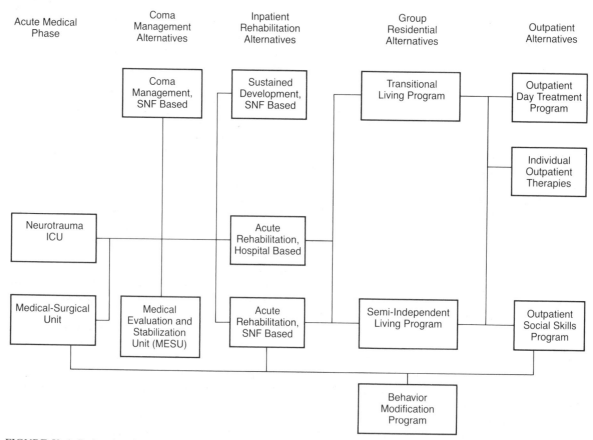

FIGURE 59–1. Referral pathways between programmatic options. Note: Chart reflects *bidirectional* patient flow. Individual cases may bypass any particular element of the network; e.g., a patient may proceed from the Trauma Stepdown Unit to group residential or from an acute rehabilitation program to an outpatient program, and so on. (Reproduced with permission from IBIS, Inc.)

incidence of between 180 to 230 significant TBIs per 100,000 for the United States have been published.

The risk of suffering a fatal or significant TBI is not randomly distributed within the population. The highest risk lies with young adult males between the ages of 15 and 24 years of age who have an incidence of up to 550 per 100,000. A strong overall association of TBI with alcohol and drug intoxication is accepted, particularly in the adolescent and young adult group.[5] Increased risk of TBI has been associated with low socioeconomic status.[6] A second peak incidence of TBI is recognized in the elderly age group; after the age of 70, the incidence again approaches the extreme rate of the young adult.[7] A less pronounced increased risk exists for the infant and very young child.

Motor vehicle accidents are the largest single cause of TBI, and TBI accounts for up to 50 per cent of traffic fatalities. For head injuries associated with coma, more than 70 per cent are secondary to motor vehicle accidents. Gunshot wounds and falls are the next leading causes. Falls are particularly prominent causes of injury for young and elderly TBI patients. Approximately 422,000 new patients with head injury were *admitted* to hospitals in the United States in 1974.[8] Estimates of physician visits with nonhospitalized patients with TBI are of a greater magnitude. Approximately 10 per cent of those hospitalized have hospital stays lasting longer than 20 days. One of every 200 persons in the United States is reported to be receiving care or is suffering from the sequelae of brain injury. For a perspective on the problem, it is useful to appreciate that TBI has 40 times the incidence and 30 times the prevalence of spinal injury. It has approximately the same order of magnitude of occurrence as stroke.

Comparison with Other Neurological Conditions

Comparison of TBI with other related forms of brain pathology is informative. It is probably only recently that such a distinction has been emphasized in the practice of clinical rehabilitation. Other conditions with certain similarities to TBI are mental retardation, stroke, and spinal cord injury.

Mental retardation is present at birth and is essentially a static condition. As such, habilitation rather than rehabilitation issues predominate in treatment. In particular, patients with mental retardation and their families have no pre-morbid level of function with which to compare the patient's current diminished functional ability, whereas the converse is true for head-injured patients and their families. A therapeutic issue for clinicians dealing with the patient with TBI is the need to deal with this inevitable pre-injury and post-injury comparison and the associated need for accommodation and grieving due to loss by the patient with TBI and the family. There are practical implications to this distinction between TBI and mental retardation. Certain treatment issues appear essentially identical for TBI and mental retardation—for example, the need for extended periods of training to allow for the slowed rate of learning or the need for life-long supportive educational and vocational settings for portions of both populations. In practice, however, efforts to engage patients with TBI into treatment programs designed for clients with mental retardation have characteristically had lack of success. Patients with TBI generally perceive themselves as normal individuals recovering from injury and have tended to resist inclusion with retarded (and other disabled) populations.

Stroke generally occurs in the older population, in which decline of function is at least expected as a natural event of that stage of life. The characteristically discrete, dense focal lesions of stroke also clinically tend to produce more complete but more circumscribed deficits than those of head injury. The characteristic lesions of blunt TBI are diffuse, multiple, and small.[9] This factor, in theory, should provide greater opportunity for partial sparing of any single functional neuronal system and for increased effectiveness of purported mechanisms of central nervous system (CNS) recovery such as collateral axonal sprouting (reactive synaptogenesis) or alternate neural pathway unmasking.[10] It is felt that these and other considerations of TBI allow increased and more extended recovery of neurological function compared with the more dense neurological injuries of stroke (or of surgical ablation and penetrating missile injuries of the central nervous system). Clinical experience confirms such prolonged and relatively increased recovery for many patients with TBI. From a strictly utilitarian perspective, since head-injured patients have an average of more than 50 years of life expectancy remaining, the total morbidity in terms of lost days of productivity after severe head injury is, therefore, proportionately larger. Any increase in functional capacity and the associated reduction in cost of care produced by efforts at rehabilitation are leveraged significantly over the lifetime of each patient. Thus, extensive and lengthy rehabilitation treatments that might not be appropriate for an elderly stroke patient may well be indicated for the patient with TBI.

Spinal cord injury shares with TBI components of extensive physical disability and dependency and the age group in which the injury primarily occurs. Many of the maturational issues of this young adult population are similar in both conditions. TBI, however, has a more variable but not immediately evident range of syndromes and outcomes than spinal cord injury, and this factor, together with the characteristic memory losses and lack of insight into the deficit of TBI patients, tends to make the process of psychological adjustment by the patient with TBI more difficult and, in some cases, nearly perpetual. Prigatano, in fact, has stated that the task of gaining understanding and acceptance of deficits is the most significant task of rehabilitation in patients with TBI.[11]

Degrees of Injury and Syndromes of Injury

TBIs constitute a continuum, and the identification and specification of individual syndromes following such injuries, therefore, are clinically convenient abstractions.

Degree of Severity

The specific deficits of each patient with TBI depend upon many factors, but none is as preeminent as the degree of severity of injury. This is so dominant a factor that clinical grouping of patients is primarily initially based on this criterion. The severity of the TBI is shown to directly correlate with the energy of the acceleration and

D. NATHAN COPE

deceleration process of impact. Other characteristics of injury, such as the involved rotational forces, impose additional contributions to the ultimate degree of injury.[12]

In practice, four basic clinical groupings are usually identified: mild, moderate, and severe head injury and the persistent vegetative state. Generally accepted definitions are not available for each of these categories, and the resulting confusion in scientific and clinical communication has been noted.[13] Nevertheless, there is a value in preserving these distinctions as concepts in clinical practice, since presentation, treatment, and outcome are principally dependent upon them.

Mild Head Injury

The mild head injury syndrome is the most frequent of all TBI syndromes. It was previously referred to as postconcussion syndrome. Mild head injury is characterized by a brief loss of consciousness at the time of injury and no persistent, hard, or focal neurological deficits but subtle neuropsychological and behavioral deficits. Until recently, it was thought that no pathoanatomical changes occurred following mild head injury and no permanent neurological deficits resulted. Recent neuropathological and neuropsychological studies have confirmed, however, that in at least a substantial proportion of these cases, definite neuroanatomical lesions are produced and permanent impairment persists.[14-16] The specific neuropathological process appears to be primarily axonal disruption that is secondary to shear forces in the brain stem reticular formation and, to some extent, in the cerebrum.[17-19] Characteristic symptoms of the syndrome include headache, dizziness, poor concentration and information processing, memory loss, fatigue, and irritability.[20]

Repeated minor injuries over time have been clearly associated with progressive loss of neurological and cognitive functions with significant atrophy of cerebral tissue.[21] Dementia pugilistica seen in boxers is a prominent clinical example of this process,[22, 23] which has been associated with other high-risk groups, e.g., jockeys and football players. Currently, the most generally accepted operational definition of mild head injury originates from work at the Medical College of Virginia. Diagnosis consists of the constellation of brief (less than 20 min) loss of consciousness, a score on the Glasgow Coma Scale of 13 or higher, no focal neurological findings, no abnormality on computed tomographic

scan or skull radiographs, and discharge from the hospital within 48 hours.

Moderate Head Injury

The moderate head injury syndrome is the least clearly differentiated condition in terms of distinct clinical characteristics. The lack of a generally accepted operational definition for this particular level of TBI has contributed to a general paucity of investigation directed toward it. The term applies, logically, to that group of patients who are placed between the mild and the severe groups. Proposed criteria for moderate head injury have included initial Glasgow Coma Scale scores ranging from 9 to 12, 10 to 12, or 8 to 10.[24] McMillan and associates have used a definition of admission to a hospital for head trauma associated with a post-traumatic amnesia lasting between 1 and 24 hours.[25] The moderate head injury syndrome, although not clearly defined, does represent a continuum connecting the minor and severe groups, and clinical experience has indicated that this category should be retained.[26]

Severe Head Injury

Severe head injury is also a multidefinition classification. The category encompasses those patients who have head injury severe enough to produce an obvious disabling deficit but who regain the capacity for conscious activity. Jennett has best characterized severe head injury. His definition includes those patients who have suffered from coma for at least six hours.[27] It is this class of patients with TBI who traditionally have undergone a sufficient amount of recovery to potentially benefit from intensive rehabilitation while also having sufficiently severe and complex deficits to require the medically supported and multidisciplinary approach of inpatient, hospital-based rehabilitation programs. Thus, most experience in the rehabilitation literature is based principally upon this severely brain-injured group. This group, however, probably represents only about 10 per cent of the total number of patients with TBI, and the appropriate caution against overgeneralization of reported outcome results, for example, needs to be maintained.

Persistent Vegetative State

A small percentage of surviving patients with TBI whose extent of injury is sufficiently severe do not regain consciousness but enter into the persistent vegetative state.[28] The condition evolves in the acutely brain-injured patient when, after some time in coma, the patient continues to demonstrate no awareness of the surroundings and neither speaks nor makes volitional movements; however, other activities, such as the sleep-wake cycle, yawning, lip-smacking, grimacing, withdrawing from noxious stimuli, and visual fixation and tracking, presumably mediated principally by lower brain structures, can and usually do resume in this condition.[29] This condition may persist for years.[30] A notable clinical problem associated with this syndrome is a not uncommon presumption of awareness and conscious perception in the vegetative patient. This misapprehension may occur with clinical staff but particularly occurs in families. Extended and unresolved grieving or insistence upon inappropriate treatments is often the result of a belief in patient awareness suggested by such automatic behaviors.

In conclusion, there is a continuum of severity in TBI, which ranges from the simple postconcussional syndrome, through a wide variety of significant neurological and psychological deficits, to prolonged coma, the persistent vegetative state, and death. As mentioned earlier, severity of injury is the single most important initial variable determining outcome.

Rating Systems

A variety of rating systems and classification schemes have been developed to describe and categorize various aspects of TBI and to help in discriminating among these multiple facets of TBI characterization.

GLASGOW COMA SCALE[31]

The most widely accepted and most demonstrably useful rating system is the Glasgow Coma Scale. This scale extends from 3 to 15 points and is designed to assess the severity of coma and impaired consciousness following TBI. Developed by Teasdale and Jennett at the University of Glasgow, it is a means of classifying and monitoring patients with severe head injury within the first two to three days of injury. Measures of three aspects of neurological functioning—eye-opening, motor capacity, and verbal response—are used to determine the total score. The lower the score, the poorer the neurological status of the patient. A

lower score correlates well with ultimate death or poorer outcomes, whereas a higher score correlates with a higher degree of ultimate neurological recovery. A score of eight or less on the scale is often considered a discriminant for those patients in coma; above the score of eight, some degree of restoration of consciousness has occurred.[32] The Glasgow Coma Scale score is simple to obtain and has proved to be accurate and reliable when obtained by a variety of health professionals. It is most widely used by emergency evacuation systems, emergency room staff, and in neurosurgical intensive care unit settings. Used sequentially, it has proved useful in following the clinical course of acutely brain-injured patients; a deteriorating coma scale score indicates a complication or an impending irreversible brain injury, such as late mass lesions and intracranial bleeding. It must, however, be appreciated that this scale has been developed for use in populations with acute injuries and becomes inaccurate as an indicator of neurological impairment during the later periods of recovery from brain injury, particularly during the rehabilitation phase.

GLASGOW OUTCOME SCALE[33]

The Glasgow Outcome Scale, also developed by Jennett's group, is meant to reliably categorize the clinical outcome of patients with TBI. In its most widely used form, it is a five-point scale, although more detailed versions have been published.[34] The five outcome categories are:

Death: self-evident criteria.

Persistent vegetative state: prolonged unconsciousness with no verbalization, no following of commands, and no meaningful interaction with environment.

Severe disability: presence of residual disabilities that prevent the patient from independent function for any 24-hour period (both physical and cognitive deficits are included).

Moderate disability: residual deficits that although significant, do not prevent an independent life style.

Good recovery: minor or no residual deficits.

RAPPAPORT DISABILITY RATING SCALE[35]

Developed by Rappaport and co-workers, the Disability Rating Scale is an effort to describe various degrees of recovery from TBI in functional terms on a single continuum. The scale ranges from 0 to 30 points: 30 representing death and 0 representing no measurable deficit. It is a compendium of several previously developed scales and includes the Glasgow Coma Scale within it. It is a

D. NATHAN COPE

significantly more finely graduated measure of functional outcome than the Glasgow Outcome Scale and, thus, provides a more discriminating way to track the course of recovery from TBI. It has been demonstrated to document a more extended length of recovery of function by patients with TBI compared with that measured by the Glasgow Outcome Scale.[36]

LEVEL OF COGNITIVE FUNCTIONING SCALE[37]

The Level of Cognitive Functioning Scale (Rancho Scale), developed by Rancho los Amigos Hospital in California, is an eight-level global measure of cognition and behavior rated as follows:

Rancho Level	Clinical Correlate
I	No response
II	Generalized response
III	Localized response
IV	Confused-agitated
V	Confused-inappropriate
VI	Confused-appropriate
VII	Automatic-appropriate
VIII	Purposeful and appropriate

Many patients progress sequentially through successive Rancho levels as they recover from TBI. This scale has proved useful in classifying the states of patients primarily based upon cognition and behavior, which have direct relevance to the type of management program and treatment approach most appropriate for that patient. It has some deficiencies in that patients do not always move sequentially through each level and nonbehavioral aspects of disability are not reflected well by this scale. Nonetheless, it is widely accepted and utilized in the treatment of brain injury.

RANGE OF SYNDROMES

Another axis upon which the patient with TBI must be placed is based upon the specific neuropathological lesions and the consequent individual deficits that the trauma and its complications produce. The various deficits seen after TBI range from purely cognitive syndromes (of memory, attention, sensory perception, and higher analytic skills) to purely physical syndromes (locked-in) with bulbar and long tract components that may closely resemble spinal cord injury and require similar treatment and rehabilitation. Such pure and

isolated physically disabled patients with TBI are, however, the exception. Almost all patients with TBI display some combination of physical and cognitive-behavioral disturbances. In each case, it is necessary to define the component deficits and determine which are most disabling and amenable to treatment. It is not feasible to prescribe an unvarying approach to rehabilitation in TBI; rather each patient's rehabilitation program must be individually designed with appropriate components of physical, cognitive, and behavioral intervention.

Pathology of Traumatic Brain Injury

Notwithstanding previous statements about the variety of lesions that may occur following blunt trauma to the brain, certain elements of injury occur with a significantly high frequency to warrant meaningful discussion about typical TBI lesions. Descriptions of these changes are given by Jennett,[38] Graham and Adams,[39] and Levin, Benton, and Grossman.[40] These pathological injuries may be divided into primary and secondary groups.

Primary Brain Injury

Primary injuries to the brain consist of diffuse and focal cerebral lesions suffered immediately at the moment of acceleration or deceleration on impact and are of two major types—cerebral contusions and axonal stretch injuries.[41] In such closed head injuries, damage, although diffusely produced by generalized shear and rotational forces, is found in various specific structures in the brain. The injury is more severe where the mechanical shearing forces are greatest, i.e., in those structures farthest from the axis of rotation. The cortex tends to be most affected, followed by the diencephalic structures, with mid-brain and brain stem structures affected least.[42]

Diffuse axonal injury, the typical neuropathological lesion of brain injury from acceleration and deceleration, was first definitively described by Stritch.[43] Diffuse axonal injury consists of mechanically induced stretching and rupturing of long axonal fiber tracts. The characteristic pathological markers for such an injury consist of axonal retraction balls and microglial clusters. Involvement is seen in ascending and descending tracts of the brain stem, including the medial lemniscal and superior cerebellar peduncles. The lesions are also present in the cerebral hemispheres.[44] Dorsal pyramidal white matter lesions constitute the gliding contusions of Lindenberg and Freytag.[45]

The cause of traumatic unconsciousness is presumed to result from shear or stretch lesions within the mesencephalic brain stem that cause impairment of the alerting or activating system of the brain[46] or, alternatively, from diffuse generalized cerebral destruction.

A second characteristic injury of TBI is cerebral contusion. Such contusions are multiple, may be quite small, and are not evident on gross pathological examination at autopsy. However, microscopic examination reveals multiple and diffuse lesions. Such contusions are characteristically located immediately below the cortical surface beneath the crests of gyri while sparing sulci.[47] As the energy of impact increases, the size and number of such lesions grow so that they eventually coalesce, ultimately leading to intracerebral hematoma. Cortical injuries are frequently produced below the site of impact (coup) or occasionally in the pole opposite the site of impact (contracoup). Because of the physicomechanical characteristics of the brain as well as specific points of anatomy of the inner table of the skull, contusions are found most frequently on the inferior or orbital pre-frontal and anteroinferior temporal lobes, irrespective of the specific site of impact.[48] Certain other specific structures are also vulnerable to injury, notably the corpus callosum, including the splenium, the fornix, the septum, and the dorsolateral quadrant of the rostral brain stem.[49] This distribution of injury in TBI has clinical significance. Lesions of anterior frontal lobe tend to be associated with characteristic deficits in the initiation of novel responses, e.g., perseveration, whereas temporal lobe lesions correlate with characteristic losses in memory function and affectual changes.[50, 51]

TBI lesions typically have a bilateral distribution but an asymmetrical density. Although the lesions are characteristically more extensive on one side of the brain, they may be routinely elicited on the other side if careful assessment is done. Vascular injury also occurs, preferentially at the junction of structures or tissues with differing mechanicoelastic properties, such as at margins of white matter and gray matter.

In minor injury, pathological change may be apparent only with microscopic examination of tissue. One clinical consequence of the small size and diffuseness of these lesions is that available neuroimaging techniques, e.g., computerized tomography and magnetic resonance imaging scans, may not show an abnormality in many mild (and some severe) cases of injury. It is now clear that the normality of such studies does not rule out significant brain injury.[52] It does appear, however, that magnetic resonance imaging is significantly superior to computed tomography in demonstrating both the diffuse long tract lesions and focal cerebral contusions of TBI that had been previously inapparent,[53, 54] and the extent and location of these lesions correlate with later neuropsychological deficits.

Secondary Brain Injury

In addition to the injuries produced by the direct action of the mechanical stresses on impact, secondary processes invariably occur following TBI that may contribute to additional damage of the central nervous system. This secondary brain damage principally is composed of a few characteristic types—ischemia, mass lesions, and increased intracranial pressure.

Ischemia may occur from a variety of mechanisms, including acute respiratory arrest, hypovolemic shock, and vascular damage. Focal ischemic damage may be due to occlusion or loss of perfusion of major vascular structures. Such occlusion may occur as a result of direct trauma. Alternatively, cerebral edema, resulting from mechanical injury to brain tissue, may cause rapid and extensive swelling of the brain, leading to elevated intracranial pressure. If such pressure is sufficiently extensive, transtentorial herniation results, with occlusion of vascular structures and destruction of cerebral matter. Cranial nerve injuries may also be a result of this process as well as from direct traction or mechanical disruption. Extensive focal vascular injury may lead to relatively predominant stroke syndromes superimposed upon the primary TBI picture.

Widespread ischemic neuronal loss also is known to occur with high frequency in TBI.[55] Certain cerebral structures prove to be particularly sensitive to ischemic insults, especially structures in the hippocampus, basal ganglia, cerebellum, and cortex.[56] Cortical ischemia often arises in watershed distributions if generalized hemodynamic insufficiency occurs. With cardiac and ventilatory arrest or other causes of profound hypoxemia, a severe diffuse cortical mantle death results. Mass lesions (subdural, epidural, and intracerebral hematomas) are not rare and contribute to further cerebral damage by similar mechanisms. It should be appreciated that in Adams' series of autopsy findings of severe head injury, more than 90 per cent of the cases showed evidence of either ischemic or pressure injury in addition to the primary traumatic changes.[57]

It is the variability in type, location, and degree of the pathological changes in TBI, as well as the obvious variability in pre-morbid brain and personality characteristics of the individual patient, that leads to the widely diverse deficits and outcomes.

Prognosis

A characteristic of TBI is that the prediction of ultimate deficit early after onset is more difficult than with many other neurological conditions. The prediction of expected outcome in any *single* case of TBI is still a very uncertain process, and this uncertainty is a significant contributor to the difficulties of clinical rehabilitation and research of this condition. In the early comatose phase of TBI, the condition of the patients cannot routinely be reliably distinguished by currently available clinical means into those who will do well and recover with minimal deficits and those who will never recover consciousness or will recover only to exhibit catastrophic neurological deficits. Patients who have a similar history, evident mechanism and severity of injury, or early clinical appearance and course often have vastly different types and severities of disabilities. These differences emerge as recovery proceeds. One patient who achieves nearly total neuromuscular recovery may be difficult to distinguish grossly from a nonimpaired individual in terms of physical function but may have a severe dementing deficit. A patient with an acute TBI who appears to be similar to other patients with TBI may have normal or near-normal cognitive recovery but also may have a mid-brain or brain-stem syndrome, resulting in motor deficits.

Each patient with TBI has a complex combination of physical, cognitive, and behavioral deficits that present a unique rehabilitation problem. This clinical variability has led, in part, to the distinctively individualized approach to rehabilitation treatment now used for TBI patients. The more prolonged recovery course of TBI also contributes to the difficulty of accurate prognosis in the individual patient. This factor, in turn, makes the assessment of efficacy of particular treatments more problematic for TBI than for other conditions.

The pathological lesions of TBI are frequently hidden within the skull, and their extent and distribution can often only be inferred. Accurate prognosis performed within the early period following injury has been accomplished with a high degree of accuracy only for gross measures of outcome, such as in relation to death or survival.[58] As the requirement for more discrete outcomes increases (and the assessment of results of rehabilitation requires such discrimination), the reliability of prognosis drops precipitously. High degrees of variability among subjects are characteristic of studies of recovery in TBI. Approaches that utilize empirically derived multivariate recovery curves to achieve more accurate early prognosis have been proposed.[59-61] To date, such multivariate approaches remain intriguing and potentially powerful but speculative. Currently, it must be accepted that no clinically useful, objective, highly reliable, prognostic system exists for determining finer distinctions of outcome.

Lacking reliable mechanisms of prognosis, accurate planning for later treatment and meaningful assessment of effectiveness of various treatment interventions remain enormously difficult. The formulation of clinical outcome estimates should best be considered probabilistic procedures. Therefore, information relating to outcome potential should always be presented to patients and families in such a manner as to reflect this uncertainty. A great deal of damage may be done, for example, when family members are informed that a comatose patient's situation does not allow the hope for rehabilitation when such an outcome is not definitely established. Extremely delayed arousal and partial recovery from extended periods of coma, for example, are known to occur.[62] In one case, delayed recovery from coma apparently began as late as six years following the onset of the injury.[63]

In spite of the lack of completely reliable prognostic indicators, a number of helpful prognostic variables have emerged and are generally accepted as correlating to some degree with outcome following TBI[64-66] and are discussed below.

Duration of Coma and Duration of Post-Traumatic Amnesia

Two of the most useful prognostic indicators are the duration of coma and post-traumatic amnesia.

One of the clearest relationships between acute status and outcome exists for duration and depth of coma,[67, 68] which has been demonstrated for children as well as for adults.[69] The duration of coma is a particularly valuable measure to assess and screen patients for need of rehabilitation services. Although the precise duration of coma may be difficult to determine after the fact in clinical settings (e.g., when rehabilitative consultation is requested), great precision generally is not required. It is usually sufficient to determine the order of magnitude of the duration of coma, i.e., whether the patient in question has been in coma for a few minutes, an hour, a day, a week, or a month. Patients whose coma persists from several weeks to several months constitute the core of the population who are in need of comprehensive rehabilitation. The expected degree of disability and the likelihood of the need for and response to rehabilitation relate closely to this factor of coma duration. A patient who is in coma for only a few hours will usually have only subtle neuropsychological and personality deficits. The patient whose coma lasts several days to several weeks generally has substantial deficits but, in most cases, has the capacity to become physically independent and perhaps to return to gainful employment. The patient in coma for a month or two is probably permanently impaired to a significant extent, both physically and psychologically. However, in such a patient, rehabilitation has the potential to produce significant gains in physical independence and self-care. Patients in coma for three or more months tend to remain essentially dependent in almost all areas of function. Although significant rehabilitation goals may exist for these patients, they usually are limited in scope. It has been pointed out, however, that significant recovery can occur after coma lasting longer than one year in a small number of cases.[70]

A question exists regarding the life expectancy of patients who enter the persistent vegetative state but who are otherwise without significant disease. This is relevant for the practical task of estimating requirements and planning resources for appropriate lifelong care. There are no data that confidently answer this question. It appears that survival in such a state is more a function of the intensity and appropriateness of the nursing and medical care provided. One long-term epidemiological study of outcome of patients with persistent vegetative state in Japan reported a 65 per cent death rate after three years. Only 7 per cent of the affected patients evolved beyond the persistent vegetative state over that period.[71]

Post-traumatic amnesia is a second clearly delineated clinical measure that has been correlated closely with overall outcome of brain injury as well as specific cognitive and psychological deficits.[72–76] Post-traumatic amnesia may be considered equivalent to anterograde amnesia. It corresponds to that period after injury in which the incorporation of new information into long-term memory does not take place. The resolution of post-traumatic amnesia clinically corresponds to the period when general confusion ends and incorporation of ongoing daily events into the working memory occurs. It has been suggested that more consistent methods of determining duration of post-traumatic amnesia may allow even a stronger correlation with outcome.[77] A recently developed standard objective means of determining the resolution of post-traumatic amnesia and the impairment of general orientation is the Galveston Orientation and Amnesia Test.[78] Points are cumulatively subtracted from a total score of 100 for errors in orientation, and the patient's recall is tested at the bedside. The normal range is from 100 to 75; borderline abnormal scores, from 74 to 66; and the abnormal range, below 66. Prolonged post-traumatic amnesia, as measured by the Galveston Orientation and Amnesia Test, has been correlated with a poor outcome.

Neurological Indicators

The extent and severity of acute neurological deficits such as impaired oculocephalic, oculovestibular, and pupillary reflex responses increase in proportion to the degree of injury to the CNS and result in a proportionally poorer outcome.[79–81] The same is true for deficits of the motor system.[82, 83] Decerebration and decortication during the acute emergency or neurosurgical phase are significant indicators of brain injury of increased severity.

Physiological Indicators

Ischemic injury, when it is clearly the major cause of deep coma, can generally be considered to reflect a worse prognosis than uncomplicated TBI, although similar neurological indicators apply.[84] Biochemical measures have been investigated and appear promising as indicators of the severity of injury. Levels of the creatine phosphokinase (CPK1) and lactic dehydrogenase (LDH1) isoenzymes relate to the severity of injury to the CNS.[85] The CK-BB isoenzyme is felt to be a specific indicator of injury of the central nervous

D. NATHAN COPE

system, and increasing levels of this enzyme correlate with delayed, more severe outcomes. Stepwise discriminant analysis using this marker and other indicators such as increased intracranial pressure have increased the accuracy of prognosis.[86] The lactate level in the cerebrospinal fluid also is related to a delayed outcome.[87] Catecholamines have been shown to increase up to fivefold above normal levels after TBI, and the degree of such elevation correlates well with degree of neurological damage and outcome.[88]

Electrophysiological Indicators

ELECTROENCEPHALOGRAM

Currently, the electroencephalogram appears to add only marginally to other acute assessment techniques in regard to increasing the accuracy of the prediction of outcome. Hansotia reviewed a series of patients with acute coma who subsequently developed the persistent vegetative state. The electroencephalogram did not differentiate coma from persistent vegetative state or the transition from one state to the other. Eventual outcome (survival) also was not indicated by criteria on the electroencephalogram, and changes in the pattern on the electroencephalogram did not correlate with clinical improvement.[89]

The confirmation of brain death, however, is still aided by the electroencephalogram, as is diagnosis of specific seizure disorders.

EVOKED POTENTIALS

Cortical evoked potentials have been extensively studied as an electrophysiological means of assessing traumatic brain injury. There have been a number of studies correlating outcome with the degree of evoked potential abnormality noted in the acute period.[90–92] The more abnormal the evoked potential of any modality (somatosensory, auditory, and visual), the poorer the resulting outcome.[93] Evoked potentials have been demonstrated to forecast the specific degree of sensorimotor deficits with greater precision than clinical assessment. It has been reported that late event–related potentials, which reflect aspects of cognitive function, may offer some advantage over neuropsychological assessment in identifying persistent subtle neurological dysfunction.[94]

Three principal clinical objectives of evaluation by evoked potentials have evolved. The first is to determine the severity of injury at an early phase and, consequently, to allow an accurate prognosis. A second purpose of evoked potentials is to investigate possible abnormalities of specific sensory pathways in patients unable to cooperate with more usual evaluation techniques, e.g., to determine whether or not visual, auditory, or somatosensory inputs are reaching cortical receptor fields in a comatose or poorly responsive patient. Finally, evoked potentials may be used to establish a psychogenic or pathophysiological cause of the symptoms in patients with mild head injuries by objectively verifying the presence or absence of electrophysiological abnormalities.[95] This latter issue frequently arises in the context of administrative or medicolegal disability determinations. A recent review of the use of evoked potentials in TBI is available.[96]

COMPUTERIZED SPECTRAL ELECTROENCEPHALOGRAPHIC ANALYSIS

Computerized spectral electroencephalographic analysis is a new approach to investigating brain injury. This spectral analysis of the electroencephalogram (neurometrics) has been shown to differentiate a variety of psychiatric and neurological conditions, including stroke, dementia, and mild cognitive impairment from normal subjects, and the magnitude of neurometric abnormality corresponds with the degree of clinical severity.[97] Preliminary study indicates that these methods may also show a high correlation with delayed outcomes in TBI. An early report of increased accuracy in predicting such an outcome has appeared.[98] These techniques may be expected to offer increased assistance to diagnosis and prognosis in the future.

BRAIN IMAGING

Skull Radiographs

It is now well recognized that skull radiography has a limited role in the evaluation of brain trauma,[99] and significant brain trauma may occur in the absence of skull fracture.

Computed Tomography

The outcome of patients with TBI correlated with the degree of abnormality shown by computed tomography scan of the brain. This is demonstrated for both acute changes and later indications of generalized cerebral loss.[100–102]

Magnetic Resonance Imaging

Magnetic resonance imaging has been correlated with outcome and can provide a definition of central nervous system detail unmatched by other imaging techniques. Bone and blood, however, may not be as well delineated as in computed tomography. On the other hand, there are reports that indicate that magnetic resonance imaging may better reflect the diffuse axonal injury of minor and moderate TBI.[103, 104]

Positron Emission Tomography

Positron emission tomography offers a method of study of both brain anatomy and physiology as well as pathophysiology,[105] which has the potential of providing significant information about structure-function relationships. Positron emission tomography has been reported to have a greater capacity to demonstrate more areas of clinical (neurological and behavioral) dysfunction than computed tomography in patients with TBI.[106] The technique has been suggested as having potential to study cerebral reorganization following damage to the brain.[107] In conclusion, combinations of computed tomography, magnetic resonance imaging, and positron emission tomography, correlated with functional measures such as neuropsychological investigations, are being used in current research and clinical approaches to delineate posttraumatic pathology and brain-behavior relationships.[108]

Age

In general, the older the patient with brain injury, the less optimistic is the outlook for that patient's recovery. The issue of age as a prognostic indicator has been addressed in numerous reports.[109–112] A high death rate, an increased duration of hospital stay, and a 20-fold increase in the rate of discharge to chronic care facilities have been reported for older patients.[113] This pessimism regarding the potential for rehabilitation of the geriatric patient may be overestimated. Some of the decreased outcomes that are suggested by statistical studies may be a result of the increased incidence of mortality and associated morbidity that occurs in older individuals in association with serious trauma rather than a direct result of the brain injury per se. Several large prospective studies of brain injury have not shown such a negative effect of age upon outcome.[114, 115]

Sex

Sex has not been shown to be a predictor of outcome,[116] although certain behavioral sequelae, such as aggression, are felt by some to be more frequent in males.

Pre-morbid Capacity

The personality and capabilities of each TBI victim that existed before the injury will contribute to the degree of functional restoration considered possible following injury. Better levels of pre-morbid education, income, and employment are clearly positive predictors of functional recovery.[117] Specific groups who do not characteristically have optimal pre-morbid functional levels have a higher risk of suffering from TBI. Individuals with impulse-control deficiencies, substance abuse problems, learning disabilities, and a previous head injury all have a significantly higher likelihood of suffering TBI. In establishing the prognosis and therapeutic goals for an individual patient, therefore, the examiner should be vigilant for any history of these problems. It may be unrealistic, for example, to attempt to return a patient with a pre-morbid learning disability to a competitive academic setting.

Socioeconomic Status

A critical element in the long-term outcome of the patient with TBI is the degree of support from the family. Some evidence exists that patients from higher economic groups have better outcomes for comparable degrees of injury.[121] Also the amount of economic support available for pursuing a long-term program of rehabilitation and for life-long maintenance of the levels of function achieved by such rehabilitation needs to be considered in treatment planning.

Cognitive Predictors

It has been noted that cognitive disabilities contribute significantly more toward the patient's total disability following TBI than related physical disabilities. This has been confirmed in a number of studies.[122–126] Associated with strictly cognitive losses in poor outcomes is the patient's denial or unawareness of disability and behavioral disturbance.[127] The prediction of outcome based on early cognitive assessment has not been thoroughly investigated, although some relationship would appear evident.[128]

D. NATHAN COPE

Although continuing progress is being made in developing more precise objective methods and algorithms for use in prognosis, the *clinical* evaluation, consisting of history, physical examination, mental examination, and social evaluation, remains the best predictor of prognosis and of the patient's suitability for rehabilitation. Also, there is no substitute for extensive clinical experience in developing the ability to make such estimates in an accurate manner.

Associated Injuries

It is evident that the high energy of the impact that results in most head injuries will also result in associated injuries to other organ systems. Perhaps one third to one half of patients with severe head injuries admitted to the hospital have a second injury elsewhere, and this frequency increases with the increasing severity of head injury. The diagnosis of such associated injuries is frequently missed or delayed. Irving reported the overall frequency of associated injuries to be 47 per cent; and the relative distribution of such associated injuries is as follows: facial, 22.5 per cent; thoracic, 10.1 per cent; abdominal, <5.0 per cent; pelvic, <5.0 per cent; spinal, 5.0 per cent; and limb, 14.6 per cent.[129] Kalisky, Morrison, and co-workers have surveyed this problem in a rehabilitation setting.[130] Table 59–2 documents the incidence and variety of such problems found in their study of a consecutive series of 180 patients with severe head injury.

Approximately 5 to 10 per cent of patients with TBI have associated spinal cord injury. Alternatively, recent reports of surveys of neurosurgical and rehabilitation populations with a primary diagnosis of spinal injury have suggested a significantly higher degree of occult brain injury or cognitive dysfunction, which in some series is greater than 50 per cent. These brain injuries have not been previously appreciated clinically.[131, 132] Such dual diagnoses have been associated with a higher incidence of mortality and morbidity[133] as well as impaired rehabilitation outcomes.[134] An essential clinical implication of these data is that all acute head-injured patients whose mechanism of injury involved a high-energy impact need a cervical and, occasionally, a complete spinal radiographic examination to rule out occult fractures and dislocations. Such studies should be done immediately at the time of initial evaluation.

TABLE 59–2. Medical Complications of Head Injury

Neurologic:	56 per cent—ventricular dilatation on computed tomography, seizure disorder, subdural hematoma or hygroma, meningitis or empyema
Gastrointestinal:	50 per cent—impaired liver function, including hepatitis, esophagitis, gastritis, ulcer disease, gastrointestinal bleeding
Genitourinary:	45 per cent—urinary tract infection, bladder dysfunction, urethral strictures
Respiratory:	34 per cent—tracheostomy site colonization, atelectasis, pneumonia, pulmonary embolus
Cardiovascular:	32 per cent—nonspecific ST and T wave changes, hypertension, thrombophlebitis, endocarditis
Dermatologic:	21 per cent—acne vulgaris, decubiti, seborrheic dermatitis, allergic rash, folliculitis
Musculoskeletal:	21 per cent—heterotopic ossification, osteomyelitis
Endocrine:	4 per cent inappropriate secretion of antidiuretic hormone, hypothyroidism, panhypopituitarism
Other problems identified:	Sepsis: 5 per cent Anemia: 2 per cent

Rehabilitation

Assessment

Given the wide variability in outcome and difficulty with prognosis, head injury has been notoriously difficult for the inexperienced physician to assess, and, consequently, the development of appropriate long-term rehabilitation plans is equally difficult.[135] Patients with TBI are frequently not cooperative during examination, or if they are cooperative, they frequently provide misleading information in their own assessment of the significant deficits present. The multiplicity and nondiscreteness of many TBI deficits are often confusing and frustrating.

It is often impractical to achieve a *comprehensive* assessment of the patient with TBI on a single initial visit. Frequently, the inexperienced physician focuses on only the most obvious deficits (e.g., contractures, dysarthrias, mobility or range-of-motion problems) or the deficits with which he or she may be most familiar (for example, gait disturbances, electrodiagnosis of peripheral neuropathy, or equipment needs). These problems may all be significant, but by failing to establish a valid priority or hierarchy of the most critical rehabilitation issues, goals most appropriate to that stage of recovery for that specific patient may be neglected. Knowing the major *disabling* deficits of TBI and keeping in mind the clinical management questions relevant to the particular patient and setting help maintain a relevant focus for such initial evaluations. Information from the initial patient assessment should be gathered with the objective of establishing a plan, if indicated, for a comprehensive evaluation. Frequently, this involves the input from a multidisciplinary team, which then allows the determination of an appropriate course of treatment. One aspect of the examination of the patient with TBI that is important in reference to setting priorities of needs is the amount of effort that should be devoted to analysis and management of cognitive, behavioral, psychiatric, and social aspects of functioning.

This comprehensive analysis often requires the assistance of neuropsychologists, psychiatrists, speech and language pathologists, and social workers, but the less formal mental status examination conducted in the office is an essential component of the examining physician's evaluation. Strub and Black have an excellent manual to be used as a guide in this aspect of examination.[136] More sensitive bedside cognitive screening instruments have recently been developed that can be applied to the assessment of patients with TBI.[137, 138] The examiner must become familiar with neurobehavioral[139] and neuropsychiatric[140] diagnoses, syndromes, and concepts relevant to TBI. A separate interview with appropriate family members also is essential to obtain their perspective on significant post-injury deficits (which frequently are different from and often more accurate than that of the patient). For the patient with an acute condition, a further purpose of the initial assessment is to obtain a baseline of significant functions against which later recovery may be compared. For the optimal development of such comprehensive treatment plans, the elements of current neurological status, pre-morbid function, socioeconomic status, and family support need to be integrated into a realistic projection of feasible rehabilitation objectives. Details of this clinical assessment process have been presented elsewhere.[141]

Methods of Rehabilitation

As mentioned earlier, the rehabilitation of the severely brain-injured patient is a long-term, multifaceted process. It involves management of ongoing and potential neurosurgical, medical, neurological, orthopedic, urological, otolaryngological, and ophthalmological conditions. The physical, cognitive, psychological, behavioral, and social deficits must also be evaluated and treated. TBI programs require the involvement of experienced members of multiple clinical disciplines, including physical, occupational, and speech therapy; rehabilitation nursing; clinical and neuropsychology; social workers; and educational and vocational counselors and teachers operating in coordinated interdisciplinary teams. It has become more prevalent for TBI rehabilitation programs (like those for other medically catastrophic conditions) to involve representatives from third-party payers as participants, or at the least as informants, of the treatment team. Such treatment lasts for many years and takes place in multiple settings. Hospital-based rehabilitation is only the initial phase for most patients.

MEDICAL REHABILITATION

The typical patient with TBI is a young adult, and pre-morbid medical problems unrelated to the trauma are rare. Nevertheless, significant medical issues are common during the initial period of rehabilitation; some persist indefinitely. It is a critical component of the rehabilitation process to manage these issues appropriately. An important point is that any additional physiological stress placed upon the patient with TBI significantly depresses function of the central nervous system. For example, it is not unusual for a patient to appear to be in prolonged coma on first examination, then rapidly to become alert and responsive when the infection has cleared or a positive nitrogen balance has been achieved by adequate nutrition. A variety of common medications also cause the same artificially depressed level of arousal. Overly pessimistic prognoses are often given due to failure to consider these additional stressors, which erroneously indicate more serious brain damage.

Sepsis is an ongoing risk in the early rehabilitation phase following TBI. As in other debilitated patients, the respiratory and genitourinary tracts are the most common sites of primary infection. Decreased arousal, indwelling catheterization, and the inability to report symptoms all contribute to the need for increased alertness to this issue on the part of medical personnel.

Gastrointestinal Disorders. Depressed levels of arousal, decreased sensation, abnormal and absent protective reflexes, impulsivity, and judgment deficits all contribute to a substantial risk of aspiration and pneumonia. Most specialized rehabilitation programs for acute TBI have developed special teams composed of nursing, physical, occupational, and speech-language therapists and dietitians who perform a thorough evaluation of the patient's swallowing and feeding capacity immediately on admission. An appropriate initial diet (often nasogastric tube feeding alone) is determined, and an aggressive feeding training program is initiated. For most patients with significant neuromuscular involvement, a cinefluoroscopy series of the swallowing sequence, performed with contrast media of various consistencies, is now recommended to identify occult aspiration,[142, 143] which is frequently missed in patients with TBI and other conditions by clinical assessment alone.[144] Feeding gastrostomy or jejunostomy may be necessary if it is apparent that prolonged delay will occur in achieving safe oral intake. Gastric hyperacidity and gastrointestinal bleeding occur following TBI,[145] which may be due to an ulcer resulting from stress. Pancreatitis may be a direct result of initial trauma but has also been primarily associated with brain injury. Pancreatic inflammation has been related to heightened intracranial pressure, hypovolemia, and steroid use.[146] Hepatic dysfunction can occur and persist as a result of direct trauma, transfusion-induced hepatitis, or drug toxicity.

Integument. Decubiti are significant complications in patients with head injury as they are for all debilitated populations. They do not appear to be as common currently as in earlier reports,[147] perhaps because of better awareness on the part of nursing and medical personnel.

Nutritional Considerations. Severe brain injury initially places increased metabolic demands on the victim; a hypermetabolic state similar to that associated with major trauma or burns is not uncommon.[148] It is not clear how long such conditions persist, but in some cases, they appear to last for many months after the onset of the injury. Provision of increased calories and protein may reduce this catabolic process[149, 150] and accelerate recovery.

Cardiovascular Disorders. Because of the generally young age of most patients with TBI, cardiovascular problems are relatively infrequent following the trauma. However, direct trauma to the thorax may cause myocardial damage or injury to great vessels, which should be looked for in the physical examination, the chest x-ray study, and the electrocardiogram. Orthostatic hypotension may be a problem in the older patient or in the

patient who has been bed-ridden for extended periods. Hypertension following head injury is an unusual but is not a rare consequence of TBI and is felt to occur on a central basis, perhaps involving excessive catecholaminergic activity,[151] a specific brain structure lesion, or an occult spinal injury with dysreflexia.[152] Elevated blood pressure has been reported to be a consequence of insidious hydrocephalus in several patients several years after the occurrence of TBI. The hypertension resolved following ventriculoperitoneal shunting.[153] In treating this problem, awareness should be maintained of the possible adverse cognitive consequences of many antihypertensive agents, and they should be avoided, if possible.[154, 155]

Endocrine Disorders. Endocrinological difficulties are not uncommon sequelae of traumatic brain injury. These difficulties are generally subsumed under various hypothalamic and hypopituitary syndromes resulting from injury to the infundibular stalk.[156–158] Such complications have been documented to occur following injury with no or very brief losses of consciousness.[159] Consequences of this injury include diabetes insipidus, hypogonadism, hypothyroidism, growth hormone deficiency, and adrenal insufficiency (the response to adrenal stimulation frequently has been reported as subnormal without clinical evidence of hypoadrenalism[160]). Another endocrinological disturbance includes hyponatremia, which is probably associated with inappropriate antidiuretic hormone secretion.[161]

NEUROLOGICAL REHABILITATION

Seizures. The incidence of post-traumatic epilepsy is variously reported to range between 5 and 50 per cent. The extent to which epilepsy develops is clearly related to the severity and characteristics of the injury. Jennett has discussed the factors of importance in the predisposition to post-traumatic seizure disorder in patients with nonpenetrating head injuries.[162] The risk factors include early seizures (occurring within the first week after injury), dural penetration, cerebral injury (e.g., penetrating injuries and intracerebral hematomas), depressed skull fractures, focal neurological signs, and post-traumatic amnesia lasting longer than 24 hours. Similar discussions on assessing the risk for penetrating brain lesions are available and support the same principles.[163] Methods for mathematically calculating the risks of seizure occurrence have been developed[164, 165] but are not generally used.

The prophylactic use of anticonvulsants in high-risk patients in order to prevent the later development of a seizure disorder has a long history but is still an area of controversy.[166, 167] Evidence regarding the efficacy of this practice is inconclusive, and clinical practice is varied.[168] In those patients with severe TBI, however, use of anticonvulsants is probably the rule; hence, most patients admitted to rehabilitation programs for acute conditions receive some form of anticonvulsant.

There are substantial adverse cognitive effects caused by the use of phenytoin and phenobarbital.[169] It is now generally accepted that carbamazepine is the anticonvulsant of choice for the long-term management of seizures associated with TBI, due to its low degree of related cognitive impairment.[170] Whether to change a patient from phenytoin or phenobarbital, which is more frequently utilized in neurosurgical settings, to carbamazepine when the patient is apparently tolerating one of the two medications well is an unanswered question at present. Changing drugs increases the risk of a toxic reaction by exposing the patient to a second agent. To continue with phenytoin or phenobarbital will routinely compound the cognitive burden of the impaired patient. Another common clinical dilemma involves the presence of elevated hepatic enzymes in a patient receiving phenytoin. The question is whether to discontinue the drug based on this indicator. Moderate enzyme elevations are known to be common with use of phenytoin and other anticonvulsants and usually indicate enzyme induction rather than hepatocyte toxicity, which does not routinely require more than monitoring.[171]

The issue of whether or not to withdraw anticonvulsant medication after the patient experiences a seizure-free interval also arises routinely. No certain guidelines are available to indicate whether such a withdrawal can be accomplished without seizure occurrence. Wallis has recently conducted a comprehensive review of the factors involved in this decision in general epileptic populations.[172] Several points need to be considered. The rate of relapse is relatively high in adults, ranging from 40 to 60 per cent, but the magnitude of the risks of anticonvulsant withdrawal, including breakthrough seizures, appears relatively small, since both status epilepticus and physical injury as a result of seizure are not frequent. Also, seizures that occur during anticonvulsant withdrawal may represent drug withdrawal seizure rather than a recurrence of epilepsy and, therefore, do not require the reinstitution of medications. No well-defined electroencephalographic indicators are available that assist in defining the risk of recurrence, although the electroencephalogram may be critical to help precisely define the seizure type. The major risks to adults during the withdrawal of medications are felt to be the impact upon driving privileges and job status if seizures recur. In patients with TBI, at least in the population with severe disability, neither driving nor competitive employment is a frequent concern, whereas the possibility of improving cognition routinely is considered to be an important goal. The rationale for attempts at anticonvulsant drug withdrawal in posttraumatic brain-injured patients may, therefore, be more compelling. Also, certain patients may benefit from anticonvulsant withdrawal relatively *early* in the post-injury period. If no documented seizures have occurred, it may be an acceptable clinical risk to perform a trial withdrawal of medication while the patient is still in the protective environment of a rehabilitation unit rather than later when the patient is in the relatively more dangerous community and home setting. In general, it is suggested that patients with TBI be offered the opportunity to undergo anticonvulsant withdrawal after a seizure-free interval lasting three months to two years following the injury.[173]

Other Neurological Conditions. Various other neurological conditions may be associated with TBI on an infrequent basis. Posthypoxic leukoencephalopathy is a potential complication of TBI when hypoxia is an associated pathologic process.[174, 175] Cerebellar ataxia and action tremor have been reported after TBI and successfully managed with beta blockade.[176] Pathological laughing and crying are also known to occur and patients have responded to the administration of antidepressants[177] and L-dopa.[178] Action myoclonus, either as a consequence of hypoxia (Lance-Adams syndrome) or of direct trauma, is a rare complication that responds to specific pharmacological interventions, including the administration of clonazepam, valproate, and 5-hydroxytryptophan.[179] Paroxysmal choreoathetosis rarely has been documented following TBI and has been managed with anticonvulsants.[180, 181] This condition must be differentiated from partial seizures. Stuttering following brain injury has also occurred and been managed with anticonvulsants.[182] Both anorexia and bulimia are not infrequent occurrences following TBI. Aggressive, creative, and persistent feeding programs usually will assist in the resolution of appetite loss, which in many cases is due to hyperesthesias and pathological protective reflexes of the oral apparatus. Bulimia following TBI has been a less frequent but more difficult management problem and may be the result of hypothalamic disturbance. It may·be a manifestation in humans of the Klüver-Bucy syndrome.[183] Successful results with the use of naltrexone in managing this condition following brain injury have recently been reported.[184]

Dementia. One concern of patients and their families is the relationship between traumatic brain injury and the subsequent development of presenile dementia. A number of studies have suggested a relationship between TBI in early life and the subsequent development of Alzheimer's dementia,[185–188] although other (less well-controlled) studies have failed to support this association.[189, 190] Certainly, a recommendation to strictly avoid activities that are likely to contribute further to brain injury is indicated for all patients with TBI; contact sports such as boxing and football and use of neurotoxic substances such as alcohol and illicit drugs should be strongly discouraged.

NEUROSURGICAL REHABILITATION

Although the neurosurgical status of patients with TBI is presumed to be stable at the time of entry into formal rehabilitation settings, certain residual issues remain that must be understood and monitored by the rehabilitation physician.[191] Many patients with TBI are left with cranial defects after craniotomy and require protective head gear until a cranioplasty can be performed, using either preserved autologous bone or synthetic material such as methyl methacrylate. If there has been an infection or foreign body retention in the central nervous system, most surgeons prefer to wait for 12 to 18 months before this repair is performed.

Mass Lesions. Intracranial collections of fluid or blood (subdural, epidural, and intracerebral hematomas and hygromas) are often late consequences of TBI.[192, 193] Beyond the first month after injury, however, the significant complications appear limited to subdural hematoma, infection, and hydrocephalus. A small number of patients who suffer *mild* injury also develop late mass lesions, which require surgical intervention, reportedly as late as 30 days after injury.[194] Subdural hematomas have been followed sequentially after TBI and have been documented to expand or rebleed as late as six months after the initial diagnosis.[195]

Hydrocephalus. Hydrocephalus is a significant consequence of TBI and may appear years after the occurrence of the injury.[196] Most commonly, hydrocephalus appears to be of the *ex vacuo* variety, which reflects primary atrophy of the cerebral mantle secondary to diffuse neuronal degeneration. This type of ventricular enlargement is quite common for severe head injury, reportedly demonstrated in up to 75 to 86 per cent of late follow-up computed tomography scans.[197, 198] This type of hydrocephalus following TBI needs to be differentiated from the dynamic hydrocephalus that reflects impaired or obstructed cerebrospinal fluid circulatory processes, either with or without increased cerebrospinal fluid pressure. The incidence of dynamic hydrocephalus is unclear, since it has been reported in as few as 0.7 per cent of head injuries.[199] Other, more selective studies of TBI have indicated incidences approaching 10 per cent.[200] Since it is a passive reflection of the initial cerebral injury, the *ex vacuo* variety of hydrocephalus needs no intervention. The dynamic form of hydrocephalus, whether characterized by elevated or normal pressure, is often thought to require ventricular shunting, although it is not possible to definitively determine beforehand which patients will benefit from such a procedure.[201]

Abscesses. Cerebral infection following TBI is a relatively rare complication. Factors that are associated with an increased incidence of infection include open cranial injuries, particularly when contamination is present; retained or implanted foreign bodies; and basilar skull fractures associated with dural tears and cerebrospinal fluid leaks, particularly when the sinuses are breached by the fracture line. Cerebral infection can appear many months following the occurrence of the injury. Other, more rare neurosurgical complications include late epidural mass lesions, persistent pneumocephalus (with risk of late meningitis), and vascular lesions (traumatic aneurysms[202] and fistulas[203]).

Overall, as many as 20 per cent of patients in a rehabilitation setting for acute TBI have been shown to have late complications that required neurosurgical intervention. These neurosurgical processes were notable for the slow and insidious manner of their appearance. Routine follow-up computed tomography scanning was recommended for patients with TBI in rehabilitation settings for acute conditions and felt to be indicated in terms of the analysis of cost-benefit and risk-benefit ratios.[204]

OTOLARYNGOLOGICAL REHABILITATION

For the severely brain-injured patient, prolonged endotracheal intubation and tracheostomy are routine. Although the anatomical integrity of the respiratory system has often been restored by the time patients enter into formal rehabilitation programs, steps should be taken during the acute phase to minimize the possible complications of tracheal stenosis and tracheomalacia. Early tracheostomy may minimize incidence of these conditions. Low pressure cuffs should be used whenever possible, and extubation or tracheostomy should not be delayed. Not infrequently, patients still rely on a tracheostomy when they enter rehabilitation. A planned and gradual weaning process by progressive reduction in tracheostomy tube sizes, intermittent plugging of the tube, and the use of tracheostomy buttons contributes to a safe extubation process. Some clinicians have suggested that endoscopy be used in all cases before extubation to rule out occult airway obstruction from granulations.[205]

ORTHOPEDIC REHABILITATION

Fractures are perhaps the most common inadequately treated condition associated with TBI, and unsatisfactory fracture healing is the most preventable complication. Aggressive operative intervention in the early period following injury is a major principle of orthopedic management.[206–208] Immediate fixation within 24 hours of injury results in improved general and orthopedic outcomes.[209] External or internal fixation of major fractures rather than casting or traction is often preferred, since the development of later agitation or severe spasticity may impede the beneficial effects of these latter methods. When done, casting should not produce flexed positions that tend to exacerbate the deformities secondary to neurological posturing. The practice of treating orthopedic problems expectantly in severely head-injured patients on the presumption that the patient will not survive is common and should be strongly resisted. Resulting functional losses due to severe contractures have been shown to be a major contributor to failed rehabilitation.[210]

Nonoperative techniques have been reported for the management of neurologically induced joint contractures. Simple positioning and the use of range-of-motion exercises are of first importance and must always be a primary goal of nursing management. Other approaches include static and dynamic splinting (including serial splint-casting)[211] and the administration of antispasmodics.[212] For isolated spasticity problems, nerve and motor-point blocks using phenol or alcohol are feasible and play a role in the diagnosis and management of specific spasticity problems.[213–215] Functional electrical stimulation has been reported to assist in physical therapy of the neuromuscularly impaired patient with TBI.[216]

The decision to undertake operative interventions to correct contractures or muscular imbalances should be made only after careful consideration. The recovery process in TBI is prolonged and not uniform. The proper surgical solution to contractures or muscle imbalance problems is different in each patient. It has been recommended that a minimum of 18 months be allowed to pass following injury before definitive surgical releases or tendon transpositions are done.[217] If these precautions are disregarded, overcorrection or other unanticipated results of surgery may occur. Exceptions to this prohibition of early surgery may apply to *simple* contractures when significant rehabilitation obstacles result from not correcting these defects. The most common example of this type of correction is the lengthening of the Achilles tendon for equinus deformity. Early performance of this procedure frequently allows patients to become safely ambulatory; conversely, extensive reconstruction of the forefoot should be deferred to prevent the possibility of complications such as the development of rocker-bottom foot.

Preoperative polyelectromyographic examination has been shown to be helpful in identifying specific pathological patterns of muscle activation and spasticity and, thereby, providing a guide for surgical intervention.[218, 219] Specific discussion of surgical considerations for the common orthopedic problems following TBI recently have been offered.[220, 221]

The management of generalized spasticity is, however, more problematic in the head-injured patient. The majority of antispasmodic medications are generally contraindicated in TBI owing to their sedative and cognition-impairing properties, and owing to the incoordination, ataxia, and generalized weakness they produce.[222] Dantrolene sodium, which acts directly upon the contractile mechanism of muscle, may be the preferred antispasmodic medication in TBI. The benzodiazepines are characteristically associated with production of antegrade amnesia and, therefore, may be particularly undesirable in the patient with TBI.[223]

Heterotopic Ossification. Heterotopic ossification occurs after TBI and is not histologically different from that seen in other predisposing conditions. It has been reported, however, to have a distinctive distribution in contrast with spinal cord injury, with heterotopic ossification more consistently periarticular and with a higher prevalence in the upper extremities. The incidence of the condition has been reported to be from 11 to 20 per cent.[224] As with this condition elsewhere in the body, proper management is unclear. It is generally accepted that moderate nontraumatic range-of-motion exercises are appropriate, as is attention to limb positioning to minimize functional deficit from any loss of range of motion that does develop. The value of aggressive ranging to the limits of toleration or performing joint mobilization under general anesthesia has not been proved. Etidronate disodium has been used for this condition after TBI, although the long-term benefit has yet to be demonstrated conclusively.[225] The consideration of any surgical approach to the resection of bone tissue must weigh the risks and benefits of such a major procedure. Surgery is justified only when the defect hinders progress toward significant functional goals. As with heterotopic ossification in other conditions, a maturation period of 12–18 months is usually recommended to allow bone maturity to occur, which is felt to minimize regrowth after resection. Regrowth of bone following excision may be more likely in more severely injured patients.[226] In certain clinical situations in which rapid mobilization has significant therapeutic and functional results, early surgical removal has been effectively done in some head injury centers.[227]

Scoliosis. Scoliosis and other problems of trunk and pelvic posture due to neuromuscular imbalance, spasticity, and abnormal patterning are common following severe TBI. It has been pointed out that prior to achieving optimal limb control and function, the stability and appropriate posture of the pelvis and trunk must be ensured.[228] Thus, attention to comfortable seating systems for wheelchair-dependent patients that provide maximum stability and position of pelvis and trunk and inhibition of pathoneurological patterns, e.g., symmetrical and asymmetrical tonic neck or flexor and extensor mass reflexes, is a routinely important initial step before functional self-care goals can be effectively approached.[229, 230]

Structural curvature of the spine secondary to neuroparalytic imbalance is a known problem in the young, growing patient. However, curves in the adult do occur and are exhibited with complaints of pain, progression, cardiopulmonary symptoms, and cosmetic deformity. Custom-fitted seating devices may prevent such progression and increase seating tolerance. Progression and pain appear to be the most common indications for surgical correction in the adult, which has been recommended for curves greater than from 60 to 100 degrees.[231] However, no reports are available on the surgical management of scoliosis specifically following acquired brain injury in the adult.

UROLOGIC REHABILITATION

Urinary tract infections are frequent complications following TBI and are usually associated with placement of indwelling catheters. Unless persistent reinfection occurs, no elaborate evaluation of the genitourinary system is usually indicated. The principal type of incontinence found following TBI indicates an uninhibited bladder, which results from direct injury to those cortical structures of sensation, awareness, judgment, and initiative that are directed toward elimination functions. It may be startling to find a patient with TBI with significant frontal injury but without motor or sensory loss who, although perfectly alert and cooperative, is routinely incontinent and who is seemingly unaware of this problem, even when cued by staff. In spite of instruction, these patients may persistently fail to initiate appropriate behaviors to manage voiding or bowel evacuation. It is not unreported, however, for detrusor-sphincter dyssynergia to occur following TBI,[232] although no prospective studies of the relative frequency of this problem are available. Such cases may reflect lower brain stem injury. Occult spinal injury must be kept in mind as a cause as well, although diffuse bilateral cerebral injury has been reported to be associated with a dyssynergic sphincter pattern on urodynamic study.[233]

The satisfactory resolution of bladder and bowel dysfunction is of critical importance in the overall success of the rehabilitation effort. Incontinence is a very effective barrier to re-entry into any type of community function and also is a highly efficient predictor of the need for placement in a long-term skilled nursing facility.

OLFACTORY REHABILITATION

Anosmia is frequent following TBI. The incidence increases as severity of injury rises and has been reported as high as 20 per cent in patients whose post-traumatic amnesia lasted more than seven days.[234] Loss of smell has been demonstrated to have a cognitive component (recognition) as well, even when frank anosmia is not present.[235]

VISUAL REHABILITATION

Visual loss can be due to injuries in multiple locations throughout the visual pathway. When the injury is to the optic nerve, little is available in the way of treatment. However, the possibility of successfully retraining patients with visual field defects due to cortical lesions has been reported,[236, 237] although these findings have not been replicated in another laboratory[238] and there is continuing discussion regarding the discrepancies involved in the disparate findings.[239] The theoretical implications of this purported restitution by training of patients with late, fixed, neurological deficits for the field of general rehabilitation of brain injury are significant.

Neuroparalytic visuomotor paresis with diplopia is a common problem following TBI. Mechanical etiologies such as muscle entrapment syndromes from edema or orbital fractures need to be ruled out rapidly. Diplopia secondary to neuroparalytic or neuroparetic etiology is more common. The common practice of alternate patching of each eye is only indicated in older children (over age of six) and adults if impairment of function or patient distress dictates its use. A therapeutic process of stimulating fusion by approximating the split images may be accomplished by partially correcting lenses made of polycarbonate. If the diplopia is persistent, specific surgical techniques are available to offer correction, particularly the adjustable suture technique. Neger has comprehensively reviewed the ophthalmological treatment of the patient with TBI.[240]

Facial Nerve. Injury to the facial nerve is not uncommon and may be peripheral or central in etiology. If severe and persistent, temporary closure of the eyelid by tarsorrhaphy may be indicated to prevent corneal ulceration while the patient recovers. Due to decreased cognitive abilities in TBI, the utility of cranial nerve transfer procedures, which require extensive postoperative neuromotor retraining of the patient for success, is marginal, and these procedures should be approached with caution in patients with TBI.

AUDITORY REHABILITATION

Cranial nerve VIII and the associated auditory apparatus are very frequently involved following TBI. Up to 70 per cent of patients admitted to a neurotrauma center following head injury demonstrated pathological involvement of the ear. Such dysfunction is frequently associated with fractures of the temporal bone. It has been recommended that a combination of direct otological examination, high-resolution computed tomography, and auditory evoked potentials is necessary to adequately evaluate the possible deficits in this system.[241]

Other injuries to the auditory-vestibular apparatus may produce the frequent sequelae of dizziness. General treatment may be effective,[242] although a treatable cause of this complaint is a perilymphatic fistula, which may resemble Ménière's disease.[243]

VELOPHARYNGEAL REHABILITATION

Velopharyngeal insufficiency is common, usually occurring secondary to associated cranial nerve injury, and contributes to feeding dysfunction and hypernasality of speech. Techniques such as palatal push backs, pharyngeal flaps, or muscle transfers have been used successfully to correct these difficulties. Extended courses of recovery of cranial nerve dysfunction are not uncommon following TBI and, therefore, definitive procedures such as velopharyngoplasty should await clear evidence of stability of the neuromuscular picture. Such operative procedures have been performed with good success in patients with TBI, however, when proper attention to technique is given. For greater degrees of palatal insufficiency, the lateral port control pharyngeal flap has been shown to be particularly useful for patients with TBI.[244] Prosthetic approaches to flaccid insufficiency, such as a palatal prosthesis, are generally not well tolerated by patients with TBI and, therefore, are less effective unless the patient's level of cognitive function and insight allow full appreciation of the need for this approach. Dysarthria and dysphagia may occur due to spasticity, flaccidity, and apraxia, which are to be expected.

Dysphonia. Dysphonia may occur following TBI secondary to CNS injury, tenth nerve involvement, or direct damage to the vocal cords from prolonged or traumatic intubation. Delayed recovery of function is possible. When recovery from dysphonia secondary to unilateral true vocal cord paralysis is excessively delayed or does not occur or, occasionally, if aspiration is a continual problem due to unilateral paralysis, improvement may be temporarily or permanently produced by a local injection of collagen[245] or Teflon paste[246] in the region of the vocal cord.

D. NATHAN COPE

REHABILITATION OF LANGUAGE FUNCTION

The presence of language disturbance following TBI is commonplace, even after relatively minor injuries. A recent study found that *no* patient suffering from a coma, regardless of how brief, was free of significant linguistic disturbance an average of one year after injury.[247] Classical aphasias of distinct types are rare in TBI, and attempts to fit observed language disturbances into these traditional patterns tend to be misleading. Aphasias after head injury have been characterized and exhibit a combined picture of mixed receptive and expressive types, with strong elements of linguistic, conceptual, or cognitive overlay.[248–250] The use of speech or communication aids such as alphabet boards and electronic communication devices (e.g., Canon, Words +, and Sharp) are occasionally helpful, but before elaborate communication aids are prescribed, a very careful assessment of the patient's cognitive and emotional capacity to use these sophisticated devices must be done.

COGNITIVE AND BEHAVIORAL DEFICITS

The cognitive and behavioral disturbances that follow TBI have proved to be major disabling features in the patient's functional recovery.[251, 252] Currently, a major focus of rehabilitation intervention is the design and implementation of cognitive retraining or remediation programs.[253–256] The rationale for these programs includes the supposition that specific deficits in cognitive functioning may be identified following various injuries to the brain; that the brain has both the ability to recover from such injuries and deficits, to a variable degree, and to acquire compensatory capabilities to replace deficits that are irrecoverable; and, finally, that the extent to which such recovery occurs is significantly dependent on specific therapeutic remediation or training interventions. Theoretical aspects of this concept are complex and are not extensively discussed here but are available elsewhere.[257, 258]

Programs designed to enhance basic attention, memory, language, and visuospatial function are representative of such cognitive retraining programs. It appears that the evidence to date to some extent supports these programs' ability to improve vigilance, attention, and visuospatial aspects of disability more than memory.[259] For example, Sivak has demonstrated the correlation of improved driving performance in patients following specific treatment for visuospatial deficit compared with that of a nonspecifically treated control group.[260] Controlled studies of general cognitive treatment approaches indicate that improved neuropsychological functioning as well as improved work and academic capability results from treatment.[261] The value of such approaches has yet to be unequivocally demonstrated, and it is unclear which patients and problems benefit from such treatment.

Stimulation of the Patient in Coma. A clinical intervention related to cognitive remediation is stimulation of the patient in coma by attempting to improve or increase the rate of recovery and arousal of the patient through increasing sensorimotor input.[262] It is hypothesized that increasing baseline stimulation to critical brain structures, presumably including the reticular activating system in particular, promotes arousal and recovery of these patients. The deleterious effects of sensory deprivation may be minimized in this way as well. No experimental confirmation of the overall efficacy of such approaches in altering the recovery pattern of such patients is available.[263] Several suggestive findings of such approaches include reports of increased arousal and improvement in findings on electroencephalograms in four patients in prolonged persistent vegetative states following dorsal column stimulation;[264] and improvement of the comatose patient's condition, as reflected in electroencephalographic and clinical studies, following sensorimotor therapy.[265] Several clinical considerations are evident in participating or recommending such programs, however, independent of the question of primary efficacy. First, such programs allow families of patients to begin earlier participation in the care of the patient with TBI. This active involvement may then facilitate realistic understanding of patient deficits and promote an appropriate grieving process. Families are known to pursue inappropriate levels of treatment for extended periods when these psychological tasks are not completed. A coma stimulation program, if used, should not only promote early involvement of the family with the patient during the rehabilitation process, therefore, but also interaction of the rehabilitation team with the family and realistic attitudes toward the patient's recovery. Conversely, inappropriate representation of these programs by professionals can promote dysfunctional expectations of recovery for the patient and family. Second, attention to maintenance of physiological systems is encouraged by the optimism engendered in the family by such programs. Third, arousal of the patient from coma, when it does occur, is presumably identified earlier by the primary caregivers, and appropriate interventions are performed. Concerns about the use of such programs, however, include the misuse of medical and economic resources, physical and emotional exhaustion of family members, and the development of excessive or unrealistic expectations for the patient's recovery by the family.[266]

PSYCHIATRIC AND PSYCHOLOGICAL REHABILITATION

Psychiatric and neuropsychological disturbances are also major reasons for the lack of success in the patient's rehabilitation and reintegration into independent community settings.[267, 268] The patient's characteristic lack of self-awareness, poor impulse control, memory deficits, and behavioral disturbances are not addressed by traditional methods of occupational, physical, speech, and nursing rehabilitation.[269] In response to the emerging recognition of such behaviors as an important issue following TBI and the need to reliably measure them, Levin and associates have developed the Neurobehavioral Rating Scale, which is designed to allow staff to reliably identify and quantify such activity demonstrated by patients with TBI.[270] These behaviorial problems may frequently impede conventional rehabilitative therapeutic approaches, which could be used to treat the patient's more traditional rehabilitation problems, by preventing meaningful patient cooperation or limiting patient understanding and learning. The patient with TBI is frequently unresponsive to usual degrees or types of motivating interventions, is disruptive of unit and therapeutic routines, and often is violent and assaultive. Interestingly, violent behavior in the population at large has been associated with individuals who have suffered significant head trauma.[271] Although physical disabilities after TBI tend to decrease in significance, psychological and behavioral difficulties have been known to frequently increase with time following injury.[272] In this sense, it may be said that "as head-injured patients get better, they get worse."

Organic aggressiveness is well known, and the pathophysiology is only partially understood. Damage to many cerebral structures may be associated with affective disturbances, including aggression.[273, 274] Dysfunction seems to most frequently involve frontal, temporal, and limbic regions, although generalized diffuse cortical loss may produce similar syndromes as well. Unless the aggressiveness is clearly the result of seizure activity, i.e., complex partial or temporal-limbic sei-

zures, the electroencephalogram is not helpful in the diagnosis of most organically related disturbances.[275] Evoked potentials may have some correlation with such behavior, perhaps associated with diminished reticular formation output that would aid in the diagnosis of the condition. Due to the common combination of residual or resolving medical and surgical problems and rehabilitation concerns associated with these behavioral disorders, rehabilitation units and staff that treat patients with TBI now require a combination of medical or surgical and psychological or psychiatric management skills. Innovative architectural approaches have freed professionals from the reliance on medications or restraints in the treatment of these patients. For example, management of the restless, agitated patient who is emerging from coma frequently requires control of the patient's attempts to leave bed or wander from the unit. Traditional approaches to this problem have involved heavy sedation or limb restraints. Newer solutions to this clinical problem include "locked" or otherwise secure seclusion rooms. The method of the architecturally secure or "locked" unit allows confused patients to freely ambulate while preventing elopement from the floor. In some cases, fabrication of a walled, padded, floor level enclosure allows the patient to move freely but with a minimum of restraints.[277] If intravenous or other tube maintenance or other medical management issues are critical, however, there should be no reluctance to adequately sedate or restrain the patient.

Behavioral Programs. For occasions when these techniques and skills of the TBI unit prove inadequate in the management of disturbed behavior, a specific type of TBI program, the behavioral program, has been developed. Behavioral programs are generally based upon learning and social principles and are structured to provide strict contingency management.[278, 279] When the behavioral disturbance following injury is too extreme to be handled with normal management capabilities in the usual rehabilitation setting, patients should ideally be transferred to such a specialized unit. Here, the most severely aggressive and dysfunctional social behaviors are eliminated through extinction and positive and negative reinforcement methods. Substantial successes have been reported in controlling even long-standing intractable patients in such centers.[280]

Nosology. Little work has been done to clarify the nosology of the psychiatric disturbances following TBI, although some early discussions are available.[281–283]

DEPRESSION. Depression following TBI undoubtedly occurs.[284, 285] The diagnosis of depression in brain-injured patients, however, remains problematic in that biological signs are difficult to differentiate from strict neurological deficits. Also, the linguistic defects of the brain-injured patient make self-reported historical evidence unreliable.[286] Suicide is not unknown,[287] although it is surprisingly infrequent considering the magnitude of loss that confronts patients with TBI. However, the specific elements of depressive syndromes following TBI remain to be elucidated. Neurochemical and neuroendocrine changes have been reported.[288] Use of insight-targeted psychodynamic treatment is frequently ineffective, at least for the patients with severe cases of TBI, due to the memory and cognitive deficits characteristic of the head-injured patient. In general, supportive and structured approaches are more appropriate, as are efforts to help the patient and family develop an appropriate and self-fulfilling social and vocational environment. Nevertheless, effective psychotherapeutic approaches have been recently described.[289] Antidepressants and electroconvulsive therapy[290] appear to be effective in the treatment for this organic depressive syndrome.

MANIA. Bipolar or manic-depressive psychosis is known to occur after a variety of organic brain lesions and is increasingly being reported following TBI.[291] Characteristics of this TBI-based manic syndrome, which seem to differentiate it from idiopathic or primary bipolar disease, include the lack of grandiosity or hallucinations, and irritability rather than euphoria.

SCHIZOPHRENIA. Schizophrenia and schizophreniform psychoses are reported after TBI, but the question of whether the rate is above the expected incidence of the population at large remains unanswered.[292] A higher rate of significant psychosis has been recently reported following severe head injury.[293]

Psychotropic Medications. The commonplace use of psychoactive medications in the treatment of organic brain syndromes, including those secondary to TBI, is not usually appreciated. It is irrefutable that extensive overuse and misuse occurs.[294, 295] Control of behavior disturbances, particularly agitated, confused, and aggressive behavior, is the most common reason for psychopharmacological treatment within the many settings in which TBI patients routinely reside, e.g., hospitals, rehabilitation facilities, skilled nursing facilities, and group residential homes. Before resorting to any psychopharmacological approach, it should be appreciated that appropriate staffing, contingency management, and staff training can significantly decrease the frequency of, or eliminate, this type of behavior.[296] Pharmacological management is common, particularly in institutions with deficiencies in staff or training. When pharmacological control of behavior is initiated, there is excessive dependency on the use of antipsychotics. There is, however, a lack of data demonstrating the efficacy of antipsychotics in managing the disruptive behaviors of the brain-injured patient short of doses that sedate (and, thereby, suppress) all behaviors, the adaptive as well as the problematic.[297]

There is growing recognition of a variety of possible alternative psychopharmacological choices for the management of such behavior disorders. These possibilities include antidepressants, lithium, beta-blockers, anticonvulsants, stimulants, and others. Specifics of the relative indications among these choices have been recently comprehensively reviewed.[298] However, clinicians using psychotropic medications for the management of behavioral disturbances following TBI must be cognizant that, at present, indications for such use are empirical. The choice of one class of drug over another may be suggested by clinical features, but the appropriateness of the choice is always subject to clinical demonstration in the individual patient. In practice, this requires utilization of some form of single-case design for each patient treated. Several reports of successful cases illustrating this technique have recently been published.[299–301] A baseline, a treatment, and a placebo or washout phase are all essential features of such an approach, as well as quantifiable, operationally defined target behaviors.[302]

Also, it is essential to appreciate that many of the effects of psychopharmacological drugs (and those of other classes of agents) have significant effects upon attention and cognition. Literature is evolving that focuses on efforts to improve cognition with specific pharmacological treatment with the cholinergic agonists, psychostimulants, antidepressants, and neuroactive peptides following TBI.[303–309] It is clear, however, that the inadvertent clinical impairment of these cognitive processes by drugs given for other purposes is much more common.[310] There is also the likelihood that psychoactive drugs may either facilitate or impair the patient's recovery from lesions of the central nervous system. Catecholaminergic blockade (particularly noradrenergic blockade) appears to impede recovery and, thus, is another relative contraindication for the use of antipsychotics and other antiadrenergic agents. Conversely, psychostimulants and other adrenergic agonists may increase the rate or degree of recovery from brain damage. Sutton, Feeney, and Hayes have recently discussed these issues.[311-313]

Length of Recovery

Coinciding with and to some extent providing theoretical support for the development of these novel categorical programs for extended treatment of TBI is an emerging new perspective toward mammalian central nervous system injury and recovery. Although it has always been known that recovery of function often occurs after brain injury, the extent of such recovery has been seen as strictly limited. Previously, the degree to which such recovery occurred was thought to be related directly and only to the severity of injury, or alternatively stated, the residual amount of the central nervous system that was preserved. Beyond maintenance of a physiologically supportive environment in which to promote neuronal survival, no other treatment was thought to improve results. This structural, "hard-wired" conception of central nervous system function limited, to some extent, ideas regarding the intensity and length of rehabilitation deemed appropriate for the brain-injured patient.

However, basic investigation into the limits of the recovery process of the central nervous system in experimental animals (specifically in mammals, including primates) has indicated that a much greater potential for recovery exists than was previously thought. The brain is now seen as able to compensate, to some variable degree, for loss of tissue from a variety of causes, and this recovery is also thought to be dependent on retraining after the injury. This newly appreciated potential is related to the concept of brain "plasticity." This concept states that rather than being an invariably fixed organ with rigid structure and function relationships, the brain is able to respond to injury by reorganization and increased functional capacity. This ability implies that rehabilitation techniques may be important in the facilitation of this reorganization and recovery of function after injury. A number of recent monographs and reviews have summarized the evidence supporting this emerging area of theory and investigation.[314-317]

This newly delineated potential for enhanced recovery through appropriate rehabilitation as well as the clinical observation that functional recovery, particularly of complex and learned behaviors,

proceeds for extensive periods (in some cases for many years) after TBI have supported the rationale for extended, graded, TBI rehabilitation programs.

Reflecting all these considerations, current "comprehensive" brain injury rehabilitation involves treatment for many years in a variety of settings from the acute hospital, to residential and day institutions, and, finally, to educational and vocational programs.[318] Patients move sequentially through various elements of this "system" of treatment programs until maximum function is achieved (see Fig. 59–1). Currently, an average acute hospital stay for a patient with severe TBI may have a duration of several months, followed by an acute hospital–based rehabilitation stay lasting 2 to 4 months, followed by 6 to 18 months in various community-based programs. There are many case reports of delayed and prolonged recovery (see earlier discussion). Varghese followed a cohort of TBI patients for two years after injury, using the Glasgow Outcome Scale, and reported that 68 per cent of patients had continued to improve over that interval.[319] Thomas and Mayer reported three cases of delayed functional recovery of head-injured patients who were hospitalized as long as four years before they first entered a rehabilitation program.[320] A report from Israel documented nine cases of significant recovery in patients who had been in comas for a year or more.[321] Such cases have demonstrated that delayed recovery does occur but suggests that such recovery reflects the alleviation of prolonged neglect. The possibility of prolonged *continued* recovery in patients who receive ongoing treatment from time of injury was suggested in a case report of such improvement during treatment over a four-year post-injury treatment program.[322]

Goals of Rehabilitation

Many of the treatment objectives used in rehabilitation for TBI are similar to those used in other chronic disabling neurological conditions. The restitution of sensorimotor capacity, mobility, capacity for self-care, and communicative functions is, of course, the routine goal of rehabilitation for TBI. Increased cognitive, behavioral, and social functions are additional aims. It is felt that recovery is more prolonged for the complex aspects of higher cognition and social skills than for the more basic motor functions or cognitive activities of memory or information processing. This should not be surprising, since even with extensive injury, the central nervous system continues to be an organ of "learning;" new tasks can be mastered, even if at a slower rate or by means of alternative cognitive strategies. In these instances, the process of rehabilitation is truly an educational one, i.e., eliciting compensation for functional losses rather than attempting to restore neuronal deficits.

Despite this perspective of an improved and less limited prognosis for TBI and the possibility of expanded long-term treatment objectives, it must be appreciated that the prospects for recovery from severe TBI often remain limited. Overall reports of return to employment after severe head injury are not encouraging. Various reports indicate that between one third to two thirds of TBI patients remain unemployed following injury.[323, 324] A two-year follow-up of patients with TBI severe enough to require referral to an inpatient rehabilitation program revealed that only about 10 per cent had returned to competitive employment.[325] A group of moderately to severely injured patients with TBI who received prolonged neuropsychological treatment had a re-employment rate of up to 65 per cent. However, this rate was noted to drop to 50 per cent over time.[326]

For the majority of patients with TBI who are injured severely enough to require comprehensive inpatient rehabilitation, some significant reduction in dependency is the most realistic and still very important goal. Assisting a TBI patient to achieve independence in self-care, feeding, cooking, or mobility in the community is extremely valued by the patient and his or her family. Any such reduction in dependency will generate tremendous savings in the cost of care over the lifetime of that patient. Associated with the goal of reducing dependency is the goal of diminishing social isolation and anomie. The lack of social sensitivity that is so characteristic of these patients requires intensive effort toward re-education and reacquisition of social skills. Late behavioral difficulties and overall deterioration have been related to the lack of supportive and rewarding social environments for these individuals; by maximizing the quality of social life, regression and dependency are minimized.

The Family of the Patient with TBI

Due to the poor social skills that are characteristic of patients with TBI and the extended period of treatment, the family becomes a critical element in supporting the patient's long-term recovery and adjustments to disability. At the same time, as a result of the need to provide this support, the burdens on families caring for these patients are enormous. Families of head-injured individuals are recognized to have distinct stresses and burdens related to the patient with TBI.[327–330] Rosenbaum and Najenson compared emotional distress in matched samples of spouses of patients with TBI and spinal cord–injured patients and reported that whereas the wives of spinal cord–injured patients achieved an increased adjustment over the year after injury, the wives of patients with TBI had *increasing* levels of distress.[331] Since families of head-injured patients have been noted to tend to deteriorate over time,[332, 333] the achievement of the maximum potential rehabilitation of the TBI patient implies the need for maintaining the family of the patient with TBI as well. It appears that patients who do not have or who cannot obtain this supportive family environment have a poorer outcome than those who do have a supportive family environment. Therefore, a major rehabilitation goal is to assist these primary care providers (spouse and families) to acquire those skills (medical, psychological economic, and social) needed to carry out their long-term task of assisting the patient with TBI. Important components of this goal are, for example, to plan for and support home-care aides or assistants or to provide families with intermittent respite from direct care responsibility.

Cost-Benefit Ratio of the Rehabilitation of Patients with TBI

Given the pervading theme that recovery from TBI proceeds for significantly more extensive periods than that for traditional rehabilitation programs, it is not unusual to find active and aggressive multidisciplinary treatment continuing for two to four years after injury.

Probably no other diagnostic entity entails a requirement for longer or more intensive treatment than that now recommended for TBI. The expense of such treatment for severe head injury is commonly in the six figure range. It is increasingly necessary to address both the evidence for efficacy and the cost-benefit ratio of such treatment. To date, the work needed to clearly answer these questions has not been completed. Although a definitive demonstration of the efficacy of this lengthy period of comprehensive treatment is difficult to obtain, there are reports that appear to support this long-term comprehensive approach to treatment[334] and that suggest that this extensive comprehensive rehabilitative effort is both efficacious and cost-efficient. In 1984, Aronow compared patients who, after sustaining TBI, were treated solely with intensive acute neurosurgical and medical care, with only random individual therapy given (N = 61), with equally severely injured patients receiving both acute care and extended comprehensive rehabilitation (N = 61). Assessment of function and dependency was performed two years after injury, and the level of care needed and associated increased costs were calculated. Annual savings in such costs for patients who were rehabilitated, compared with patients who received equivalent acute care but no rehabilitation, were at high as $11,949 each. Total annual savings for the group undergoing rehabilitation was calculated to be $335,842, and the cost of their rehabilitation was calculated to be regained after three years of such savings.[337]

The importance of initiating comprehensive rehabilitation soon after injury was demonstrated in a similar study of carefully matched patients with TBI who were placed quickly into a comprehensive acute rehabilitation program or who were delayed in admission to such a program. The length of time necessary to bring the delayed group to an equivalent level of function (and discharge from the rehabilitation program) was doubled from 43 to 89 days, with an estimated increase in cost of $40,000 per patient.[338] Similar benefits have also been reported in later transitional and day-based rehabilitation programs.[339] Cole and associates reported on their experience with a community-based, low-intensity, educationally and socially oriented program for patients with chronic disabilities from TBI who had completed all formal rehabilitation. Treatment was begun at an average of 25.7 months after injury and all patients had demonstrated an inability to function at an independent level in educational or supported work settings, yet 47 per cent of these patients attained an improved level of function within the program to enable them to move into higher levels of functioning. Cost was reported to average $3 per hour per patient, indicating that relatively nonprofessional and low-cost programs may be beneficial for extended periods after injury.[340]

The general problems in performing such research on outcome are extensive, and more definitive studies await the development of adequate indices of severity and nosology and instruments to assess outcome itself.[341]

Conclusion

The rehabilitation of the patient with TBI is a new and growing area. Many of the appropriate techniques are yet to be defined. More than in nearly any other area of rehabilitation, care of patients with TBI calls on the physiatrist to understand and utilize the full spectrum of methods in neurological and behavioral sciences, for although the physical disabilities after TBI can be significant, the psychological, psychiatric, and neurological sequelae are routinely the limiting factors in the rehabilitation of these patients. Rehabilitation medicine is only beginning the investigation into these topics and into appropriate rehabilitation approaches.

References

1. National Directory of Head Injury Rehabilitation Services, 1989 Ed. Southborough, Ma., The National Head Injury Foundation, 1989.
2. Frankowski, R. F.: The demography of head injury in the United States. In Miner, M. E., and Wagner, K. A. (Eds.): Neurotrauma: Treatment, Rehabilitation, and Related Issues, No. 1. Boston, Butterworths Publishers, 1986, pp. 1–17.
3. Anderson, D. W., and McLaurin, R. L.: The national head and spinal cord injury survey. J. Neurosurg., 53:S1–S43, 1980.
4. Jennett, B., and Teasdale, G.: Management of Head Injuries. Philadelphia, F.A. Davis Company, 1981, pp. 1–8.
5. Schwartz, R. H.: Alcohol, drugs, and head injury. Pediatrics, 78:1169, 1986.
6. Kraus, J. F., Fife, D., Ramstein, K., et al: The relationship of family income to the incidence, external causes, and outcomes of serious brain injury, San Diego County, California. AJPH 1986; 76:1345-1347.
7. Kraus, J. F., Black, M. A., Hessol, N., et al: The incidence of acute brain injury and serious impairment in a defined population. Am. J. Epidemiol., 119:186–201, 1983.
8. Anderson, D. W., McLaurin, R. L.: The national head and spinal cord injury survey. J. Neurosurg., 53:S1–S43, 1980.
9. Oppenheimer, D. R.: Microscopic lesions in the brain following head injury. J. Neurol. Neurosurg. Psychiatry, 31:299–306, 1968.
10. Bach-Y-Rita, P.: Brain plasticity as a basis of the

development of rehabilitation procedures for hemiplegia. Scand. J. Rehabil. Med., 13:73–83, 1981.

11. Prigatano, G. P., and Fordyce, D. J.: Cognitive dysfunction and psychosocial adjustment after brain injury. *In* Prigatano, G. P. (Ed.): Neuropsychological Rehabilitation after Brain Injury. Baltimore, Johns Hopkins University Press, 1986, pp. 12–14.

12. Ommaya, A. K., and Genarelli, T. A.: Cerebral concussion and traumatic unconsciousness: Correlation of experimental and clinical observations on blunt head injuries. Brain, 97:633–654, 1974.

13. Berrol, S.: Moderate Head Injury. National Invitational Conference on Traumatic Brain Injury (TBI) Research. Tyson's Corner's, VA, National Institute on Disability Rehabilitation Research (NIDRR), 1987.

14. Jane, J. A., and Gennarelli, T.: Axonal degeneration induced by experimental noninvasive minor head injury. J. Neurosurg., 62:96–100, 1985.

15. Rimel, R. W., Giordani, B., and Barth, J. T., et al: Disability caused by minor head injury. Neurosurgery, 9:221–228, 1981.

16. Rutherford, W. H., Merrett, J. D., and McDonald, J. R.: Sequelae of concussion caused by minor head injury. Lancet, i:1-4, 1977.

17. Levin, H. S., Handel, S. F., Goldman, A. M., et al: Magnetic resonance imaging after "diffuse" nonmissile head injury. Arch. Neurol., 42:963–986, 1985.

18. Jane, J. A., Rimel, R. W., Pobereskin, L. H., et al: Outcome and pathology of head injury. *In* Grussman, R. G., Gildenberg, P. L. (Eds.): Head Injury: Basic and Clinical Aspects. New York, Raven Press, 1982, pp. 229–236.

19. Povlishock, J. T., Becker, D. P., Cheng, C. L. Y., et al: Axonal change in minor head injury. J. Neuropathol. Exp. Neurol., 42:225–242, 1983.

20. Barth, J. T., Macchiocchi, S. N., Giordani, B., et al: Neuropsychological sequelae of minor head injury. Neurosurgery, 13:529–533, 1983.

21. Gronwall, D., and Wrightson, P.: Cumulative effects of concussion. Lancet, ii:995–997, 1975.

22. Report of the Board of Science and Education Working Party on Boxing. London, British Medical Association, 1984.

23. Morrison, R. G.: Medical and public health aspects of boxing. J. A. M. A., 255:2475–2480, 1986.

24. Rimel, R., Giordani, B., Barth, J., et al: Moderate head injury: completing the clinical spectrum of brain trauma. Neurosurgery, 11:344-351, 1982.

25. McMillan, T. M., and Glucksman, E. E.: The neuropsychology of moderate head injury. J. Neurol. Neurosurg. Psychiatry, 50:393–397, 1987.

26. Rimel, R. W., Giordani, B., Barth, J. T., et al: Moderate head injury: Completing the clinical spectrum of brain trauma. Neurosurgery, 11:344–351, 1982.

27. Jennett, B., and Teasdale, G.: Management of

Head Injuries. Philadelphia, F.A. Davis Company, 1981, pp. 318–319.

28. Jennett, B., and Plum F.: Persistent vegetative state after brain damage. Lancet, 1:734–737, 1972.

29. Bricolo, A., Turazzi, S., and Feriotti, G.: Prolonged post-traumatic unconsciousness. Therapeutic assets and liabilities. J. Neurosurg., 52:625–634, 1980.

30. Walshe, T. M., and Leonard, C.: Persistent vegetative state: Extension of the syndrome to include chronic disorders. Arch. Neurol., 42:1045-1052, 1985.

31. Teasdale, G., and Jennett, B.: Assessment of coma and impaired consciousness: A practical scale. Lancet, 2:81–84, 1974.

32. Jennett, B., and Teasdale, G.: Management of Head Injuries. Philadelphia, F.A. Davis Company, 1981, p. 81.

33. Jennett, B., and Bond, M.: Assessment of outcome after severe brain damage. Lancet 1:480–484, 1975.

34. Jennett, B., Snoek, J., and Bond, M. R., et al: Disability after severe head injury: Observations on the use of the Glasgow Outcome Scale. J. Neurol. Neurosurg. Psychiatry, 44:285-293, 1981.

35. Rappaport, M., Hall, K. M., Hopkins, K., et al: Disability rating scale for severe head trauma: Coma to community. Arch. Phys. Med. Rehabil., 63:118–123, 1982.

36. Hall, K., Cope, D. N., and Rappaport, M.: Glasgow outcome scale and disability rating scale: Comparative usefulness in following recovery in traumatic head injury. Arch. Phys. Med. Rehabil., 66:35–37, 1985.

37. Hagen, C., Malkmus, D., and Durham, P.: Levels of cognitive functioning. *In*: Rehabilitation of the Head Injured Adult: Comprehensive Physical Management. Downey, CA, Professional Staff Association of Rancho Los Amigos Hospital, Inc., 1979, pp. 87–88.

38. Jennett, B., and Teasdale, G.: Management of Head Injuries. Philadelphia, F.A. Davis Company, 1981, pp. 19–43.

39. Graham, D. I., Adams, J. H., and Generelli, T. A.: Pathology of brain damage in head injury. *In* Cooper, P. R. (Ed.): Head Injury, 2nd Ed. Baltimore, Williams & Wilkins, 1987.

40. Levin, H. S., Benton, A. L., and Grossman, R. G.: Neurobehavioral Consequences of Closed Head Injury. New York, Oxford University Press, 1982, pp. 3–48.

41. Adams, J. H., Mitchell, D. E., Graham, D. I., et al: Diffuse brain damage of immediate impact type: Its relationship to primary brain-stem damage in head injury. Brain, 100:489–502, 1977.

42. Ommaya, A. K., and Gennarelli, T. A.: Cerebral concussion and traumatic unconsciousness: Correlation of experimental and clinical observation on blunt head injuries. Brain, 97:633–654, 1974.

43. Stritch, S. J.: Diffuse degeneration of the cerebral white matter in severe dementia following head

injury. J. Neurol. Neurosurg. Psychiatry, 19:163–185, 1956.

44. Adams, J. H., Mitchell, D. E., Graham, D. I., et al: Diffuse brain damage of immediate impact type: Its relationship to primary brain-stem damage in head injury. Brain, 100:489–502, 1977.

45. Adams, J. H., Doyle, D., Graham, D. I., et al: Gliding contusions in nonmissile head injury in humans. Arch. Pathol. Lab. Med., 110:485–488, 1986.

46. Ommaya, A. K., and Genarelli, T. A.: Cerebral concussion and traumatic unconsciousness: Correlation of experimental and clinical observations on blunt head injuries. Brain, 97:633–654, 1974.

47. Adams, J. H., Mitchell, D. E., Graham, D. I., et al: Diffuse brain damage of immediate impact type: Its relationship to primary brain-stem damage in head injury. Brain, 100:489–502, 1977.

48. Adams, J. H., Scott, G., Parker, L. S., Graham, D. I., Doyle, D.: The contusion index. A quantitative approach to cerebral contusions in head injury. Neuropathol. Appl. Neurobiol., 6:319–324, 1980.

49. Adams, J. H., Mitchell, D. E., Graham, D. I., et al: Diffuse brain damage of immediate impact type: Its relationship to primary brain-stem damage in head injury. Brain, 100:489–502, 1977.

50. Levin, H. S., Amparo, E., Eisenberg, H. M., et. al.: Magnetic resonance imaging and computerized tomography in relation to the neurobehavioral sequelae of mild and moderate head injuries. J. Neurosurg., 66:706–713, 1987.

51. Snow, R. B., Zimmerman, R. D., Gandy, S. E., et al: Comparison of magnetic resonance imaging and computed tomography in the evaluation of head injury. Neurosurgery, 18:45–52, 1986.

52. Lobato, R. D., Sarabia, R., and Rivas, J. J., et al: Normal computerized tomography scans in severe head injury: Prognostic and clinical management implications. J. Neurosurg., 65:784–789, 1986.

53. Wilberger, J. E., Deeb, Z., and Rothfus, W.: Magnetic resonance imaging in cases of severe head injury. Neurosurgery, 20:571–576, 1987.

54. Grosswasser, Z., Reider-Groswasser, I., Soroker, N., et al: Magnetic resonance imaging in head-injured patients with normal late computed tomography scans. Surg. Neurol., 27:331–337, 1987.

55. Graham, D. I., and Adams, J. H.: Ischemic brain damage in fatal head injuries. Lancet, i:265–266, 1971.

56. Graham, D. I., Adams, J. H., and Doyle, D.: Ischemic brain damage in fatal head injuries. J. Neurol. Sci., 213–234, 1978.

57. Jennett, B., and Teasdale, G.: Management of Head Injuries. Philadelphia, F.A. Davis Company, 1981, p. 31.

58. Jennett, B., Teasdale, G., Braakman, R., et al.: Predicting outcome in individual patients after severe head injury. Lancet, 1(7696):1031-1034, 1976.

59. Artiola i Fortuny, L., and Hiorns, R. W.: Recovery curves in a visual search task. Int. Rehab. Med., 1:177–181, 1979.

60. Hiorns, R. W., and Newcombe, F.: Recovery curves: Uses and limitations. Int. Rehab. Med., 1:173-176, 1979.

61. Mackworth, N., Mackworth, J., and Cope, D. N.: Towards an interpretation of head injury recovery trends. In Berrol, S., Rappaport, M., Cope, D. N., et al (Eds.): Severe Head Trauma: A Comprehensive Medical Approach (NIHR Project 13-P-59156/9). 1982; I: VIII.

62. Arts, W. F. M., Van Dongen, H. R., Van Hof-Van Duin, J., et al: Unexpected improvement after prolonged post-traumatic vegetative state. J. Neurol. Neurosurg. Psychiatry, 48:1300–1303, 1985.

63. Tanheco, J., and Kaplan, P. E.: Physical and surgical rehabilitation of patient after 6-year coma. Arch. Phys. Med. Rehabil., 63:36–38, 1982.

64. Gilchrist, E., and Wilkinson, M.: Some factors determining prognosis in young people with severe head injuries. Arch. Neurol., 36:355–359, 1979.

65. Roberts, A. H.: Severe Accident Head Injury: An Assessment of Long-Term Prognosis. London, MacMillan Press, Ltd., 1979.

66. Klonoff, P. S., Costa, L. D., and Snow, W. G.: Predictors and indicators of quality of life in patients with closed-head injury. J. Clin. Exper. Neuropsychol., 8:469–485, 1986.

67. Young, B., Rapp, R. P., Norton, J. A., et al: Early prediction of outcome in head-injured patients. J. Neurosurg., 54:300–303, 1981.

68. Gilchrist, E., and Wilkinson, M.: Some factors determining prognosis in young people with severe head injuries. Arch. Neurol., 36:355–358, 1979.

69. Eiben, C. F., Anderson, T. P., Lockman, L., et al: Functional outcome of closed head injury in children and young adults. Arch. Phys. Med. Rehabil., 65:168–170, 1984.

70. Rosin, A. J.: Very prolonged unresponsive state following brain injury. Scand. J. Rehabil. Med., 10:33–38, 1978.

71. Higashi, K., Sakata, M., Hatano, S., et al: Epidemiological studies on patients with a persistent vegetative state. J. Neurol. Neurosurg. Psychiatry, 40:876–885, 1977.

72. Russell, W. R., and Smith, A.: Post-traumatic amnesia in closed head injury. Arch. Neurol., 5:4–17, 1961.

73. Smith, A.: Duration of impaired consciousness as an index of severity in closed head injuries: A review. Dis. Nerv. Syst., 22:69–74, 1961.

74. Russell, W. R.: The Traumatic Amnesias. London, Oxford University Press, 1971.

75. Levin, H. S., Benton, A. L., and Grossman, R. G.: Neurobehavioral Consequences of Closed Head Injuries. New York, Oxford University Press, 1982, pp. 73–79.

76. Gronwall, D., and Wrightson, P.: Delayed recovery of intellectual function after minor head injury. Lancet, ii:605–609, 1974.

77. Mandelberg, I. A.: Cognitive recovery after severe head injury. 3. WAIS verbal and performance IQs as a function of post-traumatic amnesia duration and time from injury. J. Neurol. Neurosurg. Psychiatry, 39:1001–1007, 1976.

78. Levin, H. S., O'Donnell, V. M., and Grossman, R. G.: The Galveston orientation and amnesia test. J. Nerv. Ment. Dis., 167:675–684, 1979.

79. Braakman, R., Gelpke, G. J., Habbema, J. D. F., et al: Systematic selection of prognostic features in patients with severe head injury. Neurosurgery, 6:362–370, 1980.

80. Mueller-Jensen, A., Neunzig, H.-P., and Emskotter, T.: Outcome prediction in comatose patients: Significance of reflex eye movement analysis. J. Neurol. Neurosurg. Psychiatry, 50:389–392, 1987.

81. Miller, J. D., Butterworth, J. F., Gudeman, S. K., et al: Further experience in the management of severe head injury. J. Neurosurg., 54:289–299, 1981.

82. Miller, J. D., Butterworth, J. F., Gudeman, S. K., et al: Further experience in the management of severe head injury. J. Neurosurg., 54:289–299, 1981.

83. Becker, D. P., Miller, J. D., Ward, J. D., et al: The outcome from severe head injury with early diagnosis and intensive management. J. Neurosurg., 47:491–502, 1977.

84. Levy, D. E., Caronna, J. J., and Singer, B. H.: Predicting outcome from hypoxic-ischemic coma. J. A. M. A., 253:1420–1426, 1985.

85. Bakay, R. A., and Ward, A. A.: Enzymatic changes in serum and cerebrospinal fluid in neurological injury. J. Neurosurg., 1983; 58:27-37.

86. Hans, P., Albert, A., Born, J. D., et al: Derivation of a bioclinical prognostic index in severe head injury. Intensive Care Med., 11:186–191, 1985.

87. DeSalles, A. A. F., Kontas, H. A., Becker, D. P., et al: Prognostic significance of ventricular CSF lactate in severe head injury. J. Neurosurg., 65:615–624, 1986.

88. Hamill, R. W., Woolf, P. D., McDonald, J. V., et al: Catecholamines predict outcome in traumatic brain injury. Ann. Neurol., 21:438–443, 1987.

89. Hansotia, P. L.: Persistent vegetative state: Review and report of electrodiagnostic studies in eight cases. Arch. Neurol., 42:1048–1052, 1985.

90. Greenberg, R. P., Becker, D. P., Miller, J. D., et al: Evaluation of brain function in severe human head trauma with multimodality evoked potentials. Part 2. Localization of brain dysfunction and correlation with posttraumatic neurological conditions. J. Neurosurg., 47:163–177, 1977.

91. Rappaport, M., Hall, K., Hopkins, K., et al: Evoked brain potentials and disability in brain damaged patients. Arch. Phys. Med. Rehabil., 58:333–338, 1977.

92. Anderson, D. C., Bundlie, S., and Rockswold, G. L.: Multimodality evoked potentials in closed head trauma. Arch. Neurol., 41:369–374, 1984.

93. Greenberg, R. P., Becker, D. P., Miller, J. D., et al: Evaluation of brain function in severe human head trauma with multimodality evoked potentials. Part 2: Localization of brain dysfunction and correlation with posttraumatic neurological conditions. J. Neurosurg., 47:163–177, 1977.

94. Olbrich, H. M., Nau, H. E., Lodemann, E., et al: Evoked potential assessment of mental function during recovery from severe head injury. Surg. Neurol., 26:112–118, 1986.

95. Rowe, J. M., and Carlson, C.: Brainstem auditory evoked potentials in postconcussion dizziness. Arch. Neurol., 37:679–683, 1980.

96. Newlon, P. G.: Utility of multimodality evoked potentials in cerebral injury. Neurol. Clin., 3:675–687, 1985.

97. John, E. R., Prichep, J., and Easton, F. P.: Neurometrics: Computer-assisted differential diagnosis of brain dysfunction. Science, 239:162–169, 1988.

98. Cantor, D. S., McAlaster, R., Meyer, W. I., et al: Electrophysiologic prognostic indices for recovery from head injury. (Abstract.) Washington, D.C., American Association of Neurologic Surgeons, April 24–28, 1983.

99. Masters S. J., McClean, P. M., Arcarese, J. S., et al: Skull X-ray examinations after head trauma: Recommendations by a multidisciplinary panel and validation study. N. Engl. J. Med., 316:84–91, 1987.

100. Timming, R., Orrison, W. W., and Mikula, J. A.: Computerized tomography and rehabilitation outcome after severe head trauma. Arch. Phys. Med. Rehabil., 63:154–159, 1982.

101. Van Dangen, K. J., and Braakman, R.: Late computed tomography in survivors of severe head injury. Neurosurgery, 7:14–22, 1980.

102. Kishore, P. R., Lipper, M. H., and Miller, J. D.: Post-traumatic hydrocephalus in patients with severe head injury. Neuroradiology, 16:261–265, 1978.

103. Zimmerman, R. A., Bilaniuk, L. T., Hackney, D. B., et al: Head Injury: Early results of comparing CT and high-field MR. A. J. R., 147:1215–1222, 1986.

104. Levin, H. S., Handel, S. F., and Goldman, A. M.: Magnetic resonance imaging after "diffuse" non-missile head injury. Arch. Neurol., 42:963–968, 1985.

105. Phelps, M. E., and Mazziotta, J. C.: Positron emission tomography: Human brain function and biochemistry. Science, 228:799–809, 1985.

106. Rao, N., Turski, P. A., and Polcyn, R. E.: 18F Positron emission computed tomography in closed head injury. Arch. Phys. Med. Rehabil., 65:780–785, 1984.

107. Mazziota, J. C., and Phelps, M. E.: Human sensory stimulation and deprivation: Positron emission tomographic results and strategies. Ann. Neurol., 15(suppl):S50–S60, 1984.

108. Langfitt, T. W., Obrist, W. D., Alavi, A., et al:

Computerized tomography, magnetic resonance imaging, and positron emission tomography in the study of brain trauma. J. Neurosurg., 64:760–767, 1986.

109. Becker, D. P., Miller, J. D., Ward, J. D., et al: The outcome from severe head injury with early diagnosis and intensive management. J. Neurosurg., 47:491–502, 1977.

110. Lundholm, J., Jepson, B. N., and Thornval, G.: The late neurological, psychological, and social aspects of severe traumatic coma. Scand. J. Rehab. Med., 7:97–100, 1975.

111. Eiben, C. F., Anderson, T. P., Lockman, L., et al: Functional outcome of closed head injury in children and young adults. Arch. Phys. Med. Rehabil., 65:168–179, 1984.

112. Lewin, W., Marshall, T. F., and Roberts, A. H.: Long-term outcome after severe head injury. Br. Med. J., 2:1533–1538, 1979.

113. Fife, S., Faich, G., Hollinshead, W., et al: Incidence and outcome of hospital-treated head injury in Rhode Island. Am. J. Public Health, 76:773–778, 1986.

114. Cope, D.N.: Conclusions. In Berrol, S., Rappaport, M., Cope D. N., et al (Eds.): Severe Head Trauma: A Comprehensive Medical Approach (NIHR Project 13-P-59156/9). 1982; I: IX-5.

115. Uzzell, B. P., Langfitt, T. W., and Dolinskas, C. A.: Influence of injury severity on quality of survival after head injury. Surg. Neurol., 27:419–429, 1987.

116. Carlsson, C. A., von Essen, C., and Lofgrem, J.: Factors affecting the clinical course of patients with severe head injuries. J. Neurosurg., 29:242–251, 1968.

117. Rimel, R. W., Giordani, B., Barth, J. T., et.al.: Moderate head injury: Completing the clinical spectrum of brain trauma. Neurosurgery, 11:344–351, 1982.

118. Fahy, T. J., Irving, M. H., and Millac, P.: Severe head injuries. Lancet, i:475–479, 1967.

119. Fuld, P. A.: Recovery of intellectual ability after closed head injury. Dev. Med. Child. Neurol., 19:495–502, 1977.

120. Haas, J. F., Cope, D. N., and Hall, K.: Premorbid prevalence of poor academic performance in severe head injury. J. Neurol. Neurosurg. Psychiatry, 50:52–56, 1987.

121. Kraus, J. F., Fife, D., and Ramstein, K.: The relationship of family income to the incidence, external causes, and outcomes of serious brain injury, San Diego County, California. Am. J. Public Health, 76:1345–1347, 1986.

122. Bond, M. R.: Assessment of the psychosocial outcome after severe head injury. In: CIBA Foundation Symposium: Outcomes of Severe Damage to the Central Nervous System. New York, Elsevier, 1975: 141–157.

123. Bond, M. R.: Assessment of the psychosocial out-

come of severe head injury. Acta Neurochir., 34:57–70, 1976.

124. Brooks, D. N., Aughton, M. E., Bond, M. R., et al: Cognitive sequelae in relationship to early indices of severity of brain damage after severe blunt head injury. J. Neurol. Neurosurg. Psychiatry, 43:529–534, 1980.

125. Levin, H. S., Grossman, R. G., Rose, J. E., et al: Long-term neuropsychological outcome of closed head injury. J. Neurosurg., 50:412–422, 1979.

126. Jennett, B., Snoek, J., Bond, M. R., and Brooks, N.: Disability after severe head injury: Observations on the use of the Glasgow Outcome Scale. J. Neurol. Neurosurg. Psychiatry, 44:285–293, 1981.

127. Grosswasser, Z., Mendelson, L., Stern, M. J., et al: Re-evaluation of prognostic factors in rehabilitation after severe head injury. Scand. J. Rehab. Med., 9:147–149, 1977.

128. Benton, A. L.: Thoughts on the application of neuropsychological tests, In Levin, H. S., Grafman, J., and Eisenberg, H. M.: Neurobehavioral Recovery From Head Injury. New York, Oxford University Press, 1987, p. 113.

129. Irving, M. H., and Irving, P. M.: Associated injuries in head injured patients. J. Trauma, 7:500–511, 1967.

130. Kalisky, Z., Morrison, D. P., Meyers, C. A., et al: Medical problems encountered during rehabilitation of patients with head injury. Arch. Phys. Med. Rehabil., 66:25–29, 1985.

131. Wilmot, C. B., Cope, D. N., Hall, K. M., et al: Occult head injury: its incidence in spinal cord injury. Arch. Phys. Med. Rehabil., 66:227–231, 1985.

132. Davidoff, G., Morris, J., Roth, E., et al: Closed head injury in spinal cord injured patients: retrospective study of loss of consciousness and post-traumatic amnesia. Arch. Phys. Med. Rehabil., 66:41–43, 1985.

133. Wagner, KA, Kopaniky, D. R., and Esposito, L.: Head and spinal cord injured patients: Impact of combined sequelae. Arch. Phys. Med. Rehabil. Abstr., 64:519, 1983.

134. Cope, D.N., Wilmot, C. B., and Hall, K. M.: Occult head injury in spinal cord injury: Relationship to premorbid history and learning self-care. Arch. Phys. Med. Rehabil., in press.

135. Berrol, S.: Medical assessment. In Rosenthal, S., Griffith, E. R., Bond, M. R., Miller, J. D.: Rehabilitation of the Head-Injured Adult. Philadelphia, F. A. Davis Company, 1983, pp. 231–239.

136. Strub, R. L., and Black, F. W.: The Mental Status Examination in Neurology. Philadelphia, F. A. Davis Company, 1977.

137. Kiernan, R. J., Mueller, J., Langston, J. W., et al: The neurobehavioral cognitive status examination: A brief but differentiated approach to cognitive assessment. Ann. Intern. Med., 107:481–485, 1987.

138. Schwamm, L. H., Van Dyke, C., Kiernan, R. J.,

et al: The neurobehavioral cognitive status examination: Comparison with the cognitive capacity screening examination and the mini-mental state examination in a neurosurgical population. Ann. Intern. Med., 107:486–491, 1987.

139. Mesulam, M.: Principles of Behavioral Neurology. Philadelphia, F.A. Davis Company, 1985.

140. Silver, J. M., Yudofsky, S. C., and Hales, R. E.: Neuropsychiatric aspects of traumatic brain injury. *In* Hales, R. E., and Yudofsky, S. C. (Eds.): Textbook of Neuropsychiatry. Washington, D.C., The American Psychiatric Press, 1987, pp. 191–208.

141. Cope, D. N.: The physiatric assessment of traumatic brain injury. *In* Rosenthal M., Griffith, E. R., Bond, M. R., et al (Eds.): Rehabilitation of Head Injured Adult, 2nd Edition. Philadelphia, F. A. Davis Company, in press.

142. Logeman, J. A.: Evaluation and Treatment of Swallowing Disorders. San Diego, College Hill Press, 1983.

143. Mandelstam, P., and Lieber, A.: Cineradiographic evaluation of esophagus in normal adults: Study of 146 subjects ranging in age from 21 to 90 years. Gastroenterology, 58:32–39, 1970.

144. Splaingard, M., Hutchins, B., Sulton, L., et al: Aspiration in rehabilitation patients: A blinded study of videofluoroscopy versus bedside clinical assessment. (Abstract.) Arch. Phys. Med. Rehabil., 67:622–623, 1986.

145. Kamada, T., Fusamoto, H., Kawano, S., et al: Gastrointestinal bleeding following head injury: A clinical study of 433 cases. J. Trauma, 17:44–47, 1977.

146. Eichelberger, M. R., Chatten, J., Bruce, D. A., et. al.: Acute pancreatitis and increased intracranial pressure. J. Pediatr. Surg., 16:562–570, 1981.

147. Rusk, H. A., Block, J. W., and Lowman, E. W.: Rehabilitation following traumatic brain damage; Immediate and long term follow up results in 127 cases. Med. Clin. N. Am., 53:677–684, 1969.

148. Kester, D., Caplan, R., Souba, W. W., et al: Metabolic response to trauma. Contemp. Orthop., 14:53–60, 1987.

149. Cliftos, G. L., Robertson, C. S., and Choi, S. C.: Assessment of nutritional requirements of head-injured patients. J. Neurosurg., 64:895–901, 1986.

150. Blisten, C., and Lamid, S.: Nutritional management of a patient with brain damage and SCI. Arch. Phys. Med. Rehabil., 64:382–383, 1983.

151. Robertson, C. S., Clifton, G. L., Taylor, A. A., et al: Treatment of hypertension associated with head injury. J. Neurosurg., 59:455–460, 1983.

152. Sandel, M. E., Abrams, M. D., and Horn, L. J.: Hypertension after brain injury: Case report. Arch. Phys. Med. Rehabil., 67:469–472, 1986.

153. Jackson, R. D., and Mysiw, W. J.: Systemic hypertension and hydrocephalus in closed head injury: A new association. (Abstract.) Arch. Phys. Med. Rehabil., 65:661, 1984.

154. Solomon, S., Hotchkiss, E., and Saravay, S. M.: Impairment of memory function by antihypertensive medication. Arch. Gen. Psychiatry, 40:1109–1112, 1983.

155. Glenn, M. B.: Chronic hypertension after traumatic brain injury: Pharmacologic options. J. Head Trauma Rehabil., 2:87–89, 1987.

156. Fleischer, A. S., Rudman, D., Payne, N. S., et al: Hypothalamic hypothyroidism and hypogonadism in prolonged traumatic coma. J. Neurosurg., 49:650, 1978.

157. Edwards, O. M., and Clark, J. D. A.: Post-traumatic hypopituitarism: Six cases and a review of the literature. Medicine, 65:281–290, 1986.

158. Klingbeil, G. E. G., and Cline, P.: Anterior hypopituitarism: A consequence of head injury. Arch. Phys. Med. Rehabil., 66:44–46, 1985.

159. Notman, D. D., Mortex, M. A., and Moses, A. M.: Permanent diabetes insipidus following head trauma: Observations on ten patients and an approach to diagnosis. J. Trauma, 20:599–602, 1980.

160. Barreca, T., Perria, C., Sannia, A., et al: Evaluation of anterior pituitary function in patients with post-traumatic diabetes insipidus. J. Clin. Endocrinol. Metab, 51:1279–1282, 1980.

161. Ishikawa, A., Toshikazu, S., Kaneko, K., et al: Hyponatremia responsive to fluidrocortisone acetate in elderly patients after head injury. Ann. Intern. Med., 106:187–191, 1987.

162. Jennett, B.: Post-traumatic epilepsy. *In* Rosenthal, M., Griffith, E. R., Bond, M. R., et al (Eds.): Rehabilitation of Head Injured Adult. F.A. Davis Company, Philadelphia, 1983.

163. Weiss, G. H., Salazar, A. M., Vance, S. C., et al: Predicting post-traumatic epilepsy in penetrating head injury. Arch. Neurol., 43:771–773, 1986.

164. Feeney, D. M., and Walker, A. E.: The prediction of post-traumatic epilepsy: A mathematical approach. Arch. Neurol., 36:8–12, 1979.

165. Weiss, G. H., Feeney, D. M., Caveness, W. F., et al: Prognostic factors for the occurrence of post-traumatic epilepsy. Arch. Neurol., 40:7–10, 1983.

166. Wohns, R. N. W., and Wyler, A. R.: Prophylactic phenytoin in severe head injuries. J. Neurosurg., 51:507–509, 1979.

167. Young, B., Rapp, R. P., and Norton, J. A.: Failure of prophylactically administered phenytoin to prevent early post-traumatic seizures. J. Neurosurg., 58:231–235, 1983.

168. Rapport, R. L., and Penry, J. K.: A survey of attitudes toward the pharmacological prophylaxis of post-traumatic epilepsy. J. Neurosurg., 38:159–166, 1973.

169. Reynolds, E. H., and Trimble, M. R.: Adverse neuropsychiatric effects of anticonvulsant drugs. Drugs, 29:570–581, 1985.

170. Glenn, M. B.: Anticonvulsants for prophylaxis of post-traumatic seizures. J. Head Trauma Rehabil., 1:73–74, 1986.

171. Porter, R. J., and Kelley, K. R.: Anti-epileptic

drugs and mild liver function elevation. J.A.M.A., 253:1791–1792, 1985.

172. Wallis, W. E.: Withdrawal of anticonvulsant drugs in seizure-free epileptic patients. Clin. Neuropharmacol., 10:423–433, 1987.

173. Glenn, M. B.: Anticonvulsants for prophylaxis of post-traumatic seizures. J. Head Trauma Rehabil., 1:73–74. 1986.

174. Ginsberg, M. D., Hedley-White, E. T., and Richardson, E. P.: Hypoxic ischemic leukoencephalopathy in man. Arch. Neurol., 33:5–14, 1976.

175. Wainapel, S. F., Gupta, P. C., and Matz, R.: Posthypoxic leukoencephalopathy with late recovery. Arch. Phys. Med. Rehabil., 65:201–202, 1984.

176. Ellison, P. H.: Propranolol for severe head-injury action tremor. Neurology, 28:197–199, 1978.

177. Schiffer, R. B., Herndon, R. M., and Rudick, R. A.: Treatment of pathologic laughing and weeping with amitriptyline. N. Engl. J. Med., 312:1480–1482, 1985.

178. Udaka, F., Yamao, S., Nagata, H., et al: Pathologic laughing and crying treated with levodopa. Arch. Neurol., 41:1095–1096, 1984.

179. Fahn, S.: Posthypoxic myoclonus: Literature review update. Adv. Neurol., 43:157–169, 1986.

180. Drake, M. E., Jackson, R. D., and Miller, C. A.: Paroxysmal choreoathetosis after head injury. J. Neurol. Neurosurg. Psychiatry, 49:837–843, 1986.

181. Robin, J. J.: Paroxysmal choreoathetosis following head injury. Ann. Neurol., 2:447–448, 1977.

182. Baratz, R., and Mesulam, M.: Adult-onset stuttering treated with anticonvulsants. Arch. Neurol., 38:132, 1981.

183. Gerstenbrand, F., Poewe, W., Aichner, F., et al: Kluver-Bucy Syndrome in man: Experiences with posttraumatic cases. Neurosci. Biobehav. Rev., 7:413–417, 1983.

184. Childs, A.: Naltrexone in organic bulimia: A preliminary report. Brain Injury, 1:49–55, 1987.

185. Heyman, A., Wilkenson, W. E., Stafford, J. A., et al: Alzheimer's disease: A study of epidemiologic aspects. Ann. Neurol., 15:335–341, 1984.

186. French, L. R., Schuman, L. M., Mortimer, J. A., et al: A case-control study of dementia of the Alzheimer's type. Am. J. Epidemiol., 121:414–421, 1985.

187. Sullivan, P., Petitti, D., and Barbaccia, J.: Head trauma and age of onset of dementia of the Alzheimer type. J. A. M. A., 257:2289–2290, 1987.

188. Amaducci, L. A., Fratiglioni, L., Rocca, W. A., et al: Risk factors for Alzheimer's disease (AD): A case-control study on an Italian population. Neurology, 35(Suppl 1):277, 1985.

189. Sulkava, R., Erkinjuntti, T., and Palo, J.: Head injuries in Alzheimer's disease and vascular dementia. Neurology, 35:1804, 1985.

190. Barclay, L. L., Kheyfeta, S., Zemcov, A., et al: Risk factors in Alzheimer's disease (AD): Abstracts. Thirtieth Oholo Biological Conference on Basic and Therapeutic Strategies in Alzheimer's and Other Age-related Neuropsychiatric Disorders. Eilat, Israel, 1985: 48.

191. Herz, D. A., Gregerson, M., and Pearl, L.: Rehabilitative neurosurgery. Neurosurgery, 18:311–315, 1986.

192. Koo, A., and La Roque, R.: Evaluation of head trauma by computed tomography. Radiology, 123:345–350, 1977.

193. Merino-deVillasante, J., and Taveras, J.: Computerized tomography (CT) in acute head trauma. Am. J. Roentgenol., 118:609–613, 1976.

194. Dacey, R. G., Alves, W. M., Rimel, R. W., et al: Neurosurgical complications after apparently minor head injury. J. Neurosurg., 65:203–210, 1986.

195. Yamada, H., Watanabe, T., Murata, S., et al: Developmental process of chronic subdural collections of fluid based on CT scan findings. Surg. Neurol., 13:441–448, 1980.

196. Kishore, P. R. S., Lipper, M. H., Miller, J. D., et al: Posttraumatic hydrocephalus in patients with severe head injury. Neuroradiology, 16:261–265, 1978.

197. Levin, H. S., Meyers, C. A., Grossman, R. G., et al: Ventricular enlargement after closed head injury. Arch. Neurol., 38:623–629, 1981.

198. Van Dongen, K. J., and Braakman, R.: Late computed tomography in survivors of severe head injury. Neurosurgery, 7:14–22, 1980.

199. Cardoso, E. R., and Galbraith, S.: Posttraumatic hydrocephalus—A retrospective review. Surg. Neurol., 23:261–264, 1985.

200. Cope, D. N., Date, E. S., and Mar, E. Y.: Serial computerized tomographic evaluations in traumatic head injury. Arch. Phys. Med. Rehabil., 7:483–486, 1988.

201. Cardoso, E. R., and Galbraith, S.: Posttraumatic hydrocephalus—A retrospective review. Surg. Neurol., 23:261–264, 1985.

202. Parkinson, D., and West, M. P.: Traumatic intracranial aneurysms. J. Neurosurg., 52:11–20, 1980.

203. Noterman, J., Flament-Durand, J., Hermanus, N., et al: Traumatic aneurysm of the anterior cerebral artery associated with a contralateral carotid-cavernous fistula: A case report. Neurosurgery, 17:807–810, 1985.

204. Cope, D. N., Date, E. S., and Mar, E. Y.: Serial computerized tomographic evaluations in traumatic head injury. Arch. Phys. Med. Rehabil., in press.

205. Jaffe, K. M., and Hays, R. M.: Pediatric head injury: Rehabilitative medical management. J. Head Trauma Rehabil., 1:30–40, 1986.

206. Kernohan, J., Dakin, P. K., Beacon, J. P., et al: Treatment of major skeletal injuries in patients with a severe head injury. Br. Med. J., 288:1822–1823, 1984.

207. Rhoades, M. E., and Garland, D. E.: Orthopedic prognosis of brain injured adults. Clin. Orthop., 131:104–110, 1978.

208. Garland, D. E., and Rhoades, M. E.: Orthopedic

management of brain injured adults. Clin. Orthop., 131:111–122, 1978.

209. Hanscomb, D. A.: Acute management of the multiply injured head trauma patient. J. Head Trauma Rehabil., 2:1–12, 1987.

210. Yarkony, G., and Sahgal, V.: Contractures: A major complication of craniocerebral trauma. Clin. Orthop., 219:93–96, 1987.

211. Booth, B. J., Doyle, M., and Montgomery, J.: Serial casting for the management of spasticity in the head-injured adult. Phys. Ther., 63:1960–1966, 1983.

212. Glenn, M. B.: Antispasticity medications in the patient with traumatic brain injury. J. Head Trauma Rehabil., 1:71-72, 1986.

213. Braun, R. M., Hoffer, M. M., Mooney, V., et al: Phenol nerve block in the treatment of acquired spastic hemiplegia in the upper limb. J. Bone Joint Surg. [Am.], 55A:580–585, 1973.

214. Khalili, A. A., and Betts, H. B.: Peripheral nerve block with phenol in the management of spasticity: Indications and complications. J. A. M. A., 200:1155–1157, 1967.

215. Garland, D. E., Lilling, M., and Keenan, M. A.: Percutaneous phenol blocks to motor points of spastic forearm muscles in head-injured adults. Arch. Phys. Med. Rehabil., 65:243–245, 1984.

216. Baker, L. L., Parker, K., and Sanderson, D.: Neuromuscular electrical stimulation for the head-injured patient. Phys. Ther., 63:1967–1974, 1983.

217. Garland, D. E., and Keenan, M. A.: Orthopedic strategies in the management of the adult head-injured patient. Phys. Ther., 63:2004–2009, 1983.

218. Perry, J., Waters, R. L., and Perrin, T.: Electromyographic analysis of equinovarus following stroke. Clin. Orthop., 131:47–53, 1978.

219. Avert, H. N., Haas, J. F., Mayer, N. H., et al: Polyelectromyography: A valuable physiatric tool. (Abstract.) Arch. Phys. Med. Rehabil., 66:523, 1985.

220. Botte, M. J., and Keenan, M. A.: Reconstructive surgery of the upper extremity in the patient with head trauma. J. Head Trauma Rehabil., 2:34–45, 1987.

221. Smith, C. W., and Leventhal, L.: Surgical treatment of lower extremity deformities in adult head-injured patients. J. Head Trauma Rehabil., 2:53–56, 1987.

222. Glenn, M. B., and Wroblewski, M. S.: Antispasticity medications in the patient with traumatic brain injury. J. Head Trauma Rehabil., 1:71-72, 1986.

223. Romney, D. M., and Angus, W. R.: A brief review of the effects of diazepam on memory. Psychopharmacol. Bull., 20:313–316, 1984.

224. Garland, D. E., Blum, C. E., and Waters, R. L.: Periarticular heterotopic ossification in head-injured adults: Incidence and location. J. Bone Joint Surg. [Am.], 62A:1143–1146, 1980.

225. Speilman, G., Gennarelli, T., and Rogers, R.: Disodium etidronate: Its role in preventing heterotopic ossification in severe head injuries. Arch. Phys. Med. Rehabil., 64:539–542, 1983.

226. Garland, D. E., Keenan, M. A., Smith, C. W., et al: Resurrection of heterotopic ossification in the head trauma adult. (Abstract.) Arch. Phys. Med. Rehabil., 66:536, 1985.

227. Horn, L. J.: Personal communication, 1988.

228. Fisher, B.: Effect of trunk control and alignment on limb function. J. Head Trauma Rehabil., 2:72–79, 1987.

229. Zoltan, B. B., and Ryckman, D. M.: Head injury in adults. In Pedretti, L. W. (Ed.): Occupational Therapy: Practice Skills for Physical Dysfunction, 2nd Ed. St Louis, C.V. Mosby, 1985.

230. Shaw, R.: Persistent vegetative state: Principles and techniques for seating and positioning. J. Head Trauma Rehabil., 1:31–37, 1986.

231. Swank, S., Lonstein, J. E., Moe, J. H., et al: Surgical treatment of adult scoliosis. J. Bone Joint Surg., 63:268–287, 1981.

232. Whyte, J., and Glenn, M. B.: Management of the patient in a persistent vegetative state: Current status and needed research. National Invitational Conference on Traumatic Brain Injury (TBI) Research. National Institute on Disability and Rehabilitation Research (NIDRR), Tyson's Corners, Va., 1987.

233. Khan, Z., Hertanu, J., Wen, C. Y., et al: Predictive correlation of urodynamic dysfunction and brain injury after cerebrovascular accident. J. Urol., 126:86–88, 1981.

234. Sumner, D.: Post-traumatic anosmia. Brain 87:107–120, 1964.

235. Levin, H. S., High, W. M., and Eisenberg, H. M.: Impairment of olfactory recognition after closed head injury. Brain, 108:579–591, 1985.

236. Zihl, J., and Von Cramon, D.: Restitution of visual function in patients with cerebral blindness. J. Neurol. Neurosurg. Psychiatry, 42:312–322, 1979.

237. Berrol, S., Swick, J., and Fryer, J.: Visual field retraining in brain damaged patients. (Abstr) Arch. Phys. Med. Rehabil., 61:503, 1980.

238. Balliet, R., Blood, K. M., and Bach-Y-Rita, P.: Visual field rehabilitation in the cortically blind? J. Neurol. Neurosurg. Psychiatry, 48:1113–1124, 1985.

239. Zihl, J., Von Craman, D.: Visual field rehabilitation in the cortically blind? [Letter.] J. Neurol. Neurosurg. Psychiatry 1986; 49:965-967.

240. Neger, R. E.: Ocular motility imbalance after brain injury. In Berrol, S., and Mayer, N. (Eds.): Rehabilitation Management of Traumatic Brain Injury. Baltimore, Williams & Wilkins, in press.

241. Aguilar, E. A., Hall, J. W., and Mackey-Hargadine, J.: Neuro-otologic evaluation of the patient with acute, severe head injuries: Correlations among physical findings, auditory evoked responses, and computerized tomography. Otolaryngol. Head Neck Surg., 94:211–219, 1986.

242. Childs, A.: Scopolamine effects in vestibular defensiveness. Arch. Phys. Med. Rehabil., 67:554–555, 1986.

243. Lehrer, J. F., and Poole, D. C.: Vertigo from perilymphatic fistulas. J. A. M. A. 256:1002–1003, 1986.

244. Levine, P. A., and Goode, P. L.: Lateral port control pharyngeal flap: A versatile approach to velopharyngeal insufficiency. Otolaryngol. Head Neck Surg., 90:310–314, 1982.

245. Ford, C. N., and Bless, D. M.: Clinical experience with injectable collagen for vocal fold augmentation. Laryngoscope, 96:863–869, 1986.

246. Lewy, R. B.: Teflon injection of the vocal cord: complications, errors, and precautions. Ann. Otol. Rhinol. Laryngol., 92:473-474, 1983.

247. Sarno, M. T.: Verbal impairment after closed head injury: Report on a replication study. J. Nerv. Ment. Dis., 172:475–479, 1984.

248. Hagen, C. H.: Language disorders secondary to closed head injury: Diagnosis and treatment. Top. Lang. Dis., 1:73-87, 1981.

249. Sarno, M. T.: The nature of verbal impairment after closed head injury. J. Nerv. Ment. Dis., 168:685–692, 1980.

250. Sarno, M. T., and Buonaguro, A.: Characteristics of verbal impairment in closed head injured patients. Arch. Phys. Med. Rehabil., 67:400–405, 1986.

251. Brooks, D. N., and McKinlay, W.: Personality and behavioral change after severe blunt head injury—a relative's view. J. Neurol. Neurosurg. Psychiatry, 46:336–344, 1983.

252. Bond, M. R., Brooks, D. N., and McKinlay, W.: Burdens imposed on the relatives of those with severe brain damage due to injury. Acta Neurochir. [Suppl] (Wien) 28:124–125, 1979.

253. Gloag, D.: Rehabilitation after head injury—1: Cognitive problems. Br. Med. J., 290:834–837, 1985.

254. Diller, L., Gordon, W. A.: Interventions for cognitive deficits in brain injured adults. J. Consult. Clin. Psychol., 49:822–834, 1981.

255. Cope, D. N.: Cognitive rehabilitation. West. J. Med., 144:736–737, 1986.

256. Prigatano, G. P. (Ed.): Neuropsychological Rehabilitation after Brain Injury. Baltimore, Johns Hopkins University Press, 1986.

257. Diller, L.: A model for cognitive retraining. Clin. Psychol., 29:13–15, 1976.

258. Grimm, B. H., and Bleiberg, J.: Psychological Rehabilitation in Traumatic Brain Injury. In Filskov, S. B., and Boll, T. J. (Eds.): Handbook of Clinical Neuropsychology, Vol. II. New York, John Wiley & Sons, 1986.

259. Rimmele, C. T., and Hester, R. K.: Cognitive rehabilitation after traumatic head injury. Arch. Clin. Neuropsychol., 2:353–384, 1987.

260. Sivak, M., Hill, C., Henson, D., et al: Improved driving performance following perceptual training in persons with brain damage. Arch. Phys. Med. Rehabil., 65:163–167, 1984.

261. Prigatano, G., Fordyce, D., Zeiner, H., et al: Neuropsychological rehabilitation after closed head injury in young adults. J. Neurol. Neurosurg. Psychiatry, 47:505–513, 1984.

262. LeWinn, E. B., and Dimancescu, M. D.: Environmental deprivation and enrichment in coma. [Letter.] Lancet, 2:156–157, 1978.

263. Whyte, J., and Glenn, MB: The care and rehabilitation of the patient in a persistent vegetative state. J. Head Trauma Rehabil., 1:39–53, 1986.

264. Kanno, T., Kamei, Y., Yokoyama, T., Jain, V. K.: Neurostimulation for patients in vegetative status. P. A. C. E., 10:207–208, 1987.

265. Weber, P. L.: Sensorimotor therapy: Its effect on the electroencephalograms of acute comatose patients. Arch. Phys. Med. Rehabil., 65:457–462, 1984.

266. Romano, M. D.: Family response to traumatic head injury. Scand. J. Rehabil. Med., 6:1–4, 1974.

267. Keshavan, M. S., Channabasavanna, S. M., and Narayana Reddy, G. N.: Post-traumatic psychiatric disturbances: Patterns and predictors of outcome. Br. J. Psychiatry, 157–160, 1981.

268. Grant, I., and Alves, W.: Psychiatric and psychosocial disturbances in head injury. In Levin, H. S., Grafman, J., and Eisenberg, H. M. (Eds.): Neurobehavioral Recovery from Head Injury. New York, Oxford University Press, 1987.

269. Shaw, L., Brodsky, L., and McMahon, B. T.: Neuropsychiatric intervention in the rehabilitation of head injured patients. Psychiatr. J. Univ. Ottawa, 10:237–240, 1985.

270. Levin, H. S., High, W. M., Goethe, K. E., et al: The neurobehavioral rating scale: Assessment of the behavioral sequelae of head injury by the clinician. J. Neurol. Neurosurg. Psychiatry, 50:183–193, 1987.

271. Bell, C. C.: Coma and the etiology of violence, part 2. J. Nat. Med. Assoc., 79:79–85, 1987.

272. Institute of Rehabilitation Medicine: Working Approaches to Remediation of Cognitive Deficits in Brain Damaged Persons. Rehabilitation Monograph #64, New York, Institute of Rehabilitation Medicine, NYU Medical Center, 1982.

273. Elliott, F. A.: The episodic dyscontrol syndrome and aggression. Neurol. Clin., 2:113–129, 1984.

274. Mesulam, M.-M.: Patterns on Behavioral Neuroanatomy: Association Areas, the Limbic System, and Hemispheric Specialization. In Mesulam M-M. (Ed.): Principles of Behavioral Neurology. Philadelphia, F.A. Davis Company, 1985.

275. Riley, T., and Niedermeyer, E.: Rage attacks and episodic violent behavior: Electroencephalographic findings and general considerations. Clin. Electroencephalogr., 9:131–139, 1978.

276. Cannon, P. A., and Drake, M. E.: EEG and brain stem auditory evoked potentials in brain-injured

patients with rage attacks and self-injurious behavior. Clin. Electroencephalogr., 17:169–172, 1986.

277. Kessler, L. A.: The padded patient enclosure. Neurosurgery, 17:869-870, 1985.

278. Grimm, B. H., and Bleiberg, J.: Psychological rehabilitation in traumatic brain injury. In Filskov, S. B., and Boll, T. J. (Eds.): Handbook of Clinical Neuropsychology, Vol II. New York, John Wiley & Sons, 1986.

279. Wood, R. L.: Brain Injury Rehabilitation: A Neurobehavioral Approach. Rockville, Aspen Publishers, 1987.

280. Eames, P., and Wood, R. L.: Rehabilitation after severe brain injury: A special-unit approach to behavior disorders. Int. Rehabil. Med., 7:130–133, 1985.

281. Lishman, W. A.: Brain damage in relation to psychiatric disability after head injury. Br. J. Psychiatry, 114:373–410, 1968.

282. Prigatano, G. P.: Psychiatric aspects of head injury: Problem areas and suggested guidelines for research. In Levin, H. S., Grafman, J., and Eisenberg, H. M. (Eds.): Neurobehavioral Recovery from Head Injury. New York, Oxford University Press, 1987.

283. Grant, I., and Alves, W.: Psychiatric and psychosocial disturbances in head injury. In Levin, H. S., Grafman J., and Eisenberg, H. M.: Neurobehavioral Recovery from Head Injury. New York, Oxford University Press, 1987.

284. Levin, H. S., Grossman, R. G., Rose, J. E., et al: Long-term neuropsychological outcome of closed head injury. J. Neurosurg., 80:412–422, 1979.

285. Oddy, M., Coughlin, T., Tyerman, A., et al: Social adjustment after closed head injury: A further follow-up seven years after injury. J. Neurol. Neurosurg. Psychiatry, 48:564–568, 1985.

286. Ross, E. D., and Rush, A. J.: Diagnosis and neuroanatomical correlates of depression in brain-damaged patients: Implications for a neurology of depression. Arch. Gen. Psychiatry, 38:1344–1354, 1981.

287. LaVecchio, F. A.: Assessment and management of the suicidal brain-injured adult in a rehabilitation setting: A neuropsychological approach. (Abstract.) Arch. Phys. Med. Rehabil., 65:619, 1984.

288. Peck, E., Ettigi, P., and Narasimhachari, N., et al: Neurochemical and neuroendocrine findings in post head injury onset depression. (Abstract.) Arch. Phys. Med. Rehabil., 65:645, 1984.

289. Block, S. H.: Psychotherapy of the individual with brain injury. Brain Injury, 1:203–206, 1987.

290. Ruedrich, S. L., Chu, C., and Moore, S. L.: ECT for major depression in a patient with acute brain trauma. Am. J. Psychiatry, 140:928–929, 1983.

291. Reiss, H., Schwartz, C. E., and Klerman, G. L.: Manic syndrome following head injury: Another form of secondary mania. J. Clin. Psychiatry, 48:29–30, 1987.

292. Grant, I., and Alves, W.: Psychiatric and psycho-

logical disturbances in head injury. In Levin, H. S., Grafman, J., and Eisenberg, H. M. (Eds.): Neurobehavioral Recovery from Head Injury. New York, Oxford University Press, 1987.

293. Thomsen, I. V.: Late outcome of very severe blunt head trauma: a 10-15 year second follow-up. J. Neurol. Neurosurg. Psychiatry, 47:260–268, 1984.

294. Rango, N.: Nursing home care in the United States. N. Engl. J. Med., 307:883–890, 1982.

295. Ray, W. A., Federspiel, C. F., and Schaffner, W.: A study of antipsychotic drug use in nursing homes: Epidemiologic evidence suggesting misuse. Am. J. Public Health, 70:485–491, 1980.

296. Infantino, J. A., and Musingo, S.: Assaults and injuries among staff with and without training in aggression control techniques. Hosp. Commun. Psychiatry, 36:1312–1314, 1985.

297. Cope, D. N.: Psychopharmacologic considerations in the treatment of traumatic brain injury. J. Head Trauma Rehabil., 2:1–5, 1987.

298. Cope, D.N. (Ed.): J. Head Trauma Rehabil., 2:4, 1987.

299. Haas, J. F., and Cope, D. N.: Neuropharmacologic management of behavior sequelae in head injury: A case report. Arch. Phys. Med. Rehabil., 66:472–474, 1985.

300. Evans, R. W., and Gualtieri, C. T.: Psychostimulant pharmacotherapy in traumatic brain injury. J. Head Trauma Rehabil., 2:29–33, 1987.

301. Weinberg, R. M., Auerbach, S. H., and Moore, S.: Pharmacologic treatment of cognitive deficits: A case study. Brain Injury 1987; 1:57–59.

302. Herson, M., and Barlow, D.: Single Case Experimental Designs. New York, Pergamon Press, 1976.

303. Weinberg, R. M., Auerbach, S. H., and Moore, S.: Pharmacologic treatment of cognitive deficits: A case study. Brain Injury, 1:57–59, 1987.

304. Walton, R. G.: Lecithin and physostigmine for post traumatic memory and cognitive deficits. Psychosomatics, 23:435–436, 1982.

305. Ducote, C., Moore, K., Gandonlini, J., et al: Imipramine for the treatment of akinetic mutism and arousal-attention deficits after traumatic brain injury. Presentation. Baltimore, MD, American Academy of Physical Medicine and Rehabilitation, 48th Assembly, 1986.

306. Evans, R. W., and Gualtieri, C. T.: Psychostimulant pharmacotherapy in traumatic brain injury. J. Head Trauma Rehabil., 2:29–33, 1987.

307. Winsberg, B. G., Bialer, I., Kupietz, S., et al: Effects of imipramine and dextroamphetamine on behavior of neuropsychiatrically impaired children. Am. J. Psychiatry, 128:109–115, 1979.

308. Strupp, F. J., and Levitsky, D. A.: Mnemonic role for vasopressin: The evidence for and against. Neurosci. Biobehav. Rev., 9:399–411, 1985.

309. Mysiw, W. J., and Jackson, R. D.: Tricyclic antidepressant therapy after traumatic brain injury. J. Head Trauma Rehabil., 2:34–42, 1987.

310. Cope, D. N.: The pharmacology of memory and attention. J. Head Trauma Rehabil., 1:34–42, 1986.

311. Hayes, R. L., Stonnington, H. H., and Lyeth, B. G.: Editorial: Pharmacological treatment of head injury—A new challenge. Brain Injury, 1:1–2, 1987.

312. Sutton, R. L., Weaver, M. S., and Feeney, D. M.: Drug-induced modifications of behavioral recovery following cortical trauma. J. Head Trauma Rehabil., 2:50–58, 1987.

313. Feeney, D. M., Gonzalez, A., and Law, W. A.: Amphetamines, haloperidol and experience interact to affect rate of recovery after motor cortex injury. Science, 217:855–857, 1982.

314. Finger, S., and Stein, D. G. (Eds): Brain Damage and Recovery: Research and Clinical Perspectives. New York, Academic Press, 1982.

315. Bach-y-Rita, P. (Ed.): Recovery of Function: Theoretical Considerations for Brain Injury Rehabilitation. Baltimore, University Park Press, 1980.

316. Goldman, P. S., and Lewis, M. E.: Developmental biology of brain damage and experience. In Cotman, C. (Ed): Neuronal Plasticity. New York, Raven Press, 1978.

317. Yu, J.: Functional recovery with and without training following brain damage in experimental animals: A review. Arch. Phys. Med. Rehabil., 57:38–41, 1976.

318. Cope, D. N.: Traumatic closed head injury: Status of rehabilitation treatment. Semin. Neurol., 5:212–220, 1985.

319. Varghese, G., Anderson, M., and Redford, J. B.: Recovery after brain injury: A two-year postdischarge follow-up. (Abstract.) Arch. Phys. Med. Rehabil., 60:654, 1984.

320. Thomas, G. M., and Mayer, N. H.: Delayed functional recovery from craniocerebral trauma. (Abstract.) Arch. Phys. Med. Rehabil., 60:532, 1979.

321. Najenson, T., Sazbon, J., Fiselzon, E., et al: Recovery of communication functions after prolonged coma. Scand. J. Rehabil. Med., 10:15–21, 1978.

322. Cope, D. N.: Traumatic closed head injury: status of rehabilitation treatment. Semin. Neurol., 5:212–220, 1985.

323. Gilchrist, E., and Wilkenson, M.: Some factors determining prognosis in young people with severe head injuries. Arch. Neurol., 36:355–359, 1979.

324. Oddy, M., Coughlan, T., Tyerman, A., et al: Social adjustment after closed head injury: A further follow-up seven years after injury. J. Neurol. Neurosurg. Psychiatry, 48:1564–1568, 1985.

325. Cope, D. N., and Martin, J.: Unpublished data. In Berrol, S., Cervelli, L., Cope, D. N., MacWorth, N. H., Macworth, J., Rappaport, M., Hall, K., Hopkins, H., (eds): Severe Head Trauma: A Comprehensive Medical Approach (Collaborative). (NIHR Project 13-P-59156/9). San Jose, California, 1982.

326. Prigatano, G. P., Fordyce, D. J., Zeiner, H. K., et al: The outcome of neuropsychologic rehabilitation efforts. In Fordyce, G. P.: Neuropsychological Rehabilitation after Brain Trauma. Baltimore, Johns Hopkins University Press, 1986, p. 131.

327. Brooks, D. N., and McKinely, W.: Personality and behavioral change after severe head injury—a relative's view. J. Neurol. Neurosurg. Psychiatry, 46:336–344, 1983.

328. Cunning, J. E.: Emotional aspects of head trauma in children. Rehabil. Lit., 37:335–339, 1976.

329. Lezak, M. D.: Living with the characterologically altered brain injured patient. J. Clin. Psychiatry, 39:592–598, 1978.

330. Oddy, M., Humphrey, M., and Uttley, D.: Stresses upon the relatives of head injured patients. Br. J. Psychiatry, 133:507–513, 1978.

331. Rosenbaum, M., and Najensson, T.: Changes in life patterns and symptoms of low mood as reported by wives of severely brain-injured soldiers. J. Consult. Clin. Psychol., 44:881–886, 1976.

332. Livingstone, M. G.: Assessment of need for coordinated approach in families with victims of head injury. Br. Med. J., 293:742–744, 1986.

333. Lezak, M. D.: Brain damage is a family affair. J. Clin. Exp. Neuropsychol., 10:111–123, 1988.

334. Prigatano, G. P., Fordyce, D. J., Zeiner, H. K., et al: The outcome of neuropsychological rehabilitation efforts. In Prigatano, G. P. (Ed.): Neuropsychological Rehabilitation after Brain Injury. Baltimore, Johns Hopkins University Press, 1986, pp. 119–133.

335. Haffey, W. J. (Ed.): Evaluation of outcome. J. Head Trauma Rehabil., 2:3, 1987.

336. Hall, K. M., and Cope, D. N.: The current status of head injury rehabilitation. In Miner, M. E., and Wagner, K. A. (Eds.): Neurotrauma: Treatment, Rehabilitation and Related Issues, No. 1. Boston, Butterworths, 1986.

337. Aronow, H. U.: Rehabilitation effectiveness with severe brain injury: Translating research into policy. J. Head Trauma Rehabil., 2:24–36, 1987.

338. Cope, D. N., and Hall, K. H.: Head injury rehabilitation: Benefit of early intervention. Arch. Phys. Med. Rehabil., 63:433–437, 1982.

339. Fryer, L. J., and Haffey, W. J.: Cognitive rehabilitation and community readaption: Outcomes from two program models. J. Head Trauma Rehabil., 2:51–63, 1987.

340. Cole, J. R., Cope, D. N., and Cervelli, L.: Rehabilitation of the severely brain-injured patient: A community-based, low-cost model program. Arch. Phys. Med. Rehabil., 66:38–40, 1985.

341. Diller, L., Ben-Yishay, Y.: Outcomes and evidence in neuropsychological rehabilitation in closed head injury. In Levin, H. S., Grafman, J., and Eisenberg, H. M. (Eds.): Neurobehaviorial Recovery from Head Injury. New York, Oxford University Press, 1987.

60

Neuropsychological Assessment and Training in Acute Brain Injury

JAY M. UOMOTO

New cases per year of acute brain injury occur at an alarmingly high rate, estimated to be in the range of 500,000 in the United States.[1-3] The incidence rate of between 180 and 200 cases per 100,000[3, 4] has been noted to be one and one half times the incidence of schizophrenia. The prevalence rate of traumatic brain injury has been estimated to be more than twice the incidence rate at approximately 439 cases per 100,000.[5] In an epidemiological study of San Diego County in California, Kraus and co-workers[6] found that the largest proportion of patients (72.5 per cent) fell into the "mild" level of head injury severity. Of the remaining patients, 8 per cent were classified as "moderate," 7.9 per cent were classified as "severe," and 11.5 per cent were dead on arrival. These investigators found the causes of traumatic brain injury to commonly break down into primarily five categories. Close to one half (44 per cent) of those who sustained acute brain injuries were injured as a result of motor vehicle accidents, followed by falls (21 per cent), assaults (12 per cent), sport-related accidents (10 per cent), and firearms (6 per cent). Whereas it is likely that these incidence rates have been consistent over the past decade, advances in medical technology and trauma/emergency care procedures have increased the survival rate among head trauma victims. The mortality rate of severe brain injuries is in the range of 50 per cent,[7] implying that another 50 per cent survive significant trauma. Anderson and McLaurin[8] report that by 1974 among all head injury victims they sampled, 97 per cent of those were discharged alive from their initial hospitalization. Thus, moderate and severely brain-injured patients who now receive trauma care are more often being sustained beyond initial treatment and are faced with a long and arduous process of recovery and rehabilitation.

With regard to demographics, in a study by Rimel and Jane,[9] the highest proportion of individuals sustaining head injuries is in the age range between 10 and 29 years, accounting for 62 per cent of the population they sampled. Others have shown high incidence rates among the 15- to 24-year-old age range with a decline in those rates with increasing age, rising again after age 70.[10] Adolescents and young adults are consistently overrepresented in studies of incidence rates. Males outnumber females in head injury cases by a ratio of 2:1 to 4:1.[11] Jennett and Teasdale[1] found alcohol consumption to be a frequent occurrence immediately prior to closed head injuries; 46 per cent of those admitted to primary surgical wards and 42 per cent of those with neurosurgical admissions have had alcohol associated with the head injury. No consistent relationship between socioeconomical level and cause of injury has been found, although a trend toward a higher incidence of assaults among those in lower social strata has been documented.[12] In summary, the higher proportion of those patients requiring comprehensive rehabilitation will be young males from a range of socioeconomical backgrounds with a higher likelihood of alcohol use problems.

Evidence is accumulating to show that rehabilitation efforts are beneficial to the long-term out-comes of brain-injured patients,[13] and within the past 10 years, the brain injury rehabilitation system has become more comprehensive and available, yet it is still young in its development.[14] The scope of brain injury rehabilitation is too large to cover in detail in this chapter, and therefore the focus will be on the cognitive and behavioral consequences resulting from brain injury. In particular, the importance of neuropsychological evaluation of brain-injured patients is underscored with respect to training and rehabilitation efforts. Acute brain injury will refer primarily to traumatic brain injury of a penetrating or closed type. The pathophysiology and mechanisms of traumatic brain injury are well described by several authors[15–17] and will not be covered here.

Neurobehavioral Sequelae in Brain Injury

Whenever I try to analyze anything and have to concentrate for a long time, the strain of coping with things that are not clear makes me anxious and upset. Since this can easily touch off an attack, I've quit trying to read books or burden my mind with too many ideas.
L. ZAZETSKY

A moving account of the struggles and experiences of a brain-injured patient was aptly captured by the Russian neuropsychologist Luria[18] in his compilation of writings by L. Zazetsky. It illustrates the intimate interaction between neuropsychological deficits and everyday life experiences of a patient who sustained a severe penetrating brain injury. In the context of this chapter, it is therefore important to underscore the areas that affect and are effected by cognitive impairment in the brain-injured patient.

Any discussion of the neurobehavioral consequences of brain injury cannot be made in isolation from the total clinical picture presented by such patients. A host of interactive variables and circumstances occur from the outset of brain injury that persist well beyond the initial hospitalization. Figure 60–1 illustrates the numerous areas that are involved. Each needs to be considered in rehabilitation treatment of this patient population. Cognitive and behavioral sequelae are often cited as primary problematic areas of concern and targets for rehabilitation efforts, yet the success of treatment can be contingent upon how the patient is functioning in other aspects of life.

Physical Sequelae

Among the more common physical/medical complications of traumatic brain injury (TBI) are included such problems as pyrexia, diplopia and other visual disturbances, vestibular and auditory changes,[19] as well as other fractures and contusions that are sustained in the initial injury itself. TBI patients are at risk for post-traumatic seizures, and this risk increases if the patient suffered a seizure within the first week after injury.[1] Such seizures can be a grand mal, generalized, or focal type and require prophylactic medications at least through the first year after injury. Medications such as Dilantin can add cloudiness to the patient's level of awareness and thus cause further impairment of cognition. Alternative seizure control medications such as carbamazepine may minimize the impact on cognitive impairment.[20] Finally, central nervous system damage can result in gait, balance, and ambulation problems, further complicating rehabilitation efforts. Chronic pain problems, physical deconditioning, and communicative disorders can accompany TBI and also may require extensive physical rehabilitation. As noted by Bray and colleagues,[21] the physical sequelae of TBI can limit the patient's ability to be independent and thus benefit from comprehensive rehabilitation efforts.

Cognitive Sequelae

As will be delineated later, a host of neuropsychological impairments can accompany TBI. As a general rule, the more severe and extensive the brain injury, the greater are the type, degree, and extent of cognitive impairment. Unlike focal cerebral vascular accidents, for instance, those who sustain traumatic brain injuries have more global and pervasive cognitive impairments.

Behavioral Sequelae

Among the most pervasive and difficult consequences of brain injury are the behavioral disturbances often associated with brain trauma. As will be discussed later, behavior problems such as anger outbursts, physical aggressiveness, and verbal disinhibition interact with cognitive impairment in that the patient's ability to self-modify such behaviors and the degree to which these problems respond to environmental manipulations in part depend on the degree of cognitive impairment.

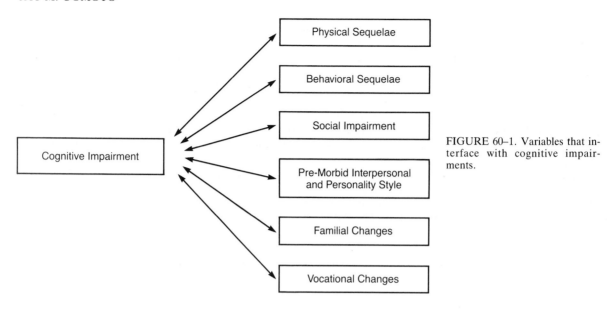

FIGURE 60–1. Variables that interface with cognitive impairments.

Social Impairment

TBI patients with significant cognitive impairment may not be able to manage social situations as they may have before injury owing to reduced capacity to deal with multiple inputs and memory deficits. A reduced ability to process information rapidly may render a patient unable to track conversations adequately, let alone to respond efficiently and appropriately in a situation that demands adept social skills. In a study undertaken by Lezak and her colleagues,[22] 42 male TBI patients were evaluated on the Portland Adaptability Inventory, an instrument that measures degree of impairment in the areas of temperament and emotionality, activities and social behavior, and physical capabilities. Their results indicated that the most persisting problems faced by patients are those of social contact, work/school involvement, and leisure, with many of these problems persisting five years after injury. They note that physical capabilities played a lesser role in the patient's social capabilities. One could postulate that cognitive and behavioral difficulties make a larger contribution to long-term outcome of social adjustment. Cognitive impairments can therefore limit the capacity of the patient to re-learn or compensate for social skill deficits. In those who also suffer expressive or receptive speech deficits, the ability of the patient to reintegrate with peers or other social contacts is further reduced.

Pre-Morbid Interpersonal and Personality Style

Many researchers have noted significant changes in personality and interpersonal functioning after brain injury.[23–26] What must also be considered in examining the impact of cognitive deficits upon patient rehabilitation and outcome are possible pre-existing personality traits and styles that are altered or exacerbated by brain injury. Rimel and co-workers[27] have found that a history of maladaptive behavior prior to injury can impact negatively upon the amount of disability after injury. For example, an individual who may be behaviorally impulsive prior to head injury may become more impulsive after injury, thus making cognitive rehabilitation a more difficult task. In another instance, a person who characterologically is compulsive and highly detail-oriented may find it extremely frustrating to cope with errors, misplacement of objects, and inefficiency in organizational skills secondary to short-term memory deficits.

Familial Changes

Family members of brain-injured patients must cope with and endure a wide spectrum of neurobehavioral impairments.[28, 29] These deficits can act as significant stressors to the integrity of the family system and cause much burden to family members.[26, 30–32] In most reports the cognitive deficits are less identified as the primary source of stress, whereas the emotional and behavioral changes are cited as more distressing. Nevertheless, cognitive impairment can be disruptive to family functioning, particularly in a situation in which the parent is brain-injured, is also responsible for managing discipline and financial affairs, and because of cognitive deficits is unable to consistently set limits with children or may become overwhelmed by household responsibilities. It is not unusual to find spouses or children fulfilling parental roles and responsibilities for the patient. Romano[31] studied family reactions to the head-injured patient and noted a phenomenon of denial of disability among family members. This took the form of verbal refusals to acknowledge the presence of changes in the patient, inappropriate responses such as lack of follow-through with compensatory strategies, and "common fantasies" that involve a belief in marked recovery in the patient in the face of little objective evidence of positive change. Such denial by family members can disrupt rehabilitation efforts and not allow the patient to fully benefit from cognitive rehabilitation treatment, thus perpetuating neuropsychological difficulties.

Vocational Changes

Due to the nature of the head-injured population's being of active working age, loss of employment and disruption of vocational/career direction often occur in TBI.[33, 34] An interplay between cognitive assets and deficits and vocational outcome is often seen. Patients may not be aware of the extent to which their cognitive capabilities differ from pre-injury levels and may be more rigid in wishing to return to their former employment. In other instances, a work history of limited transferable skills added with neuropsychological impairments can result in poor vocational outcomes for the patient with brain injury. Assessment of cognitive functions may therefore need to address questions regarding which type or class of vocational options should be pursued as well as provide some predictions about suitability of certain jobs given the patient's deficits.

In all of the preceding interactions it is essential to consider neuropsychological functioning in the context of several realms. The task of cognitive assessment is multipurpose in nature depending on the particular questions being asked of such an assessment. Neuropsychological variables cannot be considered in isolation from other realms of functioning or behavior. It can be a useful component to highlight, augment, or clarify information in these other realms. In comprehensive brain injury rehabilitation programs, neuropsychological assessment is considered a key element in structuring individual treatment programs, assisting in treatment decisions, explaining patient behavior, and predicting long-term outcome. The term *neurobehavioral* is thus a relevant and appropriate word to be used when evaluating and treating the brain-injured patient because of the interconnections between neurological and behavioral impairments.

Neuropsychological Assessment of Acute Brain Injury

General Considerations

Neuropsychological assessment is increasingly becoming a standard part of comprehensive evaluations in rehabilitative treatment programs for patients with acute brain injury. Although, historically, neuropsychology has been used for the purpose of differential diagnosis of neurological conditions, there is a growing press for using neuropsychological results in treatment-planning and strategizing interventions for those with brain injury. With the advent of more sophisticated diagnostic imaging techniques such as magnetic resonance imaging (MRI) and positron emission tomography (PET), there will likely be less need for neuropsychological testing to be used solely for diagnostic purposes. The cognitive and behavioral sequelae may persist and continue to be pervasive over the course of recovery. Therefore, neuropsychological assessment can be useful throughout the course of treatment and recovery to monitor cognitive and behavioral changes as well as provide ongoing direction for cognitive remediation and other rehabilitation components.

The field of neuropsychology is concerned with the relationship between brain function/impairment and observable behavior. The major underlying implication is that the exhibited behavior of the patient is a composite of brain functioning/integrity, psychological states, interpersonal propensities, and social contingencies. Modes of investigation in neuropsychological assessment include diagnostic interviewing, application of behavioral tests and procedures, and administration and interpretation of neuropsychological tests. Crockett, Clark, and Klonoff[35] note that neuropsychological assessment is an "active" procedure in that the methods of investigation require individual volition and effort. This is contrasted to neurological assessment that may be termed "passive" in nature, in which effort is not often required of the patient to evaluate (e.g., in CT scanning procedures). Neuropsychology has developed primarily out of the clinical psychology field and, hence, a majority of neuropsychologists are clinical psychologists by training. Individuals who refer to themselves as "clinical neuropsychologists" are usually those with specialty training in neuropsychology at the postdoctoral level and who may have obtained board status through the American Board of Professional Psychology/American Board of Clinical Neuropsychology.

The neuropsychologist is now becoming a vital member of the interdisciplinary rehabilitation team that also includes the physiatrist, speech/language pathologist, physical therapist, occupational therapist, vocational rehabilitation counselor, rehabilitation nurse, social worker, and program case manager. It is the responsibility of the neuropsychologist, whether in an inpatient, transitional living, day treatment, or outpatient setting, to provide input regarding cognitive assets/deficits and behavioral excesses/deficits to the rehabilitation team for evaluative and treatment direction purposes. This is discussed in more detail later. Further resource information regarding neuropsychology and assessment can be found in excellent texts by Filskov and Boll,[36, 37] Lezak,[38] Luria,[39] Reitan and Davison,[40] and Wedding, Horton, and Webster.[41]

Neuropsychological Assessment for the Brain-Injured Patient

There are a multiplicity of purposes for obtaining a neuropsychological assessment on a brain-injured patient. Such assessments are often setting-specific in that information needed in an inpatient setting may differ greatly from that required in a transitional living, independent living, or outpatient treatment context. For example, in an acute rehabilitation medicine unit, the questions asked in a neuropsychological evaluation may be focused on assessing the patient's ability to follow directions and remember trained skills, or the degree of cognitive ability to execute a series of instructions from a physical therapist. In the acute setting it is often helpful to obtain baseline data on cognitive assets and deficits in order to compare such findings at a later time to track degree of recovery from brain injury. In the outpatient setting, neuropsychological testing may be requested to assist the vocational rehabilitation counselor in developing a realistic vocational plan for the patient. In an independent living center context, the same neuropsychological data could be used to help determine the patient's safety in the community. For the purposes of this discussion, there are some general functions and applications that neuropsychological assessments provide across settings.

NEUROLOGICAL DIAGNOSIS

With the advent of refined diagnostic techniques, neuropsychological assessment is being less used specifically and solely for the purpose of neurological diagnosis. However, there are instances when this type of input is relevant. In progressive dementias, for example, the CT scan or MRI scan may show generalized brain atrophy, yet this may not specifically identify whether a dementia is present or what type it is. There are no medical tests at present that positively identify Alzheimer's disease,[42] and such findings can be obtained only by morphological studies post mortem. Therefore, neuropsychological testing, particularly with repeat testing intervals, can assist in identifying cognitive decline over time and thus provide evidence for a progressive dementia. Without cognitive decline, a differential between a progressive deficit and a cerebral vascular accident deficit could be suggested by the pattern of testing results. Testing can also confirm diagnostic imaging findings in that the pattern of results will correlate with lateralization and localization of brain damage. This underscores the importance of recognizing the interrelationships between brain and behavior.[43]

An area of increasing importance for the role of neuropsychological assessment is that of minor head injury. Such individuals experience brief loss of consciousness, suffer transient post-traumatic amnesia, obtain Glasgow Coma Scale[44] scores of between 13 and 15, and experience a set of neurobehavioral sequelae often referred to as a postconcussion syndrome.[45] These patients often present no abnormality on CT scans or skull radiographs[46] and may have negative neurological examinations.[47] Diffuse axonal stretching and shearing[48] may occur that cannot be identified outside of neuropathological studies upon autopsy. In these cases, the neuropsychological evaluation can sometimes document cognitive impairments that are not found by medical testing and thus lend some explanation for the behavioral sequelae that are seen in minor head injury.

Another issue in the use of neuropsychological testing is in the differential diagnosis of psychological disorders and brain damage. A common case is that of differentiating between clinical depression and brain dysfunction such as seen in dementia,[49] cerebral vascular accidents, head injury, tumors, and other conditions. Affective dysfunction is a very common concomitant to brain damage[50] and typically adds excess disability to the total clinical picture. Depression itself contributes to additional cognitive deficits in terms of decreased concentration, recent memory deficits, and slowed psychomotor responses. Part of the task of neuropsychological assessment is then to identify the presence of depression in the patient and make a determination as to the contribution of depression to cognitive deficits. Testing in this situation requires assessing a variety of cognitive functions as well as providing data on the psychological and behavioral state of the patient with brain injury.

The co-existence of alcohol/drug abuse and brain injury is not uncommon, and such dual diagnoses can pose difficult questions when one is asked to determine prognosis and develop rehabilitation strategies. Neuropsychological assessment in these cases may be necessary to differentiate deficits due to chronic alcoholism (e.g., recent memory deficits) from those attributable to acute brain injury. Whereas some trends in the pattern of test results have been shown among alcoholics[51, 52] and in drug abuse,[53] less is known about the combined effect of both brain injury and alcohol/drug abuse.

FUNCTIONAL DIAGNOSIS

Over and beyond diagnostic imaging studies, the neuropsychological assessment can provide information about the patient's cognitive abilities, in terms of both assets and deficits. Although a large part of medical practice is focused on deficit remediation, in rehabilitating the brain-injured patient it is equally important to capitalize on the patient's cognitive and behavioral assets. Thus, neuropsychological evaluations can assist in the functional diagnosis or delineation of assets and deficits to be used by the interdisciplinary rehabilitation team.

Testing results can be utilized to make predictions as to which training methods will or will not work with a particular brain-injured patient. For example, if a patient demonstrates greater difficulty in verbal recent memory ability, yet maintains good visual retention skills, the training strategy will be to "show" rather than "tell" the patient what sequence of tasks needs to be accomplished in therapy. Assessment of the speed with which a brain-impaired person processes cognitive information may yield information about the rate of learning capacity a patient possesses and thus implicate a "step-at-a-time" approach to training. By maximizing the particular strategies that best enable the patient to perform tasks, it is hoped that over the long term, costs for treatment will be reduced.

Often the neuropsychological assessment is used by other specific disciplines to assist in their assessment or treatment of the brain-injured patient. Morse and Morse[54] state that the interface between neuropsychology and other disciplines can generate clinical dilemmas. These include situations in which there is a discrepancy between poor neuropsychological test performance and good functional abilities in work situations that require those same skills that were tested. The reverse can be true with good test performance occurring in the face of poor functional skills. In these situations one may need to examine why these discrepancies exist; it also underscores the need to evaluate the patient on several fronts rather than to rely on the data of a single discipline. Neuropsychological testing is typically conducted in a controlled and structured environment that may yield results regarding the patient's full cognitive capacities at the time of the assessment. Conversely, testing is often considered stressful both emotionally and mentally since the nature of testing is to investigate maximum performance with errors being inevitable, whereas in a less stressful situation the patient's performance may actually be better. It is likely that discrepancies between testing performance and everyday abilities may be a function of different abilities being assessed in different contexts. Both sources of information are seen as important.

Functional diagnosis based on neuropsychological data may involve determining rehabilitation potential. Since comprehensive rehabilitation programs for brain-injured individuals are very costly, it is important to identify those areas that can be impacted the most by treatment and that will be of most lasting benefit to the patient. For example, if a patient's neuropsychological test results show preserved verbal expressive ability and poor complex problem-solving, such a patient may present as being of normal functioning to the casual observer. In fact this patient may not be able to implement tasks or possess the ability to solve problems and mobilize those intact verbal skills in a work or social situation. Rehabilitation should then be focused on a particular vocational or avocational goal that can capitalize on good verbal skills yet minimize the need for complex problem-solving.

A common element in brain injury rehabilitation programs is the use of cognitive remediation or cognitive retraining strategies. As will be discussed later, this involves the patient's working on compensatory and remedial strategies to improve the functional outcome of cognitive skills such as memory and problem-solving abilities. Neuropsychological assessment can yield an array of information regarding the pattern of cognitive assets that can be mobilized to assist with rebuilding other deficit areas. For example, a patient may exhibit significant attentional deficits yet may demonstrate a potential for better recent memory skill. In this case, the cognitive training strategy would be to enhance basic attention and concentration abilities through focused attention-training and the minimization of distractability.

Kay and Silver[34] remark that neuropsychological evaluation is becoming "something of a catchword in the field of vocational rehabilitation of head injured persons." They note that it is beneficial for vocational counselors to know information about several areas of the patient's neuropsychological functioning in order to develop a vocational plan that is both realistic and feasible to carry out. Cognitive capabilities, attention and concentration, capacity and speed of information processing, learning and memory, abstract thinking and problem-solving, communication skills, and visuospatial/perceptual skills of the brain-injured patient are functions that are useful for the counselor to know about the patient in order to specifically plan career and job directions. The neuropsychological evaluation can provide a component of information needed to identify a fit between the patient's assets, deficits, interests, and past and present skills and behavior with prospective job placements—certainly a most difficult task.

Finally, the neuropsychological evaluation may assist in the determination of case disposition, for example, from an acute hospitalization setting. The level and type of cognitive functioning will determine in part the type of brain injury rehabilitation

facility that may be most appropriate to refer. If the patient demonstrates excellent recovery of cognitive functions, that person may be more appropriately discharged to an outpatient or more vocationally oriented treatment setting versus another patient who exhibits significant behavioral or executive function disturbances. In the latter case, a more structured day treatment or transitional living setting may make a better disposition plan.

MONITORING PATIENT PROGRESS

Although neuropsychological evaluations can be costly, repeat testing can be useful to measure cognitive change over time. In the case of closed head injury, one expects recovery of cognitive functions over time. When decline in functioning is seen on repeat testing, the hypothesis may be more toward a dementia, malignant tumor, or other progressive neurological condition. Ideally, repeat testing can identify whether cognitive rehabilitation strategies are effective, although it is difficult to differentiate those effects due to training from those attributable to recovery. Another application is in examining the impact of medication on cognitive functioning. For example, a patient on seizure prophylaxis (e.g., Dilantin) may be tapered off of the medication, and a partial clearing of cognitive functioning may result. This could be monitored by pre- versus post-taper assessments. The same method can be employed to examine the effects of depression treatment (e.g., psychopharmacological or psychological intervention) on improving cognitive function, because depression can add attention, memory, and judgment impairment to the clinical picture of the brain-injured patient.

LITIGATION

Cases of acute brain injury will frequently go to litigation, perhaps because of the pervasive and long-term ramifications involved when a person's brain is damaged. Physical, cognitive, interpersonal, social, vocational, and recreational competencies can all be affected by brain injury and result in longstanding disability in these areas. As such, documentation of the extent of damage and issues of prognosis are standard questions raised in litigation cases. The neuropsychological evaluation can thus provide objective data regarding the cognitive status of the patient and how it may have been affected by a trauma or acquired condition. There are a number of difficult issues to address in litigation cases, such as what is a "normal" neuropsychological profile, what is the "expected" recovery curve in traumatic brain injury, what was the patient's pre-injury or pre-morbid level of functioning, and how much of the cognitive deficits seen on testing can be attributable to brain damage versus psychological overlay problems. As more research is conducted and data are gathered, neuropsychological evaluations may be able to more specifically answer these questions.

Methods of Neuropsychological Assessment

There exists a wealth of literature on methods of neuropsychological assessment and the ongoing debates as to which methods are preferred or useful and under which conditions.[36–38, 55, 56] As is true for many subspecialties in psychology, there are different orientations in the types and methods of neuropsychological assessment. When seeking a neuropsychological consultation, it is therefore important to bear in mind the different orientations to assessment. There are four major camps that are prevalent in both the research literature and clinical practice. Proponents of the *Halstead-Reitan Neuropsychological Battery* compose a large number of practitioners whose tradition began with the early work of Ward Halstead in the 1940s.[40, 57, 58] It is a fixed battery approach in that a specific set of tests is given to all patients; in this case, a set of seven standardized tests is administered, often with a number of allied procedures including the Wechsler Adult Intelligence Scale, Trailmaking Test, Sensory-Perceptual Examination, Reitan-Indiana Aphasia Screening Examination, and others. This battery as well as others has been extensively applied to brain-injured populations from which normative data have been generated.[59, 60] In a more controversial light is another fixed battery approach called the *Luria-Nebraska Neuropsychological Battery*,[61, 62] which is a set of procedures and tasks that is based on the work of the Russian neurologist A. R. Luria. Luria's work was first systematized by Anne-Lise Christensen, a neuropsychologist who developed a set of stimulus cards and tests called Luria's Neuropsychological Investigation.[63] This was further developed and standardized into its present form. The controversies around this instrument basically revolve around issues of validity, reliability, and ability to discriminate between diagnostic groups.[64–66] Arthur L. Benton, a neuropsychologist, has developed a set

of measures that may not be readily identified as a battery of tests, yet his tests deserve recognition for the types of specific information they yield.[67] The *Boston Process Approach* concerns itself with not only the standardized procedures required of test administration and interpretation, but also the way in which the patient performs to obtain scores.[68] Tests such as the Wechsler Adult Intelligence Scale (Revised) are administered in the standard fashion; however, in this approach, other methods are appended to yield further information about the process by which patients solve problems, therefore expounding further the cognitive skills and deficits that a patient may possess. Finally, there are proponents of what is referred to as the *hypothesis testing approach*. Lezak refers here to a process in which the "neuropsychological examination can be viewed as a series of experiments that generate explanatory hypotheses in the course of testing them."[38] Neuropsychological tests are thus chosen for the particular problem or hypothesis that is presented by the patient. In all of these approaches, the goal is to describe in as much detail as possible the spectrum of cognitive abilities, propensities, assets, and deficits that are both intact and damaged by brain injury. The type of method employed by a neuropsychologist is dependent on the type of training received. In the rehabilitation medicine setting, any one or combination of these approaches may be implemented, and in the hands of an experienced neuropsychologist, all can yield important data about the patient.

Reliability and Validity

Of significant importance in employing tests are issues of an instrument's reliability and validity. The issue of test construction of neuropsychological tests has been discussed in detail by Goldstein.[69] He suggests that a comprehensive battery ideally "assesses all of the major functional areas generally affected by structural brain damage." In order to do this, the battery must therefore have excellent psychometric properties such as construct, face, concurrent, and predictive validity. Moreover, tests must possess good reliability (e.g., test-retest; interrater; split-half; alternative forms), particularly since reliability sets the upper limit to validity.[70] With these issues in mind, a member of the interdisciplinary area must use judgment when considering the results of neuropsychological testing in light of each test's validity and reliability. In some cases, "homemade" tests for a specific purpose may be utilized without an appreciation of necessary psychometric issues, which can lead to drawing erroneous conclusions from the results. It should be noted that most neuropsychologists have had some training in psychometric and test construction theory and can evaluate these properties of a test.

Relevance for Everyday Functioning

Neuropsychological assessment, as stated earlier, can be used for a number of purposes, one of which is functional diagnosis. Implied in this usage is the goal of predicting everyday functioning. The ultimate goal perhaps is to be able to make accurate predictions of a brain-injured patient's ability to carry out everyday tasks and behavior from an assessment. Assessment findings should not be the only source or the primary source of information to make such predictions. For example, whereas it is important for the health care professional to be aware of a brain-injured patient's ability to plan, organize, and efficiently execute tasks in order to help make decisions about independent living,[71] other sources of information need to be taken into account. *In vivo* community assessment with observational data can be useful to augment neuropsychological information. Occupational therapy data and observations, as well as the family's and friends' reports, assist in making prognostic statements. In sum, when making predictions about global behavior such as activities of daily living, work behavior, safety skills, or independent living ability, a comprehensive analysis including neuropsychological input and other components will yield more predictive power.

Neuropsychological Components

At present, there is no agreed upon system of classifying the various neuropsychological components that are measured in an assessment. Some theoretical delineations, based primarily on the type of test (or domain that a test is purported to measure) that is considered, have been proposed.[38, 54, 72] Presented in Table 60–1 is an outline of the major cognitive areas covered and respective tests/procedures in a neuropsychological assessment with a brain-injured patient. See Lezak[38] for references regarding the majority of the individual tests listed.

GENERAL NEUROPSYCHOLOGICAL FUNCTIONING

In any assessment, a global estimate of the patient's general cognitive level is desired. Judgments can then be made as to the relative position of each individual test compared with the general index of functioning. The Halstead Impairment Index is based on the Halstead-Reitan Neuropsychological Battery, in which seven indexed tests are given (among others), and the number of tests scored in the impaired range (based on cutoff scores) determines the level of general impairment. The score ranges from 0.0 (normal range) to 1.0 (severe impairment). A recent expansion of the Impairment Index is the Neuropsychological Deficit Scale developed by Ralph M. Reitan and his colleagues.[73] This scale combines cutoff scores from several other tests and procedures from the battery to yield a total score. In many cases, the Full Scale IQ score from the Wechsler Adult Intelligence Scale (WAIS; and Revised version) is used to suggest general level of functioning. Based on age, education, and occupational background, an estimate can be made of pre-morbid or pre-injury general intellectual functioning using a regression formula and norms,[74, 75] which are then used to compare against current level of IQ. Furthermore, the Digit Symbol subtest of the WAIS has typically been seen as a measure of brain damage irrespective of the laterality of a brain lesion.[38] The General Memory Index (GMI) of the Wechsler Memory Scale—Revised can be a useful gauge of overall memory functioning in the brain-injured patient and therefore can be considered a general neuropsychological measure. The level of memory functioning on the GMI is often commensurate with IQ scores and general impairment ratings.

INTELLECTUAL FUNCTIONING

The most widely utilized test battery of intellectual functions is the WAIS and WAIS–R. Although it was not developed as a neuropsychological measure, many of the subtests are sensitive to brain damage and result in subscale profiles that are unique to brain injury. It yields both verbal and performance (nonverbal) scores that can provide useful information not only for neuropsychological purposes but also for academic planning

TABLE 60–1. Cognitive Variables Measured in Neuropsychological Assessment and Representative Tests and Procedures

VARIABLE	TEST/PROCEDURES	VARIABLE	TEST/PROCEDURES
General neuropsychological functioning	Halstead Impairment Index Neuropsychological Deficit Scale Full Scale IQ (Wechsler Adult Intelligence Scale; Revised, WAIS/WAIS–R) Digit Symbol (WAIS; WAIS–R) Symbol Digit Modalities Test General Memory Index (Wechsler Memory Scale—Revised)	Speed of cognitive processing	Trailmaking Test—Part B PASAT Digital Symbol (WAIS, WAIS–R)
		Visuospatial and perceptual-motor integration	Tactual Performance Test Performance subtests of WAIS, WAIS–R Rey-Osterreith Complex Figure Test Benton Visual Retention Test Bender-Gestalt Test Hooper Visual Organization Test
Intellectual functioning	WAIS, WAIS–R Stanford-Binet Intelligence Scale Peabody Picture Vocabulary Test Quick Test of Intelligence	Sensory and motor functioning	Reitan-Klove Sensory Perceptual Exam
Academic achievement	Wide Range Achievement Test—Revised Review of academic records		Tactual Form Recognition Finger Oscillation Test (Finger Tapping)
Attention and concentration	Digit Span (WAIS, WAIS–R) Arithmetic (WAIS, WAIS–R) Trailmaking Test—Part A Speech-Sounds Perception Test Seashore Rhythm Test Digit Vigilance Test Letter Cancellation Test Paced Auditory Serial Addition Test (PASAT) Stroop Test	Language and communication	Fingertip Number Writing Purdue Pegboard Test Trailmaking Test—Part A Boston Diagnostic Aphasia Examination Multilingual Aphasia Examination Reitan-Indiana Aphasia Examination Token Test
Memory functioning	Wechsler Memory Scale—Russell Revision Wechsler Memory Scale—Revised Selective Reminding Test Rey Auditory-Verbal Learning Test Fuld Object-Memory Evaluation Benton Visual Retention Test Sentence Repetition Rey-Osterreith Complex Figure Test Memory and Location of the Tactual Performance Test Rivermead Behavioural Memory Test	Abstraction, problem-solving, new learning, executive functioning	Boston Naming Test Controlled Oral Word Association Test Gates-MacGinitie Reading Tests Verbal subtests of WAIS, WAIS–R Category Test Wisconsin Card Sorting Test Trailmaking Test—Part B Tactual Performance Test Similarities and Comprehension subtests of WAIS, WAIS–R

and vocational rehabilitation services for brain-injured patients. Another less used battery for brain-injured patients is the Stanford-Binet Intelligence Scale; norms range from age two to young adult, and tests vary on the number of verbally loaded tests based on the age of the patient. Other ancillary measures that are good at estimating general intelligence are nonverbal response format tests such as the Peabody Picture Vocabulary Test

and the Quick Test of Intelligence These tests can be especially useful in testing the patient with an expressive aphasia.

ACADEMIC ACHIEVEMENT

In assessing the brain-injured patient, it is helpful to know what level of basic academic abilities exists. On the Wide Range Achievement Test, for example, basic spelling, reading, and arithmetic skills are assessed with scores reflecting grade-level equivalents. Such information is particularly useful to the vocational counselor who may be seeking a job placement for a brain-damaged patient that is commensurate with the academic skills that patient possesses. Because these data are rather global, academic records from elementary school to college can be used to examine strengths and weaknesses for the course of a patient's schooling. In some brain injuries, the patient may seemingly score well on intellectual and academic tests but complain of being less capable or mentally adept. Examination of records may reveal an individual who had a consistently high grade-point average, and who now may have significant academic problems, although the actual performance may be in the high-average range.

ATTENTION AND CONCENTRATION

The ability to attend to stimuli and sustain attention is an entry-level cognitive skill. Attending to small visual details and listening carefully to sounds or speech are examples of skills in this area. In Reitan's model of neuropsychological functioning,[59] attention and concentration skills are the levels of cognitive processing that lead to language and visuospatial abilities. Therefore, the ability to focus attention, sustain concentration, and block distractions will affect other cognitive abilities such as recent memory or complex problem-solving skill. Several factors can influence attention and concentration ability that may be functional in nature, such as clinical depression, excessive medication or seizure prophylaxis medication, and anxiety.

MEMORY FUNCTIONING

There are a host of memory measures with new scales being developed rather regularly. Listed in Table 60–1 are the more common measures utilized to assess brain-injured patients. Memory is a complex process that combines attentional, encoding, storage, retrieval, and recognition mechanisms. Because of the complexity of memory, guidelines have been suggested as to criteria that an adequate memory test should meet. Erickson, Poon, and Walsh-Sweeney[76] have recommended that a good memory test should assess orientation, short-term memory, delayed recall of information, and remote/long-term memory. Mateer, Sohlberg, and Crinean[77] have developed a typology of memory problems in brain-injured patients and, by

factor analysis, derived four memory components: attention/prospective memory (immediate, working memory); retrograde memory (recall of information prior to brain injury); anterograde memory (memory for episodic and semantic memory within hours of recall); and historic/overlearned memory (overlearned cultural and personal information). Several memory scales will include measures of recent verbal memory, recent visual memory, delayed recall of both verbal and visual information, and recognition memory. It is thus important to examine the literature on the test construction of each memory measure to know what construct or aspect of memory functioning is being assessed. Comparisons between memory measure scores can therefore be more accurate when similar concepts are compared. Some measures, such as the Memory and Location component of the Tactual Performance Test of the Halstead-Reitan Neuropsychological Battery, are a combination of many tasks that include incidental memory. Incidental memory is a task that involves being asked to recall information that the person was not initially asked to remember, but has done so incidentally. Other newer procedures such as the Rivermead Behavioral Memory Battery utilize a more *in vivo* approach to assessing memory by having the patient perform certain tasks within the room of the neuropsychological examination.

SPEED OF COGNITIVE PROCESSING

Brain-injured patients may not always make errors in cognitive operations or tasks; however, they may at times exhibit difficulty with processing information quickly. Rapid decision-making, or listening to a conglomeration of information and attempting to process that information rapidly, may pose problems. Many timed neuropsychological tests will tap into this cognitive processing speed component. For rehabilitation purposes, the patient's ability on these measures assists in structuring the method of instruction (e.g., step-by-step) and the context (e.g., allowing the patient time to complete a task; setting the patient up in a job station that requires less time constraints) for rehabilitation activities.

VISUOSPATIAL AND PERCEPTUAL-MOTOR INTEGRATION

These variables relate to the brain-injured patient's ability to analyze spatial relationships and make sense out of depth and space terms. Perceptual-motor integration skill refers to the ability to perceive stimuli, formulate a representation of those visual stimuli in memory, and translate those stimuli into a motor response (e.g., drawing a picture of an object that is presented visually). Several of these functions have a right hemispheric focus, with special emphasis on the right parietal regions. These functions become relevant in the return to work situation in which, for example, a brain-injured patient with visuospatial deficits may wish to do manual dexterity or fine motor coordination tasks but experiences difficulty in executing these tasks. In this case, the interdisciplinary team may opt to remediate or teach compensatory strategies for visuospatial problems, and the vocational counselor's task would be to attempt a fit between such problems and a job that minimizes the use of such functions. A problem with tests of visuospatial and perceptual-motor abilities is the confound of requiring a motor response. The peripheral motor integrity of the patient (and, in particular, of the hands) needs to be taken into account when interpreting these tests.

SENSORY AND MOTOR FUNCTIONING

In many types of brain injuries, lateralized sensory and motor deficits can occur that have a central nervous system basis. This is to be differentiated from peripheral motor and sensory difficulties that may arise out of previous or existing hand and arm injuries. The interpretation of lateralized findings comes from multiple sources on the neuropsychological examination and is not based solely on specific sensory and motor tests (e.g., speed of finger tapping comparing left and right hands; perceiving shapes of objects with both hands). Motor speed and strength can be influenced by clinical depression, and attention deficits affect the patient's ability to carry out these tests. The majority of the tests that are listed in Table 60–1 include procedures for examining right- versus left-hand differences. Dominant hand performances are compared with nondominant hand output where significant discrepancies between the two hands are interpreted in light of norms.

LANGUAGE AND COMMUNICATION

The majority of brain injury rehabilitation programs have speech/language pathologists on staff to evaluate and treat patients with language and communication deficits. The aphasias and dysarthria are by far the most common problems seen in brain injury in terms of language disorders. The neuropsychologist may or may not be involved in the assessment of language and communication functions, depending on the degree to which speech therapists are utilized. Many of the tests administered by a speech therapist are the same as those given by a neuropsychologist. Because of the complexity of language, no one test of speech or language function can describe the patient in detail. Therefore, many batteries of tests have been developed to assess the multiple aspects of speech and language abilities. As noted by Lezak,[38] the Boston Diagnostic Aphasia Examination is one of the most comprehensive batteries available to assess the aphasias and provide valuable data for rehabilitation planning. Although the WAIS and WAIS–R were not developed as speech and communication assessment devices, many of the verbal subtests can yield important information about verbal output and ability to comprehend verbal input stimuli. For rehabilitation purposes, it is often very useful to obtain information regarding the patient's verbal, auditory, and written comprehension, as well as expressive capacity.

ABSTRACTION, PROBLEM-SOLVING, NEW LEARNING, AND EXECUTIVE FUNCTIONS

A critical element of any neuropsychological evaluation is the assessment of higher-order cognitive processing, something that Lezak refers to as "executive functions."[38] In Lezak's scheme, executive functions involve goal formulating, planning, carrying out goal-directed plans, and effective performances. Stuss and Benson[78] underscore the predominant thrust of the frontal lobes as being significant for higher-order processing, where anticipation, goal selection, pre-planning, and monitoring are included in the executive functions. They note that the executive functions "represent many of the important activities that are almost universally attributed to the frontal lobes which become active in nonroutine, novel situations that require new solutions." At the behavioral level, these executive functions have correlates in terms of ability to use novel strategies to solve newly presented problems, ability to utilize abstract reasoning to inductively or deductively find solutions to problems, application of a range of solutions to problems, and ability to learn and generalize from previous learning trials and feedback. The ability to handle and cognitively process from multiple inputs (e.g., listening to verbal instructions while executing a task, coordinating eye-hand movements, and blocking out distracting stimuli) may

JAY M. UOMOTO

be considered an executive function. In sum, these functions refer to the ability to encode, integrate, process, and respond to stimuli in an organized fashion. Stuss and Benson rightly summarize that the frontal lobes operate as but a part of a total cognitive process:

The different functions of the brain do not work in isolation. When a new mental activity or preference is formed, it represents an amalgam of many nervous system attributes, actively derived from a process of trial against many relevant systems. The integration of autonomic and somatic nervous system elements, the correlation of visceral and emotional facets with verbal and nonverbal somatic information, provides an advanced level of mental control.

The assessment of executive functions is important in the total rehabilitation picture, since it is the cornerstone of determining prognosis. For example, a patient may possess excellent verbal expressive skills and maintain a high level of verbal intelligence and overlearned material, but if the patient shows significant impairment of executive functioning, that person will have great difficulty in organizing and utilizing those intact skills. The ability to integrate newly learned material and generalize across situations is an important prognosticator of whether treatment will generalize to another context. In those cases in which executive functions are significantly compromised, the rehabilitation strategy is to train the brain-injured patient in the setting in which that person will be working or living, and not to rely on generalization.

Head Injury Severity Ratings

Global indices of the severity of brain injury are used to categorize patients. They provide a basis on which to examine differences in severity among groups in memory[79] and other variables in neuropsychological recovery.[80] Two traditional methods have been used to estimate head injury severity: duration of coma and length of post-traumatic amnesia. Table 60–2 presents global cutoff points that have been proposed for each index.[81] Duration of coma can sometimes be estimated from emergency room or paramedic reports. In many cases, an hourly to daily record of Glasgow Coma Scale[44] scores exists in the medical record that assists in the estimation of severity. This scale provides a score based on eye opening response, best motor response, and best verbal response; scores range from a low of 3 to a maximum of 15. Post-traumatic

TABLE 60–2. Indices of Head Injury Severity

INDEX	LEVEL OF SEVERITY
PTA*	
less than 10 minutes	Very mild injury
10–60 minutes	Mild injury
1–24 hours	Moderate injury
1–7 days	Severe injury
greater than 7 days	Very severe injury
Coma	
0–1 hour	Mild injury
1–6 hours	Moderate injury
greater than 6 hours	Severe injury
Glasgow Coma Scale Score	
12–15	Mild injury
9–11	Moderate injury
3–8	Severe injury

*Post-traumatic amnesia.

amnesia (PTA)[82–84] refers to the time from the onset of injury to the time when continuous memory on a daily basis is reestablished. PTA can be tracked by professional staff while the patient is in the acute hospitalization or acute rehabilitation phase of treatment. In those cases in which the patient is discharged soon after trauma treatment (such as in minor head injury), ratings of PTA are mainly obtained from patient self-report, family, or friends in close proximity to the patient.

Recommendations for Neuropsychological Consultation

Whether in an acute rehabilitation or outpatient setting, the neuropsychologist is often called on to render an opinion about a patient and give recommendations for treatment and prognosis. As stated before, each neuropsychologist may have a unique orientation and preferences for tests employed in the assessment process. As such, clarification of the issues and questions at hand with a patient will yield useful data from the assessment. Neuropsychological evaluations are expensive, and thus maximum benefit from the data is important. The following are guidelines for requesting neuropsychological evaluations.

Identifying Information. Refer the neuropsychologist to relevant summaries of medical and psychosocial history or provide these data with the consultation request (which can be in the form of a letter or standard consultation form).

Diagnostic Hypotheses and Rationale. In those cases in which a differential diagnosis is being sought (e.g., depression versus cognitive impairment), it is helpful to note any impressions and rationale for possible diagnoses. In this way, specific neuropsychological or psychological tests may be included in a test battery to address the diagnostic questions.

List of Questions or Issues to be Addressed. Although this can be time-consuming, the neuropsychological evaluation or report can be tailor-made to answer particular questions that are relevant for a case. Rather than opting for the standard "assess cognitive deficits" consultation, a set of questions regarding level of intellectual functioning, ability for new learning, potential for benefiting from visual feedback modalities, or identification of maximal compensatory strategies may assist in better utilizing the evaluation in rehabilitation.

Information Regarding Logistics. This refers to including information about when a report is due, when the patient will be discharged, who will be reading the results, where the patient is located (if on an inpatient unit), who can provide collateral information, functional limitations of the patient relevant to testing (e.g., hemiparesis, spinal cord injury level and type, diplopia, unilateral neglect, pain problems, potential for anger outbursts, clinical depression, fractures in the arm or hand, aphasias, hearing loss), estimation of tolerance for full testing or interval testing, and funding for assessment.

Ancillary Data that Affect the Presentation of Neuropsychological Findings. Indicate for what purposes the results will be utilized. For example, indicate if the data will be discussed in a case conference to decide on treatment or compensatory strategies. When litigation is involved, the neuropsychologist may wish to be informed so as to prepare a report and present findings in a manner consistent with the case. The report may be used for disability ratings, which will structure the presentation of findings.[72] Test results are often of interest to family members, and thus the neuropsychologist may wish to prepare comments and explanations that address their needs.

Behavioral Sequelae and Typology

Acute brain injuries are associated with a host of behavioral problems that affect the lives of both patient and family. Cognitive and behavioral dis-

turbances persist for months and sometimes years beyond the initial injury. Consequently, those who are close to the patient (most often family members) experience psychological stress and burden.[30, 85, 86]

Interface Between Cognitive and Behavior Problems

Cognitive impairments interact with behavior disturbance in a somewhat complex fashion. Klonoff, Costa, and Snow[87] found that neuropsychological problems and initial Glasgow Coma Scale scores were significantly correlated with quality of life (e.g., activities of daily living) and social role functioning. One can postulate that such decreases in quality of life aspects in the patient can lead to poor self-concept and physical and psychological deactivation, and thus lead to behavioral problems such as anger, irritability, clinical depression, and anxiety difficulties. Recent memory problems can result in the brain-injured patient's having trouble recalling important information someone else may have imparted, leading to increased frustration and propensity to anger. Lack of awareness of cognitive and behavioral problems secondary to brain injury added to difficulties in rapidly processing information or from multiple inputs can lead to frustration, irritability, depression, and anger in the patient. Increased frustration will also make ineffective cognitive processing, which in turn may lead to more frustration; thus, a downward spiral of disability can result. Another example of the interaction between cognitive and behavioral realms is in the case of engaging the behaviorally impaired (e.g., impulsive, easily agitated) patient in cognitive remediation tasks. Such a patient may not be able to sustain the attention and concentration necessary to focus on learning compensatory strategies, as well as to exert enough self-control to employ strategies in the home or social environment.

A Typology of Behavior Disturbance

Behavioral disturbances appear to persist over a significant length of time. Lezak[22] utilized the Portland Adaptability Inventory to examine temperament and emotionality in head-injured patients over time and found anger problems to be present in 70 per cent of those patients at 49 to 60 months after injury. In that same study, there appeared to be an increase in the percentage of patients with depression in the 7- to 12-month period following injury. At four to five years, 52 per cent were bothered by depression.

In developing rehabilitation programs for brain-injured patients, it is important to recognize the impact of behavioral disturbances on both family and patient alike. Careful assessment of these problems during regular intervals in the patient's recovery assists the health care professional in structuring interventions that allow maximal community and vocational re-entry. Table 60–3 presents an outline of the major areas of behavioral disturbances seen most often in acute brain injury. Two major behavioral categories can be delineated in assessing disturbance. *Disinhibition* refers to the process of losing inhibitory controls over action and emotions. The patient may or may not be aware of a change in ability to inhibit responses, such as anger outbursts. *Deficits* refer to a paucity of action or emotion, or an absence of spontaneous behavior and initiative. Not all aspects of these behavior problems are present in each patient with brain injury, and it is difficult to predict prognosis of these difficulties. Assessment of behavioral disturbance comes from multiple sources. Family report and patient self-report are often useful to obtain, particularly in comparing similarities and differences between patient and family member. Clinician and staff observations provide data that can be compared with home or work environment settings, thus examining the impact of structured therapies on behavior as well as looking at generalization across settings of treatment. Psychometric devices to measure psychological aspects of behavior problems (e.g., depression and anxiety) are numerous and have been applied to assess head-injured patients (e.g., Dikmen and Reitan[88]). Once behavior problems are assessed and defined, treatment programs and training strategies can be developed and executed.

Training and Rehabilitation of Brain Injury

It is beyond the scope of this chapter to delineate the variations in the type of rehabilitation programs in which brain-injured patients can be involved. There are several commonalities across program and training approaches in terms of the type of rehabilitation staff and strategies employed

TABLE 60–3. A Typology of Behavioral Sequelae in Acute Brain Injury

TYPE	FEATURES
Behavioral Disinhibition	
Verbal/physical aggressiveness	Sudden and spontaneous outbursts; precipitated by minor antecedents; often short-lived; decrease or loss of learned inhibitory controls; lack of prediction in behavior/outburst
Coarse social behavior	Loss of interpersonal tact; inappropriate frankness; decreased appreciation of social cues, impact on others, and feedback; impulsive social actions; social behavior out of context for the situation
Verbal disinhibition	Overproduction of verbal output; tangential output; decreased awareness of overproduction; decreased ability to stop overproduction
Undercontrolled sexual behavior	Inappropriate attempts in developing intimate contacts or relationships; conversation with sexual innuendo and lewd remarks; inappropriate touching
Emotional dyscontrol	Emotional lability; anger outbursts; decreased ability to modify emotions; irritability; disproportionate emotional reactions to events or situations
Behavioral Deficits	
Initiation deficit	Decrease in spontaneous behaviors; limitation in creative actions; indifference to environmental stimuli; need for prompting of behavioral actions
Physical deficit	Fatigue; lethargy; psychomotor retardation; drowsiness
Affective deficit	Restricted or bland affect; anhedonia; decreased responsivitiy to humor

to train brain-injured patients in ways of coping with and compensating for their deficits. It should be noted, however, that specific programs for brain injury, from inpatient to outpatient management, are relatively new, and only now is the field beginning to proliferate. The reader is referred to texts by Edelstein and Couture,[89] Goldstein and Ruthven,[90] Prigatano,[91] Rosenthal, Griffith, Bond, and Miller,[92] Uzzell and Gross,[93] Wood,[94] and Ylvisaker and Gobble[95] for more detailed descriptions of brain injury rehabilitation. Some issues are worth highlighting to understand the nature and scope of training and rehabilitation.

Interdisciplinary Focus

With many physical disability groups, a team of rehabilitation professionals is involved in the care of the patient. The same holds for patients with brain injuries. A distinction is often made between "multidisciplinary" and "interdisciplinary." In the former, each team member works with the patient from the particular perspective of his or her discipline. For example, a physical therapist will work on range-of-motion activities with a patient who may have residual muscle weakness secondary to a brain injury. Interdisciplinary planning involves identifying common goals that a number of disciplines may share responsibility for assisting the patient to reach. For example, a brain-injured patient may exhibit verbal disinhibition, and all disciplines may be involved in helping to remediate the problem. The speech therapist and neuropsychologist may identify cues and intervention strategies to be used to modify verbal overproduction. The occupational and physical therapists will implement these cues throughout their therapies. The vocational counselor may integrate these strategies in counseling sessions and may wish to enlist the help of job station or on-the-job-training supervisors to implement the same technique, thus maximizing the opportunity for generalizing treatment. In most brain injury rehabilitation programs, team meetings are often regularly held in which common treatment goals and strategies are identified. The importance of generalizing treatment effects is critical for brain-injured patients, since they often have impaired capacities for abstract thinking and dealing with novel situations. The disciplines of physiatry, neuropsychology, clinical psychology, speech and language pathology, physical therapy, occupational therapy, social work, rehabilitation nursing, and vocational rehabilitation counseling are most often represented in brain injury rehabilitation programs. In addition, a new discipline is coming to the forefront in such programs called *case management*.

Case Management

As was mentioned earlier in this chapter, brain-injured patients can present a host of physical, emotional, and social problems that result from the injury. Because many patients require an enormous amount of treatment and training, management of the various components of the patient's treatment can be complicated. Case management includes the functions of coordinating treatment components, advocating for the patient and family to interface with other systems and agencies, assisting in the seeking of funding for treatment, coordinating written reports and dissemination of information in a timely fashion to important resources, and monitoring the process of rehabilitation to maximize treatment outcomes. Case manager positions are now being more frequently created in head injury programs across the country as the demand for coordinating and managing the problems of this population increases. The case manager is now considered a regular participating member of the interdisciplinary rehabilitation team.

Cognitive Rehabilitation

This is a highly popular concept that is now emerging in the field of brain injury rehabilitation. Cognitive rehabilitation is also known by the terms "cognitive remediation" and "cognitive retraining." There is currently no agreed upon definition of this area of training, and there exist many different strategies and philosophies about the concept. As Grimm and Bleiberg[96] note:

Contrary to its implied meaning, the term does not refer to a standard set of therapeutic activities prescribed to someone with a particular generic deficit, although certain intervention protocols reported in the literature seem to suggest just that.

They go on by quoting Gianutsos,[97] who stated that cognitive rehabilitation is

..."a service designed to remediate disorders of perceptions, memory and language in brain-injured person." Many rehabilitation programs adopt a similar slogan in their marketing efforts, despite the fact that interventions for cognitive deficits still are being developed and only recently have been subjected to the most elementary of scientific inquiry. The future very well may see the development of adequately validated cognitive retraining "packages" but we are a far cry from this at present.

There are arguments on both sides of whether cognitive remediation strategies are effective in outcome. A problem arises, however, in defining what a proper outcome may be, or by what criteria outcome is measured in the case of cognitive rehabilitation. These issues are further clouded by the fact that comprehensive rehabilitation programs include numerous other activities and therapies that may equally or more fully account for improvements in cognition. Finally, the natural recovery process from brain injury may account for changes in cognitive ability over time. For a more thorough discussion and review of various cognitive rehabilitation techniques, see Grimm and Bleiberg.[96]

There are two basic approaches in cognitive rehabilitation. In the more *curriculum-based model*, individuals with brain injury are trained and drilled on memory exercises, language, and problem-solving tasks with the basic intent of improving cognition in those areas that are impaired. Those who advocate the use of computer retraining techniques tend to approach cognitive rehabilitation from this perspective. In the *functional/goal-directed model*, the emphasis is on developing compensatory strategies to "make up the difference" for cognitive impairments. For example, if a person experiences significant compromise in recent verbal memory, the patient can be trained to use a memory book and instructed in ways to use note-taking and mnemonic devices to aid in retaining verbal material. Such strategies may be tailor-made to fit the particular situations in which the patient will need to remember information (e.g., listening to a lecture; following instructions while on the job). Such compensatory strategy training is goal-directed in that the focus is not so much on the exact cognitive impairments, but rather on those impairments that pose obstacles to significant goals in the patient's life. For example, if problem-solving abilities were impaired because of brain injury, and it interfered with the patient's desire to return to a position requiring management decisions, the patient would be trained on a particular problem-solving strategy that could be used on the job. Such a functionally based system of cognitive rehabilitation often requires an interdisciplinary effort to implement because of the broad range of vocational, independent living, social, and recreational goals that a patient may present. Grimm and Bleiberg aptly summarize the state of the art of cognitive rehabilitation:

Cognitive retraining as a therapeutic modality has yet to come of age, and, as noted with other interventions for brain-injured patients, remains at present in the technique-building phase of development. . . . As one father of a severely impaired young man commented, "J. J. became quite good at shooting down Mar-

tians. . . . If only we could teach him to tie his shoes and ask for the urinal." The point is that if this mode of treatment is to remain viable and credible, practitioners of the art must exercise professional restraint as to whom they admit for training or at least avoid false claims of effectiveness by carefully delineating the limitations in our present knowledge and the need for further research.

A Comprehensive System of Brain Injury Rehabilitation

In recognition of the high incidence of brain injury in the general population, more programs and services for this population are emerging in major metropolitan areas. Presented in Figure 60–2 is a system of rehabilitation that tracks brain-injured patients from the initial injury to the point of community and home re-entry. Ideally, all components would exist in each city, although this is dependent on economical, social, and accessibility factors. Unfortunately, funding for brain injury rehabilitation is not easily attainable and is dependent on the insurance coverage, personal assets, litigation status, and workers' compensation status of the patient. The fact that brain injury rehabilitation is a long process adds to the financial commitments that are required for such treatment. As is the case with much medical care, those who can afford treatment are the ones that can access these brain injury programs.

In the acute phase of intervention, a patient may be taken initially to an emergency room or to a designated trauma center for initial medical stabilization. Depending on the severity of injury, treatment within an intensive care unit may be required. In cases of minor head injury, many are discharged directly to their homes with instructions to return to the emergency room should problems persist. More patients are being seen with minor head injury in rehabilitation programs whose problems do persist and have developed into larger psychosocial difficulties, much like the case of chronic pain patients. Once the patient has been stabilized, admission to a neurosurgery unit or other acute hospitalization takes place. If a patient remains in a coma, a specialized coma stimulation program may be referred to; if successful, the patient would be appropriate for further structured therapy. If unsuccessful, the patient may be institutionalized in a long-term care facility or nursing home. Acute rehabilitation on an inpatient basis can start interdisciplinary treatment of some of the more gross

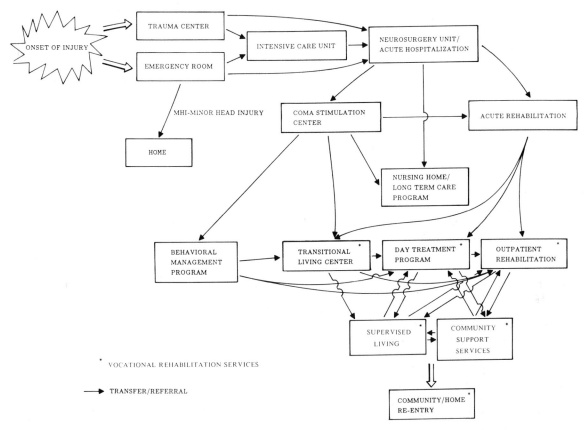

FIGURE 60–2. Brain injury rehabilitation system.

cognitive and physical sequelae of brain injury. From there the patient may be transferred to a post-acute type of program.

The level of post-acute care is ofen determined by the level of severity of brain injury as well as the functional capabilities of the patient. These can range from the most environmentally structured programs such as behavioral management facilities to more traditional outpatient programs. There are cases in which a patient may need the supervision of being in an independent living facility, where the patient lives with supportive services and receives rehabilitation at a day treatment or outpatient facility. Throughout the post-acute phase, the patient may be receiving some level of vocational services. It is hoped that should the patient progress to the level of independent living, community or home re-entry can be considered. Reintegration back into the home and work environments is often very difficult to accomplish with

the brain-injured patient, and modification in the environment is almost always inevitable. As programs and techniques improve, both in the acute and post-acute phases, it is hoped that functional outcomes of the brain-injured patient will also greatly improve.

References

1. Jennett, B., and Teasdale, G.: Management of Head Injuries. Philadelphia, F. A. Davis, 1981.
2. Caveness, W. F.: Incidence of craniocerebral trauma in the United States in 1976, and trend from 1970–1975. *In* Thompson, R. A., and Green, J. R. (Eds.): Advances in Neurology, Vol. 22. New York, Raven Press, 1979.
3. Silver, J. M., Yudofsky, S. C., and Hales, R. E.: Neuropsychiatric aspects of traumatic brain injury. *In* Hales, R. E., and Yudofsky, S. C. (Eds.): The American Psychiatric Press Textbook of Neuropsy-

chiatry. Washington, DC, American Psychiatric Association Press, 1987.

4. Kurtske, J. F.: The current neurologic burden of illness and injury in the United States. Neurology, 32:1207–1214, 1982.

5. Kalsbeck, W. D., McLaurin, R. L., Harris, B. S. H., and Miller, J. D.: The National Head and Spinal Cord Injury Survey: Major findings. J. Neurosurg., 53:519–531, 1980.

6. Kraus, J. F., Black, M. A., Hessol, N., Ley, P., Rokaw, W., Sullivan, C., Bowers, S., Knowlton, S., and Marshall, L.: The incidence of acute brain injury and serious impairment in a defined population. Am. J. Epidemiol., 119:186, 1984.

7. Editorial: Head injuries. Lancet, 1:589–591, 1978.

8. Anderson, D. W., and McLaurin, R. L. (Eds.): Report on the national head and spinal cord injury survey conducted for the National Institute of Neurological and Communicative Disorders and Stroke. J. Neurosurg. [Suppl.], 53:1–43, 1980.

9. Rimel, R. W., and Jane, J. A.: Characteristics of the head-injured patient. In Rosenthal, M., Griffith, E. R., Bond, M. R., and Miller, J. D. (Eds.): Rehabilitation of the Head Injured Adult. Philadelphia, F. A. Davis, 1983.

10. Annegers, J. F., Grabow, J. D., Kurland, L. T., and Laws, E. R.: The incidence, causes, and secular trends of head trauma in Olmstead County, Minnesota. Neurology, 30:912–919, 1980.

11. Kraus, J. F.: Injury to the head and spinal cord: The epidemiological relevance of the medical literature published from 1960 to 1978. J. Neurosurg. [Suppl.], 53:3–10, 1980.

12. Kerr, T. A., Kay, D. W. K., and Lassman, L. P.: Characteristics of patients, type of accident, and mortality in a consecutive series of head injuries admitted to a neurosurgical unit. Br. J. Prevent. Soc. Med., 25:179–185, 1971.

13. Aronow, H. U.: Rehabilitation effectiveness with severe pain injury: Translating research into policy. J. Head Trauma Rehabil., 2:24–36, 1987.

14. Burke, D.: Planning a system of care for head injuries. Brain Injury, 1:189–198, 1987.

15. Alexander, M. P.: Traumatic brain injury. In Benson, D. F., and Blumer, D. (Eds.): Psychiatric Aspects of Neurologic Disease, Vol. II. New York, Grune & Stratton, 1982.

16. Levin, H. S., Benton, A. L., and Grossman, R. C.: Neurobehavioral Consequences of Closed Head Injury. New York, Oxford University Press, 1982.

17. Cooper, P. R.: Head Injury. Baltimore, Williams & Wilkins, 1982.

18. Luria, A. R.: The Man with a Shattered World. Cambridge, Harvard University Press, 1972.

19. Namerow, N. S.: Current concepts and advances in brain injury rehabilitation. J. Neurol. Rehabil., 1:101–114, 1987.

20. Evans, R. W., and Gualtieri, C. T.: Carbamazepine: A neuropsychological and psychiatric profile. Clin. Neuropharmacol., 1:221–241, 1985.

21. Bray, L. J., Carlson, F., Humphrey, R., Mastrilli, J. P., and Valko, A. S.: Physical rehabilitation. In Ylvisaker, M., and Gobble, E. M. R. (Eds.): Community Re-entry for Head Injured Adults. Boston, College-Hill Press, 1987.

22. Lezak, M. D.: Relationships between personality disorders, social disturbances, and physical disability following traumatic brain injury. J. Head Trauma Rehabil., 2:57–70, 1987.

23. Prigatano, G. P.: Neuropsychological deficits, personality variables, and outcome. In Ylvisaker, M., and Gobble, E. M. R. (Eds.): Community Re-entry for Head Injured Adults. Boston, College-Hill Press, 1987.

24. Prigatano, G. P., Pepping, M., and Klonoff, P.: Cognitive, personality, and psychosocial factors in the neuropsychological assessment of brain-injured patients. In Uzzell, B., and Gross, Y. (Eds.): Clinical Neuropsychology of Intervention. Boston, Martinus Nijhoff, 1986.

25. Levin, H. S., and Grossman, R. G.: Behavioral sequelae of closed head injury: A quantitative study. Arch. Neurol., 35:720–727, 1978.

26. Brooks, D. N., and McKinlay, W.: Personality and behavioral change after severe blunt head injury—a relative's view. J. Neurol. Neurosurg. Psychiatry, 46:336–344, 1983.

27. Rimel, R. W., Giordani, B., Barth, J. T., and Jane, J. A.: Moderate head injury: Completing the clinical spectrum of head trauma. Neurosurgery, 11:344–350, 1982.

28. Bond, M. R.: Effects on the family system. In Rosenthal, M., Griffith, E. R., Bond, M. R., and Miller, J. D. (Eds.): Rehabilitation of the Head Injured Adult. Philadelphia, F. A. Davis, 1983.

29. Lezak, M. D.: Living with the characterologically altered brain injured patient. J. Clin. Psychiatry, 39:592–598, 1978.

30. Oddy, M., Humphrey, M., and Uttley, D.: Stresses upon the relatives of head-injured patients. Br. J. Psychiatry, 133:507–513, 1978.

31. Romano, M. D.: Family response to traumatic head injury. Scand. J. Rehabil. Med., 6:1–4, 1974.

32. Rosenbaum, M., and Najenson, T.: Changes in life patterns and symptoms of low mood as reported by wives of severely brain-injured soldiers. J. Consult. Clin. Psychol., 44:881–888, 1976.

33. Wachter, J. F., Fawber, H. L., and Scott, M. B.: Treatment aspects of vocational evaluation and placement for traumatically brain-injured adults. In Ylvisaker, M., and Gobble, E. M. R. (Eds.): Community Re-entry for Head Injured Adults. Boston, College-Hill Press, 1987.

34. Kay, T., and Silver, S. M.: The contribution of the neuropsychological evaluation to the vocational rehabilitation of the head-injured adult. J. Head Trauma Rehabil., 3:65–76, 1988.

35. Crockett, D., Clark, C., and Klonoff, H.: Introduction—an overview of neuropsychology. In Filskov,

S. B., and Boll, T. J. (Eds.): Handbook of Clinical Neuropsychology. New York, Wiley, 1981.

36. Filskov, S. B., and Boll, T. J. (Eds.): Handbook of Clinical Neuropsychology. New York, Wiley, 1981.

37. Filskov, S. B., and Boll, T. J. (Eds.): Handbook of Clinical Neuropsychology, Vol. 2. New York, Wiley, 1986.

38. Lezak, M. D.: Neuropsychological Assessment, 2nd Ed. New York, Oxford University Press, 1983.

39. Luria, A. R.: The Working Brain: An Introduction to Neuropsychology. New York, Basic Books, 1973.

40. Reitan, R. M., and Davison, L. A. (Eds.): Clinical Neuropsychology: Current Status and Applications. Washington, DC, V. H. Winston & Sons, 1974.

41. Wedding, D., Horton, A. M., and Webster, J. (Eds.): The Neuropsychology Handbook: Behavioral and Clinical Perspectives. New York, Springer, 1986.

42. Libow, C. S.: Senile dementia and "pseudosenility": Clinical diagnosis. In Eisdorfer, C., Friedel, R. O. (Eds.): Cognitive and Emotional Disturbances in the Elderly. Chicago, Year Book Medical Publishers, 1977.

43. Filskov, S. B., Grimm, B. H., and Lewis, J. A.: Brain-behavior relationships. In Filskov, S. B., Boll, T. J. (Eds.): Handbook of Clinical Neuropsychology. New York, Wiley, 1981.

44. Teasdale, G., and Jennett, B.: Assessment of coma and impaired consciousness: A practical scale. Lancet, 4:81–84, 1974.

45. Horwitz, N. H.: Postconcussion syndrome. Trauma, 2:72, 1960.

46. Rimel, R. W., Giordani, B., and Barth, J. T.: Disability caused by minor head injury. Neurosurgery, 9:221–229, 1981.

47. Schoenhuber, R., and Gentilini, M.: Auditory brain stem responses in the prognosis of late postconcussional symptoms and neuropsychological dysfunction after minor head injury. Neurosurgery, 19:532–534, 1986.

48. Gennarelli, T. A.: Mechanisms and pathophysiology of cerebral concussion. J. Head Trauma Rehabil., 1:23–29, 1986.

49. Gallagher, D., and Thompson, L. W.: Depression. In Lewinsohn, P. M., and Teri, L. (Eds.): Clinical Geropsychology: New Directions in Assessment and Treatment. New York, Pergamon Press, 1983.

50. Ruckdeschel-Hibbard, M., Gordon, W. A., and Diller, L.: Affective disturbances associated with brain damage. In Filskov, S. B., and Boll, T. J. (Eds.): Handbook of Clinical Neuropsychology, Vol. 2. New York, Wiley, 1986.

51. Brandt, J., and Butters, N.: The alcoholic Wernicke-Korsakoff syndrome and its relationship to long-term alcohol abuse. In Grant, I., and Adams, K. M. (Eds.): Neuropsychological Assessment of Neuropsychiatric Disorders. New York, Oxford University Press, 1986.

52. Ryan, C., Didario, B., Butters, N., and Adinolfi, A.: The relationship between abstinence and recovery of function in male alcoholics. J. Clin. Neuropsychol., 2:125–134, 1980.

53. Carlin, A. S.: Neuropsychological consequences of drug abuse. In Grant, I., and Adams, K. M. (Eds.): Neuropsychological Assessment of Neuropsychiatric Disorders. New York, Oxford University Press, 1986.

54. Morse, P. A., and Morse, A. R.: Functional living skills: Promoting the interaction between neuropsychology and occupational therapy. J. Head Trauma Rehabil., 3:32–44, 1988.

55. Grant, I., and Adams, K. M. (Eds.): Neuropsychological Assessment of Neuropsychiatric Disorders. New York, Oxford University Press, 1986.

56. Incagnoli, T., Goldstein, G., and Golden, C. J. (Eds.): Clinical Applications of Neuropsychological Test Batteries. New York, Plenum Press, 1986.

57. Boll, T. J.: The Halstead-Reitan Neuropsychological Battery. In Filskov, S. B., and Boll, T. J. (Eds.): Handbook of Clinical Neuropsychology. New York, Wiley, 1981.

58. Parsons, O. A.: Overview of the Halstead-Reitan Battery. In Incagnoli, T., Goldstein, G., and Golden, C. J. (Eds.): Clinical Application of Neuropsychological Test Batteries. New York, Plenum Press, 1986.

59. Reitan, R. M., and Wolfson, D.: The Halstead-Reitan Neuropsychological Test Battery: Theory and Clinical Interpretation. Tucson, AZ, Neuropsychology Press, 1985.

60. Russell, E. W., Neuringer, C., and Goldstein, G.: Assessment of Brain Damage: A Neuropsychological Key Approach. New York, Wiley, 1970.

61. Golden, C. J.: A standardized version of Luria's neuropsychological tests: A quantitative and qualitative approach to neuropsychological evaluation. In Filskov, S. B., and Boll, T. J. (Eds.): Handbook of Clinical Neuropsychology. New York, Wiley, 1981.

62. Golden, C. J., Purish, A. D., and Hammeke, T. A.: Luria-Nebraska Neuropsychological Battery: Forms I and II. Los Angeles, Western Psychological Services, 1985.

63. Christensen, A. L.: Luria's Neuropsychological Investigation. New York, Spectrum, 1975.

64. Adams, K. M.: Luria left in the lurch: Unfulfilled promises are not valid tests. J. Clin. Neuropsychol., 6:455–458, 1984.

65. Spiers, P. A.: The Luria-Nebraska Battery revisited: A theory in practice or just practicing? J. Consult. Clin. Psychol., 50:301–306, 1982.

66. Stambrook, M.: The Luria-Nebraska Neuropsychological Battery: A promise that may be partly fulfilled. J. Clin. Neuropsychol., 5:247–269, 1984.

67. Benton, A. L., Hamster, K., Varney, N., and Spreen, O.: Contributions to Neuropsychological Assessment: A Clinical Manual. New York, Oxford University Press, 1983.

68. Milberg, W. P., Hebben, N., and Kaplan, E.: The Boston Process Approach to neuropsychological as-

sessment. *In* Grant, I., and Adams, K. M. (Eds.):
Neuropsychological Assessment of Neuropsychiatric
Disorders. New York, Oxford University Press,
1986.

69. Goldstein, G.: Comprehensive neuropsychological
assessment batteries. *In* Goldstein, G., and Hersen,
M. (Eds.): Handbook of Psychological Assessment.
New York, Pergamon Press, 1984.

70. Nunnally, J. C.: Psychometric Theory, 2nd Ed. New
York, McGraw-Hill, 1978.

71. Condeluci, A., Cooperman S., and Seif, B. A.:
Independent living: Settings and supports. *In* Ylvisaker, M., and Gobble, E. M. R. (Eds.): Community Re-entry for Head Injured Adults. Boston,
College-Hill, 1987.

72. Kodimer, C.: Neuropsychological assessment and
Social Security disability: Writing meaningful reports and documentation. J. Head Trauma Rehabil.,
3:77–85, 1988.

73. Reitan, R. M., and Wolfson, D.: Development,
scoring, and validation of the Neuropsychological
Deficit Scale. *In* Reitan, R. M., and Wolfson, D.
(Eds.): Traumatic Brain Injury II: Recovery and
Rehabilitation. Tucson, AZ, Neuropsychology
Press, 1987.

74. Matarazzo, J. D., and Herman, D. O.: Relationship
of education and IQ in the WAIS-R standardization
sample. J. Consult. Clin. Psychol., 52:631–634,
1984.

75. Wilson, R. S., Rosenbaum, G., Brown, G., Rourke,
D., Whitman, D., and Grisell, J.: An index of
premorbid intelligence. J. Consult. Clin. Psychol.,
46:1554–1555, 1978.

76. Erickson, R. C., Poon, L. W., and Walsh-Sweeney,
L.: Clinical memory testing of the elderly. *In* Poon,
L. W., Fozard, J. L., and Cermak, L. S. (Eds.):
New Directions in Memory and Aging. Hillsdale,
NJ, Erlbaum, 1980.

77. Mateer, C. A., Sohlberg, M. M., and Crinean, J.:
Focus on clinical research: Perceptions of memory
functions in individuals with closed head injury. J.
Head Trauma Rehabil., 2:74–84, 1987.

78. Stuss, D. T., and Benson, D. F.: The Frontal Lobes.
New York, Raven Press, 1986.

79. Dikmen, S., Temkin, N., McLean, A., Wyler, A.,
and Machamer, J.: Memory and head injury severity. J. Neurol. Neurosurg. Psychiatry, 50:1613–1618,
1987.

80. Dikmen, S. D., Reitan, R. M., and Temkin, N. R.:
Neuropsychological recovery in head injury. Arch.
Neurol., 40:333–338, 1983.

81. Bond, M. R.: Neurobehavioral sequelae of closed
head injury. *In* Grant, I., and Adams, K. M. (Eds.):
Neuropsychological Assessment of Neuropsychiatric

Disorders. New York, Oxford University Press,
1986.

82. Russell, W. R.: Cerebral involvement in head injury. Brain, 55:549–603, 1932.

83. Fortuny, L. A. I., Briggs, M., Newcombe, F.,
Ratcliffe, G., and Thomas, C.: Measuring the duration of post-traumatic amnesia. J. Neurol. Neurosurg. Psychiatry, 43:377–379, 1980.

84. Levin, H. S., Benton, A. L., and Grossman, R. G.:
Neurobehavioral Consequences of Closed Head Injury. New York, Oxford University Press, 1982.

85. Panting, A., and Merry, P. H.: The long-term
rehabilitation of severe head injuries with particular
reference to the need for social and medical support
for the patient's family. Rehabilitation, 38:33–37,
1972.

86. Bond, M. R.: Effects on the family system. *In*
Rosenthal, M., Griffith, E. R., Bond, M. R., and
Miller, J. D. (Eds.): Rehabilitation of the Head
Injured Adult. Philadelphia, F. A. Davis, 1983.

87. Klonoff, P. S., Costa, L. D., and Snow, W. G.:
Predictors and indicators of quality of life in patients
with closed-head injury. J. Clin. Exp. Neuropsychol., 8:469–485, 1986.

88. Dikmen, S., and Reitan, R. M.: Emotional sequelae
of head injury. Ann. Neurol., 2:492–494, 1977.

89. Edelstein, B. A., and Couture, E. T. (Eds.): Behavioral Assessment and Rehabilitation of the Traumatically Brain-Damaged. New York, Plenum
Press, 1984.

90. Goldstein, G., and Ruthven, L.: Rehabilitation of
the Brain-Damaged Adult. New York, Plenum
Press, 1983.

91. Prigatano, G. P.: Neuropsychological Rehabilitation
After Brain Injury. Baltimore, Johns Hopkins University Press, 1986.

92. Rosenthal, M., Griffith, E. R., Bond, M. R., and
Miller, J. D. (Eds.): Rehabilitation of the Head
Injured Adult. Philadelphia, F. A. Davis, 1983.

93. Uzzell, B. P., and Gross, Y. (Eds.): Clinical Neuropsychology of Intervention. Boston, Martinus
Nijhoff Publishing, 1986.

94. Wood, R. L.: Brain Injury Rehabilitation: A Neurobehavioral Approach. Rockville, MD, Aspen,
1987.

95. Ylvisaker, M., and Gobble, E. M. R. (Eds.): Community Re-entry of Head Injured Adults. Boston,
College-Hill, 1987.

96. Grimm, B. H., and Bleiberg, J.: Psychological re-
habilitation in traumatic brain injury. *In* Filskov, S.
B., and Boll, T. J. (Eds.): Handbook of Clinical
Neuropsychology, Vol. 2. New York, Wiley, 1986.

97. Gianutsos, R.: What is cognitive rehabilitation? J.
Rehabil., 46:36–40, 1980.

61

Environmental Accessibility for Physically Disabled People

ALAN HOWARD WELNER

Environments provide situations that encourage meaningful, productive interactions between individuals and their surroundings. According to Ostroff, developing contexts that provide opportunities for people to develop their potential is a basic element involved in designing environments for all people.[1] Lawton[2] has advanced a conceptual framework that balances individual competence with environmental suitability, termed the Competence-Press Model. The model's major tenet is that suitable forms of environmental stimulation and support bring about maximum engagement of individuals.

Psychological theory suggests that a person's self-image depends greatly on interaction with others and with the environment. Environments for disabled people sometimes include childlike motifs and institutional settings, both of which can be psychologically debilitating as well as adversely affecting the development of a strong sense of self-worth.[3, 91–94]

Persons with disabilities often do not fare as well as nondisabled people because of physical barriers, social barriers, educational barriers, employment barriers, and attitudinal barriers.[4] The modern approach to dealing with these problems is embodied in the concept of normalization, which refers to an attitude whereby disabled people are treated as being ordinary rather than special.[5] Normalization includes promotion of barrier-free environmental design.

Those affected by environmental barriers include more than 1 million Americans who wear leg braces, 172,000 who use artificial limbs, and the 7.6 million people with heart conditions.[6] The significance of environmental barriers to elderly persons is considerable, as the ability to climb a single step is one of their most commonly lost faculties.[7] Pregnant women, people carrying heavy loads, and those with temporary disabilities are others potentially influenced by environmental barriers.[8] A recent estimate suggests that there are approximately 36 million disabled Americans.[3]

Current Practice

Efforts are made to shape the living environment so that it becomes a series of tools rather than a collection of obstacles.[19] Privacy short of isolation and independence short of unreasonable expectations are helpful concepts that may be used to plan living arrangements.[20] The best designs facilitating the disabled are unobtrusive so that those who are more competent are not made to feel dependent.[21] Where special designs and equipment are indispensable, designers and manufacturers might promote solutions and products that are esthetically pleasing.[22]

As one architect noted, "What is barrier-free for one person is a barrier for another."[19] Segments of the disabled community with particular needs may benefit from certain environmental modifications that may not be helpful to other disabled people. For example, lowering tools and surfaces into the optimal range of people using wheelchairs can be a hazard to very young children. Curb cuts, which are helpful to wheelchair users and others with difficulties in ambulation, may be problems for blind pedestrians who rely on curbs for orientation.[23] A projecting, wall-mounted drinking

1273

1274

ALAN HOWARD WELNER

TABLE 61–1. Administration of the Barrier-Free Movement at the National Level: Selected Highlights

SUPPORTIVE ORGANIZATIONS	ACCESSIBILITY CODES
American Institute of Architects[9]	American National Standard for Buildings and Facilities—Providing Accessibility and Usability for Physically Handicapped People ANSI* A117.1–1986[10]
American National Standards Institute[10]	
Architectural and Transportation Barriers Compliance Board[9]	
Environmental Design Research Association (EDRA)[11]	
National Easter Seal Society[10]	Uniform Federal Accessibility Standards†
Paralyzed Veterans of America, National Architecture and Barrier-free Design Program[12]	
Presidents Committee on Employment of the Handicapped[9]	
Barrier-free Design Center of Toronto, Ontario (Canada)[13]	
Disabled Persons' Community Resources (Ottawa, Canada)[14]	
Center on Environment for the Handicapped (London, U.K.)[15]	

*ANSI is a private, nonprofit institution that creates voluntary consensus standards and assures their regular review and updating, generally on a five-year cycle.[16]

†Some notations regarding the minimum number of applications of a standard, commonly termed "scope" requirements, are included in the Uniform Federal Accessibility Standards.[17] An example of a "scope" guideline is described in a 1985 document which states that new hotels and motels are to provide at least one guest bedroom suitable for use by a wheelchair-user for every 20 bedrooms on the principal entrance floor.[18]

fountain might well serve people using wheelchairs but prove a hazard to people who are blind. A blind person may be more comfortable in smaller spaces where most elements are within reach, whereas a person in a wheelchair maneuvers better in open spaces. A floor textured to aid blind people in guiding their feet would detract from optimal wheelchair mobility. However, both groups function better in a space with hard-surfaced floors. The sound characteristics in a room with acoustically reflective floors can be helpful to blind people in obtaining directional cues from the environment. Additionally, traction is best for wheelchairs on hard surfaces.[24]

Countermeasures Helpful to People with Mobility Impairments

WHEELCHAIRS AND SEATING

Wheelchairs have contributed significantly to improved environmental accessibility for people with impairment of mobility. Certain wheelchair dimensions have gained widespread acceptance as standard measurements[17] (Fig. 61–1).

Elements of posture and positioning in the wheelchair are of significance. Excessive elevation of the legrests can cause postural alterations resulting in excessive pressure upon the sacrum, with the attendant risk of pressure sores. Increased hip flexion, which may be achieved through modification of the seating cushion, can assist in preventing some wheelchair users from sliding out of their chair. A cushion facilitating hip extension may be required to accommodate limitations in hip flexion or to improve the drainage of urine into collection devices.[25]

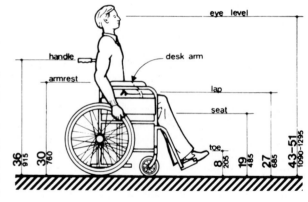

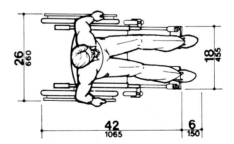

NOTE: Footrests may extend further for very large people.

FIGURE 61–1. Dimensions of adult-sized wheelchairs. (Reproduced from the Uniform Federal Accessibility Standards, 1984, with the permission of the United States Architectural and Transportation Barriers Compliance Board.)

Seating preferences of people with physical disabilities not confined to a wheelchair have been described. A significant percentage of adults with arthritis report difficulty arising from chairs, particularly those with low seats. Difficulty was attributed to stiffness as well as knee and back problems.[26] The additional movement necessitated by more pronounced knee and hip flexion angles and the increased muscle power required to overcome mechanical disadvantage that develops with progressive knee flexion[27] are other contributing factors. Alterations increasing the height of furniture is a common practice in ameliorating this difficulty. Techniques include the placement of platforms or blocks under chairs, beds, and tables, and the use of casters or cushions.[26] Electrical rising chairs, spring-assisted seats, and high chairs are other alternatives.[27] Patients with ankylosing spondylitis or low back pain prefer a firm seat; however, pain often precludes sitting for intervals longer than 30 minutes. In contrast, patients with rheumatoid arthritis favor soft upholstery.[28]

ACCESSIBLE PASSAGEWAYS
(Fig. 61–2)

Current research indicates that for normal walking, a coefficient of static friction greater than 0.4 will produce safe walking surfaces.[29] It has been reported[30] that in assessing biomechanical factors causing slipping accidents, dynamic friction is more significant than is static friction. The development of values for coefficients of static and dynamic friction for various floor surfaces appropriate to normal ambulators as well as those with impairing conditions appears to be a promising area for future fruitful study.

The relative expenditure of energy for ambulation on various surfaces is another significant area to be investigated. It appears that cardiopulmonary stresses for wheelchair locomotion are higher than for walking. In switching from tile to carpet locomotion, significant increases in energy expenditure occurred for wheelchair users that were not noted in bipedal ambulators.[31] It is hoped that additional studies of energy expenditure during ambulation will be forthcoming in the near future.

Handrails are recommended to be mounted between 30 and 34 inches (760 to 865 mm) above surfaces and have a clear space away from the adjacent wall of 1½ inches (38 mm).[17] People who have suffered strokes with hemiparesis or amputations may have only one arm with the functional capability to use a handrail. Therefore, handrails should be provided on both sides of passageways.[29]

STAIRWAYS AND RAMPS

On any given flight of stairs, all steps should have uniform riser heights and uniform tread depth. Stair treads should be no less than 11 inches (280 mm) in depth as measured from consecutive risers.

Stairs are designed best with sloping risers angulated outward to meet the leading edge of the tread, to minimize the hazard of tripping. The sloping angle of the risers is recommended to be at least 60 degrees with the horizontal. The radius of curvature at the leading edge of the tread should be no greater than 1/2 inch (13 mm). Nosings should project no more than 1.5 inches (38 mm).[17]

People with lower extremity prostheses, orthoses, or difficulties of coordination often use risers to provide guidance, support, and balance for their limbs or crutches during ascent.[29] For these reasons, open risers are discouraged on accessible stairways.

Pictures and other objects on stairway walls are discouraged, since distraction may occur. Lighting sources are provided best at both the top and bottom of stairways to minimize shadows. When carpeting is used on stairways, large patterns that could cause problems of depth perception or confusion are not recommended. Carpeting reduces the size of steps and may cause heels to catch and soles to slide, and, therefore, is to be avoided if possible. It is suggested that gradual changes in levels of lighting be provided between stairways and surrounding areas to allow time for accommodation of the eyes. These safety measures are of heightened importance for people with visual impairments and for senior citizens.[32]

Ramps are essential for users of wheelchairs if elevators or lifts are not available to connect different levels (Fig. 61–3). Disabled people not in wheelchairs sometimes have difficulty with ramps, particularly lengthy ones, and prefer to use steps. Wherever possible, a ramp should be situated within a reasonable distance of steps to allow a real choice.[33]

KITCHENS

Accessibility in kitchens is achieved by adopting an arrangement of facilities in accord with recommended accessibility standards as well as the selective utilization of specific adaptive devices to meet individual requirements.[34] There are three basic work centers in a kitchen: the stove and oven; the refrigerator and freezer; and the sink, disposal, and dishwasher. Work centers are best arranged

ALAN HOWARD WELNER

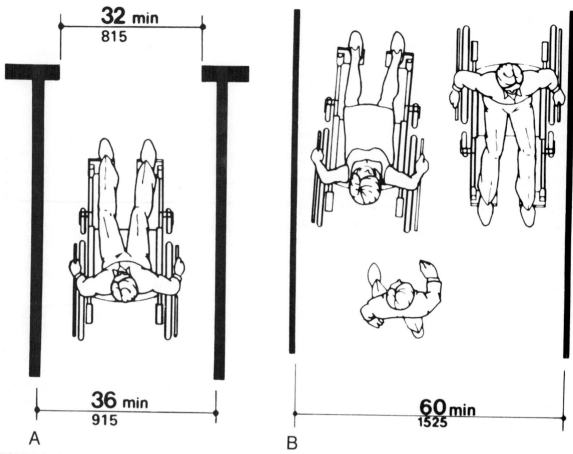

A   B

FIGURE 61–2. *A*, Minimum clear width for single wheelchair. *B*, Minimum clear width for two wheelchairs. (Reproduced from the Uniform Federal Accessibility Standards, 1984, with the permission of the United States Architectural and Transportation Barriers Compliance Board.)

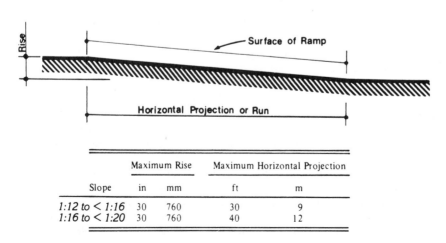

FIGURE 61–3. Components of a single ramp run and sample ramp dimensions. (Reproduced from the Uniform Federal Accessibility Standards, 1984, with the permission of the United States Architectural and Transportation Barriers Compliance Board.)

	Maximum Rise		Maximum Horizontal Projection	
Slope	in	mm	ft	m
1:12 to < 1:16	30	760	30	9
1:16 to < 1:20	30	760	40	12

following the natural sequence of food preparation. Food is first taken from the refrigerator and prepared near the sink; subsequent activity moves to the area of the stove during cooking. Work centers are best aligned following a right to left progression for right-handed people. The three work centers are most efficiently arranged in a U-shaped configuration. This basic flow pattern is consistent with methods of task simplification, which is an important theme in accessibility designs.

For the sink, it is recommended that the depth of the bowl not exceed 6½ inches (165 mm). A deeper sink may be adjusted with a slatted rack. Faucets with a single lever that controls both the temperature and the volume of flow are easiest to use.

The recommended minimum counter height is 28 inches (911 mm), which is accessible to people using wheelchairs. Provided that the thickness of the countertop does not exceed 2 inches (50 mm), the height for the recommended minimum clearance for the lower extremities of 26 inches (660 mm) will be met. Related recommendations are a clear front to back depth of 19 inches (485 mm) and width of 30 inches (760 mm) (Fig. 61–4).

RESTROOMS

Since restrooms are not considered primary or productive space in most buildings, the tendency is to design them as compactly as possible.[35] The unfortunate result is that most restrooms do not have sufficient floor area to accommodate the wheelchair. Recommendations specifically applicable to restrooms include the following: the vestibule inside the entry door should be at least 48 inches (1219 mm) deep if the door swings inward and 42 inches deep (1067 mm) if the door swings outward.[35] The recommended commode height is 17 to 19 inches (430 to 485 mm), which matches well with the 19 inch (485 mm) seat height of standard adult wheelchairs (Fig. 61–5). A bathtub seat should provide a level, secure area to facilitate transfer from a wheelchair or crutches. It is also of utility in enabling people to sit while removing orthotic or prosthetic devices. Grab bars around a commode, bathtub, or shower are placed at a height of 33 to 36 inches (840 to 915 mm). Showers offer some disabled people the possibility to wash independently and can also avoid some of the hazards of a bath.[36] Slip-resistant surfacing for appropriate areas is an important consideration.

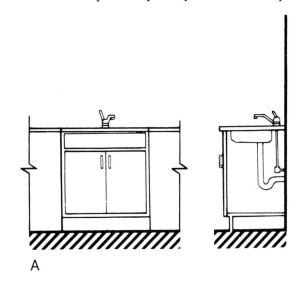

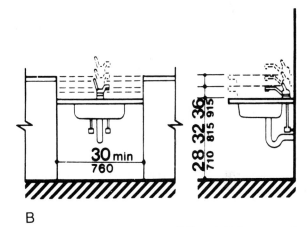

FIGURE 61–4. Kitchen sink accessibility. *A*, Before removal of cabinets and base. *B*, Minimal width for wheelchairs and variable alternatives of height for the handicapped user. (Reproduced from the Uniform Federal Accessibility Standards, 1984, with the permission of the United States Architectural and Transportation Barriers Compliance Board.)

Accessibility for Disabled Children

Children with disabilities, although normal in many spheres, may have slowed or altered development in one or more areas. The nature of the disability may cause changes that are predictable. For example, some degenerative diseases have a well-defined course. Disabling conditions may increase or decrease in severity over time. Physically disabled children may not be able to modify their responses to an inadequate environment with the same resiliency as others. For example, marginal

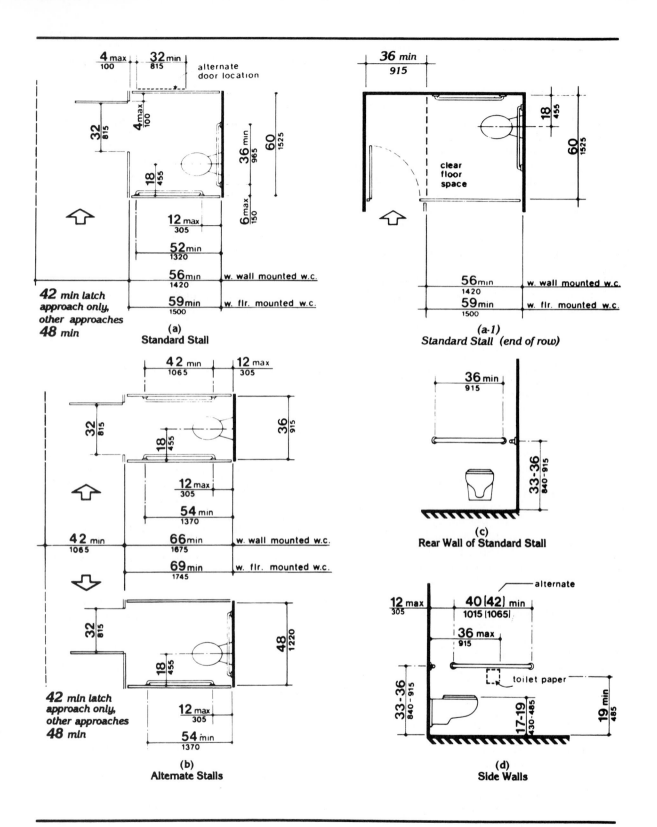

FIGURE 61–5. Restroom specifications of minimal dimensions for accessibility. (Reproduced from the Uniform Federal Accessibility Standards, 1984, with the permission of the United States Architectural and Transportation Barriers Compliance Board.)

lighting levels may present some difficulty to those with normal vision, but be disabling for children with visual impairment.

The decreased physical capabilities of children with disability often result in diminished opportunity to participate directly with their environment. The well-intentioned concern for safety and protection is sometimes emphasized to the extent that opportunities to master many basic independent interactions with the environment that are well within their capabilities are precluded. Alternatively, concerns regarding safety are of prime importance in the design of environments for all children. Those with physical disabilities, in light of their increased vulnerability, are particularly sensitive to environmental hazards.

Environmental measures that compensate for the child's deficiencies may facilitate the development of their assets. For example, children who are easily distracted or have perceptual problems benefit where spaces are clearly defined and sensory stimulation is carefully controlled. Lighting oriented on the task may assist in focusing attention.[37]

Household furnishings, particularly coffee tables, are an important hazard to children, particularly in the 12- to 36-month age range. Most children begin walking at the age of 12 months; however, stability is not achieved until approximately 2 years of age. During the learning process, youngsters stumble frequently and often attempt to stabilize themselves on nearby objects. Coffee tables are used as supports during an incipient fall. Failure to adequately grasp tables results in contact between edges of tables and, usually, children's heads. Reported injuries include lacerations, hematomas, and, occasionally, perforation of the optic globe or depressed skull fractures. Prominent supraorbital ridges protect eyes in most cases. Thus, classic "coffee table lacerations" are seen in the eyebrow region of young children.[38] The new vogue in glass furniture, particularly large coffee tables and glass doors, is becoming a major hazard in the home. Breakage of glass furnishings has been associated with serious eye injuries in children.[39] These concerns have marked significance to children with physical disabilities. Diminished ambulatory stability in a child with impaired mobility may heighten the importance of supports such as coffee tables and the hazards they pose. Children with visual impairments may be more likely to become involved in injury through untoward contact with furnishings, and the presence of glass furniture in the immediate environment heightens the risk.

Suggestions for minimizing these hazards include the placement of padding at pointed edges on furniture, or the avoidance of furnishings with pointed corners and sharp edges.[38] The use of safety glass in furniture would probably diminish environmental hazards and accident rates as well.[39]

Variety in space settings for children with disabilities is important toward the fulfillment of a well-rounded and mature social development. Environments allowing solitude as well as group activity can help a child develop a positive sense of identity and good social skills. Children with disabilities may feel particularly vulnerable in busy places. Private space offers an opportunity for decreasing stress and anxiety from public exposure.

The colorless uniformity among personal spaces allotted to residents in institutional settings has become disfavored in recent years. The expression of personal tastes within spaces allotted to individuals is encouraged. Encouragement of self-expression aids children in developing character and personal style. In addition, it has been found that children are more attentive to the care of space identified as their own.

Basic barrier-free standards for children[40] suggest a maximum height for controls, receptacles, and dispensers of 40 inches (1016 mm) from the floor. Handrails are to be placed at a height of 24 inches (610 mm) from the center of the bar to the floor. Requirements for load support for adult handrails are significantly higher than the pediatric standard. Recommendations for water fountain spigot heights are 30 inches for children (762 mm) and 36 inches (915 mm) for adults.[17] The commode height recommended for children is 15 inches (381 mm) from the floor surface to the top of the seat, whereas the adult recommendation is 17 to 19 inches (432 to 483 mm).

The United States Architectural and Transportation Barriers Compliance Board has developed recommendations relating to accessibility for physically handicapped disabled in elementary schools. Recommendations include modifications or additions to sections of the Uniform Federal Accessibility Standards to make them suitable to the dimensions and anthropometrics of children. The population specifically addressed by the recommendations is disabled children in elementary schools, grades one through six. The document was published in March 1986 and entitled *Recommendations for Accessibility to Serve Physically Handicapped Children in Elementary Schools.*[41]

Resource centers supporting progress in the design of environments for children with disabilities,

ALAN HOWARD WELNER

in addition to the organizations with broadly based holdings previously mentioned, include the Adaptive Environment Center in Boston, Massachusetts. Since 1978, this organization has served the state of Massachusetts on all aspects of designing for accessibility[42] in addition to its interest in environmental matters relating to children. Other organizations are the Handicapped Adventure Playground Association in London, England, and the International Playground Association in Sheffield, England.[37]

Outdoor Environments and Accessibility

Accessibility relating to outdoor environments has been described in some detail,[43, 44] and a number of thoughtful guidelines have been developed. Accessible facilities are best located on level sites adjacent to a firm path with a stable surface. In large measure, the nature of the surface of a path determines the accessibility of activities subserved by the access route. In order of decreasing accessibility, possible choices include concrete; asphalt; wood planking, which tends to be used over wet, fragile, or sandy areas; well-packed rock of fine grade; well-compacted pea-sized gravel; bound wood chips; coarse gravel; rock; unbound wood chips; and sand.

One classification stratifies pathways and trails for physically disabled people into five grades, with the higher grades reflecting decreased structure and greater negotiating difficulties.[43, 44]

Horticultural establishments with a particular interest in the participation of physically disabled people are located worldwide.[45]

Parking spaces for physically disabled people are to be at least 96 inches (2440 mm) wide and should have an adjacent access aisle 60 inches (1525 mm) in minimum width. Two accessible parking spaces may share a common access aisle. Parking spaces designated for physically handicapped people and accessible passenger loading zones that serve a particular building are best located on the shortest possible accessible circulation route to an accessible entrance.[17]

Accessibility and Emergency Escape

In recent years, matters relating to methods for emergency egress for physically disabled people have received increasing attention from the research community concerned with environmental design. Although much of this embryonic field remains unexplored, there appears to be some consensus regarding certain principles.

It is understood that people with disabilities sometimes require alternative means whereby they can be alerted to the presence of an emergency. Flashing lights activated simultaneously with audible systems to alert those with visual impairments are of benefit. Some corporations are providing hearing-impaired individuals with vibrating pagers that are activated in an emergency and provide a warning to evacuate. Other firms have issued two-way radios to persons confined to wheelchairs, providing means for them to be located and given instructions.

Tactile maps may help people with visual disabilities become aware of exit alternatives. Exit signs placed near floors will be below the smoke level[46] and more within the line of horizontal vision of wheelchair users. For similar reasons, arrows in carpeting or tiles of hallways indicating exit routes are of benefit.

A recent study demonstrated that relatively untrained assistants can carry a wheelchair and occupant down a stairway at an acceptable speed in event of fire. Three-person support, with one person stationed in back and the other two positioned at either side to provide support and guidance to the front portion of the wheelchair, is a safer arrangement than support by two people. However, in some situations there may not be adequate room for three people to support a wheelchair on a stairway. The wheelchair user could be transferred to a carrying chair, as used by ambulance services, requiring only two assistants for support. To permit a wheelchair-bound patient to be carried by three assistants and allow people to pass, a stairway width of 59 inches (1500 mm) is recommended,[47] as are adequate landings.

An alternative in stair design for the future might include treads of sufficient surface area to fully accommodate a wheelchair having all wheels in contact with the surface of a tread. With this modification, only one person may be required to safely assist a wheelchair-bound individual in stairway descent where access to an elevator is precluded. Enlarged treads also may make a cascade fall down multiple stairs less likely. However, treads of this magnitude may not be practical in situations where space is at a premium.

Enclosures such as a lobby or corridor protected by at least one fire door may serve as intermediate destinations for disabled people in their path of egress. Provisions should then permit safe access to a stairway separated from the fire by at least two fire doors or an elevator. Note that elevators designed for use during emergency situations operate under manual control and do not automatically respond to calls from floors.[48]

Visual Disability and the Environment

Blind people are more acutely aware of auditory as well as other sensory stimuli than are people with normal vision. The sound of breathing is one way visually disabled people recognize and localize others. Moving from one enclosed space to another can lead to changes in ear pressure, which gives blind people important cues.[49]

Blind children enjoy bouncing high-pitched sounds off ceilings and learn to angle the beams proficiently. This play develops into a method whereby blind adults can determine the height of ceilings.[50] For these reasons, blind people find music and sound systems in public interiors to be particularly helpful.[51]

Changes in floor covering, such as from tile to carpet, help blind people distinguish different areas. For example, a house recently designed for a blind person includes an uncarpeted entry niche adjacent to carpeted living areas; the sound of footsteps announces an arrival.[3] Concrete or wood is used to indicate areas clear of obstacles to blind persons; carpeting signals the presence of obstructions such as furniture. A creative alternative in the design of stairways is demonstrated in the British Liverpool Cathedral, where accessibility of those partially sighted is enhanced by virtue of the alternating black and white marble steps.[52]

Braille descriptions on handrails are of assistance. Curved rather than sharp margins on furniture, textured needlepoint artwork, and recesses for guide sticks along walls that end at wall stopping points are other commonly used design elements appreciated by visually disabled people.[51]

An adjustable length, lightweight, battery-operated electronic cane couples laser detection units to auditory and tactile signaling devices and serves to warn visually impaired users of nearby hazards during ambulation activities. Three laser beams emanate from the handle of the device. High-, medium-, and low-pitched sounds are transmitted corresponding to beams directed upward, parallel to the surface, and downward respectively. Vibra-

tory signals in the handle in the region of the index finger register events in the path of the middle beam. When beams are crossed within certain proximities, auditory and, in the case of the middle beam, vibratory cueing is initiated. The auditory device can be switched off, leaving the vibratory pathway uninterrupted.[53]

There are other considerations of significance to those with compromised vision. Modifications in signs are of benefit. Letters and numerals on signs and clocks may be designed with enlarged dimensions and placed on sharply contrasting backgrounds for maximum legibility.[54] Abbreviated rather than fully spelled words are easier to read for people with visual impairment.[55] Color is commonly used as a means for attracting attention to key elements of the environment;[56] this technique is used to benefit those with visual disability in using bright red coloring for hallway railings, best accentuated by a contrasting wall color.[57] Spatial ambiguity and fluidity is esthetically pleasing and has become a major theme in modern design. Unfortunately, it can create problems for people with visual disabilities.[3]

Developmental decrements in the human visual system are important to consider in designing environments. The diminished ability of the pupil to expand as a consequence of age-related changes is responsible for limiting the amount of light entering the aging eye. It has been estimated that by the age of 60 years, a threefold reduction in potential pupillary expansion has occurred, which requires compensation by providing increased illumination by a factor of three. Since the aging eye is more sensitive to glare, matte surfaces that minimize reflection should be used to prevent the distortion and confusion that could be produced by reflected rays. Spotlighting increases illumination needed for acuity and minimizes confusing shadows produced if all lighting is increased.[56]

Vision is an important factor in the maintenance of postural stability. Recent studies have initiated exploration of the interrelationships among visual disability, postural stability, falls, and aging. It is currently believed that visual disability may be an important factor as a cause of falls in the elderly population.[58, 59] Among elderly people, the possibility of hip fracture resulting from a fall underscores the importance of preventive measures.

Guide dogs are a recognized adjunct to improved mobility for those with visual impairments. Carefully selected and trained dogs are matched to appropriate people with due consideration to factors such as size, personal characteristics, and temperament. Generally, guide dogs are trained to stop at each curb, stairway, and wheelchair ramp. Dogs are unable to read traffic patterns or signals and must rely on the person holding the harness for instructions in this regard. The owner devotes significant time and energy to maintaining the dog, which includes daily feeding, grooming, obedience training, and a considerable amount of exercise.[60] Future directions for guide dog training and use include hearing dogs for those with auditory impairments[61] and guide dog robots.[62] Centers have been established for the purpose of providing people and dogs with the specialized training necessary to ensure the success of their collaboration. The Seeing Eye, Inc., of Morristown, New Jersey, established in 1929, was the first of such concerns in the United States and serves Puerto Rico and Canada as well as the 48 mainland states. Other guide dog schools include Guide Dogs for the Blind, Inc., San Rafael, California; International Guiding Eyes, Inc., Sylmar, California; Eye of the Pacific Guide Dogs and Mobility Services, Inc., Honolulu, Hawaii; Leader Dogs for the Blind, Rochester, Michigan; Guide Dog Foundation for the Blind, Inc., Smithtown, New York; Guiding Eyes for the Blind, Inc., Yorktown Heights, New York; and Pilot Dogs, Inc., Columbus, Ohio.[63] The British organization Guide Dogs for the Blind Association was first established with the support of Mrs. D. H. Eustis, who was instrumental in forming the first guide dog centers in Switzerland and the United States. Training centers sponsored by the association are stationed at several United Kingdom locations.[64]

Auditory Disability and the Environment

Hearing aids are used by an estimated 3 million Americans.[65] Hearing aids function best when background noise is low. When an attempt is made to hear sound originating at some distance from the user of the hearing aid, difficulties arise in that ambient sounds unrelated to the material of interest are also amplified and confuse the presentation. Similar difficulties are incurred by people with hearing impairment who do not use hearing aids.

Individuals with hearing impairment appear to benefit from listening systems that receive the sound near its source, provide amplification, deliver the amplified version to the listener's ear, and avoid extraneous sound. Four major types of assistive listening systems are available.[65]

FM Systems. In FM systems, FM transmitters are connected to a public address system and deliver signals to FM receivers equipped with earphones. Hearing aid users with a "t" switch position on their equipment may use a neck loop to receive the signal. The "t" position indicates that the hearing aid is equipped with a telecoil, which is generally used with a telephone. FM systems produce sound of excellent quality, and electrical interference is usually not a problem. Relatively little positional restriction is imposed on those using this system.

Induction Loops. Induction loops consist of a wire encircling an area. The loop receives sound transmitted by a microphone and transmits by creating a magnetic field within the loop. The signal can be received by hearing aids set at the "t" position or by special portable units. In order to receive the signal, the receiving person with an appropriate receiver must be located within the area enclosed by the loop. Unfortunately, sound quality is often uneven within the reception area. In addition, fluorescent lighting can interfere with transmission.

Infrared Systems. Infrared systems use light beams in the infrared range to carry information from a transmitter connected to a public address system. A special portable receiver is required. Receivers must be within a line of sight with the transmitter. Unfortunately, large amounts of infrared light through other sources such as sunlight, incandescent light, and fluorescent light may interfere with transmission.

AM Systems. AM systems, which sometimes may function using AM radios as receivers, allow flexibility in choice of listening locations for those using receiving equipment. Such systems are subject to the same sources of interference that affect AM radio transmission and do not function optimally in buildings with substantial amounts of structural steel.

Of increasing importance in recent years has been the advent of telecommunication devices for the deaf, abbreviated TDD. These devices permit people with hearing or speech impairment to communicate over a standard telephone without an interpreter. In this mode of telephone dialogue, both parties must be outfitted with compatible equipment.[66] TDD users type messages on a keyboard and receive messages on a display screen. The ringer can be replaced by a telephone signal light. In addition to home use, telecommunication devices are used to increase the ability of those with hearing or speech impairments to communicate in more remote locations, such as airports.[67] The Architectural and Transportation Barriers Compliance Board maintains a continually updated directory of TDD-equipped federal agency telephone numbers. Copies of the directory are available at no charge from the Board.[68]

Visual doorbell systems represent an additional technological advance of benefit to those with hearing impairment. The majority of visual call systems use ordinary filament lamps for signaling. In some circumstances a xenon beacon is of utility. It produces a bright flashing light and can therefore attract significant attention over a wide area.[69]

Environments for Disabled Senior Citizens

Disability increases significantly with age. In the United States, 46 per cent of people 65 or more years of age have chronic activity-limiting disability.[70] In addition to the environmental measures applicable to the disabled community at large, certain measures have particular importance to disabled elderly persons. Decreased capacity for processing sensory stimuli of all modalities with consequent slowed reaction times is an important consideration in arranging a well-conceived environment. An environmental setting with simple and direct spatial organization and circulation patterns[21] as well as familiar surroundings over time are of benefit to elderly persons,[20] particularly in maintaining their orientation and acclimatization. In designing facilities for elderly people with or without disabilities, rooms are best arranged in groups to simulate a family atmosphere. One authority recommends no more than 10 rooms per cluster to achieve this effect.[71]

A number of creative designs have implemented these concepts. For example, open spaces that afford a nearly complete view of several adjacent functional areas obviate dependence on memory for the location of or the pathway to an important place.[72] One modern institutional design incorporates circulation patterns deliberately routed through each living room, which provides opportunities for activity and stimulation of both circulating as well as seated residents.[71] A recently designed geriatric complex consists of separate but interconnected physical facilities that are designed to accommodate a comprehensive program of care. Accommodations range from housing for elderly people, to a skilled nursing facility, to specialized care for senile and critically ill patients. This ar-

rangement provides for ready access to higher levels of care on an outpatient or inpatient basis when the need arises. The maintenance of intracenter care, in addition to the reassuring familiarity of surroundings, helps to avoid the trauma of transferring to higher levels of care, which is often feared to be a one-way journey.[73]

Devices and Products for Improving Accessibility

Technological advances are accruing benefits to people with physical disabilities. Innovative door-handle design has produced a model that unlatches by pushing or pulling on the handle as well as with the conventional twisting motion.[3] Voice synthesizers use microprocessor technology to provide instructions to elevator passengers in special circumstances, as well as routine floor announcements to benefit those with visual disabilities. A new restroom design uses electronic sensors to operate washroom fixtures without handles, buttons, or levers. The sensors meter toilet and urinal flushing, lavatory water flow, soap dispensers, hand driers, and shower operation.[55] Bathroom fixtures designed for the convenience of people using wheelchairs include roll-in showers or bathtubs and tilt-down mirrors.[74] Electronic window controls open and close windows from a pushbutton. Input from a module located outside prompts the command module to close the windows when rain commences. Thermostatically controlled window operators will soon be available. Electronic door openers offer advantages in their allowing the use of heavier doors or doors requiring more force to operate than that 8½ to 15 pounds of pressure called for in the various codes. Adjustments available on many devices hold the door open for a pre-set time, allowing disabled people to pass unassisted.[55]

A recent report[75] notes the development of a curb-climbing aid for standard manual wheelchairs. Intended for use by paraplegic persons, it consists of bilateral ramps that the user can deploy and retrieve from the seated position using attached telescopic rods. The ramps and rods may be carried in a ready-for-use position or stowed away in a bag hung behind the wheelchair backrest.

The wheelchair cannot be accommodated on an escalator. Manufacturers have experimented with devices to correct the problem; however, it is currently generally felt that the two machines are incompatible.[76] Automated walkways that operate on level surfaces as well as on an incline are being marketed. Their landings are designed to be flush with the conveyor, facilitating their use by people with disabilities. Modern escalators are equipped with emergency stop buttons at the top and bottom landings. One design features a 1.5 to 4.0 ft (457 to 1219 mm) stopping distance with a controlled rate of deceleration.[76]

High performance indoor/outdoor wheelchairs have been developed and are being refined over time. Current parameters for performance for automated wheelchairs include an indoor maximum speed of 3.5 miles per hour (5.6 km per hour) and an outdoor maximum of 7.0 miles per hour (11.0 km per hour). The height of a wheelchair's center of gravity in relation to its small wheelbase and the abrupt changes of speed of the usual push-pull steering system are among the limiting factors for increasing wheelchair speed. It is currently suggested that wheelchairs be designed to have a minimum range of approximately 15 miles (24.0 km) with space available for larger batteries to extend the range to 20 to 25 miles (32 to 40 km).[77]

The Veterans Administration publishes a circular that lists approved add-on automobile adaptive equipment. Listed products include van lifts, hand controls, and low-effort sensitized steering/braking systems.[78]

"Kneeling devices" for buses are used to reduce the distance from curbs to the first step of the bus from the usual 10 to 13 inches to 4 to 6 inches. Typical deployment time is 2 to 3 seconds to lower and 5 to 10 seconds to raise the bus back to the normal ride height. The bus cannot be moved while in the kneeling position.[79]

The provision of a hoist may make transfers more comfortable for a person with a disability and easier to accomplish for those who assist. Electrical hoists are easier to use by an attendant, generate fewer complaints, and are more frequently in use during follow-up than are manual hoists. The more frequent breakdowns of electrical hoists as compared with manual ones do not seem to offset the successful usage of electrical models. Hammock-type slings appear more commonly prescribed for patients with Duchenne muscular dystrophy than band-type slings. The converse situation exists for patients with rheumatoid arthritis, Still's disease, ankylosing spondylitis, and thoracic or lumbar spinal cord lesions. There are instances where people changed slings after initial delivery of the hoist. The usual reason for modification was the need for greater support, particularly of the head, for those with progressive diseases. Gener-

ally, it appears that voluminous slings are disfavored when compared with smaller models if they provide sufficient support. An electrical hoist with ceiling track is particularly suitable for small rooms, since it requires no floor space either during use or for storage. However, installation may be costly, and it is easier and less expensive when incorporated into new buildings or extensions to existing buildings. Portable hoists offer the advantages of maneuverability, absence of installation costs, and ease of supply since they are generally stock items.[80]

Policy Considerations

According to a national opinion survey of attitudes and experiences of disabled Americans conducted by Louis Harris Associates, life for disabled Americans has improved dramatically in the last decade. Laws passed by the Federal government were cited as a major reason for the improvement. The report, entitled *Disabled Americans: Self Perceptions—1986*, was the first undertaken to determine how disabled people perceive their lives and opportunities. An interim report on the survey, conducted for the International Center for the Disabled in New York City, included information from screening 12,000 American households. It was noted that disabled Americans are still an extraordinarily disadvantaged group. Lack of readily accessible transportation and work sites were mentioned as major barriers to employment by disabled Americans.[81]

The financially precarious position of many with physical disabilities is particularly unfortunate in light of recent changes developing throughout the health care industry. Health care is increasingly becoming an enterprising concern. The egalitarian spirit of community service in the provision of health care appears to have faded somewhat recently in light of significant increases of cost that have become a concomitant of the many technological successes of modern medicine.

The utilitarian economic perspective appears to have impacted upon the barrier-free environmental research and development field as well. Economic responsibilities implicit in promulgation of barrier-free codes are carefully considered prior to inclusion of new standards.[55]

Although legislative support of environmental accessibility has been offered through measures such as Section 190 of the Internal Revenue Code, made permanent in 1986, which permits business establishments a tax deduction up to $35,000 for removing architectural and transportation barriers,[16] widespread implementation of these ideals does not appear likely in the near future. Disabled employees are often viewed as substandard trading partners in the exchange of goods and services for compensation, which is a significant disincentive to their being hired and maintained in employment. In support of the existence of this unfortunate attitude is a recent study which indicated that teachers perceived greater error in written English attributed to the exceptional student.[82] In addition, because of physical, social, and attitudinal barriers, people with disabilities are often unemployed or employed performing activities and receiving compensation far below their capabilities. The resultant economic and social bargaining position of disabled people is not competitive with other members of the community. It is therefore generally more profitable for private enterprise to focus their marketing efforts toward attracting nondisabled customers as well as employees. Altruistic efforts of those eager to assist people with physical disabilities are often eclipsed by the socioeconomical restraints.

Fortunately, some private concerns are embracing the barrier-free philosophy. Exemplary in this regard is the Disney Organization, which has published a booklet guiding guests to their resources for people with disabilities. Helpful measures that are made available include complimentary tape cassettes and portable tape recorders designed to assist sight-impaired guests, telephones with amplified handsets, personal units that amplify the audio in selected attractions, telecommunication devices for the deaf (TDDs), a wheelchair rental, buses with wheelchair lifts, accessible restrooms, and parking space for nonambulatory guests serviced by a motor tram that transports people with disabilities as well as their wheelchairs.[83]

Future legislative efforts to provide economic incentives to the private sector for the removal of environmental barriers appear to have some likelihood for success. For example, a business concern with a large number of potential patrons who are physically disabled might, with the aid of economic incentives, not be as concerned about the economic limitations of disabled individuals, and rather focus on the potential economic benefits that may be realized. Adequate business volume, along with economic incentives, may in selected circumstances be adequate impetus to influence utilitarian decisions toward the provision of accessibility.

As described in Lawton's conceptual model,[2] environmental accessibility results from the interaction of people with an appropriate degree of competence to negotiate a particular environment and surroundings that are sufficiently accommodating. In light of present financial conditions, an avenue to be emphasized might well be small projects such as the development of adaptive aids so that those with physical disabilities can negotiate the existing environment better. In past years, such products were considered medical items, with reimbursement commonly occurring through government channels. Government funding for these purposes was regarded as virtually limitless, and the products were provided free of charge to the consumer. Prevailing economic conditions in the health care marketplace have changed, and adaptive aids are increasingly presented as consumer goods. Competitive market influences are likely to improve the design of such items. For example, new products that blend ergonomic considerations and sculpture into the creative design of plastic molded household articles of utility to those with disabilities are being marketed.[84]

Negotiating the social and attitudinal barriers involved in environmental accessibility may be considerably more difficult than the economic problems. There is a lingering perception that people with disabilities are different, difficult, and therefore to be excluded from mainstream settings. People with disabilities are often regarded as being dangerous to nondisabled members of the community.[85]

There indeed are instances in which a given person with disabilities may be perceived as difficult. Their encumbered presentation, coupled with the all too frequent necessity for special provisions, immediately colors their social interactions with difficulty. Living with a disabling condition that imposes broad social and vocational limitations certainly may serve as a catalyst for a certain amount of difficult behavior. It must be realized that the challenges and strength of character required to adapt constructively to serious disability are highly significant. It is hoped that in the future a more forgiving spirit will develop regarding this element of disability. In addition, the presence of physical disability is not synonymous with consistently difficult conduct; prejudgment in this manner is probably unfair.

The possible danger that people with physical disabilities may pose to other members of the community is a complex issue. When meeting a person in a wheelchair, one is immediately alerted that the wheelchair user is having or has probably

ALAN HOWARD WELNER

had some significant contact with health care providers and is not enjoying excellent health. Curiosity about the nature of the impairment may be accompanied by fears of contagion that may not be well founded. People who do have extensive contact with health care providers may, in fact, be safer than random social contacts in the community in that whatever health problems the disabled person may have, related or unrelated to the disabling condition, are likely to have been identified and addressed.

Nondisabled people may perceive danger from people with physical disabilities simply because they may be aware of differences between those with and without disabilities but do not understand disability or the diversity of circumstances leading to disability. The present marketplace for health services is developing an atmosphere wherein the mysticism is being removed from medical practice, and the general public is becoming better informed regarding the nature of illness and treatment. It therefore appears likely that disabling conditions will meet with more understanding and tolerance from the community at large in the future than was assumed in the past. It is heartening to realize that as a culture we have progressed significantly since the advent of the prehistoric custom of trephining, a practice in which holes were cut in skulls of children with physical impairments to help the evil spirits escape.[86] However, the association between evil and physical disability is still noted in media presentations through the present day.[87]

Mass communication media play a key role in the portrayal of people with disabilities and are an instrumental factor to be included in efforts toward the removal of attitudinal barriers. Currently accepted terminology favors the use of the word disabled as a descriptive noun or adjective. Separation of the description of disability from the noun identifying the subject is encouraged.[88] This terminology is designed to contribute to weakening the commonly held misconception that physical disability in one sphere is, of necessity, indicative of other physical disabilities, mental deficiency, and moral compromise.[87]

Perhaps the next generation of accepted nomenclature regarding physical disability should strive to clearly define and circumscribe pertinent physical deficits. In this manner, diffuse terminology with the concomitant diffuse stigmatizing effect on individuals so designated may be avoided. Specific terminology may be particularly applicable in instances of minor, limited deficiency. Detailed descriptions may not be tactful where multiple complex deficits are involved.

Current evidence indicates that an effective media campaign to remove attitudinal barriers should include that provision of accurate information as well as allow the general population opportunity for personal contact with those who have disabilities.[89] It is hoped that the future will afford people with physical disabilities the opportunity to participate in increasing numbers in high-visibility media positions. For example, the next scriptwriting of a popular space mission adventure show might include a blind crew member who has developed a keen awareness of auditory signals, and by virtue of this developed skill can offer a unique contribution to the collective expertise of the crew. In this manner, the special proficiencies that are common concomitants of successful adaptation to major disabilities can be made known to the general population. Improved general esteem for people with disabilities and diminished attitudinal barriers would appear likely to ensue.

There is a diversity of perspectives among the various segments of the professional community attempting to improve the welfare of those with physical disabilities. Disabled people often require a significant degree of medical supervision. The emphasis on disease and scientific principles is certainly an important element in the care of physically disabled people. However, this perspective is sometimes exclusive of concepts involved in community integration and development of health using artistic and imaginative approaches of environmental design and architecture. A recent study[90] notes that students of medicine and architecture have sharply contrasting cognitive styles. Medical students favor a realist style with strengths in verbal, analytic, and sequential skills. Architectural students tend to have an idealist style, and excel in activities requiring visual-spatial and nonlinear aptitude and are adept with the holistic approach. Efforts toward a bridging of perspectives between physicians and architects who are particularly interested in the development of improved environments for people with physical disability would be a worthwhile goal for both professions. Such improved understanding and cooperation would probably result in smoother transitions between the medical care and community setting.

Conclusions

Much progress has been achieved through research and the construction of barrier-free environments. However, barriers continue to impede the integration of disabled persons into the mainstream of society. It is hoped that heightened social consciousness and increased general awareness of the needs of the physically disabled will result in improved funding to eliminate the remaining environmental barriers. Increased efforts are needed by the physically disabled members of the community as well as the professionals in rehabilitation and other interested parties to stimulate greater participation in this field by the public and private sectors.

ACKNOWLEDGMENT

The support of Dade W. Moeller, Ph.D., Professor of Environmental Science and Physiology and Associate Dean for Continuing Education, Harvard University School of Public Health, and William J. Erdman II, M.D., M.Sc., Distinguished Professor of Physical Medicine and Rehabilitation and Laurence E. Earley, M.D., Senior Associate Dean, Professor and Chairman, Department of Medicine, University of Pennsylvania School of Medicine, made this publication possible and is deeply appreciated.

Acknowledged with gratitude are the efforts of Jon T. Lang, Ph.D., Associate Professor and Chair, Urban Design Program, Graduate School of Fine Arts, University of Pennsylvania; Kevin Kieran, R.I.A.I., Instructor, Harvard University Graduate School of Design; Larry Allison, Communications Manager, and Ruth Hall Lusher, A.I.A., Architectural Barriers Specialist, United States Architectural and Transportation Barriers Compliance Board.

References

1. Ostroff, E.: Humanizing Environments. Cambridge, MA, World Guide Publishers, 1978.
2. Lawton, M. P.: An ecological theory of aging applied to elderly housing. J. Archit. Educ., 31:8–10, 1977.
3. Stephens, S.: Hidden barriers. Progressive Architecture, 59:94–95, 1978.
4. President's Committee on Employment of the Handicapped publication: MAINSTREET—Community Action for Disabled Americans—A Guide for Service Organizations. Washington, DC, U.S. Government Printing Office, #361–270/4902, 1982.
5. Langton-Lockton, S.: CEH Report. Design for Special Needs, 36:3, 1985.
6. Asher, J., and Asher, J.: How to accommodate workers in wheelchairs. Reprinted from Job Safety and Health (Oct. 1976), distributed by the President's Committee on Employment of the Handicapped. Washington, DC, U.S. Government Printing Office, #928 962, 1976.
7. Bessell, B.: Building study—Tiddington Court: Shelter for life. Design for Special Needs, 37:12–13, 1985.
8. Greer, N. R.: The state of the art of design for accessibility. Am. Inst. Arch. J., 76:58–61, 1987.
9. United States Department of Health and Human Services publication: Resource Guide—Architectural Barrier Removal. Washington, DC, U.S. Government Printing Office, #0–3ii–234/P017 (80), 1980.
10. National Easter Seal Society, President's Committee on Employment of the Handicapped, and U.S. HUD, Secretariat, American National Standard for Buildings and Facilities: Providing Accessibility and Usability for Physically Handicapped People, ANSI A117.1, 1986; available from the American National Standards Institute, Inc., 1430 Broadway, New York, NY 10018.
11. Harvey, J., and Henning, D. (Eds.): Environment Design Research Association Conference, EDRA 18:Public Environments, May 29–June 2, 1987; available from the Environmental Design Research Association, P.O. Box 23129, L'Enfant Plaza Station, Washington, DC 20024.
12. Paralyzed Veterans of America release: National Architecture and Barrier-Free Design Program in PVA Annual Report, 1987, p. 16; available from Paralyzed Veterans of America, 801 18th St., NW, Washington, DC 20006.
13. Snell, H.: Executive Director, Barrier-Free Design Center of Toronto, 150 Eglinton Ave E, Suite 400, Toronto M4P 1E8, Ontario, Canada; personal communication, 1987.
14. Ryan, J.: Barrier-Free Coordinator, Barrier Free Environment Committee of the Disabled Persons' Community Resources, 1400 Clyde, Suite 222, Nepean, Ottawa, Ontario, K2G3J2 Canada; personal communication, 1987.
15. Center on Environment for the Handicapped release: Center on Environment for the Handicapped; available from the Center.
16. United States Architectural and Transportation Barriers Compliance Board release: Access America, Fall 1986.
17. General Services Administration, Department of Defense, Department of Housing and Urban Development, U.S. Postal Service, Secretariat, Uniform Federal Accessibility Standards, published originally in the Federal Register, Aug. 7, 1984; available from the U.S. Architectural and Transportation Barriers Compliance Board, Suite 501, 1111 18th St., NW, Washington, DC 20036–3894.
18. Szitasi, V., Davies, A., and Penton, J.: Tourism—Little Chef Lodges—the better place to stop? Design for Special Needs, 44:7–9, 1987.

19. Rush, R.: Barrier-free and energy conscious. Prog. Arch., 63:150–153, 1982.
20. Hoglund, J. D.: Privacy and independence in housing for the elderly. Prog. Arch., 65:150–151, 1984.
21. Jordan, J. J.: Recognizing and designing for the special needs of the elderly. Am. Inst. Arch. J., 66:50–55, 1977.
22. Chown, E. (Ed.): Design for Special Needs, Journal of the Centre on Environment for the Handicapped of London, U.K., 35 Great Smith St., London SW1P3BJ, U.K.; personal communication, 1987.
23. Greer, N. R.: Community center for victims of four different disabilities. Am. Inst. Arch. J., 76:71, 1987.
24. Nesmith, L.: Designing for 'special populations.' Am. Inst. Arch. J., 76:62–64, 1987.
25. Nelham, R. L.: Principles and practice in the manufacture of seating for the handicapped. Physiotherapy, 70:54–58, 1984.
26. Wade, C. S., and Kramer, R. M.: The relationship between arthritic adults and furniture usage: A study. Rehabil. Lit., 45:80–84, 1984.
27. Munton, J. S., Ellis, M. I., Chamberlain, M. A., and Wright, V.: An investigation into the problems of easy chairs used by the arthritic and the elderly. Rheumatol. Rehabil., 20:164–173, 1981.
28. Atherton, J., Clarke, A. K., Chatfield, J., and Harrison, R. A.: Easy chairs for arthritic patients. Physiotherapy, 68:116, 1982.
29. Kiewel, H. D.: Ramps, stairs, and floor treatments. Access Information Bulletin; available from Paralyzed Veterans of America, 801 18th St., NW, Washington, DC 20006.
30. Tisserand, M.: Progress in the prevention of falls caused by slipping. Ergonomics, 28:1027–1042, 1985.
31. Glaser, R. M., Sawka, M. N., Wilde, S. W., Woodrow, B. K., and Suryaprasad, A. G.: Energy cost and cardiopulmonary responses for wheelchair locomotion and walking on tile and on carpet. Paraplegia, 19:220–226, 1981.
32. United States Consumer Product Safety Commission release, Fact Sheet No. 48: Older Consumers and Stairway Accidents; available from the U.S. Consumer Product Safety Commission, Washington, DC 20207.
33. Thorpe, S.: Access design sheet: 1. Ramps, a checklist for architects. Design for Special Needs, 34:17–18, 1984.
34. Orleans, P.: Kitchens. Access Information Bulletin, Nov. 1980; available from Paralyzed Veterans of America, 801 18th St., NW, Washington, DC 20006.
35. Cochran, W.: Restrooms. Access Information Bulletin, 1981; available from Paralyzed Veterans of America, 801 18th St., NW, Washington, DC 20006.
36. Thorpe, S.: Housing design sheet: II. Showers, a check-list for architects. Design for Special Needs, 44:18–19, 1987.
37. Enseki, C., and Ahern, K.: Environments for all children. Access Information Bulletin; available from Paralyzed Veterans of America, 801 18th St., NW, Washington, DC 20006.
38. Ruddy, R., Bacchi, D., and Fleisher, G.: Injuries involving household furniture: Spectrum and strategies for prevention. Ped. Emerg. Care, 1:184–186, 1985.
39. Cole, G. F., Jones, R. B., and Digby, M.: Glass furniture hazard. Arch. Dis. Child., 59:1198, 1984.
40. Capital Development Board, State of Illinois release: Illinois Accessibility Code effective May 1, 1988; available from the Capital Development Board, State of Illinois Center, 100 W Randolph St., 14th Fl., Chicago, IL 60601.
41. United States Architectural and Transportation Barriers Compliance Board release: Recommendations for Accessibility to Serve Physically Handicapped Children in Elementary Schools, March 1986.
42. Lacey, A.: Access abroad—an American dream? Design for Special Needs, 43:10–13, 1987.
43. Bunin, N. M., Jasperse, D., and Cooper, S.: A Guide to Designing Accessible Outdoor Recreation Facilities, a publication of the Heritage Conservation and Recreation Service, U.S. Department of the Interior, Lake Central Regional Office, Ann Arbor, MI, Jan. 1980.
44. Plourde, R. M.: Recreation. Access Information Bulletin, Nov. 1980; available from Paralyzed Veterans of America, 801 18th St., NW, Washington, DC 20006.
45. Center on Environment for the Handicapped of London, U.K., release: Horticulture and the Countryside for Handicapped People, proceedings of a conference held Sept. 6–7, 1984; available from the Center.
46. Smith, A. C.: Poor building designs hinder safe emergency escape by handicapped. Occup. Health Saf., 54:63–65, 1985.
47. Gartshore, D., and Sime, J.: Assisted escape—some guidelines for designers, building managers and the mobility impaired. Design for Special Needs, 42:6–9, 1987.
48. Dobinson, J.: Means of escape for disabled people: Defining a realistic approach. Design for Special Needs, 39:14–16, 1986.
49. Brodey, W.: The other than visual world of the blind. Architectural Design, 39:9–10, 1969.
50. Brodey, W.: Sound and space. Am. Inst. Arch. J., 42:58–60, 1964.
51. National Library Service for the Blind and Physical Handicapped publication: Planning Barriers-Free Libraries. Washington, DC, U.S. Government Printing Office, #0–352–614, 1981.
52. Burnaby, G.: Reviews—Building Bulletin 61: Designing for children with special educational needs— ordinary schools. Design for Special Needs, 35:20, 1984.
53. LS&S Group, Inc., release: LS&S Group, Inc. Specializing in Products for the Visually Impaired 1987–1988; available from LS&S Group, Inc., P.O. Box 673, Northbrook, IL 60065.

54. Cooper, Carlson, Duy, Ritchie, Inc., Architects and Planners, Kansas City, MO, release: Hospital clinic aids patients with permanent visual impairments. Hospitals, 56:106–107, 1982.

55. Fisher, T.: Enabling the disabled. Prog. Arch., 66:119–131, 1985.

56. Cooper, B. A., Gowland, C., and McIntosh, J.: The use of color in the environment of the elderly to enhance function. Clin. Geriatr. Med., 2:151–163, 1986.

57. Olsen, R. V., Winkel, G., and Pershing, A.: Lighting system greets and guides visitors. Hospitals, 56:56–57, 1982.

58. Archea, J. C.: Environmental factors associated with stair accidents by the elderly. Clin. Geriatr. Med., 1:555–569, 1985.

59. Cohn, T. E., and Lasley, D. J.: Visual depth illusion and falls in the elderly. Clin. Geriatr. Med., 1:601–620, 1985.

60. Warnath, C.: Guide dogs: Mobility tool and social bridge to the sighted world. J. Rehabil., 48:58–61, 1982.

61. Fogle, B., and Radcliffe, A.: Hearing dogs for the deaf. Practitioner, 227:1051–1053, 1983.

62. Tachi, S., Tanie, K., Komoriya, K., and Abe, M.: Electrocutaneous communication in a guide dog robot (MELDOG). IEEE Trans. Biomed. Eng., BME—32:461–469, 1985.

63. American Foundation for the Blind release: AFB—Directory of Agencies Serving the Visually Handicapped in the U.S., 22nd Ed. American Foundation for the Blind, Inc., 15 W 16th St, New York, NY 10011, 1984.

64. Lane, D. R.: Guide dogs for the blind. Vet. Rec., 108:470–472, 1981.

65. United States Architectural and Transportation Barriers Compliance Board release: Assistive Listening Sys, Feb. 1987.

66. United States Architectural and Transportation Barriers Compliance Board release: Telecommunication Devices for the Deaf: A Guide to Selection, Ordering, and Installation, 1985.

67. Airports Operators Council International, Inc., Pub. Access Travel: Airports, A Guide to Accessibility of Terminals, 5th Ed., Oct. 1985; available from the Airports Operators Council International, 1700 K Street, NW, Washington, DC 20006.

68. United States Architectural and Transportation Barriers Compliance Board release: Access America, Winter 1987.

69. The Royal National Institute for the Deaf publication: Visual Doorbell Systems, Oct. 1982; available from The Royal National Institute for the Deaf, 105 Gower St., London WC1E 6AH, U.K.

70. DeJong, G., and Lifchez, R.: Physical disability and public policy. Sci. Am., 248:40–49, 1983.

71. Habell, M. and Mold, F.: A new approach to designing for the elderly. J. R. Soc. Health, 106:1–4, 1986.

72. Whelihan, W. M.: Geriatric center's environment fosters interaction. Hosp. Prog., 61:50–55, 1980.

73. Blumenkranz, J., Bernhard, F., and Gottlieb, G.: Geriatric complex offers options from housing to skilled nursing hospitals. J. Am. Hosp. Assoc., 53:123–128, 1979.

74. Canty, D.: Courtyard housing sensitively designed for the disabled. Architecture, 76:72–73, 1987.

75. Szeto, A. Y. J., and White, R. N.: Evaluation of a curb-climbing aid for manual wheelchairs: Considerations of stability, effort, and safety. J. Rehabil. Res. Dev., 20:45–56, 1983.

76. Rush, R.: Designing the moving experience. Prog. Arch., 60:92–110, 1979.

77. Stout, G.: Some aspects of high performance indoor/outdoor wheelchairs. Bull. Prosthet. Res., 16:135–175, 1979.

78. Veteran's Administration release: VA Approved Add-On Automobile Adaptive Equipment, Circular 10–88–51, May 13, 1988; available from VA Prosthetics and Sensory Aids Service, Washington, DC 20420.

79. American Public Transit Association release: Public Transit: Meeting the Mobility Needs of Elderly and Disabled Persons, Oct., 1985. Available from the American Public Transit Assoc., 1225 Connecticut Ave, NW, Washington, DC 20036.

80. Haworth, R., and Nichols, P. J. R.: Hoists in the home: Their recommendation and use. Rheumatol. Rehabil., 19:42–51, 1980.

81. United States Architectural and Transportation Barriers Compliance Board release: Access America, Spring 1986.

82. Barowsky, E. I.: Effects of stereotypic expectation on evaluation of written English attributed to handicapped and nonhandicapped students. Psychol. Rep., 59:1097–1098, 1986.

83. Walt Disney World release: The Disabled Guests Guide Book, published by the Walt Disney Co. (1987); available from Walt Disney World Co., P.O. Box 10,000, Lake Buena Vista, FL 32830–1000.

84. Braidwood, S.: Age: The final frontier. Design, 426:40–45, June 1984.

85. Langton-Lockton, S.: CEH report. Design for Special Needs, 38:3, 1985.

86. Ross, R.: Civilization's treatment of the handicapped. In McDevitt, G. M. (Ed.): The Handicapped Experience: Some Humanistic Perspectives. Baltimore, University of Baltimore Press, 1979, pp. 7–13.

87. Weinberg, N., and Santana, R.: Comic books: Champions of the disabled stereotype. Rehabil. Lit., 39:327–331, 1978.

88. Research and Training Center on Independent Living release: Guidelines for Reporting and Writing about People with Disabilities; available from Media Project, Research and Training Center on Independent Living, 348 Haworth Hall, University of Kansas, Lawrence, KS 66045.

89. Gething, L.: International year of disabled persons

in Australia: Attitudes and integration. Rehabil. Lit., 47:66–70, 1986.

90. Kienholz, A., and Hritzuk, J.: Comparing students in architecture and medicine: Findings from two new measures of cognitive style. Psychol. Rep., 58:823–830, 1986.

91. Morton, D.: Bearing down on barriers. Progressive Architecture, 59:63–64, 1978.

92. Filler, M.: Extrasensory perception. Progressive Architecture, 59:82–85, 1978.

93. Dixon, J. M.: Accessible and perceivable. Progressive Architecture, 59:6, 1978.

94. Schlage Lock Co.: Release Rollock® door knob. Progressive Architecture, 59:128, 1978.

Index

Note: Page numbers in *italics* indicate ilustrations; page numbers followed by t indicate tables.